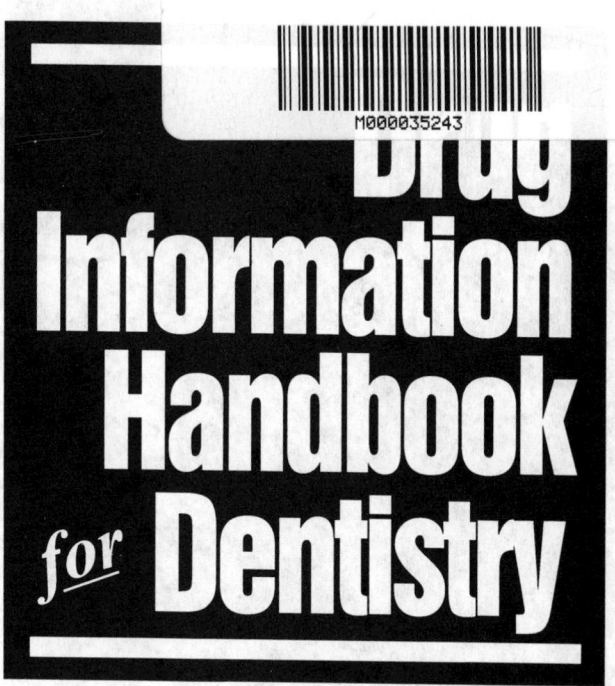

# Drug Information Handbook *for* Dentistry

5th Edition 1999-2000



lexi-comp

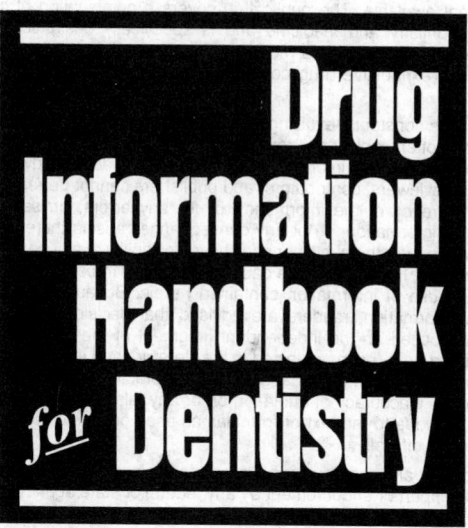

# Drug Information Handbook *for* Dentistry

**5th Edition** **1999-2000**

**Richard L. Wynn, BSPharm, PhD**
*Professor of Pharmacology*
Baltimore College of Dental Surgery
Dental School
University of Maryland at Baltimore
Baltimore, Maryland

**Timothy F. Meiller, DDS, PhD**
*Professor*
Oral Medicine and Diagnostic Sciences
Baltimore College of Dental Surgery
*Professor of Oncology*
Greenebaum Cancer Center
University of Maryland at Baltimore
Baltimore, Maryland

**Harold L. Crossley, DDS, PhD**
*Associate Professor of Pharmacology*
Baltimore College of Dental Surgery
Dental School
University of Maryland at Baltimore
Baltimore, Maryland

**LEXI-COMP INC**
**Hudson (Cleveland)**

## NOTICE

This handbook is intended to serve the user as a handy reference and not as a complete drug information resource. It does not include information on every therapeutic agent available. The publication covers a combination of commonly used drugs in dentistry and medicine and is specifically designed to present important aspects of drug data in a more concise format than is typically found in medical literature, exhaustive drug compendia, or product material supplied by manufacturers.

Drug information is constantly evolving because of ongoing research and clinical experience and is often subject to interpretation. While great care has been taken to ensure the accuracy of the information presented, the reader is advised that the authors, editors, reviewers, contributors, and publishers cannot be responsible for the continued currency of the information or for any errors, omissions, or the application of this information, or for any consequences arising therefrom. Therefore, the author(s) and/or the publisher shall have no liability to any person or entity with regard to claims, loss, or damage caused, or alleged to be caused, directly or indirectly, by the use of information contained herein. Because of the dynamic nature of drug information, readers are advised that decisions regarding drug therapy must be based on the independent judgment of the clinician, changing information about a drug (eg, as reflected in the literature and manufacturer's most current product information), and changing medical practices. The editors are not responsible for any inaccuracy of quotation or for any false or misleading implication that may arise due to the text or formulas as used or due to the quotation of revisions no longer official.

The editors, authors, and contributors have written this book in their private capacities. No official support or endorsement by any federal or state agency or pharmaceutical company is intended or inferred.

The publishers have made every effort to trace the copyright holders for borrowed material. If they have inadvertently overlooked any, they will be pleased to make the necessary arrangements at the first opportunity.

If you have any suggestions or questions regarding any information presented in this handbook, please contact our drug information pharmacist at

**1-800-837-LEXI (5394)**



This manual was produced using the FormuLex™ Program —
A complete publishing service of Lexi-Comp Inc.

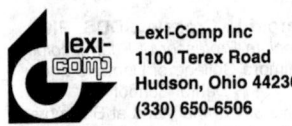

**Lexi-Comp Inc**
**1100 Terex Road**
**Hudson, Ohio 44236**
**(330) 650-6506**

ISBN 0-916589-78-1

# TABLE OF CONTENTS

# ABOUT THE AUTHORS

## Richard L. Wynn, BSPharm, PhD

Richard L. Wynn, PhD, is Professor of Pharmacology at the Baltimore College of Dental Surgery, Dental School, University of Maryland at Baltimore. Dr Wynn has served as a dental educator, researcher, and teacher of dental pharmacology and dental hygiene pharmacology for his entire professional career. He holds a BS (pharmacy; registered pharmacist, Maryland), an MS (physiology) and a PhD (pharmacology) from the University of Maryland. Dr Wynn chaired the Department of Pharmacology at the University of Maryland Dental School from 1980 to 1995. Previously, he chaired the Department of Oral Biology at the University of Kentucky College of Dentistry. He has to his credit over 180 publications including original research articles, textbooks, textbook chapters, monographs, and articles in continuing education journals. He has given over 300 continuing education seminars to dental professionals in the U.S., Canada, and Europe. Dr Wynn has been a consultant to drug industry for 17 years. His research laboratories have contributed to the development of new analgesics and anesthetics. He is a consultant to the U.S. Pharmacopeia, Dental Drugs and Products section, a consultant to the Academy of General Dentistry, a consultant to the American Dental Association, and a former consultant to the Council on Dental Education, Commission on Accreditation. He is a featured columnist and his drug review articles, entitled *Pharmacology Today*, appear in each issue of General Dentistry, a journal published by the Academy. He is currently funded by drug industry and government agencies for research on the development of new drugs. One of his primary interests continues to be keeping dental professionals informed on all aspects of drug use in dental practice.

## Timothy F. Meiller, DDS, PhD

Dr Meiller is Professor of Oral Medicine and Diagnostic Sciences at the Baltimore College of Dental Surgery and Professor of Oncology in the Program of Oncology at the Greenebaum Cancer Center, University of Maryland at Baltimore.

Dr Meiller has held his position in Oral Medicine at the Dental School for 22 years and serves as an attending faculty at the Greenebaum Cancer Center. He is a Diplomate of the American Board of Oral Medicine. He is a graduate of Johns Hopkins University and the University of Maryland Dental and Graduate Schools, holding a DDS and a PhD in Immunology/Virology. He has over 165 publications to his credit. He maintains an active general dental practice and is a consultant to the National Institutes of Health. He is currently engaged in ongoing investigations into cellular immune dysfunction in oral diseases associated with AIDS, in cancer patients, and in other medically compromised patients.

## Harold L. Crossley, DDS, PhD

Dr Crossley is Associate Professor of Pharmacology at the Baltimore College of Dental Surgery, Dental School, University of Maryland at Baltimore. A native of Rhode Island, Hal received a Bachelor of Science degree in Pharmacy from the University of Rhode Island in 1964. He later was awarded the Master of Science (1970) and Doctorate degrees (1972) in the area of Pharmacology. The University of Maryland Dental School in Baltimore awarded Dr Crossley the DDS degree in 1980. He is the Director of Conjoint Sciences and Preclinical Studies at the School of Dentistry and maintains an intramural part-time private dental practice. Dr Crossley has co-authored a number of articles dealing with law enforcement on both a local and federal level. This liaison with law enforcement agencies keeps him well-acquainted with the "drug culture". He has been appointed to the Governor's Commission on Prescription Drug Abuse and the Maryland State Dental Association's Well-Being Committee.

Drawing on this unique background, Dr Crossley has become nationally and internationally recognized as an expert on street drugs and chemical dependency as well as the clinical pharmacology of dental drugs.

# EDITORIAL ADVISORY PANEL

**Martin D. Higbee, PharmD**
*Associate Professor*
Department of Pharmacy Practice
The University of Arizona
Tucson, Arizona

**Jane Hurlburt Hodding, PharmD**
*Supervisor, Children's Pharmacy*
Miller Children's Hospital at Long Beach Memorial
Long Beach, California

**Rebecca T. Horvat, PhD**
*Assistant Professor of Pathology and Laboratory Medicine*
University of Kansas Medical Center
Kansas City, Kansas

**Naomi Ingrim, PharmD**
*Specialist in Poison Information*
Central Texas Poison Center
Temple,TX

**Carlos M. Isada, MD**
Department of Infectious Disease
Cleveland Clinic Foundation
Cleveland, Ohio

**David S. Jacobs, MD**
*President, Pathologists Chartered*
Overland Park, Kansas

**Bernard L. Kasten, Jr, MD**
*Vice-President/Medical Director*
Corning Clinical Laboratories
Teteroboro, New Jersey

**Donna M. Kraus, PharmD**
*Assistant Professor of Pharmacy Practice*
Departments of Pharmacy Practice and Pediatrics
*Clinical Pharmacist*
Pediatric Intensive Care Unit
University of Illinois at Chicago
Chicago, Illinois

**Charles Lacy, RPh, PharmD**
*Drug Information Pharmacist*
Cedars-Sinai Medical Center
Los Angeles, California

**Brenda R. Lance, RN, MSN**
*Nurse Coordinator*
Ritzman Infusion Services
Akron, Ohio

**Leonard L. Lance, RPh, BSPharm**
*Clinical Pharmacist*
Lexi-Comp Inc
Hudson, Ohio

**Jerrold B. Leikin, MD**
*Associate Director*
Emergency Services
Rush Presbyterian-St Luke's Medical Center
Chicago, Illinois

**Eugene S. Olsowka, MD, PhD**
*Pathologist*
Institute of Pathology PC
Saginaw, Michigan

## EDITORIAL ADVISORY PANEL *(Continued)*

# PREFACE TO THE FIFTH EDITION

The authors of the *Drug Information Handbook for Dentistry* are gratified that the text has received many indicators of success over these last several years. We wish to congratulate and thank the practitioners and students that have made each of the previous editions a success. Each of us have endeavored to respond to all of the comments and creative suggestions from our readership and as a result have incorporated many of these ideas into this new 5th edition.

The goals and the philosophy of the handbook remain the same as in all previous editions. Complete cross-referencing of generic, brand names, medical and oral conditions along with the therapeutic indication and example prescribing guidelines have been the basis of the text. We know the practitioners and staff members can easily access needed information.

The drug monographs now number over 1450 and the complete alphabetical index exceeds 3800 drug names. This indexing system has been the key to much of the success of this book. Clinicians can cross-reference between an oral medicine problem, a suggested drug regimen, and the important pharmacologic information necessary to move ahead with a treatment selection.

This 5th edition includes easy-to-use algorithms to help the clinician make treatment decisions in evolving areas of patient care including preprocedural antibiotics related to endocarditis and joint prostheses. New chapters on periodontal disease management and HIV infection and AIDS have been added. New drugs have been added to further explain the available combinations for pain control and treatment of common conditions such as temporomandibular dysfunction. Other topics in the text have been edited as appropriate. One very key area has been an entire chapter now dedicated to management of the human immunodeficiency virus infected (AIDS) patient. Also, the chapter on chemical dependency has been updated to include new information. Many chapters now have a section called "Frequently Asked Questions" to help us focus on real-life scenarios. The chapter on herbals and natural products has been expanded to present information on many of the most popular dietary supplements. Chapters on drug interactions and metabolism along with sections on effects of smoking and smoking cessation products have been updated.

We know that our text remains an excellent companion to complete oral medicine and medical reference libraries that each clinician should have available. We hope that it compliments the sound foundation that each dental clinician has received during their education and by building on their knowledge of oral and systemic disease we have helped them with this text to focus on therapeutic considerations. Dental office management protocols, along with prescribing guidelines, should aid the busy practitioner. The active general practitioner, the specialist, the dental hygienist, and the advanced student of dentistry or dental hygiene will be better prepared for patient care with this new 5th edition.

Timothy F. Meiller

Richard L. Wynn

Harold L. Crossley

# ACKNOWLEDGMENTS

This handbook exists in its present form as a result of the concerted efforts of many individuals, including Jack D. Bolinski, DDS, and Brad F. Bolinski who recognized the need for a comprehensive dental and medical drug compendium; the publisher and president of Lexi-Comp Inc, Robert D. Kerscher; Lynn D. Coppinger, managing editor; Barbara F. Kerscher, production manager; and David C. Marcus, director of information systems.

Other members of the Lexi-Comp staff whose contributions deserve special mention include Mark F. Bonfiglio, PharmD, director of pharmacotherapy resources; Leonard L. Lance, BSPharm, pharmacy editor; Diane M. Harbart, MT (ASCP), medical editor; Jeanne E. Wilson, production/systems liaison; Leslie J. Ruggles, Julie A. Katzen, Jennifer L. Rocky, Stacey L. Hurd, and Kathleen E. Schleicher, project managers; Alexandra J. Hart, composition specialist; Jackie L. Mizer, Ginger S. Conner,and Kathy Smith, production assistants; Tracey J. Reinecke, graphic designer; Edmund A. Harbart, vice-president, custom publishing division; Jack L. Stones, vice-president, reference publishing division; Jay L. Katzen, director of marketing and business development; Brian B. Vossler, director of sales; Jerry M. Reeves, Marc L. Long, and Patrick T. Grubb, regional sales managers; Brad F. Bolinski, Kristin M. Thompson, Matthew C. Kerscher, Tina L. Collins, Kelene A. Murphy, and Leslie G. Rodia, sales and marketing representatives; Paul A. Rhine and Jason M. Buchwald, academic account managers; Kenneth J. Hughes, manager of authoring systems; Sean M. Conrad and James M. Stacey, system analysts; Thury L. O'Connor, vice-president of technology; David J. Wasserbauer, vice-president, finance and administration; Elizabeth M. Conlon and Rebecca A. Dryhurst, accounting; and Frederick C. Kerscher, inventory and fulfillment manager.

Much of the material contained in this book was a result of pharmacy contributors throughout the United States and Canada. Lexi-Comp has assisted many medical institutions to develop hospital-specific formulary manuals that contain clinical drug information as well as dosing. Working with these clinical pharmacists, hospital pharmacy and therapeutics committees, and hospital drug information centers, Lexi-Comp has developed an evolutionary drug database that reflects the practice of pharmacy in these major institutions.

In addition, the authors wish to thank their families, friends, and colleagues who supported them in their efforts to complete this handbook.

# USE OF THE DRUG INFORMATION HANDBOOK FOR DENTISTRY

The *Drug Information Handbook for Dentistry, 5th Edition* is organized into six sections: Introductory text, drug monographs, oral medicine topics, appendix, therapeutic category index, and alphabetical index.

## INTRODUCTORY TEXT

The first section is a compilation of information pertinent to the use of this handbook.

## ALPHABETICAL LISTING OF DRUG MONOGRAPHS

The drug information section of the handbook, in which all drugs are listed alphabetically, incorporates drugs commonly prescribed in dentistry as well as medications that dental patients may currently be taking. Extensive cross-referencing (with easy visibility marked with a diamond ♦), is provided by brand names and synonyms.

Each monograph is consistent in its format and may include all or some of the following fields:

| | |
|---|---|
| Generic Name | U.S. Adopted Name |
| Pronunciation Guide | Phonetic listing of generic name |
| Related Information | Cross-reference to other pertinent drug information found elsewhere in the book |
| U.S. Brand Names | Common trade names used in the United States |
| Canadian Brand Names | Trade names found in Canada if different from the U.S. |
| Therapeutic Category | Unique systematic classification of medications |
| Synonyms | Other names or accepted abbreviations of the drug in the U.S. and Canada |
| Use | Information pertaining to appropriate dental and medical indications of the drug |
| Restrictions | DEA classification for federally scheduled controlled substances and their associated prescribing limits |
| Usual Dosage | The amount of the drug to be typically given or taken during therapy |
| Mechanism of Action | How the drug works in the body to elicit a response |
| Local Anesthetic/Vasoconstrictor Precautions | Specific information to prevent potential drug interactions related to anesthesia |
| Effects on Dental Treatment | How drug therapy affects the dental treatment/ diagnosis with suggested management approaches |
| Other Adverse Effects | Side effects grouped by percentage of incidence and body groups |
| Contraindications | Information pertaining to inappropriate use of the drug |
| Warnings/Precautions | Cautions and hazardous conditions related to use of the drug |
| Drug Interactions | A list of agents that when combined may affect the therapy |
| Drug Uptake | Information includes onset and duration of effect, absorption, time to peak serum concentration, and serum half-life |
| Pregnancy Risk Factor | Five categories established by the FDA to indicate the potential of a systemically absorbed drug for causing birth defects |
| Breast-feeding Considerations | Information pertaining to drug administration while breast-feeding |
| Dosage Forms | Information with regard to form, strength, and availability of the drug |

## USE OF THE DRUG INFORMATION HANDBOOK FOR DENTISTRY *(Continued)*

| | |
|---|---|
| Dietary Considerations | Information regarding effect of food with drug |
| Generic Available | Indicated by a "yes" or "no" |
| Comments | Additional pertinent information |
| Selected Readings | Sources and literature where the user may find additional information |

### ORAL MEDICINE TOPICS

The third section contains text on Oral Medicine topics and is divided into two major parts.

In each of the two major parts, the systemic condition or the oral disease state is described briefly, followed by the pharmacologic considerations, with which the dentist must be familiar. Selected readings have been listed for further inquiry.

Part I: **Dental Management and Therapeutic Considerations in Medically Compromised Patients** focuses on common medical conditions and their associated drug therapies with which the dentist must be familiar. Patient profiles with commonly associated drug regimens are described.

Part II: **Dental Management and Therapeutic Considerations in Patients With Specific Oral Conditions and Other Oral Medicine Topics** focus on therapies the dentist may choose to prescribe for patients suffering from oral disease or are in need of special care. Some overlap between these sections has resulted from systemic conditions that have oral manifestations and vice-versa. Cross-references to the descriptions and the monographs for individual drugs described elsewhere in this handbook allow for easy retrieval of information. Example prescriptions of selected drug therapies for each condition are presented so that the clinician can evaluate alternate approaches to treatment. Seldom is there a single drug of choice.

Those drug prescriptions listed represent prototype drugs and popular prescriptions and are examples only. The therapeutic index is available for cross-referencing if alternatives or additional drugs are sought.

### APPENDIX

The Appendix section offers a compilation of tables, guidelines, and conversion information which can often be helpful when considering patient care. This section is broken down into various sections for ease of use. The Appendix also includes descriptions of most over-the-counter drugs and oral care products. There are also presentations of drug interactions and drugs under development.

### THERAPEUTIC CATEGORY INDEX

The Therapeutic Category Index provides a useful listing by an easy-to-use therapeutic classification system.

### ALPHABETICAL INDEX

The Alphabetical Index provides a quick reference for generic, American and Canadian brand names, and major headings from the chapters. From this index, the reader can cross-reference to the drug monographs and to Oral Medicine topics.

# FDA PREGNANCY CATEGORIES

Throughout this book there is a field labeled Pregnancy Risk Factor (PRF) and the letter A, B, C, D, or X immediately following which signifies a category. The FDA has established these five categories to indicate the potential of a systemically absorbed drug for causing birth defects. The key differentiation among the categories rests upon the reliability of documentation and the risk:benefit ratio. Pregnancy Category X is particularly notable in that if any data exists that may implicate a drug as a teratogen and the risk:benefit ratio is clearly negative, the drug is contraindicated during pregnancy.

These categories are summarized as follows:

- **A** Controlled studies in pregnant women fail to demonstrate a risk to the fetus in the first trimester with no evidence of risk in later trimesters. The possibility of fetal harm appears remote.
- **B** Either animal-reproduction studies have not demonstrated a fetal risk but there are no controlled studies in pregnant women, or animal-reproduction studies have shown an adverse effect (other than a decrease in fertility) that was not confirmed in controlled studies in women in the first trimester and there is no evidence of a risk in later trimesters.
- **C** Either studies in animals have revealed adverse effects on the fetus (teratogenic or embryocidal effects or other) and there are no controlled studies in women, or studies in women and animals are not available. Drugs should be given only if the potential benefits justify the potential risk to the fetus.
- **D** There is positive evidence of human fetal risk, but the benefits from use in pregnant women may be acceptable despite the risk (eg, if the drug is needed in a life-threatening situation or for a serious disease for which safer drugs cannot be used or are ineffective).
- **X** Studies in animals or human beings have demonstrated fetal abnormalities or there is evidence of fetal risk based on human experience, or both, and the risk of the use of the drug in pregnant women clearly outweighs any possible benefit. The drug is contraindicated in women who are or may become pregnant.

# PHARMACOLOGY OF DRUG METABOLISM AND INTERACTIONS

Most drugs undergo metabolic transformation in the body prior to excretion. Drug metabolism is an enzyme-dependent process that developed as an adaptation to life on earth. Unlike fish, terrestrial vertebrates are unable to excrete lipid soluble compounds because kidney tubular reabsorption favors their retention. Excretion of these substances is accomplished in fish into the surrounding water. Although drug metabolism in humans results in the formation of compounds that are more polar in nature, it does not always result in the initial production of biologically inactive compounds. This means that a drug may stay active for some time during this metabolic process. Enzymatic modification of a parent drug can be distinguished by three basic patterns. First, an inactive parent drug may be transformed to an active compound. Second, an active parent drug may be converted to a second active compound which is subsequently converted to an inactive metabolite or by-product. Third, an inactive compound may be formed directly from an active parent drug.

The most common reaction in drug metabolism is an oxidation reaction in which oxygen in the form of a hydroxyl group is attached to the drug molecule. With oxidation, the original drug molecule is changed just enough so that the drug metabolite won't attach to the receptor that is specific for the original molecule. This chemical change may render the drug inactive and is one mechanism of terminating drug activity. The overall process is called hydroxylation and is the direct incorporation of oxygen into the substrate drug molecule. Although the liver is the primary site for these hydroxylation enzyme reactions, these systems are also present in the kidney and gastrointestinal epithelium. This process is also called oxidative drug metabolism by an oxidative enzyme system.

This oxidative enzyme system relies on a particular cytochrome and numerous isoforms known as the cytochrome P-450 system with designations CYP. Cytochrome P-450 is a complex of protein and heme that contains an iron atom in its oxidized state. Through an energy transfer cascade, cytochrome P-450 is reduced utilizing energy and reducing the iron to a ferrous form. This then binds with molecular oxygen and the cytochrome P-450 eventually reverts to its oxidized form. The oxidized drug bound through this process to the cytochrome P-450 is then released and the cytochrome is regenerated. The rate of drug biotransformation or metabolism appears to be directly related to the amounts of cytochrome P-450 in the microsomal and enzyme cascade. In fact, there is a direct correlation between these systems.

Many drugs that are currently on the market now have associated with them their relationship to the cytochrome P-450 system and a system of analyses has been developed to identify drugs that tend to interfere with the availability of cytochrome P-450 more readily than others. Also, there are numerous isoforms of these enzymes that have been identified within the system. The specific interaction of one drug with another drug's metabolism has now been elucidated through analyses of reactions. Many of the drugs that our patients may be taking may slow the metabolism of another drug. It is important to be aware that our knowledge regarding these systems is increasing on a daily basis. Examples of isoform interactions of this system are found in Tables 1-3. Drugs of common importance in dentistry are in bold. Many of the drugs used as antivirals, for instance, interfere with specific isoforms of the cytochrome P-450 system and may, therefore, interact adversely with the metabolism of other drugs which the patient may be taking.

Another area of intense interest involves smoking effects on drug's metabolism as well as the effects of smoking cessation drugs (Table 4). A review of the literature suggests that at least a dozen drugs interact with cigarette smoke in a clinically significant manner. Polycyclic aromatic hydrocarbons (PAHs) are largely responsible for enhancing drug metabolism. Cigarette smoke induces increased concentrations of the isoenzyme CYP1A2, which is responsible for the metabolism of theophylline. Theophylline is, therefore, eliminated more quickly in smokers than in nonsmokers. Cigarette smoke induces an increase in the concentration of CYP1A2, the isoenzyme responsible for the metabolism of theophylline. As a result of hepatic induction of CYP1A2, serum concentrations of theophylline have been shown to be reduced in smokers. Cigarette smoking may reduce substantially the plasma concentrations of tacrine. The manufacturer states that mean plasma tacrine concentrations in smokers are about one-third of the concentration in nonsmokers (presumably after multiple doses of tacrine).

Patients with insulin-dependent diabetes who smoke heavily may require a higher dosage of insulin than nonsmokers. Cigarette smoking may also reduce serum concentrations of flecainide. Although the mechanism of this interaction is unknown, enhanced hepatic metabolism is a possibility. Propoxyphene, a pain reliever, has been found to be less effective in heavy smokers than in nonsmokers. The mechanism for the inefficacy of propoxyphene in smokers compared with nonsmokers may be enhanced biotransformation.

Frankl and Soloff reported in a study of five young, health chronic smokers that propranolol followed by smoking significantly decreased cardiac output and significantly increased blood pressure and peripheral resistance compared with smoking alone. Steady-state concentrations of propranolol were found to be lower in smokers than in nonsmokers. Lastly, the incidence of drowsiness associated with the use of diazepam and chloridazepoxide showed that drowsiness was less likely to occur in smokers than in nonsmokers. Smoking probably acts by producing arousal of the central nervous system rather than be accelerating metabolism and reducing the concentrations of these drugs in the brain. Finally, the interaction between smoking and oral contraceptives is complex and may be deadly. Women older than 35 years of age who smoke more than 15 cigarettes daily may be at increased risk of myocardial infarction.

The norepinephrine and serotonin reuptake inhibitors as a new class of smoking cessation drugs have also received attention relative to metabolic interactions. *In vitro* studies indicate that bupropion is primarily metabolized to hydroxybupropion by the CYP2B6 isoenzyme. Therefore, the potential exists for a drug interaction between Zyban® and drugs that affect the CYP2B6 isoenzyme metabolism (eg, orphenadrine and cyclophosphamide). The hydroxybupropion metabolite of bupropion does not appear to be metabolized by the cytochrome P-450 isoenzymes. No systemic data have been collected on the metabolism of Zyban® following concomitant administration with other drugs, or alternatively, the effect of concomitant administration of Zyban® on the metabolism of other drugs.

Animal data, however, indicated that bupropion may be an inducer of drug metabolizing enzymes in humans. However, following chronic administration of bupropion, 100 mg 3 times daily to 8 healthy male volunteers for 14 days, there was no evidence of induction of its own metabolism. Because bupropion is extensively metabolized, the coadministration of other drugs may affect its clinical activity. In particular, certain drugs may induce the metabolism of bupropion (eg, carbamazepine, phenobarbital, phenytoin), while other drugs may inhibit the metabolism of bupropion (eg, cimetidine). Studies in animals demonstrate that the acute toxicity of bupropion is enhanced by the MAO inhibitor phenelzine.

Limited clinical data suggest a higher incidence of adverse experiences in patients receiving concurrent administration of bupropion and levodopa. Administration of Zyban® to patients receiving levodopa concurrently should be undertaken with caution, using small initial doses and gradual dose increases. Concurrent administration of Zyban® and agents (eg, abrupt discontinuation of benzodiazepines) that lower seizure threshold, should be undertaken only with extreme caution. Physiological changes resulting from smoking cessation itself, with or without treatment with Zyban®, may alter the pharmacokinetics of some concomitant medications, which may require dosage adjustment.

Once a drug has been metabolized in the liver, it is eliminated through several different mechanisms. One is directly through the bile and into the intestine and eventually excreted in feces. More commonly, however, the metabolites and the original drug themselves pass back into the liver from the general circulation and are carried to other organs and tissues. Eventually, these metabolites are excreted through the kidney. In the kidney, the drug and its metabolites may be filtered by the glomerulus or secreted by the renal tubules into the urine. From the kidney, some of the drug may be reabsorbed and pass back into the blood. Another organ to which the drug may be carried is the lung. If the drug or its metabolite is volatile, it can pass from the blood into the alveolar air and be eliminated in the breath. To a minor extent, drugs and metabolites can also be excreted by sweat and by the saliva. In nursing mothers, drugs are also excreted into the mother's milk.

The clinical considerations of drug metabolism may affect which other drugs can and should be administered. Drug tolerance may be a consideration in that larger doses of a drug may be necessary to obtain effect in patients in which the metabolism is extremely rapid. These interactions via cytochrome P-450 or its isoforms can be occasionally used beneficially to increase/maintain blood levels of one drug by administering a second drug. Dental clinicians should attempt to stay current on this topic of drug interactions as our knowledge evolves.

# PHARMACOLOGY OF DRUG METABOLISM AND INTERACTIONS *(Continued)*

## Table 1.
## CYTOCHROME P-450 AND DRUG INTERACTIONS

(Dental Drugs Appear in Bold)

### (Drugs Causing Inhibitory and Inductive Interaction

| Inhibitory (Enhancement of Interacting Drug Effect) | Inductive (Impairment of Interacting Drug Effect) |
|---|---|
| Amiodarone (Cordarone®) | Anticonvulsants |
| Cimetidine (Tagamet®) | Chronic ethanol use |
| **Erythromycin** | Cigarette smoking |
| Ethanol intoxication | Rifampin (Rifadin®, Rimactane®) |
| **Fluconazole** | |
| Isoniazid (Laniazid®, Nydrazid®) | |
| **Itraconazole** | |
| **Ketoconazole** | |
| Neuroleptics | |
| Oral contraceptives | |
| Psoralen dermatologics | |
| Quinidine | |
| Quinolone antibiotics | |
| SSRIs | |
| Tricyclic antidepressants | |

### LOW THERAPEUTIC INDEX DRUGS

**Hepatic Oxidation (Cytochrome P-450 Mediated Clearance)**
Antiarrhythmic drugs
Anticonvulsants
Antineoplastic/immunosuppressive drugs
Oral anticoagulants
Theophylline

### CYTOCHROME P-450 ENZYMES AND RESPECTIVE METABOLIZED DRUGS

#### Cytochrome P-450 1A2

**SUBSTRATES**
**Acetaminophen**
Acetonilide
Aminophylline
**Amitriptyline (demethylation)**
Antipyrine
Betaxolol
Caffeine
Chlorpromazine
Clomipramine (demethylation)
Clozapine
Cyclobenzaprine (demethylation)
Desipramine (demethylation)
**Diazepam**
Estradiol
Fluvoxamine
Grepafloxacin
Haloperidol
Imipramine (demethylation)
Levopromazine
Maprotiline
Methadone
Metoclopramide
Mirtazapine (hydroxylation)
Nortriptyline
Olanzapine (demethylation, hydroxylation)
Ondansetron
Phenacetin
Phenothiazines
Propafenone
Propranolol
Riluzole
Ritonavir
Ropinirole
Ropivacaine
Tacrine
Tamoxifen
Theophylline
Thioridazine
Thiothixene
Trifluoperazine
Verapamil
Warfarin (R-warfarin, minor pathway)
Zileuton
Zopiclone

**INDUCERS**
**Carbamazepine**
Charbroiled meats
Cruciferous vegetables (cabbage, brussel sprouts, broccoli, cauliflower)
Nicotine
Omeprazole
Phenobarbital
Phenytoin
Primidone
Rifampin
Ritonavir

**INHIBITORS**
Anastrozole

Cimetidine
**Ciprofloxacin**
Citalopram (weak)
**Clarithromycin**
Diethyldithiocarbamate
Diltiazem
Enoxacin
**Erythromycin**
Ethinyl estradiol
Fluvoxamine
Fluoxetine (high dose)
Grapefruit juice
Isoniazid
**Ketoconazole**
Levofloxacin
Mexiletine
Mibefradil
Norfloxacin
Paroxetine (high dose)
Ritonavir
Sertraline (weak)
Tacrine
Tert TCAs
Zileuton

### Cytochrome P-450 2A6

**Substrate**
Letrozole
Montelukast
Nicotine
Ritonavir
Tamoxifen

**INDUCERS**
Barbiturates

**INHIBITORS**
Diethyldithiocarbamate
Letrozole
Ritonavir
Tranylcypromine

### Cytochrome P-450 2B6

**Substrate**
Antipyrine
Bupropion (hydroxylation)
Cyclophosphamide
Ifosfamide
Nicotine
Orphenadrine
Tamoxifen

**INDUCERS**
Phenobarbital
Phenytoin
Primidone

**INHIBITORS**
Diethyldithiocarbamate
Orphenadrine

### Cytochrome P-450 2C (Specific isozyme has not been identified)

**SUBSTRATES**
Antipyrine
Carvedilol
Clozapine (minor)
Mestranol
Mephobarbital
Tamoxifen
Ticrynafen

**INDUCERS**
**Carbamazepine**
Phenobarbital
Phenytoin
Primidone
Sulfinpyrazone

**INHIBITORS**
Isoniazid
**Ketoconazole**
**Ketoprofen**

### Cytochrome P-450 2C8

**SUBSTRATES**
**Carbamazepine**
**Diazepam**
**Diclofenac**
**Ibuprofen**
Mephobarbital
**Naproxen (5-hydroxylation)**
Omeprazole
Paclitaxel
Retinoic acid
Tolbutamide
Warfarin (S-warfarin)

**INDUCERS**
Phenobarbital
Primidone

**INHIBITORS**
Anastrozole
Omeprazole

### Cytochrome P-450 2C9

**SUBSTRATES**
**Amitriptyline (demethylation)**
Dapsone
**Diclofenac**
**Flurbiprofen**
Fluvastatin
Glimepiride
Hexobarbital
**Ibuprofen**
Imipramine (demethylation)
Indomethacin
Irbesartan
Losartan
Mefenamic acid
**Metronidazole**
Mirtazapine
Montelukast
**Naproxen (5-hydroxylation)**
Phenytoin
Piroxicam
Ritonavir
Sildenafil citrate
Tenoxicam
Tetrahydrocannabinol
Tolbutamide
Torsemide

## PHARMACOLOGY OF DRUG METABOLISM AND INTERACTIONS *(Continued)*

Warfarin (S-warfarin)
Zafirlukast (hydroxylation)
Zileuton

**INDUCERS**
**Fluconazole**
Fluoxetine
Rifampin

**INHIBITORS**
Amiodarone
Anastrozole
Chloramphenicol
Cimetidine
**Diclofenac**
Disulfiram
**Flurbiprofen**
Fluvastatin
Fluvoxamine
**Ketoprofen**
**Metronidazole**
Omeprazole
Phenylbutazone
Ritonavir
Sulfamethoxazole-trimethoprim
Sulfaphenazole
Sulfinpyrazone
Sulfonamides
Troglitazone
Valproic acid
Warfarin (R-warfarin)
Zafirlukast

### Cytochrome P-450 2C18

**SUBSTRATES**
Dronabinol
**Naproxen**
Omeprazole
Piroxicam
Proguanil
Propranolol
Retinoic acid
Warfarin

**INHIBITORS**
Cimetidine

### Cytochrome P-450 2C19

**SUBSTRATES**
**Amitriptyline (demethylation)**
Barbiturates
Carisoprodol
Citalopram
Clomipramine (demethylation)
Desmethyldiazepam
**Diazepam (N-demethylation, minor pathway)**
Divalproex sodium
Hexobarbital
Imipramine (demethylation)
Lansoprazole
Mephenytoin
Mephobarbital
Moclobemide
Olanzapine (minor)
Omeprazole
Pentamidine
Phenytoin
Proguanil
Propranolol
Ritonavir
Topiramate
Valproic acid
Warfarin (R-warfarin)

**INDUCERS**
Rifampin

**INHIBITORS**
Cimetidine
Citalopram (weak)
Felbamate
**Fluconazole**
Fluoxetine
Fluvoxamine
Letrozole
Omeprazole
Proguanil
Ritonavir
Sertraline
Teniposide
Tolbutamide
Topiramate
Tranylcypromine
Troglitazone

### Cytochrome P-450 2D6

**SUBSTRATES**
**Amitriptyline (hydroxylation)**
Amphetamine
Betaxolol
Bisoprolol
Brofaromine
Bufurolol
Bupropion
Captopril
Carvedilol
Chlorpheniramine
Chlorpromazine
Cinnarizine
Clomipramine (hydroxylation)
Clozapine (minor pathway)
Codeine (hydroxylation, o-demethylation)
Cyclobenzaprine (hydroxylation)
Cyclophosphamide
Debrisoquin
Delavirdine
Desipramine
Dextromethorphan (o-demethylation)
Dihydrocodeine
Diphenhydramine
Dolasetron
Donepezil
Doxepin
Encainide
Fenfluramine
Flecainide
Fluoxetine (minor pathway)
Fluphenazine
Halofantrine
Haloperidol (minor pathway)

**Hydrocodone**
Hydrocortisone
Hydroxyamphetamine
Imipramine (hydroxylation)
Labetalol
Loratadine
Maprotiline
m-Chlorophenylpiperazine (m-CPP)
**Meperidine**
Methadone
Methamphetamine
Metoclopramide
Metoprolol
Mexiletine
Mianserin
Mirtazapine (hydroxylation)
Molindone
Morphine
Nortriptyline (hydroxylation)
Olanzapine (minor, hydroxymethylation)
Ondansetron
Orphenadrine
**Oxycodone**
Papaverine
Paroxetine (minor pathway)
Penbutolol
Pentazocine
Perhexiline
Perphenazine
Phenformin
Pindolol
Promethazine
Propafenone
Propranolol
Quetiapine
Remoxipride
Risperidone
Ritonavir (minor)
Ropivacaine
Selegiline
Sertindole
Sertraline (minor pathway)
Sparteine
Tamoxifen
Thioridazine
Tiagabine
Timolol
Tolterodine
Tramadol
Trazodone
Trimipramine
Tropisetron
Venlafaxine (o-desmethylation)
Yohimbine

**INHIBITORS**
Amiodarone
Chloroquine
Chlorpromazine
Cimetidine
Citalopram
Clomipramine
**Codeine**
Delavirdine
Desipramine
Dextropropoxyphene
Diltiazem
Doxorubicin
Fluoxetine
Fluphenazine
Fluvoxamine
Haloperidol
Labetalol
Lobeline
Lomustine
Methadone
Mibefradil
Moclobemide
Norfluoxetine
Paroxetine
Perphenazine
Propafenone
Quinacrine
Quinidine
Ranitidine
Risperidone (weak)
Ritonavir
Sertindole
Sertraline (weak)
Thioridazine
Valproic acid
Venlafaxine (weak)
Vinblastine
Vincristine
Vinorelbine
Yohimbine

## Cytochrome P-450 2E1

**SUBSTRATES**
**Acetaminophen**
Acetone
Aniline
Benzene
Caffeine
Chlorzoxazone
Clozapine
Dapsone
Dextromethorphan
Enflurane
Ethanol
Halothane
Isoflurane
Isoniazid
Methoxyflurane
Nitrosamine
Ondansetron
Phenol
Ritonavir
Sevoflurane
Styrene
Tamoxifen
Theophylline
Venlafaxine

**INDUCERS**
Ethanol
Isoniazid

**INHIBITORS**
Diethyldithiocarbamate (disulfiram metabolite)
Dimethyl sulfoxide
Disulfiram
Ritonavir

## Cytochrome P-450 3A3/4

**SUBSTRATES**
**Acetaminophen**
Alfentanil
Alprazolam**

## PHARMACOLOGY OF DRUG METABOLISM AND INTERACTIONS *(Continued)*

Amiodarone
**Amitriptyline**
Amlodipine
Anastrozole
Androsterone
Antipyrine
Astemizole**
Atorvastatin
Benzphetamine
Bepridil
Budesonide
Bupropion (minor)
Buspirone
Bromazepam
Bromocriptine
Busulfan
Caffeine
Cannabinoids
**Carbamazepine**
Cerivastatin
Chlorpromazine
Cimetidine
Cisapride**
Citalopram
**Clarithromycin**
**Clindamycin**
Clomipramine
Clonazepam
Clozapine
Cocaine
**Codeine (demethylation)**
Cortisol
Cortisone
Cyclobenzaprine (demethylation)
Cyclophosphamide
Cyclosporine
Dapsone
Dehydroepiandrostendione
Delavirdine
Desmethyldiazepam
**Dexamethasone**
Dextromethorphan (minor, N-demethylation)
**Diazepam (minor; hydroxylation, N-demethylation)**
Digitoxin
Diltiazem
Disopyramide
Docetaxel
Dolasetron
Donepezil
Doxorubicin
**Doxycycline**
Dronabinol
Enalapril
**Erythromycin**
Estradiol
Ethinyl estradiol
Ethosuximide
Etoposide
Felodipine
Fentanyl
Fexofenadine
Finasteride
Fluoxetine
Flutamide
Glyburide
Granisetron
Halofantrine
Hydrocortisone
Hydroxyarginine
Ifosfamide
Imipramine
Indinavir
Isradipine
**Itraconazole**
**Ketoconazole**
Lansoprazole (minor)
Letrozole
**Lidocaine**
Loratadine
Losartan
Lovastatin
Methadone
Mibefradil
**Miconazole**
**Midazolam**
Mifepristone
Mirtazapine (N-demethylation)
Montelukast
Navelbine
Nefazodone
Nelfinavir**
Nevirapine
Nicardipine
Nifedipine
Niludipine
Nimodipine
Nisoldipine
Nitrendipine
Omeprazole (sulfonation)
Ondansetron
Oral contraceptives
Orphenadrine
Paclitaxel
Pimozide**
Pravastatin
Prednisone
Progesterone
Proguanil
Propafenone
Quercetin
Quetiapine
Quinidine
Quinine
Repaglinide
Retinoic acid
Rifampin
Ritonavir**
Salmeterol
Saquinavir
Sertindole
Sertraline
Sibutramine##
Sildenafil citrate
Simvastatin
Sufentanil
Tacrolimus
Tamoxifen
Temazepam
Teniposide
Testosterone
Tetrahydrocannabinol
Theophylline
Tiagabine
Tolterodine
Toremifene
Trazodone
Tretinoin
**Triazolam****

Troglitazone
Troleandomycin
Venlafaxine (N-demethylation)
Verapamil
Vinblastine
Vincristine
Warfarin (R-warfarin)
Yohimbine
Zileuton
Zatoestron
Ziprasidone
Zolpidem**
Zonisamide

**INDUCERS**
**Carbamazepine**
**Dexamethasone**
Ethosuximide
Glucocorticoids
Griseofulvin
Nafcillin
Nelfinavir
Nevirapine
Phenobarbital
Phenylbutazone
Phenytoin
Primidone
Progesterone
Rifabutin
Rifampin
Sulfadimidine
Sulfinpyrazone
Troglitazone

**INHIBITORS**
Amiodarone
Anastrozole
**Azithromycin**
Cannabinoids
Cimetidine
**Clarithromycin****
**Clotrimazole**
Cyclosporine
Danazol
Delavirdine
**Dexamethasone**
Diethyldithiocarbamate
Diltiazem
Dirithromycin
Disulfiram
**Erythromycin****
Ethinyl estradiol
**Fluconazole (weak)**
Fluoxetine
Fluvoxamine**
Gestodene
Grapefruit juice
Indinavir
Isoniazid
**Itraconazole****
**Ketoconazole****
**Metronidazole**
Mibefradil**
Miconazole (moderate)
Nefazodone**
Nelfinavir
Nevirapine
Norfloxacin
Norfluoxetine
Omeprazole (weak)
Oxiconazole
Paroxetine (weak)
Propoxyphene
Quinidine
Quinine**
Ranitidine
Ritonavir**
Saquinavir
Sertindole
Sertraline
Troglitazone
Troleandomycin
Valproic acid (weak)
Verapamil
Zafirlukast
Zileuton

****Contraindications:**
Astemizole, cisapride, and triazolam contraindicated with nefazodone
Pimozide contraindicated with macrolide antibiotics
Alprazolam and triazolam contraindicated with ketoconazole and itraconazole
Astemizole, and cisapride contraindicated with fluvoxamine
Ritonavir contraindicated with triazolam, zolpidem, astemizole, rifabutin, quinine, clarithromycin, troleandomycin
Mibefradil contraindicated with astemizole
Nelfinavir contraindicated with rifabutin

##Do not use with SSRIs, sumatriptan, lithium, meperidine, fentanyl, dextromethorphan, or pentazocine within 2 weeks of a MAOI.

### Cytochrome P-450 3A5-7

**SUBSTRATES**
Cortisol
Ethinyl estradiol
Lovastatin
Nifedipine
Quinidine
Testosterone
**Triazolam**
Vinblastine
Vincristine

**INDUCERS**
Phenobarbital
Phenytoin
Primidone
Rifampin

**INHIBITORS**
**Clotrimazole**
**Ketoconazole**
**Metronidazole**
**Miconazole**
Troleandomycin

**Note:** Bolded entries indicate drugs used in dentistry.

# PHARMACOLOGY OF DRUG METABOLISM AND INTERACTIONS *(Continued)*

**Table 2.**
**CONTRAINDICATED MEDICATIONS AND POTENTIAL ALTERNATIVES* WHEN A PATIENT IS TAKING RITONAVIR (Norvir®)**

| Contraindicated Medications[a] | | | Potential Alternatives[b] (these alternatives may not be therapeutically equivalent) | | |
|---|---|---|---|---|---|
| **Drug Class** | **Generic Name** | **Brand Name** | **Generic Name** | **Brand Name** | **Exposed Patients** |
| Analgesic | Meperidine | Demerol® | Acetaminophen | Tylenol® | N=135 |
| | Piroxicam | Feldene® | Aspirin | | N=43 |
| Cardiovascular (antiarrhythmic) | Amiodarone | Cordarone® | Very limited clinical experience | | |
| | Encainide | Enkaid® | | | |
| | Flecainide | Tambocor® | | | |
| | Propafenone | Rythmol® | | | |
| Antimycobacterial | Rifabutin | Mycobutin® | Clarithromycin | Biaxin® | N=156[c] |
| | | | Ethambutol | Myambutol® | N=66 |
| Cardiovascular (calcium channel blocker) | Bepridil | Vascor® | Very limited clinical experience | | |
| Cold and allergy (antihistamine) | Astemizole | Hismanal® | Loratadine | Claritin® | N=36 |
| Ergot alkaloid (vasoconstrictor) | Dihydroergotamine | D.H.E. 45® | Very limited clinical experience | | |
| | Ergotamine | Various | | | |
| Gastrointestinal | Cisapride | Propulsid® | Very limited clinical experience | | |
| Psychotropic (antidepressant) | Bupropion | Wellbutrin® | Desipramine | Norpramin®[d] | |
| Psychotropic (neuroleptic) | Clozapine | Clozaril® | Very limited clinical experience | | |
| | Pimozide | Orap® | | | |
| Psychotropic (sedative/ hypnotic) | Alprazolam | Xanax® | Temazepam | Restoril® | N=40 |
| | Clorazepate | Tranxene® | Lorazepam | Ativan® | N=33 |
| | Diazepam | Valium® | | | |
| | Estazolam | ProSom™ | | | |
| | Flurazepam | Dalmane® | | | |
| | Midazolam | Versed® | | | |
| | Triazolam | Halcion® | | | |
| | Zolpidem | Ambien" | | | |

[a] See the CONTRAINDICATIONS section of the Norvir® package insert.

[b] See the PRECAUTIONS-DRUG INTERACTIONS section of the Norvir® package insert for more information.

*During clinical trials, Norvir® was given to patients concomitantly taking a variety of medications. These medications were not evaluated in drug interaction studies. The number of Norvir®-treated patients exposed to each drug is provided in the last column.

[c] Also evaluated in drug interaction study (N=22). See "Results of Drug Interaction Studies."

[d] No clinical experience with combination. Only evaluated in drug interaction study (N=14). See "Results of Drug Interaction Studies."

Norvir® has high affinity for several cytochrome P-450 (CYP) isoenzymes including CYP3A, CYP2D6, and CYP2C9. Large dose reductions (>50%) and increased therapeutic drug concentration monitoring of therapeutic and adverse effects is recommended when drugs extensively metabolized are used concomitantly with Norvir®.

## Table 3.
## DRUG INTERACTIONS WITH HIV ANTIVIRAL DRUGS

| Indinavir | Nelfinavir | Ritonavir | Saquinavir |
|---|---|---|---|
| •Inhibits cytochrome P-450 (less than ritonavir)<br>•Not recommended for concurrent use: rifampin, terfenadine, astemizole, cisapride, triazolam, midazolam, ergot alkaloids<br>•Indinavir levels increased by: ketoconazole, delavirdine<br>•Indinavir levels reduced by rifampin, rifabutin, nevirapine, grapefruit juice<br>•Didanosine: reduces indinavir absorption unless taken >2 hours apart | •Inhibits cytochrome P-450 (less than ritonavir)<br>•Nelfinavir levels reduced by rifampin, rifabutin<br>•Not recommended for concurrent use: rifampin, triazolam, midazolam, ergot alkaloids, terfenadine, astemizole, cisapride<br>•Nelfinavir decreases levels of ethinyl estradiol and norethindrone<br>•Nelfinavir increases levels of rifabutin, saquinavir, and indinavir | •Inhibits cytochrome P-450 (potent inhibitor)<br>•Ritonavir increases levels of multiple drugs that are not recommended for current use<br>•Didanosine: reduced absorption of both drugs; take >2 hours apart<br>•Ritonavir decreases levels of ethinyl estradiol, theophylline, sulfamethoxazole, and zidovudine<br>•Ritonavir increases levels of clarithromycin and desipramine | •Inhibits cytochrome P-450<br>•Saquinavir levels increased by: ritonavir, ketoconazole, grapefruit juice, nelfinavir, delavirdine<br>•Saquinavir levels reduced by: rifampin, rifabutin, phenobarbital, phenytoin, dexamethasone, carbamazepine, and nevirapine<br>•Not recommended for concurrent use: terfenadine, astemizole, cisapride, ergot alkaloids |

## Table 4.
## INTERACTIONS BETWEEN CIGARETTE SMOKE AND DRUGS

| Drug | Mechanism | Effect on Cigarette Smokers |
|---|---|---|
| Theophylline | Induction of the CYP1A2 isozyme | Smoking may lead to reduced theophylline serum concentrations and decreased clinical effect; the elimination of theophylline is considerably more rapid in smokers |
| Tacrine | Induction of the CYP1A2 isozyme | Effectiveness of tacrine in smokers may be decreased |
| Insulin | Decreased insulin absorption, which may be related to peripheral vasoconstriction | Insulin-dependent diabetics who smoke heavily may require a 15% to 30% higher dose of insulin than nonsmokers |
| Flecainide | Unknown | Smoking may reduce flecainide serum concentrations |
| Propoxyphene | Unknown | Smokers may require a higher dosage of propoxyphene to achieve analgesic effects |
| Propranolol | Increased release of catecholamines (eg, epinephrine) in smokers | Smokers taking propranolol may have increased blood pressure and heart rate relative to nonsmokers. Effects on prevention of angina pectoris and stroke should be considered |
| Diazepam; Chlordiazepoxide | Unknown; whether pharmacokinetics is altered or end-organ responsiveness is decreased is unclear | Smokers may require larger doses of diazepam and chlordiazepoxide to achieve sedative effects |

Adapted from Schein, JR, "Cigarette Smoking and Clinically Significant Drug Interactions," *Ann Pharmacother*, 1995, 29(11):1139-47.

# ALPHABETICAL LISTING OF DRUGS

- **A-200™ Shampoo [OTC]** *see* Pyrethrins *on page 867*
- **A and D™ Ointment [OTC]** *see* Vitamin A and Vitamin D *on page 1049*

## Abacavir (a BAK a veer)

**Related Information**

Systemic Viral Diseases *on page 1115*

**U.S. Brand Names** Ziagen®

**Therapeutic Category** Reverse Transcriptase Inhibitor

**Use** Treatment of HIV infections in combination with other antiretroviral agents

**Usual Dosage** Oral:

Children 3 months to 16 years: 8 mg/kilogram body weight twice daily (maximum: 300 mg twice daily) in combination with other antiretroviral agents

Adults: 300 mg twice daily in combination with other antiretroviral agents

**Mechanism of Action** Nucleoside reverse transcriptase inhibitor which interferes with HIV viral RNA dependent DNA polymerase resulting in inhibition of viral replication

**Local Anesthetic/Vasoconstrictor Precautions** No information available to require special precautions

**Effects on Dental Treatment** No effects or complications reported

**Other Adverse Effects Note**: Hypersensitivity reactions, which may be fatal, occur in ~5% of patients. Symptoms may include anaphylaxis, fever, rash, fatigue, diarrhea, abdominal pain, nausea and vomiting. Less common symptoms may include edema, lethargy, malaise, myalgia, shortness of breath, mouth ulcerations, conjunctivitis, lymphadenopathy, hepatic failure and renal failure.

Rates of adverse reactions were defined during combination therapy with lamivudine. Adverse reaction rates attributable to abacavir alone are not available.

Adults:

>10%:

Endocrine & metabolic: Hyperglycemia, hypertriglyceridemia (25%)

Gastrointestinal: Nausea (47%), vomiting (16%), diarrhea (12%), anorexia (11%), pancreatitis

1% to 10%: Central nervous system: Insomnia (7%)

Incidence unknown:

Neuromuscular & skeletal: Weakness

Miscellaneous: Elevated transaminases

Children:

>10%:

Central nervous system: Fever (19%), headache (16%)

Dermatologic: Rash (11%)

Gastrointestinal: Nausea (38%), vomiting (38%), diarrhea (16%)

1% to 10%: Gastrointestinal: Anorexia (9%)

**Drug Uptake**

Absorption: Bioavailability 83%; food may decrease absorption

Serum half-life: 1.5 hours

Time to maximum peak: 0.7-1.7 hours

**Pregnancy Risk Factor** C

**Generic Available** No

- **Abbokinase®** *see* Urokinase *on page 1035*
- **Abbreviations and Measurements** *see page 1198*

## Abciximab (ab SIK si mab)

**U.S. Brand Names** ReoPro®

**Therapeutic Category** Platelet Aggregation Inhibitor

**Synonyms** C7E3; 7E3

**Use** Adjunct to percutaneous transluminal coronary angioplasty or atherectomy (PTCA) for the prevention of acute cardiac ischemic complications in patients at high risk for abrupt closure of the treated coronary vessel

**Usual Dosage** I.V.: 0.25 mg/kg bolus followed by an infusion of 10 mcg/minute for 12 hours

**Mechanism of Action** Abciximab binds to the glycoprotein GPIIb/IIIa receptor, a major receptor involved in the common pathway for platelet aggregation. Platelet aggregation is, therefore, inhibited.

**Local Anesthetic/Vasoconstrictor Precautions** No information available to require special precautions

**Effects on Dental Treatment** No effects or complications reported

**Other Adverse Effects**

>10%:

Cardiovascular: Hypotension

Central nervous system: Pain

Gastrointestinal: Nausea
Hematologic: Major bleeding episodes
1% to 10%:
Cardiovascular: Bradycardia, peripheral edema
Hematologic: Minor bleeding episodes, thrombocytopenia, anemia
Respiratory: Pleural effusion

**Drug Interactions** Increased toxicity:
Bleeding could occur when abciximab is given with any of the following drugs:
Heparin, other anticoagulants, thrombolytics, and antiplatelet drugs
Allergic reactions: Diagnostic or therapeutic monoclonal antibodies

**Drug Uptake** Half-life: ~30 minutes

**Pregnancy Risk Factor** C

**Dosage Forms** Injection: 2 mg/mL (5 mL)

**Generic Available** No


- ♦ **Abelcet™ Injection** *see* Amphotericin B Lipid Complex *on page 81*
- ♦ **ABLC** *see* Amphotericin B Lipid Complex *on page 81*
- ♦ **Absorbine® Antifungal [OTC]** *see* Tolnaftate *on page 997*
- ♦ **Absorbine® Antifungal Foot Powder [OTC]** *see* Miconazole *on page 672*
- ♦ **Absorbine® Jock Itch [OTC]** *see* Tolnaftate *on page 997*
- ♦ **Absorbine Jr.® Antifungal [OTC]** *see* Tolnaftate *on page 997*


## Acarbose (AY car bose)

**Related Information**
Endocrine Disorders & Pregnancy *on page 1082*

**U.S. Brand Names** Precose®

**Canadian Brand Names** Pradnase®

**Therapeutic Category** Alpha-Glucosidase Inhibitor; Hypoglycemic Agent, Oral

**Use** Treatment of noninsulin-dependent diabetes mellitus (NIDDM); as monotherapy or in combination with a sulfonylurea when diet plus acarbose or a sulfonylurea does not result in adequate glycemic control

**Usual Dosage** Oral:
Adults: Dosage must be individualized on the basis of effectiveness and tolerance while not exceeding the maximum recommended dose of 100 mg 3 times/day
**Initial dose:** 25 mg 3 times/day with the first bite of each main meal
**Maintenance dose:** Should be adjusted at 4- to 8-week intervals based on 1-hour postprandial glucose levels and tolerance. Dosage may be increased from 25 mg 3 times/day to 50 mg 3 times/day. Some patients may benefit from increasing the dose to 100 mg 3 times/day. Maintenance dose ranges: 50-100 mg 3 times/day.
**Maximum dose:**
≤60 kg: 50 mg 3 times/day
>60 kg: 100 mg 3 times/day

**Patients receiving sulfonylureas:** Acarbose given in combination with a sulfonylurea will cause a further lowering of blood glucose and may increase the hypoglycemic potential of the sulfonylurea. If hypoglycemia occurs, appropriate adjustments in the dosage of these agents should be made.

Elderly: Mean steady-state AUC and maximum concentrations of acarbose were 1.5 times higher in elderly compared to young volunteers; however, these differences were not statistically significant

**Mechanism of Action** Competitive, reversible inhibition of pancreatic alpha-amylase and membrane-bound intestinal alpha-glucoside hydrolase enzymes to result in delayed glucose absorption and a lowering of postprandial hyperglycemia

**Local Anesthetic/Vasoconstrictor Precautions** No information available to require special precautions

**Effects on Dental Treatment** No effects or complications reported

**Drug Interactions** Decreased effect of acarbose if given concomitantly with any of the following drugs: Thiazides and other diuretics, corticosteroids, phenothiazines, thyroid products, estrogens, oral contraceptives, phenytoin, nicotinic acid, sympathomimetics, calcium channel-blocking drugs, isoniazid, intestinal adsorbents (eg, charcoal), digestive enzyme preparations (eg, amylase, pancreatin)

**Drug Uptake** Absorption: <2% absorbed as active drug

**Pregnancy Risk Factor** B

**Dosage Forms** Tablet: 50 mg, 100 mg

**Generic Available** No


- ♦ **Accolate®** *see* Zafirlukast *on page 1056*
- ♦ **Accupril®** *see* Quinapril *on page 871*

♦ **Accutane®** *see* Isotretinoin *on page 557*

## Acebutolol (a se BYOO toe lole)

**U.S. Brand Names** Sectral®

**Canadian Brand Names** Monitan®; Rhotral

**Therapeutic Category** Antiarrhythmic Agent, Class II; Antiarrhythmic Agent (Supraventricular & Ventricular); Beta-adrenergic Blocker, Cardioselective

**Use** Treatment of hypertension, ventricular arrhythmias, angina

**Usual Dosage** Oral:

Adults: 400-800 mg/day in 2 divided doses; maximum: 1200 mg/day

Elderly: Initial: 200-400 mg/day; dose reduction due to age related decrease in $Cl_{cr}$ will be necessary; do not exceed 800 mg/day

**Mechanism of Action** Competitively blocks $beta_1$-adrenergic receptors with little or no effect on $beta_2$-receptors except at high doses; exhibits membrane stabilizing and intrinsic sympathomimetic activity

**Local Anesthetic/Vasoconstrictor Precautions** No information available to require special precautions

**Effects on Dental Treatment** Noncardioselective beta-blockers (ie, propranolol, nadolol) enhance the pressor response to epinephrine, resulting in hypertension and bradycardia. This has not been reported for acebutolol, a cardioselective beta-blocker. Therefore, local anesthetic with vasoconstrictor can be safely used in patients medicated with acebutolol. Many nonsteroidal anti-inflammatory drugs such as ibuprofen and indomethacin can reduce the hypotensive effect of beta-blockers after 3 or more weeks of therapy with the NSAID. Short-term NSAID use (ie, 3 days) requires no special precautions in patients taking beta-blockers.

**Other Adverse Effects**

>10%: Central nervous system: Fatigue

1% to 10%:

- Cardiovascular: Chest pain, edema, bradycardia, hypotension
- Central nervous system: Headache, dizziness, insomnia, depression, abnormal dreams
- Dermatologic: Rash
- Gastrointestinal: Constipation, diarrhea, dyspepsia, nausea, flatulence
- Genitourinary: Micturition (frequency)
- Neuromuscular & skeletal: Arthralgia, myalgia
- Ocular: Abnormal vision
- Respiratory: Dyspnea, rhinitis, cough

<1%:

- Cardiovascular: Ventricular arrhythmias, heart block, heart failure, facial swelling
- Gastrointestinal: Dry mouth, anorexia
- Genitourinary: Impotence, urinary retention
- Miscellaneous: Cold extremities

**Drug Interactions**

Decreased effect of beta-blockers:

- Barbiturates (increased liver metabolism of beta-blockers to result in lower serum levels)
- NSAIDs (attenuate the hypotensive therapeutic effects of beta-blockers)
- Rifampin (increased liver metabolism of beta-blockers to result in lower serum levels)

Increased effects of beta-blockers:

- Calcium channel blockers (increase serum levels of beta-blockers by unknown mechanism to enhance hypotension)

Beta-blockers increase the effects of:

- Epinephrine (vasoconstrictor; initial hypertensive episode followed by bradycardia) only from noncardioselective type beta-blockers
- Phenylephrine (Neosynephrine®; enhanced pressor response)
- Theophylline (inhibit theophylline metabolism causing increase in serum concentrations)

**Drug Uptake**

Absorption: Oral: Well absorbed (40%)

Serum half-life: 6-7 hours average

Time to peak: 2-4 hours

**Pregnancy Risk Factor** B

**Generic Available** Yes

**Selected Readings**

Foster CA and Aston SJ, "Propranolol-Epinephrine Interaction: A Potential Disaster," *Plast Reconstr Surg*, 1983, 72(1):74-8.

Wong DG, Spence JD, Lamki L, et al, "Effect of Nonsteroidal Anti-inflammatory Drugs on Control of Hypertension of Beta-Blockers and Diuretics," *Lancet*, 1986, 1(8488):997-1001.

Wynn RL, "Dental Nonsteroidal Anti-inflammatory Drugs and Prostaglandin-Based Drug Interactions, Part Two," *Gen Dent*, 1992, 40(2):104, 106, 108.

Wynn RL, "Epinephrine Interactions With Beta-Blockers," *Gen Dent*, 1994, 42(1):16, 18.

- **Aceon®** *see* Perindopril Erbumine *on page 784*
- **Acephen® [OTC]** *see* Acetaminophen *on this page*
- **Aceta® [OTC]** *see* Acetaminophen *on this page*

## Acetaminophen (a seet a MIN oh fen)

**Related Information**

Acetaminophen and Pseudoephedrine *on page 31*
Acetaminophen, Dextromethorphan, and Pseudoephedrine *on page 32*
Butalbital Compound and Acetaminophen *on page 164*
Oral Pain *on page 1122*

**U.S. Brand Names** Acephen® [OTC]; Aceta® [OTC]; Apacet® [OTC]; Arthritis Foundation® Pain Reliever, Aspirin Free [OTC]; Aspirin Free Anacin® Maximum Strength [OTC]; Children's Silapap® [OTC]; Feverall™ [OTC]; Feverall™ Sprinkle Caps [OTC]; Genapap® [OTC]; Halenol® Childrens [OTC]; Infants Feverall™ [OTC]; Infants' Silapap® [OTC]; Junior Strength Panadol® [OTC]; Liquiprin® [OTC]; Mapap® [OTC]; Maranox® [OTC]; Neopap® [OTC]; Panadol® [OTC]; Redutemp® [OTC]; Ridenol® [OTC]; Tempra® [OTC]; Tylenol® [OTC]; Tylenol® Extended Relief [OTC]; Uni-Ace® [OTC]

**Canadian Brand Names** Abenol®; A.F. Anacin®; Atasol®; Pediatrix; Tantaphen®

**Therapeutic Category** Analgesic, Non-narcotic; Antipyretic

**Use**

Dental: Treatment of postoperative pain
Medical: Treatment of pain and fever; does not have anti-inflammatory effects

**Usual Dosage** Oral:

Children <12 years: 10-15 mg/kg/dose every 4-6 hours as needed; do not exceed 5 doses (2.6 g) in 24 hours
Adults: 325-650 mg (1-2 tablets) every 4-6 hours or 1000 mg 3-4 times/day; do not exceed 4 g/day (4000 mg)

**Mechanism of Action** Inhibits the synthesis of prostaglandins in the CNS and peripherally blocks pain impulse generation; produces antipyresis by inhibition of hypothalamic heat-regulating center

**Local Anesthetic/Vasoconstrictor Precautions** No information available to require special precautions

**Effects on Dental Treatment** No effects or complications reported

**Other Adverse Effects** No data reported

**Contraindications** Patients with known Glucose-6-phosphate dehydrogenase (G-6-PD) deficiency; hypersensitivity to acetaminophen

**Warnings/Precautions** May cause severe hepatic toxicity on overdose; use with caution in patients with alcoholic liver disease; chronic daily dosing in adults of 5-8 g of acetaminophen over several weeks or 3-4 g/day of acetaminophen for 1 year have resulted in liver damage

**Drug Interactions**

Alcohol: Chronic excessive alcohol ingestion increases the liver toxicity of high doses of acetaminophen
Cholestyramine: Cholestyramine reduces the plasma acetaminophen concentrations and probably reduces acetaminophen response
Isoniazid (INH): Acetaminophen blood levels are increased by INH; hepatotoxicity has been reported with combination of acetaminophen and INH
Phenobarbital: Barbiturates such as phenobarbital may enhance the hepatotoxic effect of large doses of acetaminophen
Phenytoin: Phenytoin may enhance the hepatotoxic potential of large doses of acetaminophen
Warfarin (Coumadin®): Acetaminophen, when given to patients taking warfarin, may cause enhanced anticoagulation

**Drug Uptake**

Onset: 1-3 hours
Duration: 3-4 hours
Serum half-life: 1-4 hours
Time to peak serum concentration: 0.5-2 hours

**Pregnancy Risk Factor** B

**Breast-feeding Considerations** May be taken while breast-feeding

**Dosage Forms**

Caplet: 160 mg, 325 mg, 500 mg
Caplet, extended: 650 mg
Capsule: 80 mg
Drops: 48 mg/mL (15 mL); 60 mg/0.6 mL (15 mL); 80 mg/0.8 mL (15 mL); 100 mg/mL (15 mL, 30 mL)
Elixir: 80 mg/5 mL, 120 mg/5 mL, 160 mg/5 mL, 167 mg/5 mL, 325 mg/5 mL
Liquid, oral: 160 mg/5 mL, 500 mg/15 mL
Solution: 100 mg/mL (15 mL); 120 mg/2.5 mL
Suppository, rectal: 80 mg, 120 mg, 125 mg, 300 mg, 325 mg, 650 mg

(Continued)

## Acetaminophen *(Continued)*

Suspension, oral: 160 mg/5 mL
Suspension, oral drops: 80 mg/0.8 mL
Tablet: 325 mg, 500 mg, 650 mg
Tablet, chewable: 80 mg, 160 mg

**Dietary Considerations** May be taken with food

**Generic Available** Yes

**Comments** Doses of acetaminophen >5 g/day for several weeks can produce severe, often fatal liver damage. Hepatotoxicity caused by acetaminophen is potentiated by chronic alcohol consumption. It has been reported that a combination of two quarts of whiskey a day with 8-10 acetaminophen tablets daily resulted in severe liver toxicity. People who consume alcohol at the same time that they use acetaminophen, even in therapeutic doses, are at risk of developing hepatotoxicity.

A study by Hylek, et al, suggested that the combination of acetaminophen with warfarin (Coumadin®) may cause enhanced anticoagulation. The following recommendations have been made by Hylek, et al, and supported by an editorial in *JAMA* by Bell.

Dose and duration of acetaminophen should be as low as possible, individualized and monitored

The study by Hylek reported the following:

For patients who reported taking the equivalent of at least 4 regular strength (325 mg) tablets for longer than a week, the odds of having an INR >6.0 were increased 10-fold above those not taking acetaminophen. Risk decreased with lower intakes of acetaminophen reaching a background level of risk at a dose of 6 or fewer 325 mg tablets per week.

**Selected Readings**

Barker JD Jr, de Carle DJ, and Anuras S, "Chronic Excessive Acetaminophen Use in Liver Damage," *Ann Intern Med*, 1977, 87(3):299-301.
Bell WR, "Acetaminophen and Warfarin: Undesirable Synergy," *JAMA*, 1998, 279(9):702-3.
Dionne RA, Campbell RA, Cooper SA, et al, "Suppression of Postoperative Pain by Preoperative Administration of Ibuprofen in Comparison to Placebo, Acetaminophen, and Acetaminophen Plus Codeine," *J Clin Pharmacol*, 1983, 23(1):37-43.
Hylek EM, Heiman H, Skates SJ, et al, "Acetaminophen and Other Risk Factors for Excessive Warfarin Anticoagulation," *JAMA*, 1998, 279(9):657-62.
Lee WM, "Drug-Induced Hepatotoxicity," *N Engl J Med*, 1995, 333(17):1118-27.
Licht H, Seeff LB, and Zimmerman HJ, "Apparent Potentiation of Acetaminophen Hepatotoxicity by Alcohol," *Ann Intern Med*, 1980, 92(4):511.
McClain CJ, et al, "Potentiation of Acetaminophen Hepatotoxicity by Alcohol," *JAMA*, 1980, 244:251.
Murphy R, Swartz R, and Watkins PB, "Severe Acetaminophen Toxicity in a Patient Receiving Isoniazid," *Ann Intern Med*, 1990, 113(110):799-800.

♦ **Acetaminophen and Butalbital Compound** *see* Butalbital Compound and Acetaminophen *on page 164*

## Acetaminophen and Codeine (a seet a MIN oh fen & KOE deen)

**Related Information**

Acetaminophen *on previous page*

**U.S. Brand Names** Capital® and Codeine; Phenaphen® With Codeine; Tylenol® With Codeine

**Canadian Brand Names** Atasol® 8, 15, 30 With Caffeine; Empracet® 30, 60; Emtec-30®; Lenoltec No 1, 2, 3, 4; Novo-Gesic-C8; Novo-Gesic-C15; Novo-Gesic-C30

**Therapeutic Category** Analgesic, Narcotic

**Use**

Dental: Treatment of postoperative pain
Medical: Relief of pain

**Restrictions** C-III; C-V; Refillable up to 5 times in 6 months

**Usual Dosage**

Children: Not recommended in pediatric dental patients
Adults: Based on codeine (30-60 mg/dose) every 4-6 hours; 1-2 tablets every 4 hours to a maximum of 12 tablets/24 hours

**Mechanism of Action**

Acetaminophen: Inhibits the synthesis of prostaglandins in the CNS and peripherally blocks pain impulse generation; produces antipyresis by inhibition of hypothalamic heat-regulating center
Codeine: Binds to opiate receptors (mu and kappa subtypes) in the CNS causing inhibition of ascending pain pathways, altering the perception of and response to pain

**Local Anesthetic/Vasoconstrictor Precautions** No information available to require special precautions

**Effects on Dental Treatment** <1% of patients may experience dry mouth

**Other Adverse Effects**
>10%:
Central nervous system: Lightheadedness, dizziness, sedation
Gastrointestinal: Nausea, vomiting
1% to 10%: Gastrointestinal: Constipation

**Contraindications** Patients with known G-6-PD deficiency; hypersensitivity to acetaminophen; hypersensitivity to codeine

**Warnings/Precautions** Use with caution in patients with hypersensitivity reactions to other phenanthrene derivative opioid agonists (morphine, hydrocodone, hydromorphone, levorphanol, oxycodone, oxymorphone); respiratory diseases including asthma, emphysema, COPD, or severe liver or renal insufficiency; some preparations contain sulfites which may cause allergic reactions; may be habit-forming

Enhanced analgesia has been seen in elderly patients on therapeutic doses of narcotics; duration of action may be increased in the elderly; the elderly may be particularly susceptible to the CNS depressant and constipating effects of narcotics

**Drug Interactions**
With codeine component: Increased toxicity of CNS depressants, phenothiazines, tricyclic antidepressants, guanabenz, MAO inhibitors (may also lead to a decrease in blood pressure)
With acetaminophen component: Refer to Acetaminophen monograph

**Drug Uptake**
Acetaminophen:
Onset: 1-3 hours
Duration: 3-4 hours
Serum half-life: 1-4 hours
Time to peak serum concentration: 0.5-2 hours
Codeine:
Onset (analgesia): Oral: 30-45 minutes
Duration: 4-6 hours
Serum half-life: 2.5-3.5 hours
Time to peak serum concentration: 1-2 hours

**Pregnancy Risk Factor** C

**Breast-feeding Considerations** Both acetaminophen and codeine may be taken while breast-feeding

**Dosage Forms**
Capsule:
#2: Acetaminophen 325 mg and codeine phosphate 15 mg (C-III)
#3: Acetaminophen 325 mg and codeine phosphate 30 mg (C-III)
#4: Acetaminophen 325 mg and codeine phosphate 60 mg (C-III)
Elixir: Acetaminophen 120 mg and codeine phosphate 12 mg per 5 mL with alcohol 7% (C-V)
Suspension, oral, alcohol free: Acetaminophen 120 mg and codeine phosphate 12 mg per 5 mL (C-V)
Tablet: Acetaminophen 500 mg and codeine phosphate 30 mg (C-III); acetaminophen 650 mg and codeine phosphate 30 mg (C-III)
Tablet:
#1: Acetaminophen 300 mg and codeine phosphate 7.5 mg (C-III)
#2: Acetaminophen 300 mg and codeine phosphate 15 mg (C-III)
#3: Acetaminophen 300 mg and codeine phosphate 30 mg (C-III)
#4: Acetaminophen 300 mg and codeine phosphate 60 mg (C-III)

**Dietary Considerations** May be taken with food

**Generic Available** Yes

**Comments** Codeine products, as with other narcotic analgesics, are recommended only for acute dosing (ie, 3 days or less). The most common adverse effect you will see in your dental patients from codeine is nausea, followed by sedation and constipation. Codeine has narcotic addiction liability, especially when given long term. Because of the acetaminophen component, this product should be used with caution in patients with alcoholic liver disease.

A study by Hylek, et al, suggested that the combination of acetaminophen with warfarin (Coumadin®) may cause enhanced anticoagulation. The following recommendations have been made by Hylek, et al, and supported by an editorial in *JAMA* by Bell.

Dose and duration of acetaminophen should be as low as possible, individualized and monitored

The study by Hylek reported the following:

For patients who reported taking the equivalent of at least 4 regular strength (325 mg) tablets for longer than a week, the odds of having an INR >6.0 were increased 10-fold above those not taking acetaminophen. Risk decreased

(Continued)

## Acetaminophen and Codeine *(Continued)*

with lower intakes of acetaminophen reaching a background level of risk at a dose of 6 or fewer 325 mg tablets per week.

**Selected Readings**

Bell WR, "Acetaminophen and Warfarin: Undesirable Synergy," *JAMA*, 1998, 279(9):702-3.
Dionne RA, "New Approaches to Preventing and Treating Postoperative Pain," *J Am Dent Assoc*, 1992, 123(6):26-34.
Dionne RA, Campbell RA, Cooper SA, et al, "Suppression of Postoperative Pain by Preoperative Administration of Ibuprofen in Comparison to Placebo, Acetaminophen, and Acetaminophen Plus Codeine," *J Clin Pharmacol*, 1983, 23(1):37-43.
Forbes JA, Butterworth GA, Burchfield WH, et al, "Evaluation of Ketorolac, Aspirin, and an Acetaminophen-Codeine Combination in Postoperative Oral Surgery Pain," *Pharmacotherapy*, 1990, 10(6 Pt 2):77S-93S.
Gobetti JP, "Controlling Dental Pain," *J Am Dent Assoc*, 1992, 123(6):47-52.
Hylek EM, Heiman H, Skates SJ, et al, "Acetaminophen and Other Risk Factors for Excessive Warfarin Anticoagulation," *JAMA*, 1998, 279(9):657-62.

## Acetaminophen and Dextromethorphan

(a seet a MIN oh fen & dex troe meth OR fan)

**U.S. Brand Names** Bayer® Select® Chest Cold Caplets [OTC]; Drixoral® Cough & Sore Throat Liquid Caps [OTC]

**Therapeutic Category** Analgesic, Non-narcotic; Antipyretic; Antitussive

**Use** Treatment of mild to moderate pain and fever; symptomatic relief of coughs caused by minor viral upper respiratory tract infections or inhaled irritants; most effective for a chronic nonproductive cough

**Usual Dosage** Oral:

Children: 10-15 mg/kg/dose every 4-6 hours as needed; do **not** exceed 5 doses in 24 hours

Adults: 325-650 mg every 4-6 hours or 1000 mg 3-4 times/day; do **not** exceed 4 g/day

**Local Anesthetic/Vasoconstrictor Precautions** No information available to require special precautions

**Effects on Dental Treatment** No effects or complications reported

**Warnings/Precautions** Research on chicken embryos exposed to concentrations of dextromethorphan relative to those typically taken by humans has shown to cause birth defects and fetal death; more study is needed, but it is suggested that pregnant women should be advised not to use dextromethorphan-containing medications

**Generic Available** Yes

**Selected Readings**

Barker JD Jr, de Carle DJ, and Anuras S, "Chronic Excessive Acetaminophen Use in Liver Damage," *Ann Intern Med*, 1977, 87(3):299-301.
Dionne RA, Campbell RA, Cooper SA, et al, "Suppression of Postoperative Pain by Preoperative Administration of Ibuprofen in Comparison to Placebo, Acetaminophen, and Acetaminophen Plus Codeine," *J Clin Pharmacol*, 1983, 23(1):37-43.
Licht H, Seeff LB, and Zimmerman HJ, "Apparent Potentiation of Acetaminophen Hepatotoxicity by Alcohol," *Ann Intern Med*, 1980, 92(4):511.

## Acetaminophen and Diphenhydramine

(a seet a MIN oh fen & dye fen HYE dra meen)

**U.S. Brand Names** Arthritis Foundation® Nighttime [OTC]; Excedrin® P.M. [OTC]; Midol® PM [OTC]

**Therapeutic Category** Analgesic, Non-narcotic

**Use** Relief of mild to moderate pain; sinus headache

**Usual Dosage** Adults: Oral: Take 2 caplets or 5 mL of liquid at bedtime or as directed by physician; do not exceed recommended dosage; not for use in children <12 years of age

**Local Anesthetic/Vasoconstrictor Precautions** No information available to require special precautions

**Effects on Dental Treatment** 1% to 10%: Dry mouth

**Generic Available** Yes

**Selected Readings**

Barker JD Jr, de Carle DJ, and Anuras S, "Chronic Excessive Acetaminophen Use in Liver Damage," *Ann Intern Med*, 1977, 87(3):299-301.
Dionne RA, Campbell RA, Cooper SA, et al, "Suppression of Postoperative Pain by Preoperative Administration of Ibuprofen in Comparison to Placebo, Acetaminophen, and Acetaminophen Plus Codeine," *J Clin Pharmacol*, 1983, 23(1):37-43.
Licht H, Seeff LB, and Zimmerman HJ, "Apparent Potentiation of Acetaminophen Hepatotoxicity by Alcohol," *Ann Intern Med*, 1980, 92(4):511.

## Acetaminophen and Phenyltoloxamine

(a seet a MIN oh fen & fen il to LOKS a meen)

**U.S. Brand Names** Percogesic® [OTC]

**Therapeutic Category** Analgesic, Non-narcotic

**Use** Relief of mild to moderate pain

**Usual Dosage** Adults: Oral: 1-2 tablets every 4 hours

**Local Anesthetic/Vasoconstrictor Precautions** No information available to require special precautions

**Effects on Dental Treatment** No effects or complications reported

**Pregnancy Risk Factor** B

**Generic Available** Yes

**Selected Readings**

Barker JD Jr, de Carle DJ, and Anuras S, "Chronic Excessive Acetaminophen Use in Liver Damage," *Ann Intern Med*, 1977, 87(3):299-301.

Dionne RA, Campbell RA, Cooper SA, et al, "Suppression of Postoperative Pain by Preoperative Administration of Ibuprofen in Comparison to Placebo, Acetaminophen, and Acetaminophen Plus Codeine," *J Clin Pharmacol*, 1983, 23(1):37-43.

Licht H, Seeff LB, and Zimmerman HJ, "Apparent Potentiation of Acetaminophen Hepatotoxicity by Alcohol," *Ann Intern Med*, 1980, 92(4):511.

## Acetaminophen and Pseudoephedrine

(a seet a MIN oh fen & soo doe e FED rin)

**U.S. Brand Names** Allerest® No Drowsiness [OTC]; Bayer® Select Head Cold Caplets [OTC]; Coldrine® [OTC]; Dristan® Cold Caplets [OTC]; Dynafed®, Maximum Strength [OTC]; Ornex® No Drowsiness [OTC]; Sinarest®, No Drowsiness [OTC]; Sine-Aid®, Maximum Strength [OTC]; Sine-Off® Maximum Strength No Drowsiness Formula [OTC]; Sinus Excedrin® Extra Strength [OTC]; Sinus-Relief® [OTC]; Sinutab® Without Drowsiness [OTC]; Tylenol® Sinus, Maximum Strength [OTC]

**Canadian Brand Names** Dristan® ND, Extra Strength

**Therapeutic Category** Decongestant/Analgesic

**Synonyms** Pseudoephedrine and Acetaminophen

**Use** Relief of mild to moderate pain; relief of congestion

**Usual Dosage** Adults: Oral: 2 tablets every 4-6 hours

**Local Anesthetic/Vasoconstrictor Precautions** No information available to require special precautions

**Effects on Dental Treatment** No effects or complications reported

**Other Adverse Effects** See individual agents

**Dosage Forms** Tablet:

Allerest® No Drowsiness; Coldrine®, Tylenol® Sinus, Maximum Strength; Ornex® No Drowsiness, Sinus-Relief®: Acetaminophen 325 mg and pseudoephedrine hydrochloride 30 mg

Bayer® Select Head Cold; Dristan® Cold; Dynafed®, Maximum Strength; Sinarest®, No Drowsiness; Sine-Aid®, Maximum Strength; Sine-Off® Maximum Strength No Drowsiness Formula; Sinus Excedrin® Extra Strength; Sinutab® Without Drowsiness; Tylenol® Sinus, Maximum Strength: Acetaminophen 500 mg and pseudoephedrine hydrochloride 30 mg

**Generic Available** Yes

## Acetaminophen, Aspirin, and Caffeine

(a seet a MIN oh fen, AS pir in, & KAF een)

**U.S. Brand Names** Excedrin®, Extra Strength [OTC]; Excedrin® Migraine [OTC]; Gelpirin® [OTC]; Goody's® Headache Powders

**Therapeutic Category** Analgesic, Non-narcotic

**Use** Relief of mild to moderate pain

**Usual Dosage** Adults: Oral: 1-2 tablets every 2-6 hours as needed for pain

**Local Anesthetic/Vasoconstrictor Precautions** No information available to require special precautions

**Effects on Dental Treatment** No effects or complications reported

**Other Adverse Effects** See individual agents

**Pregnancy Risk Factor** D

**Generic Available** Yes

**Selected Readings**

Barker JD Jr, de Carle DJ, and Anuras S, "Chronic Excessive Acetaminophen Use in Liver Damage," *Ann Intern Med*, 1977, 87(3):299-301.

Desjardins PJ, Cooper SA, Gallegos TL, et al, "The Relative Analgesic Efficacy of Propiram Fumarate, Codeine Aspirin, and Placebo in Post-Impaction Dental Pain," *J Clin Pharmacol*, 1984, 24(1):35-42.

Dionne RA, Campbell RA, Cooper SA, et al, "Suppression of Postoperative Pain by Preoperative Administration of Ibuprofen in Comparison to Placebo, Acetaminophen, and Acetaminophen Plus Codeine," *J Clin Pharmacol*, 1983, 23(1):37-43.

Forbes JA, Butterworth GA, Burchfield WH, et al, "Evaluation of Ketorolac, Aspirin, and an Acetaminophen-Codeine Combination in Postoperative Oral Surgery Pain," *Pharmacotherapy*, 1990, 10(6 Pt 2):77S-93S.

Forbes JA, Keller CK, Smith JW, et al, "Analgesic Effect of Naproxen Sodium, Codeine, a Naproxen-Codeine Combination and Aspirin on the Postoperative Pain of Oral Surgery," *Pharmacotherapy*, 1986, 6(5):211-8.

Licht H, Seeff LB, and Zimmerman HJ, "Apparent Potentiation of Acetaminophen Hepatotoxicity by Alcohol," *Ann Intern Med*, 1980, 92(4):511.

## Acetaminophen, Chlorpheniramine, and Pseudoephedrine

(a seet a MIN oh fen, klor fen IR a meen, & soo doe e FED rin)

**U.S. Brand Names** Alka-Seltzer® Plus Cold Liqui-Gels® Capsules [OTC]; Aspirin-Free Bayer® Select® Allergy Sinus Caplets [OTC]; Co-Hist® [OTC]; Sinutab® Tablets [OTC]

**Canadian Brand Names** Tylenol® Allergy & Sinus

**Therapeutic Category** Analgesic, Non-narcotic; Antihistamine/Decongestant Combination

**Use** Temporary relief of sinus symptoms

**Usual Dosage** Adults: Oral: 2 tablets every 6 hours

**Local Anesthetic/Vasoconstrictor Precautions** Use with caution since pseudoephedrine is a sympathomimetic amine which could interact with epinephrine to cause a pressor response

**Effects on Dental Treatment**

Chlorpheniramine: Prolonged use will cause significant xerostomia

Pseudoephedrine: Up to 10% of patients could experience tachycardia, palpitations, and dry mouth; use vasoconstrictor with caution

**Other Adverse Effects** See individual agents

**Pregnancy Risk Factor** B

**Generic Available** Yes

**Selected Readings**

Barker JD Jr, de Carle DJ, and Anuras S, "Chronic Excessive Acetaminophen Use in Liver Damage," *Ann Intern Med*, 1977, 87(3):299-301.

Dionne RA, Campbell RA, Cooper SA, et al, "Suppression of Postoperative Pain by Preoperative Administration of Ibuprofen in Comparison to Placebo, Acetaminophen, and Acetaminophen Plus Codeine," *J Clin Pharmacol*, 1983, 23(1):37-43.

Licht H, Seeff LB, and Zimmerman HJ, "Apparent Potentiation of Acetaminophen Hepatotoxicity by Alcohol," *Ann Intern Med*, 1980, 92(4):511.

## Acetaminophen, Dextromethorphan, and Pseudoephedrine

(a seet a MIN oh fen, deks troe meth OR fan, & soo doe e FED rin)

**U.S. Brand Names** Alka-Seltzer® Plus Flu & Body Aches Non-Drowsy Liqui-Gels® [OTC]; Comtrex® Maximum Strength Non-Drowsy [OTC]; Sudafed® Severe Cold [OTC]; Theraflu® Non-Drowsy Formula Maximum Strength [OTC]; Tylenol® Cold No Drowsiness [OTC]; Tylenol® Flu Maximum Strength [OTC]

**Canadian Brand Names** Contac® Day & Night Cold and Flu System

**Therapeutic Category** Cold Preparation

**Synonyms** Dextromethorphan, Acetaminophen, and Pseudoephedrine; Pseudoephedrine, Acetaminophen, and Dextromethorphan; Pseudoephedrine, Dextromethorphan, and Acetaminophen

**Use** Treatment of mild to moderate pain and fever; symptomatic relief of cough and congestion

**Usual Dosage** Adults: Oral: 2 tablets every 6 hours

**Local Anesthetic/Vasoconstrictor Precautions** No information available to require special precautions

**Effects on Dental Treatment** No effects or complications reported

**Other Adverse Effects** See individual agents

**Warnings/Precautions** Research on chicken embryos exposed to concentrations of dextromethorphan relative to those typically taken by humans has shown to cause birth defects and fetal death; more study is needed, but it is suggested that pregnant women should be advised not to use dextromethorphan-containing medications

**Dosage Forms** Tablet:

Alka-Seltzer® Plus Flu & Body Aches Non-Drowsy: Acetaminophen 500 mg, dextromethorphan hydrobromide 10 mg, and pseudoephedrine hydrochloride 30 mg

Tylenol® Cold No Drowsiness: Acetaminophen 325 mg, dextromethorphan hydrobromide 15 mg, and pseudoephedrine hydrochloride 30 mg

Comtrex® Maximum Strength Non-Drowsy; Sudafed® Severe Cold; Theraflu® Non-Drowsy Formula Maximum Strength; Tylenol® Flu Maximum Strength: Acetaminophen 500 mg, dextromethorphan hydrobromide 15 mg, and pseudoephedrine hydrochloride 30 mg

**Generic Available** Yes

## Acetaminophen, Isometheptene, and Dichloralphenazone

(a seet a MIN oh fen, eye soe me THEP teen, & dye KLOR al FEN a zone)

**U.S. Brand Names** Isocom®; Isopap®; Midchlor®; Midrin®; Migratine®

**Therapeutic Category** Analgesic, Non-narcotic; Antimigraine Agent

**Use** Relief of migraine and tension headache

**Usual Dosage** Adults: Oral: 2 capsules at first sign of headache, followed by 1 capsule every 60 minutes until relieved, up to 5 capsules in a 12-hour period

**Local Anesthetic/Vasoconstrictor Precautions** No information available to require special precautions

**Effects on Dental Treatment** No effects or complications reported

**Pregnancy Risk Factor** B

**Generic Available** Yes

**Comments** Should not exceed 5 g in 12 hours; may cause drowsiness; avoid alcohol and other CNS depressants

**Selected Readings**


Barker JD Jr, de Carle DJ, and Anuras S, "Chronic Excessive Acetaminophen Use in Liver Damage," *Ann Intern Med*, 1977, 87(3):299-301.

Dionne RA, Campbell RA, Cooper SA, et al, "Suppression of Postoperative Pain by Preoperative Administration of Ibuprofen in Comparison to Placebo, Acetaminophen, and Acetaminophen Plus Codeine," *J Clin Pharmacol*, 1983, 23(1):37-43.

Licht H, Seeff LB, and Zimmerman HJ, "Apparent Potentiation of Acetaminophen Hepatotoxicity by Alcohol," *Ann Intern Med*, 1980, 92(4):511.


♦ **Acetasol® HC Otic** *see* Acetic Acid, Propylene Glycol Diacetate, and Hydrocortisone *on next page*

## Acetazolamide (a set a ZOLE a mide)

**U.S. Brand Names** Diamox®; Diamox® Sequels®

**Canadian Brand Names** Acetazolam®; Apo®-Acetazolamide; Novo-Zolamide

**Therapeutic Category** Anticonvulsant, Miscellaneous; Antiglaucoma Agent; Carbonic Anhydrase Inhibitor; Diuretic, Carbonic Anhydrase Inhibitor

**Use** Lowers intraocular pressure to treat glaucoma, also as a diuretic, adjunct treatment of refractory seizures and acute altitude sickness; centrencephalic epilepsies (sustained release not recommended for anticonvulsant)

**Usual Dosage Note:** I.M. administration is not recommended because of pain secondary to the alkaline pH

Children:
- Glaucoma:
  - Oral: 8-30 mg/kg/day or 300-900 mg/m$^2$/day divided every 8 hours
  - I.M., I.V.: 20-40 mg/kg/24 hours divided every 6 hours, not to exceed 1 g/day
- Edema: Oral, I.M., I.V.: 5 mg/kg or 150 mg/m$^2$ once every day
- Epilepsy: Oral: 8-30 mg/kg/day in 1-4 divided doses, not to exceed 1 g/day; sustained release capsule is not recommended for treatment of epilepsy

Adults:
- Glaucoma:
  - Chronic simple (open-angle): Oral: 250 mg 1-4 times/day or 500 mg sustained release capsule twice daily
  - Secondary, acute (closed-angle): I.M., I.V.: 250-500 mg, may repeat in 2-4 hours to a maximum of 1 g/day
- Edema: Oral, I.M., I.V.: 250-375 mg once daily
- Epilepsy: Oral: 8-30 mg/kg/day in 1-4 divided doses, not to exceed 1 g/day; **sustained release capsule is not recommended for treatment of epilepsy**
- Altitude sickness: Oral: 250 mg every 8-12 hours (or 500 mg extended release capsules every 12-24 hours). Therapy should begin 24-48 hours before and continue during ascent and for at least 48 hours after arrival at the high altitude.
- Urine alkalinization: Oral: 5 mg/kg/dose repeated 2-3 times over 24 hours

Elderly: Oral: Initial: 250 mg twice daily; use lowest effective dose

**Mechanism of Action** Reversible inhibition of the enzyme carbonic anhydrase resulting in reduction of hydrogen ion secretion at renal tubule and an increased renal excretion of sodium, potassium, bicarbonate, and water to decrease production of aqueous humor; also inhibits carbonic anhydrase in central nervous system to retard abnormal and excessive discharge from CNS neurons

**Local Anesthetic/Vasoconstrictor Precautions** No information available to require special precautions

**Effects on Dental Treatment** Metallic taste in >10% of patients; disappears upon drug withdrawal

**Other Adverse Effects**

>10%:
- Central nervous system: Malaise
- Gastrointestinal: Anorexia, diarrhea, metallic taste
- Renal: Polyuria

<1%:
- Central nervous system: Fever, fatigue, mental depression, drowsiness
- Dermatologic: Rash

(Continued)

## Acetazolamide *(Continued)*

Endocrine & metabolic: Hyperchloremic metabolic acidosis, hypokalemia, hyperglycemia
Gastrointestinal: GI irritation, dryness of mouth, black stools
Genitourinary: Dysuria
Hematologic: Bone marrow suppression, blood dyscrasias
Neuromuscular & skeletal: Paresthesia, weakness
Ocular: Myopia
Renal: Renal calculi

**Drug Interactions** Acetazolamide increases lithium excretion and alters excretion of other drugs by alkalinization of urine (such as amphetamines, quinidine, procainamide, methenamine, phenobarbital, salicylates)

**Drug Uptake**
Onset of action:
Extended release capsule: 2 hours
I.V.: 2 minutes
Peak effect:
Extended release capsule: 3-6 hours
Tablet: 1-4 hours
I.V.: 15 minutes
Duration:
Extended release capsule: 18-24 hours
Tablet: 8-12 hours
I.V.: 4-5 hours
Serum half-life: 2.4-5.8 hours

**Pregnancy Risk Factor** C

**Generic Available** Yes

♦ **Acetic Acid and Aluminum Acetate Otic** *see* Aluminum Acetate and Acetic Acid *on page 54*

## Acetic Acid, Propylene Glycol Diacetate, and Hydrocortisone

(a SEE tik AS id, PRO pa leen GLY kole dye AS e tate, & hye droe KOR ti sone)

**U.S. Brand Names** Acetasol® HC Otic; VōSol® HC Otic

**Therapeutic Category** Otic Agent, Anti-infective

**Use** Treatment of superficial infections of the external auditory canal caused by organisms susceptible to the action of the antimicrobial, complicated by swelling

**Usual Dosage** Adults: Instill 4 drops in ear(s) 3-4 times/day

**Local Anesthetic/Vasoconstrictor Precautions** No information available to require special precautions

**Effects on Dental Treatment** No effects or complications reported

**Other Adverse Effects** Transient burning or stinging may be noticed occasionally when the solution is first instilled into the acutely inflamed ear

**Generic Available** Yes

## Acetohexamide (a set oh HEKS a mide)

**Related Information**
Endocrine Disorders & Pregnancy *on page 1082*

**U.S. Brand Names** Dymelor®

**Therapeutic Category** Antidiabetic Agent; Hypoglycemic Agent, Oral; Sulfonylurea Agent

**Use** Adjunct to diet for the management of mild to moderately severe, stable, noninsulin-dependent (type II) diabetes mellitus

**Usual Dosage** Adults: Oral (elderly patients may be more sensitive and should be started at a lower dosage initially): 250 mg to 1.5 g/day in 1-2 divided doses; doses >1.5 g/day are not recommended; if dose is ≤1 g, administer as a single daily dose

**Mechanism of Action** Believed to cause hypoglycemia by stimulating insulin release from the pancreatic beta cells; reduces glucose output from the liver (decreases gluconeogenesis); insulin sensitivity is increased at peripheral target sites (alters receptor sensitivity/receptor density); potentiates effects of ADH; may produce mild diuresis and significant uricosuric activity

**Local Anesthetic/Vasoconstrictor Precautions** No information available to require special precautions

**Effects on Dental Treatment** Use salicylates with caution in patients taking acetohexamide because of potential increased hypoglycemia. NSAIDs such as ibuprofen, naproxen and others may be safely used. Acetohexamide-dependent diabetics (noninsulin-dependent, type II) should be appointed for dental treatment in mornings to minimize chance of stress-induced hypoglycemia.

**Other Adverse Effects**

>10%:

Central nervous system: Headache, dizziness

Gastrointestinal: Constipation, diarrhea, heartburn, anorexia, epigastric fullness

1% to 10%: Dermatologic: Rash, urticaria, photosensitivity

<1%:

Endocrine & metabolic: Hypoglycemia

Hematologic: Aplastic anemia, hemolytic anemia, bone marrow suppression, thrombocytopenia, agranulocytosis

**Drug Interactions**

Monitor patient closely; large number of drugs interact with sulfonylureas

Decreased effect: Decreased hypoglycemic effect when acetohexamide is coadministered with cholestyramine, diazoxide, hydantoins, rifampin, thiazides, loop or thiazide diuretics

Increased effect: Increased hypoglycemia when acetohexamide is coadministered with salicylates or beta-adrenergic blockers; MAO inhibitors; oral anticoagulants, NSAIDs, sulfonamides, insulin, clofibrate, fenfluramine, fluconazole, gemfibrozil, $H_2$ antagonists, methyldopa, tricyclic antidepressants

**Drug Uptake**

Onset of effect: 1 hour

Peak hypoglycemic effects: 8-10 hours

Duration: 12-24 hours, prolonged with renal impairment

Serum half-life:

Parent compound: 0.8-2.4 hours

Metabolite: 5-6 hours

**Pregnancy Risk Factor** D

**Generic Available** Yes

## Acetohydroxamic Acid (a SEE toe hye droks am ik AS id)

**U.S. Brand Names** Lithostat®

**Therapeutic Category** Urinary Tract Product

**Synonyms** AHA

**Use** Adjunctive therapy in chronic urea-splitting urinary infection

**Usual Dosage** Oral:

Children: Initial: 10 mg/kg/day

Adults: 250 mg 3-4 times/day for a total daily dose of 10-15 mg/kg/day

**Local Anesthetic/Vasoconstrictor Precautions** No information available to require special precautions

**Effects on Dental Treatment** No effects or complications reported

**Pregnancy Risk Factor** X

**Generic Available** No

## Acetophenazine (a set oh FEN a zeen)

**U.S. Brand Names** Tindal®

**Therapeutic Category** Antipsychotic Agent

**Use** Management of manifestations of psychotic disorders

**Usual Dosage** Adults: Oral: 20 mg 3 times/day up to 60-120 mg/day

Hospitalized schizophrenic patients may require doses as high as 400-600 mg/day

**Mechanism of Action** Antagonizes the effects of dopamine in the basal ganglia and limbic areas of the forebrain; this activity appears responsible for the antipsychotic efficacy, as well as the production of extrapyramidal symptoms; increases the secretion of prolactin and has a marked suppressive effect on the chemoreceptor trigger zone; also produces peripheral blockade of cholinergic neurons

**Local Anesthetic/Vasoconstrictor Precautions** No information available to require special precautions

**Effects on Dental Treatment** Orthostatic hypotension and nasal congestion possible in dental patients. Since the drug is a dopamine antagonist, extrapyramidal symptoms of the TMJ is a possibility; increased motor activity of head, face, and neck may occur. This drug is also an anticholinergic causing xerostomia.

**Other Adverse Effects**

>10%:

Cardiovascular: Hypotension, orthostatic hypotension

Central nervous system: Pseudoparkinsonism, akathisia, dystonias, tardive dyskinesia (persistent), dizziness

Gastrointestinal: Constipation

Ocular: Pigmentary retinopathy

Respiratory: Nasal congestion

Miscellaneous: Decreased sweating

(Continued)

## Acetophenazine *(Continued)*

1% to 10%:
Dermatologic: Photosensitivity, skin rash
Endocrine & metabolic: Changes in menstrual cycle, changes in libido, pain in breasts
Gastrointestinal: Weight gain, nausea, vomiting, stomach pain
Genitourinary: Dysuria, ejaculatory disturbances
Neuromuscular & skeletal: Trembling of fingers

<1%:
Central nervous system: Neuroleptic malignant syndrome (NMS), impairment of temperature regulation, lowering of seizures threshold
Dermatologic: Discoloration of skin (blue-gray)
Endocrine & metabolic: Galactorrhea
Genitourinary: Priapism
Hematologic: Agranulocytosis, leukopenia
Hepatic: Cholestatic jaundice, hepatotoxicity
Ocular: Cornea and lens changes

**Drug Interactions** No data reported

**Drug Uptake**
Duration: ~24 hours, permitting daily dosing
Absorption: Tissue saturation, particularly in high lipid tissues such as the central nervous system
Serum half-life: Range: 20-40 hours

**Pregnancy Risk Factor** C

**Generic Available** No

## Acetylcholine (a se teel KOE leen)

**U.S. Brand Names** Miochol-E®

**Therapeutic Category** Cholinergic Agent, Ophthalmic; Ophthalmic Agent, Miotic

**Use** Produces complete miosis in cataract surgery, keratoplasty, iridectomy and other anterior segment surgery where rapid miosis is required

**Usual Dosage** Adults: Intraocular: 0.5-2 mL of 1% injection (5-20 mg) instilled into anterior chamber before or after securing one or more sutures

**Mechanism of Action** Causes contraction of the sphincter muscles of the iris, resulting in miosis and contraction of the ciliary muscle, leading to accommodation spasm

**Local Anesthetic/Vasoconstrictor Precautions** None

**Effects on Dental Treatment** Ophthalmic use of acetylcholine has no effect on dental treatment

**Other Adverse Effects** <1%:
Cardiovascular: Bradycardia, hypotension, flushing
Central nervous system: Headache
Ocular: Altered distance vision, decreased night vision, transient lenticular opacities
Respiratory: Dyspnea
Miscellaneous: Sweating

**Drug Interactions** No data reported

**Drug Uptake**
Onset of miosis: Occurs promptly
Duration: ~10 minutes

**Pregnancy Risk Factor** C

**Generic Available** No

## Acetylcysteine (a se teel SIS teen)

**U.S. Brand Names** Mucomyst®; Mucosil™

**Canadian Brand Names** Parvolex®

**Therapeutic Category** Antidote, Acetaminophen; Mucolytic Agent

**Use** Adjunctive mucolytic therapy in patients with abnormal or viscid mucous secretions in acute and chronic bronchopulmonary diseases; pulmonary complications of surgery and cystic fibrosis; diagnostic bronchial studies; antidote for acute acetaminophen toxicity

**Usual Dosage**
Acetaminophen poisoning: Children and Adults: Oral: 140 mg/kg; followed by 17 doses of 70 mg/kg every 4 hours; repeat dose if emesis occurs within 1 hour of administration; therapy should continue until all doses are administered even though the acetaminophen plasma level has dropped below the toxic range

Inhalation: Acetylcysteine 10% and 20% solution (Mucomyst®) (dilute 20% solution with sodium chloride or sterile water for inhalation); 10% solution may be used undiluted

Children: 3-5 mL of 20% solution or 6-10 mL of 10% solution until nebulized given 3-4 times/day

Adolescents: 5-10 mL of 10% to 20% solution until nebulized given 3-4 times/day

**Note:** Patients should receive an aerosolized bronchodilator 10-15 minutes prior to acetylcysteine

Meconium ileus equivalent: Children and Adults: 100-300 mL of 4% to 10% solution by irrigation or orally

**Mechanism of Action** Exerts mucolytic action through its free sulfhydryl group which opens up the disulfide bonds in the mucoproteins thus lowering mucous viscosity. The exact mechanism of action in acetaminophen toxicity is unknown; thought to act by providing substrate for conjugation with the toxic metabolite.

**Local Anesthetic/Vasoconstrictor Precautions** No information available to require special precautions

**Effects on Dental Treatment** Stomatitis has been reported in 1% to 10% of patients

**Other Adverse Effects**

>10%:

Gastrointestinal: Vomiting

Miscellaneous: Unpleasant odor during administration

1% to 10%:

Central nervous system: Drowsiness, chills, clamminess

Gastrointestinal: Stomatitis, nausea

Local: Irritation

Respiratory: Bronchospasm, rhinorrhea, hemoptysis

<1%: Dermatologic: Skin rash

**Drug Interactions** No data reported

**Drug Uptake**

Oral: Peak plasma levels: 1-2 hours

Onset of action: Inhalation: Mucus liquefaction occurs maximally within 5-10 minutes

Duration: Can persist for >1 hour

Serum half-life:

Reduced acetylcysteine: 2 hours

Total acetylcysteine: 5.5 hours

**Pregnancy Risk Factor** B

**Generic Available** Yes

- **Achromycin®** *see* Tetracycline *on page 965*
- **Achromycin® V** *see* Tetracycline *on page 965*
- **Acidulated Phosphate Fluoride** *see* Fluoride *on page 441*
- **Aclovate®** *see* Alclometasone *on page 44*

## Acrivastine and Pseudoephedrine

(AK ri vas teen & soo doe e FED rin)

**U.S. Brand Names** Semprex®-D

**Therapeutic Category** Antihistamine/Decongestant Combination

**Use** Temporary relief of nasal congestion, decongest sinus openings, running nose, itching of nose or throat, and itchy, watery eyes due to hay fever or other upper respiratory allergies

**Usual Dosage** Adults: 1 capsule 3-4 times/day

**Mechanism of Action**

Acrivastine is an analogue of triprolidine and it is considered to be relatively less sedating than traditional antihistamines; believed to involve competitive blockade of $H_1$-receptor sites resulting in the inability of histamine to combine with its receptor sites and exert its usual effects on target cells

Pseudoephedrine: Directly stimulates alpha-adrenergic receptors of respiratory mucosa causing vasoconstriction; directly stimulates beta-adrenergic receptors causing bronchial relaxation, increased heart rate and contractility

**Local Anesthetic/Vasoconstrictor Precautions** Use with caution since pseudoephedrine is a sympathomimetic amine which could interact with epinephrine to cause a pressor response

**Effects on Dental Treatment** Up to 10% of patients could experience tachycardia, palpitations, and dry mouth; use vasoconstrictor with caution

**Other Adverse Effects**

>10%: Central nervous system: Drowsiness, headache

1% to 10%:

Cardiovascular: Tachycardia, palpitations

Central nervous system: Nervousness, dizziness, insomnia, vertigo, lightheadedness, fatigue

Gastrointestinal: Nausea, vomiting, dry mouth, diarrhea

Genitourinary: Dysuria

(Continued)

## Acrivastine and Pseudoephedrine *(Continued)*

Neuromuscular & skeletal: Weakness
Respiratory: Pharyngitis, cough increase
Miscellaneous: Sweating
<1%:
Endocrine & metabolic: Dysmenorrhea
Gastrointestinal: Dyspepsia

**Drug Interactions** Increased toxicity with MAO inhibitors (hypertensive crisis) sympathomimetics, CNS depressants, alcohol (sedation)

**Pregnancy Risk Factor** B

**Generic Available** No

- **ACT® [OTC]** *see* Fluoride *on page 441*
- **ACT** *see* Dactinomycin *on page 294*
- **Actagen-C®** *see* Triprolidine, Pseudoephedrine, and Codeine *on page 1026*
- **Actagen® Syrup [OTC]** *see* Triprolidine and Pseudoephedrine *on page 1025*
- **Actagen® Tablet [OTC]** *see* Triprolidine and Pseudoephedrine *on page 1025*
- **Acthar®** *see* Corticotropin *on page 278*
- **Actidose-Aqua® [OTC]** *see* Charcoal *on page 219*
- **Actidose® With Sorbitol [OTC]** *see* Charcoal *on page 219*
- **Actifed® Allergy Tablet (Day) [OTC]** *see* Pseudoephedrine *on page 863*
- **Actifed® Allergy Tablet (Night) [OTC]** *see* Diphenhydramine and Pseudoephedrine *on page 339*
- **Actifed® With Codeine** *see* Triprolidine, Pseudoephedrine, and Codeine *on page 1026*
- **Actigall™** *see* Ursodiol *on page 1036*
- **Actimmune®** *see* Interferon Gamma-1b *on page 545*
- **Actinex®** *see* Masoprocol *on page 616*
- **Actinomycin D** *see* Dactinomycin *on page 294*
- **Actiq® Oral Transmucosal** *see* Fentanyl *on page 424*
- **Actisite®** *see* Tetracycline Periodontal Fibers *on page 966*
- **Activase®** *see* Alteplase *on page 52*
- **Activelle™** *see* Estradiol and Norethindrone *on page 388*
- **Actonel®** *see* Risedronate *on page 890*
- **Actron® [OTC]** *see* Ketoprofen *on page 565*
- **Acular® Ophthalmic** *see* Ketorolac Tromethamine *on page 566*
- **Acutrim® 16 Hours [OTC]** *see* Phenylpropanolamine *on page 797*
- **Acutrim® II, Maximum Strength [OTC]** *see* Phenylpropanolamine *on page 797*
- **Acutrim® Late Day [OTC]** *see* Phenylpropanolamine *on page 797*

## Acyclovir (ay SYE kloe veer)

**Related Information**

Oral Viral Infections *on page 1137*
Systemic Viral Diseases *on page 1115*

**U.S. Brand Names** Zovirax®

**Canadian Brand Names** Avirax™

**Therapeutic Category** Antiviral Agent, Oral; Antiviral Agent, Parenteral; Antiviral Agent, Topical

**Use**

Dental: Treatment of initial and prophylaxis of recurrent mucosal and cutaneous herpes simplex (HSV-1 and HSV-2) infections

Medical: In medicine, herpes simplex encephalitis, herpes zoster, genital herpes infection, varicella-zoster infections in healthy, nonpregnant persons >13 years of age, children <12 months of age who have a chronic skin or lung disorder or are receiving long-term aspirin therapy, and immunocompromised patients; for herpes zoster, acyclovir should be started within 72 hours of the appearance of the rash to be effective; acyclovir will not prevent postherpetic neuralgias

**Usual Dosage**

Dosing weight should be based on the smaller of lean body weight or total body weight

Adult determination of lean body weight (LBW) in kg:
LBW males: 50 kg + (2.3 kg x inches >5 feet)
LBW females: 45 kg + (2.3 kg x inches >5 feet)

**Treatment of herpes simplex virus infections:** I.V.

Children and Adults:
Mucocutaneous HSV infection 750 $mg/m^2$/day divided every 8 hours or 5 mg/kg/dose every 8 hours for 5-10 days
HSV encephalitis: 1500 $mg/m^2$/day divided every 8 hours for 5-10 days

I.V.: 5 mg/kg/dose every 8 hours for 5-10 days

**Treatment of herpes simplex virus infections:** Adults:

Oral: Treatment: 200 mg every 4 hours while awake (5 times/day)

Topical: ½" ribbon of ointment for a 4" square surface area every 3 hours (6 times/day)

**Treatment of varicella-zoster virus (chickenpox) infections:**

Oral:

Adults: 600-800 mg/dose every 4 hours while awake (5 times/day) for 7-10 days or 1000 mg every 6 hours for 5 days

Children: 10-20 mg/kg/dose (up to 800 mg) 4 times/day for 5 days; begin treatment within the first 24 hours of rash onset

I.V.: Children and Adults: 1500 mg/m$^2$/day divided every 8 hours or 10 mg/kg/dose every 8 hours for 7 days

**Treatment of herpes zoster infections:**

Oral:

Adults (immunocompromised): 800 mg every 4 hours (5 times/day) for 7-10 days

Children (immunocompromised): 250-600 mg/m$^2$/dose 4-5 times/day for 7-10 days

I.V.: Children and Adults (immunocompromised): 7.5 mg/kg/dose every 8 hours

**Prophylaxis in immunocompromised patients:**

Varicella zoster or herpes zoster in HIV-positive patients: Adults: Oral: 400 mg every 4 hours (5 times/day) for 7-10 days

Bone marrow transplant recipients: Children and Adults: I.V.:

Autologous patients who are HSV seropositive: 150 mg/m$^2$/dose (5 mg/kg) every 12 hours; with clinical symptoms of herpes simplex: 150 mg/m$^2$/dose every 8 hours

Autologous patients who are CMV seropositive: 500 mg/m$^2$/dose (10 mg/kg) every 8 hours; for clinically symptomatic CMV infection, consider replacing acyclovir with ganciclovir

**Prophylaxis of herpes simplex virus infections:** Adults: 200 mg 3-4 times/day or 400 mg twice daily

**Mechanism of Action** Inhibits DNA synthesis and viral replication by competing with deoxyguanosine triphosphate for viral DNA polymerase and incorporation into viral DNA

**Local Anesthetic/Vasoconstrictor Precautions** No information available to require special precautions

**Effects on Dental Treatment** No effects or complications reported

**Other Adverse Effects** 1% to 10%:

Central nervous system: Lethargy, dizziness, seizures, confusion, agitation, coma, headache

Dermatologic: Rash

Gastrointestinal: Nausea, vomiting

Neuromuscular & skeletal: Tremor

Renal: Elevated creatinine

**Contraindications** Hypersensitivity to acyclovir

**Warnings/Precautions**

Systemic: Use with caution in patients with pre-existing renal disease or in those receiving other nephrotoxic drugs concurrently; use with caution in patients with underlying neurologic abnormalities, serious hepatic or electrolyte abnormalities, or substantial hypoxia

Topical: No data reported

**Drug Interactions** Systemic: Increased CNS side effects with zidovudine and probenecid

**Drug Uptake**

Absorption: Oral: 15% to 30%

Time to peak serum concentration:

Oral: 1.5-2 hours

I.V.: Within 1 hour

Serum half-life:

Adults: 3.3 hours

Children 1-12 years: 2-3 hours

**Pregnancy Risk Factor** C

**Breast-feeding Considerations** May be taken while breast-feeding

**Dosage Forms**

Capsule: 200 mg

Powder for Injection: 500 mg (10 mL); 1000 mg (20 mL)

Ointment, topical: 5% [50 mg/g] (3 g, 15 g)

Suspension, oral (banana flavor): 200 mg/5 mL

Tablet: 400 mg, 800 mg

**Dietary Considerations** May be taken with food; food does not appear to affect absorption

(Continued)

## Acyclovir *(Continued)*

**Generic Available** Yes

- ♦ **Adagen™** *see* Pegademase Bovine *on page 769*
- ♦ **Adalat®** *see* Nifedipine *on page 720*
- ♦ **Adalat® CC** *see* Nifedipine *on page 720*

## Adapalene (a DAP a leen)

**U.S. Brand Names** Differin®

**Therapeutic Category** Acne Products

**Use** Topical treatment of acne vulgaris

**Usual Dosage** Children >12 years and Adults: Topical: Apply once daily before retiring; therapeutic results should be noticed after 8-12 weeks of treatment

**Mechanism of Action** Retinoid-like compound which is a modulator of cellular differentiation, keratinization and inflammatory processes, all of which represent important features in the pathology of acne vulgaris

**Local Anesthetic/Vasoconstrictor Precautions** No information available to require special precautions

**Effects on Dental Treatment** No effects or complications reported

**Other Adverse Effects**

>10%: Dermatologic: Erythema, scaling, dryness, pruritus, burning, pruritus or burning immediately after application

≤1% Dermatologic: Skin irritation, stinging sunburn, acne flares

**Drug Uptake** Absorption: Topical: Minimum absorption occurs

**Pregnancy Risk Factor** C

**Dosage Forms** Gel, topical (alcohol free): 0.1% (15 g, 45 g)

**Generic Available** No

- ♦ **Adapin®** *see* Doxepin *on page 351*
- ♦ **Adderall®** *see* Dextroamphetamine and Amphetamine *on page 313*
- ♦ **Adeflor®** *see* Vitamins, Multiple *on page 1051*

## Adefovir (a DEF o veer)

**Related Information**

Systemic Viral Diseases *on page 1115*

**U.S. Brand Names** Preveon®

**Therapeutic Category** Reverse Transcriptase Inhibitor

**Use** Investigational (8/1/98); treatment of HIV infections in combination with at least two other antiretroviral agents; also has some activity against hepatitis B virus and herpes viruses

**Usual Dosage** Oral:

HIV: 125 mg once daily

Hepatitis B: 125 mg once daily

**Mechanism of Action** Acyclic nucleotide reverse transcriptase inhibitor which interferes with HIV viral RNA dependent DNA polymerase resulting in inhibition of viral replication

**Local Anesthetic/Vasoconstrictor Precautions** No information available to require special precautions

**Effects on Dental Treatment** No effects or complications reported

**Other Adverse Effects**

Endocrine & metabolic: Elevation of transaminases, hot flashes

Gastrointestinal: GI symptoms

Genitourinary: Urethritis

Hematologic: Elevation of hemoglobin

**Drug Uptake** Serum half-life: 1.6 hours; 16-18 hours intracellularly

**Pregnancy Risk Factor** Not available

**Generic Available** No

- ♦ **Adenocard®** *see* Adenosine *on this page*

## Adenosine (a DEN oh seen)

**U.S. Brand Names** Adenocard®

**Therapeutic Category** Antiarrhythmic Agent (Supraventricular); Antiarrhythmic Agent, Miscellaneous

**Synonyms** 9-Beta-D-ribofuranosyladenine

**Use** Treatment of paroxysmal supraventricular tachycardia (PSVT)

**Usual Dosage Rapid I.V. push (over 1-2 seconds) via peripheral line:**

Children: Pediatric advanced life support (PALS): Treatment of SVT: 0.1 mg/kg; if not effective, give 0.2 mg/kg

Alternatively: Initial dose: 0.05 mg/kg; if not effective within 2 minutes, increase dose by 0.05 mg/kg increments every 2 minutes to a maximum dose of 0.25 mg/kg or until termination of PSVT; medium dose required: 0.15 mg/kg

Maximum single dose: 12 mg
Adults: 6 mg; if not effective within 1-2 minutes, 12 mg may be given; may repeat 12 mg bolus if needed
Maximum single dose: 12 mg

**Note:** Patients who are receiving concomitant theophylline therapy may be less likely to respond to adenosine therapy
**Note:** Higher doses may be needed for administration via peripheral versus central vein

**Mechanism of Action** Slows conduction time through the A-V node, interrupting the re-entry pathways through the A-V node, restoring normal sinus rhythm

**Local Anesthetic/Vasoconstrictor Precautions** No information available to require special precautions

**Effects on Dental Treatment** No effects or complications reported

**Other Adverse Effects**
>10%:
Cardiovascular: Flushing of face, arrhythmias, palpitations
Respiratory: Dyspnea
1% to 10%:
Cardiovascular: Chest pain
Central nervous system: Dizziness
Gastrointestinal: Nausea
Neuromuscular & skeletal: Numbness
Respiratory: Cough
<1%:
Cardiovascular: Hypotension, tightness of chest
Central nervous system: Lightheadedness, headache, apprehension, pressure in head
Dermatologic: Burning sensation
Gastrointestinal: Metallic taste, pressure in groin
Neuromuscular & skeletal: Heaviness in arms, neck and back pain
Ocular: Blurred vision
Respiratory: Hypoventilation
Miscellaneous: Sweating, tightness in throat

**Drug Uptake**
Duration: Very brief
Serum half-life: <10 seconds, thus adverse effects are usually rapidly self-limiting

**Pregnancy Risk Factor** C

**Generic Available** No

**Comments** Short action an advantage; not effective in atrial flutter, atrial fibrillation, or ventricular tachycardia

- **Adipex-P®** *see* Phentermine *on page 793*
- **Adlone®** *see* Methylprednisolone *on page 661*
- **ADR** *see* Doxorubicin *on page 353*
- **Adrenalin®** *see* Epinephrine (Dental) *on page 374*
- **Adriamycin® PFS** *see* Doxorubicin *on page 353*
- **Adriamycin® RDF** *see* Doxorubicin *on page 353*
- **Adrucil® Injection** *see* Fluorouracil *on page 443*
- **Adsorbocarpine®** *see* Pilocarpine *on page 802*
- **Adsorbonac® Ophthalmic [OTC]** *see* Sodium Chloride *on page 920*
- **Adsorbotear® Ophthalmic Solution [OTC]** *see* Artificial Tears *on page 97*
- **Advanced Formula Oxy® Sensitive Gel [OTC]** *see* Benzoyl Peroxide *on page 130*
- **Advil® [OTC]** *see* Ibuprofen *on page 522*
- **Advil® Cold & Sinus Caplets [OTC]** *see* Pseudoephedrine and Ibuprofen *on page 864*
- **Aeroaid® [OTC]** *see* Thimerosal *on page 976*
- **AeroBid®-M Oral Aerosol Inhaler** *see* Flunisolide *on page 439*
- **AeroBid® Oral Aerosol Inhaler** *see* Flunisolide *on page 439*
- **Aerolate III®** *see* Theophylline *on page 969*
- **Aerolate JR®** *see* Theophylline *on page 969*
- **Aerolate SR® S** *see* Theophylline *on page 969*
- **Aerosporin®** *see* Polymyxin B *on page 815*
- **AeroZoin® [OTC]** *see* Benzoin *on page 130*
- **Afrin® Children's Nose Drops [OTC]** *see* Oxymetazoline *on page 755*
- **Afrin® Saline Mist [OTC]** *see* Sodium Chloride *on page 920*
- **Afrin® Sinus [OTC]** *see* Oxymetazoline *on page 755*
- **Afrin® Tablet [OTC]** *see* Pseudoephedrine *on page 863*
- **Aftate® for Athlete's Foot [OTC]** *see* Tolnaftate *on page 997*

- ♦ **Aftate® for Jock Itch [OTC]** *see* Tolnaftate *on page 997*
- ♦ **Aggrastat®** *see* Tirofiban *on page 988*
- ♦ **$AgNO_3$** *see* Silver Nitrate *on page 913*
- ♦ **Agrylin™** *see* Anagrelide *on page 85*
- ♦ **AHA** *see* Acetohydroxamic Acid *on page 35*
- ♦ **AHF** *see* Antihemophilic Factor (Human) *on page 89*
- ♦ **Airet®** *see* Albuterol *on next page*
- ♦ **Akarpine®** *see* Pilocarpine *on page 802*
- ♦ **AKBeta®** *see* Levobunolol *on page 580*
- ♦ **AK-Chlor®** *see* Chloramphenicol *on page 222*
- ♦ **AK-Cide® Ophthalmic** *see* Sulfacetamide Sodium and Prednisolone *on page 940*
- ♦ **AK-Con® Ophthalmic** *see* Naphazoline *on page 703*
- ♦ **AK-Dilate® Ophthalmic Solution** *see* Phenylephrine *on page 795*
- ♦ **AK-Homatropine® Ophthalmic** *see* Homatropine *on page 499*
- ♦ **Akineton®** *see* Biperiden *on page 140*
- ♦ **AK-NaCl® [OTC]** *see* Sodium Chloride *on page 920*
- ♦ **AK-Nefrin® Ophthalmic Solution** *see* Phenylephrine *on page 795*
- ♦ **Akne-Mycin® Topical** *see* Erythromycin, Topical *on page 386*
- ♦ **AK-Neo-Dex® Ophthalmic** *see* Neomycin and Dexamethasone *on page 710*
- ♦ **AK-Pentolate®** *see* Cyclopentolate *on page 285*
- ♦ **AK-Poly-Bac® Ophthalmic** *see* Bacitracin and Polymyxin B *on page 117*
- ♦ **AK-Pred®** *see* Prednisolone *on page 832*
- ♦ **AKPro® Ophthalmic** *see* Dipivefrin *on page 341*
- ♦ **AK-Spore H.C.® Ophthalmic Ointment** *see* Bacitracin, Neomycin, Polymyxin B, and Hydrocortisone *on page 118*
- ♦ **AK-Spore H.C.® Ophthalmic Suspension** *see* Neomycin, Polymyxin B, and Hydrocortisone *on page 712*
- ♦ **AK-Spore H.C.® Otic** *see* Neomycin, Polymyxin B, and Hydrocortisone *on page 712*
- ♦ **AK-Spore® Ophthalmic Ointment** *see* Bacitracin, Neomycin, and Polymyxin B *on page 118*
- ♦ **AK-Spore® Ophthalmic Solution** *see* Neomycin, Polymyxin B, and Gramicidin *on page 712*
- ♦ **AK-Sulf® Ophthalmic** *see* Sulfacetamide Sodium *on page 939*
- ♦ **AK-Taine®** *see* Proparacaine *on page 852*
- ♦ **AKTob® Ophthalmic** *see* Tobramycin *on page 990*
- ♦ **AK-Tracin®** *see* Bacitracin *on page 117*
- ♦ **AK-Trol®** *see* Neomycin, Polymyxin B, and Dexamethasone *on page 711*
- ♦ **Akwa Tears® Solution [OTC]** *see* Artificial Tears *on page 97*
- ♦ **Alazide®** *see* Hydrochlorothiazide and Spironolactone *on page 504*
- ♦ **Albalon-A® Ophthalmic** *see* Naphazoline and Antazoline *on page 704*
- ♦ **Albalon® Liquifilm® Ophthalmic** *see* Naphazoline *on page 703*


## Albendazole (al BEN da zole)

**U.S. Brand Names** Albenza®

**Therapeutic Category** Anthelmintic

**Use** Treatment of parenchymal neurocysticercosis and cystic hydatid disease of the liver, lung, and peritoneum; albendazole may also be useful in the treatment of ascariasis, trichuriasis, enterobiasis, hookworm, strongyloidiasis, giardiasis, and microsporidiosis in AIDS

**Usual Dosage** Oral:

Children ≤2 years:

- Neurocysticercosis: 15 mg/kg for 8 days; repeat as necessary
- Hookworm, pinworm, roundworm: 200 mg as a single dose; treatment may be repeated in 3 weeks
- Strongyloidiasis and tapeworm: 200 mg/day for 3 days; treatment may be repeated in 3 weeks

Children >2 years and Adults:

- Hydatid disease: 800-1200 mg/day in divided doses for 28 days followed by a 2-week drug-free period, then repeated for a duration of therapy ranging from 1-12 months determined by the size, number, and location of cysts
- Neurocysticercosis: 15 mg/kg for 8-30 days; repeat as necessary
- Roundworm, pinworm, hookworm: 400 mg as a single dose; treatment may be repeated in 3 weeks
- Giardiasis: Strongyloidiasis and tapeworm: 400 mg/day for 3 days; treatment may be repeated in 3 weeks (giardiasis is a single course)

**Mechanism of Action** Albendazole appears to cause selective degeneration of cytoplasmic microtubules in intestinal and tegmental cells of intestinal helminths, and larvae; glycogen is depleted, glucose uptake and cholinesterase secretion are impaired, and desecratory substances accumulate intracellularly. ATP production decreases causing energy depletion, immobilization, and worm death.

**Local Anesthetic/Vasoconstrictor Precautions** No information available to require special precautions

**Effects on Dental Treatment** No effects or complications reported

**Other Adverse Effects** (Percentages of occurrence were not available for all adverse effects at the time of this writing)

Central nervous system: Dizziness, headache, fever

Dermatologic: Alopecia, rash, pruritus

Gastrointestinal: Abdominal pain, anorexia, constipation, diarrhea, dry mouth, epigastric pain, nausea, vomiting

Hematologic: Eosinophilia, neutropenia

Hepatic: Elevated LFTs, jaundice

**Drug Interactions** Carbamazepine may accelerate albendazole metabolism; dexamethasone increases plasma levels of albendazole metabolites

**Drug Uptake**

Absorption: Oral absorption is poor (<5%); may increase up to 4.5 times when administered with a fatty meal; albendazole itself is essentially undetectable in plasma; albendazole sulfoxide is probably the active agent

Serum half-life: ~8.5 hours

**Pregnancy Risk Factor** X

**Generic Available** No

♦ **Albenza®** *see* Albendazole *on previous page*

## Albuterol (al BYOO ter ole)

**Related Information**

Ipratropium and Albuterol *on page 548*

Respiratory Diseases *on page 1079*

**U.S. Brand Names** Airet®; Proventil®; Proventil® HFA; Ventolin®; Ventolin® Rotocaps®; Volmax®

**Canadian Brand Names** Apo®-Salvent; Novo-Salmol; Sabulin

**Therapeutic Category** Adrenergic Agonist Agent; Antiasthmatic; Beta$_2$-Adrenergic Agonist Agent; Bronchodilator

**Use** Bronchodilator in reversible airway obstruction due to asthma or COPD; prevention of exercise-induced bronchospasm in patients ≥12 years of age

**Usual Dosage**

Oral:

Children:

2-6 years: 0.1-0.2 mg/kg/dose 3 times/day; maximum dose not to exceed 12 mg/day (divided doses)

6-12 years: 2 mg/dose 3-4 times/day; maximum dose not to exceed 24 mg/day (divided doses)

Children >12 years and Adults: 2-4 mg/dose 3-4 times/day; maximum dose not to exceed 32 mg/day (divided doses)

Elderly: 2 mg 3-4 times/day; maximum: 8 mg 4 times/day

Inhalation MDI: 90 mcg/spray:

Children <12 years: 1-2 inhalations 4 times/day using a tube spacer

Children ≥12 years and Adults: 1-2 inhalations every 4-6 hours; maximum: 12 inhalations/day

Exercise-induced bronchospasm: 2 inhalations 15 minutes before exercising

Inhalation: Nebulization: 2.5 mg = 0.5 mL of the 0.5% inhalation solution to be diluted in 1-2.5 mL of NS **or** 0.01-0.05 mL/kg of 0.5% solution every 4-6 hours; intensive care patients may require more frequent administration; minimum dose: 0.1 mL; maximum dose: 1 mL diluted in 1-2 mL normal saline

<5 years: 1.25-2.5 mg every 4-6 hours as needed

>5 years: 2.5-5 mg every 4-6 hours as needed

**Mechanism of Action** Relaxes bronchial smooth muscle by action on beta$_2$-adrenergic receptors with little effect on heart rate

**Local Anesthetic/Vasoconstrictor Precautions** No information available to require special precautions

**Effects on Dental Treatment** No effects or complications reported

**Other Adverse Effects**

>10%:

Cardiovascular: Tachycardia, palpitations, pounding heartbeat

Gastrointestinal: GI upset, nausea

1% to 10%:

Cardiovascular: Flushing of face, hypertension or hypotension

(Continued)

## Albuterol *(Continued)*

Central nervous system: Nervousness, CNS stimulation, hyperactivity, insomnia, dizziness, lightheadedness, drowsiness, headache
Gastrointestinal: Dry mouth, heartburn, vomiting, unusual taste
Genitourinary: Dysuria
Neuromuscular & skeletal: Muscle cramping, tremor, weakness
Respiratory: Coughing
Miscellaneous: Increased sweating

<1%:
Cardiovascular: Chest pain, unusual pallor
Gastrointestinal: Loss of appetite
Respiratory: Paradoxical bronchospasm

**Drug Interactions** Increased toxicity: Cardiovascular effects may be potentiated in patients also receiving MAO inhibitors, tricyclic antidepressants, sympathomimetic agents (eg, amphetamine, dopamine, dobutamine), inhaled anesthetics (eg, enflurane)

**Drug Uptake**
Time to peak: 2-3 hours
Duration of action: 4-6 hours
Serum half-life: 2.7-5 hours

**Pregnancy Risk Factor** C

**Generic Available** Yes

- **Alcaine®** *see* Proparacaine *on page 852*

## Alclometasone (al kloe MET a sone)

**U.S. Brand Names** Aclovate®

**Therapeutic Category** Corticosteroid, Topical (Low Potency)

**Use** Treats inflammation of corticosteroid-responsive dermatosis (low potency topical corticosteroid)

**Usual Dosage** Topical: Apply a thin film to the affected area 2-3 times/day

**Mechanism of Action** Stimulates the synthesis of enzymes needed to decrease inflammation, suppress mitotic activity, and cause vasoconstriction

**Local Anesthetic/Vasoconstrictor Precautions** No information available to require special precautions

**Effects on Dental Treatment** No effects or complications reported

**Other Adverse Effects**

1% to 10%:
Dermatologic: Itching, erythema, dryness papular rashes
Local: Burning, irritation

<1%: Dermatologic: Hypertrichosis, acneiform eruptions, hypopigmentation, perioral dermatitis, maceration of skin, skin atrophy, striae, miliaria

**Drug Interactions** No data reported

**Pregnancy Risk Factor** C

**Dosage Forms**
Cream, as dipropionate: 0.05% (15 g, 45 g, 60 g)
Ointment, topical, as dipropionate: 0.05% (15 g, 45 g, 60 g)

**Generic Available** No

- **Alconefrin® Nasal Solution [OTC]** *see* Phenylephrine *on page 795*
- **Aldactazide®** *see* Hydrochlorothiazide and Spironolactone *on page 504*
- **Aldactone®** *see* Spironolactone *on page 931*
- **Aldara™** *see* Imiquimod *on page 530*

## Aldesleukin (al des LOO kin)

**U.S. Brand Names** Proleukin®

**Therapeutic Category** Antineoplastic Agent, Miscellaneous; Biological Response Modulator

**Synonyms** IL-2; Interleukin-2

**Use** Primarily investigated in tumors known to have a response to immunotherapy, such as melanoma and renal cell carcinoma; has been used in conjunction with LAK cells, TIL cells, IL-1, and interferon

**Usual Dosage** All orders should be written in million International units (million IU) (refer to individual protocols)

Adults: Metastatic renal cell carcinoma:

Treatment consists of two 5-day treatment cycles separated by a rest period. 600,000 units/kg (0.037 mg/kg)/dose administered every 8 hours by a 15-minute I.V. infusion for a total of 14 doses; following 9 days of rest, the schedule is repeated for another 14 doses, for a maximum of 28 doses per course.

**Investigational regimen:** I.V. continuous infusion: 4.5 million units/m$^2$/day in 250-1000 mL of $D_5W$ for 5 days

**Dose modification:** Hold or interrupt a dose rather than reducing dose; refer to protocol

**Retreatment:** Patients should be evaluated for response ~4 weeks after completion of a course of therapy and again immediately prior to the scheduled start of the next treatment course. Additional courses of treatment may be given to patients only if there is some tumor shrinkage following the last course and retreatment is not contraindicated. Each treatment course should be separated by a rest period of at least 7 weeks from the date of hospital discharge. Tumors have continued to regress up to 12 months following the initiation of therapy.

**Mechanism of Action** IL-2 promotes proliferation, differentiation, and recruitment of T and B cells, natural killer (NK) cells, and thymocytes; IL-2 also causes cytolytic activity in a subset of lymphocytes and subsequent interactions between the immune system and malignant cells; IL-2 can stimulate lymphokine-activated killer (LAK) cells and tumor-infiltrating lymphocytes (TIL) cells. LAK cells (which are derived from lymphocytes from a patient and incubated in IL-2) have the ability to lyse cells which are resistant to NK cells; TIL cells (which are derived from cancerous tissue from a patient and incubated in IL-2) have been shown to be 50% more effective than LAK cells.

**Local Anesthetic/Vasoconstrictor Precautions** No information available to require special precautions

**Effects on Dental Treatment** Stomatitis in >10% of patients

**Other Adverse Effects**

>10%:

Cardiovascular: Hypotension, sensory dysfunction, sinus tachycardia, arrhythmias, edema

Central nervous system: Dizziness, fever, mental status changes, fatigue, malaise, pain, chills

Dermatological: Pruritus, erythema, rash, dry skin, exfoliative dermatitis

Endocrine & metabolic: Acidosis, hypocalcemia, hypophosphatemia, hypomagnesemia

Gastrointestinal: Nausea, vomiting, weight gain, diarrhea, stomatitis, anorexia, GI bleeding

Hematological: Anemia, thrombocytopenia, leukopenia, coagulation disorders, elevated transaminases

Hepatic: Jaundice, elevated bilirubin, alkaline phosphatase, transaminases

Neuromuscular & skeletal: Weakness

Renal: Oliguria, anuria, proteinuria, elevated BUN, serum creatinine

Respiratory: Pulmonary congestion, dyspnea, pulmonary edema

1% to 10%:

Cardiovascular: Bradycardia, premature ventricular contractions (PVCs), myocardial ischemia, myocardial infarction, cardiac arrest, syncope

Central nervous system: Sensory disorders

Dermatologic: Purpura

Endocrine & metabolic: Hypokalemia, hypoproteinemia, hyponatremia, alkalosis, hypocholesterolemia

Gastrointestinal: Dyspepsia, constipation, weight loss

Hepatic: Ascites

Hematologic: Leukocytosis, eosinophilia

Local: Injection site reactions

Neuromuscular & skeletal: Arthralgia, myalgia

Renal: Hematuria, renal impairment

Respiratory: Respiratory failure, tachypnea, wheezing

<1%:

Cardiovascular: Congestive heart failure

Central nervous system: Coma, seizures

Dermatologic: Alopecia

Endocrine & metabolic: Hypothyroidism, hypercalcemia

Gastrointestinal: Pancreatitis

Neuromuscular & skeletal: Arthritis, muscle spasm

Renal: Polyuria

Miscellaneous: Allergic reactions

**Drug Uptake**

Absorption: Oral: Not absorbed

Serum half-life:

Initial: 6-13 minutes

Terminal: 20-120 minutes

**Pregnancy Risk Factor** C

**Generic Available** No

**Comments** 22 million units = 1.3 mg

(Continued)

## Aldesleukin *(Continued)*

1 Cetus Unit = 6 International Units
1.1 mg = 18 x $10^6$ International Units (or 3 x $10^6$ Cetus Units)
1 Roche Unit (Teceleukin) = 3 International Units

- **Aldoclor®** *see* Chlorothiazide and Methyldopa *on page 229*
- **Aldomet®** *see* Methyldopa *on page 658*
- **Aldoril®** *see* Methyldopa and Hydrochlorothiazide *on page 659*

## Alendronate (a LEN droe nate)

**U.S. Brand Names** Fosamax®

**Therapeutic Category** Bisphosphonate Derivative

**Use** FDA-approved: Osteoporosis in postmenopausal women; Paget's disease of the bone

**Usual Dosage** Oral:

Adults: Patients with osteoporosis or Paget's disease should receive supplemental calcium and vitamin D if dietary intake is inadequate

**Osteoporosis in postmenopausal women:** 10 mg once daily. Safety of treatment for >4 years has not been studied (extension studies are ongoing).

**Paget's disease of bone:** 40 mg once daily for 6 months

Retreatment: Relapses during the 12 months following therapy occurred in 9% of patients who responded to treatment. Specific retreatment data are not available. Retreatment with alendronate may be considered, following a 6-month post-treatment evaluation period, in patients who have relapsed based on increases in serum alkaline phosphatase, which should be measured periodically. Retreatment may also be considered in those who failed to normalize their serum alkaline phosphatase.

Elderly: No dosage adjustment is necessary

**Mechanism of Action** A bisphosphonate which inhibits bone resorption via actions on osteoclasts or on osteoclast precursors; decreases the rate of bone resorption direction, leading to an indirect decrease in bone formation

**Local Anesthetic/Vasoconstrictor Precautions** No information available to require special precautions

**Effects on Dental Treatment** No effects or complications reported

**Other Adverse Effects Note:** Incidence of adverse effects increases significantly in patients treated for Paget's disease at 40 mg/day, mostly GI adverse effects

1% to 10%:

Central nervous system: Headache (2.6%); pain (4.1%)

Gastrointestinal: Flatulence (2.6%); acid regurgitation (2%); esophagitis ulcer (1.5%); dysphagia, abdominal distention (1%)

<1%:

Dermatologic: Rash, erythema (rare)

Gastrointestinal: Gastritis (0.5%)

**Drug Uptake**

Absorption: Oral:

Male: 0.6% given in a fasting state

Female: 0.7%

Bioavailability: Reduced up to 60% with food or drink

Half-life: Terminal: Exceeds 10 years; serum concentrations cleared >95% in 6 hours

**Pregnancy Risk Factor** C

**Dosage Forms** Tablet, as sodium: 10 mg, 40 mg

**Generic Available** No

- **Alersule Forte®** *see* Chlorpheniramine, Phenylephrine, and Methscopolamine *on page 235*
- **Alesse™** *see* Ethinyl Estradiol and Levonorgestrel *on page 402*
- **Aleve® (Naproxen Sodium) (OTC)** *see* Naproxen *on page 705*
- **Alfenta®** *see* Alfentanil *on this page*

## Alfentanil (al FEN ta nil)

**Related Information**

Narcotic Agonists *on page 1223*

**U.S. Brand Names** Alfenta®

**Therapeutic Category** Analgesic, Narcotic; General Anesthetic, Intravenous

**Use** Analgesic adjunct given by continuous infusion or in incremental doses in maintenance of anesthesia with barbiturate or nitrous oxide ($N_2O$) or a primary anesthetic agent for the induction of anesthesia in patients undergoing general surgery in which endotracheal intubation and mechanical ventilation are required

**Usual Dosage** Doses should be titrated to appropriate effects; wide range of doses is dependent upon desired degree of analgesia/anesthesia

Children <12 years: Dose not established
Adults: Dose should be based on ideal body weight; see table.

**Alfentanil**

| Indication | Approximate Duration of Anesthesia (min) | Induction Period (Initial Dose) (mcg/kg) | Maintenance Period (Increments/ Infusion) | Total Dose (mcg/kg) | Effects |
|---|---|---|---|---|---|
| Incremental injection | ≤30 | 8-20 | 3-5 mcg/kg or 0.5-1 mcg/kg/ min | 8-40 | Spontaneously breathing or assisted ventilation when required. |
| | 30-60 | 20-50 | 5-15 mcg/kg | Up to 75 | Assisted or controlled ventilation required. Attenuation of response to laryngoscopy and intubation. |
| Continuous infusion | >45 | 50-75 | 0.5-3.0 mcg/kg/ min average infusion rate 1-1.5 mcg/kg/min | Dependent on duration of procedure | Assisted or controlled ventilation required. Some attenuation of response to intubation and incision, with intraoperative stability. |
| Anesthetic induction | >45 | 130-245 | 0.5-1.5 mcg/kg/ min or general anesthetic | Dependent on duration of procedure | Assisted or controlled ventilation required. Administer slowly (over three minutes). Concentration of inhalation agents reduced by 30%-50% for initial hour. |

**Mechanism of Action** Binds to opiate receptors (mu and kappa subtypes) in the CNS causing inhibition of ascending pain pathways, altering the perception of and response to pain; produces generalized CNS depression

**Local Anesthetic/Vasoconstrictor Precautions** No information available to require special precautions

**Effects on Dental Treatment** Erythromycin inhibits the liver metabolism of alfentanil resulting in increased sedation and prolonged respiratory depression

**Other Adverse Effects**

Endocrine & metabolic: Antidiuretic hormone release
Ocular: Miosis
>10%:
Cardiovascular: Bradycardia, peripheral vasodilation
Central nervous system: Drowsiness, sedation, increased intracranial pressure
Gastrointestinal: Nausea, vomiting, constipation
1% to 10%:
Cardiovascular: Cardiac arrhythmias, orthostatic hypotension
Central nervous system: Confusion, CNS depression
Ocular: Blurred vision
<1%:
Central nervous system: Convulsions, mental depression, paradoxical CNS excitation or delirium, dizziness, dysesthesia
Dermatologic: Skin rash, urticaria, itching
Gastrointestinal: Biliary tract spasm
Genitourinary: Urinary tract spasm
Respiratory: Respiratory depression, bronchospasm, laryngospasm
Miscellaneous: Physical and psychological dependence with prolonged use, cold, clammy skin

**Drug Interactions** Increased toxicity: CNS depressants (eg, benzodiazepines, barbiturates, phenothiazines, tricyclic antidepressants), erythromycin, reserpine, beta-blockers

**Drug Uptake** Serum half-life: Adults: 83-97 minutes

**Pregnancy Risk Factor** C

**Generic Available** No

**Selected Readings**

Bartkowski RR, Goldberg ME, Larijani GE, et al, "Inhibition of Alfentanil Metabolism by Erythromycin," *Clin Pharmacol Ther*, 1989, 46(1):99-102.

Bartkowski RR and McDonnell TE, "Prolonged Alfentanil Effect Following Erythromycin Administration," *Anesthesiology*, 1990, 73(3):566-8.

♦ **Alferon® N** *see* Interferon Alfa-n3 *on page 543*

## Alglucerase (al GLOO ser ase)

**U.S. Brand Names** Ceredase® Injection

**Therapeutic Category** Enzyme, Glucocerebrosidase

**Synonyms** Glucocerebrosidase

(Continued)

## Alglucerase *(Continued)*

**Use** Orphan drug for treatment of Gaucher's disease

**Usual Dosage** Usually administered as a 20-60 units/kg I.V. infusion given with a frequency ranging from 3 times/week to once every 2 weeks

**Mechanism of Action** Glucocerebrosidase is an enzyme prepared from human placental tissue. Gaucher's disease is an inherited metabolic disorder caused by the defective activity of beta-glucosidase and the resultant accumulation of glucosyl ceramide laden macrophages in the liver, bone, and spleen; acts by replacing the missing enzyme associated with Gaucher's disease.

**Local Anesthetic/Vasoconstrictor Precautions** No information available to require special precautions

**Effects on Dental Treatment** No effects or complications reported

**Other Adverse Effects**

>10%: Local: Discomfort, burning, and edema at the site of injection

<1%:

Central nervous system: Fever, chills

Gastrointestinal: Abdominal discomfort, nausea, vomiting

**Drug Uptake** Half-life, elimination: ~4-20 minutes

**Pregnancy Risk Factor** C

**Generic Available** No

- **Alkaban-AQ®** *see* Vinblastine *on page 1046*
- **Alka-Mints® [OTC]** *see* Calcium Carbonate *on page 172*
- **Alka-Seltzer® Plus Cold Liqui-Gels® Capsules [OTC]** *see* Acetaminophen, Chlorpheniramine, and Pseudoephedrine *on page 32*
- **Alka-Seltzer® Plus Flu & Body Aches Non-Drowsy Liqui-Gels® [OTC]** *see* Acetaminophen, Dextromethorphan, and Pseudoephedrine *on page 32*
- **Alkeran®** *see* Melphalan *on page 626*
- **Allbee® With C [OTC]** *see* Vitamin B Complex With Vitamin C *on page 1050*
- **Allbee® With C** *see* Vitamins, Multiple *on page 1051*
- **Allegra®** *see* Fexofenadine *on page 429*
- **Aller-Chlor® [OTC]** *see* Chlorpheniramine *on page 231*
- **Allercon® Tablet [OTC]** *see* Triprolidine and Pseudoephedrine *on page 1025*
- **Allerest® 12 Hour Capsule [OTC]** *see* Chlorpheniramine and Phenylpropanolamine *on page 233*
- **Allerest® 12 Hour Nasal Solution [OTC]** *see* Oxymetazoline *on page 755*
- **Allerest® Eye Drops [OTC]** *see* Naphazoline *on page 703*
- **Allerest® Maximum Strength [OTC]** *see* Chlorpheniramine and Pseudoephedrine *on page 233*
- **Allerest® No Drowsiness [OTC]** *see* Acetaminophen and Pseudoephedrine *on page 31*
- **Allerfrin® Syrup [OTC]** *see* Triprolidine and Pseudoephedrine *on page 1025*
- **Allerfrin® Tablet [OTC]** *see* Triprolidine and Pseudoephedrine *on page 1025*
- **Allerfrin® w/Codeine** *see* Triprolidine, Pseudoephedrine, and Codeine *on page 1026*
- **Allergan® Ear Drops** *see* Antipyrine and Benzocaine *on page 91*
- **Allergic Skin Reactions to Drugs** *see page 1267*
- **AllerMax® Oral [OTC]** *see* Diphenhydramine *on page 338*
- **Allerphed® Syrup [OTC]** *see* Triprolidine and Pseudoephedrine *on page 1025*

## Allopurinol (al oh PURE i nole)

**U.S. Brand Names** Zyloprim®

**Canadian Brand Names** Apo®-Allopurinol; Novo-Purol; Purinol®

**Therapeutic Category** Uric Acid Lowering Agent; Uricosuric Agent

**Use** Prevention of attacks of gouty arthritis and nephropathy; also used to treat secondary hyperuricemia which may occur during treatment of tumors or leukemia; prevent recurrent calcium oxalate calculi

**Usual Dosage** Oral:

Children ≤10 years: 10 mg/kg/day in 2-3 divided doses **or** 200-300 mg/m$^2$/day in 2-4 divided doses, maximum: 800 mg/24 hours

Alternative:

<6 years: 150 mg/day in 3 divided doses

6-10 years: 300 mg/day in 2-3 divided doses

Children >10 years and Adults: Daily doses >300 mg should be administered in divided doses

Myeloproliferative neoplastic disorders: 600-800 mg/day in 2-3 divided doses for prevention of acute uric acid nephropathy for 2-3 days starting 1-2 days before chemotherapy

Gout:

Mild: 200-300 mg/day

Severe: 400-600 mg/day

**Mechanism of Action** Allopurinol inhibits xanthine oxidase, the enzyme responsible for the conversion of hypoxanthine to xanthine to uric acid. Allopurinol is metabolized to oxypurinol which is also an inhibitor of xanthine oxidase; allopurinol acts on purine catabolism, reducing the production of uric acid without disrupting the biosynthesis of vital purines.

**Local Anesthetic/Vasoconstrictor Precautions** No information available to require special precautions

**Effects on Dental Treatment** No effects or complications reported

**Other Adverse Effects**

>10%: Dermatologic: Skin rash (usually maculopapular), exfoliative, urticarial or purpuric lesions

1% to 10%:

- Central nervous system: Drowsiness, chills, fever
- Dermatologic: Alopecia
- Gastrointestinal: Nausea, vomiting, diarrhea, abdominal pain, abdominal pain, dyspepsia
- Hepatic: Elevated alkaline phosphatase, AST, and ALT, hepatomegaly, hyperbilirubinemia, and jaundice; hepatic necrosis has been reported

<1%:

- Cardiovascular: Vasculitis
- Central nervous system: Headache, neuritis
- Dermatologic: Toxic epidermal necrolysis and Stevens-Johnson syndrome have been reported
- Hematologic: Bone marrow suppression has been reported in patients receiving allopurinol with other myelosuppressive agents
- Idiosyncratic: Reaction characterized by fever, chills, eosinophilia, arthralgia, nausea, and vomiting, leukopenia, leukocytosis
- Local: Thrombophlebitis
- Neuromuscular & skeletal: Peripheral neuropathy, paresthesia
- Ocular: Cataracts
- Renal: Renal impairment
- Respiratory: Epistaxis

**Drug Interactions**

Decreased effect with alcohol

Increased toxicity:

- Allopurinol prolongs half-life of oral anticoagulants
- Allopurinol increases serum half-life of theophylline
- Allopurinol may compete for excretion in renal tubule with chlorpropamide and increase chlorpropamide's serum half-life
- Allopurinol inhibits metabolism of azathioprine and mercaptopurine
- Thiazide diuretics enhance toxicity of allopurinol
- Use with ampicillin may increase the incidence of skin rash
- Urinary acidification with large amounts of vitamin C may increase kidney stone formation

**Drug Uptake**

Decreases in serum uric acid occur in 1-2 days with nadir achieved in 1-2 weeks

Absorption:

- Oral: ~80% of dose absorbed from GI tract; peak plasma concentrations are seen 30-120 minutes after administration
- Rectal: Poor and erratic

Serum half-life:

- Normal renal function:
- Parent drug: 1-3 hours
- Oxypurinol: 18-30 hours

**Pregnancy Risk Factor** C

**Generic Available** Yes


- ♦ **All-*trans*-Retinoic Acid** *see* Tretinoin, Oral *on page 1007*
- ♦ **Alomide®** *see* Lodoxamide Tromethamine *on page 597*
- ♦ **Alor® 5/500** *see* Hydrocodone and Aspirin *on page 507*
- ♦ **Alora® Transdermal** *see* Estradiol *on page 387*
- ♦ **Alpha$_1$-PI** *see* Alpha$_1$-Proteinase Inhibitor *on this page*


## Alpha$_1$-Proteinase Inhibitor (al fa won PRO tee in ase in HI bi tor)

**U.S. Brand Names** Prolastin® Injection

**Therapeutic Category** Antitrypsin Deficiency Agent

**Synonyms** Alpha$_1$-PI; Alpha$_1$-Proteinase Inhibitor, Human

**Use** Congenital alpha$_1$-antitrypsin deficiency

**Usual Dosage** Adults: I.V.: 60 mg/kg once weekly (at a rate ≥0.08 mL/kg/minute)

**Mechanism of Action** Human alpha$_1$-proteinase inhibitor is prepared from the pooled human plasma of normal donors and is intended for use in the therapy of

(Continued)

## Alpha$_1$-Proteinase Inhibitor *(Continued)*

congenital alpha$_1$-antitrypsin deficiency. Alpha$_1$-antitrypsin (AAT) is the principal protease inhibitor in the serum and exists as a single polypeptide glycoprotein. Production of AAT occurs in the liver hepatocyte and secretion occurs at a rate to maintain serum concentrations of 150-200 mg/dL. The major physiologic role of the antiprotease is that of combining with proteolytic enzymes to render them inactive. Several proteases can be inactivated by AAT including trypsin, chymotrypsin, coagulation factor XI, plasmin, thrombin, and neutrophil elastase.

**Local Anesthetic/Vasoconstrictor Precautions** No information available to require special precautions

**Effects on Dental Treatment** No effects or complications reported

**Other Adverse Effects** <1%:

Central nervous system: Dizziness, lightheadedness, fever <102°F (delayed up to 12 hours after treatment)

Hematologic: Leukocytosis

**Drug Uptake** Serum half-life, elimination (parent compound): 4.5-5.2 days

**Pregnancy Risk Factor** C

**Generic Available** No

**Comments** Sodium content of 1 L after reconstitution: 100-210 mEq

- **Alpha$_1$-Proteinase Inhibitor, Human** *see* Alpha$_1$-Proteinase Inhibitor *on previous page*
- **Alphagan®** *see* Brimonidine *on page 149*
- **Alphamul® [OTC]** *see* Castor Oil *on page 196*
- **AlphaNine® SD** *see* Factor IX Complex (Human) *on page 417*
- **Alphatrex®** *see* Betamethasone *on page 136*

## Alprazolam (al PRAY zoe lam)

**Related Information**

Patients Requiring Sedation *on page 1152*

Temporomandibular Dysfunction (TMD) *on page 1149*

**U.S. Brand Names** Xanax®

**Canadian Brand Names** Apo®-Alpraz; Novo-Alprazol; Nu-Alprax

**Therapeutic Category** Antianxiety Agent; Benzodiazepine; Tranquilizer, Minor

**Use** Treatment of anxiety; adjunct in the treatment of depression; management of panic attacks

**Usual Dosage** Oral:

Children <18 years: Safety and dose have not been established

Adults: 0.25-0.5 mg 2-3 times/day, titrate dose upward; maximum: 4 mg/day

**Mechanism of Action** Binds at stereospecific receptors at several sites within the central nervous system, including the limbic system, reticular formation; effects may be mediated through GABA

**Local Anesthetic/Vasoconstrictor Precautions** No information available to require special precautions

**Effects on Dental Treatment** Significant dry mouth will occur in over 10% of patients; normal salivary flow occurs with cessation of drug therapy

**Other Adverse Effects**

Treatment of anxiety:

>10%:

Central nervous system: Drowsiness, lightheadedness, depression, headache

Gastrointestinal: Xerostomia, constipation, diarrhea

1& to 10%:

Cardiovascular: Hypotension, tachycardia/palpitations

Central nervous system: Confusion, nervousness, dizziness, akathisia, insomnia, memory impairment

Gastrointestinal: Nausea, vomiting, weight gain/loss, increased salivation

Neuromuscular & skeletal: Rigidity, tremor

Ocular: Blurred vision

Respiratory: Nasal congestion

Treatment of panic disorder:

>10%:

Cardiovascular: Tachycardia, chest pain

Central nervous system: Insomnia, lightheadedness, headache, anxiety, fatigue, irritability, cognitive disorder, dizziness, impaired coordination

Dermatologic: Rash

Endocrine & metabolic: Decreased libido

Gastrointestinal: Nausea, vomiting, diarrhea, decreased salivation, weight loss, decreased appetite, constipation

Neuromuscular & skeletal: Dysarthria, abnormal involuntary movement

Ocular: Blurred vision

Respiratory: Nasal congestion
Miscellaneous: Diaphoresis
1% to 10%:
Cardiovascular: Syncope
Central nervous system: Confusion, memory impairment, depression
Endocrine & metabolic: Increased libido, sexual dysfunction
Gastrointestinal: Increased salivation
Neuromuscular & skeletal: Muscle stiffness, cramps, muscular twitching, weakness, muscle tone disorders
Otic: Tinnitus
Respiratory: Hyperventilation
<1%:
Central nervous system: Seizures, hallucinations, depersonalization
Gastrointestinal: Taste alteration
Hepatic: Elevated bilirubin, elevated hepatic enzymes, jaundice
Ocular: Diplopia

**Drug Interactions** Alprazolam will produce an additive CNS depressant effect when coadministered with other psychotropic medications, anticonvulsants and antihistamines; the blood level of alprazolam can be increased by cimetidine (Tagamet®) and by oral contraceptives; the clinical significance of this effect is unclear; fluvoxamine (Luvox®) can increase alprazolam plasma concentrations resulting in increased psychomotor impairment

**Drug Uptake**
Serum half-life: 12-15 hours
Time to peak serum concentration: Within 1-2 hours

**Pregnancy Risk Factor** D

**Dosage Forms** Tablet: 0.25 mg, 0.5 mg, 1 mg, 2 mg

**Dietary Considerations** May be taken with food or water to avoid gastrointestinal upset

**Generic Available** Yes

## Alprostadil (al PROS ta dill)

**U.S. Brand Names** Caverject® Injection; Edex® Injection; Muse® Pellet; Prostin VR Pediatric® Injection

**Therapeutic Category** Prostaglandin

**Synonyms** $PGE_1$; Prostaglandin $E_1$

**Use** Temporary maintenance of patency of ductus arteriosus in neonates with ductal-dependent congenital heart disease until surgery can be performed. These defects include cyanotic (eg, pulmonary atresia, pulmonary stenosis, tricuspid atresia, Fallot's tetralogy, transposition of the great vessels) and acyanotic (eg, interruption of aortic arch, coarctation of aorta, hypoplastic left ventricle) heart disease; diagnosis and treatment of erectile dysfunction of vasculogenic, psychogenic, or neurogenic etiology; adjunct in the diagnosis of erectile dysfunction

**Investigational:** Treatment of pulmonary hypertension in infants and children with congenital heart defects with left-to-right shunts

**Usual Dosage**

**Patent ductus arteriosus** (Prostin VR Pediatric®):

I.V. continuous infusion into a large vein, or alternatively through an umbilical artery catheter placed at the ductal opening: 0.05-0.1 mcg/kg/minute with therapeutic response, rate is reduced to lowest effective dosage; with unsatisfactory response, rate is increased gradually; maintenance: 0.01-0.4 mcg/kg/minute

$PGE_1$ is usually given at an infusion rate of 0.1 mcg/kg/minute, but it is often possible to reduce the dosage to 1/2 or even 1/10 without losing the therapeutic effect. The mixing schedule is shown in the table.

| Add 1 Ampul (500 mcg) to: | Concentration (mcg/mL) | Infusion Rate: mL/min/kg Needed to Infuse 0.1 mcg/kg/min | Infusion Rate: mL/kg/24 h |
|---|---|---|---|
| 250 mL | 2 | 0.05 | 72 |
| 100 mL | 5 | 0.02 | 28.8 |
| 50 mL | 10 | 0.01 | 14.4 |
| 25 mL | 20 | 0.005 | 7.2 |

Therapeutic response is indicated by increased pH in those with acidosis or by an increase in oxygenation ($pO_2$) usually evident within 30 minutes

(Continued)

## Alprostadil *(Continued)*

**Erectile dysfunction** (Caverject®):

Vasculogenic, psychogenic, or mixed etiology: Individualize dose by careful titration; usual dose: 2.5-60 mcg (doses >60 mcg are not recommended); initiate dosage titration at 2.5 mcg, increasing by 2.5 mcg to a dose of 5 mcg and then in increments of 5-10 mcg depending on the erectile response until the dose produces an erection suitable for intercourse, not lasting >1 hour; if there is absolutely no response to initial 2.5 mcg dose, the second dose may increased to 7.5 mcg, followed by increments of 5-10 mcg

Neurogenic etiology (eg, spinal cord injury): Initiate dosage titration at 1.25 mcg, increasing to a doses of 2.5 mcg and then 5 mcg; increase further in increments 5 mcg until the dose is reached that produces an erection suitable for intercourse, not lasting >1 hour

**Note:** Patient must stay in the physician's office until complete detumescence occurs; if there is no response, then the next higher dose may be given within 1 hour; if there is still no response, a 1-day interval before giving the next dose is recommended; increasing the dose or concentration in the treatment of impotence results in increasing pain and discomfort

**Mechanism of Action** Causes vasodilation by means of direct effect on vascular and ductus arteriosus smooth muscle

**Local Anesthetic/Vasoconstrictor Precautions** No information available to require special precautions

**Effects on Dental Treatment** No effects or complications reported

**Other Adverse Effects**

>10%:

Cardiovascular: Flushing
Central nervous system: Fever
Genitourinary: Penile pain
Respiratory: Apnea

1% to 10%:

Cardiovascular: Bradycardia, hypotension, hypertension, tachycardia, cardiac arrest, edema
Central nervous system: Seizures, headache, dizziness
Endocrine & metabolic: Hypokalemia
Gastrointestinal: Diarrhea
Genitourinary: Prolonged erection, penile fibrosis, penis disorder, penile rash, penile edema
Hematologic: Disseminated intravascular coagulation
Local: Injection site hematoma, injection site bruising
Neuromuscular & skeletal: Back pain
Respiratory: Upper respiratory infection, sinusitis, nasal congestion, cough
Miscellaneous: Sepsis, localized pain in structures other than the injection site, flu syndrome

**Drug Uptake** Serum half-life: 5-10 minutes

**Pregnancy Risk Factor** X

**Generic Available** No

- **AL-R® [OTC]** *see* Chlorpheniramine *on page 231*
- **Alrex™** *see* Loteprednol *on page 604*
- **Altace™** *see* Ramipril *on page 877*

## Alteplase (AL te plase)

**U.S. Brand Names** Activase®

**Canadian Brand Names** Lysatec-rt-PA®

**Therapeutic Category** Thrombolytic Agent

**Use** Management of acute myocardial infarction for the lysis of thrombi in coronary arteries; management of acute massive pulmonary embolism (PE) in adults; to improve neurologic recovery and decrease disability in adults following acute ischemic stroke, and most common type of stroke, caused by blood clots that block blood flow, treatment must start within 3 hours of the start of the stroke and only after bleeding in the brain has been ruled out by a cranial computerized tomography (CT) scan

**Usual Dosage**

Coronary artery thrombi: I.V.: Front loading dose: Total dose is 100 mg over 1.5 hours (for patients who weigh <65 kg, use 1.25 mg/kg/total dose). Add this dose to a 100 mL bag of 0.9% sodium chloride for a total volume of 200 mL. Infuse 15 mg (30 mL) over 1-2 minutes; infuse 50 mg (100 mL) over 30 minutes. Begin heparin 5000-10,000 unit bolus followed by continuous infusion of 1000 units/hour. Infuse 35 mg/hour (70 mL) for next 2 hours.

Acute pulmonary embolism: 100 mg over 2 hours

**Mechanism of Action** Initiates local fibrinolysis by binding to fibrin in a thrombus (clot) and converts entrapped plasminogen to plasmin

**Local Anesthetic/Vasoconstrictor Precautions** No information available to require special precautions

**Effects on Dental Treatment** No effects or complications reported

**Other Adverse Effects**

1% to 10%:

Cardiovascular: Hypotension
Central nervous system: Fever
Dermatologic: Bruising
Gastrointestinal: GI hemorrhage, nausea, vomiting
Genitourinary: GU hemorrhage

<1%:

Central nervous system: Intracranial hemorrhage
Gastrointestinal: Gingival hemorrhage
Hematologic: Retroperitoneal hemorrhage, rapid lysis of coronary artery thrombi by thrombolytic agents may be associated with reperfusion-related atrial and/or ventricular arrhythmias
Respiratory: Epistaxis

**Drug Interactions** Increased effect: Anticoagulants, aspirin, ticlopidine, dipyridamole, and heparin are at least additive

**Pregnancy Risk Factor** C

**Generic Available** No

♦ **ALternaGEL® [OTC]** *see* Aluminum Hydroxide *on page 55*

## Altretamine (al TRET a meen)

**U.S. Brand Names** Hexalen®

**Therapeutic Category** Antineoplastic Agent, Alkylating Agent

**Use** Palliative treatment of persistent or recurrent ovarian cancer following first-line therapy with a cisplatin- or alkylating agent-based combination

**Usual Dosage** Oral (refer to protocol):

Adults: 4-12 mg/kg/day in 3-4 divided doses for 21-90 days

Alternatively: 240-320 mg/m$^2$/day in 3-4 divided doses for 21 days, repeated every 6 weeks

Alternatively: 260 mg/m$^2$/day for 14-21 days of a 28-day cycle in 4 divided doses

**Temporarily discontinue** (for ≥14 days) & subsequently restart at 200 mg/m$^2$/day if any of the following occurs:

if GI intolerance unresponsive to symptom measures
WBC <2000/mm$^3$
granulocyte count <1000/mm$^3$
platelet count <75,000/mm$^3$
progressive neurotoxicity

**Mechanism of Action** Although altretamine clinical antitumor spectrum resembles that of alkylating agents, the drug has demonstrated activity in alkylator-resistant patients; probably requires hepatic microsomal mixed-function oxidase enzyme activation to become cytotoxic. The drug selectively inhibits the incorporation of radioactive thymidine and uridine into DNA and RNA, inhibiting DNA and RNA synthesis; metabolized to reactive intermediates which covalently bind to microsomal proteins and DNA. These reactive intermediates can spontaneously degrade to demethylated melamines and formaldehyde which are also cytotoxic.

**Local Anesthetic/Vasoconstrictor Precautions** No information available to require special precautions

**Effects on Dental Treatment** No effects or complications reported

**Other Adverse Effects**

>10%:

Central nervous system: Neurotoxicity
Gastrointestinal: Nausea, vomiting
Hematologic: Anemia, thrombocytopenia, leukopenia
Neuromuscular & skeletal: Peripheral sensory neuropathy

1% to 10%:

Central nervous system: Seizures
Gastrointestinal: Anorexia, diarrhea, stomach cramps
Hepatic: Elevated alkaline phosphatase

<1%:

Central nervous system: Dizziness, depression
Dermatologic: Rash, alopecia
Hematologic: Myelosuppression
Hepatic: Hepatotoxicity
Neuromuscular & skeletal: Tremor

**Drug Interactions**

Decreased effect: Phenobarbital may increase metabolism of altretamine

(Continued)

## Altretamine *(Continued)*

Increased toxicity: May cause severe orthostatic hypotension when administered with MAO inhibitors; cimetidine may decrease metabolism of altretamine

**Drug Uptake**

Absorption: Oral: Well absorbed (75% to 89%)
Serum half-life: 13 hours
Peak plasma levels: 0.5-3 hours after dose

**Pregnancy Risk Factor** D

**Generic Available** No

- **Alu-Cap® [OTC]** *see* Aluminum Hydroxide *on next page*
- **Aludrox® [OTC]** *see* Aluminum Hydroxide and Magnesium Hydroxide *on page 56*

## Aluminum Acetate and Acetic Acid

(a LOO mi num AS e tate & a SEE tik AS id)

**U.S. Brand Names** Otic Domeboro®

**Therapeutic Category** Otic Agent, Anti-infective

**Synonyms** Acetic Acid and Aluminum Acetate Otic; Burow's Otic

**Use** Treatment of superficial infections of the external auditory canal

**Usual Dosage** Instill 4-6 drops in ear(s) every 2-3 hours; insert saturated wick, keep moist for 24 hours

**Local Anesthetic/Vasoconstrictor Precautions** No information available to require special precautions

**Effects on Dental Treatment** No effects or complications reported

**Other Adverse Effects** 1% to 10%: Irritation

**Generic Available** Yes

## Aluminum Carbonate (a LOO mi num KAR bun ate)

**U.S. Brand Names** Basaljel® [OTC]

**Therapeutic Category** Antacid

**Use** Hyperacidity; hyperphosphatemia

**Usual Dosage** Adults: Oral:

Antacid: 2 tablets/capsules or 10 mL of suspension every 2 hours, up to 12 times/day
Hyperphosphatemia: 2 tablets/capsules or 12 mL of suspension with meals

**Local Anesthetic/Vasoconstrictor Precautions** No information available to require special precautions

**Effects on Dental Treatment** Aluminum carbonate prevents gastrointestinal absorption of tetracycline by forming a large ionized chelated molecule with the aluminum ion and tetracyclines in the stomach. Aluminum carbonate prevents GI absorption of ketoconazole and itraconazole by increasing the pH in the GI tract. Any of these drugs should be administered at least 1 hour before aluminum carbonate.

**Other Adverse Effects**

>10%: Gastrointestinal: Constipation, chalky taste, stomach cramps, fecal impaction
1% to 10%: Gastrointestinal: Nausea, vomiting, discoloration of feces (white speckles)
<1%: Endocrine & metabolic: Hypophosphatemia, hypomagnesemia

**Pregnancy Risk Factor** C

**Generic Available** Yes

## Aluminum Chloride (a LOO mi num KLOR ide)

**U.S. Brand Names** Gingi-Aid® Gingival Retraction Cord; Gingi-Aid® Solution; Hemodent® Gingival Retraction Cord

**Therapeutic Category** Astringent

**Use**

Dental: Hemostatic; gingival retraction
Medical: Hemostatic

**Mechanism of Action** Precipitates tissue and blood proteins causing a mechanical obstruction to hemorrhage from injured blood vessels

**Local Anesthetic/Vasoconstrictor Precautions** No information available to require special precautions

**Effects on Dental Treatment** No effects or complications reported

**Other Adverse Effects** No data reported

**Contraindications** No data reported

**Warnings/Precautions** Since large amounts of astringents may cause tissue irritation and possible damage, only small amounts should be applied

**Drug Interactions** No data reported

**Breast-feeding Considerations** May be taken while breast-feeding

**Dosage Forms**
Retraction cord impregnated with aqueous solution of aluminum chloride containing 1.0 mg or 2.0 mg/inch in lengths of 72 inches
Retraction cord impregnated with an aqueous 10% solution of aluminum chloride and dried, containing 0.9 mg/inch or 1.8 mg/inch in lengths of 84 inches
Aqueous solution, 10 g aluminum chloride/100 mL water packaged in 15 and 30 mL bottles

**Dietary Considerations** No data reported
**Generic Available** Yes

## Aluminum Hydroxide (a LOO mi num hye DROKS ide)

**U.S. Brand Names** ALternaGEL® [OTC]; Alu-Cap® [OTC]; Alu-Tab® [OTC]; Amphojel® [OTC]; Dialume® [OTC]; Nephrox Suspension [OTC]
**Canadian Brand Names** Basaljel®
**Therapeutic Category** Antacid; Antidote, Hyperphosphatemia
**Use** Treatment of hyperacidity; hyperphosphatemia
**Usual Dosage** Oral:
Peptic ulcer disease:
Children: 5-15 mL/dose every 3-6 hours or 1 and 3 hours after meals and at bedtime
Adults: 15-45 mL every 3-6 hours or 1 and 3 hours after meals and at bedtime
Prophylaxis against gastrointestinal bleeding:
Children: 5-15 mL/dose every 1-2 hours
Adults: 30-60 mL/dose every hour
Titrate to maintain the gastric pH >5
Hyperphosphatemia:
Children: 50-150 mg/kg/24 hours in divided doses every 4-6 hours, titrate dosage to maintain serum phosphorus within normal range
Adults: 500-1800 mg, 3-6 times/day, between meals and at bedtime
Antacid: Adults: 30 mL 1 and 3 hours postprandial and at bedtime

**Mechanism of Action** Neutralizes hydrochloride in stomach to form Al $(Cl)_3$ salt + $H_2O$
**Local Anesthetic/Vasoconstrictor Precautions** No information available to require special precautions
**Effects on Dental Treatment** Aluminum OH prevents gastrointestinal absorption of tetracycline by forming a large ionized chelated molecule with the aluminum ion and tetracyclines in the stomach. Aluminum OH prevents GI absorption of ketoconazole and itraconazole by increasing the pH in the GI tract. Any of these drugs should be administered at least 1 hour before $Al(OH)_3$.
**Other Adverse Effects**
>10%: Gastrointestinal: Constipation, chalky taste, stomach cramps, fecal impaction
1% to 10%: Gastrointestinal: Nausea, vomiting, discoloration of feces (white speckles)
<1%: Endocrine & metabolic: Hypophosphatemia, hypomagnesemia

**Drug Interactions** Decreased effect: Tetracyclines, digoxin, indomethacin, or iron salts, isoniazid, allopurinol, benzodiazepines, corticosteroids, penicillamine, phenothiazines, ranitidine, ketoconazole, itraconazole
**Pregnancy Risk Factor** C
**Generic Available** Yes

## Aluminum Hydroxide and Magnesium Carbonate

(a LOO mi num hye DROKS ide & mag NEE zhum KAR bun nate)
**U.S. Brand Names** Gaviscon® Liquid [OTC]
**Therapeutic Category** Antacid
**Use** Temporary relief of symptoms associated with gastric acidity
**Usual Dosage** Adults: Oral: 15-30 mL 4 times/day after meals and at bedtime
**Local Anesthetic/Vasoconstrictor Precautions** No information available to require special precautions
**Effects on Dental Treatment** Aluminum and magnesium ions prevent gastrointestinal absorption of tetracycline by forming a large ionized chelated molecule with the tetracyclines in the stomach. Aluminum hydroxide prevents GI absorption of ketoconazole and itraconazole by increasing the pH in the GI tract. Any of these drugs should be administered at least 1 hour before aluminum hydroxide.
**Other Adverse Effects** 1% to 10%:
Endocrine & metabolic: Hypermagnesemia, aluminum intoxication (prolonged use and concomitant renal failure), hypophosphatemia
Gastrointestinal: Constipation, diarrhea
Neuromuscular & skeletal: Osteomalacia

**Generic Available** Yes
**Comments** Sodium content per 5 mL Gaviscon® liquid: 0.6 mEq

## Aluminum Hydroxide and Magnesium Hydroxide

(a LOO mi num hye DROKS ide & mag NEE zhum hye DROK side)

**U.S. Brand Names** Aludrox® [OTC]; Maalox® [OTC]; Maalox® Therapeutic Concentrate [OTC]

**Canadian Brand Names** Diovol®, EX; Gelusil®, Extra Strength; Neutralca®-S; Univol®

**Therapeutic Category** Antacid

**Synonyms** Magnesium Hydroxide and Aluminum Hydroxide

**Use** Antacid, hyperphosphatemia in renal failure

**Usual Dosage** Oral: 5-10 mL or 1-2 tablets 4-6 times/day, between meals and at bedtime; may be used every hour for severe symptoms

**Local Anesthetic/Vasoconstrictor Precautions** No information available to require special precautions

**Effects on Dental Treatment** Aluminum and magnesium ions prevent gastrointestinal absorption of tetracycline by forming a large ionized chelated molecule with the tetracyclines in the stomach. Aluminum hydroxide prevents GI absorption of ketoconazole and itraconazole by increasing the pH in the GI tract. Any of these drugs should be administered at least 1 hour before aluminum hydroxide.

**Other Adverse Effects**

>10%: Gastrointestinal: Constipation, chalky taste, stomach cramps, fecal impaction

1% to 10%: Gastrointestinal: Nausea, vomiting, discoloration of feces (white speckles)

<1%: Endocrine & metabolic: Hypophosphatemia, hypomagnesemia

**Pregnancy Risk Factor** C

**Generic Available** Yes

**Comments** Sodium content of 5 mL (Maalox®): 1.3 mg (0.06 mEq)

## Aluminum Hydroxide and Magnesium Trisilicate

(a LOO mi num hye DROKS ide & mag NEE zhum trye SIL i kate)

**U.S. Brand Names** Gaviscon®-2 Tablet [OTC]; Gaviscon® Tablet [OTC]

**Therapeutic Category** Antacid

**Use** Temporary relief of hyperacidity

**Usual Dosage** Adults: Oral: Chew 2-4 tablets 4 times/day or as directed by physician

**Local Anesthetic/Vasoconstrictor Precautions** No information available to require special precautions

**Effects on Dental Treatment** Aluminum and magnesium ions prevent gastrointestinal absorption of tetracycline by forming a large ionized chelated molecule with the tetracyclines in the stomach. Aluminum hydroxide prevents GI absorption of ketoconazole and itraconazole by increasing the pH in the GI tract. Any of these drugs should be administered at least 1 hour before aluminum hydroxide.

**Pregnancy Risk Factor** C

**Generic Available** Yes

**Comments** Sodium content per tablet:

Gaviscon®: 0.8 mEq
Gaviscon®-2: 1.6 mEq

## Aluminum Hydroxide, Magnesium Hydroxide, and Simethicone

(a LOO mi num hye DROKS ide, mag NEE zhum hye DROKS ide, & sye METH i kone)

**U.S. Brand Names** Di-Gel® [OTC]; Gas-Ban DS® [OTC]; Maalox® Plus [OTC]; Magalox Plus® [OTC]; Mylanta® [OTC]; Mylanta®-II [OTC]

**Therapeutic Category** Antacid; Antiflatulent

**Use** Temporary relief of hyperacidity associated with gas; may also be used for indications associated with other antacids

**Usual Dosage** Adults: 15-30 mL or 2-4 tablets 4-6 times/day between meals and at bedtime; may be used every hour for severe symptoms

**Local Anesthetic/Vasoconstrictor Precautions** No information available to require special precautions

**Effects on Dental Treatment** Aluminum and magnesium ions prevent gastrointestinal absorption of tetracycline by forming a large ionized chelated molecule with the tetracyclines in the stomach. Aluminum hydroxide prevents GI absorption of ketoconazole and itraconazole by increasing the pH in the GI tract. Any of these drugs should be administered at least 1 hour before aluminum hydroxide.

**Other Adverse Effects**

>10%: Gastrointestinal: Chalky taste, stomach cramps, constipation, decreased bowel motility, fecal impaction, hemorrhoids

1% to 10%: Gastrointestinal: Nausea, vomiting, discoloration of feces (white speckles)

<1%: Endocrine & metabolic: Hypophosphatemia, hypomagnesemia, dehydration or fluid restriction

**Pregnancy Risk Factor** C

**Generic Available** Yes

**Comments** Sodium content of 5 mL:

Maalox® Plus: 1.3 mg (0.06 mEq)

Mylanta®: 0.7 mg (0.03 mEq)

Mylanta®-II: 1.14 mg (0.05 mEq)

## Aluminum Sulfate and Calcium Acetate

(a LOO mi num SUL fate & KAL see um AS e tate)

**U.S. Brand Names** Bluboro® [OTC]; Boropak® [OTC]; Domeboro® Topical [OTC]; Pedi-Boro® [OTC]

**Therapeutic Category** Topical Skin Product

**Use** Astringent wet dressing for relief of inflammatory conditions of the skin and to reduce weeping that may occur in dermatitis

**Usual Dosage** Topical: Soak affected area in the solution 2-4 times/day for 15-30 minutes or apply wet dressing soaked in the solution 2-4 times/day for 30-minute treatment periods; rewet dressing with solution every few minutes to keep it moist

**Local Anesthetic/Vasoconstrictor Precautions** No information available to require special precautions

**Effects on Dental Treatment** No effects or complications reported

**Generic Available** Yes

♦ **Alupent®** *see* Metaproterenol *on page 642*

♦ **Alu-Tab® [OTC]** *see* Aluminum Hydroxide *on page 55*

## Amantadine (a MAN ta deen)

**Related Information**

Respiratory Diseases *on page 1079*

Systemic Viral Diseases *on page 1115*

**U.S. Brand Names** Symmetrel®

**Canadian Brand Names** Endantadine®; PMS-Amantadine

**Therapeutic Category** Anti-Parkinson's Agent; Antiviral Agent, Oral

**Use** Symptomatic and adjunct treatment of parkinsonism; prophylaxis and treatment of influenza A viral infection; treatment of drug-induced extrapyramidal symptoms

**Usual Dosage**

Children:

- 1-9 years: (<45 kg): 5-9 mg/kg/day in 1-2 divided doses to a maximum of 150 mg/day
- 10-12 years: 100-200 mg/day in 1-2 divided doses
- Prophylaxis: Administer for 10-21 days following exposure if the vaccine is concurrently given or for 90 days following exposure if the vaccine is unavailable or contraindicated and re-exposure is possible

Adults:

- Parkinson's disease: 100 mg twice daily
- Influenza A viral infection: 200 mg/day in 1-2 divided doses
- Prophylaxis: Minimum 10-day course of therapy following exposure if the vaccine is concurrently give or for 90 following exposure if the vaccine is unavailable or contraindicated and re-exposure is possible

Elderly patients should take the drug in 2 daily doses rather than a single dose to avoid adverse neurologic reactions

**Mechanism of Action** As an antiviral, blocks the uncoating of influenza A virus preventing penetration of virus into host; antiparkinsonian activity may be due to its blocking the reuptake of dopamine into presynaptic neurons and causing direct stimulation of postsynaptic receptors

**Local Anesthetic/Vasoconstrictor Precautions** No information available to require special precautions

**Effects on Dental Treatment** >10% of patient experience dry mouth; prolonged use of amantadine may cause significant xerostomia

**Other Adverse Effects**

1% to 10%:

- Cardiovascular: Orthostatic hypotension, peripheral edema
- Central nervous system: Insomnia, depression, anxiety, irritability, dizziness, hallucinations, ataxia, headache, somnolence, nervousness, dream abnormality, agitation, fatigue
- Dermatologic: Livedo reticularis
- Gastrointestinal: Nausea, anorexia, constipation, diarrhea
- Respiratory: Dry nose

(Continued)

## Amantadine *(Continued)*

<1%:

Cardiovascular: Congestive heart failure, hypertension

Central nervous system: Psychosis, slurred speech, euphoria, confusion, amnesia, instances of convulsions

Dermatologic: Skin rash, eczematoid dermatitis

Endocrine & metabolic: Decreased libido

Gastrointestinal: Vomiting

Genitourinary: Urinary retention

Hematologic: Leukopenia, neutropenia

Neuromuscular & skeletal: Hyperkinesis, weakness

Ocular: Visual disturbances, oculogyric episodes

Respiratory: Dyspnea

**Drug Interactions** Anticholinergic drugs may potentiate CNS side effects of amantadine; these include trihexyphenidyl (Artane®) and benztropine (Cogentin®)

**Drug Uptake**

Onset of antidyskinetic action: Within 48 hours

Absorption: Well absorbed from GI tract

Serum half-life:

Normal renal function: 2-7 hours

End-stage renal disease: 7-10 days

Time to peak: 1-4 hours

**Pregnancy Risk Factor** C

**Generic Available** Yes

♦ **Amaphen®** *see* Butalbital Compound *on page 163*
♦ **Amaphen®** *see* Butalbital Compound and Acetaminophen *on page 164*
♦ **Amaryl®** *see* Glimepiride *on page 468*

## Ambenonium (am be NOE nee um)

**U.S. Brand Names** Mytelase® Caplets®

**Therapeutic Category** Cholinergic Agent

**Use** Treatment of myasthenia gravis

**Usual Dosage** Adults: Oral: 5-25 mg 3-4 times/day

**Local Anesthetic/Vasoconstrictor Precautions** No information available to require special precautions

**Effects on Dental Treatment** Increased salivation

**Other Adverse Effects**

>10%:

Gastrointestinal: Diarrhea, nausea, stomach cramps, increased mouth watering

Miscellaneous: Increased sweating

1% to 10%:

Genitourinary: Urge to urinate

Ocular: Small pupils, lacrimation

Respiratory: Increased bronchial secretions

<1%:

Cardiovascular: Bradycardia, A-V block

Central nervous system: Seizures, headache, dysphoria, somnolence

Local: Thrombophlebitis

Neuromuscular & skeletal: Muscle spasms, weakness

Ocular: Miosis, diplopia

Respiratory: Laryngospasm, respiratory paralysis

Miscellaneous: Hypersensitivity, hyper-reactive cholinergic responses

**Pregnancy Risk Factor** C

**Generic Available** No

♦ **Ambenyl® Cough Syrup** *see* Bromodiphenhydramine and Codeine *on page 151*
♦ **Ambi 10® [OTC]** *see* Benzoyl Peroxide *on page 130*
♦ **Ambien™** *see* Zolpidem *on page 1063*
♦ **Ambi® Skin Tone [OTC]** *see* Hydroquinone *on page 514*
♦ **AmBisome®** *see* Amphotericin B Lipid Complex *on page 81*
♦ **Amcill®** *see* Ampicillin *on page 81*

## Amcinonide (am SIN oh nide)

**Related Information**

Corticosteroids, Topical Comparison *on page 1222*

**U.S. Brand Names** Cyclocort®

**Therapeutic Category** Corticosteroid, Topical (Medium/High Potency)

**Use** Relief of the inflammatory and pruritic manifestations of corticosteroid-responsive dermatoses (high potency corticosteroid)

**Usual Dosage** Adults: Topical: Apply in a thin film 2-3 times/day

**Mechanism of Action** Stimulates the synthesis of enzymes needed to decrease inflammation, suppress mitotic activity, and cause vasoconstriction

**Local Anesthetic/Vasoconstrictor Precautions** No information available to require special precautions

**Effects on Dental Treatment** No effects or complications reported

**Other Adverse Effects**

1% to 10%: Topical: Itching, maceration of skin, skin atrophy, burning, erythema, dryness, irritation, papular rashes

<1%: Topical: Hypertrichosis, acneiform eruptions, hypopigmentation, perioral dermatitis, striae, miliaria

**Drug Interactions** No data reported

**Drug Uptake** Absorption: Adequate through intact skin; increases with skin inflammation or occlusion

**Pregnancy Risk Factor** C

**Generic Available** No

- **Amcort®** *see* Triamcinolone *on page 1010*
- **Amen®** *see* Medroxyprogesterone Acetate *on page 623*
- **Amerge®** *see* Naratriptan *on page 706*
- **Americaine® [OTC]** *see* Benzocaine *on page 128*
- **Amesec® [OTC]** *see* Aminophylline, Amobarbital, and Ephedrine *on page 65*
- **A-methaPred®** *see* Methylprednisolone *on page 661*
- **Amfepramone** *see* Diethylpropion *on page 325*
- **Amgenal® Cough Syrup** *see* Bromodiphenhydramine and Codeine *on page 151*
- **Amicar®** *see* Aminocaproic Acid *on page 62*
- **Amidate® Injection** *see* Etomidate *on page 414*

## Amifostine (am i FOS teen)

**U.S. Brand Names** Ethyol®

**Therapeutic Category** Antidote

**Synonyms** Ethiofos; Gammaphos; WR2721

**Use** Protection against cisplatin-induced nephrotoxicity in advanced ovarian cancer patients; it may also provide protection from cisplatin-induced peripheral neuropathy

**Usual Dosage** Adults: I.V. (refer to individual protocols): 910 mg/m$^2$ administered once daily as a 15-minute I.V. infusion, starting 30 minutes prior to chemotherapy

**Mechanism of Action** Prodrug that is dephosphorylated by alkaline phosphatase in tissues to a pharmacologically active free thiol metabolite that can reduce the toxic effects of cisplatin. The free thiol is available to bind to, and detoxify, reactive metabolites of cisplatin; and can also act as a scavenger of free radicals that may be generated in tissues exposed to cisplatin.

**Local Anesthetic/Vasoconstrictor Precautions** No information available to require special precautions

**Effects on Dental Treatment** Nausea/vomiting (may be severe)

**Other Adverse Effects**

>10%:

Cardiovascular: Flushing; hypotension (62%)

Central nervous system: Chills, dizziness, somnolence

Gastrointestinal: Nausea/vomiting (may be severe)

Respiratory: Sneezing

Miscellaneous: Feeling of warmth/coldness, hiccups

<1%:

Dermatologic: Mild rashes

Endocrine & metabolic: Hypocalcemia

Neuromuscular & skeletal: Rigors

**Drug Interactions** Increased toxicity: Special consideration should be given to patients receiving antihypertensive medications or other drugs that could potentiate hypotension

**Drug Uptake**

Absorption: Oral: Poor

Serum half-life: 9 minutes

**Pregnancy Risk Factor** C; amifostine at doses of 50 mg/kg has been shown to be embryotoxic in rabbits

**Generic Available** No

## Amikacin (am i KAY sin)

**U.S. Brand Names** Amikin®

**Therapeutic Category** Antibiotic, Aminoglycoside

**Use** Treatment of documented gram-negative enteric infection resistant to gentamicin and tobramycin (bone infections, respiratory tract infections, endocarditis, and septicemia); documented infection of mycobacterial organisms susceptible to amikacin including *Pseudomonas*, *Proteus*, *Serratia*, and gram-positive *Staphylococcus*

**Usual Dosage** Individualization is critical because of the low therapeutic index

**Use of ideal body weight (IBW) for determining the mg/kg/dose appears to be more accurate than dosing on the basis of total body weight (TBW)**

In morbid obesity, dosage requirement may best be estimated using a dosing weight of IBW + 0.4 (TBW - IBW)

Initial and periodic peak and trough plasma drug levels should be determined, particularly in critically ill patients with serious infections or in disease states known to significantly alter aminoglycoside pharmacokinetics (eg, cystic fibrosis, burns, or major surgery)

Once daily dosing: Higher peak serum drug concentration to MIC ratios, demonstrated aminoglycoside postantibiotic effect, decreased renal cortex drug uptake, and improved cost-time efficiency are supportive reasons for the use of once daily dosing regimens for aminoglycosides. Current research indicates these regimens to be as effective for nonlife-threatening infections, with no higher incidence of nephrotoxicity, than those requiring multiple daily doses. Doses are determined by calculating the entire day's dose via usual multiple dose calculation techniques and administering this quantity as a single dose. Doses are then adjusted to maintain mean serum concentrations above the MIC(s) of the causative organism(s). (Example: 14-35 mg/kg as a single dose/24 hours; peak (maximum) serum concentration may approximate 40-55 mcg/mL and trough (minimum) serum concentration <3 mcg/L). Further research is needed for universal recommendation in all patient populations and gram-negative disease; exceptions may include those with known high clearance (eg, children, patients with cystic fibrosis or burns who may require shorter dosage intervals) and patients with renal function impairment for whom longer than conventional dosage intervals are usually required.

Children and Adults: I.M., I.V.: 5-7.5 mg/kg/dose every 8 hours

**Mechanism of Action** Inhibits protein synthesis in susceptible bacteria by binding to ribosomal subunits

**Local Anesthetic/Vasoconstrictor Precautions** No information available to require special precautions

**Effects on Dental Treatment** No effects or complications reported

**Other Adverse Effects**

1% to 10%:

- Central nervous system: Neurotoxicity
- Otic: Ototoxicity (auditory), ototoxicity (vestibular)
- Renal: Nephrotoxicity

<1%:

- Cardiovascular: Hypotension
- Central nervous system: Headache, drowsiness, drug fever
- Dermatologic: Rash
- Gastrointestinal: Nausea, vomiting
- Hematologic: Eosinophilia
- Neuromuscular & skeletal: Paresthesia, tremor, arthralgia, weakness
- Respiratory: Dyspnea

**Drug Interactions**

Increased toxicity of aminoglycoside: Indomethacin I.V., amphotericin, loop diuretics, vancomycin, enflurane, methoxyflurane, cephalosporins

Increased toxicity of depolarizing and nondepolarizing neuromuscular blocking agents and polypeptide antibiotics with administration of aminoglycosides

**Drug Uptake**

Absorption: I.M.: May be delayed in the bedridden patient

Serum half-life (dependent on renal function):

- Adults:
  - Normal renal function: 1.4-2.3 hours
  - Anuria: End-stage renal disease: 28-86 hours

Time to peak serum concentration:

- I.M.: Within 45-120 minutes
- I.V.: Within 30 minutes following 30-minute infusion

**Pregnancy Risk Factor** C

**Generic Available** Yes

♦ **Amikin®** *see* Amikacin *on this page*

## Amiloride (a MIL oh ride)

**U.S. Brand Names** Midamor®

**Therapeutic Category** Diuretic, Potassium Sparing

**Use** Counteracts potassium loss induced by other diuretics in the treatment of hypertension or edematous conditions including CHF, hepatic cirrhosis, and hypoaldosteronism; usually used in conjunction with more potent diuretics such as thiazides or loop diuretics; investigational solution for cystic fibrosis

**Usual Dosage** Oral:

Children: Although safety and efficacy have not been established by the FDA in children, a dosage of 0.625 mg/kg/day has been used in children weighing 6-20 kg

Adults: 5-10 mg/day (up to 20 mg)

Elderly: Initial: 5 mg once daily or every other day

**Mechanism of Action** Interferes with potassium/sodium exchange (active transport) in the distal tubule, cortical collecting tubule and collecting duct by inhibiting sodium, potassium-ATPase; decreases calcium excretion; increases magnesium loss

**Local Anesthetic/Vasoconstrictor Precautions** No information available to require special precautions

**Effects on Dental Treatment** No effects or complications reported

**Other Adverse Effects**

1% to 10%:

- Central nervous system: Headache, fatigue, dizziness
- Endocrine & metabolic: Hyperkalemia, hyperchloremic metabolic acidosis, dehydration, hyponatremia, gynecomastia
- Gastrointestinal: Nausea, diarrhea, vomiting, abdominal pain, gas pain, appetite changes, constipation
- Genitourinary: Impotence
- Neuromuscular & skeletal: Muscle cramps, weakness
- Respiratory: Cough, dyspnea

<1%:

- Cardiovascular: Angina pectoris, orthostatic hypotension, arrhythmias, palpitations, chest pain
- Central nervous system: Vertigo, nervousness, insomnia, depression
- Dermatologic: Skin rash or dryness, pruritus, alopecia
- Endocrine & metabolic: Decreased libido
- Gastrointestinal: GI bleeding, thirst, heartburn, flatulence, dyspepsia
- Genitourinary: Bladder spasms, dysuria
- Hepatic: Jaundice
- Neuromuscular & skeletal: Arthralgia, tremor, neck/shoulder pain, back pain
- Ocular: Increased intraocular pressure
- Renal: Polyuria

**Drug Interactions** Increased risk of amiloride-associated hyperkalemia: Triamterene, spironolactone, angiotensin-converting enzyme (ACE) inhibitors, potassium preparations, indomethacin

**Drug Uptake**

Absorption: Oral: ~15% to 25%

- Onset: 2 hours
- Duration: 24 hours

Serum half-life:

- Normal renal function: 6-9 hours
- End-stage renal disease: 8-144 hours

Peak serum concentration: 6-10 hours

**Pregnancy Risk Factor** B

**Generic Available** Yes

## Amiloride and Hydrochlorothiazide

(a MIL oh ride & hye droe klor oh THYE a zide)

**U.S. Brand Names** Moduretic®

**Canadian Brand Names** Apo®-Amilzide; Moduret®; Novamilor; Nu-Amilzide

**Therapeutic Category** Diuretic, Combination

**Synonyms** Hydrochlorothiazide and Amiloride

**Use** Antikaliuretic diuretic, antihypertensive

**Usual Dosage** Adults: Oral: Start with 1 tablet/day, then may be increased to 2 tablets/day if needed; usually given in a single dose

**Local Anesthetic/Vasoconstrictor Precautions** No information available to require special precautions

**Effects on Dental Treatment** No effects or complications reported

**Other Adverse Effects** See individual agents

**Pregnancy Risk Factor** B

**Generic Available** Yes

♦ **2-Amino-6-Mercaptopurine** *see* Thioguanine *on page 977*

## Aminocaproic Acid (a mee noe ka PROE ik AS id)

**U.S. Brand Names** Amicar®

**Therapeutic Category** Hemostatic Agent

**Use** Treatment of excessive bleeding from fibrinolysis

**Usual Dosage** In the management of acute bleeding syndromes, oral dosage regimens are the same as the I.V. dosage regimens in adults and children

Chronic bleeding: Oral, I.V.: 5-30 g/day in divided doses at 3- to 6-hour intervals

Acute bleeding syndrome:

Children: Oral, I.V.: 100 mg/kg or 3 g/m$^2$ during the first hour, followed by continuous infusion at the rate of 33.3 mg/kg/hour or 1 g/m$^2$/hour; total dosage should not exceed 18 g/m$^2$/24 hours

Traumatic hyphema: Oral: 100 mg/kg/dose every 6-8 hours

Adults:

Oral: For elevated fibrinolytic activity, give 5 g during first hour, followed by 1-1.25 g/hour for approximately 8 hours or until bleeding stops

I.V.: Administer 4-5 g in 250 mL of diluent during first hour followed by continuous infusion at the rate of 1-1.25 g/hour in 50 mL of diluent, continue for 8 hours or until bleeding stops

Maximum daily dose: Oral, I.V.: 30 g

**Mechanism of Action** Competitively inhibits activation of plasminogen to plasmin, also, a lesser antiplasmin effect

**Local Anesthetic/Vasoconstrictor Precautions** No information available to require special precautions

**Effects on Dental Treatment** No effects or complications reported

**Other Adverse Effects**

1% to 10%:

Cardiovascular: Hypotension, bradycardia, arrhythmia

Central nervous system: Dizziness, headache, malaise, fatigue

Dermatologic: Rash

Gastrointestinal: GI irritation, nausea, cramps, diarrhea

Hematologic: Decreased platelet function, elevated serum enzymes

Neuromuscular & skeletal: Myopathy, weakness

Otic: Tinnitus

Respiratory: Nasal congestion

<1%:

Central nervous system: Convulsions

Genitourinary: Ejaculation problems

Neuromuscular & skeletal: Rhabdomyolysis

Renal: Renal failure

**Drug Interactions** No data reported

**Drug Uptake** Serum half-life: 1-2 hours

**Pregnancy Risk Factor** C

**Generic Available** Yes: Injection

**Comments** Antifibrinolytic drugs are useful to control bleeding after dental extractions in patients with hemophilia. A clinical trial reported that aminocaproic acid or tranexamic acid reduces both recurrent bleeding and the amount of clotting factor replacement therapy required. In adults, the oral dose was 50-60 mg aminocaproic acid per kg every 4 hours until dental sockets were completely healed.

**Selected Readings**

Walsh PN, Rizza CR, Matthews JM, et al, "Epsilon-Aminocaproic Acid Therapy for Dental Extractions in Haemophilia and Christmas Disease: A Double Blind Controlled Trial," *Br J Haematol*, 1971, 20(5):463-75.

♦ **Amino-Cerv™ Vaginal Cream** *see* Urea *on page 1034*

## Aminoglutethimide (a mee noe gloo TETH i mide)

**U.S. Brand Names** Cytadren®

**Therapeutic Category** Antiadrenal Agent; Antineoplastic Agent, Adjuvant

**Use** Suppression of adrenal function in selected patients with Cushing's syndrome; also used successfully in postmenopausal patients with advanced breast carcinoma and in patients with metastatic prostate carcinoma as salvage (third-line hormonal agent)

**Usual Dosage** Adults: Oral: 250 mg every 6 hours may be increased at 1- to 2-week intervals to a total of 2 g/day; give in divided doses, 2-3 times/day to reduce incidence of nausea and vomiting

**Mechanism of Action** Blocks the enzymatic conversion of cholesterol to delta-5-pregnenolone, thereby reducing the synthesis of adrenal glucocorticoids, mineralocorticoids, estrogens, aldosterone, and androgens

**Local Anesthetic/Vasoconstrictor Precautions** No information available to require special precautions

**Effects on Dental Treatment** Over 10% of patients likely to experience nausea; approximately 10% may experience orthostatic hypotension

**Other Adverse Effects** Most adverse effects will diminish in incidence and severity after the first 2-6 weeks

>10%:

Central nervous system: Headache, dizziness, drowsiness, and lethargy are frequent at the start of therapy, clumsiness
Dermatologic: Systemic lupus erythematosus, skin rash
Gastrointestinal: Nausea, vomiting, anorexia
Hepatic: Cholestatic jaundice
Neuromuscular & skeletal: Myalgia
Renal: Nephrotoxicity
Respiratory: Pulmonary alveolar damage

1% to 10%:

Cardiovascular: Hypotension and tachycardia, orthostatic hypotension
Dermatologic: Hirsutism in females
Endocrine & metabolic: Adrenocortical insufficiency
Hematologic: Rare cases of neutropenia, leukopenia, thrombocytopenia, pancytopenia, and agranulocytosis have been reported

<1%: Endocrine & metabolic: Adrenal suppression, lipid abnormalities (hypercholesterolemia), hyperkalemia, hypothyroidism, goiter

**Drug Interactions** Aminoglutethimide enhances elimination of dexamethasone resulting in reduction of steroid response; increased clearance of digitoxin after 3-8 weeks of aminoglutethimide therapy resulting in decreased effect of digitoxin; aminoglutethimide increases the metabolism of theophylline; decrease in anticoagulant response to warfarin

**Drug Uptake**

Onset of action (adrenal suppression): 3-5 days
Serum half-life: 7-15 hours; shorter following multiple administrations than following single doses (induces hepatic enzymes increasing its own metabolism)

**Pregnancy Risk Factor** D

**Generic Available** No

♦ **Amino-Opti-E® [OTC]** *see* Vitamin E *on page 1050*

## Aminophylline (am in OFF i lin)

**Related Information**

Dental Drug Interactions: Update on Drug Combinations Requiring Special Considerations *on page 1225*
Respiratory Diseases *on page 1079*
Theophylline *on page 969*

**U.S. Brand Names** Phyllocontin®; Truphylline®

**Therapeutic Category** Theophylline Derivative

**Synonyms** Theophylline Ethylenediamine

**Use** Bronchodilator in reversible airway obstruction due to asthma or COPD; increase diaphragmatic contractility; neonatal idiopathic apnea of prematurity

**Usual Dosage**

Neonates: Apnea of prematurity:

Loading dose: 5 mg/kg for one dose
Maintenance: I.V.:

0-24 days: Begin at 2 mg/kg/day divided every 12 hours and titrate to desired levels and effects
>24 days: 3 mg/kg/day divided every 12 hours; increased dosages may be indicated as liver metabolism matures (usually >30 days of life); monitor serum levels to determine appropriate dosages

Theophylline levels should be initially drawn after 3 days of therapy; repeat levels are indicated 3 days after each increase in dosage or weekly if on a stabilized dosage

Treatment of acute bronchospasm:

Loading dose (in patients not currently receiving aminophylline or theophylline): 6 mg/kg (based on aminophylline) administered I.V. over 20-30 minutes; administration rate should not exceed 25 mg/minute (aminophylline)

Approximate I.V. maintenance dosages are based upon **continuous infusions**; bolus dosing (often used in children <6 months of age) may be determined by multiplying the hourly infusion rate by 24 hours and dividing by the desired number of doses/day

6 weeks to 6 months: 0.5 mg/kg/hour
6 months to 1 year: 0.6-0.7 mg/kg/hour
1-9 years: 1-1.2 mg/kg/hour
9-12 years and young adult smokers: 0.9 mg/kg/hour

(Continued)

## Aminophylline *(Continued)*

12-16 years: 0.7 mg/kg/hour
Adults (healthy, nonsmoking): 0.7 mg/kg/hour
Older patients and patients with cor pulmonale, patients with congestive heart failure or liver failure: 0.25 mg/kg/hour
Dosage should be adjusted according to serum level measurements during the first 12- to 24-hour period; avoid using suppositories due to erratic, unreliable absorption.

Rectal: Adults: 500 mg 3 times/day

**Mechanism of Action** Causes bronchodilatation, diuresis, CNS and cardiac stimulation, and gastric acid secretion by blocking phosphodiesterase which increases tissue concentrations of cyclic adenine monophosphate (cAMP) which in turn promotes catecholamine stimulation of lipolysis, glycogenolysis, and gluconeogenesis and induces release of epinephrine from adrenal medulla cells

**Local Anesthetic/Vasoconstrictor Precautions** No information available to require special precautions

**Effects on Dental Treatment** Prescribe erythromycin with caution to patients taking theophylline products. Erythromycin will delay the normal metabolic inactivation of theophyllines leading to increased blood levels; this has resulted in nausea, vomiting and CNS restlessness

**Other Adverse Effects**

**Uncommon at serum theophylline concentrations ≤20 mcg/mL**

1% to 10%:
- Cardiovascular: Tachycardia
- Central nervous system: Nervousness, restlessness
- Gastrointestinal: Nausea, vomiting

<1%:
- Central nervous system: Insomnia, irritability, seizures
- Dermatologic: Skin rash
- Gastrointestinal: Gastric irritation
- Neuromuscular & skeletal: Tremor
- Miscellaneous: Allergic reactions

**Drug Interactions** Decreased effect/increased toxicity: Changes in diet may affect the elimination of theophylline; charcoal-broiled foods may increase elimination, reducing half-life by 50%; see table for factors affecting serum levels.

**Factors Reported to Affect Theophylline Serum Levels**

| Decreased Theophylline Level | Increased Theophylline Level |
|---|---|
| Smoking (cigarettes, marijuana) | Hepatic cirrhosis |
| High protein/low carbohydrate diet | Cor pulmonale |
| Charcoal | CHF |
| Phenytoin | Fever/viral illness |
| Phenobarbital | Propranolol |
| Carbamazepine | Allopurinol (>600 mg/d) |
| Rifampin | Erythromycin |
| I.V. isoproterenol | Cimetidine |
| Aminoglutethimide | Troleandomycin |
| Barbiturates | Ciprofloxacin |
| Hydantoins | Oral contraceptives |
| Ketoconazole | Beta blockers |
| Sulfinpyrazone | Calcium channel blockers |
| Isoniazid | Corticosteroids |
| Loop diuretics | Disulfiram |
| Sympathomimetics | Ephedrine |
| | Influenza virus vaccine |
| | Interferon |
| | Macrolides |
| | Mexiletine |
| | Quinolones |
| | Thiabendazole |
| | Thyroid hormones |
| | Carbamazepine |
| | Isoniazid |
| | Loop diuretics |

**Drug Uptake** Pharmacokinetic parameters are those of theophylline

Absorption: Oral: Depends upon dosage form
Half-life: Highly variable and dependent upon age, liver function, cardiac function, lung disease, and smoking history
Time to peak serum concentration:
Oral: 1 hour
Uncoated tablet: 2 hours
Chewable tablet: 1-1.5 hours
Enteric-coated tablet: 5 hours
I.V.: Within 30 minutes

**Pregnancy Risk Factor** C

**Dietary Considerations** Food does not appreciably affect absorption; avoid extremes of dietary protein and carbohydrate intake; limit charcoal-broiled foods

**Generic Available** Yes

**Selected Readings**

Cummins LH, et al, "Erythromycin's Effect on Theophylline Blood Levels. Correspondence," *Pediatrics*, 1977, 59:144-5.
Delaforge M and Sartori E, "In Vivo Effects of Erythromycin, Oleandomycin, and Erythralosamine Derivatives on Hepatic Cytochrome P-450," *Biochem Pharmacol*, 1990, 40(2):223-8.
Ludden TM, "Pharmacokinetic Interactions of the Macrolide Antibiotics," *Clin Pharmacokinet*, 1985, 10(1):63-79.

## Aminophylline, Amobarbital, and Ephedrine

(am in OFF i lin, am oh BAR bi tal, & e FED rin)

**U.S. Brand Names** Amesec® [OTC]

**Therapeutic Category** Antiasthmatic; Bronchodilator

**Use** Symptomatic relief of asthma

**Usual Dosage** Adults: Oral: 1 capsule every 6 hours

**Local Anesthetic/Vasoconstrictor Precautions** Use vasoconstrictors with caution since ephedrine may enhance cardiostimulation and vasopressor effects of sympathomimetics

**Effects on Dental Treatment** Prescribe erythromycin with caution to patients taking theophylline products. Erythromycin will delay the normal metabolic inactivation of theophyllines leading to increased blood levels; this has resulted in nausea, vomiting and CNS restlessness

**Other Adverse Effects** See individual agents

**Pregnancy Risk Factor** C

**Generic Available** No

♦ **Aminosalicilico, Acido** *see* Aminosalicylate Sodium *on this page*

## Aminosalicylate Sodium (a MEE noe sa LIS i late SOW dee um)

**U.S. Brand Names** Sodium P.A.S.

**Canadian Brand Names** Tubasal®

**Therapeutic Category** Antitubercular Agent; Nonsteroidal Anti-inflammatory Drug (NSAID), Oral

**Synonyms** Aminosalicilico, Acido

**Use** Treatment of tuberculosis with combination drugs

**Usual Dosage** Oral:
Children: 150-300 mg/kg/day in 3-4 equally divided doses
Adults: 150 mg/kg/day in 2-3 equally divided doses (usually 12-14 g/day)

**Mechanism of Action** Aminosalicylic acid (PAS) is a highly specific bacteriostatic agent active against *M. tuberculosis*. Most strains of *M. tuberculosis* are sensitive to a concentration of 1 µg/mL; structurally related to para-aminobenzoic acid (PABA) and its mechanism of action is thought to be similar to the sulfonamides, a competitive antagonism with PABA; disrupts plate biosynthesis in sensitive organisms

**Local Anesthetic/Vasoconstrictor Precautions** No information available to require special precautions

**Effects on Dental Treatment** NSAID formulations are known to reversibly decrease platelet aggregation via mechanisms different than observed with aspirin. The dentist should be aware of the potential of abnormal coagulation. Caution should also be exercised in the use of NSAIDs in patients already on anticoagulant therapy with drugs such as warfarin (Coumadin®).

**Other Adverse Effects**
1% to 10%: Gastrointestinal: Nausea, vomiting, diarrhea, abdominal pain
<1%:
Cardiovascular: Vasculitis
Central nervous system: Fever
Dermatologic: Skin eruptions
Endocrine & metabolic: Goiter with or without myxedema
Hematologic: Leukopenia, agranulocytosis, thrombocytopenia, hemolytic anemia
Hepatic: Jaundice, hepatitis

(Continued)

## Aminosalicylate Sodium *(Continued)*

**Drug Interactions** A small reduction in digoxin (Lanoxin®) plasma levels may result from coadministration with aminosalicylate sodium; probenecid increases the serum concentration of aminosalicylate sodium

**Drug Uptake** Absorption: Readily absorbed >90%

**Pregnancy Risk Factor** C

**Generic Available** Yes

♦ **Aminosalicylate Sodium** *see* Para-Aminosalicylate Sodium *on page 765*

## Amiodarone (a MEE oh da rone)

**Related Information**

Cardiovascular Diseases *on page 1066*

**U.S. Brand Names** Cordarone®

**Therapeutic Category** Antiarrhythmic Agent, Class III; Antiarrhythmic Agent (Supraventricular & Ventricular)

**Use** Management of resistant, life-threatening ventricular arrhythmias or supraventricular arrhythmias unresponsive to conventional therapy with less toxic agents

**Usual Dosage** Oral:

Children (calculate doses for children <1 year on body surface area):

Loading dose: 10-15 mg/kg/day or 600-800 mg/1.73 $m^2$/day for 4-14 days or until adequate control of arrhythmia or prominent adverse effects occur (this loading dose may be given in 1-2 divided doses/day); dosage should then be reduced to 5 mg/kg/day or 200-400 mg/1.73 $m^2$/day given once daily for several weeks; if arrhythmia does not recur, reduce to lowest effective dosage possible; usual daily minimal dose: 2.5 mg/kg/day; maintenance doses may be given for 5 of 7 days/week

Adults: Ventricular arrhythmias: 800-1600 mg/day in 1-2 doses for 1-3 weeks, then 600-800 mg/day in 1-2 doses for 1 month; maintenance: 400 mg/day; lower doses are recommended for supraventricular arrhythmias

**Mechanism of Action** Class III antiarrhythmic agent which inhibits adrenergic stimulation, prolongs the action potential and refractory period in myocardial tissue; decreases A-V conduction and sinus node function

**Local Anesthetic/Vasoconstrictor Precautions** No information available to require special precautions

**Effects on Dental Treatment** This drug is indicated only for life-threatening arrhythmias; dental treatment would not be a consideration during these emergencies

**Other Adverse Effects** With large dosages (≥400 mg/day), adverse reactions occur in ~75% patients and require discontinuance in 5% to 20%

>10%:

Central nervous system: Ataxia, fatigue, malaise, dizziness, headache, insomnia, nightmares

Dermatologic: Photosensitivity

Gastrointestinal: Nausea, vomiting

Neuromuscular & skeletal: Tremor, paresthesia, weakness

Respiratory: Pulmonary fibrosis (cough, fever, dyspnea, malaise), interstitial pneumonitis

Miscellaneous: Alveolitis

1% to 10%:

Cardiovascular: Congestive heart failure, cardiac arrhythmias (atropine-resistant bradycardia, heart block, sinus arrest, paroxysmal ventricular tachycardia), myocardial depression, flushing, edema

Endocrine & metabolic: Hypothyroidism or hyperthyroidism (less common), decreased libido

Gastrointestinal: Constipation, anorexia, abdominal pain, abnormal salivation, dysgeusia

Hematologic: Coagulation abnormalities

Hepatic: Abnormal liver function tests

Ocular: Visual disturbances

Miscellaneous: Abnormal smell

<1%:

Cardiovascular: Hypotension, vasculitis

Central nervous system: Pseudotumor cerebri

Dermatologic: Skin rash, alopecia, slate blue discoloration of skin

Endocrine & metabolic: Hyperglycemia, hypertriglyceridemia

Genitourinary: Epididymitis

Hematologic: Thrombocytopenia

Hepatic: Cirrhosis, severe hepatic toxicity (potentially fatal hepatitis)

Ocular: Optic neuritis, corneal microdeposits, photophobia

**Drug Interactions Cytochrome P-450 3A enzyme inhibitor**
Amiodarone appears to interfere with the hepatic metabolism of several drugs resulting in significantly increased plasma concentrations; see table.

**Amiodarone Common Drug Interactions**

| Drug | Interaction |
|---|---|
| Anticoagulants, oral | The effects of the anticoagulant is increased due to inhibition of its metabolism |
| β-adrenergic receptor antagonists | β-blocker effects are enhanced by amiodarone's inhibition of the β-blocker's hepatic metabolism |
| Calcium channel antagonists | Additive effects of both drugs resulting in a reduction in cardiac sinus conduction, atrioventricular nodal conduction and myocardial contractility |
| Digoxin | Digoxin concentrations may be increased with resultant increases in activity and potential for toxicity |
| Flecainide | Flecainide plasma concentrations are increased |
| Phenytoin | Phenytoin serum concentrations are increased due to reduction in phenytoin metabolism, with possible symptoms of phenytoin toxicity |
| Procainamide | Procainamide serum concentrations may be increased |
| Quinidine | Quinidine serum concentrations may be increased and can potentially cause fatal cardiac dysrhythmias |

**Drug Uptake**
Onset of effect: 3 days to 3 weeks after starting therapy
Peak effect: 1 week to 5 months
Duration of effect after discontinuation of therapy: 7-50 days
**Note:** Mean onset of effect and duration after discontinuation may be shorter in children versus adults
Serum half-life: Oral chronic therapy: 40-55 days (range: 26-107 days); shortened in children versus adults
**Pregnancy Risk Factor** C
**Generic Available** No

♦ **Ami-Tex LA®** *see* Guaifenesin and Phenylpropanolamine *on page 480*
♦ **Amitone® [OTC]** *see* Calcium Carbonate *on page 172*

## Amitriptyline (a mee TRIP ti leen)

**U.S. Brand Names** Elavil®
**Canadian Brand Names** Apo®-Amitriptyline; Levate®; Novo-Tryptin
**Therapeutic Category** Antidepressant, Tricyclic
**Use** Treatment of various forms of depression, often in conjunction with psychotherapy; analgesic for certain chronic and neuropathic pain, prophylaxis against migraine headaches
**Usual Dosage**
Children: Pain management: Oral: Initial: 0.1 mg/kg at bedtime, may advance as tolerated over 2-3 weeks to 0.5-2 mg/day at bedtime

Adolescents: Oral: Initial: 25-50 mg/day; may give in divided doses; increase gradually to 100 mg/day in divided doses

Adults:
Oral: 30-100 mg/day single dose at bedtime or in divided doses; dose may be gradually increased up to 300 mg/day; once symptoms are controlled, decrease gradually to lowest effective dose
I.M.: 20-30 mg 4 times/day

**Mechanism of Action** Increases the synaptic concentration of serotonin and/or norepinephrine in the central nervous system by inhibition of their reuptake at the presynaptic neuronal membrane
**Local Anesthetic/Vasoconstrictor Precautions** Use with caution; epinephrine, norepinephrine and levonordefrin have been shown to have an increased pressor response in combination with TCAs
**Effects on Dental Treatment** >10% of patients experience dry mouth; amitriptyline is the most anticholinergic and sedating of the antidepressants; pronounced effects on the cardiovascular system; long-term treatment with TCAs such as
(Continued)

## Amitriptyline *(Continued)*

amitriptyline increases the risk of caries by reducing salivation and salivary buffer capacity. In a study by Rundergren, et al, pathological alterations were observed in the oral mucosa of 72% of 58 patients; 55% had new carious lesions after taking TCAs for a median of 5½ years. Current research is investigating the use of the salivary stimulant pilocarpine (Salagen®) to overcome the xerostomia from amitriptyline.

**Other Adverse Effects** Anticholinergic effects may be pronounced; moderate to marked sedation can occur (tolerance to these effects usually occurs)

>10%:
- Central nervous system: Dizziness, drowsiness, headache
- Gastrointestinal: Constipation, increased appetite, nausea, unpleasant taste, weight gain
- Neuromuscular & skeletal: Weakness

1% to 10%:
- Cardiovascular: Hypotension, postural hypotension, arrhythmias, tachycardia, sudden death
- Central nervous system: Nervousness, restlessness, parkinsonian syndrome, insomnia, sedation, fatigue, anxiety, impaired cognitive function, seizures have occurred occasionally, extrapyramidal symptoms are possible
- Gastrointestinal: Diarrhea, heartburn
- Genitourinary: Sexual dysfunction, urinary retention
- Neuromuscular & skeletal: Tremor
- Ocular: Eye pain, blurred vision
- Miscellaneous: Excessive sweating

<1%:
- Central nervous system: Anxiety, seizures
- Dermatologic: Alopecia, photosensitivity
- Endocrine & metabolic: Breast enlargement, galactorrhea, rarely SIADH
- Genitourinary: Testicular swelling
- Hematologic: Leukopenia, eosinophilia, rarely agranulocytosis
- Hepatic: Cholestatic jaundice, elevated liver enzymes
- Ocular: Increased intraocular pressure
- Otic: Tinnitus
- Miscellaneous: Trouble with gums, decreased lower esophageal sphincter tone may cause GE reflux; allergic reactions

**Drug Interactions**

Decreased effect: Phenobarbital may increase the metabolism of amitriptyline; amitriptyline blocks the uptake of guanethidine and thus prevents the hypotensive effect of guanethidine

Increased toxicity: Clonidine has caused hypertensive crisis; amitriptyline may be additive with or may potentiate the action of other CNS depressants such as sedatives or hypnotics; with MAO inhibitors, hyperpyrexia, hypertension, tachycardia, confusion, seizures, and **deaths have been reported**; amitriptyline may increase the prothrombin time in patients stabilized on warfarin; amitriptyline potentiates the pressor and cardiac effects of sympathomimetic agents such as isoproterenol, epinephrine, etc; cimetidine and methylphenidate may decrease the metabolism of amitriptyline

Additive anticholinergic effects seen with other anticholinergic agents

**Drug Uptake**

Onset of action: 7-21 days
Serum half-life: Adults: 9-25 hours (15-hour average)
Time to peak serum concentration: Within 4 hours

**Pregnancy Risk Factor** D

**Generic Available** Yes

**Selected Readings**


Boakes AJ, Laurence DR, Teoh PC, et al, "Interactions Between Sympathomimetic Amines and Antidepressant Agents in Man," *Br Med J*, 1973, 1(849):311-5.

Jastak JT and Yagiela JA, "Vasoconstrictors and Local Anesthesia: A Review and Rationale for Use," *J Am Dent Assoc*, 1983, 107(4):623-30.

Larochelle P, Hamet P, and Enjalbert M, "Responses to Tyramine and Norepinephrine After Imipramine and Trazodone," *Clin Pharmacol Ther*, 1979, 26(1):24-30.

Mitchell JR, "Guanethidine and Related Agents. III Antagonism by Drugs Which Inhibit the Norepinephrine Pump in Man," *J Clin Invest*, 1970, 49(8):1596-604.

Rundegren J, van Dijken J, Mörnstad H, et al, "Oral Conditions in Patients Receiving Long-Term Treatment With Cyclic Antidepressant Drugs," *Swed Dent J*, 1985, 9(2):55-64.

Svedmyr N, "The Influence of a Tricyclic Antidepressive Agent (Protriptyline) on Some of the Circulatory Effects of Noradrenaline and Adrenalin® in Man," *Life Sci*, 1968, 7(1):77-84.


## Amitriptyline and Chlordiazepoxide

(a mee TRIP ti leen & klor dye az e POKS ide)

**U.S. Brand Names** Limbitrol® DS 10-25

**Therapeutic Category** Antidepressant, Tricyclic; Antipsychotic Agent

**Synonyms** Chlordiazepoxide and Amitriptyline

**Use** Treatment of moderate to severe anxiety and/or agitation and depression

**Usual Dosage** Initial: 3-4 tablets in divided doses; this may be increased to 6 tablets/day as required; some patients respond to smaller doses and can be maintained on 2 tablets

**Local Anesthetic/Vasoconstrictor Precautions** Use with caution; epinephrine, norepinephrine and levonordefrin have been shown to have an increased pressor response in combination with TCAs

**Effects on Dental Treatment**

Amitriptyline: The most anticholinergic and sedating of the antidepressants; pronounced effects on the cardiovascular system; long-term treatment with TCAs such as amitriptyline increases the risk of caries by reducing salivation and salivary buffer capacity. In a study by Rundergren, et al, pathological alterations were observed in the oral mucosa of 72% of 58 patients; 55% had new carious lesions after taking TCAs for a median of 5½ years. Current research is investigating the use of the salivary stimulant pilocarpine (Salagen®) to overcome the xerostomia from amitriptyline.

Chlordiazepoxide: Over 10% of patients will experience dry mouth which disappears with cessation of drug therapy

**Other Adverse Effects** See individual agents

**Pregnancy Risk Factor** D

**Generic Available** Yes

**Selected Readings**

Boakes AJ, Laurence DR, Teoh PC, et al, "Interactions Between Sympathomimetic Amines and Antidepressant Agents in Man," *Br Med J*, 1973, 1(849):311-5.

Jastak JT and Yagiela JA, "Vasoconstrictors and Local Anesthesia: A Review and Rationale for Use," *J Am Dent Assoc*, 1983, 107(4):623-30.

Larochelle P, Hamet P, and Enjalbert M, "Responses to Tyramine and Norepinephrine After Imipramine and Trazodone," *Clin Pharmacol Ther*, 1979, 26(1):24-30.

Mitchell JR, "Guanethidine and Related Agents. III Antagonism by Drugs Which Inhibit the Norepinephrine Pump in Man," *J Clin Invest*, 1970, 49(8):1596-604.

Rundegren J, van Dijken J, Mörnstad H, et al, "Oral Conditions in Patients Receiving Long-Term Treatment With Cyclic Antidepressant Drugs," *Swed Dent J*, 1985, 9(2):55-64.

Svedmyr N, "The Influence of a Tricyclic Antidepressive Agent (Protriptyline) on Some of the Circulatory Effects of Noradrenaline and Adrenalin in Man," *Life Sci*, 1968, 7(1):77-84.

## Amitriptyline and Perphenazine

(a mee TRIP ti leen & per FEN a zeen)

**U.S. Brand Names** Etrafon®; Triavil®

**Canadian Brand Names** Elavil Plus®; Apo®-Peram; PMS-Levazine; Proavil

**Therapeutic Category** Antidepressant, Tricyclic; Phenothiazine Derivative

**Synonyms** Perphenazine and Amitriptyline

**Use** Treatment of patients with moderate to severe anxiety and depression

**Usual Dosage** Oral: 1 tablet 2-4 times/day

**Local Anesthetic/Vasoconstrictor Precautions**

Amitriptyline: Use with caution; epinephrine, norepinephrine and levonordefrin have been shown to have an increased pressor response in combination with TCAs

Perphenazine: No information available to require special precautions

**Effects on Dental Treatment** >10% of patients experience dry mouth

Amitriptyline: The most anticholinergic and sedating of the antidepressants; pronounced effects on the cardiovascular system; long-term treatment with TCAs such as amitriptyline increases the risk of caries by reducing salivation and salivary buffer capacity. In a study by Rundergren, et al, pathological alterations were observed in the oral mucosa of 72% of 58 patients; 55% had new carious lesions after taking TCAs for a median of 5½ years. Current research is investigating the use of the salivary stimulant pilocarpine (Salagen®) to overcome the xerostomia from amitriptyline.

Perphenazine: Significant hypotension may occur, especially when the drug is administered parenterally; orthostatic hypotension is due to alpha-receptor blockade, the elderly are at greater risk for orthostatic hypotension

Tardive dyskinesia: Prevalence rate may be 40% in elderly; development of the syndrome and the irreversible nature are proportional to duration and total cumulative dose over time

Extrapyramidal reactions are more common in elderly with up to 50% developing these reactions after 60 years of age; drug-induced **Parkinson's syndrome** occurs often; **Akathisia** is the most common extrapyramidal reaction in elderly

Increased confusion, memory loss, psychotic behavior, and agitation frequently occur as a consequence of anticholinergic effects

Antipsychotic associated sedation in nonpsychotic patients is extremely unpleasant due to feelings of depersonalization, derealization, and dysphoria

(Continued)

## Amitriptyline and Perphenazine *(Continued)*

**Other Adverse Effects**

>10%:
- Central nervous system: Dizziness, drowsiness, headache
- Gastrointestinal: Constipation, increased appetite, nausea, unpleasant taste, weight gain
- Neuromuscular & skeletal: Weakness

1% to 10%:
- Cardiovascular: Arrhythmias, hypotension
- Central nervous system: Confusion, delirium, hallucinations, nervousness, restlessness, Parkinsonian syndrome, insomnia
- Endocrine & metabolic: Sexual dysfunction
- Gastrointestinal: Diarrhea, heartburn
- Genitourinary: Dysuria
- Neuromuscular & skeletal: Fine muscle tremors
- Ocular: Blurred vision, eye pain
- Miscellaneous: Excessive sweating

<1%:
- Central nervous system: Anxiety, seizures
- Dermatologic: Alopecia, photosensitivity
- Endocrine & metabolic: Breast enlargement, galactorrhea, SIADH
- Gastrointestinal: Trouble with gums, decreased lower esophageal sphincter tone may cause GE reflux
- Genitourinary: Testicular swelling
- Hematologic: Agranulocytosis, leukopenia, eosinophilia
- Hepatic: Cholestatic jaundice, elevated liver enzymes
- Ocular: Increased intraocular pressure
- Otic: Tinnitus
- Miscellaneous: Allergic reactions

**Pregnancy Risk Factor** D

**Generic Available** Yes

**Selected Readings**

Boakes AJ, Laurence DR, Teoh PC, et al, "Interactions Between Sympathomimetic Amines and Antidepressant Agents in Man," *Br Med J*, 1973, 1(849):311-5.

Jastak JT and Yagiela JA, "Vasoconstrictors and Local Anesthesia: A Review and Rationale for Use," *J Am Dent Assoc*, 1983, 107(4):623-30.

Larochelle P, Hamet P, and Enjalbert M, "Responses to Tyramine and Norepinephrine After Imipramine and Trazodone," *Clin Pharmacol Ther*, 1979, 26(1):24-30.

Mitchell JR, "Guanethidine and Related Agents. III Antagonism by Drugs Which Inhibit the Norepinephrine Pump in Man," *J Clin Invest*, 1970, 49(8):1596-604.

Rundegren J, van Dijken J, Mörnstad H, et al, "Oral Conditions in Patients Receiving Long-Term Treatment With Cyclic Antidepressant Drugs," *Swed Dent J*, 1985, 9(2):55-64.

Svedmyr N, "The Influence of a Tricyclic Antidepressive Agent (Protriptyline) on Some of the Circulatory Effects of Noradrenaline and Adrenalin in Man," *Life Sci*, 1968, 7(1):77-84.

## Amlexanox (am LEKS an oks)

**Related Information**

Oral Nonviral Soft Tissue Ulcerations or Erosions *on page 1141*

**U.S. Brand Names** Aphthasol™

**Therapeutic Category** Anti-inflammatory Agent, Locally Applied

**Use** Treatment of aphthous ulcers (ie, canker sores); has been investigated in many allergic disorders

**Usual Dosage** Administer (0.5 cm - ¼") directly on ulcers 4 times/day following oral hygiene, after meals, and at bedtime

**Mechanism of Action** As a benzopyrano-bipyridine carboxylic acid derivative, amlexanox has anti-inflammatory and antiallergic properties; it inhibits chemical mediatory release of the slow-reacting substance of anaphylaxis (SRS-A) and may have antagonistic effect son interleukin-3

**Local Anesthetic/Vasoconstrictor Precautions** Discontinue therapy if rash or contact mucositis develops

**Effects on Dental Treatment** No effects or complications reported

**Other Adverse Effects**

>1%:
- Dermatologic: Allergic contact dermatitis
- Gastrointestinal: Oral irritation

<1%: Gastrointestinal: Contact mucositis

**Contraindications** Hypersensitivity to amlexanox or components

**Drug Uptake**
- Absorption: Systemic absorption with swallowing of topical application of oral paste
- Serum half-life: 3.5 hours
- Time to peak serum concentration: 2 hours

**Pregnancy Risk Factor** B

**Dosage Forms** Paste: 5% (5 g)

**Generic Available** No

**Comments** Treatment of canker sores with amlexanox showed a 76% median reduction in ulcer size compared to a 40% reduction with placebo. Greer, et al, reported an overall mean reduction in ulcer size of 1.82 $mm^2$ for patients treated with 5% amlexanox versus an average reduction of 0.52 $mm^2$ for the control group. Recent studies in over thousands of patients have confirmed that amlexanox accelerates the resolution of pain and healing of aphthous ulcers more significantly than vehicle and no treatment.

**Selected Readings**

Binnie WH, Curro FA, Khandwala A, et al, "Amlexanox Oral Paste: A Novel Treatment That Accelerates the Healing of Aphthous Ulcers," *Compend Contin Educ Dent*, 1997, 18(11):1116-8, 1120-2, 1124.

Greer RO Jr, Lindenmuth JE, Juarez T, et al, "A Double-Blind Study of Topically Applied 5% Amlexanox in the Treatment of Aphthous Ulcers," *J Oral Maxillofac Surg*, 1993, 51(3):243-8.

Khandwala A, Van Inwegen RG, and Alfano MC, "5% Amlexanox Oral Paste, A New Treatment for Recurrent Minor Aphthous Ulcers: I. Clinical Demonstration of Acceleration of Healing and Resolution of Pain," *Oral Surg Oral Med Oral Pathol Oral Radiol Endod*, 1997, 83(2):222-30.

Khandwala A, Van Inwegen RG, Charney MR, et al, "5% Amlexanox Oral Paste, A New Treatment for Recurrent Minor Aphthous Ulcers: II. Pharmacokinetics and Demonstration of Clinical Safety," *Oral Surg Oral Med Oral Pathol Oral Radiol Endod*, 1997, 83(2):231-8.

## Amlodipine (am LOE di peen)

**Related Information**

Calcium Channel Blockers & Gingival Hyperplasia *on page 1204*
Cardiovascular Diseases *on page 1066*

**U.S. Brand Names** Norvasc®

**Therapeutic Category** Antianginal Agent; Calcium Channel Blocker

**Use** Treatment of hypertension and angina

**Usual Dosage** Adults: Oral: Initial dose: 2.5-5 mg once daily; usual dose: 5-10 mg once daily; maximum dose: 10 mg once daily

**Mechanism of Action** Inhibits calcium ion from entering the "slow channels" or select voltage-sensitive areas of vascular smooth muscle and myocardium during depolarization, producing a relaxation of coronary vascular smooth muscle and coronary vasodilation; increases myocardial oxygen delivery in patients with vasospastic angina

**Local Anesthetic/Vasoconstrictor Precautions** No information available to require special precautions

**Effects on Dental Treatment** Calcium channel blockers (CCBs) cause gingival hyperplasia in ~1% of patients. There have been fewer reports with amlodipine than with other CCBs. The hyperplasia will usually disappear with cessation of drug therapy; consultation with physician is suggested.

**Other Adverse Effects**

>10%: Cardiovascular: Peripheral edema

1% to 10%:
- Cardiovascular: Edema, flushing, palpitations
- Central nervous system: Headache, fatigue, dizziness, somnolence
- Dermatologic: Dermatitis, rash
- Endocrine & metabolic: Sexual dysfunction
- Gastrointestinal: Nausea, abdominal pain
- Neuromuscular & skeletal: Muscle cramps
- Respiratory: Dyspnea

<1%:
- Cardiovascular: Hypotension, bradycardia, arrhythmias, abnormal EKG, ventricular extrasystoles
- Dermatologic: Alopecia, petechiae
- Gastrointestinal: Weight gain, anorexia
- Neuromuscular & skeletal: Joint stiffness
- Respiratory: Nasal congestion, cough, epistaxis
- Miscellaneous: Sweating

**Drug Interactions** CYP3A3/4 enzyme substrate; hepatic enzyme inhibitor

Increased effect:
- Amlodipine and benazepril may increase hypotensive effect
- Amlodipine and cyclosporine may increase cyclosporine levels
- Beta-blockers in combination with calcium antagonists may result in increased cardiac depression
- Severe hypotension or increased fluid volume requirements have occurred with fentanyl and calcium blockers

**Drug Uptake**

Onset of action: 30-50 minutes
Peak effect: 6-12 hours
Duration: 24 hours
Absorption: Oral: Well absorbed
Serum half-life: 30-50 hours

(Continued)

## Amlodipine *(Continued)*

**Pregnancy Risk Factor** C

**Generic Available** No

**Selected Readings**

Jorgensen MG, "Prevalence of Amlodipine-Related Gingival Hyperplasia," *J Periodontol*, 1997, 68(7):676-8.

Wynn RL, "An Update on Calcium Channel Blocker-Induced Gingival Hyperplasia," *Gen Dent*, 1995, 43(3):218-22.

Wynn RL, "Calcium Channel Blockers and Gingival Hyperplasia," *Gen Dent*, 1991, 39(4):240-3.

## Amlodipine and Benazepril (am LOE di peen & ben AY ze pril)

**U.S. Brand Names** Lotrel®

**Therapeutic Category** Angiotensin-Converting Enzyme (ACE) Inhibitor; Calcium Channel Blocker

**Use** Treatment of hypertension

**Usual Dosage** Adults: Oral: 1 capsule daily

**Mechanism of Action** The mechanism through which benazepril lowers blood pressure is believed to be primarily suppression of the renin-angiotensin-aldosterone system, benazepril has an antihypertensive effect even in patients with low-renin hypertension; amlodipine is a dihydropyridine calcium antagonist that inhibits the transmembrane influx of calcium ions into vascular smooth muscle and cardiac muscle; amlodipine is a peripheral arterial vasodilator that acts directly on vascular smooth muscle to cause a reduction in peripheral vascular resistance and reduction in blood pressure

**Local Anesthetic/Vasoconstrictor Precautions** No information available to require special precautions

**Effects on Dental Treatment** Calcium channel blockers (CCBs) cause gingival hyperplasia in approximately 1% of the patients. There have been fewer reports with amlodipine than with other CCBs. The hyperplasia will usually disappear with cessation of drug therapy. Consultation with physician is suggested.

**Drug Uptake**

Absorption: Not influenced by the presence of food in the GI tract; food effects on absorption have not been studied
- Amlodipine: 64% to 90%
- Benazepril: 37%

Time to peak (plasma):
- Amlodipine: 6-12 hours
- Benazepril: 0.5-2 hours

**Pregnancy Risk Factor** C (first trimester); D (second and third trimesters)

**Generic Available** No

**Selected Readings**

Wynn RL, "An Update on Calcium Channel Blocker-Induced Gingival Hyperplasia," *Gen Dent*, 1995, 43(3):218-22.

Wynn RL, "Calcium Channel Blockers and Gingival Hyperplasia," *Gen Dent*, 1991, 39(4):240-3.

♦ **Ammonapse** *see* Sodium Phenylbutyrate *on page 923*

## Ammonia Spirit, Aromatic (a MOE nee ah SPEAR it, air oh MAT ik)

**U.S. Brand Names** Aromatic Ammonia Aspirols®

**Therapeutic Category** Respiratory Stimulant

**Use** Respiratory and circulatory stimulant, treatment of fainting

**Usual Dosage** Used as "smelling salts" to treat or prevent fainting

**Local Anesthetic/Vasoconstrictor Precautions** No information available to require special precautions

**Effects on Dental Treatment** No effects or complications reported

**Other Adverse Effects** 1% to 10%:
- Gastrointestinal: Nausea, vomiting
- Respiratory: Irritation to nasal mucosa, coughing

**Contraindications** Hypersensitivity to ammonia or any component

**Drug Interactions** No data reported

**Pregnancy Risk Factor** C

**Breast-feeding Considerations** No data reported

**Dosage Forms**
- Inhalant, crushable glass perles: 0.33 mL, 0.4 mL
- Solution: 30 mL, 60 mL, 120 mL

**Dietary Considerations** No data reported

**Generic Available** Yes

## Ammonium Chloride (a MOE nee um KLOR ide)

**Therapeutic Category** Metabolic Alkalosis Agent; Urinary Acidifying Agent

**Use** Diuretic or systemic and urinary acidifying agent; treatment of hypochloremic states

**Usual Dosage** Metabolic alkalosis: The following equations represent different methods of correction utilizing either the serum $HCO_3^-$, the serum chloride, or the base excess

**Dosing of mEq $NH_4Cl$ via the chloride-deficit method (hypochloremia):**

Dose of mEq $NH_4Cl$ = [0.2 L/kg x body weight (kg)] x [103 - observed serum chloride]; administer 100% of dose over 12 hours, then re-evaluate

**Note:** 0.2 L/kg is the estimated chloride space and 103 is the average normal serum chloride concentration

**Dosing of mEq $NH_4Cl$ via the bicarbonate-excess method (refractory hypochloremic metabolic alkalosis):**

Dose of $NH_4Cl$ = [0.5 L/kg x body weight (kg)] x (observed serum $HCO_3^-$ - 24); administer 50% of dose over 12 hours, then re-evaluate

**Note:** 0.5 L/kg is the estimated bicarbonate space and 24 is the average normal serum bicarbonate concentration

**Dosing of mEq $NH_4Cl$ via the base-excess method:**

Dose of $NH_4Cl$ = [0.3 L/kg x body weight (kg)] x measured base excess (mEq/L); administer 50% of dose over 12 hours, then re-evaluate

**Note:** 0.3 L/kg is the estimated extracellular bicarbonate and base excess is measured by the chemistry lab and reported with arterial blood gases

These equations will yield different requirements of ammonium chloride

Equation #1 is inappropriate to use if the patient has severe metabolic alkalosis without hypochloremia or if the patient has uremia

Equation #3 is the most useful for the first estimation of ammonium chloride dosage

Children: Urinary acidifying agents: Oral, I.V.: 75 mg/kg/day in 4 divided doses; maximum daily dose: 6 g

Adults: Urinary acidifying agent/diuretic:

Oral: 1-2 g every 4-6 hours

I.V.: 1.5 g/dose every 6 hours

**Mechanism of Action** Increases acidity by increasing free hydrogen ion concentration

**Local Anesthetic/Vasoconstrictor Precautions** No information available to require special precautions

**Effects on Dental Treatment** No effects or complications reported

**Other Adverse Effects** 1% to 10%:

Cardiovascular: Bradycardia

Central nervous system: Mental confusion, coma, headache

Dermatologic: Rash

Endocrine & metabolic: Metabolic acidosis secondary to hyperchloremia

Gastrointestinal: Gastric irritation, nausea, vomiting

Local: Pain at site of injection

Respiratory: Hyperventilation

**Drug Uptake** Absorption: Rapid from GI tract, complete within 3-6 hours

**Pregnancy Risk Factor** C

**Dosage Forms**

Injection: 26.75% [5 mEq/mL] (20 mL)

Tablet: 500 mg

Tablet, enteric coated: 500 mg

**Generic Available** Yes

♦ **Ammonium Lactate** *see* Lactic Acid With Ammonium Hydroxide *on page 570*

## Amobarbital (am oh BAR bi tal)

**U.S. Brand Names** Amytal®

**Canadian Brand Names** Novambarb®

**Therapeutic Category** Barbiturate; Hypnotic; Sedative

**Use**

Oral: Hypnotic in short-term treatment of insomnia, to reduce anxiety and provide sedation preoperatively

I.M., I.V.: Control status epilepticus or acute seizure episodes. Also used in catatonic, negativistic, or manic reactions and in "Amytal® Interviewing" for narcoanalysis

**Usual Dosage**

Children: Oral:

Sedation: 6 mg/kg/day divided every 6-8 hours

Insomnia: 2 mg/kg or 70 mg/m²/day in 4 equally divided doses

Hypnotic: 2-3 mg/kg

Adults:

Insomnia: Oral: 65-200 mg at bedtime

Sedation: Oral: 30-50 mg 2-3 times/day

Preanesthetic: Oral: 200 mg 1-2 hours before surgery

(Continued)

## Amobarbital *(Continued)*

Hypnotic:

Oral: 65-200 mg at bedtime

I.M., I.V.: 65-500 mg, should not exceed 500 mg I.M. or 1000 mg I.V.

**Mechanism of Action** Interferes with transmission of impulses from the thalamus to the cortex of the brain resulting in an imbalance in central inhibitory and facilitatory mechanisms

**Local Anesthetic/Vasoconstrictor Precautions** No information available to require special precautions

**Effects on Dental Treatment** No effects or complications reported

**Other Adverse Effects**

>10%:

Central nervous system: Dizziness, lightheadedness, "hangover" effect, drowsiness, CNS depression, fever

Local: Pain at injection site

1% to 10%:

Central nervous system: Confusion, mental depression, unusual excitement, nervousness, faint feeling, headache, insomnia, nightmares

Gastrointestinal: Nausea, vomiting, constipation

<1%:

Cardiovascular: Hypotension

Central nervous system: Hallucinations

Dermatologic: Skin rash, exfoliative dermatitis urticaria, Stevens-Johnson syndrome

Hematologic: Agranulocytosis, megaloblastic anemia, thrombocytopenia

Local: Thrombophlebitis

Respiratory: Respiratory depression, apnea, laryngospasm

**Drug Interactions**

Barbiturates can induce hepatic microsomal enzymes resulting in increased metabolism and, therefore, decreased effects of anticoagulants, corticosteroids, doxycycline

Increased toxicity when combined with other CNS depressants or antidepressants, respiratory and CNS depression may be additive

**Drug Uptake**

Onset of action:

I.V.: Within 5 minutes

Oral: Within 1 hour

Serum half-life, biphasic:

Initial: 40 minutes

Terminal: 20 hours

**Pregnancy Risk Factor** D

**Generic Available** Yes: Capsule

## Amobarbital and Secobarbital

(am oh BAR bi tal & see koe BAR bi tal)

**U.S. Brand Names** Tuinal®

**Therapeutic Category** Barbiturate; Hypnotic

**Synonyms** Secobarbital and Amobarbital

**Use** Short-term treatment of insomnia

**Usual Dosage** Adults: Oral: 1-2 capsules at bedtime

**Local Anesthetic/Vasoconstrictor Precautions** No information available to require special precautions

**Effects on Dental Treatment** No effects or complications reported

**Other Adverse Effects**

>10%:

Central nervous system: Dizziness, lightheadedness, drowsiness, "hangover" effect

Local: Pain at injection site

1% to 10%:

Central nervous system: Confusion, mental depression, unusual excitement, nervousness, faint feeling, headache, insomnia, nightmares

Gastrointestinal: Constipation, nausea, vomiting

<1%:

Central nervous system: Hallucinations

Cardiovascular: Hypotension

Dermatologic: Skin rash, exfoliative dermatitis, Stevens-Johnson syndrome

Hematologic: Agranulocytosis, megaloblastic anemia, thrombocytopenia

Local: Thrombophlebitis

Respiratory: Respiratory depression

**Pregnancy Risk Factor** D

**Generic Available** No

♦ **AMO Vitrax®** *see* Sodium Hyaluronate *on page 922*

## Amoxapine (a MOKS a peen)

**U.S. Brand Names** Asendin®

**Therapeutic Category** Antidepressant, Tricyclic

**Use** Treatment of neurotic and endogenous depression and mixed symptoms of anxiety and depression

**Usual Dosage** Once symptoms are controlled, decrease gradually to lowest effective dose. Maintenance dose is usually given at bedtime to reduce daytime sedation. Oral:

Children: Not established in children <16 years of age

Adolescents: Initial: 25-50 mg/day; increase gradually to 100 mg/day; may give as divided doses or as a single dose at bedtime

Adults: Initial: 25 mg 2-3 times/day, if tolerated, dosage may be increased to 100 mg 2-3 times/day; may be given in a single bedtime dose when dosage <300 mg/day

Elderly: Initial: 25 mg at bedtime increased by 25 mg weekly for outpatients and every 3 days for inpatients if tolerated; usual dose: 50-150 mg/day, but doses up to 300 mg may be necessary

Maximum daily dose:
- Inpatient: 600 mg
- Outpatient: 400 mg

**Mechanism of Action** Reduces the reuptake of serotonin and norepinephrine and blocks the response of dopamine receptors to dopamine

**Local Anesthetic/Vasoconstrictor Precautions** Use with caution; epinephrine, norepinephrine and levonordefrin have been shown to have an increased pressor response in combination with TCAs

**Effects on Dental Treatment** >10% of patients experience dry mouth; long-term treatment with TCAs such as amoxapine increases the risk of caries by reducing salivation and salivary buffer capacity

**Other Adverse Effects**

>10%:
- Central nervous system: Dizziness, drowsiness, headache
- Gastrointestinal: Constipation, increased appetite, nausea, unpleasant taste, weight gain
- Neuromuscular & skeletal: Weakness

1% to 10%:
- Cardiovascular: Arrhythmias, hypotension
- Central nervous system: Confusion, delirium, hallucinations, nervousness, restlessness, parkinsonian syndrome, insomnia, tardive dyskinesia
- Endocrine & metabolic: Sexual dysfunction
- Gastrointestinal: Diarrhea, heartburn
- Genitourinary: Dysuria
- Neuromuscular & skeletal: Fine muscle tremors
- Ocular: Blurred vision, eye pain
- Miscellaneous: Excessive sweating

<1%:
- Central nervous system: Anxiety, seizures, neuroleptic malignant syndrome
- Dermatologic: Photosensitivity, alopecia
- Endocrine & metabolic: Breast enlargement, galactorrhea, SIADH
- Gastrointestinal: Trouble with gums, decreased lower esophageal sphincter tone may cause GE reflex
- Genitourinary: Testicular swelling
- Hematologic: Agranulocytosis, leukopenia, eosinophilia
- Hepatic: Cholestatic jaundice, elevated liver enzymes
- Ocular: Increased intraocular pressure
- Otic: Tinnitus
- Miscellaneous: Allergic reactions

**Drug Interactions**

Decreased effect of clonidine, guanethidine

Increased effect of CNS depressants, sympathomimetics, anticholinergic agents

Increased toxicity of MAO inhibitors (hyperpyrexia, tachycardia, hypertension, seizures and death may occur); similar interactions as with other tricyclics may occur

**Drug Uptake**

Onset of antidepressant effect: Usually occurs after 1-2 weeks

Absorption: Oral: Rapidly and well absorbed

Serum half-life:
- Parent drug: 11-16 hours
- Active metabolite (8-hydroxy): Adults: 30 hours

Time to peak serum concentration: Within 1-2 hours

(Continued)

## Amoxapine *(Continued)*

**Pregnancy Risk Factor** C

**Generic Available** Yes

**Selected Readings**


Boakes AJ, Laurence DR, Teoh PC, et al, "Interactions Between Sympathomimetic Amines and Antidepressant Agents in Man," *Br Med J*, 1973, 1(849):311-5.

Jastak JT and Yagiela JA, "Vasoconstrictors and Local Anesthesia: A Review and Rationale for Use," *J Am Dent Assoc*, 1983, 107:623-30.

Larochelle P, Hamet P, and Enjalbert M, "Responses to Tyramine and Norepinephrine After Imipramine and Trazodone," *Clin Pharmacol Ther*, 1979, 26(1):24-30.

Mitchell JR, "Guanethidine and Related Agents. III Antagonism by Drugs Which Inhibit the Norepinephrine Pump in Man," *J Clin Invest*, 1970, 49(8):1596-604.

Rundegren J, van Dijken J, Mörnstad H, et al, "Oral Conditions in Patients Receiving Long-Term Treatment With Cyclic Antidepressant Drugs," *Swed Dent J*, 1985, 9(2):55-64.

Svedmyr N, "The Influence of a Tricyclic Antidepressive Agent (Protriptyline) on Some of the Circulatory Effects of Noradrenaline and Adrenalin® in Man," *Life Sci*, 1968, 7(1):77-84.


## Amoxicillin (a moks i SIL in)

**Related Information**


Animal and Human Bites Guidelines *on page 1164*

Antibiotic Prophylaxis, Preprocedural Guidelines for Dental Patients *on page 1097*

Cardiovascular Diseases *on page 1066*

Dentin Hypersensitivity; High Caries Index; Xerostomia *on page 1145*

Oral Bacterial Infections *on page 1128*

Periodontal Diseases *on page 1132*


**U.S. Brand Names** Amoxil®; Biomox®; Larotid®; Trimox®; Utimox®; Wymox®

**Canadian Brand Names** Apo®-Amoxi; Novamoxin®; Nu-Amoxi; Pro-Amox®

**Therapeutic Category** Antibiotic, Penicillin

**Use**

Dental: Antibiotic for standard prophylactic regimen for dental patients who are at risk

Medical: Treatment of sinusitis, otitis media, and infections caused by susceptible organisms involving the respiratory tract, skin, and urinary tract

**Usual Dosage** Subacute bacterial endocarditis prophylaxis (standard regimen):

Children: 50 mg/kg 1 hour before dental procedure with no follow-up dose needed; total children's dose should not exceed adult dose

Adults: 2 g 1 hour before dental procedure with no follow-up dose

Joint replacement prophylaxis: 2 g 1 hour before dental procedure with no follow-up dose needed

**Mechanism of Action** Interferes with bacterial cell wall synthesis during active multiplication, causing cell wall death and resultant bactericidal activity against susceptible bacteria

**Local Anesthetic/Vasoconstrictor Precautions** No information available to require special precautions

**Effects on Dental Treatment** Prolonged use of penicillins may lead to development of oral candidiasis

**Other Adverse Effects** 1% to 10%:

Central nervous system: Seizures, fever

Dermatologic: Rash (especially patients with mononucleosis)

Gastrointestinal: Diarrhea

Miscellaneous: Superinfection

**Contraindications** Hypersensitivity to amoxicillin, penicillin, or any component

**Warnings/Precautions** In patients with renal impairment, doses and/or frequency of administration should be modified in response to the degree of renal impairment; a high percentage of patients with infectious mononucleosis have developed rash during therapy with amoxicillin; a low incidence of cross-allergy with other beta-lactams and cephalosporins exists

**Drug Interactions** Efficacy of oral contraceptives may be reduced with amoxicillin; disulfiram, probenecid may cause increased amoxicillin levels; allopurinol may increase the potential for amoxicillin rash

**Drug Uptake**

Onset: Oral: Rapid and nearly complete

Time to peak serum concentration: 2 hours (capsule) and 1 hour (suspension)

Serum half-life:

Adults with normal renal function: 0.7-1.4 hours

Children: 1-2 hours

**Pregnancy Risk Factor** B

**Breast-feeding Considerations** May be taken while breast-feeding

**Dosage Forms**

Capsule, as trihydrate: 250 mg, 500 mg

Powder for oral suspension, as trihydrate: 125 mg/5 mL (5 mL, 80 mL, 100 mL, 150 mL, 200 mL); 250 mg/5 mL (5 mL, 80 mL, 100 mL, 150 mL, 200 mL)

Powder for oral suspension, drops, as trihydrate: 50 mg/mL (15 mL, 30 mL)
Tablet, chewable, as trihydrate: 125 mg, 250 mg
Tablet, film coated: 500 mg, 875 mg

**Dietary Considerations** Peak concentrations may be delayed with food; may be taken with food; may be mixed with formula, milk, or juice

**Generic Available** Yes

**Selected Readings**

Dajani AS, Taubert KA, Wilson WW, et al, "Prevention of Bacterial Endocarditis. Recommendations by the American Heart Association," *JAMA* 1997, 277(22):1794-801.

Dajani AS, Taubert KA, Wilson W, et al, "Prevention of Bacterial Endocarditis: Recommendations by the American Heart Association," *J Am Dent Assoc* 1997, 128(8):1142-51.

Wynn RL, "Amoxicillin Update," *Gen Dent*, 1991, 39(5):322,4,6.

## Amoxicillin and Clavulanate Potassium

(a moks i SIL in & klav yoo LAN ate poe TASS ee um)

**Related Information**

Animal and Human Bites Guidelines *on page 1164*
Dentin Hypersensitivity; High Caries Index; Xerostomia *on page 1145*
Oral Bacterial Infections *on page 1128*

**U.S. Brand Names** Augmentin®

**Canadian Brand Names** Clavulin®

**Therapeutic Category** Antibiotic, Penicillin

**Use**

Dental: Treatment of orofacial infections when beta-lactamase-producing staphylococci and beta-lactamase-producing *Bacteroides* are present

Medical: Treatment of otitis media, sinusitis, and infections caused by susceptible organisms involving the lower respiratory tract, skin and skin structure, and urinary tract; spectrum same as amoxicillin with additional coverage of beta-lactamase producing *B. catarrhalis*, *H. influenzae*, *N. gonorrhoeae*, and *S. aureus* (not MRSA). The expanded coverage of this combination makes it a useful alternative when penicillinase-producing bacteria are present and patients cannot tolerate alternative treatments.

**Usual Dosage** Oral:

Children <40 kg: 20-40 mg (amoxicillin)/kg/day in divided doses every 8 hours

Children >40 kg and Adults: 250-500 mg every 8 hours or 875 mg every 12 hours for at least 7 days; maximum dose: 2 g/day

**Mechanism of Action** Interferes with bacterial cell wall synthesis during active multiplication, causing cell wall death and resultant bactericidal activity against susceptible bacteria. Clavulanic acid binds and inhibits beta-lactamases that inactivate amoxicillin resulting in an antibiotic combination having an expanded spectrum of activity.

**Local Anesthetic/Vasoconstrictor Precautions** No information available to require special precautions

**Effects on Dental Treatment** Prolonged use of penicillins may lead to development of oral candidiasis

**Other Adverse Effects** <1%:

Dermatologic: Rash, urticaria
Gastrointestinal: Nausea, vomiting, diarrhea
Genitourinary: Vaginitis

**Contraindications** Known hypersensitivity to amoxicillin, clavulanic acid, or penicillin

**Warnings/Precautions** In patients with renal impairment, doses and/or frequency of administration should be modified in response to the degree of renal impairment; high percentage of patients with infectious mononucleosis have developed rash during therapy; a low incidence of cross-allergy with cephalosporins exists; incidence of diarrhea is higher than with amoxicillin alone

**Drug Interactions** Efficacy of oral contraceptives may be reduced; probenecid may cause increased amoxicillin levels; amoxicillin may increase the effect of anticoagulants

**Drug Uptake** Amoxicillin pharmacokinetics are not affected by clavulanic acid

Onset: Rapid and nearly complete

Time to peak serum concentration:

- Capsule: 2 hours
- Suspension: 1 hour

Serum half-life:

- Adults with normal renal function: ~1 hour for both agents
- Children: 1-2 hours

**Pregnancy Risk Factor** B

**Breast-feeding Considerations**

Amoxicillin: May be taken while breast-feeding
Clavulanic acid: No data reported

(Continued)

## Amoxicillin and Clavulanate Potassium *(Continued)*

**Dosage Forms**

Suspension, oral:

125 (banana flavor): Amoxicillin trihydrate 125 mg and clavulanate potassium 31.25 mg per 5 mL (75 mL, 150 mL)

200: Amoxicillin 200 mg and clavulanate potassium 28.5 mg per 5 mL (50 mL, 75 mL, 100 mL)

250 (orange flavor): Amoxicillin trihydrate 250 mg and clavulanate potassium 62.5 mg per 5 mL (75 mL, 150 mL)

400: Amoxicillin 400 mg and clavulanate potassium 57 mg per 5 mL (50 mL, 75 mL, 100 mL)

Tablet:

250: Amoxicillin trihydrate 250 mg and clavulanate potassium 125 mg

500: Amoxicillin trihydrate 500 mg and clavulanate potassium 125 mg

875: Amoxicillin trihydrate 875 mg and clavulanate potassium 125 mg

Tablet, chewable:

125: Amoxicillin trihydrate 125 mg and clavulanate potassium 31.25 mg

250: Amoxicillin trihydrate 250 mg and clavulanate potassium 62.5 mg

**Dietary Considerations** May be taken with meals or on an empty stomach; may mix with milk, formula, or juice

**Generic Available** No

**Comments** In maxillary sinus, anterior nasal cavity, and deep neck infections, beta-lactamase-producing staphylococci and beta-lactamase-producing *Bacteroides* usually are present. In these situations, antibiotics that resist the beta-lactamase enzyme are indicated. Amoxicillin and clavulanic acid is administered orally for moderate infections. Ampicillin sodium and sulbactam sodium (Unasyn®) is administered parenterally for more severe infections.

**Selected Readings**

Wynn RL and Bergman SA, "Antibiotics and Their Use in the Treatment of Orofacial Infections, Part I and Part II," *Gen Dent*, 1994, 42(5):398-402, 498-502.

♦ **Amoxil®** *see* Amoxicillin *on page 76*

## Amphetamine (am FET a meen)

**Related Information**

Dextroamphetamine and Amphetamine *on page 313*

**Therapeutic Category** Amphetamine; Central Nervous System Stimulant, Amphetamine

**Use** Treatment of narcolepsy; exogenous obesity; abnormal behavioral syndrome in children (minimal brain dysfunction); attention deficit hyperactive disorder (ADHD)

**Usual Dosage** Oral:

Narcolepsy:

Children:

6-12 years: 5 mg/day, increase by 5 mg at weekly intervals

>12 years: 10 mg/day, increase by 10 mg at weekly intervals

Adults: 5-60 mg/day in 2-3 divided doses

Attention deficit disorder: Children:

3-5 years: 2.5 mg/day, increase by 2.5 mg at weekly intervals

>6 years: 5 mg/day, increase by 5 mg at weekly intervals not to exceed 40 mg/day

Short-term adjunct to exogenous obesity: Children >12 years and Adults: 10 mg or 15 mg long-acting capsule daily, up to 30 mg/day; or 5-30 mg/day in divided doses (immediate release tablets only)

**Mechanism of Action** The amphetamines are noncatechol sympathomimetic amines with pharmacologic actions similar to ephedrine. They require breakdown by monoamine oxidase for inactivation; produce central nervous system and respiratory stimulation, a pressor response, mydriasis, bronchodilation, and contraction of the urinary sphincter; thought to have a direct effect on both alpha- and beta-receptor sites in the peripheral system, as well as release stores of norepinephrine in adrenergic nerve terminals. The central nervous system action is thought to occur in the cerebral cortex and reticular-activating system. The anorexigenic effect is probably secondary to the CNS-stimulating effect; the site of action is probably the hypothalamic feeding center

**Local Anesthetic/Vasoconstrictor Precautions** Use vasoconstriction with caution in patients taking amphetamine sulfate. Amphetamines enhance the sympathomimetic response of epinephrine and norepinephrine leading to potential hypertension and cardiotoxicity.

**Effects on Dental Treatment** No effects or complications reported

**Other Adverse Effects**

>10%:

Cardiovascular: Arrhythmia

Central nervous system: False feeling of well being, nervousness, restlessness, insomnia

1% to 10%:

Cardiovascular: Hypertension

Central nervous system: Mood or mental changes, dizziness, lightheadedness, headache

Endocrine & metabolic: Changes in libido

Gastrointestinal: Diarrhea, nausea, vomiting, stomach cramps, constipation, anorexia, weight loss, dry mouth

Ocular: Blurred vision

Miscellaneous: Increased sweating

<1%:

Cardiovascular: Chest pain

Central nervous system: CNS stimulation (severe), Tourette's syndrome, hyperthermia, seizures, paranoia

Dermatologic: Skin rash, urticaria

Miscellaneous: Tolerance and withdrawal with prolonged use

**Drug Interactions** Increased toxicity of MAO inhibitors (hyperpyrexia, hypertension, arrhythmias, seizures, cerebral hemorrhage, and death has occurred)

**Pregnancy Risk Factor** C

**Generic Available** Yes

♦ **Amphojel® [OTC]** *see* Aluminum Hydroxide *on page 55*

♦ **Amphotec®** *see* Amphotericin B Cholesteryl Sulfate Complex *on next page*

## Amphotericin B (am foe TER i sin bee)

**Related Information**

Oral Fungal Infections *on page 1134*

**U.S. Brand Names** Fungizone®

**Therapeutic Category** Antifungal Agent, Oral Nonabsorbed; Antifungal Agent, Systemic; Antifungal Agent, Topical

**Use** Treatment of severe systemic infections and meningitis caused by susceptible fungi such as *Candida* species, *Histoplasma capsulatum*, *Cryptococcus neoformans*, *Aspergillus* species, *Blastomyces dermatitidis*, *Torulopsis glabrata*, and *Coccidioides immitis*; fungal peritonitis; irrigant for bladder fungal infections; topically for cutaneous and mucocutaneous candidal infections; orally for the treatment of oral candidiasis caused by susceptible strains of *Candida albicans*

**Usual Dosage**

I.V.:

Children:

Test dose (not required): I.V.: 0.1 mg/kg/dose to a maximum of 1 mg; infuse over 30-60 minutes

Initial therapeutic dose: 0.25 mg/kg gradually increased, usually in 0.25 mg/kg increments on each subsequent day, until the desired daily dose is reached

Maintenance dose: 0.25-1 mg/kg/day given once daily; infuse over 2-6 hours. Once therapy has been established, amphotericin B can be administered on an every other day basis at 1-1.5 mg/kg/dose; cumulative dose: 1.5-2 g over 6-10 weeks

Adults:

Test dose (not required).: 1 mg infused over 20-30 minutes

Initial dose: 0.25 mg/kg administered over 2-6 hours, gradually increased on subsequent days to the desired level by 0.25 mg/kg increments per day; in critically ill patients, may initiate with 1-1.5 mg/kg/day with close observation

Maintenance dose: 0.25-1 mg/kg/day or 1.5 mg/kg over 4-6 hours every other day; do not exceed 1.5 mg/kg/day; cumulative dose: 1-4 g over 4-10 weeks

Duration of therapy varies with nature of infection: Histoplasmosis, *Cryptococcus*, or blastomycosis may be treated with total dose of 2-4 g

I.T.:

Children.: 25-100 mcg every 48-72 hours; increase to 500 mcg as tolerated

Adults: 25-300 mcg every 48-72 hours; increase to 500 mcg to 1 mg as tolerated

Oral: 1 mL (100 mg) 4 times/day

Topical: Apply to affected areas 2-4 times/day for 1-4 weeks of therapy depending on nature and severity of infection

**Mechanism of Action** Binds to ergosterol altering cell membrane permeability in susceptible fungi and causing leakage of cell components with subsequent cell death

**Local Anesthetic/Vasoconstrictor Precautions** No information available to require special precautions

(Continued)

## Amphotericin B *(Continued)*

**Effects on Dental Treatment** No effects or complications reported

**Other Adverse Effects**

>10%:

Central nervous system: Fever, chills, headache, malaise, generalized pain
Endocrine & metabolic: Hypokalemia, hypomagnesemia
Gastrointestinal: Anorexia
Hematologic: Anemia
Renal: Nephrotoxicity

1% to 10%:

Cardiovascular: Hypotension, hypertension, flushing
Central nervous system: Delirium, arachnoiditis, pain along lumbar nerves
Gastrointestinal: Nausea, vomiting
Genitourinary: Urinary retention
Hematologic: Leukocytosis, bone marrow suppression
Local: Thrombophlebitis
Neuromuscular & skeletal: Paresthesia (especially with I.T. therapy)
Renal: Renal tubular acidosis, renal failure

<1%:

Cardiovascular: Cardiac arrest
Central nervous system: Convulsions
Dermatologic: Maculopapular rash
Hematologic: Coagulation defects, thrombocytopenia, agranulocytosis, leukopenia
Hepatic: Acute liver failure
Ocular: Vision changes
Otic: Hearing loss
Renal: Anuria
Respiratory: Dyspnea

**Drug Interactions** Increased toxicity: Cyclosporine and aminoglycosides (nephrotoxicity), corticosteroids (hypokalemia)

**Drug Uptake**

Serum half-life, biphasic:
Initial: 15-48 hours
Terminal: 15 days
Time to peak: Within 1 hour following a 4- to 6-hour dose

**Pregnancy Risk Factor** B

**Dosage Forms**

Cream: 3% (20 g)
Lotion: 3% (30 mL)
Ointment, topical: 3% (20 g)
Powder for injection, lyophilized: 50 mg
Suspension, oral: 100 mg/mL (24 mL with dropper)

**Generic Available** Yes

## Amphotericin B Cholesteryl Sulfate Complex

(am foe TER i sin bee koe LOY dal dis PER shun)

**U.S. Brand Names** Amphotec®

**Therapeutic Category** Antifungal Agent

**Use** Effective in the treatment of invasive mycoses in patient refractory to or intolerant of conventional amphotericin B

**Usual Dosage** Children and Adults: 3-4 mg/kg/day I.V. (infusion of 1 mg/kg/hour); maximum: 7.5 mg/kg/day; duration of therapy is often <6 weeks

**Mechanism of Action** Binds to ergosterol altering cll membrane permeability in susceptible fungi and causing leakage of cell components with subsequent cell death

**Local Anesthetic/Vasoconstrictor Precautions** No information available to require special precautions

**Effects on Dental Treatment** No effects or complications reported

**Other Adverse Effects**

1% to 10%:

Cardiovascular: Hypotension, tachycardia
Central nervous system: Headache, chills, fever
Dermatologic: Rash
Endocrine & metabolic: Hypokalemia, hypomagnesemia
Gastrointestinal: Nausea, diarrhea, abdominal pain
Hematologic: Thrombocytopenia
Hepatic: LFT change
Neuromuscular & skeletal: Rigors
Respiratory: Dyspnea

**Note:** Amphotericin B colloidal dispersion has an improved therapeutic index compared to conventional amphotericin B, and has been used safely in patients with amphotericin B-related nephrotoxicity; however, continued decline of renal function has occurred in some patients

**Warnings/Precautions** Anaphylaxis has been reported; facilities for cardiopulmonary resuscitation should be available; infusion reactions, sometimes, severe, usually subside with continued therapy

**Drug Interactions** Increased toxicity: Cyclosporine and aminoglycosides (nephrotoxicity), corticosteroids (hypokalemia)

**Drug Uptake** Serum half-life: 28-29 hours

**Pregnancy Risk Factor** B

## Amphotericin B Lipid Complex

(am foe TER i sin bee LIP id KOM pleks)

**U.S. Brand Names** Abelcet™ Injection; AmBisome®

**Therapeutic Category** Antifungal Agent, Systemic

**Synonyms** ABLC

**Use** Treatment of aspergillosis in patients who are refractory to or intolerant of conventional amphotericin B therapy. This indication is based on results obtained primarily from emergency use studies for the treatment of aspergillosis; orphan drug status for cryptococcal meningitis

**Usual Dosage** Children and Adults: I.V.: 2.5-5 mg/kg/day as a single infusion

**Note:** Significantly higher dose of ABLC are tolerated; it appears that attaining higher doses with ABLC produce more rapid fungicidal activity *in vivo* than standard amphotericin B preparations

**Local Anesthetic/Vasoconstrictor Precautions** No information available to require special precautions

**Effects on Dental Treatment** No effects or complications reported

**Other Adverse Effects**

>10%:

- Central nervous system: Chills, fever
- Renal: Elevated serum creatinine
- Miscellaneous: Multiple organ failure

1% to 10%:

- Cardiovascular: Hypotension, cardiac arrest
- Central nervous system: Headache, pain
- Dermatologic: Rash
- Endocrine & metabolic: Hypokalemia, acidosis
- Gastrointestinal: Nausea, vomiting, diarrhea, gastrointestinal hemorrhage, abdominal pain
- Hepatic: Bilirubinemia
- Renal: Renal failure
- Respiratory: Respiratory failure, dyspnea, pneumonia

**Warnings/Precautions** Anaphylaxis has been reported with amphotericin B desoxycholate and other amphotericin B-containing drugs. Facilities for cardiopulmonary resuscitation should be available during administration due to the possibility of anaphylactic reaction. If severe respiratory distress occurs, the infusion should be immediately discontinued and the patient should not receive further infusions. During the initial dosing, the drug should be administered intravenously and under close clinical observation by medically trained personnel. Acute reactions (including fever and chills) may occur 1-2 hours after starting an intravenous infusion. These reactions are usually more common with the first few doses and generally diminish with subsequent doses.

**Pregnancy Risk Factor** B

**Dosage Forms** Injection: 50 mg; 5 mg/mL (20 mL)

**Generic Available** No

## Ampicillin (am pi SIL in)

**Related Information**

Antibiotic Prophylaxis, Preprocedural Guidelines for Dental Patients *on page 1097*

Cardiovascular Diseases *on page 1066*

Dental Drug Interactions: Update on Drug Combinations Requiring Special Considerations *on page 1225*

**U.S. Brand Names** Amcill®; Marcillin®; Omnipen®; Omnipen®-N; Polycillin-N®; Principen®; Totacillin®; Totacillin®-N

**Canadian Brand Names** Ampicin® Sodium; Apo®-Ampi Trihydrate; Jaa Amp® Trihydrate; Nu-Ampi Trihydrate; Pro-Ampi® Trihydrate; Taro-Ampicillin® Trihydrate

**Therapeutic Category** Antibiotic, Penicillin

(Continued)

## Ampicillin *(Continued)*

**Use**

Dental: Alternate antibiotic for the prevention of bacterial endocarditis in patients undergoing dental procedures. It is used in those patients unable to take oral medications

Medical: Treatment of susceptible bacterial infections (nonbeta-lactamase-producing organisms); susceptible bacterial infections caused by streptococci, pneumococci, nonpenicillinase-producing staphylococci, *Listeria*, meningococci; some strains of *H. influenzae*, *Salmonella*, *Shigella*, *E. coli*, *Enterobacter*, and *Klebsiella*

**Usual Dosage** Prevention of bacterial endocarditis in patients unable to take oral medications:

Children: 50 mg/kg I.M. or I.V. within 30 minutes before procedure; total children's dose should not exceed adult dose

Adults: I.M., I.V.: 2 g 30 minutes before procedure

Joint replacement prophylaxis: I.M., I.V.: 2 g 1 hour prior to procedure

**Mechanism of Action** Interferes with bacterial cell wall synthesis during active multiplication, causing cell wall death and resultant bactericidal activity against susceptible bacteria

**Local Anesthetic/Vasoconstrictor Precautions** No information available to require special precautions

**Effects on Dental Treatment** Prolonged use of penicillins may lead to development of oral candidiasis

**Other Adverse Effects**

>10%:

Dermatologic: Rash (appearance of a rash should be carefully evaluated to differentiate a nonallergic ampicillin rash from a hypersensitivity reaction; incidence is higher in patients with viral infections, *Salmonella* infections, lymphocytic leukemia, or patients that have hyperuricemia)

Gastrointestinal: Diarrhea, vomiting

1% to 10%: Gastrointestinal: Severe abdominal cramps and/or pain

**Contraindications** Known hypersensitivity to ampicillin or other penicillins

**Warnings/Precautions** Dosage adjustment may be necessary in patients with renal impairment; a low incidence of cross-allergy with other beta-lactams exists; high percentage of patients with infectious mononucleosis have developed rash during therapy with ampicillin. Appearance of a rash should be carefully evaluated to differentiate a nonallergic ampicillin rash from a hypersensitivity reaction. Ampicillin rash occurs in 5% to 10% of children receiving ampicillin and is a generalized dull red, maculopapular rash, generally appearing 3-14 days after the start of therapy. It normally begins on the trunk and spreads over most of the body. It may be most intense at pressure areas, elbows, and knees.

**Drug Interactions** Efficacy of oral contraceptives may be reduced with ampicillin; probenecid may cause increased penicillin levels; ampicillin may increase the effect of anticoagulants; allopurinol may increase the potential for amoxicillin (ampicillin) rash

**Drug Uptake**

Absorption: Oral: 50%

Serum half-life: Adults and Children: 1-1.8 hours

Time to peak serum concentration: Oral: Within 1-2 hours

**Pregnancy Risk Factor** B

**Breast-feeding Considerations** Excreted into breast milk in small amounts like amoxicillin which is compatible with breast-feeding

**Dosage Forms**

Capsule, as anhydrous: 250 mg, 500 mg

Capsule, as trihydrate: 250 mg, 500 mg

Powder for injection, as sodium: 125 mg, 250 mg, 500 mg, 1 g, 2 g, 10 g

Powder for oral suspension, as trihydrate: 125 mg/5 mL (5 mL unit dose, 80 mL, 100 mL, 150 mL, 200 mL); 250 mg/5 mL (5 mL unit dose, 80 mL, 100 mL, 150 mL, 200 mL); 500 mg/5 mL (5 mL unit dose, 100 mL)

Powder for oral suspension, drops, as trihydrate: 100 mg/mL (20 mL)

**Dietary Considerations** Should be taken on an empty stomach; food decreases rate and extent of absorption

**Generic Available** Yes

**Selected Readings**

Dajani AS, Taubert KA, Wilson WW, et al, "Prevention of Bacterial Endocarditis. Recommendations by the American Heart Association," *JAMA* 1997, 277(22):1794-801.

Dajani AS, Taubert KA, Wilson W, et al, "Prevention of Bacterial Endocarditis: Recommendations by the American Heart Association," *J Am Dent Assoc* 1997, 128(8):1142-51.

## Ampicillin and Probenecid (am pi SIL in & proe BEN e sid)

**U.S. Brand Names** Polycillin-PRB®; Probampacin®

**Therapeutic Category** Antibiotic, Penicillin

**Use** Uncomplicated infections caused by susceptible strains of *Neisseria gonorrhoeae* in adults

**Usual Dosage** Administer entire contents of bottle as a single one time dose

**Local Anesthetic/Vasoconstrictor Precautions** No information available to require special precautions

**Effects on Dental Treatment** >10% oral candidiasis after chronic dosing

**Other Adverse Effects**

>10%:
- Central nervous system: Headache
- Dermatologic: Rash
- Gastrointestinal: Anorexia, nausea, vomiting, diarrhea, oral candidiasis
- Neuromuscular & skeletal: Gouty arthritis (acute)

1% to 10%:
- Cardiovascular: Flushing of face
- Central nervous system: Dizziness
- Dermatologic: Skin rash, itching
- Gastrointestinal: Sore gums, severe abdominal or stomach cramps and pain
- Genitourinary: Dysuria
- Renal: Renal calculi

<1%:
- Central nervous system: Seizures
- Hematologic: Leukopenia, hemolytic anemia, aplastic anemia
- Hepatic: Hepatic necrosis
- Renal: Urate nephropathy, nephrotic syndrome
- Miscellaneous: Anaphylaxis, penicillin encephalopathy, lymphocytic leukemia

**Drug Interactions** Avoid concomitant use with ketorolac since its half-life is increased two-fold and levels and toxicity are significantly increased by probenecid; allopurinol theoretically has an additional potential for ampicillin rash

**Pregnancy Risk Factor** B

**Generic Available** Yes

## Ampicillin and Sulbactam (am pi SIL in & SUL bak tam)

**Related Information**

Dental Drug Interactions: Update on Drug Combinations Requiring Special Considerations *on page 1225*

**U.S. Brand Names** Unasyn®

**Therapeutic Category** Antibiotic, Penicillin

**Use**

Dental: Parenteral beta-lactamase-resistant antibiotic combination to treat more severe orofacial infections where beta-lactamase-producing staphylococci and beta-lactamase-producing *Bacteroides* are present

Medical: Treatment of susceptible bacterial infections involved with skin and skin structure, intra-abdominal infections, gynecological infections; spectrum is that of ampicillin plus organisms producing beta-lactamases such as *S. aureus*, *H. influenzae*, *E. coli*, *Klebsiella*, *Acinetobacter*, *Enterobacter*, and anaerobes

**Usual Dosage** Unasyn® (ampicillin/sulbactam) is a combination product. Each 3 g vial contains 2 g of ampicillin and 1 g of sulbactam. Sulbactam has very little antibacterial activity by itself, but effectively extends the spectrum of ampicillin to include beta-lactamase producing strains that are resistant to ampicillin alone. Therefore, dosage recommendations for Unasyn® are based on the ampicillin component.

I.M., I.V.:
- Children: 100-200 mg ampicillin/kg/day divided every 6 hours; maximum dose: 8 g ampicillin/day
- Adults: 1-2 g ampicillin every 6-8 hours; maximum dose: 8 g ampicillin/day

**Mechanism of Action** Interferes with bacterial cell wall synthesis during active multiplication, causing cell wall death and resultant bactericidal activity against susceptible bacteria; addition of sulbactam, a beta-lactamase inhibitor, to ampicillin extends the spectrum of ampicillin to include beta-lactamase producing organisms

**Local Anesthetic/Vasoconstrictor Precautions** No information available to require special precautions

**Effects on Dental Treatment** Prolonged use of penicillins may lead to development of oral candidiasis, some patients may experience hairy tongue

**Other Adverse Effects**

>10%: Local: Pain at injection site (I.M.)

1% to 10%:
- Dermatologic: Rash
- Gastrointestinal: Diarrhea
- Local: Pain at injection site (I.V.)

(Continued)

## Ampicillin and Sulbactam *(Continued)*

**Contraindications** Hypersensitivity to ampicillin, sulbactam or any component, or penicillins

**Warnings/Precautions** Dosage adjustment may be necessary in patients with renal impairment; a low incidence of cross-allergy with other beta-lactams exists; high percentage of patients with infectious mononucleosis have developed rash during therapy with ampicillin. Appearance of a rash should be carefully evaluated to differentiate a nonallergic ampicillin rash from a hypersensitivity reaction. Ampicillin rash occurs in 5% to 10% of children receiving ampicillin and is a generalized dull red, maculopapular rash, generally appearing 3-14 days after the start of therapy. It normally begins on the trunk and spreads over most of the body. It may be most intense at pressure areas, elbows, and knees.

**Drug Interactions** Efficacy of oral contraceptives may be reduced with ampicillin and sulbactam; probenecid results in increased amoxicillin levels; allopurinol may increase the potential for amoxicillin/ampicillin rash

**Drug Uptake**

Absorption: Oral: 50%

Duration: Ampicillin: 6 hours

Serum half-life:

- Ampicillin: 1-1.8 hours
- Sulbactam: 1-1.3 hours

Time to peak serum concentration: Ampicillin: 1-2 hours

**Pregnancy Risk Factor** B

**Breast-feeding Considerations**

Ampicillin: Excreted into breast milk in small amounts like amoxicillin which is compatible with breast-feeding

Sulbactam sodium: No data reported

**Dosage Forms** Powder for injection: 1.5 g [ampicillin sodium 1 g and sulbactam sodium 0.5 g]; 3 g [ampicillin sodium 2 g and sulbactam sodium 1 g]

**Dietary Considerations** No data reported

**Generic Available** No

**Comments** In maxillary sinus, anterior nasal cavity, and deep neck infections, beta-lactamase-producing staphylococci and beta-lactamase-producing *Bacteroides* usually are present. In these situations, antibiotics that resist the beta-lactamase enzyme should be administered. Amoxicillin and clavulanic acid is administered orally for moderate infections. Ampicillin sodium and sulbactam sodium (Unasyn®) is administered parenterally for more severe infections.

**Selected Readings**

Wynn RL and Bergman SA, "Antibiotics and Their Use in the Treatment of Orofacial Infections, Part I and Part II," *Gen Dent*, 1994, 42(5):398-402, 498-502.

♦ **AMPT** *see* Metyrosine *on page 669*

## Amrinone (AM ri none)

**U.S. Brand Names** Inocor®

**Therapeutic Category** Adrenergic Agonist Agent

**Use** Treatment of low cardiac output states (sepsis, congestive heart failure); adjunctive therapy of pulmonary hypertension; normally prescribed for patients who have not responded well to therapy with digitalis, diuretics, and vasodilators

**Usual Dosage** Dosage is based on clinical response; **Note:** Dose should not exceed 10 mg/kg/24 hours

Children and Adults: 0.75 mg/kg I.V. bolus over 2-3 minutes followed by maintenance infusion of 5-10 mcg/kg/minute; I.V. bolus may need to be repeated in 30 minutes

**Mechanism of Action** Inhibits myocardial cyclic adenosine monophosphate (cAMP) phosphodiesterase activity and increases cellular levels of cAMP resulting in a positive inotropic effect and increased cardiac output; also possesses systemic and pulmonary vasodilator effects resulting in pre- and afterload reduction; slightly increases atrioventricular conduction

**Local Anesthetic/Vasoconstrictor Precautions** No information available to require special precautions

**Effects on Dental Treatment** No effects or complications reported

**Other Adverse Effects**

1% to 10%:

- Cardiovascular: Arrhythmias, hypotension (may be infusion rate-related), ventricular and supraventricular arrhythmias
- Gastrointestinal: Nausea
- Hematologic: Thrombocytopenia (may be dose-related)

<1%:

- Cardiovascular: Chest pain
- Central nervous system: Fever
- Gastrointestinal: Vomiting, abdominal pain, anorexia

Hepatic: Hepatotoxicity
Local: Pain or burning at injection site

**Drug Interactions** No data reported

**Drug Uptake**

Onset of action: I.V.: Within 2-5 minutes
Peak effect: Within 10 minutes
Duration: Dose dependent (~30 minutes low dose, ~2 hours higher doses)
Serum half-life:
Adults, normal volunteers: 3.6 hours
Adults with CHF: 5.8 hours

**Pregnancy Risk Factor** C

**Generic Available** No

- ♦ **Amvisc®** *see* Sodium Hyaluronate *on page 922*
- ♦ **Amvisc® Plus** *see* Sodium Hyaluronate *on page 922*

## Amyl Nitrite (AM il NYE trite)

**Therapeutic Category** Vasodilator, Coronary

**Use** Coronary vasodilator in angina pectoris; adjunct in treatment of cyanide poisoning; used to produce changes in the intensity of heart murmurs

**Usual Dosage** Adults: 1-6 inhalations from one capsule are usually sufficient to produce the desired effect

**Local Anesthetic/Vasoconstrictor Precautions** No information available to require special precautions

**Effects on Dental Treatment** No effects or complications reported

**Other Adverse Effects**

1% to 10%:
Cardiovascular: Postural hypotension, cutaneous flushing of head, neck, and clavicular area
Central nervous system: Headache
<1%:
Dermatologic: Skin rash
Hematologic: Hemolytic anemia

**Drug Interactions** Increased toxicity: Alcohol

**Drug Uptake**

Onset of action: Angina relieved within 30 seconds
Duration: 3-15 minutes

**Pregnancy Risk Factor** X

**Generic Available** Yes

- ♦ **Amytal®** *see* Amobarbital *on page 73*
- ♦ **Anabolin® Injection** *see* Nandrolone *on page 703*
- ♦ **Anacin® [OTC]** *see* Aspirin *on page 100*
- ♦ **Anadrol®** *see* Oxymetholone *on page 755*
- ♦ **Anafranil®** *see* Clomipramine *on page 263*

## Anagrelide (an AG gre lide)

**U.S. Brand Names** Agrylin™

**Therapeutic Category** Platelet Aggregation Inhibitor

**Synonyms** Anagrelide Hydrochloride

**Use** Agent for essential thrombocythemia (ET); treatment of patients with thrombocythemia, secondary to myeloproliferative disorders

**Usual Dosage** Adults: Oral: 0.5 mg 4 times/day or 1 mg twice daily, maintain for ≥1 week, then adjust to the lowest effective dose to reduce and maintain platelet count <600,000 μL ideally to the normal range

**Mechanism of Action** Anagrelide appears to inhibit cyclic nucleotide phosphodiesterase and the release of arachidonic acid from phospholipase, possibly by inhibiting phospholipase A2. It also causes a dose-related reduction in platelet production, which results from decreased megakaryocyte hypermaturation. The drug disrupts the postmitotic phase of maturation.

**Local Anesthetic/Vasoconstrictor Precautions** No information available to require special precautions

**Effects on Dental Treatment** No effects or complications reported

**Drug Uptake**

Half-life, plasma: 1.3 hours
Peak serum concentrations: Oral: 1 hour

**Dosage Forms** Capsule: 0.5 mg, 1 mg

- ♦ **Anagrelide Hydrochloride** *see* Anagrelide *on this page*
- ♦ **Ana-Kit®** *see* Insect Sting Kit *on page 536*
- ♦ **Anamine® Syrup [OTC]** *see* Chlorpheniramine and Pseudoephedrine *on page 233*

- **Anaplex® Liquid [OTC]** *see* Chlorpheniramine and Pseudoephedrine *on page 233*
- **Anaprox® (Naproxen Sodium)** *see* Naproxen *on page 705*
- **Anaspaz®** *see* Hyoscyamine *on page 519*

## Anastrozole (an AS troe zole)

**U.S. Brand Names** Arimidex®

**Therapeutic Category** Antineoplastic Agent, Miscellaneous

**Use** Treatment of advanced breast cancer in postmenopausal women with disease progression following tamoxifen therapy. Patients with ER-negative disease and patients who did not respond to tamoxifen therapy rarely responded to anastrozole.

**Usual Dosage** Breast cancer: Adults: Oral (refer to individual protocols): 1 mg once daily

**Mechanism of Action** Potent and selective nonsteroidal aromatase inhibitor. It significantly lowers serum estradiol concentrations and has not detectable effect on formation of adrenal corticosteroids or aldosterone. In postmenopausal women, the principal source of circulating estrogen is conversion of adrenally generated androstenedione to estrone by aromatase in peripheral tissues.

**Local Anesthetic/Vasoconstrictor Precautions** No information available to require special precautions

**Effects on Dental Treatment** No effects or complications reported

**Other Adverse Effects**

>5%:

Cardiovascular: Flushing

Gastrointestinal: Little to mild nausea (10%), vomiting

Neuromuscular & skeletal: Increased bone and tumor pain

2% to 5%:

Cardiovascular: Hypertension

Central nervous system: Somnolence, confusion, insomnia, anxiety, nervousness, fever, malaise, accidental injury

Dermatologic: Hair thinning, pruritus

Endocrine & metabolic: Breast pain

Gastrointestinal: Weight loss

Genitourinary: Urinary tract infection

Local: Thrombophlebitis

Neuromuscular & skeletal: Myalgia, arthralgia, pathological fracture, neck pain

Respiratory: Sinusitis, bronchitis, rhinitis

Miscellaneous: Flu-like syndrome, infection

**Drug Interactions** Anastrozole inhibited *in vitro* metabolic reactions catalyzed by cytochromes P-450 1A2, 2C8/9, and 3A4, but only at relatively high concentrations. It is unlikely that coadministration of anastrozole with other drugs will result in clinically significant inhibition of cytochrome P-450-mediated metabolism of other drugs.

**Drug Uptake**

Absorption: Well absorbed from GI tract; food does not affect absorption

Serum half-life: 50 hours

**Pregnancy Risk Factor** C

**Generic Available** No

- **Anatuss® [OTC]** *see* Guaifenesin, Phenylpropanolamine, and Dextromethorphan *on page 481*
- **Anatuss® DM [OTC]** *see* Guaifenesin, Pseudoephedrine, and Dextromethorphan *on page 482*
- **Anbesol® [OTC]** *see* Benzocaine *on page 128*
- **Anbesol® Maximum Strength [OTC]** *see* Benzocaine *on page 128*
- **Ancef®** *see* Cefazolin *on page 199*
- **Ancobon®** *see* Flucytosine *on page 436*
- **Androderm® Transdermal System** *see* Testosterone *on page 961*
- **Andro/Fem® Injection** *see* Estradiol and Testosterone *on page 389*
- **Android-25®** *see* Methyltestosterone *on page 662*
- **Andro-L.A.® Injection** *see* Testosterone *on page 961*
- **Androlone®-D Injection** *see* Nandrolone *on page 703*
- **Androlone® Injection** *see* Nandrolone *on page 703*
- **Andropository® Injection** *see* Testosterone *on page 961*
- **Anergan®** *see* Promethazine *on page 847*
- **Anexsia® 5/500** *see* Hydrocodone and Acetaminophen *on page 505*
- **Anexsia® 7.5/650** *see* Hydrocodone and Acetaminophen *on page 505*
- **Anexsia® 10/660** *see* Hydrocodone and Acetaminophen *on page 505*
- **Animal and Human Bites Guidelines** *see page 1164*

## Anisotropine (an iss oh TROE peen)

**U.S. Brand Names** Valpin® 50

**Canadian Brand Names** Miradon®

**Therapeutic Category** Anticholinergic Agent; Antispasmodic Agent, Gastrointestinal

**Use** Adjunctive treatment of peptic ulcer

**Usual Dosage** Adults: Oral: 50 mg 3 times/day

**Mechanism of Action** Blocks the action of acetylcholine at parasympathetic sites in smooth muscle, secretory glands, and the CNS; increases cardiac output, dries secretions, antagonizes histamine and serotonin

**Local Anesthetic/Vasoconstrictor Precautions** No information available to require special precautions

**Effects on Dental Treatment** >10% of patients experience dry mouth; orthostatic hypotension possible

**Other Adverse Effects**

>10%:

Cardiovascular: Palpitations
Dermatologic: Dry skin
Gastrointestinal: Constipation
Respiratory: Dry nose/throat
Miscellaneous: Decreased sweating

1% to 10%:

Endocrine & metabolic: Decreased flow of breast milk
Gastrointestinal: Decreased salivary secretion

<1%:

Cardiovascular: Orthostatic hypotension
Central nervous system: Confusion, drowsiness, headache, loss of memory, fatigue
Dermatologic: Skin rash, photosensitivity
Gastrointestinal: Bloated feeling, nausea, vomiting
Genitourinary: Decreased urination
Neuromuscular & skeletal: Weakness
Ocular: Increased intraocular pain, blurred vision

**Drug Interactions** No data reported

**Drug Uptake**

Absorption: Poor (~10%) from GI tract

**Pregnancy Risk Factor** C

**Generic Available** Yes

## Anistreplase (a NISS tre plase)

**Related Information**

Cardiovascular Diseases *on page 1066*

**U.S. Brand Names** Eminase®

**Therapeutic Category** Thrombolytic Agent

**Use** Management of acute myocardial infarction (AMI) in adults; lysis of thrombi obstructing coronary arteries, reduction of infarct size; and reduction of mortality associated with AMI

**Usual Dosage** Adults: I.V.: 30 units injected over 2-5 minutes as soon as possible after onset of symptoms

**Mechanism of Action** Activates the conversion of plasminogen to plasmin by forming a complex exposing plasminogen-activating site and cleavage of a peptide bond that converts plasminogen to plasmin; plasmin being capable of thrombolysis, by degrading fibrin, fibrinogen and other procoagulant proteins into soluble fragments, effective both outside and within the formed thrombus/embolus

**Local Anesthetic/Vasoconstrictor Precautions** No information available to require special precautions

**Effects on Dental Treatment** No effects or complications reported

**Other Adverse Effects**

>10%:

Cardiovascular: Arrhythmias, hypotension, perfusion arrhythmias
Hematologic: Bleeding or oozing from cuts

1% to 10%: Anaphylactic reaction

<1%:

Central nervous system: Headache, chills
Dermatologic: Rash
Gastrointestinal: Nausea, vomiting
Hematologic: Anemia
Ocular: Eye hemorrhage
Respiratory: Bronchospasm, epistaxis
Miscellaneous: Sweating

(Continued)

## Anistreplase *(Continued)*

**Drug Interactions** Increased efficacy and bleeding potential: Anticoagulants (heparin, warfarin), antiplatelet agents (aspirin)

**Drug Uptake**

Duration: Fibrinolytic effect persists for 4-6 hours following administration

Serum half-life: 70-120 minutes

**Pregnancy Risk Factor** C

**Generic Available** No

- **Anodynos-DHC® [5/500]** *see* Hydrocodone and Acetaminophen *on page 505*
- **Anoquan®** *see* Butalbital Compound *on page 163*
- **Anoquan®** *see* Butalbital Compound and Acetaminophen *on page 164*
- **Ansaid®** *see* Flurbiprofen *on page 448*
- **Antabuse®** *see* Disulfiram *on page 344*
- **Antazoline-V® Ophthalmic** *see* Naphazoline and Antazoline *on page 704*
- **Anthra-Derm®** *see* Anthralin *on this page*

## Anthralin (AN thra lin)

**U.S. Brand Names** Anthra-Derm®; Drithocreme®; Drithocreme® HP 1%; Dritho-Scalp®; Micanol® Cream

**Canadian Brand Names** Anthraforte®; Anthranol®; Anthrascalp®

**Therapeutic Category** Antipsoriatic Agent, Topical; Keratolytic Agent

**Use** Treatment of psoriasis (quiescent or chronic psoriasis)

**Usual Dosage Adults: Topical:** Generally, apply once a day or as directed. The irritant potential of anthralin is directly related to the strength being used and each patient's individual tolerance. Always commence treatment for at least one week using the lowest strength possible.

Skin application: Apply sparingly only to psoriatic lesions and rub gently and carefully into the skin until absorbed. Avoid applying an excessive quantity which may cause unnecessary soiling and staining of the clothing or bed linen.

Scalp application: Comb hair to remove scalar debris and, after suitably parting, rub cream well into the lesions, taking care to prevent the cream from spreading onto the forehead

Remove by washing or showering; optimal period of contact will vary according to the strength used and the patient's response to treatment. Continue treatment until the skin is entirely clear (ie, when there is nothing to feel with the fingers and the texture is normal)

**Mechanism of Action** Reduction of the mitotic rate and proliferation of epidermal cells in psoriasis by inhibiting synthesis of nucleic protein from inhibition of DNA synthesis to affected areas

**Local Anesthetic/Vasoconstrictor Precautions** No information available to require special precautions

**Effects on Dental Treatment** No effects or complications reported

**Other Adverse Effects**

1% to 10%: Topical: Transient primary irritation of uninvolved skin; temporary discoloration of hair and fingernails, may stain skin, hair, or fabrics

<1%: Topical: Skin rash, excessive irritation

**Drug Interactions** Increased toxicity: Long-term use of topical corticosteroids may destabilize psoriasis, and withdrawal may also give rise to a "rebound" phenomenon, allow an interval of at least 1 week between the discontinuance of topical corticosteroids and the commencement of therapy

**Pregnancy Risk Factor** C

**Generic Available** Yes

## Anthrax Vaccine Adsorbed (AN thraks vak SEEN ad SORBED)

**Therapeutic Category** Vaccine

**Use** Recommended for individuals who may come in contact with animal products which come from anthrax endemic areas and may be contaminated with *Bacillus anthracis* spores; recommended for high-risk persons such as veterinarians and other handling potentially infected animals. Routine immunization for the general population is not recommended.

The Department of Defense is implementing an anthrax vaccination program against the biological warfare agent anthrax, which will be administered to all active duty and reserve personnel.

**Usual Dosage**

Primary immunization: S.C.: Three injections of 0.5 mL each given 2 weeks apart followed by three additional S.C. injections given at 6, 12, and 18 months

Subsequent booster injections: 0.5 mL at 1-year intervals are recommended for immunity to be maintained

**Mechanism of Action** Active immunization against *Bacillus anthracis*

**Local Anesthetic/Vasoconstrictor Precautions** No information available to require special precautions

**Effects on Dental Treatment** No effects of complications reported

**Other Adverse Effects**

>10%: Local: Mild reactions

1% to 10%: Local: Moderate reactions with inflammation and pruritus, subcutaneous nodules; all local reactions have been reversible

<1%: Central nervous system: Malaise, chills, fever, lassitude

**Pregnancy Risk Factor** C

**Dosage Forms** Injection: 5 mL (10 doses each)

- **AntibiOtic® Otic** *see* Neomycin, Polymyxin B, and Hydrocortisone *on page 712*
- **Antibiotic Prophylaxis, Preprocedural Guidelines for Dental Patients** *see page 1097*
- **Antidigoxin Fab Fragments** *see* Digoxin Immune Fab *on page 330*

## Antihemophilic Factor (Human)

(an tee hee moe FIL ik FAK tor HYU man)

**U.S. Brand Names** Hemofil® M; Humate-P®; Koāte®-HP; Koāte®-HS; Monoclate-P®; Profilate® OSD; Profilate® SD

**Therapeutic Category** Antihemophilic Agent; Blood Product Derivative

**Synonyms** AHF; Factor VIII

**Use** Management of hemophilia A in patients whom a deficiency in factor VIII has been demonstrated

**Usual Dosage** I.V.: Individualize dosage based on coagulation studies performed prior to and during treatment at regular intervals. One AHF unit is the activity present in 1 mL of normal pooled human plasma; dosage should be adjusted to actual vial size currently stocked in the pharmacy.

Hospitalized patients: 20-50 units/kg/dose; may be higher for special circumstances. Dose can be given every 12-24 hours and more frequently in special circumstances.

**Formula to approximate percentage increase in plasma antihemophilic factor:**

Units required = desired level increase (desired level - actual level) x plasma volume (mL)

Total blood volume (mL blood/kg) = 70 mL/kg (adults); 80 mL/kg (children)

Plasma volume = total blood volume (mL) x [1 - Hct (in decimals)]

Example: For a 70 kg adult with a Hct = 40% : plasma volume = [70 kg x 70 mL/kg] x [1 - 0.4] = 2940 mL

To calculate number of units of factor VIII needed to increase level to desired range (highly individualized and dependent on patient's condition):

Number of units = desired level increase [desired level - actual level] x plasma volume (in mL)

Example: For a 100% level in the above patient who has an actual level of 20% the number of units needed = [1 (for a 100% level) - 0.2] x 2940 mL = 2352 units

**Mechanism of Action** Protein (factor VIII) in normal plasma which is necessary for clot formation and maintenance of hemostasis; activates factor X in conjunction with activated factor IX; activated factor X converts prothrombin to thrombin, which converts fibrinogen to fibrin and with factor XIII forms a stable clot

**Local Anesthetic/Vasoconstrictor Precautions** No information available to require special precautions

**Effects on Dental Treatment** No effects or complications reported

**Other Adverse Effects** <1%:

Cardiovascular: Flushing, tachycardia

Central nervous system: Headache

Gastrointestinal: Nausea, vomiting

Neuromuscular & skeletal: Paresthesia

Miscellaneous: Allergic vasomotor reactions, tightness in neck or chest

**Drug Uptake** Serum half-life, biphasic: 4-24 hours with a mean of 12 hours (biphasic: 12 hours is usually used for dosing interval estimates)

**Pregnancy Risk Factor** C

**Generic Available** Yes

## Antihemophilic Factor (Porcine)

(an tee hee moe FIL ik FAK ter POR seen)

**U.S. Brand Names** Hyate®:C

**Therapeutic Category** Antihemophilic Agent

**Use** Treatment of congenital hemophiliacs with antibodies to human factor VIII:C and also for previously nonhemophiliac patients with spontaneously acquired

(Continued)

## Antihemophilic Factor (Porcine) *(Continued)*

inhibitors to human factor VIII:C; patients with inhibitors who are bleeding or who are to undergo surgery

**Usual Dosage** Clinical response should be used to assess efficacy rather than relying upon a particular laboratory value for recovery of factor VIII:C.

Initial dose:

Antibody level to human factor VIII:C <50 Bethesda units/mL: 100-150 porcine units/kg (body weight) is recommended

Antibody level to human factor VIII:C >50 Bethesda units/mL: Activity of the antibody to porcine factor VIII:C should be determined; **an antiporcine antibody level** >20 Bethesda units/mL indicates that the patient is unlikely to benefit from treatment; for lower titers, a dose of 100-150 porcine units/kg is recommended

If a patient has previously been treated with Hyate®:C, this may provide a guide to his likely response and, therefore, assist in estimation of the preliminary dose

Subsequent doses: Following administration of the initial dose, if the recovery of factor VIII:C in the patient's plasma is not sufficient, a further higher dose should be administered; if recovery after the second dose is still insufficient, a third and higher dose may prove effective

**Mechanism of Action** Factor VIII:C is the coagulation portion of the factor VIII complex in plasma. Factor VIII:C acts as a cofactor for factor IX to activate factor X in the intrinsic pathway of blood coagulation.

**Local Anesthetic/Vasoconstrictor Precautions** No information available to require special precautions

**Effects on Dental Treatment** No effects or complications reported

**Other Adverse Effects** 1% to 10%:

Central nervous system: Fever, headache, chills

Dermatologic: Skin rashes

Gastrointestinal: Nausea, vomiting

**Pregnancy Risk Factor** C

**Generic Available** No

**Comments** Sodium ion concentration is not more than 200 mmol/L; the assayed amount of activity is stated on the label, but may vary depending on the type of assay and hemophilic substrate plasma used

## Antihemophilic Factor (Recombinant)

(an tee hee moe FIL ik FAK tor ree KOM be nant)

**U.S. Brand Names** Bioclate®; Helixate®; Kogenate®; Recombinate®

**Therapeutic Category** Antihemophilic Agent

**Synonyms** Factor VIII Recombinant

**Use** Management of hemophilia A in patients whom a deficiency in factor VIII has been demonstrated

**Usual Dosage** I.V.: Individualize dosage based on coagulation studies performed prior to and during treatment at regular intervals. One AHF unit is the activity present in 1 mL of normal pooled human plasma; dosage should be adjusted to actual vial size currently stocked in the pharmacy.

Hospitalized patients: 20-50 units/kg/dose; may be higher for special circumstances; dose can be given every 12-24 hours and more frequently in special circumstances

**Formula to approximate percentage increase in plasma antihemophilic factor:**

Units required = desired level increase (desired level - actual level) x plasma volume (mL)

Total blood volume (mL blood/kg) = 70 mL/kg (adults); 80 mL/kg (children).

Plasma volume = total blood volume (mL) x [1 - Hct (in decimals)]

ie, for a 70 kg adult with a Hct = 40% : plasma volume = [70 kg x 70 mL/kg] x [1 - 0.4] = 2940 mL

To calculate number of units of factor VIII needed to increase level to desired range (highly individualized and dependent on patient's condition):

Number of units = desired level increase [desired level - actual level] x plasma volume (in mL)

ie, for a 100% level in the above patient who has an actual level of 20% the number of units needed = [1 (for a 100% level) - 0.2] x 2940 mL = 2352 units

**Local Anesthetic/Vasoconstrictor Precautions** No information available to require special precautions

**Effects on Dental Treatment** No effects or complications reported

**Other Adverse Effects** <1%:

Cardiovascular: Flushing, tachycardia

Central nervous system: Headache
Gastrointestinal: Nausea, vomiting
Neuromuscular & skeletal: Paresthesia, tightness in neck or chest
Miscellaneous: Allergic vasomotor reactions

**Pregnancy Risk Factor** C

**Generic Available** No

♦ **Antihist-1® [OTC]** *see* Clemastine *on page 257*

## Anti-inhibitor Coagulant Complex

(an tee-in HI bi tor coe AG yoo lant KOM pleks)

**U.S. Brand Names** Autoplex® T; Feiba VH Immuno®

**Therapeutic Category** Hemophilic Agent

**Use** Patients with factor VIII inhibitors who are to undergo surgery or those who are bleeding

**Usual Dosage** Dosage range: 25-100 factor VIII correctional units per kg depending on the severity of hemorrhage

**Local Anesthetic/Vasoconstrictor Precautions** No information available to require special precautions

**Effects on Dental Treatment** No effects or complications reported

**Other Adverse Effects** <1%:

Cardiovascular: Hypotension, flushing
Central nervous system: Fever, headache, chills
Dermatologic: Rash, urticaria
Hematologic: Disseminated intravascular coagulation
Miscellaneous: Anaphylaxis, indications of protein sensitivity

**Pregnancy Risk Factor** C

**Generic Available** No

♦ **Antilirium®** *see* Physostigmine *on page 801*

♦ **Antiminth® [OTC]** *see* Pyrantel Pamoate *on page 865*

## Antipyrine and Benzocaine (an tee PYE reen & BEN zoe kane)

**U.S. Brand Names** Allergan® Ear Drops; Auralgan®; Auroto®; Otocalm® Ear

**Therapeutic Category** Otic Agent, Analgesic; Otic Agent, Cerumenolytic

**Synonyms** Benzocaine and Antipyrine

**Use** Temporary relief of pain and reduction of swelling associated with acute congestive and serous otitis media, swimmer's ear, otitis externa; facilitates ear wax removal

**Usual Dosage** Otic: Fill ear canal; moisten cotton pledget, place in external ear, repeat every 1-2 hours until pain and congestion is relieved; for ear wax removal instill drops 3-4 times/day for 2-3 days

**Local Anesthetic/Vasoconstrictor Precautions** Information available to require special precautions

**Effects on Dental Treatment** No effects or complications reported

**Other Adverse Effects** <1%:

Cardiovascular: Local edema
Local: Burning, stinging, tenderness
Miscellaneous: Hypersensitivity reactions

**Pregnancy Risk Factor** C

**Generic Available** Yes

## Antirabies Serum (Equine) (an tee RAY beez SEER um EE kwine)

**Therapeutic Category** Serum

**Synonyms** ARS

**Use** Rabies prophylaxis

**Usual Dosage** 1000 units/55 lb in a single dose, infiltrate up to 50% of dose around the wound

**Local Anesthetic/Vasoconstrictor Precautions** No information available to require special precautions

**Effects on Dental Treatment** No effects or complications reported

**Other Adverse Effects** 1% to 10%:

Dermatologic: Urticaria
Local: Pain at injection site
Miscellaneous: Serum sickness

**Pregnancy Risk Factor** C

**Generic Available** No

**Comments** Because of a significantly lower incidence of adverse reactions, Rabies Immune Globulin, Human is preferred over Antirabies Serum Equine

♦ **Antispas® Injection** *see* Dicyclomine *on page 322*

## Antithrombin III (an tee THROM bin three)

**U.S. Brand Names** ATnativ®; Thrombate III™

**Therapeutic Category** Blood Product Derivative

**Synonyms** ATIII; Heparin Cofactor I

**Use** Agent for hereditary antithrombin III deficiency

**Usual Dosage** After first dose of antithrombin III, level should increase to 120% of normal; thereafter maintain at levels >80%. Generally, achieved by administration of maintenance doses once every 24 hours; initially and until patient is stabilized, measure antithrombin III level at least twice daily, thereafter once daily and always immediately before next infusion. 1 unit = quantity of antithrombin III in 1 mL of normal pooled human plasma; administration of 1 unit/1 kg raises AT-III level by 1% to 2%; assume plasma volume of 40 mL/kg

Initial dosage (units) = [desired AT-III level % - baseline AT-III level %] x body weight (kg) divided by 1%/units/kg, eg, if a 70 kg adult patient had a baseline AT-III level of 57%, the initial dose would be (120% - 57%) x 70/1%/units/kg = 4,410 units

Measure antithrombin III preceding and 30 minutes after dose to calculate *in vivo* recovery rate; maintain level within normal range for 2-8 days depending on type of surgery or procedure

**Mechanism of Action** Antithrombin III is the primary physiologic inhibitor of *in vivo* coagulation. It is an alpha$_2$-globulin. Its principal actions are the inactivation of thrombin, plasmin, and other active serine proteases of coagulation, including factors IXa, Xa, XIa, XIIa, and VIIa. The inactivation of proteases is a major step in the normal clotting process. The strong activation of clotting enzymes at the site of every bleeding injury facilitates fibrin formation and maintains normal hemostasis. Thrombosis in the circulation would be caused by active serine proteases if they were not inhibited by antithrombin III after the localized clotting process. Patients with congenital deficiency are in a prethrombotic state, even if asymptomatic, as evidenced by elevated plasma levels of prothrombin activation fragment, which are normalized following infusions of antithrombin III concentrate.

**Local Anesthetic/Vasoconstrictor Precautions** No information available to require special precautions

**Effects on Dental Treatment** No effects or complications reported

**Other Adverse Effects** <1%:

Central nervous system: Dizziness, lightheadedness, fever
Cardiovascular: Chest tightness, chest pain, vasodilatory effects, edema
Dermatologic: Urticaria
Endocrine & metabolic: Fluid overload
Gastrointestinal: Nausea, foul taste in mouth, cramps, bowel fullness
Hematologic: Hematoma formation
Ocular: Film over eye
Renal: Diuretic effects
Respiratory: Dyspnea

**Pregnancy Risk Factor** C

**Generic Available** No


- **Antithymocyte Globulin (Equine)** *see* Lymphocyte Immune Globulin *on page 608*
- **Antithymocyte Immunoglobulin** *see* Lymphocyte Immune Globulin *on page 608*
- **Anti-Tuss® Expectorant [OTC]** *see* Guaifenesin *on page 478*
- **Antivert®** *see* Meclizine *on page 620*
- **Antizol®** *see* Fomepizole *on page 453*
- **Antrizine®** *see* Meclizine *on page 620*
- **Anturane®** *see* Sulfinpyrazone *on page 945*
- **Anusol® Ointment [OTC]** *see* Pramoxine *on page 828*
- **Anxanil®** *see* Hydroxyzine *on page 518*
- **Anzemet®** *see* Dolasetron *on page 347*
- **Apacet® [OTC]** *see* Acetaminophen *on page 27*
- **Apatate® [OTC]** *see* Vitamin B Complex *on page 1050*
- **Aphrodyne™** *see* Yohimbine *on page 1056*
- **Aphthasol™** *see* Amlexanox *on page 70*
- **A.P.L.®** *see* Chorionic Gonadotropin *on page 246*
- **Aplisol®** *see* Tuberculin Purified Protein Derivative *on page 1031*
- **Aplitest®** *see* Tuberculin Purified Protein Derivative *on page 1031*
- **Aplonidine** *see* Apraclonidine *on next page*

## Apraclonidine (a pra KLOE ni deen)

**U.S. Brand Names** Iopidine®

**Therapeutic Category** Alpha$_2$-Adrenergic Agonist Agent, Ophthalmic

**Synonyms** Aplonidine; Apraclonidine Hydrochloride; p-Aminoclonidine

**Use** Prevention and treatment of postsurgical intraocular pressure elevation

**Usual Dosage** Adults: Ophthalmic: Instill 1 drop in operative eye 1 hour prior to laser surgery, second drop in eye upon completion of procedure

**Mechanism of Action** Apraclonidine is a potent alpha-adrenergic agent similar to clonidine; relatively selective for alpha$_2$-receptors but does retain some binding to alpha$_1$-receptors; appears to result in reduction of aqueous humor formation; its penetration through the blood-brain barrier is more polar than clonidine which reduces its penetration through the blood-brain barrier and suggests that its pharmacological profile is characterized by peripheral rather than central effects.

**Local Anesthetic/Vasoconstrictor Precautions** No information available to require special precautions

**Effects on Dental Treatment** No effects or complications reported

**Other Adverse Effects**

1% to 10%:

- Central nervous system: Lethargy
- Gastrointestinal: Dry mouth
- Ocular: Upper lid elevation, conjunctival blanching, mydriasis, burning and itching eyes, discomfort, conjunctival microhemorrhage, blurred vision
- Respiratory: Dry nose

<1%: Miscellaneous: Allergic response; some systemic effects have also been reported including GI, CNS, and cardiovascular symptoms (arrhythmias)

**Drug Uptake**

Onset of action: 1 hour

Maximum IOP: 3-5 hours

**Pregnancy Risk Factor** C

**Generic Available** Yes

- **Apraclonidine Hydrochloride** *see* Apraclonidine *on this page*
- **Apresazide®** *see* Hydralazine and Hydrochlorothiazide *on page 502*
- **Apresoline®** *see* Hydralazine *on page 501*
- **Aprodine® Syrup [OTC]** *see* Triprolidine and Pseudoephedrine *on page 1025*
- **Aprodine® Tablet [OTC]** *see* Triprolidine and Pseudoephedrine *on page 1025*
- **Aprodine® w/C** *see* Triprolidine, Pseudoephedrine, and Codeine *on page 1026*

## Aprotinin (a proe TYE nin)

**U.S. Brand Names** Trasylol®

**Therapeutic Category** Hemostatic Agent

**Use** Reduction or prevention of blood loss in patients undergoing coronary artery bypass surgery when a high index of suspicion of excessive bleeding potential exists; this includes open heart reoperation, pre-existing coagulopathy, operations on the great vessels, and patients whose religious beliefs prohibit blood transfusions

**Usual Dosage**

Test dose: **All** patients should receive a 1 mL I.V. test dose at least 10 minutes prior to the loading dose to assess the potential for allergic reactions

Regimen A (standard dose):
- 2 million units (280 mg) loading dose I.V. over 20-30 minutes
- 2 million units (280 mg) into pump prime volume
- 500,000 units/hour (70 mg/hour) I.V. during operation

Regimen B (low dose):
- 1 million units (140 mg) loading dose I.V. over 20-30 minutes
- 1 million units (140 mg) into pump prime volume
- 250,000 units/hour (35 mg/hour) I.V. during operation

**Mechanism of Action** Serine protease inhibitor; inhibits plasmin, kallikrein, and platelet activation producing antifibrinolytic effects; a weak inhibitor of plasma pseudocholinesterase. It also inhibits the contact phase activation of coagulation and preserves adhesive platelet glycoproteins making them resistant to damage from increased circulating plasmin or mechanical injury occurring during bypass

**Local Anesthetic/Vasoconstrictor Precautions** No information available to require special precautions

**Effects on Dental Treatment** No effects or complications reported

**Other Adverse Effects** Increase in postoperative renal dysfunction compared to placebo; anaphylactic reactions have been reported in <0.5% of cases; such reactions are more likely to occur with repeated administration

**Drug Uptake** Serum half-life: 150 minutes

**Pregnancy Risk Factor** C

(Continued)

## Aprotinin *(Continued)*

**Generic Available** No

- **Aquacare® [OTC]** *see* Urea *on page 1034*
- **Aquachloral® Supprettes®** *see* Chloral Hydrate *on page 221*
- **AquaMEPHYTON®** *see* Phytonadione *on page 801*
- **Aquaphyllin®** *see* Theophylline *on page 969*
- **AquaSite® Ophthalmic Solution [OTC]** *see* Artificial Tears *on page 97*
- **Aquasol® A [OTC]** *see* Vitamin A *on page 1048*
- **Aquasol E® [OTC]** *see* Vitamin E *on page 1050*
- **AquaTar® [OTC]** *see* Coal Tar *on page 270*
- **Aquatensen®** *see* Methyclothiazide *on page 657*
- **Aquest®** *see* Estrone *on page 393*
- **Aralen® Phosphate** *see* Chloroquine Phosphate *on page 228*
- **Aralen® Phosphate With Primaquine Phosphate** *see* Chloroquine and Primaquine *on page 227*
- **Arava™** *see* Leflunomide *on page 574*

## Ardeparin (ar dee PA rin)

**U.S. Brand Names** Normiflo®

**Therapeutic Category** Anticoagulant (Other)

**Synonyms** Ardeparin Sodium

**Use** Prevention of deep vein thrombosis (DVT) which may lead to pulmonary embolism following knee replacement surgery

**Usual Dosage** Adults: S.C.: 50 anti-Xa units every 12 hours

**Mechanism of Action** A low molecular weight heparin with antithrombotic properties; a partially depolymerized porcine mucosal heparin that has the same molecular subunits as heparin sodium, USP; acts at multiple sites in the normal coagulation system; binds to and accelerates the activity of antithrombin III, thereby inhibiting thrombosis by inactivating factor Xa and thrombin; inhibits thrombin by binding to heparin cofactor II

**Local Anesthetic/Vasoconstrictor Precautions** No information available to require special precautions

**Effects on Dental Treatment** No effects or complications reported

**Drug Uptake**

Absorption: Well absorbed

Bioavailability:

Anti-Xa: 92% ± 16%

Anti-IIa: 63% ± 19%

Peak plasma levels:

Peak anti-Xa: 0.09 ± 0.03 to 0.32 ± 0.05 units/mL after 30-100 anti-Xa units/kg single doses reached in 2.7 ± 0.6 hours

Mean anti-IIa: 0.07 ± 0.02 units/mL after 100 anti-Xa units/kg single doses reached in 3 ± 1 hours

Half-life: Anti-Xa: Longer than heparin sodium, USP

**Note:** Mean plasma clearances of ardeparin anti-Xa and anti-IIa activities in normal volunteers following a single 90 anti-Xa units/kg I.V. bolus dose are 30 ± 7 and 46 ± 16 mL/hour/kg respectively, and the mean disposition half-lives are 3.3 ± 2.4 and 1.2 ± 0.3 hours respectively

**Dosage Forms** Injection, as sodium: Anti-Xa units 5000 (0.5 mL); Anti-Xa units 10,000 (0.5 mL)

- **Ardeparin Sodium** *see* Ardeparin *on this page*
- **Aredia™** *see* Pamidronate *on page 762*
- **Arfonad®** *see* Trimethaphan Camsylate (Discontinued 4/96) *on page 1020*
- **Argesic®-SA** *see* Salsalate *on page 902*

## Arginine (AR ji neen)

**U.S. Brand Names** R-Gene®

**Therapeutic Category** Metabolic Alkalosis Agent

**Use** Pituitary function test (growth hormone); management of severe, uncompensated, metabolic alkalosis (pH ≥7.55) **after** optimizing therapy with sodium, potassium, or ammonium chloride supplements

**Usual Dosage** I.V.:

Growth hormone (pituitary function) reserve test:

Children: 500 mg (5 mL) kg/dose administered over 30 minutes

Adults: 30 g (300 mL) administered over 30 minutes

Metabolic alkalosis: Children and Adults: Usual dose: 10 g/hour

Acid required (mEq) =

[1] 0.2 (L/kg) x wt (kg) x [103 - serum chloride] (mEq/L) **or**

[2] 0.3 (L/kg) x wt (kg) x base excess (mEq/L) **or**

[3] 0.5 (L/kg) x wt (kg) x [serum $HCO_3$ - 24] (mEq/L)

Give 1/2 to 2/3 of calculated dose and re-evaluate

**Note:** Arginine hydrochloride should never be used as an alternative to chloride supplementation but used in the patient who is unresponsive to sodium chloride or potassium chloride supplementation

**Mechanism of Action**

Stimulates pituitary release of growth hormone and prolactin through origins in the hypothalamus; patients with impaired pituitary function have lower or no increase in plasma concentrations of growth hormone after administration of arginine. Arginine hydrochloride has been used for severe metabolic alkalosis due to its high chloride content.

Arginine hydrochloride has been used investigationally to treat metabolic alkalosis. Arginine contains 475 mEq of hydrogen ions and 475 mEq of chloride ions/L. Arginine is metabolized by the liver to produce hydrogen ions. It may be used in patients with relative hepatic insufficiency because arginine combines with ammonia in the body to produce urea.

**Local Anesthetic/Vasoconstrictor Precautions** No information available to require special precautions

**Effects on Dental Treatment** No effects or complications reported

**Other Adverse Effects**

1% to 10%: Rapid I.V. infusion may produce flushing, local irritation, nausea & vomiting

Central nervous system: Headache

Neuromuscular & skeletal: Numbness

<1%:

Endocrine & metabolic: Hyperglycemia, hyperkalemia, elevated serum gastrin concentration, hyperchloremia

Gastrointestinal: Abdominal pain, bloating

**Drug Uptake**

Absorption: Oral: Well absorbed

Time to peak serum concentration: Within 2 hours

**Pregnancy Risk Factor** C

**Generic Available** Yes


- ♦ **Argyrol® S.S. 20%** *see* Silver Protein, Mild *on page 914*
- ♦ **Aricept®** *see* Donepezil *on page 348*
- ♦ **Arimidex®** *see* Anastrozole *on page 86*
- ♦ **Aristocort®** *see* Triamcinolone *on page 1010*
- ♦ **Aristocort® A** *see* Triamcinolone *on page 1010*
- ♦ **Aristocort® Forte** *see* Triamcinolone *on page 1010*
- ♦ **Aristocort® Intralesional** *see* Triamcinolone *on page 1010*
- ♦ **Aristospan® Intra-Articular** *see* Triamcinolone *on page 1010*
- ♦ **Aristospan® Intralesional** *see* Triamcinolone *on page 1010*
- ♦ **Arlidin®** *see* Nylidrin *on page 734*
- ♦ **Arm-a-Med® Isoetharine** *see* Isoetharine *on page 551*
- ♦ **Arm-a-Med® Isoproterenol** *see* Isoproterenol *on page 553*
- ♦ **Arm-a-Med® Metaproterenol** *see* Metaproterenol *on page 642*
- ♦ **A.R.M.® Caplet [OTC]** *see* Chlorpheniramine and Phenylpropanolamine *on page 233*
- ♦ **Armour® Thyroid** *see* Thyroid *on page 982*
- ♦ **Aromatic Ammonia Aspirols®** *see* Ammonia Spirit, Aromatic *on page 72*
- ♦ **Arrestin®** *see* Trimethobenzamide *on page 1020*
- ♦ **ARS** *see* Antirabies Serum (Equine) *on page 91*
- ♦ **Artane®** *see* Trihexyphenidyl *on page 1018*
- ♦ **Artha-G®** *see* Salsalate *on page 902*
- ♦ **Arthritis Foundation® Nighttime [OTC]** *see* Acetaminophen and Diphenhydramine *on page 30*
- ♦ **Arthritis Foundation® Pain Reliever [OTC]** *see* Aspirin *on page 100*
- ♦ **Arthritis Foundation® Pain Reliever, Aspirin Free [OTC]** *see* Acetaminophen *on page 27*
- ♦ **Arthropan® [OTC]** *see* Choline Salicylate *on page 245*
- ♦ **Arthrotec®** *see* Diclofenac and Misoprostol *on page 321*


## Articaine Hydrochloride and Epinephrine

**Canadian Brand Names** Ultracaine DS®; Ultracaine DS Forte®

**Therapeutic Category** Local Anesthetic, Injectable

**Use** Anesthesia for infiltration and nerve block anesthesia in clinical dentistry

(Continued)

## Articaine Hydrochloride and Epinephrine *(Continued)*

**Usual Dosage** Adults:

Ultracaine DS® Forte:

Infiltration:

Volume: 0.5-2.5 mL

Total dose: 20-100 mg

Nerve block:

Volume: 0.5-3.4 mL

Total dose: 20-136 mg

Oral surgery:

Volume: 1-5.1 mL

Total dose: 40-204 mg

Ultracaine DS®:

Infiltration:

Volume: 0.5-2.5 mL

Total dose: 20-100 mg

Nerve block:

Volume: 0.5-3.4 mL

Total dose: 20-136 mg

Oral surgery:

Volume: 1-5.1 mL

Total dose: 40-204 mg

Maximum dose: 7 mg/kg

To date, Ultracaine® has not been administered to children <4 years of age, nor in doses >5 mg/kg in children between the ages of 4 and 12

**Mechanism of Action** Blocks nerve conduction by interfering with the permeability of the nerve axonal membrane to sodium ions; this results in the loss of the generation of the nerve axon potential

**Local Anesthetic/Vasoconstrictor Precautions** No information available to require special precautions

**Effects on Dental Treatment** No effects or complications reported

**Other Adverse Effects**

Cardiovascular: Myocardial depression, arrhythmias, tachycardia, bradycardia, blood pressure changes, edema

Central nervous system: Excitation, depression, nervousness, dizziness, headache, somnolence, unconsciousness, convulsions, chills

Dermal: Allergic reactions include cutaneous lesions, urticaria, itching, reddening of skin

Gastrointestinal: Vomiting, allergic reactions include nausea and diarrhea

Local: Reactions at the site of injection, swelling, burning, ischemia, tissue necrosis

Neuromuscular & skeletal: Tremors

Ocular: Visual disturbances, blurred vision, blindness, diplopia, pupillary constriction

Otic: Tinnitus

Respiratory: Allergic reactions include wheezing, acute asthmatic attacks

**Contraindications** Known hypersensitivity to any of its components and/or local anesthetics of the amide group; in the presence of inflammation and/or sepsis near the injection site; in patients with severe shock, any degree of heart block, paroxysmal tachycardia, known arrhythmia with rapid heart rate, narrow-angle glaucoma, cholinesterase deficiency, existing neurologic disease, severe hypertension; when articaine with epinephrine is used, the caution required of any vasopressor drug should be followed

**Warnings/Precautions** Articaine should be used cautiously in persons with known drug allergies or sensitivities, or suspected sensitivity to the amide-type local anesthetics. Avoid excessive premedications with sedatives, tranquilizers, and antiemetic agents. Inject slowly with frequent aspirations and if blood is aspirated, relocate needle. Articaine should be used with extreme caution in patients having a history of thyrotoxicosis or diabetes. Due to the sulfite component of the articaine preparation, hypersensitivity reactions may occur occasionally in patients with bronchial asthma.

**Drug Interactions** Solutions containing epinephrine should be used with caution, if at all, in patients taking MAO inhibitors or tricyclic antidepressants because severe prolonged hypertension may result

**Breast-feeding Considerations** Articaine is unlikely to be transferred to mother's milk since it is rapidly metabolized and eliminated

**Dosage Forms** Injection:

Ultracaine DS®: Articaine hydrochloride with epinephrine [1:200,000] and sodium metabisulfite [0.5 mg/mL] and an antioxidant and water for injection (1.7 mL [50s])

Ultracaine DS Forte®: Articaine hydrochloride 4% with epinephrine [1:100,000] and sodium metabisulfite [0.5 mg/mL] and an antioxidant and water for injection (1.7 mL) [50s]

- ♦ **Articulose-50®** *see* Prednisolone *on page 832*

## Artificial Tears (ar ti FISH il tears)

**U.S. Brand Names** Adsorbotear® Ophthalmic Solution [OTC]; Akwa Tears® Solution [OTC]; AquaSite® Ophthalmic Solution [OTC]; Bion® Tears Solution [OTC]; Comfort® Tears Solution [OTC]; Dakrina® Ophthalmic Solution [OTC]; Dry Eyes® Solution [OTC]; Dry Eye® Therapy Solution [OTC]; Dwelle® Ophthalmic Solution [OTC]; Eye-Lube-A® Solution [OTC]; HypoTears PF Solution [OTC]; HypoTears Solution [OTC]; Isopto® Plain Solution [OTC]; Isopto® Tears Solution [OTC]; Just Tears® Solution [OTC]; Lacril® Ophthalmic Solution [OTC]; Liquifilm® Forte Solution [OTC]; Liquifilm® Tears Solution [OTC]; LubriTears® Solution [OTC]; Moisture® Ophthalmic Drops [OTC]; Murine® Solution [OTC]; Murocel® Ophthalmic Solution [OTC]; Nature's Tears® Solution [OTC]; Nu-Tears® II Solution [OTC]; Nu-Tears® Solution [OTC]; OcuCoat® Ophthalmic Solution [OTC]; OcuCoat® PF Ophthalmic Solution [OTC]; Puralube® Tears Solution [OTC]; Refresh® Ophthalmic Solution [OTC]; Refresh® Plus Ophthalmic Solution [OTC]; Tear Drop® Solution [OTC]; TearGard® Ophthalmic Solution [OTC]; Teargen® Ophthalmic Solution [OTC]; Tearisol® Solution [OTC]; Tears Naturale® Free Solution [OTC]; Tears Naturale® II Solution [OTC]; Tears Naturale® Solution [OTC]; Tears Plus® Solution [OTC]; Tears Renewed® Solution [OTC]; Ultra Tears® Solution [OTC]; Viva-Drops® Solution [OTC]

**Canadian Brand Names** Teardrops®

**Therapeutic Category** Ophthalmic Agent, Miscellaneous

**Synonyms** Hydroxyethylcellulose; Polyvinyl Alcohol

**Use** Ophthalmic lubricant; for relief of dry eyes and eye irritation

**Usual Dosage** Use as needed to relieve symptoms, 1-2 drops into eye(s) 3-4 times/day

**Local Anesthetic/Vasoconstrictor Precautions** No information available to require special precautions

**Effects on Dental Treatment** No effects or complications reported

**Other Adverse Effects** 1% to 10%: Ocular: May cause mild stinging or temporary blurred vision

**Pregnancy Risk Factor** C

**Generic Available** Yes

- ♦ **A.S.A. [OTC]** *see* Aspirin *on page 100*
- ♦ **Asacol®** *see* Mesalamine *on page 638*

## Ascorbic Acid (a SKOR bik AS id)

**U.S. Brand Names** Ascorbicap® [OTC]; C-Crystals® [OTC]; Cebid® Timecelles® [OTC]; Cecon® [OTC]; Cevalin® [OTC]; Cevi-Bid® [OTC]; Ce-Vi-Sol® [OTC]; Dull-C® [OTC]; Flavorcee® [OTC]; N'ice® Vitamin C Drops [OTC]; Vita-C® [OTC]

**Canadian Brand Names** Apo®-C; Ascorbic 500; Redoxon®; Revitalose-C-1000®

**Therapeutic Category** Urinary Acidifying Agent; Vitamin, Water Soluble

**Synonyms** Cevitamic Acid

**Use** Prevention and treatment of scurvy and to acidify the urine

**Investigational use:** In large doses to decrease the severity of "colds"; dietary supplementation

**Usual Dosage** Oral, I.M., I.V., S.C.:

Recommended daily allowance (RDA):
- <6 months: 30 mg
- 6 months to 1 year: 35 mg
- 1-3 years: 40 mg
- 4-10 years: 45 mg
- 11-14 years: 50 mg
- >14 years and Adults: 60 mg

Children:
- Scurvy: 100-300 mg/day in divided doses for at least 2 weeks
- Urinary acidification: 500 mg every 6-8 hours
- Dietary supplement: 35-100 mg/day

Adults:
- Scurvy: 100-250 mg 1-2 times/day for at least 2 weeks
- Urinary acidification: 4-12 g/day in 3-4 divided doses
- Prevention and treatment of colds: 1-3 g/day
- Dietary supplement: 50-200 mg/day

**Mechanism of Action** Not fully understood; necessary for collagen formation and tissue repair; involved in some oxidation-reduction reactions as well as other (Continued)

## Ascorbic Acid *(Continued)*

metabolic pathways, such as synthesis of carnitine, steroids, and catecholamines and conversion of folic acid to folinic acid

**Local Anesthetic/Vasoconstrictor Precautions** No information available to require special precautions

**Effects on Dental Treatment** No effects or complications reported

**Other Adverse Effects**

1% to 10%: Renal: Hyperoxaluria

<1%:

Cardiovascular: Flushing, faintness

Central nervous system: Dizziness, headache, fatigue, flank pain

Gastrointestinal: Nausea, vomiting, heartburn, diarrhea

**Contraindications** Large doses during pregnancy

**Warnings/Precautions** Diabetics and patients prone to recurrent renal calculi (eg, dialysis patients) should not take excessive doses for extended periods of time

**Drug Interactions**

Decreased effect:

Aspirin decreases ascorbate levels, increases aspirin

Fluphenazine decreases fluphenazine levels

Warfarin decreases effect

Increased effect: Iron enhances absorption; oral contraceptives increase contraceptive effect

**Drug Uptake** Absorption: Oral: Readily absorbed; an active process and is thought to be dose-dependent

**Pregnancy Risk Factor** A (C if used in doses above RDA recommendation)

**Breast-feeding Considerations** Compatible

**Dosage Forms**

Capsule, timed release: 500 mg

Crystals: 4 g/teaspoonful (100 g, 500 g); 5 g/teaspoonful (180 g)

Injection: 250 mg/mL (2 mL, 30 mL); 500 mg/mL (2 mL, 50 mL)

Liquid, oral: 35 mg/0.6 mL (50 mL)

Lozenges: 60 mg

Powder: 4 g/teaspoonful (100 g, 500 g)

Solution, oral: 100 mg/mL (50 mL)

Syrup: 500 mg/5 mL (5 mL, 10 mL, 120 mL, 480 mL)

Tablet: 25 mg, 50 mg, 100 mg, 250 mg, 500 mg, 1000 mg

Tablet:

Chewable: 100 mg, 250 mg, 500 mg

Timed release: 500 mg, 1000 mg, 1500 mg

**Generic Available** Yes

- **Ascorbic Acid and Ferrous Sulfate** *see* Ferrous Sulfate and Ascorbic Acid *on page 428*
- **Ascorbicap® [OTC]** *see* Ascorbic Acid *on previous page*
- **Ascriptin® [OTC]** *see* Aspirin *on page 100*
- **Asendin®** *see* Amoxapine *on page 75*
- **Asmalix®** *see* Theophylline *on page 969*

## Asparaginase (a SPIR a ji nase)

**U.S. Brand Names** Elspar®

**Canadian Brand Names** Kidrolase®

**Therapeutic Category** Antineoplastic Agent, Miscellaneous

**Synonyms** L-asparaginase

**Use** Treatment of acute lymphocytic leukemia, lymphoma; used for induction therapy

**Usual Dosage** **Refer to individual protocols**; dose must be individualized based upon clinical response and tolerance of the patient

I.M. administration is **preferred** over I.V. administration; I.M. administration may decrease the risk of anaphylaxis

Asparaginase is available from two different microbiological sources: One is from *Escherichia coli* and the other is from *Erwinia carotovora*. The *Erwinia* is restricted to patients who have sustained anaphylaxis to the *E. coli* preparation.

I.M., I.V.: 6000 units/m$^2$ every other day for 3-4 weeks or daily doses of 1000-20,000 units/m$^2$ for 10-20 days; other induction regimens have been utilized

Desensitization should be performed before administering the first dose of asparaginase to patients who developed a positive reaction to the intradermal skin test or who are being retreated. One schedule begins with a total of 1 unit given I.V. and doubles the dose every 10 minutes until the total amount given in the planned dose for that day.

**Asparaginase Desensitization**

| Injection No. | Elspar Dose (IU) | Accumulated Total Dose |
|---|---|---|
| 1 | 1 | 1 |
| 2 | 2 | 3 |
| 3 | 4 | 7 |
| 4 | 8 | 15 |
| 5 | 16 | 31 |
| 6 | 32 | 63 |
| 7 | 64 | 127 |
| 8 | 128 | 255 |
| 9 | 256 | 511 |
| 10 | 512 | 1,023 |
| 11 | 1,024 | 2,047 |
| 12 | 2,048 | 4,095 |
| 13 | 4,096 | 8,191 |
| 14 | 8,192 | 16,383 |
| 15 | 16,384 | 32,767 |
| 16 | 32,768 | 65,535 |
| 17 | 65,536 | 131,071 |
| 18 | 131,072 | 262,143 |

For example, if a patient was to receive a total dose of 4000 units, he/she would receive injections 1 through 12 during the desensitization

**Mechanism of Action** Some malignant cells (ie, lymphoblastic leukemia cells and those of lymphocyte derivation) must acquire the amino acid asparagine from surrounding fluid such as blood, whereas normal cells can synthesize their own asparagine. asparaginase is an enzyme that deaminates asparagine to aspartic acid and ammonia in the plasma and extracellular fluid and therefore deprives tumor cells of the amino acid for protein synthesis.

There are two purified preparations of the enzyme, one from *Escherichia coli* and one from *Erwinia carotovora.* These two preparations vary slightly in the gene sequencing and have slight differences in enzyme characteristics. Both are highly specific for asparagine and have less than 10% activity for the D-isomer. The preparation from *E. coli* has had the most use in clinical and research practice.

**Local Anesthetic/Vasoconstrictor Precautions** No information available to require special precautions

**Effects on Dental Treatment** No effects or complications reported

**Other Adverse Effects**

>10%:

Gastrointestinal: Pancreatitis occurs in <15% of patients but may progress to severe hemorrhagic pancreatitis

Miscellaneous: Hypersensitivity and anaphylactic reactions occur in ~10% to 40% of patients and can be fatal. This reaction is more common in patients receiving asparaginase alone or by I.V. administration. Hypersensitivity appears rarely with the first dose and more commonly after the second or third treatment. Hypersensitivity may be treated with antihistamines and/or steroids. If an anaphylactic reaction occurs, a change in treatment to the *Erwinia* preparation may be made, since this preparation does not share antigenic cross-reactivity with the *E. coli* preparation. Note that allergic reactions to the *Erwinia* preparation may also occur and ultimately develop in 5% to 20% of patients.

1% to 10%:

Endocrine & metabolic: Hyperuricemia

Gastrointestinal: Mouth sores

<1%:

Cardiovascular: Hypotension

Central nervous system: Disorientation, drowsiness, seizures, and coma which may be due to elevated $NH_4$ levels, hyperthermia, fever, malaise, chills

Dermatologic: Urticaria, rash, pruritus

Endocrine & metabolic: Transient diabetes mellitus

Gastrointestinal: Weight loss

Hematologic: Inhibition of protein synthesis will cause a decrease in production of albumin, insulin (resulting in hyperglycemia), serum lipoprotein, antithrombin III, and clotting factors II, V, VII, VIII, IX, and X. Leg vein thrombosis. The loss of the later two proteins may result in either thrombotic or hemorrhagic events; these protein losses occur in 100% of patients.

(Continued)

## Asparaginase *(Continued)*

Hepatic: Elevated serum bilirubin, ST, alkaline phosphatase, and possible decrease in mobilization of lipids

Renal: Azotemia

Respiratory: Coughing, laryngeal spasm

**Drug Uptake**

Absorption: Not absorbed from GI tract, therefore, requires parenteral administration; I.M. administration produces peak blood levels 50% lower than those from I.V. administration (I.M. may be less immunogenic)

Serum half-life: 8-30 hours

**Pregnancy Risk Factor** C

**Generic Available** No

**Comments** Myelosuppressive effects:

WBC: Mild

Platelets: Mild

Onset (days): 7

Nadir (days): 14

Recovery (days): 21

- **A-Spas® S/L** *see* Hyoscyamine *on page 519*
- **Aspergum® [OTC]** *see* Aspirin *on this page*

## Aspirin (AS pir in)

**Related Information**

Butalbital Compound and Aspirin *on page 165*

Cardiovascular Diseases *on page 1066*

Carisoprodol and Aspirin *on page 192*

Dental Drug Interactions: Update on Drug Combinations Requiring Special Considerations *on page 1225*

Oral Pain *on page 1122*

Rheumatoid Arthritis and Osteoarthritis *on page 1092*

**U.S. Brand Names** Anacin® [OTC]; Arthritis Foundation® Pain Reliever [OTC]; A.S.A. [OTC]; Ascriptin® [OTC]; Aspergum® [OTC]; Asprimox® [OTC]; Bayer® Aspirin [OTC]; Bayer® Buffered Aspirin [OTC]; Bayer® Low Adult Strength [OTC]; Bufferin® [OTC]; Buffex® [OTC]; Cama® Arthritis Pain Reliever [OTC]; Easprin®; Ecotrin® [OTC]; Ecotrin® Low Adult Strength [OTC]; Empirin® [OTC]; Extra Strength Adprin-B® [OTC]; Extra Strength Bayer® Enteric 500 Aspirin [OTC]; Extra Strength Bayer® Plus [OTC]; Halfprin® 81® [OTC]; Regular Strength Bayer® Enteric 500 Aspirin [OTC]; St Joseph® Adult Chewable Aspirin [OTC]; ZORprin®

**Canadian Brand Names** Apo®-ASA; ASA®; Asaphen; Entrophen®; MSD® Enteric Coated ASA; Novasen

**Therapeutic Category** Analgesic, Non-narcotic; Anti-inflammatory Agent; Antipyretic; Platelet Aggregation Inhibitor

**Use**

Dental: Treatment of postoperative pain

Medical: Treatment of pain and fever; may be used as prophylaxis of myocardial infarction and transient ischemic episodes; management of rheumatoid arthritis, rheumatic fever, osteoarthritis, and gout (high dose)

Aspirin is recommended for use in men and women to treat transient ischemic attack, ischemic stroke, angina, acute myocardial infarction (MI), recurrent MI, specific revascularization procedures, and rheumatologic diseases. To minimize adverse events, low dosages (50-325 mg) are recommended for cardiac and cerebrovascular users (75-325 mg for angina and previous heart attack users).

**Usual Dosage** Analgesic: Oral:

Children: 10-15 mg/kg/dose every 4-6 hours, up to a total of 60-80 mg/kg/24 hours

Adults: 325-650 mg (1-2 tablets) every 4-6 hours, up to 4 g/day

**Mechanism of Action** Inhibits prostaglandin synthesis by decreasing the activity of the enzyme, cyclo-oxygenase, which results in decreased formation of prostaglandin precursors, acts on the hypothalamic heat-regulating center to reduce fever, blocks thromboxane synthetase action which prevents formation of the platelet-aggregating substance thromboxane $A_2$

**Local Anesthetic/Vasoconstrictor Precautions** No information available to require special precautions

**Effects on Dental Treatment** Avoid aspirin if possible, for 1 week prior to surgery because of the possibility of postoperative bleeding

**Other Adverse Effects**

>10%: Gastrointestinal: Nausea, vomiting, dyspepsia, epigastric discomfort, heartburn, stomach pains

1% to 10%: Gastrointestinal: Ulceration

Aspirin allergy (incidence is 0.2%): Asthmatic syndrome, wheezing, bronchiolar constriction

**Contraindications** Bleeding disorders (factor VII or IX deficiencies), hypersensitivity to salicylates or other NSAIDs, tartrazine dye and asthma

**Warnings/Precautions** Use with caution in patients with platelet and bleeding disorders, renal dysfunction, erosive gastritis, or peptic ulcer disease, previous nonreaction does not guarantee future safe taking of medication; do not use aspirin in children <16 years of age for chickenpox or flu symptoms due to the association with Reye's syndrome

Avoid aspirin if possible, for 1 week prior to surgery because of the possibility of postoperative bleeding; use with caution in impaired hepatic function

Elderly are a high-risk population for adverse effects from nonsteroidal anti-inflammatory agents. As much as 60% of elderly with GI complications to NSAIDs can develop peptic ulceration and/or hemorrhage asymptomatically. Also, concomitant disease and drug use contribute to the risk for GI adverse effects. Use lowest effective dose for shortest period possible. Consider renal function decline with age. Use with caution in patients with history of asthma

**Drug Interactions**

Aspirin:

- Warfarin (Coumadin®): Aspirin in normal doses increases the risk of bleeding in anticoagulate patients by inhibition of platelet function; larger doses of aspirin enhance the hypoprothrombinemic response to warfarin
- Acetazolamide (Diamox®): Aspirin increases the plasma concentration of acetazolamide by displacement from plasma protein binding sites. These have resulted in central nervous system toxicity due to higher levels of acetazolamide
- Methotrexate: Salicylates block the renal tubular secretion of methotrexate to result in methotrexate toxicity (hepatotoxicity)
- NSAIDs: Aspirin may cause a reduction in serum levels of NSAIDs

**Drug Uptake**

Absorption: Rapid

Serum half-life:

- Parent drug: 15-20 minutes
- Salicylates (dose-dependent): From 3 hours at lower doses (300-600 mg), to 5-6 hours (after 1 g) to 10 hours with higher doses

Time to peak serum concentration: ~1-2 hours

**Pregnancy Risk Factor** C (D if full-dose aspirin in 3rd trimester)

**Breast-feeding Considerations** Use cautiously due to potential adverse effects in nursing infants

**Dosage Forms**

Capsule: 356.4 mg and caffeine 30 mg

Suppository, rectal: 60 mg, 120 mg, 125 mg, 130 mg, 195 mg, 200 mg, 300 mg, 325 mg, 600 mg, 650 mg, 1.2 g

Tablet: 65 mg, 75 mg, 81 mg, 325 mg, 500 mg

Tablet: 400 mg and caffeine 32 mg

Tablet:

- Buffered: 325 mg and magnesium-aluminum hydroxide 150 mg; 325 mg, magnesium hydroxide 75 mg, aluminum hydroxide 75 mg, buffered with calcium carbonate; 325 mg and magnesium-aluminum hydroxide 75 mg
- Chewable: 81 mg
- Controlled release: 800 mg
- Delayed release: 81 mg
- Enteric coated: 81 mg, 325 mg, 500 mg, 650 mg, 975 mg
- Gum: 227.5 mg
- Timed release: 650 mg

**Dietary Considerations** Should be taken with water, food, or milk to decrease GI effects; food decreases rate but not extent of absorption (oral)

**Generic Available** Yes

**Comments** Anti-inflammatory actions of aspirin are not seen clinically at doses <3500 mg/day. Patients taking one aspirin tablet daily as an antithrombotic and who require dental surgery should be given special consideration in consultation with the physician before removal of the aspirin relative to prevention of postoperative bleeding.

**Selected Readings**

Desjardins PJ, Cooper SA, Gallegos TL, et al, "The Relative Analgesic Efficacy of Propiram Fumarate, Codeine Aspirin, and Placebo in Post-Impaction Dental Pain," *J Clin Pharmacol*, 1984, 24(1):35-42.

Forbes JA, Butterworth GA, Burchfield WH, et al, "Evaluation of Ketorolac, Aspirin, and an Acetaminophen-Codeine Combination in Postoperative Oral Surgery Pain," *Pharmacotherapy*, 1990, 10(6 Pt 2):77S-93S.

Forbes JA, Keller CK, Smith JW, et al, "Analgesic Effect of Naproxen Sodium, Codeine, a Naproxen-Codeine Combination and Aspirin on the Postoperative Pain of Oral Surgery," *Pharmacotherapy*, 1986, 6(5):211-8.

(Continued)

## Aspirin *(Continued)*

Hurlen M, Erikssen J, Smith P, et al, "Comparison of Bleeding Complications of Warfarin and Warfarin Plus Acetylsalicylic Acid: A Study in 3166 Outpatients," *J Intern Med*, 1994, 236(3):299-304.

## Aspirin and Codeine (AS pir in & KOE deen)

**Related Information**

Dental Drug Interactions: Update on Drug Combinations Requiring Special Considerations *on page 1225*

Oral Pain *on page 1122*

**U.S. Brand Names** Empirin® With Codeine

**Canadian Brand Names** Coryphen® Codeine; 222® Tablets; 282® Tablets; 292® Tablets

**Therapeutic Category** Analgesic, Narcotic

**Use**

Dental: Treatment of postoperative pain

Medical: Relief of pain

**Restrictions** C-III; Refillable up to 5 times in 6 months

**Usual Dosage** Oral:

Children: Not recommended in pediatric dental patients

Adults: 1-2 tablets every 4-6 hours as needed for pain; maximum: 12 tablets over 24 hours

**Mechanism of Action** Aspirin inhibits prostaglandin synthesis, acts on the hypothalamus heat-regulating center to reduce fever, blocks prostaglandin synthetase action which prevents formation of the platelet-aggregating substance thromboxane $A_2$; codeine binds to opiate receptors (mu and kappa subtypes) in the CNS causing inhibition of ascending pain pathways, altering the perception of and response to pain

**Local Anesthetic/Vasoconstrictor Precautions** No information available to require special precautions

**Effects on Dental Treatment** <1% of patients may experience dry mouth; avoid aspirin, if possible, for 1 week prior to surgery because of the possibility of postoperative bleeding

Use with caution in impaired hepatic function; use with caution in patients with platelet and bleeding disorders, renal dysfunction, erosive gastritis, or peptic ulcer disease, previous nonreaction does not guarantee future safe taking of medication; do not use aspirin in children <16 years of age for chickenpox or flu symptoms due to the association with Reye's syndrome

Avoid aspirin if possible, for 1 week prior to surgery because of the possibility of postoperative bleeding; use with caution in impaired hepatic function

Elderly are a high-risk population for adverse effects from nonsteroidal anti-inflammatory agents. As much as 60% of elderly with GI complications to NSAIDs can develop peptic ulceration and/or hemorrhage asymptomatically. Also, concomitant disease and drug use contribute to the risk for GI adverse effects. Use lowest effective dose for shortest period possible. Consider renal function decline with age. Use with caution in patients with history of asthma.

**Other Adverse Effects**

>10%:

- Central nervous system: Lightheadedness, dizziness, sedation, depression
- Gastrointestinal: Nausea, heartburn, stomach pains, dyspepsia, epigastric discomfort, vomiting

1% to 10%: Gastrointestinal: Ulceration, constipation

Aspirin allergy (incidence is 0.2%): Asthmatic syndrome, wheezing, bronchiolar constriction

**Contraindications** Hypersensitivity to aspirin or codeine

**Warnings/Precautions** Use with caution in patients with impaired renal function, erosive gastritis, or peptic ulcer disease

Enhanced analgesia has been seen in elderly patients on therapeutic doses of narcotics; duration of action may be increased in the elderly; the elderly may be particularly susceptible to the CNS depressant and constipating effects of narcotics

**Drug Interactions**

Aspirin:

- Warfarin (Coumadin®): Aspirin in normal doses increases the risk of bleeding in anticoagulate patients by inhibition of platelet function; larger doses of aspirin enhance the hypoprothrombinemic response to warfarin
- Acetazolamide (Diamox®): Aspirin increases the plasma concentration of acetazolamide by displacement from plasma protein binding sites. These have resulted in central nervous system toxicity due to higher levels of acetazolamide

Methotrexate: Salicylates block the renal tubular secretion of methotrexate to result in methotrexate toxicity (hepatotoxicity)

NSAIDs: Aspirin may cause a reduction in serum levels of NSAIDs

Codeine: Increased toxicity when given with CNS depressants, phenothiazines, tricyclic antidepressants (TCAs), other narcotic analgesics, MAO inhibitors

**Drug Uptake**

Aspirin:

Absorption: Rapid

Serum half-life:

Parent drug: 15-20 minutes

Salicylates (dose-dependent): From 3 hours at lower doses (300-600 mg), to 5-6 hours (after 1 g) to 10 hours with higher doses

Time to peak serum concentration: ~1-2 hours

Codeine:

Onset of effect: 0.5-1 hour

Duration of effect: 4-6 hours

Serum half-life: 2.5-3.5 hours

Time to peak serum concentration: 1-1.5 hours

**Pregnancy Risk Factor** D

**Breast-feeding Considerations**

Aspirin: Cautious use due to potential adverse effects in nursing infants

Codeine: Codeine not contraindicated with breast-feeding

**Dosage Forms** Tablet:

#2: Aspirin 325 mg and codeine phosphate 15 mg

#3: Aspirin 325 mg and codeine phosphate 30 mg

#4: Aspirin 325 mg and codeine phosphate 60 mg

**Dietary Considerations** May be taken with food or milk to minimize GI distress; food decreases rate but not extent of absorption (oral)

**Generic Available** Yes

**Comments** Codeine products, as with other narcotic analgesics, are recommended only for limited acute dosing (ie, 3 days or less). The most common adverse effect you will see in your dental patients from codeine is nausea, followed by sedation and constipation. Codeine has narcotic addiction liability, especially when given long term. The aspirin component has anticoagulant effects and can affect bleeding times.

**Selected Readings**

Dionne RA, "New Approaches to Preventing and Treating Postoperative Pain," *J Am Dent Assoc*, 1992, 123(6):26-34.

Gobetti JP, "Controlling Dental Pain," *J Am Dent Assoc*, 1992, 123(6):47-52.

## Aspirin and Meprobamate (AS pir in & me proe BA mate)

**U.S. Brand Names** Equagesic®

**Canadian Brand Names** 292 MEP®

**Therapeutic Category** Skeletal Muscle Relaxant

**Synonyms** Meprobamate and Aspirin

**Use** Adjunct to treatment of skeletal muscular disease in patients exhibiting tension and/or anxiety

**Usual Dosage** Oral: 1 tablet 3-4 times/day

**Local Anesthetic/Vasoconstrictor Precautions** No information available to require special precautions

**Effects on Dental Treatment** Avoid aspirin if possible, for 1 week prior to surgery because of the possibility of postoperative bleeding

Use with caution in impaired hepatic function; use with caution in patients with platelet and bleeding disorders, renal dysfunction, erosive gastritis, or peptic ulcer disease, previous nonreaction does not guarantee future safe taking of medication; do not use aspirin in children <16 years of age for chickenpox or flu symptoms due to the association with Reye's syndrome

Elderly are a high-risk population for adverse effects from nonsteroidal anti-inflammatory agents. As much as 60% of elderly with GI complications to NSAIDs can develop peptic ulceration and/or hemorrhage asymptomatically. Also, concomitant disease and drug use contribute to the risk for GI adverse effects. Use lowest effective dose for shortest period possible. Consider renal function decline with age. Use with caution in patients with history of asthma

**Other Adverse Effects** See individual agents

**Pregnancy Risk Factor** D

**Generic Available** Yes

**Comments** Abrupt discontinuation after sustained use (generally >10 days) may cause withdrawal symptoms

**Selected Readings**

Desjardins PJ, Cooper SA, Gallegos TL, et al, "The Relative Analgesic Efficacy of Propiram Fumarate, Codeine Aspirin, and Placebo in Post-Impaction Dental Pain," *J Clin Pharmacol*, 1984, 24(1):35-42.

(Continued)

## Aspirin and Meprobamate *(Continued)*

Forbes JA, Butterworth GA, Burchfield WH, et al, "Evaluation of Ketorolac, Aspirin, and an Acetaminophen-Codeine Combination in Postoperative Oral Surgery Pain," *Pharmacotherapy*, 1990, 10(6 Pt 2):77S-93S.

Forbes JA, Keller CK, Smith JW, et al, "Analgesic Effect of Naproxen Sodium, Codeine, a Naproxen-Codeine Combination and Aspirin on the Postoperative Pain of Oral Surgery," *Pharmacotherapy*, 1986, 6(5):211-8.

- **Aspirin Free Anacin® Maximum Strength [OTC]** *see* Acetaminophen *on page 27*
- **Aspirin-Free Bayer® Select® Allergy Sinus Caplets [OTC]** *see* Acetaminophen, Chlorpheniramine, and Pseudoephedrine *on page 32*
- **Asprimox® [OTC]** *see* Aspirin *on page 100*
- **Astelin®** *see* Azelastine *on page 113*

## Astemizole (a STEM mi zole)

**U.S. Brand Names** Hismanal®

**Therapeutic Category** Antihistamine

**Use** Perennial and seasonal allergic rhinitis and other allergic symptoms including urticaria

**Usual Dosage** Oral:

Children:

<6 years: 0.2 mg/kg/day

6-12 years: 5 mg/day

Children >12 years and Adults: 10-30 mg/day; give 30 mg on first day, 20 mg on second day, then 10 mg/day in a single dose

**Mechanism of Action** Competes with histamine for $H_1$-receptor sites on effector cells in the gastrointestinal tract, blood vessels, and respiratory tract; binds to lung receptors significantly greater than it binds to cerebellar receptors, resulting in a reduced sedative potential

**Local Anesthetic/Vasoconstrictor Precautions** No information available to require special precautions

**Effects on Dental Treatment** Up to 10% of patients taking astemizole may have significant dry mouth which will disappear with cessation of drug therapy; no erythromycin products or antifungals (ketoconazole, itraconazole) should be given since cardiotoxicities could occur (See respective monographs in Dental Drug Monographs section)

**Other Adverse Effects**

1% to 10%:

Central nervous system: Drowsiness, headache, fatigue, nervousness, dizziness

Gastrointestinal: Appetite increase, weight increase, nausea, diarrhea, abdominal pain, dry mouth

Neuromuscular & skeletal: Arthralgia

Respiratory: Pharyngitis

<1%:

Cardiovascular: Palpitations, edema

Central nervous system: Depression

Dermatologic: Angioedema, photosensitivity, rash

Hepatic: Hepatitis

Neuromuscular & skeletal: Myalgia, paresthesia

Respiratory: Bronchospasm, epistaxis, thickening of mucous

**Contraindications** Patients with severe hepatic impairment; contraindicated with coadministration of clarithromycin, troleandomycin, serotonin reuptake inhibitors, protease inhibitors, zileuton, and grapefruit juice

**Drug Interactions** Increased toxicity: CNS depressants (sedation), triazole antifungals (ie, ketoconazole, miconazole, fluconazole - torsade de pointes and other cardiotoxicities have been reported), macrolide antibiotics (ie, erythromycin, clarithromycin - cardiotoxicity)

**Drug Uptake** Long-acting, with steady-state plasma levels seen within 4-8 weeks following initiation of chronic therapy

Serum half-life: 20 hours

Time to peak serum concentration: Oral: Long-acting, with steady-state plasma levels of parent compound and metabolites seen within 4-8 weeks following initiation of chronic therapy; peak plasma levels appear in 1-4 hours following administration

**Pregnancy Risk Factor** C

**Dosage Forms** Tablet: 10 mg

**Dietary Considerations** Should be taken on an empty stomach; do not take with grapefruit juice

**Generic Available** No

- **AsthmaNefrin®** *see* Epinephrine, Racemic *on page 375*

♦ **Astramorph™ PF Injection** *see* Morphine Sulfate *on page 688*
♦ **Atacand™** *see* Candesartan *on page 179*
♦ **Atarax®** *see* Hydroxyzine *on page 518*

# Atenolol (a TEN oh lole)

**Related Information**

Cardiovascular Diseases *on page 1066*

**U.S. Brand Names** Tenormin®

**Canadian Brand Names** Apo®-Atenol; Novo-Atenol; Nu-Atenol; Taro-Atenol®

**Therapeutic Category** Antianginal Agent; Beta-adrenergic Blocker, Cardioselective

**Use** Treatment of hypertension, alone or in combination with other agents; management of angina pectoris, postmyocardial infarction patients

**Unlabeled use:** Acute alcohol withdrawal, supraventricular and ventricular arrhythmias, and migraine headache prophylaxis

**Usual Dosage**

Oral:

Children: 1-2 mg/kg/dose given daily

Adults:

Hypertension: 50 mg once daily, may increase to 100 mg/day; doses >100 mg are unlikely to produce any further benefit

Angina pectoris: 50 mg once daily, may increase to 100 mg/day; some patients may require 200 mg/day

Postmyocardial infarction: Follow I.V. dose with 100 mg/day or 50 mg twice daily for 6-9 days postmyocardial infarction

I.V.: Postmyocardial infarction: Early treatment: 5 mg slow I.V. over 5 minutes; may repeat in 10 minutes; if both doses are tolerated, may start oral atenolol 50 mg every 12 hours or 100 mg/day for 6-9 days postmyocardial infarction

**Mechanism of Action** Competitively blocks response to beta-adrenergic stimulation, selectively blocks beta$_1$-receptors with little or no effect on beta$_2$-receptors except at high doses

**Local Anesthetic/Vasoconstrictor Precautions** No information available to require special precautions

**Effects on Dental Treatment** Noncardioselective beta-blockers (ie, propranolol, nadolol) enhance the pressor response to epinephrine, resulting in hypertension and bradycardia. This has not been reported for atenolol, a cardioselective beta-blocker. Therefore, local anesthetic with vasoconstrictor can be safely used in patients medicated with atenolol. Many nonsteroidal anti-inflammatory drugs such as ibuprofen and indomethacin can reduce the hypotensive effect of beta-blockers after 3 or more weeks of therapy with the NSAID. Short-term NSAID use (ie, 3 days) requires no special precautions in patients taking beta-blockers.

**Other Adverse Effects**

1% to 10%:

Cardiovascular: Persistent bradycardia, hypotension, chest pain, edema, heart failure, second or third degree A-V block, Raynaud's phenomenon

Central nervous system: Dizziness, fatigue, insomnia, lethargy, confusion, mental impairment, depression, headache, nightmares

Gastrointestinal: Constipation, diarrhea, nausea

Genitourinary: Impotence

<1%:

Respiratory: Dyspnea (especially with large doses), wheezing

Miscellaneous: Cold extremities

**Drug Interactions**

Decreased effect of beta-blockers:

Barbiturates (increased liver metabolism of beta-blockers to result in lower serum levels)

NSAIDs (attenuate the hypotensive therapeutic effects of beta-blockers)

Rifampin (increased liver metabolism of beta-blockers to result in lower serum levels)

Increased effects of beta-blockers:

Calcium channel blockers (increase serum levels by unknown mechanism to enhance hypotension)

Beta-blockers increase the effects of:

Epinephrine (vasoconstrictor; initial hypotensive episode followed by bradycardia) only from noncardioselective type beta-blockers

Phenylephrine (Neosynephrine®; enhanced pressor response)

Theophylline (inhibit theophylline metabolism causing increase in serum concentrations)

**Drug Uptake**

Absorption: Incomplete from GI tract

(Continued)

## Atenolol *(Continued)*

Serum half-life, beta:

Adults:

Normal renal function: 6-9 hours, longer in those with renal impairment

End-stage renal disease: 15-35 hours

Time to peak: Oral: Within 2-4 hours

**Pregnancy Risk Factor** C

**Generic Available** Yes

**Selected Readings**

Foster CA and Aston SJ, "Propranolol-Epinephrine Interaction: A Potential Disaster," *Plast Reconstr Surg*, 1983, 72(1):74-8.
Wong DG, Spence JD, Lamki L, et al, "Effect of Nonsteroidal Anti-inflammatory Drugs on Control of Hypertension of Beta-Blockers and Diuretics," *Lancet*, 1986, 1(8488):997-1001.
Wynn RL, "Dental Nonsteroidal Anti-inflammatory Drugs and Prostaglandin-Based Drug Interactions-Part Two," *Gen Dent*, 1992, 40(2):104, 106, 108.
Wynn RL, "Epinephrine Interactions With Beta-Blockers," *Gen Dent*, 1994, 42(1):16, 18.

## Atenolol and Chlorthalidone (a TEN oh lole & klor THAL i done)

**U.S. Brand Names** Tenoretic®

**Therapeutic Category** Antihypertensive Agent, Combination

**Use** Treatment of hypertension with a cardioselective beta-blocker and a diuretic

**Usual Dosage** Adults: Oral: Initial: One (50) tablet once daily, then individualize dose until optimal dose is achieved

**Local Anesthetic/Vasoconstrictor Precautions** No information available to require special precautions

**Effects on Dental Treatment** Noncardioselective beta-blockers (ie, propranolol, nadolol) enhance the pressor response to epinephrine, resulting in hypertension and bradycardia. This has not been reported for atenolol, a cardioselective beta-blocker. Therefore local anesthetic with vasoconstrictor can be safely used in patients medicated with atenolol. Many nonsteroidal anti-inflammatory drugs such as ibuprofen and indomethacin can reduce the hypotensive effect of beta-blockers after 3 or more weeks of therapy with the NSAID. Short-term NSAID use (ie, 3 days) requires no special precautions in patients taking beta-blockers.

**Other Adverse Effects** See individual agents

**Pregnancy Risk Factor** D

**Generic Available** Yes

**Comments** May contain povidone as inactive ingredient

**Selected Readings**

Foster CA and Aston SJ, "Propranolol-Epinephrine Interaction: A Potential Disaster," *Plast Reconstr Surg*, 1983, 72(1):74-8.
Wong DG, Spence JD, Lamki L, et al, "Effect of Nonsteroidal Anti-inflammatory Drugs on Control of Hypertension of Beta-Blockers and Diuretics," *Lancet*, 1986, 1(8488):997-1001.
Wynn RL, "Dental Nonsteroidal Anti-inflammatory Drugs and Prostaglandin-Based Drug Interactions-Part Two," *Gen Dent*, 1992, 40(2):104, 106, 108.
Wynn RL, "Epinephrine Interactions With Beta-Blockers," *Gen Dent*, 1994, 42(1):16, 18.

♦ **ATG** *see* Lymphocyte Immune Globulin *on page 608*
♦ **Atgam®** *see* Lymphocyte Immune Globulin *on page 608*
♦ **ATIII** *see* Antithrombin III *on page 92*
♦ **Ativan®** *see* Lorazepam *on page 602*
♦ **ATnativ®** *see* Antithrombin III *on page 92*
♦ **Atolone®** *see* Triamcinolone *on page 1010*

## Atorvastatin (a TORE va sta tin)

**U.S. Brand Names** Lipitor®

**Therapeutic Category** HMG-CoA Reductase Inhibitor

**Use** Adjunct to diet for the reduction of elevated total and LDL-cholesterol levels in patients with hypercholesterolemia (Type IIa, IIb, and IIc); used in hypercholesterolemic patients without clinically evident heart disease to reduce the risk of myocardial infarction, to reduce the risk for revascularization, and reduce the risk of death due to cardiovascular causes with no increase in death from noncardiovascular diseases; as adjunctive therapy to diet for the treatment of patients with elevated serum triglyceride levels (Frederickson Type IV); also used in patients with primary dysbetalipoproteinemia (Frederickson Type III) who do not respond adequately to diet

**Usual Dosage** Adults: Oral: Initial: 10 mg once daily, titrate up to 80 mg/day if needed

**Mechanism of Action** Inhibitor of 3-hydroxy-3-methylglutaryl coenzyme A (HMG-CoA) reductase, the rate limiting enzyme in cholesterol synthesis (reduces the production of mevalonic acid from HMG-CoA); this then results in a compensatory increase in the expression of LDL receptors on hepatocyte membranes and a stimulation of LDL catabolism

**Local Anesthetic/Vasoconstrictor Precautions** No information available to require special precautions

**Effects on Dental Treatment** No effects or complications reported

**Other Adverse Effects**

>1%:

Central nervous system: Headache

Gastrointestinal: Diarrhea, flatulence, abdominal pain (2% to 3%)

Neuromuscular & skeletal: Myalgia (1% to 5%)

<1%:

Central nervous system: Giddiness, euphoria, mild confusion, impaired short-term memory

Hepatic: Mild LFT increases

Respiratory: Pharyngitis, rhinitis

**Drug Interactions**

Increased toxicity: Gemfibrozil (musculoskeletal effects such as myopathy, myalgia and/or muscle weakness accompanied by markedly elevated CK concentrations, rash and/or pruritus); clofibrate, niacin (myopathy), erythromycin, cyclosporine, oral anticoagulants (elevated PT)

Increased effect/toxicity of levothyroxine

Concurrent use of erythromycin and atorvastatin may result in rhabdomyolysis

According to manufacturer's information, there is an increased risk of muscle weakness and breakdown when using erythromycin and azole antifungals with atorvastatin

Erythromycin caused higher sustained blood levels of atorvastatin

**Drug Uptake**

Serum half-life: 14 hours (parent)

Time to peak serum concentration: 1-2 hours (maximal reduction in plasma cholesterol and triglycerides in 2 weeks)

**Pregnancy Risk Factor** X

**Generic Available** No

**Selected Readings**

"Atorvastatin Pharmacokinetic Interactions With Other CYP3A4 Substrates: Erythromycin and Ethinyl Estradiol," *Pharmacol Res*, 1996, 13:5437.

## Atovaquone (a TOE va kwone)

**Related Information**

Systemic Viral Diseases *on page 1115*

**U.S. Brand Names** Mepron™

**Therapeutic Category** Antiprotozoal

**Use** Acute oral treatment of mild to moderate *Pneumocystis carinii* pneumonia (PCP) in patients who are intolerant to co-trimoxazole

**Usual Dosage** Adults: Oral: 750 mg 2 times/day with food for 21 days

**Mechanism of Action** Mechanism has not been fully elucidated; may inhibit electron transport in mitochondria inhibiting metabolic enzymes

**Local Anesthetic/Vasoconstrictor Precautions** No information available to require special precautions

**Effects on Dental Treatment** No effects or complications reported

**Other Adverse Effects**

>10%:

Central nervous system: Headache, fever, insomnia, anxiety

Dermatologic: Rash

Gastrointestinal: Nausea, diarrhea, vomiting

Respiratory: Cough

1% to 10%:

Central nervous system: Dizziness

Dermatologic: Pruritus

Endocrine & metabolic: Hypoglycemia, hyponatremia

Gastrointestinal: Abdominal pain, constipation, anorexia, dyspepsia

Hematologic: Anemia, neutropenia, leukopenia

Hepatic: Elevated amylase and liver enzymes

Neuromuscular & skeletal: Weakness

Renal: Elevated creatinine and BUN

Miscellaneous: Oral *Monilia*

**Drug Interactions** No data reported

**Drug Uptake**

Absorption: Decreased significantly in single doses >750 mg; increased threefold when administered with a high-fat meal

Serum half-life: 2.9 days

**Pregnancy Risk Factor** C

**Generic Available** No

- **Atridox™** *see* Doxycycline Hyclate Periodontal Extended-Release Liquid *on page 356*
- **Atrohist® Plus** *see* Chlorpheniramine, Phenylephrine, Phenylpropanolamine, and Belladonna Alkaloids *on page 236*
- **Atromid-S®** *see* Clofibrate *on page 262*
- **Atropair®** *see* Atropine *on this page*

## Atropine (A troe peen)

**Related Information**

Cardiovascular Diseases *on page 1066*

**U.S. Brand Names** Atropair®; Atropine-Care®; Atropisol®; Isopto® Atropine; I-Tropine®

**Therapeutic Category** Anticholinergic Agent; Anticholinergic Agent, Ophthalmic; Antidote, Organophosphate Poisoning; Antispasmodic Agent, Gastrointestinal; Bronchodilator; Ophthalmic Agent, Mydriatic

**Use** Medical: Treatment of sinus bradycardia; management of peptic ulcer; treat exercise-induced bronchospasm; antidote for organophosphate pesticide poisoning; produce mydriasis and cycloplegia for examination of the retina and optic disc and accurate measurement of refractive errors; uveitis

**Usual Dosage** Preanesthetic: I.M., I.V., S.C.:

Children:

- <5 kg: 0.02 mg/kg/dose 30-60 minutes preop then every 4-6 hours as needed
- >5 kg: 0.01-0.02 mg/kg/dose to a maximum 0.4 mg 30-60 minutes preop; minimum dose: 0.1 mg

Adults: 0.4-0.6 mg 30-60 minutes preop and repeat every 4-6 hours as needed

**Mechanism of Action** Blocks the action of acetylcholine at parasympathetic sites in smooth muscle, secretory glands, and the CNS; increases cardiac output, dries secretions, antagonizes histamine and serotonin

**Local Anesthetic/Vasoconstrictor Precautions** No information available to require special precautions

**Effects on Dental Treatment** >10% of patients experience dry mouth

**Other Adverse Effects**

>10%:

- Dermatologic: Dry skin
- Gastrointestinal: Constipation, dry throat
- Local: Irritation at injection site
- Respiratory: Dry nose
- Miscellaneous: Decreased sweating

1% to 10%:

- Endocrine & metabolic: Decreased flow of breast milk
- Gastrointestinal: Dysphagia
- Ocular: Photosensitivity

**Contraindications** Hypersensitivity to atropine sulfate or any component; angle-closure glaucoma; tachycardia; thyrotoxicosis; obstructive disease of the GI tract; obstructive uropathy; contraindicated with clarithromycin, erythromycin, ketoconazole, fluconazole, and itraconazole

**Warnings/Precautions** Use with caution in children with spastic paralysis; use with caution in elderly patients. Low doses cause a paradoxical decrease in heart rates. Some commercial products contain sodium metabisulfite, which can cause allergic-type reactions. May accumulate with multiple inhalational administration, particularly in the elderly. Heat prostration may occur in hot weather. Use with caution in patients with autonomic neuropathy, prostatic hypertrophy, hyperthyroidism, congestive heart failure, cardiac arrhythmias, chronic lung disease, biliary tract disease.

**Drug Interactions** Decreased effect of phenothiazines, levodopa, cisapride, methacholine, haloperidol; increased anticholinergic effects of amantadine, phenothiazines, TCAs, meperidine, antihistamines, quinidine, MAO inhibitors

**Drug Uptake**

Absorption: Well absorbed from all dosage forms

Serum half-life: 2-3 hours

**Pregnancy Risk Factor** C

**Breast-feeding Considerations** May be taken while breast-feeding

**Dosage Forms** Injection: 0.05 mg/mL (5 mL); 0.1 mg/mL (5 mL, 10 mL); 0.3 mg/mL (1 mL, 30 mL); 0.4 mg/mL (1 mL, 20 mL, 30 mL); 0.5 mg/mL (1 mL, 5 mL, 30 mL); 0.8 mg/mL (0.5 mL, 1 mL); 1 mg/mL (1 mL, 10 mL)

**Dietary Considerations** No data reported

**Generic Available** Yes

- **Atropine-Care®** *see* Atropine *on this page*
- **Atropisol®** *see* Atropine *on this page*
- **Atrovent®** *see* Ipratropium *on page 547*
- **A/T/S® Topical** *see* Erythromycin, Topical *on page 386*

## Attapulgite (at a PULL gite)

**Related Information**

Oral Nonviral Soft Tissue Ulcerations or Erosions *on page 1141*

**U.S. Brand Names** Children's Kaopectate® [OTC]; Diasorb® [OTC]; Kaopectate® Advanced Formula [OTC]; Kaopectate® Maximum Strength Caplets; Rheaban® [OTC]

**Therapeutic Category** Antidiarrheal

**Use** Symptomatic treatment of diarrhea

**Usual Dosage** Oral:

Children:

<3 years: Not recommended

3-6 years: 750 mg/dose up to 2250 mg/24 hours

6-12 years: 1200-1500 mg/dose up to 4500 mg/24 hours

Adults: 1200-1500 mg after each loose bowel movement or every 2 hours; 15-30 mL up to 8 times/day, up to 9000 mg/24 hours

**Mechanism of Action** Controls diarrhea because of its absorbent action

**Local Anesthetic/Vasoconstrictor Precautions** No information available to require special precautions

**Effects on Dental Treatment** Do not give oral drugs concomitantly with Kaopectate® due to decreased GI absorption

**Other Adverse Effects** The powder, if chronically inhaled, can cause pneumoconiosis, since it contains large amounts of silica

1% to 10%: Constipation (dose related)

<1%: Fecal impaction

**Drug Interactions** Decreased GI absorption of orally administered clindamycin, tetracyclines, penicillamine, digoxin

**Drug Uptake** Absorption: Not absorbed from GI tract

**Pregnancy Risk Factor** B

**Generic Available** Yes

♦ **Attenuvax®** *see* Measles Virus Vaccine, Live *on page 619*

♦ **Augmentin®** *see* Amoxicillin and Clavulanate Potassium *on page 77*

♦ **Auralgan®** *see* Antipyrine and Benzocaine *on page 91*

## Auranofin (au RANE oh fin)

**Related Information**

Rheumatoid Arthritis and Osteoarthritis *on page 1092*

**U.S. Brand Names** Ridaura®

**Therapeutic Category** Gold Compound

**Use** Management of active stage of classic or definite rheumatoid arthritis in patients that do not respond to or tolerate other agents; psoriatic arthritis; adjunctive or alternative therapy for pemphigus

**Usual Dosage** Oral:

Children: Initial: 0.1 mg/kg/day divided daily; usual maintenance: 0.15 mg/kg/day in 1-2 divided doses; maximum: 0.2 mg/kg/day in 1-2 divided doses

Adults: 6 mg/day in 1-2 divided doses; after 3 months may be increased to 9 mg/day in 3 divided doses; if still no response after 3 months at 9 mg/day, discontinue drug

**Mechanism of Action** The exact mechanism of action of gold is unknown; gold is taken up by macrophages which results in inhibition of phagocytosis and lysosomal membrane stabilization; other actions observed are decreased serum rheumatoid factor and alterations in immunoglobulins. Additionally, complement activation is decreased, prostaglandin synthesis is inhibited, and lysosomal enzyme activity is decreased.

**Local Anesthetic/Vasoconstrictor Precautions** No information available to require special precautions

**Effects on Dental Treatment** No effects or complications reported

**Other Adverse Effects**

>10%:

Dermatologic: Itching, skin rash

Gastrointestinal: Stomatitis

Ocular: Conjunctivitis

Renal: Proteinuria

1% to 10%:

Dermatologic: Urticaria, alopecia

Gastrointestinal: Glossitis

Hematologic: Eosinophilia, leukopenia, thrombocytopenia

Renal: Hematuria

<1%:

Dermatologic: Angioedema

(Continued)

## Auranofin *(Continued)*

Gastrointestinal: Ulcerative enterocolitis, GI hemorrhage, gingivitis, metallic taste, dysphagia
Hematologic: Agranulocytosis, anemia, aplastic anemia
Hepatic: Hepatotoxicity
Neuromuscular & skeletal: Peripheral neuropathy
Respiratory: Interstitial pneumonitis

**Drug Interactions** Increased toxicity: Penicillamine, antimalarials, hydroxychloroquine, cytotoxic agents, immunosuppressants

**Pregnancy Risk Factor** C

**Generic Available** No

- **Aureomycin®** *see* Chlortetracycline *on page 241*
- **Auro® Ear Drops [OTC]** *see* Carbamide Peroxide *on page 186*
- **Aurolate®** *see* Gold Sodium Thiomalate *on page 474*

## Aurothioglucose (aur oh thye oh GLOO kose)

**Related Information**

Rheumatoid Arthritis and Osteoarthritis *on page 1092*

**U.S. Brand Names** Solganal®

**Therapeutic Category** Gold Compound

**Use** Adjunctive treatment in adult and juvenile active rheumatoid arthritis; alternative or adjunct in treatment of pemphigus; psoriatic patients who do not respond to NSAIDs

**Usual Dosage** I.M.: Doses should initially be given at weekly intervals

Children 6-12 years: Initial: 0.25 mg/kg/dose first week; increment at 0.25 mg/kg/dose increasing with each weekly dose; maintenance: 0.75-1 mg/kg/dose weekly not to exceed 25 mg/dose to a total of 20 doses, then every 2-4 weeks
Adults: 10 mg first week; 25 mg second and third week; then 50 mg/week until 800 mg to 1 g cumulative dose has been given; if improvement occurs without adverse reactions, give 25-50 mg every 2-3 weeks, then every 3-4 weeks

**Mechanism of Action** Unknown, may decrease prostaglandin synthesis or may alter cellular mechanisms by inhibiting sulfhydryl systems

**Local Anesthetic/Vasoconstrictor Precautions** No information available to require special precautions

**Effects on Dental Treatment** No effects or complications reported

**Other Adverse Effects**

>10%:
Dermatologic: Itching, skin rash, exfoliative dermatitis, reddened skin
Gastrointestinal: Gingivitis, glossitis, metallic taste, stomatitis

1% to 10%: Renal: Proteinuria

<1%:
Cardiovascular: EKG abnormalities
Central nervous system: Encephalitis, fever
Dermatologic: Alopecia
Gastrointestinal: Ulcerative enterocolitis
Genitourinary: Vaginitis
Hematologic: Agranulocytosis, aplastic anemia, eosinophilia, leukopenia, thrombocytopenia
Hepatic: Hepatotoxicity
Neuromuscular & skeletal: Peripheral neuropathy
Ocular: Conjunctivitis, corneal ulcers, iritis
Renal: Glomerulitis, hematuria, nephrotic syndrome
Respiratory: Pharyngitis, bronchitis, pulmonary fibrosis, interstitial pneumonitis
Miscellaneous: Anaphylactic shock, allergic reaction (severe)

**Drug Interactions** Increased toxicity: Penicillamine, antimalarials, hydroxychloroquine, cytotoxic agents, immunosuppressants

**Drug Uptake**

Absorption: I.M.: Erratic and slow
Serum half-life: 3-27 days (half-life dependent upon single or multiple dosing)
Time to peak serum concentration: Within 4-6 hours

**Pregnancy Risk Factor** C

**Generic Available** No

- **Auroto®** *see* Antipyrine and Benzocaine *on page 91*
- **Autoplex® T** *see* Anti-inhibitor Coagulant Complex *on page 91*
- **Avapro®** *see* Irbesartan *on page 548*
- **AVC™ Cream** *see* Sulfanilamide *on page 944*
- **AVC™ Suppository** *see* Sulfanilamide *on page 944*
- **Aveeno® Cleansing Bar [OTC]** *see* Sulfur and Salicylic Acid *on page 947*
- **Aventyl® Hydrochloride** *see* Nortriptyline *on page 732*

- **Avita® Topical** *see* Tretinoin, Topical *on page 1009*
- **Avitene®** *see* Microfibrillar Collagen Hemostat *on page 673*
- **Avlosulfon®** *see* Dapsone *on page 298*
- **Avonex™** *see* Interferon Beta-1a *on page 544*
- **Axid®** *see* Nizatidine *on page 728*
- **Axid® AR [OTC]** *see* Nizatidine *on page 728*
- **Axotal®** *see* Butalbital Compound *on page 163*
- **Aygestin®** *see* Norethindrone *on page 730*
- **Ayr® Saline [OTC]** *see* Sodium Chloride *on page 920*


## Azacitidine (ay za SYE ti deen)

**U.S. Brand Names** Mylosar®

**Therapeutic Category** Antineoplastic Agent, Miscellaneous

**Synonyms** AZA-CR; 5-Azacytidine; 5-AZC; Ladakamycin; NSC-102816

**Use** Refractory acute lymphocytic and myelogenous leukemia

**Usual Dosage** Children and Adults: I.V., S.C.: 50-200 mg/m²/day for 5-10 days, repeated at 2- to 3-week intervals **or** 75 mg/m²/day for 7 days every 4 weeks

**Local Anesthetic/Vasoconstrictor Precautions** No information available to require special precautions

**Effects on Dental Treatment** No effects or complications reported

**Other Adverse Effects** 1% to 10%:

Cardiovascular: Hypotension with rapid infusion
Central nervous system: Fever
Dermatologic: Rash
Gastrointestinal: Nausea, vomiting, diarrhea
Hematologic: Myelosuppression (granulocyte nadir: 14-17 days)
Hepatic: Hepatotoxicity
Neuromuscular & skeletal: Neuropathies (dose dependent) and neurologic toxicity

**Pregnancy Risk Factor** C

**Generic Available** No


- **AZA-CR** *see* Azacitidine *on this page*
- **Azactam®** *see* Aztreonam *on page 115*
- **5-Azacytidine** *see* Azacitidine *on this page*


## Azatadine (a ZA ta deen)

**U.S. Brand Names** Optimine®

**Therapeutic Category** Antihistamine

**Use** Treatment of perennial and seasonal allergic rhinitis and chronic urticaria

**Usual Dosage** Children >12 years and Adults: Oral: 1-2 mg twice daily

**Mechanism of Action** Azatadine is a piperidine-derivative antihistamine; has both anticholinergic and antiserotonin activity; has been demonstrated to inhibit mediator release from human mast cells *in vitro*; mechanism of this action is suggested to prevent calcium entry into the mast cell through voltage-dependent calcium channels

**Local Anesthetic/Vasoconstrictor Precautions** No information available to require special precautions

**Effects on Dental Treatment** This drug has atropine-like effects and the patient may experience drowsiness, dry mouth, nose and throat

**Other Adverse Effects**

>10%:
Central nervous system: Slight to moderate drowsiness
Respiratory: Thickening of bronchial secretions

1% to 10%:
Central nervous system: Headache, fatigue, nervousness, dizziness
Gastrointestinal: Appetite increase, weight increase, nausea, diarrhea, abdominal pain, dry mouth
Neuromuscular & skeletal: Arthralgia
Respiratory: Pharyngitis

<1%:
Cardiovascular: Palpitations, edema
Central nervous system: Depression
Dermatologic: Angioedema, photosensitivity, rash
Hepatic: Hepatitis
Neuromuscular & skeletal: Myalgia, paresthesia
Respiratory: Bronchospasm, epistaxis

**Drug Interactions** Increased effect/toxicity: Procarbazine, CNS depressants, tricyclic antidepressants, alcohol

**Drug Uptake**

Absorption: Oral: Rapid and extensive

(Continued)

## Azatadine *(Continued)*

Serum half-life: ~8.7 hours

**Pregnancy Risk Factor** B

**Generic Available** No

## Azatadine and Pseudoephedrine

(a ZA ta deen & soo doe e FED rin)

**U.S. Brand Names** Trinalin®

**Therapeutic Category** Antihistamine/Decongestant Combination

**Synonyms** Pseudoephedrine and Azatadine

**Use** Perennial and seasonal allergic rhinitis and other allergic symptoms including urticaria

**Usual Dosage** Adults: 1-2 mg twice daily

**Local Anesthetic/Vasoconstrictor Precautions**

Azatadine: No information available to require special precautions

Pseudoephedrine: Use with caution since pseudoephedrine is a sympathomimetic amine which could interact with epinephrine to cause a pressor response

**Effects on Dental Treatment**

Azatadine: This drug has atropine-like effects and the patient may experience drowsiness, dry mouth, nose and throat

Pseudoephedrine: Up to 10% of patients could experience tachycardia, palpitations, and dry mouth; use vasoconstrictor with caution

**Other Adverse Effects** See individual agents

**Pregnancy Risk Factor** C

**Generic Available** No

## Azathioprine (ay za THYE oh preen)

**U.S. Brand Names** Imuran®

**Therapeutic Category** Immunosuppressant Agent

**Use** Adjunct with other agents in prevention of rejection of solid organ transplants; also used in severe active rheumatoid arthritis unresponsive to other agents; **azathioprine is an imidazolyl derivative of 6-mercaptopurine**

**Usual Dosage I.V. dose is equivalent to oral dose**

Children and Adults: Renal transplantation: Oral, I.V.: 2-5 mg/kg/day to start, then 1-3 mg/kg/day maintenance

Adults: Rheumatoid arthritis: Oral: 1 mg/kg/day for 6-8 weeks; increase by 0.5 mg/kg every 4 weeks until response or up to 2.5 mg/kg/day

**Mechanism of Action** Antagonizes purine metabolism and may inhibit synthesis of DNA, RNA, and proteins; may also interfere with cellular metabolism and inhibit mitosis

**Local Anesthetic/Vasoconstrictor Precautions** No information available to require special precautions

**Effects on Dental Treatment** No effects or complications reported

**Other Adverse Effects** Dose reduction or temporary withdrawal allows reversal

>10%:

- Central nervous system: Fever, chills
- Gastrointestinal: Nausea, vomiting, anorexia, diarrhea
- Hematologic: Thrombocytopenia, leukopenia, anemia
- Miscellaneous: Secondary infection

1% to 10%:

- Dermatologic: Skin rash
- Hematologic: Pancytopenia
- Hepatic: Hepatotoxicity

<1%:

- Cardiovascular: Hypotension
- Dermatologic: Alopecia, rash, maculopapular rash, aphthous stomatitis
- Neuromuscular & skeletal: Arthralgias, which include myalgias, rigors
- Ocular: Retinopathy
- Respiratory: Dyspnea
- Miscellaneous: Rare hypersensitivity reactions

**Drug Interactions** Increased toxicity: Allopurinol (reduce azathioprine dose to 1/3 to 1/4 of normal dose). The use of angiotensin-converting enzyme inhibitors to control hypertension in patients on azathioprine has been reported to induce severe leukopenia.

**Drug Uptake** Serum half-life:

Parent drug: 12 minutes

6-mercaptopurine: 0.7-3 hours

End-stage renal disease: Slightly prolonged

**Pregnancy Risk Factor** D

**Generic Available** No

♦ **5-AZC** *see* Azacitidine *on page 111*

♦ **Azdone®** *see* Hydrocodone and Aspirin *on page 507*

## Azelaic Acid (a zeh LAY ik AS id)

**U.S. Brand Names** Azelex®

**Therapeutic Category** Topical Skin Product, Acne

**Use** *Acne vulgaris*: Topical treatment of mild to moderate inflammatory acne vulgaris

**Usual Dosage** Adults: Topical: After skin is thoroughly washed and patted dry, gently but thoroughly massage a thin film of azelaic acid cream into the affected areas twice daily, in the morning and evening. The duration of use can vary and depends on the severity of the acne. In the majority of patients with inflammatory lesions, improvement of the condition occurs within 4 weeks.

**Mechanism of Action** Exact mechanism is not known; *in vitro*, azelaic acid possesses antimicrobial activity against *Propionibacteriaceae acnes* and *Staphylococcus epidermis*; may decrease micromedo formation

**Local Anesthetic/Vasoconstrictor Precautions** No information available to require special precautions

**Effects on Dental Treatment** No effects or complications reported

**Other Adverse Effects**

1% to 10%:

Dermatologic: Pruritus, stinging

Local: Burning

Neuromuscular & skeletal: Paresthesia

<1%:

Dermatologic: Erythema, dryness, rash, peeling, dermatitis, contact dermatitis

Local: Irritation

**Drug Uptake**

Absorption: ~3% to 5% penetrates the stratum corneum; up to 10% is found in the epidermis and dermis; 4% is systemically absorbed

Serum half-life: Healthy subjects: 12 hours after topical dosing

**Pregnancy Risk Factor** B

**Generic Available** No

## Azelastine (a ZEL as teen)

**U.S. Brand Names** Astelin®

**Therapeutic Category** Antihistamine

**Synonyms** Azelastine Hydrochloride

**Use** Treatment of symptoms of seasonal allergic rhinitis (ie, rhinorrhea, sneezing, nasal pruritus) in adults and children >12 years of age

**Usual Dosage** Two sprays (137 mcg/spray) per nostril twice daily. Before initial use, the delivery system should be primed with 4 sprays or until a fine mist appears. If three or more days have elapsed since last use, the delivery system should be reprimed.

**Mechanism of Action** Azelastine competes with histamine for histamine$_1$-receptor sites on effector cells in the GI tract, blood vessels, and respiratory tract. This action inhibits the symptoms associated with seasonal allergic rhinitis (ie, sneezing, pruritus, increased mucus production).

**Local Anesthetic/Vasoconstrictor Precautions** No information available to require special precautions

**Effects on Dental Treatment** 2% to 10% of patients experience dry mouth; chronic use of antihistamines will inhibit salivary flows particularly in elderly patients; this may contribute to periodontal disease and oral discomfort

**Other Adverse Effects**

>10%:

Central nervous system: Headache (14.8%), somnolence (11.5%)

Gastrointestinal: Bitter taste (19.7%)

2% to 10%:

Central nervous system: Fatigue (2.3%), dizziness (2.0%)

Gastrointestinal: Dry mouth (2.8%), nausea (2.8%),weight increase (2.0%)

Respiratory: Nasal burning (4.1%), pharyngitis (3.8%), paroxysmal sneezing (3.1%), rhinitis (2.3%), epistaxis (2.0%)

<2%:

Cardiovascular: Flushing, hypertension, tachycardia

Central nervous system: Malaise, vertigo, hypoesthesia, anxiety, depersonalization, depression, nervousness, sleep disorder, abnormal thinking

Dermatological: Contact dermatitis, eczema, hair and follicle infection, furunculosis

Endocrine & metabolic: Amenorrhea, breast pain

(Continued)

## Azelastine *(Continued)*

Gastrointestinal: Constipation, gastroenteritis, glossitis, increased appetite, ulcerative stomatitis, vomiting, increased ALT, aphthous stomatitis, loss of taste perception, abdominal pain

Genitourinary: Albuminuria, polyuria

Neuromuscular & skeletal: Myalgia, temporomandibular dislocation, hyperkinesis, pain in extremities, back pain

Ocular: Conjunctivitis, eye abnormality, eye pain, water eyes

Renal: Hematuria

Respiratory: Bronchospasm, coughing, throat burning, laryngitis

Miscellaneous: Allergic reaction, herpes simplex, viral infection

**Contraindications** Patients with a known hypersensitivity to any of the components of Astelin®

**Warnings/Precautions** Azelastine causes somnolence. Caution should be exercised when performing activities that require mental alertness. Concurrent use of alcohol or other CNS depressants with azelastine should be avoided. Avoid use of azelastine with other antihistamines unless advised by a physician.

**Drug Interactions** Increased effect: Alcohol and CNS depressants cause additive somnolence and CNS impairment

**Drug Uptake**

Serum half-life: Azelastine 22 hours, desmethylazelastine 54 hours

Time to peak: 2 to 3 hours

**Pregnancy Risk Factor** C

**Dosage Forms** Spray, nasal: 137 mcg/actuation [100 actuations/bottle]

**Comments** Azelastine is absorbed systemically will cause sedation in some patients. Although this agent is clinically effective, the side effects of sedation, bitter taste, and high cost will limits its use in many patients.

♦ **Azelastine Hydrochloride** *see* Azelastine *on previous page*

♦ **Azelex®** *see* Azelaic Acid *on previous page*

## Azithromycin (az ith roe MYE sin)

**Related Information**

Antibiotic Prophylaxis, Preprocedural Guidelines for Dental Patients *on page 1097*

**U.S. Brand Names** Zithromax™

**Therapeutic Category** Antibiotic, Macrolide

**Synonyms** Z-PAKS™

**Use**

Dental: Alternate antibiotic in the treatment of common orofacial infections caused by aerobic gram-positive cocci and susceptible anaerobes; alternate antibiotic for the prevention of bacterial endocarditis in patients undergoing dental procedures

Medical: Treatment against most respiratory pathogens (eg, *S. pyogenes, S. pneumoniae, S. agalactiae*, viridans *Streptococcus, M. catarrhalis, C. trachomatis, Legionella* sp, *Mycoplasma pneumoniae, S. aureus*)

**Usual Dosage** Oral:

Children: Prevention of bacterial endocarditis: 15 mg/kg 1 hour before procedure with no follow-up dose needed; total children's dose should not exceed adult dose

Adults: 250 mg twice daily first day then 250 mg/day for 4 days; prevention of bacterial endocarditis: 500 mg 1 hour before procedure with no follow-up dose needed

**Mechanism of Action** Inhibits RNA-dependent protein synthesis at the chain elongation step; binds to the 50S ribosomal subunit resulting in blockage of transpeptidation

**Local Anesthetic/Vasoconstrictor Precautions** No information available to require special precautions

**Effects on Dental Treatment** No effects or complications reported

**Other Adverse Effects** 1% to 10%: Gastrointestinal: Diarrhea, nausea, abdominal pain, cramping, vomiting

**Contraindications** Hepatic impairment, known hypersensitivity to azithromycin, other macrolide antibiotics, or any Zithromax™ components; use with pimozide

**Warnings/Precautions** Use with caution in patients with hepatic dysfunction; hepatic impairment with or without jaundice has occurred chiefly in older children and adults; it may be accompanied by malaise, nausea, vomiting, abdominal colic, and fever; discontinue use if these occur; may mask or delay symptoms of incubating gonorrhea or syphilis, so appropriate culture and susceptibility tests should be performed prior to initiating azithromycin; pseudomembranous colitis has been reported with use of macrolide antibiotics

**Drug Interactions** Aluminum- and magnesium-containing antacids decrease serum levels of azithromycin by 24% but not total absorption; manufacturer recommends that when antacids are used, azithromycin should be taken 1-2 hours later

**Drug Uptake**

Absorption: Rapid from the GI tract

Serum half-life, terminal: 68 hours

Time to peak serum concentration: 2.3-4 hours

**Pregnancy Risk Factor** B

**Breast-feeding Considerations** No data reported

**Dosage Forms**

Capsule, as dihydrate: 250 mg

Capsule (Z-PAKS™): 6 capsules/box

Suspension, oral (single-dose packets): 1 g

**Dietary Considerations** Should be taken at least 1 hour prior to or 2 hours after a meal; should not be taken with food; food decreases rate and extent of absorption

**Generic Available** No

**Comments** Although the erythromycins inhibit the hepatic metabolism of theophylline and carbamazepine to enhance their effects, azithromycin has not been shown to inhibit the hepatic metabolism of these drugs. Clauzel, et al, reported that azithromycin did not inhibit the metabolism of theophylline after a standard 5-day regimen (500 mg on day one followed by 250 mg daily). Rapeport, et al, reported that azithromycin did not affect the blood levels of carbamazepine.

**Selected Readings**

Clauzel AM, Visier S, and Michel FB, "Efficacy and Safety of Azithromycin in Lower Respiratory Tract Infections," *Eur Respir J*, 1990, 3(Suppl 10):89S.

Dajani AS, Taubert KA, Wilson WW, et al, "Prevention of Bacterial Endocarditis. Recommendations by the American Heart Association," *JAMA*, 1997, 277(22):1794-801.

Dajani AS, Taubert KA, Wilson W, et al, "Prevention of Bacterial Endocarditis: Recommendations by the American Heart Association," *J Am Dent Assoc*, 1997, 128(8):1142-51.

Rapeport WG, Dewland PM, Muirhead DC, et al, "Lack of Interaction Between Azithromycin and Carbamazepine," *Br J Clin Pharmacol*, 1992, 30:551P.

Wynn RL, "New Erythromycins," *Gen Dent*, 1996, 44(4):304-7.

♦ **Azmacort™** *see* Triamcinolone *on page 1010*

♦ **Azo Gantanol®** *see* Sulfamethoxazole and Phenazopyridine *on page 943*

♦ **Azo Gantrisin®** *see* Sulfisoxazole and Phenazopyridine *on page 946*

♦ **Azopt®** *see* Brinzolamide *on page 150*

♦ **Azo-Standard® [OTC]** *see* Phenazopyridine *on page 788*

♦ **AZT + 3TC** *see* Zidovudine and Lamivudine *on page 1059*

## Aztreonam (AZ tree oh nam)

**U.S. Brand Names** Azactam®

**Therapeutic Category** Antibiotic, Miscellaneous

**Use** Treatment of patients with documented aerobic gram-negative bacillary infection in which beta-lactam therapy is contraindicated (eg, penicillin or cephalosporin allergy); used for urinary tract infections, lower respiratory tract infections, septicemia, skin/skin structure infections, intra-abdominal infections, and gynecological infections; as part of a multiple-drug regimen for the empirical treatment of neutropenic fever in persons with a history of beta-lactam allergy or with known multidrug-resistant organisms

**Usual Dosage**

Children >1 month: I.M., I.V.: 90-120 mg/kg/day divided every 6-8 hours

Cystic fibrosis: 50 mg/kg/dose every 6-8 hours (ie, up to 200 mg/kg/day); maximum: 6-8 g/day

Adults:

Urinary tract infection: I.M., I.V.: 500 mg to 1 g every 8-12 hours

Moderately severe systemic infections: 1 g I.V. or I.M. or 2 g I.V. every 8-12 hours

Severe systemic or life-threatening infections (especially caused by *Pseudomonas aeruginosa*): I.V.: 2 g every 6-8 hours; maximum: 8 g/day

**Mechanism of Action** Monobactam which is active only against gram-negative bacilli (unlikely cross-allergenicity with other beta-lactams); inhibits bacterial cell wall synthesis during active multiplication, causing cell wall destruction

**Local Anesthetic/Vasoconstrictor Precautions** No information available to require special precautions

**Effects on Dental Treatment** No effects or complications reported

**Other Adverse Effects**

1% to 10%:

Dermatologic: Rash

Gastrointestinal: Diarrhea, nausea, vomiting

Local: Thrombophlebitis, pain at injection site

(Continued)

## Aztreonam *(Continued)*

<1%:
- Cardiovascular: Hypotension
- Central nervous system: Seizures, confusion, headache, vertigo, insomnia, dizziness, fever
- Endocrine & metabolic: Breast tenderness
- Gastrointestinal: Pseudomembranous colitis, aphthous ulcer, dysgeusia, halitosis, numb tongue
- Genitourinary: Vaginitis
- Hepatic: Hepatitis, jaundice, elevation of liver enzymes
- Hematologic: Thrombocytopenia, eosinophilia, leukopenia, neutropenia
- Neuromuscular & skeletal: Myalgia, weakness
- Ocular: Diplopia
- Otic: Tinnitus
- Respiratory: Sneezing
- Miscellaneous: Anaphylaxis

**Drug Interactions** No data reported

**Drug Uptake**

Absorption: I.M.: Well absorbed; I.M. and I.V. doses produce comparable serum concentrations

Serum half-life:
- Normal renal function: 1.7-2.9 hours
- End-stage renal disease: 6-8 hours

Time to peak: Within 60 minutes (I.M., I.V. push) and 90 minutes (I.V. infusion)

**Pregnancy Risk Factor** B

**Generic Available** No


- ♦ **Azulfidine®** *see* Sulfasalazine *on page 944*
- ♦ **Azulfidine® EN-tabs®** *see* Sulfasalazine *on page 944*
- ♦ **Babee® Teething® [OTC]** *see* Benzocaine *on page 128*
- ♦ **B-A-C®** *see* Butalbital Compound *on page 163*
- ♦ **BAC** *see* Benzalkonium Chloride *on page 128*


## Bacampicillin (ba kam pi SIL in)

**U.S. Brand Names** Spectrobid®

**Canadian Brand Names** Penglobe®

**Therapeutic Category** Antibiotic, Penicillin

**Synonyms** Bacampicillin Hydrochloride; Carampicillin Hydrochloride

**Use** Treatment of susceptible bacterial infections involving the urinary tract, skin structure, upper and lower respiratory tract; activity is identical to that of ampicillin

**Usual Dosage** Oral:
- Children <25 kg: 25-50 mg/kg/day in divided doses every 12 hours
- Children >25 kg and Adults: 400-800 mg every 12 hours

**Mechanism of Action** Interferes with bacterial cell wall synthesis during active multiplication causing cell wall death and resultant bactericidal activity against susceptible bacteria

**Local Anesthetic/Vasoconstrictor Precautions** No information available to require special precautions

**Effects on Dental Treatment** No effects or complications reported

**Other Adverse Effects**

1% to 10%: Gastrointestinal: Gastric upset, diarrhea, nausea

<1%:
- Dermatologic: Rash
- Gastrointestinal: Pseudomembranous colitis
- Hematologic: Agranulocytosis
- Hepatic: Mild elevation in AST
- Miscellaneous: Hypersensitivity reactions

**Drug Interactions**

Decreased effect of oral contraceptives

Increased levels with probenecid; allopurinol theoretically has has an additive potential for amoxicillin/ampicillin rash

**Drug Uptake**

Serum half-life: 65 minutes, prolonged in patients with impaired renal function

Time to peak serum concentration: Area under the serum concentration time curve is 40% higher for bacampicillin than after equivalent ampicillin doses

**Pregnancy Risk Factor** B

**Generic Available** No

**Comments** Each mg of bacampicillin is equivalent to ampicillin 700 mcg


- ♦ **Bacampicillin Hydrochloride** *see* Bacampicillin *on this page*
- ♦ **Bacid® [OTC]** *see Lactobacillus acidophilus* and *Lactobacillus bulgaricus on page 570*

♦ **Baciguent® [OTC]** *see* Bacitracin *on this page*
♦ **Baci-IM®** *see* Bacitracin *on this page*
♦ **Bacillus Calmette-Guérin (BCG) Live** *see* BCG Vaccine *on page 121*

## Bacitracin (bas i TRAY sin)

**U.S. Brand Names** AK-Tracin®; Baciguent® [OTC]; Baci-IM®

**Canadian Brand Names** Bacigvent; Bacitin

**Therapeutic Category** Antibiotic, Ophthalmic; Antibiotic, Topical; Antibiotic, Miscellaneous

**Use** Treatment of susceptible bacterial infections (staphylococcal pneumonia and empyema); due to toxicity risks, systemic and irrigant uses of bacitracin should be limited to situations where less toxic alternatives would not be effective; oral administration has been successful in antibiotic-associated colitis

**Usual Dosage** Do not administer I.V.:

Children: I.M.: 800-1200 units/kg/day divided every 8 hours

Adults: Antibiotic-associated colitis: Oral: 25,000 units 4 times/day for 7-10 days

Topical: Apply 1-5 times/day

Ophthalmic, ointment: Instill 1/4" to 1/2" ribbon every 3-4 hours into conjunctival sac for acute infections, or 2-3 times/day for mild to moderate infections for 7-10 days

Irrigation, solution: 50-100 units/mL in normal saline, lactated Ringer's, or sterile water for irrigation; soak sponges in solution for topical compresses 1-5 times/day or as needed during surgical procedures

**Mechanism of Action** Inhibits bacterial cell wall synthesis by preventing transfer of mucopeptides into the growing cell wall

**Local Anesthetic/Vasoconstrictor Precautions** No information available to require special precautions

**Effects on Dental Treatment** No effects or complications reported

**Other Adverse Effects** 1% to 10%:

Cardiovascular: Hypotension, tightness of chest, swelling of lips and face

Central nervous system: Pain

Dermatologic: Rash, itching

Gastrointestinal: Anorexia, nausea, vomiting, diarrhea, rectal itching and burning

Hematologic: Blood dyscrasias

Miscellaneous: Sweating

**Drug Interactions** Increased toxicity: Nephrotoxic drugs, neuromuscular blocking agents, and anesthetics (increased neuromuscular blockade)

**Drug Uptake**

Duration of action: 6-8 hours

Absorption: Poor from mucous membranes and intact or denuded skin; rapidly absorbed following I.M. administration; not absorbed by bladder irrigation, but absorption can occur from peritoneal or mediastinal lavage

Time to peak serum concentration: I.M.: Within 1-2 hours

**Pregnancy Risk Factor** C

**Generic Available** Yes

## Bacitracin and Polymyxin B (bas i TRAY sin & pol i MIKS in bee)

**U.S. Brand Names** AK-Poly-Bac® Ophthalmic; Betadine® First Aid Antibiotics + Moisturizer [OTC]; Polysporin® Ophthalmic; Polysporin® Topical

**Canadian Brand Names** Bioderm®; Polytopic

**Therapeutic Category** Antibiotic, Ophthalmic; Antibiotic, Topical

**Use** Treatment of superficial infections caused by susceptible organisms

**Usual Dosage** Children and Adults:

Ophthalmic ointment: Instill 1/2" ribbon in the affected eye(s) every 3-4 hours for acute infections or 2-3 times/day for mild to moderate infections for 7-10 days

Topical ointment/powder: Apply to affected area 1-4 times/day; may cover with sterile bandage if needed

**Mechanism of Action** Refer to individual monographs for Bacitracin and Polymyxin B

**Local Anesthetic/Vasoconstrictor Precautions** No information available to require special precautions

**Effects on Dental Treatment** No effects or complications reported

**Other Adverse Effects** 1% to 10%: Local: Rash, itching, burning, anaphylactoid reactions, swelling and conjunctival erythema

**Drug Interactions** No data reported

**Pregnancy Risk Factor** C

**Generic Available** Yes

## Bacitracin, Neomycin, and Polymyxin B

(bas i TRAY sin, nee oh MYE sin & pol i MIKS in bee)

**U.S. Brand Names** AK-Spore® Ophthalmic Ointment; Medi-Quick® Topical Ointment [OTC]; Mycitracin® Topical [OTC]; Neomixin® Topical [OTC]; Neosporin® Ophthalmic Ointment; Neosporin® Topical Ointment [OTC]; Ocutricin® Topical Ointment; Septa® Topical Ointment [OTC]; Triple Antibiotic® Topical

**Canadian Brand Names** Neotopic

**Therapeutic Category** Antibiotic, Ophthalmic; Antibiotic, Topical

**Use** Helps prevent infection in minor cuts, scrapes and burns; short-term treatment of superficial external ocular infections caused by susceptible organisms

**Usual Dosage** Children and Adults:

Ophthalmic ointment: Instill ½" ribbon into the conjunctival sac every 3-4 hours for acute infections or 2-3 times/day for mild to moderate infections for 7-10 days

Topical: Apply 1-4 times/day to affected areas and cover with sterile bandage if necessary

**Mechanism of Action** Refer to individual monographs for Bacitracin; Neomycin Sulfate; and Polymyxin B Sulfate

**Local Anesthetic/Vasoconstrictor Precautions** No information available to require special precautions

**Effects on Dental Treatment** No effects or complications reported

**Other Adverse Effects** 1% to 10%:

Dermatologic: Allergic contact dermatitis

Local: Itching, reddening, failure to heal

**Drug Interactions** No data reported

**Pregnancy Risk Factor** C

**Generic Available** Yes

## Bacitracin, Neomycin, Polymyxin B, and Hydrocortisone

(bas i TRAY sin, nee oh MYE sin, pol i MIKS in bee & hye droe KOR ti sone)

**U.S. Brand Names** AK-Spore H.C.® Ophthalmic Ointment; Cortisporin® Ophthalmic Ointment; Cortisporin® Topical Ointment; Neotricin HC® Ophthalmic Ointment

**Therapeutic Category** Antibiotic, Ophthalmic; Antibiotic, Otic; Antibiotic, Topical; Corticosteroid, Ophthalmic; Corticosteroid, Otic; Corticosteroid, Topical (Low Potency)

**Use** Prevention and treatment of susceptible superficial topical infections

**Usual Dosage** Children and Adults:

Ophthalmic:

Ointment: Instill ½" ribbon to inside of lower lid every 3-4 hours until improvement occurs

Topical: Apply sparingly 2-4 times/day

**Mechanism of Action** Refer to individual monographs for Bacitracin, Neomycin, Polymyxin B, and Hydrocortisone

**Local Anesthetic/Vasoconstrictor Precautions** No information available to require special precautions

**Effects on Dental Treatment** No effects or complications reported

**Other Adverse Effects** 1% to 10%:

Dermatologic: Rash, generalized itching

Respiratory: Apnea

**Drug Interactions** No data reported

**Pregnancy Risk Factor** C

**Generic Available** Yes

## Bacitracin, Neomycin, Polymyxin B, and Lidocaine

(bas i TRAY sin, nee oh MYE sin, pol i MIKS in bee & LYE doe kane)

**U.S. Brand Names** Clomycin® [OTC]

**Therapeutic Category** Antibiotic, Topical

**Use** Prevention and treatment of susceptible superficial topical infections

**Local Anesthetic/Vasoconstrictor Precautions** No information available to require special precautions

**Effects on Dental Treatment** No effects or complications reported

**Generic Available** No

## Baclofen (BAK loe fen)

**U.S. Brand Names** Lioresal®

**Canadian Brand Names** Alpha-Baclofen®; PMS-Baclofen

**Therapeutic Category** Muscle Relaxant; Skeletal Muscle Relaxant

**Use** Treatment of reversible spasticity associated with multiple sclerosis or spinal cord lesions; intrathecal baclofen for the treatment of cerebral spasticity

There are a number of unlabeled uses for baclofen including, intractable hiccups, intractable pain relief, and bladder spasticity

**Usual Dosage**

Oral:

Children:

2-7 years: Initial: 10-15 mg/24 hours divided every 8 hours; titrate dose every 3 days in increments of 5-15 mg/day to a maximum of 40 mg/day

≥8 years: Maximum: 60 mg/day in 3 divided doses

Adults: 5 mg 3 times/day, may increase 5 mg/dose every 3 days to a maximum of 80 mg/day

Intrathecal:

Test dose: 50-100 mcg, doses >50 mcg should be given in 25 mcg increments, separated by 24 hours

Maintenance: After positive response to test dose, a maintenance intrathecal infusion can be administered via an implanted intrathecal pump. Initial dose via pump: Infusion at a 24-hourly rate dosed at twice the test dose.

**Mechanism of Action** Inhibits the transmission of both monosynaptic and polysynaptic reflexes at the spinal cord level, possibly by hyperpolarization of primary afferent fiber terminals, with resultant relief of muscle spasticity

**Local Anesthetic/Vasoconstrictor Precautions** No information available to require special precautions

**Effects on Dental Treatment** No effects or complications reported

**Other Adverse Effects**

>10%:

Central nervous system: Drowsiness, vertigo, dizziness, psychiatric disturbances, insomnia, slurred speech, ataxia, hypotonia

Neuromuscular & skeletal: Weakness

1% to 10%:

Cardiovascular: Hypotension

Central nervous system: Fatigue, confusion, headache, insomnia

Dermatologic: Rash

Gastrointestinal: Nausea, constipation

Renal: Polyuria

<1%:

Cardiovascular: Palpitations, chest pain, syncope

Central nervous system: Euphoria, excitement, depression, hallucinations

Gastrointestinal: Dry mouth, anorexia, taste disorder, abdominal pain, vomiting, diarrhea

Genitourinary: Enuresis, urinary retention, dysuria, impotence, inability to ejaculate, nocturia

Neuromuscular & skeletal: Paresthesia

Renal: Hematuria

Respiratory: Dyspnea

**Drug Interactions**

Increased effect of baclofen has been caused by opiate analgesics, benzodiazepines, hypertensive agents

Increased toxicity: CNS depressants and alcohol (sedation), tricyclic antidepressants (short-term memory loss), guanabenz (sedation), MAO inhibitors (decreased blood pressure, CNS, and respiratory effects)

**Drug Uptake**

Onset of action: Muscle relaxation effect requires 3-4 days

Absorption: Oral: Rapid; absorption from GI tract is thought to be dose dependent

Serum half-life: 3.5 hours

Time to peak serum concentration: Oral: Within 2-3 hours

**Pregnancy Risk Factor** C

**Dosage Forms**

Injection, intrathecal: 0.5 mg/mL, 2 mg/mL

Tablet: 10 mg, 20 mg

**Generic Available** Yes: Tablets only

- ♦ **Bactocill®** *see* Oxacillin *on page 745*
- ♦ **BactoShield® Topical [OTC]** *see* Chlorhexidine Gluconate *on page 225*
- ♦ **Bactrim™** *see* Trimethoprim and Sulfamethoxazole *on page 1021*
- ♦ **Bactrim™ DS** *see* Trimethoprim and Sulfamethoxazole *on page 1021*
- ♦ **Bactroban®** *see* Mupirocin *on page 691*
- ♦ **Bactroban® Nasal** *see* Mupirocin *on page 691*
- ♦ **Baker's P&S Topical [OTC]** *see* Phenol *on page 791*
- ♦ **Baking Soda** *see* Sodium Bicarbonate *on page 918*

## Balanced Salt Solution (BAL anced salt soe LOO shun)

**U.S. Brand Names** BSS® Ophthalmic

**Canadian Brand Names** Eye-Stream®

**Therapeutic Category** Ophthalmic Agent, Miscellaneous

**Use** Intraocular irrigating solution; also used to soothe and cleanse the eye in conjunction with hard contact lenses

**Usual Dosage** Use as needed for foreign body removal, gonioscopy and other general ophthalmic office procedures

**Local Anesthetic/Vasoconstrictor Precautions** No information available to require special precautions

**Effects on Dental Treatment** No effects or complications reported

**Generic Available** Yes


- ♦ **BAL in Oil®** *see* Dimercaprol *on page 336*
- ♦ **Balnetar® [OTC]** *see* Coal Tar, Lanolin, and Mineral Oil *on page 270*
- ♦ **Bancap®** *see* Butalbital Compound *on page 163*
- ♦ **Bancap®** *see* Butalbital Compound and Acetaminophen *on page 164*
- ♦ **Bancap HC® [5/500]** *see* Hydrocodone and Acetaminophen *on page 505*
- ♦ **Banophen® Decongestant Capsule [OTC]** *see* Diphenhydramine and Pseudoephedrine *on page 339*
- ♦ **Banophen® Oral [OTC]** *see* Diphenhydramine *on page 338*
- ♦ **Banthine®** *see* Methantheline *on page 646*
- ♦ **Barbidonna®** *see* Hyoscyamine, Atropine, Scopolamine, and Phenobarbital *on page 520*
- ♦ **Barbita®** *see* Phenobarbital *on page 790*
- ♦ **Barc® Liquid [OTC]** *see* Pyrethrins *on page 867*
- ♦ **Baridium® [OTC]** *see* Phenazopyridine *on page 788*
- ♦ **Basaljel® [OTC]** *see* Aluminum Carbonate *on page 54*
- ♦ **Base Ointment** *see* Zinc Oxide *on page 1061*


## Basiliximab

**U.S. Brand Names** Simulect®

**Therapeutic Category** Immunosuppressant Agent

**Use** Prophylaxis of acute organ rejection in renal transplantation

**Usual Dosage** I.V.:

Children: 12 mg/m² (maximum: 20 mg) within 2 hours prior to transplant surgery, followed by a second dose of 12 mg/m² (maximum: 20 mg) 4 days after transplantation

Adults: 20 mg within 2 hours prior to transplant surgery, followed by a second 20 mg dose 4 days after transplantation

**Mechanism of Action** Mouse-derived monoclonal IgG antibody which blocks the alpha-chain of the interleukin-2 (IL-2) receptor complex; this receptor is expressed on activated T lymphocytes and is a critical pathway for activating cell-mediated allograft rejection

**Local Anesthetic/Vasoconstrictor Precautions** No information available to require special precautions

**Effects on Dental Treatment** Causes gingival hypertrophy (GH) similar to that caused by cyclosporine; early reported indicate that frequency/incidence of basiliximab-induced GH not as high as cyclosporine-induced GH

**Other Adverse Effects** Administration of basiliximab did not appear to increase the incidence or severity of adverse effects in clinical trials. Adverse events were reported in 99% of both the placebo and basiliximab groups.

>10%:

- Cardiovascular: Edema, peripheral edema, hypertension
- Central nervous system: Fever, headache, dizziness, insomnia
- Dermatologic: Wound complications, acne
- Endocrine and metabolic: Hypokalemia, hyperkalemia, hyperglycemia, hyperuricemia, hypophosphatemia, hypocalcemia, hypercholesterolemia, acidosis
- Gastrointestinal: Constipation, nausea, diarrhea, abdominal pain, vomiting, dyspepsia, moniliasis, weight gain
- Genitourinary: Dysuria, urinary tract infection
- Hematologic: Anemia
- Neuromuscular and skeletal: Leg pain, back pain, tremor
- Respiratory: Dyspnea, infection (upper respiratory), coughing, rhinitis, pharyngitis
- Miscellaneous: Viral infection, asthenia

3% to 10%:

- Cardiovascular: Chest pain, cardiac failure, hypotension, arrhythmia, tachycardia, vascular disorder, generalized edema

Central nervous system: Hypoesthesia, neuropathy, agitation, anxiety, depression, malaise, fatigue, rigors
Dermatologic: Cyst, herpes infection, hypertrichosis, pruritus, rash, skin disorder, skin ulceration
Endocrine and metabolic: Dehydration, diabetes mellitus, fluid overload, hypercalcemia, hyperlipidemia, hypoglycemia, hypomagnesemia
Gastrointestinal: Flatulence, gastroenteritis, GI hemorrhage, gingival hyperplasia, melena, esophagitis, stomatitis
Genitourinary: Impotence, genital edema, albuminuria, bladder disorder, hematuria, urinary frequency, oliguria, abnormal renal function, renal tubular necrosis, ureteral disorder, urinary retention
Hematologic: Hematoma, hemorrhage, purpura, thrombocytopenia, thrombosis, polycythemia
Neuromuscular and skeletal: Arthralgia, arthropathy, cramps, fracture, hernia, myalgia, paresthesia
Ocular: Cataract, conjunctivitis, abnormal vision
Renal: Increased BUN
Respiratory: Bronchitis, bronchospasm, pneumonia, pulmonary edema, sinusitis
Miscellaneous: Accidental trauma, facial edema, sepsis, infection, increased glucocorticoids

**Drug Interactions** Basiliximab is an immunoglobulin; specific drug interactions have not been evaluated, but are not anticipated

**Drug Uptake** Half-life:
Children: 9.4 days
Adults: Mean: 7.2 days

**Pregnancy Risk Factor** B

**Dosage Forms** Powder for injection: 20 mg

♦ **Baycol™** *see* Cerivastatin *on page 217*
♦ **Bayer® Aspirin [OTC]** *see* Aspirin *on page 100*
♦ **Bayer® Buffered Aspirin [OTC]** *see* Aspirin *on page 100*
♦ **Bayer® Low Adult Strength [OTC]** *see* Aspirin *on page 100*
♦ **Bayer® Select® Chest Cold Caplets [OTC]** *see* Acetaminophen and Dextromethorphan *on page 30*
♦ **Bayer® Select Head Cold Caplets [OTC]** *see* Acetaminophen and Pseudoephedrine *on page 31*
♦ **Bayer® Select® Pain Relief Formula [OTC]** *see* Ibuprofen *on page 522*

## BCG Vaccine (bee see jee vak SEEN)

**U.S. Brand Names** TheraCys®; TICE® BCG

**Canadian Brand Names** ImmuCyst®; Oncotice™; Pacis™

**Therapeutic Category** Biological Response Modulator; Vaccine, Live Bacteria

**Synonyms** Bacillus Calmette-Guérin (BCG) Live

**Use** BCG vaccine is no longer recommended for adults at high risk for tuberculosis in the United States. BCG vaccination may be considered for infants and children who are skin test-negative to 5 tuberculin units of tuberculin and who cannot be given isoniazid preventive therapy but have close contact with untreated or ineffectively treated active tuberculosis patients or who belong to groups which other control measures have not been successful.

In the United States, tuberculosis control efforts are directed toward early identification, treatment of cases, and preventive therapy with isoniazid.

**Usual Dosage** Children >1 month and Adults:
Immunization against tuberculosis: 0.2-0.3 mL percutaneous; initial lesion usually appears after 10-14 days consisting of small red papule at injection site and reaches maximum diameter of 3 mm in 4-6 weeks; conduct postvaccinal tuberculin test in 2-3 months; if test is negative, repeat vaccination
Immunotherapy for bladder cancer: TICE® BCG vaccine 6 x $10^8$ viable organisms in 50 mL NS (preservative free) instilled into bladder and retained for 2 hours weekly for 6 weeks

**Mechanism of Action** BCG live is an attenuated strain of Bacillus Calmette-Guérin used as a biological response modifier; BCG live, when used intravesicular for treatment of bladder carcinoma *in situ,* is thought to cause a local, chronic inflammatory response involving macrophage and leukocyte infiltration of the bladder. By a mechanism not fully understood, this local inflammatory response leads to destruction of superficial tumor cells of the urothelium. Evidence of systemic immune response is also commonly seen, manifested by a positive PPD tuberculin skin test reaction, however, its relationship to clinical efficacy is not well-established. BCG is active immunotherapy which stimulates the host's immune mechanism to reject the tumor.

**Local Anesthetic/Vasoconstrictor Precautions** No information available to require special precautions
(Continued)

## BCG Vaccine *(Continued)*

**Effects on Dental Treatment** No effects or complications reported

**Other Adverse Effects**

1% to 10%:

Genitourinary: Bladder infection, dysuria, prostatitis

Renal: Polyuria

Miscellaneous: Flu-like syndrome

<1%:

Dermatologic: Skin ulceration, abscesses

Renal: Hematuria

Miscellaneous: Rarely anaphylactic shock in infants, lymphadenitis, tuberculosis in immunosuppressed patients

**Pregnancy Risk Factor** C

**Generic Available** No

**Comments** Live, attenuated vaccine

Live culture preparation of bacillus Calmette-Guérin (BCG) strain of *Mycobacterium bovis* and is a substrain of Pasteur Institute strain designed for use as active immunizing agent against tuberculosis

♦ **BCNU** *see* Carmustine *on page 193*

♦ **B Complex** *see* Vitamins, Multiple *on page 1051*

♦ **B Complex With C** *see* Vitamins, Multiple *on page 1051*

♦ **B-D Glucose® [OTC]** *see* Glucose *on page 470*

## Becaplermin (be KAP ler min)

**U.S. Brand Names** Regranex®

**Therapeutic Category** Topical Skin Product

**Use** Treatment of diabetic ulcers that occur on the lower limbs and feet

**Usual Dosage** Adults: Topical: Apply once daily; applied with a cotton swab or similar tool, as a coating over the ulcer

**Mechanism of Action** A genetically engineered form of platelet-derived growth factor, a naturally occurring protein in the body that stimulates wound healing.

**Local Anesthetic/Vasoconstrictor Precautions** No information available to require special precautions

**Effects on Dental Treatment** No effects or complications reported

**Dosage Forms** Gel, topical: 0.01%

♦ **Because® [OTC]** *see* Nonoxynol 9 *on page 728*

## Beclomethasone (be kloe METH a sone)

**Related Information**

Respiratory Diseases *on page 1079*

**U.S. Brand Names** Beclovent®; Beconase®; Beconase AQ®; Vancenase®; Vancenase® AQ; Vanceril®

**Canadian Brand Names** Beclodisk®; Becloforte®; Propaderm®

**Therapeutic Category** Anti-inflammatory Agent; Corticosteroid, Inhalant

**Use**

Oral inhalation: Treatment of bronchial asthma in patients who require chronic administration of corticosteroids

Nasal aerosol: Symptomatic treatment of seasonal or perennial rhinitis and nasal polyposis

**Usual Dosage** Nasal inhalation and oral inhalation dosage forms are not to be used interchangeably

Nasal:

Children 6-12 years: 1 spray in each nostril 3 times/day

Adults: 1 spray in each nostril 2-4 times/day

Oral inhalation:

Children 6-12 years: 1-2 inhalations 3-4 times/day; alternatively 2-4 inhalations twice daily; do not exceed 10 inhalations/day

Adults: 2 inhalations 3-4 times/day; alternatively 2-4 inhalations twice daily; do not exceed 20 inhalations/day; patients with severe asthma should be started on 12-16 inhalations/day (divided 3-4 times/day) and dose should be adjusted downward according to the patient's response

**Mechanism of Action** Controls the rate of protein synthesis, depresses the migration of polymorphonuclear leukocytes, fibroblasts, reverses capillary permeability, and lysosomal stabilization at the cellular level to prevent or control inflammation

**Local Anesthetic/Vasoconstrictor Precautions** No information available to require special precautions

**Effects on Dental Treatment** Localized infections with *Candida albicans* or *Aspergillus niger* have occurred frequently in the mouth and pharynx with repetitive use of oral inhaler of beclomethasone. Positive cultures for oral *Candida* may be present in up to 75% of patients. These infections may require treatment with appropriate antifungal therapy or discontinuance of treatment with beclomethasone inhaler.

**Other Adverse Effects**

>10%:

Local: Growth of *Candida* in the mouth, irritation and burning of the nasal mucosa

Respiratory: Cough, hoarseness

1% to 10%:

Gastrointestinal: Dry mouth

Respiratory: Epistaxis, nasal ulceration

<1%:

Central nervous system: Headache

Dermatologic: Skin rash

Gastrointestinal: Dysphagia

Respiratory: Bronchospasm, rhinorrhea, nasal congestion, sneezing, nasal septal perforations

**Drug Interactions** No data reported

**Drug Uptake**

Therapeutic effect: Within 1-4 weeks of use

Inhalation:

Absorption: Readily absorbed; quickly hydrolyzed by pulmonary esterases prior to absorption

Absorption: 90%

Serum half-life:

Initial: 3 hours

Terminal: 15 hours

**Pregnancy Risk Factor** C

**Generic Available** No

♦ **Beclovent®** *see* Beclomethasone *on previous page*

♦ **Beconase®** *see* Beclomethasone *on previous page*

♦ **Beconase AQ®** *see* Beclomethasone *on previous page*

♦ **Becotin® Pulvules®** *see* Vitamins, Multiple *on page 1051*

♦ **Beepen-VK®** *see* Penicillin V Potassium *on page 776*

♦ **Belix® Oral [OTC]** *see* Diphenhydramine *on page 338*

## Belladonna (bel a DON a)

**Therapeutic Category** Anticholinergic Agent; Antispasmodic Agent, Gastrointestinal

**Use** Decrease gastrointestinal activity in functional bowel disorders and to delay gastric emptying as well as decrease gastric secretion

**Usual Dosage** Tincture: Oral:

Children: 0.03 mL/kg 3 times/day

Adults: 0.6-1 mL 3-4 times/day

**Mechanism of Action** Belladonna is a mixture of the anticholinergic alkaloids atropine, hyoscyamine, and scopolamine (hyoscine). The belladonna alkaloids act primarily by competitive inhibition of the muscarinic actions of acetylcholine on structures innervated by postganglionic cholinergic neurons and on smooth muscle. The resulting effects include antisecretory activity on exocrine glands and intestinal mucosa and smooth muscle relaxation. The anticholinergic properties of scopolamine and atropine differ in that scopolamine has a more potent activity on the iris, ciliary body, and certain secretory glands; has more potent activity on the heart, intestine, and bronchial muscle, and a more prolonged duration of action; in contrast, hyoscyamine has actions similar to those of atropine, but is more potent in both its central and peripheral effects

**Local Anesthetic/Vasoconstrictor Precautions** No information available to require special precautions

**Effects on Dental Treatment** >10% of patients experience dry mouth

**Other Adverse Effects**

>10%:

Dermatologic: Dry skin

Gastrointestinal: Constipation

Respiratory: Dry nose, throat

Miscellaneous: Decreased sweating

1% to 10%:

Dermatologic: Increased photosensitivity

Endocrine & metabolic: Decreased flow of breast milk

Gastrointestinal: Dysphagia

(Continued)

## Belladonna *(Continued)*

<1%:

Cardiovascular: Ventricular fibrillation, tachycardia, palpitations, orthostatic hypotension

Central nervous system: Confusion, drowsiness, headache, loss of memory, fatigue, ataxia

Dermatologic: Skin rash

Gastrointestinal: Bloated feeling, nausea, vomiting

Genitourinary: Dysuria

Neuromuscular & skeletal: Weakness

Ocular: Increased intraocular pain, blurred vision

**Pregnancy Risk Factor** C

**Generic Available** Yes

## Belladonna and Opium (bel a DON a & OH pee um)

**U.S. Brand Names** B&O Supprettes®

**Canadian Brand Names** PMS-Opium & Beladonna

**Therapeutic Category** Analgesic, Narcotic

**Use** Relief of moderate to severe pain associated with rectal or bladder tenesmus that may occur in postoperative states and neoplastic situations; pain associated with ureteral spasms not responsive to non-narcotic analgesics and to space intervals between injections of opiates

**Usual Dosage** Adults: Rectal: 1 suppository 1-2 times/day, up to 4 doses/day

**Mechanism of Action** Anticholinergic alkaloids act primarily by competitive inhibition of the muscarinic actions of acetylcholine on structures innervated by postganglionic cholinergic neurons and on smooth muscle; resulting effects include antisecretory activity on exocrine glands and intestinal mucosa and smooth muscle relaxation. The opium component contains many narcotic alkaloids including morphine; its mechanism for gastric motility inhibition is primarily due to this morphine content; it results in a decrease in digestive secretions, an increase in GI muscle tone, and therefore a reduction in GI propulsion.

**Local Anesthetic/Vasoconstrictor Precautions** No information available to require special precautions

**Effects on Dental Treatment** This drug has atropine-like effects and the patient may experience drowsiness, dry mouth, nose and throat

**Other Adverse Effects**

>10%:

Dermatologic: Dry skin

Gastrointestinal: Constipation, dry mouth

Respiratory: Dry nose, throat

Miscellaneous: Decreased sweating

1% to 10%:

Dermatologic: Photosensitivity

Endocrine & metabolic: Decreased flow of breast milk

Gastrointestinal: Dysphagia

<1%:

Cardiovascular: Orthostatic hypotension, ventricular fibrillation, tachycardia, palpitations

Central nervous system: Confusion, drowsiness, headache, loss of memory, fatigue, ataxia, CNS depression

Dermatologic: Skin rash

Endocrine & metabolic: Antidiuretic hormone release

Gastrointestinal: Bloated feeling, nausea, vomiting, constipation, biliary tract spasm

Genitourinary: Dysuria, urinary retention, urinary tract spasm

Neuromuscular & skeletal: Weakness

Ocular: Increased intraocular pain, blurred vision

Respiratory: Respiratory depression

Miscellaneous: Histamine release, physical and psychological dependence, sweating

**Drug Interactions** Increased effect/toxicity: CNS depressants, tricyclic antidepressants

**Drug Uptake**

Onset of action:

Belladonna: 1-2 hours

Opium: Within 30 minutes

**Pregnancy Risk Factor** C

**Dosage Forms** Suppository:

#15 A: Belladonna extract 15 mg and opium 30 mg

#16 A: Belladonna extract 15 mg and opium 60 mg

**Generic Available** Yes

## Belladonna, Phenobarbital, and Ergotamine Tartrate

(bel a DON a, fee noe BAR bi tal, & er GOT a meen TAR trate)

**U.S. Brand Names** Bellergal-S®; Bel-Phen-Ergot S®; Phenerbel-S®

**Canadian Brand Names** Bellergal®; Bellergal® Spacetabs®

**Therapeutic Category** Ergot Alkaloid and Derivative

**Use** Management and treatment of menopausal disorders, gastrointestinal disorders and recurrent throbbing headache

**Usual Dosage** Oral: 1 tablet each morning and evening

**Local Anesthetic/Vasoconstrictor Precautions** No information available to require special precautions

**Effects on Dental Treatment** >10% of patients experience dry mouth

**Other Adverse Effects**

>10%:

- Cardiovascular: Peripheral vascular effects, local edema
- Central nervous system: Drowsiness, dizziness
- Dermatologic: Dry skin
- Gastrointestinal: Constipation, diarrhea, nausea, vomiting
- Local: Irritation at injection site
- Neuromuscular & skeletal: Paresthesia
- Respiratory: Dry nose, throat
- Miscellaneous: Decreased sweating

1% to 10%:

- Cardiovascular: Precordial distress and pain, transient tachycardia or bradycardia
- Dermatologic: Photosensitivity
- Endocrine & metabolic: Decreased flow of breast milk
- Gastrointestinal: Dysphagia
- Neuromuscular & skeletal: Myalgia, weakness in the legs

<1%:

- Cardiovascular: Orthostatic hypotension, ventricular fibrillation, tachycardia, palpitations
- Central nervous system: Confusion, headache, loss of memory, fatigue, ataxia
- Dermatologic: Skin rash
- Gastrointestinal: Bloated feeling, nausea, vomiting
- Genitourinary: Dysuria
- Neuromuscular & skeletal: Weakness
- Ocular: Increased intraocular pain, blurred vision

**Drug Interactions** CNS depressants

**Pregnancy Risk Factor** X

**Generic Available** Yes

- ♦ **Bellergal-S®** *see* Belladonna, Phenobarbital, and Ergotamine Tartrate *on this page*
- ♦ **Bel-Phen-Ergot S®** *see* Belladonna, Phenobarbital, and Ergotamine Tartrate *on this page*
- ♦ **Benadryl® Decongestant Allergy Tablet [OTC]** *see* Diphenhydramine and Pseudoephedrine *on page 339*
- ♦ **Benadryl® Injection** *see* Diphenhydramine *on page 338*
- ♦ **Benadryl® Oral [OTC]** *see* Diphenhydramine *on page 338*
- ♦ **Benadryl® Topical** *see* Diphenhydramine *on page 338*
- ♦ **Ben-Allergin-50® Injection** *see* Diphenhydramine *on page 338*
- ♦ **Ben-Aqua® [OTC]** *see* Benzoyl Peroxide *on page 130*

## Benazepril

(ben AY ze pril)

**Related Information**

Cardiovascular Diseases *on page 1066*

**U.S. Brand Names** Lotensin®

**Therapeutic Category** Angiotensin-Converting Enzyme (ACE) Inhibitor

**Use** Treatment of hypertension, either alone or in combination with other antihypertensive agents

**Usual Dosage** Adults: Oral: 20-40 mg/day as a single dose or 2 divided doses; maximum daily dose: 80 mg

**Mechanism of Action** Competitive inhibition of angiotensin I being converted to angiotensin II, a potent vasoconstrictor, through the angiotensin I-converting enzyme (ACE) activity, with resultant lower levels of angiotensin II which causes an increase in plasma renin activity and a reduction in aldosterone secretion

**Local Anesthetic/Vasoconstrictor Precautions** No information available to require special precautions

**Effects on Dental Treatment** No effects or complications reported

(Continued)

## Benazepril *(Continued)*

**Other Adverse Effects**

1% to 10%:

Central nervous system: Headache, dizziness, fatigue, somnolence, postural dizziness

Gastrointestinal: Nausea

Respiratory: Transient cough

<1%:

Cardiovascular: Hypotension, tachycardia

Central nervous system: Anxiety, insomnia, nervousness

Dermatologic: Rash, photosensitivity, angioedema

Endocrine & metabolic: Hyperkalemia

Gastrointestinal: Constipation, gastritis, vomiting, melena

Genitourinary: Impotence, urinary tract infection

Neuromuscular & skeletal: Hypertonia, paresthesia, arthralgia, arthritis, myalgia, weakness

Respiratory: Asthma, bronchitis, dyspnea, sinusitis

Miscellaneous: Sweating

**Drug Interactions** See table.

**Drug-Drug Interactions With ACEIs**

| Precipitant Drug | Drug (Category) and Effect | Description |
|---|---|---|
| Antacids | ACE Inhibitors: decreased | Decreased bioavailability of ACEIs. May be more likely with captopril. Separate administration times by 1-2 hours. |
| NSAIDs (indomethacin) | ACEIs: decreased | Reduced hypotensive effects of ACEIs. More prominent in low renin or volume dependent hypertensive patients. |
| Phenothiazines | ACEIs: increased | Pharmacologic effects of ACEIs may be increased. |
| ACEIs | Allopurinol: increased | Higher risk of hypersensitivity reaction possible when given concurrently. Three case reports of Stevens-Johnson syndrome with captopril. |
| ACEIs | Digoxin: increased | Increased plasma digoxin levels. |
| ACEIs | Lithium: increased | Increased serum lithium levels and symptoms of toxicity may occur. |
| ACEIs | Potassium preps/ potassium sparing diuretics increased | Coadministration may result in elevated potassium levels. |

**Drug Uptake**

Reduction in plasma angiotensin-converting enzyme activity: Oral:

Peak effect: 1-2 hours after administration of 2-20 mg dose

Duration of action: >90% inhibition for 24 hours has been observed after 5-20 mg dose

Reduction in blood pressure:

Peak effect after single oral dose: 2-6 hours

Maximum response With continuous therapy: 2 weeks

Absorption: Rapid (37% of each oral dose); food does not alter significantly; metabolite (benazeprilat) itself unsuitable for oral administration due to poor absorption

Serum half-life:

Parent drug: 0.6 hour

Metabolite elimination: 22 hours (from 24 hours after dosing onward)

Metabolite: 1.5-2 hours after fasting or 2-4 hours after a meal

Time to peak: 1-1.5 hours (unchanged parent drug)

**Pregnancy Risk Factor** C (first trimester); D (second and third trimesters)

**Generic Available** No

## Benazepril and Hydrochlorothiazide

(ben AY ze pril & hye droe klor oh THYE a zide)

**U.S. Brand Names** Lotensin HCT®

**Therapeutic Category** Antihypertensive Agent, Combination

**Use** Treatment of hypertension

**Usual Dosage** Dose is individualized

**Local Anesthetic/Vasoconstrictor Precautions** No information available to require special precautions

**Effects on Dental Treatment** No effects or complications reported

**Generic Available** No

## Bendroflumethiazide (ben droe floo meth EYE a zide)

**Related Information**

Cardiovascular Diseases *on page 1066*

**U.S. Brand Names** Naturetin®

**Therapeutic Category** Diuretic, Thiazide

**Use** Management of mild to moderate hypertension; treatment of edema associated with congestive heart failure, pregnancy, or nephrotic syndrome

**Usual Dosage** Oral:

Children: Initial: 0.1-0.4 mg/kg/day in 1-2 doses; maintenance dose: 0.05-0.1 mg/kg/day in 1-2 doses

Adults: 2.5-20 mg/day or twice daily in divided doses

**Mechanism of Action** Like other thiazide diuretics, it inhibits sodium, chloride, and water reabsorption in the renal distal tubules, thereby producing diuresis with a resultant reduction in plasma volume; hypothetically may reduce peripheral resistance through increased prostacyclin synthesis

**Local Anesthetic/Vasoconstrictor Precautions** No information available to require special precautions

**Effects on Dental Treatment** No effects or complications reported

**Other Adverse Effects**

1% to 10%:
- Cardiovascular: Orthostatic hypotension
- Endocrine & metabolic: Hyponatremia, hypokalemia
- Gastrointestinal: Anorexia, gastritis, diarrhea

<1%:
- Central nervous system: Somnolence
- Endocrine & metabolic: Hyperuricemia
- Gastrointestinal: Nausea, vomiting
- Hematologic: Aplastic anemia, hemolytic anemia, leukopenia, agranulocytosis, thrombocytopenia
- Hepatic: Hepatitis, hepatic function impairment
- Neuromuscular & skeletal: Paresthesia
- Renal: Polyuria, uremia
- Miscellaneous: Allergic reactions

**Drug Interactions**

Thiazides tend to elevate blood glucose in diabetics and thus may antagonize the hypoglycemic effect of antidiabetic drugs.

GI tract absorption of thiazides are impaired by cholestyramine (Questran®) and colestipol (Colestid®).

Thiazides increase plasma lithium concentrations; lithium toxicity may occur

**Pregnancy Risk Factor** D

**Generic Available** Yes


- ♦ **Benemid®** *see* Probenecid *on page 839*
- ♦ **Benoquin®** *see* Monobenzone *on page 686*
- ♦ **Benoxyl®** *see* Benzoyl Peroxide *on page 130*


## Bentoquatam (ben to KWA tam)

**U.S. Brand Names** IvyBlock®

**Therapeutic Category** Protectant, Topical

**Use** To protect the skin from rash due to exposure to poison sumac, poison ivy or poison oak

**Usual Dosage** Topical: Apply to exposed skin at least 15 minutes before potential contact and reapply every 4 hours

**Local Anesthetic/Vasoconstrictor Precautions** No information available to require special precautions

**Effects on Dental Treatment** No effects or complications reported

**Dosage Forms** Lotion: 5% (120 mL)

**Generic Available** No


- ♦ **Bentyl® Hydrochloride Injection** *see* Dicyclomine *on page 322*
- ♦ **Bentyl® Hydrochloride Oral** *see* Dicyclomine *on page 322*
- ♦ **Benylin® Cough Syrup [OTC]** *see* Diphenhydramine *on page 338*
- ♦ **Benylin DM® [OTC]** *see* Dextromethorphan *on page 314*
- ♦ **Benylin® Expectorant [OTC]** *see* Guaifenesin and Dextromethorphan *on page 479*
- ♦ **Benylin® Pediatric [OTC]** *see* Dextromethorphan *on page 314*
- ♦ **Benza® [OTC]** *see* Benzalkonium Chloride *on next page*
- ♦ **Benzac AC® Gel** *see* Benzoyl Peroxide *on page 130*
- ♦ **Benzac AC® Wash** *see* Benzoyl Peroxide *on page 130*

- **Benzac W® Gel** see Benzoyl Peroxide *on page 130*
- **Benzac W® Wash** see Benzoyl Peroxide *on page 130*
- **5-Benzagel®** see Benzoyl Peroxide *on page 130*
- **10-Benzagel®** see Benzoyl Peroxide *on page 130*

## Benzalkonium Chloride (benz al KOE nee um KLOR ide)

**Related Information**

Periodontal Diseases *on page 1132*

**U.S. Brand Names** Benza® [OTC]; Zephiran® [OTC]

**Therapeutic Category** Antibacterial, Topical

**Synonyms** BAC

**Use** Surface antiseptic and germicidal preservative

**Usual Dosage** Thoroughly rinse anionic detergents and soaps from the skin or other areas prior to use of solutions because they reduce the antibacterial activity of BAC. To protect metal instruments stored in BAC solution, add crushed Anti-Rust Tablets, 4 tablets/quart, to antiseptic solution, change solution at least once weekly. Not to be used for storage of aluminum or zinc instruments, instruments with lenses fastened by cement, lacquered catheters, or some synthetic rubber goods.

**Local Anesthetic/Vasoconstrictor Precautions** No information available to require special precautions

**Effects on Dental Treatment** No effects or complications reported

**Other Adverse Effects** 1% to 10%: Hypersensitivity

**Pregnancy Risk Factor** C

**Generic Available** Yes

- **Benzamycin®** see Erythromycin and Benzoyl Peroxide *on page 385*
- **Benzashave® Cream** see Benzoyl Peroxide *on page 130*
- **Benzedrex® [OTC]** see Propylhexedrine *on page 859*
- **Benzmethyzin** see Procarbazine *on page 842*

## Benzocaine (BEN zoe kane)

**Related Information**

Mouth Pain, Cold Sore, Canker Sore Products *on page 1253*

**U.S. Brand Names** Americaine® [OTC]; Anbesol® [OTC]; Anbesol® Maximum Strength [OTC]; Babee® Teething® [OTC]; Benzocol® [OTC]; Benzodent® [OTC]; Chiggertox® [OTC]; Cylex® [OTC]; Dermoplast® [OTC]; Foille® [OTC]; Foille® Medicated First Aid [OTC]; Hurricaine®; Lanacane® [OTC]; Maximum Strength Anbesol® [OTC]; Maximum Strength Orajel® [OTC]; Mycinettes® [OTC]; Numzitdent® [OTC]; Numzit Teething® [OTC]; Orabase®-B [OTC]; Orabase®-O [OTC]; Orajel® Brace-Aid Oral Anesthetic [OTC]; Orajel® Maximum Strength [OTC]; Orajel® Mouth-Aid [OTC]; Orasept® [OTC]; Orasol® [OTC]; Rhulicaine® [OTC]; Rid-A-Pain® [OTC]; Slim-Mint® [OTC]; Solarcaine® [OTC]; Spec-T® [OTC]; Tanac® [OTC]; Trocaine® [OTC]; Unguentine® [OTC]; Vicks Children's Chloraseptic® [OTC]; Vicks Chloraseptic® Sore Throat [OTC]; Zilactin-B® Medicated [OTC]

**Therapeutic Category** Local Anesthetic, Topical

**Use**

Dental: Ester-type topical local anesthetic for temporary relief of pain associated with toothache, minor sore throat pain and canker sore

Medical: Local anesthetic (ester derivative); temporary relief of pain associated with pruritic dermatosis, pruritus, minor burns, acute congestive and serious otitis media, swimmer's ear, otitis externa, hemorrhoids, rectal fissures, anesthetic lubricant for passage of catheters and endoscopic tubes

**Usual Dosage** Children and Adults:

Mucous membranes: Dosage varies depending on area to be anesthetized and vascularity of tissues

Oral mouth/throat preparations: Do not administer for >2 days or in children <2 years of age, unless directed by a physician; refer to specific package labeling

**Mechanism of Action** Local anesthetics bind selectively to the intracellular surface of sodium channels to block influx of sodium into the axon. As a result, depolarization necessary for action potential propagation and subsequent nerve function is prevented. The block at the sodium channel is reversible. When drug diffuses away from the axon, sodium channel function is restored and nerve propagation returns.

**Local Anesthetic/Vasoconstrictor Precautions** No information available to require special precautions

**Effects on Dental Treatment** No effects or complications reported

**Other Adverse Effects** 1% to 10%:

Dermatologic: Angioedema, contact dermatitis

Local: Burning, stinging

**Contraindications** Known hypersensitivity to benzocaine, other ester-type local anesthetics, or other components in the formulation; ophthalmic use

**Warnings/Precautions** Not intended for use when infections are present

**Drug Interactions** May antagonize actions of sulfonamides

**Drug Uptake**

Onset: ~1 minute

Duration: 15-20 minutes

Absorption: Topical: Poorly absorbed after administration to intact skin, but well absorbed from mucous membranes and traumatized skin

**Pregnancy Risk Factor** C

**Breast-feeding Considerations** No data reported

**Dosage Forms**

Mouth/throat preparations:

- Cream: 5% (10 g)
- Gel: 6.3% (7.5 g); 7.5% (7.2 g, 9.45 g, 14.1 g); 10% (6 g, 9.45 g, 10 g, 15 g); 15% (10.5 g); 20% (9.45 g, 14.1 g)
- Liquid: (3.7 mL); 5% (8.8 mL); 6.3% (9 mL, 22 mL, 14.79 mL); 10% (13 mL); 20% (13.3 mL)
- Lotion: 0.2% (15 mL); 2.5% (15 mL)
- Lozenges: 5 mg, 6 mg, 10 mg, 15 mg
- Ointment: 20% (5 g, 15 g)

Topical for mucous membranes:

- Gel: 6% (7.5 g); 20% (2.5 g, 3.75 g, 7.5 g, 30 g)
- Liquid: 20% (3.75 mL, 9 mL, 13.3 mL, 30 mL)

**Generic Available** Yes

♦ **Benzocaine and Antipyrine** *see* Antipyrine and Benzocaine *on page 91*

♦ **Benzocaine and Cetylpyridinium Chloride** *see* Cetylpyridinium and Benzocaine *on page 219*

## Benzocaine, Butyl Aminobenzoate, Tetracaine, and Benzalkonium Chloride

(BEN zoe kane, BYOO til a meen oh BENZ oh ate, TET ra kane, & benz al KOE nee um KLOR ide)

**U.S. Brand Names** Cetacaine®

**Therapeutic Category** Local Anesthetic, Topical

**Synonyms** Tetracaine Hydrochloride, Benzocaine Butyl Aminobenzoate and Benzalkonium Chloride

**Use** Topical anesthetic to control pain or gagging

**Usual Dosage** Apply to affected area for approximately 1 second or less

**Local Anesthetic/Vasoconstrictor Precautions** No information available to require special precautions

**Effects on Dental Treatment** No effects or complications reported

**Other Adverse Effects** Dose related and may result from high plasma levels

1% to 10%:

- Dermatologic: Contact dermatitis, angioedema
- Local: Burning, stinging

<1%:

- Cardiovascular: Edema
- Dermatologic: Urticaria
- Genitourinary: Urethritis
- Hematologic: Methemoglobinemia in infants
- Local: Tenderness

**Pregnancy Risk Factor** C

**Generic Available** No

## Benzocaine, Gelatin, Pectin, and Sodium Carboxymethylcellulose

(BEN zoe kane, JEL a tin, PEK tin, & SOW dee um kar box ee meth il SEL yoo lose)

**U.S. Brand Names** Orabase® With Benzocaine [OTC]

**Therapeutic Category** Local Anesthetic, Topical

**Use** Topical anesthetic and emollient for oral lesions

**Usual Dosage** Apply 2-4 times/day

**Local Anesthetic/Vasoconstrictor Precautions** No information available to require special precautions

**Effects on Dental Treatment** No effects or complications reported

**Other Adverse Effects** Dose related and may result from high plasma levels

1% to 10%:

- Dermatologic: Contact dermatitis, angioedema
- Local: Burning, stinging

(Continued)

## Benzocaine, Gelatin, Pectin, and Sodium Carboxymethylcellulose *(Continued)*

<1%:

Cardiovascular: Edema
Dermatologic: Urticaria
Gastrointestinal: Urethritis
Hematologic: Methemoglobinemia in infants
Local: Tenderness

**Pregnancy Risk Factor** C
**Generic Available** No

♦ **Benzocol® [OTC]** *see* Benzocaine *on page 128*
♦ **Benzodent® [OTC]** *see* Benzocaine *on page 128*

## Benzoic Acid and Salicylic Acid

(ben ZOE ik AS id & sal i SIL ik AS id)

**U.S. Brand Names** Whitfield's Ointment [OTC]
**Therapeutic Category** Antifungal Agent, Topical
**Synonyms** Salicylic Acid and Benzoic Acid
**Use** Treatment of athlete's foot and ringworm of the scalp
**Usual Dosage** Apply 1-4 times/day
**Local Anesthetic/Vasoconstrictor Precautions** No information available to require special precautions
**Effects on Dental Treatment** No effects or complications reported
**Generic Available** Yes

## Benzoin (BEN zoyn)

**U.S. Brand Names** AeroZoin® [OTC]; TinBen® [OTC]; TinCoBen® [OTC]
**Therapeutic Category** Pharmaceutical Aid; Protectant, Topical
**Synonyms** Gum Benjamin
**Use** Protective application for irritations of the skin; sometimes used in boiling water as steam inhalants for their expectorant and soothing action
**Usual Dosage** Apply 1-2 times/day
**Local Anesthetic/Vasoconstrictor Precautions** No information available to require special precautions
**Effects on Dental Treatment** No effects or complications reported
**Generic Available** Yes

## Benzonatate (ben ZOE na tate)

**Related Information**

Patients Undergoing Cancer Therapy *on page 1154*

**U.S. Brand Names** Tessalon® Perles
**Therapeutic Category** Antitussive; Local Anesthetic, Oral
**Use** Symptomatic relief of nonproductive cough
**Usual Dosage** Children >10 years and Adults: Oral: 100 mg 3 times/day or every 4 hours up to 600 mg/day
**Mechanism of Action** Tetracaine congener with antitussive properties; suppresses cough by topical anesthetic action on the respiratory stretch receptors
**Local Anesthetic/Vasoconstrictor Precautions** No information available to require special precautions
**Effects on Dental Treatment** No effects or complications reported
**Other Adverse Effects** 1% to 10%:

Central nervous system: Sedation, headache, dizziness
Dermatologic: Skin rash
Gastrointestinal: GI upset
Neuromuscular & skeletal: Numbness in chest
Ocular: Burning sensation in eyes
Respiratory: Nasal congestion

**Drug Interactions** No data reported
**Drug Uptake**

Onset of action: Therapeutic: Within 15-20 minutes
Duration: 3-8 hours

**Pregnancy Risk Factor** C
**Generic Available** Yes

## Benzoyl Peroxide (BEN zoe il peer OKS ide)

**U.S. Brand Names** Advanced Formula Oxy® Sensitive Gel [OTC]; Ambi 10® [OTC]; Ben-Aqua® [OTC]; Benoxyl®; Benzac AC® Gel; Benzac AC® Wash; Benzac W® Gel; Benzac W® Wash; 5-Benzagel®; 10-Benzagel®; Benzashave®

Cream; BlemErase® Lotion [OTC]; Brevoxyl® Gel; Clear By Design® Gel [OTC]; Clearsil® Maximum Strength [OTC]; Del Aqua-5® Gel; Del Aqua-10® Gel; Desquam-E™ Gel; Desquam-X® Gel; Desquam-X® Wash; Dryox® Gel [OTC]; Dryox® Wash [OTC]; Exact® Cream [OTC]; Fostex® 10% BPO Gel [OTC]; Fostex® 10% Wash [OTC]; Fostex® Bar [OTC]; Loroxide® [OTC]; Neutrogena® Acne Mask [OTC]; Oxy-5® Advanced Formula for Sensitive Skin [OTC]; Oxy-5® Tinted [OTC]; Oxy-10® Advanced Formula for Sensitive Skin [OTC]; Oxy 10® Wash [OTC]; PanOxyl®-AQ; PanOxyl® Bar [OTC]; Perfectoderm® Gel [OTC]; Peroxin A5®; Peroxin A10®; Persa-Gel®; Theroxide® Wash [OTC]; Vanoxide® [OTC]

**Canadian Brand Names** Acetoxyl®; Acnomel® B.P.5; Benzagel®; $H_2$Oxyl®; Oxyderm®; Solugel®

**Therapeutic Category** Acne Products; Topical Skin Product

**Use** Adjunctive treatment of mild to moderate acne vulgaris and acne rosacea

**Usual Dosage** Children and Adults:

Cleansers: Wash once or twice daily; control amount of drying or peeling by modifying dose frequency or concentration

Topical: Apply sparingly once daily; gradually increase to 2-3 times/day if needed. If excessive dryness or peeling occurs, reduce dose frequency or concentration; if excessive stinging or burning occurs, remove with mild soap and water; resume use the next day.

**Mechanism of Action** Releases free-radical oxygen which oxidizes bacterial proteins in the sebaceous follicles decreasing the number of anaerobic bacteria and decreasing irritating-type free fatty acids

**Local Anesthetic/Vasoconstrictor Precautions** No information available to require special precautions

**Effects on Dental Treatment** No effects or complications reported

**Other Adverse Effects** 1% to 10%: Dermatologic: Irritation, contact dermatitis, dryness, erythema, peeling, stinging

**Drug Interactions** Increased toxicity: Benzoyl peroxide potentiates adverse reactions seen with tretinoin

**Drug Uptake**

Absorption: ~5% through the skin; gels are more penetrating than creams

**Pregnancy Risk Factor** C

**Generic Available** Yes

## Benzoyl Peroxide and Hydrocortisone

(BEN zoe il peer OKS ide & hye droe KOR ti sone)

**U.S. Brand Names** Vanoxide-HC®

**Therapeutic Category** Acne Products; Corticosteroid, Topical (Low Potency); Topical Skin Product

**Use** Treatment of acne vulgaris and oily skin

**Usual Dosage** Shake well; apply thin film 1-3 times/day, gently massage into skin

**Local Anesthetic/Vasoconstrictor Precautions** No information available to require special precautions

**Effects on Dental Treatment** No effects or complications reported

**Other Adverse Effects** See individual agents

**Pregnancy Risk Factor** C

**Generic Available** No

## Benzphetamine (benz FET a meen)

**U.S. Brand Names** Didrex®

**Therapeutic Category** Anorexiant

**Use** Short-term adjunct in exogenous obesity

**Usual Dosage** Adults: Oral: 25-50 mg 2-3 times/day, preferably twice daily, midmorning and midafternoon; maximum dose: 50 mg 3 times/day

**Mechanism of Action** Noncatechol sympathomimetic amines with pharmacologic actions similar to ephedrine; require breakdown by monoamine oxidase for inactivation; produce central nervous system and respiratory stimulation, a pressor response, mydriasis, bronchodilation, and contraction of the urinary sphincter; thought to have a direct effect on both alpha- and beta-receptor sites in the peripheral system, as well as release stores of norepinephrine in adrenergic nerve terminals; central nervous system action is thought to occur in the cerebral cortex and reticular-activating system; anorexigenic effect is probably secondary to the CNS-stimulating effect; the site of action is probably the hypothalamic feeding center

**Local Anesthetic/Vasoconstrictor Precautions** Use with caution since amphetamines have actions similar to epinephrine and norepinephrine

**Effects on Dental Treatment** No effects or complications reported

(Continued)

## Benzphetamine *(Continued)*

**Other Adverse Effects**

>10%:

Cardiovascular: Arrhythmia

Central nervous system: False feeling of well being, nervousness, restlessness, insomnia

1% to 10%:

Cardiovascular: Hypertension

Central nervous system: Mood or mental changes, dizziness, lightheadedness, headache

Endocrine & metabolic: Changes in libido

Gastrointestinal: Diarrhea, nausea, vomiting, stomach cramps, constipation, anorexia, weight loss, dry mouth

Ocular: Blurred vision

Miscellaneous: Increased sweating

<1%:

Cardiovascular: Chest pain

Central nervous system: CNS stimulation (severe), Tourette's syndrome, hyperthermia, seizures, paranoia, tolerance and withdrawal with prolonged use

Dermatologic: Skin rash, urticaria

**Pregnancy Risk Factor** X

**Generic Available** No

## Benzthiazide (benz THYE a zide)

**Related Information**

Cardiovascular Diseases *on page 1066*

**U.S. Brand Names** Exna®

**Therapeutic Category** Diuretic, Thiazide

**Use** Management of mild to moderate hypertension; treatment of edema in congestive heart failure and nephrotic syndrome

**Usual Dosage** Oral:

Children: 1-4 mg/kg/day in 3 divided doses

Adults: 50-200 mg/day

**Mechanism of Action** Like other thiazide diuretics, it inhibits sodium, chloride, and water reabsorption in the renal distal tubules, thereby producing diuresis with a resultant reduction in plasma volume; hypothetically may reduce peripheral resistance through increased prostacyclin synthesis

**Local Anesthetic/Vasoconstrictor Precautions** No information available to require special precautions

**Effects on Dental Treatment** No effects or complications reported

**Other Adverse Effects**

1% to 10%:

Cardiovascular: Orthostatic hypotension

Endocrine & metabolic: Hyponatremia, hypokalemia

Gastrointestinal: Anorexia, upset stomach, diarrhea

<1%:

Central nervous system: Drowsiness

Endocrine & metabolic: Hyperuricemia

Gastrointestinal: Nausea, vomiting

Hematologic: Aplastic anemia, hemolytic anemia, leukopenia, agranulocytosis, thrombocytopenia

Hepatic: Hepatitis, hepatic function impairment

Neuromuscular & skeletal: Paresthesia

Renal: Polyuria, uremia

Miscellaneous: Allergic reactions

**Drug Interactions**

Thiazides tend to elevate blood glucose in diabetics and thus may antagonize the hypoglycemic effect of antidiabetic drugs.

GI tract absorption of thiazides are impaired by cholestyramine (Questran®) and colestipol (Colestid®).

Thiazides increase plasma lithium concentrations; lithium toxicity may occur.

**Drug Uptake**

Onset of action: Within 2 hours

Duration: 12 hours

**Pregnancy Risk Factor** D

**Generic Available** Yes

## Benztropine (BENZ troe peen)

**U.S. Brand Names** Cogentin®

**Canadian Brand Names** PMS-Benztropine

**Therapeutic Category** Anticholinergic Agent; Anti-Parkinson's Agent

**Use** Adjunctive treatment of Parkinson's disease; also used in treatment of drug-induced extrapyramidal effects (except tardive dyskinesia) and acute dystonic reactions

**Usual Dosage** Use in children <3 years of age should be reserved for life-threatening emergencies

Drug-induced extrapyramidal reaction: Oral, I.M., I.V.:

Children >3 years: 0.02-0.05 mg/kg/dose 1-2 times/day

Adults: 1-4 mg/dose 1-2 times/day

Acute dystonia: Adults: I.M., I.V.: 1-2 mg

Parkinsonism: Oral:

Adults: 0.5-6 mg/day in 1-2 divided doses; if one dose is greater, give at bedtime; titrate dose in 0.5 mg increments at 5- to 6-day intervals

Elderly: Initial: 0.5 mg once or twice daily; increase by 0.5 mg as needed at 5-6 days; maximum: 6 mg/day

**Mechanism of Action** Thought to partially block striatal cholinergic receptors to help balance cholinergic and dopaminergic activity

**Local Anesthetic/Vasoconstrictor Precautions** No information available to require special precautions

**Effects on Dental Treatment** Dry mouth, nose and throat very prevalent in patients taking this drug

**Other Adverse Effects**

>10%:

Dermatologic: Dry skin

Gastrointestinal: Constipation

Respiratory: Dry nose, throat

Miscellaneous: Decreased sweating

1% to 10%:

Dermatologic: Photosensitivity

Endocrine & metabolic: Decreased flow of breast milk

Gastrointestinal: Dysphagia

<1%:

Cardiovascular: Coma, tachycardia, orthostatic hypotension, ventricular fibrillation, palpitations

Central nervous system: Drowsiness, nervousness, hallucinations; the elderly may be at increased risk for confusion and hallucinations, headache, loss of memory, fatigue, ataxia

Dermatologic: Skin rash

Gastrointestinal: Nausea, vomiting, bloated feeling

Genitourinary: Dysuria

Neuromuscular & skeletal: Weakness

Ocular: Blurred vision, mydriasis, increased intraocular pain

**Drug Interactions**

Decreased effect: May increase gastric degradation of levodopa and decrease the amount of levodopa absorbed by delaying gastric emptying - the opposite may be true for digoxin

Increased toxicity: Central anticholinergic syndrome can occur when administered with narcotic analgesics, phenothiazines and other antipsychotics, tricyclic antidepressants, quinidine and some other antiarrhythmics, and antihistamines

**Drug Uptake**

Onset of action:

Oral: Within 1 hour

Parenteral: Within 15 minutes

Duration of action: 6-48 hours (wide range)

**Pregnancy Risk Factor** C

**Generic Available** Yes: Tablet

## Benzylpenicilloyl-polylysine (BEN zil pen i SIL oyl pol i LIE seen)

**U.S. Brand Names** Pre-Pen®

**Therapeutic Category** Diagnostic Agent, Penicillin Allergy Skin Test

**Use** Adjunct in assessing the risk of administering penicillin (penicillin or benzylpenicillin) in adults with a history of clinical penicillin hypersensitivity

**Usual Dosage** PPL is administered by a scratch technique or by intradermal injection. For initial testing, PPL should always be applied via the scratch technique. **Do not give intradermally to patients who have positive reactions to a scratch test.** PPL test alone does not identify those patients who react to a minor antigenic determinant and does not appear to predict reliably the occurrence of late reactions.

**Scratch test:** Use scratch technique with a 20-gauge needle to make 3-5 mm nonbleeding scratch on epidermis, apply a small drop of solution to scratch, rub

(Continued)

## Benzylpenicilloyl-polylysine *(Continued)*

in gently with applicator or toothpick. A positive reaction consists of a pale wheal surrounding the scratch site which develops within 10 minutes and ranges from 5-15 mm or more in diameter.

**Intradermal test:** Use intradermal test with a tuberculin syringe with a 26- to 30-gauge short bevel needle; a dose of 0.01-0.02 mL is injected intradermally. A control of 0.9% sodium chloride should be injected at least 1.5" from the PPL test site. Most skin responses to the intradermal test will develop within 5-15 minutes.

**Interpretation:**

(-) Negative: No reaction

(±) Ambiguous: Wheal only slightly larger than original bleb with or without erythematous flare and larger than control site

(+) Positive: Itching and marked increase in size of original bleb

Control site should be reactionless

**Mechanism of Action** Elicits IgE antibodies which produce type I accelerate urticarial reactions to penicillins

**Local Anesthetic/Vasoconstrictor Precautions** No information available to require special precautions

**Effects on Dental Treatment** No effects or complications reported

**Other Adverse Effects**

1% to 10%: Local: Intense local inflammatory response at skin test site

<1%:

Cardiovascular: Local edema

Local: Pruritus, erythema, wheal, urticaria

Miscellaneous: Systemic allergic reactions occur rarely

**Drug Interactions** Decreased effect: Corticosteroids and other immunosuppressive agents may inhibit the immune response to the skin test

**Pregnancy Risk Factor** C

**Generic Available** No

## Bepridil (BE pri dil)

**Related Information**

Calcium Channel Blockers & Gingival Hyperplasia *on page 1204*

Cardiovascular Diseases *on page 1066*

**U.S. Brand Names** Vascor®

**Canadian Brand Names** Bapadin®

**Therapeutic Category** Antianginal Agent; Calcium Channel Blocker

**Use** Treatment of chronic stable angina; due to side effect profile, reserve for patients who have been intolerant of other antianginal therapy; bepridil may be used alone or in combination with nitrates or beta-blockers

**Usual Dosage** Adults: Oral: Initial: 200 mg/day, then adjust dose at 10-day intervals until optimal response is achieved; maximum daily dose: 400 mg

**Mechanism of Action** Bepridil, a type 4 calcium antagonist, possesses characteristics of the traditional calcium antagonist, inhibiting calcium ion from entering the "slow channels" or select voltage-sensitive areas of vascular smooth muscle and myocardium during depolarization and producing a relaxation of coronary vascular smooth muscle and coronary vasodilation. However, bepridil may also inhibit fast sodium channels (inward) which may account for some of its side effects (eg, arrhythmias); a direct bradycardia effect of bepridil has been postulated via direct action on the S-A node.

**Local Anesthetic/Vasoconstrictor Precautions** No information available to require special precautions

**Effects on Dental Treatment** Other drugs of this class can cause gingival hyperplasia (ie, nifedipine) but there have been no reports for bepridil

**Other Adverse Effects**

>10%:

Central nervous system: Dizziness, headache

Gastrointestinal: Nausea, dyspepsia, abdominal pain, GI distress

Neuromuscular & skeletal: Weakness

1% to 10%:

Cardiovascular: Bradycardia, palpitations

Central nervous system: Nervousness

Gastrointestinal: Diarrhea, anorexia, dry mouth

Miscellaneous: Flu syndrome

<1%:

Cardiovascular: Ventricular premature contractions, hypertension, torsade de pointes, edema, syncope, prolonged Q-T intervals

Central nervous system: Fever, psychotic behavior, akathisia

Dermatologic: Rash

Endocrine & metabolic: Sexual dysfunction

Gastrointestinal: Taste change
Hematologic: Agranulocytosis
Neuromuscular & skeletal: Tremor, myalgia, arthritis
Ocular: Blurred vision
Respiratory: Nasal congestion, cough, pharyngitis
Miscellaneous: Sweating

**Drug Interactions** Bepridil increases digoxin serum concentrations by over 30% and enhances the cardiac effects of digoxin

**Drug Uptake**
Onset of action: 1 hour
Absorption: Oral: 100%
Serum half-life: 24 hours
Time to peak: 2-3 hours

**Pregnancy Risk Factor** C

**Generic Available** No

## Beractant (ber AKT ant)

**U.S. Brand Names** Survanta®

**Therapeutic Category** Lung Surfactant

**Use** Prevention and treatment of respiratory distress syndrome (RDS) in premature infants
Prophylactic therapy: Body weight <1250 g in infants at risk for developing or with evidence of surfactant deficiency
Rescue therapy: Treatment of infants with RDS confirmed by x-ray and requiring mechanical ventilation (administer as soon as possible - within 8 hours of age)

**Usual Dosage**
**Prophylactic treatment:** Give 100 mg phospholipids (4 mL/kg) intratracheally as soon as possible; as many as 4 doses may be administered during the first 48 hours of life, no more frequently than 6 hours apart. The need for additional doses is determined by evidence of continuing respiratory distress; if the infant is still intubated and requiring at least 30% inspired oxygen to maintain a $PAO_2$ ≤80 torr.
**Rescue treatment:** Administer 100 mg phospholipids (4 mL/kg) as soon as the diagnosis of RDS is made

**Mechanism of Action** Replaces deficient or ineffective endogenous lung surfactant in neonates with respiratory distress syndrome (RDS) or in neonates at risk of developing RDS. Surfactant prevents the alveoli from collapsing during expiration by lowering surface tension between air and alveolar surfaces.

**Local Anesthetic/Vasoconstrictor Precautions** No information available to require special precautions

**Effects on Dental Treatment** No effects or complications reported

**Other Adverse Effects** During the dosing procedure:
Cardiovascular: Transient bradycardia, vasoconstriction, hypotension, hypertension, pallor
Respiratory: Oxygen desaturation, endotracheal tube blockage, hypocarbia, hypercarbia, apnea, pulmonary air leaks, pulmonary interstitial emphysema
Miscellaneous: Increased probability of post-treatment nosocomial sepsis

**Drug Interactions** No data reported

**Generic Available** No

♦ **Berocca®** *see* Vitamin B Complex With Vitamin C and Folic Acid *on page 1050*
♦ **Beta-2®** *see* Isoetharine *on page 551*

## Beta-Carotene (BAY tah KARE oh teen)

**U.S. Brand Names** Max-Caro® [OTC]; Provatene® [OTC]; Solatene®

**Therapeutic Category** Vitamin, Fat Soluble

**Use** Reduces severity of photosensitivity reactions in patients with erythropoietic protoporphyria (EPP)

**Usual Dosage** Oral:
Children <14 years: 30-150 mg/day
Adults: 30-300 mg/day

**Mechanism of Action** The exact mechanism of action in erythropoietic protoporphyria has not as yet been elucidated; although patient must become carotenemic before effects are observed, there appears to be more than a simple internal light screen responsible for the drug's action. A protective effect was achieved when beta-carotene was added to blood samples. The concentrations of solutions used were similar to those achieved in treated patients. Topically applied beta-carotene is considerably less effective than systemic therapy.

**Local Anesthetic/Vasoconstrictor Precautions** No information available to require special precautions

**Effects on Dental Treatment** No effects or complications reported

(Continued)

## Beta-Carotene *(Continued)*

**Other Adverse Effects**

>10%: Dermatologic: Carotenodermia (yellowing of palms, hands, or soles of feet, and to a lesser extent the face)

<1%:

Central nervous system: Dizziness
Dermatologic: Ecchymoses
Gastrointestinal: Diarrhea
Neuromuscular & skeletal: Arthralgia

**Drug Interactions** Fulfills vitamin A requirements, do not prescribe additional vitamin A

**Pregnancy Risk Factor** C

**Dosage Forms** Capsule: 15 mg, 30 mg

**Generic Available** Yes

- **Betachron E-R® Capsule** *see* Propranolol *on page 857*
- **Betadine® [OTC]** *see* Povidone-Iodine *on page 827*
- **Betadine® First Aid Antibiotics + Moisturizer [OTC]** *see* Bacitracin and Polymyxin B *on page 117*
- **9-Beta-D-ribofuranosyladenine** *see* Adenosine *on page 40*
- **Betagan®** *see* Levobunolol *on page 580*

## Betaine Anhydrous (BAY tayne an HY drus)

**U.S. Brand Names** Cystadane®

**Therapeutic Category** Urinary Tract Product

**Use** Treatment of homocystinuria

**Usual Dosage** Oral: 6 g/day, usually give in two 3 g doses

**Local Anesthetic/Vasoconstrictor Precautions** No information available to require special precautions

**Effects on Dental Treatment** No effects or complications reported

**Pregnancy Risk Factor** C

**Generic Available** No

- **Betalin®S** *see* Thiamine *on page 975*

## Betamethasone (bay ta METH a sone)

**Related Information**

Corticosteroid Equivalencies Comparison *on page 1221*
Corticosteroids, Topical Comparison *on page 1222*
Respiratory Diseases *on page 1079*

**U.S. Brand Names** Alphatrex®; Betatrex®; Beta-Val®; Celestone®; Celestone® Soluspan®; Cel-U-Jec®; Diprolene®; Diprolene® AF; Diprosone®; Maxivate®; Teladar®; Valisone®

**Canadian Brand Names** Betnesol® [Disodium Phosphate]; Diprolene® Glycol [Dipropionate]; Occlucort®; Rhoprolene; Rhoprosone; Taro-Sone; Topilene; Topisone

**Therapeutic Category** Anti-inflammatory Agent; Corticosteroid, Systemic; Corticosteroid, Topical (Medium/High Potency)

**Use**

Dental: Treatment of a variety of oral diseases of allergic, inflammatory or autoimmune origin

Medical: Inflammatory dermatoses such as seborrheic or atopic dermatitis, neurodermatitis, anogenital pruritus, psoriasis, inflammatory phase of xerosis

**Usual Dosage**

Children:

Oral: 0.0175-0.25 mg/kg/day divided every 6-8 hours **or** 0.5-7.5 mg/m²/day divided every 6-8 hours

I.M.: 0.0175-0.125 mg base/kg/day divided every 6-12 hours **or** 0.5-7.5 mg base/m²/day divided every 6-12 hours

Adults:

Oral: 0.6-7.2 mg/day in 2-4 doses

I.M., I.V.: Betamethasone sodium phosphate: 0.6-9 mg/day divided every 12-24 hours

Topical: Apply thin film to affected skin areas once or twice daily

**Mechanism of Action** Controls the rate of protein synthesis, depresses the migration of polymorphonuclear leukocytes, fibroblasts, reverses capillary permeability, and lysosomal stabilization at the cellular level to prevent or control inflammation

**Local Anesthetic/Vasoconstrictor Precautions** No information available to require special precautions

**Effects on Dental Treatment** No effects or complications reported

**Other Adverse Effects** >10%:
Central nervous system: Insomnia
Gastrointestinal: Increased appetite, indigestion

**Contraindications** Systemic fungal infections; hypersensitivity to betamethasone or any component

**Warnings/Precautions** Use with caution in patients with hypothyroidism, cirrhosis, ulcerative colitis; do not use occlusive dressings on weeping or exudative lesions and general caution with occlusive dressings should be observed; discontinue if skin irritation or contact dermatitis should occur; do not use in patients with decreased skin circulation.

**Drug Interactions** Decreased effect of any systemic corticosteroid by barbiturates, phenytoin, rifampin

**Drug Uptake**
Absorption: Oral: Rapid
Serum half-life: Oral: 6.5 hours
Time to peak serum concentration: I.V.: Within 10-36 minutes

**Pregnancy Risk Factor** C

**Breast-feeding Considerations** No data reported

**Dosage Forms**
Base (Celestone®), Oral:
- Syrup: 0.6 mg/5 mL (118 mL)
- Tablet: 0.6 mg

Dipropionate (Diprosone®)
- Aerosol: 0.1% (85 g)
- Cream: 0.05% (15 g, 45 g)
- Lotion: 0.05% (20 mL, 30 mL, 60 mL)
- Ointment: 0.05% (15 g, 45 g)

Dipropionate augmented (Diprolene®)
- Cream: 0.05% (15 g, 45 g)
- Gel: 0.05% (15 g, 45 g)
- Lotion: 0.05% (30 mL, 60 mL)
- Ointment, topical: 0.05% (15 g, 45 g)

Valerate (Betatrex®, Valisone®)
- Cream: 0.01% (15 g, 60 g); 0.1% (15 g, 45 g, 110 g, 430 g)
- Lotion: 0.1% (20 mL, 60 mL)
- Ointment: 0.1% (15 g, 45 g)

Valerate (Beta-Val®)
- Cream: 0.01% (15 g, 60 g); 0.1% (15 g, 45 g, 110 g, 430 g)
- Lotion: 0.1% (20 mL, 60 mL)

Injection: Sodium phosphate (Celestone® Phosphate, Cel-U-Jec®): 4 mg betamethasone phosphate/mL (equivalent to 3 mg betamethasone/mL) (5 mL)

Injection, suspension: Sodium phosphate and acetate (Celestone® Soluspan®): 6 mg/mL (3 mg of betamethasone sodium phosphate and 3 mg of betamethasone acetate per mL) (5 mL)

**Dietary Considerations** May be taken with food to decrease GI distress

**Generic Available** Yes

## Betamethasone and Clotrimazole

(bay ta METH a sone & kloe TRIM a zole)

**U.S. Brand Names** Lotrisone®

**Canadian Brand Names** Lotriderm®

**Therapeutic Category** Antifungal Agent, Topical; Corticosteroid, Topical (Medium/High Potency)

**Use** Topical treatment of various dermal fungal infections

**Usual Dosage** Apply twice daily

**Local Anesthetic/Vasoconstrictor Precautions** No information available to require special precautions

**Effects on Dental Treatment** No effects or complications reported

**Other Adverse Effects** See individual agents

**Pregnancy Risk Factor** C

**Generic Available** No


♦ **Betapace®** *see* Sotalol *on page 927*
♦ **Betapen®-VK** *see* Penicillin V Potassium *on page 776*
♦ **Betasept® [OTC]** *see* Chlorhexidine Gluconate *on page 225*
♦ **Betaseron®** *see* Interferon Beta-1b *on page 544*
♦ **Betatrex®** *see* Betamethasone *on previous page*
♦ **Beta-Val®** *see* Betamethasone *on previous page*

## Betaxolol (be TAKS oh lol)

**Related Information**

Cardiovascular Diseases *on page 1066*

**U.S. Brand Names** Betoptic®; Betoptic® S; Kerlone®

**Therapeutic Category** Antiglaucoma Agent; Beta-adrenergic Blocker, Cardioselective; Beta-Adrenergic Blocker, Ophthalmic

**Use** Treatment of chronic open-angle glaucoma and ocular hypertension; management of hypertension

**Usual Dosage** Adults:

Ophthalmic: Instill 1 drop twice daily

Oral: 10 mg/day; may increase dose to 20 mg/day after 7-14 days if desired response is not achieved; initial dose in elderly patients: 5 mg/day

**Mechanism of Action** Competitively blocks $beta_1$-receptors, with little or no effect on $beta_2$-receptors; ophthalmic reduces intraocular pressure by reducing the production of aqueous humor

**Local Anesthetic/Vasoconstrictor Precautions** No information available to require special precautions

**Effects on Dental Treatment** Noncardioselective beta-blockers (ie, propranolol, nadolol) enhance the pressor response to epinephrine, resulting in hypertension and bradycardia. This has not been reported for betaxolol, a cardioselective beta-blocker. Therefore local anesthetic with vasoconstrictor can be safely used in patients medicated with betaxolol. Many nonsteroidal anti-inflammatory drugs such as ibuprofen and indomethacin can reduce the hypotensive effect of beta-blockers after 3 or more weeks of therapy with the NSAID. Short-term NSAID use (ie, 3 days) requires no special precautions in patients taking beta-blockers.

**Other Adverse Effects**

1% to 10%:

- Cardiovascular: Bradycardia, palpitations, edema, congestive heart failure
- Central nervous system: Dizziness, fatigue, lethargy, headache
- Dermatologic: Erythema, itching
- Ocular: Mild ocular stinging and discomfort, tearing, photophobia, decreased corneal sensitivity, keratitis
- Miscellaneous: Cold extremities

<1%:

- Cardiovascular: Chest pain
- Central nervous system: Nervousness, depression, hallucinations
- Hematologic: Thrombocytopenia

**Drug Interactions**

Decreased effects of beta-blockers:

- Barbiturates (increased liver metabolism of beta-blockers to result in lower serum levels)
- NSAIDs (attenuate the hypotensive therapeutic effects of beta-blockers)
- Rifampin (increased liver metabolism of beta-blockers to result in lower serum levels)

Increased effects of beta-blockers:

- Calcium channel blockers (increase serum levels by unknown mechanism to enhance hypotension)

Beta-blockers increase the effects of:

- Epinephrine (vasoconstrictor; initial hypertensive episode followed by bradycardia)
- Phenylephrine (Neosynephrine®; enhanced pressor response)
- Theophylline (inhibit theophylline metabolism causing increase in serum concentrations)

**Drug Uptake**

Onset of action: 1-1.5 hours

Duration: ≥12 hours

Absorption: Systemically absorbed

Serum half-life: 12-22 hours

Time to peak: Within 2 hours

**Pregnancy Risk Factor** C

**Generic Available** No

**Selected Readings**

Foster CA and Aston SJ, "Propranolol-Epinephrine Interaction: A Potential Disaster," *Plast Reconstr Surg*, 1983, 72(1):74-8.

Wong DG, Spence JD, Lamki L, et al, "Effect of Nonsteroidal Anti-inflammatory Drugs on Control of Hypertension of Beta-Blockers and Diuretics," *Lancet*, 1986, 1(8488):997-1001.

Wynn RL, "Dental Nonsteroidal Anti-inflammatory Drugs and Prostaglandin-Based Drug Interactions, Part Two," *Gen Dent*, 1992, 40(2):104, 106, 108.

Wynn RL, "Epinephrine Interactions With Beta-Blockers," *Gen Dent*, 1994, 42(1):16, 18.

## Bethanechol (be THAN e kole)

**U.S. Brand Names** Duvoid®; Myotonachol™; Urecholine®

**Canadian Brand Names** PMS-Bethanechol Chloride

**Therapeutic Category** Cholinergic Agent

**Use** Nonobstructive urinary retention and retention due to neurogenic bladder; treatment and prevention of bladder dysfunction caused by phenothiazines; diagnosis of flaccid or atonic neurogenic bladder; gastroesophageal reflux

**Usual Dosage**

Children:

Oral:

Abdominal distention or urinary retention: 0.6 mg/kg/day divided 3-4 times/day

Gastroesophageal reflux: 0.1-0.2 mg/kg/dose given 30 minutes to 1 hour before each meal to a maximum of 4 times/day

S.C.: 0.15-0.2 mg/kg/day divided 3-4 times/day

Adults:

Oral: 10-50 mg 2-4 times/day

S.C.: 2.5-5 mg 3-4 times/day, up to 7.5-10 mg every 4 hours for neurogenic bladder

**Mechanism of Action** Stimulates cholinergic receptors in the smooth muscle of the urinary bladder and gastrointestinal tract resulting in increased peristalsis, increased GI and pancreatic secretions, bladder muscle contraction, and increased ureteral peristaltic waves

**Local Anesthetic/Vasoconstrictor Precautions** No information available to require special precautions

**Effects on Dental Treatment** This is a cholinergic agent similar to pilocarpine and expect to see salivation and sweating in patients

**Other Adverse Effects**

Oral: <1%:

Cardiovascular: Hypotension, cardiac arrest, flushed skin

Gastrointestinal: Abdominal cramps, diarrhea, nausea, vomiting, salivation

Neuromuscular & skeletal: Vasomotor response

Respiratory: Bronchial constriction

Miscellaneous: Sweating

Subcutaneous: 1% to 10%:

Cardiovascular: Hypotension, cardiac arrest, flushed skin

Gastrointestinal: Abdominal cramps, diarrhea, nausea, vomiting, salivation

Neuromuscular & skeletal: Vasomotor response

Respiratory: Bronchial constriction

Miscellaneous: Sweating

**Drug Interactions**

Decreased effect: Procainamide, quinidine

Increased toxicity: Bethanechol and ganglionic blockers cause critical fall in blood pressure; cholinergic drugs or anticholinesterase agents

**Drug Uptake**

Onset of action:

Oral: 30-90 minutes

S.C.: 5-15 minutes

Duration of action:

Oral: Up to 6 hours

S.C.: 2 hours

Absorption: Oral: Variable

**Pregnancy Risk Factor** C

**Generic Available** Yes: Tablet

- **Betimol® Ophthalmic** *see* Timolol *on page 986*
- **Betoptic®** *see* Betaxolol *on previous page*
- **Betoptic® S** *see* Betaxolol *on previous page*
- **Bexophene®** *see* Propoxyphene and Aspirin *on page 856*
- **Biamine®** *see* Thiamine *on page 975*
- **Biavax® II** *see* Rubella and Mumps Vaccines, Combined *on page 898*
- **Biaxin™** *see* Clarithromycin *on page 256*

## Bicalutamide (bye ka LOO ta mide)

**U.S. Brand Names** Casodex®

**Therapeutic Category** Androgen; Antineoplastic Agent, Hormone

**Use** Combination therapy with a luteinizing hormone-releasing hormone (LHRH) analog for the treatment of advanced prostate cancer

**Usual Dosage** Adults: Oral: 1 tablet once daily (morning or evening), with or without food. It is recommended that bicalutamide be taken at the same time

(Continued)

## Bicalutamide *(Continued)*

each day; start treatment with bicalutamide at the same time as treatment with an LHRH analog.

**Mechanism of Action** Pure nonsteroidal antiandrogen that binds to androgen receptors; specifically a competitive inhibitor for the binding of dihydrotestosterone and testosterone; prevents testosterone stimulation of cell growth in prostate cancer

**Local Anesthetic/Vasoconstrictor Precautions** No information available to require special precautions

**Effects on Dental Treatment** No effects or complications reported

**Other Adverse Effects**

>10%: Endocrine & metabolic: Hot flashes (49%)

≥2% to <5%:

- Cardiovascular: Angina pectoris, congestive heart failure, edema
- Central nervous system: Anxiety, depression, confusion, somnolence, nervousness, fever, chills
- Dermatologic: Dry skin, pruritus, alopecia
- Endocrine & metabolic: Breast pain, diabetes mellitus, decreased libido, dehydration, gout
- Gastrointestinal: Anorexia, dyspepsia, rectal hemorrhage, xerostomia, melena, weight gain
- Genitourinary: Polyuria, urinary impairment, dysuria, urinary retention, urinary urgency
- Hepatic: Alkaline phosphatase increased
- Neuromuscular & skeletal: Myasthenia, arthritis, myalgia, leg cramps, pathological fracture, neck pain, hypertonia, neuropathy
- Renal: Creatinine increased
- Respiratory: Cough increased, pharyngitis, bronchitis, pneumonia, rhinitis, lung disorder
- Miscellaneous: Sepsis, neoplasma

**Drug Uptake**

Absorption: Rapid and complete

Serum half-life: Active enantiomer is 5.8 days

**Pregnancy Risk Factor** X

**Dosage Forms** Tablet: 50 mg

**Generic Available** No

- ♦ **Bicillin® C-R 900/300 Injection** *see* Penicillin G Benzathine and Procaine Combined *on page 774*
- ♦ **Bicillin® C-R Injection** *see* Penicillin G Benzathine and Procaine Combined *on page 774*
- ♦ **Bicillin® L-A** *see* Penicillin G Benzathine *on page 773*
- ♦ **Bicitra®** *see* Sodium Citrate and Citric Acid *on page 921*
- ♦ **BiCNU®** *see* Carmustine *on page 193*
- ♦ **Biltricide®** *see* Praziquantel *on page 830*
- ♦ **Biocef®** *see* Cephalexin *on page 214*
- ♦ **Bioclate®** *see* Antihemophilic Factor (Recombinant) *on page 90*
- ♦ **Biohist®-LA** *see* Carbinoxamine and Pseudoephedrine *on page 188*
- ♦ **Biomox®** *see* Amoxicillin *on page 76*
- ♦ **Bion® Tears Solution [OTC]** *see* Artificial Tears *on page 97*
- ♦ **Biozyme-C®** *see* Collagenase *on page 276*

## Biperiden (bye PER i den)

**U.S. Brand Names** Akineton®

**Therapeutic Category** Anti-Parkinson's Agent

**Use** Treatment of all forms of Parkinsonism including drug induced type (extrapyramidal symptoms)

**Usual Dosage** Adults:

Parkinsonism: Oral: 2 mg 3-4 times/day

Extrapyramidal:

- Oral: 2 mg 1-3 times/day
- I.M., I.V.: 2 mg every 30 minutes up to 4 doses or 8 mg/day

**Mechanism of Action** Biperiden is a weak anticholinergic agent. The beneficial effects in Parkinson's disease and neuroleptic-induced extrapyramidal reactions are believed to be due to the inhibition of striatal cholinergic receptors.

**Local Anesthetic/Vasoconstrictor Precautions** No information available to require special precautions

**Effects on Dental Treatment** Dry mouth, nose and throat very prevalent in patients taking this drug

**Other Adverse Effects**

>10%:

Dermatologic: Dry skin

Gastrointestinal: Constipation, dry mouth

Respiratory: Dry nose, throat

Miscellaneous: Decreased sweating

1% to 10%:

Dermatologic: Photosensitivity

Endocrine & metabolic: Decreased flow of breast milk

Gastrointestinal: Dysphagia

<1%:

Cardiovascular: Orthostatic hypotension, ventricular fibrillation, tachycardia, palpitations

Central nervous system: Confusion, drowsiness, headache, loss of memory, fatigue, ataxia

Dermatologic: Skin rash

Gastrointestinal: Bloated feeling, nausea, vomiting

Genitourinary: Dysuria

Neuromuscular & skeletal: Weakness

Ocular: Increased intraocular pain, blurred vision

**Drug Interactions**

Decreased effect of levodopa (↓ absorption)

Increased toxicity (central anticholinergic syndrome): Narcotic analgesics, phenothiazines, and other antipsychotics, tricyclic antidepressants, some antihistamines, quinidine, disopyramide

**Drug Uptake**

Serum half-life: 18.4-24.3 hours

Time to peak serum concentration: 1-1.5 hours

**Pregnancy Risk Factor** C

**Generic Available** No

♦ **Bisac-Evac® [OTC]** *see* Bisacodyl *on this page*

## Bisacodyl (bis a KOE dil)

**U.S. Brand Names** Bisac-Evac® [OTC]; Bisacodyl Uniserts®; Bisco-Lax® [OTC]; Carter's Little Pills® [OTC]; Clysodrast®; Dacodyl® [OTC]; Deficol® [OTC]; Dulcolax® [OTC]; Fleet® Laxative [OTC]

**Canadian Brand Names** Apo®-Bisacodyl; PMS-Bisacodyl

**Therapeutic Category** Laxative, Stimulant

**Use** Treatment of constipation; colonic evacuation prior to procedures or examination

**Usual Dosage**

Children:

Oral: >6 years: 5-10 mg (0.3 mg/kg) at bedtime or before breakfast

Rectal suppository:

<2 years: 5 mg as a single dose

>2 years: 10 mg

Adults:

Oral: 5-15 mg as single dose (up to 30 mg when complete evacuation of bowel is required)

Rectal suppository: 10 mg as single dose

Tannex:

Enema: 2.5 g in 1000 mL warm water

Barium enema: 2.5-5 g in 1000 mL barium suspension

Do not give >10 g within 72-hour period

**Mechanism of Action** Stimulates peristalsis by directly irritating the smooth muscle of the intestine, possibly the colonic intramural plexus; alters water and electrolyte secretion producing net intestinal fluid accumulation and laxation

**Local Anesthetic/Vasoconstrictor Precautions** No information available to require special precautions

**Effects on Dental Treatment** No effects or complications reported

**Other Adverse Effects** <1%:

Central nervous system: Vertigo

Endocrine & metabolic: Electrolyte and fluid imbalance (metabolic acidosis or alkalosis, hypocalcemia)

Gastrointestinal: Mild abdominal cramps, nausea, vomiting, rectal burning

**Drug Interactions** Decreased effect: Milk, antacids; decreased effect of warfarin

**Drug Uptake**

Onset of action:

Oral: 6-10 hours

Rectal: 0.25-1 hour

Absorption: Oral, rectal: <5% absorbed systemically

(Continued)

## Bisacodyl *(Continued)*

**Pregnancy Risk Factor** C
**Generic Available** Yes

- **Bisacodyl Uniserts®** *see* Bisacodyl *on previous page*
- **Bisco-Lax® [OTC]** *see* Bisacodyl *on previous page*
- **Bishydroxycoumarin** *see* Dicumarol *on page 322*
- **Bismatrol® (subsalicylate) [OTC]** *see* Bismuth *on this page*

## Bismuth (BIZ muth)

**Related Information**
Ranitidine Bismuth Citrate *on page 878*

**U.S. Brand Names** Bismatrol® (subsalicylate) [OTC]; Devrom® (subgallate) [OTC]; Pepto-Bismol® (subsalicylate) [OTC]; Pink Bismuth® (subsalicylate) [OTC]

**Therapeutic Category** Antidiarrheal

**Synonyms** Bismuth Subgallate; Bismuth Subsalicylate

**Use** Symptomatic treatment of mild, nonspecific diarrhea; indigestion, nausea, control of traveler's diarrhea (enterotoxigenic *Escherichia coli*); as an adjunct in the treatment of *Helicobacter pylori*-associated peptic ulcer disease

**Usual Dosage** Oral:
Nonspecific diarrhea: Subsalicylate:
Children: Up to 8 doses/24 hours:
3-6 years: 1/3 tablet or 5 mL every 30 minutes to 1 hour as needed
6-9 years: 2/3 tablet or 10 mL every 30 minutes to 1 hour as needed
9-12 years: 1 tablet or 15 mL every 30 minutes to 1 hour as needed
Adults: 2 tablets or 30 mL every 30 minutes to 1 hour as needed up to 8 doses/24 hours
Prevention of traveler's diarrhea: 2.1 g/day or 2 tablets 4 times/day before meals and at bedtime
Subgallate: 1-2 tablets 3 times/day with meals

**Mechanism of Action** Bismuth subsalicylate exhibits both antisecretory and antimicrobial action. This agent may provide some anti-inflammatory action as well. The salicylate moiety provides antisecretory effect and the bismuth exhibits antimicrobial directly against bacterial and viral gastrointestinal pathogens. Bismuth has some antacid properties.

**Local Anesthetic/Vasoconstrictor Precautions** No information available to require special precautions

**Effects on Dental Treatment** No effects or complications reported

**Other Adverse Effects**
>10%: Discoloration of the tongue (darkening), grayish black stools
<1%:
Central nervous system: Anxiety, confusion, slurred speech, headache, mental depression
Gastrointestinal: Impaction may occur in infants and debilitated patients
Neuromuscular & skeletal: Muscle spasms, weakness
Otic: Loss of hearing, tinnitus

**Drug Interactions**
Decreased effect: Tetracyclines and uricosurics
Increased toxicity: Aspirin, warfarin, hypoglycemics

**Drug Uptake** Absorption: Minimally absorbed across the GI tract while the salt (eg, salicylate) may be readily absorbed

**Pregnancy Risk Factor** C (D in 3rd trimester)
**Generic Available** Yes

- **Bismuth Subgallate** *see* Bismuth *on this page*
- **Bismuth Subsalicylate** *see* Bismuth *on this page*

## Bismuth Subsalicylate, Metronidazole, and Tetracycline

(BIZ muth sub sa LIS i late, me troe NI da zole, & tet ra SYE kleen)

**U.S. Brand Names** Helidac™

**Therapeutic Category** Antidiarrheal

**Use** In combination with an $H_2$-antagonist, used to treat and decrease rate of recurrence of active duodenal ulcer associated with *H. pylori* infection

**Usual Dosage** Adults: Chew 2 bismuth subsalicylate 262.4 mg tablets, swallow 1 metronidazole 250 mg tablet, and swallow 1 tetracycline 500 mg capsule plus an $H_2$-antagonist 4 times/day at meals and bedtime for 14 days; follow with 8 oz of water

**Mechanism of Action** Bismuth subsalicylate, metronidazole, and tetracycline individually have demonstrated *in vitro* activity against most susceptible strains of

*H. pylori* isolated from patients with duodenal ulcers. Resistance to metronidazole is increasing in the U.S.; an alternative regimen, not containing metronidazole, if *H. pylori* is not eradicated follow therapy.

**Local Anesthetic/Vasoconstrictor Precautions** No information available to require special precautions

**Effects on Dental Treatment** Tetracyclines are not recommended for use during pregnancy since they can cause enamel hypoplasia and permanent teeth discoloration; long-term use associated with oral candidiasis

**Other Adverse Effects** See individual monographs

>1%:

Central nervous system: Dizziness

Gastrointestinal: Nausea, diarrhea, abdominal pain, vomiting, anal discomfort, anorexia

Neuromuscular & skeletal: Paresthesia

<1%:

Central nervous system: Insomnia

Gastrointestinal: Constipation

Neuromuscular & skeletal: Weakness, pain

Respiratory: Upper respiratory infection

**Contraindications** Pregnancy or lactation; children; significant renal/hepatic impairment; hypersensitivity to salicylates, bismuth, metronidazole, tetracycline, or any component

**Warnings/Precautions** See individual monographs

**Drug Interactions** See individual monographs

Decreased effect: A theoretical reduction in tetracycline systemic absorption due to an interaction with bismuth or calcium carbonate, an excipient of bismuth subsalicylate has, as yet, been unproven to occur or to have any clinical bearing

**Drug Uptake** No data on combination; see individual monographs

**Pregnancy Risk Factor** D (tetracycline); B (metronidazole)

**Dosage Forms**

Tablet:

Bismuth subsalicylate: Chewable: 262.4 mg

Metronidazole: 250 mg

Capsule: Tetracycline: 500 mg

## Bisoprolol (bis OH proe lol)

**Related Information**

Cardiovascular Diseases *on page 1066*

**U.S. Brand Names** Zebeta®

**Therapeutic Category** Antianginal Agent; Beta-adrenergic Blocker, Cardioselective

**Use** Treatment of hypertension, alone or in combination with other agents

**Unlabeled use:** Angina pectoris, supraventricular arrhythmias, PVCs

**Usual Dosage** Oral:

Adults: 5 mg once daily, may be increased to 10 mg, and then up to 20 mg once daily, if necessary

Elderly: Initial dose: 2.5 mg/day; may be increased by 2.5-5 mg/day; maximum recommended dose: 20 mg/day

**Mechanism of Action** Selective inhibitor of $beta_1$-adrenergic receptors; competitively blocks $beta_1$-receptors, with little or no effect on $beta_2$-receptors at doses <10 mg

**Local Anesthetic/Vasoconstrictor Precautions** No information available to require special precautions

**Effects on Dental Treatment** Noncardioselective beta-blockers (ie, propranolol, nadolol) enhance the pressor response to epinephrine, resulting in hypertension and bradycardia. This has not been reported for bisoprolol, a cardioselective beta-blocker. Therefore local anesthetic with vasoconstrictor can be safely used in patients medicated with bisoprolol. Many nonsteroidal anti-inflammatory drugs such as ibuprofen and indomethacin can reduce the hypotensive effect of beta-blockers after 3 or more weeks of therapy with the NSAID. Short-term NSAID use (ie, 3 days) requires no special precautions in patients taking beta-blockers.

**Other Adverse Effects**

>10%: Central nervous system: Fatigue, lethargy

1% to 10%:

Cardiovascular: Hypotension, chest pain, heart failure, Raynaud's phenomenon, heart block, edema, bradycardia

Central nervous system: Headache, dizziness, insomnia, confusion, depression, abnormal dreams

Dermatologic: Rash

Gastrointestinal: Constipation, diarrhea, dyspepsia, nausea, flatulence, anorexia

(Continued)

## Bisoprolol *(Continued)*

Genitourinary: Micturition (frequency), impotence, urinary retention
Neuromuscular & skeletal: Arthralgia, myalgia
Ocular: Abnormal vision
Respiratory: Dyspnea, rhinitis, cough

**Drug Interactions**

Decreased effects of beta-blockers:
Barbiturates (increased liver metabolism of beta-blockers to result in lower serum levels)
NSAIDs (attenuate the hypotensive therapeutic effects of beta-blockers)
Rifampin (increased liver metabolism of beta-blockers to result in lower serum levels)

Increased effects of beta-blockers:
Calcium channel blockers (increase serum levels by unknown mechanism to enhance hypotension)

Beta-blockers increase the effects of:
Epinephrine (vasoconstrictor; initial hypertensive episode followed by bradycardia)
Phenylephrine (Neosynephrine®; enhanced pressor response)
Theophylline (inhibit theophylline metabolism causing increase in serum concentrations)

**Drug Uptake**

Absorption: Rapid and almost complete from GI tract
Serum half-life: 9-12 hours
Time to peak: 1.7-3 hours

**Pregnancy Risk Factor** C

**Generic Available** No

**Selected Readings**

Foster CA and Aston SJ, "Propranolol-Epinephrine Interaction: A Potential Disaster," *Plast Reconstr Surg*, 1983, 72(1):74-8.
Wong DG, Spence JD, Lamki L, et al, "Effect of Nonsteroidal Anti-inflammatory Drugs on Control of Hypertension of Beta-Blockers and Diuretics," *Lancet*, 1986, 1(8488):997-1001.
Wynn RL, "Dental Nonsteroidal Anti-inflammatory Drugs and Prostaglandin-Based Drug Interactions, Part Two," *Gen Dent*, 1992, 40(2):104, 106, 108.
Wynn RL, "Epinephrine Interactions With Beta-Blockers," *Gen Dent*, 1994, 42(1):16, 18.

## Bisoprolol and Hydrochlorothiazide

(bis OH proe lol & hye droe klor oh THYE a zide)

**U.S. Brand Names** Ziac™

**Therapeutic Category** Antihypertensive Agent, Combination; Diuretic, Thiazide

**Use** Treatment of hypertension

**Usual Dosage** Adults: Oral: Dose is individualized, given once daily

**Local Anesthetic/Vasoconstrictor Precautions** No information available to require special precautions

**Effects on Dental Treatment** Noncardioselective beta-blockers (ie, propranolol, nadolol) enhance the pressor response to epinephrine, resulting in hypertension and bradycardia. This has not been reported for bisoprolol, a cardioselective beta-blocker. Therefore local anesthetic with vasoconstrictor can be safely used in patients medicated with bisoprolol. Many nonsteroidal anti-inflammatory drugs such as ibuprofen and indomethacin can reduce the hypotensive effect of beta-blockers after 3 or more weeks of therapy with the NSAID. Short-term NSAID use (ie, 3 days) requires no special precautions in patients taking beta-blockers.

**Other Adverse Effects**

>10%: Central nervous system: Fatigue

1% to 10%:
Cardiovascular: Chest pain, edema, bradycardia, hypotension
Central nervous system: Headache, dizziness, depression, abnormal dreams
Dermatologic: Rash, photosensitivity
Endocrine & metabolic: Hypokalemia, fluid and electrolyte imbalances (hypocalcemia, hypomagnesemia, hyponatremia), hyperglycemia
Gastrointestinal: Constipation, diarrhea, dyspepsia, nausea, insomnia, flatulence
Genitourinary: Micturition (frequency)
Hematologic: Rarely blood dyscrasias
Neuromuscular & skeletal: Arthralgia, myalgia
Ocular: Abnormal vision
Renal: Prerenal azotemia
Respiratory: Rhinitis, cough, dyspnea

**Drug Interactions**

Decreased effect/levels with barbiturates, rifampin, sulfinpyrazone

Decreased effect of oral hypoglycemics; decreased absorption with cholestyramine and colestipol
Increased effect with furosemide and other loop diuretics
Increased toxicity/levels of lithium
Increased effect/toxicity/levels of and with flecainide
Increased levels/toxicity of lidocaine

**Pregnancy Risk Factor** C

**Generic Available** No

- **Bistropamide** *see* Tropicamide *on page 1029*

## Bitolterol (bye TOLE ter ole)

**Related Information**

Respiratory Diseases *on page 1079*

**U.S. Brand Names** Tornalate®

**Therapeutic Category** Antiasthmatic; Beta$_2$-Adrenergic Agonist Agent; Bronchodilator

**Use** Prevention and treatment of bronchial asthma and bronchospasm

**Usual Dosage** Children >12 years and Adults:

Bronchospasm: 2 inhalations at an interval of at least 1-3 minutes, followed by a third inhalation if needed

Prevention of bronchospasm: 2 inhalations every 8 hours; do not exceed 3 inhalations every 6 hours or 2 inhalations every 4 hours

**Mechanism of Action** Selectively stimulates beta$_2$-adrenergic receptors in the lungs producing bronchial smooth muscle relaxation; minor beta$_1$ activity

**Local Anesthetic/Vasoconstrictor Precautions** No information available to require special precautions

**Effects on Dental Treatment** No effects or complications reported

**Other Adverse Effects**

>10%: Neuromuscular & skeletal: Trembling

1% to 10%:
- Cardiovascular: Flushing of face, hypertension, pounding heartbeat
- Central nervous system: Dizziness, lightheadedness, nervousness
- Gastrointestinal: Dry mouth, nausea, unpleasant taste
- Respiratory: Bronchial irritation, coughing

<1%:
- Cardiovascular: Chest pain, arrhythmias, tachycardia
- Central nervous system: Insomnia
- Respiratory: Paradoxical bronchospasm

**Drug Interactions** Increased toxicity: Cardiovascular effects are potentiated in patients also receiving MAO inhibitors, tricyclic antidepressants, sympathomimetic agents (eg, amphetamine, dopamine, dobutamine), inhaled anesthetics (eg, enflurane)

**Drug Uptake**

Duration: 4-8 hours
Serum half-life: 3 hours
Time to peak serum concentration (colterol): Inhalation: Within 1 hour

**Pregnancy Risk Factor** C

**Generic Available** No

- **Black Draught® [OTC]** *see* Senna *on page 909*
- **BlemErase® Lotion [OTC]** *see* Benzoyl Peroxide *on page 130*
- **Blenoxane®** *see* Bleomycin *on this page*

## Bleomycin (blee oh MYE sin)

**U.S. Brand Names** Blenoxane®

**Therapeutic Category** Antineoplastic Agent, Antibiotic

**Synonyms** BLM; NIM

**Use** Palliative treatment of squamous cell carcinoma, testicular carcinoma, germ cell tumors, and the following lymphomas: Hodgkin's, lymphosarcoma and reticulum cell sarcoma; sclerosing agent to control malignant effusions

**Usual Dosage** Refer to individual protocols; 1 unit = 1 mg

May be administered I.M., I.V., S.C., or intracavitary

Children and Adults:

Test dose for lymphoma patients: I.M., I.V., S.C.: 1-5 units of bleomycin before the first dose; monitor vital signs every 15 minutes; wait a minimum of 1 hour before administering remainder of dose

**Single agent therapy:**

I.M./I.V./S.C.: Squamous cell carcinoma, lymphosarcoma, reticulum cell sarcoma, testicular carcinoma: 0.25-0.5 units/kg (10-20 units/m$^2$) 1-2 times/week

Continuous intravenous infusion: 15 units/m$^2$ over 24 hours daily for 4 days

(Continued)

## Bleomycin *(Continued)*

**Combination agent therapy:**
I.M./I.V.: 3-4 units/$m^2$
I.V.: ABVD: 10 units/$m^2$ on days 1 and 15
Maximum cumulative lifetime dose: 400 units

**Mechanism of Action** Inhibits synthesis of DNA; binds to DNA leading to single- and double-strand breaks; isolated from *Streptomyces verticillus*

**Local Anesthetic/Vasoconstrictor Precautions** No information available to require special precautions

**Effects on Dental Treatment** No effects or complications reported

**Other Adverse Effects**

>10%:
Cardiovascular: Raynaud's phenomenon
Central nervous system: Fever, chills
Dermatologic: Pruritic erythema
Gastrointestinal: Stomatitis, nausea, vomiting, anorexia, weight loss
Emetic potential: Moderately low (10% to 30%)
Integument: Approximately 50% of patients will develop erythema, induration, hyperkeratosis, and peeling of the skin. Hyperpigmentation, alopecia, nailbed changes may occur; this appears to be dose-related and is reversible after cessation of therapy.
Local: Pain at tumor site, phlebitis
Miscellaneous: Mild febrile reaction, mucocutaneous toxicity, patients may become febrile after intracavitary administration

1% to 10%:
Idiosyncratic: Similar to anaphylaxis and occurs in 1% of lymphoma patients; may include hypotension, confusion, fever, chills, and wheezing. May be immediate or delayed for several hours; symptomatic treatment includes volume expansion, pressor agents, antihistamines, and steroids.

<1%:
Cardiovascular: Myocardial infarction, cerebrovascular accident
Dermatologic: Skin thickening
Hepatic: Hepatotoxicity
Renal: Renal toxicity
Respiratory: Tachypnea, rales; dose-related when total dose is >400 units or with single doses >30 units. Pathogenesis is poorly understood, but may be related to damage of pulmonary, vascular, or connective tissue. Manifested as an acute or chronic interstitial pneumonitis with interstitial fibrosis, hypoxia, and death. Symptoms include cough, dyspnea, and bilateral pulmonary infiltrates noted on CXR. It is controversial whether steroids improve symptoms of bleomycin pulmonary toxicity.

**Drug Interactions**

Decreased effect:
Digitalis glycosides: May decrease plasma levels and renal excretion of digoxin
Phenytoin: Results in decreased phenytoin levels, possibly due to decreased oral absorption

Increased toxicity:
CCNU: Increased severity of leukopenia
Cisplatin: Results in delayed bleomycin elimination due to decrease in creatinine clearance secondary to cisplatin

**Drug Uptake**

Absorption: I.M. and intrapleural administration produces serum concentrations of 30% of I.V. administration; intraperitoneal and S.C. routes produce serum concentrations equal to those of I.V.
Serum half-life (biphasic): Dependent upon renal function:
Normal renal function:
Initial: 1.3 hours
Terminal: 9 hours
End-stage renal disease:
Initial: 2 hours
Terminal: 30 hours
Time to peak serum concentration: I.M.: Within 30 minutes

**Pregnancy Risk Factor** D

**Generic Available** Yes

- **Bleph®-10 Ophthalmic** *see* Sulfacetamide Sodium *on page 939*
- **Blephamide® Ophthalmic** *see* Sulfacetamide Sodium and Prednisolone *on page 940*
- **Blis-To-Sol® [OTC]** *see* Tolnaftate *on page 997*
- **BLM** *see* Bleomycin *on previous page*
- **Blocadren® Oral** *see* Timolol *on page 986*
- **Bluboro® [OTC]** *see* Aluminum Sulfate and Calcium Acetate *on page 57*

♦ **Bonine® [OTC]** *see* Meclizine *on page 620*
♦ **Bontril PDM®** *see* Phendimetrazine *on page 788*
♦ **Bontril® Slow-Release** *see* Phendimetrazine *on page 788*

## Boric Acid (BOR ik AS id)

**U.S. Brand Names** Borofax® Topical [OTC]; Dri-Ear® Otic [OTC]; Swim-Ear® Otic [OTC]

**Therapeutic Category** Pharmaceutical Aid

**Use**

Ophthalmic: Mild antiseptic used for inflamed eyelids

Otic: Prophylaxis of swimmer's ear

Topical ointment: Temporary relief of chapped, chafed, or dry skin, diaper rash, abrasions, minor burns, sunburn, insect bites, and other skin irritations

**Usual Dosage** Apply to lower eyelid 1-2 times/day

**Local Anesthetic/Vasoconstrictor Precautions** No information available to require special precautions

**Effects on Dental Treatment** No effects or complications reported

**Generic Available** Yes

**Comments** Not a corrosive substance

♦ **Borofax® Topical [OTC]** *see* Boric Acid *on this page*
♦ **Boropak® [OTC]** *see* Aluminum Sulfate and Calcium Acetate *on page 57*
♦ **B&O Supprettes®** *see* Belladonna and Opium *on page 124*
♦ **Botox®** *see* Botulinum Toxin Type A *on this page*

## Botulinum Toxin Type A (BOT yoo lin num TOKS in type aye)

**U.S. Brand Names** Botox®

**Therapeutic Category** Ophthalmic Agent, Toxin

**Use**

Treatment of strabismus and blepharospasm associated with dystonia (including benign essential blepharospasm or VII nerve disorders in patients ≥12 years of age)

**Unlabeled uses:** Treatment of hemifacial spasms, spasmodic torticollis (ie, cervical dystonia, clonic twisting of the head), oromandibular dystonia, spasmodic dysphonia (laryngeal dystonia) and other dystonias (ie, writer's cramp, focal task-specific dystonias)

Orphan drug: Treatment of dynamic muscle contracture in pediatric cerebral palsy patients

**Usual Dosage**

Strabismus: 1.25-5 units (0.05-0.15 mL) injected into any one muscle

Subsequent doses for residual/recurrent strabismus: Re-examine patients 7-14 days after each injection to assess the effect of that dose. Subsequent doses for patients experiencing incomplete paralysis of the target may be increased up to two fold the previously administered dose. Maximum recommended dose as a single injection for any one muscle is 25 units.

Blepharospasm: 1.25-2.5 units (0.05-0.10 mL) injected into the orbicularis oculi muscle

Subsequent doses: Each treatment lasts approximately 3 months. At repeat treatment sessions, the dose may be increased up to twofold if the response from the initial treatment is considered insufficient (usually defined as an effect that does not last >2 months). There appears to be little benefit obtainable from injecting >5 units per site. Some tolerance may be found if treatments are given any more frequently than every 3 months.

The cumulative dose should not exceed 200 units in a 30-day period

**Mechanism of Action** Botulinum A toxin is a neurotoxin produced by *Clostridium botulinum*, spore-forming anaerobic bacillus, which appears to affect only the presynaptic membrane of the neuromuscular junction in humans, where it prevents calcium-dependent release of acetylcholine and produces a state of denervation. Muscle inactivation persists until new fibrils grow from the nerve and form junction plates on new areas of the muscle-cell walls. The antagonist muscle shortens simultaneously ("contracture"), taking up the slack created by agonist paralysis; following several weeks of paralysis, alignment of the eye is measurably changed, despite return of innervation to the injected muscle.

**Local Anesthetic/Vasoconstrictor Precautions** No information available to require special precautions

**Effects on Dental Treatment** No effects or complications reported

**Other Adverse Effects**

>10%: Ocular: Dry eyes, lagophthalmos, ptosis, photophobia, vertical deviation

1% to 10%:

Dermatologic: Diffuse skin rash

Ocular: Swelling of eyelid, blepharospasm

(Continued)

## Botulinum Toxin Type A *(Continued)*

<1%: Ocular: Ectropion, keratitis, diplopia, entropion

**Drug Interactions** Increased effect: Botulinum toxin may be potentiated by aminoglycosides

**Drug Uptake**

Strabismus:

Onset of action: 1-2 days after injection

Duration of paralysis: 2-6 weeks

Blepharospasm:

Onset: 3 days after injection

Peak: 1-2 weeks

Duration of paralysis: 3 months

**Pregnancy Risk Factor** C

**Generic Available** No

- **BQ® Tablet [OTC]** *see* Chlorpheniramine, Phenylpropanolamine, and Acetaminophen *on page 236*
- **Breathe Free® [OTC]** *see* Sodium Chloride *on page 920*
- **Breezee® Mist Antifungal [OTC]** *see* Miconazole *on page 672*
- **Breezee® Mist Antifungal [OTC]** *see* Tolnaftate *on page 997*
- **Breonesin® [OTC]** *see* Guaifenesin *on page 478*
- **Brethaire®** *see* Terbutaline *on page 959*
- **Brethine®** *see* Terbutaline *on page 959*

## Bretylium (bre TIL ee um)

**Related Information**

Cardiovascular Diseases *on page 1066*

**U.S. Brand Names** Bretylol®

**Canadian Brand Names** Bretylate®

**Therapeutic Category** Antiarrhythmic Agent, Class III; Antiarrhythmic Agent (Supraventricular & Ventricular)

**Use** Treatment of ventricular tachycardia and fibrillation; used in the treatment of other serious ventricular arrhythmias resistant to lidocaine

**Usual Dosage (Note:** Patients should undergo defibrillation/cardioversion before and after bretylium doses as necessary)

Children:

I.M.: 2-5 mg/kg as a single dose

I.V.: Initial: 5 mg/kg, then attempt electrical defibrillation; repeat with 10 mg/kg if ventricular fibrillation persists at 15-minute intervals to maximum total of 30 mg/kg

Maintenance dose: I.M., I.V.: 5 mg/kg every 6-8 hours

Adults:

Immediate life-threatening ventricular arrhythmias, ventricular fibrillation, unstable ventricular tachycardia: Initial dose: I.V.: 5 mg/kg (undiluted) over 1 minute; if arrhythmia persists, give 10 mg/kg (undiluted) over 1 minute and repeat as necessary (usually at 15- to 30-minute intervals) up to a total dose of 30-35 mg/kg

Other life-threatening ventricular arrhythmias:

Initial dose: I.M., I.V.: 5-10 mg/kg, may repeat every 1-2 hours if arrhythmia persist; give I.V. dose (diluted) over 8-10 minutes

Maintenance dose: I.M.: 5-10 mg/kg every 6-8 hours; I.V. (diluted): 5-10 mg/kg every 6 hours; I.V. infusion (diluted): 1-2 mg/minute (little experience with doses >40 mg/kg/day)

**2 g/250 mL $D_5W$** (infusion pump should be used for I.V. infusion administration)

Rate of I.V. infusion: 1-4 mg/minute

1 mg/minute = 7 mL/hour

2 mg/minute = 15 mL/hour

3 mg/minute = 22 mL/hour

4 mg/minute = 30 mL/hour

**Mechanism of Action** Class II antiarrhythmic; after an initial release of norepinephrine at the peripheral adrenergic nerve terminals, inhibits further release by postganglionic nerve endings in response to sympathetic nerve stimulation

**Local Anesthetic/Vasoconstrictor Precautions** No information available to require special precautions

**Effects on Dental Treatment** No effects or complications reported

**Other Adverse Effects**

>10%: Cardiovascular: Hypotension (both postural and supine)

1% to 10%: Gastrointestinal: Nausea, vomiting

<1%:

Cardiovascular: Transient initial hypertension, increase in PVCs, bradycardia, angina, flushing, syncope

Central nervous system: Vertigo, confusion, hyperthermia

Dermatologic: Rash

Gastrointestinal: Diarrhea, abdominal pain

Neuromuscular & skeletal: Muscle atrophy and necrosis with repeated I.M. injections at same site

Ocular: Conjunctivitis

Renal: Renal impairment

Respiratory: Respiratory depression, nasal congestion

Miscellaneous: Hiccups

**Drug Interactions**

Increased toxicity: Other antiarrhythmic agents

Additive toxicity or effect by bretylium, pressor catecholamines, digitalis

**Drug Uptake**

Onset of antiarrhythmic effect:

I.M.: May require 2 hours

I.V.: Within 6-20 minutes

Peak effect: 6-9 hours

Duration: 6-24 hours

Serum half-life: 7-11 hours; average: 4-17 hours

**Pregnancy Risk Factor** C

**Generic Available** Yes


- ♦ **Bretylol®** *see* Bretylium *on previous page*
- ♦ **Brevicon®** *see* Ethinyl Estradiol and Norethindrone *on page 404*
- ♦ **Brevital® Sodium** *see* Methohexital *on page 651*
- ♦ **Brevoxyl® Gel** *see* Benzoyl Peroxide *on page 130*
- ♦ **Bricanyl®** *see* Terbutaline *on page 959*


## Brimonidine (bri MOE ni deen)

**U.S. Brand Names** Alphagan®

**Therapeutic Category** Alpha$_2$-Adrenergic Agonist Agent, Ophthalmic

**Use** Lowering of intraocular pressure in patients with open-angle glaucoma or ocular hypertension

**Usual Dosage** Adults: Ophthalmic: Instill 1 drop in affected eye(s) 3 times/day (approximately every 8 hours)

**Mechanism of Action** Selective for alpha$_2$-receptors; appears to result in reduction of aqueous humor formation and increase uveoscleral outflow

**Local Anesthetic/Vasoconstrictor Precautions** No information available to require special precautions

**Effects on Dental Treatment** No effects or complications reported

**Other Adverse Effects**

>10%:

Central nervous system: Headache, fatigue/drowsiness

Gastrointestinal: Xerostomia

Ocular: Ocular hyperemia, burning and stinging, blurring, foreign body sensation, conjunctival follicles, ocular allergic reactions and ocular pruritus

1% to 10%:

Central nervous system: Dizziness

Ocular: Corneal staining/erosion, photophobia, eyelid erythema, ocular ache/pain, ocular dryness, tearing, eyelid edema, conjunctival edema, blepharitis, ocular irritation, conjunctival blanching, abnormal vision, lid crusting, conjunctival hemorrhage, abnormal taste, conjunctival discharge

Respiratory: Upper respiratory symptoms

**Drug Interactions**

Increased effect:

CNS depressants (eg, alcohol, barbiturates, opiates, sedatives, anesthetics): Additive or potentiating effect

Topical beta-blockers, pilocarpine → additive decreased intraocular pressure, antihypertensives, cardiac glycosides

Decreased effect: Tricyclic antidepressants can affect the metabolism and uptake of circulating amines

**Drug Uptake**

Onset of action: 1-4 hours

Duration: 12 hours

**Pregnancy Risk Factor** B

**Dosage Forms** Solution, ophthalmic, as tartrate: 0.2% (5 mL, 10 mL)

## Brinzolamide (brin ZOH la mide)

**U.S. Brand Names** Azopt®

**Therapeutic Category** Carbonic Anhydrase Inhibitor

**Use** Lowers intraocular pressure to treat glaucoma in patients with ocular hypertension or open-angle glaucoma

**Usual Dosage** Adults: Ophthalmic: Instill 1 drop in eye(s) 3 times/day

**Mechanism of Action** Inhibition of carbonic anhydrase decreases aqueous humor secretion. This results in a reduction of intraocular pressure.

**Local Anesthetic/Vasoconstrictor Precautions** No information available to require special precautions

**Effects on Dental Treatment** Taste disturbances in 5% to 10% of patients

**Other Adverse Effects**

1% to 10%:

Dermatologic: Dermatitis (1% to 5%)

Gastrointestinal: Taste disturbances (5% to 10%)

Ocular: Blurred vision (5% to 10%), blepharitis (1% to 5%), dry eye (1% to 5%), foreign body sensation (1% to 5%), eye discharge (1% to 5%), eye pain (1% to 5%), itching of eye (1% to 5%)

Respiratory: Rhinitis

<1%:

Central nervous system: Dizziness, headache

Dermatologic: Urticaria, alopecia

Gastrointestinal: Diarrhea, nausea, xerostomia

Ocular: Diplopia, eye fatigue, lid crusting

Respiratory: Dyspnea, pharyngitis

Miscellaneous: Allergic reactions

**Drug Interactions**

Concurrent use of oral carbonic anhydrase inhibitors (CAIs) - additive effects and toxicity

High-dose salicylates may result in toxicity from CAIs

**Drug Uptake** Absorption: Topical: Into the systemic circulation

**Pregnancy Risk Factor** C

**Dosage Forms** Suspension, ophthalmic: 1% (2.5 mL, 5 mL, 10 mL, 15 mL)

**Generic Available** No

- **Brofed® Elixir [OTC]** *see* Brompheniramine and Pseudoephedrine *on page 154*
- **Bromaline® Elixir [OTC]** *see* Brompheniramine and Phenylpropanolamine *on page 153*
- **Bromanate® DC** *see* Brompheniramine, Phenylpropanolamine, and Codeine *on page 155*
- **Bromanate® Elixir [OTC]** *see* Brompheniramine and Phenylpropanolamine *on page 153*
- **Bromanyl® Cough Syrup** *see* Bromodiphenhydramine and Codeine *on next page*
- **Bromarest® [OTC]** *see* Brompheniramine *on next page*
- **Bromatapp® [OTC]** *see* Brompheniramine and Phenylpropanolamine *on page 153*
- **Brombay® [OTC]** *see* Brompheniramine *on next page*
- **Bromfed® Syrup [OTC]** *see* Brompheniramine and Pseudoephedrine *on page 154*
- **Bromfed® Tablet [OTC]** *see* Brompheniramine and Pseudoephedrine *on page 154*
- **Bromfenex®** *see* Brompheniramine and Pseudoephedrine *on page 154*
- **Bromfenex® PD** *see* Brompheniramine and Pseudoephedrine *on page 154*

## Bromocriptine (broe moe KRIP teen)

**U.S. Brand Names** Parlodel®

**Canadian Brand Names** Apo® Bromocriptine

**Therapeutic Category** Anti-Parkinson's Agent; Ergot Alkaloid and Derivative

**Use** Usually used with levodopa or levodopa/carbidopa to treat Parkinson's disease - treatment of parkinsonism in patients unresponsive or allergic to levodopa

Prolactin-secreting pituitary adenomas, acromegaly, amenorrhea/galactorrhea secondary to hyperprolactinemia in the absence of primary tumor

**The indication for prevention of postpartum lactation has been withdrawn** voluntarily by Sandoz Pharmaceuticals Corporation

**Usual Dosage** Adults: Oral:

Parkinsonism: 1.25 mg 2 times/day, increased by 2.5 mg/day in 2- to 4-week intervals (usual dose range is 30-90 mg/day in 3 divided doses), though elderly patients can usually be managed on lower doses

Hyperprolactinemia: 2.5 mg 2-3 times/day

Acromegaly: Initial: 1.25-2.5 mg increasing as necessary every 3-7 days; usual dose: 20-30 mg/day

**Mechanism of Action** Semisynthetic ergot alkaloid derivative with dopaminergic properties; inhibits prolactin secretion and can improve symptoms of Parkinson's disease by directly stimulating dopamine receptors in the corpus stratum

**Local Anesthetic/Vasoconstrictor Precautions** No information available to require special precautions

**Effects on Dental Treatment** No effects or complications reported

**Other Adverse Effects** Incidence of adverse effects is high, especially at beginning of treatment and with dosages >20 mg/day

1% to 10%:

Cardiovascular: Hypotension, Raynaud's phenomenon

Central nervous system: Mental depression, confusion, hallucinations

Gastrointestinal: Nausea, constipation, anorexia

Neuromuscular & skeletal: Leg cramps

Respiratory: Nasal congestion

<1%:

Cardiovascular: Hypertension, myocardial infarction, syncope

Central nervous system: Dizziness, drowsiness, fatigue, insomnia, headache, seizures

Gastrointestinal: Vomiting, abdominal cramps

**Drug Interactions**

Decreased effect: Amitriptyline, butyrophenones, imipramine, methyldopa, phenothiazines, reserpine, may decrease bromocriptine's efficacy at reducing prolactin

Increased toxicity: Ergot alkaloids (increased cardiovascular toxicity)

**Drug Uptake**

Serum half-life (biphasic):

Initial: 6-8 hours

Terminal: 50 hours

Time to peak serum concentration: Oral: Within 1-2 hours

**Pregnancy Risk Factor** C (See Contraindications)

**Generic Available** No

## Bromodiphenhydramine and Codeine

(brome oh dye fen HYE dra meen & KOE deen)

**U.S. Brand Names** Ambenyl® Cough Syrup; Amgenal® Cough Syrup; Bromanyl® Cough Syrup; Bromotuss® w/Codeine Cough Syrup

**Therapeutic Category** Antihistamine; Cough Preparation

**Synonyms** Codeine and Bromodiphenhydramine

**Use** Relief of upper respiratory symptoms and cough associated with allergies or common cold

**Usual Dosage** Adults: Oral: 5-10 mL every 4-6 hours

**Local Anesthetic/Vasoconstrictor Precautions** No information available to require special precautions

**Effects on Dental Treatment**

Bromodiphenhydramine: 1% to 10%: Dry mouth

Codeine: <1%: Dry mouth

**Pregnancy Risk Factor** C

**Dosage Forms** Liquid: Bromodiphenhydramine hydrochloride 12.5 mg and codeine phosphate 10 mg per 5 mL

**Generic Available** Yes

- **Bromotuss® w/Codeine Cough Syrup** *see* Bromodiphenhydramine and Codeine *on this page*
- **Bromphen® [OTC]** *see* Brompheniramine *on this page*
- **Bromphen® DC w/Codeine** *see* Brompheniramine, Phenylpropanolamine, and Codeine *on page 155*

## Brompheniramine (brome fen IR a meen)

**U.S. Brand Names** Bromarest® [OTC]; Brombay® [OTC]; Bromphen® [OTC]; Brotane® [OTC]; Chlorphed® [OTC]; Cophene-B®; Diamine T.D.® [OTC]; Dimetane® Extentabs® [OTC]; Nasahist B®; ND-Stat®

**Therapeutic Category** Antihistamine

**Use** Perennial and seasonal allergic rhinitis and other allergic symptoms including urticaria

**Usual Dosage**

Oral:

Children:

≤6 years: 0.125 mg/kg/dose given every 6 hours; maximum: 6-8 mg/day

6-12 years: 2-4 mg every 6-8 hours; maximum: 12-16 mg/day

(Continued)

## Brompheniramine *(Continued)*

Adults: 4 mg every 4-6 hours or 8 mg of sustained release form every 8-12 hours or 12 mg of sustained release every 12 hours; maximum: 24 mg/day

Elderly: Initial: 4 mg once or twice daily. **Note:** Duration of action may be 36 hours or more, even when serum concentrations are low.

I.M., I.V., S.C.:

Children ≤12 years: 0.5 mg/kg/24 hours divided every 6-8 hours

Adults: 10 mg every 6-12 hours, maximum: 40 mg/24 hours

**Mechanism of Action** Competes with histamine for $H_1$-receptor sites on effector cells in the gastrointestinal tract, blood vessels, and respiratory tract

**Local Anesthetic/Vasoconstrictor Precautions** No information available to require special precautions

**Effects on Dental Treatment** Chronic use of antihistamines will inhibit salivary flow, particularly in elderly patients; this may contribute to periodontal disease and oral discomfort

**Other Adverse Effects**

>10%:

Central nervous system: Slight to moderate drowsiness (compared with other first generation antihistamines, brompheniramine is relatively nonsedating)

Respiratory: Thickening of bronchial secretions

1% to 10%:

Central nervous system: Headache, fatigue, nervousness, dizziness

Gastrointestinal: Appetite increase, weight increase, nausea, diarrhea, abdominal pain, dry mouth

Neuromuscular & skeletal: Arthralgia

Respiratory: Pharyngitis

<1%:

Cardiovascular: Palpitations

Central nervous system: Depression

Dermatologic: Photosensitivity, rash, angioedema

Hepatic: Hepatitis

Neuromuscular & skeletal: Myalgia, paresthesia

Respiratory: Bronchospasm, epistaxis

**Drug Interactions** Increased toxicity: CNS depressants, MAO inhibitors, alcohol, tricyclic antidepressants

**Drug Uptake**

Duration: Varies with formulation

Serum half-life: 12-34 hours

Time to peak serum concentration: Oral: Within 2-5 hours

**Pregnancy Risk Factor** C

**Dosage Forms**

Elixir, as maleate: 2 mg/5 mL with 3% alcohol (120 mL, 480 mL, 4000 mL)

Injection, as maleate: 10 mg/mL (10 mL)

Tablet, as maleate: 4 mg, 8 mg, 12 mg

Tablet, sustained release, as maleate: 8 mg, 12 mg

**Generic Available** Yes

## Brompheniramine and Phenylephrine

(brome fen IR a meen & fen il EF rin)

**U.S. Brand Names** Dimetane® Decongestant Elixir [OTC]

**Therapeutic Category** Antihistamine/Decongestant Combination

**Use** Temporary relief of symptoms of seasonal and perennial allergic rhinitis, and vasomotor rhinitis, including nasal obstruction

**Usual Dosage** Children >12 years and Adults: Oral: 10 mL every 4 hours

**Local Anesthetic/Vasoconstrictor Precautions**

Brompheniramine: No information available to require special precautions

Phenylephrine: Use with caution since phenylephrine is a sympathomimetic amine which could interact with epinephrine to cause a pressor response

**Effects on Dental Treatment**

Brompheniramine: Prolonged use may decrease salivary flow

Phenylephrine: Up to 10% of patients could experience tachycardia, palpitations, and dry mouth; use vasoconstrictor with caution

**Other Adverse Effects**

>10%:

Cardiovascular: Tachycardia

Central nervous system: Slight to moderate drowsiness, nervousness, transient stimulation, insomnia

Respiratory: Thickening of bronchial secretions

1% to 10%:

Central nervous system: Headache, fatigue, nervousness, dizziness

Gastrointestinal: Appetite increase, weight increase, nausea, diarrhea, abdominal pain, dry mouth
Genitourinary: Dysuria
Neuromuscular & skeletal: Arthralgia, weakness
Respiratory: Pharyngitis
Miscellaneous: Sweating

<1%:
Cardiovascular: Edema, palpitations, hypotension
Central nervous system: Depression, sedation, paradoxical excitement, convulsions, hallucinations
Dermatologic: Angioedema, rash, photosensitivity
Genitourinary: Urinary retention
Hepatic: Hepatitis
Neuromuscular & skeletal: Myalgia, paresthesia, tremor
Ocular: Blurred vision
Respiratory: Bronchospasm, epistaxis, dyspnea

**Drug Interactions** CNS depressants, MAO inhibitors, sympathomimetics, Rauwolfia alkaloids, tricyclic antidepressants, ganglionic blocking agents, propranolol

**Pregnancy Risk Factor** C

**Dosage Forms** Elixir: Brompheniramine maleate 4 mg and phenylephrine hydrochloride 5 mg per 5 mL

**Generic Available** Yes

## Brompheniramine and Phenylpropanolamine

(brome fen IR a meen & fen il proe pa NOLE a meen)

**U.S. Brand Names** Bromaline® Elixir [OTC]; Bromanate® Elixir [OTC]; Bromatapp® [OTC]; Bromphen® Tablet [OTC]; Cold & Allergy® Elixir [OTC]; Dimaphen® Elixir [OTC]; Dimaphen® Tablets [OTC]; Dimetapp® 4-Hour Liqui-Gel Capsule [OTC]; Dimetapp® Elixir [OTC]; Dimetapp® Extentabs® [OTC]; Dimetapp® Tablet [OTC]; Genatap® Elixir [OTC]; Tamine® [OTC]; Vicks® DayQuil® Allergy Relief 4 Hour Tablet [OTC]

**Therapeutic Category** Antihistamine/Decongestant Combination

**Synonyms** Phenylpropanolamine and Brompheniramine

**Use** Temporary relief of nasal congestion, running nose, sneezing, and itchy, watery eyes

**Usual Dosage** Oral:

Children:
1-6 months: 1.25 mL 3-4 times/day
7-24 months: 2.5 mL 3-4 times/day
2-4 years: 3.75 mL 3-4 times/day
4-12 years: 5 mL 3-4 times/day

Adults: 5-10 mL 3-4 times/day or 1 regular tablet every 4 hours; sustained release: 1 tablet every 12 hours

**Local Anesthetic/Vasoconstrictor Precautions**
Brompheniramine: No information available to require special precautions
Phenylpropanolamine: Use with caution since phenylpropanolamine is a sympathomimetic amine which could interact with epinephrine to cause a pressor response

**Effects on Dental Treatment**
Brompheniramine: Prolonged use may decrease salivary flow
Phenylpropanolamine: Up to 10% of patients could experience tachycardia, palpitations, and dry mouth; use vasoconstrictor with caution

**Other Adverse Effects**

>10%:
Cardiovascular: Tachycardia
Central nervous system: Slight to moderate drowsiness, nervousness, transient stimulation, insomnia
Respiratory: Thickening of bronchial secretions

1% to 10%:
Central nervous system: Headache, fatigue, dizziness
Gastrointestinal: Appetite increase, weight increase, nausea, diarrhea, abdominal pain, dry mouth
Genitourinary: Dysuria
Neuromuscular & skeletal: Arthralgia, weakness
Respiratory: Pharyngitis
Miscellaneous: Sweating

<1%:
Central nervous system: Depression, sedation, paradoxical excitement, convulsions, hallucinations
Cardiovascular: Edema, palpitations, hypotension
Dermatologic: Angioedema, rash, photosensitivity

(Continued)

## Brompheniramine and Phenylpropanolamine *(Continued)*

Genitourinary: Urinary retention
Hepatic: Hepatitis
Neuromuscular & skeletal: Myalgia, paresthesia, tremor
Ocular: Blurred vision
Respiratory: Bronchospasm, epistaxis, dyspnea

**Drug Interactions**

Increased risk of hypertension: MAO inhibitors (hypertensive crisis, severe headache, hyperpyrexia possible), guanethidine, methyldopa

Increased toxicity with CNS depressants, sympathomimetics, TCAs, anticholinergics

Decreased decongestant activity with phenothiazines, rauwolfia alkaloids

**Pregnancy Risk Factor** B

**Dosage Forms**

Capsule (Dimetapp® 4-Hour Liqui-Gel): Brompheniramine maleate 4 mg and phenylpropanolamine hydrochloride 25 mg

Liquid (Bromaline®, Bromanate®, Cold & Allergy®, Dimaphen®, Dimetapp®, Genatap®): Brompheniramine maleate 2 mg and phenylpropanolamine hydrochloride 12.5 mg per 5 mL

Tablet (Dimaphen®, Dimetapp®, Vicks® DayQuil® Allergy Relief 4 Hour): Brompheniramine maleate 4 mg and phenylpropanolamine hydrochloride 25 mg

Tablet, sustained release: Brompheniramine maleate 12 mg and phenylpropanolamine hydrochloride 75 mg

**Generic Available** Yes

## Brompheniramine and Pseudoephedrine

(brome fen IR a meen & soo doe e FED rin)

**U.S. Brand Names** Brofed® Elixir [OTC]; Bromfed® Syrup [OTC]; Bromfed® Tablet [OTC]; Bromfenex®; Bromfenex® PD; Drixoral® Syrup [OTC]; Iofed®; Iofed® PD

**Therapeutic Category** Antihistamine/Decongestant Combination

**Use** Temporary relief of symptoms of seasonal and perennial allergic rhinitis, and vasomotor rhinitis, including nasal obstruction

**Usual Dosage** Children >12 years and Adults: Oral: 10 mL every 4-6 hours, up to 40 mL/day

**Local Anesthetic/Vasoconstrictor Precautions** Use with caution since pseudoephedrine is a sympathomimetic amine which could interact with epinephrine to cause a pressor response

**Effects on Dental Treatment**

Brompheniramine: Prolonged use may decrease salivary flow

Pseudoephedrine: Up to 10% of patients could experience tachycardia, palpitations, and dry mouth; use vasoconstrictor with caution

**Other Adverse Effects**

>10%:
Cardiovascular: Tachycardia
Central nervous system: Slight to moderate drowsiness, nervousness, transient stimulation, insomnia
Respiratory: Thickening of bronchial secretions

1% to 10%:
Central nervous system: Headache, fatigue, dizziness
Gastrointestinal: Appetite increase, weight increase, nausea, diarrhea, abdominal pain, dry mouth
Genitourinary: Dysuria
Neuromuscular & skeletal: Arthralgia, weakness
Respiratory: Pharyngitis
Miscellaneous: Sweating

<1%:
Cardiovascular: Edema, palpitations, hypotension
Central nervous system: Depression, sedation, paradoxical excitement, convulsions, hallucinations
Dermatologic: Angioedema, rash, photosensitivity
Genitourinary: Urinary retention
Hepatic: Hepatitis
Neuromuscular & skeletal: Myalgia, paresthesia, tremor
Ocular: Blurred vision
Respiratory: Bronchospasm, epistaxis, dyspnea

**Drug Interactions** CNS depressants, MAO inhibitors, sympathomimetics, Rauwolfia alkaloids, tricyclic antidepressants, ganglionic blocking agents, propranolol

**Pregnancy Risk Factor** C

**Dosage Forms**
Capsule, extended release:
Bromfenex® PD, Iofed® PD: Brompheniramine maleate 6 mg and pseudoephedrine hydrochloride 60 mg
Bromfenex®, Iofed®: Brompheniramine maleate 12 mg and pseudoephedrine hydrochloride 120 mg
Elixir:
Brofed®: Brompheniramine maleate 4 mg and pseudoephedrine hydrochloride 30 mg per 5 mL
Bromfed®: Brompheniramine maleate 2 mg and pseudoephedrine hydrochloride 30 mg per 5 mL
Drixoral®: Brompheniramine maleate 2 mg and pseudoephedrine sulfate 30 mg per 5 mL
Tablet (Bromfed®): Brompheniramine maleate 4 mg and pseudoephedrine hydrochloride 60 mg
**Generic Available** Yes

## Brompheniramine, Phenylpropanolamine, and Codeine

(brome fen IR a meen, fen il proe pa NOLE a meen, & KOE deen)
**U.S. Brand Names** Bromanate® DC; Bromphen® DC w/Codeine; Dimetane®-DC; Myphetane DC®; Poly-Histine CS®
**Therapeutic Category** Antihistamine/Decongestant Combination; Cough Preparation
**Use** Relief of coughs and upper respiratory symptoms, including nasal congestion, associated with allergy or the common cold
**Usual Dosage** Oral:
Children:
2-6 years: 2.5 mL every 4 hours
6-12 years: 5 mL every 4 hours
Children >12 years and Adults: 10 mL every 4 hours
**Local Anesthetic/Vasoconstrictor Precautions**
Brompheniramine: No information available to require special precautions
Phenylpropanolamine: Use with caution since phenylpropanolamine is a sympathomimetic amine which could interact with epinephrine to cause a pressor response
**Effects on Dental Treatment**
Brompheniramine: Prolonged use may decrease salivary flow
Codeine: <1%: Dry mouth
Phenylpropanolamine: Up to 10% of patients could experience tachycardia, palpitations, and dry mouth; use vasoconstrictor with caution
**Drug Interactions** CNS depressants, MAO inhibitors, sympathomimetics, Rauwolfia alkaloids, tricyclic antidepressants, ganglionic blocking agents, propranolol
**Pregnancy Risk Factor** C
**Dosage Forms** Liquid: Brompheniramine maleate 2 mg, phenylpropanolamine hydrochloride 12.5 mg, and codeine phosphate 10 mg per 5 mL with alcohol 0.95% (480 mL)
**Generic Available** Yes

- **Bromphen® Tablet [OTC]** *see* Brompheniramine and Phenylpropanolamine *on page 153*
- **Bronchial®** *see* Theophylline and Guaifenesin *on page 973*
- **Bronkephrine® Injection** *see* Ethylnorepinephrine *on page 410*
- **Bronkometer®** *see* Isoetharine *on page 551*
- **Bronkosol®** *see* Isoetharine *on page 551*
- **Brontex® Liquid** *see* Guaifenesin and Codeine *on page 478*
- **Brontex® Tablet** *see* Guaifenesin and Codeine *on page 478*
- **Brotane® [OTC]** *see* Brompheniramine *on page 151*
- **BSS® Ophthalmic** *see* Balanced Salt Solution *on page 120*

## Budesonide

(byoo DES oh nide)
**U.S. Brand Names** Pulmicort Turbuhaler®; Rhinocort®
**Canadian Brand Names** Entocort®; Pulmicort®
**Therapeutic Category** Anti-inflammatory Agent; Corticosteroid, Inhalant; Glucocorticoid
**Use**
Nasal: Management of symptoms of seasonal or perennial rhinitis in adults and nonallergic perennial rhinitis in adults
Oral: Indicated for the maintenance treatment of asthma as prophylactic therapy in adult and pediatric patients six years of age or older; it is also indicated for patients requiring oral corticosteroid therapy for asthma; many of those
(Continued)

## Budesonide *(Continued)*

patients may be able to reduce or eliminate their requirement for oral corticosteroids over time; is NOT indicated for the relief of acute bronchospasm.

**Usual Dosage**

Nasal:

Children <6 years: Not Recommended

Children ≥6 years and Adults: 256 mcg/day, given as either 2 sprays in each nostril in the morning and evening or 4 sprays in each nostril in the morning

Oral:

Children: 200 mcg twice daily; maximum dose: 400 mcg twice daily

Adults: 200-400 mcg twice daily; maximum dose: 800 mcg twice daily twice

**Local Anesthetic/Vasoconstrictor Precautions** No information available to require special precautions

**Effects on Dental Treatment** Localized infections with *Candida albicans* or *Aspergillus niger* have occurred frequently in the mouth and pharynx with repetitive use of oral inhaler of beclomethasone. Positive cultures for oral *Candida* may be present in up to 75% of patients. These infections may require treatment with appropriate antifungal therapy or discontinuance of treatment with beclomethasone inhaler.

**Other Adverse Effects**

>10%:

Cardiovascular: Pounding heartbeat

Central nervous system: Nervousness, headache, dizziness

Dermatologic: Itching, skin rash

Gastrointestinal: GI irritation, bitter taste

Respiratory: Coughing, upper respiratory tract infection, bronchitis, hoarseness

Miscellaneous: Oral candidiasis, increased susceptibility to infections, sweating

1% to 10%:

Central nervous system: Insomnia, psychic changes

Dermatologic: Acne, urticaria

Endocrine & metabolic: Menstrual problems

Gastrointestinal: Anorexia, dry mouth/throat, increase in appetite

Ocular: Cataracts

Respiratory: Epistaxis

Miscellaneous: Loss of smell/taste

<1%:

Gastrointestinal: Abdominal fullness

Respiratory: Bronchospasm, dyspnea

**Drug Interactions** No data reported

**Drug Uptake** Absorption: Nasal: 20% of dose delivered reaches systemic circulation

**Pregnancy Risk Factor** C

**Generic Available** No

- **Bufferin® [OTC]** *see* Aspirin *on page 100*
- **Buffex® [OTC]** *see* Aspirin *on page 100*

## Bumetanide (byoo MET a nide)

**Related Information**

Cardiovascular Diseases *on page 1066*

**U.S. Brand Names** Bumex®

**Canadian Brand Names** Burinex®

**Therapeutic Category** Diuretic, Loop

**Use** Management of edema secondary to congestive heart failure or hepatic or renal disease including nephrotic syndrome; may be used alone or in combination with antihypertensives in the treatment of hypertension; can be used in furosemide-allergic patients; (1 mg = 40 mg furosemide)

**Usual Dosage**

Children:

<6 months: Dose not established

>6 months:

Oral: Initial: 0.015 mg/kg/dose once daily or every other day; maximum dose: 0.1 mg/kg/day

I.M., I.V.: Dose not established

Adults:

Oral: 0.5-2 mg/dose 1-2 times/day; maximum: 10 mg/day

I.M., I.V.: 0.5-1 mg/dose; maximum: 10 mg/day

Continuous I.V. infusions of 0.9-1 mg/hour may be more effective than bolus dosing

**Mechanism of Action** Inhibits reabsorption of sodium and chloride in the ascending loop of Henle and proximal renal tubule, interfering with the chloride-binding cotransport system, thus causing increased excretion of water, sodium, chloride, magnesium, phosphate and calcium; it does not appear to act on the distal tubule

**Local Anesthetic/Vasoconstrictor Precautions** No information available to require special precautions

**Effects on Dental Treatment** No effects or complications reported

**Other Adverse Effects**

>10%:
- Endocrine & metabolic: Hyperuricemia, hypochloremia, hypokalemia
- Renal: Azotemia

1% to 10%:
- Central nervous system: Dizziness, encephalopathy, headache
- Endocrine & metabolic: Hyponatremia
- Neuromuscular & skeletal: Muscle cramps, weakness

<1%:
- Cardiovascular: Hypotension
- Dermatologic: Rash, pruritus
- Endocrine & metabolic: Hyperglycemia
- Gastrointestinal: Cramps, nausea, vomiting
- Hepatic: Alteration of liver function test results
- Otic: Hearing loss
- Renal: Elevated serum creatinine

**Drug Interactions**
- Additive effect: Other antihypertensive agents
- Decreased effect: Indomethacin and other NSAIDs, probenecid
- Increased effect: Lithium excretion may be decreased

**Drug Uptake**

Onset of effect:
- Oral, I.M.: 0.5-1 hour
- I.V.: 2-3 minutes

Duration of action: 6 hours

Serum half-life:
- Infants <6 months: Possibly 2.5 hours
- Children and Adults: 1-1.5 hours

**Pregnancy Risk Factor** D

**Generic Available** Yes

♦ **Bumex®** *see* Bumetanide *on previous page*
♦ **Bupap®** *see* Butalbital Compound and Acetaminophen *on page 164*
♦ **Buphenyl®** *see* Sodium Phenylbutyrate *on page 923*

## Bupivacaine (byoo PIV a kane)

**Related Information**

Oral Pain *on page 1122*

**U.S. Brand Names** Marcaine®; Sensorcaine®; Sensorcaine®-MPF

**Therapeutic Category** Dental/Local Anesthetics; Local Anesthetic, Injectable

**Use** Local anesthetic (injectable) for peripheral nerve block, infiltration, sympathetic block, caudal or epidural block, retrobulbar block

**Usual Dosage** Dose varies with procedure, depth of anesthesia, vascularity of tissues, duration of anesthesia and condition of patient. Metabisulfites (in epinephrine-containing injection); do not use solutions containing preservatives for caudal or epidural block.

Caudal block (with or without epinephrine):
- Children: 1-3.7 mg/kg
- Adults: 15-30 mL of 0.25% or 0.5%

Epidural block (other than caudal block):
- Children: 1.25 mg/kg/dose
- Adults: 10-20 mL of 0.25% or 0.5%

Peripheral nerve block: 5 mL dose of 0.25% or 0.5% (12.5-25 mg); maximum: 2.5 mg/kg (plain); 3 mg/kg (with epinephrine); up to a maximum of 400 mg/day

Sympathetic nerve block: 20-50 mL of 0.25% (no epinephrine) solution

**Mechanism of Action** Blocks both the initiation and conduction of nerve impulses by decreasing the neuronal membrane's permeability to sodium ions, which results in inhibition of depolarization with resultant blockade of conduction

**Local Anesthetic/Vasoconstrictor Precautions** No information available to require special precautions

**Effects on Dental Treatment** No effects or complications reported

**Other Adverse Effects** 1% to 10% (dose related):
- Cardiovascular: Cardiac arrest, hypotension, bradycardia, palpitations
- Central nervous system: Seizures, restlessness, anxiety, dizziness
- Gastrointestinal: Nausea, vomiting
- Neuromuscular & skeletal: Weakness
- Ocular: Blurred vision

(Continued)

## Bupivacaine *(Continued)*

Otic: Tinnitus
Respiratory: Apnea

**Contraindications** Hypersensitivity to bupivacaine hydrochloride or any component, para-aminobenzoic acid or parabens

**Warnings/Precautions** Use with caution in patients with liver disease. Some commercially available formulations contain sodium metabisulfite, which may cause allergic-type reactions. Pending further data, should not be used in children <12 years of age and the solution for spinal anesthesia should not be used in children <18 years of age. **Do not use solutions containing preservatives for caudal or epidural block**; convulsions due to systemic toxicity leading to cardiac arrest have been reported, presumably following unintentional intravascular injection. 0.75% is **not** recommended for obstetrical anesthesia.

**Drug Interactions**

Increased effect: Hyaluronidase

Increased toxicity: Beta-blockers, ergot-type oxytocics, MAO inhibitors, TCAs, phenothiazines, vasopressors

**Drug Uptake**

Onset of anesthesia (dependent on route administered): Within 4-10 minutes generally

Duration of action: 1.5-8.5 hours

Serum half-life (age dependent): Adults: 1.5-5.5 hours

**Pregnancy Risk Factor** C

**Dosage Forms**

Injection: 0.25% (10 mL, 20 mL, 30 mL, 50 mL); 0.5% (10 mL, 20 mL, 30 mL, 50 mL); 0.75% (2 mL, 10 mL, 20 mL, 30 mL)

Injection, with epinephrine (1:200,000): 0.25% (10 mL, 30 mL, 50 mL); 0.5% (1.8 mL, 3 mL, 5 mL, 10 mL, 30 mL, 50 mL); 0.75% (30 mL)

**Generic Available** Yes

## Bupivacaine and Epinephrine (byoo PIV a kane & ep i NEF rin)

**Related Information**

Oral Pain *on page 1122*

**U.S. Brand Names** Marcaine® With Epinephrine; Sensorcaine® MPF

**Canadian Brand Names** Sensorcaine® With Epinephrine

**Therapeutic Category** Dental/Local Anesthetics; Local Anesthetic, Injectable

**Use** Dental and Medical: Local anesthesia

**Usual Dosage**

Children <10 years: Dosage has not been established

Children >10 years and Adults: Infiltration and nerve block in maxillary and mandibular area: 9 mg (1.8 mL) of bupivacaine as a 0.5% solution with epinephrine 1:200,000 per injection site. A second dose may be administered if necessary to produce adequate anesthesia after allowing up to 10 minutes for onset. Up to a maximum of 90 mg of bupivacaine hydrochloride per dental appointment. The effective anesthetic dose varies with procedure, intensity of anesthesia needed, duration of anesthesia required, and physical condition of the patient; always use the lowest effective dose along with careful aspiration.

The following numbers of dental carpules (1.8 mL) provide the indicated amounts of bupivacaine hydrochloride 0.5% and epinephrine 1:200,000.

| # of Cartridges | Mg Bupivacaine (0.5%) | Mg Vasoconstrictor (Epinephrine 1:200,000) |
|---|---|---|
| 1 | 9 | 0.009 |
| 2 | 18 | 0.018 |
| 3 | 27 | 0.027 |
| 4 | 36 | 0.036 |
| 5 | 45 | 0.045 |
| 6 | 54 | 0.054 |
| 7 | 63 | 0.063 |
| 8 | 72 | 0.072 |
| 9 | 81 | 0.081 |
| 10 | 90 | 0.090 |

**Note:** Adult and children doses of bupivacaine hydrochloride with epinephrine cited from USP Dispensing Information (USP DI), 17th ed, The United States Pharmacopeial Convention, Inc, Rockville, MD, 1997, 134.

**Mechanism of Action** Local anesthetics bind selectively to the intracellular surface of sodium channels to block influx of sodium into the axon. As a result, depolarization necessary for action potential propagation and subsequent nerve function is prevented. The block at the sodium channel is reversible. When drug diffuses away from the axon, sodium channel function is restored and nerve propagation returns.

Epinephrine prolongs the duration of the anesthetic actions of bupivacaine by causing vasoconstriction (alpha adrenergic receptor agonist) of the vasculature surrounding the nerve axons. This prevents the diffusion of bupivacaine away from the nerves resulting in a longer retention in the axon

**Local Anesthetic/Vasoconstrictor Precautions** No information available to require special precautions

**Effects on Dental Treatment** No effects or complications reported

**Other Adverse Effects** Degree of adverse effects in the central nervous system and cardiovascular system are directly related to the blood levels of bupivacaine

Cardiovascular: Myocardial effects include a decrease in contraction force as well as a decrease in electrical excitability and myocardial conduction rate resulting in bradycardia and reduction in cardiac output.

Central nervous system: High blood levels result in anxiety, restlessness, disorientation, confusion, dizziness, tremors and seizures. This is followed by depression of CNS resulting in somnolence, unconsciousness and possible respiratory arrest. Nausea and vomiting may also occur. In some cases, symptoms of CNS stimulation may be absent and the primary CNS effects are somnolence and unconsciousness.

Hypersensitivity reactions: Extremely rare, but may be manifest as dermatologic reactions and edema at injection site. Asthmatic syndromes have occurred. Patients may exhibit hypersensitivity to bisulfites contained in local anesthetic solution to prevent oxidation of epinephrine. In general, patients reacting to bisulfites have a history of asthma and their airways are hyper-reactive to asthmatic syndrome.

Psychogenic reactions: It is common to misinterpret psychogenic responses to local anesthetic injection as an allergic reaction. Intraoral injections are perceived by many patients as a stressful procedure in dentistry. Common symptoms to this stress are sweating, palpitations, hyperventilation, generalized pallor and a fainting feeling.

**Contraindications** Hypersensitivity to bupivacaine

**Warnings/Precautions** Should be avoided in patients with uncontrolled hyperthyroidism

**Drug Interactions** Due to epinephrine component: With tricyclic antidepressants or MAO inhibitors could result in increased pressor response; with nonselective beta-blockers (ie, propranolol) could result in serious hypertension and reflex bradycardia

**Drug Uptake**

Onset of action: Infiltration and nerve block: 2-20 minutes

Duration:

Infiltration: 60 minutes

Nerve block: 5-7 hours

Serum half-life: 1.5-5.5 hours/adult

**Pregnancy Risk Factor** C

**Breast-feeding Considerations** Usual infiltration doses of bupivacaine with epinephrine given to nursing mothers has not been shown to affect the health of the nursing infant

**Dosage Forms** Injection: Bupivacaine hydrochloride 0.5% with epinephrine 1:200,000 (1.8 mL cartridges in boxes of 50)

**Dietary Considerations** No data reported

**Generic Available** Yes

**Selected Readings**

Ayoub ST and Coleman AE, "A Review of Local Anesthetics," *Gen Dent*, 1992, 40(4):285-7, 289-90.

Jastak JT and Yagiela JA, "Vasoconstrictors and Local Anesthesia: A Review and Rationale for Use," *J Am Dent Assoc*, 1983, 107(4):623-30.

MacKenzie TA and Young ER, "Local Anesthetic Update," *Anesth Prog*, 1993, 40(2):29-34.

Wynn RL, "Epinephrine Interactions With Beta-Blockers," *Gen Dent*, 1994, 42(1):16, 18.

Yagiela JA, "Local Anesthetics," *Anesth Prog*, 1991, 38(4-5):128-41.

♦ **Buprenex®** *see* Buprenorphine *on this page*

## Buprenorphine (byoo pre NOR feen)

**Related Information**

Narcotic Agonists *on page 1223*

**U.S. Brand Names** Buprenex®

**Therapeutic Category** Analgesic, Narcotic

**Use** Management of moderate to severe pain

**Usual Dosage** I.M., slow I.V.:

Children ≥13 years and Adults: 0.3-0.6 mg every 6 hours as needed

(Continued)

## Buprenorphine *(Continued)*

Elderly: 0.15 mg every 6 hours; elderly patients are more likely to suffer from confusion and drowsiness compared to younger patients

**Long-term use is not recommended**

**Mechanism of Action** Opiate agonist/antagonist that produces analgesia by binding to kappa and mu opiate receptors in the CNS

**Local Anesthetic/Vasoconstrictor Precautions** No information available to require special precautions

**Effects on Dental Treatment** No effects or complications reported

**Other Adverse Effects**

>10%: Central nervous system: Drowsiness

1% to 10%:

- Cardiovascular: Hypotension
- Central nervous system: Dizziness, headache
- Gastrointestinal: Vomiting, nausea
- Respiratory: Respiratory depression

<1%:

- Central nervous system: Euphoria, slurred speech, malaise
- Dermatologic: Allergic dermatitis
- Genitourinary: Urinary retention
- Neuromuscular & skeletal: Paresthesia
- Ocular: Blurred vision

**Drug Interactions** Increased toxicity: Barbiturates, benzodiazepines (increase CNS and respiratory depression)

**Drug Uptake**

Onset of analgesia: Within 10-30 minutes

Absorption: I.M., S.C.: 30% to 40%

Serum half-life: 2.2-3 hours

**Pregnancy Risk Factor** C

**Generic Available** Yes

## Bupropion (byoo PROE pee on)

**Related Information**

Vasoconstrictor Interactions With Antidepressants *on page 1277*

**U.S. Brand Names** Wellbutrin®; Wellbutrin® SR; Zyban™

**Therapeutic Category** Antidepressant, Miscellaneous

**Use** Treatment of depression; as an aid to smoking cessation treatment in smokers ≥18 years of age

**Usual Dosage** Adults: Oral: Begin at 150 mg/day for first 3 days, increase dosage to maximum 300 mg/day (150 mg twice daily) for 7-12 weeks; allow at least 8 hours between successive doses

**Mechanism of Action** Antidepressant structurally different from all other previously marketed antidepressants; like other antidepressants the mechanism of bupropion's activity is not fully understood; weak blocker of serotonin and norepinephrine re-uptake, inhibits neuronal dopamine re-uptake and is **not** a monoamine oxidase A or B inhibitor

**Local Anesthetic/Vasoconstrictor Precautions** None; this is not a tricyclic type antidepressant and will not enhance pressor response of epinephrine

**Effects on Dental Treatment** A common adverse effect is significant dry mouth (>10%); normal salivary flow will occur with cessation of drug therapy

**Other Adverse Effects**

>10%:

- Central nervous system: Agitation, insomnia, fever, headache, psychosis, confusion, anxiety, restlessness, dizziness, seizures, chills, akathisia
- Gastrointestinal: Nausea, vomiting, constipation, weight loss
- Genitourinary: Impotence
- Neuromuscular & skeletal: Tremor

1% to 10%:

- Central nervous system: Hallucinations, fatigue
- Dermatologic: Skin rash
- Ocular: Blurred vision

<1%:

- Cardiovascular: Syncope
- Central nervous system: Drowsiness

**Contraindications** In patients with a seizure disorder or with a current profile of bulimia or anorexia nervosa; contraindicated with concurrent administration of an MAO inhibitor

**Warnings/Precautions** Use of bupropion is associated with dose-dependent risk of seizures; therefore, doses of >300 mg/day should not be prescribed

**Drug Interactions**
Decreased effects: Increased clearance: Carbamazepine, phenytoin, cimetidine, phenobarbital
Increased effects: Levodopa, MAO inhibitors

**Drug Uptake**
Absorption: Rapidly absorbed from GI tract
Serum half-life: 14 hours
Time to peak serum concentration: Oral: Within 3 hours

**Pregnancy Risk Factor** B

**Dosage Forms**
Tablet (Wellbutrin®): 75 mg, 100 mg
Tablet, sustained release (Wellbutrin® SR, Zyban™): 100 mg, 150 mg

**Generic Available** No

- **Burow's Otic** *see* Aluminum Acetate and Acetic Acid *on page 54*
- **BuSpar®** *see* Buspirone *on this page*

## Buspirone (byoo SPYE rone)

**Related Information**
Patients Requiring Sedation *on page 1152*

**U.S. Brand Names** BuSpar®

**Therapeutic Category** Antianxiety Agent; Tranquilizer, Minor

**Use** Management of anxiety; has shown little potential for abuse
**Unlabeled use:** Panic attacks

**Usual Dosage** Adults: Oral: 15 mg/day (5 mg 3 times/day); may increase in increments of 5 mg/day every 2-4 days to a maximum of 60 mg/day

**Mechanism of Action** Selectively antagonizes CNS serotonin $5\text{-}HT_1A$ receptors without affecting benzodiazepine-GABA receptors; may down-regulate postsynaptic $5\text{-}HT_2$ receptors as do antidepressants

**Local Anesthetic/Vasoconstrictor Precautions** No information available to require special precautions

**Effects on Dental Treatment** No effects or complications reported

**Other Adverse Effects**
>10%:
Central nervous system: Dizziness, lightheadedness, headache, restlessness
Gastrointestinal: Nausea
1% to 10%: Central nervous system: Drowsiness
<1%:
Cardiovascular: Chest pain, tachycardia
Central nervous system: Confusion, insomnia, nightmares, sedation, disorientation, excitement, fever, ataxia
Dermatologic: Rash, urticaria
Gastrointestinal: Dry mouth, vomiting, diarrhea, flatulence
Hematologic: Leukopenia, eosinophilia
Neuromuscular & skeletal: Weakness
Ocular: Blurred vision
Otic: Tinnitus

**Drug Interactions**
Increased effects: Cimetidine may increase serum levels of buspirone resulting in increased effects
Increased toxicity: MAO inhibitors, phenothiazines, CNS depressants; increased toxicity of digoxin and haloperidol

**Drug Uptake**
Serum half-life: 2-3 hours
Time to peak serum concentration: Oral: Within 40-60 minutes

**Pregnancy Risk Factor** B

**Dosage Forms** Tablet, as hydrochloride: 5 mg, 10 mg

**Dietary Considerations** Food may decrease the absorption of buspirone, but it may also decrease the first-pass metabolism, thereby increasing the bioavailability of buspirone

**Generic Available** No

## Busulfan (byoo SUL fan)

**U.S. Brand Names** Myleran®

**Therapeutic Category** Antineoplastic Agent, Alkylating Agent

**Use** Chronic myelogenous leukemia and bone marrow disorders, such as polycythemia vera and myeloid metaplasia, conditioning regimens for bone marrow transplantation

**Usual Dosage** Oral (**refer to individual protocols**):
Children:
For remission induction of CML: 0.06-0.12 mg/kg/day **or** 1.8-4.6 mg/m²/day; titrate dosage to maintain leukocyte count above 40,000/mm³; reduce

(Continued)

## Busulfan *(Continued)*

dosage by 50% if the leukocyte count reaches 30,000-40,000/mm³; discontinue drug if counts fall to ≤20,000/mm³

BMT marrow-ablative conditioning regimen: 1 mg/kg/dose (ideal body weight) every 6 hours for 16 doses

Adults:

BMT marrow-ablative conditioning regimen: 1 mg/kg/dose (ideal body weight) every 6 hours for 16 doses

Remission:

Induction of CML: 4-8 mg/day (may be as high as 12 mg/day)

Maintenance doses: Controversial, range from 1-4 mg/day to 2 mg/week; treatment is continued until WBC reaches 10,000-20,000 cells/mm³ at which time drug is discontinued; when WBC reaches 50,000/mm³, maintenance dose is resumed

Unapproved uses:

Polycythemia vera: 2-6 mg/day

Thrombocytosis: 4-6 mg/day

**Mechanism of Action** Reacts with N-7 position of guanosine and interferes with DNA replication and transcription of RNA. Busulfan has a more marked effect on myeloid cells (and is, therefore, useful in the treatment of CML) than on lymphoid cells. The drug is also very toxic to hematopoietic stem cells (thus its usefulness in high doses in BMT preparative regimens). Busulfan exhibits little immunosuppressive activity. Interferes with the normal function of DNA by alkylation and cross-linking the strands of DNA.

**Local Anesthetic/Vasoconstrictor Precautions** No information available to require special precautions

**Effects on Dental Treatment** No effects or complications reported

**Other Adverse Effects** Fertility/carcinogenesis: Sterility, ovarian suppression, amenorrhea, azoospermia, and testicular atrophy; malignant tumors have been reported in patients on busulfan therapy

>10%:

Hematologic: Severe pancytopenia, leukopenia, thrombocytopenia, anemia, and bone marrow suppression are common and patients should be monitored closely while on therapy. Since this is a delayed effect (busulfan affects the stem cells), the drug should be discontinued temporarily at the first sign of a large or rapid fall in any blood element. Some patients may develop bone marrow fibrosis or chronic aplasia which is probably due to the busulfan toxicity. In large doses, busulfan is myeloablative and is used for this reason in BMT.

Myelosuppressive: WBC: Moderate; Platelets: Moderate; Onset (days): 7-10; Nadir (days): 14-21; Recovery (days): 28

1% to 10%:

Cardiovascular: Endocardial fibrosis

Dermatologic: Hyperpigmentation skin (busulfan tan), urticaria, erythema, alopecia

Endocrine & metabolic: Amenorrhea

Gastrointestinal: Nausea, vomiting, diarrhea; drug has little effect on the GI mucosal lining

Emetic potential: Low (<10%)

Neuromuscular & skeletal: Weakness

<1%:

Central nervous system: Generalized or myoclonic seizures and loss of consciousness have been associated with high-dose busulfan (4 mg/kg/day), blurred vision

Endocrine & metabolic: Adrenal suppression, gynecomastia, hyperuricemia

Genitourinary: Isolated cases of hemorrhagic cystitis have been reported

Hepatic: Hepatic dysfunction

Ocular: Cataracts

Respiratory: After long-term or high-dose therapy, a syndrome known as busulfan lung may occur. This syndrome is manifested by a diffuse interstitial pulmonary fibrosis and persistent cough, fever, rales, and dyspnea. May be relieved by corticosteroids.

**Drug Interactions** No data reported

**Drug Uptake**

Absorption: Rapidly and completely from the GI tract

Serum half-life:

After first dose: 3.4 hours

After last dose: 2.3 hours

Time to peak serum concentration:

Oral: Within 4 hours

I.V.: Within 5 minutes

**Pregnancy Risk Factor** D
**Generic Available** No

## Butabarbital Sodium (byoo ta BAR bi tal SOW dee um)

**U.S. Brand Names** Butalan®; Buticaps®; Butisol Sodium®
**Therapeutic Category** Barbiturate; Hypnotic; Sedative
**Use** Sedative, hypnotic
**Usual Dosage** Oral:
Children: Preop: 2-6 mg/kg/dose; maximum: 100 mg
Adults:
Sedative: 15-30 mg 3-4 times/day
Hypnotic: 50-100 mg
Preop: 50-100 mg 1-1½ hours before surgery
**Mechanism of Action** Interferes with transmission of impulses from the thalamus to the cortex of the brain resulting in an imbalance in central inhibitory and facilitatory mechanisms
**Local Anesthetic/Vasoconstrictor Precautions** No information available to require special precautions
**Effects on Dental Treatment** No effects or complications reported
**Other Adverse Effects**
>10%: Central nervous system: Dizziness, lightheadedness, drowsiness, "hang-over" effect
1% to 10%:
Central nervous system: Confusion, mental depression, unusual excitement, nervousness, faint feeling, headache, insomnia, nightmares
Gastrointestinal: Constipation, nausea, vomiting
<1%:
Cardiovascular: Hypotension
Central nervous system: Hallucinations
Dermatologic: Skin rash, exfoliative dermatitis, Stevens-Johnson syndrome, angioedema
Hematologic: Agranulocytosis, megaloblastic anemia, thrombocytopenia
Local: Thrombophlebitis
Respiratory: Respiratory depression
Miscellaneous: Dependence
**Drug Interactions**
Barbiturates can induce hepatic microsomal enzymes resulting in increased metabolism and therefore decreased effects of anticoagulants, corticosteroids, doxycycline
Increased toxicity when combined with other CNS depressants or antidepressants, respiratory and CNS depression may be additive
**Drug Uptake**
Serum half-life: 40-140 hours
Time to peak serum concentration: Oral: Within 40-60 minutes
**Pregnancy Risk Factor** D
**Generic Available** Yes

- **Butace®** *see* Butalbital Compound *on this page*
- **Butalan®** *see* Butabarbital Sodium *on this page*

## Butalbital Compound (byoo TAL bi tal KOM pound)

**Related Information**
Butalbital Compound and Acetaminophen *on next page*
Butalbital Compound and Aspirin *on page 165*
**U.S. Brand Names** Amaphen®; Anoquan®; Axotal®; B-A-C®; Bancap®; Butace®; Endolor®; Esgic®; Femcet®; Fiorgen PF®; Fioricet®; Fiorinal®; G-1®; Isollyl Improved®; Lanorinal®; Marnal®; Medigesic®; Phrenilin®; Phrenilin® Forte®; Repan®; Sedapap-10®; Triapin®; Two-Dyne®
**Canadian Brand Names** Tecnal®
**Therapeutic Category** Analgesic, Non-narcotic; Barbiturate
**Use** Relief of symptomatic complex of tension or muscle contraction headache
**Usual Dosage** Adults: Oral: 1-2 tablets or capsules every 4 hours; not to exceed 6/day
**Mechanism of Action** Butalbital, like other barbiturates, has a generalized depressant effect on the central nervous system (CNS). Barbiturates have little effect on peripheral nerves or muscle at usual therapeutic doses. However, at toxic doses serious effects on the cardiovascular system and other peripheral systems may be observed. These effects may result in hypotension or skeletal muscle weakness. While all areas of the central nervous system are acted on by barbiturates, the mesencephalic reticular activating system is extremely sensitive to their effects. Barbiturates act at synapses where gamma-aminobenzoic acid is a neurotransmitter, but they may act in other areas as well.
(Continued)

## Butalbital Compound *(Continued)*

**Local Anesthetic/Vasoconstrictor Precautions** No information available to require special precautions

**Effects on Dental Treatment** No effects or complications reported

**Other Adverse Effects**

>10%:

Central nervous system: Dizziness, lightheadedness, drowsiness, "hangover" effect

Gastrointestinal: Nausea, heartburn, stomach pains, dyspepsia, epigastric discomfort

1% to 10%:

Central nervous system: Confusion, mental depression, unusual excitement, nervousness, faint feeling, headache, insomnia, nightmares, fatigue

Dermatologic: Skin rash

Gastrointestinal: Constipation, vomiting, gastrointestinal ulceration

Hematologic: Hemolytic anemia

Neuromuscular & skeletal: Weakness

Respiratory: Dyspnea

Miscellaneous: Anaphylactic shock

<1%:

Cardiovascular: Hypotension

Central nervous system: Hallucinations, jitters

Dermatologic: Exfoliative dermatitis, Stevens-Johnson syndrome

Hematologic: Agranulocytosis, megaloblastic anemia, occult bleeding, prolongation of bleeding time, leukopenia, thrombocytopenia, iron deficiency anemia

Hepatic: Hepatotoxicity

Local: Thrombophlebitis

Renal: Impaired renal function

Respiratory: Respiratory depression, bronchospasm

**Drug Interactions**

Decreased effect: Phenothiazines, haloperidol, quinidine, cyclosporine, tricyclic antidepressants, corticosteroids, theophylline, ethosuximide, warfarin, oral contraceptives, chloramphenicol, griseofulvin, doxycycline, beta-blockers

Increased effect/toxicity: Propoxyphene, benzodiazepines, CNS depressants, valproic acid, methylphenidate, chloramphenicol

**Drug Uptake** Serum half-life: 61 hours in healthy volunteers

**Pregnancy Risk Factor** D

**Dosage Forms**

Capsule, with acetaminophen:

Amaphen®, Anoquan®, Butace®, Endolor®, Esgic®, Femcet®, G-1®, Medigesic®, Repan®, Two-Dyne®: Butalbital 50 mg, caffeine 40 mg, and acetaminophen 325 mg

Bancap®, Triapin®: Butalbital 50 mg and acetaminophen 325 mg

Phrenilin® Forte®: Butalbital 50 mg and acetaminophen 650 mg

Capsule, with aspirin: (Fiorgen PF®, Fiorinal®, Isollyl Improved®, Lanorinal®, Marnal®): Butalbital 50 mg, caffeine 40 mg, and aspirin 325 mg

Tablet, with acetaminophen:

Esgic®, Fioricet®, Repan®: Butalbital 50 mg, caffeine 40 mg, and acetaminophen 325 mg

Phrenilin®: Butalbital 50 mg and acetaminophen 325 mg

Sedapap-10®: Butalbital 50 mg and acetaminophen 650 mg

Tablet, with aspirin:

Axotal®: Butalbital 50 mg and aspirin 650 mg

B-A-C®: Butalbital 50 mg, caffeine 40 mg, and aspirin 650 mg

Fiorinal®, Isollyl Improved®, Lanorinal®, Marnal®: Butalbital 50 mg, caffeine 40 mg, and aspirin 325 mg

**Generic Available** Yes

## Butalbital Compound and Acetaminophen

(byoo TAL bi tal KOM pound & a seet a MIN oh fen)

**U.S. Brand Names** Amaphen®; Anoquan®; Bancap®; Bupap®; Endolor®; Esgic®; Esgic-Plus®; Femcet®; Fioricet®; G-1®; Medigesic®; Phrenilin®; Phrenilin® Forte®; Repan®; Sedapap-10®; Triapin®; Two-Dyne®

**Therapeutic Category** Barbiturate/Analgesic

**Synonyms** Acetaminophen and Butalbital Compound

**Use** Relief of the symptomatic complex of tension or muscle contraction headache

**Restrictions** C-III

**Usual Dosage** Adults: Oral: 1-2 tablets or capsules every 4 hours; not to exceed 6/day

**Local Anesthetic/Vasoconstrictor Precautions** No information available to require special precautions
**Effects on Dental Treatment** No effects or complications reported
**Drug Interactions** See individual agents
**Pregnancy Risk Factor** D
**Dosage Forms**
Capsule:
Amaphen®, Anoquan®, Butace®, Endolor®, Esgic®, Femcet®, G-1®, Medigesic®, Repan®, Two-Dyne®: Butalbital 50 mg, caffeine 40 mg, and acetaminophen 325 mg
Bancap®, Triapin®: Butalbital 50 mg and acetaminophen 325 mg
Phrenilin® Forte®: Butalbital 50 mg and acetaminophen 650 mg
Tablet:
Esgic®, Fioricet®, Repan®: Butalbital 50 mg, caffeine 40 mg, and acetaminophen 325 mg
Phrenilin®: Butalbital 50 mg and acetaminophen 325 mg
Sedapap-10®: Butalbital 50 mg and acetaminophen 650 mg
**Generic Available** Yes

## Butalbital Compound and Aspirin

(byoo TAL bi tal KOM pound & AS pir in)
**U.S. Brand Names** Fiorgen PF®; Fiorinal®; Isollyl® Improved; Lanorinal®
**Canadian Brand Names** Tecnal
**Therapeutic Category** Barbiturate/Analgesic
**Use** Relief of the symptomatic complex of tension or muscle contraction headache
**Restrictions** C-III (Fiorinal®)
**Usual Dosage** Adults: Oral: 1-2 tablets or capsules every 4 hours; not to exceed 6/day
**Local Anesthetic/Vasoconstrictor Precautions** No information available to require special precautions
**Effects on Dental Treatment** No effects or complications reported
**Drug Interactions** See individual agents
**Pregnancy Risk Factor** D
**Dosage Forms**
Capsule: (Fiorgen PF®, Fiorinal®, Isollyl Improved®, Lanorinal®, Marnal®): Butalbital 50 mg, caffeine 40 mg, and aspirin 325 mg
Tablet:
B-A-C®: Butalbital 50 mg, caffeine 40 mg, and aspirin 650 mg
Fiorinal®, Isollyl Improved®, Lanorinal®, Marnal®: Butalbital 50 mg, caffeine 40 mg, and aspirin 325 mg
**Generic Available** Yes

## Butalbital Compound and Codeine

(byoo TAL bi tal KOM pound & KOE deen)
**U.S. Brand Names** Fiorinal® With Codeine
**Canadian Brand Names** Fiorinal®-C 1/4, 1/2; Tecnal C1/4, C1/2
**Therapeutic Category** Analgesic, Narcotic; Barbiturate
**Synonyms** Codeine and Butalbital Compound
**Use** Mild to moderate pain when sedation is needed
**Usual Dosage** Adults: Oral: 1-2 capsules every 4 hours as needed for pain; up to 6/day
**Local Anesthetic/Vasoconstrictor Precautions** No information available to require special precautions
**Effects on Dental Treatment** <1%: Dry mouth
**Other Adverse Effects**
>10%:
Central nervous system: Dizziness, lightheadedness, drowsiness, "hangover" effect
Gastrointestinal: Nausea, heartburn, stomach pains, dyspepsia, epigastric discomfort
1% to 10%:
Central nervous system: Confusion, mental depression, unusual excitement, nervousness, faint feeling, headache, insomnia, nightmares, fatigue
Dermatologic: Skin rash
Gastrointestinal: Constipation, vomiting, gastrointestinal ulceration
Hematologic: Hemolytic anemia
Neuromuscular & skeletal: Weakness
Respiratory: Dyspnea
Miscellaneous: Anaphylactic shock
<1%:
Cardiovascular: Hypotension
(Continued)

## Butalbital Compound and Codeine *(Continued)*

Central nervous system: Hallucinations, jitters
Dermatologic: Skin rash, exfoliative dermatitis, Stevens-Johnson syndrome
Hematologic: Agranulocytosis, megaloblastic anemia, thrombocytopenia, occult bleeding, prolongation of bleeding time, leukopenia, iron deficiency anemia
Hepatic: Hepatotoxicity
Local: Thrombophlebitis
Renal: Impaired renal function
Respiratory: Respiratory depression, bronchospasm

**Warnings/Precautions** Children and teenagers should not use for chickenpox or flu symptoms before a physician is consulted about Reye's syndrome

**Pregnancy Risk Factor** C (D if used for prolonged periods or in high doses at term)

**Dosage Forms** Capsule: Butalbital 50 mg, caffeine 40 mg, aspirin 325 mg and codeine phosphate 30 mg

**Generic Available** Yes

**Comments** Abrupt discontinuation after sustained use (generally >10 days) may cause withdrawal symptoms

## Butenafine (byoo TEN a fine)

**U.S. Brand Names** Mentax®

**Therapeutic Category** Antifungal Agent, Topical

**Use** Topical treatment of tinea pedis (athlete's foot)

**Usual Dosage** Adults: Topical: Apply once daily for 4 weeks

**Mechanism of Action** Butenafine exerts antifungal activity by blocking squalene epoxidation, resulting in inhibition of ergosterol synthesis (antidermatophyte and *Sporothrix schenckii* activity). In higher concentrations, the drug disrupts fungal cell membranes (anticandidal activity).

**Local Anesthetic/Vasoconstrictor Precautions** No information available to require special precautions

**Effects on Dental Treatment** No effects or complications reported

**Other Adverse Effects**

>1%: Dermatologic: Burning, stinging, irritation, erythema, pruritus (2%)
<1%: Dermatologic: Contact dermatitis

**Drug Uptake**

Absorption: Minimal systemic absorption when topically applied
Serum half-life: 35 hours
Time to peak serum concentration: 6 hours (10 ng/mL)

**Pregnancy Risk Factor** B

**Dosage Forms** Cream, as hydrochloride: 1% (2 g, 15 g, 30 g)

♦ **Buticaps®** *see* Butabarbital Sodium *on page 163*

♦ **Butisol Sodium®** *see* Butabarbital Sodium *on page 163*

## Butoconazole (byoo toe KOE na zole)

**U.S. Brand Names** Femstat®

**Therapeutic Category** Antifungal Agent, Vaginal

**Use** Local treatment of vulvovaginal candidiasis

**Usual Dosage** Adults:

Nonpregnant: Insert 1 applicatorful (~5 g) intravaginally at bedtime for 3 days, may extend for up to 6 days if necessary
Pregnant: **Use only during second or third trimesters**

**Mechanism of Action** Increases cell membrane permeability in susceptible fungi (*Candida*)

**Local Anesthetic/Vasoconstrictor Precautions** No information available to require special precautions

**Effects on Dental Treatment** No effects or complications reported

**Other Adverse Effects**

1% to 10%: Genitourinary: Vulvar/vaginal burning
<1%:
Genitourinary: Vulvar itching, soreness, swelling, or discharge
Renal: Polyuria

**Drug Interactions** No data reported

**Drug Uptake**

Absorption: Following intravaginal application small amounts of drug are absorbed systemically (25%) within 2-8 hours
Serum half-life: 21-24 hours

**Pregnancy Risk Factor** C (For use only in 2nd or 3rd trimester)

**Dosage Forms** Cream, vaginal, as nitrate: 2% with applicator (28 g)

**Generic Available** No

## Butorphanol (byoo TOR fa nole)

**Related Information**

Narcotic Agonists *on page 1223*

**U.S. Brand Names** Stadol®; Stadol® NS

**Therapeutic Category** Analgesic, Narcotic

**Use** Management of moderate to severe pain

**Restrictions** C-IV

**Usual Dosage** Adults:

I.M.: 1-4 mg every 3-4 hours as needed

I.V.: 0.5-2 mg every 3-4 hours as needed

Nasal spray: Headache: 1 spray in 1 nostril; if adequate pain relief is not achieved within 60-90 minutes, an additional 1 spray in 1 nostril may be given (each spray gives ~1 mg of butorphanol)

**Mechanism of Action** Mixed narcotic agonist-antagonist with central analgesic actions; binds to opiate receptors in the CNS, causing inhibition of ascending pain pathways, altering the perception of and response to pain; produces generalized CNS depression

**Local Anesthetic/Vasoconstrictor Precautions** No information available to require special precautions

**Effects on Dental Treatment** No effects or complications reported

**Other Adverse Effects**

>10%: Central nervous system: Drowsiness

1% to 10%:

- Cardiovascular: Flushing of the face, hypotension
- Central nervous system: Dizziness, lightheadedness, headache
- Gastrointestinal: Anorexia, nausea, vomiting
- Genitourinary: Decreased urination
- Miscellaneous: Increased sweating

<1%:

- Cardiovascular: Bradycardia or tachycardia, hypertension
- Central nervous system: Paradoxical CNS stimulation, confusion, hallucinations, mental depression, false sense of well being, malaise, restlessness, nightmares, CNS depression
- Dermatologic: Skin rash
- Gastrointestinal: Stomach cramps, constipation, dry mouth
- Genitourinary: Painful urination
- Neuromuscular & skeletal: Weakness
- Ocular: Blurred vision
- Otic: Tinnitus
- Respiratory: Dyspnea, respiratory depression
- Miscellaneous: Dependence with prolonged use

**Drug Interactions** Increased toxicity: CNS depressants, phenothiazines, barbiturates, skeletal muscle relaxants, alfentanil, guanabenz, MAO inhibitors

**Drug Uptake**

Absorption: Rapidly and well absorbed

Serum half-life: 2.5-4 hours

**Pregnancy Risk Factor** B (D if used for prolonged periods or in high doses at term)

**Generic Available** No


- ♦ **Byclomine® Injection** *see* Dicyclomine *on page 322*
- ♦ **Bydramine® Cough Syrup [OTC]** *see* Diphenhydramine *on page 338*
- ♦ **C2B8** *see* Rituximab *on page 893*
- ♦ **C7E3** *see* Abciximab *on page 24*
- ♦ **C8-CCK** *see* Sincalide *on page 916*
- ♦ **311C90** *see* Zolmitriptan *on page 1063*


## Cabergoline (ca BER go leen)

**U.S. Brand Names** Dostinex®

**Therapeutic Category** Ergot-like Derivative

**Use** Treatment of hyperprolactinemia

**Usual Dosage** Adults: Oral: 0.25 mg twice a week; dosage may be increased by 0.25 mg twice weekly to a dose of up to 1 mg twice a week (according to the patient's prolactin level)

**Local Anesthetic/Vasoconstrictor Precautions** No information available to require special precautions

**Effects on Dental Treatment** No effects or complications reported

**Pregnancy Risk Factor** B


- ♦ **Cafatine®** *see* Ergotamine *on page 382*
- ♦ **Cafergot®** *see* Ergotamine *on page 382*

- **Cafetrate®** *see* Ergotamine *on page 382*

## Caffeine and Sodium Benzoate

(KAF een & SOW dee um BEN zoe ate)

**Therapeutic Category** Diuretic, Miscellaneous

**Synonyms** Sodium Benzoate and Caffeine

**Use** Emergency stimulant in acute circulatory failure; as a diuretic; and to relieve spinal puncture headache

**Usual Dosage**

Children: I.M., I.V., S.C.: 8 mg/kg every 4 hours as needed

Adults: I.M., I.V.: 500 mg, maximum single dose: 1 g

**Local Anesthetic/Vasoconstrictor Precautions** No information available to require special precautions

**Effects on Dental Treatment** No effects or complications reported

**Other Adverse Effects** 1% to 10%:

Cardiovascular: Tachycardia, extrasystoles, palpitations

Central nervous system: Insomnia, restlessness, nervousness, mild delirium, headache, anxiety

Gastrointestinal: Nausea, vomiting, gastric irritation

Neuromuscular & skeletal: Muscle tension following abrupt cessation of drug after regular consumption of 500-600 mg/day

Renal: Diuresis

**Pregnancy Risk Factor** C

**Generic Available** Yes

## Caffeine, Citrated (KAF een, SIT rated)

**Therapeutic Category** Central Nervous System Stimulant, Nonamphetamine; Respiratory Stimulant

**Use** Central nervous system stimulant; used in the treatment of idiopathic apnea of prematurity

**Usual Dosage** Apnea of prematurity: Oral:

Loading dose: 10-20 mg/kg as caffeine citrate (5-10 mg/kg as caffeine base). If theophylline has been administered to the patient within the previous 5 days, a full or modified loading dose (50% to 75% of a loading dose) may be given at the discretion of the physician.

Maintenance dose: 5-10 mg/kg/day as caffeine citrate (2.5-5 mg/kg/day as caffeine base) once daily starting 24 hours after the loading dose. Maintenance dose is adjusted based on patient's response, (efficacy and adverse effects), and serum caffeine concentrations.

**Local Anesthetic/Vasoconstrictor Precautions** No information available to require special precautions

**Effects on Dental Treatment** No effects or complications reported

**Pregnancy Risk Factor** B

**Generic Available** Yes

**Comments** Has several advantages over theophylline in the treatment of neonatal apnea, its half-life is about 3 times as long, allowing once daily dosing, drug levels do not need to be drawn at peak and trough; has a wider therapeutic window, allowing more room between an effective concentration and toxicity; 2 mg caffeine citrate = 1 mg caffeine base

- **Calan®** *see* Verapamil *on page 1043*
- **Calan® SR** *see* Verapamil *on page 1043*
- **Cal Carb-HD® [OTC]** *see* Calcium Carbonate *on page 172*
- **Calcibind®** *see* Cellulose Sodium Phosphate *on page 214*
- **Calci-Chew™ [OTC]** *see* Calcium Carbonate *on page 172*
- **Calciday-667® [OTC]** *see* Calcium Carbonate *on page 172*

## Calcifediol (kal si fe DYE ole)

**U.S. Brand Names** Calderol®

**Therapeutic Category** Vitamin D Analog

**Use** Treatment and management of metabolic bone disease associated with chronic renal failure

**Usual Dosage** Children and Adults: Hepatic osteodystrophy: Oral: 20-100 mcg/day or every other day; titrate to obtain normal serum calcium/phosphate levels; increase dose at 4-week intervals

**Mechanism of Action** Vitamin D analog that (along with calcitonin and parathyroid hormone) regulates serum calcium homeostasis by promoting absorption of calcium and phosphorus in the small intestine; promotes renal tubule resorption of phosphate; increases rate of accretion and resorption in bone minerals

**Local Anesthetic/Vasoconstrictor Precautions** No information available to require special precautions

**Effects on Dental Treatment** No effects or complications reported

**Other Adverse Effects**

1% to 10%:

Cardiovascular: Hypotension, cardiac arrhythmias, hypertension

Central nervous system: Irritability, headache

Dermatologic: Pruritus

Endocrine & metabolic: Polydipsia, hypermagnesemia

Gastrointestinal: Nausea, vomiting, constipation, anorexia, pancreatitis, metallic taste

Neuromuscular & skeletal: Muscle/bone pain

Ocular: Conjunctivitis, photophobia

Renal: Polyuria

<1%:

Central nervous system: Overt psychosis, seizures

Endocrine & metabolic: Calcification

Gastrointestinal: Weight loss

Hepatic: Elevated AST/ALT

**Drug Interactions**

Cholestyramine reduces intestinal absorption of fat-soluble vitamins; may impair intestinal absorption of calcifediol

Magnesium-containing antacids and calcifediol should not be used concomitantly in patients on chronic renal dialysis due to potential for hypermagnesemia

**Drug Uptake**

Absorption: Rapid from the small intestines

Serum half-life: 12-22 days

Time to peak: Within 4 hours (oral)

**Pregnancy Risk Factor** A (D if used in doses above the recommended daily allowance)

**Generic Available** No

♦ **Calciferol™** *see* Ergocalciferol *on page 380*

♦ **Calcijex™** *see* Calcitriol *on next page*

♦ **Calcimar® Injection** *see* Calcitonin *on this page*

♦ **Calci-Mix™ [OTC]** *see* Calcium Carbonate *on page 172*

## Calcipotriene (kal si POE try een)

**U.S. Brand Names** Dovonex®

**Therapeutic Category** Antipsoriatic Agent, Topical

**Use** Treatment of moderate plaque psoriasis

**Usual Dosage** Adults: Topical: Apply in a thin film to the affected skin twice daily and rub in gently and completely

**Mechanism of Action** Synthetic vitamin $D_3$ analog which regulates skin cell production and proliferation

**Local Anesthetic/Vasoconstrictor Precautions** No information available to require special precautions

**Effects on Dental Treatment** No effects or complications reported

**Other Adverse Effects**

>10%: Dermatologic: Burning, itching, skin irritation, erythema, dry skin, peeling, rash, worsening of psoriasis

1% to 10%: Dermatologic: Dermatitis

<1%:

Dermatologic: Skin atrophy, hyperpigmentation, folliculitis

Endocrine & metabolic: Hypercalcemia

**Drug Interactions** No data reported

**Pregnancy Risk Factor** C

**Dosage Forms**

Cream: 0.005% (30 g, 60 g, 100 g)

Ointment, topical: 0.005% (30 g, 60 g, 100 g)

Solution, topical: 0.005%

**Generic Available** No

## Calcitonin (kal si TOE nin)

**U.S. Brand Names** Calcimar® Injection; Cibacalcin® Injection; Miacalcin® Injection; Miacalcin® Nasal Spray; Osteocalcin® Injection; Salmonine® Injection

**Canadian Brand Names** Caltine®

**Therapeutic Category** Antidote, Hypercalcemia

**Use**

Calcitonin (salmon): Treatment of Paget's disease of bone and as adjunctive therapy for hypercalcemia; also used in postmenopausal osteoporosis

Calcitonin (human): Treatment of Paget's disease of bone

**Usual Dosage**

Children: Dosage not established

(Continued)

## Calcitonin *(Continued)*

Adults:

Paget's disease:

Salmon calcitonin: I.M., S.C.: 100 units/day to start, 50 units/day or 50-100 units every 1-3 days maintenance dose; Intranasal: 200-400 units (1-2 sprays)/day

Human calcitonin: S.C.: Initial: 0.5 mg/day (maximum: 0.5 mg twice daily); maintenance: 0.5 mg 2-3 times/week or 0.25 mg/day

Hypercalcemia: Initial: Salmon calcitonin: I.M., S.C.: 4 units/kg every 12 hours; may increase up to 8 units/kg every 12 hours to a maximum of every 6 hours

Osteogenesis imperfecta: Salmon calcitonin: I.M., S.C.: 2 units/kg 3 times/week

Postmenopausal osteoporosis: Salmon calcitonin:

I.M., S.C.: 100 units/day

Intranasal: 200 units (1 spray)/day

**Mechanism of Action** Structurally similar to human calcitonin; it directly inhibits osteoclastic bone resorption; promotes the renal excretion of calcium, phosphate, sodium, magnesium and potassium by decreasing tubular reabsorption; increases the jejunal secretion of water, sodium, potassium, and chloride

**Local Anesthetic/Vasoconstrictor Precautions** No information available to require special precautions

**Effects on Dental Treatment** No effects or complications reported

**Other Adverse Effects**

>10%:

Cardiovascular: Facial flushing

Gastrointestinal: Nausea, diarrhea, anorexia

Local: Swelling at injection site

1% to 10%: Genitourinary: Frequency of urination

<1%:

Cardiovascular: Edema

Central nervous system: Chills, headache, dizziness

Dermatologic: Skin rash, urticaria

Neuromuscular & skeletal: Paresthesia, weakness

Respiratory: Dyspnea, nasal congestion, nasal congestion

**Drug Interactions** No data reported

**Drug Uptake**

Hypercalcemia:

Onset of reduction in calcium: 2 hours

Duration of effect: 6-8 hours

Serum half-life: S.C.: 1.2 hours

**Pregnancy Risk Factor** C

**Generic Available** No

## Calcitriol (kal si TRYE ole)

**U.S. Brand Names** Calcijex™; Rocaltrol®

**Therapeutic Category** Vitamin D Analog

**Use** Management of hypocalcemia in patients on chronic renal dialysis; reduce elevated parathyroid hormone levels; decrease severity of psoriatic lesions in psoriatic vulgaris; oral solution is indicated for the management of secondary hyperparathyroidism and resultant metabolic bone disease in predialysis (moderate to severe chronic renal failure) patients (adults, neonates, and older infants).

**Usual Dosage** Individualize dosage to maintain calcium levels of 9-10 mg/dL

Renal failure:

Oral:

Children: Initial: 15 ng/kg/day; maintenance: 5-40 ng/kg/day

Adults: 0.25 mcg/day or every other day (may require 0.5-1 mcg/day)

I.V.: Adults: 0.5 mcg (0.01 mcg/kg) 3 times/week; most doses in the range of 0.5-3 mcg (0.01-0.05 mcg/kg) 3 times/week

Hypoparathyroidism/pseudohypoparathyroidism: Oral:

Children:

<1 year: 0.04-0.08 mcg/kg/day

1-6 years: Initial: 0.25 mcg/day, increase at 2- to 4-week intervals

Children >6 years and Adults: 0.5-2 mcg/day

Vitamin D-resistant rickets (familial hypophosphatemia): Oral: 2 mcg/day; initial: 15-20 ng/kg/day; maintenance: 30-60 ng/kg/day

**Mechanism of Action** Promotes absorption of calcium in the intestines and retention at the kidneys thereby increasing calcium levels in the serum; decreases excessive serum phosphatase levels, parathyroid hormone levels, and decreases bone resorption; increases renal tubule phosphate resorption

**Local Anesthetic/Vasoconstrictor Precautions** No information available to require special precautions

**Effects on Dental Treatment** No effects or complications reported

**Other Adverse Effects**

1% to 10%:

- Cardiovascular: Hypotension, cardiac arrhythmias, hypertension
- Central nervous system: Irritability, headache
- Dermatologic: Pruritus
- Endocrine & metabolic: Polydipsia
- Gastrointestinal: Nausea, vomiting, constipation, anorexia, pancreatitis, metallic taste
- Neuromuscular & skeletal: Muscle/bone pain
- Ocular: Conjunctivitis, photophobia
- Renal: Polyuria

<1%:

- Central nervous system: Overt psychosis, hyperthermia
- Endocrine & metabolic: Hypercalcemia, hypercholesterolemia
- Gastrointestinal: Weight loss
- Hepatic: Elevated LFTs
- Respiratory: Rhinorrhea

**Drug Interactions**

Cholestyramine reduces intestinal absorption of fat-soluble vitamins; may impair intestinal absorption of calcitriol

Magnesium-containing antacids and calcitriol should not be used concomitantly in patients on chronic renal dialysis due to potential for hypermagnesemia

**Drug Uptake**

Onset of action: ~2-6 hours

Duration: 3-5 days

Absorption: Oral: Rapid

Serum half-life: 3-8 hours

**Pregnancy Risk Factor** A (D if used in doses above the recommended daily allowance)

**Generic Available** No

## Calcium Acetate (KAL see um AS e tate)

**U.S. Brand Names** Calphron®; PhosLo®

**Therapeutic Category** Calcium Salt

**Use** Control of hyperphosphatemia in end-stage renal failure; calcium acetate binds phosphorus in the GI tract better than other calcium salts due to its lower solubility and subsequent reduced absorption and increased formation of calcium phosphate; calcium acetate does not promote aluminum absorption

**Usual Dosage** Adults: Oral: 2 tablets with each meal; dosage may be increased to bring serum phosphate value to <6 mg/dL; most patients require 3-4 tablets with each meal

**Mechanism of Action** Moderates nerve and muscle performance via action potential excitation threshold regulation; combines with dietary phosphate to form insoluble calcium phosphate which is excreted in feces

**Local Anesthetic/Vasoconstrictor Precautions** No information available to require special precautions

**Effects on Dental Treatment** No effects or complications reported

**Other Adverse Effects**

Mild hypercalcemia (calcium: >10.5 mg/dL) may be asymptomatic or manifest itself as constipation, anorexia, nausea, and vomiting

More severe hypercalcemia (calcium: >12 mg/dL) is associated with confusion, delirium, stupor, and coma

<1%:

- Central nervous system: Headache
- Endocrine & metabolic: Hypophosphatemia
- Gastrointestinal: Nausea, anorexia, vomiting, abdominal pain, constipation, thirst

**Drug Interactions**

Decreased effect:

- Calcium may antagonize the effects of calcium channel blockers
- May decrease the bioavailability of tetracyclines
- Renders tetracycline antibiotics inactive

Increased toxicity: Administer cautiously to a digitalized patient, may precipitate arrhythmias

**Drug Uptake** Absorption: From the GI tract requires vitamin D

**Pregnancy Risk Factor** C

**Generic Available** No

## Calcium Carbonate (KAL see um KAR bun ate)

**Related Information**

Calcium Carbonate and Magnesium Carbonate *on this page*

**U.S. Brand Names** Alka-Mints® [OTC]; Amitone® [OTC]; Cal Carb-HD® [OTC]; Calci-Chew™ [OTC]; Calciday-667® [OTC]; Calci-Mix™ [OTC]; Cal-Plus® [OTC]; Caltrate® 600 [OTC]; Caltrate, Jr.® [OTC]; Chooz® [OTC]; Dicarbosil® [OTC]; Equilet® [OTC]; Florical® [OTC]; Gencalc® 600 [OTC]; Mallamint® [OTC]; Nephro-Calci® [OTC]; Os-Cal® 500 [OTC]; Oyst-Cal 500 [OTC]; Oystercal® 500; Rolaids® Calcium Rich [OTC]; Tums® [OTC]; Tums® E-X Extra Strength Tablet [OTC]; Tums® Extra Strength Liquid [OTC]

**Canadian Brand Names** Apo®-Cal; Calcite-500; Calsan®; Pharmacal®

**Therapeutic Category** Antacid; Antidote, Hyperphosphatemia; Calcium Salt

**Use** Adjunct in prevention of postmenopausal osteoporosis, antacid, treatment and prevention of calcium depletion (osteoporosis, osteomalacia, etc); control of hyperphosphatemia in end-stage renal disease

**Usual Dosage** Oral (dosage is in terms of elemental calcium):

Recommended daily allowance (RDA):
- <6 months: 360 mg/day
- 6-12 months: 540 mg/day
- 1-10 years: 800 mg/day
- 10-18 years: 1200 mg/day
- Adults: 800 mg/day

Hypocalcemia (dose depends on clinical condition and serum calcium level):
- Children: 45-65 mg/kg/day in 4 divided doses
- Adults: 1-2 g or more/day

Adults:
- Dietary supplementation: 500 mg to 2 g divided 2-4 times/day
- To reduce bone loss with aging/osteoporosis: 1000-1500 mg/day
- Antacid: 2 tablets or 10 mL every 2 hours, up to 12 times/day

**Mechanism of Action** Moderates nerve and muscle performance via action potential excitation threshold regulation; combines with dietary phosphate to form insoluble calcium phosphate which is excreted in feces; may prevent negative calcium balance when used as a dietary supplement, or for calcium balance when used as a dietary supplement, or as treatment for osteoporosis

**Local Anesthetic/Vasoconstrictor Precautions** No information available to require special precautions

**Effects on Dental Treatment** No effects or complications reported

**Other Adverse Effects**

1% to 10%: Gastrointestinal: Constipation, flatulence

<1%:
- Cardiovascular: Hypotension, bradycardia, cardiac arrhythmias
- Central nervous system: Mood and mental changes, lethargy
- Dermatologic: Erythema
- Endocrine & metabolic: Hypercalcemia (with prolonged use), metastatic calcinosis, hypomagnesemia, hypophosphatemia, milk-alkali syndrome
- Gastrointestinal: Laxative effect, acid rebound, nausea, vomiting, GI hemorrhage, fecal impaction, elevated serum amylase
- Neuromuscular & skeletal: Myalgia
- Renal: Polyuria, renal calculi, renal dysfunction, hypercalciuria

**Drug Interactions**

Decreased effect:
- Calcium may antagonize the effects of calcium channel blockers
- May decrease the bioavailability of tetracyclines
- Renders tetracycline antibiotics inactive

Increased toxicity: Administer cautiously to a digitalized patient, may precipitate arrhythmias

**Drug Uptake** Absorption: From the GI tract requires vitamin D; calcium is absorbed in soluble, ionized form; solubility of calcium is increased in an acid environment

**Pregnancy Risk Factor** C

**Generic Available** Yes

## Calcium Carbonate and Magnesium Carbonate

(KAL see um KAR bun ate & mag NEE zhum KAR bun ate)

**U.S. Brand Names** Mylanta® Gelcaps®

**Therapeutic Category** Antacid

**Use** Hyperacidity

**Local Anesthetic/Vasoconstrictor Precautions** No information available to require special precautions

**Effects on Dental Treatment** Do not give tetracyclines concomitantly

**Drug Interactions** See individual agents
**Dosage Forms** Capsule: Calcium carbonate 311 mg and magnesium carbonate 232 mg
**Generic Available** No

## Calcium Carbonate and Simethicone
(KAL see um KAR bun ate & sye METH i kone)
**U.S. Brand Names** Titralac® Plus Liquid [OTC]
**Therapeutic Category** Antacid
**Synonyms** Simethicone and Calcium Carbonate
**Use** Relief of acid indigestion, heartburn, peptic esophagitis, hiatal hernia, and gas
**Usual Dosage** Oral: 0.5-2 g 4-6 times/day
**Local Anesthetic/Vasoconstrictor Precautions** No information available to require special precautions
**Effects on Dental Treatment** Do not give tetracycline concomitantly
**Pregnancy Risk Factor** C
**Generic Available** Yes

♦ **Calcium Channel Blockers & Gingival Hyperplasia** *see page 1204*

## Calcium Chloride (KAL see um KLOR ide)
**U.S. Brand Names** Cal Plus®
**Therapeutic Category** Calcium Salt; Electrolyte Supplement, Parenteral
**Use** Cardiac resuscitation when epinephrine fails to improve myocardial contractions, cardiac disturbances of hyperkalemia, hypocalcemia, or calcium channel blocking agent toxicity; emergent treatment of hypocalcemic tetany, treatment of hypermagnesemia
**Usual Dosage Note:** Calcium chloride is 3 times as potent as calcium gluconate
Cardiac arrest in the presence of hyperkalemia or hypocalcemia, magnesium toxicity, or calcium antagonist toxicity: I.V.:
Children: 20 mg/kg; may repeat in 10 minutes if necessary
Adults: 2-4 mg/kg (10% solution), repeated every 10 minutes
Hypocalcemia: I.V.:
Children: 10-20 mg/kg/dose (children: 1-7 mEq), repeat every 4-6 hours if needed; doses may be repeated every 1-3 days if needed
Adults: 500 mg to 1 g (7-14 mEq), repeated at 1- to 3-day intervals if necessary
Hypocalcemic tetany: I.V.:
Children: 10 mg/kg (0.5-0.7 mEq/kg) over 5-10 minutes; may repeat after 6-8 hours or follow with an infusion with a maximum dose of 200 mg/kg/day
Adults: 4.5-16 mEq may be administered until response occurs
Hypocalcemia secondary to citrated blood transfusion give 0.45 mEq **elemental** calcium for each 100 mL citrated blood infused
**Mechanism of Action** Moderates nerve and muscle performance via action potential excitation threshold regulation
**Local Anesthetic/Vasoconstrictor Precautions** No information available to require special precautions
**Effects on Dental Treatment** No effects or complications reported
**Other Adverse Effects** <1%:
Cardiovascular: Vasodilation, hypotension, bradycardia, cardiac arrhythmias, ventricular fibrillation, syncope
Central nervous system: Lethargy, coma, mania
Dermatologic: Erythema
Endocrine & metabolic: Decreased serum magnesium, hypercalcemia
Gastrointestinal: Elevated serum amylase
Local: Tissue necrosis
Neuromuscular & skeletal: Weakness
Renal: Hypercalciuria
**Drug Interactions**
Decreased effect:
Calcium may antagonize the effects of calcium channel blockers
May decrease the bioavailability of tetracyclines
Renders tetracycline antibiotics inactive
Increased toxicity: Administer cautiously to a digitalized patient, may precipitate arrhythmias
**Drug Uptake** Absorption: I.V. calcium salts are absorbed directly into the bloodstream
**Pregnancy Risk Factor** C
**Generic Available** Yes

## Calcium Citrate (KAL see um SIT rate)
**U.S. Brand Names** Citracal® [OTC]
**Therapeutic Category** Calcium Salt
(Continued)

## Calcium Citrate *(Continued)*

**Use** Adjunct in prevention of postmenopausal osteoporosis; treatment and prevention of calcium depletion

**Usual Dosage** Dosage is in terms of elemental calcium

Recommended daily allowance (RDA):

<6 months: 360 mg/day
6-12 months: 540 mg/day
1-10 years: 800 mg/day
10-18 years: 1200 mg/day
Adults: 800 mg/day

Adults: Oral: 1-2 g/day

**Mechanism of Action** Moderates nerve and muscle performance via action potential excitation threshold regulation

**Local Anesthetic/Vasoconstrictor Precautions** No information available to require special precautions

**Effects on Dental Treatment** No effects or complications reported

**Other Adverse Effects** <1%:

Central nervous system: Mental confusion, headache
Endocrine & metabolic: Hypercalcemia, milk-alkali syndrome, hypophosphatemia
Gastrointestinal: Constipation, vomiting, nausea

**Drug Interactions**

Decreased effect:

Calcium may antagonize the effects of calcium channel blockers
May decrease the bioavailability of tetracyclines
Renders tetracycline antibiotics inactive

Increased toxicity: Administer cautiously to a digitalized patient, may precipitate arrhythmias

**Drug Uptake** Absorption: From the GI tract requires vitamin D

**Pregnancy Risk Factor** C

**Generic Available** No

♦ **Calcium Disodium Edetate** *see* Edetate Calcium Disodium *on page 363*

♦ **Calcium Disodium Versenate®** *see* Edetate Calcium Disodium *on page 363*

♦ **Calcium EDTA** *see* Edetate Calcium Disodium *on page 363*

## Calcium Glubionate (KAL see um gloo BYE oh nate)

**U.S. Brand Names** Neo-Calglucon® [OTC]

**Therapeutic Category** Calcium Salt

**Use** Adjunct in prevention of postmenopausal osteoporosis; treatment and prevention of calcium depletion

**Usual Dosage** Oral:

Recommended daily allowance (RDA) (in terms of elemental calcium):

<6 months: 360 mg/day
6-12 months: 540 mg/day
1-10 years: 800 mg/day
10-18 years: 1200 mg/day
Adults: 800 mg/day

Syrup is a hyperosmolar solution; dosage is in terms of calcium glubionate

Neonatal hypocalcemia: 1200 mg/kg/day in 4-6 divided doses

Maintenance: Children: 600-2000 mg/kg/day in 4 divided doses up to a maximum of 9 g/day

Adults: 6-18 g/day in divided doses

**Mechanism of Action** Moderates nerve and muscle performance via action potential excitation threshold regulation

**Local Anesthetic/Vasoconstrictor Precautions** No information available to require special precautions

**Effects on Dental Treatment** No effects or complications reported

**Other Adverse Effects** <1%:

Central nervous system: Dizziness, headache, mental confusion
Endocrine & metabolic: Hypercalcemia, hypomagnesemia, hypophosphatemia, milk-alkali syndrome
Gastrointestinal: GI irritation, diarrhea, constipation, dry mouth
Renal: Hypercalciuria

**Drug Interactions**

Decreased effect: Calcium may antagonize the effects of calcium channel blockers; may decrease the bioavailability of tetracyclines; renders tetracycline antibiotics inactive

Increased toxicity: Administer cautiously to a digitalized patient, may precipitate arrhythmias

**Drug Uptake**

Absorption: From the GI tract requires vitamin D

**Pregnancy Risk Factor** C
**Generic Available** No

## Calcium Gluceptate (KAL see um gloo SEP tate)

**Therapeutic Category** Calcium Salt

**Use** Treatment of cardiac disturbances of hyperkalemia, hypocalcemia, or calcium channel blocker toxicity; cardiac resuscitation when epinephrine fails to improve myocardial contractions; treatment of hypermagnesemia and hypocalcemia

**Usual Dosage** I.V. (dose expressed in mg of calcium gluceptate):

Cardiac resuscitation in the presence of hypocalcemia, hyperkalemia, magnesium toxicity, or calcium channel blocker toxicity:
- Children: 110 mg/kg/dose
- Adults: 1.1-1.5 g (5-7 mL)

Hypocalcemia:
- Children: 200-500 mg/kg/day divided every 6 hours
- Adults: 500 mg to 1.1 g/dose as needed

After citrated blood administration: Children and Adults: 0.4 mEq/100 mL blood infused

**Mechanism of Action** Moderates nerve and muscle performance via action potential excitation threshold regulation

**Local Anesthetic/Vasoconstrictor Precautions** No information available to require special precautions

**Effects on Dental Treatment** No effects or complications reported

**Other Adverse Effects** <1%:
- Cardiovascular: Vasodilation, hypotension, bradycardia, cardiac arrhythmias, ventricular fibrillation, syncope
- Central nervous system: Lethargy, mania, coma
- Dermatologic: Erythema
- Endocrine & metabolic: Hypomagnesemia, hypercalcemia
- Gastrointestinal: Elevated serum amylase
- Local: Tissue necrosis
- Neuromuscular & skeletal: Weakness
- Renal: Hypercalciuria

**Drug Interactions**

Decreased effect:
- Calcium may antagonize the effects of calcium channel blockers
- May decrease the bioavailability of tetracyclines
- Renders tetracycline antibiotics inactive

Increased toxicity: Administer cautiously to digitalized patients, may precipitate arrhythmias

**Drug Uptake** Absorption: I.M. and I.V. calcium salts are absorbed directly into the bloodstream

**Pregnancy Risk Factor** C
**Generic Available** Yes

## Calcium Gluconate (KAL see um GLOO koe nate)

**U.S. Brand Names** Kalcinate®

**Therapeutic Category** Calcium Salt

**Use** Treatment and prevention of hypocalcemia; treatment of tetany, cardiac disturbances of hyperkalemia, cardiac resuscitation when epinephrine fails to improve myocardial contractions, hypocalcemia, or calcium channel blocker toxicity; calcium supplementation

**Usual Dosage** Dosage is in terms of **elemental** calcium

Recommended daily allowance (RDA):
- <6 months: 400 mg/day
- 6-12 months: 600 mg/day
- 1-10 years: 800 mg/day
- 10-18 years: 1200 mg/day
- Adults: 800 mg/day

**Calcium gluconate** electrolyte requirement in newborn period:
- Premature: 200-1000 mg/kg/24 hours
- Term:
  - 0-24 hours: 0-500 mg/kg/24 hours
  - 24-48 hours: 200-500 mg/kg/24 hours
  - 48-72 hours: 200-600 mg/kg/24 hours
  - >3 days: 200-800 mg/kg/24 hours

Hypocalcemia:
- Oral:
  - Children: 200-500 mg/kg/day divided every 6 hours
  - Adults: 500 mg to 2 g 2-4 times/day

(Continued)

## Calcium Gluconate *(Continued)*

I.V.:

Children: 200-500 mg/kg/day (children 1-7 mEq/day) as a continuous infusion or in 4 divided doses; doses may be repeated every 1-3 days if necessary

Adults: 2-15 g/24 hours as a continuous infusion or in divided doses, which may be repeated every 1-3 days if necessary

Hypocalcemic tetany: I.V.:

Children: 100-200 mg/kg/dose (0.5-0.7 mEq/kg/dose) over 5-10 minutes; may repeat every 6-8 hours **or** follow with an infusion of 500 mg/kg/day

Adults: 1-3 g (4.5-16 mEq) may be administered until therapeutic response occurs

Osteoporosis/bone loss: Oral: 1000-1500 mg in divided doses/day

Calcium antagonist toxicity, magnesium intoxication, or cardiac arrest in the presence of hyperkalemia or hypocalcemia: I.V.:

Children: Calcium chloride is recommended calcium salt; refer to calcium chloride monograph

Adults: 5-8 mL/dose and repeated as necessary at 10-minute intervals, however, calcium chloride is recommended calcium salt; refer to Calcium Chloride monograph

Hypocalcemia secondary to citrated blood infusion: I.V.: Give 0.45 mEq **elemental** calcium for each 100 mL citrated blood infused

Exchange transfusion:

Adults: 300 mg/100 mL of citrated blood exchanged

Maintenance electrolyte requirements for total parenteral nutrition: I.V.: Daily requirements: Adults: 8-16 mEq/1000 kcals/24 hours

**Mechanism of Action** Moderates nerve and muscle performance via action potential excitation threshold regulation

**Local Anesthetic/Vasoconstrictor Precautions** No information available to require special precautions

**Effects on Dental Treatment** No effects or complications reported

**Other Adverse Effects** <1%:

Cardiovascular: Vasodilation, hypotension, bradycardia, cardiac arrhythmias, ventricular fibrillation, syncope

Central nervous system: Lethargy, mania, coma

Dermatologic: Erythema

Endocrine & metabolic: Decrease serum magnesium, hypercalcemia

Gastrointestinal: Elevated serum amylase

Local: Tissue necrosis

Neuromuscular & skeletal: Weakness

Renal: Hypercalciuria

**Drug Interactions**

Decreased effect:

Calcium may antagonize the effects of calcium channel blockers

May decrease the bioavailability of tetracyclines

Renders tetracycline antibiotics inactive

Increased toxicity: Administer cautiously to a digitalized patient, may precipitate arrhythmias

**Drug Uptake** Absorption: I.M. and I.V. calcium salts are absorbed directly into the bloodstream; absorption from the GI tract requires vitamin D; calcium is absorbed in soluble, ionized form; solubility of calcium is increased in an acid environment (except calcium lactate)

**Pregnancy Risk Factor** C

**Generic Available** Yes

## Calcium Lactate (KAL see um LAK tate)

**Therapeutic Category** Calcium Salt

**Use** Adjunct in prevention of postmenopausal osteoporosis; treatment and prevention of calcium depletion

**Usual Dosage** Oral (in terms of calcium lactate)

Recommended daily allowance (RDA) (in terms of elemental calcium):

<6 months: 360 mg/day

6-12 months: 540 mg/day

1-10 years: 800 mg/day

10-18 years: 1200 mg/day

Adults: 800 mg/day

Children: 500 mg/kg/day divided every 6-8 hours

Maximum daily dose: 9 g

Adults: 1.5-3 g divided every 8 hours

**Mechanism of Action** Moderates nerve and muscle performance via action potential excitation threshold regulation

**Local Anesthetic/Vasoconstrictor Precautions** No information available to require special precautions

**Effects on Dental Treatment** No effects or complications reported

**Other Adverse Effects** <1%:

Central nervous system: Headache, mental confusion, dizziness

Endocrine & metabolic: Hypercalcemia, hypophosphatemia, hypomagnesemia, milk-alkali syndrome

Gastrointestinal: Constipation, nausea, dry mouth, vomiting

Renal: Hypercalciuria

**Drug Interactions**

Decreased effect:

Calcium may antagonize the effects of calcium channel blockers

May decrease the bioavailability of tetracyclines

Renders tetracycline antibiotics inactive

Increased toxicity: Administer cautiously to a digitalized patient, may precipitate arrhythmias

**Drug Uptake** Absorption: From the GI tract requires vitamin D

**Pregnancy Risk Factor** C

**Generic Available** Yes

- **Calcium Leucovorin** *see* Leucovorin *on page 577*
- **Calcium Pantothenate** *see* Pantothenic Acid *on page 764*

## Calcium Phosphate, Tribasic (KAL see um FOS fate tri BAY sik)

**U.S. Brand Names** Posture® [OTC]

**Therapeutic Category** Calcium Salt

**Use** Adjunct in prevention of postmenopausal osteoporosis; treatment and prevention of calcium depletion

**Usual Dosage** Oral (all doses in terms of elemental calcium):

Recommended daily allowance (RDA) (elemental calcium):

<6 months: 360 mg/day

6-12 months: 540 mg/day

1-10 years: 800 mg/day

10-18 years: 1200 mg/day

Adults: 800 mg/day

Children: 45-65 mg/kg/day

Adults: 1-2 g/day

**Mechanism of Action** Moderates nerve and muscle performance via action potential excitation threshold regulation

**Local Anesthetic/Vasoconstrictor Precautions** No information available to require special precautions

**Effects on Dental Treatment** No effects or complications reported

**Other Adverse Effects** <1%:

Endocrine & metabolic: Hypercalcemia, milk-alkali syndrome, hypophosphatemia

Gastrointestinal: Constipation, nausea, dry mouth

**Drug Interactions**

Decreased effect:

Calcium may antagonize the effects of calcium channel blockers

May decrease the bioavailability of tetracyclines

Renders tetracycline antibiotics inactive

Increased toxicity: Administer cautiously to a digitalized patient, may precipitate arrhythmias

**Pregnancy Risk Factor** C

**Generic Available** Yes

## Calcium Polycarbophil (KAL see um pol i KAR boe fil)

**U.S. Brand Names** Equalactin® Chewable Tablet [OTC]; Fiberall® Chewable Tablet [OTC]; FiberCon® Tablet [OTC]; Fiber-Lax® Tablet [OTC]; Mitrolan® Chewable Tablet [OTC]

**Therapeutic Category** Antidiarrheal; Laxative, Bulk-Producing

**Use** Treatment of constipation or diarrhea; calcium polycarbophil is supplied as the approved substitute whenever a bulk-forming laxative is ordered in a tablet, capsule, wafer, or other oral solid dosage form

**Usual Dosage** Oral:

Children:

2-6 years: 500 mg (1 tablet) 1-2 times/day, up to 1.5 g/day

6-12 years: 500 mg (1 tablet) 1-3 times/day, up to 3 g/day

Adults: 1 g 4 times/day, up to 6 g/day

**Mechanism of Action** Restoring a more normal moisture level and providing bulk in the patient's intestinal tract

(Continued)

## Calcium Polycarbophil *(Continued)*

**Local Anesthetic/Vasoconstrictor Precautions** No information available to require special precautions

**Effects on Dental Treatment** Oral medication should be given at least 1 hour prior to taking the bulk-producing laxative in order to prevent decreased absorption of medication

**Other Adverse Effects** 1% to 10%: Gastrointestinal: Abdominal fullness

**Drug Interactions** Decreased absorption of oral anticoagulants, digoxin, potassium-sparing diuretics, salicylates, tetracyclines

**Pregnancy Risk Factor** C

**Generic Available** Yes

- **Calderol®** *see* Calcifediol *on page 168*
- **Caldesene® Topical [OTC]** *see* Undecylenic Acid and Derivatives *on page 1033*

## Calfactant (cal FAC tant)

**U.S. Brand Names** Infasurf®

**Therapeutic Category** Lung Surfactant

**Use** Prevention of respiratory distress syndrome (RDS) in premature infants at high risk for RDS and for the treatment ("rescue") of premature infants who develop RDS; decreases the incidence of RDS, mortality due to RDS, and air leaks associated with RDS

**Usual Dosage** Should be administered intratracheally through a side-port adapter into the endotracheal tube; two attendants, one to instill the suspension, the other to monitor the patient and assist in positioning, facilitate the dosing; the dose (3 mL/kg) should be administered in two aliquots of 1.5 mL/kg each; after each aliquot is instilled, the infant should be positioned with either the right or the left side dependent; administration is made while ventilation is continued over 20-30 breaths for each aliquot, with small bursts timed only during the inspiratory cycles; a pause followed by evaluation of the respiratory status and repositioning should separate the two aliquots

**Mechanism of Action** Adsorbs rapidly to the surface of the air:liquid interface and modifies surface tension similarly to natural lung surfactant. A minimum surface tension of ≤3 mN/m is produced *in vitro* as measured on a pulsating bubble surfactometer. *Ex vivo*, restores the pressure volume mechanics and compliance of surfactant-deficient rat lungs. *In vivo*, improves lung compliance, respiratory gas exchange, and survival in preterm lambs with profound surfactant deficiency.

**Local Anesthetic/Vasoconstrictor Precautions** No information available to require special precautions

**Effects on Dental Treatment** No effects or complications reported

**Other Adverse Effects**

>10%:

Cardiovascular: Bradycardia (34%), cyanosis (65%)

Respiratory: Airway obstruction (39%), reflux (21%), requirement for manual ventilation (16%)

1% to 10%: Respiratory: Reintubation (1% to 10%)

**Dosage Forms** Suspension, intratracheal: 6 mL

**Generic Available** No

- **Calm-X® Oral [OTC]** *see* Dimenhydrinate *on page 335*
- **Calphron®** *see* Calcium Acetate *on page 171*
- **Cal-Plus® [OTC]** *see* Calcium Carbonate *on page 172*
- **Cal Plus®** *see* Calcium Chloride *on page 173*
- **Caltrate® 600 [OTC]** *see* Calcium Carbonate *on page 172*
- **Caltrate, Jr.® [OTC]** *see* Calcium Carbonate *on page 172*
- **Cama® Arthritis Pain Reliever [OTC]** *see* Aspirin *on page 100*
- **Campho-Phenique® [OTC]** *see* Camphor and Phenol *on this page*

## Camphor and Phenol (KAM for & FEE nole)

**U.S. Brand Names** Campho-Phenique® [OTC]

**Therapeutic Category** Topical Skin Product

**Use** Relief of pain and for minor infections

**Usual Dosage** Apply as needed

**Local Anesthetic/Vasoconstrictor Precautions** No information available to require special precautions

**Effects on Dental Treatment** No effects or complications reported

**Pregnancy Risk Factor** C

**Generic Available** Yes

## Camphor, Menthol, and Phenol (KAM for, MEN thol, & FEE nole)

**U.S. Brand Names** Sarna [OTC]

**Therapeutic Category** Topical Skin Product

**Use** Relief of dry, itching skin

**Usual Dosage** Topical: Apply as needed for dry skin

**Local Anesthetic/Vasoconstrictor Precautions** No information available to require special precautions

**Effects on Dental Treatment** No effects or complications reported

**Other Adverse Effects** 1% to 10%: Dermatologic: Burning sensation, especially on broken skin

**Pregnancy Risk Factor** C

**Generic Available** Yes

♦ **Camptosar®** *see* Irinotecan *on page 549*
♦ **Cancer Chemotherapy Regimens** *see page 1205*

## Candesartan (kan se SAR tan)

**U.S. Brand Names** Atacand™

**Therapeutic Category** Angiotensin II Antagonist

**Use** Treatment of hypertension; may be used alone or in combination with other antihypertensive agents

**Usual Dosage** Adults: Oral: Dosage must be individualized; blood pressure response is dose-related over the range of 2-32 mg; the usual recommended starting dose of 16 mg once daily when it is used as monotherapy in patients who are not volume depleted; it can be administered once or twice daily with total daily doses ranging from 8-32 mg; larger doses do not appear to have a greater effect and there is relatively little experience with such doses; most of the antihypertensive effect is present within 2 weeks and maximal blood pressure reduction is generally obtained within 4-6 weeks of treatment

No initial dosage adjustment is necessary for elderly patients (although higher concentrations ($C_{max}$) and AUC were observed in these populations), for patients with mildly impaired renal function, or for patients with mildly impaired hepatic function.

**Mechanism of Action** Angiotensin II is formed from angiotensin I in a reaction catalyzed by angiotensin-converting enzyme (ACE, kininase II). Angiotensin II is the principal pressor agent of the renin-angiotensin system, with effects that include vasoconstriction, stimulation of synthesis and release of aldosterone, cardiac stimulation, and renal reabsorption of sodium. Candesartan blocks the vasoconstrictor and aldosterone-secreting effects of angiotensin II by selectively blocking the binding of angiotensin II to the AT1 receptor in many tissues, such as vascular smooth muscle and the adrenal gland. Its action is therefore independent of the pathways for angiotensin II synthesis. Blockade of the renin-angiotensin system with ACE inhibitors, which inhibit the biosynthesis of angiotensin II from angiotensin I, is widely used in the treatment of hypertension. ACE inhibitors also inhibit the degradation of bradykinin, a reaction also catalyzed by ACE. Because candesartan does not inhibit ACE (kininase II), it does not affect the response to bradykinin. Whether this difference has clinical relevance is not yet known. Candesartan does not bind to or block other hormone receptors or ion channels known to be important in cardiovascular regulation.

**Local Anesthetic/Vasoconstrictor Precautions** No information available to require special precautions

**Effects on Dental Treatment** No effects or complications reported

**Other Adverse Effects**

1% to 10%:
- Cardiovascular: Flushing, chest pain, peripheral edema
- Central nervous system: Dizziness, lightheadedness, drowsiness, fatigue, headache
- Dermatologic: Rash
- Gastrointestinal: Nausea, diarrhea, vomiting
- Neuromuscular & skeletal: Back pain, arthralgia
- Respiratory: Upper respiratory tract infection, pharyngitis, rhinitis, bronchitis, cough, sinusitis

<1%:
- Cardiovascular: Tachycardia, palpitations, angina, myocardial infarction
- Central nervous system: Vertigo, anxiety, depression, somnolence, fever
- Dermatologic: Angioedema, rash
- Endocrine & metabolic: Hyperglycemia, hypertriglyceridemia, hyperuricemia
- Gastrointestinal: Dyspepsia, gastroenteritis
- Neuromuscular & skeletal: Paresthesias, increased CPK, myalgia, weakness
- Renal: Hematuria
- Respiratory: Epistaxis, dyspnea

(Continued)

## Candesartan *(Continued)*

Miscellaneous: Diaphoresis (increased)

**Drug Interactions** Potassium salts/supplements; candesartan is not metabolized by cytochrome P-450

**Drug Uptake**

Onset of action: 2-3 hours
Peak effect: 6-8 hours
Duration: >24 hours
Half-life (dose dependent): 9 hours
Time to peak: 3-4 hours

**Pregnancy Risk Factor** C (1st trimester); D (2nd & 3rd trimester)

**Generic Available** No

## Cantharidin (kan THAR e din)

**U.S. Brand Names** Verr-Canth™

**Canadian Brand Names** Canthacur®; Cantharone®

**Therapeutic Category** Keratolytic Agent

**Use** Removal of ordinary and periungual warts

**Usual Dosage** Apply directly to lesion, cover with nonporous tape, remove tape in 24 hours, reapply if necessary

**Local Anesthetic/Vasoconstrictor Precautions** No information available to require special precautions

**Effects on Dental Treatment** No effects or complications reported

**Pregnancy Risk Factor** C

**Generic Available** No

♦ **Cantil®** *see* Mepenzolate Bromide *on page 628*

♦ **Capastat® Sulfate** *see* Capreomycin *on next page*

## Capecitabine (ka pe SITE a been)

**U.S. Brand Names** Xeloda™

**Therapeutic Category** Antineoplastic Agent, Antimetabolite

**Use** Treatment of patients with metastatic breast cancer resistant to both paclitaxel and an anthracycline-containing chemotherapy regimen or resistant to paclitaxel and for whom further anthracycline therapy is not indicated (eg, patients who have received cumulative doses of 400 mg/m² of doxorubicin or doxorubicin equivalents). Resistance is defined as progressive disease while on treatment, with or without an initial response, or relapse within 6 months of completing treatment with an anthracycline-containing adjuvant regimen.

**Usual Dosage** Refer to individual protocols.

2510 mg/m² days 1-14 every 3 weeks
1657 mg/m² days 1-14 every 3 weeks
1331 mg/m²/day

**Mechanism of Action** Capecitabine is a prodrug of fluorouracil. It undergoes hydrolysis in the liver and tissues to form fluorouracil which is the active moiety. Fluorouracil is a fluorinated pyrimidine antimetabolite that inhibits thymidylate synthetase, blocking the methylation of deoxyuridylic acid to thymidylic acid, interfering with DNA, and to a lesser degree, RNA synthesis. Fluorouracil appears to be phase specific for the $G_1$ and S phases of the cell cycle.

**Local Anesthetic/Vasoconstrictor Precautions** No information available to require special precautions

**Effects on Dental Treatment** Relatively high incidence of stomatitis; oral candidiasis has been reported

**Other Adverse Effects**

>10%:

- Central nervous system: Fatigue (41%), fever (12%)
- Gastrointestinal: Diarrhea (57%), may be dose limiting; mild to moderate nausea (53%), vomiting (37%), stomatitis (24%), anorexia (23%), abdominal pain (20%), constipation (15%)
- Dermatologic: Palmar-plantar erythrodysesthesia (hand-and-foot syndrome) (57%), may be dose limiting; dermatitis (37%)
- Hematologic: Lymphopenia (94%), anemia (72%), neutropenia (26%), thrombocytopenia (24%)
- Hepatic: Increased bilirubin (22%)
- Neuromuscular & skeletal: Paresthesia (21%)
- Ocular: Eye irritation (15%)

1% to 10%:

- Central nervous system: Headache (9%), dizziness (8%), insomnia (8%)
- Dermatologic: Nail disorders (7%)
- Gastrointestinal: Intestinal obstruction (1.1%)
- Endocrine & metabolic: Dehydration (7%)

Neuromuscular & skeletal: Myalgia (9%)

<1%: Necrotizing enterocolitis, gastritis, colitis, duodenitis, hematemesis, GI hemorrhage, esophagitis, increased diaphoresis, photosensitization, radiation recall, chest pain, ataxia, encephalopathy, change in consciousness, cachexia, hypertriglyceridemia, dyspnea, epistaxis, bronchospasm, respiratory distress, oral candidiasis, infections, bone pain, joint stiffness, cardiomyopathy, hypotension, thrombophlebitis, DVT, lymphedema, PE, CVA, ITP, pancytopenia, confusion, nocturia, hepatic fibrosis, cholestasis, hepatitis, hypersensitivity

**Drug Interactions**

Increased effect: Taking capecitabine immediately before an aluminum hydroxide/magnesium hydroxide antacid, or a meal, increases the absorption of capecitabine

Increased toxicity: The concentration of 5-fluorouracil is increased and its toxicity may be enhanced by leucovorin. Deaths from severe enterocolitis, diarrhea, and dehydration have been reported in elderly patients receiving weekly leucovorin and fluorouracil.

**Drug Uptake**

Absorption: Rapid and extensive

Half-life: Elimination: 0.5-1 hour

**Pregnancy Risk Factor** D

**Generic Available** No

- **Capital® and Codeine** *see* Acetaminophen and Codeine *on page 28*
- **Capitrol®** *see* Chloroxine *on page 230*
- **Capoten®** *see* Captopril *on next page*
- **Capozide®** *see* Captopril and Hydrochlorothiazide *on page 183*

## Capreomycin (kap ree oh MYE sin)

**Related Information**

Nonviral Infectious Diseases *on page 1095*

**U.S. Brand Names** Capastat® Sulfate

**Therapeutic Category** Antibiotic, Miscellaneous; Antitubercular Agent

**Use** Treatment of tuberculosis in conjunction with at least one other antituberculosis agent

**Usual Dosage** I.M.:

Children: 15-20 mg/kg/day, up to 1 g/day maximum

Adults: 15-30 mg/kg/day up to 1 g/day for 60-120 days, followed by 1 g 2-3 times/week

**Mechanism of Action** Capreomycin is a cyclic polypeptide antimicrobial. It is administered as a mixture of capreomycin IA and capreomycin IB. The mechanism of action of capreomycin is not well understood. Mycobacterial species that have become resistant to other agents are usually still sensitive to the action of capreomycin. However, significant cross-resistance with viomycin, kanamycin, and neomycin occurs.

**Local Anesthetic/Vasoconstrictor Precautions** No information available to require special precautions

**Effects on Dental Treatment** No effects or complications reported

**Other Adverse Effects**

>10%:

Otic: Ototoxicity

Renal: Nephrotoxicity

1% to 10%: Hematologic: Eosinophilia

<1%:

Central nervous system: Vertigo, fever

Dermatologic: Rash

Hematologic: Leukocytosis, thrombocytopenia

Local: Pain, induration, bleeding at injection site

Otic: Tinnitus

**Drug Interactions** Additive nephrotoxicity and ototoxicity with other aminoglycosides such as streptomycin

**Drug Uptake**

Absorption: Oral: Poor absorption necessitates parenteral administration

Serum half-life: Dependent upon renal function and varies with creatinine clearance; 4-6 hours

Time to peak serum concentration: I.M.: Within 1 hour

**Pregnancy Risk Factor** C

**Generic Available** No

## Capsaicin (kap SAY sin)

**U.S. Brand Names** Capsin® [OTC]; Capzasin-P® [OTC]; Dolorac™ [OTC]; No Pain-HP® [OTC]; R-Gel® [OTC]; Zostrix® [OTC]; Zostrix®-HP [OTC]

**Therapeutic Category** Analgesic, Topical; Topical Skin Product

(Continued)

## Capsaicin *(Continued)*

**Use** FDA approved for the topical treatment of pain associated with postherpetic neuralgia, rheumatoid arthritis, osteoarthritis, diabetic neuropathy, and post-surgical pain.

**Unlabeled uses:** Treatment of pain associated with psoriasis, chronic neuralgias unresponsive to other forms of therapy, and intractable pruritus

**Usual Dosage** Children ≥2 years and Adults: Topical: Apply to affected area at least 3-4 times/day; application frequency less than 3-4 times/day prevents the total depletion, inhibition of synthesis, and transport of substance P resulting in decreased clinical efficacy and increased local discomfort

**Mechanism of Action** Induces release of substance P, the principal chemomediator of pain impulses from the periphery to the CNS, from peripheral sensory neurons; after repeated application, capsaicin depletes the neuron of substance P and prevents reaccumulation

**Local Anesthetic/Vasoconstrictor Precautions** No information available to require special precautions

**Effects on Dental Treatment** No effects or complications reported

**Other Adverse Effects**

>10%: Local: ≥30%: Transient burning on application which usually diminishes with repeated use

1% to 10%:

Local: Itching, stinging sensation, erythema

Respiratory: Cough

**Drug Interactions** No data reported

**Drug Uptake** Data following the use of topical capsaicin in humans are lacking

Onset of action: Pain relief is usually seen within 14-28 days of regular topical application; maximal response may require 4-6 weeks of continuous therapy

Duration: Several hours

**Pregnancy Risk Factor** C

**Generic Available** No

♦ **Capsin® [OTC]** *see* Capsaicin *on previous page*

## Captopril (KAP toe pril)

**Related Information**

Cardiovascular Diseases *on page 1066*

**U.S. Brand Names** Capoten®

**Canadian Brand Names** Apo®-Capto; Novo-Captopril; Nu-Capto; Syn-Captopril

**Therapeutic Category** Angiotensin-Converting Enzyme (ACE) Inhibitor

**Use** Management of hypertension and treatment of congestive heart failure

**Unlabeled use:** Hypertensive crisis, diabetic nephropathy, rheumatoid arthritis, diagnosis of anatomic renal artery stenosis, hypertension secondary to scleroderma renal crisis, diagnosis of aldosteronism, idiopathic edema, Bartter's syndrome, postmyocardial infarction for prevention of ventricular failure; increase circulation in Raynaud's phenomenon

**Usual Dosage Note:** Dosage must be titrated according to patient's response; use lowest effective dose. Oral:

Children: Initial: 0.5 mg/kg/dose; titrate upward to maximum of 6 mg/kg/day in 2-4 divided doses

Older Children: Initial: 6.25-12.5 mg/dose every 12-24 hours; titrate upward to maximum of 6 mg/kg/day

Adolescents: Initial: 12.5-25 mg/dose given every 8-12 hours; increase by 25 mg/dose to maximum of 450 mg/day

Adults:

Hypertension:

Initial dose: 12.5-25 mg 2-3 times/day; may increase by 12.5-25 mg/dose at 1- to 2-week intervals up to 50 mg 3 times/day; add diuretic before further dosage increases

Maximum dose: 150 mg 3 times/day

Congestive heart failure:

Initial dose: 6.25-12.5 mg 3 times/day in conjunction with cardiac glycoside and diuretic therapy; initial dose depends upon patient's fluid/electrolyte status

Target dose: 50 mg 3 times/day

Maximum dose: 100 mg 3 times/day

**Mechanism of Action** Competitive inhibitor of angiotensin-converting enzyme (ACE); prevents conversion of angiotensin I to angiotensin II, a potent vasoconstrictor; results in lower levels of angiotensin II which causes an increase in plasma renin activity and a reduction in aldosterone secretion

**Local Anesthetic/Vasoconstrictor Precautions** No information available to require special precautions

**Effects on Dental Treatment** No effects or complications reported

**Other Adverse Effects**

1% to 10%:

Cardiovascular: Tachycardia, chest pain, palpitations

Central nervous system: Insomnia, headache, dizziness, fatigue, malaise

Dermatologic: Rash, pruritus, alopecia

Gastrointestinal: Abdominal pain, vomiting, nausea, diarrhea, anorexia, constipation, dysgeusia

Neuromuscular & skeletal: Paresthesias

Renal: Oliguria

Respiratory: Transient cough

<1%:

Cardiovascular: Hypotension

Dermatologic: Angioedema

Endocrine & metabolic: Hyperkalemia

Gastrointestinal: Dysgeusia

Hematologic: Neutropenia, agranulocytosis

Renal: Proteinuria, elevated BUN, serum creatinine

**Drug Interactions**

Increased toxicity:

Probenecid increases blood levels of captopril

Captopril and diuretics have additive hypotensive effects; see table.

**Drug-Drug Interactions With ACEIs**

| Precipitant Drug | Drug (Category) and Effect | Description |
|---|---|---|
| Antacids | ACE Inhibitors: decreased | Decreased bioavailability of ACEIs. May be more likely with captopril. Separate administration times by 1-2 hours. |
| NSAIDs (indomethacin) | ACEIs: decreased | Reduced hypotensive effects of ACEIs. More prominent in low renin or volume dependent hypertensive patients. |
| Phenothiazines | ACEIs: increased | Pharmacologic effects of ACEIs may be increased. |
| ACEIs | Allopurinol: increased | Higher risk of hypersensitivity reaction possible when given concurrently. Three case reports of Stevens-Johnson syndrome with captopril. |
| ACEIs | Digoxin: increased | Increased plasma digoxin levels. |
| ACEIs | Lithium: increased | Increased serum lithium levels and symptoms of toxicity may occur. |
| ACEIs | Potassium preps/ potassium sparing diuretics increased | Coadministration may result in elevated potassium levels. |

Increased serum lithium levels and symptoms of lithium toxicity have been reported in patients receiving concomitant lithium and ACE inhibitor therapy. These drugs should be coadministered with caution.

**Drug Uptake**

Onset of effect: Maximal decrease in blood pressure 1-1.5 hours after dose

Duration: Dose related, may require several weeks of therapy before full hypotensive effect is seen

Absorption: Oral: 60% to 75%

Serum half-life (dependent upon renal and cardiac function):

Adults, normal: 1.9 hours

Congestive heart failure: 2.06 hours

Anuria: 20-40 hours

Time to peak: Within 1-2 hours

**Pregnancy Risk Factor** C (first trimester); D (second and third trimesters)

**Dosage Forms** Tablet: 12.5 mg, 25 mg, 50 mg, 100 mg

**Generic Available** Yes

# Captopril and Hydrochlorothiazide

(KAP toe pril & hye droe klor oh THYE a zide)

**Related Information**

Cardiovascular Diseases *on page 1066*

**U.S. Brand Names** Capozide®

**Therapeutic Category** Antihypertensive Agent, Combination

**Use** Management of hypertension and treatment of congestive heart failure

**Usual Dosage** Adults: Oral:

(Continued)

## Captopril and Hydrochlorothiazide *(Continued)*

Hypertension: Initial: 25 mg 2-3 times/day; may increase at 1- to 2-week intervals up to 150 mg 3 times/day (captopril dosages)

Congestive heart failure: 6.25-25 mg 3 times/day (maximum: 450 mg/day) (captopril dosages)

**Mechanism of Action** Captopril is a competitive inhibitor of angiotensin-converting enzyme (ACE); prevents conversion of angiotensin I to angiotensin II, a potent vasoconstrictor. This results in lower levels of angiotensin II which causes an increase in plasma renin activity and a reduction in aldosterone secretion. Hydrochlorothiazide inhibits sodium reabsorption in the distal tubules causing increased excretion of sodium and water as well as potassium and hydrogen ions.

**Local Anesthetic/Vasoconstrictor Precautions** No information available to require special precautions

**Effects on Dental Treatment** No effects or complications reported

**Other Adverse Effects**

Captopril:

1% to 10%:

Cardiovascular: Tachycardia, chest pain, palpitations

Central nervous system: Insomnia, headache, dizziness, fatigue, malaise

Dermatologic: Rash, pruritus, alopecia

Gastrointestinal: Abdominal pain, vomiting, nausea, diarrhea, anorexia, constipation, dysgeusia

Neuromuscular & skeletal: Paresthesias

Renal: Oliguria

Respiratory: Transient cough

<1%:

Cardiovascular: Hypotension

Dermatologic: Angioedema

Endocrine & metabolic: Hyperkalemia

Gastrointestinal: Dysgeusia

Hematologic: Neutropenia, agranulocytosis

Renal: Proteinuria, elevated BUN, serum creatinine

Hydrochlorothiazide:

1% to 10%: Endocrine & metabolic: Hypokalemia

<1%:

Cardiovascular: Hypotension

Dermatologic: Photosensitivity

Endocrine & metabolic: Fluid and electrolyte imbalances (hypocalcemia, hypomagnesemia, hyponatremia), hyperglycemia

Hematologic: Rarely blood dyscrasias

Renal: Prerenal azotemia

**Contraindications** Hypersensitivity to captopril, hydrochlorothiazide or any component

**Drug Interactions** Probenecid increases blood levels of captopril. Increased serum lithium levels and symptoms of lithium toxicity have been reported in patients receiving concomitant lithium and ACE inhibitor therapy. Hydrochlorothiazide decreases antidiabetic drug efficacy. Hydrochlorothiazide has been reported to increase digoxin-related cardiac arrhythmias

**Pregnancy Risk Factor** C

**Dosage Forms** Tablet:

25/15: Captopril 25 mg and hydrochlorothiazide 15 mg

25/25: Captopril 25 mg and hydrochlorothiazide 25 mg

50/15: Captopril 50 mg and hydrochlorothiazide 15 mg

50/25: Captopril 50 mg and hydrochlorothiazide 25 mg

**Generic Available** Yes

♦ **Capzasin-P® [OTC]** *see* Capsaicin *on page 181*

♦ **Carafate®** *see* Sucralfate *on page 936*

## Caramiphen and Phenylpropanolamine

(kar AM i fen & fen il proe pa NOLE a meen)

**U.S. Brand Names** Ordrine AT® Extended Release Capsule; Rescaps-D® S.R. Capsule; Tuss-Allergine® Modified T.D. Capsule; Tussogest® Extended Release Capsule

**Therapeutic Category** Antihistamine/Decongestant Combination

**Synonyms** Phenylpropanolamine and Caramiphen

**Use** Symptomatic relief of cough and nasal congestion associated with the common cold

**Usual Dosage** Oral:

Children:

2-6 years: ½ teaspoonful every 4 hours

6-12 years: 1 teaspoonful every 4 hours

Children >12 years and Adults: 1 capsule every 12 hours or 2 teaspoonfuls every 4 hours

**Local Anesthetic/Vasoconstrictor Precautions** Use with caution since phenylpropanolamine is a sympathomimetic amine which could interact with epinephrine to cause a pressor response

**Effects on Dental Treatment** Up to 10% of patients could experience tachycardia, palpitations, and dry mouth; use vasoconstrictor with caution

**Pregnancy Risk Factor** C

**Generic Available** Yes

♦ **Carampicillin Hydrochloride** *see* Bacampicillin *on page 116*

## Carbachol (KAR ba kole)

**U.S. Brand Names** Carbastat® Ophthalmic; Carboptic® Ophthalmic; Isopto® Carbachol Ophthalmic; Miostat® Intraocular

**Therapeutic Category** Antiglaucoma Agent; Cholinergic Agent, Ophthalmic; Ophthalmic Agent, Miotic

**Use** Lowers intraocular pressure in the treatment of glaucoma; cause miosis during surgery

**Usual Dosage** Adults:

Ophthalmic: Instill 1-2 drops up to 3 times/day

Intraocular: 0.5 mL instilled into anterior chamber before or after securing sutures

**Mechanism of Action** Synthetic direct-acting cholinergic agent that causes miosis by stimulating muscarinic receptors in the eye

**Local Anesthetic/Vasoconstrictor Precautions** No information available to require special precautions

**Effects on Dental Treatment** Ophthalmic use of carbachol has no effect on dental treatment

**Other Adverse Effects**

1% to 10%: Ocular: Blurred vision, eye pain

<1%:

Cardiovascular: Hypotension

Central nervous system: Headache

Gastrointestinal: Stomach cramps, diarrhea, increased peristalsis

Local: Ciliary spasm with temporary decrease of visual acuity

Ocular: Corneal clouding, persistent bullous keratopathy, postoperative keratitis, retinal detachment, transient ciliary and conjunctival injection

Respiratory: Asthma

**Drug Interactions** No data reported

**Drug Uptake**

Ophthalmic instillation:

Onset of miosis: 10-20 minutes

Duration of reduction in intraocular pressure: 4-8 hours

Intraocular administration:

Onset of miosis: Within 2-5 minutes

Duration: 24 hours

**Pregnancy Risk Factor** C

**Generic Available** No

## Carbamazepine (kar ba MAZ e peen)

**Related Information**

Dental Drug Interactions: Update on Drug Combinations Requiring Special Considerations *on page 1225*

**U.S. Brand Names** Epitol®; Tegretol®; Tegretol®-XR

**Canadian Brand Names** Apo®-Carbamazepine; Mazepine®; Novo-Carbamaz; Nu-Carbamazepine; PMS-Carbamazepine

**Therapeutic Category** Anticonvulsant, Miscellaneous

**Use**

Dental: Used to relieve pain in trigeminal neuralgia

Medical: Prophylaxis of generalized tonic-clonic, partial (especially complex partial), and mixed partial or generalized seizure disorder

**Unlabeled use:** Treat bipolar disorders and other affective disorders; resistant schizophrenia, alcohol withdrawal, restless leg syndrome, and psychotic behavior associated with dementia; may be used to relieve pain in trigeminal neuralgia or diabetic neuropathy

**Usual Dosage** Oral (dosage must be adjusted according to patient's response and serum concentrations):

Children >12 years and Adults: 200 mg twice daily to start, increase by 200 mg/day at weekly intervals until therapeutic levels achieved; usual dose: 800-1200 mg/day in 3-4 divided doses; some patients have required up to 1.6-2.4 g/day;

(Continued)

## Carbamazepine *(Continued)*

extended release tablet: 200 mg twice daily for epilepsy, initial dose: 100 mg for trigeminal neuralgia

Children <12 years: Not used in children for trigeminal neuralgia

**Mechanism of Action** In addition to anticonvulsant effects, carbamazepine has anticholinergic, antineuralgic, antidiuretic, muscle relaxant and antiarrhythmic properties; may depress activity in the nucleus ventralis of the thalamus or decrease synaptic transmission or decrease summation of temporal stimulation leading to neural discharge by limiting influx of sodium ions across cell membrane or other unknown mechanisms; stimulates the release of ADH and potentiates its action in promoting reabsorption of water; chemically related to tricyclic antidepressants

**Local Anesthetic/Vasoconstrictor Precautions** No information available to require special precautions

**Effects on Dental Treatment** Some patients may experience sore throat or mouth ulcers

**Other Adverse Effects**

Dermatologic: Rash; but does not necessarily mean the drug should be stopped

>10%:

- Central nervous system: Sedation, dizziness, fatigue, slurred speech, clumsiness, confusion
- Gastrointestinal: Nausea, vomiting
- Ocular: Blurred vision, nystagmus

**Contraindications** Hypersensitivity to carbamazepine or any component; may have cross-sensitivity with tricyclic antidepressants; should not be used in any patient with bone marrow depression, or taking MAO inhibitors

**Warnings/Precautions** MAO inhibitors should be discontinued for a minimum of 14 days before carbamazepine is begun; administer with caution to patients with history of cardiac damage or hepatic disease; potentially fatal blood cell abnormalities have been reported following treatment; early detection of hematologic change is important; advise patients of early signs and symptoms including fever, sore throat, mouth ulcers, infections, easy bruising, petechial or purpuric hemorrhage; carbamazepine is not effective in absence, myoclonic or akinetic seizures; exacerbation of certain seizure types have been seen after initiation of carbamazepine therapy in children with mixed seizure disorders. Elderly may have increased risk of SIADH-like syndrome.

**Drug Interactions** Carbamazepine may induce the metabolism of warfarin, cyclosporine, doxycycline, oral contraceptives, phenytoin, theophylline, benzodiazepines, ethosuximide, valproic acid, corticosteroids, and thyroid hormones thereby diminishing the effects of these drugs; erythromycin, isoniazid, propoxyphene, verapamil, danazol, isoniazid, diltiazem, and cimetidine may inhibit hepatic metabolism of carbamazepine with resultant increase of carbamazepine serum concentrations and toxicity

**Drug Uptake**

Absorption: Slowly absorbed from GI tract

Serum half-life:

- Initial: 18-55 hours
- Multiple dosing:
  - Adults: 12-17 hours
  - Children: 8-14 hours

Time to peak serum concentration: Unpredictable, within 4-8 hours

**Pregnancy Risk Factor** C

**Breast-feeding Considerations** May be taken while breast-feeding

**Dosage Forms**

Suspension, oral (citrus-vanilla flavor): 100 mg/5 mL (450 mL)

Tablet: 200 mg

Tablet, chewable: 100 mg

Tablet, extended release: 100 mg, 200 mg, 400 mg

**Dietary Considerations** Food increases absorption

**Generic Available** Yes: Tablet

## Carbamide Peroxide (KAR ba mide per OKS ide)

**Related Information**

Oral Rinse Products *on page 1257*

**U.S. Brand Names** Auro® Ear Drops [OTC]; Debrox® Otic [OTC]; E•R•O Ear [OTC]; Gly-Oxide® Oral [OTC]; Mollifene® Ear Wax Removing Formula [OTC]; Murine® Ear Drops [OTC]; Orajel® Perioseptic® [OTC]; Proxigel® Oral [OTC]

**Canadian Brand Names** Clamurid®

**Therapeutic Category** Anti-infective Agent, Oral; Otic Agent, Cerumenolytic

**Use** Relief of minor swelling of gums, oral mucosal surfaces, and lips including canker sores and dental irritation; emulsify and disperse ear wax

**Usual Dosage** Children and Adults:

Gel: Gently massage on affected area 4 times/day; do not drink or rinse mouth for 5 minutes after use

Oral solution (should not be used for >7 days): Oral preparation should not be used in children <3 years of age; apply several drops undiluted on affected area 4 times/day after meals and at bedtime; expectorate after 2-3 minutes **or** place 10 drops onto tongue, mix with saliva, swish for several minutes, expectorate

Otic solution (should not be used for >4 days): Tilt head sideways and instill 5-10 drops twice daily up to 4 days, tip of applicator should not enter ear canal; keep drops in ear for several minutes by keeping head tilted and placing cotton in ear

**Mechanism of Action** Carbamide peroxide releases hydrogen peroxide which serves as a source of nascent oxygen upon contact with catalase; deodorant action is probably due to inhibition of odor-causing bacteria; softens impacted cerumen due to its foaming action

**Local Anesthetic/Vasoconstrictor Precautions** No information available to require special precautions

**Effects on Dental Treatment** No effects or complications reported

**Other Adverse Effects** 1% to 10%: Local: Rash, irritation, superinfections, redness

**Drug Interactions** No data reported

**Pregnancy Risk Factor** C

**Generic Available** Yes

♦ **Carbastat® Ophthalmic** *see* Carbachol *on page 185*

## Carbenicillin (kar ben i SIL in)

**U.S. Brand Names** Geocillin®

**Canadian Brand Names** Geopen®

**Therapeutic Category** Antibiotic, Penicillin

**Use** Treatment of serious urinary tract infections and prostatitis caused by susceptible gram-negative aerobic bacilli or mixed aerobic-anaerobic bacterial infections excluding those secondary to *Klebsiella* sp and *Serratia marcescens*

**Usual Dosage** Oral:

Children: 30-50 mg/kg/day divided every 6 hours; maximum dose: 2-3 g/day

Adults: 1-2 tablets every 6 hours for urinary tract infections or 2 tablets every 6 hours for prostatitis

**Mechanism of Action** Interferes with bacterial cell wall synthesis during active multiplication

**Local Anesthetic/Vasoconstrictor Precautions** No information available to require special precautions

**Effects on Dental Treatment** Prolonged use of penicillins may lead to development of oral candidiasis

**Other Adverse Effects**

>10%: Gastrointestinal: Diarrhea

1% to 10%: Gastrointestinal: Nausea, bad taste, vomiting, flatulence, glossitis

<1%:

- Central nervous system: Headache, hyperthermia
- Dermatologic: Skin rash, urticaria
- Endocrine & metabolic: Hypokalemia
- Genitourinary: Vaginitis
- Hematologic: Anemia, thrombocytopenia, leukopenia, neutropenia, eosinophilia
- Hepatic: Elevated LFTs
- Local: Thrombophlebitis
- Ocular: Itchy eyes
- Renal: Hematuria
- Miscellaneous: Furry tongue

**Drug Interactions**

Decreased effect with administration of aminoglycosides within 1 hour; may inactivate both drugs

Increased duration of half-life with probenecid

**Drug Uptake**

Absorption: Oral: 30% to 40%

Serum half-life:

- Children: 0.8-1.8 hours
- Adults: 1-1.5 hours, prolonged to 10-20 hours with renal insufficiency

Time to peak serum concentration: Within 0.5-2 hours in patients with normal renal function; serum concentrations following oral absorption are inadequate for treatment of systemic infections

**Pregnancy Risk Factor** B

(Continued)

## Carbenicillin *(Continued)*

**Generic Available** No

## Carbidopa (kar bi DOE pa)

**U.S. Brand Names** Lodosyn®

**Therapeutic Category** Anti-Parkinson's Agent

**Use** Given with levodopa in the treatment of parkinsonism to enable a lower dosage of levodopa to be used and a more rapid response to be obtained and to decrease side-effects; for details of administration and dosage, see Levodopa; has no effect without levodopa

**Usual Dosage** Adults: Oral: 70-100 mg/day; maximum daily dose: 200 mg

**Mechanism of Action** Carbidopa is a peripheral decarboxylase inhibitor with little or no pharmacological activity when given alone in usual doses. It inhibits the peripheral decarboxylation of levodopa to dopamine; and as it does not cross the blood-brain barrier, unlike levodopa, effective brain concentrations of dopamine are produced with lower doses of levodopa. At the same time reduced peripheral formation of dopamine reduces peripheral side-effects, notably nausea and vomiting, and cardiac arrhythmias, although the dyskinesias and adverse mental effects associated with levodopa therapy tend to develop earlier.

**Local Anesthetic/Vasoconstrictor Precautions** No information available to require special precautions

**Effects on Dental Treatment** Dopaminergic therapy in Parkinson's disease includes the use of carbidopa in combination with levodopa. Carbidopa/levodopa combination is associated with orthostatic hypotension. Patients medicated with this drug combination should be carefully assisted from the chair and observed for signs of orthostatic hypotension.

**Other Adverse Effects** Adverse reactions are associated with concomitant administration with levodopa

>10%: Central nervous system: Anxiety, confusion, nervousness, mental depression

1% to 10%:
- Cardiovascular: Orthostatic hypotension, palpitations, cardiac arrhythmias
- Central nervous system: Memory loss, insomnia, fatigue, hallucinations, ataxia, dystonic movements
- Gastrointestinal: Nausea, vomiting, GI bleeding
- Ocular: Blurred vision

<1%:
- Cardiovascular: Hypertension
- Gastrointestinal: Duodenal ulcer
- Hematologic: Hemolytic anemia

**Drug Interactions** Reports of interaction with tricyclic antidepressants resulting in hypertension and dyskinesias

**Drug Uptake**

Absorption: Rapid but incomplete from GI tract

**Pregnancy Risk Factor** C

**Generic Available** No

## Carbinoxamine and Pseudoephedrine

(kar bi NOKS a meen & soo doe e FED rin)

**U.S. Brand Names** Biohist®-LA; Carbiset® Tablet; Carbiset-TR® Tablet; Carbodec® Syrup; Carbodec® Tablet; Carbodec TR® Tablet; Cardec-S® Syrup; Rondec® Drops; Rondec® Filmtab®; Rondec® Syrup; Rondec-TR®

**Therapeutic Category** Antihistamine/Decongestant Combination

**Use** Temporary relief of nasal congestion, running nose, sneezing, itching of nose or throat, and itchy, watery eyes due to the common cold, hay fever, or other respiratory allergies

**Usual Dosage** Oral:

Children:
- Drops: 1-18 months: 0.25-1 mL 4 times/day
- Syrup:
  - 18 months to 6 years: 2.5 mL 3-4 times/day
  - >6 years: 5 mL 2-4 times/day

Adults:
- Liquid: 5 mL 4 times/day
- Tablets: 1 tablet 4 times/day

**Mechanism of Action** Carbinoxamine competes with histamine for $H_1$-receptor sites on effector cells in the gastrointestinal tract, blood vessels, and respiratory tract

**Local Anesthetic/Vasoconstrictor Precautions** Pseudoephedrine is a sympathomimetic which has potential to enhance vasoconstrictor effects of epinephrine; use local anesthetic with vasoconstrictor with caution

**Effects on Dental Treatment** 1% to 10% of patients will experience dry mouth which disappears with cessation of drug therapy

**Other Adverse Effects**

>10%:

Central nervous system: Slight to moderate drowsiness
Respiratory: Thickening of bronchial secretions

1% to 10%:

Central nervous system: Headache, fatigue, nervousness, dizziness
Gastrointestinal: Appetite increase, weight gain, nausea, diarrhea, abdominal pain, dry mouth
Neuromuscular & skeletal: Arthralgia
Respiratory: Pharyngitis

<1%:

Cardiovascular: Edema, palpitations
Central nervous system: Depression
Dermatologic: Angioedema, photosensitivity, rash
Hepatic: Hepatitis
Neuromuscular & skeletal: Myalgia, paresthesia
Respiratory: Bronchospasm, epistaxis

**Drug Interactions** May enhance the effects of barbiturates, TCAs, MAO inhibitors, ethanolamine antihistamines

**Pregnancy Risk Factor** C

**Generic Available** Yes

## Carbinoxamine, Pseudoephedrine, and Dextromethorphan

(kar bi NOKS a meen, soo doe e FED rin, & deks troe meth OR fan)

**U.S. Brand Names** Carbodec® DM; Cardec® DM; Pseudo-Car® DM; Rondamine®-DM Drops; Rondec®-DM; Tussafed® Drops

**Therapeutic Category** Antihistamine/Decongestant Combination; Cough Preparation

**Use** Relief of coughs and upper respiratory symptoms, including nasal congestion, associated with allergy or the common cold

**Usual Dosage**

Infants: Drops:

1-3 months: 1/4 mL 4 times/day
3-6 months: 1/2 mL 4 times/day
6-9 months: 3/4 mL 4 times/day
9-18 months: 1 mL 4 times/day

Children 1 1/2 to 6 years: Syrup: 2.5 mL 4 times/day
Children >6 years and Adults: Syrup: 5 mL 4 times/day

**Local Anesthetic/Vasoconstrictor Precautions** Use with caution since pseudoephedrine is a sympathomimetic amine which could interact with epinephrine to cause a pressor response

**Effects on Dental Treatment** Up to 10% of patients could experience tachycardia, palpitations, and dry mouth; use vasoconstrictor with caution

**Warnings/Precautions** Research on chicken embryos exposed to concentrations of dextromethorphan relative to those typically taken by humans has shown to cause birth defects and fetal death; more study is needed, but it is suggested that pregnant women should be advised not to use dextromethorphan-containing medications

**Pregnancy Risk Factor** C (see Warnings)

**Generic Available** Yes


- **Carbiset® Tablet** *see* Carbinoxamine and Pseudoephedrine *on previous page*
- **Carbiset-TR® Tablet** *see* Carbinoxamine and Pseudoephedrine *on previous page*
- **Carbocaine®** *see* Mepivacaine *on page 632*
- **Carbocaine® 2% With Neo-Cobefrin®** *see* Mepivacaine and Levonordefrin *on page 632*
- **Carbocaine® 3%** *see* Mepivacaine Dental Anesthetic *on page 634*
- **Carbodec® DM** *see* Carbinoxamine, Pseudoephedrine, and Dextromethorphan *on this page*
- **Carbodec® Syrup** *see* Carbinoxamine and Pseudoephedrine *on previous page*
- **Carbodec® Tablet** *see* Carbinoxamine and Pseudoephedrine *on previous page*
- **Carbodec TR® Tablet** *see* Carbinoxamine and Pseudoephedrine *on previous page*


## Carbol-Fuchsin Solution (kar bol-FOOK sin soe LOO shun)

**Therapeutic Category** Antifungal Agent, Topical

**Synonyms** Castellani Paint

**Use** Treatment of superficial mycotic infections

**Usual Dosage** Apply to affected area 2-4 times/day

(Continued)

## Carbol-Fuchsin Solution *(Continued)*

**Local Anesthetic/Vasoconstrictor Precautions** No information available to require special precautions

**Effects on Dental Treatment** No effects or complications reported

**Generic Available** Yes

♦ **Carbolic Acid** *see* Phenol *on page 791*

## Carboplatin (KAR boe pla tin)

**U.S. Brand Names** Paraplatin®

**Therapeutic Category** Antineoplastic Agent, Alkylating Agent

**Synonyms** CBDCA

**Use** Palliative treatment of ovarian carcinoma; also used in the treatment of small cell lung cancer, squamous cell carcinoma of the esophagus; solid tumors of the bladder, cervix and testes; pediatric brain tumor, neuroblastoma

**Usual Dosage** IVPB, I.V. infusion, Intraperitoneal (**refer to individual protocols**):

Children:

Solid tumor: 560 mg/m$^2$ once every 4 weeks

Brain tumor: 175 mg/m$^2$ once weekly for 4 weeks with a 2-week recovery period between courses; dose is then adjusted on platelet count and neutrophil count values

Adults:

Ovarian cancer: Usual doses range from 360 mg/m$^2$ I.V. every 3 weeks single agent therapy to 300 mg/m$^2$ every 4 weeks as combination therapy

In general, however, single intermittent courses of carboplatin should not be repeated until the neutrophil count is at least 2000/mm$^3$ and the platelet count is at least 100,000/mm$^3$

**Mechanism of Action** Analogue of cisplatin which covalently binds to DNA; possible cross-linking and interference with the function of DNA

**Local Anesthetic/Vasoconstrictor Precautions** No information available to require special precautions

**Effects on Dental Treatment** No effects or complications reported

**Other Adverse Effects**

>10%:

Endocrine & metabolic: Electrolyte abnormalities such as hypocalcemia, hypomagnesemia, hyponatremia, and hypokalemia

Hepatic: Abnormal liver function tests

Hematologic: Neutropenia, leukopenia, thrombocytopenia (platelet count reaches a nadir between 14-21 days), anemia

Myelosuppressive: Dose-limiting toxicity; WBC: Severe (dose-dependent); Platelets: Severe; Nadir: 21-24 days; Recovery: 5-6 weeks

Local: Pain at injection site

Neuromuscular & skeletal: Weakness

1% to 10%:

Central nervous system: Pain

Dermatologic: Urticaria, rash, alopecia

Gastrointestinal: Emetogenic potential low (<10%), stomatitis, diarrhea, anorexia

Hematologic: Hemorrhagic complications

Neuromuscular & skeletal: Peripheral neuropathy

Otic: Ototoxicity in 1% of patients

<1%:

Central nervous system: Neurotoxicity has only been noted in patients previously treated with cisplatin

Ocular: Blurred vision

Renal: Nephrotoxicity (uncommon)

**Drug Uptake**

Serum half-life, terminal: 22-40 hours

**Pregnancy Risk Factor** D

**Generic Available** No

## Carboprost Tromethamine (KAR boe prost tro METH a meen)

**U.S. Brand Names** Hemabate™

**Therapeutic Category** Abortifacient; Prostaglandin

**Use** Termination of pregnancy

**Usual Dosage** Adults: I.M.:

Abortion: 250 mcg to start, 250 mcg at 1½-hour to 3½-hour intervals depending on uterine response; a 500 mcg dose may be given if uterine response is not adequate after several 250 mcg doses; do not exceed 12 mg total dose

Refractory postpartum uterine bleeding: Initial: 250 mcg; may repeat at 15- to 90-minute intervals to a total dose of 2 mg

Bladder irrigation for hemorrhagic cystitis (refer to individual protocols): [0.4-1.0 mg/dL as solution] 50 mL instilled into bladder 4 times/day for 1 hour

**Mechanism of Action** Carboprost tromethamine is a prostaglandin similar to prostaglandin $F_2$ alpha (dinoprost) except for the addition of a methyl group at the C-15 position. This substitution produces longer duration of activity than dinoprost; carboprost stimulates uterine contractility which usually results in expulsion of the products of conception and is used to induce abortion between 13-20 weeks of pregnancy. Hemostasis at the placentation site is achieved through the myometrial contractions produced by carboprost.

**Local Anesthetic/Vasoconstrictor Precautions** No information available to require special precautions

**Effects on Dental Treatment** No effects or complications reported

**Other Adverse Effects**

>10%: Gastrointestinal: Nausea

1% to 10%: Cardiovascular: Flushing

<1%:

Cardiovascular: Hypertension, hypotension

Central nervous system: Drowsiness, vertigo, nervousness, fever, headache, dystonia, vasovagal syndrome

Endocrine & metabolic: Breast tenderness

Gastrointestinal: Dry mouth, vomiting, diarrhea, hematemesis, taste alterations

Genitourinary: Bladder spasms

Neuromuscular & skeletal: Myalgia

Ocular: Blurred vision

Respiratory: Coughing, asthma, respiratory distress

Miscellaneous: Septic shock, hiccups

**Pregnancy Risk Factor** X

**Generic Available** No

- **Carboptic® Ophthalmic** *see* Carbachol *on page 185*
- **Carbose D** *see* Carboxymethylcellulose *on this page*

## Carboxymethylcellulose (kar boks ee meth il SEL yoo lose)

**U.S. Brand Names** Cellufresh® [OTC]; Celluvisc® [OTC]

**Therapeutic Category** Ophthalmic Agent, Miscellaneous

**Synonyms** Carbose D

**Use** Preservative-free artificial tear substitute

**Usual Dosage** Adults: Ophthalmic: Instill 1-2 drops into eye(s) 3-4 times/day

**Local Anesthetic/Vasoconstrictor Precautions** No information available to require special precautions

**Effects on Dental Treatment** No effects or complications reported

**Generic Available** Yes

- **Cardec® DM** *see* Carbinoxamine, Pseudoephedrine, and Dextromethorphan *on page 189*
- **Cardec-S® Syrup** *see* Carbinoxamine and Pseudoephedrine *on page 188*
- **Cardene®** *see* Nicardipine *on page 717*
- **Cardene® SR** *see* Nicardipine *on page 717*
- **Cardilate®** *see* Erythrityl Tetranitrate *on page 383*
- **Cardio-Green®** *see* Indocyanine Green *on page 533*
- **Cardioquin®** *see* Quinidine *on page 873*
- **Cardiovascular Diseases** *see page 1066*
- **Cardizem® CD** *see* Diltiazem *on page 334*
- **Cardizem® Injectable** *see* Diltiazem *on page 334*
- **Cardizem® SR** *see* Diltiazem *on page 334*
- **Cardizem® Tablet** *see* Diltiazem *on page 334*
- **Cardura®** *see* Doxazosin *on page 351*
- **Carisoprodate** *see* Carisoprodol, Aspirin, and Codeine *on next page*

## Carisoprodol (kar i soe PROE dole)

**Related Information**

Carisoprodol and Aspirin *on next page*

**U.S. Brand Names** Soma®; Soma® Compound

**Therapeutic Category** Muscle Relaxant; Skeletal Muscle Relaxant

**Synonyms** Isomeprobamate

**Use**

Dental: Treatment of muscle spasm associated with acute temporomandibular joint pain

Medical: Skeletal muscle relaxant

**Usual Dosage** Adults: Oral: 350 mg 3-4 times/day; take last dose at bedtime; compound: 1-2 tablets 4 times/day

(Continued)

## Carisoprodol *(Continued)*

**Mechanism of Action** Precise mechanism is not yet clear, but many effects have been ascribed to its central depressant actions
**Local Anesthetic/Vasoconstrictor Precautions** No information available to require special precautions
**Effects on Dental Treatment** No effects or complications reported
**Other Adverse Effects**
>10%: Central nervous system: Drowsiness
1% to 10%: Central nervous system: Dizziness, lightheadedness
**Contraindications** Acute intermittent porphyria, hypersensitivity to carisoprodol, meprobamate or any component
**Warnings/Precautions** Use with caution in renal and hepatic dysfunction
**Drug Interactions** Alcohol, CNS depressants, phenothiazines
**Drug Uptake**
Onset of action: Within 30 minutes
Duration: 4-6 hours
Serum half-life: 8 hours
Time to peak serum concentration: 4 hours
**Pregnancy Risk Factor** C
**Breast-feeding Considerations** No data reported
**Dosage Forms** Tablet:
Soma®: 350 mg
Soma® Compound: Carisoprodol 200 mg and aspirin 325 mg
**Dietary Considerations** No data reported
**Generic Available** Yes

## Carisoprodol and Aspirin (kar i soe PROE dole & AS pir in)

**U.S. Brand Names** Soma® Compound
**Therapeutic Category** Skeletal Muscle Relaxant
**Use** Skeletal muscle relaxant
**Usual Dosage** Adults: Oral: 1-2 tablets 4 times/day
**Local Anesthetic/Vasoconstrictor Precautions** No information available to require special precautions
**Effects on Dental Treatment** Avoid aspirin if possible, for 1 week prior to surgery because of the possibility of postoperative bleeding

Use with caution in impaired hepatic function; use with caution in patients with platelet and bleeding disorders, renal dysfunction, erosive gastritis, or peptic ulcer disease, previous nonreaction does not guarantee future safe taking of medication; do not use aspirin in children <16 years of age for chickenpox or flu symptoms due to the association with Reye's syndrome

Elderly are a high-risk population for adverse effects from nonsteroidal anti-inflammatory agents. As much as 60% of elderly with GI complications to NSAIDs can develop peptic ulceration and/or hemorrhage asymptomatically. Also, concomitant disease and drug use contribute to the risk for GI adverse effects. Use lowest effective dose for shortest period possible. Consider renal function decline with age. Use with caution in patients with history of asthma
**Drug Interactions** See individual agents
**Pregnancy Risk Factor** C
**Dosage Forms** Tablet: Carisoprodol 200 mg and aspirin 325 mg
**Generic Available** Yes

## Carisoprodol, Aspirin, and Codeine

(kar i soe PROE dole, AS pir in, and KOE deen)
**U.S. Brand Names** Soma® Compound w/Codeine
**Therapeutic Category** Skeletal Muscle Relaxant
**Synonyms** Carisoprodate; Isobamate
**Use** Skeletal muscle relaxant
**Restrictions** C-III
**Usual Dosage** Adults: Oral: 1 or 2 tablets 4 times/day
**Local Anesthetic/Vasoconstrictor Precautions** No information available to require special precautions
**Effects on Dental Treatment** Avoid aspirin, if possible, for 1 week prior to surgery because of the possibility of postoperative bleeding
**Pregnancy Risk Factor** C
**Dosage Forms** Tablet: Carisoprodol 200 mg, aspirin 325 mg, and codeine phosphate 16 mg
**Generic Available** No

♦ **Carmol® [OTC]** *see* Urea *on page 1034*
♦ **Carmol-HC® Topical** *see* Urea and Hydrocortisone *on page 1034*

## Carmustine (kar MUS teen)

**U.S. Brand Names** BiCNU®

**Therapeutic Category** Antineoplastic Agent, Alkylating Agent (Nitrosourea)

**Synonyms** BCNU

**Use** Brain tumors, multiple myeloma, Hodgkin's disease, and non-Hodgkin's lymphomas; some activity in malignant melanoma

**Usual Dosage** I.V. (**refer to individual protocols**):

Children: 200-250 mg/m² every 4-6 weeks as a single dose

Adults: 150-200 mg/m² every 6 weeks as a single dose or divided into daily injections on 2 successive days; next dose is to be determined based on hematologic response to the previous dose. See table.

**Suggested Carmustine Dose Following Initial Dose**

| Nadir After Prior Dose | | % of Prior Dose to Be Given |
|---|---|---|
| Leukocytes/mm³ | Platelets/mm³ | |
| >4000 | >100,000 | 100 |
| 3000-3999 | 75,000-99,999 | 100 |
| 2000-2999 | 25,000-74,999 | 70 |
| <2000 | <25,000 | 50 |

Primary brain cancer: 150-200 mg/m² every 6-8 weeks

Autologous BMT: All of the following doses are fatal without BMT

Combination therapy: Up to 300-900 mg/m²

Single agent therapy: Up to 1200 mg/m² (fatal necrosis is associated with doses >2 g/m²)

**Mechanism of Action** Interferes with the normal function of DNA by alkylation and cross-linking the strands of DNA, and by possible protein modification

**Local Anesthetic/Vasoconstrictor Precautions** No information available to require special precautions

**Effects on Dental Treatment** No effects or complications reported

**Other Adverse Effects**

>10%:

Gastrointestinal: Nausea and vomiting occur within 2-4 hours after drug injection; dose-related

Emetic potential: <200 mg: Moderately high (60% to 90%); ≥200 mg: High (>90%)

Local: Pain at injection site

1% to 10%:

Cardiovascular: Facial flushing

Dermatologic: Alopecia

Gastrointestinal: Stomatitis, diarrhea, anorexia

Hematologic: Anemia

<1%:

Central nervous system: Ataxia, dizziness

Dermatologic: Hyperpigmentation, dermatitis, facial flushing is probably due to the ethanol used in reconstitution

Hematologic: Myelosuppressive: Delayed, occurs 4-6 weeks after administration and is dose-related; usually persists for 1-2 weeks; thrombocytopenia is usually more severe than leukopenia. Myelofibrosis and preleukemic syndromes are being reported. WBC: Moderate; Platelets: Severe; Onset (days): 14; Nadir (days): 21-35; Recovery (days): 42-50.

Hepatic: Reversible toxicity, elevated LFTs in 20%

Local: Burning at injection site

Ocular: Retinal hemorrhages, ocular toxicity

Pulmonary: Fibrosis occurs mostly in patients treated with prolonged total doses >1400 mg/m² or with bone marrow transplantation doses. Risk factors include a history of lung disease, concomitant bleomycin, or radiation therapy. PFTs should be conducted prior to therapy and monitored. Patients with predicted FVC or $DL_{co}$ <70% are at a higher risk.

Renal: Azotemia, decrease in kidney size, renal failure

**Drug Uptake**

Absorption: Highly lipid soluble

Serum half-life (biphasic):

Initial: 1.4 minutes

Secondary: 20 minutes (active metabolites may persist for days and have a plasma half-life of 67 hours)

**Pregnancy Risk Factor** D

**Generic Available** No

- **Carnation Instant Breakfast® [OTC]** *see* Enteral Nutritional Products *on page 371*
- **Carnitor® Injection** *see* Levocarnitine *on page 580*
- **Carnitor® Oral** *see* Levocarnitine *on page 580*

## Carteolol (KAR tee oh lole)

**Related Information**

Cardiovascular Diseases *on page 1066*

**U.S. Brand Names** Cartrol®; Ocupress®

**Therapeutic Category** Antianginal Agent; Antiglaucoma Agent; Beta-adrenergic Blocker, Noncardioselective; Beta-Adrenergic Blocker, Ophthalmic

**Use** Management of hypertension; treatment of chronic open-angle glaucoma and intraocular hypertension

**Usual Dosage** Adults:

Oral: 2.5 mg as a single daily dose, with a maintenance dose normally 2.5-5 mg once daily; maximum daily dose: 10 mg; doses >10 mg do not increase response and may in fact decrease effect

Ophthalmic: Instill 1 drop in affected eye(s) twice daily; see Additional Information

**Mechanism of Action** Competitively blocks $beta_1$-adrenergic receptors with little or no effect on $beta_2$-receptors except at high doses; exhibits membrane stabilizing and intrinsic sympathomimetic activity

**Local Anesthetic/Vasoconstrictor Precautions** No information available to require special precautions

**Effects on Dental Treatment** Noncardioselective beta-blockers (ie, propranolol, nadolol) enhance the pressor response to epinephrine, resulting in hypertension and bradycardia. This has not been reported for carteolol, a cardioselective beta-blocker. Therefore, local anesthetic with vasoconstrictor can be safely used in patients medicated with carteolol. Many nonsteroidal anti-inflammatory drugs such as ibuprofen and indomethacin can reduce the hypotensive effect of beta-blockers after 3 or more weeks of therapy with the NSAID. Short-term NSAID use (ie, 3 days) requires no special precautions in patients taking beta-blockers

**Other Adverse Effects**

1% to 10%:

Cardiovascular: Congestive heart failure, arrhythmia

Central nervous system: Mental depression, headache, dizziness

Neuromuscular & skeletal: Back pain, arthralgia

<1%:

Cardiovascular: Bradycardia, chest pain, mesenteric arterial thrombosis, A-V block, persistent bradycardia, hypotension, edema, Raynaud's phenomenon

Central nervous system: Fatigue, insomnia, lethargy, nightmares, confusion

Dermatologic: Purpura

Endocrine & metabolic: Hyperglycemia

Gastrointestinal: Ischemic colitis, constipation, nausea, diarrhea

Genitourinary: Impotence

Hematologic: Thrombocytopenia

Respiratory: Bronchospasm

Miscellaneous: Cold extremities

**Drug Interactions**

Decreased effect of beta-blockers:

Barbiturates (increased liver metabolism of beta-blockers to result in lower serum levels)

NSAIDs (attenuate the hypotensive therapeutic effects of beta-blockers)

Rifampin (increased liver metabolism of beta-blockers to result in lower serum levels)

Increased effects of beta-blockers:

Calcium channel blockers (increased serum levels of beta-blockers by unknown mechanism to enhance hypotension)

Beta-blockers increase the effects of:

Epinephrine (vasoconstrictor; initial hypertensive episode followed by bradycardia) only from noncardioselective type beta-blockers

Phenylephrine (Neosynephrine®; enhanced pressor response)

Theophylline (inhibit theophylline metabolism causing increase in serum concentrations)

**Drug Uptake**

Onset of effect: Oral: 1-1.5 hours

Peak effect: 2 hours

Duration: 12 hours

Absorption: Oral: 80%

Serum half-life: 6 hours

**Pregnancy Risk Factor** C

**Generic Available** No

**Selected Readings**

Foster CA and Aston SJ, "Propranolol-Epinephrine Interaction: A Potential Disaster," *Plast Reconstr Surg*, 1983, 72(1):74-8.

Wong DG, Spence JD, Lamki L, et al, "Effect of Nonsteroidal Anti-inflammatory Drugs on Control of Hypertension of Beta-Blockers and Diuretics," *Lancet*, 1986, 1(8488):997-1001.

Wynn RL, "Dental Nonsteroidal Anti-inflammatory Drugs and Prostaglandin-Based Drug Interactions, Part Two," *Gen Dent*, 1992, 40(2):104, 106, 108.

Wynn RL, "Epinephrine Interactions With Beta-Blockers," *Gen Dent*, 1994, 42(1):16, 18.

♦ **Carter's Little Pills® [OTC]** *see* Bisacodyl *on page 141*

♦ **Cartia® XT** *see* Diltiazem *on page 334*

♦ **Cartrol®** *see* Carteolol *on previous page*

## Carvedilol (KAR ve dil ole)

**Related Information**

Cardiovascular Diseases *on page 1066*

**U.S. Brand Names** Coreg®

**Therapeutic Category** Beta-adrenergic Blocker, Noncardioselective

**Use** Management of hypertension; can be used alone or in combination with other agents, especially thiazide-type diuretics

**Usual Dosage** Adults: Oral:

Hypertension: 6.25 mg twice daily; if tolerated, dose should be maintained for 1-2 weeks, then increased to 12.5 mg twice daily; dosage may be increased to a maximum of 25 mg twice daily after 1-2 weeks; reduce dosage if heart rate drops <55 beats/minute

Congestive heart failure: 12.5-50 mg twice daily

Angina pectoris: 25-50 mg twice daily

Idiopathic cardiomyopathy: 6.25-25 mg twice daily

**Mechanism of Action** As a racemic mixture, carvedilol has nonselective beta-adrenoreceptor and alpha-adrenergic blocking activity at equal potency. No intrinsic sympathomimetic activity has been documented. Associated effects include reduction of cardiac output, exercise- or beta agonist-induced tachycardia, reduction of reflex orthostatic tachycardia, vasodilation, decreased peripheral vascular resistance (especially in standing position), decreased renal vascular resistance, reduced plasma renin activity, and increased levels of atrial natriuretic peptide.

**Local Anesthetic/Vasoconstrictor Precautions** Use with caution; epinephrine has interacted with nonselective beta-blockers to result in initial hypertensive episode followed by bradycardia

**Effects on Dental Treatment** Noncardioselective beta-blockers (ie, propranolol, nadolol) enhance the pressor response to epinephrine, resulting in hypertension and bradycardia. Many nonsteroidal anti-inflammatory drugs such as ibuprofen and indomethacin can reduce the hypotensive effect of beta-blockers after 3 or more weeks of therapy with the NSAID. Short-term NSAID use (ie, 3 days) requires no special precautions in patients taking beta-blockers.

**Other Adverse Effects**

1% to 10%:

- Cardiovascular: Bradycardia, postural hypotension, edema
- Central nervous system: Dizziness, somnolence, insomnia, fatigue
- Gastrointestinal: Diarrhea, abdominal pain
- Neuromuscular & skeletal: Back pain
- Respiratory: Rhinitis, pharyngitis, dyspnea

<1%:

- Cardiovascular: A-V block, extrasystoles, hypertension, hypotension, palpitations, peripheral ischemia, syncope
- Central nervous system: Ataxia, vertigo, depression, nervousness, malaise
- Dermatologic: Pruritus, rash
- Endocrine & metabolic: Decreased male libido, hypercholesterolemia, hyperglycemia, hyperuricemia
- Gastrointestinal: Constipation, flatulence, dry mouth
- Genitourinary: Impotence
- Hematologic: Anemia, leukopenia
- Hepatic: Hyperbilirubinemia, elevated LFTs
- Neuromuscular & skeletal: Paresthesia, myalgia, weakness
- Ocular: Abnormal vision
- Otic: Tinnitus
- Respiratory: Asthma, cough
- Miscellaneous: Increased sweating

**Drug Uptake**

Absorption: Rapid; food decreases the rate but not the extent of absorption; administration with food minimizes risks of orthostatic hypotension

Serum half-life: 7-10 hours

**Pregnancy Risk Factor** C

**Generic Available** No

- **Casanthranol and Docusate** *see* Docusate and Casanthranol *on page 347*

## Cascara Sagrada (kas KAR a sah GRAH dah)

**Therapeutic Category** Laxative, Stimulant

**Use** Temporary relief of constipation; sometimes used with milk of magnesia ("black and white" mixture)

**Usual Dosage Note:** Cascara sagrada fluid extract is 5 times more potent than cascara sagrada aromatic fluid extract.

Oral (aromatic fluid extract):
- Children 2-11 years: 2.5 mL/day (range: 1-3 mL) as needed
- Children ≥12 years and Adults: 5 mL/day (range: 2-6 mL) as needed at bedtime (1 tablet as needed at bedtime)

**Mechanism of Action** Direct chemical irritation of the intestinal mucosa resulting in an increased rate of colonic motility and change in fluid and electrolyte secretion

**Local Anesthetic/Vasoconstrictor Precautions** No information available to require special precautions

**Effects on Dental Treatment** No effects or complications reported

**Other Adverse Effects** 1% to 10%:
- Cardiovascular: Faintness
- Endocrine & metabolic: Electrolyte and fluid imbalance
- Gastrointestinal: Abdominal cramps, nausea, diarrhea
- Genitourinary: Discolors urine reddish pink or brown

**Drug Interactions** Decreased effect of oral anticoagulants

**Drug Uptake**
Onset of action: 6-10 hours

**Pregnancy Risk Factor** C

**Generic Available** Yes

- **Casodex®** *see* Bicalutamide *on page 139*
- **Castellani Paint** *see* Carbol-Fuchsin Solution *on page 189*

## Castor Oil (KAS tor oyl)

**U.S. Brand Names** Alphamul® [OTC]; Emulsoil® [OTC]; Fleet® Flavored Castor Oil [OTC]; Neoloid® [OTC]; Purge® [OTC]

**Therapeutic Category** Laxative, Stimulant

**Use** Preparation for rectal or bowel examination or surgery; rarely used to relieve constipation; also applied to skin as emollient and protectant

**Usual Dosage** Oral:

Liquid:
- Children 2-11 years: 5-15 mL as a single dose
- Children ≥12 years and Adults: 15-60 mL as a single dose

Emulsified:
- 36.4%:
  - Children <2 years: 5-15 mL/dose
  - Children 2-11 years: 7.5-30 mL/dose
  - Children ≥12 years and Adults: 30-60 mL/dose
- 60% to 67%:
  - Children <2 years: 1.25-5 mL
  - Children 2-12 years: 5-15 mL
  - Adults: 15-45 mL
- 95%, mix with 1/2 to 1 full glass liquid:
  - Children: 5-10 mL
  - Adults: 15-60 mL

**Mechanism of Action** Acts primarily in the small intestine; hydrolyzed to ricinoleic acid which reduces net absorption of fluid and electrolytes and stimulates peristalsis

**Local Anesthetic/Vasoconstrictor Precautions** No information available to require special precautions

**Effects on Dental Treatment** No effects or complications reported

**Other Adverse Effects**

1% to 10%:
- Central nervous system: Dizziness
- Endocrine & metabolic: Electrolyte disturbance
- Gastrointestinal: Abdominal cramps, nausea, diarrhea

<1%: Pelvic congestion

**Drug Interactions** No data reported

**Drug Uptake** Onset of action: Oral: 2-6 hours

**Pregnancy Risk Factor** X

**Generic Available** Yes

- **Cataflam® Oral** *see* Diclofenac *on page 320*

- **Catapres® Oral** *see* Clonidine *on page 265*
- **Catapres-TTS® Transdermal** *see* Clonidine *on page 265*
- **Caverject® Injection** *see* Alprostadil *on page 51*
- **CBDCA** *see* Carboplatin *on page 190*
- **CCNU** *see* Lomustine *on page 598*
- **C-Crystals® [OTC]** *see* Ascorbic Acid *on page 97*
- **2-CdA** *see* Cladribine *on page 255*
- **CDDP** *see* Cisplatin *on page 252*
- **Cebid® Timecelles® [OTC]** *see* Ascorbic Acid *on page 97*
- **Ceclor®** *see* Cefaclor *on this page*
- **Ceclor® CD** *see* Cefaclor *on this page*
- **Cecon® [OTC]** *see* Ascorbic Acid *on page 97*
- **Cedax®** *see* Ceftibuten *on page 207*
- **CeeNU® Oral** *see* Lomustine *on page 598*
- **Ceepryn® [OTC]** *see* Cetylpyridinium *on page 219*


## Cefaclor (SEF a klor)

**U.S. Brand Names** Ceclor®; Ceclor® CD

**Canadian Brand Names** Apo®-Cefaclor

**Therapeutic Category** Antibiotic, Cephalosporin (Second Generation)

**Use**

Dental: An alternate antibiotic to treat orofacial infections in patients allergic to penicillins; susceptible bacteria including aerobic gram-positive bacteria and anaerobes

Medical: Infections in the medical patient caused by susceptible organisms including *Staphylococcus aureus* and *H. influenzae*; treatment of otitis media, sinusitis, and infections involving the respiratory tract, skin and skin structure, bone and joint, and urinary tract

**Usual Dosage** Oral:

Children >1 month: 20-40 mg/kg/day divided every 8-12 hours; maximum dose: 2 g/day (twice daily option is for treatment of otitis media or pharyngitis)

Adults: 250-500 mg every 8 hours (or daily dose can be given in 2 divided doses) for at least 7 days

**Mechanism of Action** Inhibits bacterial cell wall synthesis by binding to one or more of the penicillin-binding proteins (PBPs) which in turn inhibits the final transpeptidation step of peptidoglycan synthesis in bacterial cell walls, thus inhibiting cell wall biosynthesis. Bacteria eventually lyse due to ongoing activity of cell wall autolytic enzymes (autolysins and murein hydrolases) while cell wall assembly is arrested.

**Local Anesthetic/Vasoconstrictor Precautions** No information available to require special precautions

**Effects on Dental Treatment** No effects or complications reported

**Other Adverse Effects** 1% to 10%: Gastrointestinal: Pseudomembranous colitis, diarrhea

**Contraindications** Hypersensitivity to cefaclor, any component, or cephalosporins

**Warnings/Precautions** Modify dosage in patients with severe renal impairment; prolonged use may result in superinfection; a low incidence in cross-hypersensitivity to penicillins exists

**Drug Interactions** Probenecid may decrease cephalosporin elimination; furosemide, aminoglycosides may be a possible additive to nephrotoxicity

**Drug Uptake**

Absorption: Oral: Well absorbed, acid stable

Serum half-life: 0.5-1 hour

Time to peak serum concentration:

- Capsule: 60 minutes
- Suspension: 45 minutes

**Pregnancy Risk Factor** B

**Breast-feeding Considerations** Excreted into breast milk in small amounts like other cephalosporins

**Dosage Forms**

Capsule: 250 mg, 500 mg

Powder for oral suspension (strawberry flavor): 125 mg/5 mL (75 mL, 150 mL); 187 mg/5 mL (50 mL, 100 mL); 250 mg/5 mL (75 mL, 150 mL); 375 mg/5 mL (50 mL, 100 mL)

Tablet, extended release: 375 mg, 500 mg

**Dietary Considerations** May be taken with food, however, there is delayed absorption

**Generic Available** Yes

(Continued)

## Cefaclor *(Continued)*

**Comments** Patients allergic to penicillins can use a cephalosporin; the incidence of cross-reactivity between penicillins and cephalosporins is 1% when the allergic reaction to penicillin is delayed. Cefaclor is effective against anaerobic bacteria, but the sensitivity of alpha-hemolytic *Streptococcus* vary; approximately 10% of strains are resistant. Nearly 70% are intermediately sensitive. If the patient has a history of immediate reaction to penicillin, the incidence of cross-reactivity is 20%; cephalosporins are contraindicated in these patients.

**Selected Readings**

Saxon A, Beall GN, Rohr AS, et al, "Immediate Hypersensitivity Reactions to Beta-Lactam Antibiotics," *Ann Intern Med*, 1987, 107(2):204-15.

## Cefadroxil (sef a DROKS il)

**Related Information**

Antibiotic Prophylaxis, Preprocedural Guidelines for Dental Patients *on page 1097*

**U.S. Brand Names** Duricef®

**Therapeutic Category** Antibiotic, Cephalosporin (First Generation)

**Use**

Dental: Alternative antibiotic for prevention of bacterial endocarditis. Individuals allergic to amoxicillin (penicillins) may receive cefadroxil provided they have not had an immediate, local, or systemic IgE-mediated anaphylactic allergic reaction to penicillin.

Medical: Treatment of susceptible bacterial infections, including those caused by group A beta-hemolytic *Streptococcus*

**Usual Dosage** Oral:

Children: 30 mg/kg/day divided twice daily up to a maximum of 2 g/day
- Prophylaxis: 50 mg/kg orally 1 hour before procedure with no follow-up dose needed

Adults: 1-2 g/day in 2 divided doses
- Prophylaxis: 2 g 1 hour before procedure with no follow-up dose needed

**Mechanism of Action** Inhibits bacterial cell wall synthesis by binding to one or more of the penicillin-binding proteins (PBPs) which in turn inhibits the final transpeptidation step of peptidoglycan synthesis in bacterial cell walls, thus inhibiting cell wall biosynthesis. Bacteria eventually lyse due to ongoing activity of cell wall autolytic enzymes (autolysins and murein hydrolases) while cell wall assembly is arrested.

**Local Anesthetic/Vasoconstrictor Precautions** No information available to require special precautions

**Effects on Dental Treatment** No effects or complications reported

**Other Adverse Effects**

1% to 10%: Gastrointestinal: Diarrhea

<1%:
- Central nervous system: Fatigue, chills
- Dermatologic: Maculopapular and erythematous rash
- Gastrointestinal: Dyspepsia, pseudomembranous colitis, nausea, vomiting, heartburn, gastritis, bloating
- Hematologic: Neutropenia
- Miscellaneous: Superinfections

**Drug Interactions** Increased effect: High-dose probenecid decreases renal clearance of cephalosporins

**Drug Uptake**

Absorption: Oral: Rapid and well absorbed from GI tract
Serum half-life: 1-2 hours; 20-24 hours in renal failure
Time to peak serum concentration: Within 70-90 minutes

**Pregnancy Risk Factor** B

**Breast-feeding Considerations** Excreted into breast milk in small amounts like other cephalosporins

**Dosage Forms**

Capsule, as monohydrate: 500 mg
Suspension, oral, as monohydrate: 125 mg/5 mL, 250 mg/5 mL, 500 mg/5 mL (50 mL, 100 mL)
Tablet, as monohydrate: 1 g

**Generic Available** Yes

**Selected Readings**

"Advisory Statement. Antibiotic Prophylaxis for Dental Patients With Total Joint Replacements. American Dental Association; American Academy of Orthopedic Surgeons," *J Am Dent Assoc*, 1997, 128(7):1004-8.

Dajani AS, Taubert KA, Wilson WW, et al, "Prevention of Bacterial Endocarditis. Recommendations by the American Heart Association," *JAMA*, 1997, 277(22):1794-801.

Dajani AS, Taubert KA, Wilson W, et al, "Prevention of Bacterial Endocarditis: Recommendations by the American Heart Association," *J Am Dent Assoc*, 1997, 128(8):1142-51.

Donowitz GR and Mandell GL, "Drug Therapy. Beta-Lactam Antibiotics (1)," *N Engl J Med*, 1988, 318(7):419-26.

Donowitz GR and Mandell GL, "Drug Therapy. Beta-Lactam Antibiotics (2)," *N Engl J Med*, 1988, 318(8):490-500.

Gustaferro CA and Steckelberg JM, "Cephalosporin Antimicrobial Agents and Related Compounds," *Mayo Clin Proc*, 1991, 66(10):1064-73.

♦ **Cefadyl®** *see* Cephapirin *on page 216*

## Cefamandole (sef a MAN dole)

**U.S. Brand Names** Mandol®

**Therapeutic Category** Antibiotic, Cephalosporin (Second Generation)

**Use** Treatment of susceptible bacterial infection; mainly respiratory tract, skin and skin structure, bone and joint, urinary tract and gynecologic, as well as, septicemia

**Usual Dosage** I.M., I.V.:

Children: 100-150 mg/kg/day in divided doses every 4-6 hours

Adults: 4-12 g/24 hours divided every 4-6 hours or 500-1000 mg every 4-8 hours; maximum: 2 g/dose

**Mechanism of Action** Inhibits bacterial cell wall synthesis by binding to one or more of the penicillin-binding proteins (PBPs) which in turn inhibits the final transpeptidation step of peptidoglycan synthesis in bacterial cell walls, thus inhibiting cell wall biosynthesis. Bacteria eventually lyse due to ongoing activity of cell wall autolytic enzymes (autolysins and murein hydrolases) while cell wall assembly is arrested.

**Local Anesthetic/Vasoconstrictor Precautions** No information available to require special precautions

**Effects on Dental Treatment** No effects or complications reported

**Other Adverse Effects**

1% to 10%: Gastrointestinal: Diarrhea

<1%:

- Central nervous system: CNS irritation, seizures, fever
- Dermatologic: Rash, urticaria
- Gastrointestinal: Abdominal cramps, pseudomembraneous colitis
- Hematologic: Eosinophilia, hypoprothrombinemia, leukopenia, thrombocytopenia
- Hepatic: Transient elevation of liver enzymes, cholestatic jaundice
- Local: Pain at injection site
- Miscellaneous: Superinfections

**Drug Interactions**

Disulfiram-like reaction has been reported when taken within 72 hours of alcohol consumption

Increased effect: High-dose probenecid decreases renal clearance of cephalosporins

**Drug Uptake**

Serum half-life: 30-60 minutes

Time to peak serum concentration:

- I.M.: Within 1-2 hours
- I.V.: Within 10 minutes

**Pregnancy Risk Factor** B

**Generic Available** No

♦ **Cefanex®** *see* Cephalexin *on page 214*

## Cefazolin (sef A zoe lin)

**Related Information**

Animal and Human Bites Guidelines *on page 1164*

**U.S. Brand Names** Ancef®; Kefzol®; Zolicef®

**Therapeutic Category** Antibiotic, Cephalosporin (First Generation)

**Use**

Dental: Alternative antibiotic for prevention of bacterial endocarditis when parenteral administration is needed. Individuals allergic to amoxicillin (penicillins) may receive cefazolin provided they have not had an immediate, local, or systemic IgE-mediated anaphylactic allergic reaction to penicillin. Alternate antibiotic for premedication in patients not allergic to penicillin who may be at potential increased risk of hematogenous total joint infection when parenteral administration is needed.

Medical: Treatment of gram-positive bacilli and cocci (except enterococcus); some gram-negative bacilli including *E. coli*, *Proteus*, and *Klebsiella* may be susceptible

**Usual Dosage** I.M., I.V.:

Children >1 month: 50-100 mg/kg/day divided every 8 hours; maximum: 6 g/day

SBE prophylaxis: 25 mg/kg I.M. or I.V. within 30 minutes before procedure

(Continued)

## Cefazolin *(Continued)*

Adults: 1-2 g every 8 hours, depending on severity of infection; maximum dose: 12 g/day

SBE prophylaxis: 1 g I.M. or I.V. within 30 minutes before procedure

Joint replacement prophylaxis: I.M., I.V.: 1 g one hour before procedure

**Mechanism of Action** Inhibits bacterial cell wall synthesis by binding to one or more of the penicillin-binding proteins (PBPs) which in turn inhibits the final transpeptidation step of peptidoglycan synthesis in bacterial cell walls, thus inhibiting cell wall biosynthesis. Bacteria eventually lyse due to ongoing activity of cell wall autolytic enzymes (autolysins and murein hydrolases) while cell wall assembly is arrested.

**Local Anesthetic/Vasoconstrictor Precautions** No information available to require special precautions

**Effects on Dental Treatment** No effects or complications reported

**Other Adverse Effects**

1% to 10%: Gastrointestinal: Diarrhea

<1%:

- Central nervous system: CNS irritation, seizures, confusion, fever
- Dermatologic: Rash, urticaria
- Hematologic: Leukopenia, thrombocytopenia, neutropenia
- Hepatic: Transient elevation of liver enzymes, cholestatic jaundice
- Miscellaneous: Superinfections

**Drug Interactions**

Increased effect: High-dose probenecid decreases renal clearance of cephalosporins

**Drug Uptake**

Serum half-life: 90-150 minutes (prolonged with renal impairment)

Time to peak serum concentration:

- I.M.: Within 0.5-2 hours
- I.V.: Within 5 minutes

**Pregnancy Risk Factor** B

**Dosage Forms**

Infusion, premixed, as sodium, in $D_5W$ (frozen) (Ancef®): 500 mg (50 mL); 1 g (50 mL)

Injection, as sodium (Kefzol®): 500 mg, 1 g

Powder for injection, as sodium (Ancef®, Zolicef®): 250 mg, 500 mg, 1 g, 5 g, 10 g, 20 g

**Generic Available** Yes

**Selected Readings**

"Advisory Statement. Antibiotic Prophylaxis for Dental Patients With Total Joint Replacements. American Dental Association; American Academy of Orthopedic Surgeons," *J Am Dent Assoc*, 1997, 128(7):1004-8.

Dajani AS, Taubert KA, Wilson WW, et al, "Prevention of Bacterial Endocarditis. Recommendations by the American Heart Association," *JAMA*, 1997, 277(22):1794-801.

Dajani AS, Taubert KA, Wilson W, et al, "Prevention of Bacterial Endocarditis: Recommendations by the American Heart Association," *J Am Dent Assoc*, 1997, 128(8):1142-51.

Donowitz GR and Mandell GL, "Drug Therapy. Beta-Lactam Antibiotics (1)," *N Engl J Med*, 1988, 318(7):419-26.

Donowitz GR and Mandell GL, "Drug Therapy. Beta-Lactam Antibiotics (2)," *N Engl J Med*, 1988, 318(8):490-500.

Gustaferro CA and Steckelberg JM, "Cephalosporin Antimicrobial Agents and Related Compounds," *Mayo Clin Proc*, 1991, 66(10):1064-73.

## Cefdinir (SEF di ner)

**U.S. Brand Names** Omnicef®

**Therapeutic Category** Antibiotic, Cephalosporin (Third Generation)

**Synonyms** CFDN

**Use** Treatment of community-acquired pneumonia, acute exacerbations of chronic bronchitis, acute bacterial otitis media, acute maxillary sinusitis, pharyngitis/tonsillitis, and uncomplicated skin and skin structure infections.

**Usual Dosage** Oral:

Children (otitis media with effusion): 7 mg/kg orally twice daily or 14 mg/kg orally once daily

Adults and Adolescent: 300 mg orally twice daily. An oral dose of 600 mg once daily has been used in streptococcal pharyngitis.

**Mechanism of Action** Inhibits bacterial cell wall synthesis by binding to one or more of the penicillin-binding proteins (PBPs) which in turn inhibits the final transpeptidation step of peptidoglycan synthesis in bacterial cell walls, thus inhibiting cell wall biosynthesis. Bacteria eventually lyse due to ongoing activity of cell wall autolytic enzymes (autolysins and murein hydrolases) while cell wall assembly is arrested.

**Local Anesthetic/Vasoconstrictor Precautions** No information available to require special precautions

**Effects on Dental Treatment** No effects or complications reported
**Drug Uptake** Half-life: 100 minutes
**Dosage Forms**
Capsule: 300 mg
Suspension, oral: 125 mg/5 mL (60 mL, 100 mL)

## Cefepime (SEF e pim)

**U.S. Brand Names** Maxipime®
**Therapeutic Category** Antibiotic, Cephalosporin (Fourth Generation)
**Use** Treatment of respiratory tract infections (including bronchitis and pneumonia), cellulitis and other skin and soft tissue infections, and urinary tract infections; considered a fourth generation cephalosporin because it has good gram-negative coverage similar to third generation cephalosporins, but better gram-positive coverage
**Usual Dosage** I.V.:
Children: Unlabeled: 50 mg/kg every 8 hours; maximum dose: 2 g
Adults:
Most infections: 1-2 g every 12 hours for 5-10 days; higher doses or more frequent administration may be required in pseudomonal infections
Urinary tract infections, uncomplicated: 500 mg every 12 hours
**Mechanism of Action** Inhibits bacterial cell wall synthesis by binding to one or more of the penicillin-binding proteins (PBPs) which in turn inhibits the final transpeptidation step of peptidoglycan synthesis in bacterial cell walls, thus inhibiting cell wall biosynthesis. Bacterial eventually lyse due to ongoing activity of cell wall autolytic enzymes (autolysis and murein hydrolases) while cell wall assembly is arrested.
**Local Anesthetic/Vasoconstrictor Precautions** No information available to require special precautions
**Effects on Dental Treatment** No effects or complications reported
**Warnings/Precautions** Modify dosage in patients with severe renal impairment; prolonged use may result in superinfection; a low incidence of cross-hypersensitivity to penicillins exists
**Drug Interactions**
Increased effect: High-dose probenecid decreases clearance
Increased toxicity: Aminoglycosides increase nephrotoxic potential
**Drug Uptake**
Absorption: I.M.: Rapid and complete; $T_{max}$: 0.5-1.5 hours
Serum half-life: 2 hours
**Pregnancy Risk Factor** C
**Generic Available** No

## Cefixime (sef IKS eem)

**Related Information**
Nonviral Infectious Diseases *on page 1095*
**U.S. Brand Names** Suprax®
**Therapeutic Category** Antibiotic, Cephalosporin (Third Generation)
**Use** Treatment of urinary tract infections, otitis media, respiratory infections due to susceptible organisms including *S. pneumoniae* and *Pyogenes*, *H. influenzae* and many *Enterobacteriaceae*; documented poor compliance with other oral antimicrobials; outpatient therapy of serious soft tissue or skeletal infections due to susceptible organisms; single-dose oral treatment of uncomplicated cervical/urethral gonorrhea due to *N. gonorrhoeae*
**Usual Dosage** Oral:
Children: 8 mg/kg/day in 1-2 divided doses; maximum dose: 400 mg/day
Children >50 kg or >12 years and Adults: 400 mg/day in 1-2 divided doses
Uncomplicated cervical/urethral gonorrhea due to *N. gonorrhoeae*: 400 mg as a single dose
**Mechanism of Action** Inhibits bacterial cell wall synthesis by binding to one or more of the penicillin-binding proteins (PBPs) which in turn inhibits the final transpeptidation step of peptidoglycan synthesis in bacterial cell walls, thus inhibiting cell wall biosynthesis. Bacteria eventually lyse due to ongoing activity of cell wall autolytic enzymes (autolysins and murein hydrolases) while cell wall assembly is arrested.
**Local Anesthetic/Vasoconstrictor Precautions** No information available to require special precautions
**Effects on Dental Treatment** No effects or complications reported
**Other Adverse Effects**
1% to 10%: Gastrointestinal: Diarrhea (up to 15% of children), abdominal pain, nausea, dyspepsia, flatulence, pseudomembranous colitis
<1%:
Central nervous system: Headache, dizziness, fever
(Continued)

## Cefixime *(Continued)*

Dermatologic: Rash, urticaria, pruritus
Genitourinary: Vaginitis
Hematologic: Thrombocytopenia, leukopenia, eosinophilia
Hepatic: Transient elevation of LFTs
Renal: Transient elevation of BUN or creatinine

**Drug Interactions**
Increased effect: High-dose probenecid decreases renal clearance of cephalosporins

**Drug Uptake**
Absorption: Oral: 40% to 50%
Half-life:
Normal renal function: 3-4 hours
Renal failure: Up to 11.5 hours
Time to peak serum concentration: Within 2-6 hours

**Pregnancy Risk Factor** B

**Generic Available** No

♦ **Cefizox®** *see* Ceftizoxime *on page 208*

## Cefmetazole (sef MET a zole)

**U.S. Brand Names** Zefazone®

**Therapeutic Category** Antibiotic, Cephalosporin (Second Generation)

**Use** Second generation cephalosporin with an antibacterial spectrum similar to cefoxitin, useful on many aerobic and anaerobic gram-positive and gram-negative bacteria

**Usual Dosage** Adults: I.V.:
Infections: 2 g every 6-12 hours for 5-14 days
Prophylaxis: 2 g 30-90 minutes before surgery **or** 1 g 30-90 minutes before surgery; repeat 8 and 16 hours later

**Mechanism of Action** Inhibits bacterial cell wall synthesis by binding to one or more of the penicillin-binding proteins (PBPs) which in turn inhibits the final transpeptidation step of peptidoglycan synthesis in bacterial cell walls, thus inhibiting cell wall biosynthesis. Bacteria eventually lyse due to ongoing activity of cell wall autolytic enzymes (autolysins and murein hydrolases) while cell wall assembly is arrested.

**Local Anesthetic/Vasoconstrictor Precautions** No information available to require special precautions

**Effects on Dental Treatment** No effects or complications reported

**Other Adverse Effects**
1% to 10%:
Dermatologic: Rash
Gastrointestinal: Diarrhea, nausea
<1%:
Cardiovascular: Shock, hypotension
Central nervous system: Headache, fever
Endocrine & metabolic: Hot flashes
Gastrointestinal: Epigastric pain, pseudomembraneous colitis
Genitourinary: Vaginitis
Hematologic: Bleeding
Local: Pain at injection site, phlebitis
Respiratory: Respiratory distress, dyspnea, epistaxis
Miscellaneous: Alteration of color, candidiasis

**Drug Interactions** Increased effect: High-dose probenecid decreases renal clearance of cephalosporins

**Drug Uptake** Serum half-life: 72 minutes

**Pregnancy Risk Factor** B

**Generic Available** No

♦ **Cefobid®** *see* Cefoperazone *on next page*

♦ **Cefol® Filmtab®** *see* Vitamins, Multiple *on page 1051*

## Cefonicid (se FON i sid)

**U.S. Brand Names** Monocid®

**Therapeutic Category** Antibiotic, Cephalosporin (Second Generation)

**Use** Treatment of susceptible bacterial infection; mainly respiratory tract, skin and skin structure, bone and joint, urinary tract and gynecologic, as well as, septicemia; second generation cephalosporin

**Usual Dosage** Adults: I.M., I.V.: 0.5-2 g every 24 hours
Prophylaxis: Preop: 1 g/hour

**Mechanism of Action** Inhibits bacterial cell wall synthesis by binding to one or more of the penicillin-binding proteins (PBPs) which in turn inhibits the final transpeptidation step of peptidoglycan synthesis in bacterial cell walls, thus inhibiting cell wall biosynthesis. Bacteria eventually lyse due to ongoing activity of cell wall autolytic enzymes (autolysins and murein hydrolases) while cell wall assembly is arrested.

**Local Anesthetic/Vasoconstrictor Precautions** No information available to require special precautions

**Effects on Dental Treatment** No effects or complications reported

**Other Adverse Effects**

1% to 10%:
- Hematologic: Elevated platelets and eosinophils
- Hepatic: Liver function alterations
- Local: Pain at injection site

<1%:
- Central nervous system: Fever, headache
- Dermatologic: Skin rash
- Gastrointestinal: Nausea, diarrhea, abdominal pain, pseudomembranous colitis
- Hepatic: Transient elevations in liver enzymes
- Renal: Transient elevations in BUN or creatinine

**Drug Interactions** Increased effect: High-dose probenecid decreases renal clearance of cephalosporins

**Drug Uptake** Serum half-life: 6-7 hours

**Pregnancy Risk Factor** B

**Generic Available** No

## Cefoperazone (sef oh PER a zone)

**U.S. Brand Names** Cefobid®

**Therapeutic Category** Antibiotic, Cephalosporin (Third Generation)

**Use** Treatment of susceptible bacterial infection; mainly respiratory tract, skin and skin structure, bone and joint, urinary tract and gynecologic, as well as, septicemia

**Usual Dosage** I.M., I.V.:

Children: 100-150 mg/kg/day divided every 8-12 hours; up to 12 g/day

Adults: 2-4 g/day in divided doses every 12 hours; up to 12 g/day

**Mechanism of Action** Inhibits bacterial cell wall synthesis by binding to one or more of the penicillin-binding proteins (PBPs) which in turn inhibits the final transpeptidation step of peptidoglycan synthesis in bacterial cell walls, thus inhibiting cell wall biosynthesis. Bacteria eventually lyse due to ongoing activity of cell wall autolytic enzymes (autolysins and murein hydrolases) while cell wall assembly is arrested.

**Local Anesthetic/Vasoconstrictor Precautions** No information available to require special precautions

**Effects on Dental Treatment** No effects or complications reported

**Other Adverse Effects**

1% to 10%: Gastrointestinal: Diarrhea

<1%:
- Dermatologic: Maculopapular and erythematous rash
- Gastrointestinal: Dyspepsia, pseudomembranous colitis, nausea, vomiting
- Hematologic: Bleeding
- Local: Pain and induration at injection site

**Drug Interactions** Increased effect: High-dose probenecid decreases renal clearance of cephalosporins

**Drug Uptake**

Serum half-life: 2 hours, higher with hepatic disease or biliary obstruction

Time to peak serum concentration:
- I.M.: Within 1-2 hours
- I.V.: Within 15-20 minutes (serum levels 2-3 times the serum levels following I.M. administration)

**Pregnancy Risk Factor** B

**Generic Available** No

♦ **Cefotan®** *see* Cefotetan *on next page*

## Cefotaxime (sef oh TAKS eem)

**U.S. Brand Names** Claforan®

**Therapeutic Category** Antibiotic, Cephalosporin (Third Generation)

**Use** Treatment of susceptible infection in respiratory tract, skin and skin structure, bone and joint, urinary tract, gynecologic as well as septicemia, and documented or suspected meningitis

**Usual Dosage** I.M., I.V.:

Children 1 month to 12 years:

<50 kg: 100-150 mg/kg/day in divided doses every 6-8 hours

(Continued)

## Cefotaxime *(Continued)*

Meningitis: 200 mg/kg/day in divided doses every 6 hours
>50 kg: Moderate to severe infection: 1-2 g every 6-8 hours; life-threatening infection: 2 g/dose every 4 hours; maximum dose: 12 g/day
Children >12 years and Adults: 1-2 g every 6-8 hours (up to 12 g/day)

**Mechanism of Action** Inhibits bacterial cell wall synthesis by binding to one or more of the penicillin-binding proteins (PBPs) which in turn inhibits the final transpeptidation step of peptidoglycan synthesis in bacterial cell walls, thus inhibiting cell wall biosynthesis. Bacteria eventually lyse due to ongoing activity of cell wall autolytic enzymes (autolysins and murein hydrolases) while cell wall assembly is arrested.

**Local Anesthetic/Vasoconstrictor Precautions** No information available to require special precautions

**Effects on Dental Treatment** No effects or complications reported

**Other Adverse Effects**

1% to 10%:
- Central nervous system: Fever
- Dermatologic: Rash, pruritus
- Gastrointestinal: Colitis, diarrhea, nausea, vomiting
- Hematologic: Eosinophilia
- Local: Pain at injection site

<1%:
- Central nervous system: Headache
- Gastrointestinal: Pseudomembranous colitis
- Hematologic: Transient neutropenia, thrombocytopenia
- Hepatic: Transient elevation of liver enzymes
- Local: Phlebitis
- Renal: Transient elevation of BUN and creatinine

**Drug Interactions**
Increased effect: High-dose probenecid decreases renal clearance of cephalosporins

**Drug Uptake**
Serum half-life:
Cefotaxime:
Adults: 1-1.5 hours (prolonged with renal and/or hepatic impairment)
Desacetylcefotaxime: 1.5-1.9 hours (prolonged with renal impairment)
Time to peak serum concentration: I.M.: Within 30 minutes

**Pregnancy Risk Factor** B

**Generic Available** No

## Cefotetan (SEF oh tee tan)

**Related Information**
Animal and Human Bites Guidelines *on page 1164*

**U.S. Brand Names** Cefotan®

**Therapeutic Category** Antibiotic, Cephalosporin (Second Generation)

**Use** Treatment of susceptible bacterial infection; mainly respiratory tract, skin and skin structure, bone and joint, urinary tract and gynecologic, as well as, septicemia, similar spectrum to cefoxitin

**Usual Dosage** I.M., I.V.:
Children: 20-40 mg/kg/dose every 12 hours
Adults: 1-6 g/day in divided doses every 12 hours, 1-2 g may be given every 24 hours for urinary tract infection

**Mechanism of Action** Inhibits bacterial cell wall synthesis by binding to one or more of the penicillin-binding proteins (PBPs) which in turn inhibits the final transpeptidation step of peptidoglycan synthesis in bacterial cell walls, thus inhibiting cell wall biosynthesis. Bacteria eventually lyse due to ongoing activity of cell wall autolytic enzymes (autolysins and murein hydrolases) while cell wall assembly is arrested.

**Local Anesthetic/Vasoconstrictor Precautions** No information available to require special precautions

**Effects on Dental Treatment** No effects or complications reported

**Other Adverse Effects**

1% to 10%:
- Gastrointestinal: Diarrhea
- Hepatic: Hepatic enzyme elevation
- Miscellaneous: Hypersensitivity reactions

<1%:
- Central nervous system: Fever
- Dermatologic: Rash, pruritus
- Gastrointestinal: Nausea, vomiting, antibiotic-associated colitis

Hematologic: Prolongation of bleeding time or prothrombin time, neutropenia, thrombocytopenia

Local: Phlebitis

**Drug Interactions** Increased effect: High-dose probenecid decreases renal clearance of cephalosporins

**Drug Uptake**

Serum half-life: 1.5-3 hours

Time to peak serum concentration: I.M.: Within 1.5-3 hours

**Pregnancy Risk Factor** B

**Generic Available** No

## Cefoxitin (se FOKS i tin)

**U.S. Brand Names** Mefoxin®

**Therapeutic Category** Antibiotic, Cephalosporin (Second Generation)

**Use** Less active against staphylococci and streptococci than first generation cephalosporins, but active against anaerobes including *Bacteroides fragilis*; active against gram-negative enteric bacilli including *E. coli*, *Klebsiella*, and *Proteus*; used predominantly for respiratory tract, skin and skin structure, bone and joint, urinary tract and gynecologic as well as septicemia; surgical prophylaxis; intra-abdominal infections and other mixed infections

**Usual Dosage** I.M., I.V.:

Children >3 months:

Mild-moderate infection: 80-100 mg/kg/day in divided doses every 4-6 hours

Severe infection: 100-160 mg/kg/day in divided doses every 4-6 hours

Maximum dose: 12 g/day

Adults: 1-2 g every 6-8 hours (I.M. injection is painful); up to 12 g/day

**Mechanism of Action** Inhibits bacterial cell wall synthesis by binding to one or more of the penicillin-binding proteins (PBPs) which in turn inhibits the final transpeptidation step of peptidoglycan synthesis in bacterial cell walls, thus inhibiting cell wall biosynthesis. Bacteria eventually lyse due to ongoing activity of cell wall autolytic enzymes (autolysins and murein hydrolases) while cell wall assembly is arrested.

**Local Anesthetic/Vasoconstrictor Precautions** No information available to require special precautions

**Effects on Dental Treatment** No effects or complications reported

**Other Adverse Effects**

1% to 10%: Gastrointestinal: Diarrhea

<1%:

Cardiovascular: Hypotension

Central nervous system: Fever

Dermatologic: Rash, exfoliative dermatitis

Gastrointestinal: Nausea, vomiting, pseudomembranous colitis

Hematologic: Transient leukopenia, thrombocytopenia, anemia, eosinophilia

Hepatic: Elevation in serum AST concentration

Local: Thrombophlebitis

Renal: Elevations in serum creatinine and/or BUN

Respiratory: Dyspnea

**Drug Interactions** Increased effect: High-dose probenecid decreases renal clearance of cephalosporins

**Drug Uptake**

Serum half-life: 45-60 minutes, increases significantly with renal insufficiency

Time to peak serum concentration:

I.M.: Within 20-30 minutes

I.V.: Within 5 minutes

**Pregnancy Risk Factor** B

**Generic Available** No

## Cefpodoxime (sef pode OKS eem)

**U.S. Brand Names** Vantin®

**Therapeutic Category** Antibiotic, Cephalosporin (Second Generation)

**Use** Treatment of susceptible acute, community-acquired pneumonia caused by *S. pneumoniae* or nonbeta-lactamase producing *H. influenzae*; acute uncomplicated gonorrhea caused by *N. gonorrhoeae*; uncomplicated skin and skin structure infections caused by *S. aureus* or *S. pyogenes*; acute otitis media caused by *S. pneumoniae, H. influenzae,* or *M. catarrhalis*; pharyngitis or tonsillitis; and uncomplicated urinary tract infections caused by *E. coli*, *Klebsiella*, and *Proteus*

**Usual Dosage** Oral:

Children >5 months to 12 years:

Acute otitis media: 10 mg/kg/day as a single dose or divided every 12 hours (400 mg/day)

Pharyngitis/tonsillitis: 10 mg/kg/day in 2 divided doses (maximum: 200 mg/day)

(Continued)

## Cefpodoxime *(Continued)*

Children ≥13 years and Adults:
Acute community-acquired pneumonia and bacterial exacerbations of chronic bronchitis: 200 mg every 12 hours for 14 days and 10 days, respectively
Skin and skin structure: 400 mg every 12 hours for 7-14 days
Uncomplicated gonorrhea (male and female) and rectal gonococcal infections (female): 200 mg as a single dose
Pharyngitis/tonsillitis: 100 mg every 12 hours for 10 days
Uncomplicated urinary tract infection: 100 mg every 12 hours for 7 days

**Mechanism of Action** Inhibits bacterial cell wall synthesis by binding to one or more of the penicillin-binding proteins (PBPs) which in turn inhibits the final transpeptidation step of peptidoglycan synthesis in bacterial cell walls, thus inhibiting cell wall biosynthesis. Bacteria eventually lyse due to ongoing activity of cell wall autolytic enzymes (autolysins and murein hydrolases) while cell wall assembly is arrested.

**Local Anesthetic/Vasoconstrictor Precautions** No information available to require special precautions

**Effects on Dental Treatment** No effects or complications reported

**Other Adverse Effects**
1% to 10%: Gastrointestinal: Diarrhea
<1%:
Central nervous system: Headache
Dermatologic: Diaper rash
Gastrointestinal: Nausea, vomiting, abdominal pain, pseudomembranous colitis
Genitourinary: Vaginal fungal infections

**Drug Interactions**
Decreased effect: Antacids and $H_2$-receptor antagonists (reduce absorption and serum concentration of cefpodoxime)
Increased effect: Probenecid may decrease cephalosporin elimination

**Drug Uptake**
Absorption: Oral: Rapidly and well absorbed (50%), acid stable; enhanced in the presence of food or low gastric pH
Serum half-life: 2.2 hours (prolonged with renal impairment)

**Pregnancy Risk Factor** B

**Dosage Forms**
Granules for oral suspension, as proxetil (lemon creme flavor): 50 mg/5 mL (100 mL); 100 mg/5 mL (100 mL)
Tablet, film coated, as proxetil: 100 mg, 200 mg

**Dietary Considerations** May be taken with food, however, there is delayed absorption

**Generic Available** No

## Cefprozil (sef PROE zil)

**U.S. Brand Names** Cefzil®

**Therapeutic Category** Antibiotic, Cephalosporin (Second Generation)

**Use** Infections causes by susceptible organisms including *S. pneumoniae*, *S. aureus*, *S. pyogenes*; treatment of otitis media and infections involving the respiratory tract and skin and skin structure

**Usual Dosage** Oral:
Children >6 months to 12 years: 7.5-15 mg/kg every 12 hours for 10 days
Pharyngitis/tonsillitis:
Children 2-12 years: 15 mg/kg/day divided every 12 hours; maximum: 1 g/day
Children >13 years and Adults: 250-500 mg every 12-24 hours for 10-14 days

**Mechanism of Action** Inhibits bacterial cell wall synthesis by binding to one or more of the penicillin-binding proteins (PBPs) which in turn inhibits the final transpeptidation step of peptidoglycan synthesis in bacterial cell walls, thus inhibiting cell wall biosynthesis. Bacteria eventually lyse due to ongoing activity of cell wall autolytic enzymes (autolysins and murein hydrolases) while cell wall assembly is arrested.

**Local Anesthetic/Vasoconstrictor Precautions** No information available to require special precautions

**Effects on Dental Treatment** No effects or complications reported

**Other Adverse Effects**
1% to 10%:
Central nervous system: Dizziness
Dermatologic: Diaper rash, genital pruritus
Gastrointestinal: Diarrhea, nausea, vomiting, abdominal pain
Genitourinary: Vaginitis
Hematologic: Eosinophilia
Hepatic: Elevation of AST and ALT, elevation of alkaline phosphatase

Miscellaneous: Superinfection

<1%:

Central nervous system: Headache, insomnia, confusion

Dermatologic: Rash, urticaria

Hematologic: Prolonged PT

Hepatic: Cholestatic jaundice

Neuromuscular & skeletal: Arthralgia

Renal: Elevated BUN and serum creatinine

**Drug Interactions**

Increased effect: Probenecid may decrease cephalosporin elimination

**Drug Uptake**

Absorption: Oral: Well absorbed (94%)

Serum half-life, elimination: 1.3 hours (normal renal function)

Peak serum levels: 1.5 hours (fasting state)

**Pregnancy Risk Factor** B

**Dosage Forms**

Powder for oral suspension, as anhydrous: 125 mg/5 mL (50 mL, 75 mL, 100 mL); 250 mg/5 mL (50 mL, 75 mL, 100 mL)

Tablet, as anhydrous: 250 mg, 500 mg

**Dietary Considerations** May be taken with food, however, there is delayed absorption

**Generic Available** No

## Ceftazidime (SEF tay zi deem)

**U.S. Brand Names** Ceptaz™; Fortaz®; Tazicef®; Tazidime®

**Canadian Brand Names** Ceptaz™

**Therapeutic Category** Antibiotic, Cephalosporin (Third Generation)

**Use** Treatment of documented susceptible *Pseudomonas aeruginosa* infection; *Pseudomonas* infection in patients at risk of developing aminoglycoside-induced nephrotoxicity and/or ototoxicity; empiric therapy of febrile, granulocytopenic patients

**Usual Dosage** I.M., I.V.:

Children 1 month to 12 years: 30-50 mg/kg/dose every 8 hours; maximum dose: 6 g/day

Adults: 1-2 g every 8-12 hours

Urinary tract infections: 250-500 mg every 12 hours

**Mechanism of Action** Inhibits bacterial cell wall synthesis by binding to one or more of the penicillin-binding proteins (PBPs) which in turn inhibits the final transpeptidation step of peptidoglycan synthesis in bacterial cell walls, thus inhibiting cell wall biosynthesis. Bacteria eventually lyse due to ongoing activity of cell wall autolytic enzymes (autolysins and murein hydrolases) while cell wall assembly is arrested.

**Local Anesthetic/Vasoconstrictor Precautions** No information available to require special precautions

**Effects on Dental Treatment** No effects or complications reported

**Other Adverse Effects**

1% to 10%:

Gastrointestinal: Diarrhea

Local: Pain at injection site

<1%:

Central nervous system: Fever, headache, dizziness

Dermatologic: Rash, angioedema

Gastrointestinal: Nausea, vomiting, pseudomembranous colitis

Hematologic: Eosinophilia, thrombocytosis, transient leukopenia, hemolytic anemia

Hepatic: Transient elevation in liver enzymes

Local: Phlebitis

Neuromuscular & skeletal: Paresthesia

Renal: Transient elevation in BUN and creatinine

Miscellaneous: Candidiasis

**Drug Interactions** Increased effect: High-dose probenecid decreases renal clearance of cephalosporins

**Drug Uptake**

Serum half-life: 1-2 hours (prolonged with renal impairment)

Time to peak serum concentration: I.M.: Within 1 hour

**Pregnancy Risk Factor** B

**Generic Available** No

## Ceftibuten (sef TYE byoo ten)

**U.S. Brand Names** Cedax®

**Therapeutic Category** Antibiotic, Cephalosporin (Third Generation)

(Continued)

## Ceftibuten *(Continued)*

**Use** Oral cephalosporin for bronchitis, otitis media, and strep throat

**Usual Dosage** Oral:

Children <12 years: 9 mg/kg/day for 10 days; maximum daily dose: 400 mg

Children ≥12 years and Adults: 400 mg once daily for 10 days; maximum: 400 mg

**Mechanism of Action** Inhibits bacterial cell wall synthesis by binding to one or more of the penicillin-binding proteins (PBPs) which in turn inhibits the final transpeptidation step of peptidoglycan synthesis in bacterial cell walls, thus inhibiting cell wall biosynthesis. Bacteria eventually lyse due to ongoing activity of cell wall autolytic enzymes (autolysins and murein hydrolases) while cell wall assembly is arrested.

**Local Anesthetic/Vasoconstrictor Precautions** No information available to require special precautions

**Effects on Dental Treatment** No effects or complications reported

**Other Adverse Effects**

1% to 10%: Gastrointestinal: Diarrhea

<1%:

- Central nervous system: Dizziness, fatigue, headache
- Dermatologic: Rash
- Gastrointestinal: Nausea, vomiting, pseudomembranous colitis
- Hematologic: Transient neutropenia, anemia
- Hepatic: Transient elevation in LFTs

**Contraindications** Hypersensitivity to ceftibuten, any component, or cephalosporins

**Warnings/Precautions** Modify dosage in patients with severe renal impairment, prolonged use may result in superinfection; a low incidence of cross-hypersensitivity to penicillins exist

**Drug Interactions**

Increased effect: High-dose probenecid decreases clearance

Increased toxicity: Aminoglycosides increase nephrotoxic potential

**Drug Uptake**

Absorption: Rapid; food decreases peak concentrations

Serum half-life: 2 hours

Time to peak serum concentration: Within 2-3 hours

**Pregnancy Risk Factor** B

**Dosage Forms**

Capsule: 400 mg

Powder for oral suspension (cherry flavor): 90 mg/5 mL (30 mL, 60 mL, 120 mL); 180 mg/5 mL (30 mL, 60 mL, 120 mL)

**Dietary Considerations** Take without regard to food

**Generic Available** No

**Comments** In clinical trials, ceftibuten once or twice daily was at least as effective as cefaclor or ciprofloxacin for treatment of acute bacterial exacerbations of bronchitis, as effective as amoxicillin/clavulanic acid or cefaclor for otitis media, as effective as penicillin for pharyngitis, and as effective as trimethoprim-sulfamethoxazole for urinary tract infections

♦ **Ceftin®** *see* Cefuroxime *on page 210*

## Ceftizoxime (sef ti ZOKS eem)

**U.S. Brand Names** Cefizox®

**Therapeutic Category** Antibiotic, Cephalosporin (Third Generation)

**Use** Treatment of susceptible nonpseudomonal gram-negative rod infections or mixed gram-negative and anaerobic infections; predominantly respiratory tract, skin and skin structure, bone and joint, urinary tract and gynecologic, as well as septicemia

**Usual Dosage** I.M., I.V.:

Children ≥6 months: 150-200 mg/kg/day divided every 6-8 hours (maximum of 12 g/24 hours)

Adults: 1-2 g every 8-12 hours, up to 2 g every 4 hours or 4 g every 8 hours for life-threatening infections

**Mechanism of Action** Inhibits bacterial cell wall synthesis by binding to one or more of the penicillin-binding proteins (PBPs) which in turn inhibits the final transpeptidation step of peptidoglycan synthesis in bacterial cell walls, thus inhibiting cell wall biosynthesis. Bacteria eventually lyse due to ongoing activity of cell wall autolytic enzymes (autolysins and murein hydrolases) while cell wall assembly is arrested.

**Local Anesthetic/Vasoconstrictor Precautions** No information available to require special precautions

**Effects on Dental Treatment** No effects or complications reported

**Other Adverse Effects**

1% to 10%:
- Central nervous system: Fever
- Dermatologic: Rash, pruritus
- Hematologic: Eosinophilia, thrombocytosis
- Hepatic: Transient elevation of AST, ALT, and alkaline phosphatase
- Local: Pain, burning at injection site

<1%:
- Genitourinary: Vaginitis
- Hematologic: Anemia, leukopenia, neutropenia, thrombocytopenia
- Hepatic: Elevation of bilirubin
- Neuromuscular & skeletal: Numbness
- Renal: Transient elevations of BUN and creatinine

**Drug Interactions**

Increased effect: High-dose probenecid decreases renal clearance of cephalosporins

**Drug Uptake**

Serum half-life: 1.6 hours, increases to 25 hours when $Cl_{cr}$ falls to <10 mL/minute

Time to peak serum concentration: I.M.: Within 0.5-1 hour

**Pregnancy Risk Factor** B

**Generic Available** No

## Ceftriaxone (sef trye AKS one)

**Related Information**

Animal and Human Bites Guidelines *on page 1164*

Nonviral Infectious Diseases *on page 1095*

**U.S. Brand Names** Rocephin®

**Therapeutic Category** Antibiotic, Cephalosporin (Third Generation)

**Use** Treatment of lower respiratory tract infections, skin and skin structure infections, bone and joint infections, intra-abdominal and urinary tract infections, sepsis and meningitis due to susceptible organisms; documented or suspected infection due to susceptible organisms in home care patients and patients without I.V. line access; treatment of documented or suspected gonococcal infection or chancroid; emergency room management of patients at high risk for bacteremia, periorbital or buccal cellulitis, salmonellosis or shigellosis, and pneumonia of unestablished etiology (<5 years of age)

**Usual Dosage** I.M., I.V.:

Children: 50-75 mg/kg/day in 1-2 divided doses every 12-24 hours; maximum: 2 g/24 hours
- Meningitis: 100 mg/kg/day divided every 12-24 hours, up to a maximum of 4 g/24 hours; loading dose of 75 mg/kg/dose may be given at start of therapy
- Uncomplicated gonococcal infections, sexual assault, and STD prophylaxis: I.M.: 125 mg as a single dose
- Complicated gonococcal infections:
  - <45 kg: 50 mg/kg/day once daily; maximum: 1 g/day; for ophthalmia, peritonitis, arthritis, or bacteremia: 50-100 mg/kg/day divided every 12-24 hours; maximum: 2 g/day for meningitis or endocarditis
  - >45 kg: 1 g/day once daily for disseminated gonococcal infections; 1-2 g dose every 12 hours for meningitis or endocarditis
- Acute epididymitis: I.M.: 250 mg in a single dose

Adults: 1-2 g every 12-24 hours (depending on the type and severity of infection); maximum dose: 2 g every 12 hours for treatment of meningitis
- Uncomplicated gonorrhea: I.M.: 250 mg as a single dose

**Mechanism of Action** Inhibits bacterial cell wall synthesis by binding to one or more of the penicillin-binding proteins (PBPs) which in turn inhibits the final transpeptidation step of peptidoglycan synthesis in bacterial cell walls, thus inhibiting cell wall biosynthesis. Bacteria eventually lyse due to ongoing activity of cell wall autolytic enzymes (autolysins and murein hydrolases) while cell wall assembly is arrested.

**Local Anesthetic/Vasoconstrictor Precautions** No information available to require special precautions

**Effects on Dental Treatment** No effects or complications reported

**Other Adverse Effects**

1% to 10%:
- Dermatologic: Rash
- Gastrointestinal: Diarrhea
- Hematologic: Eosinophilia, thrombocytosis, leukopenia
- Hepatic: Elevations of SGOT [AST], SGPT [ALT]
- Local: Pain at injection site
- Renal: Elevations of BUN

<1%:
- Cardiovascular: Flushing

(Continued)

## Ceftriaxone *(Continued)*

Central nervous system: Fever, chills, headache, dizziness
Dermatologic: Pruritus
Gastrointestinal: Nausea, vomiting, dysgeusia
Genitourinary: Presence of casts in urine, vaginitis
Hematologic: Anemia, hemolytic anemia, neutropenia, lymphopenia, thrombocytopenia
Hepatic: Elevations of alkaline phosphatase and bilirubin
Local: Phlebitis
Renal: Elevation of creatinine
Miscellaneous: Moniliasis, sweating

**Drug Interactions** Increased effect: High-dose probenecid decreases renal clearance of cephalosporins

**Drug Uptake**
Serum half-life: Normal renal and hepatic function: 5-9 hours
Time to peak serum concentration:
I.M.: Within 1-2 hours
I.V.: Within minutes

**Pregnancy Risk Factor** B

**Generic Available** No

## Cefuroxime (se fyoor OKS eem)

**U.S. Brand Names** Ceftin®; Kefurox®; Zinacef®

**Therapeutic Category** Antibiotic, Cephalosporin (Second Generation)

**Use** Treatment of infections caused by staphylococci, group B streptococci, *H. influenzae* (type A and B), *E. coli*, *Enterobacter*, *Salmonella*, and *Klebsiella*; treatment of susceptible infections of the lower respiratory tract, otitis media, urinary tract, skin and soft tissue, bone and joint, sepsis and gonorrhea

**Usual Dosage**
Children:
Pharyngitis, tonsillitis: Oral:
Suspension: 20 mg/kg/day (maximum: 500 mg/day) in 2 divided doses
Tablet: 125 mg every 12 hours
Acute otitis media, impetigo: Oral:
Suspension: 30 mg/kg/day (maximum: 1 g/day) in 2 divided doses
Tablet: 250 mg every 12 hours
I.M., I.V.: 75-150 mg/kg/day divided every 8 hours; maximum dose: 6 g/day
Meningitis: Not recommended (doses of 200-240 mg/kg/day divided every 6-8 hours have been used); maximum dose: 9 g/day
Adults:
Oral: 250-500 mg twice daily; uncomplicated urinary tract infection: 125-250 mg every 12 hours
I.M., I.V.: 750 mg to 1.5 g/dose every 8 hours or 100-150 mg/kg/day in divided doses every 6-8 hours; maximum: 6 g/24 hours

**Mechanism of Action** Inhibits bacterial cell wall synthesis by binding to one or more of the penicillin-binding proteins (PBPs) which in turn inhibits the final transpeptidation step of peptidoglycan synthesis in bacterial cell walls, thus inhibiting cell wall biosynthesis. Bacteria eventually lyse due to ongoing activity of cell wall autolytic enzymes (autolysins and murein hydrolases) while cell wall assembly is arrested.

**Local Anesthetic/Vasoconstrictor Precautions** No information available to require special precautions

**Effects on Dental Treatment** No effects or complications reported

**Other Adverse Effects**
1% to 10%:
Hematologic: Decreased hemoglobin and hematocrit, eosinophilia
Hepatic: Transient rise in SGOT [AST], SGPT [ALT], and alkaline phosphatase
Local: Thrombophlebitis
<1%:
Central nervous system: Dizziness, fever, headache
Dermatologic: Rash
Gastrointestinal: Nausea, vomiting, diarrhea, stomach cramps, colitis, GI bleeding
Genitourinary: Vaginitis
Hematologic: Transient neutropenia and leukopenia
Hepatic: Transient increase in liver enzymes
Local: Pain at the injection site
Renal: Elevated creatinine and/or BUN

**Drug Interactions** Increased effect: High-dose probenecid decreases clearance of cefuroxime

**Drug Uptake**
Absorption: Increased when given with or shortly after food or infant formula
Serum half-life:
Adults: 1-2 hours (prolonged in renal impairment)
I.M.: Within 15-60 minutes
I.V.: 2-3 minutes

**Pregnancy Risk Factor** B

**Dosage Forms**
Infusion, as sodium, premixed (frozen) (Zinacef®): 750 mg (50 mL); 1.5 g (50 mL)
Powder for injection, as sodium: 750 mg, 1.5 g, 7.5 g
Powder for injection, as sodium (Kefurox®, Zinacef®): 750 mg, 1.5 g, 7.5 g
Powder for oral suspension, as axetil (tutti-frutti flavor) (Ceftin®): 125 mg/5 mL (50 mL, 100 mL, 200 mL)
Tablet, as axetil (Ceftin®): 125 mg, 250 mg, 500 mg

**Dietary Considerations** May be taken with food, however, bioavailability is increased with food

**Generic Available** Yes

♦ **Cefzil®** *see* Cefprozil *on page 206*
♦ **Celebrex®** *see* Celecoxib *on this page*

## Celecoxib

**Related Information**
Rheumatoid Arthritis and Osteoarthritis *on page 1092*

**U.S. Brand Names** Celebrex®

**Therapeutic Category** Selective Cyclooxygenase-2 Inhibitor

**Use** Relief of the signs and symptoms of osteoarthritis; relief of the signs and symptoms of rheumatoid arthritis in adults

**Usual Dosage** Adults: Oral:
Osteoarthritis: 200 mg/day as a single dose or in divided dose twice daily
Rheumatoid arthritis: 100-200 mg twice daily
Elderly: No specific dosing adjustment is recommended; however, the AUC in elderly patients may be increased by 50% as compared to younger subjects. Use the lowest recommended dose in patients weighing <50 kg.

**Mechanism of Action** Inhibits prostaglandin synthesis by decreasing the activity of the enzyme, cyclo-oxygenase-2 (COX-2), which results in decreased formation of prostaglandin precursors. Celecoxib does not inhibit cyclo-oxygenase-1 (COX-1) at therapeutic concentrations.

**Local Anesthetic/Vasoconstrictor Precautions** No information available to require special precautions

**Effects on Dental Treatment** Nonselective NSAIDs are known to reversibly decrease platelet aggregation via mechanisms different than observed with aspirin. According to the manufacturer, celecoxib, at single dose up to 800 mg and multiple doses of 600 mg twice daily, had no effect on platelet aggregation or bleeding time. Comparative NSAIDs (naproxen 500 mg twice daily, ibuprofen 800 mg three times daily or diclofenac 75 mg twice daily) significantly reduced platelet aggregation and prolonged the bleeding times.

**Other Adverse Effects**
>10%: Central nervous system: Headache (15.8%)
2% to 10%:
Cardiovascular: Peripheral edema (2.1%)
Central nervous system: Insomnia (2.3%), dizziness (2%)
Dermatologic : Skin rash (2.2%)
Gastrointestinal: Dyspepsia (8.8%), diarrhea (5.6%), abdominal pain (4.1%), nausea (3.5%), flatulence (2.2%)
Neuromuscular & skeletal: Back pain (2.8%)
Respiratory: Upper respiratory tract infection (8.1%), sinusitis (5%), pharyngitis (2.3%), rhinitis (2%)
Miscellaneous: Accidental injury (2.9%)
0.1% to 2%:
Cardiovascular: Hypertension (aggravated), chest pain, myocardial infarction, palpitation, tachycardia, facial edema, peripheral edema
Central nervous system: Migraine, vertigo, hypoesthesia, fatigue, fever, pain, hypotonia, anxiety, depression, nervousness, somnolence
Dermatologic: Alopecia, dermatitis, photosensitivity, pruritus, rash (maculopapular), rash (erythematous), dry skin, urticaria
Endocrine & metabolic: Hot flashes, diabetes mellitus, hyperglycemia, hypercholesterolemia, breast pain, dysmenorrhea, menstrual disturbances, hypokalemia
Gastrointestinal: Constipation, tenesmus, diverticulitis, eructation, esophagitis, gastroenteritis, vomiting, gastroesophageal reflux, hemorrhoids, hiatal
(Continued)

## Celecoxib *(Continued)*

hernia, melena, stomatitis, anorexia, increased appetite, taste disturbance, dry mouth, tooth disorder, weight gain

Genitourinary: Prostate disorder, vaginal bleeding, vaginitis, monilial vaginitis, dysuria, cystitis, urinary frequency, incontinence, urinary tract infection,

Hepatic: Elevated transaminases, increased alkaline phosphatase

Hematologic: Anemia, thrombocytopenia, ecchymosis

Neuromuscular & skeletal: Leg cramps, increased CPK, neck stiffness, arthralgia, myalgia, bone disorder, fracture, synovitis, tendonitis, neuralgia, paresthesia, neuropathy, weakness

Ocular: Glaucoma, blurred vision, cataract, conjunctivitis, eye pain

Otic: Deafness, tinnitus, earache, otitis media

Renal: Increased BUN, increased creatinine, albuminuria, hematuria, renal calculi

Respiratory: Bronchitis, bronchospasm, cough, dyspnea, laryngitis, pneumonia, epistaxis

Miscellaneous: Allergic reactions, flu-like syndrome, breast cancer, herpes infection, bacterial infection, moniliasis, viral infection, increased diaphoresis

<0.1% (limited to severe): Congestive heart failure, ventricular fibrillation, pulmonary embolism, syncope, cerebrovascular accident, gangrene, thrombophlebitis, thrombocytopenia, ataxia, acute renal failure, intestinal obstruction, pancreatitis, intestinal perforation, gastrointestinal bleeding, colitis, esophageal perforation, sepsis, sudden death

**Warnings/Precautions** Gastrointestinal irritation, ulceration, bleeding, and perforation may occur with NSAIDs (it is unclear whether celecoxib is associated with rates of these events which are similar to nonselective NSAIDs). Use with caution in patients with a history of GI disease (bleeding or ulcers), decreased renal function, hepatic disease, congestive heart failure, hypertension, or asthma. Anaphylactoid reactions may occur, even with no prior exposure to celecoxib. Use caution in patients with known or suspected deficiency of cytochrome P-450 isoenzyme 2C9.

**Drug Interactions**

Decreased effect: Efficacy of thiazide diuretics, loop diuretics (furosemide), or ACE-inhibitors may be diminished by celecoxib

Increased effect: Celecoxib is a cytochrome oxidase P-450 isoenzyme 2C9 substrate and an inhibitor of isoenzyme 2D6. Inhibitors of isoenzyme 2C9 may result in significant increases in celecoxib concentrations. Coadministration of drugs by 2D6 may result in increased serum concentrations of these agents. Fluconazole increases celecoxib concentrations two-fold. Lithium concentrations may be increased by celecoxib. Celecoxib may be used with low-dose aspirin, however rates of gastrointestinal bleeding may be increased with coadministration. Celecoxib has not been shown to alter warfarin effects, although bleeding complications may be increased.

**Drug Uptake**

Serum half-life: 11 hours

Time to peak: 3 hours

**Pregnancy Risk Factor** C (D after 34 weeks gestation or close to delivery)

**Dosage Forms** Capsule: 100 mg, 200 mg

**Comments** According to the manufacturer, two out of 5,285 patients (0.04%) experienced significant upper GI bleeding, at 14 and 32 days after initiation of dosing. Approximately 40% of the 5,285 patients were in studies that required them to be free of ulcers by endoscopy at entry into the study. As a result, the manufacturer stressed that it is unclear if the study population is representative of the general population. As of this printing, long-term studies comparing the incidence of serious upper GI adverse effects in patients taking celecoxib compared to other nonselective NSAIDs had not been reported. Celecoxib does not appear to inhibit platelet aggregation at recommended doses. Reports have shown that celecoxib does not generally affect platelet counts, prothrombin time or partial thromboplastin time (PTT).

Cross-reactivity, including bronchospasm, between aspirin and other NSAIDs has been reported in aspirin-sensitive patients. The manufacturer suggests that celecoxib should not be administered to patients with this type of aspirin sensitivity and should be used with caution in patients with pre-existing asthma.

The manufacturer studied the effect of celecoxib on the anticoagulant effect of warfarin and found no alteration of anticoagulant effect, as determined by prothrombin time, in patients taking 2 mg to 5 mg daily. However, the manufacturer has issued a caution when using celecoxib with warfarin since those patients are at increased risk of bleeding complications.

A literature report suggested that the enzyme COX-2 (cyclo-oxygenase type 2) is a major source of systemic prostacyclin biosynthesis in humans. Prostacyclin is involved in blood vessel dilation and inhibition of blood clotting. In view of the fact that celecoxib inhibits the COX-2 enzyme, prostacyclin production could be suppressed. The resultant effects on hemostasis are unknown at this time.

**Selected Readings**

McAdam BF, et al, "Systemic Biosynthesis of Prostacyclin by Cyclo-oxygenase (COX)-2: The Human Pharmacology of a Selective Inhibitor of COX-2. Proceedings of the National Academy of Science," 1999, 96:272-7.

♦ **Celestone®** *see* Betamethasone *on page 136*
♦ **Celestone® Soluspan®** *see* Betamethasone *on page 136*
♦ **Celexa®** *see* Citalopram *on page 254*
♦ **CellCept®** *see* Mycophenolate *on page 694*
♦ **Cellufresh® [OTC]** *see* Carboxymethylcellulose *on page 191*

## Cellulose, Oxidized (SEL yoo lose, OKS i dyzed)

**U.S. Brand Names** Oxycel®; Surgicel®

**Therapeutic Category** Hemostatic Agent

**Use** Temporary packing for the control of capillary, venous, or small arterial hemorrhage

**Usual Dosage** Minimal amounts of an appropriate size are laid on the bleeding site

**Local Anesthetic/Vasoconstrictor Precautions** No information available to require special precautions

**Effects on Dental Treatment** No effects or complications reported

**Other Adverse Effects** 1% to 10%:

Central nervous system: Headache
Respiratory: Nasal burning or stinging, sneezing (rhinological procedures)
Miscellaneous: Encapsulation of fluid, foreign body reactions (with or without) infection

**Contraindications** Do not apply as packing or wadding as a hemostatic agents; do not use for packing or implantation in fractures or laminectomies; do not use to control hemorrhage from large arteries or on nonhemorrhagic serous oozing surfaces

**Warnings/Precautions** By swelling, oxidized cellulose may cause nerve damage by pressure in bony confine (ie, optic nerve and chiasm); always remove from these sites of application or do not use at all (see contraindications); do not autoclave, do not moisten with water or saline (lessens hemostatic effect). Avoid wadding or packing tightly; do not use after application of $AgNO_3$ or other escharotic agents.

**Drug Interactions** No data reported

**Pregnancy Risk Factor** No data reported

**Breast-feeding Considerations** No data reported

**Dosage Forms**

Pad (Oxycel®): 3" x 3", 8 ply
Pledget (Oxycel®): 2" x 1" x 1"
Strip:
  Oxycel®:
    18" x 2", 4 ply
    5" x ½", 4 ply
    36" x ½", 4 ply
  Surgicel®:
    2" x 14"
    4" x 8"
    2" x 3"
    ½" x 2"

**Dietary Considerations** No data reported

**Generic Available** No

## Cellulose, Oxidized Regenerated

(SEL yoo lose, OKS i dyzed re JEN er aye ted)

**U.S. Brand Names** Surgicel® Absorbable Hemostat

**Therapeutic Category** Hemostatic Agent

**Use**

Dental: To control bleeding created during dental surgery
Medical: Hemostatic

**Usual Dosage** Minimal amounts of the fabric strip are laid on the bleeding site or held firmly against the tissues until hemostasis occurs

**Mechanism of Action** Cellulose, oxidized regenerated is saturated with blood at the bleeding site and swells into a brownish or black gelatinous mass which aids in the formation of a clot. When used in small amounts, it is absorbed from the sites of implantation with little or no tissue reaction.

(Continued)

## Cellulose, Oxidized Regenerated *(Continued)*

**Local Anesthetic/Vasoconstrictor Precautions** No information available to require special precautions

**Effects on Dental Treatment** No effects or complications reported

**Other Adverse Effects** No data reported

**Contraindications** Not to be used as packing or wadding unless it is removed after hemostasis occurs; not to be used for implantation in bone defects

**Warnings/Precautions** Autoclaving causes physical breakdown of the product. Closing the material in a contaminated wound without drainage may lead to complications. The material should not be moistened before insertion since the hemostatic effect is greater when applied dry. The material should not be impregnated with anti-infective agents. Its hemostatic effect is not enhanced by the addition of thrombin. The material may be left in situ when necessary but it is advisable to remove it once hemostasis is achieved.

**Drug Interactions** No data reported

**Breast-feeding Considerations** No data reported

**Dosage Forms** Knitted fabric strips: Envelopes in a size of ½" x 2"

**Dietary Considerations** No data reported

**Generic Available** No

**Comments** Oxidized regenerated cellulose is prepared by the controlled oxidation of regenerated cellulose. The fabric is white with a pale yellow cast and has a faint, caramel-like aroma. A slight discoloration may occur with age but this does not effect its hemostatic actions.

## Cellulose Sodium Phosphate (sel yoo lose SOW dee um FOS fate)

**U.S. Brand Names** Calcibind®

**Therapeutic Category** Urinary Tract Product

**Synonyms** CSP; Sodium Cellulose Phosphate

**Use** Adjunct to dietary restriction to reduce renal calculi formation in absorptive hypercalciuria type I

**Usual Dosage** Adults: Oral: 5 g 3 times/day with meals; decrease dose to 5 g with main meal and 2.5 g with each of two other meals when urinary calcium declines to <150 mg/day

**Local Anesthetic/Vasoconstrictor Precautions** No information available to require special precautions

**Effects on Dental Treatment** No effects or complications reported

**Pregnancy Risk Factor** C

**Generic Available** No


- **Celluvisc® [OTC]** *see* Carboxymethylcellulose *on page 191*
- **Celontin®** *see* Methsuximide *on page 656*
- **Cel-U-Jec®** *see* Betamethasone *on page 136*
- **Cenafed® [OTC]** *see* Pseudoephedrine *on page 863*
- **Cenafed® Plus Tablet [OTC]** *see* Triprolidine and Pseudoephedrine *on page 1025*
- **Cena-K®** *see* Potassium Chloride *on page 822*
- **Cenolate®** *see* Sodium Ascorbate *on page 917*
- **Centrax®** *see* Prazepam *on page 829*
- **Cēpacol® Anesthetic Troches [OTC]** *see* Cetylpyridinium and Benzocaine *on page 219*
- **Cēpacol® Troches [OTC]** *see* Cetylpyridinium *on page 219*
- **Cēpastat® [OTC]** *see* Phenol *on page 791*


## Cephalexin (sef a LEKS in)

**Related Information**


Antibiotic Prophylaxis, Preprocedural Guidelines for Dental Patients *on page 1097*

Dental Drug Interactions: Update on Drug Combinations Requiring Special Considerations *on page 1225*

Oral Bacterial Infections *on page 1128*


**U.S. Brand Names** Biocef®; Cefanex®; Keflex®; Keftab®

**Canadian Brand Names** Apo®-Cephalex; Novo-Lexin; Nu-Cephalex

**Therapeutic Category** Antibiotic, Cephalosporin (First Generation)

**Use**

Dental: An alternate antibiotic to treat orofacial infections in patients allergic to penicillins; susceptible bacteria including aerobic gram-positive bacteria and anaerobes. Also, an alternate antibiotic for prevention of bacterial endocarditis; individuals allergic to amoxicillin (penicillins) may receive cephalexin provided they have not had an immediate, local, or systemic IgE-mediated anaphylactic allergic reaction to penicillin. Also, antibiotic for premedication in patients not allergic to penicillin who may be at potential increased risk of hematogenous total joint infection.

Medical: Treatment of susceptible bacterial infections in the medical patient, including those caused by group A beta-hemolytic *Streptococcus*, *Staphylococcus*, *Klebsiella pneumoniae*, *E. coli*, *Proteus mirabilis*, and *Shigella*; predominantly used for lower respiratory tract, urinary tract, skin and soft tissue, and bone and joint

**Usual Dosage** Oral:

Children: 25-50 mg/kg/day every 6 hours; severe infections: 50-100 mg/kg/day in divided doses every 6 hours; maximum: 3 g/24 hours

SBE prophylaxis: 50 mg/kg orally 1 hour before procedure with no follow-up dose needed; total children's dose not to exceed adult dose

Adults: 250-1000 mg every 6 hours; maximum: 4 g/day

SBE prophylaxis: 2 g 1 hour before procedure with no follow-up dose needed

Joint prosthesis prophylaxis: Oral: 2 g 1 hour before procedure

**Mechanism of Action** Inhibits bacterial cell wall synthesis by binding to one or more of the penicillin-binding proteins (PBPs) which in turn inhibits the final transpeptidation step of peptidoglycan synthesis in bacterial cell walls, thus inhibiting cell wall biosynthesis. Bacteria eventually lyse due to ongoing activity of cell wall autolytic enzymes (autolysins and murein hydrolases) while cell wall assembly is arrested.

**Local Anesthetic/Vasoconstrictor Precautions** No information available to require special precautions

**Effects on Dental Treatment** No effects or complications reported

**Other Adverse Effects** 1% to 10%: Gastrointestinal: Diarrhea

**Contraindications** Hypersensitivity to cephalexin, any component, or cephalosporins

**Warnings/Precautions** Modify dosage in patients with severe renal impairment; prolonged use may result in superinfection; a low incidence of cross-hypersensitivity to penicillins exists

**Drug Interactions**

Increased effect: Probenecid may decrease cephalosporin elimination

Increased toxicity: Aminoglycosides may be a possible additive to nephrotoxicity

**Drug Uptake**

Duration: 6 hours

Absorption:

Adults: Rapid

Children: Delayed in young children

Serum half-life: Adults: 0.5-1.2 hours (prolonged with renal impairment)

Time to peak serum concentration: Oral: Within 1 hour

**Pregnancy Risk Factor** B

**Breast-feeding Considerations** Excreted into breast milk in small amounts like other cephalosporins

**Dosage Forms**

Capsule, as monohydrate: 250 mg, 500 mg

Powder for oral suspension, as monohydrate: 125 mg/5 mL (5 mL unit dose, 60 mL, 100 mL, 200 mL); 250 mg/5 mL (5 mL unit dose, 100 mL, 200 mL)

Suspension, oral, as monohydrate, pediatric: 100 mg/mL [5 mg/drop] (10 mL)

Tablet, as monohydrate: 250 mg, 500 mg, 1 g

Tablet, as hydrochloride: 500 mg

**Dietary Considerations** Should be taken on an empty stomach (ie, 1 hour prior to, or 2 hours after meals) to increase total absorption

**Generic Available** Yes

**Comments** Cephalexin is effective against anaerobic bacteria, but the sensitivity of alpha-hemolytic *Streptococcus* vary; approximately 10% of strains are resistant. Nearly 70% are intermediately sensitive. Patients allergic to penicillins can use a cephalosporin; the incidence of cross-reactivity between penicillins and cephalosporins is 1% when the allergic reaction to penicillin is delayed. If the patient has a history of immediate reaction to penicillin, the incidence of cross-reactivity is 20%; cephalosporins are contraindicated in these patients.

**Selected Readings**

"Advisory Statement. Antibiotic Prophylaxis for Dental Patients With Total Joint Replacements. American Dental Association; American Academy of Orthopedic Surgeons," *J Am Dent Assoc*, 1997, 128(7):1004-8.

Dajani AS, Taubert KA, Wilson WW, et al, "Prevention of Bacterial Endocarditis. Recommendations by the American Heart Association," *JAMA* 1997, 277(22):1794-801.

Dajani AS, Taubert KA, Wilson W, et al, "Prevention of Bacterial Endocarditis: Recommendations by the American Heart Association," *J Am Dent Assoc* 1997, 128(8):1142-51.

Saxon A, Beall GN, Rohr AS, et al, "Immediate Hypersensitivity Reactions to Beta-Lactam Antibiotics," *Ann Intern Med*, 1987, 107(2):204-15.

## Cephalothin (sef A loe thin)

**U.S. Brand Names** Keflin®

**Canadian Brand Names** Ceporacin®

**Therapeutic Category** Antibiotic, Cephalosporin (First Generation)

**Use** Treatment of susceptible bacterial infections, including those caused by group A beta-hemolytic *Streptococcus*; respiratory, genitourinary, gastrointestinal, skin and soft tissue, bone and joint infections; septicemia; cephalexin is the oral equivalent

**Usual Dosage** I.M., I.V.:

Children: 75-125 mg/kg/day divided every 4-6 hours; maximum dose: 10 g in a 24-hour period

Adults: 500 mg to 2 g every 4-6 hours

**Mechanism of Action** Inhibits bacterial cell wall synthesis by binding to one or more of the penicillin-binding proteins (PBPs) which in turn inhibits the final transpeptidation step of peptidoglycan synthesis in bacterial cell walls, thus inhibiting cell wall biosynthesis. Bacteria eventually lyse due to ongoing activity of cell wall autolytic enzymes (autolysins and murein hydrolases) while cell wall assembly is arrested.

**Local Anesthetic/Vasoconstrictor Precautions** No information available to require special precautions

**Effects on Dental Treatment** No effects or complications reported

**Other Adverse Effects**

1% to 10%: Gastrointestinal: Nausea, vomiting, diarrhea

<1%:

- Dermatologic: Maculopapular and erythematous rash
- Gastrointestinal: Dyspepsia, pseudomembranous colitis
- Hematologic: Bleeding
- Local: Pain and induration at injection site

**Drug Interactions** Increased effect: High-dose probenecid decreases renal clearance of cephalothin

**Drug Uptake**

Serum half-life: 30-60 minutes

Time to peak serum concentration:

- I.M.: Within 30 minutes
- I.V.: Within 15 minutes

**Pregnancy Risk Factor** B

**Generic Available** Yes

## Cephapirin (sef a PYE rin)

**U.S. Brand Names** Cefadyl®

**Therapeutic Category** Antibiotic, Cephalosporin (First Generation)

**Use** Treatment of infections when caused by susceptible strains including group A beta-hemolytic *Streptococcus*; used in serious respiratory, genitourinary, gastrointestinal, skin and soft tissue, bone and joint infections; septicemia; endocarditis; identical to cephalothin

**Usual Dosage** I.M., I.V.:

Children: 10-20 mg/kg/dose every 6 hours up to 4 g/24 hours

Adults: 500 mg to 1 g every 6 hours up to 12 g/day

**Mechanism of Action** Inhibits bacterial cell wall synthesis by binding to one or more of the penicillin-binding proteins (PBPs) which in turn inhibits the final transpeptidation step of peptidoglycan synthesis in bacterial cell walls, thus inhibiting cell wall biosynthesis. Bacteria eventually lyse due to ongoing activity of cell wall autolytic enzymes (autolysins and murein hydrolases) while cell wall assembly is arrested.

**Local Anesthetic/Vasoconstrictor Precautions** No information available to require special precautions

**Effects on Dental Treatment** No effects or complications reported

**Other Adverse Effects**

1% to 10%: Gastrointestinal: Diarrhea

<1%:

- Central nervous system: CNS irritation, seizures, fever
- Dermatologic: Rash, urticaria
- Hematologic: Leukopenia, thrombocytopenia
- Hepatic: Transient elevation of liver enzymes

**Drug Interactions** Increased effect: High-dose probenecid decreases renal clearance of cephalosporins

**Drug Uptake**

Serum half-life: 36-60 minutes

Time to peak serum concentration:

- I.M.: Within 30 minutes
- I.V.: Within 5 minutes

**Pregnancy Risk Factor** B

**Generic Available** No

## Cephradine (SEF ra deen)

**Related Information**

Antibiotic Prophylaxis, Preprocedural Guidelines for Dental Patients *on page 1097*

**U.S. Brand Names** Velosef®

**Therapeutic Category** Antibiotic, Cephalosporin (First Generation)

**Use** Treatment of susceptible bacterial infections, including those caused by group A beta-hemolytic *Streptococcus*; used in in respiratory, genitourinary, gastrointestinal, skin and soft tissue, bone and joint infections. Also, antibiotic for premedication in patients not allergic to penicillin who may be at potential increased risk of hematogenous total joint infection.

**Usual Dosage** Oral:

Children ≥9 months: 25-50 mg/kg/day in divided doses every 6 hours

Adults: 250-500 mg every 6-12 hours

Joint prosthesis prophylaxis: 2 g 1 hour before procedure

**Mechanism of Action** Inhibits bacterial cell wall synthesis by binding to one or more of the penicillin-binding proteins (PBPs) which in turn inhibits the final transpeptidation step of peptidoglycan synthesis in bacterial cell walls, thus inhibiting cell wall biosynthesis. Bacteria eventually lyse due to ongoing activity of cell wall autolytic enzymes (autolysins and murein hydrolases) while cell wall assembly is arrested.

**Local Anesthetic/Vasoconstrictor Precautions** No information available to require special precautions

**Effects on Dental Treatment** No effects or complications reported

**Other Adverse Effects**

1% to 10%: Gastrointestinal: Diarrhea

<1%:

Dermatologic: Rash

Gastrointestinal: Nausea, vomiting, pseudomembranous colitis

Renal: Elevated BUN and creatinine

**Contraindications** Hypersensitivity to cephradine, any component, or cephalosporins

**Warnings/Precautions** Prolonged use may result in superinfection; use with caution in patients with a history of colitis; reduce dose in patients with renal dysfunction; a low incidence of cross-hypersensitivity with penicillins exists

**Drug Interactions** No data reported

**Drug Uptake**

Absorption: Oral is faster than I.M. but well absorbed from all routes

Serum half-life: 1-2 hours

Time to peak serum concentration: Oral, I.M.: Within 1-2 hours

**Pregnancy Risk Factor** B

**Dosage Forms**

Capsule: 250 mg, 500 mg

Powder for oral suspension: 125 mg/5 mL (5 mL, 100 mL, 200 mL); 250 mg/5 mL (5 mL, 100 mL, 200 mL)

**Generic Available** Yes

**Selected Readings**

"Advisory Statement. Antibiotic Prophylaxis for Dental Patients With Total Joint Replacements. American Dental Association; American Academy of Orthopedic Surgeons," *J Am Dent Assoc*, 1997, 128(7):1004-8.

Donowitz GR and Mandell GL, "Drug Therapy. Beta-Lactam Antibiotics (1)," *N Engl J Med*, 1988, 318(7):419-26.

Donowitz GR and Mandell GL, "Drug Therapy. Beta-Lactam Antibiotics (2)," *N Engl J Med*, 1988, 318(8):490-500.

Gustaferro CA and Steckelberg JM, "Cephalosporin Antimicrobial Agents and Related Compounds," *Mayo Clin Proc*, 1991, 66(10):1064-73.

♦ **Cephulac®** *see* Lactulose *on page 571*

♦ **Ceptaz™** *see* Ceftazidime *on page 207*

♦ **Cerebyx®** *see* Fosphenytoin *on page 458*

♦ **Ceredase® Injection** *see* Alglucerase *on page 47*

♦ **Cerezyme®** *see* Imiglucerase *on page 527*

## Cerivastatin (se ree va STAT in)

**U.S. Brand Names** Baycol™

**Therapeutic Category** HMG-CoA Reductase Inhibitor

**Synonyms** Cerivastatin Sodium

**Use** Adjunct to dietary therapy to for the reduction of elevated total and LDL cholesterol levels in patients with primary hypercholesterolemia and mixed

(Continued)

## Cerivastatin *(Continued)*

dyslipidemia when the response to dietary restriction of saturated fat and cholesterol and other nonpharmacological measures alone has been inadequate

**Usual Dosage** Adults: Oral: 0.3 mg once daily in the evening; may be taken with or without food

**Mechanism of Action** As an HMG-CoA reductase inhibitor, cerivastatin competitively inhibits 3-hydroxyl-3-methylglutaryl coenzyme A (HMG-CoA) reductase, the enzyme that catalyzes the rate-limiting step in cholesterol biosynthesis

**Local Anesthetic/Vasoconstrictor Precautions** No information available to require special precautions

**Effects on Dental Treatment** No effects or complications reported

**Drug Interactions** Concurrent use of erythromycin and HMG-CoA reductase inhibitors may result in rhabdomyolysis. The administration of erythromycin with cerivastatin produced a 50% increase in the area under the serum concentration curve for cerivastatin.

**Drug Uptake** Half-life: 2-3 hours

**Pregnancy Risk Factor** X

**Dosage Forms** Tablet, as sodium: 0.2 mg, 0.3 mg

- **Cerivastatin Sodium** *see* Cerivastatin *on previous page*
- **Cerose-DM® [OTC]** *see* Chlorpheniramine, Phenylephrine, and Dextromethorphan *on page 234*
- **Cerubidine®** *see* Daunorubicin Hydrochloride *on page 299*
- **Cerumenex®** *see* Triethanolamine Polypeptide Oleate-Condensate *on page 1016*
- **Cervidil® Vaginal Insert** *see* Dinoprostone *on page 337*
- **Cesamet®** *see* Nabilone *on page 695*
- **Cetacaine®** *see* Benzocaine, Butyl Aminobenzoate, Tetracaine, and Benzalkonium Chloride *on page 129*
- **Cetamide® Ophthalmic** *see* Sulfacetamide Sodium *on page 939*
- **Cetapred® Ophthalmic** *see* Sulfacetamide Sodium and Prednisolone *on page 940*

## Cetirizine (se TI ra zeen)

**U.S. Brand Names** Zyrtec®

**Canadian Brand Names** Reactine™

**Therapeutic Category** Antihistamine

**Synonyms** Cetirizine Hydrochloride; P-071; UCB-P071

**Use** Perennial and seasonal allergic rhinitis and other allergic symptoms including chronic idiopathic urticaria

**Usual Dosage** Children ≥12 years and Adults: Oral: 5-10 mg once daily, depending upon symptom severity

**Mechanism of Action** Competes with histamine for $H_1$-receptor sites on effector cells in the gastrointestinal tract, blood vessels, and respiratory tract

**Local Anesthetic/Vasoconstrictor Precautions** No information available to require special precautions

**Effects on Dental Treatment** No effects or complications reported

**Other Adverse Effects**

>10%: Central nervous system: Headache has been reported to occur in 10% to 12% of patients, drowsiness has been reported in as much as 26% of patients on high doses

1% to 10%:

Central nervous system: Fatigue, dizziness

Gastrointestinal: Dry mouth

<1%: Central nervous system: Depression

**Contraindications** Hypersensitivity to cetirizine, hydroxyzine, or any component

**Warnings/Precautions** Cetirizine should be used cautiously in patients with hepatic or renal dysfunction, the elderly and in nursing mothers. Doses >10 mg/day may cause significant drowsiness

**Drug Interactions** Increased toxicity: CNS depressants, anticholinergics

**Drug Uptake**

Onset of effect: Within 15-30 minutes

Absorption: Oral: Rapid

Serum half-life: 8-11 hours

Time to peak serum concentration: Within 30-60 minutes

**Pregnancy Risk Factor** B

**Generic Available** No

- **Cetirizine Hydrochloride** *see* Cetirizine *on this page*

## Cetylpyridinium (SEE til peer i DI nee um)

**U.S. Brand Names** Ceepryn® [OTC]; Cēpacol® Troches [OTC]

**Therapeutic Category** Local Anesthetic

**Synonyms** Cetylpyridinium Chloride

**Use** Temporary relief of sore throat

**Usual Dosage** Children >6 years and Adults: Oral: Dissolve 1 lozenge in the mouth every 2 hours as needed

**Local Anesthetic/Vasoconstrictor Precautions** No information available to require special precautions

**Effects on Dental Treatment** No effects or complications reported

**Pregnancy Risk Factor** C

**Dosage Forms**

Troches, as chloride: 1:1500 (24s)

Mouthwash, as chloride: 0.05% and alcohol 14% (180 mL)

**Generic Available** Yes

## Cetylpyridinium and Benzocaine

(SEE til peer i DI nee um & BEN zoe kane)

**U.S. Brand Names** Cēpacol® Anesthetic Troches [OTC]

**Therapeutic Category** Local Anesthetic, Oral

**Synonyms** Benzocaine and Cetylpyridinium Chloride

**Use** Symptomatic relief of sore throat

**Usual Dosage** Use as needed for sore throat

**Local Anesthetic/Vasoconstrictor Precautions** No information available to require special precautions

**Effects on Dental Treatment** No effects or complications reported

**Pregnancy Risk Factor** C

**Generic Available** Yes

- **Cetylpyridinium Chloride** *see* Cetylpyridinium *on this page*
- **Cevalin® [OTC]** *see* Ascorbic Acid *on page 97*
- **Cevi-Bid® [OTC]** *see* Ascorbic Acid *on page 97*
- **Ce-Vi-Sol® [OTC]** *see* Ascorbic Acid *on page 97*
- **Cevitamic Acid** *see* Ascorbic Acid *on page 97*
- **CFDN** *see* Cefdinir *on page 200*
- **Charcoaid® [OTC]** *see* Charcoal *on this page*

## Charcoal (CHAR kole)

**U.S. Brand Names** Actidose-Aqua® [OTC]; Actidose® With Sorbitol [OTC]; Charcoaid® [OTC]; Charcocaps® [OTC]; Insta-Char® [OTC]; Liqui-Char® [OTC]; SuperChar® [OTC]

**Therapeutic Category** Antidiarrheal; Antidote, Adsorbent; Antiflatulent

**Use** Emergency treatment in poisoning by drugs and chemicals; repetitive doses for gastric dialysis in uremia to adsorb various waste products, and repetitive doses have proven useful to enhance the elimination of certain drugs (eg, theophylline, phenobarbital, and aspirin)

**Usual Dosage** Oral:

Acute poisoning:

Charcoal with sorbitol: Single-dose:

Children 1-12 years: 1-2 g/kg/dose or 15-30 g or approximately 5-10 times the weight of the ingested poison; 1 g adsorbs 100-1000 mg of poison; the use of repeat oral charcoal with sorbitol doses is not recommended. In young children, sorbitol should be repeated no more than 1-2 times/day.

Adults: 30-100 g

Charcoal in water:

Single-dose:

Children 1-12 years: 15-30 g or 1-2 g/kg

Adults: 30-100 g or 1-2 g/kg

Multiple-dose:

Children 1-12 years: 20-60 g or 0.5-1 g/kg every 2-6 hours until clinical observations, serum drug concentration have returned to a subtherapeutic range, or charcoal stool apparent

Adults: 20-60 g or 0.5-1 g/kg every 2-6 hours

Gastric dialysis: Adults: 20-50 g every 6 hours for 1-2 days

Intestinal gas, diarrhea, GI distress: Adults: 520-975 mg after meals or at first sign of discomfort; repeat as needed to a maximum dose of 4.16 g/day

**Mechanism of Action** Adsorbs toxic substances or irritants, thus inhibiting GI absorption; adsorbs intestinal gas; the addition of sorbitol results in hyperosmotic laxative action causing catharsis

(Continued)

## Charcoal *(Continued)*

**Local Anesthetic/Vasoconstrictor Precautions** No information available to require special precautions

**Effects on Dental Treatment** No effects or complications reported

**Other Adverse Effects**

>10%: Gastrointestinal: Vomiting, diarrhea with sorbitol, constipation, stools will turn black

<1%: Gastrointestinal: Swelling of abdomen

**Drug Interactions** Do not administer concomitantly with syrup of ipecac; do not mix with milk, ice cream, or sherbet

**Drug Uptake** Absorption: Not absorbed from GI tract

**Pregnancy Risk Factor** C

**Generic Available** Yes


- ♦ **Charcocaps® [OTC]** *see* Charcoal *on previous page*
- ♦ **Chealamide®** *see* Edetate Disodium *on page 363*
- ♦ **Chemical Dependency and Smoking Cessation** *see page 1158*
- ♦ **Chenix®** *see* Chenodiol *on this page*
- ♦ **Chenodeoxycholic Acid** *see* Chenodiol *on this page*


## Chenodiol (kee noe DYE ole)

**U.S. Brand Names** Chenix®

**Therapeutic Category** Bile Acid; Gallstone Dissolution Agent

**Synonyms** Chenodeoxycholic Acid

**Use** Oral dissolution of cholesterol gallstones in selected patients

**Usual Dosage** Adults: Oral: 13-16 mg/kg/day in 2 divided doses, starting with 250 mg twice daily the first 2 weeks and increasing by 250 mg/day each week thereafter until the recommended or maximum tolerated dose is achieved

**Mechanism of Action** Chenodiol is a primary acid excreted into bile, normally constituting one-third of the total biliary bile acids. Synthesis of chenodiol is regulated by the relative composition and flux of cholesterol and bile acids through the hepatocyte by a negative feedback effect on the rate-limiting enzymes for synthesis of cholesterol (HMGCoA reductase) and bile acids (cholesterol 7 alpha-hydroxyl).

**Local Anesthetic/Vasoconstrictor Precautions** No information available to require special precautions

**Effects on Dental Treatment** No effects or complications reported

**Other Adverse Effects**

>10%:

Gastrointestinal: Diarrhea (mild), biliary pain

Miscellaneous: Aminotransferase increases

1% to 10%:

Endocrine & metabolic: Increases in cholesterol and LDL cholesterol

Gastrointestinal: Dyspepsia

<1%:

Gastrointestinal: Diarrhea (severe), cramps, nausea, vomiting, flatulence, constipation

Hematologic: Leukopenia

Hepatic: Intrahepatic cholestasis, higher cholecystectomy rates

**Contraindications** Presence of known hepatocyte dysfunction or bile ductal abnormalities; a gallbladder confirmed as nonvisualizing after two consecutive single doses of dye; radiopaque stones; gallstone complications or compelling reasons for gallbladder surgery; inflammatory bowel disease or active gastric or duodenal ulcer; pregnancy

**Warnings/Precautions** Chenodiol is hepatotoxic in animal models including subhuman Primates; chenodiol should be discontinued if aminotransferases exceed 3 times the upper normal limit; chenodiol may contribute to colon cancer in otherwise susceptible individuals

**Drug Interactions** Decreased effect: Antacids, cholestyramine, colestipol, oral contraceptives

**Pregnancy Risk Factor** X

**Dosage Forms** Tablet, film coated: 250 mg

**Generic Available** No


- ♦ **Cheracol®** *see* Guaifenesin and Codeine *on page 478*
- ♦ **Cheracol® D [OTC]** *see* Guaifenesin and Dextromethorphan *on page 479*
- ♦ **Chibroxin™** *see* Norfloxacin *on page 731*
- ♦ **Chiggertox® [OTC]** *see* Benzocaine *on page 128*
- ♦ **Children's Advil® Oral Suspension [OTC]** *see* Ibuprofen *on page 522*
- ♦ **Children's Hold® [OTC]** *see* Dextromethorphan *on page 314*
- ♦ **Children's Kaopectate® [OTC]** *see* Attapulgite *on page 109*

- **Children's Motrin® Oral Suspension [OTC]** *see* Ibuprofen *on page 522*
- **Children's Silapap® [OTC]** *see* Acetaminophen *on page 27*
- **Children's Silfedrine® [OTC]** *see* Pseudoephedrine *on page 863*
- **Children's Vitamins** *see* Vitamins, Multiple *on page 1051*
- **Chlo-Amine® [OTC]** *see* Chlorpheniramine *on page 231*
- **Chlorafed® Liquid [OTC]** *see* Chlorpheniramine and Pseudoephedrine *on page 233*

## Chloral Hydrate (KLOR al HYE drate)

**U.S. Brand Names** Aquachloral® Supprettes®

**Canadian Brand Names** Novo-Chlorhydrate; PMS-Chloral Hydrate

**Therapeutic Category** Hypnotic; Sedative

**Use**

Dental: Sedative/hypnotic for dental procedures

Medical: Short-term sedative and hypnotic (<2 weeks), sedative/hypnotic for diagnostic procedures; sedative prior to EEG evaluations

**Restrictions** C-IV; Refillable up to 5 times in 6 months

**Usual Dosage**

Children: Preoperative sedation: Oral: 50-75 mg/kg/dose 30-60 minutes prior to procedure with no follow-up dose; dose should not exceed 1000 mg

Adults: Very rarely used in adults as preoperative sedative in dentistry

Sedation, anxiety: 250 mg 3 times/day

Hypnotic: 500-1000 mg at bedtime or 30 minutes prior to procedure, not to exceed 2 g/24 hours

**Mechanism of Action** Central nervous system depressant effects are due to its active metabolite trichloroethanol, mechanism unknown

**Local Anesthetic/Vasoconstrictor Precautions** No information available to require special precautions

**Effects on Dental Treatment** No effects or complications reported

**Other Adverse Effects**

>10%: Gastrointestinal: Gastric irritation, nausea, vomiting, diarrhea

1% to 10%:

Central nervous system: Clumsiness, hallucinations, drowsiness, "hangover" effect

Dermatologic: Rash, urticaria

**Contraindications** Hypersensitivity to chloral hydrate or any component; hepatic or renal impairment; gastritis or ulcers; severe cardiac disease

**Warnings/Precautions** Use with caution in patients with porphyria; use with caution in neonates, drug may accumulate with repeated use, prolonged use in neonates associated with hyperbilirubinemia; tolerance to hypnotic effect develops, therefore, not recommended for use >2 weeks; taper dosage to avoid withdrawal with prolonged use; trichloroethanol (TCE), a metabolite of chloral hydrate, is a carcinogen in mice; there is no data in humans. Chloral hydrate is considered a second line hypnotic agent in adults and elderly.

**Drug Interactions** May potentiate effects of warfarin, central nervous system depressants, alcohol; vasodilation reaction (flushing, tachycardia, etc) may occur with concurrent use of alcohol; concomitant use of furosemide (I.V.) may result in flushing, sweating, and blood pressure changes

**Drug Uptake**

Duration of effect: 4-8 hours

Absorption: Oral: Rapid

Serum half-life: Active metabolite: 8-11 hours

Time to peak serum concentration: Within 0.5-1 hour

**Pregnancy Risk Factor** C

**Breast-feeding Considerations** May be taken while breast-feeding

**Dosage Forms**

Capsule: 250 mg, 500 mg

Suppository, rectal: 324 mg, 500 mg, 648 mg

Syrup: 250 mg/5 mL (10 mL); 500 mg/5 mL (5 mL, 10 mL, 480 mL)

**Dietary Considerations** May be taken with chilled liquid to mask taste

**Generic Available** Yes

## Chlorambucil (klor AM byoo sil)

**U.S. Brand Names** Leukeran®

**Therapeutic Category** Antineoplastic Agent, Alkylating Agent (Nitrogen Mustard)

**Use** Management of chronic lymphocytic leukemia (CLL), Hodgkin's and non-Hodgkin's lymphoma; breast and ovarian carcinoma, testicular carcinoma, choriocarcinoma; Waldenström's macroglobulinemia, and nephrotic syndrome unresponsive to conventional therapy

**Usual Dosage** Oral (**refer to individual protocols**):

(Continued)

## Chlorambucil *(Continued)*

Children:

General short courses: 0.1-0.2 mg/kg/day **or** 4.5 mg/m²/day for 3-6 weeks for remission induction (usual: 4-10 mg/day); maintenance therapy: 0.03-0.1 mg/kg/day (usual: 2-4 mg/day)

Nephrotic syndrome: 0.1-0.2 mg/kg/day every day for 5-15 weeks with low-dose prednisone

Chronic lymphocytic leukemia (CLL):

Biweekly regimen: Initial: 0.4 mg/kg/dose every 2 weeks; increase dose by 0.1 mg/kg every 2 weeks until a response occurs and/or myelosuppression occurs

Monthly regimen: Initial: 0.4 mg/kg, increase dose by 0.2 mg/kg every 4 weeks until a response occurs and/or myelosuppression occurs

Malignant lymphomas:

Non-Hodgkin's lymphoma: 0.1 mg/kg/day

Hodgkin's lymphoma: 0.2 mg/kg/day

Adults: 0.1-0.2 mg/kg/day **or** 3-6 mg/m²/day for 3-6 weeks, then adjust dose on basis of blood counts. Pulse dosing has been used in CLL as intermittent, biweekly, or monthly doses of 0.4 mg/kg and increased by 0.1 mg/kg until the disease is under control or toxicity ensues. An alternate regimen is 14 mg/m²/day for 5 days, repeated every 21-28 days.

**Mechanism of Action** Interferes with DNA replication and RNA transcription by alkylation and cross-linking the strands of DNA

**Local Anesthetic/Vasoconstrictor Precautions** No information available to require special precautions

**Effects on Dental Treatment** No effects or complications reported

**Other Adverse Effects**

>10%:

Hematologic: Myelosuppressive: Use with caution when receiving radiation; bone marrow suppression frequently occurs and occasionally bone marrow failure has occurred; blood counts should be monitored closely while undergoing treatment; leukopenia, thrombocytopenia, anemia. WBC: Moderate; Platelets: Moderate; Onset (days): 7; Nadir (days): 10-14; Recovery (days): 28.

Secondary malignancies: Increased incidence of AML

1% to 10%:

Dermatologic: Skin rashes

Endocrine & metabolic: Menstrual changes, hyperuricemia

Gastrointestinal: Diarrhea, oral ulceration are infrequent

Emetic potential: Low (<10%)

<1%:

Central nervous system: Confusion, agitation, ataxia, hallucination; rarely generalized or focal seizures, drug fever

Dermatologic: Rash, skin hypersensitivity

Fertility impairment: Has caused chromosomal damage in man, oligospermia, both reversible and permanent sterility have occurred in both sexes; can produce amenorrhea in females, oligospermia

Hematologic: Leukopenia, thrombocytopenia

Hepatic: Hepatic necrosis, hepatotoxicity

Neuromuscular & skeletal: Peripheral neuropathy, tremors, muscular twitching, weakness

Ocular: Keratitis

Respiratory: Pulmonary fibrosis

**Drug Uptake**

Absorption: 70% to 80%

Serum half-life: 90 minutes to 2 hours

**Pregnancy Risk Factor** D

**Generic Available** No

## Chloramphenicol (klor am FEN i kole)

**U.S. Brand Names** AK-Chlor®; Chloromycetin®; Chloroptic®; Ophthochlor®

**Canadian Brand Names** Diochloram; Pentamycetin®; Sopamycetin

**Therapeutic Category** Antibiotic, Ophthalmic; Antibiotic, Otic; Antibiotic, Miscellaneous

**Use** Treatment of serious infections due to organisms resistant to other less toxic antibiotics or when its penetrability into the site of infection is clinically superior to other antibiotics to which the organism is sensitive; useful in infections caused by *Bacteroides, H. influenzae, Neisseria meningitidis, Salmonella,* and *Rickettsia*

**Usual Dosage**

Meningitis: Oral, I.V.: Children: 75-100 mg/kg/day divided every 6 hours

Other infections: Oral, I.V.:

Children: 50-75 mg/kg/day divided every 6 hours; maximum daily dose: 4 g/day

Adults: 50-100 mg/kg/day in divided doses every 6 hours; maximum daily dose: 4 g/day

Ophthalmic: Children and Adults: Instill 1-2 drops or 1.25 cm (1/2" of ointment every 3-4 hours); increase interval between applications after 48 hours to 2-3 times/day

Otic solution: Instill 2-3 drops into ear 3 times/day

Topical: Gently rub into the affected area 1-4 times/day

**Mechanism of Action** Reversibly binds to 50S ribosomal subunits of susceptible organisms preventing amino acids from being transferred to growing peptide chains thus inhibiting protein synthesis

**Local Anesthetic/Vasoconstrictor Precautions** No information available to require special precautions

**Effects on Dental Treatment** No effects or complications reported

**Other Adverse Effects**

<1%:

Central nervous system: Nightmares, headache

Dermatologic: Rash

Gastrointestinal: Diarrhea, stomatitis, enterocolitis, nausea, vomiting

Hematologic: Bone marrow suppression, aplastic anemia

Neuromuscular & skeletal: Peripheral neuropathy

Ocular: Optic neuritis

Miscellaneous: Gray baby syndrome

**Three (3) major toxicities associated with chloramphenicol include:**

Aplastic anemia, an idiosyncratic reaction which can occur with any route of administration; usually occurs 3 weeks to 12 months after initial exposure to chloramphenicol

Bone marrow suppression is thought to be dose-related with serum concentrations >25 µg/mL and reversible once chloramphenicol is discontinued; anemia and neutropenia may occur during the first week of therapy

Gray baby syndrome is characterized by circulatory collapse, cyanosis, acidosis, abdominal distention, myocardial depression, coma, and death; reaction appears to be associated with serum levels ≥50 µg/mL; may result from drug accumulation in patients with impaired hepatic or renal function

**Drug Interactions**

Decreased effect: Phenobarbital and rifampin may decrease concentration of chloramphenicol

Increased toxicity: Chloramphenicol inhibits the metabolism of chlorpropamide, phenytoin, oral anticoagulants

**Drug Uptake**

Serum half-life: (Prolonged with markedly reduced liver function or combined liver/kidney dysfunction):

Normal renal function: 1.6-3.3 hours

End-stage renal disease: 3-7 hours

Cirrhosis: 10-12 hours

Time to peak serum concentration: Oral: Within 0.5-3 hours

**Pregnancy Risk Factor** C

**Generic Available** Yes

## Chloramphenicol and Prednisolone

(klor am FEN i kole & pred NIS oh lone)

**U.S. Brand Names** Chloroptic-P® Ophthalmic

**Therapeutic Category** Antibiotic, Ophthalmic; Corticosteroid, Ophthalmic

**Use** Topical anti-infective and corticosteroid for treatment of ocular infections

**Usual Dosage** Ophthalmic: Instill 1-2 drops in eye(s) 2-4 times/day

**Local Anesthetic/Vasoconstrictor Precautions** No information available to require special precautions

**Effects on Dental Treatment** No effects or complications reported

**Pregnancy Risk Factor** C

**Generic Available** No

## Chloramphenicol, Polymyxin B, and Hydrocortisone

(klor am FEN i kole, pol i MIKS in bee, & hye droe KOR ti sone)

**U.S. Brand Names** Ophthocort® Ophthalmic

**Therapeutic Category** Antibiotic, Ophthalmic

**Use** Topical anti-infective and corticosteroid for treatment of ocular infections

**Usual Dosage** Apply 1/2" ribbon every 3-4 hours until improvement occurs

**Local Anesthetic/Vasoconstrictor Precautions** No information available to require special precautions

**Effects on Dental Treatment** No effects or complications reported

(Continued)

## Chloramphenicol, Polymyxin B, and Hydrocortisone *(Continued)*

**Pregnancy Risk Factor** C

**Generic Available** No

- **Chloraseptic® Oral [OTC]** *see* Phenol *on page 791*
- **Chlorate® [OTC]** *see* Chlorpheniramine *on page 231*

## Chlordiazepoxide (klor dye az e POKS ide)

**U.S. Brand Names** Libritabs®; Librium®; Mitran®; Reposans-10®

**Canadian Brand Names** Apo®-Chlordiazepoxide; Corax®; Medilium®; Novo-Poxide; Solium®

**Therapeutic Category** Benzodiazepine; Hypnotic; Sedative

**Use** Approved for anxiety, may be useful for acute alcohol withdrawal symptoms

**Usual Dosage**

Children:

<6 years: Not recommended

>6 years: Anxiety: Oral, I.M.: 0.5 mg/kg/24 hours divided every 6-8 hours

Adults:

Anxiety:

Oral: 15-100 mg divided 3-4 times/day

I.M., I.V.: Initial: 50-100 mg followed by 25-50 mg 3-4 times/day as needed

Preoperative anxiety: I.M.: 50-100 mg prior to surgery

Alcohol withdrawal symptoms: Oral, I.V.: 50-100 mg to start, dose may be repeated in 2-4 hours as necessary to a maximum of 300 mg/24 hours

**Mechanism of Action** Benzodiazepines appear to potentiate the effects of GABA and other inhibitory transmitters by binding to specific benzodiazepine receptor sites; benzodiazepine anxiolytic sedative that produces CNS depression at the subcortical level, except at high doses, whereby it works at the cortical level

**Local Anesthetic/Vasoconstrictor Precautions** No information available to require special precautions

**Effects on Dental Treatment** >10% of patients will experience dry mouth which disappears with cessation of drug therapy

**Other Adverse Effects**

>10%:

Cardiovascular: Chest pain

Central nervous system: Drowsiness, fatigue, lightheadedness, memory impairment, insomnia, anxiety, depression, headache, impaired coordination

Dermatologic: Skin eruptions, rash

Endocrine & metabolic: Decreased libido

Gastrointestinal: Nausea, constipation, vomiting, diarrhea, increased or decreased appetite

Neuromuscular & skeletal: Dysarthria

Ocular: Blurred vision

Miscellaneous: Decreased salivation, sweating

1% to 10%:

Cardiovascular: Hypotension, tachycardia, edema, syncope

Central nervous system: Confusion, mental impairment, nervousness, dizziness, akathisia

Dermatologic: Dermatitis

Gastrointestinal: Weight gain or loss, increased salivation

Neuromuscular & skeletal: Rigidity, tremor, muscle cramps

Otic: Tinnitus

Respiratory: Nasal congestion, hyperventilation

<1%:

Endocrine & metabolic: Menstrual irregularities

Hematologic: Blood dyscrasias

Neuromuscular & skeletal: Depressed reflexes

Miscellaneous: Drug dependence

**Drug Interactions** Potentiation of chlordiazepoxide-induced sedation may occur with alcohol and sedative-hypnotics

**Drug Uptake**

Serum half-life: 6.6-25 hours

End-stage renal disease: 5-30 hours

Cirrhosis: 30-63 hours

Time to peak serum concentration:

Oral: Within 2 hours

I.M.: Results in lower peak plasma levels than oral

**Pregnancy Risk Factor** D

**Dosage Forms**

Capsule, as hydrochloride: 5 mg, 10 mg, 25 mg
Powder for injection, as hydrochloride: 100 mg
Tablet: 5 mg, 10 mg, 25 mg

**Generic Available** Yes

- **Chlordiazepoxide and Amitriptyline** *see* Amitriptyline and Chlordiazepoxide *on page 68*
- **Chlordiazepoxide and Clidinium** *see* Clidinium and Chlordiazepoxide *on page 258*
- **Chloresium® [OTC]** *see* Chlorophyll *on next page*

## Chlorhexidine Gluconate (klor HEKS i deen GLOO koe nate)

**Related Information**

Dentin Hypersensitivity; High Caries Index; Xerostomia *on page 1145*
Oral Nonviral Soft Tissue Ulcerations or Erosions *on page 1141*
Periodontal Diseases *on page 1132*

**U.S. Brand Names** BactoShield® Topical [OTC]; Betasept® [OTC]; Dyna-Hex® Topical [OTC]; Exidine® Scrub [OTC]; Hibiclens® Topical [OTC]; Hibistat® Topical [OTC]; Peridex® Oral Rinse; Periochip®; PerioGard®

**Canadian Brand Names** Bactigras® (Chlorhexidine Acetate); Hibidil® 1:2000; Hibitane® Skin Cleanser; Oro-Clense

**Therapeutic Category** Antibacterial, Oral Rinse; Antibiotic, Topical; Antimicrobial Mouth Rinse; Antiplaque Agent

**Use**

Dental:

Antibacterial dental rinse; chlorhexidine is active against gram-positive and gram-negative organisms, facultative anaerobes, aerobes, and yeast

Chip, for periodontal pocket insertion; indicated as an adjunct to scaling and root planing procedures for reduction of pocket depth in patients with adult periodontitis; may be used as part of a periodontal maintenance program

Medical: Skin cleanser for surgical scrub, cleanser for skin wounds, germicidal hand rinse

**Usual Dosage** Periodontal chip: Adults: One chip is inserted into a periodontal pocket with a probing pocket depth ≥5 mm. Up to 8 chips may be inserted in a single visit. Treatment is recommended every 3 months in pockets with a remaining depth ≥5 mm. If dislodgment occurs 7 days or more after placement, the subject is considered to have had the full course of treatment. If dislodgment occurs within 48 hours, a new chip should be inserted.

Insertion of periodontal chip: Pocket should be isolated and surrounding area dried prior to chip insertion. The chip should be grasped using forceps with the rounded edges away from the forceps. The chip should be inserted into the periodontal pocket to its maximum depth. It may be maneuvered into position using the tips of the forceps or a flat instrument. The chip biodegrades completely and does not need to be removed. Patients should avoid dental floss at the site of Periochip® insertion for 10 days after placement because flossing might dislodge the chip.

**Mechanism of Action** The bactericidal effect of chlorhexidine is a result of the binding of this cationic molecule to negatively charged bacterial cell walls and extramicrobial complexes. At low concentrations, this causes an alteration of bacterial cell osmotic equilibrium and leakage of potassium and phosphorous resulting in a bacteriostatic effect. At high concentrations of chlorhexidine, the cytoplasmic contents of the bacterial cell precipitate and result in cell death.

**Local Anesthetic/Vasoconstrictor Precautions** No information available to require special precautions

**Effects on Dental Treatment** Swelling of face has been reported

**Other Adverse Effects**

>10%: Increase of tartar on teeth, changes in taste. Staining of oral surfaces (mucosa, teeth, dorsum of tongue) may be visible as soon as 1 week after therapy begins and is more pronounced when there is a heavy accumulation of unremoved plaque and when teeth fillings have rough surfaces. Stain does not have a clinically adverse effect but because removal may not be possible, patients with anterior restoration should be advised of the potential permanency of the stain.

1% to 10%: Tongue irritation, oral irritation

<1%: Respiratory: Nasal congestion, dyspnea

Chlorhexidine periodontal chip (Periochip®): In clinical trials, adverse reactions were similar to those reported with placement of a placebo chip. Most oral pain or sensitivity occurred after the first chip placement, was limited to the first week, and resolved spontaneously. Reactions occurred less frequently with subsequent chip placement at 3 and 6 months. Events reported with a frequency >1% included: toothache (50.7%), upper respiratory infection

(Continued)

## Chlorhexidine Gluconate *(Continued)*

(28.4%), headache (27.1%), sinusitis (13.8%), bronchitis (6.2%), back pain (6.7%), abscess (5.8%), pain (4.9%), allergy (4%), gum hyperplasia (3.6%), pharyngitis (3.6%), dyspepsia (3.1%), arthrosis (2.7%), ulcerative stomatitis (2.2%), and tendonitis (2.2%). Gingival bleeding was reported in 1% of patients in both the treatment and placebo groups. The frequency of tooth disorders, including cracked/broken/fractured teeth, mobile teeth, and lost crowns, bridges or fillings was 6.2% in the chlorhexidine group and 6.8% in the placebo group.

**Warnings/Precautions** Use of periodontal chip has not been studied in patients with an acutely abscessed periodontal pocket and is not recommended

**Drug Interactions** No data reported

**Drug Uptake** Periochip® releases chlorhexidine *in vitro* in a biphasic manner, initially releasing approximately 40% of the chlorhexidine within the first 24 hours and then releasing the remaining chlorhexidine for 7-10 days

**Pregnancy Risk Factor** B

**Breast-feeding Considerations** No data reported

**Dosage Forms**

Foam, topical, with isopropyl alcohol 4% (BactoShield®): 4% (180 mL)

Liquid, topical, with isopropyl alcohol 4%:

Dyna-Hex® Skin Cleanser: 2% (120 mL, 240 mL, 480 mL, 960 mL, 4000 mL); 4% (120 mL, 240 mL, 480 mL, 4000 mL)

BactoShield® 2: 2% (960 mL)

BactoShield®, Betasept®, Exidine® Skin Cleanser, Hibiclens® Skin Cleanser: 4% (15 mL, 120 mL, 240 mL, 480 mL, 960 mL, 4000 mL)

Rinse:

Oral (mint flavor) (Peridex®, PerioGard®): 0.12% with alcohol 11.6% (480 mL)

Topical (Hibistat® Hand Rinse): 0.5% with isopropyl alcohol 70% (120 mL, 240 mL)

Sponge/Brush (Hibiclens®): 4% with isopropyl alcohol 4% (22 mL)

Wipes (Hibistat®): 0.5% (50s)

**Generic Available** Yes

♦ **2-Chlorodeoxyadenosine** *see* Cladribine *on page 255*

♦ **Chloroethane** *see* Ethyl Chloride *on page 410*

♦ **Chloromycetin®** *see* Chloramphenicol *on page 222*

## Chlorophyll (KLOR oh fil)

**U.S. Brand Names** Chloresium® [OTC]; Derifil® [OTC]; Nullo® [OTC]; PALS® [OTC]

**Therapeutic Category** Gastrointestinal Agent, Miscellaneous; Topical Skin Product

**Synonyms** Chlorophyllin

**Use** Topically promotes normal healing, relieves pain and swelling, and reduces malodors in wounds, burns, surface ulcers, abrasions and skin irritations; used orally to control fecal and urinary odors in colostomy, ileostomy, or incontinence

**Usual Dosage**

Topical: Apply generously and cover with gauze, linen, or other appropriate dressing; do not change dressings more often than every 48-72 hours

Oral: Children >12 years and Adults: 1-2 tablets/day; may increase to 3 tablets/day

Ostomy: Take tablets orally or place in the appliance

**Local Anesthetic/Vasoconstrictor Precautions** No information available to require special precautions

**Effects on Dental Treatment** No effects or complications reported

**Other Adverse Effects** 1% to 10%: Gastrointestinal: Mild diarrhea, green stools

**Generic Available** No

♦ **Chlorophyllin** *see* Chlorophyll *on this page*

## Chloroprocaine (klor oh PROE kane)

**Related Information**

Oral Pain *on page 1122*

**U.S. Brand Names** Nesacaine®; Nesacaine®-MPF

**Therapeutic Category** Dental/Local Anesthetics; Local Anesthetic, Injectable

**Use** Infiltration anesthesia and peripheral and epidural anesthesia

**Usual Dosage** Dosage varies with anesthetic procedure, the area to be anesthetized, the vascularity of the tissues, depth of anesthesia required, degree of muscle relaxation required, and duration of anesthesia; range: 1.5-25 mL of 2% to 3% solution; single adult dose should not exceed 800 mg

Infiltration and peripheral nerve block: 1% to 2%

Infiltration, peripheral and central nerve block, including caudal and epidural block: 2% to 3%, without preservatives

**Mechanism of Action** Chloroprocaine HCl is benzoic acid, 4-amino-2-chloro-2-(diethylamino) ethyl ester monohydrochloride. Chloroprocaine is an ester-type local anesthetic, which stabilizes the neuronal membranes and prevents initiation and transmission of nerve impulses thereby affecting local anesthetic actions. Local anesthetics including chloroprocaine, reversibly prevent generation and conduction of electrical impulses in neurons by decreasing the transient increase in permeability to sodium. The differential sensitivity generally depends on the size of the fiber; small fibers are more sensitive than larger fibers and require a longer period for recovery. Sensory pain fibers are usually blocked first, followed by fibers that transmit sensations of temperature, touch, and deep pressure. High concentrations block sympathetic somatic sensory and somatic motor fibers. The spread of anesthesia depends upon the distribution of the solution. This is primarily dependent on the volume of drug injected.

**Local Anesthetic/Vasoconstrictor Precautions** No information available to require special precautions

**Effects on Dental Treatment** No effects or complications reported

**Other Adverse Effects** <1%:

Cardiovascular: Myocardial depression, hypotension, bradycardia, cardiovascular collapse, edema

Central nervous system: Anxiety, restlessness, disorientation, confusion, seizures, drowsiness, unconsciousness, chills, shivering

Dermatologic: Urticaria

Gastrointestinal: Nausea, vomiting

Local: Transient stinging or burning at injection site

Neuromuscular & skeletal: Tremor

Ocular: Blurred vision

Otic: Tinnitus

Respiratory: Respiratory arrest

Miscellaneous: Anaphylactoid reactions

**Drug Interactions** PABA (from ester-type anesthetics) may inhibit sulfonamides

**Drug Uptake**

Onset of action: 6-12 minutes

Duration: 30-60 minutes

**Pregnancy Risk Factor** C

**Dosage Forms** Injection, as hydrochloride:

Preservative free (Nesacaine®-MPF): 2% (30 mL); 3% (30 mL)

With preservative (Nesacaine®): 1% (30 mL); 2% (30 mL)

**Generic Available** No

♦ **Chloroptic®** *see* Chloramphenicol *on page 222*

♦ **Chloroptic-P® Ophthalmic** *see* Chloramphenicol and Prednisolone *on page 223*

## Chloroquine and Primaquine (KLOR oh kwin & PRIM a kween)

**U.S. Brand Names** Aralen® Phosphate With Primaquine Phosphate

**Therapeutic Category** Antimalarial Agent

**Use** Prophylaxis of malaria, regardless of species, in all areas where the disease is endemic

**Usual Dosage** Oral: Start at least 1 day before entering the endemic area; continue for 8 weeks after leaving the endemic area

Children: For suggested weekly dosage (based on body weight), see table:

| Weight | | Chloroquine Base (mg) | Primaquine Base (mg) | Dose* (mL) |
|---|---|---|---|---|
| lb | kg | | | |
| 10-15 | 4.5-6.8 | 20 | 3 | 2.5 |
| 16-25 | 7.3-11.4 | 40 | 6 | 5 |
| 26-35 | 11.8-15.9 | 60 | 9 | 7.5 |
| 36-45 | 16.4-20.5 | 80 | 12 | 10 |
| 46-55 | 20.9-25 | 100 | 15 | 12.5 |
| 56-100 | 25.4-45.4 | 150 | 22.5 | ½ tablet |
| 100+ | >45.4 | 300 | 45 | 1 tablet |

*Dose based on liquid containing approximately 40 mg of chloroquine base and 6 mg primaquine base per 5 mL, prepared from chloroquine phosphate with primaquine phosphate tablets.

Adults: 1 tablet/week on the same day each week

**Mechanism of Action** Chloroquine concentrates within parasite acid vesicles and raises internal pH resulting in inhibition of parasite growth; may involve aggregates of ferriprotoporphyrin IX acting as chloroquine receptors causing (Continued)

## Chloroquine and Primaquine *(Continued)*

membrane damage; may also interfere with nucleoprotein synthesis. Primaquine eliminates the primary tissue exoerythrocytic forms of *P. falciparum*; disrupts mitochondria and binds to DNA.

**Local Anesthetic/Vasoconstrictor Precautions** No information available to require special precautions

**Effects on Dental Treatment** No effects or complications reported

**Other Adverse Effects**

1% to 10%: Gastrointestinal: Diarrhea, nausea

<1%:

- Cardiovascular: Hypotension, EKG changes
- Central nervous system: Fatigue, personality changes, headache
- Dermatologic: Pruritus, hair bleaching
- Gastrointestinal: Anorexia, vomiting, stomatitis
- Hematologic: Blood dyscrasias
- Ocular: Retinopathy, blurred vision

**Drug Interactions**

Decreased absorption if administered concomitantly with kaolin and magnesium trisilicate

Increased toxicity/levels with cimetidine

**Drug Uptake** Absorption: Oral: Both drugs are readily absorbed

**Pregnancy Risk Factor** C

**Generic Available** No

## Chloroquine Phosphate (KLOR oh kwin FOS fate)

**U.S. Brand Names** Aralen® Phosphate

**Therapeutic Category** Amebicide; Antimalarial Agent

**Use** Suppression or chemoprophylaxis of malaria; treatment of uncomplicated or mild-moderate malaria; extraintestinal amebiasis; rheumatoid arthritis; discoid lupus erythematosus, scleroderma, pemphigus

**Usual Dosage** Oral (**dosage expressed in terms of mg of base**):

Suppression or prophylaxis of malaria:

- Children: Administer 5 mg base/kg/week on the same day each week (not to exceed 300 mg base/dose); begin 1-2 weeks prior to exposure; continue for 4-6 weeks after leaving endemic area; if suppressive therapy is not begun prior to exposure, double the initial loading dose to 10 mg base/kg and give in 2 divided doses 6 hours apart, followed by the usual dosage regimen
- Adults: 300 mg/week (base) on the same day each week; begin 1-2 weeks prior to exposure; continue for 4-6 weeks after leaving endemic area; if suppressive therapy is not begun prior to exposure, double the initial loading dose to 600 mg base and give in 2 divided doses 6 hours apart, followed by the usual dosage regimen

Acute attack:

- Children: 10 mg/kg on day 1, followed by 5 mg/kg 6 hours later and 5 mg/kg on days 2 and 3
- Adults: 600 mg on day 1, followed by 300 mg 6 hours later, followed by 300 mg on days 2 and 3

Extraintestinal amebiasis:

- Children: 10 mg/kg once daily for 2-3 weeks (up to 300 mg base/day)
- Adults: 600 mg base/day for 2 days followed by 300 mg base/day for at least 2-3 weeks

**Mechanism of Action** Binds to and inhibits DNA and RNA polymerase; interferes with metabolism and hemoglobin utilization by parasites; inhibits prostaglandin effects; chloroquine concentrates within parasite acid vesicles and raises internal pH resulting in inhibition of parasite growth; may involve aggregates of ferriprotoporphyrin IX acting as chloroquine receptors causing membrane damage; may also interfere with nucleoprotein synthesis

**Local Anesthetic/Vasoconstrictor Precautions** No information available to require special precautions

**Effects on Dental Treatment** No effects or complications reported

**Other Adverse Effects**

1% to 10%: Gastrointestinal: Nausea, diarrhea

<1%:

- Cardiovascular: Hypotension, EKG changes
- Central nervous system: Fatigue, personality changes, headache
- Dermatologic: Pruritus, hair bleaching
- Gastrointestinal: Anorexia, vomiting, stomatitis
- Hematologic: Blood dyscrasias
- Ocular: Retinopathy, blurred vision

**Drug Interactions**

Decreased absorption if administered concomitantly with kaolin and magnesium trisilicate

Increased toxicity/levels with cimetidine

**Drug Uptake**

Absorption: Oral: Rapid (~89%)

Serum half-life: 3-5 days

Time to peak serum concentration: Within 1-2 hours

**Pregnancy Risk Factor** C

**Generic Available** Yes

## Chlorothiazide (klor oh THYE a zide)

**Related Information**

Cardiovascular Diseases *on page 1066*

**U.S. Brand Names** Diurigen®; Diuril®

**Therapeutic Category** Diuretic, Thiazide

**Use** Management of mild to moderate hypertension, or edema associated with congestive heart failure, pregnancy, or nephrotic syndrome in patients unable to take oral hydrochlorothiazide, when a thiazide is the diuretic of choice

**Usual Dosage** I.V. form not recommended for children and should only be used in adults if unable to take oral in emergency situations:

Children >6 months:

- Oral: 20 mg/kg/day in 2 divided doses
- I.V.: 4 mg/kg/day

Adults:

- Oral: 500 mg to 2 g/day divided in 1-2 doses
- I.V.: 100-500 mg/day

Elderly: Oral: 500 mg once daily **or** 1 g 3 times/week

**Mechanism of Action** Inhibits sodium reabsorption in the distal tubules causing increased excretion of sodium and water as well as potassium and hydrogen ions, magnesium, phosphate, calcium

**Local Anesthetic/Vasoconstrictor Precautions** No information available to require special precautions

**Effects on Dental Treatment** No effects or complications reported

**Other Adverse Effects**

1% to 10%: Endocrine & metabolic: Hypokalemia, hyponatremia

<1%:

- Cardiovascular: Arrhythmia, weak pulse, orthostatic hypotension
- Central nervous system: Dizziness, vertigo, headache, fever
- Dermatologic: Rash, photosensitivity
- Endocrine & metabolic: Hypochloremic alkalosis, hyperglycemia, hyperlipidemia, hyperuricemia
- Hematologic: Rarely blood dyscrasias, leukopenia, agranulocytosis, aplastic anemia
- Neuromuscular & skeletal: Paresthesias
- Renal: Prerenal azotemia

**Drug Interactions**

Decreased absorption of thiazides with cholestyramine resins; chlorothiazide causes a decreased effect of oral hypoglycemics

Increased toxicity: Digitalis glycosides, lithium (decreased clearance), probenecid

**Drug Uptake**

Onset of diuresis: Oral: 2 hours

Duration of diuretic action:

- Oral: 6-12 hours
- I.V.: ~2 hours

Absorption: Oral: Poor

Serum half-life: 1-2 hours

**Pregnancy Risk Factor** D

**Generic Available** Yes: Tablet

## Chlorothiazide and Methyldopa

(klor oh THYE a zide & meth il DOE pa)

**U.S. Brand Names** Aldoclor®

**Canadian Brand Names** Supres®

**Therapeutic Category** Antihypertensive Agent, Combination

**Synonyms** Methyldopa and Chlorothiazide

**Use** Treatment of hypertension

**Usual Dosage** Oral: 1 tablet 2-3 times/day for first 48 hours, then adjust

**Local Anesthetic/Vasoconstrictor Precautions** No information available to require special precautions

(Continued)

## Chlorothiazide and Methyldopa *(Continued)*

**Effects on Dental Treatment** No effects or complications reported
**Pregnancy Risk Factor** D
**Generic Available** No

## Chlorothiazide and Reserpine

(klor oh THYE a zide & re SER peen)
**U.S. Brand Names** Diupres-250®; Diupres-500®
**Therapeutic Category** Antihypertensive Agent, Combination
**Synonyms** Reserpine and Chlorothiazide
**Use** Management of hypertension
**Usual Dosage** Oral: 1-2 tablets 1-2 times/day
**Local Anesthetic/Vasoconstrictor Precautions** No information available to require special precautions
**Effects on Dental Treatment** No effects or complications reported
**Pregnancy Risk Factor** D
**Generic Available** Yes

## Chlorotrianisene (klor oh trye AN i seen)

**Related Information**
Endocrine Disorders & Pregnancy *on page 1082*
**U.S. Brand Names** TACE®
**Therapeutic Category** Estrogen Derivative
**Use** Treat inoperable prostatic cancer; management of atrophic vaginitis, female hypogonadism, vasomotor symptoms of menopause
**Usual Dosage** Adults: Oral:
- Atrophic vaginitis: 12-25 mg/day in 28-day cycles (21 days on and 7 days off)
- Female hypogonadism: 12-25 mg cyclically for 21 days. May be followed by I.M. progesterone 100 mg or 5 days of oral progestin; next course may begin on day 5 of induced uterine bleeding.
- Postpartum breast engorgement: 12 mg 4 times/day for 7 days or 50 mg every 6 hours for 6 doses; give first dose within 8 hours after delivery
- Vasomotor symptoms associated with menopause: 12-25 mg cyclically for 30 days; one or more courses may be prescribed
- Prostatic cancer (inoperable/progressing): 12-25 mg/day

**Mechanism of Action** Diethylstilbestrol derivative with similar estrogenic actions
**Local Anesthetic/Vasoconstrictor Precautions** No information available to require special precautions
**Effects on Dental Treatment** No effects or complications reported
**Other Adverse Effects**
- >10%:
  - Cardiovascular: Peripheral edema
  - Endocrine & metabolic: Enlargement of breasts (female and male), breast tenderness
  - Gastrointestinal: Nausea, anorexia, bloating
- 1% to 10%:
  - Central nervous system: Headache
  - Endocrine & metabolic: Increased libido (female), decreased libido (male)
  - Gastrointestinal: Vomiting, diarrhea
- <1%:
  - Cardiovascular: Hypertension, thromboembolism, myocardial infarction, edema
  - Central nervous system: Depression, dizziness, anxiety, stroke
  - Dermatologic: Chloasma, melasma, rash
  - Endocrine & metabolic: Breast tumors, amenorrhea, alterations in frequency and flow of menses, decreased glucose tolerance, hypertriglyceridemia, elevated LDL
  - Gastrointestinal: GI distress
  - Hepatic: Cholestatic jaundice
  - Ocular: Intolerance to contact lenses
  - Miscellaneous: Increased susceptibility to *Candida* infection

**Drug Interactions** No data reported
**Drug Uptake**
Onset of therapeutic effect: Commonly occurs within 14 days of therapy
**Pregnancy Risk Factor** X
**Generic Available** No

## Chloroxine (klor OKS een)

**U.S. Brand Names** Capitrol®
**Therapeutic Category** Antiseborrheic Agent, Topical; Shampoos

**Use** Treatment of dandruff or seborrheic dermatitis of the scalp

**Usual Dosage** Use twice weekly, massage into wet scalp, avoid contact with eyes, lather should remain on the scalp for approximately 3 minutes, then rinsed; application should be repeated and the scalp rinsed thoroughly

**Local Anesthetic/Vasoconstrictor Precautions** No information available to require special precautions

**Effects on Dental Treatment** No effects or complications reported

**Pregnancy Risk Factor** C

**Generic Available** No

- **Chlorphed® [OTC]** *see* Brompheniramine *on page 151*
- **Chlorphed®-LA Nasal Solution [OTC]** *see* Oxymetazoline *on page 755*

## Chlorphenesin (klor FEN e sin)

**U.S. Brand Names** Maolate®

**Canadian Brand Names** Mycil®

**Therapeutic Category** Muscle Relaxant; Skeletal Muscle Relaxant

**Use** Adjunctive treatment of discomfort in short-term, acute, painful musculoskeletal conditions

**Usual Dosage** Adults: Oral: 800 mg 3 times/day, then adjusted to lowest effective dosage, usually 400 mg 4 times/day for up to a maximum of 2 months

**Local Anesthetic/Vasoconstrictor Precautions** No information available to require special precautions

**Effects on Dental Treatment** No effects or complications reported

**Other Adverse Effects**

>10%: Central nervous system: Somnolence

1% to 10%:

- Cardiovascular: Tachycardia, flushing of face, tightness in chest, syncope
- Central nervous system: Mental depression, dizziness, lightheadedness, headache, paradoxical stimulation
- Dermatologic: Angioedema
- Gastrointestinal: Stomach cramps, nausea, vomiting
- Neuromuscular & skeletal: Trembling
- Ocular: Burning of eyes
- Respiratory: Dyspnea
- Miscellaneous: Allergic fever, hiccups

<1%:

- Central nervous system: Ataxia
- Dermatologic: Skin rash, urticaria, erythema multiforme
- Hematologic: Aplastic anemia, leukopenia, eosinophilia
- Ocular: Blurred vision

**Pregnancy Risk Factor** C

**Generic Available** No

## Chlorpheniramine (klor fen IR a meen)

**Related Information**

Dentin Hypersensitivity; High Caries Index; Xerostomia *on page 1145*

Oral Bacterial Infections *on page 1128*

**U.S. Brand Names** Aller-Chlor® [OTC]; AL-R® [OTC]; Chlo-Amine® [OTC]; Chlorate® [OTC]; Chlor-Pro® [OTC]; Chlor-Trimeton® [OTC]; Phenetron®; Telachlor®; Teldrin® [OTC]

**Canadian Brand Names** Chlor-Tripolon®

**Therapeutic Category** Antihistamine

**Use** Perennial and seasonal allergic rhinitis and other allergic symptoms including urticaria

**Usual Dosage**

Children: Oral: 0.35 mg/kg/day in divided doses every 4-6 hours

- 2-6 years: 1 mg every 4-6 hours, not to exceed 6 mg in 24 hours
- 6-12 years: 2 mg every 4-6 hours, not to exceed 12 mg/day or sustained release 8 mg at bedtime

Children >12 years and Adults: Oral: 4 mg every 4-6 hours, not to exceed 24 mg/day or sustained release 8-12 mg every 8-12 hours, not to exceed 24 mg/day

Adults: Allergic reactions: I.M., I.V., S.C.: 10-20 mg as a single dose; maximum recommended dose: 40 mg/24 hours

Elderly: 4 mg once or twice daily. **Note:** Duration of action may be 36 hours or more when serum concentrations are low.

**Mechanism of Action** Competes with histamine for $H_1$-receptor sites on effector cells in the gastrointestinal tract, blood vessels, and respiratory tract

**Local Anesthetic/Vasoconstrictor Precautions** No information available to require special precautions

(Continued)

## Chlorpheniramine *(Continued)*

**Effects on Dental Treatment** Chronic use of antihistamines will inhibit salivary flow, particularly in elderly patients; this may contribute to periodontal disease and oral discomfort

**Other Adverse Effects**

Genitourinary: Urinary retention
Ocular: Diplopia
Renal: Polyuria

>10%:

- Central nervous system: Slight to moderate drowsiness
- Respiratory: Thickening of bronchial secretions

1% to 10%:

- Central nervous system: Headache, excitability, fatigue, nervousness, dizziness
- Gastrointestinal: Nausea, dry mouth, diarrhea, abdominal pain, appetite increase, weight gain
- Neuromuscular & skeletal: Arthralgia, weakness
- Respiratory: Pharyngitis

<1%:

- Cardiovascular: Palpitations
- Central nervous system: Depression
- Dermatologic: Dermatitis, photosensitivity, angioedema
- Hepatic: Hepatitis
- Neuromuscular & skeletal: Myalgia, paresthesia
- Respiratory: Bronchospasm, epistaxis

**Drug Interactions** Sedative effects of chlorpheniramine are enhanced by other CNS depressants, MAO inhibitors, alcohol, and tricyclic antidepressants

**Drug Uptake** Serum half-life: 20-24 hours

**Pregnancy Risk Factor** B

**Dosage Forms**

Capsule, as maleate: 12 mg
Capsule, as maleate, timed release: 8 mg, 12 mg
Injection, as maleate: 10 mg/mL (1 mL, 30 mL); 100 mg/mL (2 mL)
Syrup, as maleate: 2 mg/5 mL (120 mL, 473 mL)
Tablet, as maleate: 4 mg, 8 mg, 12 mg
Tablet, as maleate:
- Chewable: 2 mg
- Timed release: 8 mg, 12 mg

**Dietary Considerations** May be taken with food or water

**Generic Available** Yes

## Chlorpheniramine and Acetaminophen

(klor fen IR a meen & a seet a MIN oh fen)

**U.S. Brand Names** Coricidin® [OTC]

**Therapeutic Category** Analgesic, Non-narcotic; Antihistamine

**Use** Symptomatic relief of congestion, headache, aches and pains of colds and flu

**Usual Dosage** Adults: Oral: 2 tablets every 4 hours, up to 20/day

**Local Anesthetic/Vasoconstrictor Precautions** No information available to require special precautions

**Effects on Dental Treatment** Chronic use of antihistamines will inhibit salivary flow, particularly in elderly patients; this may contribute to periodontal disease and oral discomfort

**Generic Available** Yes

## Chlorpheniramine and Phenylephrine

(klor fen IR a meen & fen il EF rin)

**U.S. Brand Names** Dallergy-D® Syrup; Ed A-Hist® Liquid; Histatab® Plus Tablet [OTC]; Histor-D® Syrup; Rolatuss® Plain Liquid; Ru-Tuss® Liquid

**Therapeutic Category** Antihistamine/Decongestant Combination

**Synonyms** Phenylephrine and Chlorpheniramine

**Use** Temporary relief of nasal congestion and eustachian tube congestion as well as runny nose, sneezing, itching of nose or throat, itchy and watery eyes

**Usual Dosage** Oral:

Children:
- 2-5 years: 2.5 mL every 4 hours
- 6-12 years: 5 mL every 4 hours

Adults: 10 mL every 4 hours

**Local Anesthetic/Vasoconstrictor Precautions** Use with caution since phenylephrine is a sympathomimetic amine which could interact with epinephrine to cause a pressor response

**Effects on Dental Treatment**
Chlorpheniramine: Prolonged use will cause significant xerostomia
Phenylephrine: Up to 10% of patients could experience tachycardia, palpitations, and dry mouth; use vasoconstrictor with caution; prolonged use will cause significant xerostomia

**Pregnancy Risk Factor** C
**Generic Available** Yes

## Chlorpheniramine and Phenylpropanolamine

(klor fen IR a meen & fen il proe pa NOLE a meen)

**U.S. Brand Names** Allerest® 12 Hour Capsule [OTC]; A.R.M.® Caplet [OTC]; Chlor-Rest® Tablet [OTC]; Demazin® Syrup [OTC]; Genamin® Cold Syrup [OTC]; Ornade® Spansule®; Resaid®; Rescon Liquid [OTC]; Silaminic® Cold Syrup [OTC]; Temazin® Cold Syrup [OTC]; Thera-Hist® Syrup [OTC]; Triaminic® Allergy Tablet [OTC]; Triaminic® Cold Tablet [OTC]; Triaminic® Syrup [OTC]; Tri-Nefrin® Extra Strength Tablet [OTC]; Triphenyl® Syrup [OTC]

**Canadian Brand Names** Chlor-Tripolon® Decongestant; Contac.C®; Coricidin®; Corsym®

**Therapeutic Category** Antihistamine/Decongestant Combination

**Synonyms** Phenylpropanolamine and Chlorpheniramine

**Use** Symptomatic relief of nasal congestion, runny nose, sneezing, itchy nose or throat, and itchy or watery eyes due to the common cold or allergic rhinitis

**Usual Dosage**
Children <12 years: 5 mL every 3-4 hours
Children >12 years and Adults: 1 capsule every 12 hours or 5-10 mL every 3-4 hours

**Local Anesthetic/Vasoconstrictor Precautions** Use with caution since phenylpropanolamine is a sympathomimetic amine which could interact with epinephrine to cause a pressor response

**Effects on Dental Treatment**
Chlorpheniramine: Prolonged use will cause significant xerostomia
Phenylpropanolamine: Up to 10% of patients could experience tachycardia, palpitations, and dry mouth; use vasoconstrictor with caution; prolonged use will cause significant xerostomia

**Pregnancy Risk Factor** C
**Generic Available** Yes

## Chlorpheniramine and Pseudoephedrine

(klor fen IR a meen & soo doe e FED rin)

**U.S. Brand Names** Allerest® Maximum Strength [OTC]; Anamine® Syrup [OTC]; Anaplex® Liquid [OTC]; Chlorafed® Liquid [OTC]; Chlor-Trimeton® 4 Hour Relief Tablet [OTC]; Co-Pyronil® 2 Pulvules® [OTC]; Deconamine® SR; Deconamine® Syrup [OTC]; Deconamine® Tablet [OTC]; Fedahist® Tablet [OTC]; Hayfebrol® Liquid [OTC]; Histalet® Syrup [OTC]; Klerist-D® Tablet [OTC]; Pseudo-Gest Plus® Tablet [OTC]; Rhinosyn® Liquid [OTC]; Rhinosyn-PD® Liquid [OTC]; Ryna® Liquid [OTC]; Sudafed® Plus® Liquid [OTC]; Sudafed® Plus® Tablet [OTC]

**Therapeutic Category** Antihistamine/Decongestant Combination

**Synonyms** Pseudoephedrine and Chlorpheniramine

**Use** Relief of nasal congestion associated with the common cold, hay fever, and other allergies, sinusitis, eustachian tube blockage, and vasomotor and allergic rhinitis

**Usual Dosage** Oral:
Capsule: One every 12 hours
Tablet: One 3-4 times/day

**Local Anesthetic/Vasoconstrictor Precautions** Use with caution since pseudoephedrine is a sympathomimetic amine which could interact with epinephrine to cause a pressor response

**Effects on Dental Treatment**
Chlorpheniramine: Prolonged use will cause significant xerostomia
Pseudoephedrine: Up to 10% of patients could experience tachycardia, palpitations, and dry mouth; use vasoconstrictor with caution; prolonged use will cause significant xerostomia

**Pregnancy Risk Factor** C
**Generic Available** Yes

## Chlorpheniramine, Ephedrine, Phenylephrine, and Carbetapentane

(klor fen IR a meen, e FED rin, fen il EF rin, & kar bay ta PEN tane)

**U.S. Brand Names** Rentamine®; Rynatuss® Pediatric Suspension; Tri-Tannate® Plus

**Therapeutic Category** Antihistamine/Decongestant Combination

(Continued)

## Chlorpheniramine, Ephedrine, Phenylephrine, and Carbetapentane *(Continued)*

**Use** Symptomatic relief of cough

**Usual Dosage** Children:

<2 years: Titrate dose individually

2-6 years: 2.5-5 mL every 12 hours

>6 years: 5-10 mL every 12 hours

**Local Anesthetic/Vasoconstrictor Precautions**

Ephedrine: Use vasoconstrictors with caution since ephedrine may enhance cardiostimulation and vasopressor effects of sympathomimetics

Phenylephrine: Use with caution since phenylephrine is a sympathomimetic amine which could interact with epinephrine to cause a pressor response

**Effects on Dental Treatment**

Chlorpheniramine: Prolonged use will cause significant xerostomia

Ephedrine: No effects or complications reported

Phenylephrine: Up to 10% of patients could experience tachycardia, palpitations, and dry mouth; use vasoconstrictor with caution

**Pregnancy Risk Factor** C

**Generic Available** Yes

## Chlorpheniramine, Phenindamine, and Phenylpropanolamine

(klor fen IR a meen, fen IN dah meen, & fen il proe pa NOLE a meen)

**U.S. Brand Names** Nolamine®

**Therapeutic Category** Antihistamine/Decongestant Combination

**Use** Upper respiratory and nasal congestion

**Usual Dosage** Adults: Oral: 1 tablet every 8-12 hours

**Local Anesthetic/Vasoconstrictor Precautions** Use with caution since phenylpropanolamine is a sympathomimetic amine which could interact with epinephrine to cause a pressor response

**Effects on Dental Treatment**

Chlorpheniramine: Prolonged use will cause significant xerostomia

Phenylpropanolamine: Up to 10% of patients could experience tachycardia, palpitations, and dry mouth; use vasoconstrictor with caution

**Generic Available** No

## Chlorpheniramine, Phenylephrine, and Codeine

(klor fen IR a meen, fen il EF rin, & KOE deen)

**U.S. Brand Names** Pediacof®; Pedituss®

**Therapeutic Category** Antihistamine/Decongestant Combination; Cough Preparation

**Use** Symptomatic relief of rhinitis, nasal congestion and cough due to colds or allergy

**Usual Dosage** Children 6 months to 12 years: 1.25-10 mL every 4-6 hours

**Local Anesthetic/Vasoconstrictor Precautions** Use with caution since phenylephrine is a sympathomimetic amine which could interact with epinephrine to cause a pressor response

**Effects on Dental Treatment**

Chlorpheniramine: Prolonged use will cause significant xerostomia

Codeine: <1%: Dry mouth

Phenylephrine: Up to 10% of patients could experience tachycardia, palpitations, and dry mouth; use vasoconstrictor with caution; prolonged use will cause significant xerostomia

**Generic Available** No

## Chlorpheniramine, Phenylephrine, and Dextromethorphan

(klor fen IR a meen, fen il EF rin, & deks troe meth OR fan)

**U.S. Brand Names** Cerose-DM® [OTC]

**Therapeutic Category** Antihistamine/Decongestant Combination; Cough Preparation

**Use** Temporary relief of cough due to minor throat and bronchial irritation; relieves nasal congestion, runny nose and sneezing

**Usual Dosage** Adults: Oral: 5-10 mL 4 times/day

**Local Anesthetic/Vasoconstrictor Precautions**

Chlorpheniramine, Dextromethorphan: No information available to require special precautions

Phenylephrine: Use with caution since phenylephrine is a sympathomimetic amine which could interact with epinephrine to cause a pressor response

**Effects on Dental Treatment**

Chlorpheniramine: Prolonged use will cause significant xerostomia

Dextromethorphan: No effects or complications reported

Phenylephrine: Up to 10% of patients could experience tachycardia, palpitations, and dry mouth; use vasoconstrictor with caution; prolonged use will cause significant xerostomia

**Warnings/Precautions** Research on chicken embryos exposed to concentrations of dextromethorphan relative to those typically taken by humans has shown to cause birth defects and fetal death; more study is needed, but it is suggested that pregnant women should be advised not to use dextromethorphan-containing medications

**Generic Available** No

## Chlorpheniramine, Phenylephrine, and Methscopolamine

(klor fen IR a meen, fen il EF rin, & meth skoe POL a meen)

**U.S. Brand Names** Alersule Forte®; D.A.II® Tablet; Dallergy®; Dura-Vent/DA®; Extendryl® SR; Histor-D® Timecelles®

**Therapeutic Category** Antihistamine/Decongestant Combination

**Use** Relieves nasal congestion, runny nose and sneezing

**Usual Dosage** Adults: Oral: 1 capsule every 12 hours

**Local Anesthetic/Vasoconstrictor Precautions** Use with caution since phenylephrine is a sympathomimetic amine which could interact with epinephrine to cause a pressor response

**Effects on Dental Treatment**

Chlorpheniramine: Prolonged use will cause significant xerostomia

Methscopolamine: Anticholinergic side effects can cause a reduction of saliva production or secretion contributes to discomfort and dental disease (ie, caries, oral candidiasis and periodontal disease)

Phenylephrine: Up to 10% of patients could experience tachycardia, palpitations, and dry mouth; use vasoconstrictor with caution

**Generic Available** Yes

## Chlorpheniramine, Phenylephrine, and Phenylpropanolamine

(klor fen IR a meen, fen il EF rin, & fen il proe pa NOLE a meen)

**U.S. Brand Names** Hista-Vadrin® Tablet

**Therapeutic Category** Antihistamine/Decongestant Combination

**Use** Symptomatic relief of rhinitis and nasal congestion due to colds or allergy

**Usual Dosage** Adults: Oral: 1 tablet every 6 hours

**Local Anesthetic/Vasoconstrictor Precautions** Use with caution since phenylephrine and phenylpropanolamine are sympathomimetic amines which could interact with epinephrine to cause a pressor response

**Effects on Dental Treatment** Up to 10% of patients could experience tachycardia, palpitations, and dry mouth; use vasoconstrictor with caution; prolonged use will cause significant xerostomia

**Pregnancy Risk Factor** C

**Generic Available** Yes

## Chlorpheniramine, Phenylephrine, and Phenyltoloxamine

(klor fen IR a meen, fen il EF rin, & fen il tole LOKS a meen)

**U.S. Brand Names** Comhist®; Comhist® LA

**Therapeutic Category** Antihistamine/Decongestant Combination

**Use** Symptomatic relief of rhinitis and nasal congestion due to colds or allergy

**Usual Dosage** Oral: 1 capsule every 8-12 hours or 1-2 tablets 3 times/day

**Local Anesthetic/Vasoconstrictor Precautions** Use with caution since phenylephrine is a sympathomimetic amine which could interact with epinephrine to cause a pressor response

**Effects on Dental Treatment**

Chlorpheniramine: Prolonged use will cause significant xerostomia

Phenylephrine: Up to 10% of patients could experience tachycardia, palpitations, and dry mouth; use vasoconstrictor with caution

**Pregnancy Risk Factor** C

**Generic Available** No

## Chlorpheniramine, Phenylephrine, Phenylpropanolamine, and Belladonna Alkaloids

(klor fen IR a meen, fen il EF rin, fen il proe pa NOLE a meen, & bel a DON a AL ka loydz)

**U.S. Brand Names** Atrohist® Plus; Phenahist-TR®; Phenchlor® S.H.A.; Ru-Tuss®; Stahist®

**Therapeutic Category** Cold Preparation

**Synonyms** Phenylephrine, Chlorpheniramine, Phenylpropanolamine, and Belladonna Alkaloids; Phenylpropanolamine, Chlorpheniramine, Phenylephrine, and Belladonna Alkaloids

**Use** Relief of symptoms resulting from irritation of sinus, nasal, and upper respiratory tract tissues, including nasal congestion, watering eyes, and postnasal drip; this product contains anticholinergic agents and should be reserved for patients who do not respond to other antihistamine/decongestants

**Usual Dosage** Children ≥12 years and Adults: Oral: 1 tablet morning and evening, swallowed whole

**Local Anesthetic/Vasoconstrictor Precautions** Use with caution since phenylpropanolamine & phenylephrine are sympathomimetic amines which could interact with epinephrine to cause a pressor response

**Effects on Dental Treatment**

Chlorpheniramine: Prolonged use will cause significant xerostomia

Phenylephrine, Phenylpropanolamine: Up to 10% of patients could experience tachycardia, palpitations, and dry mouth; use vasoconstrictor with caution

**Pregnancy Risk Factor** C

**Dosage Forms** Tablet, sustained release: Chlorpheniramine 8 mg, phenylephrine 25 mg, phenylpropanolamine 50 mg, hyoscyamine 0.19 mg, atropine 0.04 mg, and scopolamine 0.01 mg

**Generic Available** Yes

## Chlorpheniramine, Phenylpropanolamine, and Acetaminophen

(klor fen IR a meen, fen il proe pa NOLE a meen, & a seet a MIN oh fen)

**U.S. Brand Names** BQ® Tablet [OTC]; Congestant D® [OTC]; Coricidin D® [OTC]; Dapacin® Cold Capsule [OTC]; Duadacin® Capsule [OTC]; Tylenol® Cold Effervescent Medication Tablet [OTC]

**Therapeutic Category** Analgesic, Non-narcotic; Antihistamine/Decongestant Combination

**Use** Symptomatic relief of nasal congestion and headache from colds/sinus congestion

**Usual Dosage** Adults: Oral: 2 tablets every 4 hours, up to 12 tablets/day

**Local Anesthetic/Vasoconstrictor Precautions** Use with caution since phenylpropanolamine is a sympathomimetic amine which could interact with epinephrine to cause a pressor response

**Effects on Dental Treatment**

Acetaminophen: No effects or complications reported

Chlorpheniramine: Prolonged use will cause significant xerostomia

Phenylpropanolamine: Up to 10% of patients could experience tachycardia, palpitations, and dry mouth; use vasoconstrictor with caution

**Generic Available** Yes

## Chlorpheniramine, Phenylpropanolamine, and Dextromethorphan

(klor fen IR a meen, fen il proe pa NOLE a meen, & deks troe meth OR fan)

**U.S. Brand Names** Triaminicol® Multi-Symptom Cold Syrup [OTC]

**Therapeutic Category** Antihistamine/Decongestant Combination; Cough Preparation

**Use** Provides relief of runny nose, sneezing, suppresses cough, promotes nasal and sinus drainage

**Usual Dosage** Oral:

Children 6-12 years: 5 mL every 4 hours

Adults: 10 mL every 4 hours

**Local Anesthetic/Vasoconstrictor Precautions** Use with caution since phenylpropanolamine is a sympathomimetic amine which could interact with epinephrine to cause a pressor response

**Effects on Dental Treatment**

Chlorpheniramine: Prolonged use will cause significant xerostomia

Dextromethorphan: No effects or complications reported

Phenylpropanolamine: Up to 10% of patients could experience tachycardia, palpitations, and dry mouth; use vasoconstrictor with caution; prolonged use will cause significant xerostomia

**Warnings/Precautions** Research on chicken embryos exposed to concentrations of dextromethorphan relative to those typically taken by humans has shown to cause birth defects and fetal death; more study is needed, but it is suggested that pregnant women should be advised not to use dextromethorphan-containing medications

**Pregnancy Risk Factor** C (see Warnings)

**Generic Available** Yes

**Comments** Alcohol free

## Chlorpheniramine, Phenyltoloxamine, Phenylpropanolamine, and Phenylephrine

(klor fen IR a meen, fen il tole LOKS a meen, fen il proe pa NOLE a meen & fen il EF rin)

**U.S. Brand Names** Naldecon®; Naldelate®; Nalgest®; Nalspan®; New Decongestant®; Par Decon®; Tri-Phen-Chlor®; Uni-Decon®

**Therapeutic Category** Antihistamine/Decongestant Combination

**Use** Symptomatic treatment of nasal and eustachian tube congestion associated with sinusitis and acute upper respiratory infection; symptomatic relief of perennial and allergic rhinitis

**Usual Dosage** Oral:

Children:

- 3-6 months: 1/4 mL (pediatric drops) every 3-4 hours
- 6-12 months: 2.5 mL (pediatric syrup) or 1/2 mL (pediatric drops) every 3-4 hours
- 1-6 years: 5 mL (pediatric syrup) or 1 mL (pediatric drops) every 3-4 hours
- 6-12 years: 2.5 mL (syrup) or 10 mL (pediatric syrup) or 1/2 tablet every 3-4 hours

Children >12 years and Adults: 5 mL (syrup) or 1 tablet every 3-4 hours

**Local Anesthetic/Vasoconstrictor Precautions** Use with caution since phenylpropanolamine & phenylephrine are sympathomimetic amines which could interact with epinephrine to cause a pressor response

**Effects on Dental Treatment**

Chlorpheniramine: Prolonged use will cause significant xerostomia

Phenylephrine, Phenylpropanolamine: Up to 10% of patients could experience tachycardia, palpitations, and dry mouth; use vasoconstrictor with caution

**Pregnancy Risk Factor** C

**Generic Available** Yes

## Chlorpheniramine, Pseudoephedrine, and Codeine

(klor fen IR a meen, soo doe e FED rin, & KOE deen)

**U.S. Brand Names** Codehist® DH; Decohistine® DH; Dihistine® DH; Ryna-C® Liquid

**Therapeutic Category** Antihistamine/Decongestant Combination; Cough Preparation

**Use** Temporary relief of cough associated with minor throat or bronchial irritation or nasal congestion due to common cold, allergic rhinitis, or sinusitis

**Usual Dosage** Oral:

Children:

- 25-50 lb: 1.25-2.50 mL every 4-6 hours, up to 4 doses in 24-hour period
- 50-90 lb: 2.5-5 mL every 4-6 hours, up to 4 doses in 24-hour period

Adults: 10 mL every 4-6 hours, up to 4 doses in 24-hour period

**Local Anesthetic/Vasoconstrictor Precautions** Use with caution since pseudoephedrine is a sympathomimetic amine which could interact with epinephrine to cause a pressor response

**Effects on Dental Treatment**

Chlorpheniramine: Prolonged use will cause significant xerostomia

Codeine: <1%: Dry mouth

Pseudoephedrine: Up to 10% of patients could experience tachycardia, palpitations, and dry mouth; use vasoconstrictor with caution

**Other Adverse Effects** 1% to 10%:

Cardiovascular: Hypotension

Central nervous system: Sedation, dizziness, drowsiness, increased intracranial pressure

Gastrointestinal: Constipation, biliary tract spasm

Genitourinary: Urinary tract spasm

Miscellaneous: Physical or psychological dependence with continued use

**Pregnancy Risk Factor** C

**Generic Available** Yes

## Chlorpheniramine, Pyrilamine, and Phenylephrine

(klor fen IR a meen, pye RIL a meen, & fen il EF rin)

**U.S. Brand Names** Rhinatate® Tablet; R-Tannamine® Tablet; R-Tannate® Tablet; Rynatan® Pediatric Suspension; Rynatan® Tablet; Tanoral® Tablet; Triotann® Tablet; Tri-Tannate® Tablet

**Therapeutic Category** Antihistamine/Decongestant Combination

**Use** Symptomatic relief of nasal congestion associated with upper respiratory tract condition

**Usual Dosage** Children:

<2 years: Titrate dose individually
2-6 years: 2.5-5 mL every 12 hours
>6 years: 5-10 mL every 12 hours

**Local Anesthetic/Vasoconstrictor Precautions** Use with caution since phenylephrine is a sympathomimetic amine which could interact with epinephrine to cause a pressor response

**Effects on Dental Treatment**

Chlorpheniramine: Prolonged use will cause significant xerostomia
Phenylephrine: Up to 10% of patients could experience tachycardia, palpitations, and dry mouth; use vasoconstrictor with caution

**Pregnancy Risk Factor** C

**Generic Available** Yes

## Chlorpheniramine, Pyrilamine, Phenylephrine, and Phenylpropanolamine

(klor fen IR a meen, pye RIL a meen, fen il EF rin, & fen il proe pa NOLE a meen)

**U.S. Brand Names** Histalet Forte® Tablet

**Therapeutic Category** Antihistamine/Decongestant Combination

**Use** Symptomatic relief of rhinitis and nasal congestion due to colds or allergy

**Usual Dosage** Adults: Oral: 1 tablet 2-3 times/day

**Local Anesthetic/Vasoconstrictor Precautions** Use with caution since phenylephrine & phenylpropanolamine are sympathomimetic amines which could interact with epinephrine to cause a pressor response

**Effects on Dental Treatment**

Chlorpheniramine: Prolonged use will cause significant xerostomia
Phenylephrine, Phenylpropanolamine: Up to 10% of patients could experience tachycardia, palpitations, and dry mouth; use vasoconstrictor with caution

**Pregnancy Risk Factor** C

**Generic Available** Yes

♦ **Chlor-Pro® [OTC]** *see* Chlorpheniramine *on page 231*

## Chlorpromazine (klor PROE ma zeen)

**U.S. Brand Names** Ormazine; Thorazine®

**Canadian Brand Names** Apo®-Chlorpromazine; Chlorprom®; Chlorpromanyl®; Largactil®; Novo-Chlorpromazine

**Therapeutic Category** Antiemetic; Antipsychotic Agent; Phenothiazine Derivative

**Use** Treatment of psychoses, nausea and vomiting; Tourette's syndrome; mania; intractable hiccups (adults); behavioral problems (children)

**Usual Dosage**

Children >6 months:
- Psychosis:
  - Oral: 0.5-1 mg/kg/dose every 4-6 hours; older children may require 200 mg/day or higher
  - I.M., I.V.: 0.5-1 mg/kg/dose every 6-8 hours; maximum dose for <5 years (22.7 kg): 40 mg/day; maximum for 5-12 years (22.7-45.5 kg): 75 mg/day
- Nausea and vomiting:
  - Oral: 0.5-1 mg/kg/dose every 4-6 hours as needed
  - I.M., I.V.: 0.5-1 mg/kg/dose every 6-8 hours; maximum dose for <5 years (22.7 kg): 40 mg/day; maximum for 5-12 years (22.7-45.5 kg): 75 mg/day
  - Rectal: 1 mg/kg/dose every 6-8 hours as needed

Adults:
- Psychosis:
  - Oral: Range: 30-800 mg/day in 1-4 divided doses, initiate at lower doses and titrate as needed; usual dose: 200 mg/day; some patients may require 1-2 g/day
  - I.M., I.V.: Initial: 25 mg, may repeat (25-50 mg) in 1-4 hours, gradually increase to a maximum of 400 mg/dose every 4-6 hours until patient is controlled; usual dose: 300-800 mg/day
- Intractable hiccups: Oral, I.M.: 25-50 mg 3-4 times/day

Nausea and vomiting:
Oral: 10-25 mg every 4-6 hours
I.M., I.V.: 25-50 mg every 4-6 hours
Rectal: 50-100 mg every 6-8 hours

Elderly (nonpsychotic patient; dementia behavior): Initial: 10-25 mg 1-2 times/day; increase at 4- to 7-day intervals by 10-25 mg/day. Increase dose intervals (bid, tid, etc) as necessary to control behavior response or side effects; maximum daily dose: 800 mg; gradual increases (titration) may prevent some side effects or decrease their severity.

**Mechanism of Action** Blocks postsynaptic mesolimbic dopaminergic receptors in the brain; exhibits a strong alpha-adrenergic blocking effect and depresses the release of hypothalamic and hypophyseal hormones; believed to depress the reticular-activating system, thus affecting basal metabolism, body temperature, wakefulness, vasomotor tone, and emesis

**Local Anesthetic/Vasoconstrictor Precautions** Most pharmacology textbooks state that in presence of phenothiazines, systemic doses of epinephrine paradoxically decrease the blood pressure. This is the so called "epinephrine reversal" phenomenon. This has never been observed when epinephrine is given by infiltration as part of the anesthesia procedure.

**Effects on Dental Treatment** Significant hypotension may occur, especially when the drug is administered parenterally; orthostatic hypotension is due to alpha-receptor blockade, the elderly are at greater risk for orthostatic hypotension

Tardive dyskinesia: Prevalence rate may be 40% in elderly; development of the syndrome and the irreversible nature are proportional to duration and total cumulative dose over time

Extrapyramidal reactions are more common in elderly with up to 50% developing these reactions after 60 years of age; drug-induced **Parkinson's syndrome** occurs often; **Akathisia** is the most common extrapyramidal reaction in elderly

Increased confusion, memory loss, psychotic behavior, and agitation frequently occur as a consequence of anticholinergic effects

Antipsychotic associated sedation in nonpsychotic patients is extremely unpleasant due to feelings of depersonalization, derealization, and dysphoria

**Other Adverse Effects**

>10%:
- Cardiovascular: Hypotension (especially with I.V. use), tachycardia, arrhythmias, orthostatic hypotension
- Central nervous system: Pseudoparkinsonism, akathisia, dystonias, tardive dyskinesia (persistent), dizziness
- Gastrointestinal: Constipation
- Ocular: Pigmentary retinopathy
- Respiratory: Nasal congestion
- Miscellaneous: Decreased sweating

1% to 10%:
- Dermatologic: Pruritus, rash, photosensitivity
- Endocrine & metabolic: Amenorrhea, galactorrhea, gynecomastia, changes in libido, pain in breasts
- Gastrointestinal: GI upset, nausea, vomiting, stomach pain, weight gain, dry mouth
- Genitourinary: Dysuria, ejaculatory disturbances, urinary retention
- Neuromuscular & skeletal: Trembling of fingers
- Ocular: Blurred vision

<1%:
- Central nervous system: Sedation, drowsiness, restlessness, anxiety, extrapyramidal reactions, seizures, altered central temperature regulation, lowering of seizures threshold, neuroleptic malignant syndrome (NMS)
- Dermatologic: Discoloration of skin (blue-gray)
- Genitourinary: Priapism
- Hematologic: Agranulocytosis (more often in women between 4th and 10th weeks of therapy), leukopenia (usually in patients with large doses for prolonged periods)
- Hepatic: Cholestatic jaundice, hepatotoxicity
- Ocular: Cornea and lens changes
- Miscellaneous: Anaphylactoid reactions

**Warnings/Precautions** Safety in children <6 months of age has not been established; use with caution in patients with seizures, bone marrow depression, or severe liver disease

**Drug Interactions** Increased toxicity: Additive effects with other CNS depressants

(Continued)

## Chlorpromazine *(Continued)*

**Drug Uptake**

Serum half-life, biphasic:

Initial: 2 hours

Terminal: 30 hours

**Pregnancy Risk Factor** C

**Generic Available** Yes

## Chlorpropamide (klor PROE pa mide)

**Related Information**

Endocrine Disorders & Pregnancy *on page 1082*

**U.S. Brand Names** Diabinese®

**Canadian Brand Names** Apo®-Chlorpropamide; Novo-Propamide

**Therapeutic Category** Antidiabetic Agent; Hypoglycemic Agent, Oral; Sulfonylurea Agent

**Use** Control blood sugar in adult onset, noninsulin-dependent diabetes (type II); **unlabeled use:** Neurogenic diabetes insipidus

**Usual Dosage** Oral: The dosage of chlorpropamide is variable and should be individualized based upon the patient's response

Initial dose:

Adults: 250 mg/day in mild to moderate diabetes in middle-aged, stable diabetic

Elderly: 100-125 mg/day in older patients

Maintenance dose: 100-250 mg/day; severe diabetics may require 500 mg/day; avoid doses >750 mg/day

**Mechanism of Action** Stimulates insulin release from the pancreatic beta cells; reduces glucose output from the liver; insulin sensitivity is increased at peripheral target sites

**Local Anesthetic/Vasoconstrictor Precautions** No information available to require special precautions

**Effects on Dental Treatment** Chlorpropamide-dependent diabetics (noninsulin dependent, Type II) should be appointed for dental treatment in morning in order to minimize chance of stress-induced hypoglycemia

**Other Adverse Effects**

>10%:

Central nervous system: Headache, dizziness

Gastrointestinal: Anorexia, constipation, heartburn, epigastric fullness, nausea, vomiting, diarrhea

1% to 10%: Dermatologic: Skin rash, urticaria, photosensitivity

<1%:

Cardiovascular: Edema

Endocrine & metabolic: Hypoglycemia, hyponatremia, SIADH

Hematologic: Blood dyscrasias, aplastic anemia, hemolytic anemia, bone marrow suppression, thrombocytopenia, agranulocytosis

Hepatic: Cholestatic jaundice

**Drug Interactions**

Excessive ethanol intake may lead to hypoglycemia; "antabuse-like" reaction may occur in patients taking chlorpropamide

Salicylates may enhance the hypoglycemic response to chlorpropamide due to increased plasma levels of chlorpropamide by displacing from plasma proteins

Thiazide diuretics will increase blood glucose leading to increased requirements of chlorpropamide

**Drug Uptake**

Peak effect: Oral: Within 6-8 hours

Serum half-life: 30-42 hours; prolonged in the elderly or with renal disease

Time to peak serum concentration: Within 3-4 hours

**Pregnancy Risk Factor** C

**Generic Available** Yes

## Chlorprothixene (klor proe THIKS een)

**U.S. Brand Names** Taractan®

**Therapeutic Category** Antipsychotic Agent

**Use** Management of psychotic disorders

**Usual Dosage**

Children >6 years: Oral: 10-25 mg 3-4 times/day

Adults:

Oral: 25-50 mg 3-4 times/day, to be increased as needed; doses exceeding 600 mg/day are rarely required

I.M.: 25-50 mg up to 3-4 times/day

**Mechanism of Action** The mechanism of action for chlorprothixene, like other thioxanthenes and phenothiazines, is not fully understood. The sites of action appear to be the reticular activating system of the midbrain, the limbic system, the hypothalamus, and the globus pallidus and corpus striatum. The mechanism appears to be one or more of a combination of postsynaptic blockade of adrenergic, dopaminergic, or serotonergic receptor sites, metabolic inhibition of oxidative phosphorylation, or decrease in the excitability of neuronal membranes.

**Local Anesthetic/Vasoconstrictor Precautions** No information available to require special precautions

**Effects on Dental Treatment** Over 10% of dental patients may experience tardive dyskinesia and Parkinson-like syndromes; orthostatic hypotension is induced by chlorprothixene in over 10% of patients

**Other Adverse Effects**

>10%:
- Cardiovascular: Hypotension, orthostatic hypotension
- Central nervous system: Pseudoparkinsonism, akathisia, dystonias, tardive dyskinesia (persistent), dizziness
- Gastrointestinal: Constipation
- Ocular: Pigmentary retinopathy
- Respiratory: Nasal congestion
- Miscellaneous: Decreased sweating

1% to 10%:
- Dermatologic: Photosensitivity, skin rash
- Endocrine & metabolic: Changes in menstrual cycle, changes in libido, pain in breasts
- Gastrointestinal: Weight gain, nausea, vomiting, stomach pain
- Genitourinary: Dysuria, ejaculatory disturbances
- Neuromuscular & skeletal: Trembling of fingers

<1%:
- Central nervous system: Neuroleptic malignant syndrome (NMS)
- Dermatologic: discoloration of skin (blue-gray)
- Endocrine & metabolic: Galactorrhea
- Genitourinary: Priapism
- Hematologic: Agranulocytosis, leukopenia
- Hepatic: Cholestatic jaundice, hepatotoxicity
- Ocular: Cornea and lens changes, pigmentary retinopathy
- Miscellaneous: Impairment of temperature regulation lowering of seizures threshold

**Drug Interactions**

Decreased effect of guanethidine

Increased effect/toxicity: Alcohol, CNS depressants

**Pregnancy Risk Factor** C

**Generic Available** No

♦ **Chlor-Rest® Tablet [OTC]** *see* Chlorpheniramine and Phenylpropanolamine *on page 233*

## Chlortetracycline (klor tet ra SYE kleen)

**U.S. Brand Names** Aureomycin®

**Therapeutic Category** Antibiotic, Ophthalmic; Antibiotic, Tetracycline Derivative

**Use**

Ophthalmic: Treatment of superficial ocular infections involving the conjunctiva or cornea due to strains of susceptible microorganisms

Topical: Treatment of superficial infections of the skin due to susceptible organisms, also infection prophylaxis in minor skin abrasions

**Usual Dosage**

Ophthalmic:
- Acute infections: Instill ½" (1.25 cm) every 3-4 hours until improvement
- Mild to moderate infections: Instill ½" (1.25 cm) 2-3 times/day

Topical: Apply 1-4 times/day, cover with sterile bandage if needed

**Mechanism of Action** Inhibits bacterial protein synthesis by binding with the 30S and possibly the 50S ribosomal subunit(s) of susceptible bacteria; may also cause alterations in the cytoplasmic membrane; usually bacteriostatic, may be bactericidal

**Local Anesthetic/Vasoconstrictor Precautions** No information available to require special precautions

**Effects on Dental Treatment** No effects or complications reported

**Other Adverse Effects**

1% to 10%: Dermatologic: Faint yellowing of skin

<1%: Dermatologic: Redness, swelling, irritation, photosensitivity

**Drug Interactions** No data reported

(Continued)

## Chlortetracycline *(Continued)*

**Pregnancy Risk Factor** D

**Dosage Forms** Ointment:
- Ophthalmic: 1% [10 mg/g] (3.5 g)
- Topical: 3% (14.2 g, 30 g)

**Generic Available** Yes

## Chlorthalidone (klor THAL i done)

**Related Information**

Cardiovascular Diseases *on page 1066*

**U.S. Brand Names** Hygroton®; Thalitone®

**Canadian Brand Names** Apo®-Chlorthalidone; Novo-Thalidone; Uridon®

**Therapeutic Category** Diuretic, Thiazide

**Use** Management of mild to moderate hypertension, used alone or in combination with other agents; treatment of edema associated with congestive heart failure, nephrotic syndrome, or pregnancy. Recent studies have found chlorthalidone effective in the treatment of isolated systolic hypertension in the elderly.

**Usual Dosage** Oral:
- Children: 2 mg/kg/dose 3 times/week or 1-2 mg/kg/day
- Adults: 25-100 mg/day or 100 mg 3 times/week
- Elderly: Initial: 12.5-25 mg/day or every other day; there is little advantage to using doses >25 mg/day

**Mechanism of Action** Sulfonamide-derived diuretic that inhibits sodium and chloride reabsorption in the cortical-diluting segment of the ascending loop of Henle

**Local Anesthetic/Vasoconstrictor Precautions** No information available to require special precautions

**Effects on Dental Treatment** No effects or complications reported

**Other Adverse Effects**
- 1% to 10%: Endocrine & metabolic: Hypokalemia
- <1%:
  - Cardiovascular: Hypotension
  - Dermatologic: Photosensitivity
  - Endocrine & metabolic: Fluid and electrolyte imbalances (hypocalcemia, hypomagnesemia, hyponatremia), hyperglycemia
  - Hematologic: Rarely blood dyscrasias
  - Renal: Prerenal azotemia

**Drug Interactions**
- Decreased absorption of thiazides with cholestyramine resins; chlorthalidone may cause a decreased effect of oral hypoglycemics
- Increased toxicity: Digitalis glycosides, lithium (decreased clearance), probenecid

**Drug Uptake**
- Peak effect: 2-6 hours
- Absorption: Oral: 65%
- Serum half-life: 35-55 hours; may be prolonged with renal impairment, with anuria: 81 hours

**Pregnancy Risk Factor** D

**Generic Available** Yes

♦ **Chlor-Trimeton® [OTC]** *see* Chlorpheniramine *on page 231*

♦ **Chlor-Trimeton® 4 Hour Relief Tablet [OTC]** *see* Chlorpheniramine and Pseudoephedrine *on page 233*

## Chlorzoxazone (klor ZOKS a zone)

**Related Information**

Temporomandibular Dysfunction (TMD) *on page 1149*

**U.S. Brand Names** Flexaphen®; Paraflex®; Parafon Forte™ DSC

**Therapeutic Category** Centrally Acting Skeletal Muscle Relaxant; Muscle Relaxant; Skeletal Muscle Relaxant

**Use**
- Dental: Treatment of muscle spasm with acute temporomandibular joint pain
- Medical: Treatment of muscle spasm associated with acute painful musculoskeletal conditions

**Usual Dosage** Oral:
- Children: 20 mg/kg/day or 600 mg/m²/day in 3-4 divided doses
- Adults: 250-500 mg 3-4 times/day up to 750 mg 3-4 times/day

**Mechanism of Action** Acts on the spinal cord and subcortical levels by depressing polysynaptic reflexes

**Local Anesthetic/Vasoconstrictor Precautions** No information available to require special precautions

**Effects on Dental Treatment** No effects or complications reported

**Other Adverse Effects**

>10%: Central nervous system: Drowsiness

1% to 10%:

Cardiovascular: Tachycardia, tightness in chest, flushing of face, syncope

Central nervous system: Mental depression, dizziness, lightheadedness, headache, paradoxical stimulation

Dermatologic: Angioedema

Gastrointestinal: Nausea, vomiting, stomach cramps

Neuromuscular & skeletal: Trembling

Ocular: Burning of eyes

Respiratory: Dyspnea

Miscellaneous: Hiccups, allergic fever

**Drug Interactions** Alcohol, CNS depressants

**Drug Uptake**

Onset of action: Within 1 hour

**Pregnancy Risk Factor** C

**Breast-feeding Considerations** No data reported

**Dosage Forms**

Caplet (Parafon Forte™ DSC): 500 mg

Capsule (Flexaphen®, Mus-Lax®): 250 mg with acetaminophen 300 mg

Tablet: Paraflex®: 250 mg

**Dietary Considerations** No data reported

**Generic Available** Yes

♦ **Cholac®** *see* Lactulose *on page 571*

♦ **Cholan-HMB®** *see* Dehydrocholic Acid *on page 302*

## Cholecalciferol (kole e kal SI fer ole)

**U.S. Brand Names** Delta-D®

**Therapeutic Category** Vitamin D Analog

**Synonyms** $D_3$

**Use** Dietary supplement, treatment of vitamin D deficiency or prophylaxis of deficiency

**Usual Dosage** Adults: Oral: 400-1000 units/day

**Local Anesthetic/Vasoconstrictor Precautions** No information available to require special precautions

**Effects on Dental Treatment** No effects or complications reported

**Other Adverse Effects**

1% to 10%:

Cardiovascular: Hypotension, cardiac arrhythmias, hypertension

Central nervous system: Irritability, headache

Dermatologic: Pruritus

Endocrine & metabolic: Polydypsia

Gastrointestinal: Nausea, vomiting, anorexia, pancreatitis, metallic taste

Neuromuscular & skeletal: Bone pain, myalgia

Ocular: Conjunctivitis, photophobia

Renal: Polyuria

<1%:

Central nervous system: Overt psychosis

Gastrointestinal: Weight loss

**Pregnancy Risk Factor** C

**Generic Available** No

**Comments** Cholecalciferol 1 mg = 40,000 units of vitamin D activity

♦ **Choledyl®** *see* Oxtriphylline *on page 749*

## Cholera Vaccine (KOL er a vak SEEN)

**Therapeutic Category** Vaccine, Inactivated Bacteria

**Use** Primary immunization for cholera prophylaxis

**Usual Dosage**

Children:

6 months to 4 years: Two 0.2 mL doses I.M./S.C. 1 week to 1 month apart; booster doses (0.2 mL I.M./S.C.) every 6 months

5-10 years: Two 0.3 mL doses I.M./S.C. or two 0.2 mL intradermal doses 1 week to 1 month apart; booster doses (0.3 mL I.M./S.C. or 0.2 mL I.D.) every 6 months

Children ≥10 years and Adults: Two 0.5 mL doses given I.M./S.C. or two 0.2 mL doses I.D. 1 week to 1 month apart; booster doses (0.5 mL I.M. or S.C. or 0.2 mL I.D.) every 6 months

**Mechanism of Action** Inactivated vaccine producing active immunization

(Continued)

## Cholera Vaccine *(Continued)*

**Local Anesthetic/Vasoconstrictor Precautions** No information available to require special precautions

**Effects on Dental Treatment** No effects or complications reported

**Other Adverse Effects** >10%:
- Cardiovascular: Swelling
- Central nervous system: Malaise, fever, headache, pain
- Dermatologic: Tenderness, erythema
- Local: Induration at injection site

**Pregnancy Risk Factor** C

**Generic Available** No

**Comments** Inactivated bacteria vaccine

## Cholestyramine Resin (koe LES tir a meen REZ in)

**Related Information**

Cardiovascular Diseases *on page 1066*

**U.S. Brand Names** Prevalite®; Questran®; Questran® Light

**Canadian Brand Names** PMS-Cholestyramine

**Therapeutic Category** Lipid Lowering Drugs

**Use** Adjunct in the management of primary hypercholesterolemia; pruritus associated with elevated levels of bile acids; diarrhea associated with excess fecal bile acids; binding toxicologic agents; pseudomembraneous colitis

**Usual Dosage** Oral (dosages are expressed in terms of anhydrous resin):
- Powder:
  - Children: 240 mg/kg/day in 3 divided doses; need to titrate dose depending on indication
  - Adults: 4 g 1-6 times/day to a maximum of 16-32 g/day
- Tablet: Adults: Initial: 4 g once or twice daily; maintenance: 8-16 g/day in 2 divided doses

**Mechanism of Action** Forms a nonabsorbable complex with bile acids in the intestine, releasing chloride ions in the process; inhibits enterohepatic reuptake of intestinal bile salts and thereby increases the fecal loss of bile salt-bound low density lipoprotein cholesterol

**Local Anesthetic/Vasoconstrictor Precautions** No information available to require special precautions

**Effects on Dental Treatment** No effects or complications reported

**Other Adverse Effects**
- 1% to 10%: Gastrointestinal: Constipation
- <1%:
  - Dermatologic: Rash; irritation of perianal area, skin, or tongue
  - Endocrine & metabolic: Hyperchloremic acidosis
  - Gastrointestinal: Nausea, vomiting, abdominal distention and pain, malabsorption of fat-soluble vitamins, intestinal obstruction, steatorrhea
  - Hematologic: Hypoprothrombinemia (secondary to vitamin K deficiency)
  - Renal: Elevated urinary calcium excretion

**Drug Interactions** Decreased effect: Decreased absorption (oral) of digitalis glycosides, warfarin, thyroid hormones, thiazide diuretics, propranolol, phenobarbital, amiodarone, methotrexate, NSAIDs, and other drugs by binding to the drug in the intestine

**Drug Uptake**
- Absorption: Not absorbed from the GI tract
- Peak effect: 21 days

**Pregnancy Risk Factor** C

**Generic Available** Yes

## Choline Magnesium Trisalicylate

(KOE leen mag NEE zhum trye sa LIS i late)

**Related Information**

Rheumatoid Arthritis and Osteoarthritis *on page 1092*

**U.S. Brand Names** Trilisate®

**Therapeutic Category** Analgesic, Non-narcotic; Anti-inflammatory Agent; Nonsteroidal Anti-inflammatory Drug (NSAID), Oral; Salicylate

**Use** Management of osteoarthritis, rheumatoid arthritis, and other arthritis; salicylate salts may not inhibit platelet aggregation and, therefore, should not be substituted for aspirin in the prophylaxis of thrombosis

**Usual Dosage** Oral (based on total salicylate content):
- Children <37 kg: 50 mg/kg/day given in 2 divided doses
- Adults: 500 mg to 1.5 g 2-3 times/day; usual maintenance dose: 1-4.5 g/day

**Mechanism of Action** Inhibits prostaglandin synthesis; acts on the hypothalamus heat-regulating center to reduce fever; blocks the generation of pain impulses

**Local Anesthetic/Vasoconstrictor Precautions** No information available to require special precautions

**Effects on Dental Treatment** NSAID formulations are known to reversibly decrease platelet aggregation via mechanisms different than observed with aspirin. The dentist should be aware of the potential of abnormal coagulation. Caution should also be exercised in the use of NSAIDs in patients already on anticoagulant therapy with drugs such as warfarin (Coumadin®).

**Other Adverse Effects**

>10%: Gastrointestinal: Nausea, heartburn, stomach pains, dyspepsia, epigastric discomfort

1% to 10%:

Central nervous system: Fatigue
Dermatologic: Skin rash
Gastrointestinal: Gastrointestinal ulceration
Hematologic: Hemolytic anemia
Neuromuscular & skeletal: Weakness
Respiratory: Dyspnea
Miscellaneous: Anaphylactic shock

<1%:

Central nervous system: Insomnia, nervousness, jitters
Hematologic: Occult bleeding, prolongation of bleeding time, leukopenia, thrombocytopenia, iron deficiency anemia
Hepatic: Hepatotoxicity
Renal: Impaired renal function
Respiratory: Bronchospasm

**Drug Interactions**

Decreased effect with antacids
Increased effect of warfarin

**Drug Uptake**

Absorption: Absorbed from the stomach and small intestine
Serum half-life: Dose-dependent ranging from 2-3 hours at low doses to 30 hours at high doses
Time to peak serum concentration: ~2 hours

**Pregnancy Risk Factor** C

**Generic Available** Yes

## Choline Salicylate (KOE leen sa LIS i late)

**U.S. Brand Names** Arthropan® [OTC]

**Canadian Brand Names** Teejel®

**Therapeutic Category** Analgesic, Non-narcotic; Anti-inflammatory Agent; Nonsteroidal Anti-inflammatory Drug (NSAID), Oral; Salicylate

**Use** Temporary relief of pain of rheumatoid arthritis, rheumatic fever, osteoarthritis, and other conditions for which oral salicylates are recommended; useful in patients in which there is difficulty in administering doses in a tablet or capsule dosage form, because of the liquid dosage form

**Usual Dosage** Children >12 years and Adults: Oral: 5 mL (870 mg) every 3-4 hours, if necessary, but not more than 6 doses in 24 hours
Rheumatoid arthritis: 870-1740 mg (5-10 mL) up to 4 times/day

**Mechanism of Action** Inhibits prostaglandin synthesis; acts on the hypothalamus heat-regulating center to reduce fever; blocks the generation of pain impulses

**Local Anesthetic/Vasoconstrictor Precautions** No information available to require special precautions

**Effects on Dental Treatment** NSAID formulations are known to reversibly decrease platelet aggregation via mechanisms different than observed with aspirin. The dentist should be aware of the potential of abnormal coagulation. Caution should also be exercised in the use of NSAIDs in patients already on anticoagulant therapy with drugs such as warfarin (Coumadin®).

**Other Adverse Effects**

>10%: Gastrointestinal: Nausea, heartburn, stomach pains, dyspepsia, epigastric discomfort

1% to 10%:

Central nervous system: Fatigue
Dermatologic: Skin rash
Gastrointestinal: Gastrointestinal ulceration
Hematologic: Hemolytic anemia
Neuromuscular & skeletal: Weakness
Respiratory: Dyspnea
Miscellaneous: Anaphylactic shock

<1%:

Central nervous system: Insomnia, nervousness, jitters

(Continued)

## Choline Salicylate *(Continued)*

Hematologic: Occult bleeding, prolongation of bleeding time, leukopenia, thrombocytopenia, iron deficiency anemia
Hepatic: Hepatotoxicity
Renal: Impaired renal function
Respiratory: Bronchospasm

**Drug Interactions**
Decreased effect with antacids
Increased effect of warfarin

**Drug Uptake**
Absorption: From the stomach and small intestine within ~2 hours
Serum half-life: Dose-dependent ranging from 2-3 hours at low doses to 30 hours at high doses
Time to peak serum concentration: 1-2 hours

**Pregnancy Risk Factor** C
**Generic Available** No

♦ **Choline Theophyllinate** *see* Oxtriphylline *on page 749*
♦ **Choloxin®** *see* Dextrothyroxine *on page 314*

## Chondroitin Sulfate-Sodium Hyaluronate

(kon DROY tin SUL fate-SOW de um hye a loo ROE nate)

**U.S. Brand Names** Viscoat®
**Therapeutic Category** Ophthalmic Agent, Viscoelastic
**Synonyms** Sodium Hyaluronate-Chrondroitin Sulfate
**Use** Surgical aid in anterior segment procedures, protects corneal endothelium and coats intraocular lens thus protecting it
**Usual Dosage** Carefully introduce (using a 27-gauge needle or cannula) into anterior chamber after thoroughly cleaning the chamber with a balanced salt solution
**Mechanism of Action** Functions as a tissue lubricant and is thought to play an important role in modulating the interactions between adjacent tissues
**Local Anesthetic/Vasoconstrictor Precautions** No information available to require special precautions
**Effects on Dental Treatment** No effects or complications reported
**Other Adverse Effects** 1% to 10%: Increased intraocular pressure (transient)
**Drug Uptake** Absorption: Following intravitreous injection, diffusion occurs slowly
**Pregnancy Risk Factor** C
**Generic Available** No

♦ **Chooz® [OTC]** *see* Calcium Carbonate *on page 172*
♦ **Chorex®** *see* Chorionic Gonadotropin *on this page*

## Chorionic Gonadotropin (kor ee ON ik goe NAD oh troe pin)

**U.S. Brand Names** A.P.L.®; Chorex®; Choron®; Gonic®; Pregnyl®; Profasi® HP
**Therapeutic Category** Gonadotropin; Ovulation Stimulator
**Use** Induces ovulation and pregnancy in anovulatory, infertile females; treatment of hypogonadotropic hypogonadism, prepubertal cryptorchidism
**Usual Dosage** I.M.:

Children:

Prepubertal cryptorchidism (not due to anatomical obstruction): 4000 units 3 times/week for 3 weeks

**or**

5000 units every other day for 4 injections

**or**

15 injections of 500-1000 units over a period of 6 weeks

**or**

500 units 3 times per week for 4-6 weeks. If unsuccessful, start another course 1 month later, giving 1000 units/injection.

Hypogonadotropic hypogonadism in males: 500-1000 units 3 times/week for 3 weeks, followed by the same dose twice weekly for 3 weeks

**or**

1000-2000 units 3 times/week

**or**

4000 units 3 times/week for 6-9 months; reduce dose to 2000 units 3 times/week for an additional 3 months

Adults:

Use with menotropins to stimulate spermatogenesis: 5000 units 3 times/week for 4-6 months. With the beginning of menotropins therapy, hCG dose is continued at 2000 2 times/week.

Induction of ovulation and pregnancy: 5000-10,000 units one day following last dose of menotropins

**Mechanism of Action** Stimulates production of gonadal steroid hormones by causing production of androgen by the testis; as a substitute for luteinizing hormone (LH) to stimulate ovulation

**Local Anesthetic/Vasoconstrictor Precautions** No information available to require special precautions

**Effects on Dental Treatment** No effects or complications reported

**Other Adverse Effects**

1% to 10%:

Central nervous system: Mental depression, fatigue

Endocrine & metabolic: Pelvic pain, ovarian cysts, enlargement of breasts, precocious puberty

Local: Pain at the injection site

Neuromuscular & skeletal: Premature closure of epiphyses

<1%:

Cardiovascular: Peripheral edema

Central nervous system: Irritability, restlessness, headache

Endocrine & metabolic: Ovarian hyperstimulation syndrome, gynecomastia

**Drug Interactions** No data reported

**Drug Uptake** Half-life, biphasic:

Initial: 11 hours

Terminal: 23 hours

**Pregnancy Risk Factor** C

**Generic Available** Yes

- **Choron®** *see* Chorionic Gonadotropin *on previous page*
- **Chromagen® OB [OTC]** *see* Vitamins, Multiple *on page 1051*
- **Chroma-Pak®** *see* Trace Metals *on page 1001*
- **Chromium** *see* Trace Metals *on page 1001*
- **Chronulac®** *see* Lactulose *on page 571*
- **Chymodiactin®** *see* Chymopapain *on this page*

## Chymopapain (KYE moe pa pane)

**U.S. Brand Names** Chymodiactin®

**Therapeutic Category** Enzyme, Intradiscal; Enzyme, Proteolytic

**Use** Alternative to surgery in patients with herniated lumbar intervertebral disks

**Usual Dosage** Adults: 2000-4000 units/disc with a maximum cumulative dose not to exceed 8000 units for patients with multiple disc herniations

**Mechanism of Action** Chymopapain, when injected into the disc center, causes hydrolysis of the mucal mucopolysaccharide protein complex into acid polysaccharide, polypeptides, and amino acids. Subsequently, the water trapping properties of the nucleus pulposus are destroyed which permanently diminishes the pressure within the disc. The adjacent structures including the annulus fibrosus are not affected by chymopapain.

**Local Anesthetic/Vasoconstrictor Precautions** No information available to require special precautions

**Effects on Dental Treatment** No effects or complications reported

**Other Adverse Effects**

>10%: Neuromuscular & skeletal: Back pain

1% to 10%:

Central nervous system: Dizziness, headache

Gastrointestinal: Nausea

Neuromuscular & skeletal: Weakness in legs

<1%:

Central nervous system: CNS hemorrhage, seizures

Dermatologic: Allergic dermatitis

Gastrointestinal: Paralytic ileus

Local: Thrombophlebitis

Ocular: Conjunctivitis

Respiratory: Rhinorrhea, dyspnea

Miscellaneous: Anaphylaxis

**Pregnancy Risk Factor** C

**Generic Available** No

- **Cibacalcin® Injection** *see* Calcitonin *on page 169*

## Ciclopirox (sye kloe PEER oks)

**U.S. Brand Names** Loprox®

**Therapeutic Category** Antifungal Agent, Topical

**Use** Treatment of tinea pedis (athlete's foot), tinea cruris (jock itch), tinea corporis (ringworm), cutaneous candidiasis, and tinea versicolor (pityriasis)

(Continued)

## Ciclopirox *(Continued)*

**Usual Dosage** Children >10 years and Adults: Apply twice daily, gently massage into affected areas; if no improvement after 4 weeks of treatment, re-evaluate the diagnosis

**Mechanism of Action** Inhibiting transport of essential elements in the fungal cell causing problems in synthesis of DNA, RNA, and protein

**Local Anesthetic/Vasoconstrictor Precautions** No information available to require special precautions

**Effects on Dental Treatment** No effects or complications reported

**Other Adverse Effects** 1% to 10%:

Central nervous system: Pain

Local: Irritation, redness, or burning; worsening of clinical condition

**Drug Interactions** No data reported

**Drug Uptake**

Absorption: <2% absorbed through intact skin

Serum half-life: 1.7 hours

**Pregnancy Risk Factor** B

**Dosage Forms**

Cream, topical, as olamine: 1% (15 g, 30 g, 90 g)

Lotion, as olamine: 1% (30 mL)

**Generic Available** No

## Cidofovir (si DOF o veer)

**U.S. Brand Names** Vistide®

**Therapeutic Category** Antiviral Agent, Parenteral

**Use** Treatment of CMV retinitis in patients with acquired immunodeficiency syndrome (AIDS)

**Usual Dosage**

Induction treatment: 5 mg/kg once weekly for 2 consecutive weeks

Maintenance treatment: 5 mg/kg administered once every 2 weeks

**Probenecid must be administered orally with each dose of cidofovir**

Probenecid dose: 2 g 3 hours prior to cidofovir dose, 1 g 2 hours and 8 hours after completion of the infusion; patients should also receive 1 L of normal saline intravenously prior to each infusion of cidofovir; saline should be infused over 1-2 hours

**Mechanism of Action** Cidofovir is converted to cidofovir diphosphate which is the active intracellular metabolite; cidofovir diphosphate suppresses CMV replication by selective inhibition of viral DNA synthesis. Incorporation of cidofovir into growing viral DNA chain results in reductions in the rate of viral DNA synthesis.

**Local Anesthetic/Vasoconstrictor Precautions** No information available to require special precautions

**Effects on Dental Treatment** No effects or complications reported

**Other Adverse Effects**

>10%:

Central nervous system: Fever, headache, chills

Dermatologic: Rash, alopecia

Gastrointestinal: Nausea, vomiting, diarrhea, anorexia, abdominal pain

Hematologic: Neutropenia, anemia

Neuromuscular & skeletal: Weakness

Ocular: Ocular hypotony

Renal: Proteinuria, elevated creatinine

Respiratory: Dyspnea

Miscellaneous: Infections

<10%:

Cardiovascular: Hypotension, tachycardia

Central nervous system: Anxiety, hallucinations, depression, convulsion, somnolence, malaise

Dermatologic: Acne, skin discoloration/dryness, pruritus, urticaria

Endocrine & metabolic: Hyperglycemia, hyperlipidemia, hypocalcemia, hypokalemia, dehydration

Gastrointestinal: Colitis, GI distress, stomatitis

Genitourinary: Urinary incontinence, glycosuria

Hematologic: Thrombocytopenia

Hepatic: Elevated LFTs

Neuromuscular & skeletal: Skeletal pain, myalgia, arthralgia, neuropathy

Ocular: Ocular symptoms

Renal: Hematuria

Respiratory: Respiratory symptoms

Miscellaneous: Allergic reaction, sarcoma, sepsis

**Warnings/Precautions** Dose-dependent nephrotoxicity is a major dose-limiting toxicity related to cidofovir. Cidofovir is not recommended for use in patients with creatinine >1.5 mg/dL or creatinine clearance <55 mL/minute; in these benefits, consideration should be made of potential benefits vs risks. Dose adjustment or discontinuation may be required for changes in renal function while on therapy; renal function secondary to cidofovir is not always reversible. Neutropenia and metabolic acidosis (Fanconi syndrome) have been reported; administration of cidofovir must be accompanied by oral probenecid and intravenous saline prehydration.

**Drug Interactions** Probenecid may decrease metabolism or tubular excretion of drugs such as AZT, acyclovir, benzodiazepines, acetaminophen, ACE inhibitors, barbiturates, loop diuretics, famotidine, NSAIDs, and theophylline; avoid concomitant administration with other nephrotoxic agents

**Drug Uptake** The following pharmacokinetic data is based on a combination of cidofovir administered with probenecid:

Serum half-life: ~2.6 hours (nonintracellular)

**Pregnancy Risk Factor** C

**Generic Available** No

**Comments** Cidofovir preparation should be performed in a class two laminar flow biologic safety cabinet and personnel should be wearing surgical gloves and a closed front surgical gown with knit cuffs; appropriate safety equipment is recommended for preparation, administration, and disposal of cidofovir. If cidofovir contacts skin, wash and flush thoroughly with water.

**Selected Readings**

Hitchcock MJ, Jaffe HS, Martin JC, et al, "Cidofovir, A New Agent With Potent Anti-Herpesvirus Activity," *Antiviral Chemistry & Chemotherapy*, 1996, 7:115-27.

♦ **Ciloxan™** *see* Ciprofloxacin *on next page*

## Cimetidine (sye MET i deen)

**Related Information**

Dental Drug Interactions: Update on Drug Combinations Requiring Special Considerations *on page 1225*

**U.S. Brand Names** Tagamet®; Tagamet® HB [OTC]

**Canadian Brand Names** Apo®-Cimetidine; Novo-Cimetine; Nu-Cimet; Peptol®

**Therapeutic Category** Histamine $H_2$ Antagonist

**Use** Short-term treatment of active duodenal ulcers and benign gastric ulcers; long-term prophylaxis of duodenal ulcer; gastric hypersecretory states; gastroesophageal reflux; prevention of upper GI bleeding in critically ill patients.

**Usual Dosage**

Children: Oral, I.M., I.V.: 20-40 mg/kg/day in divided doses every 4 hours

Adults: Short-term treatment of active ulcers:

Oral: 300 mg 4 times/day or 800 mg at bedtime or 400 mg twice daily for up to 8 weeks

I.M., I.V.: 300 mg every 6 hours or 37.5 mg/hour by continuous infusion; I.V. dosage should be adjusted to maintain an intragastric pH ≥5

Patients with an active bleed: Give cimetidine as a continuous infusion (see above)

Duodenal ulcer prophylaxis: Oral: 400-800 mg at bedtime

Gastric hypersecretory conditions: Oral, I.M., I.V.: 300-600 mg every 6 hours; dosage not to exceed 2.4 g/day

**Mechanism of Action** Competitive inhibition of histamine at $H_2$-receptors of the gastric parietal cells resulting in reduced gastric acid secretion, gastric volume and hydrogen ion concentration reduced

**Local Anesthetic/Vasoconstrictor Precautions** No information available to require special precautions

**Effects on Dental Treatment** No effects or complications reported

**Other Adverse Effects**

1% to 10%:

Central nervous system: Dizziness, agitation, headache, drowsiness

Gastrointestinal: Diarrhea, nausea, vomiting

<1%:

Cardiovascular: Bradycardia, hypotension, tachycardia

Central nervous system: Confusion, fever

Dermatologic: Rash

Endocrine & metabolic: Gynecomastia, swelling of breasts, decreased sexual ability

Hematologic: Neutropenia, agranulocytosis, thrombocytopenia

Hepatic: Elevated AST and ALT

Neuromuscular & skeletal: Myalgia

Renal: Elevated creatinine

(Continued)

## Cimetidine *(Continued)*

**Drug Interactions** Inhibits liver metabolism of many drugs resulting in potential for increased toxicity of those drugs; these include warfarin anticoagulants, phenytoin, propranolol, nifedipine, diazepam, tricyclic antidepressants, theophylline, and metronidazole

**Drug Uptake**

Serum half-life: Adults (with normal renal function): 2 hours

Time to peak serum concentration: Oral: Within 1-2 hours

**Pregnancy Risk Factor** B

**Generic Available** Yes

♦ **Cinobac® Pulvules®** *see* Cinoxacin *on this page*

## Cinoxacin (sin OKS a sin)

**U.S. Brand Names** Cinobac® Pulvules®

**Therapeutic Category** Antibiotic, Quinolone

**Use** Treatment of urinary tract infections

**Usual Dosage** Children >12 years and Adults: 1 g/day in 2-4 doses for 7-14 days

**Mechanism of Action** Inhibits microbial synthesis of DNA with resultant problems in protein synthesis

**Local Anesthetic/Vasoconstrictor Precautions** No information available to require special precautions

**Effects on Dental Treatment** No effects or complications reported

**Other Adverse Effects**

1% to 10%:

- Central nervous system: Headache, dizziness
- Gastrointestinal: Heartburn, abdominal pain, GI bleeding, belching, flatulence, anorexia, nausea

<1%:

- Central nervous system: Insomnia, confusion
- Gastrointestinal: Diarrhea
- Hematologic: Thrombocytopenia
- Ocular: Photophobia
- Otic: Tinnitus

**Drug Interactions** Decreased effect: Decreased urine levels with probenecid; decreased absorption with aluminum-, magnesium-, calcium-containing antacids

**Drug Uptake**

Absorption: Oral: Rapid and complete; food decreases peak levels by 30% but not total amount absorbed

Serum half-life: 1.5 hours, prolonged in renal impairment

Time to peak serum concentration: Oral: Within 2-3 hours

**Pregnancy Risk Factor** B

**Generic Available** Yes

♦ **Cipro™** *see* Ciprofloxacin *on this page*

## Ciprofloxacin (sip roe FLOKS a sin)

**Related Information**

Nonviral Infectious Diseases *on page 1095*

**U.S. Brand Names** Ciloxan™; Cipro™

**Therapeutic Category** Antibiotic, Ophthalmic; Antibiotic, Quinolone

**Use**

Dental: Useful as a single agent or in combination with metronidazole in the treatment of periodontitis associated with the presence of *Actinobacillus actinomycetemcomitans*, (AA) as well as enteric rods/pseudomonads

Medical: Treatment of documented or suspected pseudomonal infection (eg, home care patients); documented multidrug resistant gram-negative organisms; documented infectious diarrhea due to *Campylobacter jejuni*, *Shigella*, or *Salmonella*; osteomyelitis caused by susceptible organisms in which parenteral therapy is not feasible; used ophthalmically for superficial ocular infections (corneal ulcers, conjunctivitis) due to strains of microorganisms susceptible to ciprofloxacin

**Usual Dosage** Adults: Oral: 250-750 mg every 12 hours, depending on severity of infection and susceptibility; in treatment of periodontitis, ciprofloxacin and metronidazole 500 mg each twice daily for 8 days

**Mechanism of Action** Inhibits DNA-gyrase in susceptible organisms; inhibits relaxation of supercoiled DNA and promotes breakage of double-stranded DNA

**Local Anesthetic/Vasoconstrictor Precautions** No information available to require special precautions

**Effects on Dental Treatment** <1% of patients experience painful oral mucosa, oral candidiasis, oral ulceration, or mouth dryness

**Other Adverse Effects** 1% to 10%:
Central nervous system: Headache, restlessness
Dermatologic: Rash
Gastrointestinal: Nausea, diarrhea, vomiting, abdominal pain

**Contraindications** Hypersensitivity to ciprofloxacin, any component or other quinolones

**Warnings/Precautions** Not recommended in children <18 years of age; has caused transient arthropathy in children; CNS stimulation may occur (tremor, restlessness, confusion, and very rarely hallucinations or seizures). Use with caution in patients with known or suspected CNS disorders.

**Drug Interactions** Decreased absorption with antacids containing aluminum, magnesium, and/or calcium (by up to 98% if given at the same time); quinolones cause increased levels of caffeine, warfarin, cyclosporine, and theophylline; azlocillin, cimetidine, probenecid increases quinolone levels

**Drug Uptake**
Absorption: Oral: Rapid
Serum half-life: 3-5 hours in patients with normal renal function
Time to peak serum concentration: Oral: Within 0.5-2 hours

**Pregnancy Risk Factor** C

**Breast-feeding Considerations** Not compatible; can resume breast-feeding 48 hours after the last dose

**Dosage Forms**
Infusion, in $D_5W$: 400 mg (200 mL)
Infusion, in NS or $D_5W$: 200 mg (100 mL)
Injection: 200 mg (20 mL); 400 mg (40 mL)
Tablet: 250 mg, 500 mg, 750 mg

**Dietary Considerations** Dairy foods decrease ciprofloxacin concentration, use caution with xanthine-containing foods and beverages; food delays absorption but total absorption remains unchanged

**Generic Available** Yes

**Selected Readings**

Rams TE and Slots J, "Antibiotics in Periodontal Therapy: An Update," *Compendium*, 1992, 13(12):1130, 1132, 1134.

## Ciprofloxacin and Hydrocortisone

(sip roe FLOKS a sin & hye droe KOR ti sone)

**U.S. Brand Names** Cipro™ HC Otic

**Therapeutic Category** Antibiotic/Corticosteroid, Otic

**Use** Treatment of acute otitis externa, sometimes known as "swimmer's ear"

**Usual Dosage** Children >1 year and Adults: Otic: The recommended dosage for all patients is 3 drops of the suspension in the affected ear twice daily for 7 days; twice-daily dosing schedule is more convenient for patients than that of existing treatments with hydrocortisone, which are typically administered 3-4 times/day; a twice-daily dosage schedule may be especially helpful for parents and caregivers of young children

**Local Anesthetic/Vasoconstrictor Precautions** No information available to require special precautions

**Effects on Dental Treatment** No effects or complications reported

**Dosage Forms** Suspension, otic: Ciprofloxacin hydrochloride 0.2% and hydrocortisone 1%

♦ **Cipro™ HC Otic** *see* Ciprofloxacin and Hydrocortisone *on this page*

## Cisapride (SIS a pride)

**Related Information**
Endocrine Disorders & Pregnancy *on page 1082*

**U.S. Brand Names** Propulsid®

**Canadian Brand Names** Prepulsid®

**Therapeutic Category** Antiemetic; Gastrointestinal Agent, Prokinetic

**Use** Treatment of nocturnal symptoms of gastroesophageal reflux disease (GERD), also demonstrated effectiveness for gastroparesis, refractory constipation, and nonulcer dyspepsia

**Usual Dosage** Oral:
Children: 0.15-0.3 mg/kg/dose 3-4 times/day; maximum: 10 mg/dose
Adults: Initial: 10 mg 4 times/day at least 15 minutes before meals and at bedtime; in some patients the dosage will need to be increased to 20 mg to obtain a satisfactory result

**Mechanism of Action** Enhances the release of acetylcholine at the myenteric plexus. *In vitro* studies have shown cisapride to have serotonin-4 receptor agonistic properties which may increase gastrointestinal motility and cardiac rate; increases lower esophageal sphincter pressure and lower esophageal peristalsis; accelerates gastric emptying of both liquids and solids
(Continued)

## Cisapride *(Continued)*

**Local Anesthetic/Vasoconstrictor Precautions** No information available to require special precautions

**Effects on Dental Treatment** No effects or complications reported

**Other Adverse Effects**

>5%:

Central nervous system: Headache

Dermatologic: Rash

Gastrointestinal: Diarrhea, GI cramping, dyspepsia, flatulence, nausea, dry mouth

Respiratory: Rhinitis

<5%:

Cardiovascular: Tachycardia

Central nervous system: Extrapyramidal effects, drowsiness, fatigue, seizures, insomnia, anxiety

Hematologic: Thrombocytopenia, pancytopenia, leukopenia, granulocytopenia, aplastic anemia

Hepatic: Elevated LFTs

Respiratory: Sinusitis, coughing, upper respiratory tract infection

Miscellaneous: Increased incidence of viral infection

**Drug Interactions** CYP3A3/4 enzyme substrate

Cisapride is contraindicated in patients taking clarithromycin, erythromycin, ketoconazole, fluconazole, and itraconazole. Cisapride accelerates gastric emptying; this could affect the absorption of other drugs given simultaneously. Serious cardiac arrhythmias including ventricular tachycardia, ventricular fibrillation, torsade de pointes, and QT prolongation have been reported in patients taking cisapride. Many of these patients also took drugs expected to increase cisapride blood levels by inhibiting the cytochrome P450 3A4 enzymes that metabolize cisapride. These drugs include clarithromycin, erythromycin, ketoconazole, fluconazole, and itraconazole; some of these events were fatal.

Decreased effect: Atropine, digoxin

Increased toxicity: Warfarin, diazepam increased levels, cimetidine, and ranitidine, CNS depressants

**Drug Uptake**

Onset of action: 0.5-1 hour

Serum half-life: 6-12 hours

**Pregnancy Risk Factor** C

**Generic Available** No

## Cisplatin (SIS pla tin)

**U.S. Brand Names** Platinol®; Platinol®-AQ

**Therapeutic Category** Antineoplastic Agent, Alkylating Agent

**Synonyms** CDDP

**Use** Management of metastatic testicular or ovarian carcinoma, advanced bladder cancer, osteosarcoma, Hodgkin's and non-Hodgkin's lymphoma, head or neck cancer, cervical cancer, lung cancer, brain tumors, neuroblastoma; used alone or in combination with other agents

**Usual Dosage** I.V. (**refer to individual protocols**):

An estimated $Cl_{cr}$ should be on all cisplatin chemotherapy orders along with other patient parameters (ie, patient's height, weight, and body surface area). Pharmacy and nursing staff should check the $Cl_{cr}$ on the order and determine the appropriateness of cisplatin dosing.

It is recommended that a 24-hour urine creatinine clearance be checked prior to a patient's first dose of cisplatin and periodically thereafter (ie, after every 2-3 cycles of cisplatin)

Pretreatment hydration with 1-2 L of fluid is recommended prior to cisplatin administration; adequate hydration and urinary output (>100 mL/hour) should be maintained for 24 hours after administration

**If the dose prescribed is a reduced dose, then this should be indicated on the chemotherapy order**

Children: Various dosage schedules range from 30-100 mg/m² once every 2-3 weeks; may also dose similar to adult dosing

Osteogenic sarcoma or neuroblastoma: 90 mg/m² once every 3 weeks or 30 mg/m² once weekly

Recurrent brain tumors: 60 mg/m² once daily for 2 consecutive days every 3-4 weeks

Adults:

Head and neck cancer: 100-150 mg/m² every 3-4 weeks

Testicular cancer: 10-20 mg/m²/day for 5 days repeated every 3-4 weeks

Metastatic ovarian cancer: 50 mg/m² every 3 weeks

Intraperitoneal: cisplatin has been administered intraperitoneal with systemic sodium thiosulfate for ovarian cancer; doses up to 90-270 mg/m$^2$ have been administered and retained for 4 hours before draining

**Mechanism of Action** Inhibits DNA synthesis by the formation of DNA cross-links; denatures the double helix; covalently binds to DNA bases and disrupts DNA function; may also bind to proteins; the *cis*-isomer is 14 times more cytotoxic than the *trans*-isomer; both forms cross-link DNA but cis-platinum is less easily recognized by cell enzymes and, therefore, not repaired. Cisplatin can also bind two adjacent guanines on the same strand of DNA producing intrastrand cross-linking and breakage

**Local Anesthetic/Vasoconstrictor Precautions** No information available to require special precautions

**Effects on Dental Treatment** No effects or complications reported

**Other Adverse Effects**

>10%:

Endocrine & metabolic: Hyperuricemia

Gastrointestinal: Cisplatin is one of the most emetogenic agents used in cancer chemotherapy; nausea and vomiting occur in 76% to 100% of patients and is dose related. Prophylactic antiemetics should always be prescribed; nausea and vomiting may last up to 1 week after therapy.

Emetic potential: <75 mg: Moderately high (60% to 90%); ≥75 mg: High (>90%)

Hematologic: Myelosuppressive effects: Mild with moderate doses, mild to moderate with high-dose therapy; WBC: Mild; Platelets: Mild; Onset (days): 10; Nadir (days): 14-23; Recovery (days): 21-39

Local: Extravasation: May cause thrombophlebitis and tissue damage if infiltrated; may use sodium thiosulfate as antidote, but consult hospital policy for guidelines

Nephrotoxicity: Related to elimination, protein binding, and uptake of cisplatin. Two types of nephrotoxicity: Acute renal failure and chronic renal insufficiency.

Acute renal failure and azotemia is a dose-dependent process and can be minimized with proper administration and prophylaxis. Damage to the proximal tubules by the aquation products of cisplatin is suspected to cause the toxicity. It is manifested as elevated BUN and creatinine, oliguria, protein wasting, and potassium, calcium, and magnesium wasting.

Chronic renal dysfunction can develop in patients receiving multiple courses of cisplatin. This occurs with slow release of the platinum ion from tissues, which then accumulates in the distal tubules. Manifestations of this toxicity are varied and can include sodium and water wasting, nephropathy, decreased $Cl_{cr}$, and magnesium wasting.

Recommendations for minimizing nephrotoxicity include:

Prepare cisplatin in saline-containing vehicles

Vigorous hydration (125-150 mL/hour) before, during, and after cisplatin administration

Simultaneous administration of either mannitol or furosemide

Avoid other nephrotoxic agents (aminoglycosides, amphotericin, etc)

Otic: Ototoxicity, manifested as high frequency hearing loss (especially pronounced in children)

Miscellaneous: Anaphylactic reaction occurs within minutes after administration and can be controlled with epinephrine, antihistamines, and steroids

1% to 10%:

Gastrointestinal: Anorexia

Local: Pain at injection site

<1%:

Cardiovascular: Bradycardia, arrhythmias

Dermatologic: Mild alopecia

Endocrine & metabolic: SIADH, hypomagnesemia, hypocalcemia, hypokalemia, hypophosphatemia

Gastrointestinal: Mouth sores

Hepatic: Elevation of liver enzymes

Local: Phlebitis

Neurotoxicity: Peripheral neuropathy is dose- and duration-dependent. The mechanism is through axonal degeneration with subsequent damage to the long sensory nerves. Toxicity can first be noted at doses of 200 mg/m$^2$, with measurable toxicity at doses >350 mg/m$^2$. This process is irreversible and progressive with continued therapy. Baseline audiography should be performed.

Ocular: Optic neuritis, blurred vision, papilledema

**Drug Uptake**

Serum half-life:

Initial: 20-30 minutes

(Continued)

## Cisplatin *(Continued)*

Beta: 1 hour
Terminal: ~24 hours
Secondary half-life: 44-73 hours

**Pregnancy Risk Factor** D

**Generic Available** No

**Comments** Sodium content (10 mg): 35.4 mg (1.54 mEq)

## Citalopram (sye TAL oh pram)

**U.S. Brand Names** Celexa®

**Therapeutic Category** Antidepressant

**Synonyms** Nitalapram

**Use** Treatment of depression; currently being evaluated for use in the treatment of dementia, smoking cessation, alcohol abuse, obsessive-compulsive disorder, and diabetic neuropathy

**Usual Dosage** Oral: 20 mg once daily, in the morning or evening. Dose is generally increased to 40 mg once daily. Doses should be increased by 20 mg at intervals of not less than 1 week. Doses >40 mg/day are not generally recommended, although some patients may respond to doses up to 60 mg/day.

Elderly or hepatically impaired patients: Initial dose of 20 mg is recommended; increase dose to 40 mg/day only in nonresponders

Maintenance: Generally, patients are maintained on the dose required for acute stabilization. If side effects are bothersome, dose reduction by 20 mg/day may be considered.

**Mechanism of Action** Inhibits CNS neuronal reuptake of serotonin, which enhances serotonergic activity. Activity as an antidepressant has been presumed to be associated with this effect. Has limited or no affinity for histamine, dopamine, acetylcholine (muscarinic), GABA, benzodiazepine, and adrenergic (alpha- and beta-) receptors. Antagonism of these receptors is believed to be associated with sedative, anticholinergic and cardiovascular adverse effects of tricyclic antidepressants.

**Local Anesthetic/Vasoconstrictor Precautions** Although caution should be used in patients taking tricyclic antidepressants, no interactions have been reported with vasoconstrictors and fluoxetine, a nontricyclic antidepressant which acts to increase serotonin

**Effects on Dental Treatment** Dry mouth in >10% of patients; premarketing trials reported abnormal taste

**Other Adverse Effects**

>10%:

Central nervous system: Somnolence (18%), insomnia (15%)
Gastrointestinal: Nausea (21%), dry mouth (20%)
Miscellaneous: Increased diaphoresis (11%)

1% to 10%:

Central nervous system: Fatigue (5%), anxiety (4%), agitation (3%), yawning (2%), fever (2%)
Endocrine/metabolic: Dysmenorrhea (3%), decreased libido (males 3.8%, females 1.3%), anorgasmia (females 1.1%)
Gastrointestinal: Diarrhea (8%), dyspepsia (5%), vomiting (4%), anorexia (4%), abdominal pain (3%)
Genitourinary: Ejaculation disorder (6%), impotence (3%)
Neuromuscular/skeletal: Tremor (8%), arthralgia (2%), myalgia (2%)
Respiratory: Upper respiratory tract infection (5%), rhinitis (5%), sinusitis (3%)

The following events had an incidence >2% in clinical trials but the incidence on placebo was greater than or equal to the incidence on citalopram: Headache, asthenia, dizziness, constipation, palpitation, abnormal vision, sleep disorder, nervousness, pharyngitis, micturition disorder, back pain

The following treatment emergent effects were also noted at a frequency ≥1% in premarketing trials: Migraine, impaired concentration, confusion, hypotension, postural hypotension, tachycardia, suicide attempt, rash, pruritus, weight gain or loss, abnormal taste, increased appetite, amenorrhea, paresthesia, abnormal accommodation, cough

Several cases of hyponatremia and SIADH have been reported with citalopram. As with other antidepressants, hypomania/mania may be activated in a small proportion of patients with major affective disorders.

**Drug Interactions** **Extensive metabolism via CYP450 isoenzymes 3A4 and 2C19.** Decreases in citalopram clearance are possible when used with inhibitors of these isoenzymes (including ketoconazole, itraconazole, fluconazole, and erythromycin). Citalopram is also a weak inhibitor of CYP450 isoenzymes 1A2, 2D6, and 2C19.

Caution when use with other CNS active agents. See Contraindications and Warnings regarding the use of MAO inhibitors. Cimetidine increases AUC by 43%, lithium may enhance serotonergic effects, and carbamazepine may increase clearance of citalopram via enzyme induction. Citalopram may increase the serum concentration of metoprolol. Serum concentrations of imipramine metabolite (desipramine) may be increased.

**Drug Uptake**

Serum half-life: 24-48 hours; average 35 hours (doubled in patients with hepatic impairment)

Time to peak serum concentration: 1-6 hours, average within 4 hours

**Pregnancy Risk Factor** C

**Dosage Forms** Tablet, as hydrobromide: 20 mg, 40 mg

- ♦ **Citanest Forte® With Epinephrine** *see* Prilocaine With Epinephrine *on page 836*
- ♦ **Citanest Plain 4% Injection** *see* Prilocaine *on page 835*
- ♦ **Citracal® [OTC]** *see* Calcium Citrate *on page 173*
- ♦ **Citrate of Magnesia** *see* Magnesium Citrate *on page 611*
- ♦ **Citric Acid and d-gluconic Acid Irrigant** *see* Citric Acid Bladder Mixture *on this page*

## Citric Acid Bladder Mixture (SI trik AS id BLAD dur MIKS chur)

**U.S. Brand Names** Renacidin®

**Therapeutic Category** Irrigating Solution

**Synonyms** Citric Acid and d-gluconic Acid Irrigant; Hemiacidrin

**Use** Preparing solutions for irrigating indwelling urethral catheters; to dissolve or prevent formation of calcifications

**Usual Dosage** 30-60 mL of 10% (sterile) solution 2-3 times/day by means of a rubber syringe

**Local Anesthetic/Vasoconstrictor Precautions** No information available to require special precautions

**Effects on Dental Treatment** No effects or complications reported

**Pregnancy Risk Factor** C

**Generic Available** Yes

- ♦ **Citrotein® [OTC]** *see* Enteral Nutritional Products *on page 371*
- ♦ **Citrovorum Factor** *see* Leucovorin *on page 577*
- ♦ **Citrucel® [OTC]** *see* Methylcellulose *on page 658*

## Cladribine (KLA dri been)

**U.S. Brand Names** Leustatin™

**Therapeutic Category** Antineoplastic Agent, Antimetabolite

**Synonyms** 2-CdA; 2-Chlorodeoxyadenosine

**Use** Hairy cell and chronic lymphocytic leukemias

**Usual Dosage** I.V.:

Children:

Acute leukemia:

The safety and effectiveness of cladribine in children have not been established; in a phase I study involving patients 1-21 years of age with relapsed acute leukemia, cladribine was administered by continuous intravenous infusion at doses ranging from 3-10.7 mg/m²/day for 5 days (0.5-2 times the dose recommended in HCL). Investigators reported beneficial responses in this study; the dose-limiting toxicity was severe myelosuppression with profound neutropenia and thrombocytopenia.

Continuous intravenous infusion: 15-18 mg/m²/day for 5 days

Adults:

Hairy cell leukemia:

Continuous intravenous infusion: 0.09-0.1 mg/kg/day continuous infusion for 7 consecutive days

Continuous intravenous infusion: 4 mg/m²/day for 7 days

Non-Hodgkin's lymphoma: Continuous intravenous infusion: 0.1 mg/kg/day for 7 days

**Mechanism of Action** A purine nucleoside analogue; prodrug which is activated via phosphorylation by deoxycytidine kinase to a 5′-triphosphate derivative. This active form incorporates into susceptible cells and into DNA to result in the breakage of DNA strand and shutdown of DNA synthesis and also results in a depletion of nicotinamide adenine dinucleotide and adenosine triphosphate (ATP). The induction of strand breaks results in a drop in the cofactor nicotinamide adenine dinucleotide and disruption of cell metabolism. ATP is depleted to deprive cells of an important source of energy. Cladribine is able to kill resting as well as dividing cells, unlike most other cytotoxic drugs.

(Continued)

## Cladribine *(Continued)*

**Local Anesthetic/Vasoconstrictor Precautions** No information available to require special precautions

**Effects on Dental Treatment** No effects or complications reported

**Other Adverse Effects**

>10%:

Bone marrow suppression: Commonly observed in patients treated with cladribine, especially at high doses; at the initiation of treatment, however, most patients in clinical studies had hematologic impairment as a result of HCL. During the first 2 weeks after treatment initiation, mean platelet counts decline and subsequently increased with normalization of mean counts by day 12. Absolute neutrophil counts and hemoglobin declined and subsequently increased with normalization of mean counts by week 5 and week 6.

Central nervous system: Fatigue, headache

Dermatologic: Rash

Fever: Temperature ≥101°F has been associated with the use of cladribine in approximately 66% of patients in the first month of therapy. Although 69% of patients developed fevers, less than 33% of febrile events were associated with documented infection.

Gastrointestinal: Nausea and vomiting are not severe with cladribine at any dose level. Most cases of nausea were mild, not accompanied by vomiting and did not require treatment with antiemetics. In patients requiring antiemetics, nausea was easily controlled most often by chlorpromazine.

Local: Injection site reactions

1% to 10%:

Cardiovascular: Edema, tachycardia

Central nervous system: Dizziness, insomnia, chills, malaise, pain

Dermatologic: Pruritus, erythema

Gastrointestinal: Constipation, abdominal pain

Neuromuscular & skeletal: Arthralgia, myalgia, trunk pain, weakness

Miscellaneous: Sweating

**Drug Uptake** Serum half-life: Biphasic:

Alpha: 25 minutes

Beta: 6.7 hours

Terminal, mean (normal renal function): 5.4 hours

**Pregnancy Risk Factor** D

**Generic Available** No

♦ **Claforan®** *see* Cefotaxime *on page 203*

## Clarithromycin (kla RITH roe mye sin)

**Related Information**

Antibiotic Prophylaxis, Preprocedural Guidelines for Dental Patients *on page 1097*

Respiratory Diseases *on page 1079*

**U.S. Brand Names** Biaxin™

**Therapeutic Category** Antibiotic, Macrolide

**Use**

Dental: Alternate antibiotic in the treatment of common orofacial infections caused by aerobic gram-positive cocci and susceptible anaerobes; alternate antibiotic for the prevention of bacterial endocarditis in patients undergoing dental procedures

Medical: Treatment against most respiratory pathogens (eg, *S. pyogenes*, *S. pneumoniae*, *S. agalactiae*, viridans *Streptococcus*, *M. catarrhalis*, *C. trachomatis*, *Legionella* sp, *Mycoplasma pneumoniae*, *S. aureus*). Clarithromycin is highly active (MICs ≤0.25 mcg/mL) against *H. influenzae*, the combination of clarithromycin and its metabolite demonstrate an additive effect. Additionally, clarithromycin has shown activity against *C. pneumoniae* (including strain TWAR) and *M. avium* infection.

**Usual Dosage** Oral:

Children: Prevention of bacterial endocarditis: 15 mg/kg orally 1 hour before procedure; total children's dose should not exceed adult dose

Adults: 250-500 mg every 12 hours for 7 days; prevention of bacterial endocarditis: 500 mg 1 hour before procedure

**Mechanism of Action** Exerts its antibacterial action by binding to 50S ribosomal subunit resulting in inhibition of protein synthesis. The 14-OH metabolite of clarithromycin is twice as active as the parent compound.

**Local Anesthetic/Vasoconstrictor Precautions** No information available to require special precautions

**Effects on Dental Treatment** No effects or complications reported

**Other Adverse Effects** 1% to 10%:
Central nervous system: Headache
Gastrointestinal: Diarrhea, nausea, dysgeusia, dyspepsia, abdominal pain

**Contraindications** Hypersensitivity to clarithromycin, erythromycin, or any macrolide antibiotic; use with pimozide

**Warnings/Precautions** In presence of severe renal impairment with or without coexisting hepatic impairment, decreased dosage or prolonged dosing interval may be appropriate; antibiotic associated colitis has been reported with use of clarithromycin; elderly patients have experienced increased incidents of adverse effects due to known age-related decreases in renal function

**Drug Interactions** Clarithromycin increases serum theophylline levels by as much as 20% and significantly increases carbamazepine levels. Patients taking cisapride and given clarithromycin may experience toxic increases in cisapride blood levels. When coadministered with astemizole, could result in cardiotoxicity. Clarithromycin produces small increases in ritonavir and indinavir serum concentrations that are unlikely to produce toxicity. Both ritonavir and indinavir significantly increase clarithromycin concentrations. The clinical significance of this effect is unknown. Clarithromycin increases cyclosporine serum levels. Toxic cyclosporine concentrations and renal toxicity may result.

**Note:** While other drug interactions (digoxin, anticoagulants, ergotamine, triazolam) known to occur with erythromycin have not been reported in clinical trials with clarithromycin, concurrent use of these drugs should be monitored closely

**Drug Uptake**
Absorption: Rapid; highly stable in the presence of gastric acid (unlike erythromycin)
Serum half-life, elimination: 3-4 hours with a 250 mg dose; 5-7 hours with a 500 mg dose
Time to peak serum concentration: Oral: 2-4 hours

**Pregnancy Risk Factor** C

**Breast-feeding Considerations** No data reported; however, erythromycins may be taken while breast-feeding

**Dosage Forms**
Granules for oral suspension: 125 mg/5 mL (100 mL, 200 mL); 250 mg/5 mL (100 mL, 200 mL)
Tablet, film coated: 250 mg, 500 mg

**Dietary Considerations** May be taken with or without meals; may be taken with milk; food delays absorption; total absorption remains unchanged

**Generic Available** No

**Comments** *Helicobacter pylori* induced gastric ulcers: Combination regimen with bismuth subsalicylate, tetracycline, clarithromycin, and an $H_2$ receptor antagonist; or combination of omeprazole and clarithromycin. Adult dosage: Oral: 250 mg twice daily to 500 mg 3 times/day.

**Selected Readings**
Dajani AS, Taubert KA, Wilson WW, et al, "Prevention of Bacterial Endocarditis. Recommendations by the American Heart Association," *JAMA* 1997, 277(22):1794-801.
Dajani AS, Taubert KA, Wilson W, et al, "Prevention of Bacterial Endocarditis: Recommendations by the American Heart Association," *J Am Dent Assoc* 1997, 128(8):1142-51.
"Pimozide (Orap) Contraindicated With Clarithromycin (Biaxin™) and Other Macrolide Antibiotics," *FDA Medical Bulletin*, October 1996, 3.
Wynn RL, "New Erythromycins," *Gen Dent*, 1996, 44(4):304-7.

♦ **Claritin®** *see* Loratadine *on page 600*
♦ **Claritin-D®** *see* Loratadine and Pseudoephedrine *on page 601*
♦ **Claritin-D 24-Hour®** *see* Loratadine and Pseudoephedrine *on page 601*
♦ **Clear Away® Disc [OTC]** *see* Salicylic Acid *on page 900*
♦ **Clear By Design® Gel [OTC]** *see* Benzoyl Peroxide *on page 130*
♦ **Clear Eyes® [OTC]** *see* Naphazoline *on page 703*
♦ **Clearsil® Maximum Strength [OTC]** *see* Benzoyl Peroxide *on page 130*
♦ **Clear Tussin® 30** *see* Guaifenesin and Dextromethorphan *on page 479*

## Clemastine (KLEM as teen)

**U.S. Brand Names** Antihist-1® [OTC]; Tavist®; Tavist®-1 [OTC]

**Therapeutic Category** Antihistamine

**Use** Perennial and seasonal allergic rhinitis and other allergic symptoms including urticaria

**Usual Dosage** Oral:
Children: <12 years: 0.4-1 mg twice daily
Children >12 years and Adults: 1.34 mg twice daily to 2.68 mg 3 times/day; do not exceed 8.04 mg/day; lower doses should be considered in patients >60 years

**Mechanism of Action** Competes with histamine for $H_1$-receptor sites on effector cells in the gastrointestinal tract, blood vessels, and respiratory tract
(Continued)

## Clemastine *(Continued)*

**Local Anesthetic/Vasoconstrictor Precautions** No information available to require special precautions

**Effects on Dental Treatment** No effects or complications reported

**Other Adverse Effects**

>10%:
- Central nervous system: Slight to moderate drowsiness
- Respiratory: Thickening of bronchial secretions

1% to 10%:
- Central nervous system: Headache, fatigue, nervousness, increased dizziness
- Gastrointestinal: Appetite increase, nausea, diarrhea, abdominal pain, dry mouth
- Neuromuscular & skeletal: Arthralgia
- Respiratory: Pharyngitis

<1%:
- Cardiovascular: Edema, palpitations
- Central nervous system: Depression
- Dermatologic: Angioedema, photosensitivity, rash
- Hepatic: Hepatitis
- Neuromuscular & skeletal: Myalgia, paresthesia
- Respiratory: Bronchospasm, epistaxis

**Drug Interactions** May interact with other sedatives to cause drowsiness; these include alcohol and tranquilizers

**Drug Uptake** Absorption: Almost 100% from GI tract

**Pregnancy Risk Factor** C

**Generic Available** Yes

## Clemastine and Phenylpropanolamine

(KLEM as teen & fen il proe pa NOLE a meen)

**U.S. Brand Names** Tavist-D®

**Therapeutic Category** Antihistamine/Decongestant Combination

**Use** Symptomatic relief of allergic rhinitis; pruritus of the eyes, nose or throat, lacrimation and nasal congestion

**Usual Dosage** Children >12 years and Adults: Oral: 1 tablet every 12 hours

**Local Anesthetic/Vasoconstrictor Precautions** Use with caution since phenylpropanolamine is a sympathomimetic amine which could interact with epinephrine to cause a pressor response

**Effects on Dental Treatment** Up to 10% of patients could experience tachycardia, palpitations, and dry mouth; use vasoconstrictor with caution

**Pregnancy Risk Factor** B

**Dosage Forms** Tablet: Clemastine fumarate 1.34 mg and phenylpropanolamine hydrochloride 75 mg

**Generic Available** No

♦ **Cleocin HCl®** *see* Clindamycin *on this page*

♦ **Cleocin Pediatric®** *see* Clindamycin *on this page*

♦ **Cleocin Phosphate®** *see* Clindamycin *on this page*

## Clidinium and Chlordiazepoxide

(kli DI nee um & klor dye az e POKS ide)

**U.S. Brand Names** Clindex®; Librax®

**Canadian Brand Names** Apo®-Chlorax; Corium®; ProChlorax

**Therapeutic Category** Antispasmodic Agent, Gastrointestinal

**Synonyms** Chlordiazepoxide and Clidinium

**Use** Adjunct treatment of peptic ulcer, treatment of irritable bowel syndrome

**Usual Dosage** Oral: 1-2 capsules 3-4 times/day, before meals or food and at bedtime

**Local Anesthetic/Vasoconstrictor Precautions** No information available to require special precautions

**Effects on Dental Treatment** No effects or complications reported

**Pregnancy Risk Factor** D

**Generic Available** Yes

**Comments** After extended therapy, abrupt discontinuation should be avoided and a gradual dose tapering schedule followed

♦ **Climara® Transdermal** *see* Estradiol *on page 387*

## Clindamycin (klin da MYE sin)

**Related Information**

Animal and Human Bites Guidelines *on page 1164*

Antibiotic Prophylaxis, Preprocedural Guidelines for Dental Patients *on page 1097*

Cardiovascular Diseases *on page 1066*
Oral Bacterial Infections *on page 1128*
Periodontal Diseases *on page 1132*

**U.S. Brand Names** Cleocin HCl®; Cleocin Pediatric®; Cleocin Phosphate®

**Canadian Brand Names** Dalacin® C [Hydrochloride]

**Therapeutic Category** Acne Products; Antibiotic, Anaerobic; Antibiotic, Miscellaneous

**Use**

Dental: Alternate antibiotic, when amoxicillin cannot be used, for the standard regimen for prevention of bacterial endocarditis in patients undergoing dental procedures; an alternative to penicillin VK and erythromycin for treating orofacial infections; alternate antibiotic for prophylaxis for dental patients with total joint replacement

Medical: Treatment against aerobic and anaerobic streptococci (except enterococci), most staphylococci, *Bacteroides* sp and *Actinomyces*; used topically in treatment of severe acne, vaginally for *Gardnerella vaginalis*, alternate treatment for toxoplasmosis

**Usual Dosage**

Children:

Prevention of bacterial endocarditis: 20 mg/kg orally 1 hour before procedure with no follow-up dose needed; for patients allergic to penicillin and unable to take oral medications: 20 mg/kg I.V. within 30 minutes before procedure

Orofacial infections: 8-25 mg/kg in 3-4 equally divided doses

Adults:

Prevention of bacterial endocarditis in patients unable to take amoxicillin: Oral: 600 mg 1 hour before procedure with no follow-up dose needed; for patients allergic to penicillin and unable to take oral medications: 600 mg I.V. within 30 minutes before procedure

Orofacial infections: 150-450 mg every 6 hours for at least 7 days; maximum dose: 1.8 g/day

Patients with prosthesis allergic to penicillin: Oral: 600 mg 1 hour before procedure

Patients with prosthesis allergic to penicillin and unable to take oral medication: I.V.: 600 mg 1 hour before procedure

**Mechanism of Action** Reversibly binds to 50S ribosomal subunits preventing peptide bond formation thus inhibiting bacterial protein synthesis; bacteriostatic or bactericidal depending on drug concentration, infection site, and organism

**Local Anesthetic/Vasoconstrictor Precautions** No information available to require special precautions

**Effects on Dental Treatment** No effects or complications reported

**Other Adverse Effects**

>10%: Gastrointestinal: Diarrhea

1% to 10%:

Dermatologic: Rashes

Gastrointestinal: Pseudomembranous colitis, nausea, vomiting

**Contraindications** Hypersensitivity to clindamycin or any component; previous pseudomembranous colitis, hepatic impairment

**Warnings/Precautions** Dosage adjustment may be necessary in patients with severe hepatic dysfunction; no change necessary with renal insufficiency; can cause severe and possibly fatal colitis; use with caution in patients with a history of pseudomembranous colitis; discontinue drug if significant diarrhea, abdominal cramps, or passage of blood and mucus occurs

**Drug Interactions** Increased duration of neuromuscular blockade from tubocurarine, pancuronium; increased risk for renal toxicity with gentamicin

**Drug Uptake**

Absorption: 90% absorbed rapidly from GI tract following oral administration

Serum half-life: Adults: 1.6-5.3 hours, average: 2-3 hours

Time to peak serum concentration: Oral: Within 60 minutes

**Pregnancy Risk Factor** B

**Breast-feeding Considerations** May be taken while breast-feeding

**Dosage Forms**

Capsule, as hydrochloride: 75 mg, 150 mg, 300 mg

Granules for oral solution, as palmitate: 75 mg/5 mL (100 mL)

Infusion, as phosphate, in $D_5W$: 300 mg (50 mL); 600 mg (50 mL)

Injection, as phosphate: 150 mg/mL (2 mL, 4 mL, 6 mL, 50 mL, 60 mL)

**Dietary Considerations** Peak concentrations may be delayed with food; may be taken with food

**Generic Available** Yes

**Comments** Clindamycin has not been shown to interfere with oral contraceptive activity; however, it reduces GI microflora, thus, oral contraceptive users should be advised to use additional methods of birth control. About 1% of clindamycin

(Continued)

## Clindamycin *(Continued)*

users develop pseudomembranous colitis. Symptoms may occur 2-9 days after initiation of therapy; however, it has never occurred with the 1-dose regimen of clindamycin used to prevent bacterial endocarditis.

**Selected Readings**

"Advisory Statement. Antibiotic Prophylaxis for Dental Patients With Total Joint Replacements. American Dental Association; American Academy of Orthopedic Surgeons," *J Am Dent Assoc*, 1997, 128(7):1004-8.

Dajani AS, Taubert KA, Wilson WW, et al, "Prevention of Bacterial Endocarditis. Recommendations by the American Heart Association," *JAMA* 1997, 277(22):1794-801.

Dajani AS, Taubert KA, Wilson W, et al, "Prevention of Bacterial Endocarditis: Recommendations by the American Heart Association," *J Am Dent Assoc* 1997, 128(8):1142-51.

Wynn RL and Bergman SA, "Antibiotics and Their Use in the Treatment of Orofacial Infections, Part I and Part II," *Gen Dent*, 1994, 42(5):398-402, 498-502.

Wynn RL, "Clindamycin: An Often Forgotten but Important Antibiotic," *AGD Impact*, 1994, 22:10.

♦ **Clindex®** *see* Clidinium and Chlordiazepoxide *on page 258*

♦ **Clinoril®** *see* Sulindac *on page 948*

## Clioquinol (klye oh KWIN ole)

**U.S. Brand Names** Vioform® [OTC]

**Therapeutic Category** Antifungal Agent, Topical

**Use** Used topically in the treatment of tinea pedis, tinea cruris, and skin infections caused by dermatophytic fungi (ring worm)

**Usual Dosage** Children and Adults: Topical: Apply 2-3 times/day; do not use for longer than 7 days

**Mechanism of Action** Chelates bacterial surface and trace metals needed for bacterial growth

**Local Anesthetic/Vasoconstrictor Precautions** No information available to require special precautions

**Effects on Dental Treatment** No effects or complications reported

**Other Adverse Effects** 1% to 10%:

Dermatologic: Skin irritation, rash

Neuromuscular & skeletal: Peripheral neuropathy

Ocular: Optic atrophy

**Drug Interactions** No data reported

**Drug Uptake**

Absorption: With an occlusive dressing, up to 40% of dose can be absorbed systemically during a 12-hour period; absorption is enhanced when applied under diapers

Serum half-life: 11-14 hours

**Pregnancy Risk Factor** C

**Generic Available** Yes: Cream

## Clioquinol and Hydrocortisone

(klye oh KWIN ole & hye droe KOR ti sone)

**U.S. Brand Names** Corque® Topical; Pedi-Cort V® Creme

**Therapeutic Category** Antifungal Agent, Topical; Corticosteroid, Topical (Low Potency)

**Synonyms** Hydrocortisone and Clioquinol; Iodochlorhydroxyquin and Hydrocortisone

**Use** Contact or atopic dermatitis; eczema; neurodermatitis; anogenital pruritus; mycotic dermatoses; moniliasis

**Usual Dosage** Apply in a thin film 3-4 times/day

**Local Anesthetic/Vasoconstrictor Precautions** No information available to require special precautions

**Effects on Dental Treatment** No effects or complications reported

**Pregnancy Risk Factor** C

**Generic Available** Yes

## Clobetasol (kloe BAY ta sol)

**Related Information**

Corticosteroids, Topical Comparison *on page 1222*

Oral Nonviral Soft Tissue Ulcerations or Erosions *on page 1141*

**U.S. Brand Names** Temovate®

**Canadian Brand Names** Dermasone; Dermovate®; Gen-Clobetasol; Novo-Clobetasol

**Therapeutic Category** Corticosteroid, Topical (Very High Potency)

**Use** Short-term relief of inflammation of moderate to severe corticosteroid-responsive dermatosis (very high potency topical corticosteroid)

**Usual Dosage** Adults: Topical: Apply twice daily for up to 2 weeks with no more than 50 g/week

**Mechanism of Action** Stimulates the synthesis of enzymes needed to decrease inflammation, suppress mitotic activity, and cause vasoconstriction

**Local Anesthetic/Vasoconstrictor Precautions** No information available to require special precautions

**Effects on Dental Treatment** No effects or complications reported

**Other Adverse Effects**

1% to 10%:

Dermatologic: Erythema, papular rashes

Local: Itching, burning, dryness, irritation

<1%: Dermatologic: Hypertrichosis, acneiform eruptions, hypopigmentation, perioral dermatitis, maceration of skin, skin atrophy, striae, miliaria

**Drug Interactions** No data reported

**Drug Uptake** Absorption: Percutaneous absorption variable and dependent upon many factors including vehicle used, integrity of epidermis, dose, and use of occlusive dressings

**Pregnancy Risk Factor** C

**Generic Available** Yes

## Clocortolone (kloe KOR toe lone)

**Related Information**

Corticosteroids, Topical Comparison *on page 1222*

**U.S. Brand Names** Cloderm®

**Therapeutic Category** Corticosteroid, Topical (Medium Potency)

**Use** Inflammation of corticosteroid-responsive dermatoses (medium potency topical corticosteroid)

**Usual Dosage** Adults: Apply sparingly and gently; rub into affected area from 1-4 times/day

**Mechanism of Action** Stimulates the synthesis of enzymes needed to decrease inflammation, suppress mitotic activity, and cause vasoconstriction

**Local Anesthetic/Vasoconstrictor Precautions** No information available to require special precautions

**Effects on Dental Treatment** No effects or complications reported

**Other Adverse Effects**

1% to 10%:

Dermatologic: Erythema, papular rashes

Local: Itching, burning,

<1%: Dermatologic: Hypertrichosis, acneiform eruptions, hypopigmentation, perioral dermatitis, maceration of skin, skin atrophy, striae, miliaria

**Drug Interactions** No data reported

**Drug Uptake** Absorption: Percutaneous absorption is variable and dependent upon many factors including vehicle used, integrity of epidermis, dose, and use of occlusive dressings

**Pregnancy Risk Factor** C

**Generic Available** No

♦ **Cloderm®** *see* Clocortolone *on this page*

## Clofazimine (kloe FA zi meen)

**U.S. Brand Names** Lamprene®

**Therapeutic Category** Antibiotic, Miscellaneous

**Use** Treatment of dapsone-resistant leprosy; multibacillary dapsone-sensitive leprosy; erythema nodosum leprosum; *Mycobacterium avium* - intracellular (MAI) infections

**Usual Dosage** Oral:

Children: Leprosy: 1 mg/kg/day every 24 hours in combination with dapsone and rifampin

Adults:

Dapsone-resistant leprosy: 100 mg/day in combination with one or more antileprosy drugs for 3 years; then alone 100 mg/day

Dapsone-sensitive multibacillary leprosy: 100 mg/day in combination with two or more antileprosy drugs for at least 2 years and continue until negative skin smears are obtained, then institute single drug therapy with appropriate agent

Erythema nodosum leprosum: 100-200 mg/day for up to 3 months or longer then taper dose to 100 mg/day when possible

Pyoderma gangrenosum: 300-400 mg/day for up to 12 months

**Mechanism of Action** Binds preferentially to mycobacterial DNA to inhibit mycobacterial growth; also has some anti-inflammatory activity through an unknown mechanism

**Local Anesthetic/Vasoconstrictor Precautions** No information available to require special precautions

(Continued)

## Clofazimine *(Continued)*

**Effects on Dental Treatment** No effects or complications reported

**Other Adverse Effects**

>10%:

Dermatologic: Dry skin, pink to brownish-black discoloration of the skin
Gastrointestinal: Abdominal pain, nausea, vomiting, diarrhea
Ocular: Pink to brownish-black discoloration of the conjunctiva

1% to 10%:

Dermatologic: Rash, pruritus
Endocrine & metabolic: Elevated blood sugar
Gastrointestinal: Discoloration of feces/sputum
Genitourinary: Discoloration of urine
Ocular: Irritation of the eyes
Miscellaneous: Discoloration of sweat

**Drug Interactions** No data reported

**Drug Uptake**

Absorption: Oral: 45% to 70% absorbed slowly
Serum half-life:
Terminal: 8 days
Tissue: 70 days
Time to peak serum concentration: 1-6 hours with chronic therapy

**Pregnancy Risk Factor** C

**Generic Available** No

## Clofibrate (kloe FYE brate)

**U.S. Brand Names** Atromid-S®

**Canadian Brand Names** Abitrate®; Claripex®; Novo-Fibrate

**Therapeutic Category** Lipid Lowering Drugs

**Use** Adjunct to dietary therapy in the management of hyperlipidemias associated with high triglyceride levels (types III, IV, V); primarily lowers triglycerides and very low density lipoprotein

**Usual Dosage** Adults: Oral: 500 mg 4 times/day; some patients may respond to lower doses

**Mechanism of Action** Mechanism is unclear but thought to reduce cholesterol synthesis and triglyceride hepatic-vascular transference

**Local Anesthetic/Vasoconstrictor Precautions** No information available to require special precautions

**Effects on Dental Treatment** No effects or complications reported

**Other Adverse Effects**

>10%: Gastrointestinal: Nausea

1% to 10%: Gastrointestinal: Diarrhea, vomiting, dyspepsia, flatulence, abdominal distress

<1%:

Cardiovascular: Angina, cardiac arrhythmias
Central nervous system: Headache, dizziness, fatigue
Dermatologic: Skin rash, urticaria, pruritus, alopecia
Gastrointestinal: Gallstones
Genitourinary: Impotence
Hematologic: Leukopenia, anemia, eosinophilia, agranulocytosis
Hepatic: Elevated liver function test
Neuromuscular & skeletal: Muscle cramping, aching, myalgia, weakness
Renal: Renal toxicity, rhabdomyolysis-induced renal failure
Miscellaneous: Dry, brittle hair

**Drug Interactions**

Increased effect:

Warfarin: Clofibrate increases the hypoprothrombinemic effect of warfarin. The mechanism has not been established, but serious bleeding episodes have occurred in some patients receiving both drugs

Sulfonylureas: Clofibrate may enhance the effects of the sulfonylurea-type oral hypoglycemics by displacement from plasma protein binding sites

**Drug Uptake**

Absorption: Occurs completely; intestinal transformation is required to activate the drug
Serum half-life: 6-24 hours, increases significantly with reduced renal function; with anuria: 110 hours
Time to peak serum concentration: Within 3-6 hours

**Pregnancy Risk Factor** C

**Generic Available** Yes

♦ **Clomid®** *see* Clomiphene *on next page*

## Clomiphene (KLOE mi feen)

**U.S. Brand Names** Clomid®; Milophene®; Serophene®

**Therapeutic Category** Ovulation Stimulator

**Use** Treatment of ovulatory failure in patients desiring pregnancy

**Unlabeled use:** Male infertility

**Usual Dosage** Adults: Oral:

Males (infertility): 25 mg/day for 25 days with 5 days rest, or 100 mg every Monday, Wednesday, Friday

Females (ovulatory failure): Oral: 50 mg/day for 5 days (first course); start the regimen on or about the fifth day of cycle; if ovulation occurs do not increase dosage; if not, increase next course to 100 mg/day for 5 days. Three courses of therapy are an adequate therapeutic trial. Further treatment is not recommended in patients who do not exhibit ovulation.

**Mechanism of Action** Induces ovulation by stimulating the release of pituitary gonadotropins

**Local Anesthetic/Vasoconstrictor Precautions** No information available to require special precautions

**Effects on Dental Treatment** No effects or complications reported

**Other Adverse Effects**

>10%: Endocrine & metabolic: Hot flashes, ovarian enlargement

1% to 10%:

- Cardiovascular: Thromboembolism
- Central nervous system: Mental depression, headache
- Endocrine & metabolic: Breast enlargement (males), abnormal menstrual flow
- Gastrointestinal: Distention, bloating, nausea, vomiting
- Hepatic: Hepatotoxicity
- Ocular: Blurring of vision, diplopia, floaters, after-images, phosphenes, photophobia

<1%:

- Central nervous system: Insomnia, fatigue
- Dermatologic: Alopecia (reversible)
- Gastrointestinal: Weight gain
- Renal: Polyuria

**Drug Interactions** No data reported

**Drug Uptake** Serum half-life: 5-7 days

**Pregnancy Risk Factor** X

**Generic Available** No

## Clomipramine (kloe MI pra meen)

**U.S. Brand Names** Anafranil®

**Canadian Brand Names** Apo®-Clomipramine

**Therapeutic Category** Antidepressant, Tricyclic

**Use** Treatment of obsessive-compulsive disorder (OCD); may also relieve depression, panic attacks, and chronic pain

**Usual Dosage** Oral: Initial:

Children: 25 mg/day and gradually increase, as tolerated, to a maximum of 3 mg/kg/day or 200 mg/day, whichever is smaller

Adults: 25 mg/day and gradually increase, as tolerated, to 100 mg/day the first 2 weeks, may then be increased to a total of 250 mg/day maximum

**Mechanism of Action** Clomipramine appears to affect serotonin uptake while its active metabolite, desmethylclomipramine, affects norepinephrine uptake

**Local Anesthetic/Vasoconstrictor Precautions** Use with caution; epinephrine, norepinephrine and levonordefrin have been shown to have an increased pressor response in combination with TCAs

**Effects on Dental Treatment** >10% of patients experience dry mouth; long-term treatment with TCAs such as clomipramine increases the risk of caries by reducing salivation and salivary buffer capacity

**Other Adverse Effects**

>10%:

- Central nervous system: Dizziness, drowsiness, headache
- Gastrointestinal: Constipation, increased appetite, nausea, unpleasant taste, weight gain
- Neuromuscular & skeletal: Weakness

1% to 10%:

- Cardiovascular: Arrhythmias, hypotension
- Central nervous system: Confusion, delirium, hallucinations, nervousness, restlessness, parkinsonian syndrome, insomnia
- Endocrine & metabolic: Sexual dysfunction
- Gastrointestinal: Diarrhea, heartburn
- Genitourinary: Dysuria
- Neuromuscular & skeletal: Fine muscle tremors

(Continued)

## Clomipramine *(Continued)*

Ocular: Blurred vision, eye pain
Miscellaneous: Excessive sweating

<1%:
Central nervous system: Anxiety, seizures
Dermatologic: Alopecia, photosensitivity
Endocrine & metabolic: Breast enlargement, galactorrhea, SIADH
Gastrointestinal: Trouble with gums, decreased lower esophageal sphincter tone may cause GE reflux
Genitourinary: Testicular swelling
Hematologic: Agranulocytosis, leukopenia, eosinophilia
Hepatic: Cholestatic jaundice, elevated liver enzymes
Ocular: Increased intraocular pressure
Otic: Tinnitus
Miscellaneous: Allergic reactions

**Drug Interactions**

Decreased effect: Phenobarbital may increase the metabolism of clomipramine; clomipramine blocks the uptake of guanethidine and thus prevents the hypotensive effect of guanethidine

Increased toxicity: Tricyclic antidepressants, such as clomipramine, can inhibit the antihypertensive to clonidine resulting in hypertension; clomipramine may be additive with or may potentiate the action of other CNS depressants such as sedatives or hypnotics; with MAO inhibitors, hyperpyrexia, hypertension, tachycardia, confusion, and seizures. Clomipramine may increase the prothrombin time in patients stabilized on warfarin; clomipramine may potentiate the pressor and cardiac effects of sympathomimetic agents such as isoproterenol, epinephrine, etc; cimetidine and methylphenidate may decrease the metabolism of clomipramine

Additive anticholinergic effects seen with other anticholinergic agents

**Drug Uptake**

Absorption: Oral: Rapid
Serum half-life: 20-30 hours

**Pregnancy Risk Factor** C

**Generic Available** Yes

**Selected Readings**

Boakes AJ, Laurence DR, Teoh PC, et al, "Interactions Between Sympathomimetic Amines and Antidepressant Agents in Man," *Br Med J*, 1973, 1(849):311-5.

Jastak JT and Yagiela JA, "Vasoconstrictors and Local Anesthesia: A Review and Rationale for Use," *J Am Dent Assoc*, 1983, 107(4):623-30.

Larochelle P, Hamet P, and Enjalbert M, "Responses to Tyramine and Norepinephrine After Imipramine and Trazodone," *Clin Pharmacol Ther*, 1979, 26(1):24-30.

Mitchell JR, "Guanethidine and Related Agents. III Antagonism by Drugs Which Inhibit the Norepinephrine Pump in Man," *J Clin Invest*, 1970, 49(8):1596-604.

Rundegren J, van Dijken J, Mörnstad H, et al, "Oral Conditions in Patients Receiving Long-Term Treatment With Cyclic Antidepressant Drugs," *Swed Dent J*, 1985, 9(2):55-64.

Svedmyr N, "The Influence of a Tricyclic Antidepressive Agent (Protriptyline) on Some of the Circulatory Effects of Noradrenaline and Adrenalin® in Man," *Life Sci*, 1968, 7(1):77-84.

◆ **Clomycin® [OTC]** *see* Bacitracin, Neomycin, Polymyxin B, and Lidocaine *on page 118*

## Clonazepam (kloe NA ze pam)

**U.S. Brand Names** Klonopin™

**Canadian Brand Names** PMS-Clonazepam; Rivotril®

**Therapeutic Category** Anticonvulsant, Benzodiazepine

**Use** Prophylaxis of petit mal, petit mal variant (Lennox-Gastaut), akinetic, and myoclonic seizures

**Unlabeled use:** Restless legs syndrome, neuralgia, multifocal tic disorder, parkinsonian dysarthria, acute manic episodes, and adjunct therapy for schizophrenia

**Usual Dosage** Oral:

Children <10 years or 30 kg:
Initial daily dose: 0.01-0.03 mg/kg/day (maximum: 0.05 mg/kg/day) given in 2-3 divided doses; increase by no more than 0.5 mg every third day until seizures are controlled or adverse effects seen
Usual maintenance dose: 0.1-0.2 mg/kg/day divided 3 times/day; not to exceed 0.2 mg/kg/day

Adults:
Initial daily dose: Do not exceed 1.5 mg given in 3 divided doses; may increase by 0.5-1 mg every third day until seizures are controlled or adverse effects seen
Usual maintenance dose: 0.05-0.2 mg/kg; do not exceed 20 mg/day

**Mechanism of Action** Suppresses the spike-and-wave discharge in absence seizures by depressing nerve transmission in the motor cortex

**Local Anesthetic/Vasoconstrictor Precautions** No information available to require special precautions

**Effects on Dental Treatment** No effects or complications reported

**Other Adverse Effects**

>10%:

Cardiovascular: Tachycardia

Central nervous system: Somnolence (50%), ataxia (30%), fatigue, depression, amnesia, lightheadedness, insomnia, anxiety, headache

Dermatologic: Rash

Gastrointestinal: Constipation, diarrhea, nausea, vomiting

Neuromuscular & skeletal: Dysarthria

Ocular: Blurred vision

Miscellaneous: Diaphoresis

1% to 10%:

Cardiovascular: Syncope, hypotension

Central nervous system: Confusion

Dermatologic: Dermatitis

Gastrointestinal: Weight gain or loss, increased salivation

Neuromuscular & skeletal: Rigidity, tremor, muscle cramps/weakness

Otic: Tinnitus

Respiratory: Nasal congestion

**Drug Interactions** No significant interactions have been reported

**Drug Uptake**

Onset of effect: 20-60 minutes

Duration: Up to 6-8 hours in infants and young children, up to 12 hours in adults

Absorption: Oral: Well absorbed

Serum half-life:

Children: 22-33 hours

Adults: 19-50 hours

Time to peak serum concentration: Oral: 1-3 hours

Steady-state: 5-7 days

**Pregnancy Risk Factor** C

**Generic Available** Yes

## Clonidine (KLOE ni deen)

**Related Information**

Cardiovascular Diseases *on page 1066*

**U.S. Brand Names** Catapres® Oral; Catapres-TTS® Transdermal; Duraclon® Injection

**Canadian Brand Names** Apo®-Clonidine; Dixarit®; Novo-Clonidine; Nu-Clonidine

**Therapeutic Category** Alpha-Adrenergic Blockers - Central-Acting (Alpha$_2$-Agonists)

**Use** Management of mild to moderate hypertension; either used alone or in combination with other antihypertensives; not recommended for first-line therapy for hypertension; also used for heroin withdrawal and in smoking cessation therapy; other uses may include prophylaxis of migraines, glaucoma, paralytic ileus, and diabetes-associated diarrhea

**Usual Dosage**

Oral:

Children: Initial: 5-10 mcg/kg/day in divided doses every 8-12 hours; increase gradually at 5- to 7-day intervals to 25 mcg/kg/day in divided doses every 6 hours; maximum: 0.9 mg/day

Clonidine tolerance test (test of growth hormone release from pituitary): 0.15 mg/m$^2$ or 4 mcg/kg as single dose

Adults: Initial dose: 0.1 mg twice daily, usual maintenance dose: 0.2-1.2 mg/day in 2-4 divided doses; maximum recommended dose: 2.4 mg/day

Nicotine withdrawal symptoms: 0.1 mg twice daily to maximum of 0.4 mg/day for 3-4 weeks

Elderly: Initial: 0.1 mg once daily at bedtime, increase gradually as needed

Transdermal: Apply once every 7 days; for initial therapy start with 0.1 mg and increase by 0.1 mg at 1- to 2-week intervals; dosages >0.6 mg do not improve efficacy

**Mechanism of Action** Stimulates alpha$_2$-adrenoreceptors in the brain stem, thus activating an inhibitory neuron, resulting in reduced sympathetic outflow, producing a decrease in vasomotor tone and heart rate

**Local Anesthetic/Vasoconstrictor Precautions** No information available to require special precautions

**Effects on Dental Treatment** >10% of patients experience significant dry mouth

(Continued)

## Clonidine *(Continued)*

**Other Adverse Effects**

>10%:

Central nervous system: Drowsiness, dizziness

Gastrointestinal: Constipation

1% to 10%:

Cardiovascular: Orthostatic hypotension

Central nervous system: Nervousness, agitation, mental depression, headache, fatigue

Dermatologic: Rash

Endocrine & metabolic: Decreased sexual activity, loss of libido

Gastrointestinal: Nausea, vomiting

Genitourinary: Nocturia, impotence

Hepatic: Abnormal liver function tests

Neuromuscular & skeletal: Weakness

<1%:

Cardiovascular: Palpitations, tachycardia, bradycardia, Raynaud's phenomenon, congestive heart failure

Central nervous system: Insomnia, vivid dreams, delirium, fever

Dermatologic: Pruritus, urticaria, alopecia

Endocrine & metabolic: Gynecomastia

Gastrointestinal: Weight gain

Genitourinary: Difficulty in micturition, urinary retention

Ocular: Burning of the eyes, blurred vision

**Drug Interactions**

Tricyclic antidepressants antagonize hypotensive effects of clonidine; this could result in hypertension

Increased toxicity: Beta-blockers may potentiate bradycardia in patients receiving clonidine and may increase the rebound hypertension of withdrawal; discontinue beta-blocker several days before clonidine is tapered

**Drug Uptake**

Onset of effect: Oral: 0.5-1 hour; $T_{max}$: 2-4 hours

Duration: 6-10 hours

Serum half-life: Adults:

Normal renal function: 6-20 hours

Renal impairment: 18-41 hours

**Pregnancy Risk Factor** C

**Generic Available** Yes: Tablet

## Clonidine and Chlorthalidone (KLOE ni deen & klor THAL i done)

**U.S. Brand Names** Combipres®

**Therapeutic Category** Antihypertensive Agent, Combination

**Use** Management of mild to moderate hypertension

**Usual Dosage** Oral: 1 tablet 1-2 times/day

**Local Anesthetic/Vasoconstrictor Precautions** No information available to require special precautions

**Effects on Dental Treatment** No effects or complications reported

**Pregnancy Risk Factor** C

**Generic Available** No

## Clopidogrel (kloh PID oh grel)

**Related Information**

Cardiovascular Diseases *on page 1066*

**U.S. Brand Names** Plavix®

**Therapeutic Category** Platelet Aggregation Inhibitor

**Synonyms** Clopidogrel Bisulfate

**Use** The reduction of atherosclerotic events (myocardial infarction, stroke, vascular deaths) in patients with atherosclerosis documented by recent myocardial infarctions, recent stroke or established peripheral arterial disease

**Usual Dosage** Adults: Oral: 75 mg once daily

**Mechanism of Action** Blocks the ADP receptor and in so doing, prevents the binding of fibrinogen to that site. Clopidrogel, however, does not alter the receptor, which suggests that it prevents the binding of fibrinogen in an indirect manner. This drug reduces the number of functional ADP receptors. The effect of clopidrogel continues for several days after discontinuing the drug and it effects decrease proportionally to platelet renewal.

**Local Anesthetic/Vasoconstrictor Precautions** No information available to require special precautions

**Effects on Dental Treatment** If a patient is to undergo elective surgery and an antiplatelet effect is not desired, clopidogrel should be discontinued 7 days prior to surgery

**Contraindications** In patients with active pathologic bleeding or who have shown hypersensitivity to the drug or any component of the drug and should be used with caution in patients with severe liver disease

**Drug Interactions**

Naproxen: In healthy volunteers receiving naproxen, concomitant administration of clopidogrel was associated with increased occult gastrointestinal blood loss

NSAIDs: Manufacturers warning states that NSAIDs and clopidogrel should be coadministered with caution

**Drug Uptake**

Onset:

Maximal effect on bleeding time: 5-6 days

Maximal effect on platelet function: 3-7 days

Half-life, elimination: ~8 hours (carboxylic acid derivative)

Time to peak serum concentration: Oral: ~1 hour

**Dosage Forms** Tablet, as bisulfate: 75 mg

♦ **Clopidogrel Bisulfate** *see* Clopidogrel *on previous page*

## Clorazepate (klor AZ e pate)

**U.S. Brand Names** Gen-XENE®; Tranxene®

**Canadian Brand Names** Apo®-Clorazepate; Novo-Clopate

**Therapeutic Category** Anticonvulsant, Benzodiazepine; Benzodiazepine; Sedative

**Use** Treatment of generalized anxiety and panic disorders; management of alcohol withdrawal; adjunct anticonvulsant in management of partial seizures

**Usual Dosage** Oral:

Children 9-12 years: Anticonvulsant: Initial: 3.75-7.5 mg/dose twice daily; increase dose by 3.75 mg at weekly intervals, not to exceed 60 mg/day in 2-3 divided doses

Children >12 years and Adults: Anticonvulsant: Initial: Up to 7.5 mg/dose 2-3 times/day; increase dose by 7.5 mg at weekly intervals; not to exceed 90 mg/day

Adults:

Anxiety: 7.5-15 mg 2-4 times/day, or given as single dose of 11.25 or 22.5 mg at bedtime

Alcohol withdrawal: Initial: 30 mg, then 15 mg 2-4 times/day on first day; maximum daily dose: 90 mg; gradually decrease dose over subsequent days

**Mechanism of Action** Facilitates gamma aminobutyric acid (GABA)-mediated transmission inhibitory neurotransmitter action, depresses subcortical levels of CNS

**Local Anesthetic/Vasoconstrictor Precautions** No information available to require special precautions

**Effects on Dental Treatment** Many patients will experience drowsiness and dry mouth while taking clorazepate which will disappear with cessation of drug therapy; orthostatic hypotension is possible; it is suggested that narcotic analgesics not be given for pain control to patients taking clorazepate because of enhanced sedation

**Other Adverse Effects**

>10%: Central nervous system: Drowsiness

1% to 10%:

Central nervous system: Confusion, nervousness, dizziness, headache

Gastrointestinal: Xerostomia

Ocular: Blurred vision

<1%:

Cardiovascular: Decreased systolic blood pressure

Hematologic: Decreased hematocrit

Hepatic: Abnormal LFTs

Renal: Abnormal kidney function tests

**Drug Interactions** Increased effect: Cimetidine, CNS depressants, alcohol

**Drug Uptake**

Serum half-life: Adults:

Desmethyldiazepam: 48-96 hours

Oxazepam: 6-8 hours

Time to peak serum concentration: Oral: Within 1 hour

**Pregnancy Risk Factor** D

**Generic Available** Yes

♦ **Clorpactin® WCS-90** *see* Oxychlorosene *on page 750*

## Clotrimazole (kloe TRIM a zole)

**Related Information**

Oral Fungal Infections *on page 1134*

(Continued)

## Clotrimazole *(Continued)*

**U.S. Brand Names** Gyne-Lotrimin® 3; Mycelex® Troche

**Canadian Brand Names** Canesten® Topical, Vaginal; Clotrimaderm; Myclo-Derm®; Myclo-Gyne®

**Therapeutic Category** Antifungal Agent, Oral Nonabsorbed; Antifungal Agent, Topical; Antifungal Agent, Vaginal

**Use**

Dental: Treatment of susceptible fungal infections, including oropharyngeal candidiasis; limited data suggests that the use of clotrimazole troches may be effective for prophylaxis against oropharyngeal candidiasis in neutropenic patients

Medical: Treatment of susceptible fungal infections including dermatophytoses, superficial mycoses, and cutaneous candidiasis, as well as vulvovaginal candidiasis

**Usual Dosage** Children >3 years and Adults: 10 mg troche dissolved slowly 5 times/day for 14 consecutive days

**Mechanism of Action** Binds to phospholipids in the fungal cell membrane altering cell wall permeability resulting in loss of essential intracellular elements

**Local Anesthetic/Vasoconstrictor Precautions** No information available to require special precautions

**Effects on Dental Treatment** No effects or complications reported

**Other Adverse Effects**

>10%: Hepatic: Abnormal liver function tests

1% to 10%:

Gastrointestinal: Nausea and vomiting may occur in patients on clotrimazole troches

Local: Mild burning, irritation, stinging to skin or vaginal area

**Contraindications** Hypersensitivity to clotrimazole or any component

**Warnings/Precautions** Clotrimazole should not be used for treatment of systemic fungal infection; safety and effectiveness of clotrimazole lozenges (troches) in children <3 years of age have not been established

**Drug Interactions** Increased cyclosporine levels can occur; enhanced hypoglycemic effects with sulfonylureas

**Drug Uptake**

Duration: Up to 3 hours

Absorption: Oral: Poor

Time to peak serum concentration: Oral topical administration: Salivary levels occur within 3 hours following 30 minutes of dissolution time in the mouth

**Pregnancy Risk Factor** B; C (oral)

**Breast-feeding Considerations** No data reported

**Dosage Forms** Troche, oral (Mycelex®): 10 mg

**Dietary Considerations** No data reported

**Generic Available** Yes

## Cloxacillin (kloks a SIL in)

**U.S. Brand Names** Cloxapen®; Tegopen®

**Canadian Brand Names** Apo®-Cloxi; Novo-Cloxin; Nu-Cloxi; Orbenin®; Taro-Cloxacillin®

**Therapeutic Category** Antibiotic, Penicillin

**Use**

Dental: Treatment of susceptible orofacial infections, notably penicillinase-producing staphylococci

Medical: Treatment of susceptible bacterial infections in the medical patient, notably penicillinase-producing staphylococci causing respiratory tract, skin and skin structure, bone and joint, urinary tract infections, endocarditis, septicemia, and meningitis

**Usual Dosage** Oral:

Children <20 kg: 50-100 mg/kg/day in divided doses every 6 hours

Children >20 kg and Adults: 250-500 mg every 6 hours for at least 7 days

**Mechanism of Action** Inhibits bacterial cell wall synthesis by binding to one or more of the penicillin-binding proteins (PBPs) which in turn inhibits the final transpeptidation step of peptidoglycan synthesis in bacterial cell walls, thus inhibiting cell wall biosynthesis. Bacteria eventually lyse due to ongoing activity of cell wall autolytic enzymes (autolysins and murein hydrolases) while cell wall assembly is arrested.

**Local Anesthetic/Vasoconstrictor Precautions** No information available to require special precautions

**Effects on Dental Treatment** Prolonged use of penicillins may lead to development of oral candidiasis

**Other Adverse Effects** 1% to 10%:
Gastrointestinal: Nausea, diarrhea
Hematologic: Agranulocytosis
Hepatic: Elevations of AST and ALT
Renal: Hematuria
Miscellaneous: Serum sickness-like reactions

**Contraindications** Hypersensitivity to cloxacillin or any component, or penicillins

**Warnings/Precautions** Monitor PTT if patient concurrently on warfarin, elimination of drug is slow in renally impaired; use with caution in patients allergic to cephalosporins due to a low incidence of cross-hypersensitivity

**Drug Interactions** Efficacy of oral contraceptives may be reduced; disulfiram, probenecid may increase cloxacillin levels; cloxacillin may increase the effect of anticoagulants

**Drug Uptake**
Absorption: Oral: ~50%
Serum half-life: 0.5-1.5 hours
Time to peak serum concentration: Oral: Within 0.5-2 hours

**Pregnancy Risk Factor** B

**Breast-feeding Considerations** No data reported; however, other penicillins may be taken while breast-feeding

**Dosage Forms**
Capsule, as sodium: 250 mg, 500 mg
Powder for oral suspension, as sodium: 125 mg/5 mL (100 mL, 200 mL)

**Dietary Considerations** Should be taken 1 hour before or 2 hours after meals with water

**Generic Available** Yes

**Comments** Although cloxacillin is a penicillin antibiotic indicated for infections caused by penicillinase-secreting staph, amoxicillin with clavulanic acid is considered the drug of choice for these types of orofacial infections

♦ **Cloxapen®** *see* Cloxacillin *on previous page*

## Clozapine (KLOE za peen)

**U.S. Brand Names** Clozaril®

**Therapeutic Category** Antipsychotic Agent

**Use** Management of schizophrenic patients

**Usual Dosage** Adults: Oral: 25 mg once or twice daily initially and increased, as tolerated to a target dose of 300-450 mg/day after 2 weeks, but may require doses as high as 600-900 mg/day

**Mechanism of Action** Clozapine is a weak dopamine$_1$ and dopamine$_2$ receptor blocker; in addition, it blocks the serotonin$_2$, alpha-adrenergic, and histamine $H_1$ central nervous system receptors

**Local Anesthetic/Vasoconstrictor Precautions** Most pharmacology textbooks state that in presence of phenothiazines, systemic doses of epinephrine paradoxically decrease the blood pressure. This is the so called "epinephrine reversal" phenomenon. This has never been observed when epinephrine is given by infiltration as part of the anesthesia procedure.

**Effects on Dental Treatment** Many patients may experience orthostatic hypotension with clozapine; precautions should be taken; do not use atropine-like drugs for xerostomia in patients taking clozapine because of significant potentiation

**Other Adverse Effects**
>10%:
Cardiovascular: Tachycardia, hypotension, orthostatic hypotension
Central nervous system: Fever, headache, drowsiness
Gastrointestinal: Constipation, nausea, vomiting, unusual weight gain
1% to 10%:
Cardiovascular: EKG changes, hypertension
Central nervous system: Agitation, akathisia
Gastrointestinal: Abdominal discomfort, heartburn, dry mouth
Ocular: Blurred vision
Miscellaneous: Increased sweating
<1%:
Central nervous system: Insomnia, seizures, tardive dyskinesia, neuroleptic malignant syndrome
Genitourinary: Dysuria, impotence
Hematologic: Agranulocytosis, eosinophilia, granulocytopenia, leukopenia, thrombocytopenia
Neuromuscular & skeletal: Rigidity, tremor

**Drug Interactions**
Decreased effect with phenytoin
Increased effect of CNS depressants, guanabenz, anticholinergics
(Continued)

## Clozapine *(Continued)*

Increased toxicity with cimetidine, MAO inhibitors, neuroleptics, TCAs

Clozapine may significantly potentiate the hypotensive effects of antihypertensive drugs and the anticholinergic effects of atropine-type drugs. In medical emergencies, the administration of epinephrine should be avoided in the treatment of drug-induced hypotension because of a possible reverse epinephrine effect. There are no data to suggest any interaction between clozapine and the use of vasoconstrictors in local anesthesia.

**Pregnancy Risk Factor** B

**Generic Available** No

♦ **Clozaril®** *see* Clozapine *on previous page*

♦ **Clysodrast®** *see* Bisacodyl *on page 141*

## Coal Tar (KOLE tar)

**U.S. Brand Names** AquaTar® [OTC]; Denorex® [OTC]; DHS® Tar [OTC]; Duplex® T [OTC]; Estar® [OTC]; Fototar® [OTC]; Neutrogena® T/Derm; Oxipor® VHC [OTC]; Pentrax® [OTC]; Polytar® [OTC]; psoriGel® [OTC]; T/Gel® [OTC]; Zetar® [OTC]

**Canadian Brand Names** Balnetar®; Ionil-T® Plus

**Therapeutic Category** Antipsoriatic Agent, Topical; Antiseborrheic Agent, Topical

**Synonyms** Crude Coal Tar; LCD; Pix Carbonis

**Use** Topically for controlling dandruff, seborrheic dermatitis, or psoriasis

**Usual Dosage**

Bath: Add appropriate amount to bath water, for adults usually 60-90 mL of a 5% to 20% solution or 15-25 mL of 30% lotion; soak 5-20 minutes, then pat dry; use once daily to 3 days

Shampoo: Rub shampoo onto wet hair and scalp, rinse thoroughly; repeat; leave on 5 minutes; rinse thoroughly; apply twice weekly for the first 2 weeks then once weekly or more often if needed

Skin: Apply to the affected area 1-4 times/day; decrease frequency to 2-3 times/week once condition has been controlled

Scalp psoriasis: Tar oil bath or coal tar solution may be painted sparingly to the lesions 3-12 hours before each shampoo

Psoriasis of the body, arms, legs: Apply at bedtime; if thick scales are present, use product with salicylic acid and apply several times during the day

**Local Anesthetic/Vasoconstrictor Precautions** No information available to require special precautions

**Effects on Dental Treatment** No effects or complications reported

**Other Adverse Effects** 1% to 10%: Dermatologic: Dermatitis, folliculitis

**Pregnancy Risk Factor** C

**Generic Available** Yes

**Comments** Avoid exposure to sunlight for 24 hours after use; may stain clothing and skin

## Coal Tar and Salicylic Acid (KOLE tar & sal i SIL ik AS id)

**U.S. Brand Names** X-seb® T [OTC]

**Canadian Brand Names** Polytar® AF; P&S™ Plus Tar Gel; Sebcur/T®

**Therapeutic Category** Antipsoriatic Agent, Topical; Antiseborrheic Agent, Topical

**Use** Seborrheal dermatitis; dandruff

**Usual Dosage** Use as shampoo twice weekly

**Local Anesthetic/Vasoconstrictor Precautions** No information available to require special precautions

**Effects on Dental Treatment** No effects or complications reported

**Pregnancy Risk Factor** C

**Generic Available** Yes

## Coal Tar, Lanolin, and Mineral Oil

(KOLE tar, LAN oh lin, & MIN er al oyl)

**U.S. Brand Names** Balnetar® [OTC]

**Therapeutic Category** Antipsoriatic Agent, Topical; Antiseborrheic Agent, Topical

**Use** Psoriasis; seborrheal dermatitis; atopic dermatitis; eczematoid dermatitis

**Usual Dosage** Add to bath water, soak for 5-20 minutes then pat dry

**Local Anesthetic/Vasoconstrictor Precautions** No information available to require special precautions

**Effects on Dental Treatment** No effects or complications reported

**Generic Available** Yes

♦ **Cobalamin** *see* Cyanocobalamin *on page 282*

## Cocaine (koe KANE)

**Therapeutic Category** Local Anesthetic, Topical

**Use** Topical anesthesia (ester derivative) for mucous membranes

**Usual Dosage** Dosage depends on the area to be anesthetized, tissue vascularity, technique of anesthesia, and individual patient tolerance; use the lowest dose necessary to produce adequate anesthesia should be used, not to exceed 1 mg/kg. Use reduced dosages for children, elderly, or debilitated patients.

Topical application (ear, nose, throat, bronchoscopy): Concentrations of 1% to 4% are used; concentrations >4% are not recommended because of potential for increased incidence and severity of systemic toxic reactions

**Mechanism of Action** Blocks both the initiation and conduction of nerve impulses by decreasing the neuronal membrane's permeability to sodium ions, which results in inhibition of depolarization with resultant blockade of conduction; interferes with the uptake of norepinephrine by adrenergic nerve terminals producing vasoconstriction

**Local Anesthetic/Vasoconstrictor Precautions** Although plain local anesthetic is not contraindicated, vasoconstrictor is absolutely contraindicated in any patient under the influence of or within 2 hours of cocaine use

**Effects on Dental Treatment** See comments below

**Other Adverse Effects**

>10%:

- Central nervous system: CNS stimulation
- Local: Loss of smell/taste, chronic rhinitis, nasal congestion

1% to 10%:

- Cardiovascular: Bradycardia with low doses, tachycardia with moderate doses, hypertension, cardiac arrhythmias
- Central nervous system: Nervousness, restlessness, euphoria, excitement, hallucination, seizures
- Gastrointestinal: Vomiting
- Neuromuscular & skeletal: Tremors and clonic-tonic reactions
- Ocular: Sloughing of the corneal epithelium, ulceration of the cornea
- Respiratory: Tachypnea, respiratory failure

**Drug Interactions** Increased toxicity: MAO inhibitors

**Drug Uptake** Following topical administration to mucosa:

- Onset of action: Within 1 minute
- Peak action: Within 5 minutes
- Duration: ≥30 minutes, depending on dosage administered
- Absorption: Well absorbed through mucous membranes; limited by drug-induced vasoconstriction; enhanced by inflammation
- Serum half-life: 75 minutes

**Pregnancy Risk Factor** C (X if nonmedicinal use)

**Dosage Forms**

- Powder, as hydrochloride: 5 g, 25 g
- Solution, topical, as hydrochloride: 4% [40 mg/mL] (2 mL, 4 mL, 10 mL); 10% [100 mg/mL] (4 mL, 10 mL)
- Solution, topical, viscous, as hydrochloride: 4% [40 mg/mL] (4 mL, 10 mL); 10% [100 mg/mL] (4 mL, 10 mL)
- Tablet, soluble, for topical solution, as hydrochloride: 135 mg

**Generic Available** Yes

**Comments** The cocaine user, regardless of how the cocaine was administered, presents the potential of life-threatening situation in the dental operatory. The patient under the influence of cocaine could be compared to a car going 100 miles per hour. Blood pressure is elevated and heart rate is likely increased. The use of a local anesthetic with epinephrine in such a patient may result in a medical emergency. Such patients can be identified by their jitteriness, irritability, talkativeness, tremors, and short abrupt speech patterns. These same signs and symptoms may also be seen in a normal dental patient with preoperative dental anxiety; therefore, the dentist must be particularly alert in order to identify the potential cocaine abuser. If a patient is suspected, they should never be given a local anesthetic with vasoconstrictor for fear of exacerbating the cocaine-induced sympathetic response. Life-threatening episodes of cardiac arrhythmias and hypertensive crises have been reported when local anesthetic with vasoconstrictor was administered to a patient under the influence of cocaine. No local anesthetic used by any dentist can interfere with, nor test positive by cocaine in any urine testing screen. Therefore, the dentist needn't be concerned with any false drug use accusations associated with dental anesthesia.

♦ **Codafed® Expectorant** *see* Guaifenesin, Pseudoephedrine, and Codeine *on page 482*

♦ **Codamine®** *see* Hydrocodone and Phenylpropanolamine *on page 510*

- **Codamine® Pediatric** *see* Hydrocodone and Phenylpropanolamine *on page 510*
- **Codehist® DH** *see* Chlorpheniramine, Pseudoephedrine, and Codeine *on page 237*

## Codeine (KOE deen)

**Related Information**

Dental Drug Interactions: Update on Drug Combinations Requiring Special Considerations *on page 1225*

Narcotic Agonists *on page 1223*

**Canadian Brand Names** Codeine Contin®; Linctus Codeine Blac; Linctus With Codeine Phosphate; Paveral Stanley Syrup With Codeine Phosphate

**Therapeutic Category** Analgesic, Narcotic; Antitussive

**Synonyms** Methylmorphine

**Use**

Dental: Treatment of postoperative pain

Medical: Relief of pain

**Restrictions** C-II; Nonrefillable

**Usual Dosage** Oral:

Children: Not recommended in pediatric dental patients

Adults: 30 mg/dose; range: 15-60 mg every 4-6 hours as needed; maximum: 360 mg/24 hours

**Mechanism of Action** Binds to opiate receptors (mu and kappa subtypes) in the CNS causing inhibition of ascending pain pathways, altering the perception of and response to pain

**Local Anesthetic/Vasoconstrictor Precautions** No information available to require special precautions

**Effects on Dental Treatment** <1% of patients experience dry mouth

**Other Adverse Effects**

>10%:

Central nervous system: Lightheadedness, dizziness, sedation

Gastrointestinal: Nausea, vomiting

1% to 10%: Gastrointestinal: Constipation

**Contraindications** Hypersensitivity to codeine

**Warnings/Precautions** Use with caution in patients with hypersensitivity reactions to other phenanthrene derivative opioid agonists (morphine, hydrocodone, hydromorphone, levorphanol, oxycodone, oxymorphone); respiratory diseases including asthma, emphysema, COPD, or severe liver or renal insufficiency; some preparations contain sulfites which may cause allergic reactions; may be habit-forming

Enhanced analgesia has been seen in elderly patients on therapeutic doses of narcotics; duration of action may be increased in the elderly; the elderly may be particularly susceptible to the CNS depressant and constipating effects of narcotics

**Drug Interactions** Increased toxicity of CNS depressants, phenothiazines, tricyclic antidepressants, guanabenz, MAO inhibitors (may also lead to a decrease in blood pressure)

**Drug Uptake**

Onset of effect: Analgesia: 30-45 minutes

Duration of effect: 4-6 hours

Serum half-life: 2.5-3.5 hours

Time to peak serum concentration: 1-2 hours

**Pregnancy Risk Factor** C (D if used for prolonged periods or in high doses at term)

**Breast-feeding Considerations** May be taken while breast-feeding

**Dosage Forms**

Injection, as phosphate: 30 mg (1 mL, 2 mL); 60 mg (1 mL, 2 mL)

Solution, oral: 15 mg/5 mL

Tablet, as sulfate: 15 mg, 30 mg, 60 mg

Tablet, as phosphate, soluble: 30 mg, 60 mg

Tablet, as sulfate, soluble: 15 mg, 30 mg, 60 mg

**Dietary Considerations** May be taken with food or water to minimize GI distress

**Generic Available** Yes

**Comments** It is recommended that codeine not be used as the sole entity for analgesia because of moderate efficacy along with relatively high incidence of nausea, sedation, and constipation. In addition, codeine has some narcotic addiction liability. Codeine in combination with acetaminophen or aspirin is recommended. Maximum effective analgesic dose of codeine is 60 mg (1 grain). Beyond 60 mg increases respiratory depression only.

**Selected Readings**

Desjardins PJ, Cooper SA, Gallegos TL, et al, "The Relative Analgesic Efficacy of Propiram Fumarate, Codeine, Aspirin, and Placebo in Post-Impaction Dental Pain," *J Clin Pharmacol*, 1984, 24(1):35-42.

Forbes JA, Keller CK, Smith JW, et al, "Analgesic Effect of Naproxen Sodium, Codeine, a Naproxen-Codeine Combination and Aspirin on the Postoperative Pain of Oral Surgery," *Pharmacotherapy*, 1986, 6(5):211-8.

- ♦ **Codeine and Bromodiphenhydramine** *see* Bromodiphenhydramine and Codeine *on page 151*
- ♦ **Codeine and Butalbital Compound** *see* Butalbital Compound and Codeine *on page 165*
- ♦ **Codiclear® DH** *see* Hydrocodone and Guaifenesin *on page 508*
- ♦ **Codoxy®** *see* Oxycodone and Aspirin *on page 753*
- ♦ **Cogentin®** *see* Benztropine *on page 132*
- ♦ **Co-Gesic® [5/500]** *see* Hydrocodone and Acetaminophen *on page 505*
- ♦ **Cognex®** *see* Tacrine *on page 950*
- ♦ **Co-Hist® [OTC]** *see* Acetaminophen, Chlorpheniramine, and Pseudoephedrine *on page 32*
- ♦ **Colace® [OTC]** *see* Docusate *on page 346*

## Colchicine (KOL chi seen)

**Therapeutic Category** Anti-inflammatory Agent; Uricosuric Agent

**Use** Treat acute gouty arthritis attacks and to prevent recurrences of such attacks; management of familial Mediterranean fever

**Usual Dosage**

Prophylaxis of familial Mediterranean fever: Oral:
- Children:
  - ≤5 years: 0.5 mg/day
  - >5 years: 1-1.5 mg/day in 2-3 divided doses
- Adults: 1-2 mg/day in 2-3 divided doses

Gouty arthritis, acute attacks: Adults:
- Oral: Initial: 0.5-1.2 mg, then 0.5-0.6 mg every 1-2 hours or 1-1.2 mg every 2 hours until relief or GI side effects (nausea, vomiting, or diarrhea) occur to a maximum total dose of 8 mg; wait 3 days before initiating another course of therapy
- I.V.: Initial: 1-3 mg, then 0.5 mg every 6 hours until response, not to exceed 4 mg/day; if pain recurs, it may be necessary to administer a daily dose of 1-2 mg for several days, however, do not give more colchicine by any route for at least 7 days after a full course of I.V. therapy (4 mg), transfer to oral colchicine in a dose similar to that being given I.V.

Gouty arthritis, prophylaxis of recurrent attacks: Adults: Oral: 0.5-0.6 mg/day or every other day

**Mechanism of Action** Decreases leukocyte motility, decreases phagocytosis in joints and lactic acid production, thereby reducing the deposition of urate crystals that perpetuates the inflammatory response

**Local Anesthetic/Vasoconstrictor Precautions** No information available to require special precautions

**Effects on Dental Treatment** No effects or complications reported

**Other Adverse Effects**

- >10%: Gastrointestinal: Nausea, vomiting, diarrhea, abdominal pain
- 1% to 10%:
  - Dermatologic: Alopecia
  - Gastrointestinal: Anorexia
- <1%:
  - Dermatologic: Rash
  - Genitourinary: Azoospermia
  - Hematologic: Bone marrow suppression, agranulocytosis, aplastic anemia
  - Hepatic: Hepatotoxicity
  - Neuromuscular & skeletal: Myopathy, peripheral neuritis

**Drug Interactions** Decreased effect: Vitamin $B_{12}$ absorption may be reduced

**Drug Uptake**

- Onset of effect:
  - Oral: Relief of pain and inflammation occurs after 24-48 hours
  - I.V.: 6-12 hours
- Serum half-life: 12-30 minutes
- Time to peak serum concentration: Oral: Within 0.5-2 hours declining for the next 2 hours before increasing again due to enterohepatic recycling

**Pregnancy Risk Factor** C (oral)/D (parenteral)

**Generic Available** Yes: Tablet

## Colchicine and Probenecid (KOL chi seen & proe BEN e sid)

**Therapeutic Category** Uricosuric Agent

**Synonyms** Probenecid and Colchicine

**Use** Treatment of chronic gouty arthritis when complicated by frequent, recurrent acute attacks of gout

**Usual Dosage** Adults: Oral: 1 tablet daily for 1 week, then 1 tablet twice daily thereafter

**Local Anesthetic/Vasoconstrictor Precautions** No information available to require special precautions

**Effects on Dental Treatment** No effects or complications reported

**Other Adverse Effects** 1% to 10%:

- Cardiovascular: Flushing
- Central nervous system: Headache, dizziness
- Dermatologic: Rash, alopecia
- Gastrointestinal: Anorexia, nausea, vomiting, diarrhea, abdominal pain
- Hematologic: Anemia, leukopenia, aplastic anemia, agranulocytosis
- Hepatic: Hepatic necrosis, hepatotoxicity
- Neuromuscular & skeletal: Peripheral neuritis, myopathy
- Renal: Nephrotic syndrome, uric acid stones, polyuria
- Miscellaneous: Hypersensitivity reactions

**Pregnancy Risk Factor** C oral/D parenteral

**Generic Available** Yes

**Comments** Do not initiate therapy until an acute gouty attack has subsided

- ♦ **Cold & Allergy® Elixir [OTC]** *see* Brompheniramine and Phenylpropanolamine *on page 153*
- ♦ **Coldlac-LA®** *see* Guaifenesin and Phenylpropanolamine *on page 480*
- ♦ **Coldloc®** *see* Guaifenesin, Phenylpropanolamine, and Phenylephrine *on page 481*
- ♦ **Coldrine® [OTC]** *see* Acetaminophen and Pseudoephedrine *on page 31*
- ♦ **Colestid®** *see* Colestipol *on this page*

## Colestipol (koe LES ti pole)

**Related Information**

Cardiovascular Diseases *on page 1066*

**U.S. Brand Names** Colestid®

**Therapeutic Category** Lipid Lowering Drugs

**Use** Adjunct in management of primary hypercholesterolemia; regression of arteriolosclerosis; relief of pruritus associated with elevated levels of bile acids; possibly used to decrease plasma half-life of digoxin in toxicity

**Usual Dosage** Adults: Oral: 5-30 g/day in divided doses 2-4 times/day

**Mechanism of Action** Binds with bile acids to form an insoluble complex that is eliminated in feces; it thereby increases the fecal loss of bile acid-bound low density lipoprotein cholesterol

**Local Anesthetic/Vasoconstrictor Precautions** No information available to require special precautions

**Effects on Dental Treatment** No effects or complications reported

**Other Adverse Effects**

>10%: Gastrointestinal: Constipation

1% to 10%: Gastrointestinal: Abdominal pain and distention, belching, flatulence, nausea, vomiting, diarrhea

<1%:

- Central nervous system: Headache, dizziness, anxiety, vertigo, drowsiness, fatigue
- Dermatologic: Dermatitis, urticaria
- Endocrine & metabolic: Elevated serum phosphorous and chloride with decrease of sodium and potassium
- Gastrointestinal: Peptic ulceration, GI irritation and bleeding, anorexia
- Hepatic: Cholelithiasis, cholecystitis
- Neuromuscular & skeletal: Arthralgia, arthritis, weakness
- Respiratory: Dyspnea

**Drug Interactions** Decreased absorption of tetracycline, vitamins A, D, E and K, digitalis glycosides, warfarin, thyroid hormones, thiazide diuretics, propranolol, phenobarbital, amiodarone, methotrexate, NSAIDs, and other drugs by binding to the drug in the intestine

**Drug Uptake** Absorption: Oral: Not absorbed

**Pregnancy Risk Factor** C

**Generic Available** No

## Colfosceril Palmitate (kole FOS er il PALM i tate)

**U.S. Brand Names** Exosurf® Neonatal™

**Therapeutic Category** Lung Surfactant

**Synonyms** Dipalmitoylphosphatidylcholine; DPPC; Synthetic Lung Surfactant

**Use** Neonatal respiratory distress syndrome (RDS):

Prophylactic therapy: Infants at risk for developing RDS with body weight <1350 g; infants with evidence of pulmonary immaturity with body weight >1350 g

Rescue therapy: Treatment of infants with RDS based on respiratory distress not attributable to any other causes and chest radiographic findings consistent with RDS

**Usual Dosage** For intratracheal use only

Prophylactic treatment: Give 5 mL/kg (as two 2.5 mL/kg half-doses) as soon as possible; the second and third doses should be administered at 12 and 24 hours later to those infants remaining on ventilators

Rescue treatment: Give 5 mL/kg (as two 2.5 mL/kg half-doses) as soon as the diagnosis of RDS is made; the second 5 mL/kg (as two 2.5 mL/kg half-doses) dose should be administered 12 hours later

**Mechanism of Action** Replaces deficient or ineffective endogenous lung surfactant in neonates with respiratory distress syndrome (RDS) or in neonates at risk of developing RDS; reduces surface tension and stabilizes the alveoli from collapsing

**Local Anesthetic/Vasoconstrictor Precautions** No information available to require special precautions

**Effects on Dental Treatment** No effects or complications reported

**Other Adverse Effects** 1% to 10%: Respiratory: Pulmonary hemorrhage, apnea, mucous plugging, decrease in transcutaneous $O_2$ >20%

**Drug Uptake**

Absorption: Intratracheal: Absorbed from the alveolus

**Generic Available** No

♦ **Colgate Total® Toothpaste** *see* Triclosan and Fluoride *on page 1014*

## Colistimethate (koe lis ti METH ate)

**U.S. Brand Names** Coly-Mycin® M Parenteral

**Therapeutic Category** Antibiotic, Miscellaneous

**Use** Treatment of infections due to sensitive strains of certain gram-negative bacilli

**Usual Dosage** Children and Adults: I.M., I.V.: 2.5-5 mg/kg/day in 2-4 divided doses

**Local Anesthetic/Vasoconstrictor Precautions** No information available to require special precautions

**Effects on Dental Treatment** No effects or complications reported

**Other Adverse Effects** 1% to 10%:

Central nervous system: Vertigo, slurring of speech

Dermatologic: Urticaria

Gastrointestinal: GI upset

Renal: Decreased urine output

Respiratory: Respiratory arrest

**Pregnancy Risk Factor** B

**Generic Available** No

## Colistin (koe LIS tin)

**U.S. Brand Names** Coly-Mycin® S Oral

**Therapeutic Category** Antibiotic, Miscellaneous; Antidiarrheal

**Synonyms** Polymyxin E

**Use** Treat diarrhea in infants and children caused by susceptible organisms, especially *E. coli* and *Shigella*

**Usual Dosage** Diarrhea: Children: Oral: 5-15 mg/kg/day in 3 divided doses given every 8 hours

**Mechanism of Action** A polypeptide antibiotic that binds to and damages the bacterial cell membrane

**Local Anesthetic/Vasoconstrictor Precautions** No information available to require special precautions

**Effects on Dental Treatment** No effects or complications reported

**Other Adverse Effects** <1%:

Gastrointestinal: Nausea, vomiting

Neuromuscular & skeletal: Neuromuscular blockade

Renal: Nephrotoxicity

Respiratory: Respiratory arrest

Miscellaneous: Hypersensitivity reactions, superinfections

(Continued)

## Colistin *(Continued)*

**Drug Uptake**

Absorption: Oral: Slightly absorbed from GI tract (adults); unpredictable absorption occurs in infants, can lead to significant serum levels

Serum half-life: 2.8-4.8 hours, prolonged in renal insufficiency; with anuria: 48-72 hours

**Pregnancy Risk Factor** C

**Generic Available** No

## Colistin, Neomycin, and Hydrocortisone

(koe LIS tin, nee oh MYE sin & hye droe KOR ti sone)

**U.S. Brand Names** Coly-Mycin® S Otic Drops

**Therapeutic Category** Antibiotic, Miscellaneous; Corticosteroid, Otic; Otic Agent, Anti-infective

**Use** Treatment of superficial and susceptible bacterial infections of the external auditory canal; for treatment of susceptible bacterial infections of mastoidectomy and fenestration cavities

**Usual Dosage**

Children: 3 drops in affected ear 3-4 times/day

Adults: 4 drops in affected ear 3-4 times/day

**Local Anesthetic/Vasoconstrictor Precautions** No information available to require special precautions

**Effects on Dental Treatment** No effects or complications reported

**Pregnancy Risk Factor** C

**Generic Available** No

♦ **CollaCote®** *see* Collagen, Absorbable *on this page*

## Collagen, Absorbable (KOL la jen, ab SORB able)

**U.S. Brand Names** CollaCote®; CollaPlug®; CollaTape®

**Therapeutic Category** Hemostatic Agent

**Use**

Dental: To control bleeding created during dental surgery

Medical: Hemostatic

**Usual Dosage** Children and Adults: A sufficiently large dressing should be selected so as to completely cover the oral wound

**Mechanism of Action** The highly porous sponge structure absorbs blood and wound exudate. The collagen component causes aggregation of platelets which bind to collagen fibrils. The aggregated platelets degranulate, releasing coagulation factors that promote the formation of fibrin.

**Local Anesthetic/Vasoconstrictor Precautions** No information available to require special precautions

**Effects on Dental Treatment** No effects or complications reported

**Other Adverse Effects** No data reported

**Contraindications** No data reported

**Warnings/Precautions** Should not be used on infected or contaminated wounds

**Drug Interactions** No data reported

**Breast-feeding Considerations** May be taken while breast-feeding

**Dosage Forms** Wound dressings: 1" x 3", 3/4" x 1 1/2", 3/8" x 3/4"

**Dietary Considerations** No data reported

**Generic Available** Yes

**Comments** The dressing should be applied over the wound and held in place with moderate pressure. The period of time necessary to apply pressure will vary with the degree of bleeding. In general, 2-5 minutes should be sufficient to achieve hemostasis. At the end of the procedure, the dressing can be removed, replaced or left in situ, any excess dressing should be removed prior to wound closure.

## Collagenase (KOL la je nase)

**U.S. Brand Names** Biozyme-C®; Santyl®

**Therapeutic Category** Enzyme, Topical Debridement

**Use** Promotes debridement of necrotic tissue in dermal ulcers and severe burns

**Usual Dosage** Topical: Apply once daily

**Mechanism of Action** Collagenase is an enzyme derived from the fermentation of *Clostridium histolyticum* and differs from other proteolytic enzymes in that its enzymatic action has a high specificity for native and denatured collagen. Collagenase will not attack collagen in healthy tissue or newly formed granulation tissue. In addition, it does not act on fat, fibrin, keratin, or muscle.

**Local Anesthetic/Vasoconstrictor Precautions** No information available to require special precautions

**Effects on Dental Treatment** No effects or complications reported

**Other Adverse Effects**
1% to 10%: Local: Irritation
<1%: Local: Pain and burning may occur at site of application

**Drug Interactions** Decreased effect: Enzymatic activity is inhibited by detergents, benzalkonium chloride, hexachlorophene, nitrofurazone, tincture of iodine, and heavy metal ions (silver and mercury)

**Pregnancy Risk Factor** C

**Generic Available** No

- **CollaPlug®** *see* Collagen, Absorbable *on previous page*
- **CollaTape®** *see* Collagen, Absorbable *on previous page*
- **Collyrium Fresh® Ophthalmic [OTC]** *see* Tetrahydrozoline *on page 967*
- **Colovage®** *see* Polyethylene Glycol-Electrolyte Solution *on page 815*
- **Coly-Mycin® M Parenteral** *see* Colistimethate *on page 275*
- **Coly-Mycin® S Oral** *see* Colistin *on page 275*
- **Coly-Mycin® S Otic Drops** *see* Colistin, Neomycin, and Hydrocortisone *on previous page*
- **CoLyte®** *see* Polyethylene Glycol-Electrolyte Solution *on page 815*
- **CombiPatch®** *see* Estradiol and Norethindrone *on page 388*
- **Combipres®** *see* Clonidine and Chlorthalidone *on page 266*
- **Combivent®** *see* Ipratropium and Albuterol *on page 548*
- **Combivir®** *see* Zidovudine and Lamivudine *on page 1059*
- **Comfort® Ophthalmic [OTC]** *see* Naphazoline *on page 703*
- **Comfort® Tears Solution [OTC]** *see* Artificial Tears *on page 97*
- **Comhist®** *see* Chlorpheniramine, Phenylephrine, and Phenyltoloxamine *on page 235*
- **Comhist® LA** *see* Chlorpheniramine, Phenylephrine, and Phenyltoloxamine *on page 235*
- **Common Oral-Facial Infections and Antibiotics for Treatment** *see page 1268*
- **Compazine®** *see* Prochlorperazine *on page 843*
- **Compound W® [OTC]** *see* Salicylic Acid *on page 900*
- **Compoz® Gel Caps [OTC]** *see* Diphenhydramine *on page 338*
- **Compoz® Nighttime Sleep Aid [OTC]** *see* Diphenhydramine *on page 338*
- **Comtrex® Maximum Strength Non-Drowsy [OTC]** *see* Acetaminophen, Dextromethorphan, and Pseudoephedrine *on page 32*
- **Condylox®** *see* Podofilox *on page 812*
- **Conex® [OTC]** *see* Guaifenesin and Phenylpropanolamine *on page 480*
- **Congess® Jr** *see* Guaifenesin and Pseudoephedrine *on page 481*
- **Congess® Sr** *see* Guaifenesin and Pseudoephedrine *on page 481*
- **Congestac®** *see* Guaifenesin and Pseudoephedrine *on page 481*
- **Congestant D® [OTC]** *see* Chlorpheniramine, Phenylpropanolamine, and Acetaminophen *on page 236*
- **Constilac®** *see* Lactulose *on page 571*
- **Constulose®** *see* Lactulose *on page 571*
- **Contac® Cough Formula Liquid [OTC]** *see* Guaifenesin and Dextromethorphan *on page 479*
- **Control® [OTC]** *see* Phenylpropanolamine *on page 797*
- **Controlled Substances** *see page 1269*
- **Contuss®** *see* Guaifenesin, Phenylpropanolamine, and Phenylephrine *on page 481*
- **Contuss® XT** *see* Guaifenesin and Phenylpropanolamine *on page 480*
- **Cool Mint Listerine® Antiseptic [OTC]** *see* Mouthwash, Antiseptic *on page 690*
- **Copaxone®** *see* Glatiramer Acetate *on page 468*
- **Cophene-B®** *see* Brompheniramine *on page 151*
- **Cophene XP®** *see* Hydrocodone, Pseudoephedrine, and Guaifenesin *on page 511*
- **Copolymer-1** *see* Glatiramer Acetate *on page 468*
- **Copper** *see* Trace Metals *on page 1001*
- **Co-Pyronil® 2 Pulvules® [OTC]** *see* Chlorpheniramine and Pseudoephedrine *on page 233*
- **Cordarone®** *see* Amiodarone *on page 66*
- **Cordran®** *see* Flurandrenolide *on page 447*
- **Cordran® SP** *see* Flurandrenolide *on page 447*
- **Coreg®** *see* Carvedilol *on page 195*
- **Corgard®** *see* Nadolol *on page 696*
- **Coricidin® [OTC]** *see* Chlorpheniramine and Acetaminophen *on page 232*

- **Coricidin D® [OTC]** *see* Chlorpheniramine, Phenylpropanolamine, and Acetaminophen *on page 236*
- **Corlopam®** *see* Fenoldopam *on page 423*
- **Corque® Topical** *see* Clioquinol and Hydrocortisone *on page 260*
- **Cortatrigen® Otic** *see* Neomycin, Polymyxin B, and Hydrocortisone *on page 712*
- **Cortef®** *see* Hydrocortisone *on page 511*
- **Corticaine® Topical** *see* Dibucaine and Hydrocortisone *on page 318*
- **Corticosteroid Equivalencies Comparison** *see page 1221*
- **Corticosteroids, Topical Comparison** *see page 1222*

## Corticotropin (kor ti koe TROE pin)

**U.S. Brand Names** Acthar®; H.P. Acthar® Gel

**Therapeutic Category** Adrenal Corticosteroid

**Use** Acute exacerbations of multiple sclerosis; diagnostic aid in adrenocortical insufficiency, severe muscle weakness in myasthenia gravis; cosyntropin is preferred over corticotropin for diagnostic test of adrenocortical insufficiency (cosyntropin is less allergenic and test is shorter in duration)

**Usual Dosage** Injection has a rapid onset and duration of activity of approximately 2 hours; the repository injection has a slower onset, but may sustain effects for ≤3 days

Children:

Anti-inflammatory/immunosuppressant:

I.M., I.V., S.C. (aqueous): 1.6 units/kg/day or 50 units/m²/day divided every 6-8 hours

I.M. (gel): 0.8 units/kg/day or 25 units/m²/day divided every 12-24 hours

Infantile spasms: Various regimens have been used. Some neurologists recommend low-dose ACTH (5-40 units/day) for short periods (1-6 weeks), while others recommend larger doses of ACTH (40-160 units/day) for long periods of treatment (3-12 months). Well designed comparative dosing studies are needed. Example of low dose regimen:

Initial: I.M. (gel): 20 units/day for 2 weeks, if patient responds, taper and discontinue; if patient does not respond, increase dose to 30 units/day for 4 weeks then taper and discontinue

I.M. usual dose (gel): 20-40 units/day or 5-8 units/kg/day in 1-2 divided doses; range: 5-160 units/day

Oral prednisone (2 mg/kg/day) was as effective as I.M. ACTH gel (20 units/day) in controlling infantile spasms

Adults: Acute exacerbation of multiple sclerosis: I.M.: 80-120 units/day for 2-3 weeks

Diagnostic purposes: I.V.: 10-25 units in 500 mL 5% dextrose in water infused over 8 hours

Repository injection: I.M., S.C.: 40-80 units every 24-72 hours

**Mechanism of Action** Stimulates the adrenal cortex to secrete adrenal steroids (including hydrocortisone, cortisone), androgenic substances, and a small amount of aldosterone

**Local Anesthetic/Vasoconstrictor Precautions** No information available to require special precautions

**Effects on Dental Treatment** No effects or complications reported

**Other Adverse Effects**

>10%:

Central nervous system: Insomnia, nervousness

Gastrointestinal: Increased appetite, indigestion

1% to 10%:

Endocrine & metabolic: Diabetes mellitus

Neuromuscular & skeletal: Arthralgia

Ocular: Cataracts

Respiratory: Epistaxis

<1%:

Central nervous system: Seizures, mood swings, headache, delirium, hallucinations, euphoria

Dermatologic: Skin atrophy, bruising, hyperpigmentation, acne, hirsutism

Endocrine & metabolic: Amenorrhea, sodium and water retention, Cushing's syndrome, hyperglycemia, bone growth suppression

Gastrointestinal: Abdominal distention, ulcerative esophagitis, pancreatitis

Neuromuscular & skeletal: Muscle wasting

Miscellaneous: Hypersensitivity reactions

**Drug Interactions** Decreased effect: Spironolactone, hydrocortisone, cortisone; can antagonize the effects of anticholinesterases (eg, neostigmine)

**Pregnancy Risk Factor** C

**Generic Available** Yes

## Cortisone Acetate (KOR ti sone AS e tate)

**Related Information**

Corticosteroid Equivalencies Comparison *on page 1221*
Respiratory Diseases *on page 1079*

**U.S. Brand Names** Cortone® Acetate

**Therapeutic Category** Adrenal Corticosteroid; Anti-inflammatory Agent; Corticosteroid, Systemic

**Use** Management of adrenocortical insufficiency

**Usual Dosage** If possible, administer glucocorticoids before 9 AM to minimize adrenocortical suppression; dosing depends upon the condition being treated and the response of the patient; supplemental doses may be warranted during times of stress in the course of withdrawing therapy

Children:
- Anti-inflammatory or immunosuppressive:
  - Oral: 2.5-10 mg/kg/day **or** 20-300 mg/m²/day in divided doses every 6-8 hours
  - I.M.: 1-5 mg/kg/day **or** 14-375 mg/m²/day in divided doses every 12-24 hours
- Physiologic replacement:
  - Oral: 0.5-0.75 mg/kg/day **or** 20-25 mg/m²/day in divided doses every 8 hours
  - I.M.: 0.25-0.35 mg/kg/day once daily **or** 12.5 mg/m²/day
- Stress coverage for surgery: I.M.: 1 and 2 days before preanesthesia, and 1-3 days after surgery: 50-62.5 mg/m²/day; 4 days after surgery: 31-50 mg/m²/day; 5 days after surgery, resume presurgical corticosteroid dose.

Adults: Oral, I.M.: 25-300 mg/day in divided doses every 12-24 hours

**Mechanism of Action** Decreases inflammation by suppression of migration of polymorphonuclear leukocytes and reversal of increased capillary permeability

**Local Anesthetic/Vasoconstrictor Precautions** No information available to require special precautions

**Effects on Dental Treatment** A compromised immune response may occur if patient has been taking systemic cortisone; the need for corticosteroid coverage in these patients should be considered before any dental treatment; consult with physician

**Other Adverse Effects**

>10%:
- Central nervous system: Insomnia, nervousness
- Gastrointestinal: Increased appetite, indigestion

1% to 10%:
- Dermatologic: Hirsutism
- Endocrine & metabolic: Diabetes mellitus
- Gastrointestinal: Peptic ulcer, nausea, vomiting
- Neuromuscular & skeletal: Muscle weakness, osteoporosis, fractures, arthralgia
- Ocular: Cataracts, glaucoma
- Respiratory: Epistaxis

<1%:
- Cardiovascular: Edema, hypertension
- Central nervous system: Mood swings, vertigo, seizures, headache, psychoses, pseudotumor cerebri, delirium, hallucinations, euphoria
- Dermatologic: Acne, skin atrophy, hyperpigmentation, bruising
- Endocrine & metabolic: Cushing's syndrome, pituitary-adrenal axis suppression, growth suppression, glucose intolerance, hypokalemia, alkalosis, amenorrhea, sodium and water retention, hyperglycemia
- Gastrointestinal: Abdominal distention, ulcerative esophagitis, pancreatitis
- Neuromuscular & skeletal: Muscle wasting
- Miscellaneous: Hypersensitivity reactions

**Drug Interactions**

Decreased effect:
- Barbiturates, phenytoin, rifampin causes decreased cortisone effects
- Cortisone causes decreased warfarin effects
- Cortisone causes decreased effects of salicylates

Increased effect: Estrogens (increased cortisone effects)

Increased toxicity:
- Cortisone + NSAIDs causes increased ulcerogenic potential
- Cortisone causes increased potassium deletion due to diuretics

**Drug Uptake**

Peak effect:
- Oral: Within 2 hours
- I.M.: Within 20-48 hours

Duration of action: 30-36 hours

Absorption: Slow rate of absorption

Serum half-life: 30 minutes to 2 hours

(Continued)

## Cortisone Acetate *(Continued)*

End-stage renal disease: 3.5 hours

**Pregnancy Risk Factor** D

**Dosage Forms**

Injection: 50 mg/mL (10 mL)

Tablet: 5 mg, 10 mg, 25 mg

**Dietary Considerations** Limit caffeine; may need diet with increased potassium, pyridoxine, vitamin C, vitamin D, folate, calcium, and phosphorus and decreased sodium; may be taken with food to decrease GI distress

**Generic Available** Yes

- **Cortisporin® Ophthalmic Ointment** *see* Bacitracin, Neomycin, Polymyxin B, and Hydrocortisone *on page 118*
- **Cortisporin® Ophthalmic Suspension** *see* Neomycin, Polymyxin B, and Hydrocortisone *on page 712*
- **Cortisporin® Otic** *see* Neomycin, Polymyxin B, and Hydrocortisone *on page 712*
- **Cortisporin® Topical Cream** *see* Neomycin, Polymyxin B, and Hydrocortisone *on page 712*
- **Cortisporin® Topical Ointment** *see* Bacitracin, Neomycin, Polymyxin B, and Hydrocortisone *on page 118*
- **Cortone® Acetate** *see* Cortisone Acetate *on previous page*
- **Cortrosyn®** *see* Cosyntropin *on this page*
- **Corvert®** *see* Ibutilide *on page 524*
- **Cosmegen®** *see* Dactinomycin *on page 294*

## Cosyntropin (koe sin TROE pin)

**U.S. Brand Names** Cortrosyn®

**Canadian Brand Names** Synacthen® Depot

**Therapeutic Category** Adrenal Corticosteroid

**Use** Diagnostic test to differentiate primary adrenal from secondary (pituitary) adrenocortical insufficiency

**Usual Dosage**

Adrenocortical insufficiency: I.M., I.V. (over 2 minutes): Peak plasma cortisol concentrations usually occur 45-60 minutes after cosyntropin administration

Children <2 years: 0.125 mg

Children >2 years and Adults: 0.25 mg

When greater cortisol stimulation is needed, an I.V. infusion may be used:

Children >2 years and Adults: 0.25 mg administered at 0.04 mg/hour over 6 hours

Congenital adrenal hyperplasia evaluation: 1 mg/m²/dose up to a maximum of 1 mg

**Mechanism of Action** Stimulates the adrenal cortex to secrete adrenal steroids (including hydrocortisone, cortisone), androgenic substances, and a small amount of aldosterone

**Local Anesthetic/Vasoconstrictor Precautions** No information available to require special precautions

**Effects on Dental Treatment** No effects or complications reported

**Other Adverse Effects**

1% to 10%:

Cardiovascular: Flushing

Central nervous system: Mild fever

Dermatologic: Pruritus

Gastrointestinal: Chronic pancreatitis

<1%: Hypersensitivity reactions

**Drug Interactions** No data reported

**Drug Uptake** Time to peak serum concentration: Within 1 hour (plasma cortisol levels rise in healthy individuals within 5 minutes of administration I.M. or I.V. push)

**Pregnancy Risk Factor** C

**Generic Available** No

- **Cotazym®** *see* Pancrelipase *on page 763*
- **Cotazym-S®** *see* Pancrelipase *on page 763*
- **Cotrim®** *see* Trimethoprim and Sulfamethoxazole *on page 1021*
- **Cotrim® DS** *see* Trimethoprim and Sulfamethoxazole *on page 1021*
- **Co-trimoxazole** *see* Trimethoprim and Sulfamethoxazole *on page 1021*
- **Coumadin®** *see* Warfarin *on page 1053*
- **Covera-HS®** *see* Verapamil *on page 1043*
- **Cozaar®** *see* Losartan *on page 603*
- **CP-99,219-27** *see* Trovafloxacin/Alatrofloxacin *on page 1030*

- ♦ **Creon®** *see* Pancreatin *on page 763*
- ♦ **Creon® 10** *see* Pancrelipase *on page 763*
- ♦ **Creon® 20** *see* Pancrelipase *on page 763*
- ♦ **Creo-Terpin® [OTC]** *see* Dextromethorphan *on page 314*
- ♦ **Cresylate®** *see* m-Cresyl Acetate *on page 618*
- ♦ **Crinone™ Vaginal Gel** *see* Progesterone *on page 846*
- ♦ **Criticare HN® [OTC]** *see* Enteral Nutritional Products *on page 371*
- ♦ **Crixivan®** *see* Indinavir *on page 533*


## Cromolyn Sodium (KROE moe lin SOW dee um)

**Related Information**

Respiratory Diseases *on page 1079*

**U.S. Brand Names** Gastrocrom®; Intal®; Nasalcrom®

**Canadian Brand Names** Novo-Cromolyn; Opticrom®; PMS-Sodium Cromoglycate; Rynacrom®

**Therapeutic Category** Inhalation, Miscellaneous

**Synonyms** Sodium Cromoglycate

**Use** Adjunct in the prophylaxis of allergic disorders, including rhinitis, giant papillary conjunctivitis, and asthma; inhalation product may be used for prevention of exercise-induced bronchospasm; systemic mastocytosis, food allergy, and treatment of inflammatory bowel disease; **cromolyn is a prophylactic drug with no benefit for acute situations**

**Usual Dosage** Not effective for immediate relief of symptoms in acute asthmatic attacks; must be used at regular intervals for 2-4 weeks to be effective

Children:

Inhalation (taper frequency to the lowest effective dose, ie, 4 times/day → 3 times/day → twice daily):

Initial dose: Metered spray: >5 years: 2 inhalations 4 times/day by metered spray

Initial dose: Nebulization solution: >2 years: 20 mg 4 times/day

Prevention of exercise-induced bronchospasm: Metered spray: >5 years: Single dose of 2 inhalations (aerosol) just prior to (10 minutes to 1 hour) exercise

Nasal: >6 years: Instill 1 spray in each nostril 3-4 times/day

Children 2-12 years: Oral: 100 mg 4 times/day 15-20 minutes before meals, not to exceed 40 mg/kg/day

Children >12 years and Adults: Oral: 200 mg 4 times/day 15-20 minutes before meal, up to 400 mg 4 times/day

Adults:

Inhalation: Metered spray: 2 inhalations 4 times/day

Nasal: Instill 1 spray in each nostril 3-4 times/day

Ophthalmic: Instill 1-2 drops 4-6 times/day into each eye

**Mechanism of Action** Prevents the mast cell release of histamine, leukotrienes and slow-reacting substance of anaphylaxis by inhibiting degranulation after contact with antigens

**Local Anesthetic/Vasoconstrictor Precautions** No information available to require special precautions

**Effects on Dental Treatment** No effects or complications reported

**Other Adverse Effects**

>10%: Local: Hoarseness, coughing, unpleasant taste (inhalation aerosol)

1% to 10%:

Dermatologic: Angioedema

Gastrointestinal: Dry mouth

Genitourinary: Dysuria

Respiratory: Sneezing, nasal congestion

<1%:

Central nervous system: Dizziness, headache

Dermatologic: Rash, urticaria

Gastrointestinal: Nausea, vomiting, diarrhea

Local: Nasal burning

Neuromuscular & skeletal: Arthralgia

Ocular: Ocular stinging, lacrimation

Respiratory: Wheezing, throat irritation, eosinophilic pneumonia, pulmonary infiltrates

Miscellaneous: Anaphylactic reactions

**Drug Interactions** No data reported

**Drug Uptake**

Absorption:

Inhalation: ~8% of dose reaches the lungs upon inhalation of the powder and is well absorbed

Oral: Only 0.5% to 2% of dose absorbed

(Continued)

## Cromolyn Sodium *(Continued)*

Serum half-life: 80-90 minutes

Time to peak serum concentration: Inhalation: Within 15 minutes

**Pregnancy Risk Factor** B

**Generic Available** Yes

## Crotamiton (kroe TAM i tonn)

**U.S. Brand Names** Eurax®

**Therapeutic Category** Antipruritic, Topical; Scabicidal Agent

**Use** Treatment of scabies and symptomatic treatment of pruritus

**Usual Dosage** Topical:

Scabicide: Children and Adults: Wash thoroughly and scrub away loose scales, then towel dry; apply a thin layer and massage drug onto skin of the entire body from the neck to the toes (with special attention to skin folds, creases, and interdigital spaces). Repeat application in 24 hours. Take a cleansing bath 48 hours after the final application. Treatment may be repeated after 7-10 days if live mites are still present.

Pruritus: Massage into affected areas until medication is completely absorbed; repeat as necessary

**Mechanism of Action** Crotamiton has scabicidal activity against *Sarcoptes scabiei*; mechanism of action unknown

**Local Anesthetic/Vasoconstrictor Precautions** No information available to require special precautions

**Effects on Dental Treatment** No effects or complications reported

**Other Adverse Effects** <1%: Local: Pruritus, irritation, contact dermatitis, warm sensation

**Drug Interactions** No data reported

**Pregnancy Risk Factor** C

**Generic Available** No


- **Crude Coal Tar** *see* Coal Tar *on page 270*
- **Crystamine®** *see* Cyanocobalamin *on this page*
- **Crysti 1000®** *see* Cyanocobalamin *on this page*
- **Crysticillin® A.S.** *see* Penicillin G Procaine *on page 775*
- **Crystodigin®** *see* Digitoxin *on page 328*
- **CSP** *see* Cellulose Sodium Phosphate *on page 214*
- **Cuprimine®** *see* Penicillamine *on page 772*
- **Curretab®** *see* Medroxyprogesterone Acetate *on page 623*
- **Cutivate™** *see* Fluticasone *on page 450*


## Cyanocobalamin (sye an oh koe BAL a min)

**U.S. Brand Names** Crystamine®; Crysti 1000®; Cyanoject®; Cyomin®

**Canadian Brand Names** Rubramin®

**Therapeutic Category** Vitamin, Water Soluble

**Synonyms** Cobalamin

**Use**

Dental: Vitamin $B_{12}$ deficiency

Medical: Treatment of pernicious anemia; increased $B_{12}$ requirements due to pregnancy, thyrotoxicosis, hemorrhage, malignancy, liver or kidney disease

**Usual Dosage** I.M. or deep S.C. (oral is not generally recommended due to poor absorption and I.V. is not recommended due to more rapid elimination):

Recommended daily allowance (RDA):

Children: 0.3-2 mcg

Adults: 2 mcg

Pernicious anemia, congenital (if evidence of neurologic involvement): 1000 mcg/day for at least 2 weeks; maintenance: 50 mcg/month

Children: 30-50 mcg/day for 2 or more weeks (to a total dose of 1000-5000 mcg), then follow with 100 mcg month as maintenance dosage

Adults: 100 mcg/day for 6-7 days; if improvement, give same dose on alternate days for 7 doses; then every 3-4 days for 2-3 weeks; once hematologic values have returned to normal, maintenance dosage: 100 mcg/month. **Note:** Use only parenteral therapy as oral therapy is not dependable.

Vitamin $B_{12}$ deficiency:

Children: 100 mcg/day for 10-15 days (total dose of 1-1.5 mg), then once or twice weekly for several months; may taper to 60 mcg every month

Adults: Initial: 30 mcg/day for 5-10 days; maintenance: 100-200 mcg/month

**Mechanism of Action** Coenzyme for various metabolic functions, including fat and carbohydrate metabolism and protein synthesis, used in cell replication and hematopoiesis

**Local Anesthetic/Vasoconstrictor Precautions** No information available to require special precautions

**Effects on Dental Treatment** No effects or complications reported

**Other Adverse Effects** 1% to 10%:

Dermatologic: Itching

Gastrointestinal: Diarrhea

**Contraindications** Hypersensitivity to cyanocobalamin or any component, cobalt; patients with hereditary optic nerve atrophy

**Warnings/Precautions** I.M. route used to treat pernicious anemia; vitamin $B_{12}$ deficiency for >3 months results in irreversible degenerative CNS lesions; treatment of vitamin $B_{12}$ megaloblastic anemia may result in severe hypokalemia, sometimes, fatal, when anemia corrects due to cellular potassium requirements. $B_{12}$ deficiency masks signs of polycythemia vera; vegetarian diets may result in $B_{12}$ deficiency; pernicious anemia occurs more often in gastric carcinoma than in general population.

**Drug Interactions**

Aminosalicylic acid may reduce therapeutic action of vitamin $B_{12}$

Chloramphenicol may decrease the hematologic effect of vitamin $B_{12}$ in patients with pernicious anemia

Colchicine and prolonged alcohol (>2 weeks) use may decrease absorption of vitamin $B_{12}$

**Drug Uptake** Absorption: Absorbed from the terminal ileum in the presence of calcium; for absorption to occur gastric "intrinsic factor" must be present to transfer the compound across the intestinal mucosa

**Pregnancy Risk Factor** A (C if dose exceeds RDA recommendation)

**Dosage Forms**

Gel, nasal (Ener-B®): 400 mcg/0.1 mL

Injection: 30 mcg/mL (30 mL); 100 mcg/mL (1 mL, 10 mL, 30 mL); 1000 mcg/mL (1 mL, 10 mL, 30 mL)

Tablet [OTC]: 25 mcg, 50 mcg, 100 mcg, 250 mcg, 500 mcg, 1000 mcg

**Generic Available** Yes

- **Cyanoject®** *see* Cyanocobalamin *on previous page*
- **Cyclan®** *see* Cyclandelate *on this page*

## Cyclandelate (sye KLAN de late)

**U.S. Brand Names** Cyclan®; Cyclospasmol®

**Therapeutic Category** Vasodilator, Peripheral

**Use** Considered as "possibly effective" for adjunctive therapy in peripheral vascular disease and possibly senility due to cerebrovascular disease or multi-infarct dementia; migraine prophylaxis, vertigo, tinnitus, and visual disturbances secondary to cerebrovascular insufficiency and diabetic peripheral polyneuropathy

**Usual Dosage** Adults: Oral: Initial: 1.2-1.6 g/day in divided doses before meals and at bedtime until response; maintenance therapy: 400-800 mg/day in 2-4 divided doses; start with lowest dose in elderly due to hypotensive potential; decrease dose by 200 mg decrements to achieve minimal maintenance dose; improvement can usually be seen over weeks of therapy and prolonged use; short courses of therapy are usually ineffective and not recommended

**Mechanism of Action** Cyclandelate, 3,3,5-trimethylcyclohexyl mandelate is a vasodilator that exerts a direct, papaverine-like action on smooth muscles, particularly that found within the blood vessels. Animal data indicate that cyclandelate also has antispasmodic properties; exhibits no adrenergic stimulation or blocking action; action exceeds that of papaverine; mild calcium channel blocking agent, may benefit in mild hypercalcemia; calcium channel blocking activity may explain some of its pharmacologic effects (enhanced blood flow) and inhibition of platelet aggregation.

**Local Anesthetic/Vasoconstrictor Precautions** No information available to require special precautions

**Effects on Dental Treatment** No effects or complications reported

**Other Adverse Effects** <1%:

Cardiovascular: Flushing of face, tachycardia

Central nervous system: Headache, pain, dizziness

Gastrointestinal: Belching, heartburn

Neuromuscular & skeletal: Paresthesia, weakness

**Drug Interactions** No data reported

**Pregnancy Risk Factor** C

**Generic Available** Yes

## Cyclizine (SYE kli zeen)

**U.S. Brand Names** Marezine® [OTC]

**Canadian Brand Names** Marzine®

(Continued)

## Cyclizine *(Continued)*

**Therapeutic Category** Antiemetic; Antihistamine

**Use** Prevention and treatment of nausea, vomiting, and vertigo associated with motion sickness; control of postoperative nausea and vomiting

**Usual Dosage**

Children 6-12 years:

- Oral: 25 mg up to 3 times/day
- I.M.: Not recommended

Adults:

- Oral: 50 mg taken 30 minutes before departure, may repeat in 4-6 hours if needed, up to 200 mg/day
- I.M.: 50 mg every 4-6 hours as needed

**Mechanism of Action** Cyclizine is a piperazine derivative with properties of histamines. The precise mechanism of action in inhibiting the symptoms of motion sickness is not known. It may have effects directly on the labyrinthine apparatus and central actions on the labyrinthine apparatus and on the chemoreceptor trigger zone. Cyclizine exerts a central anticholinergic action.

**Local Anesthetic/Vasoconstrictor Precautions** No information available to require special precautions

**Effects on Dental Treatment** >10% of patients will experience dry mouth

**Other Adverse Effects**

>10%: Central nervous system: Drowsiness

1% to 10%:

- Central nervous system: Headache
- Dermatologic: Dermatitis
- Gastrointestinal: Nausea
- Ocular: Diplopia
- Renal: Polyuria, urinary retention

**Drug Interactions** Increased effect/toxicity with CNS depressants, alcohol

**Pregnancy Risk Factor** B

**Generic Available** No

## Cyclobenzaprine (sye kloe BEN za preen)

**Related Information**

Temporomandibular Dysfunction (TMD) *on page 1149*

**U.S. Brand Names** Flexeril®

**Canadian Brand Names** Novo-Cycloprine

**Therapeutic Category** Muscle Relaxant; Skeletal Muscle Relaxant

**Use**

Dental: Treatment of muscle spasm associated with acute temporomandibular joint pain

Medical: Treatment of muscle spasm associated with acute painful musculoskeletal conditions; supportive therapy in tetanus

**Usual Dosage** Oral: **Note:** Do not use longer than 2-3 weeks

Children: Dosage has not been established

Adults: 20-40 mg/day in 2-4 divided doses; maximum dose: 60 mg/day

**Mechanism of Action** Centrally acting skeletal muscle relaxant pharmacologically related to tricyclic antidepressants; reduces tonic somatic motor activity influencing both alpha and gamma motor neurons

**Local Anesthetic/Vasoconstrictor Precautions** No information available to require special precautions

**Effects on Dental Treatment** >10% of patient experience dry mouth

**Other Adverse Effects**

>10%: Central nervous system: Drowsiness, dizziness, lightheadedness

1% to 10%:

- Cardiovascular: Swelling of face, lips, syncope
- Gastrointestinal: Bloated feeling
- Neuromuscular & skeletal: Problems in speaking, muscle weakness
- Ocular: Blurred vision

**Contraindications** Hypersensitivity to cyclobenzaprine or any component; do not use concomitantly or within 14 days of MAO inhibitors; hyperthyroidism, congestive heart failure, arrhythmias

**Warnings/Precautions** Cyclobenzaprine shares the toxic potentials of the tricyclic antidepressants and the usual precautions of tricyclic antidepressant therapy should be observed; use with caution in patients with urinary hesitancy or angle-closure glaucoma

**Drug Interactions** Do not use concomitantly or within 14 days after MAO inhibitors; because of chemical similarities to the tricyclic antidepressants, may have additive toxicities; because of cyclobenzaprine's anticholinergic action, use with caution in patients receiving these agents; alcohol, barbiturates, and other CNS depressants may be enhanced by cyclobenzaprine

**Drug Uptake**
Absorption: Oral: Completely
Onset of action: Commonly occurs within 1 hour
Duration: 12-24 hours
Serum half-life: 1-3 days
Time to peak serum concentration: Within 3-8 hours
**Pregnancy Risk Factor** B
**Breast-feeding Considerations** No data reported
**Dosage Forms** Tablet, as hydrochloride: 10 mg
**Dietary Considerations** No data reported
**Generic Available** Yes

- **Cyclocort®** *see* Amcinonide *on page 58*
- **Cyclogyl®** *see* Cyclopentolate *on this page*
- **Cyclomydril® Ophthalmic** *see* Cyclopentolate and Phenylephrine *on this page*

## Cyclopentolate (sye kloe PEN toe late)

**U.S. Brand Names** AK-Pentolate®; Cyclogyl®; I-Pentolate®
**Canadian Brand Names** Marzine®
**Therapeutic Category** Anticholinergic Agent, Ophthalmic; Ophthalmic Agent, Mydriatic
**Use** Diagnostic procedures requiring mydriasis and cycloplegia
**Usual Dosage**
Children: Instill 1 drop of 0.5%, 1%, or 2% in eye followed by 1 drop of 0.5% or 1% in 5 minutes, if necessary
Adults: Instill 1 drop of 1% followed by another drop in 5 minutes; 2% solution in heavily pigmented iris
**Mechanism of Action** Prevents the muscle of the ciliary body and the sphincter muscle of the iris from responding to cholinergic stimulation, causing mydriasis and cycloplegia
**Local Anesthetic/Vasoconstrictor Precautions** No information available to require special precautions
**Effects on Dental Treatment** No effects or complications reported
**Other Adverse Effects** 1% to 10%:
Cardiovascular: Tachycardia
Central nervous system: Restlessness, hallucinations, psychosis, hyperactivity, seizures, incoherent speech, ataxia
Dermatologic: Burning sensation
Ocular: Increase in intraocular pressure, loss of visual accommodation
Miscellaneous: Allergic reaction
**Drug Uptake**
Peak effect:
Cycloplegia: 25-75 minutes
Mydriasis: 30-60 minutes
Duration: Recovery takes up to 24 hours
**Pregnancy Risk Factor** C
**Generic Available** Yes
**Comments** Pilocarpine ophthalmic drops applied after the examination may reduce recovery time to 3-6 hours

## Cyclopentolate and Phenylephrine
(sye kloe PEN toe late & fen il EF rin)

**U.S. Brand Names** Cyclomydril® Ophthalmic
**Therapeutic Category** Anticholinergic/Adrenergic Agonist
**Synonyms** Phenylephrine and Cyclopentolate
**Use** Induce mydriasis greater than that produced with cyclopentolate HCl alone
**Usual Dosage** Ophthalmic: Instill 1 drop every 5-10 minutes, not to exceed 3 instillations
**Local Anesthetic/Vasoconstrictor Precautions** No information available to require special precautions
**Effects on Dental Treatment** No effects or complications reported
**Pregnancy Risk Factor** C
**Dosage Forms** Solution, ophthalmic: Cyclopentolate hydrochloride 0.2% and phenylephrine hydrochloride 1% (2 mL, 5 mL)
**Generic Available** No

## Cyclophosphamide (sye kloe FOS fa mide)

**U.S. Brand Names** Cytoxan®; Neosar®
**Canadian Brand Names** Procytox®
(Continued)

## Cyclophosphamide *(Continued)*

**Therapeutic Category** Antineoplastic Agent, Alkylating Agent (Nitrogen Mustard)

**Use** Treatment of Hodgkin's and non-Hodgkin's lymphoma, Burkitt's lymphoma, chronic lymphocytic leukemia, chronic granulocytic leukemia, AML, ALL, mycosis fungoides, breast cancer, multiple myeloma, neuroblastoma, retinoblastoma, rhabdomyosarcoma, Ewing's sarcoma; testicular, endometrium and ovarian, and lung cancer, and as a conditioning regimen for BMT; prophylaxis of rejection for kidney, heart, liver, and BMT transplants, severe rheumatoid disorders, nephrotic syndrome, Wegener's granulomatosis, idiopathic pulmonary hemosideroses, myasthenia gravis, multiple sclerosis, systemic lupus erythematosus, lupus nephritis, autoimmune hemolytic anemia, idiopathic thrombocytic purpura, macroglobulinemia, and antibody-induced pure red cell aplasia

**Usual Dosage Refer to individual protocols**

Patients with compromised bone marrow function may require a 33% to 50% reduction in initial loading dose

Children: I.V.:
- Neuroblastomas/sarcomas: 3 g/m$^2$/day for 2 days or 2 g/m$^2$/day for 3 days
- SLE: 500-750 mg/m$^2$ every month; maximum dose: 1 g/m$^2$
- JRA/vasculitis: 10 mg/kg every 2 weeks

Children and Adults:
- Oral: 50-100 mg/m$^2$/day as continuous therapy or 400-1000 mg/m$^2$ in divided doses over 4-5 days as intermittent therapy
- I.V.:
  - Single doses: 400-1800 mg/m$^2$ (30-50 mg/kg) per treatment course (1-5 days) which can be repeated at 2- to 4-week intervals
  - Maximum single dose without BMT is 7 g/m$^2$ (190 mg/kg) single agent therapy
  - Continuous daily doses: 60-120 mg/m$^2$ (1-2.5 mg/kg) per day
  - Autologous BMT: IVPB: 50 mg/kg/dose for 4 days or 60 mg/kg/dose for 2 days; total dose is usually divided over 2-4 days

Nephrotic syndrome: Oral: 2-3 mg/kg/day every day for up to 12 weeks when corticosteroids are unsuccessful

**Mechanism of Action** Interferes with the normal function of DNA by alkylation and cross-linking the strands of DNA, and by possible protein modification; cyclophosphamide also possesses potent immunosuppressive activity; note that cyclophosphamide must be metabolized to its active form in the liver

**Local Anesthetic/Vasoconstrictor Precautions** No information available to require special precautions

**Effects on Dental Treatment** No effects or complications reported

**Other Adverse Effects**

>10%:
- Dermatologic: Alopecia is frequent, but hair will regrow although it may be of a different color or texture. Hair loss usually occurs 3 weeks after therapy.
- Fertility: May cause sterility; interferes with oogenesis and spermatogenesis; may be irreversible in some patients; gonadal suppression (amenorrhea)
- Gastrointestinal: Nausea and vomiting occur more frequently with larger doses, usually beginning 6-10 hours after administration; also seen are anorexia, diarrhea, stomatitis, mucositis
  - Emetic potential: Oral: Low (<10%); <1 g: Moderate (30% to 60%); ≥1 g: High (>90%)
- Hepatic: Jaundice seen occasionally

1% to 10%:
- Cardiovascular: Facial flushing
- Central nervous system: Headache
- Dermatologic: Skin rash
- Hematologic: Anemia
  - Myelosuppressive: Thrombocytopenia occurs less frequently than with mechlorethamine; WBC: Moderate; Platelets: Moderate; Onset (days): 7; Nadir (days): 10-14; Recovery (days): 21

<1%:
- Cardiovascular: High-dose therapy may cause cardiac dysfunction manifested as congestive heart failure; cardiac necrosis or hemorrhagic myocarditis has occurred rarely, but is fatal. Cyclophosphamide may also potentiate the cardiac toxicity of anthracyclines.
- Central nervous system: Dizziness
- Dermatologic: Darkening of skin/fingernails
- Endocrine & metabolic: Hyperglycemia, hypokalemia, distortion, hyperuricemia
- Genitourinary: Acute hemorrhagic cystitis is believed to be a result of chemical irritation of the bladder by acrolein, a cyclophosphamide metabolite. Acute hemorrhagic cystitis occurs in 7% to 12% of patients, and has been reported

in up to 40% of patients. Hemorrhagic cystitis can be severe and even fatal. Patients should be encouraged to drink plenty of fluids (3-4 L/day) during therapy, void frequently, and avoid taking the drug at nighttime. If large I.V. doses are being administered, I.V. hydration should be given during therapy. The administration of mesna or continuous bladder irrigation may also be warranted.

Hepatic: Hepatic toxicity

Renal: SIADH has occurred with I.V. doses >50 mg/kg; renal tubular necrosis has also occurred, but usually resolves after the discontinuation of therapy

Respiratory: Nasal congestion occurs when given in large I.V. doses; patients experience runny eyes, rhinorrhea, sinus congestion, and sneezing during or immediately after the infusion; interstitial pulmonary fibrosis with prolonged high dosage has occurred

Secondary malignancy: Has developed with cyclophosphamide alone or in combination with other antineoplastics; both bladder carcinoma and acute leukemia are well documented

**Drug Interactions**

Decreased effect: Digoxin: Cyclophosphamide may reduce digoxin serum levels

Increased toxicity:

Allopurinol may cause an increase in bone marrow depression and may result in significant elevations of cyclophosphamide cytotoxic metabolites

Anesthetic agents: Cyclophosphamide reduces serum pseudocholinesterase concentrations and may prolong the neuromuscular blocking activity of succinylcholine; use with caution with halothane, nitrous oxide, and succinylcholine

Chloramphenicol results in prolonged cyclophosphamide half-life to increase toxicity

Cimetidine inhibits hepatic metabolism of drugs and may reduce the activation of cyclophosphamide

Doxorubicin: Cyclophosphamide may enhance cardiac toxicity of anthracyclines

Phenobarbital and phenytoin induce hepatic enzymes and cause a more rapid production of cyclophosphamide metabolites with a concurrent decrease in the serum half-life of the parent compound

Tetrahydrocannabinol results in enhanced immunosuppression in animal studies

Thiazide diuretics: Leukopenia may be prolonged

**Pregnancy Risk Factor** D

**Generic Available** No

## Cycloserine (sye kloe SER een)

**Related Information**

Nonviral Infectious Diseases *on page 1095*

**U.S. Brand Names** Seromycin® Pulvules®

**Therapeutic Category** Antibiotic, Miscellaneous; Antitubercular Agent

**Use** Adjunctive treatment in pulmonary or extrapulmonary tuberculosis; treatment of acute urinary tract infections caused by *E. coli* or *Enterobacter* sp when less toxic conventional therapy has failed or is contraindicated

**Usual Dosage** Some of the neurotoxic effects may be relieved or prevented by the concomitant administration of pyridoxine

Tuberculosis: Oral:

Children: 10-20 mg/kg/day in 2 divided doses up to 1000 mg/day for 18-24 months

Adults: Initial: 250 mg every 12 hours for 14 days, then give 500 mg to 1 g/day in 2 divided doses for 18-24 months (maximum daily dose: 1 g)

**Mechanism of Action** Inhibits bacterial cell wall synthesis by competing with amino acid (D-alanine) for incorporation into the bacterial cell wall; bacteriostatic or bactericidal

**Local Anesthetic/Vasoconstrictor Precautions** No information available to require special precautions

**Effects on Dental Treatment** No effects or complications reported

**Other Adverse Effects**

1% to 10%: Central nervous system: Drowsiness, headache

<1%:

Cardiovascular: Cardiac arrhythmias

Central nervous system: Dizziness, vertigo, seizures, confusion, psychosis, paresis, coma

Dermatologic: Rash

Endocrine & metabolic: Vitamin $B_{12}$ deficiency, folate deficiency

Hepatic: Elevated liver enzymes

Neuromuscular & skeletal: Tremor

(Continued)

## Cycloserine *(Continued)*

**Drug Interactions** Increased toxicity: Alcohol, isoniazid, ethionamide increase toxicity of cycloserine; cycloserine inhibits the hepatic metabolism of phenytoin

**Drug Uptake**

Absorption: Oral: ~70% to 90% from the GI tract

Serum half-life: 10 hours in patients with normal renal function

Time to peak serum concentration: Oral: Within 3-4 hours

**Pregnancy Risk Factor** C

**Generic Available** No

♦ **Cyclospasmol®** *see* Cyclandelate *on page 283*

## Cyclosporine (SYE kloe spor een)

**U.S. Brand Names** Neoral® Oral; Sandimmune® Injection; Sandimmune® Oral

**Therapeutic Category** Immunosuppressant Agent

**Use** Immunosuppressant which may be used with azathioprine and/or corticosteroids to prolong organ and patient survival in kidney, liver, heart, and bone marrow transplants

**Usual Dosage** Children and Adults (oral dosage is ~3 times the I.V. dosage); **dosage should be based on ideal body weight:**

I.V.:

Initial: 5-6 mg/kg/day beginning 4-12 hours prior to organ transplantation; patients should be switched to oral cyclosporine as soon as possible; dose should be infused over 2-24 hours

Maintenance: 2-10 mg/kg/day in divided doses every 8-12 hours; dose should be adjusted to maintain whole blood HPLC trough concentrations in the reference range

Oral: Solution or soft gelatin capsule (Sandimmune®):

Initial: 14-18 mg/kg/day, beginning 4-12 hours prior to organ transplantation

Maintenance: 5-15 mg/kg/day divided every 12-24 hours; maintenance dose is usually tapered to 3-10 mg/kg/day

Focal segmental glomerulosclerosis: Initial: 3 mg/kg/day divided every 12 hours

Dosing considerations of cyclosporine, see table.

**Cyclosporine**

| Condition | Cyclosporine |
|---|---|
| Switch from I.V. to oral therapy | Threefold increase in dose |
| T-tube clamping | Decrease dose; increase availability of bile facilitates absorption of CsA |
| Pediatric patients | About 2-3 times higher dose compared to adults |
| Liver dysfunction | Decrease I.V. dose; increase oral dose |
| Renal dysfunction | Decrease dose to decrease levels if renal dysfunction is related to the drug |
| Dialysis | Not removed |
| Inhibitors of hepatic metabolism | Decrease dose |
| Inducers of hepatic metabolism | Monitor drug level; may need to increase dose |

Oral: Solution or soft gelatin capsule in a microemulsion (Neoral®): Based on the organ transplant population:

Initial: Same as the initial dose for solution or soft gelatin capsule (listed above)

**or**

Renal: 9 mg/kg/day (range: 6-12 mg/kg/day)

Liver: 8 mg/kg/day (range: 4-12 mg/kg/day)

Heart: 7 mg/kg/day (range: 4-10 mg/kg/day)

**Note:** A 1:1 ratio conversion from Sandimmune® to Neoral® has been recommended initially; however, lower doses of Neoral® may be required after conversion to prevent overdose. Total daily doses should be adjusted based on the cyclosporine trough blood concentration and clinical assessment of organ rejection. CsA blood trough levels should be determined prior to conversion. After conversion to Neoral®, CsA trough levels should be monitored every 4-7 days

**Mechanism of Action** Inhibition of production and release of interleukin II and inhibits interleukin II-induced activation of resting T-lymphocytes

**Local Anesthetic/Vasoconstrictor Precautions** No information available to require special precautions

**Effects on Dental Treatment** Gingival hypertrophy

**Other Adverse Effects**

>10%:

Cardiovascular: Hypertension
Dermatologic: Hirsutism
Gastrointestinal: Gingival hypertrophy
Neuromuscular & skeletal: Tremor
Renal: Nephrotoxicity

1% to 10%:

Central nervous system: Seizure, headache
Dermatologic: Acne
Gastrointestinal: Abdominal discomfort, nausea, vomiting
Neuromuscular & skeletal: Leg cramps

<1%:

Cardiovascular: Hypotension, tachycardia, flushing
Central nervous system: Sensitivity to temperature extremes
Endocrine & metabolic: Hyperkalemia, hypomagnesemia, hyperuricemia
Gastrointestinal: Pancreatitis
Hepatic: Hepatotoxicity
Neuromuscular & skeletal: Myositis, paresthesias
Respiratory: Respiratory distress, sinusitis
Miscellaneous: Anaphylaxis, warmth, increased susceptibility to infection

**Drug Interactions**

Decreased effect: Rifampin, phenytoin, phenobarbital decreases plasma concentration of cyclosporine

Increased toxicity: Erythromycin, clarithromycin, ketoconazole, fluconazole, and itraconazole increase plasma concentration of cyclosporine

**Drug Uptake**

Absorption: Oral:

Solution or soft gelatin capsule (Sandimmune®): Erratically and incompletely absorbed; dependent on the presence of food, bile acids, and GI motility; larger oral doses of cyclosporine are needed in pediatric patients versus adults due to a shorter bowel length resulting in limited intestinal absorption

Solution in microemulsion or soft gelatin capsule in a microemulsion are bioequivalent (Neoral®): Erratically and incompletely absorbed; increased absorption, up to 30% when compared to Sandimmune®; absorption is less dependent on food intake, bile, or GI motility when compared to Sandimmune®

Serum half-life:

Solution or soft gelatin capsule (Sandimmune®): Biphasic, alpha phase: 1.4 hours and terminal phase 6-24 hours (prolonged in patients with hepatic dysfunction)

Solution or soft gelatin capsule in a microemulsion (Neoral®): 8.4 hours, lower in pediatric patients versus adults due to the higher metabolism rate

Time to peak serum concentration:

Oral solution or capsule (Sandimmune®): 2-6 hours; some patients have a second peak at 5-6 hours

Oral solution or capsule in a microemulsion (Neoral®): 1.5-2 hours (in renal transplant patients)

**Pregnancy Risk Factor** C

**Generic Available** No

**Comments** Cyclosporine serum levels are likely to be increased with clarithromycin or erythromycin administration. Toxic cyclosporine concentrations and renal toxicity may result. Clarithromycin inhibits the CYP3A4 enzyme which metabolizes cyclosporine. Azithromycin (Zithromycin®) and dirithromycin (Dynabac®) are unlikely to interact with cyclosporine.

**Selected Readings**

Ferrari SL, Goffin E, Mourad M, et al, "The Interaction Between Clarithromycin and Cyclosporine in Kidney Transplant Recipients," *Transplantation*, 1994, 58(6):725-7.

Harnett JD, Parfrey PS, Paul MD, et al, "Erythromycin-Cyclosporine Interaction in Renal Transplant Recipients," *Transplantation*, 1987, 43(2):316-8.

♦ **Cycofed® Pediatric** *see* Guaifenesin, Pseudoephedrine, and Codeine *on page 482*
♦ **Cycrin®** *see* Medroxyprogesterone Acetate *on page 623*
♦ **Cyklokapron® Injection** *see* Tranexamic Acid *on page 1004*
♦ **Cyklokapron® Oral** *see* Tranexamic Acid *on page 1004*
♦ **Cylert®** *see* Pemoline *on page 770*
♦ **Cylex® [OTC]** *see* Benzocaine *on page 128*
♦ **Cyomin®** *see* Cyanocobalamin *on page 282*

## Cyproheptadine (si proe HEP ta deen)

**U.S. Brand Names** Periactin®

**Canadian Brand Names** PMS-Cyproheptadine

(Continued)

## Cyproheptadine *(Continued)*

**Therapeutic Category** Antihistamine

**Use** Perennial and seasonal allergic rhinitis and other allergic symptoms including urticaria; its off-labeled uses have included appetite stimulation, blepharospasm, cluster headaches, migraine headaches, Nelson's syndrome, pruritus, schizophrenia, spinal cord damage associated spasticity, and tardive dyskinesia

**Usual Dosage** Oral:

Children: 0.25 mg/kg/day in 2-3 divided doses or 8 mg/m²/day in 2-3 divided doses

2-6 years: 2 mg every 8-12 hours (not to exceed 12 mg/day)

7-14 years: 4 mg every 8-12 hours (not to exceed 16 mg/day)

Adults: 4-20 mg/day divided every 8 hours (not to exceed 0.5 mg/kg/day) in patients with significant hepatic dysfunction

**Mechanism of Action** A potent antihistamine and serotonin antagonist, competes with histamine for $H_1$-receptor sites on effector cells in the gastrointestinal tract, blood vessels, and respiratory tract

**Local Anesthetic/Vasoconstrictor Precautions** No information available to require special precautions

**Effects on Dental Treatment** No effects or complications reported

**Other Adverse Effects**

>10%:

Central nervous system: Slight to moderate drowsiness

Respiratory: Thickening of bronchial secretions

1% to 10%:

Central nervous system: Headache, fatigue, nervousness, dizziness

Gastrointestinal: Appetite stimulation, nausea, diarrhea, abdominal pain, dry mouth

Neuromuscular & skeletal: Arthralgia

Respiratory: Pharyngitis

<1%:

Cardiovascular: Tachycardia, palpitations, edema

Central nervous system: Sedation, CNS stimulation, seizures, depression

Dermatologic: Photosensitivity, rash, angioedema

Hematologic: Hemolytic anemia, leukopenia, thrombocytopenia

Hepatic: Hepatitis

Neuromuscular & skeletal: Myalgia, paresthesia

Respiratory: Bronchospasm, epistaxis

Miscellaneous: Allergic reactions

**Drug Interactions** Increased toxicity: MAO inhibitors cause hallucinations

**Pregnancy Risk Factor** B

**Generic Available** Yes

♦ **Cystadane®** *see* Betaine Anhydrous *on page 136*

♦ **Cystagon®** *see* Cysteamine *on this page*

## Cysteamine (sis TEE a meen)

**U.S. Brand Names** Cystagon®

**Therapeutic Category** Antiurolithic

**Use** Nephropathic cystinosis in children and adults

**Usual Dosage** Initiate therapy with ¼ to ⅛ of maintenance dose; titrate slowly upward over 4-6 weeks

Children <12 years: Oral: Maintenance: 1.3 g/m²/day divided into 4 doses

Children >12 years and Adults (>110 lb): 2 g/day in 4 divided doses; dosage may in increased to 1.95 g/m²/day if cystine levels are <1 nmol/½ cystine/mg protein, although intolerance and incidence of adverse events may be increased

**Mechanism of Action** Reacts with cystine in the lysosome to convert it to cysteine and to a cysteine-cysteamine mixed disulfide, both of which can then exit the lysosome in patients with cystinosis, an inherited defect of lysosomal transport

**Local Anesthetic/Vasoconstrictor Precautions** No information available to require special precautions

**Effects on Dental Treatment** No effects or complications reported

**Other Adverse Effects**

5% to 10%:

Central nervous system: Fever, lethargy

Dermatologic: Rash

Gastrointestinal: Vomiting, anorexia, diarrhea

<5%:

Cardiovascular: Hypertension

Central nervous system: Somnolence, encephalopathy, headache, seizures, ataxia, confusion, dizziness, jitteriness, nervousness, impaired cognition, emotional changes, hallucinations, nightmares
Dermatologic: Urticaria
Endocrine & metabolic: Dehydration
Gastrointestinal: Bad breath, abdominal pain, dyspepsia, constipation, gastroenteritis, duodenitis, duodenal ulceration
Hematologic: Anemia, leukopenia
Hepatic: Abnormal LFTs
Neuromuscular & skeletal: Tremor, hyperkinesia
Otic: Decreased hearing

**Pregnancy Risk Factor** C

**Generic Available** No

## Cysteine (SIS teen)

**Therapeutic Category** Nutritional Supplement

**Use** Total parenteral nutrition of infants as an additive to meet the I.V. amino acid requirements

**Usual Dosage** Combine 500 mg of cysteine with 12.5 g of amino acid, then dilute with 50% dextrose

**Local Anesthetic/Vasoconstrictor Precautions** No information available to require special precautions

**Effects on Dental Treatment** No effects or complications reported

**Generic Available** Yes

♦ **Cystospaz®** *see* Hyoscyamine *on page 519*
♦ **Cystospaz-M®** *see* Hyoscyamine *on page 519*
♦ **Cytadren®** *see* Aminoglutethimide *on page 62*

## Cytarabine (sye TARE a been)

**U.S. Brand Names** Cytosar-U®

**Therapeutic Category** Antineoplastic Agent, Antimetabolite

**Use** Ara-C is one of the most active agents in leukemia; also active against lymphoma, meningeal leukemia, and meningeal lymphoma; has little use in the treatment of solid tumors

**Usual Dosage** I.V. bolus, IVPB, and continuous intravenous infusion doses of cytarabine are very different. Bolus doses are relatively well tolerated since the drug is rapidly metabolized; continuous infusion uniformly results in myelosuppression. Refer to individual protocols.

Children and Adults:
Induction remission:
I.V.: 200 mg/m²/day for 5 days at 2-week intervals
100-200 mg/m²/day for 5- to 10-day therapy course or every day until remission
I.T.: 5-75 mg/m² every 2-7 days until CNS findings normalize
**or**
<1 year: 20 mg
1-2 years: 30 mg
2-3 years: 50 mg
>3 years: 70 mg

Maintenance remission:
I.V.: 70-200 mg/m²/day for 2-5 days at monthly intervals
I.M., S.C.: 1-1.5 mg/kg single dose for maintenance at 1- to 4-week intervals
High-dose therapies:
Doses as high as 1-3 g/m² have been used for refractory or secondary leukemias or refractory non-Hodgkin's lymphoma
Doses of 3 g/m² every 12 hours for up to 12 doses have been used
Bone marrow transplant: 1.5 g/m² continuous infusion over 48 hours

**Mechanism of Action** Inhibition of DNA synthesis; cell cycle-specific for the S phase of cell division; cytosine gains entry into cells by a carrier process, and then must be converted to its active compound; cytosine acts as an analog and is incorporated into DNA; however, the primary action is inhibition of DNA polymerase resulting in decreased DNA synthesis and repair; degree of its cytotoxicity correlates linearly with its incorporation into DNA; therefore, incorporation into the DNA is responsible for drug activity and toxicity

**Local Anesthetic/Vasoconstrictor Precautions** No information available to require special precautions

**Effects on Dental Treatment** No effects or complications reported

(Continued)

## Cytarabine *(Continued)*

**Other Adverse Effects**

Central nervous system: Has produced seizures when given I.T.; cerebellar syndrome (or cerebellar toxicity), manifested as ataxia, dysarthria, and dysdiadochokinesia, has been reported to be dose-related. This may or may not be reversible.

High-dose therapy toxicities: Cerebellar toxicity, conjunctivitis (make sure the patient is on steroid eye drops during therapy), corneal keratitis, hyperbilirubinemia, pulmonary edema, pericarditis, and tamponade

>10%:

Central nervous system: Fever, rash

Dermatologic: Oral/anal ulceration

Gastrointestinal: Nausea, vomiting, diarrhea, and mucositis which subside quickly after discontinuing the drug; GI effects may be more pronounced with divided I.V. bolus doses than with continuous infusion

Emetic potential: ≤20 mg: Moderately low (10% to 30%); 250 mg to 1 g: Moderately high (60% to 90%); >1 g: High (>90%)

Hematologic: Bleeding

Myelosuppressive: Occurs within the first week of treatment and lasts for 10-14 days; primarily manifested as granulocytopenia, but anemia can also occur. WBC: Severe; Platelets: Severe; Onset (days): 4-7; Nadir (days): 14-18; Recovery (days): 21-28

Hepatic: Hepatic dysfunction, mild jaundice and acute increase in transaminases can be produced

Local: Thrombophlebitis

1% to 10%:

Cardiovascular: Cardiomegaly

Central nervous system: Dizziness, headache, somnolence, confusion, neuritis, malaise

Dermatologic: Skin freckling, itching, alopecia

Genitourinary: Urinary retention

Local: Cellulitis at injection site

Neuromuscular & skeletal: Myalgia, bone pain, peripheral neuropathy

Respiratory: Syndrome of sudden respiratory distress progressing to pulmonary edema, pneumonia

Miscellaneous: Sepsis

**Drug Interactions**

Decreased effect of gentamicin, flucytosine; decreased digoxin oral tablet absorption

Increased toxicity: Alkylating agents and radiation; purine analogs; methotrexate

**Drug Uptake**

Absorption: Because high concentrations of cytidine deaminase are in the GI mucosa and liver, three- to tenfold higher doses than I.V. would need to be given orally; therefore, the oral route is not used

Serum half-life:

Initial: 7-20 minutes

Terminal: 0.5-2.6 hours

**Pregnancy Risk Factor** D

**Generic Available** Yes


- **Cytomel®** *see* Liothyronine *on page 592*
- **Cytosar-U®** *see* Cytarabine *on previous page*
- **Cytotec®** *see* Misoprostol *on page 680*
- **Cytovene®** *see* Ganciclovir *on page 462*
- **Cytoxan®** *see* Cyclophosphamide *on page 285*
- **$D_3$** *see* Cholecalciferol *on page 243*
- **D-3-Mercaptovaline** *see* Penicillamine *on page 772*


## Dacarbazine (da KAR ba zeen)

**U.S. Brand Names** DTIC-Dome®

**Therapeutic Category** Antineoplastic Agent, Miscellaneous

**Synonyms** DIC; Dimethyl Triazeno Imidazol Carboxamide; DTIC; Imidazole Carboxamide

**Use** Singly or in various combination therapy to treat malignant melanoma, Hodgkin's disease, soft-tissue sarcomas (fibrosarcomas, rhabdomyosarcoma), islet cell carcinoma, medullary carcinoma of the thyroid, and neuroblastoma

**Usual Dosage** I.V. (**refer to individual protocols**):

Children:

Pediatric solid tumors: 200-470 mg/m²/day over 5 days every 21-28 days

Pediatric neuroblastoma: 800-900 mg/m² as a single dose on day 1 of therapy every 3-4 weeks in combination therapy

Hodgkin's disease: 375 mg/m$^2$ on days 1 and 15 of treatment course, repeat every 28 days

Adults:

Malignant melanoma: 2-4.5 mg/kg/day for 10 days, repeat in 4 weeks **or** may use 250 mg/m$^2$/day for 5 days, repeat in 3 weeks

Hodgkin's disease: 150 mg/m$^2$/day for 5 days, repeat every 4 weeks **or** 375 mg/m$^2$ on day 1, repeat in 15 days of each 28-day cycle in combination with other agents **or** 375 mg/m$^2$ repeated in 15 days of each 28-day cycle

**Mechanism of Action** Alkylating agent which forms methylcarbonium ions that attack nucleophilic groups in DNA; cross-links strands of DNA resulting in the inhibition of DNA, RNA, and protein synthesis, but the exact mechanism of action is still unclear; originally developed as a purine antimetabolite, but it does not interfere with purine synthesis; metabolism by the host is necessary for activation of dacarbazine, then the methylated species acts by alkylation of nucleic acids; dacarbazine is active in all phases of the cell cycle

**Local Anesthetic/Vasoconstrictor Precautions** No information available to require special precautions

**Effects on Dental Treatment** No effects or complications reported

**Other Adverse Effects**

>10%:

Central nervous system: Polyneuropathy, headache, and seizures have been reported

Extravasation: Dacarbazine is a vesicant; may cause tissue necrosis after extravasation; apply ice and consult extravasation policy if this occurs

Gastrointestinal: Moderate to severe nausea and vomiting in 90% of patients and lasting up to 12 hours after administration; nausea and vomiting are dose-related and occur more frequently when given as a one-time dose, as opposed to a less intensive 5-day course; diarrhea may also occur

Emetic potential: <500 mg: Moderately high (60% to 90%); ≥500 mg: High (>90%)

Local: Pain and burning at infusion site

Hematologic: Myelosuppressive effects: Mild to moderate is common and dose-related; leukopenia and thrombocytopenia may be delayed 2-3 weeks and may be the dose-limiting toxicity; WBC: Mild (primarily leukocytes); Platelets: Mild; Onset (days): 7; Nadir (days): 10-14; Recovery (days): 21-28

Neuromuscular & skeletal: Weakness

Ocular: Blurred vision

1% to 10%:

Cardiovascular: Facial flushing

Dermatologic: Alopecia, rash

Gastrointestinal: Anorexia, metallic taste

Hematologic: Myelosuppression

Neuromuscular & skeletal: Paresthesias

Flu-like effects: Fever, malaise, headache, myalgia, and sinus congestion may last up to several days after administration

<1%:

Cardiovascular: Orthostatic hypotension

Dermatologic: Photosensitivity reactions

Gastrointestinal: Stomatitis, diarrhea

Hepatic: Hepatotoxicity, elevated LFTs

Miscellaneous: Mild immunosuppression, anaphylaxis

**Drug Uptake**

Onset of action: I.V.: 18-24 days

Absorption: Oral administration demonstrates slow and variable absorption; preferable to administer by I.V. route

Serum half-life (biphasic):

Initial: 20-40 minutes

Terminal: 5 hours

**Pregnancy Risk Factor** C

**Generic Available** Yes

## Daclizimab (da KLIK si mab)

**U.S. Brand Names** Zenapax®

**Therapeutic Category** Immunosuppressant Agent

**Use** Prevent rejection of kidney transplants

**Usual Dosage** I.V.: 1 mg/kg over a 15-minute period

**Mechanism of Action** Inhibits the binding of IL-2 to the high affinity IL-2 receptor, thus suppressing T-cell activity against allografts. Its active ingredient, daclizimab, a humanized monoclonal antibody, binds to the alpha subunit of the high affinity interleukin-2 receptor (IL-2R) which is expressed on activated T-cells.

(Continued)

## Dacliximab *(Continued)*

**Local Anesthetic/Vasoconstrictor Precautions** No information available to require special precautions

**Effects on Dental Treatment** No effects or complications reported

**Drug Uptake**

Volume of central compartment: 2.5 L

Volume of peripheral compartment: 3.4 L

Estimated half-life (terminal elimination): 20 days (480 hours)

♦ **Dacodyl® [OTC]** *see* Bisacodyl *on page 141*

## Dactinomycin (dak ti noe MYE sin)

**U.S. Brand Names** Cosmegen®

**Therapeutic Category** Antineoplastic Agent, Antibiotic

**Synonyms** ACT; Actinomycin D

**Use** Management, either alone or in combination with other treatment modalities of Wilms' tumor, rhabdomyosarcoma, neuroblastoma, retinoblastoma, Ewing's sarcoma, trophoblastic neoplasms, testicular carcinoma, and other malignancies

**Usual Dosage Refer to individual protocols**

**Calculation of the dosage for obese or edematous patients should be on the basis of surface area in an effort to relate dosage to lean body mass**

Children >6 months and Adults: I.V.:

15 mcg/kg/day **or** 400-600 mcg/m$^2$/day (maximum: 500 mcg) for 5 days, may repeat every 3-6 weeks **or**

2.5 mg/m$^2$ given in divided doses over 1-week period and repeated at 2-week intervals **or**

0.75-2 mg/m$^2$ as a single dose given at intervals of 1-4 weeks have been used

**Mechanism of Action** Binds to the guanine portion of DNA intercalating between guanine and cytosine base pairs inhibiting DNA and RNA synthesis and protein synthesis; product of *Streptomyces parvullus* (a yeast species)

**Local Anesthetic/Vasoconstrictor Precautions** No information available to require special precautions

**Effects on Dental Treatment** No effects or complications reported

**Other Adverse Effects**

>10%:

Dermatologic: Alopecia (reversible), hyperpigmentation of skin

Central nervous system: Unusual fatigue

Extravasation: An irritant and should be administered through a rapidly running I.V. line; extravasation can lead to tissue necrosis, pain, and ulceration

Gastrointestinal: Severe nausea and vomiting occur in most patients and persist for up to 24 hours; stomatitis, anorexia, abdominal pain, and diarrhea, esophagitis

Hematologic: Myelosuppressive: Dose-limiting toxicity; anemia, aplastic anemia, agranulocytosis, pancytopenia; WBC: Moderate; Platelets: Moderate; Onset (days): 7; Nadir (days): 14-21; Recovery (days): 21-28

1% to 10%: Gastrointestinal: Mucositis

<1%:

Central nervous system: Fever

Dermatologic: Skin eruptions, acne

Endocrine & metabolic: Hyperuricemia, hypocalcemia

Hepatic: Hepatitis, liver function test abnormalities Anaphylactoid reaction

**Drug Uptake**

Serum half-life: 36 hours

Time to peak serum concentration: I.V.: Within 2-5 minutes

**Pregnancy Risk Factor** C

**Generic Available** No

♦ **D.A.II® Tablet** *see* Chlorpheniramine, Phenylephrine, and Methscopolamine *on page 235*

♦ **Dairy Ease® [OTC]** *see* Lactase *on page 569*

♦ **Dakin's Solution** *see* Sodium Hypochlorite Solution *on page 922*

♦ **Dakrina® Ophthalmic Solution [OTC]** *see* Artificial Tears *on page 97*

♦ **Dalalone L.A.®** *see* Dexamethasone *on page 308*

♦ **Dalgan®** *see* Dezocine *on page 315*

♦ **Dallergy®** *see* Chlorpheniramine, Phenylephrine, and Methscopolamine *on page 235*

♦ **Dallergy-D® Syrup** *see* Chlorpheniramine and Phenylephrine *on page 232*

♦ **Dalmane®** *see* Flurazepam *on page 448*

## Dalteparin (dal TE pa rin)

**U.S. Brand Names** Fragmin®

**Canadian Brand Names** Fragmin™

**Therapeutic Category** Anticoagulant (Other)

**Use** Prevention of deep vein thrombosis which may lead to pulmonary embolism, in patients requiring abdominal surgery who are at risk for thromboembolism complications (ie, patients >40 years of age, obese, patients with malignancy, history of deep vein thrombosis or pulmonary embolism, and surgical procedures requiring general anesthesia and lasting longer than 30 minutes)

**Usual Dosage** Adults: S.C.:

Low-moderate risk patients: 2500 units 1-2 hours prior to surgery, then once daily for 5-10 days postoperatively

High risk patients: 5000 units 1-2 hours prior to surgery and then once daily for 5-10 days postoperatively

**Mechanism of Action** Low molecular weight heparin analog with a molecular weight of 4000-6000 daltons; the commercial product contains 3% to 15% heparin with a molecular weight <3000 daltons, 65% to 78% with a molecular weight of 3000-8000 daltons and 14% to 26% with a molecular weight >8000 daltons; while dalteparin has been shown to inhibit both factor Xa and factor IIa (thrombin), the antithrombotic effect of dalteparin is characterized by a higher ratio of antifactor Xa to antifactor IIa activity (ratio = 4)

**Local Anesthetic/Vasoconstrictor Precautions** No information available to require special precautions

**Effects on Dental Treatment** No effects or complications reported

**Other Adverse Effects** 1% to 10%:

Central nervous system: Allergic fever

Dermatologic: Pruritus, rash, bullous eruption, skin necrosis

Hematologic: Bleeding, thrombocytopenia, wound hematoma

Local: Pain at injection site, injection site hematoma, injection site reactions

Miscellaneous: Anaphylactoid reactions, allergic reactions

**Drug Interactions** Increased toxicity: Caution should be used when using aspirin, other platelet inhibitors, and oral anticoagulants in combination with dalteparin due to an increased risk of bleeding

**Drug Uptake**

Peak serum concentrations: 4 hours

Half-life, elimination: 2-5 hours (route dependent)

**Pregnancy Risk Factor** B

**Dosage Forms** Injection: Prefilled syringe: Anti-cactor Xa 2500 units per 0.2 mL; anti-cactor Xa 5000 units per 0.2 mL

**Generic Available** No

♦ **Damason-P®** *see* Hydrocodone and Aspirin *on page 507*

## Danaparoid (da NAP a roid)

**U.S. Brand Names** Orgaran®

**Therapeutic Category** Anticoagulant (Other)

**Synonyms** Danaparoid Sodium

**Use** Prophylaxis of postoperative deep vein thrombosis (DVT)

**Usual Dosage** S.C.:

Children: Safety and effectiveness have not been established

Adults: 750 anti-Xa units twice daily; beginning 1-4 hours before surgery and then not sooner than 2 hours after surgery and every 12 hours until the risk of DVT has diminished, the average duration of therapy is 7-10 days

**Mechanism of Action** Prevents fibrin formation in coagulation pathway via thrombin generation inhibition by anti-Xa and anti-IIa effects.

**Local Anesthetic/Vasoconstrictor Precautions** No information available to require special precautions

**Effects on Dental Treatment** No effects or complications reported

**Other Adverse Effects** 1% to 10%:

Cardiovascular: Peripheral edema, generalized edema

Central nervous system: Fever, insomnia, headache, dizziness

Dermatologic: Rash, pruritus

Gastrointestinal: Nausea, constipation, vomiting

Genitourinary: Urinary tract infections, urinary retention

Hematologic: Anemia, hemorrhage, hematoma

Local: Injection site pain

Neuromuscular & skeletal: Joint disorder, weakness

**Warnings/Precautions** Do not administer intramuscularly; use with extreme caution in patients with a history of bacterial endocarditis, hemorrhagic stroke, recent CNS or ophthalmological surgery, bleeding diathesis, uncontrolled arterial hypertension, or a history of recent gastrointestinal ulceration and hemorrhage.

(Continued)

## Danaparoid *(Continued)*

Danaparoid shows a low cross-sensitivity with antiplatelet antibodies in individuals with type II heparin-induced thrombocytopenia. This product contains sodium sulfite which may cause allergic-type reactions, including anaphylactic symptoms and life-threatening asthmatic episodes in susceptible people; this is seen more frequently in asthmatics.

**Drug Interactions** Increased toxicity with oral anticoagulants, platelet inhibitors

**Drug Uptake**

Onset of effect: Maximum anti-factor Xa and antithrombin (anti-factor IIa) activities occur 2-5 hours after S.C. administration

Serum half-life, plasma: Mean terminal half-life: ~24 hours

**Pregnancy Risk Factor** B

**Generic Available** No

♦ **Danaparoid Sodium** *see* Danaparoid *on previous page*

## Danazol (DA na zole)

**U.S. Brand Names** Danocrine®

**Canadian Brand Names** Cyclomen®

**Therapeutic Category** Androgen

**Use** Treatment of endometriosis, fibrocystic breast disease, and hereditary angioedema

**Usual Dosage** Adults: Oral:

Endometriosis: 100-400 mg twice daily for 3-6 months (may extend to 9 months)
Fibrocystic breast disease: 50-200 mg twice daily for 2-6 months
Hereditary angioedema: 400-600 mg/day in 2-3 divided doses

**Mechanism of Action** Suppresses pituitary output of follicle-stimulating hormone and luteinizing hormone that causes regression and atrophy of normal and ectopic endometrial tissue; decreases rate of growth of abnormal breast tissue; reduces attacks associated with hereditary angioedema by increasing levels of C4 component of complement

**Local Anesthetic/Vasoconstrictor Precautions** No information available to require special precautions

**Effects on Dental Treatment** No effects or complications reported

**Other Adverse Effects**

>10%:
- Cardiovascular: Fluid retention, edema
- Dermatologic: Oily skin, acne, hirsutism
- Endocrine & metabolic: Irregular menstrual periods, decreased breast size
- Gastrointestinal: Weight gain
- Hematologic: Breakthrough bleeding
- Hepatic: Hepatic impairment
- Miscellaneous: Voice deepening

1% to 10%:
- Endocrine & metabolic: Virilization, androgenic effects, amenorrhea, hypoestrogenism
- Neuromuscular & skeletal: Weakness

<1%:
- Central nervous system: Dizziness, headache
- Dermatologic: Skin rashes, photosensitivity
- Gastrointestinal: Pancreatitis, bleeding gums
- Genitourinary: Monilial vaginitis, testicular atrophy, enlarged clitoris
- Hepatic: Cholestatic jaundice
- Neuromuscular & skeletal: Carpal tunnel syndrome
- Miscellaneous: Benign intracranial hypertension

**Drug Interactions** Danazol has prolonged the prothrombin times in patients taking warfarin; anticoagulant effects are enhanced; danazol has increased the serum concentrations of carbamazepine (Tegretol®) leading to dizziness, nausea, drowsiness, and ataxia

**Drug Uptake**

Onset of therapeutic effect: Within 4 weeks following daily doses

Serum half-life: 4.5 hours (variable)

Time to peak serum concentration: Within 2 hours

**Pregnancy Risk Factor** X

**Generic Available** Yes

♦ **Danocrine®** *see* Danazol *on this page*

♦ **Dantrium®** *see* Dantrolene *on next page*

## Dantrolene (DAN troe leen)

**U.S. Brand Names** Dantrium®

**Therapeutic Category** Antidote, Malignant Hyperthermia; Hyperthermia, Treatment; Muscle Relaxant; Skeletal Muscle Relaxant

**Use** Treatment of spasticity associated with spinal cord injury, stroke, cerebral palsy, or multiple sclerosis; also used as treatment of malignant hyperthermia

**Usual Dosage**

Spasticity: Oral:

Children: Initial: 0.5 mg/kg/dose twice daily, increase frequency to 3-4 times/day at 4- to 7-day intervals, then increase dose by 0.5 mg/kg to a maximum of 3 mg/kg/dose 2-4 times/day up to 400 mg/day

Adults: 25 mg/day to start, increase frequency to 2-4 times/day, then increase dose by 25 mg every 4-7 days to a maximum of 100 mg 2-4 times/day or 400 mg/day

Malignant hyperthermia: Children and Adults:

Oral: 4-8 mg/kg/day in 4 divided doses

Preoperative prophylaxis: Begin 1-2 days prior to surgery with last dose 3-4 hours prior to surgery

I.V.: 1 mg/kg; may repeat dose up to cumulative dose of 10 mg/kg (mean effective dose is 2.5 mg/kg), then switch to oral dosage

Preoperative: 2.5 mg/kg ~1¼ hours prior to anesthesia and infused over 1 hour with additional doses as needed and individualized

**Mechanism of Action** Acts directly on skeletal muscle by interfering with release of calcium ion from the sarcoplasmic reticulum; prevents or reduces the increase in myoplasmic calcium ion concentration that activates the acute catabolic processes associated with malignant hyperthermia

**Local Anesthetic/Vasoconstrictor Precautions** No information available to require special precautions

**Effects on Dental Treatment** No effects or complications reported

**Other Adverse Effects**

>10%:

Central nervous system: Drowsiness, dizziness, lightheadedness, fatigue,

Dermatologic: Rash

Gastrointestinal: Diarrhea (mild), nausea, vomiting

Neuromuscular & skeletal: Weakness

1% to 10%:

Cardiovascular: Pleural effusion with pericarditis

Central nervous system: Chills, fever, headache, insomnia, nervousness, mental depression

Gastrointestinal: Diarrhea (severe), constipation, anorexia, stomach cramps

Ocular: Blurred vision

Respiratory: Respiratory depression

<1%:

Central nervous system: Seizures, confusion

Hepatic: Hepatitis

**Drug Interactions** When given simultaneously dantrolene has increased the toxicity of the following drugs: Estrogens (hepatotoxicity), CNS depressants (sedation), MAO inhibitors, phenothiazines, clindamycin (increased neuromuscular blockade), verapamil (hyperkalemia and cardiac depression), warfarin, clofibrate and tolbutamide

**Drug Uptake**

Absorption: Slow and incomplete from GI tract

Serum half-life: 8.7 hours

**Pregnancy Risk Factor** C

**Generic Available** No

◆ **Dapacin® Cold Capsule [OTC]** *see* Chlorpheniramine, Phenylpropanolamine, and Acetaminophen *on page 236*

## Dapiprazole (DA pi pray zole)

**U.S. Brand Names** Rēv-Eyes™

**Therapeutic Category** Alpha-Adrenergic Blocking Agent, Ophthalmic

**Use** Reverse dilation due to drugs (adrenergic or parasympathomimetic) after eye exams

**Usual Dosage** Adults: Administer 2 drops followed 5 minutes later by an additional 2 drops applied to the conjunctiva of each eye; should not be used more frequently than once a week in the same patient

**Mechanism of Action** Dapiprazole is a selective alpha-adrenergic blocking agent, exerting effects primarily on alpha$_1$-adrenoceptors. It induces miosis via relaxation of the smooth dilator (radial) muscle of the iris, which causes pupillary constriction. It is devoid of cholinergic effects. Dapiprazole also partially reverses the cycloplegia induced with parasympatholytic agents such as tropicamide. (Continued)

## Dapiprazole *(Continued)*

Although the drug has no significant effect on the ciliary muscle *per se*, it may increase accommodative amplitude, therefore relieving the symptoms of paralysis of accommodation.

**Local Anesthetic/Vasoconstrictor Precautions** No information available to require special precautions

**Effects on Dental Treatment** No effects or complications reported

**Other Adverse Effects**

>10%:

- Central nervous system: Headache
- Ocular: Conjunctival injection, burning sensation in the eyes, lid edema, ptosis, lid erythema, chemosis, itching, punctate keratitis, corneal edema, photophobia

1% to 10%: Ocular: Dry eyes, blurring of vision, tearing of eye

**Drug Interactions** No data reported

**Pregnancy Risk Factor** B

**Generic Available** No

## Dapsone (DAP sone)

**Related Information**

HIV Infection and AIDS *on page 1085*

**U.S. Brand Names** Avlosulfon®

**Therapeutic Category** Antibiotic, Sulfone

**Use** Treatment of leprosy and dermatitis herpetiformis (infections caused by *Mycobacterium leprae*), alternative agent for *Pneumocystis carinii* pneumonia prophylaxis (given alone) and treatment (given with trimethoprim)

**Usual Dosage** Oral:

Leprosy:

- Children: 1-2 mg/kg/24 hours, up to a maximum of 100 mg/day
- Adults: 50-100 mg/day for 3-10 years
- Dermatitis herpetiformis: Adults: Start at 50 mg/day, increase to 300 mg/day, or higher to achieve full control, reduce dosage to minimum level as soon as possible
- Prophylaxis of *Pneumocystis carinii* pneumonia: Children >1 month: 1 mg/kg/day; maximum: 100 mg
- Treatment of *Pneumocystis carinii* pneumonia: Adults: 100 mg/day in combination with trimethoprim (20 mg/kg/day) for 21 days

**Mechanism of Action** Dapsone is a sulfone antimicrobial. The mechanism of action of the sulfones is similar to that of the sulfonamides. Sulfonamides are competitive antagonists of para-aminobenzoic acid (PABA) and prevent normal bacterial utilization of PABA for the synthesis of folic acid.

**Local Anesthetic/Vasoconstrictor Precautions** No information available to require special precautions

**Effects on Dental Treatment** No effects or complications reported

**Other Adverse Effects**

1% to 10%:

- Hematologic: Dose-related hemolysis, methemoglobinemia with cyanosis
- Miscellaneous: Reactional states

<1%:

- Central nervous system: Insomnia, headache
- Dermatologic: Exfoliative dermatitis
- Gastrointestinal: Nausea, vomiting
- Hematologic: Hemolytic anemia, methemoglobinemia, leukopenia, agranulocytosis
- Hepatic: Hepatitis, cholestatic jaundice
- Neuromuscular & skeletal: Peripheral neuropathy
- Ocular: Blurred vision
- Otic: Tinnitus

**Drug Interactions**

Dapsone has decreased the effects of para-aminobenzoic acid and rifampin

Dapsone has increased the effects of folic acid antagonists

**Drug Uptake**

Absorption: Oral: Well absorbed

Serum half-life, elimination: 30 hours (range: 10-50 hours)

**Pregnancy Risk Factor** C

**Generic Available** Yes

♦ **Daranide®** *see* Dichlorphenamide *on page 319*

♦ **Daraprim®** *see* Pyrimethamine *on page 868*

♦ **Daricon®** *see* Oxyphencyclimine *on page 758*

♦ **Darvocet-N®** *see* Propoxyphene and Acetaminophen *on page 855*

- ♦ **Darvocet-N® 100** *see* Propoxyphene and Acetaminophen *on page 855*
- ♦ **Darvon®** *see* Propoxyphene *on page 854*
- ♦ **Darvon® Compound-65 Pulvules®** *see* Propoxyphene and Aspirin *on page 856*
- ♦ **Darvon-N®** *see* Propoxyphene *on page 854*
- ♦ **Daunomycin** *see* Daunorubicin Hydrochloride *on this page*


# Daunorubicin Citrate (Liposomal)

(daw noe ROO bi sin SI trate lip po SOE mal)

**U.S. Brand Names** DaunoXome®

**Therapeutic Category** Antineoplastic Agent, Anthracycline; Antineoplastic Agent, Antibiotic

**Use** Advanced HIV-associated Kaposi's sarcoma; first-line cytotoxic therapy for advanced HIV-associated Kaposi's sarcoma

**Usual Dosage** Adults: I.V.: 40 mg/m$^2$ over 1 hour; repeat every 2 weeks; continue treatment until there is evidence of progressive disease

**Mechanism of Action** Liposomal daunorubicin contains an aqueous solution of the citrate salt of daunorubicin encapsulated with lipid vesicles (liposomes) composed of a lipid bilayer of distearoylphosphatidylcholine and cholesterol (2:1 molar ratio). This liposomal daunorubicin is formulated to maximum the selectivity of daunorubicin for solid tumors *in situ*; refer to Daunorubicin monograph.

**Local Anesthetic/Vasoconstrictor Precautions** No information available to require special precautions

**Effects on Dental Treatment** No effects or complications reported

**Other Adverse Effects**

>10%:

Central nervous system: Fatigue, headache
Gastrointestinal: Abdominal pain, anorexia, diarrhea, nausea, vomiting
Hematologic: Neutropenia
Neuromuscular & skeletal: Neuropathy
Respiratory: Cough, dyspnea, rhinitis
Miscellaneous: Infection

5% to 10%:

Cardiovascular: Hypertension, palpitations, syncope, tachycardia, chest pain, edema
Central nervous system: Depression, dizziness, insomnia, malaise
Dermatologic: Alopecia, pruritus
Endocrine & metabolic: Hot flashes
Gastrointestinal: Constipation, stomatitis, tenesmus
Neuromuscular & skeletal: Arthralgia, myalgia
Ocular: Abnormal vision
Respiratory: Sinusitis

**Contraindications** Hypersensitivity to previous doses or any constituents of the product

**Warnings/Precautions**

The U.S. Food and Drug Administration (FDA) currently recommends that procedures for proper handling and disposal of antineoplastic agents be considered.

The primary toxicity is myelosuppression, especially off the granulocytic series, which may be severe, with much less marked effects on platelets and erythroid series. Potential cardiac toxicity, particularly in patients who have received prior anthracyclines or who have pre-existing cardiac disease, may occur. Refer to Daunorubicin monograph.

Although grade 3-4 injection site inflammation has been reported in patients treated with the liposomal daunorubicin, no instances of local tissue necrosis were observed with extravasation. However, refer to daunorubicin monograph and avoid extravasation.

Reduce dosage in patients with impaired hepatic function. Hyperuricemia can be induced secondary to rapid lysis of leukemic cells. As a precaution, administer allopurinol prior to initiating antileukemic therapy.

**Drug Uptake** Serum half-life: 4.4 hours

**Pregnancy Risk Factor** D

**Dosage Forms** Injection: 2 mg/mL (equivalent to 50 mg daunorubicin base) (1 mL, 4 mL, 10 mL unit packs)

**Generic Available** No

# Daunorubicin Hydrochloride

(daw noe ROO bi sin hye droe KLOR ide)

**U.S. Brand Names** Cerubidine®

**Therapeutic Category** Antineoplastic Agent, Antibiotic

**Synonyms** Daunomycin; DNR; Rubidomycin Hydrochloride

**Use** In combination with other agents in the treatment of leukemias (ALL, AML)

(Continued)

## Daunorubicin Hydrochloride *(Continued)*

**Usual Dosage** I.V. (**refer to individual protocols**):

Children:

ALL Combination therapy: Remission induction: 25-45 mg/m$^2$ on day 1 every week for 4 cycles **or** 30-45 mg/m$^2$/day for 3 days

In children <2 years or <0.5 m$^2$, daunorubicin should be based on weight - mg/kg: 1 mg/kg per protocol with frequency dependent on regimen employed

Cumulative dose should not exceed 300 mg/m$^2$ in children >2 years or 10 mg/kg in children <2 years

Adults: 30-60 mg/m$^2$/day for 3-5 days, repeat dose in 3-4 weeks

Single agent induction for AML: 60 mg/m$^2$/day for 3 days; repeat every 3-4 weeks

Combination therapy induction for AML: 45 mg/m$^2$/day for 3 days of the first course of induction therapy; subsequent courses: Every day for 2 days

ALL combination therapy: 45 mg/m$^2$/day for 3 days

Cumulative dose should not exceed 400-600 mg/m$^2$

**Mechanism of Action** Inhibition of DNA and RNA synthesis, by intercalating between DNA base pairs and by steric obstruction; is not cell cycle-specific for the S phase of cell division; daunomycin is preferred over doxorubicin for the treatment of ANLL because of its dose-limiting toxicity (myelosuppression) is not of concern in the therapy of this disease; has less mucositis associated with its use

**Local Anesthetic/Vasoconstrictor Precautions** No information available to require special precautions

**Effects on Dental Treatment** No effects or complications reported

**Other Adverse Effects**

>10%:

Dermatologic: Alopecia (reversible)

Gastrointestinal: Mild nausea or vomiting occurs in 50% of patients within the first 24 hours; stomatitis may occur 3-7 days after administration, but is not as severe as that caused by doxorubicin

Genitourinary: Discoloration of urine (red)

1% to 10%:

Cardiovascular: Congestive heart failure

Endocrine & metabolic: Hyperuricemia

Gastrointestinal: GI ulceration, diarrhea

Hematologic: Myelosuppressive: Dose-limiting toxicity, occurs in all patients; leukopenia is more significant than thrombocytopenia; WBC: Severe; Platelets: Severe; Onset (days): 7; Nadir (days): 14; Recovery (days): 21-28

Local: Extravasation: Daunorubicin is a vesicant; infiltration can cause severe inflammation, tissue necrosis, and ulceration; if the drug is infiltrated, consult institutional policy, apply ice to the area, and elevate the limb

<1%:

Cardiovascular: Pericarditis/myocarditis

Central nervous system: Chills

Dermatologic: Skin rash, urticaria

Hepatic: Elevation in serum bilirubin, AST, and alkaline phosphatase

Miscellaneous: Fertility impairment, pigmentation changes in nailbeds

**Drug Uptake** Serum half-life: 14-20 hours

**Pregnancy Risk Factor** D

**Generic Available** No

- **DaunoXome®** *see* Daunorubicin Citrate (Liposomal) *on previous page*
- **Daypro™** *see* Oxaprozin *on page 747*
- **Dayto Himbin®** *see* Yohimbine *on page 1056*
- **DC 240® Softgels® [OTC]** *see* Docusate *on page 346*
- **DCF** *see* Pentostatin *on page 782*
- **DDAVP®** *see* Desmopressin Acetate *on page 306*
- **Debrisan® [OTC]** *see* Dextranomer *on page 312*
- **Debrox® Otic [OTC]** *see* Carbamide Peroxide *on page 186*
- **Decadron®** *see* Dexamethasone *on page 308*
- **Decadron®-LA** *see* Dexamethasone *on page 308*
- **Deca-Durabolin® Injection** *see* Nandrolone *on page 703*
- **Decaject-L.A.®** *see* Dexamethasone *on page 308*
- **Decholin®** *see* Dehydrocholic Acid *on page 302*
- **Declomycin®** *see* Demeclocycline *on page 303*
- **Decofed® Syrup [OTC]** *see* Pseudoephedrine *on page 863*
- **Decohistine® DH** *see* Chlorpheniramine, Pseudoephedrine, and Codeine *on page 237*

- **Decohistine® Expectorant** *see* Guaifenesin, Pseudoephedrine, and Codeine *on page 482*
- **Deconamine® SR** *see* Chlorpheniramine and Pseudoephedrine *on page 233*
- **Deconamine® Syrup [OTC]** *see* Chlorpheniramine and Pseudoephedrine *on page 233*
- **Deconamine® Tablet [OTC]** *see* Chlorpheniramine and Pseudoephedrine *on page 233*
- **Deconsal® II** *see* Guaifenesin and Pseudoephedrine *on page 481*
- **Deconsal® Sprinkle®** *see* Guaifenesin and Phenylephrine *on page 480*
- **Defen-LA®** *see* Guaifenesin and Pseudoephedrine *on page 481*

## Deferoxamine (de fer OKS a meen)

**U.S. Brand Names** Desferal® Mesylate

**Therapeutic Category** Antidote, Aluminum Toxicity; Antidote, Iron Toxicity

**Use** Acute iron intoxication; chronic iron overload secondary to multiple transfusions; diagnostic test for iron overload; used investigationally in the treatment of aluminum accumulation in renal failure; iron overload secondary to congenital anemias; hemochromatosis; removal of corneal rust rings following surgical removal of foreign bodies

**Usual Dosage**

Children:

Acute iron intoxication (I.M. is preferred route for patients not in shock). Treat until urine is no longer pink salmon colored:

I.M.: 50 mg/kg/dose every 6 hours to a maximum of 6 g/day

I.V.: 15 mg/kg/hour; maximum: 6 g/day

Chronic iron overload:

I.M., I.V.: 50 mg/kg/dose to a maximum of 6 g/24 hours or 2 g/dose; do not exceed 15 mg/kg/hour I.V.

S.C.: 20-40 mg/kg/day over 8-12 hours (via a portable, controlled infusion device)

Aluminum-induced bone disease: 20-40 mg/kg every hemodialysis treatment, frequency dependent on clinical status of the patient

Adults:

Acute iron intoxication: (I.M. is preferred route for patients not in shock). Treat until urine is no longer pink salmon colored:

I.M., I.V.: 1 g stat, then 0.5 g every 4 hours for 2 doses, then 0.5 g every 4-12 hours up to 6 g/day; do not exceed 15 mg/kg/hour I.V.

Chronic iron overload:

I.M.: 0.5-1 g every day

I.V.: 2 g after each unit of blood infusion at 15 mg/kg/hour

S.C.: 1-2 g every day over 8-24 hours

**Mechanism of Action** Complexes with trivalent ions (ferric ions) to form ferrioxamine, which are removed by the kidneys

**Local Anesthetic/Vasoconstrictor Precautions** No information available to require special precautions

**Effects on Dental Treatment** No effects or complications reported

**Other Adverse Effects**

1% to 10%: Local: Pain and induration at injection site

<1%:

Cardiovascular: Flushing, hypotension, tachycardia, shock, swelling

Central nervous system: Fever

Dermatologic: Erythema, urticaria, pruritus, rash, cutaneous wheal formation

Gastrointestinal: Abdominal discomfort, diarrhea

Neuromuscular & skeletal: Leg cramps

Ocular: Blurred vision, cataracts

Otic: Hearing loss

Miscellaneous: Anaphylaxis

**Drug Interactions** No data reported

**Drug Uptake**

Absorption: Oral: <15%

Serum half-life:

Parent drug: 6.1 hours

Ferrioxamine: 5.8 hours

**Pregnancy Risk Factor** C

**Generic Available** No

- **Deficol® [OTC]** *see* Bisacodyl *on page 141*
- **Degas® [OTC]** *see* Simethicone *on page 915*
- **Degest® 2 Ophthalmic [OTC]** *see* Naphazoline *on page 703*

## Dehydrocholic Acid (dee hye droe KOE lik AS id)

**U.S. Brand Names** Cholan-HMB®; Decholin®

**Canadian Brand Names** Dycholium®

**Therapeutic Category** Bile Acid; Laxative, Hydrocholeretic

**Use** Relief of constipation; adjunct to various biliary tract conditions

**Usual Dosage** Children >12 years and Adults: 250-500 mg 2-3 times/day after meals up to 1.5 g/day

**Local Anesthetic/Vasoconstrictor Precautions** No information available to require special precautions

**Effects on Dental Treatment** No effects or complications reported

**Other Adverse Effects** 1% to 10%: Gastrointestinal: Dehydration, diarrhea, abdominal cramps

**Pregnancy Risk Factor** C

**Generic Available** Yes


- **Dekasol-L.A.®** *see* Dexamethasone *on page 308*
- **Deladumone® Injection** *see* Estradiol and Testosterone *on page 389*
- **Del Aqua-5® Gel** *see* Benzoyl Peroxide *on page 130*
- **Del Aqua-10® Gel** *see* Benzoyl Peroxide *on page 130*
- **Delatest® Injection** *see* Testosterone *on page 961*
- **Delatestryl® Injection** *see* Testosterone *on page 961*


## Delavirdine (de la VIR deen)

**Related Information**

HIV Infection and AIDS *on page 1085*

**U.S. Brand Names** Rescriptor®

**Therapeutic Category** Antiviral Agent, Oral

**Synonyms** U-90152S

**Use** Treatment of HIV-1 infection in combination with appropriate antiretrovirals

**Usual Dosage** Adults: Oral: 400 mg 3 times/day

**Mechanism of Action** Delavirdine binds directly to reverse transcriptase, blocking RNA-dependent and DNA-dependent DNA polymerase activities

**Local Anesthetic/Vasoconstrictor Precautions** No information available to require special precautions

**Effects on Dental Treatment** No effects or complications reported

**Drug Uptake**

Absorption: Rapid

Half-life: Approximately 5.8 hours

Time to peak: Approximately 1 hour

**Pregnancy Risk Factor** C

**Dosage Forms** Tablet: 100 mg


- **Delfen® [OTC]** *see* Nonoxynol 9 *on page 728*
- **Del-Mycin® Topical** *see* Erythromycin, Topical *on page 386*
- **Delsym® [OTC]** *see* Dextromethorphan *on page 314*
- **Delta-Cortef®** *see* Prednisolone *on page 832*
- **Delta-D®** *see* Cholecalciferol *on page 243*
- **Deltasone®** *see* Prednisone *on page 833*
- **Delta-Tritex®** *see* Triamcinolone *on page 1010*
- **Demadex®** *see* Torsemide *on page 1000*
- **Demazin® Syrup [OTC]** *see* Chlorpheniramine and Phenylpropanolamine *on page 233*


## Demecarium (dem e KARE ee um)

**U.S. Brand Names** Humorsol®

**Therapeutic Category** Antiglaucoma Agent; Cholinergic Agent, Ophthalmic; Ophthalmic Agent, Miotic

**Use** Management of chronic simple glaucoma, chronic and acute angle-closure glaucoma; strabismus

**Usual Dosage** Children and Adults: Ophthalmic:

Glaucoma: Instill 1 drop into eyes twice weekly to a maximum dosage of 1 or 2 drops twice daily for up to 4 months

Strabismus:

Diagnosis: Instill 1 drop daily for 2 weeks, then 1 drop every 2 days for 2-3 weeks. If eyes become straighter, an accommodative factor is demonstrated.

Therapy: Instill not more than 1 drop at a time in both eyes every day for 2-3 weeks. Then reduce dosage to 1 drop every other day for 3-4 weeks and re-evaluate. Continue at 1 drop every 2 days to 1 drop twice a week and evaluate the patient's condition every 4-12 weeks. If improvement continues, reduce dose to 1 drop once a week and eventually off of medication. Discontinue therapy after 4 months if control of the condition still requires 1 drop every 2 days.

**Mechanism of Action** Cholinesterase inhibitor (anticholinesterase) which causes acetylcholine to accumulate at cholinergic receptor sites and produces effects equivalent to excessive stimulation of cholinergic receptors. Demecarium mainly acts by inhibiting true (erythrocyte) cholinesterase and causes a reduction in intraocular pressure due to facilitation of outflow of aqueous humor; the reduction is likely to be particularly marked in eyes in which the pressure is elevated.

**Local Anesthetic/Vasoconstrictor Precautions** No information available to require special precautions

**Effects on Dental Treatment** No effects or complications reported

**Other Adverse Effects**

1% to 10%: Ocular: Stinging, burning, myopia, visual blurring

<1%:

Cardiovascular: Bradycardia, hypotension, flushing

Gastrointestinal: Nausea, vomiting, diarrhea

Neuromuscular & skeletal: Weakness

Ocular: Retinal detachment, miosis, twitching eyelids, watering eyes

Respiratory: Dyspnea

Miscellaneous: Sweating

**Drug Interactions** No data reported

**Pregnancy Risk Factor** C

**Generic Available** No

## Demeclocycline (dem e kloe SYE kleen)

**U.S. Brand Names** Declomycin®

**Therapeutic Category** Antibiotic, Tetracycline Derivative

**Use** Treatment of susceptible bacterial infections (acne, gonorrhea, pertussis and urinary tract infections) caused by both gram-negative and gram-positive organisms; used when penicillin is contraindicated (other agents are preferred); treatment of chronic syndrome of inappropriate secretion of antidiuretic hormone (SIADH)

**Usual Dosage** Oral:

Children ≥8 years: 8-12 mg/kg/day divided every 6-12 hours

Adults: 150 mg 4 times/day or 300 mg twice daily

Uncomplicated gonorrhea (penicillin sensitive): 600 mg stat, 300 mg every 12 hours for 4 days (3 g total)

SIADH: 900-1200 mg/day or 13-15 mg/kg/day divided every 6-8 hours initially, then decrease to 0.6-0.9 g/day

**Mechanism of Action** Inhibits protein synthesis by binding with the 30S and possibly the 50S ribosomal subunit(s) of susceptible bacteria; may also cause alterations in the cytoplasmic membrane

**Local Anesthetic/Vasoconstrictor Precautions** No information available to require special precautions

**Effects on Dental Treatment** Tetracycline's are not recommended for use during pregnancy or in children ≤8 years of age since they have been reported to cause enamel hypoplasia and permanent teeth discoloration. The use of tetracycline's should only be used in these patients if other agents are contraindicated or alternative antimicrobials will not eradicate the organism. Long-term use associated with oral candidiasis.

**Other Adverse Effects**

1% to 10%:

Dermatologic: Photosensitivity

Gastrointestinal: Nausea, diarrhea

<1%:

Cardiovascular: Pericarditis

Central nervous system: Increased intracranial pressure, bulging fontanels in infants

Dermatologic: Dermatologic effects, pruritus, exfoliative dermatitis

Endocrine & metabolic: Diabetes insipidus syndrome

Gastrointestinal: Vomiting, esophagitis, anorexia, abdominal cramps

Neuromuscular & skeletal: Paresthesia

Renal: Acute renal failure, azotemia

Miscellaneous: Superinfections, anaphylaxis, pigmentation of nails

**Drug Interactions**

Decreased effect with antacids (aluminum, calcium, zinc, or magnesium), bismuth salts, sodium bicarbonate, barbiturates, carbamazepine, hydantoins

Decreased effect of oral contraceptives

Increased effect of warfarin

**Drug Uptake**

Onset of action for diuresis in SIADH: Several days

(Continued)

## Demeclocycline *(Continued)*

Absorption: ~50% to 80% from GI tract; food and dairy products reduce absorption
Serum half-life: Reduced renal function: 10-17 hours
Time to peak serum concentration: Oral: Within 3-6 hours

**Pregnancy Risk Factor** D

**Dosage Forms**
Capsule, as hydrochloride: 150 mg
Tablet, as hydrochloride: 150 mg, 300 mg

**Dietary Considerations** Should be taken 1 hour before or 2 hours after food or milk with plenty of fluid

**Generic Available** No


- ♦ **Demerol®** *see* Meperidine *on page 629*
- ♦ **4-demethoxydaunorubicin** *see* Idarubicin *on page 525*
- ♦ **Demser®** *see* Metyrosine *on page 669*
- ♦ **Demulen®** *see* Ethinyl Estradiol and Ethynodiol Diacetate *on page 400*
- ♦ **Denavir™** *see* Penciclovir *on page 771*
- ♦ **Denorex® [OTC]** *see* Coal Tar *on page 270*
- ♦ **Dental Drug Interactions: Update on Drug Combinations Requiring Special Considerations** *see page 1225*
- ♦ **Dental Office Emergencies** *see page 1174*
- ♦ **Dentifrice Products** *see page 1242*
- ♦ **Dentin Hypersensitivity; High Caries Index; Xerostomia** *see page 1145*
- ♦ **Dentipatch®** *see* Lidocaine Transoral *on page 590*
- ♦ **Denture Adhesive Products** *see page 1250*
- ♦ **Denture Cleanser Products** *see page 1252*
- ♦ **Deoxycoformycin** *see* Pentostatin *on page 782*
- ♦ **2′-deoxycoformycin** *see* Pentostatin *on page 782*
- ♦ **Depacon®** *see* Valproic Acid and Derivatives *on page 1037*
- ♦ **Depakene®** *see* Valproic Acid and Derivatives *on page 1037*
- ♦ **Depakote®** *see* Valproic Acid and Derivatives *on page 1037*
- ♦ **depAndrogyn® Injection** *see* Estradiol and Testosterone *on page 389*
- ♦ **depAndro® Injection** *see* Testosterone *on page 961*
- ♦ **Depen®** *see* Penicillamine *on page 772*
- ♦ **depGynogen® Injection** *see* Estradiol *on page 387*
- ♦ **depMedalone®** *see* Methylprednisolone *on page 661*
- ♦ **Depo®-Estradiol Injection** *see* Estradiol *on page 387*
- ♦ **Depogen® Injection** *see* Estradiol *on page 387*
- ♦ **Depoject®** *see* Methylprednisolone *on page 661*
- ♦ **Depo-Medrol®** *see* Methylprednisolone *on page 661*
- ♦ **Deponit®** *see* Nitroglycerin *on page 725*
- ♦ **Depopred®** *see* Methylprednisolone *on page 661*
- ♦ **Depo-Provera®** *see* Medroxyprogesterone Acetate *on page 623*
- ♦ **Depo-Testadiol® Injection** *see* Estradiol and Testosterone *on page 389*
- ♦ **Depotest® Injection** *see* Testosterone *on page 961*
- ♦ **Depotestogen® Injection** *see* Estradiol and Testosterone *on page 389*
- ♦ **Depo®-Testosterone Injection** *see* Testosterone *on page 961*
- ♦ **Deproist® Expectorant with Codeine** *see* Guaifenesin, Pseudoephedrine, and Codeine *on page 482*
- ♦ **Derifil® [OTC]** *see* Chlorophyll *on page 226*
- ♦ **Derma-Smoothe/FS®** *see* Fluocinolone *on page 440*
- ♦ **Dermatop®** *see* Prednicarbate *on page 832*
- ♦ **Dermoplast® [OTC]** *see* Benzocaine *on page 128*
- ♦ **Desferal® Mesylate** *see* Deferoxamine *on page 301*


## Desipramine (des IP ra meen)

**U.S. Brand Names** Norpramin®; Pertofrane®

**Canadian Brand Names** PMS-Desipramine

**Therapeutic Category** Antidepressant, Tricyclic

**Use** Treatment of various forms of depression, often in conjunction with psychotherapy; analgesic adjunct in chronic pain, peripheral neuropathies

**Usual Dosage** Oral:
Children 6-12 years: 10-30 mg/day or 1-5 mg/kg/day in divided doses; do not exceed 5 mg/kg/day
Adolescents: Initial: 25-50 mg/day; gradually increase to 100 mg/day in single or divided doses; maximum: 150 mg/day

Adults: Initial: 75 mg/day in divided doses; increase gradually to 150-200 mg/day in divided or single dose; maximum: 300 mg/day

Elderly: Initial: 10-25 mg/day; increase by 10-25 mg every 3 days for inpatients and every week for outpatients if tolerated; usual maintenance dose: 75-100 mg/day, but doses up to 300 mg/day may be necessary

**Mechanism of Action** Traditionally believed to increase the synaptic concentration of norepinephrine in the central nervous system by inhibition of reuptake by the presynaptic neuronal membrane. However, additional receptor effects have been found including desensitization of adenyl cyclase, down regulation of beta-adrenergic receptors, and down regulation of serotonin receptors.

**Local Anesthetic/Vasoconstrictor Precautions** Use with caution; epinephrine, norepinephrine and levonordefrin have been shown to have an increased pressor response in combination TCAs

**Effects on Dental Treatment** >10% of patients experience dry mouth; long-term treatment with TCAs increases the risk of caries by reducing salivation and salivary buffer capacity

**Other Adverse Effects**

>10%:

Central nervous system: Dizziness, drowsiness, headache

Gastrointestinal: Constipation, increased appetite, nausea, unpleasant taste, weight gain

1% to 10%:

Cardiovascular: Arrhythmias, hypotension,

Central nervous system: Confusion, delirium, hallucinations, nervousness, restlessness, parkinsonian syndrome, insomnia

Endocrine & metabolic: Sexual dysfunction

Gastrointestinal: Diarrhea, heartburn

Genitourinary: Dysuria

Neuromuscular & skeletal: Fine muscle tremors, weakness

Ocular: Blurred vision, eye pain

Miscellaneous: Excessive sweating

<1%:

Central nervous system: Anxiety, seizures

Dermatologic: Alopecia, photosensitivity

Endocrine & metabolic: Breast enlargement, galactorrhea, SIADH

Gastrointestinal: Trouble with gums, decreased lower esophageal sphincter tone may cause GE reflux

Genitourinary: Testicular swelling

Hematologic: Agranulocytosis, leukopenia, eosinophilia

Hepatic: Cholestatic jaundice, elevated liver enzymes

Ocular: Increased intraocular pressure

Otic: Tinnitus

Miscellaneous: Allergic reactions

**Drug Interactions**

Decreased effect: Phenobarbital may increase the metabolism, of desipramine; desipramine blocks the uptake of guanethidine and thus prevents the hypotensive effect of guanethidine

Increased toxicity: Clonidine causes hypertensive crisis; desipramine may be additive with or may potentiate the action of other CNS depressants such as sedatives or hypnotics; with MAO inhibitors, hyperpyrexia, hypertension, tachycardia, confusion, and seizures. Desipramine may increase the prothrombin time in patients stabilized on warfarin; desipramine may potentiate the pressor and cardiac effects of sympathomimetic agents such as isoproterenol, epinephrine, etc; cimetidine and methylphenidate may decrease the metabolism of desipramine

Additive anticholinergic effects seen with other anticholinergic agents

**Drug Uptake**

Onset of action: 1-3 weeks (maximum antidepressant effects: after >2 weeks)

Absorption: Well absorbed (90%) from GI tract

Serum half-life: Adults: 12-57 hours

**Pregnancy Risk Factor** C

**Generic Available** Yes: Tablet

**Selected Readings**

Boakes AJ, Laurence DR, Teoh PC, et al, "Interactions Between Sympathomimetic Amines and Antidepressant Agents in Man," *Br Med J*, 1973, 1(849):311-5.

Jastak JT and Yagiela JA, "Vasoconstrictors and Local Anesthesia: A Review and Rationale for Use," *J Am Dent Assoc*, 1983, 107(4):623-30.

Larochelle P, Hamet P, and Enjalbert M, "Responses to Tyramine and Norepinephrine After Imipramine and Trazodone," *Clin Pharmacol Ther*, 1979, 26(1):24-30.

Mitchell JR, "Guanethidine and Related Agents. III Antagonism by Drugs Which Inhibit the Norepinephrine Pump in Man," *J Clin Invest*, 1970, 49(8):1596-604.

Rundegren J, van Dijken J, Mörnstad H, et al, "Oral Conditions in Patients Receiving Long-Term Treatment With Cyclic Antidepressant Drugs," *Swed Dent J*, 1985, 9(2):55-64.

(Continued)

## Desipramine *(Continued)*

Svedmyr N, "The Influence of a Tricyclic Antidepressive Agent (Protriptyline) on Some of the Circulatory Effects of Noradrenaline and Adrenalin® in Man," *Life Sci*, 1968, 7(1):77-84.

♦ **Desitin® Topical [OTC]** *see* Zinc Oxide, Cod Liver Oil, and Talc *on page 1061*

## Desmopressin Acetate (des moe PRES in AS e tate)

**U.S. Brand Names** DDAVP®; Stimate™

**Canadian Brand Names** Octostim®

**Therapeutic Category** Antihemophilic Agent; Hemostatic Agent; Vasopressin Analog, Synthetic

**Use** Treatment of diabetes insipidus and controlling bleeding in mild hemophilia, von Willebrand disease, and thrombocytopenia (eg, uremia)

**Usual Dosage** Dilute I.V. dose in 50 mL 0.9% sodium chloride and infuse over 15-30 minutes

Children:

Diabetes insipidus: 3 months to 12 years: Intranasal: Initial: 5 mcg/day divided 1-2 times/day; range: 5-30 mcg/day di ided 1-2 times/day

Von Willebrand disease, thrombocytopathies, hemophilia: >3 months:

Intranasal: 2-4 mcg/kg/dose

I.V.: 0.3 mcg/kg by slow infusion over 15-30 minutes; usually tachyphylaxis occurs after 2-3 doses in 24 hours, recovery of response may take 48-72 hours

Nocturnal enuresis: ≥6 years: Intranasal: Initial: 20 mcg at bedtime; range: 10-40 mcg

Adults:

Diabetes insipidus: I.V., S.C.: 2-4 mcg/day in 2 divided doses or 1/10 of the maintenance intranasal dose; intranasal: 5-40 mcg/day 1-3 times/day

Von Willebrand disease, thrombocytopathies, hemophilia:

Intranasal: 2-4 mcg/kg/dose

I.V.: 0.3 mcg/kg by slow infusion over 15-30 minutes; usually tachyphylaxis occurs after 2-3 doses in 24 hours; recovery of responsiveness may take 48-72 hours

Oral: Begin therapy 12 hours after the last intranasal dose for patients previously on intranasal therapy

Children: Initial: 0.05 mg; fluid restrictions required in children to prevent hyponatremia and water intoxication

Adults: 0.05 mg twice daily; adjust individually to optimal therapeutic dose. Total daily dose should be increased or decreased (range: 0.1-1.2 mg divided 2-3 times/day) as needed to obtain adequate antidiuresis.

**Mechanism of Action** Enhances reabsorption of water in the kidneys by increasing cellular permeability of the collecting ducts; possibly causes smooth muscle constriction with resultant vasoconstriction; raises plasma levels of von Willebrand factor and factor VIII

**Local Anesthetic/Vasoconstrictor Precautions** No information available to require special precautions

**Effects on Dental Treatment** No effects or complications reported

**Other Adverse Effects**

1% to 10%:

Cardiovascular: Facial flushing

Central nervous system: Headache, dizziness

Gastrointestinal: Nausea, abdominal cramps

Genitourinary: Vulval pain

Local: Pain at the injection site

Respiratory: Nasal congestion

<1%:

Cardiovascular: Hypertension

Endocrine & metabolic: Hyponatremia, water intoxication

**Drug Interactions** No data reported

**Drug Uptake**

Intranasal administration:

Onset of ADH effects: Within 1 hour

Peak effect: Within 1-5 hours

Duration: 5-21 hours

I.V. infusion:

Onset of increased factor VIII activity: Within 15-30 minutes

Peak effect: 90 minutes to 3 hours

Absorption: Nasal: Slow; 10% to 20%

Serum half-life: Elimination (terminal): 75 minutes

**Pregnancy Risk Factor** B

**Generic Available** No

- **Desogen®** *see* Ethinyl Estradiol and Desogestrel *on page 399*
- **Desogestrel and Ethinyl Estradiol** *see* Ethinyl Estradiol and Desogestrel *on page 399*

## Desonide (DES oh nide)

**U.S. Brand Names** DesOwen®; Tridesilon®

**Canadian Brand Names** Desocort®

**Therapeutic Category** Corticosteroid, Topical (Low Potency)

**Use** Adjunctive therapy for inflammation in acute and chronic corticosteroid responsive dermatosis (low potency corticosteroid)

**Usual Dosage** Children and Adults: Topical: Apply 2-4 times/day sparingly

**Mechanism of Action** Stimulates the synthesis of enzymes needed to decrease inflammation, suppress mitotic activity, and cause vasoconstriction

**Local Anesthetic/Vasoconstrictor Precautions** No information available to require special precautions

**Effects on Dental Treatment** No effects or complications reported

**Other Adverse Effects** <1%:

Dermatologic: Itching, dry skin, folliculitis, hypertrichosis, acneiform eruptions, hypopigmentation, perioral dermatitis, allergic contact dermatitis, skin maceration, skin atrophy, striae

Local: Burning, irritation, miliaria

Miscellaneous: Secondary infection

**Drug Interactions** No data reported

**Drug Uptake**

Onset of effect: Commonly noted within 7 days of continued therapy

Absorption: Topical absorption extensive from the scalp, face, axilla and scrotum; adequate through epidermis on appendages; absorption can be increased with occlusion or the addition of penetrants (eg, urea, DMSO)

**Pregnancy Risk Factor** C

**Dosage Forms**

Cream, topical: 0.05% (15 g, 60 g)

Lotion: 0.05% (60 mL, 120 mL)

Ointment, topical: 0.05% (15 g, 60 g)

**Generic Available** Yes

- **DesOwen®** *see* Desonide *on this page*

## Desoximetasone (des oks i MET a sone)

**Related Information**

Corticosteroids, Topical Comparison *on page 1222*

**U.S. Brand Names** Topicort®; Topicort®-LP

**Therapeutic Category** Corticosteroid, Topical (High Potency)

**Use** Relieves inflammation and pruritic symptoms of corticosteroid-responsive dermatosis [medium to high potency topical corticosteroid]

**Usual Dosage** Topical:

Children: Apply sparingly in a very thin film to affected area 1-2 times/day

Adults: Apply sparingly in a thin film twice daily

**Mechanism of Action** Stimulates the synthesis of enzymes needed to decrease inflammation, suppress mitotic activity, and cause vasoconstriction

**Local Anesthetic/Vasoconstrictor Precautions** No information available to require special precautions

**Effects on Dental Treatment** No effects or complications reported

**Other Adverse Effects** <1%: Topical: Burning, itching, irritation, dryness, folliculitis, hypertrichosis, acneiform eruptions, hypopigmentation, perioral dermatitis, allergic contact dermatitis, skin maceration, secondary infection, skin atrophy, striae, miliaria

**Drug Interactions** No data reported

**Drug Uptake** Absorption: Topical: Extensive from the scalp, face, axilla, and scrotum and adequate through epidermis on appendages; absorption can be increased with occlusion or the addition of penetrants

**Pregnancy Risk Factor** C

**Generic Available** Yes

- **Desoxyn®** *see* Methamphetamine *on page 645*
- **Desoxyribonuclease and Fibrinolysin** *see* Fibrinolysin and Desoxyribonuclease *on page 430*
- **Desquam-E™ Gel** *see* Benzoyl Peroxide *on page 130*
- **Desquam-X® Gel** *see* Benzoyl Peroxide *on page 130*
- **Desquam-X® Wash** *see* Benzoyl Peroxide *on page 130*
- **Desyrel®** *see* Trazodone *on page 1007*
- **Detrol™** *see* Tolterodine *on page 997*

- **Detussin® Expectorant** *see* Hydrocodone, Pseudoephedrine, and Guaifenesin *on page 511*
- **Devrom® (subgallate) [OTC]** *see* Bismuth *on page 142*
- **Dexacidin®** *see* Neomycin, Polymyxin B, and Dexamethasone *on page 711*

## Dexamethasone (deks a METH a sone)

**Related Information**

Corticosteroid Equivalencies Comparison *on page 1221*
Corticosteroids, Topical Comparison *on page 1222*
Neomycin, Polymyxin B, and Dexamethasone *on page 711*
Oral Nonviral Soft Tissue Ulcerations or Erosions *on page 1141*
Respiratory Diseases *on page 1079*

**U.S. Brand Names** Dalalone L.A.®; Decadron®; Decadron®-LA; Decaject-L.A.®; Dekasol-L.A.®; Dexasone L.A.®; Dexone®; Dexone L.A.®; Hexadrol®; I-Methasone®; Solurex L.A.®

**Therapeutic Category** Antiemetic; Anti-inflammatory Agent; Corticosteroid, Inhalant; Corticosteroid, Ophthalmic; Corticosteroid, Systemic; Corticosteroid, Topical (Low Potency)

**Use**

Dental: Treatment of a variety of oral diseases of allergic, inflammatory or autoimmune origin

Medical: Systemically and locally for chronic swelling, allergic, hematologic, neoplastic, and autoimmune diseases; may be used in management of cerebral edema, septic shock, as a diagnostic agent, antiemetic

**Usual Dosage**

Children: Anti-inflammatory immunosuppressant: Oral, I.M., I.V. (injections should be given as sodium phosphate): 0.08-0.3 mg/kg/day or 2.5-10 mg/m²/day in divided doses every 6-12 hours

Adults: Anti-inflammatory:

Oral, I.M., I.V. (injections should be given as sodium phosphate): 0.5-9 mg/day in divided doses every 6-12 hours
I.M. (as acetate): 8-16 mg; may repeat in 1-3 weeks
Intralesional (as acetate): 0.8-1.6 mg
Topical: Apply a thin film to affected area once or twice daily

**Mechanism of Action** Decreases inflammation by suppression of migration of polymorphonuclear leukocytes and reversal of increased capillary permeability; suppresses normal immune response

**Local Anesthetic/Vasoconstrictor Precautions** No information available to require special precautions

**Effects on Dental Treatment** No effects or complications reported

**Other Adverse Effects** >10%:

Central nervous system: Insomnia, nervousness
Gastrointestinal: Increased appetite, indigestion

**Contraindications** Active untreated infections; viral, fungal, or tuberculosis; diseases of the eye

**Warnings/Precautions** Fatalities have occurred due to adrenal insufficiency in asthmatic patients during and after transfer from systemic corticosteroids to aerosol steroids; aerosol steroids do **not** provide the systemic steroid needed to treat patients having trauma, surgery, or infections; use with caution in patients with hypothyroidism, cirrhosis, hypertension, congestive heart failure, ulcerative colitis, thromboembolic disorders. Because of the risk of adverse effects, systemic corticosteroids should be used cautiously in the elderly in the smallest possible dose and for the shortest possible time.

**Drug Interactions** Barbiturates, phenytoin, rifampin cause decrease in dexamethasone effects; dexamethasone decreases effect of salicylates, vaccines, toxoids

**Drug Uptake**

Absorption: Rapid and complete
Duration of metabolic effect: Can last for 72 hours; acetate is a long-acting repository preparation with a prompt onset of action
Serum half-life:
Normal renal function: 1.8-3.5 hours
Biological half-life: 36-54 hours
Time to peak serum concentration:
Oral: Within 1-2 hours
I.M.: Within 8 hours

**Pregnancy Risk Factor** C

**Breast-feeding Considerations** No data reported

**Dosage Forms**

Elixir: 0.5 mg/5 mL (5 mL, 20 mL, 100 mL, 120 mL, 237 mL, 240 mL, 500 mL)
Injection, as acetate suspension: 8 mg/mL (1 mL, 5 mL); 16 mg/mL (1 mL, 5 mL)

Injection, as sodium phosphate: 4 mg/mL (1 mL, 5 mL, 10 mL, 25 mL, 30 mL); 10 mg/mL (1 mL, 10 mL); 20 mg/mL (5 mL); 24 mg/mL (5 mL, 10 mL)
Solution, oral:
Concentrate: 0.5 mg/0.5 mL (30 mL) (30% alcohol)
Oral: 0.5 mg/5 mL (5 mL, 20 mL, 500 mL)
Tablet: 0.25 mg, 0.5 mg, 0.75 mg, 1 mg, 1.5 mg, 2 mg, 4 mg, 6 mg
Tablet, therapeutic pack: 6 x 1.5 mg; 8 x 0.75 mg

**Dietary Considerations** May be taken with meals to decrease GI upset; limit caffeine; may need diet with increased potassium, pyridoxine, vitamin C, vitamin D, folate, calcium, and phosphorus

**Generic Available** Yes

- ♦ **Dexamethasone and Neomycin** *see* Neomycin and Dexamethasone *on page 710*
- ♦ **Dexasone L.A.®** *see* Dexamethasone *on previous page*
- ♦ **Dexasporin®** *see* Neomycin, Polymyxin B, and Dexamethasone *on page 711*
- ♦ **Dexatrim® Pre-Meal [OTC]** *see* Phenylpropanolamine *on page 797*

## Dexbrompheniramine and Pseudoephedrine

(deks brom fen EER a meen & soo doe e FED rin)

**U.S. Brand Names** Disobrom® [OTC]; Disophrol® Chronotabs® [OTC]; Disophrol® Tablet [OTC]; Drixomed®; Drixoral® [OTC]

**Therapeutic Category** Antihistamine/Decongestant Combination

**Synonyms** Pseudoephedrine and Dexbrompheniramine

**Use** Relief of symptoms of upper respiratory mucosal congestion in seasonal and perennial nasal allergies, acute rhinitis, rhinosinusitis and eustachian tube blockage

**Usual Dosage** Children >12 years and Adults: Oral: 1 tablet every 12 hours, may require 1 tablet every 8 hours

**Local Anesthetic/Vasoconstrictor Precautions** Use with caution since pseudoephedrine is a sympathomimetic amine which could interact with epinephrine to cause a pressor response

**Effects on Dental Treatment** Up to 10% of patients could experience tachycardia, palpitations, and dry mouth; use vasoconstrictor with caution

**Pregnancy Risk Factor** B

**Generic Available** Yes

- ♦ **Dexchlor®** *see* Dexchlorpheniramine *on this page*

## Dexchlorpheniramine (deks klor fen EER a meen)

**U.S. Brand Names** Dexchlor®; Poladex®; Polaramine®

**Therapeutic Category** Antihistamine

**Use** Perennial and seasonal allergic rhinitis and other allergic symptoms including urticaria

**Usual Dosage** Oral:
Children:
2-5 years: 0.5 mg every 4-6 hours (do not use timed release)
6-11 years: 1 mg every 4-6 hours or 4 mg timed release at bedtime
Adults: 2 mg every 4-6 hours or 4-6 mg timed release at bedtime or every 8-10 hours

**Mechanism of Action** Competes with histamine for $H_1$-receptor sites on effector cells in the gastrointestinal tract, blood vessels, and respiratory tract

**Local Anesthetic/Vasoconstrictor Precautions** No information available to require special precautions

**Effects on Dental Treatment** Up to 10% of patients will complain of significant dry mouth and drowsiness. This will disappear with cessation of drug therapy.

**Other Adverse Effects**
>10%:
Central nervous system: Slight to moderate drowsiness
Respiratory: Thickening of bronchial secretions
1% to 10%:
Central nervous system: Headache, fatigue, nervousness, dizziness
Gastrointestinal: Appetite increase, weight gain, nausea, diarrhea, abdominal pain, dry mouth
Neuromuscular & skeletal: Arthralgia
Respiratory: Pharyngitis
<1%:
Cardiovascular: Edema, palpitations
Central nervous system: Depression
Dermatologic: Angioedema, photosensitivity, rash
Hepatic: Hepatitis
Neuromuscular & skeletal: Myalgia, paresthesia
Respiratory: Bronchospasm, epistaxis
(Continued)

## Dexchlorpheniramine *(Continued)*

**Drug Interactions** Alcohol and other sedative drugs will potentiate the sedative effects of dexchlorpheniramine

**Drug Uptake**

Duration: 3-6 hours

Absorption: Well absorbed from GI tract

**Pregnancy Risk Factor** B

**Generic Available** Yes

- **Dexedrine®** *see* Dextroamphetamine *on page 312*
- **Dexferrum® Injection** *see* Iron Dextran Complex *on page 550*
- **Dexone®** *see* Dexamethasone *on page 308*
- **Dexone L.A.®** *see* Dexamethasone *on page 308*

## Dexpanthenol (deks PAN the nole)

**U.S. Brand Names** Ilopan®; Ilopan-Choline®; Panthoderm® [OTC]

**Therapeutic Category** Gastrointestinal Agent, Stimulant

**Use** Prophylactic use to minimize paralytic ileus, treatment of postoperative distention

**Usual Dosage**

Children and Adults: Relief of itching and aid in skin healing: Topical: Apply to affected area 1-2 times/day

Adults:

Relief of gas retention: Oral: 2-3 tablets 3 times/day

Prevention of postoperative ileus: I.M.: 250-500 mg stat, repeat in 2 hours, followed by doses every 6 hours until danger passes

Paralyzed ileus: I.M.: 500 mg stat, repeat in 2 hours, followed by doses every 6 hours, if needed

**Mechanism of Action** A pantothenic acid B vitamin analog that is converted to coenzyme A internally; coenzyme A is essential to normal fatty acid synthesis, amino acid synthesis and acetylation of choline in the production of the neurotransmitter, acetylcholine

**Local Anesthetic/Vasoconstrictor Precautions** No information available to require special precautions

**Effects on Dental Treatment** No effects or complications reported

**Other Adverse Effects** <1%:

Cardiovascular: Slight drop in blood pressure

Dermatologic: Dermatitis, urticaria

Gastrointestinal: Vomiting, diarrhea, hyperperistalsis

Hematologic: Prolonged bleeding time

Local: Irritation

Neuromuscular & skeletal: Paresthesia

Respiratory: Dyspnea

**Drug Interactions** Increased/prolonged effect of succinylcholine (do not administer within 1 hour)

**Drug Uptake**

Absorption: Well absorbed

**Pregnancy Risk Factor** C

**Generic Available** Yes

## Dexrazoxane (deks ray ZOKS ane)

**U.S. Brand Names** Zinecard®

**Canadian Brand Names** Zinecard®

**Therapeutic Category** Cardioprotective Agent

**Use** Reduction of the incidence and severity of cardiomyopathy associated with doxorubicin administration in women with metastatic breast cancer who have received a cumulative doxorubicin dose of 300 mg/m$^2$ and who would benefit from continuing therapy with doxorubicin. It is not recommended for use with the initiation of doxorubicin therapy.

**Usual Dosage** Adults: I.V.: The recommended dosage ratio of dexrazoxane:doxorubicin is 10:1 (eg, 500 mg/m$^2$ dexrazoxane:50 mg/m$^2$ doxorubicin). Administer the reconstituted solution by slow I.V. push or rapid IV infusion from a bag. After completing the infusion, and prior to a total elapsed time of 30 minutes (from the beginning of the dexrazoxane infusion), give the I.V. injection of doxorubicin.

**Mechanism of Action** Derivative of EDTA and potent intracellular chelating agent. The mechanism of cardioprotectant activity is not fully understood. Appears to be converted intracellularly to a ring-opened chelating agent that interferes with iron-mediated free radical generation thought to be responsible, in part, for anthracycline-induced cardiomyopathy.

**Local Anesthetic/Vasoconstrictor Precautions** No information available to require special precautions

**Effects on Dental Treatment** No effects or complications reported

**Other Adverse Effects** The adverse experiences are likely attributable to the FAC regimen, with the exception of pain on injection that was observed mainly with dexrazoxane. Patients receiving FAC with dexrazoxane experienced more severe leukopenia, granulocytopenia, and thrombocytopenia at nadir than patients receiving FAC without dexrazoxane; but recovery counts were similar for the two groups.

1% to 2%: Dermatologic: Urticaria, recall skin reaction, extravasation

**Drug Interactions** Decreased effect: There is some evidence that the use of dexrazoxane concurrently with the initiation of FAC therapy interferes with the antitumor efficacy of the regimen, and this use is not recommended

**Drug Uptake** Serum half-life: 2.1-2.5 hours

**Pregnancy Risk Factor** C

**Dosage Forms** Powder for injection, lyophilized: 250 mg, 500 mg (10 mg/mL when reconstituted)

**Generic Available** No

## Dextran (DEKS tran)

**U.S. Brand Names** Gentran®; LMD®; Macrodex®; Rheomacrodex®

**Canadian Brand Names** Hyskon®

**Therapeutic Category** Plasma Volume Expander

**Synonyms** Dextran 40; Dextran 70; Dextran, High Molecular Weight; Dextran, Low Molecular Weight

**Use** Fluid replacement and blood volume expander used in the treatment of hypovolemia, shock, or near shock states

**Usual Dosage** I.V.: (requires an infusion pump):

Children: Total dose should not be >20 mL/kg during first 24 hours

Adults: 500-1000 mL at rate of 20-40 mL/minute; if therapy continues beyond 24 hours, total daily dosage should not exceed 10 mL/kg and therapy should not continue beyond 5 days

**Mechanism of Action** Produces plasma volume expansion by virtue of its highly colloidal starch structure, similar to albumin

**Local Anesthetic/Vasoconstrictor Precautions** No information available to require special precautions

**Effects on Dental Treatment** No effects or complications reported

**Other Adverse Effects** <1%:

Cardiovascular: Mild hypotension, tightness of chest
Central nervous system: Fever
Dermatologic: Urticaria
Gastrointestinal: Nausea, vomiting
Neuromuscular & skeletal: Arthralgia
Respiratory: Nasal congestion, wheezing
Miscellaneous: Anaphylaxis

**Drug Uptake** Onset of action: I.V.: Within minutes to 1 hour (depending upon the molecular weight polysaccharide administered), infusion volume expansion occurs

**Pregnancy Risk Factor** C

**Generic Available** Yes

**Comments** Dextran 40 is known as low molecular weight dextran (LMD®) and has an average molecular weight of 40,000; dextran 75 has an average molecular weight of 75,000

## Dextran 1 (DEKS tran won)

**U.S. Brand Names** Promit®

**Therapeutic Category** Plasma Volume Expander

**Use** Prophylaxis of serious anaphylactic reactions to I.V. infusion of dextran

**Usual Dosage** I.V. (time between dextran 1 and dextran solution should not exceed 15 minutes):

Children: 0.3 mL/kg 1-2 minutes before I.V. infusion of dextran

Adults: 20 mL 1-2 minutes before I.V. infusion of dextran

**Mechanism of Action** Binds to dextran-reactive immunoglobulin without bridge formation and no formation of large immune complexes

**Local Anesthetic/Vasoconstrictor Precautions** No information available to require special precautions

**Effects on Dental Treatment** No effects or complications reported

**Other Adverse Effects** <1%:

Cardiovascular: Mild hypotension, tightness of chest
Central nervous system: Fever
Dermatologic: Urticaria
(Continued)

## Dextran 1 *(Continued)*

Gastrointestinal: Nausea, vomiting
Local: Cutaneous reactions
Neuromuscular & skeletal: Arthralgia
Respiratory: Nasal congestion, wheezing

**Pregnancy Risk Factor** C

**Dosage Forms** Injection: 150 mg/mL (20 mL)

**Generic Available** No

- **Dextran 40** *see* Dextran *on previous page*
- **Dextran 70** *see* Dextran *on previous page*
- **Dextran, High Molecular Weight** *see* Dextran *on previous page*
- **Dextran, Low Molecular Weight** *see* Dextran *on previous page*

## Dextranomer (deks TRAN oh mer)

**U.S. Brand Names** Debrisan® [OTC]

**Therapeutic Category** Topical Skin Product

**Use** Clean exudative ulcers and wounds such as venous stasis ulcers, decubitus ulcers, and infected traumatic and surgical wounds; no controlled studies have found dextranomer to be more effective than conventional therapy

**Usual Dosage** Debride and clean wound prior to application; apply to affected area once or twice daily in a 1/4" layer; apply a dressing and seal on all four sides; removal should be done by irrigation

**Mechanism of Action** Dextranomer is a network of dextran-sucrose beads possessing a great many exposed hydroxy groups; when this network is applied to an exudative wound surface, the exudate is drawn by capillary forces generated by the swelling of the beads, with vacuum forces producing an upward flow of exudate into the network

**Local Anesthetic/Vasoconstrictor Precautions** No information available to require special precautions

**Effects on Dental Treatment** No effects or complications reported

**Other Adverse Effects** 1% to 10%:

Local: Transitory pain, blistering
Dermatologic: Maceration may occur, erythema
Hematologic: Bleeding

**Drug Interactions** No data reported

**Pregnancy Risk Factor** C

**Generic Available** No

## Dextroamphetamine (deks troe am FET a meen)

**Related Information**

Dextroamphetamine and Amphetamine *on next page*

**U.S. Brand Names** Dexedrine®

**Therapeutic Category** Amphetamine; Anorexiant; Central Nervous System Stimulant, Amphetamine

**Use** Narcolepsy, exogenous obesity, abnormal behavioral syndrome in children (minimal brain dysfunction), attention deficit hyperactive disorder (ADHD)

**Usual Dosage** Oral:

Children:

Narcolepsy: 6-12 years: Initial: 5 mg/day, may increase at 5 mg increments in weekly intervals until side effects appear; maximum dose: 60 mg/day

Attention deficit disorder:

3-5 years: Initial: 2.5 mg/day given every morning; increase by 2.5 mg/day in weekly intervals until optimal response is obtained, usual range: 0.1-0.5 mg/kg/dose every morning with maximum of 40 mg/day

≥6 years: 5 mg once or twice daily; increase in increments of 5 mg/day at weekly intervals until optimal response is reached, usual range: 0.1-0.5 mg/kg/dose every morning (5-20 mg/day) with maximum of 40 mg/day

Children >12 years and Adults:

Narcolepsy: Initial: 10 mg/day, may increase at 10 mg increments in weekly intervals until side effects appear; maximum: 60 mg/day

Exogenous obesity: 5-30 mg/day in divided doses of 5-10 mg 30-60 minutes before meals

**Mechanism of Action** Blocks reuptake of dopamine and norepinephrine from the synapse, thus increases the amount of circulating dopamine and norepinephrine in cerebral cortex to reticular activating system; inhibits the action of monoamine oxidase and causes catecholamines to be released

**Local Anesthetic/Vasoconstrictor Precautions** Use vasoconstriction with caution in patients taking dextroamphetamine. Amphetamines enhance the sympathomimetic response of epinephrine and norepinephrine leading to potential hypertension and cardiotoxicity.

**Effects on Dental Treatment** Up to 10% of patients taking dextroamphetamines may present with hypertension. The use of local anesthetic without vasoconstrictor is recommended in these patients.

**Other Adverse Effects**

>10%:

Cardiovascular: Arrhythmia

Central nervous system: False feeling of well being, nervousness, restlessness, insomnia

1% to 10%:

Cardiovascular: Hypertension

Central nervous system: Mood or mental changes, dizziness, lightheadedness, headache

Endocrine & metabolic: Changes in libido

Gastrointestinal: Diarrhea, nausea, vomiting, stomach cramps, constipation, anorexia, weight loss, dry mouth

Ocular: Blurred vision

Miscellaneous: Increased sweating

<1%:

Cardiovascular: Chest pain

Central nervous system: CNS stimulation (severe), Tourette's syndrome, hyperthermia, seizures, paranoia

Dermatologic: Skin rash, urticaria

Miscellaneous: Tolerance and withdrawal with prolonged use

**Drug Interactions**

Adrenergic blockers are inhibited by amphetamines

Amphetamines enhance the activity of tricyclic or sympathomimetic agents

MAO Inhibitors slow the metabolism of amphetamines

Amphetamines will counteract the sedative effects of antihistamines

Amphetamines potentiate the analgesic effects of meperidine

**Drug Uptake**

Onset of action: 1-1.5 hours

Serum half-life: Adults: 34 hours (pH dependent)

Time to peak serum concentration: Oral: Within 3 hours

**Pregnancy Risk Factor** C

**Generic Available** Yes

## Dextroamphetamine and Amphetamine

(deks troe am FET a meen & am FET a meen)

**U.S. Brand Names** Adderall®

**Therapeutic Category** Amphetamine

**Use** Treatment of narcolepsy; exogenous obesity; abnormal behavioral syndrome in children (minimal brain dysfunction); attention deficit hyperactive disorder (ADHD)

**Usual Dosage** Oral:

Narcolepsy:

Children:

6-12 years: 5 mg/day, increase by 5 mg at weekly intervals

>12 years: 10 mg/day, increase by 10 mg at weekly intervals

Adults: 5-60 mg/day in 2-3 divided doses

Attention deficit disorder: Children:

3-5 years: 2.5 mg/day, increase by 2.5 mg at weekly intervals

>6 years: 5 mg/day, increase by 5 mg at weekly intervals not to exceed 40 mg/day

Short-term adjunct to exogenous obesity: Children >12 years and Adults: 5-30 mg/day in divided doses

**Local Anesthetic/Vasoconstrictor Precautions** Use vasoconstriction with caution in patients taking dextroamphetamine. Amphetamines enhance the sympathomimetic response of epinephrine and norepinephrine leading to potential hypertension and cardiotoxicity.

**Effects on Dental Treatment** Up to 10% of patients taking dextroamphetamines may present with hypertension. The use of local anesthetic without vasoconstrictor is recommended in these patients.

**Other Adverse Effects** See individual agents

**Drug Interactions** See individual agents

**Dosage Forms** Tablet:

10 mg [dextroamphetamine sulfate 2.5 mg, dextroamphetamine saccharate 2.5 mg and amphetamine aspartate 2.5 mg, amphetamine sulfate 2.5 mg]

20 mg [dextroamphetamine sulfate 5 mg, dextroamphetamine saccharate 5 mg and amphetamine aspartate 5 mg, amphetamine sulfate 5 mg]

**Generic Available** No

## Dextromethorphan (deks troe meth OR fan)

**Related Information**

Acetaminophen, Dextromethorphan, and Pseudoephedrine *on page 32*
Guaifenesin, Pseudoephedrine, and Dextromethorphan *on page 482*

**U.S. Brand Names** Benylin DM® [OTC]; Benylin® Pediatric [OTC]; Children's Hold® [OTC]; Creo-Terpin® [OTC]; Delsym® [OTC]; Drixoral® Cough Liquid Caps [OTC]; Hold® DM [OTC]; Pertussin® CS [OTC]; Pertussin® ES [OTC]; Robitussin® Cough Calmers [OTC]; Robitussin® Pediatric [OTC]; Scot-Tussin DM® Cough Chasers [OTC]; Silphen DM® [OTC]; St. Joseph® Cough Suppressant [OTC]; Sucrets® Cough Calmers [OTC]; Suppress® [OTC]; Trocal® [OTC]; Vicks Formula 44® [OTC]; Vicks Formula 44® Pediatric Formula [OTC]

**Canadian Brand Names** Balminil-DM®

**Therapeutic Category** Antitussive

**Use** Symptomatic relief of coughs caused by minor viral upper respiratory tract infections or inhaled irritants; most effective for a chronic nonproductive cough

**Usual Dosage** Oral:

Children:

- <2 years: Use only as directed by a physician
- 2-6 years (syrup): 2.5-7.5 mg every 4-8 hours; extended release is 15 mg twice daily (maximum: 30 mg/24 hours)
- 6-12 years: 5-10 mg every 4 hours or 15 mg every 6-8 hours; extended release is 30 mg twice daily (maximum: 60 mg/24 hours)

Children >12 years and Adults: 10-30 mg every 4-8 hours or 30 mg every 6-8 hours; extended release is 60 mg twice daily (maximum: 120 mg/24 hours)

**Mechanism of Action** Chemical relative of morphine lacking narcotic properties except in overdose; controls cough by depressing the medullary cough center

**Local Anesthetic/Vasoconstrictor Precautions** No information available to require special precautions

**Effects on Dental Treatment** No effects or complications reported

**Other Adverse Effects** <1%:

Central nervous system: Drowsiness, dizziness, coma
Gastrointestinal: Nausea, GI upset, constipation
Respiratory: Respiratory depression

**Warnings/Precautions** Research on chicken embryos exposed to concentrations of dextromethorphan relative to those typically taken by humans has shown to cause birth defects and fetal death; more study is needed, but it is suggested that pregnant women should be advised not to use dextromethorphan-containing medications

**Drug Interactions** No data reported

**Drug Uptake**

Onset of antitussive action: Within 15-30 minutes
Duration: Up to 6 hours

**Pregnancy Risk Factor** C (see Warnings)

**Generic Available** Yes

- ♦ **Dextromethorphan, Acetaminophen, and Pseudoephedrine** *see* Acetaminophen, Dextromethorphan, and Pseudoephedrine *on page 32*
- ♦ **Dextromethorphan, Guaifenesin, and Pseudoephedrine** *see* Guaifenesin, Pseudoephedrine, and Dextromethorphan *on page 482*
- ♦ **Dextrose, Levulose and Phosphoric Acid** *see* Phosphorated Carbohydrate Solution *on page 800*

## Dextrothyroxine (deks troe thye ROKS een)

**U.S. Brand Names** Choloxin®

**Therapeutic Category** Lipid Lowering Drugs

**Use** Reduction of elevated serum cholesterol

**Usual Dosage** Oral:

Children: 0.05 mg/kg/day, increase at 1-month intervals by 0.05 mg/kg/day to a maximum of 0.4 mg/kg/day or 4 mg/day

Adults: 1-2 mg/day, increase at 1-2 mg at intervals of 4 weeks, up to a maximum of 8 mg/day

**Mechanism of Action** Unclear mechanism, thought to increase the liver breakdown of cholesterol

**Local Anesthetic/Vasoconstrictor Precautions** No information available to require special precautions

**Effects on Dental Treatment** No effects or complications reported

**Other Adverse Effects** <1%:

Cardiovascular: Myocardial infarction, angina, arrhythmias
Central nervous system: Insomnia, headache
Dermatologic: Alopecia, skin rash
Gastrointestinal: Weight loss

Neuromuscular & skeletal: Tremor, paresthesia
Ocular: Visual disturbances
Otic: Tinnitus
Miscellaneous: Sweating

**Drug Interactions**
Decreased effect of beta-blockers, digitalis, hypoglycemics; decreased effect with cholestyramine
Increased effect of anticoagulants

**Drug Uptake**
Absorption: Poorly absorbed from GI tract (25%)
Serum half-life: 18 hours

**Pregnancy Risk Factor** C

**Generic Available** No

- **Dey-Dose® Isoproterenol** *see* Isoproterenol *on page 553*
- **Dey-Dose® Metaproterenol** *see* Metaproterenol *on page 642*
- **Dey-Lute® Isoetharine** *see* Isoetharine *on page 551*

## Dezocine (DEZ oh seen)

**Related Information**
Narcotic Agonists *on page 1223*

**U.S. Brand Names** Dalgan®

**Therapeutic Category** Analgesic, Narcotic

**Use** Relief of moderate to severe postoperative, acute renal and ureteral colic, and cancer pain

**Usual Dosage** Adults (not recommended for patients <18 years):
I.M.: Initial: 5-20 mg; may be repeated every 3-6 hours as needed; maximum: 120 mg/day and 20 mg/dose
I.V.: Initial: 2.5-10 mg; may be repeated every 2-4 hours as needed

**Mechanism of Action** Binds to opiate receptors in the CNS, causing inhibition of ascending pain pathways, altering the perception of and response to pain; produces generalized CNS depression; it is a mixed agonist-antagonist that appears to bind selectively to CNS $\mu$ and $\Delta$ opiate receptors

**Local Anesthetic/Vasoconstrictor Precautions** No information available to require special precautions

**Effects on Dental Treatment** No effects or complications reported

**Other Adverse Effects**
1% to 10%:
Central nervous system: Sedation, dizziness, vertigo
Gastrointestinal: Nausea, vomiting
Local: Injection site reactions
<1%:
Cardiovascular: Hypotension, palpitations, bradycardia, peripheral vasodilation
Central nervous system: Increased intracranial pressure, CNS depression, drowsiness
Endocrine & metabolic: Antidiuretic hormone release
Gastrointestinal: Constipation, biliary tract spasm
Genitourinary: Urinary tract spasm
Ocular: Miosis
Respiratory: Respiratory depression
Miscellaneous: Histamine release, physical and psychological dependence with prolonged use

**Drug Interactions** Increased effect with CNS depressants

**Drug Uptake**
Onset of analgesia: Within 15-30 minutes
Duration of analgesia: 4-6 hours
Serum half-life: 2.6-2.8 hours

**Pregnancy Risk Factor** C

**Generic Available** No

- **DFMO** *see* Eflornithine *on page 365*
- **DHAD** *see* Mitoxantrone *on page 682*
- **DHC Plus®** *see* Dihydrocodeine Compound *on page 331*
- **D.H.E. 45® Injection** *see* Dihydroergotamine *on page 332*
- **DHS® Tar [OTC]** *see* Coal Tar *on page 270*
- **DHS Zinc® [OTC]** *see* Pyrithione Zinc *on page 869*
- **DHT™** *see* Dihydrotachysterol *on page 333*
- **Diaβeta®** *see* Glyburide *on page 471*
- **Diabetic Tussin DM® [OTC]** *see* Guaifenesin and Dextromethorphan *on page 479*
- **Diabetic Tussin® EX [OTC]** *see* Guaifenesin *on page 478*

- **Diabinese®** *see* Chlorpropamide *on page 240*
- **Dialose® [OTC]** *see* Docusate *on page 346*
- **Dialose® Plus Capsule [OTC]** *see* Docusate and Casanthranol *on page 347*
- **Dialume® [OTC]** *see* Aluminum Hydroxide *on page 55*
- **Diamine T.D.® [OTC]** *see* Brompheniramine *on page 151*
- **Diamox®** *see* Acetazolamide *on page 33*
- **Diamox® Sequels®** *see* Acetazolamide *on page 33*
- **Diaparene® [OTC]** *see* Methylbenzethonium Chloride *on page 658*
- **Diapid®** *see* Lypressin *on page 609*
- **Diar-aid® [OTC]** *see* Loperamide *on page 599*
- **Diasorb® [OTC]** *see* Attapulgite *on page 109*
- **Diastat® Rectal Delivery System** *see* Diazepam *on this page*
- **Diazemuls® Injection** *see* Diazepam *on this page*


## Diazepam (dye AZ e pam)

**Related Information**

Dental Drug Interactions: Update on Drug Combinations Requiring Special Considerations *on page 1225*

Patients Requiring Sedation *on page 1152*

Temporomandibular Dysfunction (TMD) *on page 1149*

**U.S. Brand Names** Diastat® Rectal Delivery System; Diazemuls® Injection; Diazepam Intensol®; Dizac® Injectable Emulsion; Valium® Injection; Valium® Oral

**Canadian Brand Names** Apo®-Diazepam; Diazemuls®; E Pam®; Meval®; Novo-Dipam; PMS-Diazepam; Vivol®

**Therapeutic Category** Antianxiety Agent; Anticonvulsant, Benzodiazepine; Benzodiazepine; Muscle Relaxant; Sedative; Skeletal Muscle Relaxant; Tranquilizer, Minor

**Use**

Dental: Oral medication for preoperative dental anxiety; sedative component in I.V. conscious sedation in oral surgery patients; skeletal muscle relaxant

Medical: In medicine, management of general anxiety disorders, panic disorders, and provide preoperative sedation, light anesthesia, and amnesia; treatment of status epilepticus, alcohol withdrawal symptoms; used as a skeletal muscle relaxant

**Restrictions** C-IV; Refillable up to 5 times in 6 months

**Usual Dosage**

Children: Oral:

Conscious sedation for procedures: 0.2-0.3 mg/kg (maximum: 10 mg) 45-60 minutes prior to procedure

Sedation or muscle relaxation or anxiety: 0.12-0.8 mg/kg/day in divided doses every 6-8 hours the day before the procedure

Adults:

Oral: Preop sedation/antianxiety: 2-10 mg 2 times/day the day before the procedure; 2-10 mg morning of procedure if needed

I.V.: Conscious sedation: 5-15 mg titrated slowly to effect

**Mechanism of Action** Depresses all levels of the CNS, including the limbic and reticular formation, probably through the increased action of gamma-aminobutyric acid (GABA), which is a major inhibitory neurotransmitter in the brain

**Local Anesthetic/Vasoconstrictor Precautions** No information available to require special precautions

**Effects on Dental Treatment** >10% of patients experience dry mouth or changes in salivation

**Other Adverse Effects**

>10%:

Central nervous system: Drowsiness, ataxia, amnesia, slurred speech, lightheadedness

Local: Phlebitis, pain with injection

1% to 10%: Central nervous system: Confusion, dizziness

**Contraindications** Hypersensitivity to diazepam or any component; there may be a cross-sensitivity with other benzodiazepines; do not use in a comatose patient, in those with pre-existing CNS depression, respiratory depression, narrow-angle glaucoma, or severe uncontrolled pain; do not use in pregnant women

**Warnings/Precautions** Use with caution in patients receiving other CNS depressants, patients with low albumin, hepatic dysfunction, and in the elderly and young infants. Due to its long-acting metabolite, diazepam is not considered a drug of choice in the elderly; long-acting benzodiazepines have been associated with falls in the elderly.

**Drug Interactions** Enzyme inducers may increase the metabolism of diazepam; CNS depressants (alcohol, barbiturates, opioids) may enhance sedation and respiratory depression; cimetidine may decrease the metabolism of diazepam; cisapride can significantly increase diazepam levels; valproic acid may displace diazepam from binding sites which may result in an increase in sedative effects; selective serotonin reuptake inhibitors (eg, fluoxetine, sertraline, paroxetine) have greatly increased diazepam levels by altering its clearance

**Drug Uptake**

Absorption: Oral: 85% to 100%, more reliable than I.M.

Serum half-life:

Parent drug: Adults: 20-50 hours, increased half-life in neonates, elderly, and those with severe hepatic disorders

Active major metabolite (desmethyldiazepam): 50-100 hours, can be prolonged in neonates

Time to peak serum concentration: 0.5-2 hours

**Pregnancy Risk Factor** D

**Breast-feeding Considerations** Not compatible

**Dosage Forms**

Gel, rectal delivery system (Diastat®):

Pediatric rectal tip (4.4 cm): 5 mg/mL (2.5 mg, 5 mg, 10 mg) [twin packs]

Adult rectal tip (6 cm): 5 mg/mL (10 mg, 15 mg, 20 mg) [twin packs]

Injection: 5 mg/mL (1 mL, 2 mL, 5 mL, 10 mL)

Injection, emulsified:

Dizac®: 5 mg/mL (3 mL)

Diazemuls®: 5 mg/mL (2 mL)

Solution, oral (wintergreen-spice flavor): 5 mg/5 mL (5 mL, 10 mL, 500 mL)

Solution, oral concentrate (Diazepam Intensol®): 5 mg/mL (30 mL)

Tablet: 2 mg, 5 mg, 10 mg

**Dietary Considerations** May be taken with food or water

**Generic Available** Yes

♦ **Diazepam Intensol®** *see* Diazepam *on previous page*

## Diazoxide (dye az OKS ide)

**U.S. Brand Names** Hyperstat® I.V.; Proglycem®

**Therapeutic Category** Antihypertensive Agent; Antihypoglycemic Agent

**Use**

Oral: Hypoglycemia related to islet cell adenoma, carcinoma, hyperplasia, or adenomatosis, nesidioblastosis, leucine sensitivity, or extrapancreatic malignancy

I.V.: Emergency lowering of blood pressure

**Usual Dosage**

Hypertension: Children and Adults: I.V.: 1-3 mg/kg up to a maximum of 150 mg in a single injection; repeat dose in 5-15 minutes until blood pressure adequately reduced; repeat administration at intervals of 4-24 hours; monitor the blood pressure closely; do not use longer than 10 days

Hyperinsulinemic hypoglycemia: Oral: **Note:** Use lower dose listed as initial dose

Children and Adults: 3-8 mg/kg/day in divided doses every 8-12 hours

**Mechanism of Action** Inhibits insulin release from the pancreas; produces direct smooth muscle relaxation of the peripheral arterioles which results in decrease in blood pressure and reflex increase in heart rate and cardiac output

**Local Anesthetic/Vasoconstrictor Precautions** No information available to require special precautions

**Effects on Dental Treatment** No effects or complications reported

**Other Adverse Effects**

1% to 10%:

Cardiovascular: Hypotension

Central nervous system: Dizziness

Gastrointestinal: Nausea, vomiting

Neuromuscular & skeletal: Weakness

<1%:

Cardiovascular: Tachycardia, flushing

Central nervous system: Seizures, headache, extrapyramidal symptoms and development of abnormal facies with chronic oral use

Dermatologic: Rash, hirsutism

Endocrine & metabolic: Hyperglycemia, ketoacidosis, sodium and water retention, hyperuricemia, inhibition of labor

Gastrointestinal: Anorexia, constipation

Hematologic: Leukopenia, thrombocytopenia

Local: Pain, burning, cellulitis/phlebitis upon extravasation

**Drug Interactions**

Decreased effect: Diazoxide may increase phenytoin metabolism or free fraction

Increased toxicity:

Diuretics and hypotensive agents may potentiate diazoxide adverse effects

(Continued)

## Diazoxide *(Continued)*

Diazoxide may decrease warfarin protein binding

**Drug Uptake**

Hyperglycemic effect: Oral:

Onset of action: Within 1 hour

Duration (normal renal function): 8 hours

Hypotensive effect: I.V.:

Peak: Within 5 minutes

Duration: Usually 3-12 hours

Serum half-life:

Children: 9-24 hours

Adults: 20-36 hours

End-stage renal disease: >30 hours

**Pregnancy Risk Factor** C

**Generic Available** Yes: Injection

- **Dibent® Injection** *see* Dicyclomine *on page 322*
- **Dibenzyline®** *see* Phenoxybenzamine *on page 792*

## Dibucaine (DYE byoo kane)

**U.S. Brand Names** Nupercainal® [OTC]

**Therapeutic Category** Local Anesthetic, Topical

**Use**

Dental: Amide derivative local anesthetic for minor skin conditions

Medical: Fast, temporary relief of pain and itching due to hemorrhoids, minor burns

**Usual Dosage** Children and Adults: Topical: Apply gently to the affected areas; no more than 30 g for adults or 7.5 g for children should be used in any 24-hour period

**Mechanism of Action** Local anesthetics bind selectively to the intracellular surface of sodium channels to block influx of sodium into the axon. As a result, depolarization necessary for action potential propagation and subsequent nerve function is prevented. The block at the sodium channel is reversible. When drug diffuses away from the axon, sodium channel function is restored and nerve propagation returns.

**Local Anesthetic/Vasoconstrictor Precautions** No information available to require special precautions

**Effects on Dental Treatment** No effects or complications reported

**Other Adverse Effects** 1% to 10%:

Local: Burning

Dermatologic: Angioedema, contact dermatitis

**Contraindications** Known hypersensitivity to amide-type anesthetics, ophthalmic use

**Warnings/Precautions** Avoid use in sensitive individuals

**Drug Interactions** No data reported

**Drug Uptake**

Onset of action: Within 15 minutes

Duration: 2-4 hours

Absorption: Poor through intact skin, but well absorbed through mucous membranes and excoriated skin

**Pregnancy Risk Factor** C

**Breast-feeding Considerations** No data reported; however, topical administration is probably compatible

**Dosage Forms**

Cream, topical: 0.5% (45 g)

Ointment, topical: 1% (30 g, 60 g, 454 g)

**Generic Available** Yes

## Dibucaine and Hydrocortisone

(DYE byoo kane & hye droe KOR ti sone)

**U.S. Brand Names** Corticaine® Topical

**Therapeutic Category** Corticosteroid, Topical (Low Potency); Local Anesthetic, Topical

**Synonyms** Hydrocortisone and Dibucaine

**Use** Relief of the inflammatory and pruritic manifestations of corticosteroid-responsive dermatoses and for external anal itching

**Usual Dosage** Topical: Apply to affected areas 2-4 times/day

**Local Anesthetic/Vasoconstrictor Precautions** No information available to require special precautions

**Effects on Dental Treatment** No effects or complications reported

**Pregnancy Risk Factor** C

**Generic Available** Yes

- ♦ **DIC** *see* Dacarbazine *on page 292*
- ♦ **Dicarbosil® [OTC]** *see* Calcium Carbonate *on page 172*

## Dichlorodifluoromethane and Trichloromonofluoromethane

(dye klor oh dye flor oh METH ane & tri klor oh mon oh flor oh METH ane)

**Related Information**

Temporomandibular Dysfunction (TMD) *on page 1149*

**U.S. Brand Names** Fluori-Methane®

**Therapeutic Category** Local Anesthetic, Topical

**Use**

Dental: Topical application in the management of myofascial pain, restricted motion, and muscle spasm

Medical: For the control of pain associated with injections

**Usual Dosage** Invert bottle over treatment area approximately 12" away from site of application; open dispenseal spring valve completely, allowing liquid to flow in a stream from the bottle. The rate of spraying is approximately 10 cm/second and should be continued until entire muscle has been covered.

**Local Anesthetic/Vasoconstrictor Precautions** No information available to require special precautions

**Effects on Dental Treatment** No effects or complications reported

**Other Adverse Effects** No data reported

**Contraindications** In individuals with a history of hypersensitivity to dichlorofluoromethane and/or trichloromonofluoromethane; should not be used on patients having vascular impairment of the extremities

**Warnings/Precautions** For external use only; care should be taken to minimize inhalation of vapors, especially with application to head and neck; avoid contact with eyes; should not be applied to the point of frost formation

**Drug Interactions** No data reported

**Drug Uptake** No data reported

**Breast-feeding Considerations** No data reported

**Dosage Forms** Spray: 4 oz amber glass bottles; calibrated fine spray and calibrated medium spray

**Generic Available** No

**Comments** Dichlorodifluoromethane and trichloromonofluoromethane are not classified as carcinogens; based on animal studies and human experience, these fluorocarbons pose no hazard to man relative to systemic toxicity, carcinogenicity, mutagenicity, or teratogenicity when occupational exposures are <1000 ppm over an 8-hour time weighted average.

- ♦ **Dichlorotetrafluoroethane and Ethyl Chloride** *see* Ethyl Chloride and Dichlorotetrafluoroethane *on page 410*

## Dichlorphenamide (dye klor FEN a mide)

**U.S. Brand Names** Daranide®

**Therapeutic Category** Antiglaucoma Agent; Carbonic Anhydrase Inhibitor; Diuretic, Carbonic Anhydrase Inhibitor

**Synonyms** Diclofenamide

**Use** Adjunct in treatment of open-angle glaucoma and perioperative treatment for angle-closure glaucoma

**Usual Dosage** Adults: Oral: 100-200 mg to start followed by 100 mg every 12 hours until desired response is obtained; maintenance dose: 25-50 mg 1-3 times/day

**Local Anesthetic/Vasoconstrictor Precautions** No information available to require special precautions

**Effects on Dental Treatment** No effects or complications reported

**Other Adverse Effects**

>10%:

- Central nervous system: Fatigue, malaise
- Gastrointestinal: Diarrhea, anorexia, metallic taste
- Renal: Polyuria

1% to 10%:

- Central nervous system: Mental depression, somnolence
- Renal: Renal calculi

<1%:

- Central nervous system: Fever
- Dermatologic: Rash
- Endocrine & metabolic: Hyperchloremic metabolic acidosis, hypokalemia, hyperglycemia
- Gastrointestinal: Black stools, GI irritation, dryness of the mouth

(Continued)

## Dichlorphenamide *(Continued)*

Genitourinary: Dysuria
Hematologic: Blood dyscrasias, bone marrow suppression
Neuromuscular & skeletal: Paresthesias
Ocular: Myopia

**Pregnancy Risk Factor** C

**Generic Available** No

## Diclofenac (dye KLOE fen ak)

**Related Information**

Rheumatoid Arthritis and Osteoarthritis *on page 1092*

**U.S. Brand Names** Cataflam® Oral; Voltaren® Ophthalmic; Voltaren® Oral; Voltaren-XR® Oral

**Canadian Brand Names** Apo®-Diclo; Novo-Difenac®; Novo-Difenac®-SR; Nu-Diclo; Voltaren Rapide®

**Therapeutic Category** Analgesic, Non-narcotic; Anti-inflammatory Agent; Nonsteroidal Anti-inflammatory Drug (NSAID), Ophthalmic; Nonsteroidal Anti-inflammatory Drug (NSAID), Oral

**Use** Acute treatment of mild to moderate pain; acute and chronic treatment of rheumatoid arthritis, ankylosing spondylitis, and osteoarthritis; used for juvenile rheumatoid arthritis, gout, dysmenorrhea; ophthalmic solution for the treatment of postoperative swelling in patients who have undergone cataract extraction and for the treatment of photophobia in patients undergoing incisional refractive surgery

**Usual Dosage** Adults:

Oral:

Analgesia (Cataflam®): Starting dose: 50 mg 3 times/day
Rheumatoid arthritis: 150-200 mg/day in 2-4 divided doses (100 mg/day of sustained release product)
Osteoarthritis: 100-150 mg/day in 2-3 divided doses (100-200 mg/day of sustained release product)
Ankylosing spondylitis: 100-125 mg/day in 4-5 divided doses

Ophthalmic: Instill 1 drop into affected eye 4 times/day beginning 24 hours after cataract surgery and continuing for 2 weeks

**Mechanism of Action** Inhibits prostaglandin synthesis by decreasing the activity of the enzyme, cyclo-oxygenase, which results in decreased formation of prostaglandin precursors

**Local Anesthetic/Vasoconstrictor Precautions** No information available to require special precautions

**Effects on Dental Treatment** NSAID formulations are known to reversibly decrease platelet aggregation via mechanisms different than observed with aspirin. The dentist should be aware of the potential of abnormal coagulation. Caution should also be exercised in the use of NSAIDs in patients already on anticoagulant therapy with drugs such as warfarin (Coumadin®).

**Other Adverse Effects**

>10%:

Dermatologic: Skin rash
Gastrointestinal: Abdominal cramps, heartburn, indigestion, nausea

1% to 10%:

Cardiovascular: Angina pectoris, arrhythmias
Central nervous system: Dizziness, nervousness
Dermatologic: Skin rash, itching
Gastrointestinal: GI ulceration, vomiting
Genitourinary: Vaginal bleeding
Otic: Tinnitus

<1%:

Cardiovascular: Chest pain, congestive heart failure, hypertension, tachycardia
Central nervous system: Convulsions, forgetfulness, mental depression, drowsiness, insomnia
Dermatologic: Urticaria, exfoliative dermatitis, erythema multiforme, Stevens-Johnson syndrome, angioedema
Gastrointestinal: Stomatitis
Genitourinary: Cystitis
Hematologic: Agranulocytosis, anemia, pancytopenia, leukopenia, thrombocytopenia
Hepatic: Hepatitis
Neuromuscular & skeletal: Peripheral neuropathy, trembling, weakness
Ocular: Blurred vision, change in vision
Otic: Decreased hearing
Renal: Interstitial nephritis, nephrotic syndrome, renal impairment
Respiratory: Wheezing, laryngeal edema, dyspnea, epistaxis

Miscellaneous: Anaphylaxis, increased sweating

**Drug Interactions**

Decreased effect with aspirin; decreased effect of thiazides, furosemide

Increased toxicity of digoxin, methotrexate, cyclosporine, lithium, insulin, sulfonylureas, potassium-sparing diuretics, aspirin

**Drug Uptake**

Onset of action: Cataflam® has a more rapid onset of action than does the sodium salt (Voltaren®), because it is absorbed in the stomach instead of the duodenum

Serum half-life: 2 hours

Time to peak serum concentration:

Cataflam®: Within 1 hour

Voltaren®: Within 2 hours

**Pregnancy Risk Factor** B

**Dosage Forms**

Solution, ophthalmic, as sodium (Voltaren®): 0.1% (2.5 mL, 5 mL)

Tablet, enteric coated, as sodium: 25 mg, 50 mg, 75 mg

Voltaren®: 25 mg, 50 mg, 75 mg

Tablet, extended release, as sodium (Voltaren-XR®): 100 mg

Tablet, as potassium (Cataflam®): 50 mg

**Dietary Considerations** May be taken with food to decrease GI distress

**Generic Available** Yes: Tablet

## Diclofenac and Misoprostol

**U.S. Brand Names** Arthrotec®

**Therapeutic Category** Analgesic, Non-narcotic; Prostaglandin

**Use** The diclofenac component is indicated for the treatment of osteoarthritis and rheumatoid arthritis; the misoprostol component is indicated for the prophylaxis of NSAID-induced gastric and duodenal ulceration

**Usual Dosage** Adults: Oral: 1 tablet to be taken with food, 2-3 times/day; tablets should be swallowed whole, not chewed

**Mechanism of Action** See individual agents

**Local Anesthetic/Vasoconstrictor Precautions** No information available to require special precautions

**Effects on Dental Treatment** No effects or complications reported

**Warnings/Precautions** Use in premenopausal women; should not be used in premenopausal women unless they use effective contraception and have been advised of the risks of taking the product if pregnant

**Drug Uptake** The pharmacokinetic profiles of diclofenac and misoprostol administered as a combination product is similar to the profiles when the two drugs are administered as separate tablets. No pharmacokinetic interaction between the two drugs has been observed following multiple doses.

**Pregnancy Risk Factor** X

**Dosage Forms** Tablet: Diclofenac 50 mg and misoprostol 200 mcg; diclofenac 75 mg and misoprostol 200 mcg

♦ **Diclofenamide** *see* Dichlorphenamide *on page 319*

## Dicloxacillin (dye kloks a SIL in)

**Related Information**

Oral Bacterial Infections *on page 1128*

**U.S. Brand Names** Dycill®; Dynapen®; Pathocil®

**Therapeutic Category** Antibiotic, Penicillin

**Use**

Dental: Treatment of susceptible orofacial infections, notably penicillinase-producing staph

Medical: Treatment of systemic infections in the medical patient such as pneumonia, skin and soft tissue infections, and osteomyelitis caused by penicillinase-producing staphylococci

**Usual Dosage** Oral:

Children >40 kg and Adults: 250-500 mg every 6 hours for at least 7 days

Children <40 kg: 125-150 mg/kg/day divided every 6 hours

**Mechanism of Action** Interferes with bacterial cell wall synthesis during active multiplication, causing cell wall death and resultant bactericidal activity against susceptible bacteria

**Local Anesthetic/Vasoconstrictor Precautions** No information available to require special precautions

**Effects on Dental Treatment** Prolonged use of penicillins may lead to development of oral candidiasis

**Other Adverse Effects** 1% to 10%: Gastrointestinal: Diarrhea

**Contraindications** Known hypersensitivity to dicloxacillin, penicillin, or any components

(Continued)

## Dicloxacillin *(Continued)*

**Warnings/Precautions** Monitor PT if patient concurrently on warfarin; elimination of drug is slow in neonates; use with caution in patients allergic to cephalosporins; bad taste of suspension may make compliance difficult

**Drug Interactions** Efficacy of oral contraceptives may be reduced; disulfiram, probenecid causes increased penicillin levels; increased effect of anticoagulants

**Drug Uptake**

Absorption: 35% to 76% from GI tract; food decreases rate and extent of absorption

Serum half-life: 0.6-0.8 hours

Time to peak serum concentration: Within 0.5-2 hours

**Pregnancy Risk Factor** B

**Breast-feeding Considerations** No data reported; however, other penicillins may be taken while breast-feeding

**Dosage Forms**

Capsule, as sodium: 125 mg, 250 mg, 500 mg

Powder for oral suspension, as sodium: 62.5 mg/5 mL (80 mL, 100 mL, 200 mL)

**Dietary Considerations** Should be taken with water 1 hour before or 2 hours after meals on an empty stomach

**Generic Available** Yes

**Comments** Although dicloxacillin is a penicillin antibiotic indicated for infections caused by penicillinase secreting staph, amoxicillin with clavulanic acid is considered the drug of choice for these types of orofacial infections

## Dicumarol (dye KOO ma role)

**Related Information**

Cardiovascular Diseases *on page 1066*

**Therapeutic Category** Anticoagulant (Warfarin-like)

**Synonyms** Bishydroxycoumarin

**Use** Prophylaxis and treatment of thromboembolic disorders

**Usual Dosage** Adults: Oral: 25-200 mg/day based on prothrombin time (PT) determinations

**Mechanism of Action** Interferes with hepatic synthesis of vitamin K-dependent coagulation factors (II, VII, IX, X)

**Local Anesthetic/Vasoconstrictor Precautions** No information available to require special precautions

**Effects on Dental Treatment** Signs of dicumarol overdose may first appear as bleeding from gingival tissue; consultation with prescribing physician is advisable prior to surgery to determine temporary dose reduction or withdrawal of medication

**Other Adverse Effects**

1% to 10%:

- Dermatologic: Skin lesions, alopecia, skin necrosis
- Gastrointestinal: Anorexia, nausea, vomiting, stomach cramps, diarrhea
- Hematologic: Hemorrhage; leukopenia, unrecognized bleeding sites (eg, colon cancer) may be uncovered by anticoagulation
- Respiratory: Hemoptysis

<1%:

- Central nervous system: Fever
- Dermatologic: Skin rash, discolored toes (blue or purple)
- Gastrointestinal: Mouth ulcers
- Hematologic: Agranulocytosis
- Hepatic: Hepatotoxicity
- Renal: Renal damage

**Drug Interactions** See Warfarin

**Pregnancy Risk Factor** D

**Dosage Forms** Tablet: 25 mg, 50 mg, 100 mg

**Dietary Considerations** Avoid proteolytic enzymes (papain), fried/boiled onions & soybean oil

**Generic Available** Yes

## Dicyclomine (dye SYE kloe meen)

**U.S. Brand Names** Antispas® Injection; Bentyl® Hydrochloride Injection; Bentyl® Hydrochloride Oral; Byclomine® Injection; Dibent® Injection; Di-Spaz® Injection; Di-Spaz® Oral; Or-Tyl® Injection

**Canadian Brand Names** Bentylol®; Formulex®

**Therapeutic Category** Antispasmodic Agent, Gastrointestinal

**Synonyms** Dicycloverine Hydrochloride

**Use** Treatment of functional disturbances of GI motility such as irritable bowel syndrome

**Unlabeled use:** Urinary incontinence

**Usual Dosage**

Oral:

Children: 10 mg/dose 3-4 times/day

Adults: Begin with 80 mg/day in 4 equally divided doses, then increase up to 160 mg/day

I.M. **(should not be used I.V.)**: Adults: 80 mg/day in 4 divided doses (20 mg/dose)

**Mechanism of Action** Blocks the action of acetylcholine at parasympathetic sites in smooth muscle, secretory glands and the CNS

**Local Anesthetic/Vasoconstrictor Precautions** No information available to require special precautions

**Effects on Dental Treatment** >10% of patients experience dry mouth

**Other Adverse Effects**

>10%:

Dermatologic: Dry skin

Gastrointestinal: Constipation

Local: Injection site reactions

Respiratory: Dry nose, throat

Miscellaneous: Decreased sweating

1% to 10%:

Dermatologic: Photosensitivity

Endocrine & metabolic: Decreased flow of breast milk

Gastrointestinal: Dysphagia

Ocular: Blurred vision

<1%:

Cardiovascular: Orthostatic hypotension, tachycardia, palpitations

Central nervous system: Confusion, drowsiness, headache, lightheadedness, loss of memory, fatigue, seizures, coma, nervousness, excitement, insomnia

Dermatologic: Skin rash

Gastrointestinal: Bloated feeling, nausea, vomiting

Genitourinary: Dysuria, urinary retention

Neuromuscular & skeletal: Muscular hypotonia, weakness

Ocular: Increased intraocular pain

Respiratory: Asphyxia, respiratory distress

**Drug Interactions**

Decreased effect: Phenothiazines, anti-Parkinson's drugs, haloperidol, sustained release dosage forms; decreased effect with antacids

Increased toxicity: Anticholinergics, amantadine, narcotic analgesics, type I antiarrhythmics, antihistamines, phenothiazines, TCAs

**Drug Uptake**

Onset of effect: 1-2 hours

Duration: Up to 4 hours

Absorption: Oral: Well absorbed

Serum half-life:

Initial phase: 1.8 hours

Terminal phase: 9-10 hours

**Pregnancy Risk Factor** B

**Generic Available** Yes

## Didanosine (dye DAN oh seen)

**Related Information**

HIV Infection and AIDS *on page 1085*

Systemic Viral Diseases *on page 1115*

**U.S. Brand Names** Videx®

**Therapeutic Category** Antiviral Agent, Oral

**Use** Treatment of advanced HIV infection in patients who are intolerant of zidovudine therapy or who have demonstrated significant clinical or immunologic deterioration during zidovudine therapy

**Usual Dosage** Oral (administer on an empty stomach):

Children: 180 mg/m²/day divided every 12 hours **or** dosing is based on body surface area (m²): See table.

**Didanosine — Pediatric Dosing**

| Body Surface Area (m²) | Dosing (Tablets) (mg bid) |
|---|---|
| ≤0.4 | 25 |
| 0.5-0.7 | 50 |
| 0.8-1 | 75 |
| 1.1-1.4 | 100 |

(Continued)

## Didanosine *(Continued)*

Adults: Dosing is based on patient weight: See table.

**Didanosine — Adult Dosing**

| Patient Weight (kg) | Dosing (Tablets) (mg bid) |
|---|---|
| 35-49 | 125 |
| 50-74 | 200 |
| ≥75 | 300 |

**Note:** Children >1 year and Adults should receive 2 tablets per dose and children <1 year should receive 1 tablet per dose for adequate buffering and absorption; tablets should be chewed

**Mechanism of Action** Didanosine, a purine nucleoside analogue and the deamination product of dideoxyadenosine (ddA), inhibits HIV replication *in vitro* in both T cells and monocytes. Didanosine is converted within the cell to the mono-, di-, and triphosphates of ddA. These ddA triphosphates act as substrate and inhibitor of HIV reverse transcriptase substrate and inhibitor of HIV reverse transcriptase thereby blocking viral DNA synthesis and suppressing HIV replication.

**Local Anesthetic/Vasoconstrictor Precautions** No information available to require special precautions

**Effects on Dental Treatment** No effects or complications reported

**Other Adverse Effects**

>10%:
- Central nervous system: Anxiety, headache, irritability, insomnia, restlessness
- Gastrointestinal: Abdominal pain, nausea, diarrhea
- Neuromuscular & skeletal: Peripheral neuropathy

1% to 10%:
- Central nervous system: Depression
- Dermatologic: Rash, pruritus
- Gastrointestinal: Pancreatitis

<1%:
- Central nervous system: Seizures
- Hematologic: Anemia, granulocytopenia, leukopenia, thrombocytopenia
- Hepatic: Hepatitis
- Ocular: Retinal depigmentation
- Renal: Renal impairment
- Miscellaneous: Hypersensitivity

**Drug Interactions** Drugs whose absorption depends on the level of acidity in the stomach such as ketoconazole, itraconazole, and dapsone should be administered at least 2 hours prior to didanosine

Decreased effect: Didanosine may decrease absorption of quinolones or tetracyclines, didanosine should be held during PCP treatment with pentamidine

Increased toxicity: Concomitant administration of other drugs which have the potential to cause peripheral neuropathy or pancreatitis may increase the risk of these toxicities

**Drug Uptake**

Absorption: Subject to degradation by the acidic pH of the stomach; buffered to resist the acidic pH; as much as 50% reduction in the peak plasma concentration is observed in the presence of food

Serum half-life:
- Children and Adolescents: 0.8 hour
- Adults:
  - Normal renal function: 1.5 hours; however, its active metabolite ddATP has an intracellular half-life >12 hours *in vitro*; this permits the drug to be dosed at 12-hour intervals; total body clearance averages 800 mL/minute
  - Impaired renal function: Half-life is increased, with values ranging from 2.5-5 hours

**Pregnancy Risk Factor** B

**Generic Available** No

♦ **Didrex®** *see* Benzphetamine *on page 131*
♦ **Didronel®** *see* Etidronate Disodium *on page 413*

## Dienestrol (dye en ES trole)

**U.S. Brand Names** DV® Vaginal Cream; Ortho®-Dienestrol Vaginal

**Therapeutic Category** Estrogen Derivative

**Use** Symptomatic management of atrophic vaginitis or kraurosis vulvae in postmenopausal women

**Usual Dosage** Adults: Vaginal: Insert 1 applicatorful once or twice daily for 1-2 weeks and then 1/2 of that dose for 1-2 weeks; maintenance dose: 1 applicatorful 1-3 times/week for 3-6 months

**Mechanism of Action** Increases the synthesis of DNA, RNA, and various proteins in target tissues; reduces the release of gonadotropin-releasing hormone from the hypothalamus; reduces FSH and LH release from the pituitary

**Local Anesthetic/Vasoconstrictor Precautions** No information available to require special precautions

**Effects on Dental Treatment** No effects or complications reported

**Other Adverse Effects**

1% to 10%:

- Cardiovascular: Peripheral edema
- Endocrine & metabolic: Breast tenderness, breast enlargement
- Gastrointestinal: Anorexia, abdominal cramping

<1%:

- Cardiovascular: Hypertension, thromboembolism, myocardial infarction
- Central nervous system: Stroke, migraine, dizziness, anxiety, depression, headache
- Dermatologic: Chloasma, melasma, rash
- Endocrine & metabolic: Decreased glucose tolerance, alterations in frequency and flow of menses, breast tenderness or enlargement, elevated triglycerides and LDL
- Gastrointestinal: Nausea, GI distress
- Hepatic: Cholestatic jaundice
- Miscellaneous: Increased susceptibility to *Candida* infection

**Drug Interactions** No data reported

**Drug Uptake**

Time to peak serum concentration: Topical: Within 3-4 hours

**Pregnancy Risk Factor** X

**Generic Available** No

♦ **Dietary Supplements** *see* Enteral Nutritional Products *on page 371*

## Diethylpropion (dye eth il PROE pee on)

**U.S. Brand Names** Tenuate®; Tenuate® Dospan®

**Canadian Brand Names** Nobesine®

**Therapeutic Category** Anorexiant

**Synonyms** Amfepramone

**Use** Short-term adjunct in exogenous obesity

**Usual Dosage** Adults: Oral:

Tablet: 25 mg 3 times/day before meals or food

Tablet, controlled release: 75 mg at midmorning

**Mechanism of Action** Diethylpropion is used as an anorexiant agent possessing pharmacological and chemical properties similar to those of amphetamines. The mechanism of action of diethylpropion in reducing appetite appears to be secondary to CNS effects, specifically stimulation of the hypothalamus to release catecholamines into the central nervous system; anorexiant effects are mediated via norepinephrine and dopamine metabolism. An increase in physical activity and metabolic effects (inhibition of lipogenesis and enhancement of lipolysis) may also contribute to weight loss.

**Local Anesthetic/Vasoconstrictor Precautions** Use vasoconstrictor with caution in patients taking diethylpropion. Amphetamine-like drugs such as diethylpropion enhance the sympathomimetic response of epinephrine and norepinephrine leading to potential hypertension and cardiotoxicity.

**Effects on Dental Treatment** Up to 10% of patients may present with hypertension. The use of local anesthetic without vasoconstrictor is recommended in these patients.

**Other Adverse Effects**

>10%:

- Cardiovascular: Hypertension
- Central nervous system: Euphoria, nervousness, insomnia

1% to 10%:

- Central nervous system: Confusion, mental depression
- Endocrine & metabolic: Changes in libido
- Gastrointestinal: Nausea, vomiting, restlessness, constipation
- Hematologic: Blood dyscrasias
- Neuromuscular & skeletal: Tremor
- Ocular: Blurred vision

<1%:

- Cardiovascular: Tachycardia, arrhythmias

(Continued)

## Diethylpropion *(Continued)*

Central nervous system: Depression, headache
Dermatologic: Alopecia
Gastrointestinal: Diarrhea, abdominal cramps
Genitourinary: Dysuria
Neuromuscular & skeletal: Myalgia
Renal: Polyuria
Respiratory: Dyspnea
Miscellaneous: Increased sweating

**Drug Interactions**
Decreased effect of guanethidine; decreased effect with phenothiazines
Increased effect/toxicity with MAO inhibitors (hypertensive crisis), CNS depressants, general anesthetics (arrhythmias), sympathomimetics

**Pregnancy Risk Factor** B
**Generic Available** Yes

## Diethylstilbestrol (dye eth il stil BES trole)

**U.S. Brand Names** Stilphostrol®
**Canadian Brand Names** Honvol®
**Therapeutic Category** Estrogen Derivative
**Use** Palliative treatment of inoperable metastatic prostatic carcinoma and postmenopausal inoperable, progressing breast cancer
**Usual Dosage** Adults:
Male:
Prostate carcinoma (inoperable, progressing): Oral: 1-3 mg/day
Diphosphate: Inoperable progressing prostate cancer:
Oral: 50 mg 3 times/day; increase up to 200 mg or more 3 times/day; maximum daily dose: 1 g
I.V.: Give 0.5 g, dissolved in 250 mL of saline or $D_5W$, administer slowly the first 10-15 minutes then adjust rate so that the entire amount is given in 1 hour; repeat for ≥5 days depending on patient response, then repeat 0.25-0.5 g 1-2 times for one week or change to oral therapy
Female: Postmenopausal inoperable, progressing breast carcinoma: Oral: 15 mg/day

**Mechanism of Action** Competes with estrogenic and androgenic compounds for binding onto tumor cells and thereby inhibits their effects on tumor growth
**Local Anesthetic/Vasoconstrictor Precautions** No information available to require special precautions
**Effects on Dental Treatment** No effects or complications reported
**Other Adverse Effects**
>10%:
Cardiovascular: Peripheral edema
Endocrine & metabolic: Enlargement of breasts (female and male), breast tenderness
Gastrointestinal: Nausea, anorexia, bloating
1% to 10%:
Central nervous system: Headache
Endocrine & metabolic: Increased libido (female), decreased libido (male)
Gastrointestinal: Vomiting, diarrhea
<1%:
Cardiovascular: Hypertension, thromboembolism, myocardial infarction, edema
Central nervous system: Stroke, depression, dizziness, anxiety
Dermatologic: Chloasma, melasma, rash
Endocrine & metabolic: Breast tumors, amenorrhea, alterations in frequency and flow of menses, elevated triglycerides and LDL
Gastrointestinal: GI distress
Hepatic: Cholestatic jaundice
Ocular: Intolerance to contact lenses
Miscellaneous: Decreased glucose tolerance, increased susceptibility to *Candida* infection

**Drug Interactions** No data reported
**Pregnancy Risk Factor** X
**Generic Available** Yes

## Difenoxin and Atropine (dye fen OKS in & A troe peen)

**U.S. Brand Names** Motofen®
**Therapeutic Category** Antidiarrheal
**Use** Treatment of diarrhea

**Usual Dosage** Adults: Oral: Initial: 2 tablets, then 1 tablet after each loose stool; 1 tablet every 3-4 hours, up to 8 tablets in a 24-hour period; if no improvement after 48 hours, continued administration is not indicated

**Local Anesthetic/Vasoconstrictor Precautions** No information available to require special precautions

**Effects on Dental Treatment** No effects or complications reported

**Other Adverse Effects**

1% to 10%:

Central nervous system: Dizziness, drowsiness, lightheadedness, headache

Gastrointestinal: Nausea, vomiting, dry mouth, epigastric distress

<1%:

Central nervous system: Confusion

Gastrointestinal: Constipation

Ocular: Blurred vision

**Pregnancy Risk Factor** C

**Generic Available** No

♦ **Differin®** *see* Adapalene *on page 40*

## Diflorasone (dye FLOR a sone)

**Related Information**

Corticosteroids, Topical Comparison *on page 1222*

**U.S. Brand Names** Florone®; Florone® E; Maxiflor®; Psorcon™

**Therapeutic Category** Corticosteroid, Topical (High Potency)

**Use** Relieves inflammation and pruritic symptoms of corticosteroid-responsive dermatosis (high to very high potency topical corticosteroid)

Maxiflor™: High potency topical corticosteroid

Psorcon™: Very high potency topical corticosteroid

**Usual Dosage** Topical: Apply ointment sparingly 1-3 times/day; apply cream sparingly 2-4 times/day

**Mechanism of Action** Decreases inflammation by suppression of migration of polymorphonuclear leukocytes and reversal of increased capillary permeability

**Local Anesthetic/Vasoconstrictor Precautions** No information available to require special precautions

**Effects on Dental Treatment** No effects or complications reported

**Other Adverse Effects** <1%:

Local: Burning, itching, folliculitis, dryness, maceration

Neuromuscular & skeletal: Muscle atrophy, arthralgia

Miscellaneous: Secondary infection

**Drug Interactions** No data reported

**Drug Uptake** Absorption: Topical: Negligible, around 1% reaches dermal layers or systemic circulation; occlusive dressings increase absorption percutaneously

**Pregnancy Risk Factor** C

**Dosage Forms**

Cream, as diacetate: 0.05% (15 g, 30 g, 60 g)

Ointment, topical, as diacetate: 0.05% (15 g, 30 g, 60 g)

**Generic Available** No

♦ **Diflucan®** *see* Fluconazole *on page 434*

## Diflunisal (dye FLOO ni sal)

**Related Information**

Dental Drug Interactions: Update on Drug Combinations Requiring Special Considerations *on page 1225*

Oral Pain *on page 1122*

Rheumatoid Arthritis and Osteoarthritis *on page 1092*

**U.S. Brand Names** Dolobid®

**Canadian Brand Names** Apo®-Diflunisal; Novo-Diflunisal; Nu-Diflunisal

**Therapeutic Category** Analgesic, Non-narcotic; Nonsteroidal Anti-inflammatory Drug (NSAID), Oral

**Use**

Dental: Treatment of postoperative pain

Medical: Management of pain and inflammatory disorders usually including rheumatoid arthritis and osteoarthritis

**Usual Dosage** Adults: Oral: 500-1000 mg followed by 250-500 mg every 8-12 hours; maximum daily dose: 1.5 g

**Mechanism of Action** Inhibits prostaglandin synthesis by decreasing the activity of the enzyme, cyclo-oxygenase, which results in decreased formation of prostaglandin precursors

**Local Anesthetic/Vasoconstrictor Precautions** No information available to require special precautions

(Continued)

## Diflunisal *(Continued)*

**Effects on Dental Treatment** NSAID formulations are known to reversibly decrease platelet aggregation via mechanisms different than observed with aspirin. The dentist should be aware of the potential of abnormal coagulation. Caution should also be exercised in the use of NSAIDs in patients already on anticoagulant therapy with drugs such as warfarin (Coumadin®).

**Other Adverse Effects**

>10%:

Cardiovascular: Fluid retention

Central nervous system: Headache

1% to 10%: Gastrointestinal: GI ulceration

**Contraindications** Hypersensitivity to diflunisal or any component, may be a cross-sensitivity with other nonsteroidal anti-inflammatory agents including aspirin; should not be used in patients with active GI bleeding

**Warnings/Precautions** Peptic ulceration and GI bleeding have been reported; platelet function and bleeding time are inhibited; ophthalmologic effects; impaired renal function, use lower dosage; peripheral edema; possibility of Reye's syndrome; may cause elevated liver function tests

**Drug Interactions** Decreased effect with antacids; increased effect/toxicity of digoxin, methotrexate, anticoagulants, phenytoin, sulfonylureas, sulfonamides, lithium, indomethacin, hydrochlorothiazide, acetaminophen

**Drug Uptake**

Absorption: Rapid and complete

Onset of effect: Within 1 hour

Duration of effect: 8-12 hours

Serum half-life: 8-12 hours

Time to peak serum concentration: Within 2-3 hours

**Pregnancy Risk Factor** C (first and second trimester); D (third trimester)

**Breast-feeding Considerations** Diflunisal is excreted in breast milk, however, there is no specific data regarding use during lactation

**Dosage Forms** Tablet: 250 mg, 500 mg

**Dietary Considerations** Should be taken with food to decrease GI distress

**Generic Available** Yes

**Comments** The advantage of diflunisal as a pain reliever is its 12-hour duration of effect. In many cases, this long effect will ensure a full night sleep during the postoperative pain period.

**Selected Readings**

Brooks PM and Day RO, "Nonsteroidal Anti-inflammatory Drugs-Differences and Similarities," *N Engl J Med,* 1991, 324(24):1716-25.

Dionne RA, "New Approaches to Preventing and Treating Postoperative Pain," *J Am Dent Assoc,* 1992, 123(6):26-34.

Forbes JA, Butterworth GA, Burchfield WH, et al, "A 12-Hour Evaluation of the Analgesic Efficacy of Diflunisal, Zomepirac Sodium, Aspirin, and Placebo in Postoperative Oral Surgery Pain," *Pharmacotherapy,* 1983, 3(2 Pt 2):38S-46S.

Forbes JA, Calderazzo JP, Bowser MW, et al, "A 12-Hour Evaluation of the Analgesic Efficacy of Diflunisal, Aspirin, and Placebo in Postoperative Dental Pain," *J Clin Pharmacol,* 1982, 22(2-3):89-96.

Gobetti JP, "Controlling Dental Pain," *J Am Dent Assoc,* 1992, 123(6):47-52.

♦ **Di-Gel® [OTC]** *see* Aluminum Hydroxide, Magnesium Hydroxide, and Simethicone *on page 56*

♦ **Digepepsin®** *see* Pancreatin *on page 763*

♦ **Digibind®** *see* Digoxin Immune Fab *on page 330*

## Digitoxin (di ji TOKS in)

**Related Information**

Cardiovascular Diseases *on page 1066*

**U.S. Brand Names** Crystodigin®

**Canadian Brand Names** Digitaline®

**Therapeutic Category** Antiarrhythmic Agent (Supraventricular); Antiarrhythmic Agent, Miscellaneous; Cardiac Glycoside

**Use** Treatment of congestive heart failure, atrial fibrillation, atrial flutter, paroxysmal atrial tachycardia, and cardiogenic shock

**Usual Dosage** Oral:

Children: Doses are very individualized; **when recommended,** digitalizing dose is as follows:

<1 year: 0.045 mg/kg

1-2 years: 0.04 mg/kg

>2 years: 0.03 mg/kg which is equivalent to 0.75 mg/mm²

Maintenance: Approximately ¹/₁₀ of the digitalizing dose

Adults: Oral:

Rapid loading dose: Initial: 0.6 mg followed by 0.4 mg and then 0.2 mg at intervals of 4-6 hours

Slow loading dose: 0.2 mg twice daily for a period of 4 days followed by a maintenance dose
Maintenance: 0.05-0.3 mg/day
Most common dose: 0.15 mg/day

**Mechanism of Action** Digitalis binds to and inhibits magnesium and adenosine triphosphate dependent sodium and potassium ATPase thereby increasing the influx of calcium ions, from extracellular to intracellular cytoplasm due to the inhibition of sodium and potassium ion movement across the myocardial membranes; this increase in calcium ions results in a potentiation of the activity of the contractile heart muscle fibers and an increase in the force of myocardial contraction (positive inotropic effect); digitalis may also increase intracellular entry of calcium via slow calcium channel influx; stimulates release and blocks re-uptake of norepinephrine; decreases conduction through the S-A and A-V nodes

**Local Anesthetic/Vasoconstrictor Precautions** Use vasoconstrictor with caution due to risk of cardiac arrhythmias with digitoxin

**Effects on Dental Treatment** Sensitive gag reflex may cause difficulty in taking a dental impression

**Other Adverse Effects**

1% to 10%: Gastrointestinal: Anorexia, nausea, vomiting

<1%:

- Cardiovascular: Sinus bradycardia, A-V block, S-A block, atrial or nodal ectopic beats, ventricular arrhythmias, bigeminy, trigeminy, atrial tachycardia with A-V block
- Central nervous system: Drowsiness, headache, fatigue, lethargy, vertigo, disorientation
- Endocrine & metabolic: Hyperkalemia with acute toxicity
- Gastrointestinal: Feeding intolerance, abdominal pain, diarrhea
- Neuromuscular & skeletal: Neuralgia
- Ocular: Blurred vision, halos, yellow or green vision, diplopia, photophobia, flashing lights

**Drug Interactions**

Decreased effect/levels of digitoxin/digoxin: Antacids (magnesium, aluminum), cholestyramine, colestipol, kaolin/pectin, aminosalicylic acid, metoclopramide, sulfasalazine

Decreased effect/levels of digitoxin only (eg, increased metabolism): Aminoglutethimide, barbiturates, hydantoins, rifampin, phenylbutazone, thyroid replacement

Increased effect/toxicity/levels of digitoxin/digoxin: Amiodarone, nifedipine, quinidine, quinine, verapamil, nondepolarizing muscle relaxants, succinylcholine, potassium-losing diuretics

Concomitant use of digitoxin and sympathomimetics increases the risk of cardiac arrhythmias

**Drug Uptake**

Absorption: 90% to 100%
Serum half-life: 7-8 days
Time to peak: 8-12 hours

**Pregnancy Risk Factor** C

**Generic Available** Yes

## Digoxin (di JOKS in)

**Related Information**

Cardiovascular Diseases *on page 1066*

**U.S. Brand Names** Lanoxicaps®; Lanoxin®

**Canadian Brand Names** Novo-Digoxin

**Therapeutic Category** Antiarrhythmic Agent (Supraventricular); Antiarrhythmic Agent, Miscellaneous; Cardiac Glycoside

**Use** Treatment of congestive heart failure and to slow the ventricular rate in tachyarrhythmias such as atrial fibrillation, atrial flutter, and supraventricular tachycardia (paroxysmal atrial tachycardia); cardiogenic shock

**Usual Dosage** When changing from oral (tablets or liquid) or I.M. to I.V. therapy, dosage should be reduced by 20% to 25%. See table.

**Mechanism of Action**

Congestive heart failure: Inhibition of the sodium/potassium ATPase pump which acts to increase the intracellular sodium-calcium exchange to increase intracellular calcium leading to increased contractility

Supraventricular arrhythmias: Direct suppression of the A-V node conduction to increase effective refractory period and decrease conduction velocity - positive inotropic effect, enhanced vagal tone, and decreased ventricular rate to fast atrial arrhythmias. Atrial fibrillation may decrease sensitivity and increase tolerance to higher serum digoxin concentrations.

**Dosage Recommendations for Digoxin**

| Age | Total Digitalizing Dose† (mcg/kg)* | | Daily Maintenance Dose‡ (mcg/kg*) | |
|---|---|---|---|---|
| | P.O. | I.V. or I.M. | P.O. | I.V. or I.M. |
| Preterm infant* | 20-30 | 15-25 | 5-7.5 | 4-6 |
| Full-term infant* | 25-35 | 20-30 | 6-10 | 5-8 |
| 1 mo - 2 y* | 35-60 | 30-50 | 10-15 | 7.5-12 |
| 2-5 y* | 30-40 | 25-35 | 7.5-10 | 6-9 |
| 5-10 y* | 20-35 | 15-30 | 5-10 | 4-8 |
| >10 y* | 10-15 | 8-12 | 2.5-5 | 2-3 |
| Adults | 0.75-1.5 mg | 0.5-1 mg | 0.125-0.5 mg | 0.1-0.4 mg |

†Give one-half of the total digitalizing dose (TDD) in the initial dose, then give one-quarter of the TDD in each of two subsequent doses at 8- to 12-hour intervals. Obtain EKG 6 hours after each dose to assess potential toxicity.

*Based on lean body weight and normal renal function for age. Decrease dose in patients with ↓ renal function; digitalizing dose often not recommended in infants and children.

‡Divided every 12 hours in infants and children <10 years of age. Given once daily to children >10 years of age and adults.

**Local Anesthetic/Vasoconstrictor Precautions** Use vasoconstrictor with caution due to risk of cardiac arrhythmias with digoxin

**Effects on Dental Treatment** Sensitive gag reflex may cause difficulty in taking a dental impression

**Other Adverse Effects**

1% to 10%: Gastrointestinal: Anorexia, nausea, vomiting

<1%:

Cardiovascular: Sinus bradycardia, A-V block, S-A block, atrial or nodal ectopic beats, ventricular arrhythmias, bigeminy, trigeminy, atrial tachycardia with A-V block

Central nervous system: Drowsiness, headache, fatigue, lethargy, vertigo, disorientation

Endocrine & metabolic: Hyperkalemia with acute toxicity

Gastrointestinal: Feeding intolerance, abdominal pain, diarrhea

Neuromuscular & skeletal: Neuralgia

Ocular: Blurred vision, halos, yellow or green vision, diplopia, photophobia, flashing lights

**Drug Interactions**

Decreased effect/levels of digitoxin/digoxin: Antacids (magnesium, aluminum), cholestyramine, colestipol, kaolin/pectin, aminosalicylic acid, metoclopramide, sulfasalazine

Decreased effect/levels of digitoxin only (eg, increased metabolism): Aminoglutethimide, barbiturates, hydantoins, rifampin, phenylbutazone, thyroid replacement

Increased effect/toxicity/levels of digitoxin/digoxin: Amiodarone, nifedipine, quinidine, quinine, verapamil, nondepolarizing muscle relaxants, succinylcholine, potassium-losing diuretics

Concomitant use of digitoxin and sympathomimetics increase the risk of cardiac arrhythmias

**Drug Uptake**

Onset of action:

Oral: 1-2 hours

I.V.: 5-30 minutes

Peak effect:

Oral: 2-8 hours

I.V.: 1-4 hours

Duration: Adults: 3-4 days both forms

Absorption: By passive nonsaturable diffusion in the upper small intestine; food may delay, but does not affect extent of digoxin absorption

Serum half-life: Dependent upon age, renal and cardiac function:

Children: 35 hours

Adults: 38-48 hours

Adults, anephric: 4-6 days

Time to peak serum concentration: Oral: Within 1 hour

**Pregnancy Risk Factor** C

**Generic Available** Yes: Tablet

## Digoxin Immune Fab (di JOKS in i MYUN fab)

**U.S. Brand Names** Digibind®

**Therapeutic Category** Antidote, Digoxin

**Synonyms** Antidigoxin Fab Fragments

**Use** Digoxin immune Fab are specific antibodies for the treatment of digitalis intoxication in carefully selected patients; use in life-threatening ventricular arrhythmias secondary to digoxin, acute digoxin ingestion (ie, >10 mg in adults or >4 mg in children), hyperkalemia (serum potassium >5 mEq/L) in the setting of digoxin toxicity

**Usual Dosage** Each vial of Digibind® will bind approximately 0.6 mg of digoxin or digitoxin

I.V.: To determine the dose of digoxin immune Fab, first determine the total body load of digoxin (TBL using either an approximation of the amount ingested or a postdistribution serum digoxin concentration). If neither ingestion amount or serum level is known: Adult dosage is 20 vials (800 mg) I.V. infusion.

**Mechanism of Action** Binds with molecules of digoxin or digitoxin and then is excreted by the kidneys and removed from the body

**Local Anesthetic/Vasoconstrictor Precautions** No information available to require special precautions

**Effects on Dental Treatment** No effects or complications reported

**Other Adverse Effects** <1%:

Cardiovascular: Worsening of low cardiac output or congestive heart failure, rapid ventricular response in patients with atrial fibrillation as digoxin is withdrawn, facial edema and redness

Endocrine & metabolic: Hypokalemia

Dermatologic: Urticarial rash

Miscellaneous: Allergic reactions

**Contraindications** Hypersensitivity to sheep products

**Drug Uptake**

Onset of action: I.V.: Improvement in signs and symptoms occur within 2-30 minutes

Serum half-life: 15-20 hours; prolonged in patients with renal impairment

**Pregnancy Risk Factor** C

**Dosage Forms** Powder for injection, lyophilized: 40 mg

**Generic Available** No

◆ **Dihistine® DH** *see* Chlorpheniramine, Pseudoephedrine, and Codeine *on page 237*

◆ **Dihistine® Expectorant** *see* Guaifenesin, Pseudoephedrine, and Codeine *on page 482*

## Dihydrocodeine Compound (dye hye droe KOE deen KOM pound)

**Related Information**

Oral Pain *on page 1122*

**U.S. Brand Names** DHC Plus®; Synalgos®-DC

**Therapeutic Category** Analgesic, Narcotic

**Use**

Dental: Management of postoperative pain

Medical: Management of mild to moderate pain from medical conditions

**Restrictions** C-III; Refillable up to 5 times in 6 months

**Usual Dosage** Oral:

Children: Not recommended

Adults: 1-2 capsules every 4-6 hours as needed for pain; maximum dose: 12 capsules/day

**Mechanism of Action** Dihydrocodeine binds to opiate receptors (mu and kappa subtypes) in the CNS causing inhibition of ascending pain pathways, altering the perception of and response to pain; produces generalized CNS depression; causes cough suppression by direct central action in the medulla; produces generalized CNS depression

Acetaminophen inhibits the synthesis of prostaglandins in the CNS and peripherally blocks pain impulse generation; produces antipyresis from inhibition of hypothalamic heat-regulating center

Aspirin inhibits prostaglandin synthesis by decreasing the activity of the enzyme, cyclo-oxygenase, which results in decreased formation of prostaglandin precursors acts on the hypothalamic heat-regulating center to reduce fever, blocks thromboxane synthetase action which prevents formation of the platelet-aggregating substance thromboxane $A_2$

**Local Anesthetic/Vasoconstrictor Precautions** No information available to require special precautions

**Effects on Dental Treatment** Use with caution in patients with platelet and bleeding disorders, renal dysfunction, erosive gastritis, or peptic ulcer disease, previous nonreaction does not guarantee future safe taking of medication; do not use aspirin in children <16 years of age for chickenpox or flu symptoms due to the association with Reye's syndrome

(Continued)

## Dihydrocodeine Compound *(Continued)*

Avoid aspirin if possible, for 1 week prior to surgery because of the possibility of postoperative bleeding; use with caution in impaired hepatic function

Elderly are a high-risk population for adverse effects from nonsteroidal anti-inflammatory agents. As much as 60% of elderly with GI complications to NSAIDs can develop peptic ulceration and/or hemorrhage asymptomatically. Also, concomitant disease and drug use contribute to the risk for GI adverse effects. Use lowest effective dose for shortest period possible. Consider renal function decline with age. Use with caution in patients with history of asthma

**Other Adverse Effects**

>10%:

Central nervous system: Lightheadedness, dizziness, sedation

Gastrointestinal: Nausea, heartburn, stomach pains, dyspepsia, vomiting

1% to 10%: Gastrointestinal: Ulceration, constipation

**Contraindications** Hypersensitivity to acetaminophen or aspirin; hypersensitivity to other phenanthrene derivative opioid agonists (morphine, hydrocodone, hydromorphone, levorphanol, oxycodone, oxymorphone)

**Warnings/Precautions** Respiratory diseases including asthma, emphysema, COPD, or severe liver or renal insufficiency; some preparations contain sulfites which may cause allergic reactions; may be habit-forming; dextromethorphan has equivalent antitussive activity but has much lower toxicity in accidental overdose

Enhanced analgesia has been seen in elderly patients on therapeutic doses of narcotics; duration of action may be increased in the elderly; the elderly may be particularly susceptible to the CNS depressant and constipating effects of narcotics

**Drug Interactions**

Dihydrocodeine component: MAO inhibitors cause increased adverse symptoms

Acetaminophen component: Refer to Acetaminophen monograph

Aspirin component: Refer to Aspirin monograph

**Drug Uptake**

Onset of action: 10-30 minutes

Duration: Oral: 4-6 hours

Serum half-life: 3.8 hours

Time to peak serum concentration: 30-60 minutes

**Pregnancy Risk Factor** B (D if used for prolonged periods or in high doses at term)

**Breast-feeding Considerations**

Acetaminophen: May be taken while breast-feeding

Aspirin: Use cautiously due to potential adverse effects in nursing infants

Dihydrocodeine: No data reported

**Dosage Forms** Capsule:

DHC Plus®: Dihydrocodeine bitartrate 16 mg, acetaminophen 356.4 mg, and caffeine 30 mg

Synalgos®-DC: Dihydrocodeine bitartrate 16 mg, aspirin 356.4 mg, and caffeine 30 mg

**Dietary Considerations** Should be taken with food

**Generic Available** Yes

**Comments** Dihydrocodeine products, as with other narcotic analgesics, are recommended only for acute dosing (ie, 3 days or less). The most common adverse effect you will see in your dental patients from dihydrocodeine is nausea, followed by sedation and constipation. Dihydrocodeine has narcotic addiction liability, especially when given long term. Dihydrocodeine with aspirin could have anticoagulant effects and could possibly affect bleeding times. Dihydrocodeine with acetaminophen should be used with caution in patients with alcoholic liver disease.

## Dihydroergotamine (dye hye droe er GOT a meen)

**U.S. Brand Names** D.H.E. 45® Injection; Migranal® Nasal Spray

**Therapeutic Category** Ergot Alkaloid and Derivative

**Use**

Injection: Aborts or prevents vascular headaches; also as an adjunct for DVT prophylaxis for hip surgery, for orthostatic hypotension, xerostomia secondary to antidepressant use, and pelvic congestion with pain;

Nasal spray: Acute treatment of migraine headaches with or without aura; is not indicated for prophylactic therapy or for the management of hemiplegic or basilar migraine

**Usual Dosage** Adults:

I.M.: 1 mg at first sign of headache; repeat hourly to a maximum dose of 3 mg total

I.V.: Up to 2 mg maximum dose for faster effects; maximum dose: 6 mg/week

**Mechanism of Action** Ergot alkaloid alpha-adrenergic blocker directly stimulates vascular smooth muscle to vasoconstrict peripheral and cerebral vessels; also has effects on serotonin receptors

**Local Anesthetic/Vasoconstrictor Precautions** No information available to require special precautions

**Effects on Dental Treatment** >10% of patients experience dry mouth

**Other Adverse Effects**

>10%:

Cardiovascular: Localized edema, peripheral vascular effects
Central nervous system: Drowsiness, dizziness
Gastrointestinal: Diarrhea, nausea, vomiting
Neuromuscular & skeletal: Paresthesia

1% to 10%:

Cardiovascular: Precordial distress and pain, transient tachycardia or bradycardia
Neuromuscular & skeletal: Myalgia in the extremities, weakness in the legs

**Drug Interactions**

Increased effect of heparin
Increased toxicity with erythromycin, clarithromycin, nitroglycerin, propranolol, troleandomycin

**Drug Uptake**

Onset of action: Within 15-30 minutes
Duration: 3-4 hours
Serum half-life: 1.3-3.9 hours
Time to peak serum concentration: I.M.: Within 15-30 minutes

**Pregnancy Risk Factor** X

**Generic Available** Yes

♦ **Dihydrohydroxycodeinone** *see* Oxycodone *on page 750*

## Dihydrotachysterol (dye hye droe tak IS ter ole)

**U.S. Brand Names** DHT™; Hytakerol®

**Therapeutic Category** Vitamin D Analog

**Use** Treatment of hypocalcemia associated with hypoparathyroidism; prophylaxis of hypocalcemic tetany following thyroid surgery

**Usual Dosage** Oral:

Hypoparathyroidism:

Young Children: Initial: 1-5 mg/day for 4 days, then 0.1-0.5 mg/day
Older Children and Adults: Initial: 0.8-2.4 mg/day for several days followed by maintenance doses of 0.2-1 mg/day

Nutritional rickets: 0.5 mg as a single dose or 13-50 mcg/day until healing occurs
Renal osteodystrophy: Maintenance: 0.25-0.6 mg/24 hours adjusted as necessary to achieve normal serum calcium levels and promote bone healing

**Mechanism of Action** Synthetic analogue of vitamin D with a faster onset of action; stimulates calcium and phosphate absorption from the small intestine, promotes secretion of calcium from bone to blood; promotes renal tubule resorption of phosphate

**Local Anesthetic/Vasoconstrictor Precautions** No information available to require special precautions

**Effects on Dental Treatment** No effects or complications reported

**Other Adverse Effects**

>10%:

Endocrine & metabolic: Hypercalcemia, hypercalciuria
Renal: Elevated serum creatinine

<1%:

Central nervous system: Convulsions
Endocrine & metabolic: Polydipsia
Gastrointestinal: Nausea, vomiting, anorexia, weight loss
Hematologic: Anemia
Neuromuscular & skeletal: Metastatic calcification, weakness
Renal: Renal damage, polyuria

**Drug Interactions**

Decreased effect/levels of vitamin D: Cholestyramine, colestipol, mineral oil
Increased toxicity: Thiazide diuretics increase calcium

**Drug Uptake**

Peak hypercalcemic effect: Within 2-4 weeks
Duration: Can be as long as 9 weeks
Absorption: Well absorbed from the GI tract

**Pregnancy Risk Factor** A (D if used in doses above the recommended daily allowance)

**Generic Available** Yes

## Dihydroxyaluminum Sodium Carbonate

(dye hye DROKS i a LOO mi num SOW dee um KAR bun ate)

**U.S. Brand Names** Rolaids® [OTC]

**Therapeutic Category** Antacid

**Use** Symptomatic relief of upset stomach associated with hyperacidity

**Usual Dosage** Oral: Chew 1-2 tablets as needed

**Local Anesthetic/Vasoconstrictor Precautions** No information available to require special precautions

**Effects on Dental Treatment** No effects or complications reported

**Dosage Forms** Tablet, chewable: 334 mg

**Generic Available** Yes

- **Dihydroxypropyl Theophylline** *see* Dyphylline *on page 361*
- **Dilacor™ XR** *see* Diltiazem *on this page*
- **Dilantin®** *see* Phenytoin *on page 799*
- **Dilantin® With Phenobarbital** *see* Phenytoin With Phenobarbital *on page 800*
- **Dilatrate®-SR** *see* Isosorbide Dinitrate *on page 555*
- **Dilaudid®** *see* Hydromorphone *on page 513*
- **Dilaudid-5®** *see* Hydromorphone *on page 513*
- **Dilaudid-HP®** *see* Hydromorphone *on page 513*
- **Dilocaine®** *see* Lidocaine *on page 586*
- **Dilor®** *see* Dyphylline *on page 361*

## Diltiazem (dil TYE a zem)

**Related Information**

Calcium Channel Blockers & Gingival Hyperplasia *on page 1204*
Cardiovascular Diseases *on page 1066*
Enalapril and Diltiazem *on page 368*

**U.S. Brand Names** Cardizem® CD; Cardizem® Injectable; Cardizem® SR; Cardizem® Tablet; Cartia® XT; Dilacor™ XR; Tiamate®; Tiazac™

**Canadian Brand Names** Apo®-Diltiaz; Novo-Diltazem; Nu-Diltiaz; Syn-Diltiazem

**Therapeutic Category** Antianginal Agent; Calcium Channel Blocker

**Use**

Capsule: Hypertension (alone or in combination); chronic stable angina or angina from coronary artery spasm

Injection: Atrial fibrillation or atrial flutter; paroxysmal supraventricular tachycardias (PSVT)

**Usual Dosage** Adults:

Oral: 30-120 mg 3-4 times/day; dosage should be increased gradually, at 1- to 2-day intervals until optimum response is obtained; usual maintenance dose: 240-360 mg/day

Sustained-release capsules:

**Cardizem® SR**: Initial: 60-120 mg twice daily; adjust to maximum antihypertensive effect (usually within 14 days); usual range: 240-360 mg/day

**Cardizem® CD, Tiazac™:** Hypertension: Total daily dose of short-acting administered once daily or initially 180 or 240 mg once daily; adjust to maximum effect (usually within 14 days); maximum: 360 mg/day; usual range: 240-360 mg/day

Cardizem® CD: Angina: Initial: 120-180 mg once daily; maximum: 480 mg once/day

**Dilacor™ XR:**

Hypertension: 180-240 mg once daily; maximum: 540 mg/day; usual range: 180-480 mg/day; use lower dose in elderly

Angina: Initial: 120 mg/day; titrate slowly over 7-14 days up to 480 mg/day, as needed

**Diltiazem — I.V. Dosage and Administration**

| | |
|---|---|
| **Initial Bolus Dose** | 0.25 mg/kg actual body weight over 2 min (average adult dose: 20 mg) |
| **Repeat Bolus Dose** may be administered after 15 min if the response is inadequate | 0.35 mg/kg actual body weight over 2 min (average adult dose: 25 mg) |
| **Continuous Infusion** Infusions >24 h or infusion rates >15 mg/h are not recommended due to potential accumulation of metabolites and increased toxicity | Initial infusion rate of 10 mg/h; rate may be increased in 5 mg/h increments up to 15 mg/h as needed; some patients may respond to an initial rate of 5 mg/h |

**Note**: Hypertensive or anginal patients treated with other formulations of diltiazem sustained release can be safely switched to Dilacor™ XR at the nearest equivalent total daily dose; subsequent titration may be needed

I.V. (requires an infusion pump): See table.

If Cardizem® injectable is administered by continuous infusion for >24 hours, the possibility of decreased diltiazem clearance, prolonged elimination half-life, and increased diltiazem and/or diltiazem metabolite plasma concentrations should be considered

**Conversion from I.V. diltiazem to oral diltiazem:** Start oral approximately 3 hours after bolus dose

**Oral dose (mg/day) is approximately equal to [rate (mg/hour) x 3 + 3] x 10**

3 mg/hour = 120 mg/day
5 mg/hour = 180 mg/day
7 mg/hour = 240 mg/day
11 mg/hour = 360 mg/day (maximum recommended dose)

**Mechanism of Action** Inhibits calcium ion from entering the "slow channels" or select voltage-sensitive areas of vascular smooth muscle and myocardium during depolarization, producing a relaxation of coronary vascular smooth muscle and coronary vasodilation; increases myocardial oxygen delivery in patients with vasospastic angina

**Local Anesthetic/Vasoconstrictor Precautions** No information available to require special precautions

**Effects on Dental Treatment** Calcium channel blockers cause gingival hyperplasia in approximately 1% of patients. There have been fewer reports with diltiazem than with other CCBs. The hyperplasia will usually disappear with cessation of drug therapy. Consultation with physician is suggested.

**Other Adverse Effects**

>10%: Central nervous system: Headache

1% to 10%:

Cardiovascular: Bradycardia, A-V block (first degree), edema, EKG abnormality
Central nervous system: Dizziness
Gastrointestinal: Nausea, vomiting
Neuromuscular & skeletal: Weakness

<1%:

Cardiovascular: A-V block (second degree), angina
Central nervous system: Abnormal dreams, amnesia, depression, insomnia, nervousness
Dermatologic: Urticaria, photosensitivity, alopecia, purpura
Gastrointestinal: Anorexia, constipation, diarrhea, dysgeusia, dyspepsia
Hematologic: Hemolytic anemia, leukopenia thrombocytopenia
Neuromuscular & skeletal: Paresthesia, tremor, gait abnormality
Ocular: Amblyopia, retinopathy
Respiratory: Pharyngitis, cough increase
Miscellaneous: Flu syndrome

**Drug Interactions** Increased toxicity/effect/levels:

$H_2$-blockers cause increased bioavailability of diltiazem
Beta-blockers cause increased cardiac depressant effects on A-V conduction
Diltiazem increases serum levels and effects/toxicity of carbamazepine, cyclosporin, digitalis, quinidine, and theophylline

**Drug Uptake**

Onset of action: Oral: 30-60 minutes (including sustained release)
Absorption: 80% to 90%
Time to peak serum concentration:
Short-acting tablets: Within 2-3 hours
Sustained release: 6-11 hours

**Pregnancy Risk Factor** C

**Generic Available** Yes

♦ **Dimacol® Caplets [OTC]** *see* Guaifenesin, Pseudoephedrine, and Dextromethorphan *on page 482*

♦ **Dimaphen® Elixir [OTC]** *see* Brompheniramine and Phenylpropanolamine *on page 153*

♦ **Dimaphen® Tablets [OTC]** *see* Brompheniramine and Phenylpropanolamine *on page 153*

## Dimenhydrinate (dye men HYE dri nate)

**U.S. Brand Names** Calm-X® Oral [OTC]; Dimetabs® Oral; Dinate® Injection; Dramamine® Oral [OTC]; Dymenate® Injection; Hydrate® Injection; TripTone® Caplets® [OTC]

**Canadian Brand Names** Apo®-Dimenhydrinate; Gravol®; PMS-Dimenhydrinate®; Travel Aid®; Travel Tabs®

**Therapeutic Category** Antiemetic; Antihistamine

(Continued)

## Dimenhydrinate *(Continued)*

**Use** Treatment and prevention of nausea, vertigo, and vomiting associated with motion sickness

**Usual Dosage**

Children:

Oral:

2-5 years: 12.5-25 mg every 6-8 hours, maximum: 75 mg/day

6-12 years: 25-50 mg every 6-8 hours, maximum: 150 mg/day

I.M.: 1.25 mg/kg or 37.5 mg/m$^2$ 4 times/day, not to exceed 300 mg/day

Adults: Oral, I.M., I.V.: 50-100 mg every 4-6 hours, not to exceed 400 mg/day

**Mechanism of Action** Competes with histamine for $H_1$-receptor sites on effector cells in the gastrointestinal tract, blood vessels, and respiratory tract; blocks chemoreceptor trigger zone, diminishes vestibular stimulation, and depresses labyrinthine function through its central anticholinergic activity

**Local Anesthetic/Vasoconstrictor Precautions** No information available to require special precautions

**Effects on Dental Treatment** Up to 10% of patients will complain of significant dry mouth and drowsiness. This will disappear with cessation of drug therapy.

**Other Adverse Effects**

>10%:

Central nervous system: Slight to moderate drowsiness

Respiratory: Thickening of bronchial secretions

1% to 10%:

Central nervous system: Headache, fatigue, nervousness, dizziness

Gastrointestinal: Appetite increase, weight gain, nausea, diarrhea, abdominal pain, dry mouth

Neuromuscular & skeletal: Arthralgia

Respiratory: Pharyngitis

<1%:

Cardiovascular: Edema, palpitations, hypotension

Central nervous system: Depression, paradoxical CNS stimulation

Dermatologic: Angioedema, photosensitivity, rash

Gastrointestinal: Anorexia

Hepatic: Hepatitis,

Local: Pain at the injection site

Neuromuscular & skeletal: Myalgia, paresthesia

Ocular: Blurred vision

Otic: Tinnitus

Renal: Polyuria

Respiratory: Bronchospasm, epistaxis

**Drug Interactions**

Increased effect/toxicity with CNS depressants, anticholinergics, TCAs, MAO inhibitors

Increased toxicity of antibiotics, especially aminoglycosides (ototoxicity)

**Drug Uptake**

Onset of action: Oral: Within 15-30 minutes

Absorption: Well absorbed from GI tract

**Pregnancy Risk Factor** B

**Generic Available** Yes

## Dimercaprol (dye mer KAP role)

**U.S. Brand Names** BAL in Oil®

**Therapeutic Category** Antidote, Arsenic Toxicity; Antidote, Gold Toxicity; Antidote, Lead Toxicity; Antidote, Mercury Toxicity

**Use** Antidote to gold, arsenic, and mercury poisoning; adjunct to edetate calcium disodium in lead poisoning

**Usual Dosage** Children and Adults: Deep I.M.:

Mild arsenic and gold poisoning: 2.5 mg/kg/dose every 6 hours for 2 days, then every 12 hours on the third day, and once daily thereafter for 10 days

Severe arsenic and gold poisoning: 3 mg/kg/dose every 4 hours for 2 days then every 6 hours on the third day, then every 12 hours thereafter for 10 days

Mercury poisoning: Initial: 5 mg/kg followed by 2.5 mg/kg/dose 1-2 times/day for 10 days

Lead poisoning (use with edetate calcium disodium):

Mild: 3 mg/kg/dose every 4 hours for 5-7 days

Severe and acute encephalopathy: 4 mg/kg/dose initially alone then every 4 hours in combination of edetate calcium disodium

**Mechanism of Action** Sulfhydryl group combines with ions of various heavy metals to form relatively stable, nontoxic, soluble chelates which are excreted in urine

**Local Anesthetic/Vasoconstrictor Precautions** No information available to require special precautions

**Effects on Dental Treatment** No effects or complications reported

**Other Adverse Effects**

>10%:

Cardiovascular: Hypertension, tachycardia

Central nervous system: Convulsions

1% to 10%: Gastrointestinal: Nausea, vomiting

<1%:

Central nervous system: Nervousness, fever, headache

Gastrointestinal: Salivation

Hematologic: Transient neutropenia

Local: Pain at the injection site

Ocular: Blepharospasm

Renal: Nephrotoxicity

Miscellaneous: Burning sensation of the lips, mouth, throat, eyes, and penis

**Drug Interactions** Toxic complexes with iron, cadmium, selenium, or uranium

**Drug Uptake**

Time to peak serum concentration: 0.5-1 hour

**Pregnancy Risk Factor** C

**Generic Available** No

- **Dimetabs® Oral** *see* Dimenhydrinate *on page 335*
- **Dimetane®-DC** *see* Brompheniramine, Phenylpropanolamine, and Codeine *on page 155*
- **Dimetane® Decongestant Elixir [OTC]** *see* Brompheniramine and Phenylephrine *on page 152*
- **Dimetane® Extentabs® [OTC]** *see* Brompheniramine *on page 151*
- **Dimetapp® 4-Hour Liqui-Gel Capsule [OTC]** *see* Brompheniramine and Phenylpropanolamine *on page 153*
- **Dimetapp® Elixir [OTC]** *see* Brompheniramine and Phenylpropanolamine *on page 153*
- **Dimetapp® Extentabs® [OTC]** *see* Brompheniramine and Phenylpropanolamine *on page 153*
- **Dimetapp® Sinus Caplets [OTC]** *see* Pseudoephedrine and Ibuprofen *on page 864*
- **Dimetapp® Tablet [OTC]** *see* Brompheniramine and Phenylpropanolamine *on page 153*
- **β,β-Dimethylcysteine** *see* Penicillamine *on page 772*
- **Dimethyl Triazeno Imidazol Carboxamide** *see* Dacarbazine *on page 292*
- **Dinate® Injection** *see* Dimenhydrinate *on page 335*

## Dinoprostone (dye noe PROST one)

**U.S. Brand Names** Cervidil® Vaginal Insert; Prepidil® Vaginal Gel; Prostin $E_2$® Vaginal Suppository

**Therapeutic Category** Abortifacient; Prostaglandin

**Synonyms** $PGE_2$; Prostaglandin $E_2$

**Use**

Gel: Promote cervical ripening prior to labor induction; usage for gel include any patient undergoing induction of labor with an unripe cervix, most commonly for pre-eclampsia, eclampsia, postdates, diabetes, intrauterine growth retardation, and chronic hypertension

Suppositories: Terminate pregnancy from 12th through 28th week of gestation; evacuate uterus in cases of missed abortion or intrauterine fetal death; manage benign hydatidiform mole

**Usual Dosage**

Abortifacient: Insert 1 suppository high in vagina, repeat at 3- to 5-hour intervals until abortion occurs up to 240 mg (maximum dose); continued administration for longer than 2 days is not advisable

Cervical ripening:

Gel:

Intracervical: 0.25-1 mg

Intravaginal: 2.5 mg

Suppositories: Intracervical: 2-3 mg

**Mechanism of Action** A synthetic prostaglandin $E_2$ abortifacient that stimulates uterine contractions similar to those seen during natural labor

**Local Anesthetic/Vasoconstrictor Precautions** No information available to require special precautions

**Effects on Dental Treatment** No effects or complications reported

**Other Adverse Effects**

>10%:

Central nervous system: Headache

(Continued)

## Dinoprostone *(Continued)*

Gastrointestinal: Vomiting, diarrhea, nausea

1% to 10%:

Cardiovascular: Bradycardia

Central nervous system: Fever

Neuromuscular & skeletal: Back pain

<1%:

Cardiovascular: Hypotension, cardiac arrhythmias, syncope, flushing, tightness of the chest

Central nervous system: Vasomotor and vasovagal reactions, dizziness, chills, pain

Endocrine & metabolic: Hot flashes

Respiratory: Wheezing, dyspnea, coughing, bronchospasm

Miscellaneous: Shivering

**Drug Interactions** Increased effect of oxytocics

**Drug Uptake**

Onset of effect (uterine contractions): Within 10 minutes

Duration: Up to 2-3 hours

Absorption: Vaginal: Slow following administration

**Pregnancy Risk Factor** X

**Dosage Forms**

Insert, vaginal (Cervidil®): 10 mg

Gel, endocervical: 0.5 mg in 3 g syringes [each package contains a 10-mm and 20-mm shielded catheter]

Suppository, vaginal: 20 mg

**Generic Available** No

## Dinoprost Tromethamine (DYE noe prost tro METH a meen)

**U.S. Brand Names** Prostin $F_2$ Alpha®

**Therapeutic Category** Prostaglandin

**Synonyms** $PGF_{2\alpha}$; Prostaglandin $F_2$ Alpha

**Use** Abort 2nd trimester pregnancy

**Usual Dosage** 40 mg (8 mL) via transabdominal tap; if abortion not completed in 24 hours, another 10-40 mg may be administered

**Local Anesthetic/Vasoconstrictor Precautions** No information available to require special precautions

**Effects on Dental Treatment** No effects or complications reported

**Pregnancy Risk Factor** X

**Dosage Forms** Injection: 5 mg/mL (4 mL, 8 mL)

**Generic Available** No


- ♦ **Diocto® [OTC]** *see* Docusate *on page 346*
- ♦ **Diocto C® [OTC]** *see* Docusate and Casanthranol *on page 347*
- ♦ **Diocto-K® [OTC]** *see* Docusate *on page 346*
- ♦ **Diocto-K Plus® [OTC]** *see* Docusate and Casanthranol *on page 347*
- ♦ **Dioctolose Plus® [OTC]** *see* Docusate and Casanthranol *on page 347*
- ♦ **Dioeze® [OTC]** *see* Docusate *on page 346*
- ♦ **Dioval® Injection** *see* Estradiol *on page 387*
- ♦ **Diovan™** *see* Valsartan *on page 1039*
- ♦ **Dipalmitoylphosphatidylcholine** *see* Colfosceril Palmitate *on page 275*
- ♦ **Dipentum®** *see* Olsalazine *on page 739*
- ♦ **Diphen® Cough [OTC]** *see* Diphenhydramine *on this page*
- ♦ **Diphenhist® [OTC]** *see* Diphenhydramine *on this page*


## Diphenhydramine (dye fen HYE dra meen)

**Related Information**


Diphenhydramine and Pseudoephedrine *on next page*

Oral Nonviral Soft Tissue Ulcerations or Erosions *on page 1141*

Oral Viral Infections *on page 1137*

Patients Undergoing Cancer Therapy *on page 1154*


**U.S. Brand Names** AllerMax® Oral [OTC]; Banophen® Oral [OTC]; Belix® Oral [OTC]; Benadryl® Injection; Benadryl® Oral [OTC]; Benadryl® Topical; Ben-Allergin-50® Injection; Benylin® Cough Syrup [OTC]; Bydramine® Cough Syrup [OTC]; Compoz® Gel Caps [OTC]; Compoz® Nighttime Sleep Aid [OTC]; Diphen® Cough [OTC]; Diphenhist® [OTC]; Dormarex® 2 Oral [OTC]; Dormin® Oral [OTC]; Genahist® Oral; Hydramyn® Syrup [OTC]; Hyrexin-50® Injection; Maximum Strength Nytol® [OTC]; Miles Nervine® Caplets [OTC]; Nytol® Oral [OTC]; Phendry® Oral [OTC]; Siladryl® Oral [OTC]; Silphen® Cough [OTC]; Sleep-eze 3® Oral [OTC]; Sleepinal® [OTC]; Sleepwell 2-nite® [OTC]; Sominex® Oral [OTC]; Tusstat® Syrup; Twilite® Oral [OTC]; Uni-Bent® Cough Syrup; 40 Winks® [OTC]

**Canadian Brand Names** Allerdryl®; Allernix®; Nytol® Extra Strength

**Therapeutic Category** Antidote, Hypersensitivity Reactions; Antihistamine; Sedative

**Use**

Dental: Symptomatic relief of allergic symptoms caused by histamine release which include nasal allergies and allergic dermatosis; also to produce local anesthesia through infiltration of mucous membranes

Medical: Can be used for mild nighttime sedation; prevention of motion sickness and as an antitussive; has antinauseant and topical anesthetic properties; treatment of phenothiazine-induced dystonic reactions

**Usual Dosage** Oral:

Children >10 kg: 12.5-25 mg 3-4 times/day; maximum daily dose: 300 mg

Adults: 25-50 mg every 6-8 hours

**Mechanism of Action** Competes with histamine for $H_1$-receptor sites on effector cells in the gastrointestinal tract, blood vessels, and respiratory tract

**Local Anesthetic/Vasoconstrictor Precautions** No information available to require special precautions

**Effects on Dental Treatment** Chronic use of antihistamines will inhibit salivary flow, particularly in elderly patients; this may contribute to periodontal disease and oral discomfort

**Other Adverse Effects** >10%: Central nervous system: Slight to moderate drowsiness

**Contraindications** Hypersensitivity to diphenhydramine or any component; should not be used in acute attacks of asthma

**Warnings/Precautions** Use with caution in patients with angle-closure glaucoma, peptic ulcer, urinary tract obstruction, hyperthyroidism; some preparations contain sodium bisulfite; elixir contains alcohol; diphenhydramine has high sedative and anticholinergic properties, so it may not be considered the antihistamine of choice for prolonged use in the elderly

**Drug Interactions** CNS depressants worsens CNS and respiratory depression, monoamine oxidase inhibitors may cause increased anticholinergic effects; elixir should not be given to patients taking drugs that can cause disulfiram reactions (ie, metronidazole, chlorpropamide) due to high alcohol content

**Drug Uptake**

Absorption: Oral: 40% to 60% reaches systemic circulation due to first-pass metabolism

Maximum sedative effect: 1-3 hours

Duration of action: 4-7 hours

Serum half-life:

- Elderly: 13.5 hours
- Adults: 2-8 hours

Time to peak serum concentration: 2-4 hours

**Pregnancy Risk Factor** C

**Breast-feeding Considerations** No data reported

**Dosage Forms**

Capsule, as hydrochloride: 25 mg, 50 mg

Cream, as hydrochloride: 1%, 2%

Elixir, as hydrochloride: 12.5 mg/5 mL (5 mL, 10 mL, 20 mL, 120 mL, 480 mL, 3780 mL)

Injection, as hydrochloride: 10 mg/mL (10 mL, 30 mL); 50 mg/mL (1 mL, 10 mL)

Lotion, as hydrochloride: 1% (75 mL)

Solution, topical spray, as hydrochloride: 1% (60 mL)

Syrup, as hydrochloride: 12.5 mg/5 mL (5 mL, 120 mL, 240 mL, 480 mL, 3780 mL)

Tablet, as hydrochloride: 25 mg, 50 mg

**Dietary Considerations** May be taken with food or water

**Generic Available** Yes

**Comments** 25-50 mg of diphenhydramine orally every 4-6 hours can be used to treat mild dermatologic manifestations of allergic reactions to penicillin and other antibiotics; used as local anesthetic in patients allergic to all other local anesthetics; used for infiltration only; should never be used for block anesthesia because of irritative qualities of vehicle. A 50:50 mixture of diphenhydramine liquid (12.5 mg/5 mL) in Kaopectate® or Maalox® is used as a local application for recurrent aphthous ulcers; swish 1 tablespoonful for 2 minutes 4 times/day.

# Diphenhydramine and Pseudoephedrine

(dye fen HYE dra meen & soo doe e FED rin)

**U.S. Brand Names** Actifed® Allergy Tablet (Night) [OTC]; Banophen® Decongestant Capsule [OTC]; Benadryl® Decongestant Allergy Tablet [OTC]

**Therapeutic Category** Antihistamine/Decongestant Combination

(Continued)

## Diphenhydramine and Pseudoephedrine *(Continued)*

**Use** Relief of symptoms of upper respiratory mucosal congestion in seasonal and perennial nasal allergies, acute rhinitis, rhinosinusitis, and eustachian tube blockage

**Usual Dosage** Adults: Oral: 1 capsule or tablet every 4-6 hours, up to 4/day

**Local Anesthetic/Vasoconstrictor Precautions** Use with caution since pseudoephedrine is a sympathomimetic amine which could interact with epinephrine to cause a pressor response

**Effects on Dental Treatment** Chronic use of antihistamines will inhibit salivary flow, particularly in elderly patients; this may contribute to periodontal disease and oral discomfort

**Other Adverse Effects** See individual agents

**Drug Interactions** See individual agents

**Dosage Forms**

Capsule: Diphenhydramine hydrochloride 25 mg and pseudoephedrine hydrochloride 60 mg

Tablet:

Actifed® Allergy (Night): Diphenhydramine hydrochloride 25 mg and pseudoephedrine hydrochloride 30 mg

Benadryl® Decongestant Allergy: Diphenhydramine hydrochloride 25 mg and pseudoephedrine hydrochloride 60 mg

**Generic Available** Yes

## Diphenidol (dye FEN i dole)

**U.S. Brand Names** Vontrol®

**Therapeutic Category** Antiemetic

**Use** Control of nausea and vomiting; peripheral vertigo and associated nausea and vomiting, Ménière's disease, and middle and inner ear surgery

**Usual Dosage** Oral:

Children: 0.88 mg/kg, children weighing 50-100 pounds the dose in 25 mg given no more often than every 4 hours; total dose in 24 hours should not exceed 5.5 mg/kg

Adults: 25 mg every 4 hours

**Local Anesthetic/Vasoconstrictor Precautions** No information available to require special precautions

**Effects on Dental Treatment** No effects or complications reported

**Other Adverse Effects**

>10%: Central nervous system: Drowsiness

1% to 10%:

Central nervous system: Dizziness, headache, nervousness, insomnia

Gastrointestinal: Dry mouth, heartburn

Neuromuscular & skeletal: Weakness

Ocular: Blurred vision

<1%: Central nervous system: Confusion, hallucinations

**Pregnancy Risk Factor** C

**Generic Available** No

## Diphenoxylate and Atropine (dye fen OKS i late & A troe peen)

**U.S. Brand Names** Logen®; Lomanate®; Lomotil®; Lonox®

**Therapeutic Category** Antidiarrheal

**Use** Treatment of diarrhea

**Usual Dosage** Oral:

Children (use with caution in young children due to variable responses): Liquid: 0.3-0.4 mg of diphenoxylate/kg/day in 2-4 divided doses **or**

<2 years: Not recommended

2-5 years: 2 mg of diphenoxylate 3 times/day

5-8 years: 2 mg of diphenoxylate 4 times/day

8-12 years: 2 mg of diphenoxylate 5 times/day

Adults: 15-20 mg/day of diphenoxylate in 3-4 divided doses; maintenance: 5-15 mg/day in 2-3 divided doses

**Mechanism of Action** Diphenoxylate inhibits excessive GI motility and GI propulsion; commercial preparations contain a subtherapeutic amount of atropine to discourage abuse

**Local Anesthetic/Vasoconstrictor Precautions** No information available to require special precautions

**Effects on Dental Treatment** Up to 10% of patients will complain of significant dry mouth and drowsiness. This will disappear with cessation of drug therapy.

**Other Adverse Effects**

1% to 10%:

Central nervous system: Nervousness, restlessness, dizziness, drowsiness, headache, mental depression

Gastrointestinal: Paralytic ileus, dry mouth
Genitourinary: Urinary retention, dysuria
Ocular: Blurred vision
Respiratory: Respiratory depression

<1%:
Cardiovascular: Tachycardia
Central nervous system: Sedation, euphoria, hyperthermia
Dermatologic: Pruritus, urticaria
Gastrointestinal: Nausea, vomiting, abdominal discomfort, pancreatitis, stomach cramps
Neuromuscular & skeletal: Muscle cramps, weakness
Miscellaneous: Increased sweating

**Drug Interactions** Increased toxicity: MAO inhibitors (hypertensive crisis), CNS depressants, antimuscarinics (paralytic ileus); may prolong half-life of drugs metabolized in liver

**Drug Uptake**
Onset of action: Within 45-60 minutes
Duration: 3-4 hours
Absorption: Oral: Well absorbed
Serum half-life: Diphenoxylate: 2.5 hours
Time to peak serum concentration: 2 hours

**Pregnancy Risk Factor** C
**Generic Available** Yes

- **Diphenylan Sodium®** *see* Phenytoin *on page 799*
- **Diphtheria $CRM_{197}$ Protein Conjugate** *see Haemophilus* b Conjugate Vaccine *on page 486*
- **Diphtheria Toxoid Conjugate** *see Haemophilus* b Conjugate Vaccine *on page 486*

## Dipivefrin (dye PI ve frin)

**U.S. Brand Names** AKPro® Ophthalmic; Propine® Ophthalmic
**Canadian Brand Names** DPE™; Optho-Dipivefrin™
**Therapeutic Category** Adrenergic Agonist Agent, Ophthalmic; Antiglaucoma Agent; Ophthalmic Agent, Vasoconstrictor
**Use** Reduces elevated intraocular pressure in chronic open-angle glaucoma; also used to treat ocular hypertension, low tension, and secondary glaucomas
**Usual Dosage** Adults: Ophthalmic: Instill 1 drop every 12 hours into the eyes
**Mechanism of Action** Dipivefrin is a prodrug of epinephrine which is the active agent that stimulates alpha- and/or beta-adrenergic receptors increasing aqueous humor outflow
**Local Anesthetic/Vasoconstrictor Precautions** No information available to require special precautions
**Effects on Dental Treatment** No effects or complications reported
**Other Adverse Effects**

1% to 10%:
Central nervous system: Headache
Local: Burning, stinging
Ocular: Ocular congestion, photophobia, mydriasis, blurred vision, ocular pain, bulbar conjunctival follicles, blepharoconjunctivitis, cystoid macular edema

<1%: Cardiovascular: Arrhythmias, hypertension

**Drug Interactions** Increased or synergistic effect when used with other agents to lower intraocular pressure

**Drug Uptake**
Ocular pressure effect:
Onset of action: Within 30 minutes
Duration: ≥12 hours
Mydriasis:
Onset of action: May occur within 30 minutes
Duration: Several hours
Absorption: Rapid into the aqueous humor

**Pregnancy Risk Factor** B
**Generic Available** Yes

- **Diprivan® Injection** *see* Propofol *on page 853*
- **Diprolene®** *see* Betamethasone *on page 136*
- **Diprolene® AF** *see* Betamethasone *on page 136*
- **Diprosone®** *see* Betamethasone *on page 136*

## Dipyridamole (dye peer ID a mole)

**U.S. Brand Names** Persantine®

**Canadian Brand Names** Apo®-Dipyridamole FC; Apo®-Dipyridamole SC; Novo-Dipiradol

**Therapeutic Category** Platelet Aggregation Inhibitor

**Use** Maintains patency after surgical grafting procedures including coronary artery bypass; used with warfarin to decrease thrombosis in patients after artificial heart valve replacement; used with aspirin to prevent coronary artery thrombosis; in combination with aspirin or warfarin to prevent other thromboembolic disorders. Dipyridamole may also be given 2 days prior to open heart surgery to prevent platelet activation by extracorporeal bypass pump and as a diagnostic agent in CAD.

**Usual Dosage**

Oral:

Children: 3-6 mg/kg/day in 3 divided doses

Doses of 4-10 mg/kg/day have been used investigationally to treat proteinuria in pediatric renal disease

Adults: 75-400 mg/day in 3-4 divided doses

I.V.: 0.14 mg/kg/minute for 4 minutes; maximum dose: 60 mg

**Mechanism of Action** Inhibits the activity of adenosine deaminase and phosphodiesterase, which causes an accumulation of adenosine, adenine nucleotides, and cyclic AMP; these mediators then inhibit platelet aggregation and may cause vasodilation; may also stimulate release of prostacyclin or $PGD_2$; causes coronary vasodilation

**Local Anesthetic/Vasoconstrictor Precautions** No information available to require special precautions

**Effects on Dental Treatment** No effects or complications reported

**Other Adverse Effects**

>10%:

Cardiovascular: Exacerbation of angina pectoris

Central nervous system: Dizziness

1% to 10%:

Cardiovascular: Hypotension, hypertension, tachycardia

Central nervous system: Headache

Dermatologic: Rash

Gastrointestinal: Abdominal distress

Respiratory: Dyspnea

<1%:

Cardiovascular: Vasodilatation, flushing, syncope, edema

Central nervous system: Migraine

Neuromuscular & skeletal: Hypertonia, weakness

Respiratory: Rhinitis, hyperventilation, pleural pain

Miscellaneous: Allergic reaction

**Drug Interactions** No data reported

**Drug Uptake**

Absorption: Readily absorbed from GI tract but variable

Serum half-life, terminal: 10-12 hours

Time to peak serum concentration: 2-2.5 hours

**Pregnancy Risk Factor** C

**Generic Available** Yes

## Dirithromycin (dye RITH roe mye sin)

**U.S. Brand Names** Dynabac®

**Therapeutic Category** Antibiotic, Macrolide

**Use** Treatment of mild to moderate upper and lower respiratory tract infections, infections of the skin and skin structure, and sexually transmitted diseases due to susceptible strains

**Usual Dosage** Adults: Oral: 500 mg once daily for 7-14 days (14 days required for treatment of community-acquired pneumonia due to *Legionella*, *Mycoplasma*, or *S. pneumoniae*; 10 days is recommended for treatment of *S. pyogenes* pharyngitis/tonsillitis)

**Mechanism of Action** After being converted during intestinal absorption to its active form, erthromycylamine, dirithromycin inhibits protein synthesis by binding to the 50S ribosomal subunits of susceptible microorganisms

**Local Anesthetic/Vasoconstrictor Precautions** No information available to require special precautions

**Effects on Dental Treatment** No effects or complications reported

**Other Adverse Effects**

Central nervous system: Headache, dizziness

Dermatologic: Skin rash, urticaria

Gastrointestinal: Abdominal pain, nausea, diarrhea, vomiting, dyspepsia, flatulence

Hepatic: Elevated LFTs, alkaline phosphatase

Neuromuscular & skeletal: Weakness

Renal: Nephrotoxicity

**Contraindications** Hypersensitivity to any macrolide or component of dirithromycin; the FDA has issued a contraindication with pimozide (Orap®), clarithromycin, and other macrolide antibiotics

**Warnings/Precautions** Contrary to potential serious consequences with other macrolides (eg, cardiac arrhythmias), the combination of terfenadine and dirithromycin has not shown alteration of terfenadine metabolism; however, caution should be taken during coadministration of dirithromycin and terfenadine

**Drug Interactions** Increased effect: Absorption of dirithromycin is slightly enhanced with concomitant antacids and $H_2$ antagonists; dirithromycin may, like erythromycin, increase the effect of alfentanil, anticoagulants, bromocriptine, carbamazepine, cyclosporine, digoxin, disopyramide, ergots, methylprednisolone, and triazolam

**Drug Uptake**

Absorption: Rapidly absorbed and nonenzymatically hydrolyzed to erythromycylamine; $T_{max}$: 4 hours

Serum half-life: 8 hours (range: 2-36 hours)

**Pregnancy Risk Factor** C

**Dosage Forms** Tablet, enteric coated: 250 mg

**Generic Available** No

**Selected Readings**

"Pimozide (Orap) Contraindicated With Clarithromycin (Biaxin™) and Other Macrolide Antibiotics," *FDA Medical Bulletin*, October 1996, 3.

♦ **Disalcid®** *see* Salsalate *on page 902*

♦ **Disanthrol® [OTC]** *see* Docusate and Casanthranol *on page 347*

♦ **Disobrom® [OTC]** *see* Dexbrompheniramine and Pseudoephedrine *on page 309*

♦ **Disonate® [OTC]** *see* Docusate *on page 346*

♦ **Disophrol® Chronotabs® [OTC]** *see* Dexbrompheniramine and Pseudoephedrine *on page 309*

♦ **Disophrol® Tablet [OTC]** *see* Dexbrompheniramine and Pseudoephedrine *on page 309*

## Disopyramide (dye soe PEER a mide)

**Related Information**

Cardiovascular Diseases *on page 1066*

**U.S. Brand Names** Norpace®

**Canadian Brand Names** Rythmodan®, -LA

**Therapeutic Category** Antiarrhythmic Agent, Class I-A; Antiarrhythmic Agent (Supraventricular & Ventricular)

**Use** Suppression and prevention of unifocal and multifocal premature, ventricular premature complexes, coupled ventricular tachycardia; effective in the conversion of atrial fibrillation, atrial flutter, and paroxysmal atrial tachycardia to normal sinus rhythm and prevention of the reoccurrence of these arrhythmias after conversion by other methods

**Usual Dosage** Oral:

Children:

- <1 year: 10-30 mg/kg/24 hours in 4 divided doses
- 1-4 years: 10-20 mg/kg/24 hours in 4 divided doses
- 4-12 years: 10-15 mg/kg/24 hours in 4 divided doses
- 12-18 years: 6-15 mg/kg/24 hours in 4 divided doses

Adults:

- <50 kg: 100 mg every 6 hours or 200 mg every 12 hours (controlled release)
- >50 kg: 150 mg every 6 hours or 300 mg every 12 hours (controlled release); if no response, may increase to 200 mg every 6 hours; maximum dose required for patients with severe refractory ventricular tachycardia is 400 mg every 6 hours

**Mechanism of Action** Class IA antiarrhythmic: Decreases myocardial excitability and conduction velocity; reduces disparity in refractory between normal and infarcted myocardium; possesses anticholinergic, peripheral vasoconstrictive, and negative inotropic effects

**Local Anesthetic/Vasoconstrictor Precautions** No information available to require special precautions

**Effects on Dental Treatment** No effects or complications reported

**Other Adverse Effects**

>10%: Genitourinary: Urinary retention/hesitancy

(Continued)

## Disopyramide *(Continued)*

1% to 10%:
Cardiovascular: Chest pains, congestive heart failure, hypotension
Endocrine & metabolic: Hypokalemia
Gastrointestinal: Stomach pain, bloating, dry mouth
Neuromuscular & skeletal: Muscle weakness
Ocular: Blurred vision

<1%:
Cardiovascular: Syncope and conduction disturbances including A-V block, widening QRS complex and lengthening of Q-T interval
Central nervous system: Fatigue, malaise, nervousness, acute psychosis, depression, dizziness, headache, pain
Dermatologic: Generalized rashes
Endocrine & metabolic: Hypoglycemia, may initiate contractions of pregnant uterus, hyperkalemia may enhance toxicities, elevated cholesterol and triglycerides
Gastrointestinal: Constipation, nausea, vomiting, diarrhea, gas, anorexia, weight gain
Hepatic: Hepatic cholestasis, elevated liver enzymes
Neuromuscular & skeletal: Weakness
Ocular: Dry eyes
Respiratory: Dyspnea, dry nose, throat

**Drug Interactions**
Decreased effect with hepatic microsomal enzyme-inducing agents (ie, phenytoin, phenobarbital, rifampin)
Increased effect/levels/toxicity with erythromycin; increased levels of digoxin

**Drug Uptake**
Onset of action: 0.5-3.5 hours
Duration of effect: 1.5-8.5 hours
Absorption: 60% to 83%
Serum half-life: Adults: 4-10 hours, increased half-life with hepatic or renal disease

**Pregnancy Risk Factor** C
**Generic Available** Yes

- **Disotate®** *see* Edetate Disodium *on page 363*
- **Di-Spaz® Injection** *see* Dicyclomine *on page 322*
- **Di-Spaz® Oral** *see* Dicyclomine *on page 322*

## Disulfiram (dye SUL fi ram)

**U.S. Brand Names** Antabuse®
**Therapeutic Category** Aldehyde Dehydrogenase Inhibitor Agent; Antialcoholic Agent
**Use** Management of chronic alcoholism
**Usual Dosage** Adults: Oral: Do not administer until the patient has abstained from alcohol for at least 12 hours
Initial: 500 mg/day as a single dose for 1-2 weeks; maximum daily dose is 500 mg
Average maintenance dose: 250 mg/day; range: 125-500 mg; duration of therapy is to continue until the patient is fully recovered socially and a basis for permanent self control has been established; maintenance therapy may be required for months or even years
**Mechanism of Action** Disulfiram is a thiuram derivative which interferes with aldehyde dehydrogenase. When taken concomitantly with alcohol, there is an increase in serum acetaldehyde levels. High acetaldehyde causes uncomfortable symptoms including flushing, nausea, thirst, palpitations, chest pain, vertigo, and hypotension. This reaction is the basis for disulfiram use in postwithdrawal long-term care of alcoholism.
**Local Anesthetic/Vasoconstrictor Precautions** No information available to require special precautions
**Effects on Dental Treatment** No effects or complications reported
**Other Adverse Effects**
>10%: Central nervous system: Drowsiness
1% to 10%:
Central nervous system: Headache, fatigue, mood changes, neurotoxicity
Dermatologic: Skin rash
Gastrointestinal: Metallic or garlic-like aftertaste
Genitourinary: Impotence

<1%:
Endocrine & metabolic: Disulfiram reaction with alcohol (flushing, sweating, cardiovascular collapse, myocardial infarction, vertigo, seizures, headache, nausea, vomiting, dyspnea, chest pain, death)

Hepatic: Hepatitis, encephalopathy

**Drug Interactions**

Increased effect: Diazepam, chlordiazepoxide

Increased toxicity:

Alcohol and disulfiram: Antabuse® reaction

Tricyclic antidepressants, metronidazole, isoniazid: Encephalopathy

Disulfiram has caused increases in serum levels of phenytoin and warfarin leading to phenytoin toxicity and enhanced anticoagulation

**Drug Uptake**

Full effect: 12 hours

Duration: May persist for 1-2 weeks after last dose

Absorption: Rapid from GI tract

**Pregnancy Risk Factor** C

**Generic Available** Yes

- ♦ **Dital®** *see* Phendimetrazine *on page 788*
- ♦ **Ditropan®** *see* Oxybutynin *on page 749*
- ♦ **Ditropan® XL** *see* Oxybutynin *on page 749*
- ♦ **Diucardin®** *see* Hydroflumethiazide *on page 512*
- ♦ **Diupres-250®** *see* Chlorothiazide and Reserpine *on page 230*
- ♦ **Diupres-500®** *see* Chlorothiazide and Reserpine *on page 230*
- ♦ **Diurigen®** *see* Chlorothiazide *on page 229*
- ♦ **Diuril®** *see* Chlorothiazide *on page 229*
- ♦ **Dizac® Injectable Emulsion** *see* Diazepam *on page 316*
- ♦ **Dizmiss® [OTC]** *see* Meclizine *on page 620*
- ♦ **DNR** *see* Daunorubicin Hydrochloride *on page 299*
- ♦ **Doan's®, Original [OTC]** *see* Magnesium Salicylate *on page 613*

## Dobutamine (doe BYOO ta meen)

**U.S. Brand Names** Dobutrex®

**Therapeutic Category** Adrenergic Agonist Agent

**Use** Short-term management of patients with cardiac decompensation

**Usual Dosage** I.V. infusion:

Children: 2.5-15 mcg/kg/minute, titrate to desired response

Adults: 2.5-15 mcg/kg/minute; maximum: 40 mcg/kg/minute, titrate to desired response

**Infusion Rates of Various Dilutions of Dobutamine**

| Desired Delivery Rate (mcg/kg/min) | Infusion Rate (mL/kg/min) | |
|---|---|---|
| | 500 mcg/mL* | 1000 mcg/mL† |
| 2.5 | 0.005 | 0.0025 |
| 5.0 | 0.01 | 0.005 |
| 7.5 | 0.015 | 0.0075 |
| 10.0 | 0.02 | 0.01 |
| 12.5 | 0.025 | 0.0125 |
| 15.0 | 0.03 | 0.015 |

* 500 mg per liter or 250 mg per 500 mL of diluent.

†1000 mg per liter or 250 mg per 250 mL of diluent.

**Mechanism of Action** Stimulates $beta_1$-adrenergic receptors, causing increased contractility and heart rate, with little effect on $beta_2$- or alpha-receptors

**Local Anesthetic/Vasoconstrictor Precautions** No information available to require special precautions

**Effects on Dental Treatment** No effects or complications reported

**Other Adverse Effects**

>10%:

Cardiovascular: Ectopic heartbeats, tachycardia, chest pain, angina, palpitations, hypertension; in higher doses ventricular tachycardia or arrhythmias may be seen; patients with atrial fibrillation or flutter are at risk of developing a rapid ventricular response

1% to 10%:

Cardiovascular: Premature ventricular beats, chest pain, angina, palpitations

Central nervous system: Headache

Gastrointestinal: Nausea, vomiting

Neuromuscular & skeletal: Mild leg cramps, paresthesia

Respiratory: Dyspnea

**Drug Interactions**

Decreased effect: Beta-adrenergic blockers (increased peripheral resistance)

(Continued)

## Dobutamine *(Continued)*

Increased toxicity: General anesthetics (ie, halothane or cyclopropane) and usual doses of dobutamine have resulted in ventricular arrhythmias in animals

**Drug Uptake**

Onset of action: I.V.: 1-10 minutes
Serum half-life: 2 minutes

**Pregnancy Risk Factor** C

**Generic Available** Yes

♦ **Dobutrex**® *see* Dobutamine *on previous page*

## Docetaxel (doe se TAKS el)

**U.S. Brand Names** Taxotere®

**Therapeutic Category** Antineoplastic Agent, Miscellaneous

**Use** FDA-approved: Treatment of patients with locally advanced or metastatic breast cancer who have progressed during anthracycline-based therapy or have relapsed during anthracycline-based adjuvant therapy

**Investigational:** Treatment of nonsmall cell lung cancer, gastric, pancreatic, head and neck, ovarian, soft tissue sarcoma, and melanoma

**Usual Dosage** Adults: I.V.: 60-100 mg/m² administered over 1 hour every 3 weeks

**Local Anesthetic/Vasoconstrictor Precautions** No information available to require special precautions

**Effects on Dental Treatment** No effects or complications reported

**Other Adverse Effects**

**Irritant chemotherapy**

>10%:

Central nervous system: Fever
Dermatologic: Alopecia
Gastrointestinal: Nausea, vomiting, diarrhea, stomatitis
Hematologic: Neutropenia, leukopenia, thrombocytopenia, anemia
Neuromuscular & skeletal: Myalgia

1% to 10%: Cardiovascular: Severe fluid retention: poorly tolerated peripheral edema, generalized edema, pleural effusion requiring urgent drainage, dyspnea at rest, cardiac tamponade or pronounced abdominal distention (due to ascites)

>1%: Miscellaneous: Hypersensitivity reactions

**Drug Interactions** Cytochrome P-450 substrate

Increased toxicity: Possibility of an inhibition of metabolism in patients treated with ketoconazole, erythromycin, and cyclosporine

**Drug Uptake** Administered by I.V. infusion and exhibits linear pharmacokinetics at the recommended dosage range

Half-life; α, β, and γ phases are 4 minutes, 36 minutes, and 11.1 hours, respectively

**Pregnancy Risk Factor** D

**Dosage Forms** Injection: 40 mg/mL (0.5 mL, 2 mL)

**Generic Available** No

## Docusate (DOK yoo sate)

**U.S. Brand Names** Colace® [OTC]; DC 240® Softgels® [OTC]; Dialose® [OTC]; Diocto® [OTC]; Diocto-K® [OTC]; Dioeze® [OTC]; Disonate® [OTC]; DOK® [OTC]; DOS® Softgel® [OTC]; D-S-S® [OTC]; Kasof® [OTC]; Modane® Soft [OTC]; Pro-Cal-Sof® [OTC]; Regulax SS® [OTC]; Sulfalax® [OTC]; Surfak® [OTC]

**Canadian Brand Names** Albert® Docusate; Colax-C®; PMS-Docusate Calcium; Regulex®; Selax®; SoFlax™

**Therapeutic Category** Laxative, Surfactant; Stool Softener

**Use** Stool softener in patients who should avoid straining during defecation and constipation associated with hard, dry stools; prophylaxis for straining (Valsalva) following myocardial infarction. A safe agent to be used in elderly; some evidence that doses <200 mg are ineffective; stool softeners are unnecessary if stool is well hydrated or "mushy" and soft; shown to be ineffective used long-term.

**Usual Dosage** Docusate salts are interchangeable; the amount of sodium, calcium, or potassium per dosage unit is clinically insignificant

Children <3 years: Oral: 10-40 mg/day in 1-4 divided doses
Children: Oral:
3-6 years: 20-60 mg/day in 1-4 divided doses
6-12 years: 40-150 mg/day in 1-4 divided doses
Adolescents and Adults: Oral: 50-500 mg/day in 1-4 divided doses
Older Children and Adults: Rectal: Add 50-100 mg of docusate liquid to enema fluid (saline or water); give as retention or flushing enema

**Mechanism of Action** Reduces surface tension of the oil-water interface of the stool resulting in enhanced incorporation of water and fat allowing for stool softening

**Local Anesthetic/Vasoconstrictor Precautions** No information available to require special precautions

**Effects on Dental Treatment** No effects or complications reported

**Other Adverse Effects** 1% to 10%: Gastrointestinal: Intestinal obstruction, diarrhea, abdominal cramping, throat irritation

**Drug Interactions**

Decreased effect of Coumadin®, aspirin

Increased toxicity with mineral oil

**Drug Uptake** Onset of action: 12-72 hours

**Pregnancy Risk Factor** C

**Generic Available** Yes

## Docusate and Casanthranol (DOK yoo sate & ka SAN thra nole)

**U.S. Brand Names** Dialose® Plus Capsule [OTC]; Diocto C® [OTC]; Diocto-K Plus® [OTC]; Dioctolose Plus® [OTC]; Disanthrol® [OTC]; DSMC Plus® [OTC]; Genasoft® Plus [OTC]; Peri-Colace® [OTC]; Pro-Sof® Plus [OTC]; Regulace® [OTC]; Silace-C® [OTC]

**Therapeutic Category** Laxative, Surfactant; Stool Softener

**Synonyms** Casanthranol and Docusate; DSS With Casanthranol

**Use** Treatment of constipation generally associated with dry, hard stools and decreased intestinal motility

**Usual Dosage** Oral:

Children: 5-15 mL of syrup at bedtime or 1 capsule at bedtime

Adults: 1-2 capsules or 15-30 mL syrup at bedtime, may be increased to 2 capsules or 30 mL twice daily or 3 capsules at bedtime

**Local Anesthetic/Vasoconstrictor Precautions** No information available to require special precautions

**Effects on Dental Treatment** No effects or complications reported

**Other Adverse Effects** 1% to 10%:

Dermatologic: Rash

Gastrointestinal: Intestinal obstruction, diarrhea, abdominal cramping, throat irritation

**Pregnancy Risk Factor** C

**Generic Available** Yes

♦ **DOK® [OTC]** *see* Docusate *on previous page*

♦ **Dolacet® [5/500]** *see* Hydrocodone and Acetaminophen *on page 505*

## Dolasetron (dol A se tron)

**U.S. Brand Names** Anzemet®

**Therapeutic Category** Antiemetic; Selective 5-$HT_3$ Receptor Antagonist

**Synonyms** Dolasetron Mesylate

**Use**

Oral: The prevention of nausea and vomiting associated with moderately-emetogenic cancer chemotherapy, including initial and repeat courses; the prevention of postoperative nausea and vomiting.

Parenteral: The prevention of nausea and vomiting associated with initial and repeat courses of emetogenic cancer chemotherapy, including high dose cisplatin; the prevention of postoperative nausea and vomiting; as with other antiemetics, routine prophylaxis is not recommended for patients in whom there is little expectation that nausea and/or vomiting will occur postoperatively; in patients where nausea and/or vomiting must be avoided postoperatively, injection is recommended even where the incidence of postoperative nausea and/or vomiting is low; the treatment of postoperative nausea and/or vomiting

**Usual Dosage**

Oral:

Prevention of cancer chemotherapy-induced nausea and vomiting:

Children (2-16 years): 1.8 mg/kg given within one hour before chemotherapy, up to a maximum of 100 mg; safety and effectiveness in pediatric patients under 2 years of age have not been established

Adults: 100 mg given within one hour before chemotherapy

Use in the elderly, renal failure patients, or hepatically impaired patients: No dosage adjustment is recommended

Prevention of postoperative nausea and vomiting:

Children (2-16 years): 1.2 mg/kg given within two hours before surgery, up to a maximum of 100 mg; safety and effectiveness in pediatric patients under 2 years of age have not been established

Adults: 100 mg within two hours before surgery

(Continued)

## Dolasetron *(Continued)*

Use in the elderly, renal failure patients, or hepatically impaired patients: No dosage adjustment is recommended

I.V.:

Prevention of cancer chemotherapy-induced nausea and vomiting

Adults: From clinical trials, the dose is 1.8 mg/kg given as a single dose approximately 30 minutes before chemotherapy; alternatively, for most patients, a fixed dose of 100 mg can be administered over 30 seconds.

Children (2-16 years): 1.8 mg/kg given as a single dose approximately 30 minutes before chemotherapy, up to a maximum of 100 mg; safety and effectiveness in pediatric patients under 2 years of age have not been established.

Injection mixed in apple or apple-grape juice may be used for oral dosing of pediatric patients. When injection is administered orally, the recommended dosage in pediatric patients 2 to 16 years of age is 1.8 mg/kg up to a maximum 100 mg dose given within 1 hour before chemotherapy. The diluted product may be kept up to 2 hours at room temperature before use.

Use in the elderly, in renal failure patients, or in hepatically impaired patients: No dosage adjustment is recommended.

Prevention of postoperative nausea and/or vomiting

Adults: 12.5 mg given as a single dose approximately 15 minutes before the cessation of anesthesia (prevention) or as soon as nausea or vomiting presents (treatment).

Children (2-16 years): 0.35 mg/kg, with a maximum dose of 12.5 mg, given as a single dose approximately 15 minutes before the cessation of anesthesia or as soon as nausea or vomiting presents. Safety and effectiveness in pediatric patients under 2 years of age have not been established. Injection mixed in apple or apple-grape juice may be used for oral dosing of pediatric patients; dosage in pediatric patients 2 to 16 years is 1.2 mg/kg up to a maximum 100-mg dose given before surgery.

**Mechanism of Action** Dolasetron is a pseudopelletierine derived serotonin antagonist. Serotonin antagonists block the serotonin receptors in the chemoreceptor trigger zone and in the gastrointestinal tract. Once the receptor site is blocked, antagonism of the chemotherapy induced nausea and vomiting that occurs.

**Local Anesthetic/Vasoconstrictor Precautions** No information available to require special precautions

**Effects on Dental Treatment** No effects or complications reported

**Drug Uptake** Half-life: elimination:

Dolasetron: 10 minutes

MDL 74,156: 8 hours

**Comments** A single I.V. dose of dolasetron mesylate (1.8 or 2.4 mg/kg) has comparable safety and efficacy to a single 32-mg IV dose of ondansetron in patients receiving cisplatin chemotherapy.

- **Dolasetron Mesylate** *see* Dolasetron *on previous page*
- **Dolene®** *see* Propoxyphene *on page 854*
- **Dolobid®** *see* Diflunisal *on page 327*
- **Dolophine®** *see* Methadone *on page 644*
- **Dolorac™ [OTC]** *see* Capsaicin *on page 181*
- **Domeboro® Topical [OTC]** *see* Aluminum Sulfate and Calcium Acetate *on page 57*
- **Dome Paste Bandage** *see* Zinc Gelatin *on page 1061*

## Donepezil (don EH pa zil)

**U.S. Brand Names** Aricept®

**Therapeutic Category** Acetylcholinesterase Inhibitor

**Use** Treatment of mild to moderate dementia of the Alzheimer's type

**Usual Dosage** Adults: Initial: 5 mg/day at bedtime; may increase to 10 mg/day at bedtime after 4-6 weeks

**Mechanism of Action** Donepezil enhances cholinergic function by increasing the concentration of acetylcholine through reversible inhibition of its hydrolysis by acetylcholinesterase; there is no evidence that donepezil alters the course of the underlying dementing process

**Local Anesthetic/Vasoconstrictor Precautions** No information available to require special precautions

**Effects on Dental Treatment** No effects or complications reported

**Other Adverse Effects**

>10%:

Central nervous system: Headache

Gastrointestinal: Nausea, diarrhea

1% to 10%:

Cardiovascular: Syncope, chest pain

Central nervous system: Fatigue, insomnia, dizziness, depression, abnormal dreams, somnolence

Dermatologic: Bruising

Gastrointestinal: Anorexia, vomiting, weight loss

Genitourinary: Polyuria

Neuromuscular & skeletal: Muscle cramps, arthritis, body pain

**Warnings/Precautions** Use with caution in patients with sick sinus syndrome or other supraventricular cardiac conduction abnormalities, in patients with seizures or asthma; avoid use in nursing mothers

**Drug Interactions** Increased effects of succinylcholine, cholinesterase inhibitors, or cholinergic agonists (bethanechol). Concomitant NSAIDs may increase the risk of gastrointestinal bleeding.

**Drug Uptake**

Absorption: Well absorbed

Half-life: 70 hours

Time to peak plasma concentration: 3-4 hours

**Pregnancy Risk Factor** C

**Dosage Forms** Tablet: 5 mg, 10 mg

**Generic Available** No

- **Donnamar®** *see* Hyoscyamine *on page 519*
- **Donnapectolin-PG®** *see* Hyoscyamine, Atropine, Scopolamine, Kaolin, Pectin, and Opium *on page 522*
- **Donnatal®** *see* Hyoscyamine, Atropine, Scopolamine, and Phenobarbital *on page 520*
- **Donnazyme®** *see* Pancreatin *on page 763*
- **Dopar®** *see* Levodopa *on page 581*
- **Dopram® Injection** *see* Doxapram *on next page*
- **Doral®** *see* Quazepam *on page 869*
- **Dormarex® 2 Oral [OTC]** *see* Diphenhydramine *on page 338*
- **Dormin® Oral [OTC]** *see* Diphenhydramine *on page 338*

## Dornase Alfa (DOOR nase AL fa)

**U.S. Brand Names** Pulmozyme®

**Therapeutic Category** Enzyme

**Use** Management of cystic fibrosis patients to reduce the frequency of respiratory infections that require parenteral antibiotics, and to improve pulmonary function

**Usual Dosage** Children >5 years and Adults: Inhalation: 2.5 mg once daily through selected nebulizers in conjunction with a Pulmo-Aide® or a Pari-Proneb® compressor

**Mechanism of Action** The hallmark of cystic fibrosis lung disease is the presence of abundant, purulent airway secretions composed primarily of highly polymerized DNA. The principal source of this DNA is the nuclei of degenerating neutrophils, which is present in large concentrations in infected lung secretions. The presence of this DNA produces a viscous mucous that may contribute to the decreased mucociliary transport and persistent infections that are commonly seen in this population. Dornase alfa is a deoxyribonuclease (DNA) enzyme produced by recombinant gene technology. Dornase selectively cleaves DNA, thus reducing mucous viscosity and as a result, airflow in the lung is improved and the risk of bacterial infection may be decreased.

**Local Anesthetic/Vasoconstrictor Precautions** No information available to require special precautions

**Effects on Dental Treatment** No effects or complications reported

**Other Adverse Effects**

>10%:

Respiratory: Pharyngitis

Miscellaneous: Voice alteration

1% to 10%:

Cardiovascular: Chest pain

Dermatologic: Rash

Ocular: Conjunctivitis

Respiratory: Laryngitis, cough, dyspnea, hemoptysis, rhinitis, hoarse throat, wheezing

**Drug Interactions** No data reported

**Drug Uptake** Following nebulization, enzyme levels are measurable in the sputum within 15 minutes and decline rapidly thereafter

**Pregnancy Risk Factor** B

**Generic Available** No

- **Doryx®** *see* Doxycycline *on page 355*

## Dorzolamide (dor ZOLE a mide)

**U.S. Brand Names** Trusopt®

**Therapeutic Category** Antiglaucoma Agent; Carbonic Anhydrase Inhibitor

**Use** Lower intraocular pressure to treat glaucoma

**Usual Dosage** Adults: Glaucoma: Instill 1 drop in the affected eye(s) 3 times/day

**Local Anesthetic/Vasoconstrictor Precautions** No information available to require special precautions

**Effects on Dental Treatment** No effects or complications reported

**Other Adverse Effects**

Central nervous system: Headache, fatigue (infrequent)
Dermatologic: Rash
Gastrointestinal: Bitter taste (~25%), nausea
Genitourinary: Urolithiasis
Neuromuscular & skeletal: Weakness (infrequent)
Ocular: Burning, stinging, or discomfort immediately following administration (~33%); iridocyclitis (rare); superficial punctate keratitis (10% to 15%); signs and symptoms of ocular allergic reaction (~10%); blurred vision, tearing, dryness (1% to 5%); photophobia (~1% to 5%)

**Drug Uptake**

Peak effect: 2 hours
Duration: 8-12 hours
Absorption: Systemically absorbed, however, detailed absorption characteristics and pharmacokinetic data are unavailable
Serum half-life: Terminal RBC half-life of 147 days

**Pregnancy Risk Factor** C

**Generic Available** No

♦ **DOS® Softgel® [OTC]** *see* Docusate *on page 346*
♦ **Dostinex®** *see* Cabergoline *on page 167*
♦ **Dovonex®** *see* Calcipotriene *on page 169*

## Doxapram (DOKS a pram)

**U.S. Brand Names** Dopram® Injection

**Therapeutic Category** Central Nervous System Stimulant, Nonamphetamine; Respiratory Stimulant

**Use** Respiratory and CNS stimulant; idiopathic apnea of prematurity refractory to xanthines

**Usual Dosage** Not for use in newborns since doxapram contains a significant amount of benzyl alcohol (0.9%)

Neonatal apnea (apnea of prematurity): I.V.:
Initial: 1-1.5 mg/kg/hour
Maintenance: 0.5-2.5 mg/kg/hour, titrated to the lowest rate at which apnea is controlled

Adults: Respiratory depression following anesthesia: I.V.:
Initial: 0.5-1 mg/kg; may repeat at 5-minute intervals; maximum total dose: 2 mg/kg
I.V. infusion: Initial: 5 mg/minute until adequate response or adverse effects seen; decrease to 1-3 mg/minute; usual total dose: 0.5-4 mg/kg; maximum: 300 mg

**Mechanism of Action** Stimulates respiration through action on respiratory center in medulla or indirectly on peripheral carotid chemoreceptors

**Local Anesthetic/Vasoconstrictor Precautions** No information available to require special precautions

**Effects on Dental Treatment** No effects or complications reported

**Other Adverse Effects**

1% to 10%:
Cardiovascular: Ectopic beats, hypotension, vasoconstriction, tachycardia, anginal pain, palpitations
Central nervous system: Headache
Gastrointestinal: Nausea, vomiting
Respiratory: Dyspnea

<1%:
Cardiovascular: Hypertension (dose related), arrhythmias, flushing
Central nervous system: CNS stimulation, restlessness, lightheadedness, jitters, hallucinations, irritability, seizures, extremely high fever
Gastrointestinal: Abdominal distention, retching
Hematologic: Hemolysis
Local: Phlebitis
Neuromuscular & skeletal: Tremor, hyper-reflexia
Ocular: Mydriasis, lacrimation
Respiratory: Coughing, laryngospasm

Miscellaneous: Sweating, feeling of warmth

**Drug Uptake**

Onset of action (respiratory stimulation): I.V.: Within 20-40 seconds

Peak effect: Within 1-2 minutes

Duration: 5-12 minutes

Serum half-life: Adults: 3.4 hours (mean half-life)

**Pregnancy Risk Factor** B

**Generic Available** No

**Comments** Initial studies suggest a therapeutic range of at least 1.5 mg/L; toxicity becomes frequent at serum levels >5 mg/L

## Doxazosin (doks AYE zoe sin)

**Related Information**

Cardiovascular Diseases *on page 1066*

**U.S. Brand Names** Cardura®

**Therapeutic Category** Alpha-Adrenergic Blockers - Peripheral-Acting ($Alpha_1$-Blockers)

**Use** Treatment of hypertension, severe congestive heart failure (in conjunction with diuretics and cardiac glycosides)

**Unlabeled use:** Symptoms of benign prostatic hypertrophy

**Usual Dosage** Oral:

Adults: 1 mg once daily in morning or evening; may be increased to 2 mg once daily; thereafter titrate upwards, if needed, over several weeks, balancing therapeutic benefit with doxazosin-induced postural hypotension; maximum dose for hypertension: 16 mg/day, for BPH: 8 mg/day

Elderly: Initial: 0.5 mg once daily

**Mechanism of Action** Competitively inhibits postsynaptic alpha-adrenergic receptors which results in vasodilation of veins and arterioles and a decrease in total peripheral resistance and blood pressure; approximately 50% as potent on a weight by weight basis as prazosin

**Local Anesthetic/Vasoconstrictor Precautions** No information available to require special precautions

**Effects on Dental Treatment** No effects or complications reported

**Other Adverse Effects**

>10%: Central nervous system: Dizziness

1% to 10%:

Cardiovascular: Palpitations, arrhythmia

Central nervous system: Vertigo, nervousness, somnolence, anxiety

Endocrine & metabolic: Decreased libido

Gastrointestinal: Nausea, vomiting, dry mouth, diarrhea, constipation

Neuromuscular & skeletal: Shoulder, neck, back pain

Ocular: Abnormal vision

Respiratory: Rhinitis

<1%:

Cardiovascular: Hypotension, tachycardia

Central nervous system: Depression

Gastrointestinal: Abdominal discomfort, flatulence

Genitourinary: Incontinence

Ocular: Conjunctivitis

Otic: Tinnitus

Renal: Polyuria

Respiratory: Dyspnea, sinusitis, epistaxis

**Drug Interactions** Increased effect with diuretics and antihypertensive medications (especially beta-blockers)

**Drug Uptake** Increased age does not significantly affect pharmacokinetics of doxazosin

Half-life: 22 hours

Time to peak serum concentration: 2-3 hours

**Pregnancy Risk Factor** B

**Generic Available** No

## Doxepin (DOKS e pin)

**U.S. Brand Names** Adapin®; Sinequan®

**Canadian Brand Names** Apo®-Doxepin; Novo-Doxepin; Triadapin®

**Therapeutic Category** Antianxiety Agent; Antidepressant, Tricyclic; Tranquilizer, Minor

**Use** Treatment of various forms of depression, usually in conjunction with psychotherapy; treatment of anxiety disorders; analgesic for certain chronic and neuropathic pain

(Continued)

## Doxepin *(Continued)*

**Usual Dosage** Oral (entire daily dose may be given at bedtime):

Adolescents: Initial: 25-50 mg/day in single or divided doses; gradually increase to 100 mg/day

Adults: Initial: 30-150 mg/day at bedtime or in 2-3 divided doses; may gradually increase up to 300 mg/day; single dose should not exceed 150 mg; select patients may respond to 25-50 mg/day

**Mechanism of Action** Increases the synaptic concentration of serotonin and/or norepinephrine in the central nervous system by inhibition of their reuptake by the presynaptic neuronal membrane

**Local Anesthetic/Vasoconstrictor Precautions** Use with caution; epinephrine, norepinephrine and levonordefrin have been shown to have an increased pressor response in combination with TCAs

**Effects on Dental Treatment** >10% of patients experience dry mouth; long-term treatment with TCAs increases the risk of caries by reducing salivation and salivary buffer capacity

**Other Adverse Effects**

>10%:

- Central nervous system: Sedation, drowsiness, dizziness, headache
- Gastrointestinal: Constipation, increased appetite, nausea, unpleasant taste, weight gain

1% to 10%:

- Cardiovascular: Hypotension, arrhythmias
- Central nervous system: Confusion, delirium, hallucinations, nervousness, restlessness, parkinsonian syndrome, insomnia
- Endocrine & metabolic: Sexual dysfunction
- Gastrointestinal: Diarrhea, heartburn
- Genitourinary: Dysuria
- Neuromuscular & skeletal: Fine muscle tremors, weakness
- Ocular: Blurred vision, eye pain
- Miscellaneous: Excessive sweating

<1%:

- Central nervous system: Anxiety, seizures
- Dermatologic: Alopecia, dermal photosensitivity
- Endocrine & metabolic: Breast enlargement, galactorrhea, SIADH
- Gastrointestinal: Trouble with gums, decreased lower esophageal sphincter tone may cause GE reflux
- Genitourinary: Urinary retention, testicular swelling
- Hematologic: Agranulocytosis, leukopenia, eosinophilia
- Hepatic: Hepatitis, cholestatic jaundice and elevated liver enzymes
- Ocular: Increased intraocular pressure
- Otic: Tinnitus
- Miscellaneous: Allergic reactions

**Drug Interactions**

Decreased effect: Phenobarbital may increase the metabolism of doxepin; doxepin blocks the uptake of guanethidine and thus prevents the hypotensive effect of guanethidine

Increased toxicity: Clonidine causes hypertensive crisis; doxepin may be additive with or may potentiate the action of other CNS depressants such as sedatives or hypnotics; with MAO inhibitors, hyperpyrexia, hypertension, tachycardia, confusion, and seizures. Doxepin may increase the prothrombin time in patients stabilized on warfarin; doxepin may potentiate the pressor and cardiac effects of sympathomimetic agents such as isoproterenol, epinephrine, etc; cimetidine and methylphenidate may decrease the metabolism of doxepin

Additive anticholinergic effects seen with other anticholinergic agents

**Drug Uptake**

Serum half-life: Adults: 6-8 hours

**Pregnancy Risk Factor** C (oral); (B topical)

**Generic Available** Yes

**Selected Readings**


Boakes AJ, Laurence DR, Teoh PC, et al, "Interactions Between Sympathomimetic Amines and Antidepressant Agents in Man," *Br Med J*, 1973, 1(849):311-5.

Jastak JT and Yagiela JA, "Vasoconstrictors and Local Anesthesia: A Review and Rationale for Use," *J Am Dent Assoc*, 1983, 107(4):623-30.

Larochelle P, Hamet P, and Enjalbert M, "Responses to Tyramine and Norepinephrine After Imipramine and Trazodone," *Clin Pharmacol Ther*, 1979, 26(1):24-30.

Mitchell JR, "Guanethidine and Related Agents. III Antagonism by Drugs Which Inhibit the Norepinephrine Pump in Man," *J Clin Invest*, 1970, 49(8):1596-604.

Rundegren J, van Dijken J, Mörnstad H, et al, "Oral Conditions in Patients Receiving Long-Term Treatment With Cyclic Antidepressant Drugs," *Swed Dent J*, 1985, 9(2):55-64.

Svedmyr N, "The Influence of a Tricyclic Antidepressive Agent (Protriptyline) on Some of the Circulatory Effects of Noradrenaline and Adrenalin® in Man," *Life Sci*, 1968, 7(1):77-84.


♦ **Doxil®** *see* Doxorubicin (Liposomal) *on page 354*

♦ **Doxil® Injection** *see* Doxorubicin *on this page*

## Doxorubicin (doks oh ROO bi sin)

**U.S. Brand Names** Adriamycin® PFS; Adriamycin® RDF; Doxil® Injection; Rubex®

**Therapeutic Category** Antineoplastic Agent, Antibiotic

**Synonyms** ADR; Hydroxydaunomycin Hydrochloride

**Use** Treatment of various solid tumors including ovarian, breast, and bladder tumors; various lymphomas and leukemias (ANL, ALL), soft tissue sarcomas, neuroblastoma, osteosarcoma

**Usual Dosage Refer to individual protocols**

I.V. (patient's ideal weight should be used to calculate body surface area):

Children: 35-75 mg/m$^2$ as a single dose, repeat every 21 days; **or** 20-30 mg/m$^2$ once weekly; **or** 60-90 mg/m$^2$ given as a continuous infusion over 96 hours every 3-4 weeks

Adults: 60-75 mg/m$^2$ as a single dose, repeat every 21 days **or** other dosage regimens like 20-30 mg/m$^2$/day for 2-3 days, repeat in 4 weeks **or** 20 mg/m$^2$ once weekly

The lower dose regimen should be given to patients with decreased bone marrow reserve, prior therapy or marrow infiltration with malignant cells

Currently the maximum cumulative dose is 550 mg/m$^2$ or 450 mg/m$^2$ in patients who have received RT to the mediastinal areas; a baseline MUGA should be performed prior to initiating treatment. If the LVEF is <30% to 40%, therapy should not be instituted; LVEF should be monitored during therapy.

Doxorubicin has also been administered intraperitoneal (phase I in refractory ovarian cancer patients) and intra-arterially.

**Mechanism of Action** Doxorubicin works through inhibition of topoisomerase-II at the point of DNA cleavage. A second mechanism of action is the production of free radicals (the hydroxy radical OH) by doxorubicin, which in turn can destroy DNA and cancerous cells. Doxorubicin is also a very powerful iron chelator, equal to deferoxamine. The iron-doxorubicin complex can bind DNA and cell membranes rapidly and produce free radicals that immediately cleave the DNA and cell membranes. Inhibits DNA and RNA synthesis by intercalating between DNA base pairs and by steric obstruction; active throughout entire cell cycle.

**Local Anesthetic/Vasoconstrictor Precautions** No information available to require special precautions

**Effects on Dental Treatment** No effects or complications reported

**Other Adverse Effects**

>10%:

Dermatologic: Alopecia

Gastrointestinal: Acute nausea and vomiting may be seen in 21% to 55% of patients; mucositis, ulceration, and necrosis of the colon, anorexia, and diarrhea

Emetic potential: ≤20 mg: Moderately low (10% to 30%); >20 mg or <75 mg: Moderate (30% to 60%); ≥75 mg: Moderately high (60% to 90%)

Hematologic: Myelosuppressive: 60% to 80% of patients will have leukopenia; dose-limiting toxicity; WBC: Moderate; Platelets: Moderate; Onset (days): 7; Nadir (days): 10-14; Recovery (days): 21-28

Local: Extravasation: Doxorubicin is one of the most notorious vesicants. Infiltration can cause severe inflammation, tissue necrosis, and ulceration. If the drug is infiltrated, consult institutional policy, apply ice to the area, and elevate the limb. Can have ongoing tissue destruction secondary to propagation of free radicals; may require debridement.

Radiation recall: Noticed in patients who have had prior irradiation; reactions include redness, warmth, erythema, and dermatitis in the radiation port. Can progress to severe desquamation and ulceration. Occurs 5-7 days after doxorubicin administration; local therapy with topical corticosteroids and cooling have given the best relief.

1% to 10%: Erythematous streaking along the vein if administered too rapidly

Cardiac toxicity: Dose-limiting and related to cumulative dose; usually a maximum total lifetime dose of 450-550 mg/m$^2$ is administered; although, it has been demonstrated that if given by continuous infusion in breast cancer patients, higher doses may be tolerated. Cardiac tissue seems to be very sensitive to damage by free radicals produced by doxorubicin. Patients may present with acute toxicity (arrhythmias, heart block, pericarditis-myocarditis) which may be fatal. More commonly, chronic toxicity is seen, in which patients present with signs of congestive heart failure. Several methods of monitoring cardiac toxicity have been utilized, including myocardial biopsy (expensive and hazardous procedure).

<1%: Allergic reaction, anaphylaxis

Miscellaneous: Fever, chills, urticaria, conjunctivitis

(Continued)

## Doxorubicin *(Continued)*

**Drug Uptake**

Absorption: Oral: Poor, <50%

Serum half-life, triphasic:

Primary: 30 minutes

Secondary: 3-3.5 hours for metabolites

Terminal: 17-30 hours for doxorubicin and its metabolites

**Pregnancy Risk Factor** D

**Generic Available** Yes

♦ **Doxorubicin Hydrochloride (Liposomal)** *see* Doxorubicin (Liposomal) *on this page*

## Doxorubicin (Liposomal) (doks oh ROO bi sin lip pah SOW mal)

**U.S. Brand Names** Doxil®

**Therapeutic Category** Antineoplastic Agent, Anthracycline; Antineoplastic Agent, Antibiotic

**Synonyms** Doxorubicin Hydrochloride (Liposomal)

**Use** Treatment of AIDS-related Kaposi's sarcoma in patients with disease that has progressed on prior combination chemotherapy or in patients who are intolerant to such therapy

Off-label use: Breast cancer, ovarian cancer, and solid tumors

**Usual Dosage Refer to individual protocols**

I.V. (patient's ideal weight should be used to calculate body surface area): 20 mg/$m^2$ over 30 minutes, once every 3 weeks, for as long as patients respond satisfactorily and tolerate treatment.

**Mechanism of Action** Doxil® is doxorubicin hydrochloride encapsulated in long-circulating STEALTH® liposomes. Liposomes are microscopic vesicles composed of a phospholipid bilayer that are capable of encapsulating active drugs. Doxorubicin works through inhibition of topoisomerase-II at the point of DNA cleavage. A second mechanism of action is the production of free radicals (the hydroxy radical OH) by doxorubicin, which in turn can destroy DNA and cancerous cells. Doxorubicin is also a very powerful iron chelator, equal to deferoxamine. The iron-doxorubicin complex can bind DNA and cell membranes rapidly and produce free radicals that immediately cleave the DNA and cell membranes. Inhibits DNA and RNA synthesis by intercalating between DNA base pairs and by steric obstruction; active throughout entire cell cycle.

**Local Anesthetic/Vasoconstrictor Precautions** No information available to require special precautions

**Effects on Dental Treatment** No effects or complications reported

**Other Adverse Effects** Information on adverse events is based on the experience reported in 753 patients with AIDS-related Kaposi's sarcoma enrolled in four studies

>10%:

Extravasation: Doxorubicin is one of the most notorious vesicants. Infiltration can cause severe inflammation, tissue necrosis, and ulceration. If the drug is infiltrated, consult institutional policy, apply ice to the area, and elevate the limb. Can have ongoing tissue destruction secondary to propagation of free radicals; may require debridement.

1% to 10%:

Cardiovascular: Cardiac toxicity (9.7%): Cardiomyopathy, congestive heart failure, arrhythmia, pericardial effusion, tachycardia, facial flushing

Dermatologic: Hyperpigmentation of nail beds, erythematous streaking along the vein if administered too rapidly

Endocrine & metabolic: Hyperuricemia

<1%:

Hypersensitivity: Allergic reaction, anaphylaxis, fever, chills, urticaria

Ocular: Conjunctivitis

**Contraindications** Hypersensitivity to doxorubicin or the components of Doxil®

**Drug Interactions**

No formal drug interaction studies have been conducted with doxorubicin hydrochloride liposome injection, however, may interact with drugs known to interact with the conventional formulation of doxorubicin hydrochloride

Decreased effect: Doxorubicin may decrease digoxin plasma levels and renal excretion

Increased effect: Allopurinol may enhance the antitumor activity of doxorubicin (animal data only)

Increased toxicity:

Cyclophosphamide enhances the cardiac toxicity of doxorubicin by producing additional myocardial cell damage

Mercaptopurine enhances toxicities

Streptozocin greatly enhances leukopenia and thrombocytopenia

Verapamil alters the cellular distribution of doxorubicin; may result in increased cell toxicity by inhibition of the P-glycoprotein pump

**Pregnancy Risk Factor** D

**Dosage Forms** Injection, as hydrochloride: 2 mg/mL (10 mL)

**Generic Available** No

- **Doxy®** *see* Doxycycline *on this page*
- **Doxychel®** *see* Doxycycline *on this page*

# Doxycycline (doks i SYE kleen)

**Related Information**

Animal and Human Bites Guidelines *on page 1164*

Nonviral Infectious Diseases *on page 1095*

Periodontal Diseases *on page 1132*

**U.S. Brand Names** Doryx®; Doxy®; Doxychel®; Periostat™; Vibramycin®; Vibra-Tabs®

**Canadian Brand Names** Apo®-Doxy; Apo®-Doxy Tabs; Doxycin; Doxytec; Novo-Doxylin; Nu-Doxycycline

**Therapeutic Category** Antibiotic, Tetracycline Derivative

**Use**

Dental: Treatment of periodontitis associated with presence of *Actinobacillus actinomycetemcomitans* (AA)

Periostat™ capsules are indicated for use as an adjunct to scaling and root planing to promote attachment level gain and to reduce pocket depth in adult periodontitis

Medical: Principally in the treatment of infections caused by susceptible *Rickettsia, Chlamydia*, and *Mycoplasma* along with uncommon susceptible gram-negative and gram-positive organisms; alternative to mefloquine for malaria prophylaxis

**Unapproved use:** Treatment for syphilis in penicillin-allergic patients; sclerosing agent for pleural effusions

**Usual Dosage** Adults: Oral:

Medical: 100 mg/day for 21 days or until improvement

Dental: As adjunctive treatment for periodontitis: 20 mg twice daily at least 1 hour before morning and evening meals for up to 9 months

**Mechanism of Action** Inhibits protein synthesis by binding with the 30S and possibly the 50S ribosomal subunit(s) of susceptible bacteria; may also cause alterations in the cytoplasmic membrane.

Additional proposed mechanism of low dose doxycycline (Periostat™): It has been shown to inhibit collagenase activity *in vitro*. Also, it has been shown that doxycycline reduces the elevated collagenase activity in the gingival crevicular fluid of patients with periodontal disease.

**Local Anesthetic/Vasoconstrictor Precautions** No information available to require special precautions

**Effects on Dental Treatment** Opportunistic "superinfection" with *Candida albicans*; tetracycline's are not recommended for use during pregnancy or in children ≤8 years of age since they have been reported to cause enamel hypoplasia and permanent teeth discoloration. The use of tetracycline's should only be used in these patients if other agents are contraindicated or alternative antimicrobials will not eradicate the organism. Long-term use associated with oral candidiasis.

**Other Adverse Effects**

>10%: Discoloration of teeth in children

<1%: Gastrointestinal: Nausea, diarrhea

Rare adverse effects of tetracyclines: Glossitis, vomiting, dysphagia, hepatotoxicity, esophageal ulceration (if capsule forms are taken before lying down), rash, anaphylaxis, exfoliative dermatitis, photosensitivity, exacerbations of SLE, hemolytic anemia, neutropenia and thrombocytopenia

Adverse effects in clinical trials with Periostat™ occurring at a frequency greater than placebo included common cold, nausea, dyspepsia, joint pain, diarrhea, rash, menstrual cramp, acid indigestion, pain, and bronchitis

**Contraindications** Hypersensitivity to doxycycline, tetracycline or any component; children <8 years of age; severe hepatic dysfunction

**Warnings/Precautions** Do not use during pregnancy - use of tetracyclines during tooth development may cause permanent discoloration of the teeth and enamel hypoplasia; prolonged use may result in superinfection, including oral or vaginal candidiasis; photosensitivity reaction may occur with this drug; avoid prolonged exposure to sunlight or tanning equipment

(Continued)

## Doxycycline *(Continued)*

Additional specific warnings for Periostat™: Effectiveness has not been established in patients with coexistent oral candidiasis; use with caution in patients with a history or predisposition to oral candidiasis

**Drug Interactions** Iron and bismuth subsalicylate may decrease doxycycline bioavailability; barbiturates, phenytoin, and carbamazepine decrease doxycycline's half-life; increased effect of warfarin. Concurrent use of tetracycline may render oral contraceptives less effective. Concurrent use of tetracycline and Penthrane® has been reported to result in fatal renal toxicity.

**Drug Uptake**

Absorption: Oral: 90% to 100%

Half-life, serum: 12-15 hours (usually increases to 22-24 hours with multiple dosing)

Time to peak serum concentration: Within 1.5-4 hours

Systemic absorption from dental subgingival gel may occur, but is limited by the slow rate of dissolution from this formulation over 7 days.

**Pregnancy Risk Factor** D

**Breast-feeding Considerations** May be taken while breast-feeding

**Dosage Forms**

Capsule, as hyclate:
- Periostat™: 20 mg
- Doxychel®, Vibramycin®: 50 mg
- Doxy®, Doxychel®, Vibramycin®: 100 mg

Capsule, coated pellets, as hyclate (Doryx®): 100 mg

Powder for injection, as hyclate (Doxy®, Doxychel®, Vibramycin® IV): 100 mg, 200 mg

Powder for oral suspension, as monohydrate (raspberry flavor) (Vibramycin®): 25 mg/5 mL (60 mL)

Syrup, as calcium (raspberry-apple flavor) (Vibramycin®): 50 mg/5 mL (30 mL, 473 mL)

Tablet, as hyclate
- Doxychel®: 50 mg
- Doxychel®, Vibra-Tabs®: 100 mg

**Dietary Considerations** May be taken with food, milk, or water

**Generic Available** Yes

**Selected Readings**

Golub LM, Ciancio S, Ramamurthy NS, et al, "Low-Dose Doxycycline Therapy: Effect on Gingival and Crevicular Fluid Collagenase Activity in Humans," *J Periodontal Res*, 1990, 25(6):321-30.

Golub LM, Lee HM, Greenwald RA, et al, "A Matrix Metalloproteinase Inhibitor Reduces Bone-Type Collagen Degradation Fragments and Specific Collagenases in Gingival Crevicular Fluid During Adult Periodontitis," *Inflamm Res*, 1997, 46(8):310-9.

Golub LM, Sorsa T, Lee HM, et al, "Doxycycline Inhibits Neutrophil (PMN)-Type Matrix Metalloproteinases in Human Adult Periodontitis Gingiva," *J Clin Periodontol*, 1995, 22(2):100-9.

Rams TE and Slots J, "Antibiotics in Periodontal Therapy: An Update," *Compendium*, 1992, 13(12):1130, 1132, 1134.

## Doxycycline Hyclate Periodontal Extended-Release Liquid

**U.S. Brand Names** Atridox™

**Therapeutic Category** Antibiotic, Tetracycline Derivative

**Use**

Dental: Treatment of periodontitis associated with presence of *Actinobacillus actinomycetemcomitans* (AA)

Atridox™ gel is indicated for the treatment of adult periodontitis for a gain in clinical attachment, reduction in probing depth, and reduction in bleeding on probing

**Usual Dosage** Adults: Subgingival application: Dose depends on size, shape and number of pockets treated. Contains 50 mg doxycycline per 500 mg of formulation in each final blended syringe product. Application may be repeated four months after initial treatment.

Atridox™ subgingival controlled-release product: The delivery system consists of 2 separate syringes in a single pouch. Syringe A contains 450 mg of a bioabsorbable polymer gel; syringe B contains doxycycline hyclate 50 mg. To prepare for instillation, couple syringe A to syringe B. Inject contents of syringe A (purple stripe) into syringe B, then push contents back into syringe A. Repeat this mixing cycle at a rate of one cycle per second for 100 cycles. If syringes are stored prior to use (a maximum of 3 days), repeat mixing cycle 10 times before use. After appropriate mixing, contents should be in syringe A. Holding syringes vertically, with syringe A at the bottom, pull back on the syringe A plunger, allowing contents to flow down barrel for several seconds. Uncouple syringes and attach enclosed blunt cannula to syringe A. Local anesthesia is not required for placement. Cannula tip may be bent to resemble periodontal probe and used to explore pocket. Express product from syringe until pocket is filled. To separate tip from formulation, turn tip towards the tooth and press against tooth surface to achieve separation. An appropriate dental instrument may be used to pack gel into the pocket. Pockets may be covered with either Coe-pak™ or Octyldent™ dental adhesive.

**Mechanism of Action** Inhibits protein synthesis by binding with the 30S and possibly the 50S ribosomal subunit(s) of susceptible bacteria; may also cause alterations in the cytoplasmic membrane

Doxycycline inhibits collagenase *in vitro* and has been shown to inhibit collagenase in the gingival crevicular fluid in adults with periodontitis

**Local Anesthetic/Vasoconstrictor Precautions** No information available to require special precautions

**Effects on Dental Treatment** Mechanical oral hygiene procedures (ie, toothbrushing, flossing) should be avoided in any treated area for 7 days

**Other Adverse Effects**

>10%: Discoloration of teeth in children

<1%: Gastrointestinal: Nausea, diarrhea

Rare adverse effects of tetracyclines: Glossitis, vomiting, dysphagia, hepatotoxicity, esophageal ulceration (if capsule forms are taken before lying down), rash, anaphylaxis, exfoliative dermatitis, photosensitivity, exacerbations of SLE, hemolytic anemia, neutropenia and thrombocytopenia

Doxycycline periodontal gel (Atridox™): The adverse effects reported in clinical trials were similar in incidence between doxycycline-containing product and vehicle alone. In addition, these effects were comparable to standard therapies including scaling and root planing or oral hygiene. Events associated with application reported with an incidence >1% included: gum discomfort (18.1%), toothache (14.3%), periodontal abscess (9.9%), tooth sensitivity (7.7%), broken tooth (5.1%), tooth mobility (2%), endodontic abscess (1.5%) and jaw pain (1.1%). Systemic adverse events included headache (27.3%), muscle aches (6.6%), diarrhea (3.3%), upset stomach (3.6%), and nausea (1.8%). Although there is no known relationship between doxycycline and hypertension, unspecified essential hypertension was noted in 1.6% of the doxycycline gel group, as compared to 0.2% in the vehicle group. Allergic reactions to the vehicle were also reported in two patients.

**Contraindications** Hypersensitivity to doxycycline, tetracycline or any component; children <8 years of age; severe hepatic dysfunction

**Warnings/Precautions** Do not use during pregnancy - use of tetracyclines during tooth development may cause permanent discoloration of the teeth and enamel hypoplasia; prolonged use may result in superinfection, including oral or vaginal candidiasis; photosensitivity reaction may occur with this drug; avoid prolonged exposure to sunlight or tanning equipment

Additional specific warnings for doxycycline gel (Atridox™) for subgingival application: This product has not been evaluated or tested in immunocompromised patients, in patients with oral candidiasis, or in conditions characterized by severe periodontal defects with little remaining periodontium. May result in overgrowth of nonsusceptible organisms, including fungi. Effects of treatment >6 months have not been evaluated. Has not been evaluated for use in regeneration of alveolar bone

**Drug Interactions** Iron and bismuth subsalicylate may decrease doxycycline bioavailability; barbiturates, phenytoin, and carbamazepine decrease doxycycline's half-life; increased effect of warfarin. Concurrent use of tetracycline may render oral contraceptives less effective. Concurrent use of tetracycline and Penthrane® has been reported to result in fatal renal toxicity.

**Drug Uptake** Systemic absorption from dental subgingival gel may occur, but is limited by the slow rate of dissolution from this formulation over 7 days.

**Pregnancy Risk Factor** D

**Dosage Forms** Gel, for subgingival application (Atridox™): 50 mg in each 500 mg of blended formulation; 2-syringe system contains doxycycline syringe (50 mg) and delivery system syringe (450 mg) along with a blunt cannula

**Dietary Considerations** May be taken with food, milk, or water

**Generic Available** No

- **D-Penicillamine** *see* Penicillamine *on page 772*
- **DPPC** *see* Colfosceril Palmitate *on page 275*
- **Dramamine® II [OTC]** *see* Meclizine *on page 620*
- **Dramamine® Oral [OTC]** *see* Dimenhydrinate *on page 335*
- **Dri-Ear® Otic [OTC]** *see* Boric Acid *on page 147*
- **Drisdol®** *see* Ergocalciferol *on page 380*
- **Dristan® Cold Caplets [OTC]** *see* Acetaminophen and Pseudoephedrine *on page 31*

- ♦ **Dristan® Long Lasting Nasal Solution [OTC]** *see* Oxymetazoline *on page 755*
- ♦ **Dristan® Saline Spray [OTC]** *see* Sodium Chloride *on page 920*
- ♦ **Dristan® Sinus Caplets [OTC]** *see* Pseudoephedrine and Ibuprofen *on page 864*
- ♦ **Drithocreme®** *see* Anthralin *on page 88*
- ♦ **Drithocreme® HP 1%** *see* Anthralin *on page 88*
- ♦ **Dritho-Scalp®** *see* Anthralin *on page 88*
- ♦ **Drixomed®** *see* Dexbrompheniramine and Pseudoephedrine *on page 309*
- ♦ **Drixoral® [OTC]** *see* Dexbrompheniramine and Pseudoephedrine *on page 309*
- ♦ **Drixoral® Cough & Congestion Liquid Caps [OTC]** *see* Pseudoephedrine and Dextromethorphan *on page 864*
- ♦ **Drixoral® Cough Liquid Caps [OTC]** *see* Dextromethorphan *on page 314*
- ♦ **Drixoral® Cough & Sore Throat Liquid Caps [OTC]** *see* Acetaminophen and Dextromethorphan *on page 30*
- ♦ **Drixoral® Non-Drowsy [OTC]** *see* Pseudoephedrine *on page 863*
- ♦ **Drixoral® Syrup [OTC]** *see* Brompheniramine and Pseudoephedrine *on page 154*


## Dronabinol (droe NAB i nol)

**Related Information**

Chemical Dependency and Smoking Cessation *on page 1158*

**U.S. Brand Names** Marinol®

**Therapeutic Category** Antiemetic

**Use** When conventional antiemetics fail to relieve the nausea and vomiting associated with cancer chemotherapy, AIDS-related anorexia

**Usual Dosage** Oral:

Children: NCI protocol recommends 5 mg/m² starting 6-8 hours before chemotherapy and every 4-6 hours after to be continued for 12 hours after chemotherapy is discontinued

Adults: 5 mg/m² 1-3 hours before chemotherapy, then give 5 mg/m²/dose every 2-4 hours after chemotherapy for a total of 4-6 doses/day; dose may be increased up to a maximum of 15 mg/m²/dose if needed (dosage may be increased by 2.5 mg/m² increments)

Appetite stimulant (AIDS-related): Initial: 2.5 mg twice daily (before lunch and dinner); titrate up to a maximum of 20 mg/day

**Mechanism of Action** Not well defined, probably inhibits the vomiting center in the medulla oblongata

**Local Anesthetic/Vasoconstrictor Precautions** No information available to require special precautions

**Effects on Dental Treatment** No effects or complications reported

**Other Adverse Effects**

>10%: Central nervous system: Drowsiness, dizziness, detachment, anxiety, difficulty concentrating, mood change

1% to 10%:

Cardiovascular: Orthostatic hypotension, tachycardia

Central nervous system: Depression, headache, vertigo, hallucinations, memory lapse, ataxia

Gastrointestinal: Dry mouth

Neuromuscular & skeletal: Paresthesia, weakness

<1%:

Cardiovascular: Syncope

Central nervous system: Nightmares, speech difficulties

Gastrointestinal: Diarrhea

Neuromuscular & skeletal: Muscular pains

Otic: Tinnitus

Miscellaneous: Sweating

**Drug Interactions** Increased toxicity (drowsiness) with alcohol, barbiturates, benzodiazepines

**Drug Uptake**

Absorption: Oral: Erratic

Serum half-life: 19-24 hours

Time to peak serum concentration: Within 2-3 hours

**Pregnancy Risk Factor** B

**Generic Available** Yes

## Droperidol (droe PER i dole)

**U.S. Brand Names** Inapsine®

**Therapeutic Category** Antiemetic; Antipsychotic Agent

**Use** Tranquilizer and antiemetic in surgical and diagnostic procedures; antiemetic for cancer chemotherapy; preoperative medication; has good antiemetic effect as well as sedative and antianxiety effects

**Usual Dosage** Titrate carefully to desired effect

Children 2-12 years:

Premedication: I.M.: 0.1-0.15 mg/kg; smaller doses may be sufficient for control of nausea or vomiting

Adjunct to general anesthesia: I.V. induction: 0.088-0.165 mg/kg

Nausea and vomiting: I.M., I.V.: 0.05-0.06 mg/kg/dose every 4-6 hours as needed

Adults:

Premedication: I.M.: 2.5-10 mg 30 minutes to 1 hour preoperatively

Adjunct to general anesthesia: I.V. induction: 0.22-0.275 mg/kg; maintenance: 1.25-2.5 mg/dose

Alone in diagnostic procedures: I.M.: Initial: 2.5-10 mg 30 minutes to 1 hour before; then 1.25-2.5 mg if needed

Nausea and vomiting: I.M., I.V.: 2.5-5 mg/dose every 3-4 hours as needed

**Mechanism of Action** Alters the action of dopamine in the CNS, at subcortical levels, to produce sedation; reduces emesis by blocking dopamine stimulation of the chemotrigger zone

**Local Anesthetic/Vasoconstrictor Precautions** Manufacturer's information states that droperidol may block vasopressor activity of epinephrine. This has not been observed during use of epinephrine as a vasoconstrictor in local anesthesia.

**Effects on Dental Treatment** Significant hypotension may occur, especially when the drug is administered parenterally; orthostatic hypotension is due to alpha-receptor blockade, the elderly are at greater risk for orthostatic hypotension

Tardive dyskinesia: Prevalence rate may be 40% in elderly; development of the syndrome and the irreversible nature are proportional to duration and total cumulative dose over time

Extrapyramidal reactions are more common in elderly with up to 50% developing these reactions after 60 years of age; drug-induced **Parkinson's syndrome** occurs often; **akathisia** is the most common extrapyramidal reaction in elderly

Increased confusion, memory loss, psychotic behavior, and agitation frequently occur as a consequence of anticholinergic effects

Antipsychotic associated sedation in nonpsychotic patients is extremely unpleasant due to feelings of depersonalization, derealization, and dysphoria

**Other Adverse Effects**

>10%:

Cardiovascular: Mild to moderate hypotension, tachycardia

Central nervous system: Postoperative drowsiness

1% to 10%:

Cardiovascular: Hypertension

Central nervous system: Extrapyramidal reactions

Respiratory: Respiratory depression

<1%:

Central nervous system: Dizziness, chills, shivering, postoperative hallucinations

Respiratory: Laryngospasm, bronchospasm

**Drug Interactions** Increased toxicity: CNS depressants, fentanyl and other analgesics increased blood pressure; conduction anesthesia decreased blood pressure; epinephrine decreased blood pressure; atropine, lithium

**Drug Uptake** Following parenteral administration:

Duration: 2-4 hours, may extend to 12 hours

Serum half-life: Adults: 2.3 hours

**Pregnancy Risk Factor** C

**Generic Available** Yes

- **Droxia®** *see* Hydroxyurea *on page 517*
- **Dr Scholl's Athlete's Foot [OTC]** *see* Tolnaftate *on page 997*
- **Dr Scholl's® Disk [OTC]** *see* Salicylic Acid *on page 900*
- **Dr Scholl's Maximum Strength Tritin [OTC]** *see* Tolnaftate *on page 997*
- **Dr Scholl's® Wart Remover [OTC]** *see* Salicylic Acid *on page 900*
- **Drugs Associated With Adverse Hematologic Effects** *see page 1270*
- **Dry Eyes® Solution [OTC]** *see* Artificial Tears *on page 97*
- **Dry Eye® Therapy Solution [OTC]** *see* Artificial Tears *on page 97*
- **Dryox® Gel [OTC]** *see* Benzoyl Peroxide *on page 130*
- **Dryox® Wash [OTC]** *see* Benzoyl Peroxide *on page 130*
- **DSMC Plus® [OTC]** *see* Docusate and Casanthranol *on page 347*

- **D-S-S® [OTC]** *see* Docusate *on page 346*
- **DSS With Casanthranol** *see* Docusate and Casanthranol *on page 347*
- **DTIC** *see* Dacarbazine *on page 292*
- **DTIC-Dome®** *see* Dacarbazine *on page 292*
- **Duadacin® Capsule [OTC]** *see* Chlorpheniramine, Phenylpropanolamine, and Acetaminophen *on page 236*
- **Dulcolax® [OTC]** *see* Bisacodyl *on page 141*
- **Dull-C® [OTC]** *see* Ascorbic Acid *on page 97*
- **DuoCet™ [5/500]** *see* Hydrocodone and Acetaminophen *on page 505*
- **Duo-Cyp® Injection** *see* Estradiol and Testosterone *on page 389*
- **DuoFilm® [OTC]** *see* Salicylic Acid *on page 900*
- **Duofilm® Solution** *see* Salicylic Acid and Lactic Acid *on page 900*
- **Duo-Medihaler® Aerosol** *see* Isoproterenol and Phenylephrine *on page 554*
- **DuoPlant® Gel [OTC]** *see* Salicylic Acid *on page 900*
- **Duo-Trach®** *see* Lidocaine *on page 586*
- **Duotrate®** *see* Pentaerythritol Tetranitrate *on page 777*
- **DuP 753** *see* Losartan *on page 603*
- **Duphalac®** *see* Lactulose *on page 571*
- **Duplex® T [OTC]** *see* Coal Tar *on page 270*
- **Duraclon® Injection** *see* Clonidine *on page 265*
- **Duradyne DHC® [5/500]** *see* Hydrocodone and Acetaminophen *on page 505*
- **Duraflor® Cavity Varnish** *see* Fluoride *on page 441*
- **Duragesic® Transdermal** *see* Fentanyl *on page 424*
- **Dura-Gest®** *see* Guaifenesin, Phenylpropanolamine, and Phenylephrine *on page 481*
- **Duralone®** *see* Methylprednisolone *on page 661*
- **Duramist® Plus [OTC]** *see* Oxymetazoline *on page 755*
- **Duramorph® Injection** *see* Morphine Sulfate *on page 688*
- **Duranest® With Epinephrine** *see* Etidocaine With Epinephrine *on page 411*
- **Duratest® Injection** *see* Testosterone *on page 961*
- **Duratestrin® Injection** *see* Estradiol and Testosterone *on page 389*
- **Durathate® Injection** *see* Testosterone *on page 961*
- **Duration® Nasal Solution [OTC]** *see* Oxymetazoline *on page 755*
- **Duratuss-G®** *see* Guaifenesin *on page 478*
- **Dura-Vent®** *see* Guaifenesin and Phenylpropanolamine *on page 480*
- **Dura-Vent/DA®** *see* Chlorpheniramine, Phenylephrine, and Methscopolamine *on page 235*
- **Duricef®** *see* Cefadroxil *on page 198*
- **Duvoid®** *see* Bethanechol *on page 139*
- **DV® Vaginal Cream** *see* Dienestrol *on page 324*
- **Dwelle® Ophthalmic Solution [OTC]** *see* Artificial Tears *on page 97*
- **Dyazide®** *see* Hydrochlorothiazide and Triamterene *on page 504*
- **Dycill®** *see* Dicloxacillin *on page 321*
- **Dyclone®** *see* Dyclonine *on this page*

## Dyclonine (DYE kloe neen)

**Related Information**

Oral Viral Infections *on page 1137*

**U.S. Brand Names** Dyclone®

**Therapeutic Category** Local Anesthetic, Oral

**Use**

Dental: Use topically for temporary relief of pain associated with oral mucosa

Medical: Local anesthetic prior to laryngoscopy, bronchoscopy, or endotracheal intubation

**Usual Dosage** Use the lowest dose needed to provide effective anesthesia

Children and Adults: Topical solution:

Mouth sores: 5-10 mL of 0.5% or 1% to oral mucosa (swab or swish and then spit) 3-4 times/day as needed; maximum single dose: 200 mg (40 mL of 0.5% solution or 20 mL of 1% solution)

Bronchoscopy: Use 2 mL of the 1% solution or 4 mL of the 0.5% solution sprayed onto the larynx and trachea every 5 minutes until the reflex has been abolished

**Mechanism of Action** Blocks impulses at peripheral nerve endings in skin and mucous membranes by altering cell membrane permeability to ionic transfer

**Local Anesthetic/Vasoconstrictor Precautions** No information available to require special precautions

**Effects on Dental Treatment** No effects or complications reported

**Other Adverse Effects** <1%:
Cardiovascular: Hypotension, bradycardia, cardiac arrest
Central nervous system: Excitation, drowsiness, nervousness, dizziness, seizures
Local: Slight irritation and stinging may occur when applied
Ocular: Blurred vision
Respiratory: Respiratory arrest
Miscellaneous: Allergic reactions

**Drug Interactions** No data reported
**Pregnancy Risk Factor** C
**Breast-feeding Considerations** No data reported
**Generic Available** No

- **Dymelor®** *see* Acetohexamide *on page 34*
- **Dymenate® Injection** *see* Dimenhydrinate *on page 335*
- **Dynabac®** *see* Dirithromycin *on page 342*
- **Dynacin® Oral** *see* Minocycline *on page 677*
- **DynaCirc®** *see* Isradipine *on page 558*
- **Dynafed®, Maximum Strength [OTC]** *see* Acetaminophen and Pseudoephedrine *on page 31*
- **Dyna-Hex® Topical [OTC]** *see* Chlorhexidine Gluconate *on page 225*
- **Dynapen®** *see* Dicloxacillin *on page 321*

## Dyphylline (DYE fi lin)

**U.S. Brand Names** Dilor®; Lufyllin®
**Therapeutic Category** Bronchodilator; Theophylline Derivative
**Synonyms** Dihydroxypropyl Theophylline
**Use** Bronchodilator in reversible airway obstruction due to asthma or COPD
**Usual Dosage**
Children: I.M.: 4.4-6.6 mg/kg/day in divided doses
Adults:
Oral: Up to 15 mg/kg 4 times/day, individualize dosage
I.M.: 250-500 mg, do not exceed total dosage of 15 mg/kg every 6 hours

**Local Anesthetic/Vasoconstrictor Precautions** No information available to require special precautions
**Effects on Dental Treatment** Do not prescribe any erythromycin product to patients taking theophylline products. Erythromycin will delay the normal metabolic inactivation of theophyllines leading to increased blood levels; this has resulted in nausea, vomiting and CNS restlessness
**Other Adverse Effects**
Uncommon at serum theophylline concentrations ≤20 mcg/mL
1% to 10%:
Cardiovascular: Tachycardia
Central nervous system: Nervousness, restlessness
Gastrointestinal: Nausea, vomiting
<1%:
Central nervous system: Insomnia, irritability, seizures
Dermatologic: Skin rash
Gastrointestinal: Gastric irritation
Neuromuscular & skeletal: Tremor
Miscellaneous: Allergic reactions

**Pregnancy Risk Factor** C
**Generic Available** Yes
**Comments** This drug is rarely used today. Requires a special laboratory measuring procedure rather than the standard theophylline assay. Saliva levels are approximately equal to 60% of plasma levels; charcoal-broiled foods may increase elimination, reducing half-life by 50%; cigarette smoking may require an increase of dosage by 50% to 100%. Because different salts of theophylline have different theophylline content, various salts are not equivalent.

- **Dyrenium®** *see* Triamterene *on page 1012*
- **Dyrexan-OD®** *see* Phendimetrazine *on page 788*
- **7E3** *see* Abciximab *on page 24*
- **Easprin®** *see* Aspirin *on page 100*

## Echothiophate Iodide (ek oh THYE oh fate EYE oh dide)

**U.S. Brand Names** Phospholine Iodide®
**Therapeutic Category** Antiglaucoma Agent; Ophthalmic Agent, Miotic
**Use** Reverses toxic CNS effects caused by anticholinergic drugs; used as miotic in treatment of glaucoma; accommodative esotropia
(Continued)

## Echothiophate Iodide *(Continued)*

**Usual Dosage** Adults:

Ophthalmic: Glaucoma: Instill 1 drop twice daily into eyes with 1 dose just prior to bedtime; some patients have been treated with 1 dose daily or every other day

Accommodative esotropia:

Diagnosis: Instill 1 drop of 0.125% once daily into both eyes at bedtime for 2-3 weeks

Treatment: Use lowest concentration and frequency which gives satisfactory response, with a maximum dose of 0.125% once daily, although more intensive therapy may be used for short periods of time

**Mechanism of Action** Produces miosis and changes in accommodation by inhibiting cholinesterase, thereby preventing the breakdown of acetylcholine; acetylcholine is, therefore, allowed to continuously stimulate the iris and ciliary muscles of the eye

**Local Anesthetic/Vasoconstrictor Precautions** No information available to require special precautions

**Effects on Dental Treatment** No effects or complications reported

**Other Adverse Effects**

1% to 10%: Ocular: Stinging, burning, myopia, visual blurring

<1%:

Cardiovascular: Bradycardia, hypotension, flushing

Gastrointestinal: Nausea, vomiting, diarrhea

Ocular: Retinal detachment, muscle weakness, browache, miosis, twitching eyelids, watering eyes

Respiratory: Dyspnea

Miscellaneous: Sweating

**Drug Interactions** Increased toxicity: Carbamate or organophosphate insecticides and pesticides; succinylcholine; systemic acetylcholinesterases may increase neuromuscular effects

**Drug Uptake**

Onset of action:

Miosis: 10-30 minutes

Intraocular pressure decrease: 4-8 hours

Peak intraocular pressure decrease: 24 hours

Duration: Up to 1-4 weeks

**Pregnancy Risk Factor** C

**Generic Available** No

♦ **E-Complex-600® [OTC]** *see* Vitamin E *on page 1050*

## Econazole (e KONE a zole)

**U.S. Brand Names** Spectazole™

**Canadian Brand Names** Ecostatin®

**Therapeutic Category** Antifungal Agent, Topical

**Use** Topical treatment of tinea pedis (athlete's foot), tinea cruris (jock itch), tinea corporis (ringworm), tinea versicolor, and cutaneous candidiasis

**Usual Dosage** Children and Adults: Topical:

Tinea pedis, tinea cruris, tinea corporis, tinea versicolor: Apply sufficient amount to cover affected areas once daily

Cutaneous candidiasis: Apply sufficient quantity twice daily (morning and evening)

Duration of treatment: Candidal infections and tinea cruris, versicolor, and corporis should be treated for 2 weeks and tinea pedis for 1 month; occasionally, longer treatment periods may be required

**Mechanism of Action** Alters fungal cell wall membrane permeability; may interfere with RNA and protein synthesis, and lipid metabolism

**Local Anesthetic/Vasoconstrictor Precautions** No information available to require special precautions

**Effects on Dental Treatment** No effects or complications reported

**Other Adverse Effects** 1% to 10%: Local: Pruritus, erythema, burning, stinging

**Drug Interactions** No data reported

**Drug Uptake** Absorption: Topical: <10%

**Pregnancy Risk Factor** C

**Dosage Forms** Cream: 1% in water miscible base (15 g, 30 g, 85 g)

**Generic Available** No

♦ **Econopred®** *see* Prednisolone *on page 832*

♦ **Econopred® Plus** *see* Prednisolone *on page 832*

♦ **Ecotrin® [OTC]** *see* Aspirin *on page 100*

♦ **Ecotrin® Low Adult Strength [OTC]** *see* Aspirin *on page 100*

♦ **Ed A-Hist® Liquid** *see* Chlorpheniramine and Phenylephrine *on page 232*

◆ **Edathamil Disodium** *see* Edetate Disodium *on this page*

◆ **Edecrin®** *see* Ethacrynic Acid *on page 395*

## Edetate Calcium Disodium

(ED e tate KAL see um dye SOW dee um)

**U.S. Brand Names** Calcium Disodium Versenate®

**Therapeutic Category** Antidote, Lead Toxicity

**Synonyms** Calcium Disodium Edetate; Calcium EDTA

**Use** Treatment of acute and chronic lead poisoning; used as an aid in the diagnosis of lead poisoning

**Usual Dosage**

Children: I.M. (preferred route of administration as rapid I.V. infusion may be lethal), I.V., S.C.:

**Asymptomatic lead poisoning:** (Blood lead concentration >55 mcg/dL or blood lead concentrations of 25-55 mcg/dL with blood erythrocyte protoporphyrin concentrations ≥35 mcg/dL and positive mobilization test) or **symptomatic lead poisoning without encephalopathy** with lead level <100 mcg/dL: 1 g/m²/day I.M./I.V. in divided doses every 8-12 hours for 3-5 days (usually 5 days) with dimercaprol; maximum: 1 g/24 hours or 50 mg/kg/day

**Symptomatic lead poisoning with encephalopathy** with lead level >100 mcg/dL (treatment with calcium EDTA and dimercaprol is preferred): 250 mg/m² I.M. or intermittent I.V. infusion 4 hours after dimercaprol, then at 4-hour intervals thereafter for 5 days (1.5 g/m²/day); dose (1.5 g/m²/day) can also be given as a single I.V. continuous infusion over 12-24 hours/day for 5 days; maximum: 1 g/24 hours or 75 mg/kg/day

**Note:** Course of therapy may be repeated in 2-3 weeks until blood lead level is normal

Adults: Treatment: I.M., I.V.: 2-4 g/day or 1.5 g/m²/day in divided doses every 12-24 hours for 5 days; may repeat course one time after at least 2 days (usually after 2 weeks) not more than 2 courses of therapy are recommended

**Mechanism of Action** Calcium is displaced by divalent and trivalent heavy metals, forming a nonionizing soluble complex that is excreted in urine

**Local Anesthetic/Vasoconstrictor Precautions** No information available to require special precautions

**Effects on Dental Treatment** No effects or complications reported

**Other Adverse Effects**

1% to 10%: Renal: Renal tubular necrosis

<1%:

Cardiovascular: Hypotension, arrhythmias

Central nervous system: Fever, headache, chills

Dermatologic: Skin lesions

Endocrine & metabolic: Hypercalcemia

Gastrointestinal: Nausea, vomiting

Hematologic: Transient marrow suppression

Local: Pain at injection site following I.M. injection, thrombophlebitis following I.V. infusion (when concentration >0.5%)

Neuromuscular & skeletal: Numbness, paresthesia

Ocular: Lacrimation

Renal: Proteinuria, microscopic hematuria

Respiratory: Sneezing, nasal congestion

**Contraindications** Severe renal disease, anuria

**Drug Interactions** Decreased effect: Do not use simultaneously with zinc insulin preparations; do not mix in the same syringe with dimercaprol

**Drug Uptake**

Absorption: I.M., S.C.: Well absorbed

Serum half-life:

I.M.: 1.5 hours

I.V.: 20 minutes

**Pregnancy Risk Factor** C

**Dosage Forms** Injection: 200 mg/mL (5 mL)

**Generic Available** No

## Edetate Disodium (ED e tate dye SOW dee um)

**U.S. Brand Names** Chealamide®; Disotate®; Endrate®

**Therapeutic Category** Antidote, Hypercalcemia; Chelating Agent, Parenteral

**Synonyms** Edathamil Disodium; EDTA; Sodium Edetate

**Use** Emergency treatment of hypercalcemia; control digitalis-induced cardiac dysrhythmias (ventricular arrhythmias)

**Usual Dosage** Hypercalcemia: I.V.:

(Continued)

## Edetate Disodium *(Continued)*

Children: 40-70 mg/kg/day slow infusion over 3-4 hours or more to a maximum of 3 g/24 hours; administer for 5 days and allow 5 days between courses of therapy

Adults: 50 mg/kg/day over 3 or more hours to a maximum of 3 g/24 hours; a suggested regimen of 5 days followed by 2 days without drug and repeated courses up to 15 total doses

**Mechanism of Action** Chelates with divalent or trivalent metals to form a soluble complex that is then eliminated in urine

**Local Anesthetic/Vasoconstrictor Precautions** No information available to require special precautions

**Effects on Dental Treatment** No effects or complications reported

**Other Adverse Effects**

Rapid I.V. administration or excessive doses may cause a sudden drop in serum calcium concentration which may lead to hypocalcemic tetany, seizures, arrhythmias, and death from respiratory arrest. Do **not** exceed recommended dosage and rate of administration.

1% to 10%: Gastrointestinal: Nausea, vomiting, abdominal cramps, diarrhea

<1%:

- Cardiovascular: Arrhythmias, transient hypotension, acute tubular necrosis
- Central nervous system: Seizures, fever, headache, tetany, chills
- Dermatologic: Eruptions, dermatologic lesions
- Endocrine & metabolic: Hypomagnesemia, hypokalemia
- Hematologic: Anemia
- Local: Thrombophlebitis, pain at the site of injection
- Neuromuscular & skeletal: Paresthesia may occur, back pain, muscle cramps
- Renal: Nephrotoxicity
- Respiratory: Death from respiratory arrest

**Contraindications** Severe renal failure or anuria

**Drug Interactions** Increased effect of insulin (edetate disodium may decrease blood glucose concentrations and reduce insulin requirements in diabetic patients treated with insulin)

**Drug Uptake** Serum half-life: 20-60 minutes

**Pregnancy Risk Factor** C

**Dosage Forms** Injection: 150 mg/mL (20 mL)

**Generic Available** Yes

**Comments** Sodium content of 1 g: 5.4 mEq

♦ **Edex® Injection** *see* Alprostadil *on page 51*
♦ **ED-SPAZ®** *see* Hyoscyamine *on page 519*
♦ **EDTA** *see* Edetate Disodium *on previous page*
♦ **E.E.S.® Oral** *see* Erythromycin *on page 383*

## Efavirenz

**U.S. Brand Names** Sustiva™

**Therapeutic Category** Non-nucleoside Reverse Transciptase Inhibitor

**Use** Treatment of HIV-1 infections in combination with at least two other antiretroviral agents; also has some activity against hepatitis B virus and herpes viruses

**Usual Dosage** Oral: Dosing at bedtime is recommended to limit central nervous system effects; should not be used as single-agent therapy

Children: Dosage is based on body weight

- 10 kg to <15 kg: 200 mg
- 15 kg to <20 kg: 250 mg
- 20 kg to <25 kg: 300 mg
- 25 kg to <32.5 kg: 350 mg
- 32.5 kg to <40 kg: 400 mg
- ≥40 kg: 600 mg

Adults: 600 mg once daily

**Local Anesthetic/Vasoconstrictor Precautions** No information available to require special precautions

**Effects on Dental Treatment** Dry mouth and taste disturbance in <2% of patients

**Other Adverse Effects**

1% to 10%:

- Central nervous system: Dizziness (2% to 10%), inability to concentrate (0% to 9%), insomnia (0% to 7%), headache (5% to 6%) abnormal dreams (0% to 4%), somnolence (0% to 3%), depression (0% to 2%), anorexia (0% to 5%), nervousness (0% to 2%), fatigue (2% to 7%), hypoesthesia (1% to 2%)
- Dermatologic: Rash (5% to 20%), pruritus (0% to 2%)

Gastrointestinal: Nausea (0% to 12%), vomiting (0% to 7%), diarrhea (2% to 12%), dyspepsia (0% to 4%), elevated transaminases (2% to 3%), abdominal pain (0% to 3%), flatulence (0% to 1%)
Genitourinary: Renal calculus (0% to 1%), hematuria (0% to 1%)
Miscellaneous: Increased sweating (0% to 2%)

<2%:
Cardiovascular: Edema (peripheral), syncope, flushing, palpitations, tachycardia
Central nervous system: Fever, pain, malaise, ataxia, depression, seizures, hallucinations, psychosis, depersonalization, amnesia, anxiety, apathy, emotional lability, agitation, confusion, euphoria, impaired coordination, migraine, speech disorder, vertigo
Dermatologic: Alopecia, eczema, folliculitis, skin exfoliation, urticaria
Endocrine & metabolic: Cholesterol and triglycerides (increased), hot flashes
Gastrointestinal: Pancreatitis, taste disturbance
Hepatic: Hepatitis
Local: Thrombophlebitis
Neuromuscular & skeletal: Asthenia, neuralgia, paresthesia, peripheral neuropathy, tremor, arthralgia, myalgia
Ocular: Abnormal vision, diplopia
Otic: Tinnitus
Respiratory: Asthma
Miscellaneous: Alcohol intolerance, allergic reaction, parosmia

Pediatric patients: Rash (40%), diarrhea (39%), fever (26%), cough (25%), nausea/vomiting (16%), central nervous system reactions (9%)

**Drug Interactions**

Increased effect: May inhibit cytochrome 450 isoenzyme 3A4, 2C9 and 2C19; coadministration with medications metabolized by these enzymes may lead to increased concentration-related effects. Astemizole, cisapride, midazolam, triazolam and ergot alkaloids may result in life-threatening toxicities. The AUC of nelfinavir is increased (20%); AUC of both ritonavir and efavirenz are increased by 20% during concurrent therapy. The AUC of ethinyl estradiol is increased 37% by efavirenz (clinical significance unknown). May increase effect of warfarin.

Decreased effect: May induce cytochrome P-450 isoenzyme 3A4. Other inducers of this enzyme (including phenobarbital, rifampin and rifabutin) may decrease serum concentrations of efavirenz. Concentrations of indinavir may be reduced; dosage increase to 1000 mg 3 times/day is recommended. Concentrations of saquinavir may be decreased (use as sole protease inhibitor is not recommended). Plasma concentrations of clarithromycin are decreased (clinical significance unknown). May decrease effect of warfarin.

**Drug Uptake**

Absorption: Increased 50% by fatty meals
Half-life: Single dose: 52-76 hours; after multiple doses: 40-55 hours
Time to peak concentration: 3-8 hours

**Pregnancy Risk Factor** C

**Dosage Forms** Capsule: 50 mg, 100 mg, 200 mg

**Dietary Considerations** Avoid high-fat meals when taking this medication. May be taken with or without food

- **Effer-K™** *see* Potassium Bicarbonate and Potassium Citrate, Effervescent *on page 821*
- **Effer-Syllium® [OTC]** *see* Psyllium *on page 865*
- **Effexor®** *see* Venlafaxine *on page 1043*
- **Efidac/24® [OTC]** *see* Pseudoephedrine *on page 863*

## Eflornithine (ee FLOR ni theen)

**U.S. Brand Names** Ornidyl® Injection

**Therapeutic Category** Antiprotozoal

**Synonyms** DFMO; Eflornithine Hydrochloride

**Use** Treatment of meningoencephalitic stage of *Trypanosoma brucei gambiense* infection (sleeping sickness)

**Usual Dosage** Adults: I.V. infusion: 100 mg/kg/dose given every 6 hours (over at least 45 minutes) for 14 days

**Mechanism of Action** Eflornithine exerts antitumor and antiprotozoal effects through specific, irreversible ("suicide") inhibition of the enzyme ornithine decarboxylase (ODC). ODC is the rate-limiting enzyme in the biosynthesis of putrescine, spermine, and spermidine, the major polyamines in nucleated cells. Polyamines are necessary for the synthesis of DNA, RNA, and proteins and are, therefore, necessary for cell growth and differentiation. Although many microorganisms and higher plants are able to produce polyamines from alternate biochemical pathways, all mammalian cells depend on ornithine decarboxylase

(Continued)

## Eflornithine *(Continued)*

to produce polyamines. Eflornithine inhibits ODC and rapidly depletes animal cells of putrescine and spermidine; the concentration of spermine remains the same or may even increase. Rapidly dividing cells appear to most susceptible to the effects of eflornithine.

**Local Anesthetic/Vasoconstrictor Precautions** No information available to require special precautions

**Effects on Dental Treatment** No effects or complications reported

**Other Adverse Effects**

>10%: Hematologic: Anemia, leukopenia, thrombocytopenia

1% to 10%:

Central nervous system: Seizures, dizziness
Dermatologic: Alopecia
Gastrointestinal: Vomiting, diarrhea
Hematologic: Eosinophilia
Otic: Hearing impairment

<1%:

Cardiovascular: Facial edema
Central nervous system: Headache
Gastrointestinal: Abdominal pain, anorexia
Neuromuscular & skeletal: Weakness

**Drug Uptake**

Absorption: Oral: ~60% readily absorbed
Half-life: 3-4 hours

**Pregnancy Risk Factor** C

**Generic Available** No

- **Eflornithine Hydrochloride** *see* Eflornithine *on previous page*
- **Efodine® [OTC]** *see* Povidone-Iodine *on page 827*
- **Efudex® Topical** *see* Fluorouracil *on page 443*
- **Elase-Chloromycetin® Topical** *see* Fibrinolysin and Desoxyribonuclease *on page 430*
- **Elase® Topical** *see* Fibrinolysin and Desoxyribonuclease *on page 430*
- **Elavil®** *see* Amitriptyline *on page 67*
- **Eldepryl®** *see* Selegiline *on page 908*
- **Eldercaps® [OTC]** *see* Vitamins, Multiple *on page 1051*
- **Eldopaque® [OTC]** *see* Hydroquinone *on page 514*
- **Eldopaque Forte®** *see* Hydroquinone *on page 514*
- **Eldoquin® [OTC]** *see* Hydroquinone *on page 514*
- **Eldoquin® Forte®** *see* Hydroquinone *on page 514*
- **Electrolyte Lavage Solution** *see* Polyethylene Glycol-Electrolyte Solution *on page 815*
- **Elimite™** *see* Permethrin *on page 785*
- **Elixophyllin®** *see* Theophylline *on page 969*
- **Elmiron®** *see* Pentosan Polysulfate Sodium *on page 781*
- **Elocon®** *see* Mometasone Furoate *on page 686*
- **Elspar®** *see* Asparaginase *on page 98*
- **Eltroxin™** *see* Levothyroxine *on page 585*
- **Emcyt®** *see* Estramustine *on page 389*
- **Emecheck® [OTC]** *see* Phosphorated Carbohydrate Solution *on page 800*
- **Emetrol® [OTC]** *see* Phosphorated Carbohydrate Solution *on page 800*
- **Emgel™ Topical** *see* Erythromycin, Topical *on page 386*
- **Eminase®** *see* Anistreplase *on page 87*
- **Emko® [OTC]** *see* Nonoxynol 9 *on page 728*
- **EMLA® Cream** *see* Lidocaine and Prilocaine *on page 589*
- **EMLA® Disc** *see* Lidocaine and Prilocaine *on page 589*
- **Empirin® [OTC]** *see* Aspirin *on page 100*
- **Empirin® With Codeine** *see* Aspirin and Codeine *on page 102*
- **Emulsoil® [OTC]** *see* Castor Oil *on page 196*
- **E-Mycin® Oral** *see* Erythromycin *on page 383*

## Enalapril (e NAL a pril)

**Related Information**

Cardiovascular Diseases *on page 1066*
Enalapril and Diltiazem *on page 368*
Enalapril and Felodipine *on page 368*

**U.S. Brand Names** Vasotec®

**Canadian Brand Names** Apo®-Enalapril

**Therapeutic Category** Angiotensin-Converting Enzyme (ACE) Inhibitor

**Use** Management of mild to severe hypertension and congestive heart failure

**Unlabeled use:** Hypertensive crisis, diabetic nephropathy, rheumatoid arthritis, diagnosis of anatomic renal artery stenosis, hypertension secondary to scleroderma renal crisis, diagnosis of aldosteronism, idiopathic edema, Bartter's syndrome, postmyocardial infarction for prevention of ventricular failure

**Usual Dosage** Use lower listed initial dose in patients with hyponatremia, hypovolemia, severe congestive heart failure, decreased renal function, or in those receiving diuretics

Children:

Investigational initial oral doses of **enalapril**: 0.1 mg/kg/day increasing as needed over 2 weeks to 0.5 mg/kg/day have been used to treat severe congestive heart failure in infants

Investigational I.V. doses of **enalaprilat**: 5-10 mcg/kg/dose administered every 8-24 hours have been used for the treatment of neonatal hypertension; monitor patients carefully; select patients may require higher doses

Adults:

Oral: **Enalapril**

Hypertension: 2.5-5 mg/day then increase as required, usual therapeutic dose for hypertension: 10-40 mg/day in 1-2 divided doses; usual therapeutic dose for heart failure: 5-20 mg/day

Heart failure: As adjunct with diuretics and digitalis, initiate with 2.5 mg once or twice daily (usual range: 5-20 mg/day in 2 divided doses; maximum: 40 mg)

Asymptomatic left ventricular dysfunction: 2.5 mg twice daily, titrated as tolerated to 20 mg/day

I.V.: **Enalaprilat**

Hypertension: 1.25 mg/dose, given over 5 minutes every 6 hours; doses as high as 5 mg/dose every 6 hours have been tolerated for up to 36 hours. **Note:** If patients are concomitantly receiving diuretic therapy, begin with 0.625 mg I.V. over 5 minutes; if the effect is not adequate after 1 hour, repeat the dose and administer 1.25 mg at 6-hour intervals thereafter; if adequate, administer 0.625 mg I.V. every 6 hours

Conversion from I.V. to oral therapy if not concurrently on diuretics: 5 mg once daily; subsequent titration as needed; if concurrently receiving diuretics and responding to 0.625 mg I.V. every 6 hours, initiate with 2.5 mg/day

**Mechanism of Action** Competitive inhibitor of angiotensin-converting enzyme (ACE); prevents conversion of angiotensin I to angiotensin II, a potent vasoconstrictor; results in lower levels of angiotensin II which causes an increase in plasma renin activity and a reduction in aldosterone secretion

**Local Anesthetic/Vasoconstrictor Precautions** No information available to require special precautions

**Effects on Dental Treatment** No effects or complications reported

**Drug-Drug Interactions With ACEIs**

| Precipitant Drug | Drug (Category) and Effect | Description |
|---|---|---|
| Antacids | ACE Inhibitors: decreased | Decreased bioavailability of ACEIs. May be more likely with captopril. Separate administration times by 1-2 hours. |
| NSAIDs (indomethacin) | ACEIs: decreased | Reduced hypotensive effects of ACEIs. More prominent in low renin or volume dependent hypertensive patients. |
| Phenothiazines | ACEIs: increased | Pharmacologic effects of ACEIs may be increased. |
| ACEIs | Allopurinol: increased | Higher risk of hypersensitivity reaction possible when given concurrently. Three case reports of Stevens-Johnson syndrome with captopril. |
| ACEIs | Digoxin: increased | Increased plasma digoxin levels. |
| ACEIs | Lithium: increased | Increased serum lithium levels and symptoms of toxicity may occur. |
| ACEIs | Potassium preps/ potassium sparing diuretics increased | Coadministration may result in elevated potassium levels. |

**Other Adverse Effects**

1% to 10%:

Cardiovascular: Chest pain, palpitations, tachycardia, syncope

(Continued)

## Enalapril *(Continued)*

Central nervous system: Insomnia, headache dizziness, fatigue, malaise
Dermatologic: Rash
Gastrointestinal: Dysgeusia, abdominal pain, vomiting, nausea, diarrhea, anorexia, constipation
Neuromuscular & skeletal: Paresthesia, weakness
Respiratory: Bronchitis, cough, dyspnea

<1%:

Cardiovascular: Angina pectoris, flushing
Dermatologic: Alopecia, erythema multiforme, pruritus, Stevens-Johnson syndrome, urticaria, angioedema
Endocrine & metabolic: Hypoglycemia, hyperkalemia
Genitourinary: Impotence
Hematologic: Agranulocytosis, neutropenia, anemia
Neuromuscular & skeletal: Myalgia
Ocular: Blurred vision
Otic: Tinnitus
Renal: Oliguria
Respiratory: Asthma, bronchospasm
Miscellaneous: Sweating

**Drug Interactions** See table.

**Drug Uptake**

Oral:

Onset of action: ~1 hour
Duration: 12-24 hours

Absorption: Oral: 55% to 75%

Serum half-life:

Enalapril: Adults:

Healthy: 2 hours
With congestive heart failure: 3.4-5.8 hours

Enalaprilat:

Infants 6 weeks to 8 months: 6-10 hours
Adults: 35-38 hours

Time to peak serum concentration: Oral:

Enalapril: Within 0.5-1.5 hours
Enalaprilat (active): Within 3-4.5 hours

**Pregnancy Risk Factor** C (first trimester); D (second and third trimesters)

**Generic Available** No

## Enalapril and Diltiazem (e NAL a pril & dil TYE a zem)

**U.S. Brand Names** Teczem®

**Therapeutic Category** Antihypertensive Agent, Combination

**Use** Combination drug for treatment of hypertension

**Local Anesthetic/Vasoconstrictor Precautions** No information available to require special precautions

**Effects on Dental Treatment** Calcium channel blockers cause gingival hyperplasia in approximately 1% of patients. There have been fewer reports with felodipine than with other CCBs. The hyperplasia will disappear with cessation of drug therapy. Consultation with physician is suggested.

**Dosage Forms** Tablet, extended release: Enalapril maleate 5 mg and diltiazem maleate 180 mg

**Generic Available** No

## Enalapril and Felodipine (e NAL a pril & fe LOE di peen)

**U.S. Brand Names** Lexxel™

**Therapeutic Category** Antihypertensive Agent, Combination

**Use** Treatment of hypertension

**Usual Dosage** Adults: Oral: 1 tablet daily

**Mechanism of Action** See individual agents

**Local Anesthetic/Vasoconstrictor Precautions** No information available to require special precautions

**Effects on Dental Treatment** Calcium channel blockers cause gingival hyperplasia in approximately 1% of patients. There have been fewer reports with felodipine than with other CCBs. The hyperplasia will disappear with cessation of drug therapy. Consultation with physician is suggested.

**Other Adverse Effects** See individual agents

**Drug Interactions** See individual agents

**Dosage Forms** Tablet, extended release: Enalapril maleate 5 mg and felodipine 5 mg

## Enalapril and Hydrochlorothiazide
(e NAL a pril & hye droe klor oh THYE a zide)

**Related Information**

Cardiovascular Diseases *on page 1066*

**U.S. Brand Names** Vaseretic® 5-12.5; Vaseretic® 10-25

**Canadian Brand Names** Vaseretic®

**Therapeutic Category** Antihypertensive Agent, Combination

**Use** Treatment of hypertension

**Usual Dosage** Oral: Dose is individualized

**Local Anesthetic/Vasoconstrictor Precautions** No information available to require special precautions

**Effects on Dental Treatment** No effects or complications reported

**Pregnancy Risk Factor** C (first trimester); D (second and third trimesters)

**Generic Available** No

- **Enbrel®** *see* Etanercept *on page 395*

## Encainide (en KAY nide)

**Related Information**

Cardiovascular Diseases *on page 1066*

**U.S. Brand Names** Enkaid®

**Therapeutic Category** Antiarrhythmic Agent, Class I-C; Antiarrhythmic Agent (Supraventricular & Ventricular)

**Use** Ventricular arrhythmias; supraventricular arrhythmias

**Usual Dosage** Adults: Oral: 25 mg every 8 hours; may increase to 35 mg every 8 hours after 3-5 days if needed; increase to 50 mg every 8 hours in another 3-5 days if response is not achieved

**Local Anesthetic/Vasoconstrictor Precautions** No information available to require special precautions

**Effects on Dental Treatment** No effects or complications reported

**Other Adverse Effects**

>10%:

Central nervous system: Dizziness

Ocular: Blurred vision

1% to 10%:

Central nervous system: Headache

Cardiovascular: Chest pain congestive heart failure, ventricular tachycardia

Gastrointestinal: Vomiting

Neuromuscular & skeletal: Weakness

Otic: Tinnitus

<1%: Neuromuscular & skeletal: Tremor

**Pregnancy Risk Factor** B

**Generic Available** No

**Comments** Based on adverse outcomes noted with encainide in the CAST trial, the FDA recommends that use of encainide be limited to patients with life-threatening ventricular arrhythmias

- **Encare® [OTC]** *see* Nonoxynol 9 *on page 728*
- **Endal®** *see* Guaifenesin and Phenylephrine *on page 480*
- **End Lice® Liquid [OTC]** *see* Pyrethrins *on page 867*
- **Endocrine Disorders & Pregnancy** *see page 1082*
- **Endolor®** *see* Butalbital Compound *on page 163*
- **Endolor®** *see* Butalbital Compound and Acetaminophen *on page 164*
- **Endrate®** *see* Edetate Disodium *on page 363*
- **Enduron®** *see* Methyclothiazide *on page 657*
- **Enduronyl®** *see* Methyclothiazide and Deserpidine *on page 657*
- **Enduronyl® Forte** *see* Methyclothiazide and Deserpidine *on page 657*
- **Engerix-B®** *see* Hepatitis B Vaccine *on page 495*
- **Enhanced-potency Inactivated Poliovirus Vaccine** *see* Poliovirus Vaccine, Inactivated *on page 813*
- **Enisyl® [OTC]** *see* L-Lysine *on page 597*
- **Enkaid®** *see* Encainide *on this page*
- **Enomine®** *see* Guaifenesin, Phenylpropanolamine, and Phenylephrine *on page 481*
- **Enovid®** *see* Mestranol and Norethynodrel *on page 641*

## Enoxacin (en OKS a sin)

**U.S. Brand Names** Penetrex™

**Therapeutic Category** Antibiotic, Quinolone

(Continued)

## Enoxacin *(Continued)*

**Use** Treatment of complicated and uncomplicated urinary tract infections caused by susceptible gram-negative and gram-positive bacteria

**Usual Dosage** Adults: Oral: 400 mg twice daily

**Mechanism of Action** Exerts a broad spectrum antimicrobial effect. The primary target of the fluoroquinolones is DNA gyrase (topoisomerase II) an essential bacterial enzyme that maintains the superhelical structure of DNA. DNA gyrase is required for DNA replication and transcription, DNA repair, recombination, and transposition.

**Local Anesthetic/Vasoconstrictor Precautions** No information available to require special precautions

**Effects on Dental Treatment** No effects or complications reported

**Other Adverse Effects**

1% to 10%: Gastrointestinal: Nausea, vomiting

<1%:

- Central nervous system: Restlessness, dizziness, confusion, seizures, headache
- Dermatologic: Rash
- Gastrointestinal: Diarrhea, GI bleeding
- Hematologic: Anemia
- Hepatic: Elevated liver enzymes
- Neuromuscular & skeletal: Tremor, arthralgia
- Renal: Elevated serum creatinine and BUN, acute renal failure

**Drug Interactions**

Decreased effect with antacids (magnesium, aluminum), iron and zinc salts, sucralfate, bismuth salts

Increased toxicity/levels of warfarin, cyclosporine, digoxin, caffeine; increased levels with cimetidine

**Drug Uptake**

Absorption: 98%

Serum half-life: 3-6 hours (average)

**Pregnancy Risk Factor** C

**Generic Available** No

## Enoxaparin (e noks ah PAIR in)

**U.S. Brand Names** Lovenox®

**Therapeutic Category** Anticoagulant (Other)

**Synonyms** Enoxaparin Sodium

**Use** Prophylaxis and treatment of thromboembolic disorders (deep vein thrombosis) which may lead to pulmonary embolism, following hip replacement therapy or total knee replacement; inpatient treatment of acute deep vein thrombosis with or without pulmonary embolism, when administered in conjunction with warfarin sodium, and outpatient treatment of acute deep vein thrombosis without pulmonary embolism when administered in conjunction with warfarin sodium

**Usual Dosage** S.C.:

Children: In one dose-finding study, children >2 months of age required 1 mg/kg twice daily for treatment of thrombotic disease

Adults:

- Prophylaxis: 30 mg twice daily; first dose within 12 hours after orthopedic surgery and every 12 hours for 3 days (including day of surgery); after 3 days, switch to adjusted dose heparin
- A single daily dose of 40 mg has been found to be equally effective in patients undergoing orthopedic or gynecologic surgical procedures
- Abdominal surgery: 40 mg once daily; first dose beginning 2 hours before surgery and continuing for a maximum of 12 days (usual: 10 days)
- Treatment of DVT: 1 mg/kg twice daily

**Mechanism of Action** Standard heparin consists of components with molecular weights ranging from 4000 to 30,000 daltons with a mean of 16,000 daltons. Heparin acts as an anticoagulant by enhancing the inhibition rate of clotting proteases by antithrombin III impairing normal hemostasis and inhibition of factor Xa. Low molecular weight heparins have a small effect on the activated partial thromboplastin time and strongly inhibit factor Xa. Enoxaparin is derived from porcine heparin that undergoes benzylation followed by alkaline depolymerization. The average molecular weight of enoxaparin is 4500 daltons which is distributed as (≤20%) 2000 daltons, (≥68%) 2000-8000 daltons, and (≤15%) >8000 daltons. Enoxaparin has a higher ratio of anti-factor Xa to anti-factor IIa activity than unfractionated heparin.

**Local Anesthetic/Vasoconstrictor Precautions** No information available to require special precautions

**Effects on Dental Treatment** No effects or complications reported

**Other Adverse Effects**
1% to 10%:
Central nervous system: Fever, confusion, pain
Dermatologic: Erythema, bruising
Gastrointestinal: Nausea
Hematologic: Hemorrhage, thrombocytopenia, hypochromic anemia, hematoma
Local: Irritation

At the recommended doses, single injections of enoxaparin do not significantly influence platelet aggregation or affect global clotting time (ie, prothrombin time or activated partial thromboplastin time)

**Warnings/Precautions** Do not administer intramuscularly; use with extreme caution in patients with a history of heparin-induced thrombocytopenia; bacterial endocarditis, hemorrhagic stroke, recent CNS or ophthalmological surgery, bleeding diathesis, uncontrolled arterial hypertension, or a history of recent gastrointestinal ulceration and hemorrhage. Elderly and patients with renal insufficiency may show delayed elimination of enoxaparin; avoid use in lactation.

**Drug Interactions** Increased toxicity with oral anticoagulants, platelet inhibitors

**Drug Uptake**
Onset of effect: Maximum antifactor Xa and antithrombin (antifactor IIa) activities occur 3-5 hours after S.C. administration
Duration: Following a 40 mg dose, significant antifactor Xa activity persists in plasma for ~12 hours
Half-life, plasma: Low molecular weight heparin is 2-4 times longer than standard heparin independent of the dose

**Pregnancy Risk Factor** B

**Dosage Forms** Injection, as sodium, preservative free: 30 mg/0.3 mL; 40 mg/0.4 mL

**Generic Available** No

- **Enoxaparin Sodium** *see* Enoxaparin *on previous page*
- **Ensure® [OTC]** *see* Enteral Nutritional Products *on this page*
- **Ensure Plus® [OTC]** *see* Enteral Nutritional Products *on this page*

## Enteral Nutritional Products

**U.S. Brand Names** Carnation Instant Breakfast® [OTC]; Citrotein® [OTC]; Criticare HN® [OTC]; Ensure® [OTC]; Ensure Plus® [OTC]; Isocal® [OTC]; Magnacal® [OTC]; Microlipid™ [OTC]; Osmolite® HN [OTC]; Pedialyte® [OTC]; Polycose® [OTC]; Portagen® [OTC]; Pregestimil® [OTC]; Propac™ [OTC]; Soyalac® [OTC]; Vital HN® [OTC]; Vitaneed™ [OTC]; Vivonex® [OTC]; Vivonex® T.E.N. [OTC]

**Canadian Brand Names** Citrisource®; Citrotein®; Glucerna™; Isocal® with Fibre; Isosource®; Nutrisource™; Optifast® 900; Palmocare®; Pediasure™; Resource®; Sandosource™ Peptide; Sustacal®; Tolerex®; Travasol®; Vital® HN; Vivonex® Plus

**Therapeutic Category** Nutritional Supplement

**Synonyms** Dietary Supplements

**Local Anesthetic/Vasoconstrictor Precautions** No information available to require special precautions

**Effects on Dental Treatment** No effects or complications reported

**Dosage Forms**
Liquid (Magnacal®): Calcium and sodium caseinate, maltodextrin, sucrose, partially hydrogenated soy oil, soy lecithin
Powder (Vivonex® T.E.N.): Amino acids, predigested carbohydrates, safflower oil

**Generic Available** Yes

- **Entertainer's Secret® Spray [OTC]** *see* Saliva Substitute *on page 901*
- **Entex®** *see* Guaifenesin, Phenylpropanolamine, and Phenylephrine *on page 481*
- **Entex® LA** *see* Guaifenesin and Phenylpropanolamine *on page 480*
- **Entex® PSE** *see* Guaifenesin and Pseudoephedrine *on page 481*
- **Enulose®** *see* Lactulose *on page 571*
- **Enzone®** *see* Pramoxine and Hydrocortisone *on page 828*

## Ephedrine (e FED rin)

**U.S. Brand Names** Kondon's Nasal® [OTC]; Pretz-D® [OTC]

**Therapeutic Category** Adrenergic Agonist Agent

**Use** Treatment of bronchial asthma, nasal congestion, acute bronchospasm, idiopathic orthostatic hypotension

**Usual Dosage**
Children:
Oral, S.C.: 3 mg/kg/day or 25-100 mg/m²/day in 4-6 divided doses every 4-6 hours

(Continued)

## Ephedrine *(Continued)*

I.M., slow I.V. push: 0.2-0.3 mg/kg/dose every 4-6 hours

Adults:

Oral: 25-50 mg every 3-4 hours as needed

I.M., S.C.: 25-50 mg, parenteral adult dose should not exceed 150 mg in 24 hours

I.V.: 5-25 mg/dose slow I.V. push repeated after 5-10 minutes as needed, then every 3-4 hours not to exceed 150 mg/24 hours

**Mechanism of Action** Releases tissue stores of epinephrine and thereby produces an alpha- and beta-adrenergic stimulation; longer acting and less potent than epinephrine

**Local Anesthetic/Vasoconstrictor Precautions** Use vasoconstrictors with caution since ephedrine may enhance cardiostimulation and vasopressor effects of sympathomimetics such as epinephrine

**Effects on Dental Treatment** No effects or complications reported

**Other Adverse Effects**

>10%: Central nervous system: CNS stimulating effects, nervousness, anxiety, apprehension, fear, tension, agitation, excitation, restlessness, irritability, insomnia, hyperactivity

1% to 10%:

Cardiovascular: Hypertension, tachycardia, palpitations, elevation or depression of blood pressure, unusual pallor

Central nervous system: Dizziness, headache

Gastrointestinal: Dry mouth, nausea, anorexia, GI upset, vomiting

Genitourinary: Painful urination

Neuromuscular & skeletal: Trembling, tremor (more common in the elderly), weakness

Miscellaneous: Increased sweating

<1%:

Cardiovascular: Chest pain, arrhythmias

Respiratory: Dyspnea

**Drug Interactions**

Decreased effect: Alpha- and beta-adrenergic blocking agents decrease ephedrine vasopressor effects

Increased toxicity: Additive cardiostimulation with other sympathomimetic agents; theophylline leads to cardiostimulation; MAO inhibitors or atropine lead to increased blood pressure; cardiac glycosides or general anesthetics lead to increased cardiac stimulation

**Drug Uptake** Oral:

Duration of action: 3-6 hours

Serum half-life: 2.5-3.6 hours

**Pregnancy Risk Factor** C

**Generic Available** Yes

♦ **Ephedrine, Theophylline and Phenobarbital** *see* Theophylline, Ephedrine, and Phenobarbital *on page 974*

♦ **E-Pilo-x® Ophthalmic** *see* Pilocarpine and Epinephrine *on page 804*

♦ **Epinal®** *see* Epinephryl Borate *on page 376*

## Epinephrine (ep i NEF rin)

**Related Information**

Dental Drug Interactions: Update on Drug Combinations Requiring Special Considerations *on page 1225*

Respiratory Diseases *on page 1079*

**Therapeutic Category** Adrenergic Agonist Agent; Antidote, Hypersensitivity Reactions; Antiglaucoma Agent; Bronchodilator

**Use** Treatment of bronchospasms, anaphylactic reactions, cardiac arrest, management of open-angle (chronic simple) glaucoma

**Usual Dosage**

Bronchodilator:

Children: S.C.: 10 mcg/kg (0.01 mL/kg of 1:1000) (single doses not to exceed 0.5 mg); injection suspension (1:200): 0.005 mL/kg/dose (0.025 mg/kg/dose) to a maximum of 0.15 mL (0.75 mg for single dose) every 8-12 hours

Adults:

I.M., S.C. (1:1000): 0.1-0.5 mg every 10-15 minutes to 4 hours

Suspension (1:200) S.C.: 0.1-0.3 mL (0.5-1.5 mg)

I.V.: 0.1-0.25 mg (single dose maximum: 1 mg)

Cardiac arrest:
Children: Asystole or pulseless arrest:
I.V., intraosseous: First dose: 0.01 mg/kg (0.1 mL/kg of a 1:10,000 solution); subsequent doses: 0.1 mg/kg (0.1 mL/kg of a 1:1000 solution); doses as high as 0.2 mg/kg may be effective; repeat every 3-5 minutes
Intratracheal: 0.1 mg/kg (0.1 mL/kg of a 1:1000 solution); doses as high as 0.2 mg/kg may be effective
Adults: Asystole:
I.V.: 1 mg every 3-5 minutes; if this approach fails, alternative regimens include: Intermediate: 2-5 mg every 3-5 minutes; Escalating: 1 mg, 3 mg, 5 mg at 3-minute intervals; High: 0.1 mg/kg every 3-5 minutes
Intratracheal: Although optimal dose is unknown, doses of 2-2.5 times the I.V. dose may be needed

Bradycardia: Children:
I.V.: 0.01 mg/kg (0.1 mL/kg of 1:10,000 solution) every 3-5 minutes as needed (maximum: 1 mg/10 mL)
Intratracheal: 0.1 mg/kg (0.1 mL/kg of 1:1000 solution every 3-5 minutes); doses as high as 0.2 mg/kg may be effective

Refractory hypotension (refractory to dopamine/dobutamine): I.V. infusion administration requires the use of an infusion pump:
Children: Infusion rate 0.1-4 mcg/kg/minute
Adults: I.V. infusion: 1 mg in 250 mL NS/$D_5W$ at 0.1-1 mcg/kg/minute; titrate to desired effect

Hypersensitivity reaction:
Children: S.C.: 0.01 mg/kg every 15 minutes for 2 doses then every 4 hours as needed (single doses not to exceed 0.5 mg)
Adults: I.M., S.C.: 0.2-0.5 mg every 20 minutes to 4 hours (single dose maximum: 1 mg)

Nebulization:
Children <2 years: 0.25 mL of 1:1000 diluted in 3 mL NS with treatments ordered individually
Children >2 years and Adolescents: 0.5 mL of 1:1000 concentration diluted in 3 mL NS
Children >2 years and Adults (racemic epinephrine):
<10 kg: 2 mL of 1:8 dilution over 15 minutes every 1-4 hours
10-15 kg: 2 mL of 1:6 dilution over 15 minutes every 1-4 hours
15-20 kg: 2 mL of 1:4 dilution over 15 minutes every 1-4 hours
>20 kg: 2 mL of 1:3 dilution over 15 minutes every 1-4 hours
Adults: Instill 8-15 drops into nebulizer reservoirs; administer 1-3 inhalations 4-6 times/day

Ophthalmic: Instill 1-2 drops in eye(s) once or twice daily

Intranasal: Children ≥6 years and Adults: Apply locally as drops or spray or with sterile swab

**Mechanism of Action** Stimulates alpha-, $beta_1$-, and $beta_2$-adrenergic receptors resulting in relaxation of smooth muscle of the bronchial tree, cardiac stimulation, and dilation of skeletal muscle vasculature; small doses can cause vasodilation via $beta_2$-vascular receptors; large doses may produce constriction of skeletal and vascular smooth muscle; decreases production of aqueous humor and increases aqueous outflow; dilates the pupil by contracting the dilator muscle

**Local Anesthetic/Vasoconstrictor Precautions** No information available to require special precautions

**Effects on Dental Treatment** No effects or complications reported

**Other Adverse Effects**
>10%:
Cardiovascular: Tachycardia (parenteral), pounding heartbeat
Central nervous system: Nervousness, restlessness
1% to 10%:
Cardiovascular: Flushing, hypertension, unusual pallor
Central nervous system: Headache, dizziness, lightheadedness, insomnia
Gastrointestinal: Nausea, vomiting
Neuromuscular & skeletal: Trembling, weakness
Miscellaneous: Increased sweating

**Contraindications** Hypersensitivity to epinephrine or any component; cardiac arrhythmias, angle-closure glaucoma

**Warnings/Precautions** Use with caution in elderly patients, patients with diabetes mellitus, cardiovascular diseases (angina, tachycardia, myocardial infarction), thyroid disease, or cerebral arteriosclerosis, Parkinson's; some products contain sulfites as antioxidants. Rapid I.V. infusion may cause death from cerebrovascular hemorrhage or cardiac arrhythmias. Oral inhalation of epinephrine is **not** the preferred route of administration.
(Continued)

## Epinephrine *(Continued)*

**Drug Interactions** Increased cardiac irritability if administered concurrently with halogenated inhalational anesthetics, beta-blocking agents, alpha-blocking agents

**Drug Uptake**

Onset of bronchodilation:

Subcutaneous: Within 5-10 minutes

Inhalation: Within 1 minute

Conjunctival instillation:

Onset of effect: Intraocular pressures fall within 1 hour

Peak effect: Within 4-8 hours

Duration of ocular effect: 12-24 hours

Absorption: Orally ingested doses are rapidly metabolized in the GI tract and liver; pharmacologically active concentrations are not achieved

**Pregnancy Risk Factor** C

**Breast-feeding Considerations** No data reported

**Dosage Forms**

Aerosol, oral:

Bitartrate (AsthmaHaler®, Bronitin®, Medihaler-Epi®, Primatene® Suspension): 0.3 mg/spray [epinephrine base 0.16 mg/spray] (10 mL, 15 mL, 22.5 mL)

Bronkaid®: 0.5% (10 mL, 15 mL, 22.5 mL)

Primatene®: 0.2 mg/spray (15 mL, 22.5 mL)

Auto-injector:

EpiPen®: Delivers 0.3 mg I.M. of epinephrine 1:1000 (2 mL)

EpiPen® Jr.: Delivers 0.15 mg I.M. of epinephrine 1:2000 (2 mL)

Injection (Adrenalin®): 0.01 mg/mL [1:100,000] (5 mL); 0.1 mg/mL [1:10,000] (3 mL, 10 mL); 1 mg/mL [1:1000] (1 mL, 2 mL, 30 mL)

Solution:

Inhalation:

Adrenalin®: 1% [10 mg/mL, 1:100] (7.5 mL)

AsthmaNefrin®, microNefrin®, Nephron®: Racepinephrine 2% [epinephrine base 1.125%] (7.5 mL, 15 mL, 30 mL)

Vaponefrin®: Racepinephrine 2% [epinephrine base 1%] (15 mL, 30 mL)

Nasal (Adrenalin®): 0.1% [1 mg/mL, 1:1000] (30 mL)

Ophthalmic, as base (Epifrin®): 0.5% (15 mL); 1% (15 mL); 2% (15 mL)

Ophthalmic, as hydrochloride: 0.1% (1 mL)

Glaucon®: 1% (10 mL); 2% (10 mL)

Topical (Adrenalin®): 0.1% [1 mg/mL, 1:1000] (30 mL, 10 mL)

Suspension for injection (Sus-Phrine®): 5 mg/mL [1:200] (0.3 mL, 5 mL)

**Dietary Considerations** No data reported

**Generic Available** Yes

## Epinephrine (Dental) (ep i NEF rin DEN tal)

**Related Information**

Dental Drug Interactions: Update on Drug Combinations Requiring Special Considerations *on page 1225*

Respiratory Diseases *on page 1079*

**U.S. Brand Names** Adrenalin®; Sus-Phrine®

**Therapeutic Category** Adrenergic Agonist Agent; Antidote, Hypersensitivity Reactions

**Use** Dental: Emergency drug for treatment of anaphylactic reactions; used as vasoconstrictor to prolong local anesthesia

**Usual Dosage** Hypersensitivity reaction:

Children: S.C.: 0.01 mg/kg every 15 minutes for 2 doses then every 4 hours as needed (single doses not to exceed 0.5 mg)

Adults: I.M., S.C.: 0.2-0.5 mg every 20 minutes to 4 hours (single dose maximum: 1 mg)

**Mechanism of Action** Stimulates alpha-, $beta_1$-, and $beta_2$-adrenergic receptors resulting in relaxation of smooth muscle of the bronchial tree, cardiac stimulation, and dilation of skeletal muscle vasculature; small doses can cause vasodilation via $beta_2$-vascular receptors; large doses may produce constriction of skeletal and vascular smooth muscle; decreases production of aqueous humor and increases aqueous outflow; dilates the pupil by contracting the dilator muscle

**Local Anesthetic/Vasoconstrictor Precautions** No information available to require special precautions

**Effects on Dental Treatment** No effects or complications reported

**Other Adverse Effects** No data reported

**Contraindications** Hypersensitivity to epinephrine or any component; cardiac arrhythmias, angle-closure glaucoma

**Warnings/Precautions** Use with caution in elderly patients, patients with diabetes mellitus, cardiovascular diseases (angina, tachycardia, myocardial infarction), thyroid disease, or cerebral arteriosclerosis, Parkinson's; some products contain sulfites as antioxidants. Rapid I.V. infusion may cause death from cerebrovascular hemorrhage or cardiac arrhythmias. Oral inhalation of epinephrine is **not** the preferred route of administration.

**Drug Interactions** Increased cardiac irritability if administered concurrently with halogenated inhalational anesthetics, beta-blocking agents, alpha-blocking agents

**Drug Uptake** Absorption: Not absorbed orally

**Pregnancy Risk Factor** C

**Breast-feeding Considerations** Usual infiltration doses of epinephrine given to nursing mothers has not been shown to affect the health of the nursing infant

**Dosage Forms**

Injection:

Adrenalin®: 0.01 mg/mL [1:100,000] (5 mL); 0.1 mg/mL [1:10,000] (3 mL, 10 mL); 1 mg/mL [1:1000] (1 mL, 2 mL, 30 mL)

Suspension (Sus-Phrine®): 5 mg/mL [1:200] (0.3 mL, 5 mL)

Solution, topical (Adrenalin®): 0.1% [1 mg/mL, 1:1000] (30 mL, 10 mL)

**Dietary Considerations** No data reported

**Generic Available** Yes

## Epinephrine, Racemic (ep i NEF rin, ra SEE mik)

**U.S. Brand Names** AsthmaNefrin®; microNefrin®; Nephron®; S-2®; Vaponefrin®

**Therapeutic Category** Vasoconstrictor

**Local Anesthetic/Vasoconstrictor Precautions** No information available to require special precautions

**Effects on Dental Treatment** No effects or complications reported

**Other Adverse Effects** No data reported

**Drug Interactions** No data reported

**Drug Uptake**

Absorption: Not absorbed orally

Onset of bronchodilation:

Subcutaneous: Within 5-10 minutes

Inhalation: Within 1 minute

**Breast-feeding Considerations** No data reported

**Dosage Forms** Solution, inhalation:

AsthmaNefrin®, microNefrin®, Nephron®, S-2®: Racepinephrine 2.25% [epinephrine base 1.125%] (7.5 mL, 15 mL, 30 mL)

Vaponefrin®: Racepinephrine 2% [epinephrine base 1%] (15 mL, 30 mL)

**Dietary Considerations** No data reported

**Generic Available** Yes

## Epinephrine, Racemic and Aluminum Potassium Sulfate

(ep i NEF rin, ra SEE mik and a LOO mi num poe TASS ee um SUL fate)

**U.S. Brand Names** Van R Gingibraid®

**Therapeutic Category** Astringent; Vasoconstrictor

**Use**

Dental: Gingival retraction

Medical: None

**Usual Dosage** Pass the impregnated yarn around the neck of the tooth and place into gingival sulcus; normal tissue moisture, water, or gingival retraction solutions activate impregnated yarn. Limit use to one quadrant of the mouth at a time; recommended use is for 3-8 minutes in the mouth.

**Mechanism of Action** Epinephrine stimulates $alpha_1$ adrenergic receptors to cause vasoconstriction in blood vessels in gingiva; aluminum potassium sulfate, precipitates tissue and blood proteins

**Local Anesthetic/Vasoconstrictor Precautions** No information available to require special precautions

**Effects on Dental Treatment** Tissue retraction around base of the tooth (therapeutic effect)

**Other Adverse Effects** No data reported

**Contraindications** Patients with cardiovascular disease, hyperthyroidism, or diabetes; patients sensitive to epinephrine; do not apply to areas of heavy or deep bleeding or over exposed bone

**Warnings/Precautions** Caution should be exercised whenever using gingival retraction cords with epinephrine since it delivers vasoconstrictor doses of racemic epinephrine to patients; the general medical history should be thoroughly evaluated before using in any patient

**Drug Interactions** No data reported

**Drug Uptake** No data reported

(Continued)

## Epinephrine, Racemic and Aluminum Potassium Sulfate *(Continued)*

**Breast-feeding Considerations** No data reported

**Dosage Forms** Yarn, saturated in solution of 8% racemic epinephrine and 7% aluminum potassium sulfate; yarn labeled type "0e" contains 0.20±0.10 mg epinephrine per inch; "1e" contains 0.40±0.20 mg per inch; "2e" contains 0.60±0.20 mg per inch

**Dietary Considerations** No data reported

**Generic Available** No

## Epinephryl Borate (ep i NEF ril BOR ate)

**U.S. Brand Names** Epinal®

**Therapeutic Category** Adrenergic Agonist Agent, Ophthalmic; Antiglaucoma Agent; Ophthalmic Agent, Vasoconstrictor

**Use** Reduces elevated intraocular pressure in chronic open-angle glaucoma

**Usual Dosage** Adults: Ophthalmic: Instill 1 drop into the eyes once or twice daily

**Local Anesthetic/Vasoconstrictor Precautions** No information available to require special precautions

**Effects on Dental Treatment** No effects or complications reported

**Generic Available** No

- **Epitol®** *see* Carbamazepine *on page 185*
- **Epivir®** *see* Lamivudine *on page 571*
- **Epivir®-HBV™** *see* Lamivudine *on page 571*
- **EPO** *see* Epoetin Alfa *on this page*

## Epoetin Alfa (e POE e tin AL fa)

**U.S. Brand Names** Epogen®; Procrit®

**Canadian Brand Names** Eprex®

**Therapeutic Category** Recombinant Human Erythropoietin

**Synonyms** EPO; Erythropoietin; *r*HuEPO-α

**Use** Anemia associated with end-stage renal disease; anemia related to therapy with AZT-treated HIV-infected patients; anemia in cancer patients receiving chemotherapy; anemia of prematurity

**Usual Dosage** Individuals with anemia due to iron deficiency, sickle cell disease, autoimmune hemolytic anemia, and bleeding, generally have appropriate endogenous EPO levels to drive erythropoiesis and would not ordinarily be candidates for EPO therapy.

In patients on dialysis, epoetin alfa usually has been administered as an IVP 3 times/week. While the administration is independent of the dialysis procedure, it may be administered into the venous line at the end of the dialysis procedure to obviate the need for additional venous access; in patients with CRF not on dialysis, epoetin alfa may be given either as an IVP or S.C. injection.

**Children and Adults: Dosing recommendations:**

Dosing schedules need to be individualized and careful monitoring of patients receiving the drug is mandatory

*r*HuEPO-α may be ineffective if other factors such as iron or $B_{12}$/folate deficiency limit marrow response

IVP, S.C.:

**Chronic renal failure patients:**

**Initial dose:** 50-100 units/kg 3 times/week

**Dose should be reduced** when the hematocrit reaches the target range of 30% to 36% or a hematocrit increase >4% points over any 2-week period

**Dose should be held** if the hematocrit exceeds 36% and until the hematocrit decreases to the target range (30% to 36%).

**Dose should be increased** not more frequently than once a month, unless clinically indicated. After any dose adjustment, the hematocrit should be determined twice weekly for at least 2-6 weeks. If a hematocrit increase of 5-6 points is not achieved after a 8-week period and iron stores are adequate, the dose may be incrementally increased. Further increases may be made at 4-6 week intervals until the desired response is obtained.

**Maintenance dose:** Should be individualized to maintain the hematocrit within the 30% to 33% target range. The median maintenance dose in phase III studies in chronic renal failure patients on dialysis was 75 units/kg 3 times/week (range 12.5-525 units/kg 3 times/week).

Epoetin doses of 75-150 units/kg/week have been shown to maintain hematocrits of 36% to 38% for up to 6 months in patients with chronic renal failure not requiring dialysis

**Zidovudine-treated HIV patients:** Prior to beginning epoetin alfa, serum erythropoietin levels should be determined. Available evidence suggest that patients receiving zidovudine with endogenous serum erythropoietin levels >500 mIU/mL are unlikely to respond to therapy with epoetin alfa.

**Initial dose:** For patients with serum erythropoietin levels <500 mIU/mL who are receiving a dose of zidovudine ≤4,200 mg/week: 100 units/kg 3 times/week for 8 weeks.

**Dose should be held** if the hematocrit is >40% until the hematocrit drops to 36%. The dose should be reduced by 25% when the treatment is resumed and then titrated to maintain the desired hematocrit.

**Dose should be reduced** if the initial dose of epoetin alfa includes a rapid rise in hematocrit (>4% points in any 2-week period).

**Increase dose** by 50-100 units/kg if the response is not satisfactory in terms of reducing transfusion requirements or increasing hematocrit after 8 weeks of therapy. Response should be evaluated every 4-8 weeks thereafter and the dose adjusted and the dose adjusted accordingly by 50-100 units/kg increments 3 times/week. If patients have not responded satisfactorily to a dose of 300 units/kg 3 times/week, it is unlikely that they will respond to higher doses.

**Maintenance dose:** Dose should be titrated to maintain target hematocrit range: 36% to 40%

**Cancer patients on chemotherapy:** Although no specific serum erythropoietin level can be stipulated above which patients would be unlikely to respond to epoetin alfa therapy, treatment of patients with grossly elevated serum erythropoietin levels (>200 mIU/mL) is not recommended

**Initial dose:** 150 units/kg 3 times/week

**Increase dose:** Response should be evaluated every 8 weeks thereafter and the dose adjusted and the dose adjusted accordingly by 50-100 units/kg increments 3 times/week up to 300 units/kg 3 times/week if the response is not satisfactory. If patients have not responded satisfactorily to a dose of 300 units/kg 3 times/week, it is unlikely that they will respond to higher doses.

**Dose should be held** if the hematocrit is >40% until the hematocrit drops to 36%. The dose should be reduced by 25% when the treatment is resumed and then titrated to maintain the desired hematocrit.

**Dose should be reduced** if the initial dose of epoetin alfa includes a rapid rise in hematocrit (>4% points in any 2-week period), the dose should be reduced

**Maintenance dose:** Dose should be titrated to maintain target hematocrit range: 36% to 40%

**Mechanism of Action** Induces erythropoiesis by stimulating the division and differentiation of committed erythroid progenitor cells; induces the release of reticulocytes from the bone marrow into the blood stream, where they mature to erythrocytes. There is a dose response relationship with this effect. This results in an increase in reticulocyte counts followed by a rise in hematocrit and hemoglobin levels.

**Local Anesthetic/Vasoconstrictor Precautions** No information available to require special precautions

**Effects on Dental Treatment** No effects or complications reported

**Other Adverse Effects**

1% to 10%:
- Cardiovascular: Hypertension, chest pain, edema
- Central nervous system: Fatigue, headache, dizziness, seizures
- Dermatologic: Rash
- Gastrointestinal: Nausea, vomiting, diarrhea
- Hematologic: Clotted access
- Neuromuscular & skeletal: Arthralgias, weakness

<1%:
- Cardiovascular: Myocardial infarction, CVA/TIA
- Miscellaneous: Hypersensitivity reactions

**Drug Uptake**

Onset of action: Several days

Peak effect: 2-3 weeks

Serum half-life: Circulating: 4-13 hours in patients with chronic renal failure; 20% shorter in patients with normal renal function

Time to peak serum concentrations: S.C.: 2-8 hours

**Pregnancy Risk Factor** C

**Generic Available** No

**Comments** Epogen® reimbursement hotline number for information regarding coverage of epoetin alfa is 1-800-2-PAY-EPO. ProCrit™ reimbursement hotline is 1-800-441-1366.

♦ **Epogen®** *see* Epoetin Alfa *on previous page*

## Epoprostenol (e poe PROST en ole)

**U.S. Brand Names** Flolan® Injection

**Therapeutic Category** Antihypertensive Agent; Platelet Aggregation Inhibitor

(Continued)

## Epoprostenol *(Continued)*

**Use** Long-term intravenous treatment of primary pulmonary hypertension (PPH)

**Usual Dosage** I.V.: The drug is administered by continuous intravenous infusion via a central venous catheter using an ambulatory infusion pump; during dose ranging it may be administered peripherally

**Acute dose ranging:** The initial infusion rate should be 2 ng/kg/minute by continuous I.V. and increased in increments of 2 ng/kg/minute every 15 minutes or longer until dose-limiting effects are elicited (such as chest pain, anxiety, dizziness, changes in heart rate, dyspnea, nausea, vomiting, headache, hypotension and/or flushing)

**Continuous chronic infusion:** Initial: 4 ng/kg/minute **less** than the maximum-tolerated infusion rate determined during acute dose ranging.

If maximum-tolerated infusion rate is <5 ng/kg/minute the chronic infusion rate should be 1/2 the maximum-tolerated acute infusion rate

**Dosage adjustments:** Dose adjustments in the chronic infusion rate should be based on persistence, recurrence or worsening of patient symptoms of pulmonary hypertension

If symptoms persist or recur after improving, the infusion rate should be increased by 1-2 ng/kg/minute increments, every 15 minutes or greater; following establishment of a new chronic infusion rate, the patient should be observed and vital signs monitored.

**Preparation of Infusion**

| To make 100 mL of solution with concentration: | Directions: |
|---|---|
| 3000 ng/mL | Dissolve one 0.5 mg vial with 6 mL supplied diluent, withdraw 3 mL and add to sufficient diluent to make a total of 100 mL |
| 5000 ng/mL | Dissolve one 0.5 mg vial with 5 mL supplied diluent, withdraw entire vial contents and add a sufficient volume of diluent to make a total of 100 mL |
| 10,000 ng/mL | Dissolve two 0.5 mg vials each with 5 mL supplied diluent, withdraw entire vial contents and add a sufficient volume of diluent to make a total of 100 mL |
| 15,000 ng/mL | Dissolve one 1.5 mg vial with 5 mL supplied diluent, withdraw entire vial contents and add a sufficient volume of diluent to make a total of 100 mL |

**Local Anesthetic/Vasoconstrictor Precautions** No information available to require special precautions

**Effects on Dental Treatment** No effects or complications reported

**Drug Uptake**

Steady state levels are reached in about 15 minutes with continuous infusions

Serum half-life: 2.7-6 minutes

**Pregnancy Risk Factor** X

**Generic Available** No

## Eprosartan (ep roe SAR tan)

**U.S. Brand Names** Teveten®

**Therapeutic Category** Angiotensin II Antagonist

**Use** For use in the management of essential hypertension

**Usual Dosage** Oral: 400-800 mg once daily, or 200-400 mg twice daily

**Mechanism of Action** Angiotensin II is formed from angiotensin I in a reaction catalyzed by angiotensin-converting enzyme (ACE, kininase II). Angiotensin II is the principal pressor agent of the renin-angiotensin system, with effects that include vasoconstriction, stimulation of synthesis and release of aldosterone, cardiac stimulation, and renal reabsorption of sodium. Eprosartan blocks the vasoconstrictor and aldosterone-secreting effects of angiotensin II by selectively blocking the binding of angiotensin II to the AT1 receptor in many tissues, such as vascular smooth muscle and the adrenal gland. Its action is therefore independent of the pathways for angiotensin II synthesis. Blockade of the renin-angiotensin system with ACE inhibitors, which inhibit the biosynthesis of angiotensin II from angiotensin I, is widely used in the treatment of hypertension. ACE inhibitors also inhibit the degradation of bradykinin, a reaction also catalyzed by ACE. Because eprosartan does not inhibit ACE (kininase II), it does not affect the response to bradykinin. Whether this difference has clinical relevance is not yet known. Eprosartan does not bind to or block other hormone receptors or ion channels known to be important in cardiovascular regulation.

**Local Anesthetic/Vasoconstrictor Precautions** No information available to require special precautions

**Effects on Dental Treatment** No effects or complications reported

**Drug Uptake**

Half-life: 5-7 hours

Time to peak serum concentration: 1-3 hours; clearance: 7.9 L/hour

- **Epsom Salts** *see* Magnesium Sulfate *on page 613*
- **EPT** *see* Teniposide *on page 956*

## Eptifibatide (ep TIF i ba tide)

**Related Information**

Cardiovascular Diseases *on page 1066*

**U.S. Brand Names** Integrilin®

**Therapeutic Category** Platelet Aggregation Inhibitor

**Use** Treatment of patients with acute coronary syndrome (UA/NQMI), including patients who are to be managed medically and those undergoing percutaneous coronary intervention (PCI); it has been shown to decrease the rate of a combined endpoint of death or new myocardial infarction. For the treatment of patients undergoing PCI, it has been shown to decrease the rate of a combined endpoint of death, new myocardial infarction, or need for urgent intervention.

**Usual Dosage** Adults: I.V.:

Acute coronary syndrome: Bolus of 180 mcg/kg as soon as possible following diagnosis, followed by a continuous infusion of 2 mcg/kg/minute until hospital discharge or initiation of CABG surgery, up to 72 hours. If a patient is to undergo a percutaneous coronary intervention (PCI) while receiving eptifibatide, consideration can be given to decreasing the infusion rate to 0.5 mcg/kg/minute (the infusion rate in IMPACT II) at the time of the procedure. Infusion should be continued for an additional 20-24 hours after the procedure, allowing for up to 96 hours of therapy.

Percutaneous coronary intervention (PCI) in patients not presenting with an acute coronary syndrome: Bolus of 135 mcg/kg administered immediately before the initiation of PCI followed by a continuous infusion of 0.5 mcg/kg/minute for 20-24 hours. In the IMPACT II Study, there was little experience in patients weighing more than 143 kg.

**Mechanism of Action** Eptifibatide is a cyclic heptapeptide which blocks the glycoprotein IIb/IIa receptor, the binding site for fibrinogen, von Willebrand factor, and other ligands. Inhibition of binding at this final common receptor reversibly blocks platelet aggregation and prevents thrombosis.

**Local Anesthetic/Vasoconstrictor Precautions** No information available to require special precautions

**Effects on Dental Treatment** Bleeding may occur while patient is medicated with eptifibatide. Platelet function is restored in about 4 hours following discontinuation.

**Other Adverse Effects** Bleeding is the major drug-related adverse effect. TIMI criteria for major bleeding events correspond to a decrease in hemoglobin >5 g/dL or intracranial bleeding. Criteria for minor bleeding events include: 1) spontaneous bleeding observed as gross hematurias or hematemesis, 2) observed blood loss (spontaneous or nonspontaneous) with a decrease in hemoglobin >3 g/dL accompanied by coffee ground emesis, heme-positive melena, retroperitoneal bleeding, or hematoma, or 3) patients with a decrease in hemoglobin >4 g/dL with no bleeding site identified. Major bleeding was reported in 4.4% to 10.5%, minor bleeding was reported in 10.5% to 14.2%, bleeding which required transfusion was reported in 5.5% to 12.8%.

Cardiovascular: Hypotension
Local: Injection site reaction
Neuromuscular & skeletal: Back pain

1% to 10%: Hematologic: Thrombocytopenia (2.8% to 3.2%)
<1%:
- Central nervous system: Intracranial hemorrhage (0.5% to 0.7%)
- Miscellaneous: Anaphylaxis (0.4% to 0.6%)

**Drug Interactions** Drugs which affect hemostasis: Thrombolytics, oral anticoagulants, nonsteroidal anti-inflammatory agents, dipyridamole, ticlopidine, clopidogrel; avoid concomitant use of other IIb/IIIA inhibitors

**Drug Uptake**

Onset of action: Within 1 hour

Half-life: 2.5 hours

Reversibility: Platelet function is restored in about 4 hours following discontinuation

**Pregnancy Risk Factor** B

**Generic Available** No

- **Equagesic®** *see* Aspirin and Meprobamate *on page 103*
- **Equalactin® Chewable Tablet [OTC]** *see* Calcium Polycarbophil *on page 177*
- **Equanil®** *see* Meprobamate *on page 635*
- **Equilet® [OTC]** *see* Calcium Carbonate *on page 172*
- **Ercaf®** *see* Ergotamine *on page 382*
- **Ergamisol®** *see* Levamisole *on page 579*

## Ergocalciferol (er goe kal SIF e role)

**U.S. Brand Names** Calciferol™; Drisdol®

**Canadian Brand Names** Ostoforte®; Radiostol®

**Therapeutic Category** Vitamin D Analog

**Use** Treatment of refractory rickets, hypophosphatemia, hypoparathyroidism

**Usual Dosage** Oral dosing is preferred

Dietary supplementation (each mcg = 40 USP units):
- Healthy Children: 10 mcg/day (400 units)
- Adults: 10 mcg/day (400 units)

Renal failure:
- Children: 100-1000 mcg/day (4000-40,000 units)
- Adults: 500 mcg/day (20,000 units)

Hypoparathyroidism:
- Children: 1.25-5 mg/day (50,000-200,000 units) and calcium supplements
- Adults: 625 mcg to 5 mg/day (25,000-200,000 units) and calcium supplements

Vitamin D-dependent rickets:
- Children: 75-125 mcg/day (3000-5000 units); maximum: 1500 mcg/day
- Adults: 250 mcg to 1.5 mg/day (10,000-60,000 units)

Nutritional rickets and osteomalacia:
- Children and Adults (with normal absorption): 25-125 mcg/day (1000-5000 units)
- Children with malabsorption: 250-625 mcg/day (10,000-25,000 units)
- Adults with malabsorption: 250-7500 mcg (10,000-300,000 units)

Vitamin D-resistant rickets:
- Children: Initial: 1000-2000 mcg/day (40,000-80,000 units) with phosphate supplements; daily dosage is increased at 3- to 4-month intervals in 250-500 mcg (10,000-20,000 units) increments
- Adults: 250-1500 mcg/day (10,000-60,000 units) with phosphate supplements

**Mechanism of Action** Stimulates calcium and phosphate absorption from the small intestine, promotes secretion of calcium from bone to blood; promotes renal tubule phosphate resorption

**Local Anesthetic/Vasoconstrictor Precautions** No information available to require special precautions

**Effects on Dental Treatment** No effects or complications reported

**Other Adverse Effects**

1% to 10%:
- Cardiovascular: Hypotension, cardiac arrhythmias, hypertension
- Central nervous system: Irritability, headache
- Dermatologic: Pruritus
- Endocrine & metabolic: Polydipsia
- Gastrointestinal: Nausea, vomiting, anorexia, pancreatitis, metallic taste
- Neuromuscular & skeletal: Bone pain, myalgia
- Ocular: Conjunctivitis, photophobia
- Renal: Polyuria

<1%:
- Central nervous system: Overt psychosis
- Gastrointestinal: Weight loss

**Drug Interactions**

Decreased effect: Cholestyramine, colestipol, mineral oil causes decreased oral absorption

Increased effect: Thiazide diuretics causes increased vitamin D effects

Increased toxicity: Cardiac glycosides causes increased toxicity

**Drug Uptake**

Peak effect: In ~1 month following daily doses

Absorption: Readily absorbed from GI tract; absorption requires intestinal presence of bile

**Pregnancy Risk Factor** A (C if dose exceeds RDA recommendation)

**Generic Available** Yes

## Ergoloid Mesylates (ER goe loid MES i lates)

**U.S. Brand Names** Germinal®; Hydergine®; Hydergine® LC

**Therapeutic Category** Ergot Alkaloid and Derivative

**Use** Treatment of cerebrovascular insufficiency in primary progressive dementia, Alzheimer's dementia, and senile onset

**Usual Dosage** Adults: Oral: 1 mg 3 times/day up to 4.5-12 mg/day; up to 6 months of therapy may be necessary

**Mechanism of Action** Ergoloid mesylates do not have the vasoconstrictor effects of the natural ergot alkaloids; exact mechanism in dementia is unknown; originally classed as peripheral and cerebral vasodilator, now considered a "metabolic enhancer"; there is no specific evidence which clearly establishes the mechanism by which ergoloid mesylate preparations produce mental effects, nor is there conclusive evidence that the drug particularly affects cerebral arteriosclerosis or cerebrovascular insufficiency

**Local Anesthetic/Vasoconstrictor Precautions** No information available to require special precautions

**Effects on Dental Treatment** No effects or complications reported

**Other Adverse Effects**

1% to 10%:

Gastrointestinal: Transient nausea

Miscellaneous: Sublingual irritation

<1%:

Cardiovascular: Bradycardia, orthostatic hypotension, flushing, syncope

Central nervous system: Headache

Dermatologic: Skin rash

Gastrointestinal: Anorexia, nausea, vomiting, stomach cramps

Ocular: Blurred vision

Respiratory: Nasal congestion

**Drug Interactions** Increased toxicity with dopamine

**Drug Uptake**

Absorption: Rapid yet incomplete

Serum half-life: 3.5 hours

Time to peak serum concentration: Within 1 hour

**Pregnancy Risk Factor** C

**Generic Available** Yes

♦ **Ergomar®** *see* Ergotamine *on next page*

♦ **Ergometrine Maleate** *see* Ergonovine *on this page*

## Ergonovine (er goe NOE veen)

**U.S. Brand Names** Ergotrate® Maleate

**Therapeutic Category** Ergot Alkaloid and Derivative

**Synonyms** Ergometrine Maleate

**Use** Prevention and treatment of postpartum and postabortion hemorrhage caused by uterine atony or subinvolution

**Usual Dosage** Adults:

Oral: 1-2 tablets (0.2-0.4 mg) every 6-12 hours for up to 48 hours

I.M., I.V. (I.V. should be reserved for emergency use only): 0.2 mg, repeat dose in 2-4 hours as needed

**Mechanism of Action** Ergot alkaloid alpha-adrenergic agonist directly stimulates vascular smooth muscle to vasoconstrict peripheral and cerebral vessels; may also have antagonist effects on serotonin

**Local Anesthetic/Vasoconstrictor Precautions** No information available to require special precautions

**Effects on Dental Treatment** No effects or complications reported

**Other Adverse Effects**

1% to 10%: Gastrointestinal: Nausea, vomiting

<1%:

Cardiovascular: Palpitations, bradycardia, transient chest pain, hypertension, cerebrovascular accidents

Central nervous system: Seizures, dizziness, headache

Local: Thrombophlebitis

Otic: Tinnitus

Respiratory: Dyspnea

Miscellaneous: Sweating

**Drug Interactions** No data reported

**Drug Uptake**

Onset of effect:

Oral: Within 5-15 minutes

I.M.: Within 2-5 minutes

Duration: Uterine effects persist for 3 hours, except when given I.V., then effects persist for ~45 minutes

**Pregnancy Risk Factor** X

**Generic Available** No

## Ergotamine (er GOT a meen)

**U.S. Brand Names** Cafatine®; Cafergot®; Cafetrate®; Ercaf®; Ergomar®; Wigraine®

**Canadian Brand Names** Ergomar®; Gynergen®

**Therapeutic Category** Adrenergic Blocking Agent; Ergot Alkaloid and Derivative

**Use** Abort or prevent vascular headaches, such as migraine or cluster

**Usual Dosage** Adults:

Oral:

Cafergot®: 2 tablets at onset of attack; then 1 tablet every 30 minutes as needed; maximum: 6 tablets per attack; do not exceed 10 tablets/week

Ergostat®: 1 tablet under tongue at first sign, then 1 tablet every 30 minutes, 3 tablets/24 hours, 5 tablets/week

Rectal (Cafergot® suppositories, Wigraine® suppositories, Cafatine® suppositories): 1 at first sign of an attack; follow with second dose after 1 hour, if needed; maximum dose: 2 per attack; do not exceed 5/week

**Mechanism of Action** Has partial agonist and/or antagonist activity against tryptaminergic, dopaminergic and alpha-adrenergic receptors depending upon their site; is a highly active uterine stimulant; it causes constriction of peripheral and cranial blood vessels and produces depression of central vasomotor centers

**Local Anesthetic/Vasoconstrictor Precautions** No information available to require special precautions

**Effects on Dental Treatment** >10% of patients experience dry mouth

**Other Adverse Effects**

>10%:

Cardiovascular: Tachycardia, bradycardia, arterial spasm, claudication and vasoconstriction; rebound headache may occur with sudden withdrawal of the drug in patients on prolonged therapy; localized edema, peripheral vascular effects

Central nervous system: Drowsiness, dizziness

Gastrointestinal: Nausea, vomiting, diarrhea

1% to 10%:

Cardiovascular: Transient tachycardia or bradycardia, precordial distress and pain

Gastrointestinal: Abdominal pain

Neuromuscular & skeletal: Weakness in the legs, myalgia, muscle pains in the extremities, paresthesia

**Drug Interactions** Increased toxicity:

Propranolol: One case of severe vasoconstriction with pain and cyanosis has been reported

Erythromycin, troleandomycin, and other macrolide antibiotics: Monitor for signs of ergot toxicity

**Drug Uptake**

Absorption: Oral, rectal: Erratic; enhanced by caffeine coadministration

Time to peak serum concentration: Within 0.5-3 hours following coadministration with caffeine

**Pregnancy Risk Factor** X

**Generic Available** Yes

♦ **Ergotrate® Maleate** *see* Ergonovine *on previous page*

♦ **E•R•O Ear [OTC]** *see* Carbamide Peroxide *on page 186*

## Erwinia Asparaginase (ehr WIN ee ah a SPAIR a ji nase)

**Therapeutic Category** Antineoplastic Agent, Miscellaneous

**Synonyms** NSC-106977; Porton Asparaginase

**Use** Acute lymphocytic leukemia (ALL) in patients sensitive to *E. coli* asparaginase

**Local Anesthetic/Vasoconstrictor Precautions** No information available to require special precautions

**Effects on Dental Treatment** No effects or complications reported

**Dosage Forms** Injection: 10,000 units

**Generic Available** No

♦ **Eryc® Oral** *see* Erythromycin *on next page*

♦ **Eryderm® Topical** *see* Erythromycin, Topical *on page 386*

♦ **Erygel® Topical** *see* Erythromycin, Topical *on page 386*

♦ **Erymax® Topical** *see* Erythromycin, Topical *on page 386*

♦ **EryPed® Oral** *see* Erythromycin *on next page*

♦ **Ery-Tab® Oral** *see* Erythromycin *on next page*

## Erythrityl Tetranitrate (e RI thri til te tra NYE trate)

**Related Information**

Cardiovascular Diseases *on page 1066*

**U.S. Brand Names** Cardilate®

**Therapeutic Category** Antianginal Agent; Nitrate; Vasodilator, Coronary

**Use** Prophylaxis and long-term treatment of frequent or recurrent anginal pain and reduced exercise tolerance associated with angina pectoris

**Usual Dosage** Adults: Oral: 5 mg under the tongue or in the buccal pouch 3 times/day or 10 mg before meals or food, chewed 3 times/day, increasing in 2-3 days if needed; dosages of up to 100 mg/day are tolerated; some patients may need bedtime doses if they experience nocturnal symptoms

**Mechanism of Action** Erythrityl tetranitrate, like other organic nitrates, induces vasodilation by dephosphorylation of the myosin light chain in smooth muscles. This is accomplished by activation of guanylate cyclase, which eventually stimulates a cyclic GMP-dependent protein kinase that alters the phosphorylation of the myosin. Venodilation causes peripheral blood pooling, which decreases venous return to the heart, central venous pressure, and pulmonary capillary wedge pressure. A reduction in pulmonary vascular resistance occurs secondary to pulmonary arteriolar dilation and afterload may be decreased by a lowering of systemic arterial pressure.

**Local Anesthetic/Vasoconstrictor Precautions** No information available to require special precautions

**Effects on Dental Treatment** No effects or complications reported

**Other Adverse Effects**

>10%: Central nervous system: Headache

1% to 10%: Cardiovascular: Tachycardia, hypotension, flushing

<1%:

- Central nervous system: Restlessness, dizziness
- Gastrointestinal: Nausea, vomiting, diarrhea
- Hematologic: Methemoglobinemia
- Neuromuscular & skeletal: Weakness

**Pregnancy Risk Factor** C

**Generic Available** No

**Comments** Doses up to 100 mg are generally well tolerated; headache may occur when increasing doses; should headache occur, reduce dose for 2-3 days; may use analgesics to treat headache

♦ **Erythrocin® Oral** *see* Erythromycin *on this page*

## Erythromycin (er ith roe MYE sin)

**Related Information**

Cardiovascular Diseases *on page 1066*

Dental Drug Interactions: Update on Drug Combinations Requiring Special Considerations *on page 1225*

Oral Bacterial Infections *on page 1128*

Oral Viral Infections *on page 1137*

Respiratory Diseases *on page 1079*

**U.S. Brand Names** E.E.S.® Oral; E-Mycin® Oral; Eryc® Oral; EryPed® Oral; Ery-Tab® Oral; Erythrocin® Oral; Ilosone® Oral; PCE® Oral

**Canadian Brand Names** Apo®-Erythro E-C; Diomycin; Erybid™; Erythro-Base®; Novo-Rythro Encap; PMS-Erythromycin

**Therapeutic Category** Antibiotic, Macrolide; Antibiotic, Ophthalmic

**Use**

Dental: An alternative to penicillin VK for treating orofacial infections

Medical: Treatment of susceptible bacterial infections in the medical patient including *M. pneumoniae, Legionella pneumophila,* diphtheria, pertussis, chancroid, *Chlamydia,* and *Campylobacter* gastroenteritis; used in conjunction with neomycin for decontaminating the bowel

**Unlabeled use:** Gastroparesis

**Usual Dosage** Orofacial infections:

Children: Base and ethylsuccinate: 30-50 mg/kg/day divided every 6-8 hours; do not exceed 2 g/day

Adults:

- Stearate or base: 250-500 mg every 6 hours for at least 7 days
- Ethylsuccinate: 400-800 mg every 6 hours for at least 7 days

**Mechanism of Action** Inhibits RNA-dependent protein synthesis at the chain elongation step; binds to the 50S ribosomal subunit resulting in blockage of transpeptidation

**Local Anesthetic/Vasoconstrictor Precautions** No information available to require special precautions

**Effects on Dental Treatment** 1% to 10% of patients experience oral candidiasis

(Continued)

## Erythromycin *(Continued)*

**Other Adverse Effects**

>10%: Gastrointestinal: Abdominal pain, cramping, nausea, vomiting

1% to 10%:

Gastrointestinal: Oral candidiasis

Hepatic: Cholestatic jaundice

Local: Phlebitis at the injection site

Miscellaneous: Hypersensitivity reactions

**Contraindications** Hepatic impairment, known hypersensitivity to erythromycin or its components; use with pimozide

**Warnings/Precautions** Hepatic impairment with or without jaundice has occurred, it may be accompanied by malaise, nausea, vomiting, abdominal colic, and fever; discontinue use if these occur; avoid using erythromycin lactobionate in neonates since formulations may contain benzyl alcohol which is associated with toxicity in neonates

**Drug Interactions** Cytochrome P-450 IIIA enzyme inhibitor

Increased toxicity:

Erythromycin decreases clearance of carbamazepine, cyclosporine, and triazolam

Erythromycin may decrease theophylline clearance and increase theophylline's half-life by up to 60% (patients on high-dose theophylline and erythromycin or who have received erythromycin for >5 days may be at higher risk)

May potentiate anticoagulant effect of warfarin

Concurrent use of erythromycin and lovastatin may result in rhabdomyolysis

**Drug Uptake**

Absorption: Variable but better with salt forms than with base form; 18% to 45% absorbed orally; due to differences in absorption, **200 mg erythromycin ethylsuccinate produces the same serum levels as 125 mg of erythromycin base** hours for the ethylsuccinate

Serum half-life: 1.5-2 hours (peak)

Time to peak serum concentration: 4 hours for the base, 30 minutes to 2.5

**Pregnancy Risk Factor** B

**Breast-feeding Considerations** May be taken while breast-feeding

**Dosage Forms**

Erythromycin base:

Capsule, delayed release: 250 mg

Capsule, delayed release, enteric coated pellets (Eryc®): 250 mg

Tablet, delayed release: 333 mg

Tablet, enteric coated (E-Mycin®, Ery-Tab®, E-Base®): 250 mg, 333 mg, 500 mg

Tablet, film coated: 250 mg, 500 mg

Tablet, polymer coated particles (PCE®): 333 mg, 500 mg

Erythromycin estolate:

Capsule (Ilosone® Pulvules®): 250 mg

Suspension, oral (Ilosone®): 125 mg/5 mL (480 mL); 250 mg/5 mL (480 mL)

Tablet (Ilosone®): 500 mg

Erythromycin ethylsuccinate:

Granules for oral suspension (EryPed®): 400 mg/5 mL (60 mL, 100 mL, 200 mL)

Powder for oral suspension (E.E.S.®): 200 mg/5 mL (100 mL, 200 mL)

Suspension, oral (E.E.S.®, EryPed®): 200 mg/5 mL (5 mL, 100 mL, 200 mL, 480 mL); 400 mg/5 mL (5 mL, 60 mL, 100 mL, 200 mL, 480 mL)

Suspension, oral [drops] (EryPed®): 100 mg/2.5 mL (50 mL)

Tablet (E.E.S.®): 400 mg

Tablet, chewable (EryPed®): 200 mg

Erythromycin gluceptate: Injection: 1000 mg (30 mL)

Erythromycin lactobionate: Powder for injection: 500 mg, 1000 mg

Erythromycin stearate: Tablet, film coated (Eramycin®, Erythrocin®): 250 mg, 500 mg

**Dietary Considerations** Erythromycin has decreased absorption with food; avoid milk and acidic beverages 1 hour before or after a dose; ethylsuccinate, estolate, and enteric coated products are **not** affected by food; ethylsuccinate may be better absorbed with food

**Generic Available** Yes

**Comments** Many patients cannot tolerate erythromycin because of abdominal pain and nausea; the mechanism of this adverse effect appears to be the motilin agonistic properties of erythromycin in the GI tract. For these patients, clindamycin is indicated as the alternative antibiotic for treatment of orofacial infections.

Erythromycin has been used as a prokinetic agent to improve gastric emptying time and intestinal motility. In adults, 200 mg was infused I.V. initially followed by 250 mg orally 3 times/day 30 minutes before meals. In children, erythromycin 3 mg/kg I.V. has been infused over 60 minutes initially followed by 20 mg/kg/day orally in 3-4 divided doses before meals or before meals and at bedtime.

HMG-CoA reductase inhibitors, also known as the statins, effectively decrease the hepatic cholesterol biosynthesis resulting in the reduction of blood LDL-cholesterol concentrations. The AUC of atorvastatin (Lipitor®) was increased 33% by erythromycin administration (Yang, et al). Combination of erythromycin and lovastatin (Mevacor®) has been associated with rhabdomyolysis (Ayanian, et al). The administration of erythromycin with cerivastatin (Baycol™) produced a 50% increase in area under the concentration curve for cerivastatin. The mechanism of erythromycin is inhibiting the CYP3A4 metabolism of atorvastatin, lovastatin, and cerivastatin. Simvastatin (Zocor®) would likely be affected in a similar manner by the coadministration of erythromycin. Clarithromycin (Biaxin™) may exert a similar effect as erythromycin on atorvastatin, lovastatin, cerivastatin, and simvastatin. Erythromycin 3 times/day had no effect on pravastatin (Pravachol®) plasma concentrations (Bottorff, et al).

**Selected Readings**


Ayanian JZ, Fuchs CS, and Stone RM, "Lovastatin and Rhabdomyolysis," *Ann Intern Med*, 1988, 109(8):682-3.

Bottorff MB, et al, "Differences in Metabolism of Lovastatin and Pravastatin as Assessed by CYP3A4 Inhibition With Erythromycin," *Pharmacotherapy*, 1997, 17:41.

"Pimozide (Orap) Contraindicated With Clarithromycin (Biaxin™) and Other Macrolide Antibiotics," *FDA Medical Bulletin*, October 1996, 3.

Wynn RL and Bergman SA, "Antibiotics and Their Use in the Treatment of Orofacial Infections, Part I and Part II," *Gen Dent*, 1994, 42(5):398-402, 498-502.

Wynn RL, "Current Concepts of the Erythromycins," *Gen Dent*, 1991, 39(6):408,10-1.

Yang BB, et al, "Atorvastatin Pharmacokinetic Interactions With Other CYP3A4 Substrates: Erythromycin and Ethinyl Estradiol," *Pharm Res*, 1996, 13:S437.


## Erythromycin and Benzoyl Peroxide

(er ith roe MYE sin & BEN zoe il per OKS ide)

**U.S. Brand Names** Benzamycin®

**Canadian Brand Names** Benzamycin®

**Therapeutic Category** Acne Products

**Use** Topical control of acne vulgaris

**Usual Dosage** Apply twice daily, morning and evening

**Local Anesthetic/Vasoconstrictor Precautions** No information available to require special precautions

**Effects on Dental Treatment** No effects or complications reported

**Pregnancy Risk Factor** C

**Generic Available** No

## Erythromycin and Sulfisoxazole

(er ith roe MYE sin & sul fi SOKS a zole)

**U.S. Brand Names** Eryzole®; Pediazole®

**Therapeutic Category** Antibiotic, Macrolide; Antibiotic, Sulfonamide Derivative

**Use** Treatment of susceptible bacterial infections of the upper and lower respiratory tract, otitis media in children caused by susceptible strains of *Haemophilus influenzae*, and other infections in patients allergic to penicillin

**Usual Dosage** Oral (dosage recommendation is based on the product's erythromycin content):

Children ≥2 months: 50 mg/kg/day erythromycin and 150 mg/kg/day sulfisoxazole in divided doses every 6 hours; not to exceed 2 g erythromycin/day or 6 g sulfisoxazole/day for 10 days

Adults: 400 mg erythromycin and 1200 mg sulfisoxazole every 6 hours

**Mechanism of Action** Erythromycin inhibits bacterial protein synthesis; sulfisoxazole competitively inhibits bacterial synthesis of folic acid from para-aminobenzoic acid

**Local Anesthetic/Vasoconstrictor Precautions** No information available to require special precautions

**Effects on Dental Treatment** No effects or complications reported

**Other Adverse Effects**

>10%: Gastrointestinal: Abdominal pain, cramping, nausea, vomiting

1% to 10%:
- Gastrointestinal: Oral candidiasis
- Hepatic: Cholestatic jaundice
- Local: Phlebitis at the injection site
- Miscellaneous: Hypersensitivity reactions

<1%:
- Cardiovascular: Ventricular arrhythmias
- Central nervous system: Fever, headache

(Continued)

## Erythromycin and Sulfisoxazole *(Continued)*

Dermatologic: Skin rash, Stevens-Johnson syndrome, toxic epidermal necrolysis
Gastrointestinal: Hypertrophic pyloric stenosis, diarrhea
Hematologic: Eosinophilia, agranulocytosis, aplastic anemia
Hepatic: Hepatic necrosis
Local: Thrombophlebitis
Renal: Toxic nephrosis, crystalluria

**Drug Interactions** Increased effect/toxicity/levels of alfentanil, anticoagulants, astemizole, terfenadine, loratadine, bromocriptine, carbamazepine, cyclosporine, digoxin, disopyramide, theophylline, triazolam, and warfarin

**Drug Uptake**
Erythromycin ethylsuccinate:
Absorption: Well absorbed from GI tract
Serum half-life: 1-1.5 hours
Sulfisoxazole acetyl:
Absorption: Readily absorbed
Serum half-life: 6 hours, prolonged in renal impairment

**Pregnancy Risk Factor** C

**Generic Available** Yes

## Erythromycin, Topical (er ith roe MYE sin TOP i kal)

**U.S. Brand Names** Akne-Mycin® Topical; A/T/S® Topical; Del-Mycin® Topical; Emgel™ Topical; Eryderm® Topical; Erygel® Topical; Erymax® Topical; E-Solve-2® Topical; ETS-2%® Topical; Ilotycin® Ophthalmic; Staticin® Topical; T-Stat® Topical

**Therapeutic Category** Acne Products; Antibiotic, Topical

**Use** Topical treatment of acne vulgaris

**Usual Dosage**
Neonates:
Ophthalmic: Prophylaxis of neonatal gonococcal or chlamydial conjunctivitis: 0.5-1 cm ribbon of ointment should be instilled into each conjunctival sac
Children and Adults:
Ophthalmic: Instill one or more times daily depending on the severity of the infection
Topical: Apply 2% solution over the affected area twice daily after the skin has been thoroughly washed and patted dry

**Local Anesthetic/Vasoconstrictor Precautions** No information available to require special precautions

**Effects on Dental Treatment** No effects or complications reported

**Other Adverse Effects** 1% to 10%: Dermatologic: Erythema, desquamation, dryness, pruritus

**Pregnancy Risk Factor** B

**Generic Available** Yes

- **Erythropoietin** *see* Epoetin Alfa *on page 376*
- **Eryzole®** *see* Erythromycin and Sulfisoxazole *on previous page*
- **Esclim®** *see* Estradiol *on next page*
- **Esgic®** *see* Butalbital Compound *on page 163*
- **Esgic®** *see* Butalbital Compound and Acetaminophen *on page 164*
- **Esgic-Plus®** *see* Butalbital Compound and Acetaminophen *on page 164*
- **Esidrix®** *see* Hydrochlorothiazide *on page 503*
- **Eskalith®** *see* Lithium *on page 596*
- **E-Solve-2® Topical** *see* Erythromycin, Topical *on this page*
- **Esoterica® Facial [OTC]** *see* Hydroquinone *on page 514*
- **Esoterica® Regular [OTC]** *see* Hydroquinone *on page 514*
- **Esoterica® Sensitive Skin Formula [OTC]** *see* Hydroquinone *on page 514*
- **Esoterica® Sunscreen [OTC]** *see* Hydroquinone *on page 514*
- **Estar® [OTC]** *see* Coal Tar *on page 270*

## Estazolam (es TA zoe lam)

**U.S. Brand Names** ProSom™

**Therapeutic Category** Benzodiazepine; Hypnotic; Sedative

**Use** Short-term management of insomnia; there has been little experience with this drug in the elderly, but because of its lack of active metabolites, it is a reasonable choice when a benzodiazepine hypnotic is indicated

**Usual Dosage** Adults: Oral: 1 mg at bedtime, some patients may require 2 mg; start at doses of 0.5 mg in debilitated or small elderly patients

**Mechanism of Action** Benzodiazepines may exert their pharmacologic effect through potentiation of the inhibitory activity of GABA. Benzodiazepines do not alter the synthesis, release, reuptake, or enzymatic degradation of GABA.

**Local Anesthetic/Vasoconstrictor Precautions** No information available to require special precautions

**Effects on Dental Treatment** Significant xerostomia occurs in up to 10% of patients. Disappears with cessation of drug therapy.

**Other Adverse Effects**

>10%:

Central nervous system: Somnolence

Neuromuscular & skeletal: Weakness

1% to 10%:

Central nervous system: "Hangover" feeling, abnormal thinking, anxiety

Gastrointestinal: Dyspepsia

Neuromuscular & skeletal: Hypokinesis

Respiratory: Cold symptoms, pharyngitis, asthma, cough, dyspnea, rhinitis

<1%:

Cardiovascular: Syncope

Central nervous system: Agitation, amnesia, apathy, seizure, sleep disorder, stupor, ataxia, neuritis

Dermatologic: Urticaria, acne, dry skin, photosensitivity

Endocrine & metabolic: Decreased libido

Gastrointestinal: Increased/decreased appetite, flatulence, gastritis, enterocolitis, melena, mouth ulceration

Genitourinary: Nocturia, urinary incontinence

Hematologic: Agranulocytosis

Hepatic: Elevated AST

Neuromuscular & skeletal: Twitching, decreased reflexes

Renal: Hematuria, oliguria

Respiratory: Epistaxis, laryngitis

**Drug Interactions**

Decreased effect: Enzyme inducers may increase the metabolism of estazolam

Increased toxicity: CNS depressants may increase CNS adverse effects; cimetidine may decrease metabolism of estazolam

**Drug Uptake** Studies have shown that the elderly are more sensitive to the effects of benzodiazepines as compared to younger adults

Half-life: 10-24 hours (no significant changes in the elderly)

Peak serum levels: 0.5-1.6 hours

**Pregnancy Risk Factor** X

**Generic Available** Yes

- **Estinyl®** *see* Ethinyl Estradiol *on page 399*
- **Estivin® II Ophthalmic [OTC]** *see* Naphazoline *on page 703*
- **Estrace® Oral** *see* Estradiol *on this page*
- **Estraderm® Transdermal** *see* Estradiol *on this page*

## Estradiol (es tra DYE ole)

**Related Information**

Endocrine Disorders & Pregnancy *on page 1082*

**U.S. Brand Names** Alora® Transdermal; Climara® Transdermal; depGynogen® Injection; Depo®-Estradiol Injection; Depogen® Injection; Dioval® Injection; Esclim®; Estrace® Oral; Estraderm® Transdermal; Estra-L® Injection; Estring®; Estro-Cyp® Injection; Gynogen L.A.® Injection; Valergen® Injection; Vivelle™ Transdermal

**Therapeutic Category** Estrogen Derivative

**Use** Treatment of atrophic vaginitis, atrophic dystrophy of vulva, menopausal symptoms, female hypogonadism, ovariectomy, primary ovarian failure, inoperable breast cancer, inoperable prostatic cancer, mild to severe vasomotor symptoms associated with menopause

**Usual Dosage** Adults (all dosage needs to be adjusted based upon the patient's response):

Male:

Prostate cancer: Valerate: I.M.: ≥30 mg or more every 1-2 weeks

Prostate cancer (androgen-dependent, inoperable, progressing): Oral: 10 mg 3 times/day for at least 3 months

Female:

Breast cancer (inoperable, progressing): Oral: 10 mg 3 times/day for at least 3 months

Osteoporosis prevention: Oral: 0.5 mg/day in a cyclic regimen (3 weeks on and 1 week off of drug)

(Continued)

## Estradiol *(Continued)*

Hypogonadism, moderate to severe vasomotor symptoms:
Oral: 1-2 mg/day in a cyclic regimen for 3 weeks on drug, then 1 week off drug
Moderate to severe vasomotor symptoms:
I.M.: Cypionate: 1-5 mg every 3-4 weeks
I.M.: Valerate: 10-20 mg every 4 weeks
Postpartum breast engorgement: I.M.: Valerate: 10-25 mg at end of first stage of labor
Transdermal: Apply 0.05 mg patch initially (titrate dosage to response) applied twice weekly in a cyclic regimen, for 3 weeks on drug and 1 week off drug in patients with an intact uterus and continuously in patients without a uterus
Atrophic vaginitis, kraurosis vulvae: Vaginal: Insert 2-4 g/day for 2 weeks then gradually reduce to 1/2 the initial dose for 2 weeks followed by a maintenance dose of 1 g 1-3 times/week

**Mechanism of Action** Increases the synthesis of DNA, RNA, and various proteins in target tissues; reduces the release of gonadotropin-releasing hormone from the hypothalamus; reduces FSH and LH release from the pituitary

**Local Anesthetic/Vasoconstrictor Precautions** No information available to require special precautions

**Effects on Dental Treatment** No effects or complications reported

**Other Adverse Effects**

>10%:
Cardiovascular: Peripheral edema
Endocrine & metabolic: Enlargement of breasts (female and male), breast tenderness
Gastrointestinal: Nausea, anorexia, bloating

1% to 10%:
Central nervous system: Headache
Endocrine & metabolic: Increased libido (female), decreased libido (male)
Gastrointestinal: Vomiting, diarrhea

<1%:
Cardiovascular: Hypertension, edema, thromboembolic disorders, myocardial infarction
Central nervous system: Depression, dizziness, anxiety, stroke
Dermatologic: Chloasma, melasma, rash
Endocrine & metabolic: Hypercalcemia, folate deficiency, change in menstrual flow, breast tumors, amenorrhea, decreased glucose tolerance, elevated triglycerides and LDL
Gastrointestinal: GI distress
Hepatic: Cholestatic jaundice
Local: Pain at injection site
Ocular: Intolerance to contact lenses
Miscellaneous: Increased susceptibility to *Candida* infection

**Drug Interactions**

Decreased effect: Rifampin decreases estrogen serum concentrations
Increased toxicity: Hydrocortisone increases corticosteroid toxic potential; increases potential for thromboembolic events with anticoagulants

**Drug Uptake**

Absorption: Readily absorbed through skin and GI tract; reabsorbed from bile in GI tract and enterohepatically recycled
Serum half-life: 50-60 minutes

**Pregnancy Risk Factor** X

**Generic Available** Yes

## Estradiol and Norethindrone (es tra DYE ole & nor eth IN drone)

**U.S. Brand Names** Activelle™; CombiPatch®

**Therapeutic Category** Estrogen Derivative

**Use** Treatment of moderate to severe vasomotor symptoms associated with the menopause; treatment of vulvar and vaginal atrophy; transdermal patch used in women with an intact uterus, treatment of moderate-to-severe vasomotor symptoms associated with menopause, treatment of vulvar and vaginal atrophy, treatment of hypoestrogenism due to hypogonadism, castration, or primary ovarian failure.

**Usual Dosage** Adults: Oral: 1 tablet daily

**Local Anesthetic/Vasoconstrictor Precautions** No information available to require special precautions

**Effects on Dental Treatment** No effects or complications reported

**Other Adverse Effects**

>10%:
Cardiovascular: Peripheral edema

Endocrine & metabolic: Enlargement of breasts, breast tenderness
Gastrointestinal: Nausea, anorexia, bloating

1% to 10%:
Central nervous system: Headache
Endocrine & metabolic: Increased libido
Gastrointestinal: Vomiting, diarrhea

<1%:
Cardiovascular: Hypertension, thromboembolism, stroke, myocardial infarction, edema
Central nervous system: Depression, dizziness, anxiety
Dermatologic: Chloasma, melasma, rash
Endocrine & metabolic: Decreased glucose tolerance, breast tumors, amenorrhea, alterations in frequency and flow of menses, increased triglycerides and LDL
Gastrointestinal: GI distress
Hepatic: Cholestatic jaundice
Ocular: Intolerance to contact lenses
Miscellaneous: Increased susceptibility to *Candida* infection

Minimize these effects by adjusting the estrogen/progestin balance or dosage. The table categorizes products by both their estrogenic and progestational potencies; because overall activity is influenced by the interaction of components, it is difficult to precisely classify products; placement in the table is only approximate. Differences between products within a group are probably not clinically significant.

**Drug Uptake**
Absorption: Well absorbed through the GI tract
Time to peak: 5-8 hours

**Pregnancy Risk Factor** X

**Generic Available** No

## Estradiol and Testosterone (es tra DYE ole & tes TOS ter one)

**U.S. Brand Names** Andro/Fem® Injection; Deladumone® Injection; depAndrogyn® Injection; Depo-Testadiol® Injection; Depotestogen® Injection; Duo-Cyp® Injection; Duratestrin® Injection; Valertest No.1® Injection

**Therapeutic Category** Estrogen and Androgen Combination

**Synonyms** Testosterone and Estradiol

**Use** Vasomotor symptoms associated with menopause; postpartum breast engorgement

**Usual Dosage** Adults: All dosage needs to be adjusted based upon the patient's response

**Local Anesthetic/Vasoconstrictor Precautions** No information available to require special precautions

**Effects on Dental Treatment** No effects or complications reported

**Pregnancy Risk Factor** X

**Generic Available** No

♦ **Estradurin®** *see* Polyestradiol *on page 814*
♦ **Estra-L® Injection** *see* Estradiol *on page 387*

## Estramustine (es tra MUS teen)

**U.S. Brand Names** Emcyt®

**Therapeutic Category** Antineoplastic Agent, Hormone (Estrogen/Nitrogen Mustard)

**Use** Palliative treatment of prostatic carcinoma (progressive or metastatic)

**Usual Dosage** Adults: Oral: 14 mg/kg/day (range: 10-16 mg/kg/day) in 3-4 divided doses for 30-90 days; some patients have been maintained for >3 years on therapy

**Mechanism of Action** Mechanism is not completely clear, thought to act as an alkylating agent and as estrogen

**Local Anesthetic/Vasoconstrictor Precautions** No information available to require special precautions

**Effects on Dental Treatment** No effects or complications reported

**Other Adverse Effects**

>10%:
Cardiovascular: Edema
Endocrine & metabolic: Decreased libido, breast tenderness, breast enlargement
Gastrointestinal: Diarrhea, nausea
Hepatic: Mild elevations in AST (SGOT) or LDH
Respiratory: Dyspnea

1% to 10%:
Cardiovascular: Myocardial infarction

(Continued)

## Estramustine *(Continued)*

Central nervous system: Insomnia, lethargy
Gastrointestinal: Anorexia, flatulence
Hematologic: Leukopenia
Local: Thrombophlebitis
Neuromuscular & skeletal: Leg cramps
Respiratory: Pulmonary embolism

<1%:
Cardiovascular: Cardiac arrest
Central nervous system: Night sweats, depression
Dermatologic: Pigment changes
Endocrine & metabolic: Hypercalcemia, hot flashes
Otic: Tinnitus

**Drug Interactions** Decreased effect: Milk products and calcium-rich foods/drugs may impair the oral absorption of estramustine phosphate sodium

**Drug Uptake**
Absorption: Oral: Well absorbed (75%)
Serum half-life: 20 hours
Time to peak serum concentration: Within 2-3 hours

**Pregnancy Risk Factor** C

**Generic Available** No

- **Estratab®** *see* Estrogens, Esterified *on page 392*
- **Estratest® H.S. Oral** *see* Estrogens and Methyltestosterone *on next page*
- **Estratest® Oral** *see* Estrogens and Methyltestosterone *on next page*
- **Estring®** *see* Estradiol *on page 387*
- **Estro-Cyp® Injection** *see* Estradiol *on page 387*

## Estrogens and Medroxyprogesterone

(ES troe jenz & me DROKS ee proe JES te rone)

**Related Information**
Endocrine Disorders & Pregnancy *on page 1082*

**U.S. Brand Names** Premphase™; Prempro™

**Therapeutic Category** Estrogen and Progestin Combination

**Use** Women with an intact uterus for the treatment of moderate to severe vasomotor symptoms associated with the menopause; treatment of atrophic vaginitis; primary ovarian failure; osteoporosis prophylactic

**Usual Dosage** Oral:

Premphase™: 1 maroon tablet/day for 28 days and 1 light purple tablet to be taken with the maroon tablet on days 15-28; for patients with moderate to severe vasomotor symptoms and vulvar and vaginal atrophy associated with menopause, re-evaluate patients at 3- and 6-month intervals to determine if treatment is still necessary; for prevention of osteoporosis, monitor patients for signs of endometrial cancer; rule out malignancy if unexplained vaginal bleeding occurs

Prempro™: Dosage as above with the exception that the white 2.5 mg Cycrin® tablet (medroxyprogesterone acetate) is taken on a daily basis with the maroon Premarin® tablet (conjugated estrogen) and not just on days 15-28

**Local Anesthetic/Vasoconstrictor Precautions** No information available to require special precautions

**Effects on Dental Treatment** No effects or complications reported

**Other Adverse Effects**

>10%:
Cardiovascular: Peripheral edema
Endocrine & metabolic: Changes in menstrual flow, amenorrhea, enlargement of breasts, breast tenderness, breakthrough bleeding, spotting
Gastrointestinal: Anorexia, nausea, bloating
Local: Pain at injection site
Neuromuscular & skeletal: Weakness

1% to 10%:
Cardiovascular: Edema
Central nervous system: Mental depression, fever, insomnia, headache
Dermatologic: Melasma or chloasma, allergic rash with or without pruritus
Endocrine & metabolic: Changes in cervical erosion and secretions, increased libido
Gastrointestinal: Weight gain or loss, vomiting, diarrhea
Hepatic: Cholestatic jaundice
Local: Thrombophlebitis
Respiratory: Pulmonary thrombosis and embolism

<1%:
Cardiovascular: Hypertension, thromboembolism, myocardial infarction

Central nervous system: Dizziness, anxiety, stroke
Dermatologic: Rash
Endocrine & metabolic: Breast tumors, amenorrhea, decreased glucose tolerance, elevated triglycerides and LDL
Gastrointestinal: GI distress
Ocular: Intolerance to contact lenses
Miscellaneous: Increased susceptibility to *Candida* infection

**Generic Available** Yes

## Estrogens and Methyltestosterone

(ES troe jenz & meth il tes TOS te rone)

**Related Information**

Endocrine Disorders & Pregnancy *on page 1082*

**U.S. Brand Names** Estratest® H.S. Oral; Estratest® Oral; Premarin® With Methyltestosterone Oral

**Therapeutic Category** Estrogen and Androgen Combination

**Use** Atrophic vaginitis; hypogonadism; primary ovarian failure; vasomotor symptoms of menopause; prostatic carcinoma; osteoporosis prophylactic

**Usual Dosage** Adults: Females: Oral: Lowest dose that will control symptoms should be chosen, normally given 3 weeks on and 1 week off

**Mechanism of Action**

Conjugated estrogens: Combination of the sodium salts of the sulfate esters of estrogenic substances, representing the average composition of material obtained from pregnant mare's urine. The primary preparation utilized is Premarin®; however, other generic products are available. Premarin® contains 50% to 65% estrone sodium sulfate, 20% to 35% equilin sodium sulfate, and 17 alpha-dihydroequilin, together with smaller amounts of 17 alpha-estradiol, equilenin, and 17 alpha-dihydroequilenin, all as salts of the sulfate ester. Estrogens are important for developing secondary sex characteristics. Estrogens promote growth in development of the vagina, uterus, fallopian tubes, and enlargement of the breast. Eventually, they stimulate and limit linear skeletal growth. Estrogens have widespread effects on metabolism such as transporting proteins and electrolyte balance.

Testosterone: It has been reported that androgens increase protein anabolism and decrease protein catabolism; however, nitrogen balance is only improved when androgen therapy is accompanied by adequate caloric and protein intake. Testosterone and related androgens cause retention of phosphorous, potassium, sodium, and nitrogen, and decrease renal excretion of calcium. Production of red blood cells secondary to erythropoietic factor stimulation has been reported with androgen administration.

**Local Anesthetic/Vasoconstrictor Precautions** No information available to require special precautions

**Effects on Dental Treatment** No effects or complications reported

**Drug Uptake**

Conjugated estrogens:
Absorption: Readily absorbed from GI tract

Testosterone:
Duration of therapeutic effect: Depends upon route of administration and which testosterone ester used; slow absorption extends duration of activity; I.M. administration usually lasts for 2-4 weeks
Absorption: I.M.: Absorbed slowly allowing for dosing intervals of 2-4 weeks
Half-life: I.M.: ~8 days

**Pregnancy Risk Factor** X

**Generic Available** No

## Estrogens, Conjugated (ES troe jenz KON joo gate ed)

**Related Information**

Dental Drug Interactions: Update on Drug Combinations Requiring Special Considerations *on page 1225*
Endocrine Disorders & Pregnancy *on page 1082*

**U.S. Brand Names** Premarin®

**Canadian Brand Names** C.E.S.™; Congest

**Therapeutic Category** Estrogen Derivative

**Use** Atrophic vaginitis; hypogonadism; primary ovarian failure; vasomotor symptoms of menopause; prostatic carcinoma; osteoporosis prophylactic

**Usual Dosage** Adults:

Male: Prostate cancer: Oral: 1.25-2.5 mg 3 times/day
Female:
Hypogonadism: Oral: 2.5-7.5 mg/day for 20 days, off 10 days and repeat until menses occur
Abnormal uterine bleeding:
Oral: 2.5-5 mg/day for 7-10 days; then decrease to 1.25 mg/day for 2 weeks

(Continued)

## Estrogens, Conjugated *(Continued)*

I.M., I.V.: 25 mg every 6-12 hours until bleeding stops
Moderate to severe vasomotor symptoms: Oral: 0.625-1.25 mg/day
Postpartum breast engorgement: Oral: 3.75 mg every 4 hours for 5 doses, then 1.25 mg every 4 hours for 5 days
Atrophic vaginitis, kraurosis vulvae: Vaginal: 2-4 g instilled/day 3 weeks on and 1 week off
Osteoporosis: Oral: 0.625 mg/day chronically
Uremic bleeding: I.V.: 0.6 mg/kg/dose daily for 5 days

**Mechanism of Action** Increases the synthesis of DNA, RNA, and various proteins in target tissues; reduces the release of gonadotropin-releasing hormone from the hypothalamus; reduces FSH and LH release from the pituitary

**Local Anesthetic/Vasoconstrictor Precautions** No information available to require special precautions

**Effects on Dental Treatment** No effects or complications reported

**Other Adverse Effects**

>10%:
- Cardiovascular: Peripheral edema
- Endocrine & metabolic: Breast tenderness, hypercalcemia, enlargement of breasts
- Gastrointestinal: Nausea, anorexia, bloating

1% to 10%:
- Central nervous system: Headache
- Endocrine & metabolic: Increased libido
- Gastrointestinal: Vomiting, diarrhea
- Local: Pain at injection site

<1%:
- Cardiovascular: Hypertension, edema, thromboembolic disorder, myocardial infarction, hypertension
- Central nervous system: Depression, dizziness, anxiety, stroke
- Dermatologic: Chloasma, melasma, rash
- Endocrine & metabolic: Breast tumors, amenorrhea, alterations in frequency and flow of menses, decreased glucose tolerance, elevated triglycerides and LDL
- Gastrointestinal: GI distress
- Hepatic: Cholestatic jaundice
- Ocular: Intolerance to contact lenses
- Miscellaneous: Increased susceptibility to *Candida* infection

**Drug Interactions**

Decreased effect: Rifampin decreases estrogen serum concentrations
Increased toxicity: Anticoagulants: Increases potential for thromboembolic events with anticoagulants

**Drug Uptake** Absorption: Readily absorbed from GI tract

**Pregnancy Risk Factor** X

**Generic Available** No

## Estrogens, Esterified (ES troe jenz, es TER i fied)

**Related Information**

Dental Drug Interactions: Update on Drug Combinations Requiring Special Considerations *on page 1225*
Endocrine Disorders & Pregnancy *on page 1082*

**U.S. Brand Names** Estratab®; Menest®

**Canadian Brand Names** Neo-Estrone®

**Therapeutic Category** Estrogen Derivative

**Use** Atrophic vaginitis; hypogonadism; primary ovarian failure; vasomotor symptoms of menopause; prostatic carcinoma; osteoporosis prophylactic

**Usual Dosage** Adults: Oral:

Male: Prostate cancer (inoperable, progressing): 1.25-2.5 mg 3 times/day
Female:
Hypogonadism: 2.5-7.5 mg/day for 20 days, off 10 days and repeat until menses occur
Moderate to severe vasomotor symptoms: 0.3-1.25 mg/day
Breast cancer (inoperable, progressing): 10 mg 3 times/day for at least 3 months

**Mechanism of Action** Primary effects on the interphase DNA-protein complex (chromatin) by binding to a receptor (usually located in the cytoplasm of a target cell) and initiating translocation of the hormone-receptor complex to the nucleus

**Local Anesthetic/Vasoconstrictor Precautions** No information available to require special precautions

**Effects on Dental Treatment** No effects or complications reported

**Other Adverse Effects**

>10%:

Cardiovascular: Peripheral edema

Endocrine & metabolic: Enlargement of breasts, breast tenderness

Gastrointestinal: Nausea, anorexia, bloating

1% to 10%:

Central nervous system: Headache

Endocrine & metabolic: Increased libido

Gastrointestinal: Vomiting, diarrhea

<1%:

Cardiovascular: Hypertension, thromboembolism, myocardial infarction, edema

Central nervous system: Stroke, depression, dizziness, anxiety

Dermatologic: Chloasma, melasma, rash

Endocrine & metabolic: Breast tumors, amenorrhea, alterations in frequency and flow of menses, decreased glucose tolerance, elevated triglycerides and LDL

Gastrointestinal: GI distress

Hepatic: Cholestatic jaundice

Ocular: Intolerance to contact lenses

Miscellaneous: Increased susceptibility to *Candida* infection

**Drug Interactions**

Decreased effect: Rifampin decreases estrogen serum concentrations

Increased toxicity:

Anticoagulants: Increases potential for thromboembolic events with anticoagulants

**Drug Uptake** Absorption: Readily absorbed from GI tract

**Pregnancy Risk Factor** X

**Generic Available** No

## Estrone (ES trone)

**Related Information**

Endocrine Disorders & Pregnancy *on page 1082*

**U.S. Brand Names** Aquest®; Kestrone®

**Canadian Brand Names** Femogen®; Neo-Estrone®; Oestrilin®

**Therapeutic Category** Estrogen Derivative

**Use** Hypogonadism; primary ovarian failure; vasomotor symptoms of menopause; prostatic carcinoma; inoperable breast cancer, kraurosis vulvae, abnormal uterine bleeding due to hormone imbalance

**Usual Dosage** Adults: I.M.:

Male: Prostatic carcinoma: 2-4 mg 2-3 times/week

Female:

Senile vaginitis and kraurosis vulvae: 0.1-0.5 mg 2-3 times/week

Breast cancer (inoperable, progressing): 5 mg 3 or more times/week

Primary ovarian failure, hypogonadism: 0.1-1 mg/week, up to 2 mg/week in single or divided doses

Abnormal uterine bleeding: 2.5 mg/day for several days

**Mechanism of Action** Estrone is a natural ovarian estrogenic hormone that is available as an aqueous mixture of water insoluble estrone and water soluble estrone potassium sulfate; all estrogens, including estrone, act in a similar manner; there is no evidence that there are biological differences among various estrogen preparations other than their ability to bind to cellular receptors inside the target cells

**Local Anesthetic/Vasoconstrictor Precautions** No information available to require special precautions

**Effects on Dental Treatment** No effects or complications reported

**Other Adverse Effects**

>10%:

Cardiovascular: Peripheral edema

Endocrine & metabolic: Enlargement of breasts, breast tenderness

Gastrointestinal: Nausea, anorexia, bloating

1% to 10%:

Central nervous system: Headache

Endocrine & metabolic: Increased libido

Gastrointestinal: Vomiting, diarrhea

<1%:

Cardiovascular: Hypertension, thromboembolism, myocardial infarction, edema

Central nervous system: Stroke, depression, dizziness, anxiety

Dermatologic: Chloasma, melasma, rash

(Continued)

## Estrone *(Continued)*

Endocrine & metabolic: Breast tumors, amenorrhea, alterations in frequency and flow of menses, decreased glucose tolerance, elevated triglycerides and LDL
Gastrointestinal: GI distress
Hepatic: Cholestatic jaundice
Ocular: Intolerance to contact lenses
Miscellaneous: Increased susceptibility to *Candida* infection

**Drug Interactions**
Decreased effect: Rifampin decreases estrogen serum concentrations
Increased toxicity:
Anticoagulants: Increases potential for thromboembolic events with anticoagulants

**Drug Uptake** Absorption: Readily absorbed from the GI tract
**Pregnancy Risk Factor** X
**Generic Available** Yes

## Estropipate (ES troe pih pate)

**Related Information**
Endocrine Disorders & Pregnancy *on page 1082*

**U.S. Brand Names** Ogen®; Ortho-Est®
**Canadian Brand Names** Estrouis®
**Therapeutic Category** Estrogen Derivative
**Use** Atrophic vaginitis; hypogonadism; primary ovarian failure; vasomotor symptoms of menopause; osteoporosis prophylactic
**Usual Dosage** Adults: Female:
Moderate to severe vasomotor symptoms: Oral: 0.625-5 mg/day
Hypogonadism or primary ovarian failure: Oral: 1.25-7.5 mg/day for 3 weeks followed by an 8- to 10-day rest period
Osteoporosis prevention: Oral: 0.625 mg/day for 25 days of a 31-day cycle
Atrophic vaginitis or kraurosis vulvae: Vaginal: Instill 2-4 g/day 3 weeks on and 1 week off

**Mechanism of Action** Crystalline estrone that has been solubilized as the sulfate and stabilized with piperazine. Primary effects on the interphase DNA-protein complex (chromatin) by binding to a receptor (usually located in the cytoplasm of a target cell) and initiating translocation of the hormone receptor complex to the nucleus.

**Local Anesthetic/Vasoconstrictor Precautions** No information available to require special precautions
**Effects on Dental Treatment** No effects or complications reported
**Other Adverse Effects**
>10%:
Cardiovascular: Peripheral edema
Endocrine & metabolic: Enlargement of breasts, breast tenderness
Gastrointestinal: Nausea, anorexia, bloating
1% to 10%:
Central nervous system: Headache
Endocrine & metabolic: Increased libido
Gastrointestinal: Vomiting, diarrhea
<1%:
Cardiovascular: Hypertension, thromboembolism, myocardial infarction, edema
Central nervous system: Stroke, depression, dizziness, anxiety
Dermatologic: Chloasma, melasma, rash
Endocrine & metabolic: Breast tumors, amenorrhea, alterations in frequency and flow of menses, decreased glucose tolerance, elevated triglycerides and LDL
Gastrointestinal: GI distress
Hepatic: Cholestatic jaundice
Ocular: Intolerance to contact lenses
Miscellaneous: Increased susceptibility to *Candida* infection

**Drug Interactions**
Decreased effect: Rifampin decreases estrogen serum concentrations
Increased toxicity: Anticoagulants: Increases potential for thromboembolic events with anticoagulants

**Drug Uptake** Absorption: Estrone is not orally active due to enzymatic degradation in the gut and liver; addition of piperazine moiety increases oral absorption
**Pregnancy Risk Factor** X
**Generic Available** Yes

♦ **Estrostep® 21** *see* Ethinyl Estradiol and Norethindrone *on page 404*

♦ **Estrostep® Fe** *see* Ethinyl Estradiol and Norethindrone *on page 404*
♦ **Estrovis®** *see* Quinestrol *on page 872*

## Etanercept

**Related Information**

Rheumatoid Arthritis and Osteoarthritis *on page 1092*

**U.S. Brand Names** Enbrel®

**Therapeutic Category** Antirheumatic, Disease Modifying

**Use** Reduction in signs and symptoms of moderately to severely active rheumatoid arthritis in patients who have had an inadequate response to one or more disease-modifying antirheumatic drugs (DMARDs).

**Usual Dosage** S.C.:
- Children: 0.4 mg/kg (maximum: 25 mg dose)
- Adult: 25 mg given twice weekly; if the physician determines that it is appropriate, patients may self-inject after proper training in injection technique
- Elderly: Although greater sensitivity of some elderly patients cannot be ruled out, no overall differences in safety or effectiveness were observed

**Mechanism of Action** Etanercept is a recombinant DNA-derived protein composed of tumor necrosis factor receptor (TNFR) linked to the Fc portion of human IgG1. Etanercept binds tumor necrosis factor (TNF) and blocks its interaction with cell surface receptors. TNF plays an important role in the inflammatory processes of rheumatoid arthritis (RA) and the resulting joint pathology.

**Local Anesthetic/Vasoconstrictor Precautions** No information available to require special precautions

**Effects on Dental Treatment** No effects or complications reported

**Other Adverse Effects** Events reported include those >3% with incidence higher than placebo

>10%:
- Central nervous system: Headache (17%)
- Local: Injection site reaction (37%)
- Respiratory: Respiratory tract infection (38%), upper respiratory tract infection (29%), rhinitis (12%)
- Miscellaneous: Infection (35%), positive ANA (11%), positive anti-double stranded DNA antibodies (15% by RIA, 3% by *Crithidia lucilae* assay)

>3% to 10%:
- Central nervous system: Dizziness (7%)
- Dermatologic: Rash (5%)
- Gastrointestinal: Abdominal pain (5%), dyspepsia (4%)
- Neuromuscular and skeletal: Weakness (5%)
- Respiratory: Pharyngitis (7%), respiratory disorder (5%), sinusitis (3%)

<3%: Malignancies, serious infection, heart failure, myocardial infarction, myocardial ischemia, cerebral ischemia, hypertension, hypotension, cholecystitis, pancreatitis, gastrointestinal hemorrhage, bursitis, depression, dyspnea

Pediatric patients (JRA): The percentages of patients reporting abdominal pain (17%) and vomiting (14.5%) was higher than in adult RA. Two patients developed varicella infection associated with aseptic meningitis which resolved without complications (see Warnings/Precautions).

**Drug Interactions** Specific drug interaction studies have not been conducted with etanercept

**Drug Uptake**
- Serum half-life: 115 hours (98-300 hours)
- Time to peak: 72 hours (48-96 hours)

**Pregnancy Risk Factor** B

**Dosage Forms** Powder for injection: 25 mg

## Ethacrynic Acid (eth a KRIN ik AS id)

**Related Information**

Cardiovascular Diseases *on page 1066*

**U.S. Brand Names** Edecrin®

**Therapeutic Category** Diuretic, Loop

**Use** Management of edema associated with congestive heart failure; hepatic cirrhosis or renal disease; short-term management of ascites due to malignancy, idiopathic edema, and lymphedema

**Usual Dosage** I.V. formulation should be diluted in $D_5W$ or NS (1 mg/mL) and infused over several minutes

Children:
- Oral: 1 mg/kg/dose once daily; increase at intervals of 2-3 days as needed, to a maximum of 3 mg/kg/day
- I.V.: 1 mg/kg/dose, (maximum: 50 mg/dose); repeat doses not routinely recommended; however, if indicated, repeat doses every 8-12 hours

(Continued)

## Ethacrynic Acid *(Continued)*

Adults:

Oral: 50-100 mg/day in 1-2 divided doses; may increase in increments of 25-50 mg at intervals of several days to a maximum of 400 mg/24 hours

I.V.: 0.5-1 mg/kg/dose (maximum: 100 mg/dose); repeat doses not routinely recommended; however, if indicated, repeat doses every 8-12 hours

**Mechanism of Action** Inhibits reabsorption of sodium and chloride in the ascending loop of Henle and distal renal tubule, interfering with the chloride-binding cotransport system, thus causing increased excretion of water, sodium, chloride, magnesium, and calcium

**Local Anesthetic/Vasoconstrictor Precautions** No information available to require special precautions

**Effects on Dental Treatment** No effects or complications reported

**Other Adverse Effects**

>10%: Diarrhea

1% to 10%:

- Cardiovascular: Orthostatic hypotension
- Central nervous system: Headache
- Endocrine & metabolic: Hyponatremia, hypochloremic alkalosis, hypokalemia
- Gastrointestinal: Loss of appetite
- Ocular: Blurred vision
- Otic: Ototoxicity

<1%:

- Central nervous system: Nervousness
- Dermatologic: Skin rash
- Endocrine & metabolic: Hyperuricemia, gout
- Gastrointestinal: Gastrointestinal bleeding, pancreatitis, stomach cramps
- Hepatic: Hepatic dysfunction, abnormal LFTs
- Hematologic: Leukopenia, agranulocytosis, thrombocytopenia
- Local: Local irritation
- Renal: Renal injury, hematuria

**Drug Interactions**

Increased effect:

- Hypotensive agents causes additive decrease in blood pressure
- Drugs affected by or causing potassium depletion cause additive decrease in potassium
- Increased nephrotoxic potential with aminoglycosides
- Digoxin increases cardiotoxic potential leading to arrhythmias
- Increased warfarin anticoagulant effects; increased lithium levels

Decreased effect:

- Probenecid decreases diuretic effects
- Decreased effectiveness of antidiabetic agents

**Drug Uptake**

Onset of diuretic effect:

- Oral: Within 30 minutes
- I.V.: 5 minutes

Peak effect:

- Oral: 2 hours
- I.V.: 30 minutes

Duration of action:

- Oral: 12 hours
- I.V.: 2 hours

Absorption: Oral: Rapid

Serum half-life: Normal renal function: 2-4 hours

**Pregnancy Risk Factor** B

**Generic Available** No

## Ethambutol (e THAM byoo tole)

**Related Information**

Nonviral Infectious Diseases *on page 1095*

**U.S. Brand Names** Myambutol®

**Canadian Brand Names** Etibi®

**Therapeutic Category** Antitubercular Agent

**Use** Treatment of tuberculosis and other mycobacterial diseases in conjunction with other antituberculosis agents; only indicated when patients are from areas where drug-resistant M. tuberculosis is endemic, in HIV-infected elderly patients, and when drug-resistant M. tuberculosis is suspected

**Usual Dosage** Oral:

Ethambutol is generally not recommended in children whose visual acuity cannot be monitored (<6 years of age). However, ethambutol should be considered for all children with organisms resistant to other drugs, when susceptibility to ethambutol has been demonstrated, or susceptibility is likely.

**Note:** A four-drug regimen (isoniazid, rifampin, pyrazinamide, and either streptomycin or ethambutol) is preferred for the initial, empiric treatment of TB. When the drug susceptibility results are available, the regimen should be altered as appropriate.

**Patients with tuberculosis and without HIV infection:**

**OPTION 1:** Isoniazid resistance rate <4%: Administer daily isoniazid, rifampin, and pyrazinamide for 8 weeks followed by isoniazid and rifampin daily or directly observed therapy (DOT) 2-3 times/week for 16 weeks. If isoniazid resistance rate is not documented, ethambutol or streptomycin should also be administered until susceptibility to isoniazid or rifampin is demonstrated. Continue treatment for at least 6 months or 3 months beyond culture conversion.

**OPTION 2:** Administer daily isoniazid, rifampin, pyrazinamide, and either streptomycin or ethambutol for 2 weeks followed by DOT 2 times/week administration of the same drugs for 6 weeks, and subsequently, with isoniazid and rifampin DOT 2 times/week administration for 16 weeks

**OPTION 3:** Administer isoniazid, rifampin, pyrazinamide, and either ethambutol or streptomycin by DOT 3 times/week for 6 months

**Patients with TB and with HIV infection:** Administer any of the above OPTIONS 1, 2 or 3; however, treatment should be continued for a total of 9 months and at least 6 months beyond culture conversion

**Note:** Some experts recommend that the duration of therapy should be extended to 9 months for patients with disseminated disease, miliary disease, disease involving the bones or joints, or tuberculosis lymphadenitis

Children (>6 years) and Adults:
Daily therapy: 15-25 mg/kg/day (maximum: 2.5 g/day)
Directly observed therapy (DOT): Twice weekly: 50 mg/kg (maximum: 2.5 g)
DOT: 3 times/week: 25-30 mg/kg (maximum: 2.5 g)

**Mechanism of Action** Suppresses mycobacteria multiplication by interfering with RNA synthesis

**Local Anesthetic/Vasoconstrictor Precautions** No information available to require special precautions

**Effects on Dental Treatment** No effects or complications reported

**Other Adverse Effects**

1% to 10%:
Central nervous system: Headache, confusion, disorientation
Endocrine & metabolic: Acute gout or hyperuricemia
Gastrointestinal: Abdominal pain, anorexia, nausea, vomiting

<1%:
Central nervous system: Malaise, mental confusion, fever
Dermatologic: Rash, pruritus
Hepatic: Abnormal liver function tests
Neuromuscular & skeletal: Peripheral neuritis
Ocular: Optic neuritis
Miscellaneous: Anaphylaxis

**Drug Interactions** Decreased absorption with aluminum salts

**Drug Uptake**
Absorption: Oral: ~80%
Serum half-life: 2.5-3.6 hours
End-stage renal disease: 7-15 hours
Time to peak serum concentration: 2-4 hours

**Pregnancy Risk Factor** B

**Generic Available** No

♦ **Ethamolin®** *see* Ethanolamine Oleate *on this page*
♦ **ETH and C** *see* Terpin Hydrate and Codeine *on page 960*

## Ethanolamine Oleate (ETH a nol a meen OH lee ate)

**U.S. Brand Names** Ethamolin®

**Therapeutic Category** Sclerosing Agent

**Synonyms** Monoethanolamine

**Use** Mild sclerosing agent used for bleeding esophageal varices

**Usual Dosage** Adults: 1.5-5 mL per varix, up to 20 mL total or 0.4 mL/kg; patients with severe hepatic dysfunction should receive less than recommended maximum dose

**Mechanism of Action** Derived from oleic acid and similar in physical properties to sodium morrhuate; however, the exact mechanism of the hemostatic effect used in endoscopic injection sclerotherapy is not known. Intravenously injected ethanolamine oleate produces a sterile inflammatory response resulting in

(Continued)

## Ethanolamine Oleate *(Continued)*

fibrosis and occlusion of the vein; a dose-related extravascular inflammatory reaction occurs when the drug diffuses through the venous wall. Autopsy results indicate that variceal obliteration occurs secondary to mural necrosis and fibrosis. Thrombosis appears to be a transient reaction.

**Local Anesthetic/Vasoconstrictor Precautions** No information available to require special precautions

**Effects on Dental Treatment** No effects or complications reported

**Other Adverse Effects**

1% to 10%:

- Central nervous system: Fever
- Gastrointestinal: Esophageal ulcer, esophageal stricture
- Neuromuscular & skeletal: Retrosternal pain
- Respiratory: Pleural effusion, pneumonia

<1%:

- Local: Injection necrosis
- Renal: Acute renal failure
- Respiration: Aspiration
- Miscellaneous: Anaphylaxis

**Drug Interactions** No data reported

**Pregnancy Risk Factor** C

**Generic Available** No

♦ **Ethaquin®** *see* Ethaverine *on this page*

♦ **Ethatab®** *see* Ethaverine *on this page*

## Ethaverine (eth AV er een)

**U.S. Brand Names** Ethaquin®; Ethatab®; Ethavex-100®; Isovex®

**Therapeutic Category** Vasodilator

**Use** Peripheral and cerebral vascular insufficiency associated with arterial spasm

**Usual Dosage** Adults: Oral: 100 mg 3 times/day

**Local Anesthetic/Vasoconstrictor Precautions** No information available to require special precautions

**Effects on Dental Treatment** No effects or complications reported

**Other Adverse Effects** <1%:

- Cardiovascular: Flushing of the face, tachycardia, hypotension
- Central nervous system: Depression, dizziness, vertigo, drowsiness, sedation, lethargy, headache
- Dermatologic: Pruritus
- Gastrointestinal: Dry mouth, nausea, constipation
- Hepatic: Hepatic hypersensitivity
- Miscellaneous: Sweating

**Generic Available** Yes

♦ **Ethavex-100®** *see* Ethaverine *on this page*

## Ethchlorvynol (eth klor VI nole)

**U.S. Brand Names** Placidyl®

**Therapeutic Category** Hypnotic; Sedative

**Use** Short-term management of insomnia

**Usual Dosage** Adults: Oral: 500-1000 mg at bedtime

**Mechanism of Action** Causes nonspecific depression of the reticular activating system

**Local Anesthetic/Vasoconstrictor Precautions** No information available to require special precautions

**Effects on Dental Treatment** No effects or complications reported

**Other Adverse Effects**

>10%:

- Central nervous system: Dizziness
- Gastrointestinal: Indigestion, nausea, stomach pain, unpleasant aftertaste
- Neuromuscular & skeletal: Weakness
- Ocular: Blurred vision

1% to 10%:

- Central nervous system: Nervousness, excitement, clumsiness, confusion, drowsiness (daytime)
- Dermatologic: Skin rash

<1%:

- Cardiovascular: Bradycardia
- Central nervous system: Hyperthermia, slurred speech
- Hepatic: Cholestatic jaundice
- Neuromuscular & skeletal: Trembling, weakness (severe)
- Respiratory: Dyspnea

**Drug Interactions**
Decreased effect of oral anticoagulants
Increased toxicity (CNS depression) with alcohol, CNS depressants, MAO inhibitors, TCAs (delirium)
**Drug Uptake**
Onset of action: 15-60 minutes
Duration: 5 hours
Absorption: Rapid from GI tract
Serum half-life: 10-20 hours
Time to peak serum concentration: 2 hours
**Pregnancy Risk Factor** C
**Generic Available** No

## Ethinyl Estradiol (ETH in il es tra DYE ole)

**Related Information**
Endocrine Disorders & Pregnancy *on page 1082*
**U.S. Brand Names** Estinyl®
**Therapeutic Category** Estrogen Derivative
**Use** Hypogonadism; primary ovarian failure; vasomotor symptoms of menopause; prostatic carcinoma; breast cancer
**Usual Dosage** Adults: Oral:
Male: Prostatic cancer (inoperable, progressing): 0.15-2 mg/day for palliation
Female:
Hypogonadism: 0.05 mg 1-3 times/day for 2 weeks of a theoretical menstrual cycle followed by progesterone for 3-6 months
Vasomotor symptoms: 0.02-0.05 mg for 21 days, off 7 days and repeat
Breast cancer (inoperable, progressing): 1 mg 3 times/day for palliation
**Mechanism of Action** Increases the synthesis of DNA, RNA, and various proteins in target tissues; reduces the release of gonadotropin-releasing hormone from the hypothalamus; reduces FSH and LH release from the pituitary
**Local Anesthetic/Vasoconstrictor Precautions** No information available to require special precautions
**Effects on Dental Treatment** No effects or complications reported
**Other Adverse Effects**
>10%:
Cardiovascular: Peripheral edema
Endocrine & metabolic: Enlargement of breasts, breast tenderness
Gastrointestinal: Nausea, anorexia, bloating
1% to 10%:
Central nervous system: Headache
Endocrine & metabolic: Increased libido
Gastrointestinal: Vomiting, diarrhea
<1%:
Cardiovascular: Hypertension, thromboembolism, myocardial infarction, edema
Central nervous system: Stroke, depression, dizziness, anxiety
Dermatologic: Chloasma, melasma, rash
Endocrine & metabolic: Breast tumors, amenorrhea, alterations in frequency and flow of menses, decreased glucose tolerance, elevated triglycerides and LDL
Gastrointestinal: GI distress
Hepatic: Cholestatic jaundice
Ocular: Intolerance to contact lenses
Miscellaneous: Increased susceptibility to *Candida* infection
**Drug Interactions**
Decreased effect: Rifampin decreases estrogen serum concentrations
Increased toxicity: Anticoagulants: Increases potential for thromboembolic events with anticoagulants
**Drug Uptake**
Absorption: Absorbed well from GI tract
**Pregnancy Risk Factor** X
**Generic Available** No

## Ethinyl Estradiol and Desogestrel

(ETH in il es tra DYE ole & des oh JES trel)
**U.S. Brand Names** Desogen®; Mircette®; Ortho-Cept®
**Therapeutic Category** Contraceptive, Oral
**Synonyms** Desogestrel and Ethinyl Estradiol
**Use** Prevention of pregnancy
(Continued)

## Ethinyl Estradiol and Desogestrel *(Continued)*

**Usual Dosage**

Contraception: Oral: 1 tablet daily, beginning on day 5 of menstrual cycle (first day of menstrual flow is day 1). With 21-tablet packages, new dosing cycle begins 7 days after last tablet taken. With 28-tablet packages, dosage is 1 tablet daily without interruption; extra tablets are placebos. If next menstrual period does not begin on schedule, rule out pregnancy before starting new dosing cycle. If menstrual period begins, start new dosing cycle 7 days after last tablet was taken. If all doses have been taken on schedule and one menstrual period is missed, continue dosing cycle. If two consecutive menstrual periods are missed, pregnancy test is required before new dosing cycle is started.

One dose missed: Take as soon as remembered or take 2 tablets next day

Two doses missed: Take 2 tablets as soon as remembered or 2 tablets next 2 days

Three doses missed: Begin new compact of tablets starting on day 1 of next cycle

**Mechanism of Action** Combination oral contraceptives inhibit ovulation via a negative feedback mechanism on the hypothalamus, which alters the normal pattern of gonadotropin secretion of a follicle-stimulating hormone (FSH) and luteinizing hormone by the anterior pituitary. The follicular phase FSH and midcycle surge of gonadotropins are inhibited. In addition, oral contraceptives produce alterations in the genital tract, including changes in the cervical mucus, rendering it unfavorable for sperm penetration even if ovulation occurs. Changes in the endometrium may also occur, producing an unfavorable environment for nidation. Oral contraceptive drugs may alter the tubal transport of the ova through the fallopian tubes. Progestational agents may also alter sperm fertility.

**Local Anesthetic/Vasoconstrictor Precautions** No information available to require special precautions

**Effects on Dental Treatment** When prescribing antibiotics, patient must be warned to use supplemental methods of birth control if on oral contraceptives

**Pregnancy Risk Factor** X

**Generic Available** No

## Ethinyl Estradiol and Ethynodiol Diacetate

(ETH in il es tra DYE ole & e thye noe DYE ole dye AS e tate)

**Related Information**

Endocrine Disorders & Pregnancy *on page 1082*

**U.S. Brand Names** Demulen®; Zovia®

**Therapeutic Category** Contraceptive, Oral

**Use** Prevention of pregnancy; treatment of hypermenorrhea, endometriosis, female hypogonadism

**Usual Dosage** Adults: Female: Oral:

For 21-tablet cycle packs, with 21 active tablets (28-day packs have 21 active tablets and 7 inert tablets): Take 1 tablet daily starting on the fifth day of menstrual cycle, with day 1 being the first day of menstruation; begin taking a new cycle pack on the eighth day after taking the last tablet from the previous pack

With 28-tablet packages, dosage is 1 tablet daily without interruption; extra tablets are placebos or contain iron. If next menstrual period does not begin on schedule, rule out pregnancy before starting new dosing cycle. If menstrual period begins, start new dosing cycle 7 days after last tablet was taken. If all doses have been taken on schedule and one menstrual period is missed, continue dosing cycle. If two consecutive menstrual periods are missed, pregnancy test is required before new dosing cycle is started.

One dose missed: Take as soon as remembered or take 2 tablets next day

Two doses missed: Take 2 tablets as soon as remembered or 2 tablets next 2 days

Three doses missed: Begin new compact of tablets starting on day 1 of next cycle

**Mechanism of Action** Combination oral contraceptives inhibit ovulation via a negative feedback mechanism on the hypothalamus, which alters the normal pattern of gonadotropin secretion of a follicle-stimulating hormone (FSH) and luteinizing hormone by the anterior pituitary. The follicular phase FSH and midcycle surge of gonadotropins are inhibited. In addition, oral contraceptives produce alterations in the genital tract, including changes in the cervical mucus, rendering it unfavorable for sperm penetration even if ovulation occurs. Changes in the endometrium may also occur, producing an unfavorable environment for nidation. Oral contraceptive drugs may alter the tubal transport of the ova through the fallopian tubes. Progestational agents may also alter sperm fertility.

**Local Anesthetic/Vasoconstrictor Precautions** No information available to require special precautions

**Effects on Dental Treatment** When prescribing antibiotics, patient must be warned to use supplemental methods of birth control if on oral contraceptives

**Other Adverse Effects**

>10%:
- Cardiovascular: Peripheral edema
- Endocrine & metabolic: Enlargement of breasts, breast tenderness
- Gastrointestinal: Nausea, anorexia, bloating

1% to 10%:
- Central nervous system: Headache
- Endocrine & metabolic: Increased libido
- Gastrointestinal: Vomiting, diarrhea

<1%:
- Cardiovascular: Hypertension, thromboembolism, myocardial infarction, edema
- Central nervous system: Depression, dizziness, anxiety, stroke
- Dermatologic: Chloasma, melasma, rash
- Endocrine & metabolic: Decreased glucose tolerance, breast tumors, amenorrhea, alterations in frequency and flow of menses, elevated triglycerides and LDL
- Gastrointestinal: GI distress
- Hepatic: Cholestatic jaundice
- Ocular: Intolerance to contact lenses
- Miscellaneous: Increased susceptibility to *Candida* infection

See tables.

**Achieving Proper Hormonal Balance in an Oral Contraceptive**

| Estrogen | | Progestin | |
|---|---|---|---|
| **Excess** | **Deficiency** | **Excess** | **Deficiency** |
| Nausea, bloating<br>Cervical mucorrhea, polyposis<br>Melasma<br>Migraine headache<br>Breast fullness or tenderness<br>Edema<br>Hypertension | Early or midcycle breakthrough bleeding<br>Increased spotting<br>Hypomenorrhea | Increased appetite<br>Weight gain<br>Tiredness, fatigue<br>Hypomenorrhea<br>Acne, oily scalp*<br>Hair loss, hirsutism*<br>Depression<br>Monilial vaginitis<br>Breast regression | Late breakthrough bleeding<br>Amenorrhea<br>Hypermenorrhea |

*Result of androgenic activity of progestins.

**Pharmacological Effects of Progestins Used in Oral Contraceptives**

| | Progestin | Estrogen | Antiestrogen | Androgen |
|---|---|---|---|---|
| Norgestrel/levonorgestrel | +++ | 0 | ++ | +++ |
| Ethynodiol diacetate | ++ | +* | +* | + |
| Norethindrone acetate | + | + | +++ | + |
| Norethindrone | + | +* | +* | + |
| Norethynodrel | + | +++ | 0 | 0 |

*Has estrogenic effect at low doses; may have antiestrogenic effect at higher doses.

+++ = pronounced effect
++ = moderate effect
+ = slight effect
0 = no effect

**Drug Interactions**

Decreased effect of oral contraceptives with barbiturates, hydantoins - phenytoin, rifampin, antibiotics - penicillins, tetracyclines, griseofulvin

Increased toxicity of acetaminophen, anticoagulants, benzodiazepines, caffeine, corticosteroids, metoprolol, theophylline, tricyclic antidepressants

**Drug Uptake** Ethinyl estradiol:

Absorption: Absorbed well from GI tract

Serum half-life, terminal: 5-14 hours

**Pregnancy Risk Factor** X

**Generic Available** Yes

## Ethinyl Estradiol and Fluoxymesterone

(eth i nil es tra DYE ole & floo oks i MES te rone)

**Therapeutic Category** Androgen; Estrogen Derivative

**Synonyms** Fluoxymesterone and Estradiol

**Use** Moderate to severe vasomotor symptoms of menopause, postpartum breast engorgement

**Usual Dosage** Oral: 1-2 tablets at bedtime given cyclically, 3 weeks on and 1 week off

**Local Anesthetic/Vasoconstrictor Precautions** No information available to require special precautions

**Effects on Dental Treatment** When prescribing antibiotics, patient must be warned to use supplemental methods of birth control if on oral contraceptives

**Other Adverse Effects** 1% to 10%:

- Cardiovascular: Hypertension, thromboembolism, myocardial infarction, edema
- Central nervous system: Depression, migraine, dizziness, anxiety, headache, stroke
- Dermatologic: Chloasma, melasma, rash
- Endocrine & metabolic: Decreased glucose tolerance, alterations in frequency and flow of menses, breast tenderness or enlargement, hypertriglyceridemia, elevated LDL
- Gastrointestinal: Nausea, GI distress
- Hepatic: Cholestatic jaundice
- Miscellaneous: Increased susceptibility to *Candida* infection

**Pregnancy Risk Factor** X

**Generic Available** No

## Ethinyl Estradiol and Levonorgestrel

(ETH in il es tra DYE ole & LEE voe nor jes trel)

**Related Information**

Endocrine Disorders & Pregnancy *on page 1082*

**U.S. Brand Names** Alesse™; Levlen®; Levlite®; Levora®; Nordette®; Preven®; Tri-Levlen®; Triphasil®

**Therapeutic Category** Contraceptive, Oral

**Use** Prevention of pregnancy; treatment of hypermenorrhea, endometriosis, female hypogonadism

**Usual Dosage** Adults: Female: Oral:

Contraception: 1 tablet daily, beginning on day 5 of menstrual cycle (first day of menstrual flow is day 1). With 20-tablet and 21-tablet packages, new dosing cycle begins 7 days after last tablet taken. With 28-tablet packages, dosage is 1 tablet daily without interruption; extra tablets are placebos or contain iron. If next menstrual period does not begin on schedule, rule out pregnancy before starting new dosing cycle. If menstrual period begins, start new dosing cycle 7 days after last tablet was taken. If all doses have been taken on schedule and one menstrual period is missed, continue dosing cycle. If two consecutive menstrual periods are missed, pregnancy test is required before new dosing cycle is started.

- One dose missed: Take as soon as remembered or take 2 tablets next day
- Two doses missed: Take 2 tablets as soon as remembered or 2 tablets next 2 days
- Three doses missed: Begin new compact of tablets starting on day 1 of next cycle

Triphasic oral contraceptive (Tri-Levlen®, Triphasil®): 1 tablet/day in the sequence specified by the manufacturer

**Mechanism of Action** Combination oral contraceptives inhibit ovulation via a negative feedback mechanism on the hypothalamus, which alters the normal pattern of gonadotropin secretion of a follicle-stimulating hormone (FSH) and luteinizing hormone by the anterior pituitary. The follicular phase FSH and midcycle surge of gonadotropins are inhibited. In addition, oral contraceptives produce alterations in the genital tract, including changes in the cervical mucus, rendering it unfavorable for sperm penetration even if ovulation occurs. Changes in the endometrium may also occur, producing an unfavorable environment for nidation. Oral contraceptive drugs may alter the tubal transport of the ova through the fallopian tubes. Progestational agents may also alter sperm fertility.

**Local Anesthetic/Vasoconstrictor Precautions** No information available to require special precautions

**Effects on Dental Treatment** When prescribing antibiotics, patient must be warned to use additional methods of birth control if taking oral contraceptives

**Other Adverse Effects**

>10%:

- Cardiovascular: Peripheral edema
- Endocrine & metabolic: Enlargement of breasts, breast tenderness

Gastrointestinal: Nausea, anorexia, bloating

1% to 10%:

Central nervous system: Headache

Endocrine & metabolic: Increased libido

Gastrointestinal: Vomiting, diarrhea

<1%:

Cardiovascular: Hypertension, thromboembolism, myocardial infarction, edema

Central nervous system: Depression, dizziness, anxiety, stroke

Dermatologic: Chloasma, melasma, rash

Endocrine & metabolic: Decreased glucose tolerance, breast tumors, amenorrhea, alterations in frequency and flow of menses, hypertriglyceridemia, elevated LDL

Gastrointestinal: GI distress

Hepatic: Cholestatic jaundice

Ocular: Intolerance to contact lenses

Miscellaneous: Increased susceptibility to *Candida* infection

See tables.

### Achieving Proper Hormonal Balance in an Oral Contraceptive

| Estrogen | | Progestin | |
|---|---|---|---|
| **Excess** | **Deficiency** | **Excess** | **Deficiency** |
| Nausea, bloating | Early or midcycle breakthrough bleeding | Increased appetite | Late breakthrough bleeding |
| Cervical mucorrhea, polyposis | Increased spotting | Weight gain | Amenorrhea |
| Melasma | Hypomenorrhea | Tiredness, fatigue | Hypermenorrhea |
| Migraine headache | | Hypomenorrhea | |
| Breast fullness or tenderness | | Acne, oily scalp* | |
| Edema | | Hair loss, hirsutism* | |
| Hypertension | | Depression | |
| | | Monilial vaginitis | |
| | | Breast regression | |

*Result of androgenic activity of progestins.

### Pharmacological Effects of Progestins Used in Oral Contraceptives

| | Progestin | Estrogen | Antiestrogen | Androgen |
|---|---|---|---|---|
| Norgestrel/levonorgestrel | +++ | 0 | ++ | +++ |
| Ethynodiol diacetate | ++ | +* | +* | + |
| Norethindrone acetate | + | + | +++ | + |
| Norethindrone | + | +* | +* | + |
| Norethynodrel | + | +++ | 0 | 0 |

*Has estrogenic effect at low doses; may have antiestrogenic effect at higher doses.

+++ = pronounced effect

++ = moderate effect

+ = slight effect

0 = no effect

**Warnings/Precautions** Use of any progestin during the first 4 months of pregnancy is not recommended; use with caution in patients with asthma, seizure disorders, migraine, cardiac, renal or hepatic impairment, cerebrovascular disorders or history of breast cancer, past and present thromboembolic disease, smokers >35 years of age

**Drug Interactions** Ethinyl estradiol is a CYP3A3/4 and 3A5-7 enzyme substrate; CYP1A2 enzyme inhibitor

Decreased effect of oral contraceptives with barbiturates, hydantoins - phenytoin, rifampin, antibiotics - penicillins, tetracyclines, griseofulvin

Increased toxicity of acetaminophen, anticoagulants, benzodiazepines, caffeine, corticosteroids, metoprolol, theophylline, tricyclic antidepressants

**Drug Uptake**

Ethinyl estradiol:

Absorption: Absorbed well from GI tract

Levonorgestrel:

Serum half-life, terminal: 11-45 hours

Time to peak: 0.5-2 hours

**Pregnancy Risk Factor** X

**Dosage Forms** Tablet:

Alesse™, Levlite®: Ethinyl estradiol 0.02 mg and levonorgestrel 0.1 mg (21s, 28s)

(Continued)

## Ethinyl Estradiol and Levonorgestrel *(Continued)*

Levlen®, Levora®, Nordette®: Ethinyl estradiol 0.03 mg and levonorgestrel 0.15 mg (21s, 28s)

Preven®: Ethinyl estradiol 0.05 mg and levonorgestrel 0.25 mg (4s)

Tri-Levlen®, Triphasil®: Phase 1 (6 brown tablets): Ethinyl estradiol 0.03 mg and levonorgestrel 0.05 mg; Phase 2 (5 white tablets): Ethinyl estradiol 0.04 mg and levonorgestrel 0.075 mg; Phase 3 (10 yellow tablets): Ethinyl estradiol 0.03 mg and levonorgestrel 0.125 mg (21s, 28s)

**Generic Available** Yes

## Ethinyl Estradiol and Norethindrone

(ETH in il es tra DYE ole & nor eth IN drone)

**Related Information**

Endocrine Disorders & Pregnancy *on page 1082*

**U.S. Brand Names** Brevicon®; Estrostep® 21; Estrostep® Fe; Genora® 0.5/35; Genora® 1/35; Jenest-28™; Loestrin®; Modicon™; N.E.E.® 1/35; Nelova™ 0.5/35E; Nelova™ 10/11; Norethin™ 1/35E; Norinyl® 1+35; Ortho-Novum® 1/35; Ortho-Novum® 7/7/7; Ortho-Novum® 10/11; Ovcon® 35; Ovcon® 50; Tri-Norinyl®

**Canadian Brand Names** Ortho®0.5/35; Synphasic®

**Therapeutic Category** Contraceptive, Oral

**Use** Prevention of pregnancy; treatment of hypermenorrhea, endometriosis, female hypogonadism

**Usual Dosage** Adults: Female: Oral:

For 21-tablet cycle packs, with 21 active tablets (28-day packs have 21 active tablets and 7 inert tablets): Take 1 tablet daily starting on the fifth day of menstrual cycle, with day 1 being the first day of menstruation; begin taking a new cycle pack on the eighth day after taking the last tablet from the previous pack

With 28-tablet packages, dosage is 1 tablet daily without interruption; extra tablets are placebos or contain iron. If next menstrual period does not begin on schedule, rule out pregnancy before starting new dosing cycle. If menstrual period begins, start new dosing cycle 7 days after last tablet was taken. If all doses have been taken on schedule and one menstrual period is missed, continue dosing cycle. If two consecutive menstrual periods are missed, pregnancy test is required before new dosing cycle is started.

One dose missed: Take as soon as remembered or take 2 tablets next day

Two doses missed: Take 2 tablets as soon as remembered or 2 tablets next 2 days

Three doses missed: Begin new compact of tablets starting on day 1 of next cycle

Biphasic oral contraceptive (Jenest™-28, Ortho-Novum™ 10/11, Nelova™ 10/11): 1 color tablet/day for 10 days, then next color tablet for 11 days

Triphasic oral contraceptive (Ortho-Novum™ 7/7/7, Tri-Norinyl®, Triphasil®): 1 tablet/day in the sequence specified by the manufacturer

**Mechanism of Action** Combination oral contraceptives inhibit ovulation via a negative feedback mechanism on the hypothalamus, which alters the normal pattern of gonadotropin secretion of a follicle-stimulating hormone (FSH) and luteinizing hormone by the anterior pituitary. The follicular phase FSH and midcycle surge of gonadotropins are inhibited. In addition, oral contraceptives produce alterations in the genital tract, including changes in the cervical mucus, rendering it unfavorable for sperm penetration even if ovulation occurs. Changes in the endometrium may also occur, producing an unfavorable environment for nidation. Oral contraceptive drugs may alter the tubal transport of the ova through the fallopian tubes. Progestational agents may also alter sperm fertility.

**Local Anesthetic/Vasoconstrictor Precautions** No information available to require special precautions

**Effects on Dental Treatment** When prescribing antibiotics, patient must be warned to use additional methods of birth control if taking oral contraceptives

**Other Adverse Effects**

>10%:

- Cardiovascular: Peripheral edema
- Endocrine & metabolic: Enlargement of breasts, breast tenderness
- Gastrointestinal: Nausea, anorexia, bloating

1% to 10%:

- Central nervous system: Headache
- Endocrine & metabolic: Increased libido
- Gastrointestinal: Vomiting, diarrhea

<1%:

- Cardiovascular: Hypertension, thromboembolism, myocardial infarction, edema
- Central nervous system: Depression, dizziness, anxiety, stroke

Dermatologic: Chloasma, melasma, rash
Endocrine & metabolic: Decreased glucose tolerance, breast tumors, amenorrhea, alterations in frequency and flow of menses, elevated triglycerides and LDL
Gastrointestinal: GI distress
Hepatic: Cholestatic jaundice
Ocular: Intolerance to contact lenses
Miscellaneous: Increased susceptibility to *Candida* infection

See tables.

**Achieving Proper Hormonal Balance in an Oral Contraceptive**

| Estrogen | | Progestin | |
|---|---|---|---|
| **Excess** | **Deficiency** | **Excess** | **Deficiency** |
| Nausea, bloating<br>Cervical mucorrhea, polyposis<br>Melasma<br>Migraine headache<br>Breast fullness or tenderness<br>Edema<br>Hypertension | Early or midcycle breakthrough bleeding<br>Increased spotting<br>Hypomenorrhea | Increased appetite<br>Weight gain<br>Tiredness, fatigue<br>Hypomenorrhea<br>Acne, oily scalp*<br>Hair loss, hirsutism*<br>Depression<br>Monilial vaginitis<br>Breast regression | Late breakthrough bleeding<br>Amenorrhea<br>Hypermenorrhea |

*Result of androgenic activity of progestins.

**Pharmacological Effects of Progestins Used in Oral Contraceptives**

| | Progestin | Estrogen | Antiestrogen | Androgen |
|---|---|---|---|---|
| Norgestrel/levonorgestrel | +++ | 0 | ++ | +++ |
| Ethynodiol diacetate | ++ | +* | +* | + |
| Norethindrone acetate | + | + | +++ | + |
| Norethindrone | + | +* | +* | + |
| Norethynodrel | + | +++ | 0 | 0 |

*Has estrogenic effect at low doses; may have antiestrogenic effect at higher doses.
+++ = pronounced effect
++ = moderate effect
\+ = slight effect
0 = no effect

**Warnings/Precautions** Use of any progestin during the first 4 months of pregnancy is not recommended; in patients with a history of thromboembolism, stroke, myocardial infarction (especially >40 years of age who smoke), liver tumor, hypertension, cardiac, renal or hepatic insufficiency; risk of cardiovascular side effects increases in those women who smoke cigarettes and in women >35 years of age

**Drug Interactions** Ethinyl estradiol is a CYP3A3/4 and 3A5-7 enzyme substrate; CYP1A2 enzyme inhibitor
Decreased effect:
Potential contraceptive failure with barbiturates, hydantoins, and rifampin
Concomitant penicillins, tetracyclines, or other antibiotics may lead to contraceptive failure
Increased toxicity:
Increased toxicity of carbamazepine, tricyclic antidepressants, and corticosteroids
Increased thromboembolic potential with oral anticoagulants

**Drug Uptake**
Ethinyl estradiol:
Absorption: Absorbed well from GI tract
Norethindrone:
Serum half-life, terminal: 5-14 hours
Time to peak: Oral: 0.5-4 hours

**Pregnancy Risk Factor** X

**Dosage Forms** Tablet:
Brevicon®, Genora® 0.5/35, Modicon™, Nelova™ 0.5/35E: Ethinyl estradiol 0.035 mg and norethindrone 0.5 mg (21s, 28s)
Estrostep®:
Triangular tablet (white): Ethinyl estradiol 0.02 mg and norethindrone acetate 1 mg
(Continued)

## Ethinyl Estradiol and Norethindrone *(Continued)*

Square tablet (white): Ethinyl estradiol 0.03 mg and norethindrone acetate 1 mg

Round tablet (white): Ethinyl estradiol 0.035 mg and norethindrone acetate 1 mg

Estrostep® Fe:

Triangular tablet (white): Ethinyl estradiol 0.02 mg and norethindrone acetate 1 mg

Square tablet (white): Ethinyl estradiol 0.03 mg and norethindrone acetate 1 mg

Round tablet (white): Ethinyl estradiol 0.035 mg and norethindrone acetate 1 mg

Brown tablet: Ferrous fumarate 75 mg

Loestrin® 1.5/30: Ethinyl estradiol 0.03 mg and norethindrone acetate 1.5 mg (21s)

Loestrin® Fe 1.5/30: Ethinyl estradiol 0.03 mg and norethindrone acetate 1.5 mg with ferrous fumarate 75 mg in 7 inert tablets (28s)

Loestrin® 1/20: Ethinyl estradiol 0.02 mg and norethindrone acetate 1 mg (21s)

Loestrin® Fe 1/20: Ethinyl estradiol 0.02 mg and norethindrone acetate 1 mg with ferrous fumarate 75 mg in 7 inert tablets (28s)

Genora® 1/35, N.E.E.® 1/35, Nelova® 1/35E, Norethin™ 1/35E, Norinyl® 1+35, Ortho-Novum® 1/35: Ethinyl estradiol 0.035 mg and norethindrone 1 mg (21s, 28s)

Jenest-28™: Phase 1 (7 white tablets): Ethinyl estradiol 0.035 mg and norethindrone 0.5 mg; Phase 2 (14 peach tablets): Ethinyl estradiol 0.035 mg and norethindrone 1 mg and 7 green inert tablets (28s)

Ortho-Novum® 7/7/7: Phase 1 (7 white tablets): Ethinyl estradiol 0.035 mg and norethindrone 0.5 mg; Phase 2 (7 light peach tablets): Ethinyl estradiol 0.035 mg and norethindrone 0.75 mg; Phase 3 (7 peach tablets): Ethinyl estradiol 0.035 mg and norethindrone 1 mg (21s, 28s)

Ortho-Novum® 10/11: Phase 1 (10 white tablets): Ethinyl estradiol 0.035 mg and norethindrone 0.5 mg; Phase 2 (11 dark yellow tablets): Ethinyl estradiol 0.035 mg and norethindrone 1 mg (21s, 28s)

Ovcon® 35: Ethinyl estradiol 0.035 mg and norethindrone 0.4 mg (21s, 28s)

Ovcon® 50: Ethinyl estradiol 0.050 mg and norethindrone 1 mg (21s, 28s)

Tri-Norinyl®: Phase 1 (7 blue tablets): Ethinyl estradiol 0.035 mg and norethindrone 0.5 mg; Phase 2 (9 green tablets): Ethinyl estradiol 0.035 mg and norethindrone 1 mg; Phase 3 (5 blue tablets): Ethinyl estradiol 0.035 mg and norethindrone 0.5 mg (21s, 28s)

**Generic Available** Yes

## Ethinyl Estradiol and Norgestimate

(ETH in il es tra DYE ole & nor JES ti mate)

**U.S. Brand Names** Ortho-Cyclen®; Ortho Tri-Cyclen®

**Therapeutic Category** Contraceptive, Oral

**Synonyms** Norgestimate and Ethinyl Estradiol

**Use** Prevention of pregnancy

**Usual Dosage**

Contraception: Oral: 1 tablet daily, beginning on day 5 of menstrual cycle (first day of menstrual flow is day 1). With 21-tablet packages, new dosing cycle begins 7 days after last tablet taken. With 28-tablet packages, dosage is 1 tablet daily without interruption; extra tablets are placebos or contain iron. If next menstrual period does not begin on schedule, rule out pregnancy before starting new dosing cycle. If menstrual period begins, start new dosing cycle 7 days after last tablet was taken. If all doses have been taken on schedule and one menstrual period is missed, continue dosing cycle. If two consecutive menstrual periods are missed, pregnancy test is required before new dosing cycle is started.

One dose missed: Take as soon as remembered or take 2 tablets next day

Two doses missed: Take 2 tablets as soon as remembered or 2 tablets next 2 days

Three doses missed: Begin new compact of tablets starting on day 1 of next cycle

Triphasic oral contraceptive: 1 tablet/day in the sequence specified by the manufacturer

**Mechanism of Action** Combination oral contraceptives inhibit ovulation via a negative feedback mechanism on the hypothalamus, which alters the normal pattern of gonadotropin secretion of a follicle-stimulating hormone (FSH) and luteinizing hormone by the anterior pituitary. The follicular phase FSH and midcycle surge of gonadotropins are inhibited. In addition, oral contraceptives produce alterations in the genital tract, including changes in the cervical mucus, rendering it unfavorable for sperm penetration even if ovulation occurs. Changes in the endometrium may also occur, producing an unfavorable environment for nidation. Oral contraceptive drugs may alter the tubal transport of the ova through the fallopian tubes. Progestational agents may also alter sperm fertility.

**Local Anesthetic/Vasoconstrictor Precautions** No information available to require special precautions

**Effects on Dental Treatment** When prescribing antibiotics, patient must be warned to use supplemental methods of birth control if on oral contraceptives

**Pregnancy Risk Factor** X

**Generic Available** No

## Ethinyl Estradiol and Norgestrel

(ETH in il es tra DYE ole & nor JES trel)

**U.S. Brand Names** Lo/Ovral®; Ovral®

**Therapeutic Category** Contraceptive, Oral

**Use** Prevention of pregnancy; treatment of hypermenorrhea, endometriosis, female hypogonadism; postcoital contraception

**Usual Dosage** Adults: Female: Oral: Contraception: 1 tablet daily, beginning on day 5 of menstrual cycle (first day of menstrual flow is day 1). With 20-tablet and 21-tablet packages, new dosing cycle begins 7 days after last tablet taken; with 28-tablet packages, dosage is 1 tablet daily without interruption; extra tablets are placebos or contain iron. If next menstrual period does not begin on schedule, rule out pregnancy before starting new dosing cycle; if menstrual period begins, start new dosing cycle 7 days after last tablet was taken; if all doses have been taken on schedule and one menstrual period is missed, continue dosing cycle; if two consecutive menstrual periods are missed, pregnancy test is required before new dosing cycle is started.

One dose missed: Take as soon as remembered or take 2 tablets next day

Two doses missed: Take 2 tablets as soon as remembered or 2 tablets next 2 days

Three doses missed: Begin new compact of tablets starting on day 1 of next cycle

"Morning After" pill: Postcoital contraception (Ovral®): 2 tablets at initial visit and 2 tablets 12 hours later

**Mechanism of Action** Combination oral contraceptives inhibit ovulation via a negative feedback mechanism on the hypothalamus, which alters the normal pattern of gonadotropin secretion of a follicle-stimulating hormone (FSH) and luteinizing hormone by the anterior pituitary. The follicular phase FSH and midcycle surge of gonadotropins are inhibited. In addition, oral contraceptives produce alterations in the genital tract, including changes in the cervical mucus, rendering it unfavorable for sperm penetration even if ovulation occurs. Changes in the endometrium may also occur, producing an unfavorable environment for nidation. Oral contraceptive drugs may alter the tubal transport of the ova through the fallopian tubes. Progestational agents may also alter sperm fertility.

**Local Anesthetic/Vasoconstrictor Precautions** No information available to require special precautions

**Effects on Dental Treatment** When prescribing antibiotics, patient must be warned to use supplemental methods of birth control if on oral contraceptives

**Other Adverse Effects**

>10%:

Cardiovascular: Peripheral edema

Endocrine & metabolic: Enlargement of breasts, breast tenderness

Gastrointestinal: Nausea, anorexia, bloating

1% to 10%:

Central nervous system: Headache

Endocrine & metabolic: Increased libido

Gastrointestinal: Vomiting, diarrhea

<1%:

Cardiovascular: Hypertension, thromboembolism, myocardial infarction, edema

Central nervous system: Depression, dizziness, anxiety, stroke

Dermatologic: Chloasma, melasma, rash

Endocrine & metabolic: Decreased glucose tolerance, breast tumors, amenorrhea, alterations in frequency and flow of menses, elevated triglycerides and LDL

Gastrointestinal: GI distress

Hepatic: Cholestatic jaundice

Ocular: Intolerance to contact lenses

Miscellaneous: Increased susceptibility to *Candida* infection

See tables.

(Continued)

## Ethinyl Estradiol and Norgestrel *(Continued)*

**Achieving Proper Hormonal Balance in an Oral Contraceptive**

| Estrogen | | Progestin | |
|---|---|---|---|
| **Excess** | **Deficiency** | **Excess** | **Deficiency** |
| Nausea, bloating<br>Cervical mucorrhea, polyposis<br>Melasma<br>Migraine headache<br>Breast fullness or tenderness<br>Edema<br>Hypertension | Early or midcycle breakthrough bleeding<br>Increased spotting<br>Hypomenorrhea | Increased appetite<br>Weight gain<br>Tiredness, fatigue<br>Hypomenorrhea<br>Acne, oily scalp*<br>Hair loss, hirsutism*<br>Depression<br>Monilial vaginitis<br>Breast regression | Late breakthrough bleeding<br>Amenorrhea<br>Hypermenorrhea |

*Result of androgenic activity of progestins.

**Pharmacological Effects of Progestins Used in Oral Contraceptives**

| | Progestin | Estrogen | Antiestrogen | Androgen |
|---|---|---|---|---|
| Norgestrel/levonorgestrel | +++ | 0 | ++ | +++ |
| Ethynodiol diacetate | ++ | +* | +* | + |
| Norethindrone acetate | + | + | +++ | + |
| Norethindrone | + | +* | +* | + |
| Norethynodrel | + | +++ | 0 | 0 |

*Has estrogenic effect at low doses; may have antiestrogenic effect at higher doses.

+++ = pronounced effect

++ = moderate effect

+ = slight effect

0 = no effect

**Drug Interactions**

Decreased effect of oral contraceptives with barbiturates, hydantoins - phenytoin, rifampin, antibiotics - penicillins, tetracyclines, griseofulvin

Increased toxicity of acetaminophen, anticoagulants, benzodiazepines, caffeine, corticosteroids, metoprolol, theophylline, tricyclic antidepressants

**Drug Uptake**

Ethinyl estradiol: Absorption: Absorbed well from GI tract

Norgestrel:

Serum half-life, terminal: 11-45 hours

Time to peak: 0.5-2 hours

**Pregnancy Risk Factor** X

**Generic Available** Yes

♦ **Ethiofos** *see* Amifostine *on page 59*

## Ethionamide (e thye on AM ide)

**Related Information**

Nonviral Infectious Diseases *on page 1095*

**U.S. Brand Names** Trecator®-SC

**Therapeutic Category** Antitubercular Agent

**Use** Treatment of tuberculosis and other mycobacterial diseases, in conjunction with other antituberculosis agents, when first-line agents have failed or resistance has been demonstrated

**Usual Dosage** Oral:

Children: 15-20 mg/kg/day in 2 divided doses, not to exceed 1 g/day

Adults: 500-1000 mg/day in 1-3 divided doses

**Mechanism of Action** Inhibits peptide synthesis

**Local Anesthetic/Vasoconstrictor Precautions** No information available to require special precautions

**Effects on Dental Treatment** No effects or complications reported

**Other Adverse Effects**

>10%: Gastrointestinal: Anorexia, nausea, vomiting

1% to 10%:

Cardiovascular: Postural hypotension

Central nervous system: Psychiatric disturbances

Gastrointestinal: Metallic taste

Hepatic: Hepatitis, jaundice

Neuromuscular & skeletal: Peripheral neuritis

<1%:

Central nervous system: Drowsiness, dizziness, seizures, headache

Dermatologic: Rash

Endocrine & metabolic: Hypothyroidism or goiter, hypoglycemia, gynecomastia

Gastrointestinal: Stomatitis, abdominal pain, diarrhea

Hematologic: Thrombocytopenia

Ocular: Optic neuritis

**Drug Interactions** No data reported

**Drug Uptake**

Serum half-life: 2-3 hours

Time to peak serum concentration: Oral: Within 3 hours

**Pregnancy Risk Factor** C

**Generic Available** No

♦ **Ethmozine®** *see* Moricizine *on page 687*

## Ethosuximide (eth oh SUKS i mide)

**U.S. Brand Names** Zarontin®

**Therapeutic Category** Anticonvulsant, Succinimide

**Use** Management of absence (petit mal) seizures, myoclonic seizures, and akinetic epilepsy; considered to be drug of choice for simple absence seizures

**Usual Dosage** Oral:

Children 3-6 years: Initial: 250 mg/day (or 15 mg/kg/day) in 2 divided doses; increase every 4-7 days; usual maintenance dose: 15-40 mg/kg/day in 2 divided doses

Children >6 years and Adults: Initial: 250 mg twice daily; increase by 250 mg as needed every 4-7 days up to 1.5 g/day in 2 divided doses; usual maintenance dose: 20-40 mg/kg/day in 2 divided doses

**Mechanism of Action** Increases the seizure threshold and suppresses paroxysmal spike-and-wave pattern in absence seizures; depresses nerve transmission in the motor cortex

**Local Anesthetic/Vasoconstrictor Precautions** No information available to require special precautions

**Effects on Dental Treatment** No effects or complications reported

**Other Adverse Effects**

>10%:

Central nervous system: Ataxia, drowsiness, sedation, dizziness, lethargy, euphoria, hallucinations, insomnia, agitation, behavioral changes, headache

Dermatologic: Stevens-Johnson syndrome

Gastrointestinal: Weight loss, nausea, vomiting, anorexia, abdominal pain

Miscellaneous: Hiccups, SLE

1% to 10%:

Central nervous system: Aggressiveness, mental depression, nightmares, fatigue

Neuromuscular & skeletal: Weakness

<1%:

Central nervous system: Paranoid psychosis

Dermatologic: Rashes, urticaria, exfoliative dermatitis

Hematologic: Leukopenia, aplastic anemia, thrombocytopenia, agranulocytosis, pancytopenia

**Drug Interactions**

Decreased effect: Phenytoin, carbamazepine, primidone, phenobarbital may increase the hepatic metabolism of ethosuximide

Increased toxicity: Isoniazid may inhibit hepatic metabolism with a resultant increase in ethosuximide serum concentrations

**Drug Uptake**

Serum half-life:

Children: 30 hours

Adults: 50-60 hours

Time to peak serum concentration:

Capsule: Within 2-4 hours

Syrup: <2-4 hours

**Pregnancy Risk Factor** C

**Generic Available** Yes

## Ethotoin (ETH oh toyn)

**U.S. Brand Names** Peganone®

**Therapeutic Category** Anticonvulsant, Hydantoin

**Synonyms** Ethylphenylhydantoin

**Use** Generalized tonic-clonic or complex-partial seizures

(Continued)

## Ethotoin *(Continued)*

**Usual Dosage** Oral:

Children: 30-60 mg/kg/day or 250 mg twice daily, may be increased up to 2-3 g/day

Adults: 250 mg 4 times/day after meals, may be increased up to 3 g/day in divided doses 4 times/day

**Local Anesthetic/Vasoconstrictor Precautions** No information available to require special precautions

**Effects on Dental Treatment** No effects or complications reported

**Other Adverse Effects**

>10%:

Central nervous system: Psychiatric changes, slurred speech, drowsiness, dizziness

Gastrointestinal: Constipation, nausea, vomiting

Neuromuscular & skeletal: Trembling

1% to 10%:

Central nervous system: Headache, insomnia

Dermatologic: Skin rash

Gastrointestinal: Anorexia, weight loss

Hematologic: Leukopenia

Hepatic: Hepatitis

Renal: Elevated serum creatinine

<1%:

Cardiovascular: Hypotension, bradycardia, cardiac arrhythmias, cardiovascular collapse

Central nervous system: Confusion, fever, ataxia

Dermatologic: Stevens-Johnson syndrome

Gastrointestinal: Gingival hyperplasia

Hematologic: Blood dyscrasias

Local: Thrombophlebitis, venous irritation and pain

Neuromuscular & skeletal: Paresthesia, peripheral neuropathy

Ocular: Diplopia, nystagmus, blurred vision

Miscellaneous: Lymphadenopathy, SLE-like syndrome

**Pregnancy Risk Factor** D

**Generic Available** No

## Ethyl Chloride (ETH il KLOR ide)

**Therapeutic Category** Local Anesthetic, Topical

**Synonyms** Chloroethane

**Use** Local anesthetic in minor operative procedures and to relieve pain caused by insect stings and burns, and irritation caused by myofascial and visceral pain syndromes

**Usual Dosage** Dosage varies with use

**Local Anesthetic/Vasoconstrictor Precautions** No information available to require special precautions

**Effects on Dental Treatment** No effects or complications reported

**Other Adverse Effects** 1% to 10%: Mucous membrane irritation, freezing may alter skin pigment

**Pregnancy Risk Factor** C

**Generic Available** Yes

**Comments** Spray for a few seconds to the point of frost formation when the tissue becomes white; avoid prolonged spraying of skin beyond this point

## Ethyl Chloride and Dichlorotetrafluoroethane

(ETH il KLOR ide & dye klor oh te tra floo or oh ETH ane)

**U.S. Brand Names** Fluro-Ethyl® Aerosol

**Therapeutic Category** Local Anesthetic, Topical

**Synonyms** Dichlorotetrafluoroethane and Ethyl Chloride

**Use** Topical refrigerant anesthetic to control pain associated with minor surgical procedures, dermabrasion, injections, contusions, and minor strains

**Usual Dosage** Press gently on side of spray valve allowing the liquid to emerge as a fine mist approximately 2" to 4" from site of application

**Local Anesthetic/Vasoconstrictor Precautions** No information available to require special precautions

**Effects on Dental Treatment** No effects or complications reported

**Pregnancy Risk Factor** C

**Generic Available** No

## Ethylnorepinephrine (eth il nor ep i NEF rin)

**U.S. Brand Names** Bronkephrine® Injection

**Therapeutic Category** Adrenergic Agonist Agent; Bronchodilator

**Use** Bronchial asthma and reversible bronchospasm

**Usual Dosage** I.M., S.C.:

Children: Usually 0.1-0.5 mL, varies according to weight

Adults: 0.5-1 mL

**Local Anesthetic/Vasoconstrictor Precautions** No information available to require special precautions

**Effects on Dental Treatment** No effects or complications reported

**Other Adverse Effects**

>10%:

Cardiovascular: Tachycardia, pounding heart beat

Central nervous system: Nervousness

Gastrointestinal: Nausea

Neuromuscular & skeletal: Trembling, tremor

1% to 10%:

Cardiovascular: Flushing of face, hypertension or hypotension

Central nervous system: Dizziness, lightheadedness, drowsiness, headache, insomnia

Gastrointestinal: Dry mouth, heartburn, vomiting, unusual taste

Genitourinary: Dysuria

Neuromuscular & skeletal: Muscle cramping, weakness

Respiratory: Coughing

Miscellaneous: Increased sweating

<1%:

Cardiovascular: Chest pain, vasoconstriction, cerebral hemorrhage, cardiac arrhythmias, palpitations, angina, cardiac arrest, sudden death, syncope, unusual pallor

Central nervous system: Fear, anxiety, restlessness, confusion, irritability, psychotic states

Endocrine & metabolic: Altered glucose metabolism

Gastrointestinal: Loss of appetite, hypersalivation

Genitourinary: Urinary retention

Local: Extravasation results in tissue necrosis

Respiratory: Paradoxical bronchospasm, pulmonary edema, dyspnea

Miscellaneous: Sweating

**Pregnancy Risk Factor** C

**Generic Available** No

♦ **Ethylphenylhydantoin** *see* Ethotoin *on page 409*

♦ **Ethyol®** *see* Amifostine *on page 59*

## Etidocaine With Epinephrine (e TI doe kane)

**Related Information**

Oral Pain *on page 1122*

**U.S. Brand Names** Duranest® With Epinephrine

**Therapeutic Category** Dental/Local Anesthetics; Local Anesthetic, Injectable

**Use** Dental: An amide-type local anesthetic for local infiltration anesthesia; injection near nerve trunks to produce nerve block

**Usual Dosage**

Children <10 years: Dosage has not been established

Children >10 years and Adults: Dental infiltration and nerve block: 15-75 mg (1-5 mL) as a 1.5% solution; up to a maximum of 5.5 mg/kg of body weight but not to exceed 400 mg/injection of etidocaine hydrochloride with epinephrine 1:200,000. The effective anesthetic dose varies with procedure, intensity of anesthesia needed, duration of anesthesia required, and physical condition of the patient. Always use the lowest effective dose along with careful aspiration.

| # of Cartridges | Mg Etidocaine (1.5%) | Mg Vasoconstrictor (Epinephrine 1:200,000) |
|---|---|---|
| 1 | 27 | 0.009 |
| 2 | 54 | 0.018 |
| 3 | 81 | 0.027 |
| 4 | 108 | 0.036 |
| 5 | 135 | 0.045 |
| 6 | 162 | 0.054 |
| 7 | 189 | 0.063 |
| 8 | 216 | 0.072 |
| 9 | 243 | 0.081 |
| 10 | 270 | 0.090 |

(Continued)

## Etidocaine With Epinephrine *(Continued)*

The numbers of dental carpules (1.8 mL) in the table provide the indicated amounts of etidocaine hydrochloride 1.5% and epinephrine 1:200,000.

**Note:** Adult and children doses of etidocaine hydrochloride with epinephrine cited from USP Dispensing Information (USP DI), 17th ed, The United States Pharmacopeial Convention, Inc, Rockville, MD, 1997, 136.

**Mechanism of Action** Local anesthetics bind selectively to the intracellular surface of sodium channels to block influx of sodium into the axon. As a result, depolarization necessary for action potential propagation and subsequent nerve function is prevented. The block at the sodium channel is reversible. When drug diffuses away from the axon, sodium channel function is restored and nerve propagation is subsequently restored.

Epinephrine prolongs the duration of the anesthetic actions of etidocaine by causing vasoconstriction (alpha adrenergic receptor agonist) of the vasculature surrounding the nerve axons. This prevents the diffusion of lidocaine away from the nerves resulting in a longer retention in the axon.

**Local Anesthetic/Vasoconstrictor Precautions** No information available to require special precautions

**Effects on Dental Treatment** No effects or complications reported

**Other Adverse Effects** Degree of adverse effects in the central nervous system and cardiovascular system are directly related to the blood levels of etidocaine. The effects below are more likely to occur after systemic administration rather than infiltration.

Cardiovascular: Myocardial effects include a decrease in contraction force as well as a decrease in electrical excitability and myocardial conduction rate resulting in bradycardia and reduction in cardiac output.

Central nervous system: High blood levels result in anxiety, restlessness, disorientation, confusion, dizziness, tremors and seizures. This is followed by depression of CNS resulting in somnolence, unconsciousness and possible respiratory arrest. Nausea and vomiting may also occur. In some cases, symptoms of CNS stimulation may be absent and the primary CNS effects are drowsiness and unconsciousness.

Hypersensitivity reactions: Extremely rare, but may be manifest as dermatologic reactions and edema at injection site. Asthmatic syndromes have occurred. Patients may exhibit hypersensitivity to bisulfites contained in local anesthetic solution to prevent oxidation of epinephrine. In general, patients reacting to bisulfites have a history of asthma and their airways are hyper-reactive to asthmatic syndrome

Psychogenic reactions: It is common to misinterpret psychogenic responses to local anesthetic injection as an allergic reaction. Intraoral injections are perceived by many patients as a stressful procedure in dentistry. Common symptoms to this stress are sweating, palpitations, hyperventilation, generalized pallor and a fainting feeling.

**Contraindications** Hypersensitivity to local anesthetics of the amide-type

**Warnings/Precautions** Should be avoided in patients with uncontrolled hyperthyroidism. Should be used in minimal amounts in patients with significant cardiovascular problems (because of epinephrine component). Aspirate the syringe after tissue penetration and before injection to minimize chance of direct vascular injection.

**Drug Interactions** Due to epinephrine component, use with tricyclic antidepressants or MAO inhibitors could result in increased pressor response; use with nonselective beta-blockers (ie, propranolol) could result in serious hypertension and reflex bradycardia

**Drug Uptake**

Onset of action: Maxillary infiltration and inferior alveolar nerve block: 3-5 minutes

Duration after infiltration or nerve block: 5-10 hours

Serum half-life: 2.7 hours

**Pregnancy Risk Factor** B

**Breast-feeding Considerations** Usual infiltration doses of etidocaine hydrochloride with epinephrine given to nursing mothers has not been shown to affect the health of the nursing infant

**Dosage Forms** Etidocaine Hydrochloride 1.5% with epinephrine 1:200,000 cartridges, 1.8 mL, in 100 cartridge boxes

**Dietary Considerations** No data reported

**Generic Available** No

**Selected Readings**

Ayoub ST and Coleman AE, "A Review of Local Anesthetics," *Gen Dent*, 1992, 40(4):285-7, 289-90.

Jastak JT and Yagiela JA, "Vasoconstrictors and Local Anesthesia: A Review and Rationale for Use," *J Am Dent Assoc*, 1983, 107(4):623-30.

MacKenzie TA and Young ER, "Local Anesthetic Update," *Anesth Prog*, 1993, 40(2):29-34.

Wynn RL, "Epinephrine Interactions With Beta-Blockers," *Gen Dent*, 1994, 42(1):16, 18.
Wynn RL, "Recent Research on Mechanisms of Local Anesthetics," *Gen Dent*, 1995, 43(4):316-8.
Yagiela JA, "Local Anesthetics," *Anesth Prog*, 1991, 38(4-5):128-41.

## Etidronate Disodium (e ti DROE nate dye SOW dee um)

**U.S. Brand Names** Didronel®

**Therapeutic Category** Antidote, Hypercalcemia; Bisphosphonate Derivative

**Use** Symptomatic treatment of Paget's disease and heterotopic ossification due to spinal cord injury or after total hip replacement, hypercalcemia associated with malignancy

**Usual Dosage** Adults:

Paget's disease: Oral: 5 mg/kg/day given every day for no more than 6 months; may give 10 mg/kg/day for up to 3 months; daily dose may be divided if adverse GI effects occur

Heterotopic ossification with spinal cord injury: 20 mg/kg/day for 2 weeks, then 10 mg/kg/day for 10 weeks (this dosage has been used in children, however, treatment >1 year has been associated with a rachitic syndrome)

Hypercalcemia associated with malignancy:

I.V. (Dilute dose in at least 250 mL NS): 7.5 mg/kg/day for 3 days; there should be at least 7 days between courses of treatment

Oral: Start 20 mg/kg/day on the last day of infusion and continue for 30-90 days

**Mechanism of Action** Decreases bone resorption by inhibiting osteocystic osteolysis; decreases mineral release and matrix or collagen breakdown in bone

**Local Anesthetic/Vasoconstrictor Precautions** No information available to require special precautions

**Effects on Dental Treatment** No effects or complications reported

**Other Adverse Effects**

1% to 10%:

Central nervous system: Fever, convulsions

Endocrine & metabolic: Hypophosphatemia, hypomagnesemia, fluid overload

Neuromuscular & skeletal: Bone pain

Respiratory: Dyspnea

<1%:

Dermatologic: Angioedema, skin rash

Gastrointestinal: Occult blood in stools, dysgeusia

Neuromuscular & skeletal: Pain, increased risk of fractures

Renal: Nephrotoxicity

Miscellaneous: Hypersensitivity reactions

**Drug Interactions** No data reported

**Drug Uptake**

Onset of therapeutic effect: Within 1-3 months of therapy

Duration: Can persist for 12 months without continuous therapy

Absorption: Dependent upon dose administered

**Pregnancy Risk Factor** B (oral)/C (parenteral)

**Generic Available** No

## Etodolac (ee toe DOE lak)

**Related Information**

Rheumatoid Arthritis and Osteoarthritis *on page 1092*

**U.S. Brand Names** Lodine®; Lodine® XL

**Therapeutic Category** Analgesic, Non-narcotic; Nonsteroidal Anti-inflammatory Drug (NSAID), Oral

**Use**

Dental: Management of postoperative pain

Medical: Acute and long-term use in the management of signs and symptoms of osteoarthritis and management of pain, not approved for use in rheumatoid arthritis

**Usual Dosage** Adults: Oral: Single dose of 76-100 mg is comparable to the analgesic effect of aspirin 650 mg; in patients ≥65 years, no substantial differences in the pharmacokinetics or side-effects profile were seen compared with the general population

Acute pain: 200-400 mg every 6-8 hours, as needed, not to exceed total daily doses of 1200 mg; for patients weighing <60 kg, total daily dose should not exceed 20 mg/kg/day; extended release dose: one tablet daily

**Mechanism of Action** Inhibits prostaglandin synthesis by decreasing the activity of the enzyme, cyclo-oxygenase, which results in decreased formation of prostaglandin precursors

**Local Anesthetic/Vasoconstrictor Precautions** No information available to require special precautions

**Effects on Dental Treatment** NSAID formulations are known to reversibly decrease platelet aggregation via mechanisms different than observed with aspirin. The dentist should be aware of the potential of abnormal coagulation.

(Continued)

## Etodolac *(Continued)*

Caution should also be exercised in the use of NSAIDs in patients already on anticoagulant therapy with drugs such as warfarin (Coumadin®).

**Other Adverse Effects** >10%:

Central nervous system: Dizziness
Dermatologic: Rash
Gastrointestinal: Abdominal cramps, heartburn, indigestion, nausea

**Contraindications** Hypersensitivity to etodolac, aspirin, or other NSAIDs

**Warnings/Precautions** Use with caution in patients with congestive heart failure, hypertension, decreased renal or hepatic function, history of GI disease, or those receiving anticoagulants

**Drug Interactions** Decreased effect with aspirin; increased effect/toxicity with aspirin (GI irritation), probenecid; increased effect/toxicity of lithium (nausea), methotrexate, digoxin, cyclosporin (nephrotoxicity), warfarin (bleeding)

**Drug Uptake**

Onset of effect: 0.5 hours following single dose of 200-400 mg
Duration of effect: 4-6 hours
Serum half-life: 7 hours
Time to peak serum concentration: 1 hour

**Pregnancy Risk Factor** C

**Breast-feeding Considerations** No data reported

**Dosage Forms**

Capsule: 200 mg, 300 mg
Tablet: 400 mg
Tablet, extended release: 400 mg, 600 mg

**Dietary Considerations** May be taken with food to decrease GI distress

**Generic Available** Yes

**Selected Readings**

Brooks PM and Day RO, "Nonsteroidal Anti-inflammatory Drugs - Differences and Similarities," *N Engl J Med*, 1991, 324(24):1716-25.

Tucker PW, Smith JR, and Adams DF, "A Comparison of 2 Analgesic Regimens for the Control of Postoperative Periodontal Discomfort," *J Periodontol*, 1996, 67(2):125-9.

## Etomidate (e TOM i date)

**U.S. Brand Names** Amidate® Injection

**Therapeutic Category** General Anesthetic, Intravenous

**Use** Induction of general anesthesia

**Usual Dosage** Children >10 years and Adults: I.V.: 0.2-0.6 mg/kg over a period of 30-60 seconds for induction of anesthesia

**Mechanism of Action** Ultrashort-acting nonbarbiturate hypnotic used for the induction of anesthesia; chemically, it is a carboxylated imidazole and has been shown to produce a rapid induction of anesthesia with minimal cardiovascular and respiratory effects

**Local Anesthetic/Vasoconstrictor Precautions** No information available to require special precautions

**Effects on Dental Treatment** No effects or complications reported

**Other Adverse Effects**

>10%:

Gastrointestinal: Nausea, vomiting
Local: Pain at injection site
Neuromuscular & skeletal: Transient skeletal movements
Ocular: Uncontrolled eye movements

1% to 10%: Hiccups

<1%:

Cardiovascular: Hypertension, hypotension, tachycardia, bradycardia, arrhythmias
Respiratory: Hyperventilation, hypoventilation, apnea, laryngospasm

**Warnings/Precautions** Consider exogenous corticosteroid replacement in patients undergoing severe stress

**Pregnancy Risk Factor** C

**Dosage Forms** Injection: 2 mg/mL (10 mL, 20 mL)

**Generic Available** No

♦ **Etopophos® Injection** *see* Etoposide *on this page*

## Etoposide (e toe POE side)

**U.S. Brand Names** Etopophos® Injection; Toposar® Injection; VePesid® Injection; VePesid® Oral

**Therapeutic Category** Antineoplastic Agent, Mitotic Inhibitor

**Use** Treatment of lymphomas, ANLL, lung, testicular, bladder, and prostate carcinoma, hepatoma, rhabdomyosarcoma, uterine carcinoma, neuroblastoma, mycosis fungoides, Kaposi's sarcoma, histiocytosis, gestational trophoblastic disease, Ewing's sarcoma, Wilms' tumor, and brain tumors

**Usual Dosage Refer to individual protocols**

Oral: Twice the I.V. dose rounded to the nearest 50 mg given once daily if total dose ≤400 mg or in divided doses if >400 mg

Children: I.V.: 60-120 $mg/m^2$/day for 3-5 days every 3-6 weeks

AML:

Remission induction: 150 $mg/m^2$/day for 2-3 days for 2-3 cycles

Intensification or consolidation: 250 $mg/m^2$/day for 3 days, courses 2-5

Conditioning regimen for allogeneic BMT: 60 mg/kg/dose as a single dose

Adults:

Small cell lung cancer:

Oral: Twice the I.V. dose rounded to the nearest 50 mg given once daily if

I.V.: 35 $mg/m^2$/day for 4 days or 50 $mg/m^2$/day for 5 days every 3-4 weeks

total dose ≤400 mg/day or in divided doses if >400 mg/day

IVPB: 200-250 $mg/m^2$ repeated every 7 weeks

Continuous intravenous infusion: 500 $mg/m^2$ over 24 hours every 3 weeks

Testicular cancer:

IVPB: 50-100 $mg/m^2$/day for 5 days repeated every 3-4 weeks

I.V.: 100 $mg/m^2$ every other day for 3 doses repeated every 3-4 weeks

BMT/relapsed leukemia: I.V.: 2.4-3.5 $g/m^2$ or 25-70 mg/kg administered over 4-36 hours

**Mechanism of Action** Inhibits mitotic activity; inhibits cells from entering prophase; inhibits DNA synthesis. Initially thought to be mitotic inhibitors similar to podophyllotoxin, but actually have no effect on microtubule assembly. However, later shown to induce DNA strand breakage and inhibition of topoisomerase II (an enzyme which breaks and repairs DNA); etoposide acts in late S or early G2 phases.

**Local Anesthetic/Vasoconstrictor Precautions** No information available to require special precautions

**Effects on Dental Treatment** No effects or complications reported

**Other Adverse Effects**

>10%:

Dermatologic: Alopecia (reversible)

Gastrointestinal: Anorexia; occasional diarrhea and infrequent nausea and vomiting at standard doses; severe mucositis occurs with high (BMT) doses

Emetic potential: Moderately low (10% to 30%)

Hematologic: Myelosuppressive: Principal dose-limiting toxicity of VP-16. White blood cell count nadir is 5-15 days after administration and is more frequent than thrombocytopenia. Recovery is usually within 24-28 days and cumulative toxicity has not been noted with VP-16 as a single agent. No difference in toxicity is seen when VP-16 is administered over a 24-hour period or over 2 hours on 5 consecutive days. WBC: Mild to severe; Platelets: Mild; Onset (days): 10; Nadir (days): 14-16; Recovery (days): 21-28

1% to 10%:

Central nervous system: Unusual fatigue

Gastrointestinal: Stomatitis, diarrhea, abdominal pain, hepatitic dysfunction

Hypotension: Related to drug infusion time; may be related to vehicle used in the I.V. preparation (polysorbate 80 plus polyethylene glycol). Best to administer the drug over 1 hour.

<1%:

Cardiovascular: Tachycardia

Central nervous system: Neurotoxicity, somnolence, fatigue, fever, headache

Irritant chemotherapy: thrombophlebitis has been reported

Hepatic: Toxic hepatitis (with high-dose therapy)

Neuromuscular & skeletal: Peripheral neuropathy

Miscellaneous: Reports of flushing or bronchospasm, which did not reoccur in one report if patients were pretreated with corticosteroids and antihistamines

**Drug Interactions** Increased toxicity:

Warfarin may cause increases prothrombin time with concurrent use

Methotrexate: Alteration of MTX transport has been found as a slow efflux of MTX and its polyglutamated form out of the cell, leading to intercellular accumulation of MTX

Calcium antagonists: Increases the rate of VP-16-induced DNA damage and cytotoxicity *in vitro*

Carmustine: Reports of frequent hepatic dysfunction with hyperbilirubinemia, ascites, and thrombocytopenia

Cyclosporine: Additive cytotoxic effects on tumor cells

**Drug Uptake**

Absorption: Oral: 32% to 57%

Serum half-life: Terminal: 4-15 hours

Children: 6-8 hours with normal renal and hepatic function

(Continued)

## Etoposide *(Continued)*

Time to peak serum concentration: Oral: 1-1.5 hours

**Pregnancy Risk Factor** D

**Generic Available** Yes

- **Etrafon®** *see* Amitriptyline and Perphenazine *on page 69*

## Etretinate (e TRET i nate)

**U.S. Brand Names** Tegison®

**Therapeutic Category** Antipsoriatic Agent, Systemic

**Use** Treatment of severe recalcitrant psoriasis in patients intolerant of or unresponsive to standard therapies

**Usual Dosage** Adults: Oral: Individualized; Initial: 0.75-1 mg/kg/day in divided doses, increase by 0.25 mg/kg/day at weekly intervals up to 1.5 mg/kg/day; maintenance dose established after 8-10 weeks of therapy 0.5-0.75 mg/kg/day

**Mechanism of Action** Unknown; related to retinoic acid and retinol (vitamin A)

**Local Anesthetic/Vasoconstrictor Precautions** No information available to require special precautions

**Effects on Dental Treatment** >10% of patients experience dry mouth

**Other Adverse Effects**

>10%:

Central nervous system: Fatigue, headache, fever
Dermatologic: Chapped lips, alopecia
Endocrine & metabolic: Hypercholesterolemia, hypertriglyceridemia
Gastrointestinal: Nausea, appetite change, sore tongue
Neuromuscular & skeletal: Hyperostosis, bone pain, arthralgia
Ocular: Eye irritation
Respiratory: Epistaxis

1% to 10%:

Cardiovascular: Edema
Central nervous system: Dizziness, lethargy
Hepatic: Hepatitis
Neuromuscular & skeletal: Myalgia
Ocular: Blurred vision
Otic: Otitis externa
Respiratory: Dyspnea

<1%:

Cardiovascular: Syncope
Central nervous system: Amnesia, confusion, pseudotumor cerebri, depression
Dermatologic: Urticaria
Gastrointestinal: Mouth ulcers, diarrhea, constipation, flatulence, weight loss, gingival bleeding
Endocrine & metabolic: Gout
Genitourinary: Dysuria
Local: Phlebitis
Neuromuscular & skeletal: Hyperkinesia, hypertonia
Ocular: Photophobia
Otic: Ear infection
Renal: Polyuria, kidney stones
Respiratory: Rhinorrhea

**Drug Interactions**

Increased effect: Milk increases absorption of etretinate
Increased toxicity: Additive toxicity with vitamin A

**Drug Uptake**

Absorption: Oral: Absorbed from small intestine; absorption enhanced when coadministered with whole milk or a high lipid meal (highly lipophilic)
Serum half-life: 4-8 days (with multiple doses)

**Pregnancy Risk Factor** X

**Generic Available** No

- **ETS-2%® Topical** *see* Erythromycin, Topical *on page 386*
- **Eudal-SR®** *see* Guaifenesin and Pseudoephedrine *on page 481*
- **Eulexin®** *see* Flutamide *on page 450*
- **Eurax®** *see* Crotamiton *on page 282*
- **Eutron®** *see* Methyclothiazide and Pargyline *on page 658*
- **Evac-Q-Mag® [OTC]** *see* Magnesium Citrate *on page 611*
- **Evalose®** *see* Lactulose *on page 571*
- **Everone® Injection** *see* Testosterone *on page 961*
- **Evista®** *see* Raloxifene *on page 876*
- **E-Vitamin® [OTC]** *see* Vitamin E *on page 1050*
- **Exact® Cream [OTC]** *see* Benzoyl Peroxide *on page 130*

- **Excedrin®, Extra Strength [OTC]** *see* Acetaminophen, Aspirin, and Caffeine *on page 31*
- **Excedrin® Migraine [OTC]** *see* Acetaminophen, Aspirin, and Caffeine *on page 31*
- **Excedrin® P.M. [OTC]** *see* Acetaminophen and Diphenhydramine *on page 30*
- **Exelderm®** *see* Sulconazole *on page 938*
- **Exidine® Scrub [OTC]** *see* Chlorhexidine Gluconate *on page 225*
- **Exna®** *see* Benzthiazide *on page 132*
- **Exosurf® Neonatal™** *see* Colfosceril Palmitate *on page 275*
- **Exsel®** *see* Selenium Sulfide *on page 909*
- **Extendryl® SR** *see* Chlorpheniramine, Phenylephrine, and Methscopolamine *on page 235*
- **Extra Action Cough Syrup [OTC]** *see* Guaifenesin and Dextromethorphan *on page 479*
- **Extra Strength Adprin-B® [OTC]** *see* Aspirin *on page 100*
- **Extra Strength Bayer® Enteric 500 Aspirin [OTC]** *see* Aspirin *on page 100*
- **Extra Strength Bayer® Plus [OTC]** *see* Aspirin *on page 100*
- **Extra Strength Doan's® [OTC]** *see* Magnesium Salicylate *on page 613*
- **Eye-Lube-A® Solution [OTC]** *see* Artificial Tears *on page 97*
- **Eye-Sed® [OTC]** *see* Zinc Supplements *on page 1062*
- **Eye-Sed® Ophthalmic [OTC]** *see* Zinc Sulfate *on page 1062*
- **Eyesine® Ophthalmic [OTC]** *see* Tetrahydrozoline *on page 967*
- **Ezide®** *see* Hydrochlorothiazide *on page 503*

## Factor IX Complex (Human) (FAK ter nyne KOM pleks HYU man)

**U.S. Brand Names** AlphaNine® SD; Konÿne® 80; Mononine®; Profilnine® Heat-Treated; Proplex® SX-T; Proplex® T

**Therapeutic Category** Antihemophilic Agent; Blood Product Derivative

**Use** To control bleeding in patients with Factor IX deficiency (Hemophilia B or Christmas Disease); prevention/control of bleeding in hemophilia A patients with inhibitors to factor VIII; Proplex® T is indicated to prevent or control bleeding due to factor VII deficiency

**Usual Dosage** Children and Adults: Dosage is expressed in units of factor IX activity and must be individualized. I.V. only:

**Factor VII deficiency: Highly individualized**

0.5 unit/kg x body weight (kg) x desired increase (%)

For example, for a 70 kg adult to increase level by 25%:

0.5 unit/kg x 70 kg x 25 = 875 units

**Factor IX deficiency: Highly individualized**

1 unit/kg x body weight (in kg) x desired increase (%)

For example, to increase the level by 25% in a 70 kg adult:

1 unit x 70 kg x 25 = 1,750 units

**Formula for units required to raise blood level %:**

Total blood volume (mL blood/kg) = 70 mL/kg (adults), 80 mL/kg (children)

Plasma volume = total blood volume (mL) x [1 - Hct (in decimals)]

For example, for a 70 kg adult with a Hct = 40%: Plasma volume = [70 kg x 70 mL/kg] x [1 - 0.4] = 2940 mL

To calculate number of units needed to increase level to desired range (highly individualized and dependent on patient's condition):

Number of units = desired level increase [desired level - actual level] x plasma volume (in mL)

For example, for a 100% level in the above patient who has an actual level of 20%: Number of units needed = [1 (for a 100% level) - 0.2] x 2940 mL = 2,352 units

| | Minor Spontaneous Hemorrhage, Prophylaxis | Major Trauma or Surgery |
|---|---|---|
| Desired levels of factor IX for hemostasis | 15%-25% | 25%-50% |
| Initial loading dose to achieve desired level | <20-30 units/kg | <75 units/kg |
| Frequency of dosing | Once; repeated in 24 h if necessary | q18-30h, depending on half-life and measured factor IX levels |
| Duration of treatment | Once; repeated if necessary | Up to 10 days, depending upon nature of insult |

(Continued)

## Factor IX Complex (Human) *(Continued)*

As a general rule, the level of factor IX required for treatment of different conditions is shown in the table.

**Factor VIII inhibitor patients:** 75 units/kg/dose; may be given every 6-12 hours

**Anticoagulant overdosage:** I.V.: 15 units/kg

**Mechanism of Action** Replaces deficient clotting factor including factor X; hemophilia B, or Christmas disease, is an X-linked recessively inherited disorder of blood coagulation characterized by insufficient or abnormal synthesis of the clotting protein factor IX. Factor IX is a vitamin K-dependent coagulation factor which is synthesized in the liver. Factor IX is activated by factor XIa in the intrinsic coagulation pathway. Activated factor IX (IXa), in combination with factor VII:C activates factor X to Xa, resulting ultimately in the conversion of prothrombin to thrombin and the formation of a fibrin clot. The infusion of exogenous factor IX to replace the deficiency present in hemophilia B temporarily restores hemostasis.

**Local Anesthetic/Vasoconstrictor Precautions** No information available to require special precautions

**Effects on Dental Treatment** No effects or complications reported

**Other Adverse Effects**

1% to 10%: Following rapid administration: Transient fever, chills, headache, flushing, paresthesia

<1%:

Cardiovascular: Thrombosis following high dosages in hemophilia B patients

Central nervous system: Somnolence

Dermatologic: Urticaria

Hematologic: Disseminated intravascular coagulation

Miscellaneous: Tightness in chest and neck

**Drug Uptake** Serum half-life:

VII component: Cleared rapidly from the serum in two phases; initial: 4-6 hours; terminal: 22.5 hours

IX component: 24 hours

**Pregnancy Risk Factor** C

**Generic Available** No

**Comments** Factor VII and IX units are listed per vial and per lot to lot variation

- **Factor VIII** *see* Antihemophilic Factor (Human) *on page 89*
- **Factor VIII Recombinant** *see* Antihemophilic Factor (Recombinant) *on page 90*

## Famciclovir (fam SYE kloe veer)

**Related Information**

Systemic Viral Diseases *on page 1115*

**U.S. Brand Names** Famvir™

**Therapeutic Category** Antiviral Agent, Oral

**Use** Management of acute herpes zoster (shingles); treatment of recurrent mucocutaneous herpes simplex infections in HIV-infected patients

**Usual Dosage** Adults: Oral:

Acute herpes zoster: 500 mg every 8 hours for 7 days

Recurrent herpes simplex in immunocompetent patients: 125 mg twice daily for 5 days

**Mechanism of Action** After undergoing rapid biotransformation to the active compound, penciclovir, famciclovir is phosphorylated by viral thymidine kinase in HSV-1, HSV-2, and VZV-infected cells to a monophosphate form; this is then converted to penciclovir triphosphate and competes with deoxyguanosine triphosphate to inhibit HSV-2 polymerase (ie, herpes viral DNA synthesis/replication is selectively inhibited)

**Local Anesthetic/Vasoconstrictor Precautions** No information available to require special precautions

**Effects on Dental Treatment** No effects or complications reported

**Other Adverse Effects**

>10%:

Central nervous system: Headache

Gastrointestinal: Nausea

1% to 10%:

Central nervous system: Fatigue, fever, dizziness, somnolence

Gastrointestinal: Diarrhea, vomiting, constipation, anorexia, abdominal pain

Neuromuscular & skeletal: Rigors, paresthesia

**Drug Interactions** Famciclovir administration produces a small increase in digoxin's peak plasma concentration; however, this change is not likely to enhance the patient response to digoxin

**Drug Uptake**

Absorption: Food decreases the maximum peak concentration and delays the time to peak; AUC remains the same

Serum half-life: Penciclovir: 2-3 hours (10, 20, and 7 hours in HSV-1, HSV-2, and VZV-infected cells); linearly decreased with reductions in renal failure

**Pregnancy Risk Factor** B

**Dosage Forms** Tablet: 125 mg, 250 mg, 500 mg

**Dietary Considerations** May be taken with food or on an empty stomach

**Generic Available** No

**Selected Readings**

Pue MA, et al, "An Investigation of the Potential Interaction Between Digoxin and Famciclovir in Healthy Male Volunteers," *Br J Clin Pharmacol*, 1993, 36:177P.

## Famotidine (fa MOE ti deen)

**U.S. Brand Names** Pepcid®; Pepcid® AC Acid Controller [OTC]

**Canadian Brand Names** Apo®-Famotidine; Novo-Famotidine; Nu-Famotidine

**Therapeutic Category** Histamine $H_2$ Antagonist

**Use** Therapy and treatment of duodenal ulcer, gastric ulcer, control gastric pH in critically ill patients, symptomatic relief in gastritis, gastroesophageal reflux, active benign ulcer, and pathological hypersecretory conditions; relief and prevention of heartburn, acid indigestion, and sour stomach from food and beverages

**Usual Dosage**

Children: Oral, I.V.: Doses of 1-2 mg/kg/day have been used; maximum dose: 40 mg

Adults:

Oral:

Duodenal ulcer, gastric ulcer: 40 mg/day at bedtime for 4-8 weeks

Hypersecretory conditions: Initial: 20 mg every 6 hours, may increase up to 160 mg every 6 hours

GERD: 20 mg twice daily for 6 weeks

I.V.: 20 mg every 12 hours

**Mechanism of Action** Competitive inhibition of histamine at $H_2$ receptors of the gastric parietal cells, which inhibits gastric acid secretion

**Local Anesthetic/Vasoconstrictor Precautions** No information available to require special precautions

**Effects on Dental Treatment** No effects or complications reported

**Other Adverse Effects**

1% to 10%:

Central nervous system: Dizziness, headache

Gastrointestinal: Constipation, diarrhea

<1%:

Cardiovascular: Bradycardia, tachycardia, palpitations, hypertension

Central nervous system: Fever, fatigue, seizures, insomnia, drowsiness

Dermatologic: Acne, pruritus, urticaria, dry skin

Gastrointestinal: Abdominal discomfort, flatulence, belching, anorexia

Hematologic: Agranulocytosis, neutropenia, thrombocytopenia

Hepatic: Elevated AST, ALT

Neuromuscular & skeletal: Paresthesia, weakness

Renal: Elevated BUN, creatinine, proteinuria

Respiratory: Bronchospasm

Miscellaneous: Allergic reaction

**Drug Interactions** Decreased effect of ketoconazole, itraconazole

**Drug Uptake**

Onset of GI effect: Oral: Within 1 hour

Duration: 10-12 hours

Serum half-life: 2.5-3.5 hours; increases with renal impairment, oliguric patients: 20 hours

Time to peak serum concentration: Oral: Within 1-3 hours

**Pregnancy Risk Factor** B

**Generic Available** No

♦ **Famvir™** *see* Famciclovir *on previous page*

♦ **Fansidar®** *see* Sulfadoxine and Pyrimethamine *on page 942*

♦ **Fareston®** *see* Toremifene *on page 1000*

♦ **Fastin®** *see* Phentermine *on page 793*

## Fat Emulsion (fat e MUL shun)

**U.S. Brand Names** Intralipid®; Liposyn®; Nutrilipid®; Soyacal®

**Therapeutic Category** Caloric Agent; Intravenous Nutritional Therapy

**Synonyms** Intravenous Fat Emulsion

(Continued)

## Fat Emulsion *(Continued)*

**Use** Source of calories and essential fatty acids for patients requiring parenteral nutrition of extended duration

**Usual Dosage** Fat emulsion should not exceed 60% of the total daily calories

Children: Initial dose: 0.5-1 g/kg/day, increase by 0.5 g/kg/day to a maximum of 3-4 g/kg/day; maximum rate of infusion: 0.25 g/kg/hour (1.25 mL/kg/hour of 20% solution)

Adolescents and Adults: Initial dose: 1 g/kg/day, increase by 0.5-1 g/kg/day to a maximum of 2.5 g/kg/day of 10% and 3 g/kg/day of 20%; maximum rate of infusion: 0.25 g/kg/hour (1.25 mL/kg/hour of 20% solution); do not exceed 50 mL/hour (20%) or 100 mL/hour (10%)

**Note:** At the onset of therapy, the patient should be observed for any immediate allergic reactions such as dyspnea, cyanosis, and fever. Slower initial rates of infusion may be used for the first 10-15 minutes of the infusion (eg, 0.1 mL/minute of 10% or 0.05 mL/minute of 20% solution).

Prevention of fatty acid deficiency (8% to 10% of total caloric intake): 0.5-1 g/kg/24 hours

Children: 5-10 mL/kg/day at 0.1 mL/minute then up to 100 mL/hour

Adults: 500 mL twice weekly at rate of 1 mL/minute for 30 minutes, then increase to 500 mL over 4-6 hours

Can be used in both children and adults on a daily basis as a caloric source in TPN

**Mechanism of Action** Essential for normal structure and function of cell membranes

**Local Anesthetic/Vasoconstrictor Precautions** No information available to require special precautions

**Effects on Dental Treatment** No effects or complications reported

**Other Adverse Effects**

>10%: Local: Thrombophlebitis

1% to 10%: Endocrine & metabolic: Hyperlipemia

<1%:

Cardiovascular: Cyanosis, flushing, chest pain
Gastrointestinal: Nausea, vomiting, diarrhea
Hepatic: Hepatomegaly
Respiratory: Dyspnea
Miscellaneous: Sepsis

**Drug Uptake**

Serum half-life: 0.5-1 hour

**Pregnancy Risk Factor** B/C

**Generic Available** Yes

- **FC1157a** *see* Toremifene *on page 1000*
- **Fedahist® Expectorant [OTC]** *see* Guaifenesin and Pseudoephedrine *on page 481*
- **Fedahist® Expectorant Pediatric [OTC]** *see* Guaifenesin and Pseudoephedrine *on page 481*
- **Fedahist® Tablet [OTC]** *see* Chlorpheniramine and Pseudoephedrine *on page 233*
- **Feiba VH Immuno®** *see* Anti-inhibitor Coagulant Complex *on page 91*

## Felbamate (FEL ba mate)

**U.S. Brand Names** Felbatol®

**Therapeutic Category** Anticonvulsant, Miscellaneous

**Use** Not a first-line agent; reserved for patients who do not adequately respond to alternative agents and whose epilepsy is so severe that benefit outweighs risk of liver failure or aplastic anemia; used as monotherapy and adjunctive therapy in patients ≥14 years of age with partial seizures with and without secondary generalization; adjunctive therapy in children ≥2 years of age who have partial and generalized seizures associated with Lennox-Gastaut syndrome

**Usual Dosage**

Monotherapy: Children >14 years and Adults:

Initial: 1200 mg/day in divided doses 3 or 4 times/day; titrate previously untreated patients under close clinical supervision, increasing the dosage in 600 mg increments every 2 weeks to 2400 mg/day based on clinical response and thereafter to 3600 mg/day in clinically indicated

Conversion to monotherapy: Initiate at 1200 mg/day in divided doses 3 or 4 times/day, reduce the dosage of the concomitant anticonvulsant(s) by 20% to 33% at the initiation of felbamate therapy; at week 2, increase the felbamate dosage to 2400 mg/day while reducing the dosage of the other anticonvulsant(s) up to an additional 33% of their original dosage; at week 3, increase the felbamate dosage up to 3600 mg/day and continue to reduce the dosage of the other anticonvulsant(s) as clinically indicated

Adjunctive therapy: Children with Lennox-Gastaut and ages 2-14 years:

Week 1:

Felbamate: 15 mg/kg/day divided 3-4 times/day

Concomitant anticonvulsant(s): Reduce original dosage by 20% to 30%

Week 2:

Felbamate: 30 mg/kg/day divided 3-4 times/day

Concomitant anticonvulsant(s): Reduce original dosage up to an additional 33%

Week 3:

Felbamate: 45 mg//kg/day divided 3-4 times/day

Concomitant anticonvulsant(s): Reduce dosage as clinically indicated

Adjunctive therapy: Children >14 years and Adults:

Week 1:

Felbamate: 1200 mg/day initial dose

Concomitant anticonvulsant(s): Reduce original dosage by 20% to 33%

Week 2:

Felbamate: 2400 mg/day (Therapeutic range)

Concomitant anticonvulsant(s): Reduce original dosage by up to an additional 33%

Week 3:

Felbamate: 3600 mg/day (Therapeutic range)

Concomitant anticonvulsant(s): Reduce original dosage as clinically indicated

**Mechanism of Action** Mechanism of action is unknown but has properties in common with other marketed anticonvulsants; has weak inhibitory effects on GABA-receptor binding, benzodiazepine receptor binding, and is devoid of activity at the MK-801 receptor binding site of the NMDA receptor-ionophore complex.

**Local Anesthetic/Vasoconstrictor Precautions** No information available to require special precautions

**Effects on Dental Treatment** No effects or complications reported

**Other Adverse Effects**

>10%:

Central nervous system: Anxiety, headache, fatigue, dizziness

Gastrointestinal: Nausea, diarrhea, anorexia, vomiting, constipation

Respiratory: Cough

1% to 10%:

Central nervous system: Somnolence, insomnia, ataxia, depression or behavior changes, clouded sensorium, lethargy, slurred speech

Dermatologic: Acne, skin rash

Gastrointestinal: Weight gain

Neuromuscular & skeletal: Muscle twitches

Ocular: Blurred vision, diplopia, uncontrollable eye movements

<1%:

Dermatologic: Alopecia

Gastrointestinal: Gum bleeding or hyperplasia

**Drug Uptake**

Absorption: Oral: Rapidly and almost completely absorbed after oral administration, food has no effect upon the tablet's absorption

Peak serum concentrations: Within 3 hours

Half-life: 20-23 hours average

**Pregnancy Risk Factor** C

**Generic Available** No

**Comments** Monotherapy has not been associated with gingival hyperplasia, impaired concentration, weight gain, or abnormal thinking

♦ **Felbatol®** *see* Felbamate *on previous page*

♦ **Feldene®** *see* Piroxicam *on page 810*

## Felodipine (fe LOE di peen)

**Related Information**

Calcium Channel Blockers & Gingival Hyperplasia *on page 1204*

Cardiovascular Diseases *on page 1066*

Enalapril and Felodipine *on page 368*

**U.S. Brand Names** Plendil®

**Canadian Brand Names** Renedil®

**Therapeutic Category** Calcium Channel Blocker

**Use** Treatment of hypertension, congestive heart failure

(Continued)

## Felodipine *(Continued)*

**Usual Dosage** Adults: Oral: 5-10 mg once daily; increase by 5 mg at 2-week intervals, as needed, to a maximum of 20 mg/day (Elderly: Begin with 2.5 mg/day)

**Mechanism of Action** Inhibits calcium ions from entering the select voltage-sensitive areas or "slow channels" of vascular smooth muscle and myocardium during depolarization, producing a relaxation of coronary vascular smooth muscle and coronary vasodilation; increases myocardial oxygen delivery in patients with vasospastic angina

**Local Anesthetic/Vasoconstrictor Precautions** No information available to require special precautions

**Effects on Dental Treatment** Calcium channel blockers cause gingival hyperplasia in approximately 1% of patients. There have been fewer reports with felodipine than with other CCBs. The hyperplasia will disappear with cessation of drug therapy. Consultation with physician is suggested.

**Other Adverse Effects**

>10%: Cardiovascular: Peripheral edema

1% to 10%:

- Cardiovascular: Chest pain, tachycardia
- Central nervous system: Dizziness, lightheadedness
- Dermatologic: Skin rash
- Gastrointestinal: Constipation, diarrhea

<1%:

- Cardiovascular: Hypotension, arrhythmia, bradycardia, palpitations
- Central nervous system: Mental depression, headache
- Gastrointestinal: Gingival hyperplasia, dry mouth, nausea
- Hepatic: Marked elevations in liver function tests
- Ocular: Blurred vision
- Respiratory: Dyspnea

**Drug Interactions** Increased toxicity/effect/levels:

Calcium channel blockers (CCB) and $H_2$-blockers such as cimetidine cause increased bioavailability CCB

Beta-blockers cause increased depressant effects on A-V conduction

**Drug Uptake**

Onset of effect: 2-5 hours

Duration: 16-24 hours

Absorption: 100%; absolute: 20% due to first-pass effect

Serum half-life: 11-16 hours

**Pregnancy Risk Factor** C

**Generic Available** No

**Selected Readings**

Lombardi T, Fiore-Donno G, Belser U, et al, "Felodipine-Induced Gingival Hyperplasia: A Clinical and Histologic Study," *J Oral Pathol Med*, 1991, 20(2):89-92.

Young PC, Turiansky GW, Sau P, et al, "Felodipine-Induced Gingival Hyperplasia," *Cutis*, 1998, 62(1):41-3.

- **Femara™** *see* Letrozole *on page 577*
- **Femcet®** *see* Butalbital Compound *on page 163*
- **Femcet®** *see* Butalbital Compound and Acetaminophen *on page 164*
- **Femguard®** *see* Sulfabenzamide, Sulfacetamide, and Sulfathiazole *on page 939*
- **Femiron® [OTC]** *see* Ferrous Fumarate *on page 426*
- **Femizol-M® [OTC]** *see* Miconazole *on page 672*
- **Femstat®** *see* Butoconazole *on page 166*
- **Fenesin™** *see* Guaifenesin *on page 478*
- **Fenesin DM®** *see* Guaifenesin and Dextromethorphan *on page 479*

## Fenofibrate (fen oh FYE brate)

**U.S. Brand Names** Lipidil®; Tricor®

**Canadian Brand Names** Apo®-Fenofibrate

**Therapeutic Category** Lipid Lowering Drugs

**Use** Adjunct to dietary therapy for the treatment of adults with very high elevations of serum triglyceride levels (types IV and V hyperlipidemia) who are at risk of pancreatitis and who do not respond adequately to a determined dietary effort; its efficacy can be enhanced by combination with other hypolipidemic agents that have a different mechanism of action; safety and efficacy may be greater than that of clofibrate

**Usual Dosage** Oral:

Children >10 years: 5 mg/kg/day

Adults: 100 mg 3 times/day with meals or 200 mg in the morning and 100 mg in the evening

**Mechanism of Action** Fenofibric acid is believed to increase VLDL catabolism by enhancing the synthesis of lipoprotein lipase; as a result of a decrease in VLDL levels, total plasma triglycerides are reduced by 30% to 60% (VLDL contains ~60% triglycerides and 10% to 15% cholesterol); apolipoprotein B, which stabilizes the structure of VLDL and LDL, decreases in a parallel fashion and plasma cholesterol levels decrease by fenofibrate's effect on LDL levels and cholesterol synthesis; modest increase in HDL occurs in some hypertriglyceridemic patients since it is involved in the storage and transport of cholesterol ester and apolipoproteins

**Local Anesthetic/Vasoconstrictor Precautions** No information available to require special precautions

**Effects on Dental Treatment** No effects or complications reported

**Other Adverse Effects**

>10%: Gastrointestinal: Nausea, gastric discomfort

1% to 10%:

Dermatologic: Skin reactions

Gastrointestinal: Constipation, diarrhea

<1%:

Central nervous system: Dizziness, headache, fatigue, insomnia

Hepatic: Transient elevation in LFTs

Neuromuscular & skeletal: Arthralgia, myalgia

**Drug Interactions**

Increased hypolipidemic effect: Cholestyramine, colestipol will add to the hypolipidemic effect of fenofibrate

**Drug Uptake**

Peak effect: 4-6 hours

Absorption: 60% to 90% when given with meals

Serum half-life: Fenofibrate: 21 hours (30 hours in elderly, 44-54 hours in hepatic impairment)

**Pregnancy Risk Factor** C

**Generic Available** No

## Fenoldopam (fe NOL doe pam)

**U.S. Brand Names** Corlopam®

**Therapeutic Category** Antihypertensive Agent

**Synonyms** Fenoldopam Mesylate

**Use Investigational** in U.S.: Severe hypertension; congestive heart failure

**Usual Dosage**

Oral: 100 mg 2-4 times daily

I.V.: Severe hypertension: Initial: 0.1 mcg/kg/minute; may be increased in increments of 0.05-0.2 mcg/kg/minute; maximal infusion rate: 1.6 mcg/kg/minute

**Mechanism of Action** A selective dopamine agonist ($D_1$-receptors) with vasodilitary properties; 6 times as potent as dopamine in producing vasodilitation

**Local Anesthetic/Vasoconstrictor Precautions** No information available to require special precautions

**Effects on Dental Treatment** No effects or complications reported

**Other Adverse Effects**

Cardiovascular: Fibrillation (atrial), hypotension, edema, tachycardia, facial flushing, asymptomatic T wave flattening on EKG, flutter (atrial), chest pain, angina

Central nervous system: Headache, dizziness

Gastrointestinal: Nausea, vomiting, diarrhea

Ocular: Intraocular pressure (increased)

**Contraindications** Previous hypersensitive reaction to fenoldopam

**Warnings/Precautions** Use with caution in patients with cirrhosis, unstable angina or glaucoma

**Drug Uptake**

Onset of action: I.V.: 15 minutes

Duration:

Oral: 2-4 hours

I.V.: 1 hour

Absorption: Oral: Poor

Distribution: $V_d$: 0.6 L/kg

Half-life: I.V.: 9.8 minutes

Metabolism: Hepatic to multiple metabolites; the 8-sulfate metabolite may have some activity

Elimination: Renal

♦ **Fenoldopam Mesylate** *see* Fenoldopam *on this page*

## Fenoprofen (fen oh PROE fen)

**Related Information**

Rheumatoid Arthritis and Osteoarthritis *on page 1092*

**U.S. Brand Names** Nalfon®

**Therapeutic Category** Analgesic, Non-narcotic; Anti-inflammatory Agent; Nonsteroidal Anti-inflammatory Drug (NSAID), Oral

**Use** Symptomatic treatment of acute and chronic rheumatoid arthritis and osteoarthritis; relief of mild to moderate pain

**Usual Dosage** Adults: Oral:

Rheumatoid arthritis: 300-600 mg 3-4 times/day up to 3.2 g/day

Mild to moderate pain: 200 mg every 4-6 hours as needed

**Mechanism of Action** Inhibits prostaglandin synthesis by decreasing the activity of the enzyme, cyclo-oxygenase, which results in decreased formation of prostaglandin precursors

**Local Anesthetic/Vasoconstrictor Precautions** No information available to require special precautions

**Effects on Dental Treatment** NSAID formulations are known to reversibly decrease platelet aggregation via mechanisms different than observed with aspirin. The dentist should be aware of the potential of abnormal coagulation. Caution should also be exercised in the use of NSAIDs in patients already on anticoagulant therapy with drugs such as warfarin (Coumadin®).

**Other Adverse Effects**

>10%:

- Central nervous system: Dizziness
- Dermatologic: Skin rash
- Gastrointestinal: Abdominal cramps, heartburn, indigestion, nausea

1% to 10%:

- Central nervous system: Headache, nervousness
- Dermatologic: Itching
- Endocrine & metabolic: Fluid retention
- Gastrointestinal: Vomiting
- Otic: Tinnitus

<1%:

- Cardiovascular: Congestive heart failure, hypertension, arrhythmias, tachycardia
- Central nervous system: Confusion, hallucinations, aseptic meningitis, mental depression, drowsiness, insomnia
- Dermatologic: Urticaria, erythema multiforme, toxic epidermal necrolysis, Stevens-Johnson syndrome, angioedema
- Endocrine & metabolic: Polydipsia, hot flashes
- Gastrointestinal: Gastritis, GI ulceration
- Genitourinary: Cystitis
- Hematologic: Agranulocytosis, anemia, hemolytic anemia, bone marrow suppression, leukopenia, thrombocytopenia
- Hepatic: Hepatitis
- Neuromuscular & skeletal: Peripheral neuropathy
- Ocular: Toxic amblyopia, blurred vision, conjunctivitis, dry eyes
- Otic: Decreased hearing
- Renal: Polyuria, acute renal failure
- Respiratory: Allergic rhinitis, dyspnea, epistaxis

**Drug Interactions**

Decreased effect with phenobarbital

Increased effect/toxicity of phenytoin, sulfonamides, sulfonylureas

Increased toxicity with salicylates, oral anticoagulants

**Drug Uptake**

Absorption: Rapid (to 80%) from upper GI tract

Serum half-life: 2.5-3 hours

Time to peak serum concentration: Within 2 hours

**Pregnancy Risk Factor** B (D if used in the 3rd trimester or near delivery)

**Generic Available** Yes

## Fentanyl (FEN ta nil)

**Related Information**

Narcotic Agonists *on page 1223*

**U.S. Brand Names** Actiq® Oral Transmucosal; Duragesic® Transdermal; Fentanyl Oralet®; Sublimaze® Injection

**Therapeutic Category** Analgesic, Narcotic; General Anesthetic, Intravenous

**Use**

Dental: Adjunct in preoperative intravenous conscious sedation in patients undergoing dental surgery

Medical: In medicine, adjunct to general or regional anesthesia; management of chronic pain (transdermal product)

**Restrictions** C-II; Nonrefillable

**Usual Dosage**

Children 1-12 years:

Sedation for minor procedures/analgesia:

I.M., I.V.: 1-2 mcg/kg/dose

Transmucosal (lozenge): 5 mcg/kg if child is not fearful; fearful children and some younger children may require doses of 5-15 mcg/kg (which also carries an increased risk of hypoventilation); drug effect begins within 10 minutes, with sedation beginning shortly thereafter

Children >12 years and Adults:

Sedation for minor procedures/analgesia:

I.M., I.V.: 0.5-1 mcg/kg/dose; higher doses are used for major procedures

Transmucosal (lozenge): 5 mcg/kg, suck on lozenge vigorously approximately 20-40 minutes before the start of procedure, drug effect begins within 10 minutes, with sedation beginning shortly thereafter

Preoperative sedation: I.M., I.V.: 50-100 mcg/dose

Pain control: Transdermal fentanyl is not to be used for acute dosing in treatment of dental pain

**Mechanism of Action** Binds to opiate receptors (mu and kappa subtypes) in the CNS causing inhibition of ascending pain pathways, altering the perception of and response to pain; produces generalized CNS depression

**Local Anesthetic/Vasoconstrictor Precautions** No information available to require special precautions

**Effects on Dental Treatment** No effects or complications reported

**Other Adverse Effects** >10%:

Cardiovascular: Hypotension, bradycardia

Central nervous system: CNS depression, drowsiness, sedation

Gastrointestinal: Nausea, vomiting, constipation

Respiratory: Respiratory depression

1% to 10%:

Cardiovascular: Cardiac arrhythmias, orthostatic hypotension

Central nervous system: Confusion, CNS depression

Gastrointestinal: Biliary tract spasm

Ocular: Miosis

<1%:

Cardiovascular: Circulatory depression

Central nervous system: Convulsions, dysesthesia, paradoxical CNS excitation or delirium, dizziness

Dermatologic: Erythema, pruritus, rash, hives, itching, cold, clammy skin

Endocrine & metabolic: ADH release

Gastrointestinal: Biliary tract spasm

Genitourinary: Urinary tract spasm

Respiratory: Bronchospasm, laryngospasm

Miscellaneous: Physical and psychological dependence with prolonged use

**Contraindications** Hypersensitivity to fentanyl or any component; increased intracranial pressure; severe respiratory depression; severe liver or renal insufficiency

Transmucosal is contraindicated in unmonitored settings where a risk of unrecognized hypoventilation exists or in treating acute or chronic pain

**Warnings/Precautions** Fentanyl shares the toxic potentials of opiate agonists, and precautions of opiate agonist therapy should be observed; use with caution in patients with bradycardia; rapid I.V. infusion may result in skeletal muscle and chest wall rigidity → impaired ventilation → respiratory distress → apnea, bronchoconstriction, laryngospasm; inject slowly over 3-5 minutes; nondepolarizing skeletal muscle relaxant may be required.

Enhanced analgesia has been seen in elderly patients on therapeutic doses of narcotics; duration of action may be increased in the elderly; the elderly may be particularly susceptible to the CNS depressant and constipating effects of narcotics

**Drug Interactions** Increased toxicity of CNS depressants, phenothiazines, tricyclic antidepressants may potentiate fentanyl's adverse effects

**Drug Uptake**

Onset of effect (respiratory depressant effect may last longer than analgesic effect):

I.M.: Analgesia: 7-15 minutes

I.V.: Analgesia: Almost immediate

Transmucosal (lozenge): 5-15 minutes with a maximum reduction in activity/apprehension

(Continued)

## Fentanyl *(Continued)*

Duration of effect:
- I.M.: 1-2 hours
- I.V.: 0.5-1 hour
- Transmucosal: Related to blood level of drug

Serum half-life: 2-4 hours; transmucosal: 5-15 hours

**Pregnancy Risk Factor** B (D if used for prolonged periods or in high doses at term)

**Breast-feeding Considerations** Not contraindicated

**Dosage Forms**

Injection, as citrate: 0.05 mg/mL (2 mL, 5 mL, 10 mL, 20 mL, 50 mL)

Lozenge, oral transmucosal:
- Fentanyl Oralet® (raspberry flavored): 200 mcg, 300 mcg, 400 mcg
- Actiq® Oral Transmucosal: 200 mcg, 400 mcg, 600 mcg, 800 mcg, 1200 mcg, 1600 mcg

Transdermal system: 25 mcg/hour [10 $cm^2$]; 50 mcg/hour [20 $cm^2$]; 75 mcg/hour [30 $cm^2$]; 100 mcg/hour [40 $cm^2$] (all available in 5s)

**Dietary Considerations** No data reported

**Generic Available** Injection: Yes

**Comments** Transdermal fentanyl should not be used as a pain reliever in dentistry due to danger of hypoventilation

- **Fentanyl Oralet®** *see* Fentanyl *on page 424*
- **Feosol® [OTC]** *see* Ferrous Sulfate *on next page*
- **Feostat® [OTC]** *see* Ferrous Fumarate *on this page*
- **Ferancee® [OTC]** *see* Ferrous Sulfate and Ascorbic Acid *on page 428*
- **Feratab® [OTC]** *see* Ferrous Sulfate *on next page*
- **Fergon® [OTC]** *see* Ferrous Gluconate *on next page*
- **Fer-In-Sol® [OTC]** *see* Ferrous Sulfate *on next page*
- **Fer-Iron® [OTC]** *see* Ferrous Sulfate *on next page*
- **Fero-Grad 500® [OTC]** *see* Ferrous Sulfate and Ascorbic Acid *on page 428*
- **Fero-Gradumet® [OTC]** *see* Ferrous Sulfate *on next page*
- **Ferospace® [OTC]** *see* Ferrous Sulfate *on next page*
- **Ferralet® [OTC]** *see* Ferrous Gluconate *on next page*
- **Ferralyn® Lanacaps® [OTC]** *see* Ferrous Sulfate *on next page*
- **Ferra-TD® [OTC]** *see* Ferrous Sulfate *on next page*
- **Ferromar® [OTC]** *see* Ferrous Sulfate and Ascorbic Acid *on page 428*
- **Ferro-Sequels® [OTC]** *see* Ferrous Fumarate *on this page*

## Ferrous Fumarate (FER us FYOO ma rate)

**U.S. Brand Names** Femiron® [OTC]; Feostat® [OTC]; Ferro-Sequels® [OTC]; Fumasorb® [OTC]; Fumerin® [OTC]; Hemocyte® [OTC]; Ircon® [OTC]; Nephro-Fer™ [OTC]; Span-FF® [OTC]

**Canadian Brand Names** Palafer®

**Therapeutic Category** Iron Salt

**Use** Prevention and treatment of iron deficiency anemias

**Usual Dosage** Oral **(dose expressed in terms of elemental iron):**

Children:
- Severe iron deficiency anemia: 4-6 mg Fe/kg/day in 3 divided doses
- Mild to moderate iron deficiency anemia: 3 mg Fe/kg/day in 1-2 divided doses
- Prophylaxis: 1-2 mg Fe/kg/day

Adults:
- Iron deficiency: 60-100 mg twice daily up to 60 mg 2 times/day
- Prophylaxis: 60-100 mg/day
- To avoid GI upset, start with a single daily dose and increase by 1 tablet/day each week or as tolerated until desired daily dose is achieved

Elderly: 200 mg 3-4 times/day

**Mechanism of Action** Replaces iron found in hemoglobin, myoglobin, and enzymes; allows the transportation of oxygen via hemoglobin

**Local Anesthetic/Vasoconstrictor Precautions** No information available to require special precautions

**Effects on Dental Treatment** Do not prescribe tetracyclines simultaneously with iron since GI tract absorption of both tetracycline and iron may be inhibited

**Other Adverse Effects**

>10%: Gastrointestinal: Stomach cramping, constipation, nausea, vomiting, dark stools

1% to 10%:
- Gastrointestinal: Heartburn, diarrhea, staining of teeth
- Genitourinary: Discolored urine

<1%: Ocular: Contact irritation

**Drug Interactions**

Decreased effect: Absorption of oral preparation of iron and tetracyclines are decreased when both of these drugs are given together; concurrent administration of antacids may decrease iron absorption; iron may decrease absorption of penicillamine when given at the same time; response to iron therapy may be delayed in patients receiving chloramphenicol

Milk may decrease absorption of iron

Increased effect: Current administration of ≥200 mg vitamin C per 30 mg elemental iron increases absorption of oral iron

**Drug Uptake**

Onset of hematologic response (essentially the same to either oral or parenteral iron salts): Red blood cell form and color changes within 3-10 days

Peak reticulocytosis: Within 5-10 days; hemoglobin values increase within 2-4 weeks

Absorption: Iron is absorbed in the duodenum and upper jejunum; in persons with normal iron stores 10% of an oral dose is absorbed, this is increased to 20% to 30% in persons with inadequate iron stores; food and achlorhydria will decrease absorption

**Pregnancy Risk Factor** A

**Generic Available** Yes

## Ferrous Gluconate (FER us GLOO koe nate)

**U.S. Brand Names** Fergon® [OTC]; Ferralet® [OTC]; Simron® [OTC]

**Canadian Brand Names** Apo®-Ferrous Gluconate

**Therapeutic Category** Iron Salt

**Use** Prevention and treatment of iron deficiency anemias

**Usual Dosage** Oral **(dose expressed in terms of elemental iron):**

Children:

- Severe iron deficiency anemia: 4-6 mg Fe/kg/day in 3 divided doses
- Mild to moderate iron deficiency anemia: 3 mg Fe/kg/day in 1-2 divided doses
- Prophylaxis: 1-2 mg Fe/kg/day

Adults:

- Iron deficiency: 60 mg twice daily up to 60 mg 4 times/day
- Prophylaxis: 60 mg/day

**Mechanism of Action** Replaces iron found in hemoglobin, myoglobin, and enzymes; allows the transportation of oxygen via hemoglobin

**Local Anesthetic/Vasoconstrictor Precautions** No information available to require special precautions

**Effects on Dental Treatment** Do not prescribe tetracyclines simultaneously with iron since GI tract absorption of both tetracycline and iron may be inhibited

**Other Adverse Effects**

>10%: Gastrointestinal: Stomach cramping, constipation, nausea, vomiting, dark stools

1% to 10%:

- Gastrointestinal: Heartburn, diarrhea, staining of teeth
- Genitourinary: Discolored urine

<1%: Ocular: Contact irritation

**Drug Interactions** Absorption of oral preparation of iron and tetracyclines is decreased when both of these drugs are given together; concurrent administration of antacids may decrease iron absorption; iron may decrease absorption of penicillamine when given at the same time. Response to iron therapy may be delayed in patients receiving chloramphenicol. Concurrent administration of ≥ 200 mg vitamin C/30 mg elemental iron increases absorption of oral iron; milk may decrease absorption of iron.

**Drug Uptake** Onset of hematologic response (essentially the same to either oral or parenteral iron salts): Red blood cells form and color changes within 3-10 days, peak reticulocytosis occurs in 5-10 days, and hemoglobin values increase within 2-4 weeks

**Pregnancy Risk Factor** A

**Generic Available** Yes

## Ferrous Sulfate (FER us SUL fate)

**U.S. Brand Names** Feosol® [OTC]; Feratab® [OTC]; Fer-In-Sol® [OTC]; Fer-Iron® [OTC]; Fero-Gradumet® [OTC]; Ferospace® [OTC]; Ferralyn® Lanacaps® [OTC]; Ferra-TD® [OTC]; Mol-Iron® [OTC]; Slow FE® [OTC]

**Canadian Brand Names** Apo®-Ferrous Sulfate; PMS-Ferrous® Sulfate

**Therapeutic Category** Iron Salt

**Use** Prevention and treatment of iron deficiency anemias

**Usual Dosage** Oral:

Children **(dose expressed in terms of elemental iron):**

- Severe iron deficiency anemia: 4-6 mg Fe/kg/day in 3 divided doses

(Continued)

## Ferrous Sulfate *(Continued)*

Mild to moderate iron deficiency anemia: 3 mg Fe/kg/day in 1-2 divided doses
Prophylaxis: 1-2 mg Fe/kg/day up to a maximum of 15 mg/day
Adults **(dose expressed in terms of ferrous sulfate)**:
Iron deficiency: 300 mg twice daily up to 300 mg 4 times/day or 250 mg (extended release) 1-2 times/day
Prophylaxis: 300 mg/day

**Mechanism of Action** Replaces iron, found in hemoglobin, myoglobin, and other enzymes; allows the transportation of oxygen via hemoglobin

**Local Anesthetic/Vasoconstrictor Precautions** No information available to require special precautions

**Effects on Dental Treatment** Do not prescribe tetracyclines simultaneously with iron since GI tract absorption of both tetracycline and iron may be inhibited

**Other Adverse Effects**

>10%: Gastrointestinal: GI irritation, epigastric pain, nausea, dark stool, vomiting, stomach cramping, constipation

1% to 10%:

Gastrointestinal: Heartburn, diarrhea, liquid preparations may temporarily stain the teeth

Genitourinary: Discolored urine

<1%: Ocular: Contact irritation

**Drug Interactions**

Decreased effect: Absorption of oral preparation of iron and tetracyclines are decreased when both of these drugs are given together; concurrent administration of antacids may decrease iron absorption; iron may decrease absorption of penicillamine when given at the same time; response to iron therapy may be delayed in patients receiving chloramphenicol; milk may decrease absorption of iron

Increased effect: Concurrent administration of ≥200 mg vitamin C per 30 mg elemental Fe increases absorption of oral iron

**Drug Uptake**

Onset of hematologic response (essentially the same to either oral or parenteral iron salts): Red blood cell form and color changes within 3-10 days

Peak reticulocytosis: Occurs in 5-10 days, and hemoglobin values increase within 2-4 weeks

Absorption: Iron is absorbed in the duodenum and upper jejunum; in persons with normal serum iron stores, 10% of an oral dose is absorbed; this is increased to 20% to 30% in persons with inadequate iron stores. Food and achlorhydria will decrease absorption

**Pregnancy Risk Factor** A

**Generic Available** Yes

## Ferrous Sulfate and Ascorbic Acid

(FER us SUL fate & a SKOR bik AS id)

**U.S. Brand Names** Ferancee® [OTC]; Fero-Grad 500® [OTC]; Ferromar® [OTC]

**Therapeutic Category** Iron Salt; Vitamin

**Synonyms** Ascorbic Acid and Ferrous Sulfate

**Use** Treatment of iron deficiency in nonpregnant adults; treatment and prevention of iron deficiency in pregnant adults

**Usual Dosage** Adults: Oral: 1 tablet daily

**Local Anesthetic/Vasoconstrictor Precautions** No information available to require special precautions

**Effects on Dental Treatment** Do not prescribe tetracyclines simultaneously with iron since GI tract absorption of both tetracycline and iron may be inhibited

**Generic Available** Yes

## Ferrous Sulfate, Ascorbic Acid, and Vitamin B-Complex

(FER us SUL fate, a SKOR bik AS id, & VYE ta min bee KOM pleks)

**U.S. Brand Names** Iberet®-Liquid [OTC]

**Therapeutic Category** Iron Salt; Vitamin

**Use** Conditions of iron deficiency with an increased needed for B-complex vitamins and vitamin C

**Usual Dosage** Oral:

Children 1-3 years: 5 mL twice daily after meals

Children >4 years and Adults: 10 mL 3 times/day after meals

**Local Anesthetic/Vasoconstrictor Precautions** No information available to require special precautions

**Effects on Dental Treatment** Do not prescribe tetracyclines simultaneously with iron since GI tract absorption of both tetracycline and iron may be inhibited

**Generic Available** Yes

## Ferrous Sulfate, Ascorbic Acid, Vitamin B-Complex, and Folic Acid

(FER us SUL fate, a SKOR bik AS id, VYE ta min bee KOM pleks, & FOE lik AS id)

**U.S. Brand Names** Iberet-Folic-500®

**Therapeutic Category** Iron Salt; Vitamin

**Use** Treatment of iron deficiency and prevention of concomitant folic acid deficiency where there is an associated deficient intake or increased need for B-complex vitamins

**Usual Dosage** Adults: Oral: 1 tablet daily

**Local Anesthetic/Vasoconstrictor Precautions** No information available to require special precautions

**Effects on Dental Treatment** Do not prescribe tetracyclines simultaneously with iron since GI tract absorption of both tetracycline and iron may be inhibited

**Pregnancy Risk Factor** A

**Generic Available** Yes

♦ **Fertinex® Injection** *see* Urofollitropin *on page 1034*

♦ **Feverall™ [OTC]** *see* Acetaminophen *on page 27*

♦ **Feverall™ Sprinkle Caps [OTC]** *see* Acetaminophen *on page 27*

## Fexofenadine (feks oh FEN a deen)

**U.S. Brand Names** Allegra®

**Therapeutic Category** Antihistamine

**Use** Nonsedating antihistamine indicated for the relief of seasonal allergic rhinitis

**Usual Dosage** Children ≥12 years and Adults: Oral: 1 capsule (60 mg) twice daily

**Mechanism of Action** Fexofenadine is an active metabolite of terfenadine and like terfenadine it competes with histamine for $H_1$-receptor sites on effector cells in the gastrointestinal tract, blood vessels and respiratory tract; it appears that fexofenadine does not cross the blood brain barrier to any appreciable degree, resulting in a reduced potential for sedation

**Local Anesthetic/Vasoconstrictor Precautions** No information available to require special precautions

**Effects on Dental Treatment** No effects or complications reported

**Other Adverse Effects** 1% to 10%:

Central nervous system: Drowsiness (1.3%), fatigue (1.3%)
Endocrine & metabolic: Dysmenorrhea (1.5%)
Gastrointestinal: Nausea (1.5%), dyspepsia (1.3%)
Miscellaneous: Viral infection (2.5%)

**Contraindications** Hypersensitivity to fexofenadine or any components of its formulation

**Drug Interactions** Fexofenadine levels have increased with erythromycin (82% higher) and with ketoconazole (135% higher); this has not been associated with any increased incidence of side effects

In two separate studies, fexofenadine 120 mg twice daily (high doses) was coadministered with standard doses of erythromycin or ketoconazole to healthy volunteers and although fexofenadine peak plasma concentrations increased, no differences in adverse events or QTc intervals were observed. **It remains unknown if a similar interaction occurs with other azole antifungal agents (eg, itraconazole) or other macrolide antibiotics (eg, clarithromycin).**

**Drug Uptake**

Onset of action: 60 minutes
Duration of antihistaminic effect: At least 12 hours
Half-life: 14.4 hours
Time to peak serum concentration: ~2.6 hours after oral administration

**Pregnancy Risk Factor** C

**Dosage Forms** Capsule, as hydrochloride: 60 mg

**Generic Available** No

**Selected Readings**

Day JH, et al, "Onset of Action, Efficacy and Safety of a Single Dose of 60 mg and 120 mg Fexofenadine HCl for Ragweed Allergy Using Controlled Antigen Exposure in an Environmental Exposure Unit," *J Allergy Clin Immunol*, 1996, 97(1 Pt 3):1007.

"Fexofenadine," *Med Lett Drugs Ther*, 1996, 38(986):95-6.

Markham A and Wagstaff AJ, "Fexofenadine," *Drugs*, 1998, 55(2):269-74 (discussion 275-6).

Simons FE, Bergman JN, Watson WT, et al, "The Clinical Pharmacology of Fexofenadine in Children," *J Allergy Clin Immunol*, 1996, 98(6 Pt 1):1062-4.

♦ **Fiberall® Chewable Tablet [OTC]** *see* Calcium Polycarbophil *on page 177*

♦ **Fiberall® Powder [OTC]** *see* Psyllium *on page 865*

♦ **Fiberall® Wafer [OTC]** *see* Psyllium *on page 865*

- ♦ **FiberCon® Tablet [OTC]** *see* Calcium Polycarbophil *on page 177*
- ♦ **Fiber-Lax® Tablet [OTC]** *see* Calcium Polycarbophil *on page 177*

## Fibrinolysin and Desoxyribonuclease

(fye brin oh LYE sin & des oks i rye boe NOO klee ase)

**U.S. Brand Names** Elase-Chloromycetin® Topical; Elase® Topical

**Therapeutic Category** Enzyme, Topical Debridement

**Synonyms** Desoxyribonuclease and Fibrinolysin

**Use** Debriding agent; cervicitis; and irrigating agent in infected wounds

**Usual Dosage**

Ointment: 2-3 times/day

Wet dressing: 3-4 times/day

**Local Anesthetic/Vasoconstrictor Precautions** No information available to require special precautions

**Effects on Dental Treatment** No effects or complications reported

**Pregnancy Risk Factor** C

**Generic Available** No

## Filgrastim (fil GRA stim)

**U.S. Brand Names** Neupogen® Injection

**Therapeutic Category** Colony Stimulating Factor

**Synonyms** G-CSF; Granulocyte Colony Stimulating Factor

**Use** To reduce the duration of neutropenia and the associated risk of infection in patients with nonmyeloid malignancies receiving myelosuppressive chemotherapeutic regimens associated with a significant incidence of severe neutropenia with fever; it has also been used in AIDS patients on zidovudine and in patients with noncancer chemotherapy-induced neutropenia

**Usual Dosage** Children and Adults: administered S.C. or I.V. as a single daily infusion over 20-30 minutes

Myelosuppressive chemotherapy: 5 mcg/kg/day S.C. or I.V. Doses may be increased in increments of 5 mcg/kg for each chemotherapy cycle, according to the duration and severity of the absolute neutrophil count (ANC) nadir. In phase III trials, efficacy was observed at doses of 4-6 mcg/kg/day. Discontinue therapy if the ANC count is >10,000/mm$^3$ after the ANC nadir has occurred following the expected chemotherapy-induced neutrophil nadir. Some cancer centers are stopping therapy at an ANC of 2500. Duration of therapy needed to attenuate chemotherapy-induced neutropenia may be dependent on the myelosuppressive potential of the chemotherapy regimen employed. Duration of therapy in clinical studies has ranged from 2 weeks to 3 years.

Bone marrow transplant patients: 10 mcg/kg/day as an I.V. infusion of 4 or 24 hours or as continuous 24-hour S.C. infusion. Administer first dose at least 24 hours after cytotoxic chemotherapy and at least 24 hours after bone marrow infusion.

**Filgrastim Dose Based on Neutrophil Response**

| Absolute Neutrophil Count | Filgrastim Dose Adjustment |
|---|---|
| When ANC >1000/mm$^3$ for 3 consecutive days | Reduce to 5 mcg/kg/day |
| If ANC remains >1000/mm$^3$ for 3 more consecutive days | Discontinue filgrastim |
| If ANC decreases to <1000/mm$^3$ | Resume at 5 mcg/kg/day |

Severe chronic neutropenia:

Congenital neutropenia: 6 mcg/kg twice daily S.C.

Idiopathic/cyclic neutropenia: 5 mcg/kg/day S.C.

Chronic daily administration is required to maintain clinical benefit. Adjust dose based on the patients' clinical course as well as ANC. In phase III studies, the target ANC was 1,500-10,000/mm$^3$. Reduce the dose of the ANC is persistently >10,000/mm$^3$.

Premature discontinuation of G-CSF therapy prior to the time of recovery from the expected neutrophil is generally not recommended. A transient increase in neutrophil counts is typically seen 1-2 days after initiation of therapy.

**Mechanism of Action** Stimulates the production, maturation, and activation of neutrophils, G-CSF activates neutrophils to increase both their migration and cytotoxicity. Natural proteins which stimulate hematopoietic stem cells to proliferate, prolong cell survival, stimulate cell differentiation, and stimulate functional activity of mature cells. CSFs are produced by a wide variety of cell types. Specific mechanisms of action are not yet fully understood, but possibly work by a second-messenger pathway with resultant protein production. See table.

| Proliferation/Differentiation | G-CSF (Filgrastim) | GM-CSF (Sargramostim) |
|---|---|---|
| Neutrophils | Yes | Yes |
| Eosinophils | No | Yes |
| Macrophages | No | Yes |
| Neutrophil migration | Enhanced | Inhibited |

**Local Anesthetic/Vasoconstrictor Precautions** No information available to require special precautions

**Effects on Dental Treatment** No effects or complications reported

**Other Adverse Effects** Effects are generally mild and dose related

>10%:

- Central nervous system: Neutropenic fever
- Dermatologic: Alopecia
- Gastrointestinal: Nausea, vomiting, diarrhea, mucositis
- Medullary bone pain (24% incidence): This occurs most commonly in lower back pain, posterior iliac crest, and sternum and is controlled with non-narcotic analgesics
- Splenomegaly: This occurs more commonly in patients with cyclic neutropenia/ congenital agranulocytosis who received S.C. injections for a prolonged (>14 days) period of time; ~33% of these patients experience subclinical splenomegaly (detected by MRI or CT scan); ~3% of these patients experience clinical splenomegaly

1% to 10%:

- Cardiovascular: Chest pain
- Central nervous system: Headache
- Dermatologic: Rash
- Endocrine & metabolic: Fluid retention
- Gastrointestinal: Anorexia, stomatitis, constipation, sore throat
- Hematologic: Leukocytosis
- Local: Pain at injection site
- Neuromuscular & skeletal: Weakness
- Respiratory: Dyspnea, cough

<1%:

- Cardiovascular: Transient supraventricular arrhythmia, pericarditis
- Local: Thrombophlebitis
- Hypersensitivity: Anaphylactic reaction

**Drug Uptake**

- Onset of action: Rapid elevation in neutrophil counts within the first 24 hours, reaching a plateau in 3-5 days
- Duration: ANC decreases by 50% within 2 days after discontinuing G-CSF; white counts return to the normal range in 4-7 days
- Absorption: S.C.: 100% absorbed; peak plasma levels can be maintained for up to 12 hours
- Serum half-life: 1.8-3.5 hours
- Time to peak serum concentration: S.C.: Within 2-6 hours

**Pregnancy Risk Factor** C

**Generic Available** No

**Comments** Reimbursement hotline: 1-800-28-AMGEN

♦ **Filibon® [OTC]** *see* Vitamins, Multiple *on page 1051*

## Finasteride (fi NAS teer ide)

**U.S. Brand Names** Propecia®; Proscar®

**Therapeutic Category** Antiandrogen; Urinary Tract Product

**Use** Early data indicate that finasteride is useful in the treatment of symptomatic benign prostatic hyperplasia (BPH); male pattern baldness or androgenetic alopecia

**Unlabeled use:** Adjuvant monotherapy after radical prostatectomy in the treatment of prostatic cancer

**Usual Dosage** Adults: Male:

- Benign prostatic hyperplasia: Oral: 5 mg/day as a single dose; clinical responses occur within 12 weeks to 6 months of initiation of therapy; long-term administration is recommended for maximal response
- Male pattern baldness: One tablet daily

**Mechanism of Action** Finasteride is a 4-azo analog of testosterone and is a competitive inhibitor of both tissue and hepatic 5-alpha reductase. This results in inhibition of the conversion of testosterone to dihydrotestosterone and markedly suppresses serum dihydrotestosterone levels; depending on dose and duration, serum testosterone concentrations may or may not increase. Testosterone-

(Continued)

## Finasteride *(Continued)*

dependent processes such as fertility, muscle strength, potency, and libido are not affected by finasteride.

**Local Anesthetic/Vasoconstrictor Precautions** No information available to require special precautions

**Effects on Dental Treatment** No effects or complications reported

**Other Adverse Effects** 1% to 10%:

Endocrine & metabolic: Decreased libido

Genitourinary: <4% incidence of impotence, decreased volume of ejaculate

**Drug Interactions** No data reported

**Drug Uptake**

Onset of clinical effect: Within 12 weeks to 6 months of ongoing therapy

Duration of action:

After a single oral dose as small as 0.5 mg: 65% depression of plasma dihydrotestosterone levels persists 5-7 days

After 6 months of treatment with 5 mg/day: Circulating dihydrotestosterone levels are reduced to castrate levels without significant effects on circulating testosterone; levels return to normal within 14 days of discontinuation of treatment

Absorption: Oral: Extent may be reduced if administered with food

Time to peak serum concentration: Oral: 2-6 hours

Serum half-life, serum: Parent drug: ~5-17 hours (mean: 1.9 fasting, 4.2 with breakfast)

Serum half-life:

Elderly: 8 hours

Adults: 6 hours (3-16)

**Pregnancy Risk Factor** X

**Generic Available** No

- **Fiorgen PF®** *see* Butalbital Compound *on page 163*
- **Fiorgen PF®** *see* Butalbital Compound and Aspirin *on page 165*
- **Fioricet®** *see* Butalbital Compound *on page 163*
- **Fioricet®** *see* Butalbital Compound and Acetaminophen *on page 164*
- **Fiorinal®** *see* Butalbital Compound *on page 163*
- **Fiorinal®** *see* Butalbital Compound and Aspirin *on page 165*
- **Fiorinal® With Codeine** *see* Butalbital Compound and Codeine *on page 165*
- **Flagyl®** *see* Metronidazole *on page 667*
- **Flarex®** *see* Fluorometholone *on page 443*
- **Flatulex® [OTC]** *see* Simethicone *on page 915*
- **Flavorcee® [OTC]** *see* Ascorbic Acid *on page 97*

## Flavoxate (fla VOKS ate)

**U.S. Brand Names** Urispas®

**Therapeutic Category** Antispasmodic Agent, Urinary

**Use** Antispasmodic used to provide symptomatic relief of dysuria, nocturia, suprapubic pain, urgency, and incontinence

**Usual Dosage** Children >12 years and Adults: Oral: 100-200 mg 3-4 times/day; reduce the dose when symptoms improve

**Mechanism of Action** Synthetic antispasmodic with similar actions to that of propantheline; it exerts a direct relaxant effect on smooth muscles via phosphodiesterase inhibition, providing relief to a variety of smooth muscle spasms; it is especially useful for the treatment of bladder spasticity, whereby it produces an increase in urinary capacity

**Local Anesthetic/Vasoconstrictor Precautions** No information available to require special precautions

**Effects on Dental Treatment** >10% of patients experience dry mouth

**Other Adverse Effects**

>10%:

Central nervous system: Drowsiness

Respiratory: Dry throat

1% to 10%:

Cardiovascular: Tachycardia, palpitations

Central nervous system: Nervousness, fatigue, vertigo, headache, drowsiness, fever

Gastrointestinal: Constipation, nausea, vomiting

<1%:

Central nervous system: Confusion (especially in the elderly)

Dermatologic: Skin rash

Hematologic: Leukopenia

Ocular: Increased intraocular pressure

**Drug Interactions** No data reported
**Drug Uptake** Onset of action: 55-60 minutes
**Pregnancy Risk Factor** B
**Generic Available** No

## Flecainide (fle KAY nide)

**Related Information**
Cardiovascular Diseases *on page 1066*

**U.S. Brand Names** Tambocor™

**Therapeutic Category** Antiarrhythmic Agent, Class I-C; Antiarrhythmic Agent (Supraventricular & Ventricular)

**Use** Prevention and suppression of documented life-threatening ventricular arrhythmias (ie, sustained ventricular tachycardia); controlling symptomatic, disabling supraventricular tachycardias in patients without structural heart disease in whom other agents fail

**Usual Dosage** Oral:
Children:
Initial: 3 mg/kg/day or 50-100 mg/m²/day in 3 divided doses
Usual: 3-6 mg/kg/day or 100-150 mg/m²/day in 3 divided doses; up to 11 mg/kg/day or 200 mg/m²/day for uncontrolled patients with subtherapeutic levels
Adults:
Life-threatening ventricular arrhythmias:
Initial: 100 mg every 12 hours
Increase by 50-100 mg/day (given in 2 doses/day) every 4 days; maximum: 400 mg/day
For patients receiving 400 mg/day who are not controlled and have trough concentrations <0.6 μg/mL, dosage may be increased to 600 mg/day
Prevention of paroxysmal supraventricular arrhythmias in patients with disabling symptoms but no structural heart disease:
Initial: 50 mg every 12 hours
Increase by 50 mg twice daily at 4-day intervals; maximum: 300 mg/day

**Mechanism of Action** Class IC antiarrhythmic; slows conduction in cardiac tissue by altering transport of ions across cell membranes; causes slight prolongation of refractory periods; decreases the rate of rise of the action potential without affecting its duration; increases electrical stimulation threshold of ventricle, HIS-Purkinje system; possesses local anesthetic and moderate negative inotropic effects

**Local Anesthetic/Vasoconstrictor Precautions** No information available to require special precautions

**Effects on Dental Treatment** No effects or complications reported

**Other Adverse Effects**
>10%:
Central nervous system: Dizziness
Ocular: Visual disturbances
Respiratory: Dyspnea
1% to 10%:
Cardiovascular: Palpitations, chest pain, edema, tachycardia
Central nervous system: Headache, fatigue, fever
Dermatologic: Rash
Gastrointestinal: Nausea, constipation, abdominal pain
Neuromuscular & skeletal: Tremor, weakness
<1%:
Cardiovascular: Bradycardia, heart block, elevated P-R, QRS duration, worsening ventricular arrhythmias, congestive heart failure
Central nervous system: Nervousness, hypoesthesia
Dermatologic: Alopecia
Hematologic: Blood dyscrasias
Hepatic: Possible hepatic dysfunction
Neuromuscular & skeletal: Paresthesia

**Drug Interactions**
Increased toxicity:
Alkalinizing agents (high dose antacids, cimetidine, carbonic anhydrase inhibitors or sodium bicarbonate) may decrease flecainide clearance
Beta-adrenergic blockers, disopyramide, verapamil (possible additive negative inotropic effects)
Digoxin, amiodarone (increased plasma concentrations)
Decreased toxicity: Smoking and acid urine (increases flecainide clearance)

**Drug Uptake**
Absorption: Oral: Rapid
Serum half-life:
Children: 8 hours
Adults: 7-22 hours, increased with congestive heart failure or renal dysfunction
(Continued)

## Flecainide *(Continued)*

End-stage renal disease: 19-26 hours
Time to peak serum concentration: Within 1.5-3 hours

**Pregnancy Risk Factor** C

**Generic Available** No

- **Fleet® Babylax® Rectal [OTC]** *see* Glycerin *on page 472*
- **Fleet® Enema [OTC]** *see* Sodium Phosphates *on page 923*
- **Fleet® Flavored Castor Oil [OTC]** *see* Castor Oil *on page 196*
- **Fleet® Laxative [OTC]** *see* Bisacodyl *on page 141*
- **Fleet® Pain Relief [OTC]** *see* Pramoxine *on page 828*
- **Fleet® Phospho®-Soda [OTC]** *see* Sodium Phosphates *on page 923*
- **Flexaphen®** *see* Chlorzoxazone *on page 242*
- **Flexeril®** *see* Cyclobenzaprine *on page 284*
- **Flolan® Injection** *see* Epoprostenol *on page 377*
- **Flomax®** *see* Tamsulosin *on page 953*
- **Flonase®** *see* Fluticasone *on page 450*
- **Florical® [OTC]** *see* Calcium Carbonate *on page 172*
- **Florinef® Acetate** *see* Fludrocortisone Acetate *on page 437*
- **Florone®** *see* Diflorasone *on page 327*
- **Florone® E** *see* Diflorasone *on page 327*
- **Floropryl®** *see* Isoflurophate *on page 552*
- **Florvite®** *see* Vitamins, Multiple *on page 1051*
- **Flovent®** *see* Fluticasone *on page 450*
- **Floxin® Oral** *see* Ofloxacin *on page 737*
- **Floxin® Otic** *see* Ofloxacin *on page 737*

## Floxuridine (floks YOOR i deen)

**U.S. Brand Names** FUDR®

**Canadian Brand Names** Fludara®

**Therapeutic Category** Antineoplastic Agent, Antimetabolite

**Synonyms** Fluorodeoxyuridine

**Use** Palliative management of carcinomas of head, neck, and brain as well as liver, gallbladder, and bile ducts

**Usual Dosage** Adults (refer to individual protocols):

Intra-arterial: Primarily by an implantable pump: 0.1-0.6 mg/kg/day continuous intra-arterial administration for 14 days then heparinized saline is given for 14 days; toxicity requires dose reduction

I.V.: 0.5-1 mg/kg/day for 6-15 days

**Mechanism of Action** Mechanism of action and pharmacokinetics are very similar to 5-FU; FUDR® is the deoxyribonucleotide of 5-FU. Inhibits DNA and RNA synthesis via formation of carbonium ions; cross-links strands of DNA, causing an imbalance of growth and cell death

**Local Anesthetic/Vasoconstrictor Precautions** No information available to require special

**Effects on Dental Treatment** No effects or complications reported

**Other Adverse Effects**

>10%: Gastrointestinal: GI hemorrhage, stomatitis, esophagopharyngitis, diarrhea, gastritis

1% to 10%:
- Gastrointestinal: Anorexia, glossitis
- Dermatologic: Alopecia, dermatitis, rash

<1%:
- Cardiovascular: Myocardial ischemia, angina
- Central nervous system: Lethargy, acute cerebellar syndrome, confusion, euphoria, fever
- Hematologic: Severe hematologic toxicity, leukopenia, thrombocytopenia, pancytopenia, agranulocytosis
- Neuromuscular & skeletal: Weakness
- Ocular: Photophobia
- Miscellaneous: Anaphylaxis

**Pregnancy Risk Factor** D

**Generic Available** No

## Fluconazole (floo KOE na zole)

**Related Information**

Oral Fungal Infections *on page 1134*

**U.S. Brand Names** Diflucan®

**Therapeutic Category** Antifungal Agent, Systemic

**Use** Oral fluconazole should be used in persons able to tolerate oral medications; parenteral fluconazole should be reserved for patients who are both unable to take oral medications and are unable to tolerate amphotericin B (eg, due to hypersensitivity or renal insufficiency)

Dental: Treatment of susceptible fungal infections in the oral cavity including candidiasis, oral thrush, and chronic mucocutaneous candidiasis; treatment of esophageal and oropharyngeal candidiasis caused by *Candida* species; treatment of severe, chronic mucocutaneous candidiasis caused by *Candida* species

Medical: Vaginal candidiasis unresponsive to nystatin or clotrimazole; treatment of hepatosplenic candidiasis; treatment of other *Candida* infections in persons unable to tolerate amphotericin B; treatment of cryptococcal infections; secondary prophylaxis for cryptococcal meningitis in persons with AIDS; antifungal prophylaxis in allogeneic bone marrow transplant recipients

**Usual Dosage** The daily dose of fluconazole is the same for oral and I.V. administration

Children: Efficacy of fluconazole has not been established in children; a small number of patients from 3-13 years of age have been treated with fluconazole using doses of 3-6 mg/kg/day once daily. Doses as high as 12 mg/kg/day once daily have been used to treat candidiasis in immunocompromised children; 10-12 mg/kg/day has been used prophylactically against fungal infections in pediatric bone marrow transplant patients.

Adults: Oral, I.V.: See table for once daily dosing.

| Indication | Day 1 | Daily Therapy | Minimum Duration of Therapy |
|---|---|---|---|
| Oropharyngeal candidiasis | 200 mg | 100 mg | 14 d |
| Esophageal candidiasis | 200 mg | 100 mg | 21 d |
| Systemic candidiasis | 400 mg | 200 mg | 28 d |
| Cryptococcal meningitis | | | 10-12 wk after CSF culture becomes negative |
| acute | 400 mg | 200 mg | |
| relapse | 200 mg | 200 mg | |

**Mechanism of Action** Interferes with cytochrome P-450 activity, decreasing ergosterol synthesis (principal sterol in fungal cell membrane) and inhibiting cell membrane formation

**Local Anesthetic/Vasoconstrictor Precautions** No information available to require special precautions

**Effects on Dental Treatment** No effects or complications reported

**Other Adverse Effects** 1% to 10%:

Central nervous system: Headache

Dermatologic: Skin rash

Gastrointestinal: Nausea, vomiting, abdominal pain, diarrhea

**Contraindications** Known hypersensitivity to fluconazole or other azoles

**Warnings/Precautions** Should be used with caution in patients with renal and hepatic dysfunction or previous hepatotoxicity from other azole derivatives. Patients who develop abnormal liver function tests during fluconazole therapy should be monitored closely and discontinued if symptoms consistent with liver disease develop.

**Drug Interactions** Cytochrome P-450 IIIA4 enzyme inhibitor and cytochrome P-450 IIC enzyme inhibitor

Rifampin decreases concentrations of fluconazole; fluconazole may increase cyclosporine levels when high doses used; may increase phenytoin serum concentration; fluconazole may also inhibit warfarin metabolism; coadministration with cisapride may cause toxic increases in cisapride blood levels; coadministration with astemizole could result in cardiotoxicity

**Drug Uptake**

Absorption: >90%

Serum half-life: 25-30 hours with normal renal function

Time to peak serum concentration: Oral: Within 2-4 hours

**Pregnancy Risk Factor** C

**Breast-feeding Considerations** Probably safe (not absorbed orally)

**Dosage Forms**

Injection: 2 mg/mL (100 mL, 200 mL)

Powder for oral suspension: 10 mg/mL (35 mL); 40 mg/mL (35 mL)

Tablet: 50 mg, 100 mg, 150 mg, 200 mg

**Dietary Considerations** No data reported

**Generic Available** No

## Flucytosine (floo SYE toe seen)

**U.S. Brand Names** Ancobon®

**Canadian Brand Names** Ancotil®

**Therapeutic Category** Antifungal Agent, Systemic

**Synonyms** 5-Flurocytosine

**Use** Adjunctive treatment of susceptible fungal infections (usually *Candida* or *Cryptococcus*); in combination with amphotericin B, fluconazole, or itraconazole; synergy with amphotericin B for fungal infections (*Aspergillus*)

**Usual Dosage** Children and Adults: Oral: 50-150 mg/kg/day in divided doses every 6 hours

**Mechanism of Action** Penetrates fungal cells and is converted to fluorouracil which competes with uracil interfering with fungal RNA and protein synthesis

**Local Anesthetic/Vasoconstrictor Precautions** No information available to require special precautions

**Effects on Dental Treatment** No effects or complications reported

**Other Adverse Effects**

1% to 10%:
- Dermatologic: Skin rash
- Gastrointestinal: Abdominal pain, diarrhea, loss of appetite, nausea, vomiting
- Hematologic: Anemia, leukopenia, thrombocytopenia
- Hepatic: Hepatitis, jaundice

<1%:
- Cardiovascular: Cardiac arrest
- Central nervous system: Confusion, hallucinations, dizziness, drowsiness, headache, parkinsonism, psychosis, ataxia
- Dermatologic: Photosensitivity
- Endocrine & metabolic: Temporary growth failure, hypoglycemia, hypokalemia
- Hematologic: Bone marrow suppression
- Hepatic: Elevated liver enzymes
- Neuromuscular & skeletal: Paresthesia
- Otic: Hearing loss
- Respiratory: Respiratory arrest

**Drug Interactions** Increased effect/toxicity (enterocolitis) with concurrent amphotericin administration

**Drug Uptake**

Absorption: Oral: 75% to 90%

Serum half-life: 3-8 hours
- Anuria: May be as long as 200 hours
- End-stage renal disease: 75-200 hours

Time to peak serum concentration: Within 2-6 hours

**Pregnancy Risk Factor** C

**Generic Available** No

♦ **Fludara®** *see* Fludarabine *on this page*

## Fludarabine (floo DARE a been)

**U.S. Brand Names** Fludara®

**Therapeutic Category** Antineoplastic Agent, Antimetabolite

**Use** Treatment of B-cell chronic lymphocytic leukemia unresponsive to previous therapy with an alkylating agent containing regimen. Fludarabine has been tested in patients with refractory acute lymphocytic leukemia and acute nonlymphocytic leukemia, but required a highly toxic dose to achieve response.

**Usual Dosage** I.V.:

Children:
- Acute leukemia: 10 mg/m$^2$ bolus over 15 minutes followed by continuous infusion of 30.5 mg/m$^2$/day over 5 days **or**
- 10.5 mg/m$^2$ bolus over 15 minutes followed by 30.5 mg/m$^2$/day over 48 hours followed by cytarabine has been used in clinical trials
- Solid tumors: 9 mg/m$^2$ bolus followed by 27 mg/m$^2$/day continuous infusion over 5 days

Adults:
- Chronic lymphocytic leukemia: 20-25 mg/m$^2$/day over a 30-minute period for 5 days; 5-day courses are repeated every 28-35 days days
- Non-Hodgkin's lymphoma: Loading dose: 20 mg/m$^2$ followed by 30 mg/m$^2$/day for 48 hours

**Mechanism of Action** Fludarabine is analogous to that of Ara-C and Ara-A. Following systemic administration, FAMP is rapidly dephosphorylated to 2-fluoro-Ara-A. 2-Fluoro-Ara-A enters the cell by a carrier-mediated transport process, then is phosphorylated intracellularly by deoxycytidine kinase to form the active metabolite 2-fluoro-Ara-ATP. 2-Fluoro-Ara-ATP inhibits DNA synthesis by inhibition of DNA polymerase and ribonucleotide reductase.

**Local Anesthetic/Vasoconstrictor Precautions** No information available to require special precautions

**Effects on Dental Treatment** No effects or complications reported

**Other Adverse Effects**

>10%:

Cardiovascular: Edema

Central nervous system: Fever, chills, fatigue, pain

Dermatologic: Rash

Gastrointestinal: Mild nausea, vomiting, diarrhea, stomatitis, GI bleeding

Genitourinary: Urinary infection

Hematologic: Myelosuppression: Dose-limiting toxicity; myelosuppression may not be related to cumulative dose; Granulocyte nadir: 13 days (3-25); Platelet nadir: 16 days (2-32); WBC nadir: 8 days; Recovery: 5-7 weeks

Neuromuscular & skeletal: Paresthesia, myalgia, weakness

Respiratory: Manifested as dyspnea and a nonproductive cough; lung biopsy has shown pneumonitis in some patients, pneumonia

Miscellaneous: Infection

1% to 10%:

Cardiovascular: Congestive heart failure

Central nervous system: Malaise, headache

Dermatologic: Alopecia

Endocrine & metabolic: Hyperglycemia

Gastrointestinal: Anorexia

Otic: Hearing loss

<1%:

Central nervous system: Reported with higher dose levels; most patients shown to have CNS demyelination; somnolence also noted; severe neurotoxicity

Endocrine & metabolic: Metabolic acidosis

Gastrointestinal: Metallic taste

Hepatic: Reversible hepatotoxicity

Renal: Renal failure, hematuria, elevated serum creatinine

Respiratory: Interstitial pneumonitis

Miscellaneous: Tumor lysis syndrome

**Drug Uptake**

Absorption: Oral preparation is under study

Serum half-life, elimination: 2-fluoro-vidarabine: 9 hours

**Pregnancy Risk Factor** D

**Generic Available** No

## Fludrocortisone Acetate (floo droe KOR ti sone AS e tate)

**U.S. Brand Names** Florinef® Acetate

**Therapeutic Category** Mineralocorticoid

**Use** Partial replacement therapy for primary and secondary adrenocortical insufficiency in Addison's disease; treatment of salt-losing adrenogenital syndrome

**Usual Dosage** Adults: Oral: 0.1-0.2 mg/day with ranges of 0.1 mg 3 times/week to 0.2 mg/day

**Mechanism of Action** Promotes increased reabsorption of sodium and loss of potassium from renal distal tubules

**Local Anesthetic/Vasoconstrictor Precautions** No information available to require special precautions

**Effects on Dental Treatment** No effects or complications reported

**Other Adverse Effects** 1% to 10%:

Cardiovascular: Hypertension, edema, congestive heart failure

Central nervous system: Convulsions, headache, dizziness

Dermatologic: Acne, rash, bruising

Endocrine & metabolic: Hypokalemic alkalosis, suppression of growth, hyperglycemia, HPA suppression

Gastrointestinal: Peptic ulcer

Neuromuscular & skeletal: Muscle weakness

Ocular: Cataracts

Miscellaneous: Sweating

**Drug Interactions**

Decreased corticosteroid effects by rifampin, barbiturates, and hydantoins

**Drug Uptake**

Absorption: Rapid and complete from GI tract, partially absorbed through skin

Serum half-life:

Plasma: 30-35 minutes

Biological: 18-36 hours

Time to peak serum concentration: Within 1.7 hours

**Pregnancy Risk Factor** C

**Generic Available** No

♦ **Flumadine®** *see* Rimantadine *on page 889*

## Flumazenil (FLO may ze nil)

**U.S. Brand Names** Romazicon™

**Canadian Brand Names** Anexate®

**Therapeutic Category** Antidote, Benzodiazepine

**Use** Benzodiazepine antagonist - reverses sedative effects of benzodiazepines used in general anesthesia; for management of benzodiazepine overdose; flumazenil does **not** antagonize the CNS effects of other GABA agonists (such as ethanol, barbiturates, or general anesthetics), **does not** reverse narcotics

**Usual Dosage** See table.

**Flumazenil**

| | |
|---|---|
| *Pediatric Dosage*<br>Further studies are needed<br>Pediatric dosage for **reversal of conscious sedation:** Intravenously through a freely running intravenous infusion into a large vein to minimize pain at the injection site | |
| Initial dose | 0.01 mg/kg over 15 seconds (maximum dose of 0.2 mg) |
| Repeat doses | 0.005-0.01 mg/kg (maximum dose of 0.2 mg) repeated at 1-minute intervals |
| Maximum total cumulative dose | 1 mg |
| Pediatric dosage for **management of benzodiazepine overdose** Intravenously through a freely running intravenous infusion into a large vein to minimize pain at the injection site | |
| Initial dose | 0.01 mg/kg (maximum dose: 0.2 mg) |
| Repeat doses | 0.01 mg/kg (maximum dose of 0.2 mg) repeated at 1-minute intervals |
| Maximum total cumulative dose | 1 mg |
| In place of repeat bolus doses, follow-up continuous infusions of 0.005-0.01 mg/kg/hour have been used; further studies are needed | |
| *Adult Dosage*<br>Adult dosage for **reversal of conscious sedation:** Intravenously through a freely running intravenous infusion into a large vein to minimize pain at the injection site | |
| Initial dose | 0.2 mg intravenously over 15 seconds |
| Repeat doses | If desired level of consciousness is not obtained, 0.2 mg may be repeated at 1-minute intervals |
| Maximum total cumulative dose | 1 mg (usual dose: 0.6-1 mg)<br>**In the event of resedation:** repeat doses may be given at 20-minute intervals with maximum of 1 mg/dose and 3 mg/hour |
| Adult dosage for **suspected benzodiazepine overdose:** Intravenously through a freely running intravenous infusion into a large vein to minimize pain at the injection site | |
| Initial dose | 0.2 mg intravenously over 30 seconds |
| Repeat doses | 0.5 mg over 30 seconds repeated at 1-minute intervals |
| Maximum total cumulative dose | 3 mg (usual dose: 1-3 mg)<br>Patients with a partial response at 3 mg may require additional titration up to a total dose of 5 mg. If a patient has not responded 5 minutes after cumulative dose of 5 mg, the major cause of sedation is not likely due to benzodiazepines. **In the event of resedation:** may repeat doses at 20-minute intervals with maximum of 1 mg/dose and 3 mg/hour |

Resedation: Repeated doses may be given at 20-minute intervals as needed; repeat treatment doses of 1 mg (at a rate of 0.5 mg/minute) should be given at any time and no more than 3 mg should be given in any hour. After intoxication with high doses of benzodiazepines, the duration of a single dose of flumazenil is not expected to exceed 1 hour; if desired, the period of wakefulness may be prolonged with repeated low intravenous doses of flumazenil, or by an infusion of 0.1-0.4 mg/hour. Most patients with benzodiazepine overdose will respond to a cumulative dose of 1-3 mg and doses >3 mg do not reliably produce additional effects. Rarely, patients with a partial response at 3 mg may require additional titration up to a total dose of 5 mg. **If a patient has not responded 5 minutes after receiving a cumulative dose of 5 mg, the major cause of sedation is not likely to be due to benzodiazepines.**

**Mechanism of Action** Antagonizes the effect of benzodiazepines on the GABA/benzodiazepine receptor complex. Flumazenil is benzodiazepine specific and does not antagonize other nonbenzodiazepine GABA agonists (including ethanol, barbiturates, general anesthetics); flumazenil does not reverse the effects of opiates

**Local Anesthetic/Vasoconstrictor Precautions** No information available to require special precautions

**Effects on Dental Treatment** No effects or complications reported

**Other Adverse Effects**

>10%:

Central nervous system: Dizziness

Gastrointestinal: Vomiting, nausea

1% to 10%:

Central nervous system: Headache, malaise, anxiety, nervousness, insomnia, abnormal crying, euphoria, depression

Endocrine & metabolic: Hot flashes

Gastrointestinal: Dry mouth

Local: Pain at injection site

Neuromuscular & skeletal: Tremor, weakness

Respiratory: Dyspnea, hyperventilation

Miscellaneous: Increased sweating disorders

<1%:

Cardiovascular: Bradycardia, tachycardia, chest pain, hypertension, ventricular extrasystoles, altered blood pressure (increases and decreases)

Central nervous system: Anxiety and sensation of coldness, generalized convulsions, withdrawal syndrome, shivering, somnolence

Otic: Abnormal hearing

Miscellaneous: Thick tongue, hiccups

**Drug Interactions** Increased toxicity:

Use with caution in overdosage involving mixed drug overdose

Toxic effects may emerge (especially with cyclic antidepressants) with the reversal of the benzodiazepine effect by flumazenil

**Drug Uptake**

Onset of action: 1-3 minutes; 80% response within 3 minutes

Peak effect: 6-10 minutes

Duration: Resedation occurs usually within 1 hour; duration is related to dose given and benzodiazepine plasma concentrations; reversal effects of flumazenil may wear off before effects of benzodiazepine

Serum half-life, adults:

Alpha: 7-15 minutes

Terminal: 41-79 minutes

**Pregnancy Risk Factor** C

**Dosage Forms** Injection: 0.1 mg/mL (5 mL, 10 mL)

**Generic Available** No

## Flunisolide (floo NIS oh lide)

**Related Information**

Respiratory Diseases *on page 1079*

**U.S. Brand Names** AeroBid®-M Oral Aerosol Inhaler; AeroBid® Oral Aerosol Inhaler; Nasalide® Nasal Aerosol; Nasarel® Nasal Spray

**Canadian Brand Names** Bronalide®; Rhinalar®; Rhinaris®-F; Syn-Flunisolide

**Therapeutic Category** Anti-inflammatory Agent; Corticosteroid, Inhalant

**Use** Steroid-dependent asthma; nasal solution is used for seasonal or perennial rhinitis

**Usual Dosage**

Children >6 years:

Oral inhalation: 2 inhalations twice daily (morning and evening) up to 4 inhalations/day

Nasal: 1 spray each nostril twice daily (morning and evening), not to exceed 4 sprays/day each nostril

Adults:

Oral inhalation: 2 inhalations twice daily (morning and evening) up to 8 inhalations/day maximum

Nasal: 2 sprays each nostril twice daily (morning and evening); maximum dose: 8 sprays/day in each nostril

**Mechanism of Action** Decreases inflammation by suppression of migration of polymorphonuclear leukocytes and reversal of increased capillary permeability; does not depress hypothalamus

**Local Anesthetic/Vasoconstrictor Precautions** No information available to require special precautions

**Effects on Dental Treatment** No effects or complications reported

(Continued)

## Flunisolide *(Continued)*

**Other Adverse Effects**

>10%:

Cardiovascular: Pounding heartbeat

Central nervous system: Dizziness, headache, nervousness

Dermatologic: Itching, skin rash

Endocrine & metabolic: Adrenal suppression, menstrual problems

Gastrointestinal: GI irritation, anorexia

Local: Nasal burning, nasal congestion, nasal dryness, sore throat, bitter taste, *Candida* infections of the nose or pharynx, atrophic rhinitis

Respiratory: Sneezing, coughing, upper respiratory tract infection, bronchitis

Miscellaneous: Increased susceptibility to infections

1% to 10%:

Central nervous system: Insomnia, psychic changes

Dermatologic: Acne, urticaria

Gastrointestinal: Increase in appetite, dry mouth/throat, ageusia

Ocular: Cataracts

Respiratory: Epistaxis,

Miscellaneous: Sweating, loss of smell

<1%:

Gastrointestinal: Abdominal fullness

Respiratory: Bronchospasm, dyspnea

**Drug Interactions** No data reported

**Drug Uptake**

Absorption: Nasal inhalation: ~50%

Serum half-life: 1.8 hours

**Pregnancy Risk Factor** C

**Generic Available** No

## Fluocinolone (floo oh SIN oh lone)

**Related Information**

Corticosteroids, Topical Comparison *on page 1222*

**U.S. Brand Names** Derma-Smoothe/FS®; Fluonid®; Flurosyn®; FS Shampoo®; Synalar®; Synalar-HP®; Synemol®

**Canadian Brand Names** Lidemol®

**Therapeutic Category** Corticosteroid, Topical (Medium Potency)

**Use** Relief of susceptible inflammatory dermatosis [low, medium, high potency topical corticosteroid]

**Usual Dosage** Children and Adults: Topical: Apply a thin layer to affected area 2-4 times/day

**Mechanism of Action** A synthetic corticosteroid which differs structurally from triamcinolone acetonide in the presence of an additional fluorine atom in the 6-alpha position on the steroid nucleus. The mechanism of action for all topical corticosteroids is not well defined, however, is believed to be a combination of three important properties: anti-inflammatory activity, immunosuppressive properties, and antiproliferative actions.

**Local Anesthetic/Vasoconstrictor Precautions** No information available to require special precautions

**Effects on Dental Treatment** No effects or complications reported

**Other Adverse Effects** <1%:

Dermatologic: Acne, hypopigmentation, allergic dermatitis, maceration of the skin, skin atrophy, folliculitis, hypertrichosis

Endocrine & metabolic: HPA suppression, Cushing's syndrome, growth retardation

Local: Burning, itching, irritation, dryness

Miscellaneous: Secondary infection

**Drug Interactions** No data reported

**Drug Uptake** Absorption: Dependent on strength of preparation, amount applied,and nature of skin at application site; ranges from ~1% in thick stratum corneum areas (palms, soles, elbows, etc) to 36% in areas of thinnest stratum corneum (face, eyelids, etc); increased absorption in areas of skin damage, inflammation, or occlusion

**Pregnancy Risk Factor** C

**Generic Available** Yes

## Fluocinonide (floo SIN oh nide)

**Related Information**

Corticosteroids, Topical Comparison *on page 1222*

Oral Nonviral Soft Tissue Ulcerations or Erosions *on page 1141*

**U.S. Brand Names** Lidex®; Lidex-E®

**Canadian Brand Names** Lyderm; Lydonide; Tiamol®; Topactin®; Topsyn®

**Therapeutic Category** Corticosteroid, Topical (High Potency)

**Use** Anti-inflammatory, antipruritic, relief of inflammatory and pruritic manifestations [high potency topical corticosteroid]

**Usual Dosage** Children and Adults: Topical: Apply thin layer to affected area 2-4 times/day depending on the severity of the condition

**Mechanism of Action** Not well defined for all topical corticosteroids; however, is felt to be a combination of three important properties: anti-inflammatory activity, immunosuppressive properties, and antiproliferative actions.

**Local Anesthetic/Vasoconstrictor Precautions** No information available to require special precautions

**Effects on Dental Treatment** No effects or complications reported

**Other Adverse Effects** <1%:

Central nervous system: Intracranial hypertension

Dermatologic: Acne, hypopigmentation, allergic dermatitis, maceration of the skin, skin atrophy

Endocrine & metabolic: HPA suppression, Cushing's syndrome, growth retardation

Local: Burning, itching, irritation, dryness, folliculitis, hypertrichosis

Miscellaneous: Secondary infection

**Drug Interactions** No data reported

**Drug Uptake** Absorption: Dependent on amount applied and nature of skin at application site; ranges from ~1% in areas of thick stratum corneum (palms, soles, elbows, etc) to 36% in areas of thin stratum corneum (face, eyelids, etc); absorption is increased in areas of skin damage, inflammation, or occlusion

**Pregnancy Risk Factor** C

**Dosage Forms**

Cream: 0.05% (15 g, 30 g, 60 g, 120 g)

Anhydrous, emollient (Lidex®): 0.05% (15 g, 30 g, 60 g, 120 g)

Aqueous, emollient (Lidex-E®): 0.05% (15 g, 30 g, 60 g, 120 g)

Gel, topical: 0.05% (15 g, 60 g)

Lidex®: 0.05% (15 g, 30 g, 60 g, 120 g)

Ointment, topical: 0.05% (15 g, 30 g, 60 g)

Lidex®: 0.05% (15 g, 30 g, 60 g, 120 g)

Solution, topical: 0.05% (20 mL, 60 mL)

Lidex®: 0.05% (20 mL, 60 mL)

**Generic Available** Yes

♦ **Fluogen®** *see* Influenza Virus Vaccine *on page 536*
♦ **Fluonid®** *see* Fluocinolone *on previous page*
♦ **Fluoracaine® Ophthalmic** *see* Proparacaine and Fluorescein *on page 852*
♦ **Fluor-A-Day®** *see* Fluoride *on this page*

# Fluoride (FLOR ide)

**Related Information**

Dentin Hypersensitivity; High Caries Index; Xerostomia *on page 1145*

Patients Undergoing Cancer Therapy *on page 1154*

**U.S. Brand Names** ACT® [OTC]; Duraflor® Cavity Varnish; Fluor-A-Day®; Fluorigard® [OTC]; Fluorinse®; Fluoritab®; Flura-Drops®; Flura-Loz®; Gel-Kam®; Gel-Tin® [OTC]; Karidium®; Karigel®; Karigel®-N; Listermint® with Fluoride [OTC]; Luride®; Luride® Lozi-Tab®; Luride®-SF Lozi-Tab®; Minute-Gel®; Pediaflor®; Pharmaflur®; Phos-Flur®; Point-Two®; PreviDent®; Stop® [OTC]; Thera-Flur®; Thera-Flur-N®

**Therapeutic Category** Fluoride; Mineral, Oral; Mineral, Oral Topical

**Synonyms** Acidulated Phosphate Fluoride; Sodium Fluoride; Stannous Fluoride

**Use** Dental: Prevention of dental caries

**Fluoride Ion**

| Fluoride Content of Drinking Water | Daily Dose, Oral (mg) |
|---|---|
| **<0.3 ppm** | |
| Birth - 6 mo | None |
| 6 mo - 3 y | 0.25 |
| 3-6 y | 0.5 |
| 6 y | 1.0 |
| **0.3-0.7 ppm** | |
| Birth - 6 mo | 0 |
| 6 mo - 3 y | 0.125 |
| 3-6 y | 0.25 |
| 6 y | 0.5 |

(Continued)

## Fluoride *(Continued)*

**Usual Dosage** Oral:

Recommended daily fluoride supplement (2.2 mg of sodium fluoride is equivalent to 1 mg of fluoride ion): See table.

Dental rinse or gel:

- Adults: 10 mL rinse or apply to teeth and spit daily after brushing
- Children 6-12 years: 5-10 mL rinse or apply to teeth and spit daily after brushing

**Mechanism of Action** Promotes remineralization of decalcified enamel; inhibits the cariogenic microbial process in dental plaque; increases tooth resistance to acid dissolution

**Local Anesthetic/Vasoconstrictor Precautions** No information available to require special precautions

**Effects on Dental Treatment** No effects or complications reported

**Other Adverse Effects** <1%:

Dermatologic: Rash

Gastrointestinal: Nausea, vomiting, products containing stannous fluoride may stain the teeth

**Contraindications** Hypersensitivity to fluoride or any component, or when fluoride content of drinking water exceeds 0.7 ppm

**Warnings/Precautions** Prolonged ingestion with excessive doses may result in dental fluorosis and osseous changes; do **not** exceed recommended dosage; some products contain tartrazine

**Drug Interactions** Decreased effect/absorption with magnesium-, aluminum-, and calcium-containing products

**Drug Uptake**

Absorption: Rapid and complete from GI tract; calcium, iron, or magnesium may delay absorption

Time to peak serum concentration: 30-60 minutes

**Pregnancy Risk Factor** C

**Breast-feeding Considerations** No data reported

**Dosage Forms** Fluoride ion content listed in brackets

**Prescription only (Rx) products:**

Drops, oral, as sodium: 0.275 mg/drop [0.125 mg/drop]
- Fluoritab®, Flura-Drops®: 0.55 mg/drop [0.25 mg/drop] (22.8 mL, 24 mL)
- Karidium®, Luride®: 0.275 mg/drop [0.125 mg/drop] (30 mL, 60 mL)
- Pediaflor®: 1.1 mg/mL [0.5 mg/mL] (50 mL)

Gel-Drops (Thera-Flur® [lime flavor], Thera-Flur-N®): 1.1% [0.55%] (24 mL)

Gel, topical:
- Acidulated phosphate fluoride (Minute-Gel® [spearmint, strawberry, grape, apple-cinnamon, cherry cola & bubblegum flavor]): 1.23% (480 mL)
- Sodium fluoride:
  - Karigel® [orange flavor]: 1.1% [0.5%]
  - Karigel®-N: 1.1% [0.5%]
  - PreviDent® ([mint, berry, cherry & fruit sherbet flavors]): 1.1% [0.5%] (24 g, 30 g, 60 g, 120 g, 130 g, 250 g)
- Stannous fluoride (Gel-Kam®) (cinnamon flavor): 0.4% [0.1%] (65 g, 105 g, 122 g)

Lozenge, as sodium (Flura-Loz® [raspberry flavor]): 2.2 mg [1 mg]

Rinse, topical, as sodium:
- Fluorinse®, Point-Two®: 0.2% [0.09%] (240 mL, 480 mL, 3780 mL)

Solution, oral, as sodium (Phos-Flur® [cherry, cinnamon, grape & wintergreen flavors]): 0.44 mg/mL [0.2 mg/mL] (250 mL, 500 mL, 3780 mL)

Tablet, as sodium:
- Chewable: 1.1 mg [0.5 mg]; 2.2 mg [1 mg]
  - Fluor-A-Day®: 0.55 mg [0.25 mg]
  - Fluor-A-Day®, Fluoritab®, Luride® Lozi-Tab®, Pharmaflur®: 1.1 mg [0.5 mg]
  - Fluor-A-Day®, Fluoritab®, Karidium®, Luride® Lozi-Tab®, Luride®-SF Lozi-Tab®, Pharmaflur®: 2.2 mg [1 mg]
- Oral: Flura®, Karidium®: 2.2 mg [1 mg]

Varnish (Duraflor®): 5% [50 mg/mL] (10 mL)

**Over-the-counter (OTC) products:**

Gel, topical:
- Stannous fluoride:
  - Gel-Tin® (lime, grape, cinnamon, raspberry, mint, and orange flavor),
  - Stop® (grape, cinnamon, bubblegum, piña colada & mint flavor): 0.4% [0.1%] (60 g, 120 g)

Rinse, topical, as sodium:
- ACT®, Fluorigard®: 0.05% [0.02%] (90 mL, 180 mL, 300 mL, 360 mL, 480 mL)

Listermint® with Fluoride: 0.02% [0.01%] (180 mL, 300 mL, 360 mL, 480 mL, 540 mL, 720 mL, 960 mL, 1740 mL)

**Dietary Considerations** Do not administer with milk; do **not** allow eating or drinking for 30 minutes after use

**Generic Available** Yes

**Comments** Neutral pH fluoride preparations are preferred in patients with oral mucositis to reduce tissue irritation; long-term use of acidulated fluorides has been associated with enamel demineralization and damage to porcelain crowns

- **Fluorigard® [OTC]** *see* Fluoride *on page 441*
- **Fluori-Methane®** *see* Dichlorodifluoromethane and Trichloromonofluoromethane *on page 319*
- **Fluorinse®** *see* Fluoride *on page 441*
- **Fluoritab®** *see* Fluoride *on page 441*
- **Fluorodeoxyuridine** *see* Floxuridine *on page 434*

## Fluorometholone (flure oh METH oh lone)

**Related Information**

Corticosteroids, Topical Comparison *on page 1222*

**U.S. Brand Names** Flarex®; Fluor-Op®; FML®; FML® Forte

**Therapeutic Category** Anti-inflammatory Agent, Ophthalmic; Corticosteroid, Ophthalmic

**Use** Inflammatory conditions of the eye, including keratitis, iritis, cyclitis, and conjunctivitis

**Usual Dosage** Children >2 years and Adults: Ophthalmic:

Ointment: May be applied every 4 hours in severe cases; 1-3 times/day in mild to moderate cases

Solution: Instill 1-2 drops into conjunctival sac every hour during day, every 2 hours at night until favorable response is obtained, then use 1 drop every 4 hours; for mild to moderate inflammation, instill 1-2 drops into conjunctival sac 2-4 times/day

**Mechanism of Action** Decreases inflammation by suppression of migration of polymorphonuclear leukocytes and reversal of increased capillary permeability

**Local Anesthetic/Vasoconstrictor Precautions** No information available to require special precautions

**Effects on Dental Treatment** No effects or complications reported

**Other Adverse Effects**

1% to 10%: Ocular: Blurred vision

<1%: Ocular: Stinging, burning, increased intraocular pressure, open-angle glaucoma, defect in visual acuity and field of vision, cataracts

**Drug Interactions** No data reported

**Drug Uptake** Absorption: Into aqueous humor with slight systemic absorption

**Pregnancy Risk Factor** C

**Generic Available** No

- **Fluor-Op®** *see* Fluorometholone *on this page*
- **Fluoroplex® Topical** *see* Fluorouracil *on this page*

## Fluorouracil (flure oh YOOR a sil)

**U.S. Brand Names** Adrucil® Injection; Efudex® Topical; Fluoroplex® Topical

**Therapeutic Category** Antineoplastic Agent, Antimetabolite

**Synonyms** 5-Fluorouracil; 5-FU

**Use** Treatment of carcinoma of stomach, colon, rectum, breast, and pancreas; also used topically for management of multiple actinic keratoses and superficial basal cell carcinomas

**Usual Dosage** **Refer to individual protocols**

**All dosages are based on the patient's actual weight. However, the estimated lean body mass (dry weight) is used if the patient is obese or if there has been a spurious weight gain due to edema, ascites or other forms of abnormal fluid retention.**

Children and Adults:

I.V.: Initial: 400-500 mg/m²/day (12 mg/kg/day; maximum: 800 mg/day) for 4-5 days either as a single daily I.V. push or 4-day continuous intravenous infusion

I.V.: Maintenance dose regimens:

200-250 mg/m² (6 mg/kg) every other day for 4 days repeated in 4 weeks

500-600 mg/m² (15 mg/kg) weekly as a continuous intravenous infusion or I.V. push

I.V.: Concomitant with leucovorin:

370 mg/m²/day for 5 days

500-1000 mg/m² every 2 weeks

600 mg/m²/week for 6 weeks

(Continued)

## Fluorouracil *(Continued)*

Although the manufacturer recommends no daily dose >800 mg, higher doses of up to 2 g/day are routinely administered by continuous intravenous infusion; by continuous intravenous infusion, higher daily doses have been successfully used

Topical:

Actinic or solar keratosis: Apply twice daily for 2-6 weeks

Superficial basal cell carcinomas: Apply 5% twice daily for at least 3-6 weeks and up to 10-12 weeks

**Mechanism of Action** A pyrimidine antimetabolite that interferes with DNA synthesis by blocking the methylation of deoxyuricytic acid; 5-FU rapidly enters the cell and is activated to the nucleotide level; there it inhibits thymidylate synthetase (TS), or is incorporated into RNA (most evident during the GI phase of the cell cycle). The reduced folate cofactor is required for tight binding to occur between the 5-FdUMP and TS.

**Local Anesthetic/Vasoconstrictor Precautions** No information available to require special precautions

**Effects on Dental Treatment** No effects or complications reported

**Other Adverse Effects** Toxicity depends on route and duration of infusion

Irritant chemotherapy

>10%:

Dermatologic: Dermatitis, alopecia

Gastrointestinal (route and schedule dependent): Heartburn, stomatitis, nausea, vomiting, esophagitis, anorexia, and diarrhea; bolus dosing produces milder GI problems, while continuous infusion tends to produce severe mucositis and diarrhea; emesis is moderate, occurring in 30% to 60% of patients, and responds well to phenothiazines and dexamethasone

Emetic potential: <1000 mg: Moderately low (10% to 30%); ≥1000 mg: Moderate (30% to 60%)

1% to 10%:

Dermatologic: Dry skin

Gastrointestinal: GI ulceration

Hematologic: Myelosuppressive: Granulocytopenia occurs around 9-14 days after 5-FU and thrombocytopenia around 7-17 days. The marrow recovers after 22 days. Myelosuppression tends to be more pronounced in patients receiving bolus dosing of 5-FU. WBC: Mild to moderate; Platelets: Mild; Onset (days): 7-10; Nadir (days): 14; Recovery (days): 21

<1%:

Cardiovascular: Chest pain, EKG changes similar to ischemic changes, and possibly cardiac enzyme abnormalities. Usually occurs within the first 2 days of therapy, and may resolve with nitroglycerin and calcium channel blockers. May be due to coronary vessel vasospasm induced by 5-FU.

Central nervous system: Headache, cerebellar ataxia, tingling of hands, somnolence, and ataxia are seen primarily in intracarotid arterial infusions for head and neck tumors; this is believed to be caused by fluorocitrate, a neurotoxic metabolite of the parent compound

Dermatologic: Hyperpigmentation of nailbeds, face, hands, and veins used in infusion; photosensitization with UV light; palmar-plantar syndrome; hand-foot syndrome, pruritic maculopapular rash

Hematologic: Coagulopathy

Hepatic: Hepatotoxicity

Neuromuscular & skeletal: Paresthesia

Ocular: Conjunctivitis, tear duct stenosis, excessive lacrimation, visual disturbances

Respiratory: Dyspnea

**Drug Uptake**

Absorption: Oral: Erratic and rarely used

Serum half-life (biphasic): Initial: 6-20 minutes; doses of 400-600 mg/m$^2$ produce drug concentrations above the threshold for cytotoxicity for normal tissue and remain there for 6 hours; 2 metabolites, FdUMP and FUTP, have prolonged half-lives depending on the type of tissue; the clinical effect of these metabolites has not been determined

**Pregnancy Risk Factor** D (injection); X (topical)

**Generic Available** Yes: Injection

**Comments** Myelosuppressive effects:

WBC: Mild

Platelets: Mild

Onset (days): 7-10

Nadir (days): 9-14

Recovery (days): 21

♦ **5-Fluorouracil** *see* Fluorouracil *on previous page*

## Fluoxetine (floo OKS e teen)

**Related Information**

Vasoconstrictor Interactions With Antidepressants *on page 1277*

**U.S. Brand Names** Prozac®

**Therapeutic Category** Antidepressant, Selective Serotonin Reuptake Inhibitor

**Use** Treatment of major depression

**Usual Dosage** Oral:

Children <18 years: Dose and safety not established; preliminary experience in children 6-14 years using initial doses of 20 mg/day have been reported

Adults: 20 mg/day in the morning; may increase after several weeks by 20 mg/day increments; maximum: 80 mg/day; doses >20 mg should be divided into morning and noon doses

Usual dosage range:

20-80 mg/day for depression and OCD

20-60 mg/day for obesity

60-80 mg/day for bulimia nervosa

**Note:** Lower doses of 5 mg/day have been used for initial treatment

Elderly: Some patients may require an initial dose of 10 mg/day with dosage increases of 10 and 20 mg every several weeks as tolerated; should not be taken at night unless patient experiences sedation

**Mechanism of Action** Inhibits CNS neuron serotonin uptake; minimal or no effect on reuptake of norepinephrine or dopamine; does not significantly bind to alpha-adrenergic, histamine or cholinergic receptors; may therefore be useful in patients at risk from sedation, hypotension, and anticholinergic effects of tricyclic antidepressants

**Local Anesthetic/Vasoconstrictor Precautions** Although caution should be used in patients taking tricyclic antidepressants, no interactions have been reported with vasoconstrictors and fluoxetine, a nontricyclic antidepressant which acts to increase serotonin

**Effects on Dental Treatment** >10% of patients experience dry mouth

**Other Adverse Effects** Predominant adverse effects are CNS and GI

>10%:

Central nervous system: Headache, nervousness, insomnia, drowsiness

Gastrointestinal: Nausea, diarrhea

1% to 10%:

Central nervous system: Anxiety, dizziness, fatigue, sedation

Dermatologic: Rash, pruritus

Endocrine & metabolic: SIADH, hypoglycemia, hyponatremia (elderly or volume-depleted patients)

Gastrointestinal: Anorexia, dyspepsia, constipation

Neuromuscular & skeletal: Tremor

Miscellaneous: Excessive sweating

<1%:

Central nervous system: Extrapyramidal reactions (rare), suicidal ideation

Ocular: Visual disturbances

Miscellaneous: Anaphylactoid reactions, allergies

**Drug Interactions**

Increased/decreased effect of lithium (both increases and decreases level has been reported)

Increased toxicity of diazepam, trazodone via decreased clearance; increased toxicity with MAO inhibitors (hyperpyrexia, tremors, seizures, delirium, coma)

Displace protein bound drugs

**Drug Uptake**

Peak antidepressant effect: After >4 weeks

Absorption: Oral: Well absorbed

Serum half-life: Adults: 2-3 days; due to long half-life, resolution of adverse reactions after discontinuation may be slow

Time to peak serum concentration: Within 4-8 hours

**Pregnancy Risk Factor** B

**Generic Available** No

**Selected Readings**

Wynn RL, "New Antidepressant Medications," *Gen Dent*, 1997, 45(1):24-8.

## Fluoxymesterone (floo oks i MES te rone)

**U.S. Brand Names** Halotestin®

**Therapeutic Category** Androgen

**Use** Replacement of endogenous testicular hormone; in female used as palliative treatment of breast cancer, postpartum breast engorgement

**Usual Dosage** Adults: Oral:

Male:

Hypogonadism: 5-20 mg/day

(Continued)

## Fluoxymesterone *(Continued)*

Delayed puberty: 2.5-20 mg/day for 4-6 months

Female:

Inoperable breast carcinoma: 10-40 mg/day in divided doses for 1-3 months

Breast engorgement: 2.5 mg after delivery, 5-10 mg/day in divided doses for 4-5 days

**Mechanism of Action** Synthetic androgenic anabolic hormone responsible for the normal growth and development of male sex organs and maintenance of secondary sex characteristics; stimulates RNA polymerase activity resulting in an increase in protein production; increases bone development

**Local Anesthetic/Vasoconstrictor Precautions** No information available to require special precautions

**Effects on Dental Treatment** No effects or complications reported

**Other Adverse Effects**

>10%:

Males: Priapism

Females: Menstrual problems (amenorrhea), virilism, breast soreness

Cardiovascular: Edema

Dermatologic: Acne

1% to 10%:

Males: Prostatic carcinoma, hirsutism (increase in pubic hair growth), impotence, testicular atrophy

Gastrointestinal: GI irritation, nausea, vomiting, prostatic hypertrophy

Hepatic: Hepatic dysfunction

<1%:

Males: Gynecomastia

Females: Amenorrhea

Endocrine & metabolic: Hypercalcemia

Hematologic: Leukopenia, polycythemia

Hepatic: Hepatic necrosis, cholestatic hepatitis

Miscellaneous: Hypersensitivity reactions

**Drug Interactions**

Decreased blood glucose concentrations and insulin requirements in patients with diabetes

Increased effect of oral anticoagulants

**Drug Uptake**

Absorption: Oral: Rapid

Serum half-life: 10-100 minutes

**Pregnancy Risk Factor** X

**Generic Available** Yes

- **Fluoxymesterone and Estradiol** *see* Ethinyl Estradiol and Fluoxymesterone *on page 402*

## Fluphenazine (floo FEN a zeen)

**U.S. Brand Names** Permitil®; Prolixin®; Prolixin Decanoate®; Prolixin Enanthate®

**Canadian Brand Names** Apo®-Fluphenazine; Modecate®; Modecate® Enanthate; Moditen® Hydrochloride; PMS-Fluphenazine

**Therapeutic Category** Antipsychotic Agent; Phenothiazine Derivative

**Use** Management of manifestations of psychotic disorders

**Usual Dosage** Adults:

Oral: 0.5-10 mg/day in divided doses at 6- to 8-hour intervals; some patients may require up to 40 mg/day

I.M.: 2.5-10 mg/day in divided doses at 6- to 8-hour intervals (parenteral dose is $^1/_3$ to $^1/_2$ the oral dose for the hydrochloride salts)

I.M., S.C. (decanoate): 12.5 mg every 3 weeks

Conversion from hydrochloride to decanoate I.M. 0.5 mL (12.5 mg) decanoate every 3 weeks is approximately equivalent to 10 mg hydrochloride/day

I.M., S.C. (enanthate): 12.5-25 mg every 3 weeks

**Mechanism of Action** Blocks postsynaptic mesolimbic dopaminergic $D_1$ and $D_2$ receptors in the brain; exhibits a strong alpha-adrenergic blocking and anticholinergic effect, depresses the release of hypothalamic and hypophyseal hormones; believed to depress the reticular activating system thus affecting basal metabolism, body temperature, wakefulness, vasomotor tone, and emesis

**Local Anesthetic/Vasoconstrictor Precautions** Most pharmacology textbooks state that in presence of phenothiazines, systemic doses of epinephrine paradoxically decrease the blood pressure. This is the so called "epinephrine reversal" phenomenon. This has never been observed when epinephrine is given by infiltration as part of the anesthesia procedure.

**Effects on Dental Treatment** Orthostatic hypotension and nasal congestion possible in dental patients. Since the drug is a dopamine antagonist, extrapyramidal symptoms of the TMJ a possibility.

**Other Adverse Effects**

>10%:

Cardiovascular: Orthostatic hypotension, hypotension, tachycardia, arrhythmias

Central nervous system: Parkinsonian symptoms, akathisia, dystonias, tardive dyskinesia (persistent), dizziness

Gastrointestinal: Constipation

Ocular: Pigmentary retinopathy

Respiratory: Nasal congestion

Miscellaneous: Decreased sweating

1% to 10%:

Dermatologic: Photosensitivity, skin rash

Endocrine & metabolic: Changes in menstrual cycle pain in breasts, amenorrhea, galactorrhea, gynecomastia, changes in libido

Gastrointestinal: Weight gain, nausea, vomiting, stomach pain

Genitourinary: Dysuria, ejaculatory disturbances

Neuromuscular & skeletal: Trembling of fingers

<1%:

Central nervous system: Sedation, drowsiness, restlessness, anxiety, extrapyramidal reactions, pseudoparkinsonian signs and symptoms, seizures, altered central temperature regulation

Dermatologic: Hyperpigmentation, pruritus, discoloration of skin (blue-gray)

Endocrine & metabolic: Galactorrhea

Gastrointestinal: Dry mouth

Genitourinary: Priapism, urinary retention

Hematologic: Agranulocytosis (more often in women between 4th and 10th weeks of therapy); leukopenia (usually in patients with large doses for prolonged periods)

Hepatic: Cholestatic jaundice, hepatotoxicity

Ocular: Retinal pigmentation, cornea and lens changes, blurred vision

**Drug Interactions**

Decreased effect: Barbiturate levels and decreased fluphenazine effectiveness when given together

Increased toxicity: With ethanol, effects of both drugs may be increased; EPSEs and other CNS effects may be increased when coadministered with lithium; may potentiate the effects of narcotics including respiratory depression

**Drug Uptake**

Following I.M. or S.C. administration (derivative dependent):

Decanoate (lasts the longest and requires more time for onset):

Onset of action: 24-72 hours

Hydrochloride salt (acts quickly and persists briefly):

Onset of action: Within 1 hour

Duration: 6-8 hours

Serum half-life: Derivative dependent:

Enanthate: 84-96 hours

Hydrochloride: 33 hours

Decanoate: 163-232 hours

**Pregnancy Risk Factor** C

**Generic Available** Yes

♦ **Flura-Drops®** *see* Fluoride *on page 441*

♦ **Flura-Loz®** *see* Fluoride *on page 441*

## Flurandrenolide (flure an DREN oh lide)

**Related Information**

Corticosteroids, Topical Comparison *on page 1222*

**U.S. Brand Names** Cordran®; Cordran® SP

**Canadian Brand Names** Drenison®

**Therapeutic Category** Corticosteroid, Topical (Medium Potency)

**Use** Inflammation of corticosteroid-responsive dermatoses [medium potency topical corticosteroid]

**Usual Dosage** Topical:

Children:

Ointment, cream: Apply sparingly 1-2 times/day

Tape: Apply once daily

Adults: Cream, lotion, ointment: Apply sparingly 2-3 times/day

**Mechanism of Action** Decreases inflammation by suppression of migration of polymorphonuclear leukocytes and reversal of increased capillary permeability

**Local Anesthetic/Vasoconstrictor Precautions** No information available to require special precautions

**Effects on Dental Treatment** No effects or complications reported

(Continued)

## Flurandrenolide *(Continued)*

**Other Adverse Effects** <1%:

Systemic: HPA suppression, Cushing's syndrome, growth retardation, burning, secondary infection

Topical: Burning, itching, irritation, dryness, folliculitis, hypertrichosis, acneiform eruptions, hypopigmentation, perioral dermatitis, allergic contact dermatitis, skin atrophy, striae, miliaria, intracranial hypertension, acne, maceration of the skin

**Drug Interactions** No data reported

**Drug Uptake** Absorption: Adequate with intact skin

**Pregnancy Risk Factor** C

**Generic Available** Yes: Lotion

## Flurazepam (flure AZ e pam)

**U.S. Brand Names** Dalmane®

**Canadian Brand Names** Apo®-Flurazepam; Novo-Flupam; PMS-Flupam; Somnol®; Som Pam®

**Therapeutic Category** Benzodiazepine; Hypnotic; Sedative

**Use** Short-term treatment of insomnia

**Usual Dosage** Oral:

Children:

<15 years: Dose not established

>15 years: 15 mg at bedtime

Adults: 15-30 mg at bedtime

**Mechanism of Action** Depresses all levels of the CNS, including the limbic and reticular formation, probably through the increased action of gamma-aminobutyric acid (GABA), which is a major inhibitory neurotransmitter in the brain

**Local Anesthetic/Vasoconstrictor Precautions** No information available to require special precautions

**Effects on Dental Treatment** >10% of patients experience dry mouth

**Other Adverse Effects**

>10%:

Cardiovascular: Tachycardia, chest pain

Central nervous system: Drowsiness, fatigue, lightheadedness, memory impairment, insomnia, anxiety, depression, headache, impaired coordination

Dermatologic: Rash

Endocrine & metabolic: Decreased libido

Gastrointestinal: Constipation, decreased salivation, nausea, vomiting, diarrhea, increased or decreased appetite

Neuromuscular & skeletal: Dysarthria

Ocular: Blurred vision

Miscellaneous: Sweating

1% to 10%:

Cardiovascular: Syncope, hypotension

Central nervous system: Confusion, nervousness, dizziness, akathisia

Dermatologic: Dermatitis

Gastrointestinal: Weight gain or loss, increased salivation

Neuromuscular & skeletal: Rigidity, tremor, muscle cramps

Otic: Tinnitus

Respiratory: Hyperventilation, nasal congestion

<1%:

Endocrine & metabolic: Menstrual irregularities

Hematologic: Blood dyscrasias

Neuromuscular & skeletal: Reflex slowing

Miscellaneous: Drug dependence

**Drug Interactions**

Decreased effect with enzyme inducers

Increased toxicity with other CNS depressants and cimetidine

**Drug Uptake**

Onset of hypnotic effect: 15-20 minutes

Peak: 3-6 hours

Duration of action: 7-8 hours

Serum half-life: Adults: 40-114 hours

**Pregnancy Risk Factor** X

**Generic Available** Yes

## Flurbiprofen (flure BI proe fen)

**Related Information**

Dental Drug Interactions: Update on Drug Combinations Requiring Special Considerations *on page 1225*

Rheumatoid Arthritis and Osteoarthritis *on page 1092*

Temporomandibular Dysfunction (TMD) *on page 1149*

**U.S. Brand Names** Ansaid®

**Canadian Brand Names** Apo®-Flurbiprofen; Froben®; Froben-SR®; Novo-Flurprofen; Nu-Flurprofen

**Therapeutic Category** Analgesic, Non-narcotic; Nonsteroidal Anti-inflammatory Drug (NSAID), Oral

**Use**

Dental: Management of postoperative pain

Medical: Acute or long-term treatment of signs and symptoms of rheumatoid arthritis and osteoarthritis; ophthalmic preparation indicated for inhibition of intraoperative miosis

**Usual Dosage** Adults: Oral: 200-300 mg/day in 2, 3, or 4 divided doses

**Mechanism of Action** Inhibits prostaglandin synthesis by decreasing the activity of the enzyme, cyclo-oxygenase, which results in decreased formation of prostaglandin precursors

**Local Anesthetic/Vasoconstrictor Precautions** No information available to require special precautions

**Effects on Dental Treatment** <1% of patients experience dry mouth; NSAID formulations are known to reversibly decrease platelet aggregation via mechanisms different than observed with aspirin. The dentist should be aware of the potential of abnormal coagulation. Caution should also be exercised in the use of NSAIDs in patients already on anticoagulant therapy with drugs such as warfarin (Coumadin®).

**Other Adverse Effects** >10%:

Central nervous system: Dizziness

Dermatologic: Rash

Gastrointestinal: Abdominal cramps, heartburn, indigestion, nausea

**Contraindications** Hypersensitivity to flurbiprofen or any component

**Warnings/Precautions** Should be used with caution in patients affected by inhibition of platelet aggregation

**Drug Interactions** Has caused bleeding in combination with anticoagulants; when given concurrently with aspirin, has resulted in 50% lower serum levels of flurbiprofen

**Drug Uptake**

Onset of effect: Within 1 hour

Duration of effect: 6-8 hours

Absorption: Rapid and nearly complete

Serum half-life: 6.5 hours

Time to peak serum concentration: 1.5 hours

**Pregnancy Risk Factor** C

**Breast-feeding Considerations** No data reported

**Dosage Forms** Tablet (Ansaid®): 50 mg, 100 mg

**Dietary Considerations** Can be taken with food, milk, or antacid to decrease GI effects; food alters rate of absorption but not amount

**Generic Available** Yes

**Comments** Flurbiprofen is a chiral NSAID with the S-(+) enantiomer possessing most of the beneficial anti-inflammatory activity; both the S-(+) and R-(-) enantiomers possess analgesic activity. All flurbiprofen preparations are marketed as the racemic mixture (equal parts of each enantiomer). Flurbiprofen may be effective in the treatment of periodontal disease. Animal studies have shown flurbiprofen in topical form to be effective in reducing loss of attachment and bone loss. Flurbiprofen as with other NSAIDs can be administered preoperatively in the patient undergoing dental surgery in order to delay the onset and severity of postoperative pain. Doses which have been used are 100 mg twice daily the day before procedure, and 50-100 mg 30 minutes before the procedure.

**Selected Readings**

Bragger U, Muhle T, Fourmousis I, et al, "Effect of the NSAID Flurbiprofen on Remodelling After Periodontal Surgery," *J Periodontal Res*, 1997, 32(7):575-82.

Cooper SA and Kupperman A, "The Analgesic Efficacy of Flurbiprofen Compared to Acetaminophen With Codeine," *J Clin Dent*, 1991, 2(3):70-4.

Cooper SA, Mardirossian G, and Miles M, "Analgesic Relative Potency Assay Comparing Flurbiprofen 50, 100, and 150 mg, Aspirin 600 mg, and Placebo in Postsurgical Dental Pain," *Clin J Pain*, 1988, 4:175-81.

Dionne RA, "Suppression of Dental Pain by the Preoperative Administration of Flurbiprofen," *Am J Med*, 1986, 80(3A):41-9.

Dionne RA, Snyder J, and Hargreaves KM, "Analgesic Efficacy of Flurbiprofen in Comparison With Acetaminophen, Acetaminophen Plus Codeine, and Placebo After Impacted Third Molar Removal," *J Oral Maxillofac Surg*, 1994, 52(9):919-24.

Forbes JA, Yorio CC, Selinger LR, et al, "An Evaluation of Flurbiprofen, Aspirin, and Placebo in Postoperative Oral Surgery Pain," *Pharmacotherapy*, 1989, 9(2):66-73.

Gallardo F and Rossi E, "Analgesic Efficacy of Flurbiprofen as Compared to Acetaminophen and Placebo After Periodontal Surgery," *J Periodontol*, 1990, 61(4):224-7.

Jeffcoat MK, Reddy MS, Haigh S, et al, "A Comparison of Topical Ketorolac, Systemic Flurbiprofen, and Placebo for the Inhibition of Bone Loss in Adult Periodontitis," *J Periodontol*, 1995, 66(5):329-38.

(Continued)

## Flurbiprofen *(Continued)*

Jeffcoat MK, Reddy MS, Wang IC, et al, "The Effect of Systemic Flurbiprofen on Bone Supporting Dental Implants," *J Am Dent Assoc*, 1995, 126(3):305-11.

Malmberg AB and Yaksh TL, "Antinociception Produced by Spinal Delivery of the S and R Enantiomers of Flurbiprofen in the Formalin Test," *Eur J Pharmacol*, 1994, 256(2):205-9.

- **5-Flurocytosine** *see* Flucytosine *on page 436*
- **Fluro-Ethyl® Aerosol** *see* Ethyl Chloride and Dichlorotetrafluoroethane *on page 410*
- **Flurosyn®** *see* Fluocinolone *on page 440*

## Flutamide (FLOO ta mide)

**U.S. Brand Names** Eulexin®

**Canadian Brand Names** Novo-Flutamide

**Therapeutic Category** Antiandrogen

**Use** In combination with LHRH agonistic analogs for the treatment of metastatic prostatic carcinoma

**Usual Dosage** Adults: Oral: 2 capsules every 8 hours for a total daily dose of 750 mg

**Mechanism of Action** Nonsteroidal antiandrogen that inhibits androgen uptake or inhibits binding of androgen in target tissues

**Local Anesthetic/Vasoconstrictor Precautions** No information available to require special precautions

**Effects on Dental Treatment** No effects or complications reported

**Other Adverse Effects**

>10%:

Gastrointestinal: Nausea, vomiting, diarrhea

Genitourinary: Impotence

Endocrine & metabolic: Loss of libido, hot flashes

1% to 10%:

Endocrine & metabolic: Gynecomastia

Gastrointestinal: Anorexia

Neuromuscular & skeletal: Numbness in extremities

<1%:

Cardiovascular: Hypertension, edema

Central nervous system: Drowsiness, nervousness, confusion

Hepatic: Hepatitis

**Drug Uptake**

Absorption: Rapid and complete

Serum half-life: 5-6 hours

**Pregnancy Risk Factor** D

**Generic Available** No

**Comments** To achieve benefit to combination therapy, both drugs need to be started simultaneously

- **Flutex®** *see* Triamcinolone *on page 1010*

## Fluticasone (floo TIK a sone)

**U.S. Brand Names** Cutivate™; Flonase®; Flovent®

**Therapeutic Category** Corticosteroid, Topical (Medium Potency)

**Use**

Intranasal: Management of seasonal and perennial allergic rhinitis in patients ≥12 years of age; perennial nonallergic rhinitis for ages ≥4 years of age

Topical: Relief of inflammation and pruritus associated with corticosteroid-responsive dermatoses [medium potency topical corticosteroid]

**Usual Dosage**

Adolescents:

Topical: Apply sparingly in a thin film twice daily

Intranasal: Initially 1 spray (50 mcg/spray) per nostril once daily. Patients not adequately responding or patients with more severe symptoms may use 2 sprays (200 mcg) per nostril. Depending on response, dosage may be reduced to 100 mcg daily. Total daily dosage should not exceed 4 sprays (200 mcg)/day.

Adults:

Topical: Apply sparingly in a thin film twice daily

Intranasal: Initially 2 sprays (50 mcg/spray) per nostril once daily. After the first few days, dosage may be reduced to 1 spray per nostril once daily for maintenance therapy. Maximum total daily dose should not exceed 4 sprays (200 mcg)/day.

**Mechanism of Action** Fluticasone belongs to a new group of corticosteroids which utilizes a fluorocarbothioate ester linkage at the 17 carbon position; extremely potent vasoconstrictive and anti-inflammatory activity; has a weak hypothalamic -pituitary- adrenocortical axis (HPA) inhibitory potency when applied topically, which gives the drug a high therapeutic index. The mechanism of action for all topical corticosteroids is not well defined, however, is believed to be a combination of three important properties: anti-inflammatory activity, immunosuppressive properties, and antiproliferative actions.

**Local Anesthetic/Vasoconstrictor Precautions** No information available to require special precautions

**Effects on Dental Treatment** No effects or complications reported

**Other Adverse Effects** <1%:

Dermatologic: Acne, hypopigmentation, allergic dermatitis, maceration of the skin, skin atrophy, folliculitis, hypertrichosis

Endocrine & metabolic: HPA suppression, Cushing's syndrome, growth retardation

Local: Burning, itching, irritation, dryness

Miscellaneous: Secondary infection

**Drug Interactions** No data reported

**Pregnancy Risk Factor** C

**Dosage Forms**

Spray, aerosol, oral inhalation (Flovent®): 44 mcg/actuation (7.9 g = 60 actuations or 13 g = 120 actuations), 110 mcg/actuation (13 g = 120 actuations); 220 mcg/actuation (13 g = 120 actuations)

Spray, intranasal (Flonase®): 50 mcg/actuation (9 g = 60 actuations, 16 g = 120 actuations)

Topical (Cutivate™):

Cream: 0.05% (15 g, 30 g, 60 g)

Ointment: 0.005% (15 g, 60 g )

**Generic Available** No

## Fluvastatin (FLOO va sta tin)

**Related Information**

Cardiovascular Diseases *on page 1066*

**U.S. Brand Names** Lescol®

**Therapeutic Category** HMG-CoA Reductase Inhibitor; Lipid Lowering Drugs

**Use** Adjunct to dietary therapy to decrease elevated serum total and LDL cholesterol concentrations in primary hypercholesterolemia

**Usual Dosage** Adults: Oral:

Initial dose: 20 mg at bedtime

Usual dose: 20-40 mg at bedtime

**Note:** Splitting the 40 mg dose into a twice/daily regimen may provide a modest improvement in LDL response; maximum response occurs within 4-6 weeks; decrease dose and monitor effects carefully in patients with hepatic insufficiency

**Mechanism of Action** Acts by competitively inhibiting 3-hydroxyl-3-methylglutaryl-coenzyme A (HMG-CoA) reductase, the enzyme that catalyzes the reduction of HMG-CoA to mevalonate; this is an early rate-limiting step in cholesterol biosynthesis. HDL is increased while total, LDL and VLDL cholesterols, apolipoprotein B, and plasma triglycerides are decreased

**Local Anesthetic/Vasoconstrictor Precautions** No information available to require special precautions

**Effects on Dental Treatment** No effects or complications reported

**Other Adverse Effects** 1% to 1%:

Central nervous system: Headache, dizziness, insomnia

Dermatologic: Rash

Gastrointestinal: Dyspepsia, diarrhea, nausea, vomiting, constipation, flatulence

Neuromuscular & skeletal: Back pain, abdominal pain, myalgia, arthropathy

Miscellaneous: Cold symptoms

**Drug Interactions**

Anticoagulant effect of warfarin may be increased

Concurrent use of erythromycin and HMG-CoA reductase inhibitors may result in rhabdomyolysis

**Drug Uptake** Serum half-life: 1.2 hours

**Pregnancy Risk Factor** X

**Generic Available** No

## Fluvoxamine (floo VOKS ah meen)

**U.S. Brand Names** Luvox®

**Canadian Brand Names** Apo®-Fluvoxamine

**Therapeutic Category** Antidepressant, Selective Serotonin Reuptake Inhibitor

**Use** Treatment of obsessive-compulsive disorder (OCD); effective in the treatment of major depression; may be useful for the treatment of panic disorder

(Continued)

## Fluvoxamine *(Continued)*

**Usual Dosage**

Adults: Initial: 50 mg at bedtime; adjust in 50 mg increments at 4- to 7-day intervals; usual dose range: 100-300 mg/day; divide total daily dose into 2 doses; give larger portion at bedtime

Elderly or hepatic impairment: Reduce dose, titrate slowly

**Mechanism of Action** Inhibits CNS neuron serotonin uptake; minimal or no effect on reuptake of norepinephrine or dopamine; does not significantly bind to alpha-adrenergic, histamine or cholinergic receptors

**Local Anesthetic/Vasoconstrictor Precautions** Although caution should be used in patients taking tricyclic antidepressants, no interactions have been reported with vasoconstrictors and fluvoxamine, a nontricyclic antidepressant which acts to increase serotonin

**Effects on Dental Treatment** No effects or complications reported

**Other Adverse Effects**

>10%: Gastrointestinal: Nausea

1% to 10%:

- Cardiovascular: Palpitations
- Central nervous system: Somnolence, headache, insomnia, dizziness, nervousness, mania, hypomania, vertigo, abnormal thinking, agitation, anxiety, malaise, amnesia
- Endocrine & metabolic: Decreased libido
- Gastrointestinal: Dry mouth, abdominal pain, vomiting, dyspepsia, constipation, diarrhea, dysgeusia, anorexia
- Neuromuscular & skeletal: Tremors, weakness
- Miscellaneous: Sweating

<1%:

- Central nervous system: Seizures, extrapyramidal reactions
- Dermatologic: Toxic epidermal necrolysis
- Hematologic: Thrombocytopenia
- Hepatic: Hepatic dysfunction
- Renal: Elevated serum creatinine

**Drug Interactions** Because fluvoxamine inhibits cytochrome P-450 isozymes IA2, IIC9, IIIA4, and possibly IID6, it is associated with numerous significant drug interactions

Increased toxicity: Terfenadine and astemizole are both metabolized by the cytochrome P-450 IIIA4 isozyme, increased levels of these drugs have been associated with prolongation of the Q-T interval and potentially fatal, torsade de pointes ventricular arrhythmias. Since fluvoxamine inhibits the enzyme responsible for their clearance, the concomitant use of these agents is contraindicated.

Potentiates triazolam and alprazolam (dose should be reduced by at least 50%), hypertensive crisis with MAO inhibitors, theophylline (doses should be reduced by 1/3 and plasma levels monitored), warfarin (reduce its dose and monitor PT/INR), carbamazepine (monitor levels), tricyclic antidepressants (monitor effects and reduce doses accordingly), methadone, beta-blockers (reduce dose of propranolol or metoprolol), diltiazem. Caution with other benzodiazepines, phenytoin, lithium, clozapine, alcohol, other CNS drugs, quinidine, ketoconazole.

**Drug Uptake**

Half-life: ~15 hours

Time to peak plasma concentration: 3-8 hours

**Pregnancy Risk Factor** C

**Generic Available** No

**Selected Readings**

Wynn RL, "New Antidepressant Medications," *Gen Dent*, 1997, 45(1):24-8.

♦ **Fluzone®** *see* Influenza Virus Vaccine *on page 536*
♦ **FML®** *see* Fluorometholone *on page 443*
♦ **FML® Forte** *see* Fluorometholone *on page 443*
♦ **FML-S® Ophthalmic Suspension** *see* Sulfacetamide Sodium and Fluorometholone *on page 939*
♦ **Foille® [OTC]** *see* Benzocaine *on page 128*
♦ **Foille® Medicated First Aid [OTC]** *see* Benzocaine *on page 128*
♦ **Folex® PFS** *see* Methotrexate *on page 651*

## Folic Acid (FOE lik AS id)

**U.S. Brand Names** Folvite®

**Canadian Brand Names** Apo®-Folic; Flodine®; Novo-Folacid

**Therapeutic Category** Vitamin, Water Soluble

**Use**

Dental: Treatment of megaloblastic and macrocytic anemias due to folate deficiency

Medical: Dietary supplement to prevent neural tube defects

**Usual Dosage** Oral, I.M., I.V., S.C.:

Children: Initial: 1 mg/day
- Deficiency: 0.5-1 mg/day
- Maintenance dose:
  - <4 years: Up to 0.3 mg/day
  - >4 years: 0.4 mg/day

Adults: Initial: 1 mg/day
- Deficiency: 1-3 mg/day
- Maintenance dose: 0.5 mg/day
- Women of childbearing age, pregnant, and lactating women: 0.8 mg/day

**Mechanism of Action** Folic acid is necessary for formation of a number of coenzymes in many metabolic systems, particularly for purine and pyrimidine synthesis; required for nucleoprotein synthesis and maintenance in erythropoiesis; stimulates WBC and platelet production in folate deficiency anemia

**Local Anesthetic/Vasoconstrictor Precautions** No information available to require special precautions

**Effects on Dental Treatment** No effects or complications reported

**Other Adverse Effects** <1%:

Cardiovascular: Slight flushing

Central nervous system: General malaise

Dermatologic: Pruritus, rash

Respiratory: Bronchospasm

Miscellaneous: Allergic reaction

**Contraindications** Pernicious, aplastic, or normocytic anemias

**Warnings/Precautions** Doses >0.1 mg/day may obscure pernicious anemia with continuing irreversible nerve damage progression. Resistance to treatment may occur with depressed hematopoiesis, alcoholism, deficiencies of other vitamins. Injection contains benzyl alcohol (1.5%) as preservative (use care in administration to neonates).

**Drug Interactions** Decreased effect: In folate-deficient patients, folic acid therapy may increase phenytoin metabolism. Phenytoin, primidone, para-aminosalicylic acid, and sulfasalazine may decrease serum folate concentrations and cause deficiency. Oral contraceptives may also impair folate metabolism producing depletion, but the effect is unlikely to cause anemia or megaloblastic changes. Concurrent administration of chloramphenicol and folic acid may result in antagonism of the hematopoietic response to folic acid.

**Drug Uptake**

Peak effect: Oral: Within 0.5-1 hour

Absorption: In the proximal part of the small intestine

**Pregnancy Risk Factor** A (C if dose exceeds RDA recommendation)

**Breast-feeding Considerations** May be taken while breast-feeding

**Dosage Forms**

Injection, as sodium folate: 5 mg/mL (10 mL); 10 mg/mL (10 mL)
- Folvite®: 5 mg/mL (10 mL)

Tablet: 0.1 mg, 0.4 mg, 0.8 mg, 1 mg
- Folvite®: 1 mg

**Generic Available** Yes

♦ **Folinic Acid** *see* Leucovorin *on page 577*

## Follitropin Alpha (foe li TRO pin AL fa)

**U.S. Brand Names** Gonal-F®

**Therapeutic Category** Ovulation Stimulator

**Use** Induction of ovulation in the anovulatory infertile patient in whom the cause of infertility is functional and not caused by primary ovarian failure

**Usual Dosage** Adults (women): S.C.: Initially 75 units/day for the first cycle; an incremental dose adjustment of up to 37.5 units may be considered after 14 days; treatment duration should not exceed 35 days unless an E2 rise indicates follicular development

**Local Anesthetic/Vasoconstrictor Precautions** No information available to require special precautions

**Effects on Dental Treatment** No effects or complications reported

**Dosage Forms** Injection: 75 FSH units, 150 FSH units

♦ **Folvite®** *see* Folic Acid *on previous page*

## Fomepizole (foe ME pi zole)

**U.S. Brand Names** Antizol®

**Therapeutic Category** Antidote

(Continued)

## Fomepizole *(Continued)*

**Synonyms** 4-Methylpyrazole; 4-MP

**Use** Ethylene glycol and methanol toxicity; may be useful in propylene glycol; unclear whether it is useful in disulfiram-ethanol reactions

**Usual Dosage** Oral: 15 mg/kg followed by 5 mg/kg in 12 hours and then 10 mg/kg every 12 hours until levels of toxin are not present

One other protocol (from France) suggests an infusion of 10-20 mg/kg before dialysis and intravenous infusion of 1-1.5 mg/kg/hour during hemodialysis

META (methylpyrazole for toxic alcohol) study in U.S. (investigational): Loading I.V. dose of 15 mg/kg followed by 10 mg/kg I.V. every 12 hours for 48 hours; continue treatment until methanol or ethylene glycol levels are <20 mg/dL; supplemental doses required during dialysis; contact your local poison center regarding this study

**Mechanism of Action** Complexes and inactivates alcohol dehydrogenase thus preventing formation of the toxic metabolites of the alcohols

**Local Anesthetic/Vasoconstrictor Precautions** No information available to require special precautions

**Effects on Dental Treatment** No effects or complications reported

**Drug Interactions** Inhibitory effects on alcohol dehydrogenase are increased in presence of ethanol; ethanol also decreases metabolism of 4-MP; 4-MPO induces cytochrome P-450 mixed function oxidases *in vitro*; 4-MP may worsen the ethanol-chlorohydrate central nervous system interaction

**Drug Uptake**

Maximum effect: 1.5-2 hours

Absorption: Oral: Readily absorbed

Distribution: $V_d$: 0.6-0.7 L/kg; unknown distribution, probably very similar to ethanol

Protein binding: Negligible

Elimination: Nonlinear elimination; at suggested therapeutic doses of 10-20 mg/kg the apparent elimination rate is 4-5 µmol/L/hour; 4-MP is dialyzable

**Selected Readings**


Borron SW and Baud FJ, "Intravenous 4-Methylpyrazole as an Antidote for Diethylene Glycol and Triethylene Glycol Poisoning: A Case Report," *Vet Hum Toxicol*, 1997, 37(1): 26-8.

Brent J, McMartin K, Phillips S, et al, "4-Methylpyrazole (Fomepizole) Therapy of Ethylene G. Poisoning: Preliminary Results of the Meta Trial," *J Toxicol Clin Toxicol*, 1997, 35(5):507.

Brent J, McMartin K, Phillips SP, et al, "4-Methylpyrazole (Fomepizole) Therapy of Methanol Poisoning: Preliminary Results of the Meta Trial," *J Toxicol Clin Toxicol*, 1997, 35(5):507.

Hung O, Kaplan J, Hoffman R, et al, "Improved Understanding of the Ethanol-Chloral Hydrate Interaction Using 4-MP," *J Toxicol Clin Toxicol*, 1997, 35(5):507-8.

Jacobsen D and McMartin KE, "Antidotes for Methanol and Ethylene Glycol Poisoning," *J Toxicol Clin Toxicol*, 1997, 35(2):127-43.

Jacobsen D and McMartin K, "4-Methylpyrazole - Present Status," *J Toxicol Clin Toxicol*, 1996, 34(4):379-81.

Jacobsen D, Ostensen J, Bredesen L, et al, "4-Methylpyrazole (4-MP) Is Effectively Removed by Haemodialysis in the Pig Model," *Hum Exp Toxicol*, 1996, 15(6):494-6.

Jacobsen D, Sebastian CS, Barron SK, et al, "Effects of 4-Methylpyrazole, Methanol/Ethylene Glycol Antidote in Healthy Humans," *J Emerg Med*, 1990, 8(4):455-61.

Jobard E, Harry P, Turcant A, et al, "4-Methylpyrazole and Hemodialysis in Ethylene Glycol Poisoning," *J Toxicol Clin Toxicol*, 1996, 34(4):373-7.

McMartin KE and Heath A, "Treatment of Ethylene Glycol Poisoning With Intravenous 4-Methylpyrazole," *N Engl J Med*, 1989, 320(2):125.


## Fomivirsen

**U.S. Brand Names** Vitravene®

**Therapeutic Category** Antiviral Agent, Ophthalmic

**Use** Treatment of cytomegalovirus (CMV) retinitis; CMV can affect one or both eyes in patients with acquired immunodeficiency syndrome (AIDS) who cannot take other treatment(s) for CMV retinitis or who did not respond to other treatments for CMV retinitis; the diagnosis should be made after a comprehensive eye exam, including indirect ophthalmoscopy

**Usual Dosage** Treatment consists of two phases:

Phase I (induction phase): One injection (6.6 mg) every other week for 2 doses

Phase II (maintenance phase): One injection (6.6 mg) once every 4 weeks

**Local Anesthetic/Vasoconstrictor Precautions** No information available to require special precautions

**Effects on Dental Treatment** No effects or complications reported

**Other Adverse Effects** Ophthalmic: Abnormal vision; swelling around the eye; blurred vision; cataract bleeding in and around the eye; decreased visual sharpness, clearness; reduced color vision; eye pain; objects in the field of vision (floaters); increased eye pressure; sensitivity to light; retinal detachment; swelling of the retina; bleeding of the retina; color changes of the retina

**Warnings/Precautions** Only works in the eye in which it is injected and does not treat CMV elsewhere in the body. Because CMV may be in other parts of the body and not only in the treated eye, a physician should monitor patient for CMV in the untreated eye or CMV elsewhere in the body (eg, pneumonitis, colitis); not recommended if there has been treatment within the last 2-4 weeks with cidofovir because of the increased risk of eye inflammation

**Dosage Forms** Injection, intravitreal: 6.6 mg

- **Formula Q® [OTC]** *see* Quinine *on page 874*
- **5-Formyl Tetrahydrofolate** *see* Leucovorin *on page 577*
- **Fortaz®** *see* Ceftazidime *on page 207*
- **Fosamax®** *see* Alendronate *on page 46*

## Foscarnet (fos KAR net)

**Related Information**

Systemic Viral Diseases *on page 1115*

**U.S. Brand Names** Foscavir®

**Therapeutic Category** Antiviral Agent, Parenteral

**Use** Approved indications in adult patients:

Herpesvirus infections suspected to be caused by acyclovir (HSV, VZV) or ganciclovir (CMV) resistant strains (this occurs almost exclusively in persons with advanced AIDS who have received prolonged treatment for a herpesvirus infection)

CMV retinitis in persons with AIDS

Other CMV infections in persons unable to tolerate ganciclovir

**Usual Dosage**

Adolescents and Adults: I.V.:

Induction treatment: 60 mg/kg/dose every 8 hours for 14-21 days

Maintenance therapy: 90-120 mg/kg/day as a single infusion

See table.

**Dose Adjustment for Renal Impairment**

The induction dose of foscarnet should be adjusted according to creatinine clearance as follows:

| Creatinine Clearance (mL/min/kg) | Foscarnet Induction Dose (mg/kg q8h) |
|---|---|
| 1.6 | 60 |
| 1.5 | 57 |
| 1.4 | 53 |
| 1.3 | 49 |
| 1.2 | 46 |
| 1.1 | 42 |
| 1 | 39 |
| 0.9 | 35 |
| 0.8 | 32 |
| 0.7 | 28 |
| 0.6 | 25 |
| 0.5 | 21 |
| 0.4 | 18 |

The maintenance dose of foscarnet should be adjusted according to creatinine clearance as follows:

| Creatinine Clearance (mL/min/kg) | Foscarnet Maintenance Dose (mg/kg/day) |
|---|---|
| 1.4 | 90-120 |
| 1.2-1.4 | 78-104 |
| 1-1.2 | 75-100 |
| 0.8-1 | 71-94 |
| 0.6-0.8 | 63-84 |
| 0.4-0.6 | 57-75 |

**Mechanism of Action** Pyrophosphate analogue which acts as a noncompetitive inhibitor of many viral RNA and DNA polymerases as well as HIV reverse transcriptase. Inhibitory effects occur at concentrations which do not affect host cellular DNA polymerases; however, some human cell growth suppression has been observed with high *in vitro* concentrations. Similar to ganciclovir, foscarnet is a virostatic agent. Foscarnet does not require activation by thymidine kinase.

**Local Anesthetic/Vasoconstrictor Precautions** No information available to require special precautions

**Effects on Dental Treatment** No effects or complications reported

(Continued)

## Foscarnet *(Continued)*

**Other Adverse Effects**

>10%:

Central nervous system: Fever, headache, seizures
Gastrointestinal: Nausea, diarrhea, vomiting
Hematologic: Anemia
Renal: Abnormal renal function, decreased creatinine clearance

1% to 10%:

Central nervous system: Fatigue, malaise, dizziness, hypoesthesia, depression, confusion, anxiety
Dermatologic: Rash
Endocrine & metabolic: Electrolyte imbalance
Gastrointestinal: Anorexia
Hematologic: Granulocytopenia, leukopenia
Local: Injection site pain
Neuromuscular & skeletal: Paresthesia, involuntary muscle contractions, rigors, neuropathy, weakness
Ocular: Vision abnormalities
Respiratory: Coughing, dyspnea
Miscellaneous: Sepsis, increased sweating

<1%:

Cardiovascular: Cardiac failure, bradycardia, arrhythmias, cerebral edema, leg edema, peripheral edema, syncope, substernal chest pain
Central nervous system: Hypothermia, abnormal crying, malignant fever, vertigo, coma, speech disorders
Endocrine & metabolic: Gynecomastia, decreased gonadotropins
Hepatic: Cholecystitis, cholelithiasis, hepatitis, hepatosplenomegaly, ascites
Neuromuscular & skeletal: Abnormal gait, dyskinesia, hypertonia
Ocular: Nystagmus
Miscellaneous: Vocal cord paralysis

**Drug Interactions** No data reported

**Drug Uptake**

Absorption: Oral: Poorly absorbed; I.V. therapy is needed for the treatment of viral infections in AIDS patients
Serum half-life: ~3 hours

**Pregnancy Risk Factor** C

**Generic Available** No

♦ **Foscavir®** *see* Foscarnet *on previous page*

## Fosfomycin (fos foe MYE sin)

**U.S. Brand Names** Monurol™

**Therapeutic Category** Antibiotic, Miscellaneous

**Synonyms** Fosfomycin Tromethamine

**Use** Treatment of uncomplicated urinary tract infections

**Usual Dosage** Adults: Urinary tract infections: Oral:

Female: Single dose of 3 g in 4 oz of water
Male: 3 g once daily for 2-3 days for complicated urinary tract infections

**Mechanism of Action** As a phosphonic acid derivative, fosfomycin inhibits bacterial wall synthesis (bactericidal) by inactivating the enzyme, pyruvyl transferase, which is critical in the synthesis of cell walls by bacteria; the tromethamine salt is preferable to the calcium salt due to its superior absorption; many gram-positive and gram-negative organisms are inhibited staphylococci, pneumococci, *E. coli, Salmonella, Shigella, H. influenzae, Neisseria* spp, and some strains of *P. aeruginosa*, indole-negative *Proteus*, and *Providencia*; *B. fragilis*, and anaerobic g (-) cocci are resistant; *in vitro* synergism occurs with penicillins, cephalosporins, aminoglycosides, erythromycin, and tetracyclines

**Local Anesthetic/Vasoconstrictor Precautions** No information available to require special precautions

**Effects on Dental Treatment** No effects or complications reported

**Other Adverse Effects**

>1%:

Central nervous system: Headache
Dermatologic: Rash
Gastrointestinal: Diarrhea (2% to 8%), nausea, vomiting, epigastric discomfort, anorexia

<1%:

Central nervous system: Dizziness, drowsiness, fatigue
Dermatologic: Pruritus

**Drug Interactions** Decreased effect: Food decreases absorption significantly; antacids or calcium salts may cause precipitate formation and decrease fosfomycin absorption

**Drug Uptake**

Absorption: Well absorbed

Serum half-life: 4-8 hours; prolonged in renal failure (50 hours with $Cl_{cr}$ <10 mL/minute)

Time to peak serum concentration: 2 hours

**Pregnancy Risk Factor** B

♦ **Fosfomycin Tromethamine** *see* Fosfomycin *on previous page*

# Fosinopril (foe SIN oh pril)

**Related Information**

Cardiovascular Diseases *on page 1066*

**U.S. Brand Names** Monopril®

**Therapeutic Category** Angiotensin-Converting Enzyme (ACE) Inhibitor

**Use** Treatment of hypertension, either alone or in combination with other antihypertensive agents; congestive heart failure

**Usual Dosage** Adults: Oral:

Hypertension: Initial: 10 mg/day; increase to a maximum dose of 80 mg/day; most patients are maintained on 20-40 mg/day; may need to divide the dose into two if trough effect is inadequate; discontinue the diuretic, if possible 2-3 days before initiation of therapy; resume diuretic therapy carefully, if needed.

Heart failure: Initial: 10 mg/day (5 mg if renal dysfunction present) and increase, as needed, to a maximum of 40 mg once daily over several weeks; usual dose: 20-40 mg/day; if hypotension, orthostasis, or azotemia occur during titration, consider decreasing concomitant diuretic dose, if any

**Mechanism of Action** Competitive inhibitor of angiotensin-converting enzyme (ACE); prevents conversion of angiotensin I to angiotensin II, a potent vasoconstrictor; results in lower levels of angiotensin II which causes an increase in plasma renin activity and a reduction in aldosterone secretion; a CNS mechanism may also be involved in hypotensive effect as angiotensin II increases adrenergic outflow from CNS; vasoactive kallikreins may be decreased in conversion to active hormones by ACE inhibitors, thus reducing blood pressure

**Local Anesthetic/Vasoconstrictor Precautions** No information available to require special precautions

**Effects on Dental Treatment** No effects or complications reported

**Drug-Drug Interactions With ACEIs**

| Precipitant Drug | Drug (Category) and Effect | Description |
|---|---|---|
| Antacids | ACE Inhibitors: decreased | Decreased bioavailability of ACEIs. May be more likely with captopril. Separate administration times by 1-2 hours. |
| NSAIDs (indomethacin) | ACEIs: decreased | Reduced hypotensive effects of ACEIs. More prominent in low renin or volume dependent hypertensive patients. |
| Phenothiazines | ACEIs: increased | Pharmacologic effects of ACEIs may be increased. |
| ACEIs | Allopurinol: increased | Higher risk of hypersensitivity reaction possible when given concurrently. Three case reports of Stevens-Johnson syndrome with captopril. |
| ACEIs | Digoxin: increased | Increased plasma digoxin levels. |
| ACEIs | Lithium: increased | Increased serum lithium levels and symptoms of toxicity may occur. |
| ACEIs | Potassium preps/ potassium sparing diuretics increased | Coadministration may result in elevated potassium levels. |

**Other Adverse Effects**

1% to 10%:

- Cardiovascular: Orthostatic hypotension
- Central nervous system: Headache, dizziness, fatigue
- Endocrine & metabolic: Sexual dysfunction
- Gastrointestinal: Diarrhea, nausea, vomiting
- Respiratory: Cough

<1%:

- Cardiovascular: Syncope
- Central nervous system: Vertigo, insomnia
- Dermatologic: Angioedema, rash
- Endocrine & metabolic: Hypoglycemia, hyperkalemia
- Gastrointestinal: Dysgeusia
- Genitourinary: Impotence

(Continued)

## Fosinopril *(Continued)*

Hematologic: Neutropenia, agranulocytosis, anemia
Neuromuscular & skeletal: Muscle cramps
Renal: Deterioration in renal function

**Drug Interactions**
Fosinopril and diuretics have additive hypotensive effects; see table.

**Drug Uptake**
Absorption: 36%
Serum half-life, serum (fosinoprilat): 12 hours
Time to peak serum concentration: ~3 hours

**Pregnancy Risk Factor** C (first trimester); D (second and third trimesters)

**Generic Available** No

## Fosphenytoin (FOS fen i toyn)

**U.S. Brand Names** Cerebyx®

**Therapeutic Category** Anticonvulsant, Hydantoin

**Use** Indicated for short-term parenteral administration when other means of phenytoin administration are unavailable, inappropriate or deemed less advantageous; the safety and effectiveness of fosphenytoin in this use has not been systematically evaluated for more than 5 days; may be used for the control of generalized convulsive status epilepticus and prevention and treatment of seizures occurring during neurosurgery

**Usual Dosage The dose, concentration in solutions, and infusion rates for fosphenytoin are expressed as phenytoin sodium equivalents; fosphenytoin should always be prescribed and dispensed in phenytoin sodium equivalents**

Status epilepticus: I.V.: Adults: Loading dose: Phenytoin equivalent 15-20 mg/kg I.V. administered at 100-150 mg/minute

Nonemergent loading and maintenance dosing: I.V. or I.M.: Adults:
Loading dose: Phenytoin equivalent 10-20 mg/kg I.V. or I.M. (max I.V. rate 150 mg/minute)
Initial daily maintenance dose: Phenytoin equivalent 4-6 mg/kg/day I.V. or I.M.

I.M. or I.V. substitution for oral phenytoin therapy: May be substituted for oral phenytoin sodium at the same total daily dose, however, Dilantin® capsules are ~90% bioavailable by the oral route; phenytoin, supplied as fosphenytoin, is 100% bioavailable by both the I.M. and I.V. routes; for this reason, plasma phenytoin concentrations may increase when I.M. or I.V. fosphenytoin is substituted for oral phenytoin sodium therapy; in clinical trials I.M. fosphenytoin was administered as a single daily dose utilizing either 1 or 2 injection sites; some patients may require more frequent dosing

**Local Anesthetic/Vasoconstrictor Precautions** No information available to require special precautions

**Effects on Dental Treatment** No effects or complications reported

**Other Adverse Effects**

I.V. administration (maximum dose/rate):
Body as whole: Pelvic pain (4.4%), weakness (2.2%), back pain (2.2%), headache (2.2%)
Cardiovascular: I.V.: Hypotension (7.7%), vasodilation (5.6%), tachycardia (2.2%)
Central nervous system: Dizziness (31%), drowsiness (20%), ataxia (11%), stupor (7.7%), extrapyramidal syndrome (4.4%), agitation (3.3%), hypesthesia (2.2%), vertigo (2.2%), brain edema (2.2%), impaired coordination (4.4%)
Dermatologic: Pruritus (48.9%)
Gastrointestinal: Nausea (8.9%), tongue disorder (4.4%), dry mouth (4.4%), vomiting (2.2%), taste perversion (3.3%)
Neuromuscular & skeletal: Paresthesia (4.4%), dysarthria (2.2%), tremor (3.3%)
Ocular: Diplopia (3.3%), amblyopia (2.2%), nystagmus (44%)
Otic: Tinnitus (8.9%), deafness (2.2%)

I.M. administration (substitute for oral phenytoin):
Body as a whole: Headache (8.9%), weakness (3.9%), accidental injury (3.4%)
Central nervous system: Ataxia (8.4%), drowsiness (6.7%), dizziness (5%)
Dermatologic: Pruritus (2.8%)
Gastrointestinal: Nausea (4.5%), vomiting (2.8%)
Dermatologic: Bruising (7.3%)
Neuromuscular & skeletal: Tremor (9.5%), paresthesia (3.9%), incoordination (7.8%), reflexes decreased (2.8%)
Ocular: Nystagmus (15%)

Other ≤1%:

Cardiovascular: Hypertension, cardiac arrest, syncope, cerebral hemorrhage, palpitations, sinus bradycardia, atrial flutter, bundle branch block, cardiomegaly, cerebral infarct, postural hypotension, pulmonary embolus, QT interval prolongation, thrombophlebitis, ventricular extrasystoles, congestive heart failure

Central nervous system: Migraine

Dermatologic: Rash, maculopapular rash, urticaria, skin discoloration, contact dermatitis, pustular rash, skin nodule, petechia

Endocrine & metabolic: Hypokalemia, hyperglycemia, hypophosphatemia, alkalosis, acidosis, dehydration, hyperkalemia, ketosis

Hematologic/lymphatic: Thrombocytopenia, anemia, leukocytosis, cyanosis, hypochromic anemia, leukopenia, lymphadenopathy

Hepatic: Acute hepatotoxicity, acute hepatic failure

Miscellaneous: Sweating

**Warnings/Precautions** Doses of fosphenytoin are expressed as their phenytoin sodium equivalent; antiepileptic drugs should not be abruptly discontinued; hypotension may occur, especially after I.V. administration at high doses and high rates of administration, administration of phenytoin has been associated with atrial and ventricular conduction depression and ventricular fibrillation, careful cardiac monitoring is needed when administering I.V. loading doses of fosphenytoin; use with caution in patients with hypotension and severe myocardial insufficiency; discontinue if skin rash or lymphadenopathy occurs; acute hepatotoxicity associated with a hypersensitivity syndrome characterized by fever, skin eruptions and lymphadenopathy has been reported to occur within the first 2 months of treatment

**Drug Interactions** No drugs are known to interfere with the conversion of fosphenytoin to phenytoin; phenytoin may decrease the serum concentration or effectiveness of valproic acid, ethosuximide, felbamate, benzodiazepines, carbamazepine, lamotrigine, primidone, warfarin, oral contraceptives, corticosteroids, cyclosporine, theophylline, chloramphenicol, rifampin, doxycycline, quinidine, mexiletine, disopyramide, dopamine, or nondepolarizing skeletal muscle relaxants; phenytoin may increase phenobarbital and primidone levels; protein binding of phenytoin can be affected by valproic acid or salicylates; serum phenytoin concentrations may be increased by cimetidine, felbamate, ethosuximide, methsuximide, chloramphenicol, disulfiram, fluconazole, omeprazole, isoniazid, trimethoprim, or sulfonamides and decreased by rifampin, cisplatin, vinblastine, bleomycin, folic acid

**Drug Uptake**

Fosphenytoin is a prodrug of phenytoin and its anticonvulsant effects are attributable to phenytoin

Conversion to phenytoin: Following I.V. administration conversion half-life is 15 minutes; following I.M. administration peak phenytoin levels are reached in 3 hours

**Pregnancy Risk Factor** D

**Generic Available** No


- **Fostex® [OTC]** *see* Sulfur and Salicylic Acid *on page 947*
- **Fostex® 10% BPO Gel [OTC]** *see* Benzoyl Peroxide *on page 130*
- **Fostex® 10% Wash [OTC]** *see* Benzoyl Peroxide *on page 130*
- **Fostex® Bar [OTC]** *see* Benzoyl Peroxide *on page 130*
- **Fototar® [OTC]** *see* Coal Tar *on page 270*
- **Fragmin®** *see* Dalteparin *on page 295*
- **Freezone® Solution [OTC]** *see* Salicylic Acid *on page 900*
- **Fresh Burst Listerine® Antiseptic [OTC]** *see* Mouthwash, Antiseptic *on page 690*
- **FS Shampoo®** *see* Fluocinolone *on page 440*
- **5-FU** *see* Fluorouracil *on page 443*
- **FUDR®** *see* Floxuridine *on page 434*
- **Fulvicin® P/G** *see* Griseofulvin *on page 477*
- **Fulvicin-U/F®** *see* Griseofulvin *on page 477*
- **Fumasorb® [OTC]** *see* Ferrous Fumarate *on page 426*
- **Fumerin® [OTC]** *see* Ferrous Fumarate *on page 426*
- **Fungizone®** *see* Amphotericin B *on page 79*
- **Fungoid® AF Topical Solution [OTC]** *see* Undecylenic Acid and Derivatives *on page 1033*
- **Fungoid® Creme** *see* Miconazole *on page 672*
- **Fungoid® Tincture** *see* Miconazole *on page 672*
- **Furacin®** *see* Nitrofurazone *on page 724*
- **Furadantin®** *see* Nitrofurantoin *on page 724*

## Furazolidone (fyoor a ZOE li done)

**U.S. Brand Names** Furoxone®

**Therapeutic Category** Antibiotic, Miscellaneous; Antidiarrheal; Antiprotozoal

**Use** Treatment of bacterial or protozoal diarrhea and enteritis caused by susceptible organisms *Giardia lamblia* and *Vibrio cholerae*

**Usual Dosage** Oral:

Children >1 month: 5-8 mg/kg/day in 4 divided doses for 7 days, not to exceed 400 mg/day or 8.8 mg/kg/day

Adults: 100 mg 4 times/day for 7 days

**Mechanism of Action** Inhibits several vital enzymatic reactions causing antibacterial and antiprotozoal action

**Local Anesthetic/Vasoconstrictor Precautions** No information available to require special precautions

**Effects on Dental Treatment** No effects or complications reported

**Other Adverse Effects**

>10%: Genitourinary: Dark yellow to brown discoloration of urine

1% to 10%:

Central nervous system: Headache

Gastrointestinal: Abdominal pain, diarrhea, nausea, vomiting

<1%:

Cardiovascular: Orthostatic hypotension

Central nervous system: Fever, dizziness, drowsiness, malaise

Dermatologic: Skin rash

Endocrine & metabolic: Hypoglycemia, disulfiram-like reaction after alcohol ingestion, leukopenia

Hematologic: Agranulocytosis, hemolysis in patients with G-6-PD deficiency

Neuromuscular & skeletal: Arthralgia

**Drug Interactions**

Increased effect with indirectly acting sympathomimetic amines such as ephedrine and phenylephrine, tricyclic antidepressants, tyramine-containing foods, MAO inhibitors, meperidine, anorexiants, dextromethorphan, fluoxetine, paroxetine, sertraline, trazodone

Increased effect/toxicity of levodopa

Disulfiram-like reaction with alcohol

**Drug Uptake** Absorption: Oral: Poor

**Pregnancy Risk Factor** C

**Generic Available** No

## Furosemide (fyoor OH se mide)

**Related Information**

Cardiovascular Diseases *on page 1066*

**U.S. Brand Names** Lasix®

**Canadian Brand Names** Apo®-Furosemide; Furoside®; Novo-Semide; Uritol®

**Therapeutic Category** Diuretic, Loop

**Use** Management of edema associated with congestive heart failure and hepatic or renal disease; used alone or in combination with antihypertensives in treatment of hypertension

**Usual Dosage**

Children:

Oral: 1-2 mg/kg/dose increased in increments of 1 mg/kg/dose with each succeeding dose until a satisfactory effect is achieved to a maximum of 6 mg/kg/dose no more frequently than 6 hours

I.M., I.V.: 1 mg/kg/dose, increasing by each succeeding dose at 1 mg/kg/dose at intervals of 6-12 hours until a satisfactory response up to 6 mg/kg/dose

Adults:

Oral: 20-80 mg/dose initially increased in increments of 20-40 mg/dose at intervals of 6-8 hours; usual maintenance dose interval is twice daily or every day

I.M., I.V.: 20-40 mg/dose, may be repeated in 1-2 hours as needed and increased by 20 mg/dose with each succeeding dose up to 1000 mg/day; usual dosing interval: 6-12 hours

Continuous I.V. infusion: Initial I.V. bolus dose of 0.1 mg/kg followed by continuous I.V. infusion doses of 0.1 mg/kg/hour doubled every 2 hours to a maximum of 0.4 mg/kg/hour if urine output is <1 mL/kg/hour have been found to be effective and result in a lower daily requirement of furosemide than with intermittent dosing. Other studies have used 20-160 mg/hour continuous I.V. infusion

Elderly: Oral, I.M., I.V.: Initial: 20 mg/day; increase slowly to desired response

**Mechanism of Action** Inhibits reabsorption of sodium and chloride in the ascending loop of Henle and distal renal tubule, interfering with the chloride-binding cotransport system, thus causing increased excretion of water, sodium, chloride, magnesium, and calcium

**Local Anesthetic/Vasoconstrictor Precautions** No information available to require special precautions

**Effects on Dental Treatment** No effects or complications reported

**Other Adverse Effects**

>10%:
- Cardiovascular: Orthostatic hypotension
- Central nervous system: Dizziness

1% to 10%:
- Central nervous system: Headache
- Dermatologic: Photosensitivity
- Endocrine & metabolic: Electrolyte imbalance (hypokalemia, hyponatremia, hypochloremia, hypercalciuria, hyperuricemia), alkalosis, dehydration
- Gastrointestinal: Diarrhea, loss of appetite, stomach cramps or pain
- Ocular: Blurred vision

<1%:
- Dermatologic: Skin rash
- Endocrine & metabolic: Gout
- Gastrointestinal: Pancreatitis, nausea
- Genitourinary: Prerenal azotemia
- Hepatic: Hepatic dysfunction
- Hematologic: Agranulocytosis, leukopenia, anemia, thrombocytopenia
- Local: Redness at injection site
- Ocular: Xanthopsia
- Otic: Ototoxicity
- Renal: Nephrocalcinosis, interstitial nephritis

**Drug Interactions**

Decreased effect:
- Furosemide interferes with hypoglycemic effect of antidiabetic agents
- Indomethacin may reduce natriuretic and hypotensive effects of furosemide

Increased effect: Effects of antihypertensive agents may be enhanced by furosemide

Increased toxicity:
- Furosemide inhibits renal clearance of lithium resulting in risk of lithium toxicity
- Concomitant use of furosemide with aminoglycoside antibiotics or other ototoxic drugs should be avoided

**Drug Uptake**

Onset of diuresis:
- Oral: Within 30-60 minutes
- I.M.: 30 minutes
- I.V.: Within 5 minutes

Peak effect: Oral: Within 1-2 hours

Duration:
- Oral: 6-8 hours
- I.V.: 2 hours

Absorption: Oral: 60% to 67%

Serum half-life:
- Normal renal function: 0.5-1.1 hours
- End-stage renal disease: 9 hours

**Pregnancy Risk Factor** C

**Generic Available** Yes

♦ **Furoxone®** *see* Furazolidone *on previous page*
♦ **G-1®** *see* Butalbital Compound *on page 163*
♦ **G-1®** *see* Butalbital Compound and Acetaminophen *on page 164*

## Gabapentin (GA ba pen tin)

**U.S. Brand Names** Neurontin®

**Therapeutic Category** Anticonvulsant, Miscellaneous

**Use** Adjunct for treatment of drug-refractory partial and secondarily generalized seizures in adults with epilepsy; not effective for absence seizures

**Usual Dosage** If gabapentin is discontinued or if another anticonvulsant is added to therapy, it should be done slowly over a minimum of 1 week

Children >12 years and Adults: Oral:
- Initial: 300 mg on day 1 (at bedtime to minimize sedation), then 300 mg twice daily on day 2, and then 300 mg 3 times/day on day 3
- Total daily dosage range: 900-1800 mg/day administered in 3 divided doses at 8-hour intervals

**Mechanism of Action** Exact mechanism of action is not known, but does have properties in common with other anticonvulsants; although structurally related to GABA, it does not interact with GABA receptors

(Continued)

## Gabapentin *(Continued)*

**Local Anesthetic/Vasoconstrictor Precautions** No information available to require special precautions

**Effects on Dental Treatment** No effects or complications reported

**Other Adverse Effects**

>10%: Central nervous system: Somnolence, dizziness, abnormal coordination, fatigue

1% to 10%:

Cardiovascular: Peripheral edema

Central nervous system: Nervousness, amnesia, depression, anxiety

Dermatologic: Pruritus

Gastrointestinal: Dyspepsia, dry mouth/throat, nausea, constipation, appetite stimulation (weight gain)

Genitourinary: Impotence

Hematologic: Leukopenia

Neuromuscular & skeletal: Back pain, myalgia, dysarthria, tremor, abnormal coordination

Ocular: Diplopia, blurred vision, nystagmus

Respiratory: Rhinitis, bronchospasm

Miscellaneous: Hiccups

**Drug Interactions**

Gabapentin does not modify plasma concentrations of standard anticonvulsant medications (ie, valproic acid, carbamazepine, phenytoin, or phenobarbital)

Decreased effect: Antacids reduce the bioavailability of gabapentin by 20%

Increased toxicity: Cimetidine may decrease clearance of gabapentin; gabapentin may increase levels of norethindrone by 13%

**Drug Uptake**

Absorption: Oral: 50% to 60%

Serum half-life: 5-6 hours

**Pregnancy Risk Factor** C

**Generic Available** No

- **Gabitril®** *see* Tiagabine *on page 983*
- **Gamastan®** *see* Immune Globulin, Intramuscular *on page 530*
- **Gamimune® N** *see* Immune Globulin, Intravenous *on page 531*
- **Gammagard®** *see* Immune Globulin, Intravenous *on page 531*
- **Gammagard® S/D** *see* Immune Globulin, Intravenous *on page 531*
- **Gammaphos** *see* Amifostine *on page 59*
- **Gammar®** *see* Immune Globulin, Intramuscular *on page 530*
- **Gammar®-P I.V.** *see* Immune Globulin, Intravenous *on page 531*
- **Gamulin® Rh** *see* $Rh_o$(D) Immune Globulin *on page 884*

## Ganciclovir (gan SYE kloe veer)

**Related Information**

Systemic Viral Diseases *on page 1115*

**U.S. Brand Names** Cytovene®; Vitrasert®

**Therapeutic Category** Antiviral Agent, Parenteral

**Use** Treatment of CMV retinitis in immunocompromised individuals, including patients with acquired immunodeficiency syndrome; treatment of CMV pneumonia in marrow transplant recipients AIDS patients and organ transplant recipients with CMV colitis, pneumonitis, and multiorgan involvement; bone marrow transplant patients when given in combination with IVIG or CMV hyperimmune globulin

Oral: Alternative to the I.V. formulation for maintenance treatment of CMV retinitis in immunocompromised patients, including patients with AIDS, in whom retinitis is stable following appropriate induction therapy and for whom the risk of more rapid progression is balanced by the benefit associated with avoiding daily I.V. infusions

**Usual Dosage**

Slow I.V. infusion (dosing is based on total body weight):

Children >3 months and Adults:

Induction therapy: 5 mg/kg/dose every 12 hours for 14-21 days followed by maintenance therapy

Maintenance therapy: 5 mg/kg/day as a single daily dose for 7 days/week or 6 mg/kg/day for 5 days/week

Oral: 1000 mg 3 times/day with food **or** 500 mg 6 times/day with food

**Mechanism of Action** Ganciclovir is phosphorylated to a substrate which competitively inhibits the binding of deoxyguanosine triphosphate to DNA polymerase resulting in inhibition of viral DNA synthesis

**Local Anesthetic/Vasoconstrictor Precautions** No information available to require special precautions

**Effects on Dental Treatment** No effects or complications reported

**Other Adverse Effects**

>10%:

Central nervous system: Headache

Hematologic: Granulocytopenia, thrombocytopenia

1% to 10%:

Central nervous system: Confusion, fever

Dermatologic: Rash

Hematologic: Anemia

Hepatic: Abnormal liver function values

Miscellaneous: Sepsis

<1%:

Cardiovascular: Arrhythmia, hypertension, hypotension, edema

Central nervous system: Ataxia, dizziness, nervousness, psychosis, malaise, coma

Dermatologic: Alopecia, pruritus, urticaria

Gastrointestinal: Nausea, vomiting, diarrhea, abdominal pain

Hematologic: Eosinophilia, hemorrhage

Local: Inflammation or pain at injection site

Neuromuscular & skeletal: Paresthesia, tremor

Ocular: Retinal detachment

Respiratory: Dyspnea

**Drug Interactions** Increased toxicity:

Zidovudine, immunosuppressive agents leads to increased hematologic toxicity

Imipenem/cilastatin leads to increased seizure potential

Probenecid: The renal clearance of ganciclovir is decreased in the presence of probenecid

**Drug Uptake**

Absorption: Oral: Absolute bioavailability under fasting conditions: 5% and following food: 6% to 9%; following fatty meal: 28% to 31%

Serum half-life: 1.7-5.8 hours; increases with impaired renal function

End-stage renal disease: 3.6 hours

**Pregnancy Risk Factor** C

**Generic Available** No

- **Gantanol®** *see* Sulfamethoxazole *on page 943*
- **Gantrisin®** *see* Sulfisoxazole *on page 946*
- **Garamycin®** *see* Gentamicin *on page 466*
- **Gas-Ban DS® [OTC]** *see* Aluminum Hydroxide, Magnesium Hydroxide, and Simethicone *on page 56*
- **Gas Relief®** *see* Simethicone *on page 915*
- **Gastrocrom®** *see* Cromolyn Sodium *on page 281*
- **Gastrosed™** *see* Hyoscyamine *on page 519*
- **Gas-X® [OTC]** *see* Simethicone *on page 915*
- **Gaviscon®-2 Tablet [OTC]** *see* Aluminum Hydroxide and Magnesium Trisilicate *on page 56*
- **Gaviscon® Liquid [OTC]** *see* Aluminum Hydroxide and Magnesium Carbonate *on page 55*
- **Gaviscon® Tablet [OTC]** *see* Aluminum Hydroxide and Magnesium Trisilicate *on page 56*
- **G-CSF** *see* Filgrastim *on page 430*
- **Gee Gee® [OTC]** *see* Guaifenesin *on page 478*

## Gelatin, Absorbable (JEL a tin, ab SORB a ble)

**U.S. Brand Names** Gelfoam® Topical

**Therapeutic Category** Hemostatic Agent

**Use**

Dental: Adjunct to provide hemostasis in oral and dental surgery

Medical: In medicine, adjunct to provide hemostasis in surgery; open prostatic surgery

**Usual Dosage** Hemostasis: Apply packs or sponges dry or saturated with sodium chloride. When applied dry, hold in place with moderate pressure. When applied wet, squeeze to remove air bubbles. The powder is applied as a paste prepared by adding approximately 4 mL of sterile saline solution to the powder.

**Local Anesthetic/Vasoconstrictor Precautions** No information available to require special precautions

**Effects on Dental Treatment** No effects or complications reported

**Other Adverse Effects** 1% to 10%: Local: Infection and abscess formation

(Continued)

## Gelatin, Absorbable *(Continued)*

**Contraindications** Should not be used in closure of skin incisions since they may interfere with the healing of skin edges

**Warnings/Precautions** Do not sterilize by heat; do not use in the presence of infection

**Drug Interactions** No data reported

**Pregnancy Risk Factor** No data reported

**Breast-feeding Considerations** No data reported

**Dosage Forms**

Packs:

Size 2 cm (40 cm x 2 cm) (1s)

Size 6 cm (40 cm x 6 cm) (6s)

Packs, dental:

Size 2 (10 mm x 20 mm x 7 mm) (15s)

Size 4 (20 mm x 20 mm x 7 mm) (15s)

**Generic Available** No

## Gelatin, Pectin, and Methylcellulose

(JEL a tin, PEK tin, & meth il SEL yoo lose)

**U.S. Brand Names** Orabase® Plain [OTC]

**Therapeutic Category** Protectant, Topical

**Use** Temporary relief from minor oral irritations

**Usual Dosage** Press small dabs into place until the involved area is coated with a thin film; do not try to spread onto area; may be used as often as needed

**Local Anesthetic/Vasoconstrictor Precautions** No information available to require special precautions

**Effects on Dental Treatment** No effects or complications reported

**Generic Available** No

- **Gelfoam® Topical** *see* Gelatin, Absorbable *on previous page*
- **Gel-Kam®** *see* Fluoride *on page 441*
- **Gelpirin® [OTC]** *see* Acetaminophen, Aspirin, and Caffeine *on page 31*
- **Gel-Tin® [OTC]** *see* Fluoride *on page 441*
- **Gelucast®** *see* Zinc Gelatin *on page 1061*

## Gemcitabine (jem SIT a been)

**U.S. Brand Names** Gemzar®

**Therapeutic Category** Antineoplastic Agent, Miscellaneous

**Synonyms** Gemcitabine Hydrochloride

**Use** Treatment of patients with inoperable pancreatic cancer; in combination with cisplatin for the first-line treatment of patients with inoperable, locally advanced (stage IIIA or IIIB) or metastatic (stage IV) nonsmall cell lung cancer

**Usual Dosage** Adults: I.V.: 1000 mg/m$^2$ once weekly for up to 7 weeks (or until toxicity necessitates reducing or holding a dose), followed by a week of rest from treatment. Subsequent cycles should consist of infusions once weekly for 3 consecutive weeks out of every 4 weeks.

**Mechanism of Action** Nucleoside analogue that primarily kills cells undergoing DNA synthesis (S-phase) and blocks the progression of cells through the G1/S-phase boundary

**Local Anesthetic/Vasoconstrictor Precautions** No information available to require special precautions

**Effects on Dental Treatment** No effects or complications reported

**Other Adverse Effects** >10%:

Cardiovascular: Peripheral edema

Central nervous system: Fever

Dermatologic: Rash, alopecia

Gastrointestinal: Nausea, vomiting, constipation, diarrhea, stomatitis

Hematologic: Anemia, leukopenia, neutropenia, thrombocytopenia

Hepatic: Elevated liver enzymes (ALT, AST, alkaline phosphatase) and bilirubin

Neuromuscular & skeletal: Pain

Renal: Proteinuria, hematuria, elevated BUN

Respiratory: Dyspnea

Miscellaneous: Infection

**Warnings/Precautions** The U.S. Food & Drug Administration (FDA) recommends that procedures for proper handling and disposal of antineoplastic agents be considered. Prolongation of the infusion time >60 minutes and more frequent than weekly dosing have been shown to increase toxicity. Gemcitabine can suppress bone marrow function manifested by leukopenia, thrombocytopenia and anemia, and myelosuppression is usually the dose-limiting ototoxicity. The incidence of fever is 41% and gemcitabine may cause fever in the absence of clinical infection. Rash has been reported in 30% of patients - typically a macular or finely granular maculopapular pruritic eruption of mild-moderate severity involving the trunk and extremities. Gemcitabine should be used with caution in patients with pre-existing renal impairment (mild proteinuria and hematuria were commonly reported; hemolytic uremic syndrome has been reported) and hepatic impairment (associated with transient elevations of serum transaminases in $^2/_3$ of patients - but no evidence of increasing hepatic toxicity).

**Drug Uptake** Serum half-life: 42-94 minutes

**Pregnancy Risk Factor** D

**Generic Available** No

- **Gemcitabine Hydrochloride** *see* Gemcitabine *on previous page*

## Gemfibrozil (jem FI broe zil)

**Related Information**

Cardiovascular Diseases *on page 1066*

**U.S. Brand Names** Lopid®

**Canadian Brand Names** Apo®-Gemfibrozil; Nu-Gemfibrozil

**Therapeutic Category** Lipid Lowering Drugs

**Use** Treatment of hypertriglyceridemia in types IV and V hyperlipidemia for patients who are at greater risk for pancreatitis and who have not responded to dietary intervention; reduction of coronary heart disease in type IIB patients who have low HDL cholesterol, increased LDL cholesterol, and increased triglycerides

**Usual Dosage** Adults: Oral: 1200 mg/day in 2 divided doses, 30 minutes before breakfast and dinner

**Mechanism of Action** The exact mechanism of action of gemfibrozil is unknown, however, several theories exist regarding the VLDL effect; it can inhibit lipolysis and decrease subsequent hepatic fatty acid uptake as well as inhibit hepatic secretion of VLDL; together these actions decrease serum VLDL levels; increases HDL cholesterol; the mechanism behind HDL elevation is currently unknown

**Local Anesthetic/Vasoconstrictor Precautions** No information available to require special precautions

**Effects on Dental Treatment** No effects or complications reported

**Other Adverse Effects**

>10%:

Gastrointestinal: Dyspepsia, abdominal pain

Hepatic: Cholelithiasis

1% to 10%:

Central nervous system: Fatigue, vertigo, headache

Dermatologic: Eczema, rash

Gastrointestinal: Diarrhea, nausea, vomiting, constipation, acute appendicitis

<1%:

Cardiovascular: Atrial fibrillation

Central nervous system: Hypesthesia, dizziness, drowsiness, mental depression

Gastrointestinal: Flatulence

Neuromuscular & skeletal: Paresthesia

Ocular: Blurred vision

**Drug Interactions** Increased toxicity:

Gemfibrozil may potentiate the effects of warfarin

Manufacturer warns against the use of gemfibrozil with concomitant lovastatin therapy

**Drug Uptake**

Absorption: Well absorbed

Serum half-life: 1.4 hours

Time to peak serum concentration: Within 1-2 hours

**Pregnancy Risk Factor** B

**Generic Available** Yes

- **Gemzar®** *see* Gemcitabine *on previous page*
- **Genabid®** *see* Papaverine *on page 764*
- **Genac® Tablet [OTC]** *see* Triprolidine and Pseudoephedrine *on page 1025*
- **Genagesic®** *see* Guaifenesin and Phenylpropanolamine *on page 480*
- **Genahist® Oral** *see* Diphenhydramine *on page 338*
- **Genamin® Cold Syrup [OTC]** *see* Chlorpheniramine and Phenylpropanolamine *on page 233*
- **Genamin® Expectorant [OTC]** *see* Guaifenesin and Phenylpropanolamine *on page 480*
- **Genapap® [OTC]** *see* Acetaminophen *on page 27*
- **Genasoft® Plus [OTC]** *see* Docusate and Casanthranol *on page 347*
- **Genaspor® [OTC]** *see* Tolnaftate *on page 997*

- **Genatap® Elixir [OTC]** *see* Brompheniramine and Phenylpropanolamine *on page 153*
- **Genatuss® [OTC]** *see* Guaifenesin *on page 478*
- **Genatuss DM® [OTC]** *see* Guaifenesin and Dextromethorphan *on page 479*
- **Gencalc® 600 [OTC]** *see* Calcium Carbonate *on page 172*
- **Geneye® Ophthalmic [OTC]** *see* Tetrahydrozoline *on page 967*
- **Gen-K®** *see* Potassium Chloride *on page 822*
- **Genora® 0.5/35** *see* Ethinyl Estradiol and Norethindrone *on page 404*
- **Genora® 1/35** *see* Ethinyl Estradiol and Norethindrone *on page 404*
- **Genora® 1/50** *see* Mestranol and Norethindrone *on page 639*
- **Genotropin® Injection** *see* Human Growth Hormone *on page 499*
- **Genpril® [OTC]** *see* Ibuprofen *on page 522*

## Gentamicin (jen ta MYE sin)

**Related Information**

Cardiovascular Diseases *on page 1066*

**U.S. Brand Names** Garamycin®

**Therapeutic Category** Antibiotic, Aminoglycoside; Antibiotic, Ophthalmic; Antibiotic, Topical

**Use** Treatment of susceptible bacterial infections, normally gram-negative organisms including *Pseudomonas, Proteus, Serratia,* and gram-positive *Staphylococcus*; treatment of bone infections, respiratory tract infections, skin and soft tissue infections, as well as abdominal and urinary tract infections, endocarditis, and septicemia; used topically to treat superficial infections of the skin or ophthalmic infections caused by susceptible bacteria

**Usual Dosage** Individualization is critical because of the low therapeutic index

**Use of ideal body weight (IBW) for determining the mg/kg/dose appears to be more accurate than dosing on the basis of total body weight (TBW).**

In morbid obesity, dosage requirement may best be estimated using a dosing weight of IBW + 0.4 (TBW - IBW)

Initial and periodic peak and trough plasma drug levels should be determined, particularly in critically ill patients with serious infections or in disease states known to significantly alter aminoglycoside pharmacokinetics (eg, cystic fibrosis, burns, or major surgery)

Once daily dosing: Higher peak serum drug concentration to MIC ratios, demonstrated aminoglycoside postantibiotic effect, decreased renal cortex drug uptake, and improved cost-time efficiency are supportive reasons for the use of once daily dosing regimens for aminoglycosides. Current research indicates these regimens to be as effective for nonlife-threatening infections, with no higher incidence of nephrotoxicity, than those requiring multiple daily doses. Doses are determined by calculating the entire day's dose via usual multiple dose calculation techniques and administering this quantity as a single dose. Doses are then adjusted to maintain mean serum concentrations above the MIC(s) of the causative organism(s). (Example: 4.0-4.5 mg/kg as a single dose; expected $Cp_{max}$: 10-20 mcg/mL and $Cp_{min}$: <1 mcg/mL). Further research is needed for universal recommendation in all patient populations and gram-negative disease; exceptions may include those with known high clearance (eg, children, patients with cystic fibrosis, or burns who may require shorter dosage intervals) and patients with renal function impairment for whom longer than conventional dosage intervals are usually required.

Neonates: I.M., I.V.:
- 0-4 weeks:
  - <1200 g: 2.5 mg/kg/dose every 18-24 hours
  - 1200-2000 g, 0-4 weeks: 2.5 mg/kg/dose every 12-18 hours
  - >2000 g: 2.5 mg/kg/dose every 12 hours
- Postnatal age >7 days:
  - 1200-2000 g: 2.5 mg/kg/dose every 8-12 hours
  - >2000 g: 2.5 mg/kg/dose every 8 hours

Newborns: Intrathecal: 1 mg every day

Infants and Children <5 years: I.M., I.V.: 2.5 mg/kg/dose every 8 hours*
- Cystic fibrosis: 2.5 mg/kg/dose every 6 hours

Children >5 years: I.M., I.V.: 1.5-2.5 mg/kg/dose every 8 hours*

*Some patients may require larger or more frequent doses (eg, every 6 hours) if serum levels document the need (ie, cystic fibrosis or febrile granulocytopenic patients)

Intrathecal: >3 months: 1-2 mg/day

Adults: I.M., I.V.:
- Severe life-threatening infections: 2-2.5 mg/kg/dose
- Urinary tract infections: 1.5 mg/kg/dose
- Synergy (for gram-positive infections): 1 mg/kg/dose

Children and Adults:
Intrathecal: 4-8 mg/day
Ophthalmic:
Ointment: Instill ½" (1.25 cm) 2-3 times/day to every 3-4 hours
Solution: Instill 1-2 drops every 2-4 hours, up to 2 drops every hour for severe infections
Topical: Apply 3-4 times/day to affected area

**Mechanism of Action** Interferes with bacterial protein synthesis by binding to 30S and 50S ribosomal subunits resulting in a defective bacterial cell membrane

**Local Anesthetic/Vasoconstrictor Precautions** No information available to require special precautions

**Effects on Dental Treatment** Increased salivation has been reported

**Other Adverse Effects**

>10%:
Central nervous system: Neurotoxicity (vertigo, ataxia, gait instability)
Otic: Ototoxicity (auditory), ototoxicity (vestibular)
Renal: Nephrotoxicity, decreased creatinine clearance
1% to 10%: Dermatologic: Itching, redness, rash, swelling

**Contraindications** Hypersensitivity to gentamicin or other aminoglycosides

**Warnings/Precautions**

Not intended for long-term therapy due to toxic hazards associated with extended administration; pre-existing renal insufficiency, vestibular or cochlear impairment, myasthenia gravis, hypocalcemia, conditions which depress neuromuscular transmission

Parenteral aminoglycosides are associated with significant nephrotoxicity or ototoxicity; the ototoxicity may be directly proportional to the amount of drug given and the duration of treatment; tinnitus or vertigo are indications of vestibular injury and impending hearing loss; renal damage is usually reversible

**Drug Interactions** Penicillins, cephalosporins, amphotericin B, loop diuretics may increase nephrotoxic potential; neuromuscular blocking agents may increase neuromuscular blockade. Clindamycin (Cleocin®) may increase the risk of renal toxicity following gentamicin administration.

**Drug Uptake**

Absorption: Oral: Not absorbed
Serum half-life: Adults: 1.5-3 hours
Time to peak serum concentration:
I.M.: Within 30-90 minutes
I.V.: 30 minutes after a 30-minute infusion

**Pregnancy Risk Factor** C

**Breast-feeding Considerations** No data reported; however, gentamicin is not absorbed orally and other aminoglycosides may be taken while breast-feeding

**Dosage Forms**

Injection: 40 mg/mL (1 mL, 2 mL, 10 mL, 20 mL)
Injection, pediatric: 10 mg/mL (2 mL)

**Generic Available** Yes

♦ **Gentamicin and Prednisolone** *see* Prednisolone and Gentamicin *on page 833*

## Gentian Violet (JEN shun VYE oh let)

**Therapeutic Category** Antibacterial, Topical; Antifungal Agent, Topical

**Use** Treatment of cutaneous or mucocutaneous infections caused by *Candida albicans* and other superficial skin infections - antibacterial and antifungal dye

**Usual Dosage** Children and Adults: Topical: Apply 0.5% to 2% locally with cotton to lesion 2-3 times/day for 3 days, do not swallow and avoid contact with eyes

**Mechanism of Action** Topical antiseptic/germicide effective against some vegetative gram-positive bacteria, particularly *Staphylococcus* sp, and some yeast; it is much less effective against gram-negative bacteria and is ineffective against acid-fast bacteria

**Local Anesthetic/Vasoconstrictor Precautions** No information available to require special precautions

**Effects on Dental Treatment** No effects or complications reported

**Other Adverse Effects** 1% to 10%:

Local: Esophagitis, burning, irritation, vesicle formation, ulceration of mucous membranes
Systemic: Sensitivity reactions, laryngitis, tracheitis, laryngeal obstruction

**Drug Interactions** No data reported

**Pregnancy Risk Factor** C

**Generic Available** Yes

♦ **Gentran®** *see* Dextran *on page 311*

♦ **Gen-XENE®** *see* Clorazepate *on page 267*

- **Geocillin®** *see* Carbenicillin *on page 187*
- **Geref® Injection** *see* Sermorelin Acetate *on page 910*
- **German Measles Vaccine** *see* Rubella Virus Vaccine, Live *on page 899*
- **Germinal®** *see* Ergoloid Mesylates *on page 380*
- **Gevrabon® [OTC]** *see* Vitamin B Complex *on page 1050*
- **GG-Cen® [OTC]** *see* Guaifenesin *on page 478*
- **Gingi-Aid® Gingival Retraction Cord** *see* Aluminum Chloride *on page 54*
- **Gingi-Aid® Solution** *see* Aluminum Chloride *on page 54*


## Glatiramer Acetate (gla TIR a mer AS e tate)

**U.S. Brand Names** Copaxone®

**Therapeutic Category** Biological, Miscellaneous

**Synonyms** Copolymer-1

**Use** Relapsing-remitting type multiple sclerosis; studies indicate that it reduces the frequency of attacks and the severity of disability; appears to be most effective for patients with minimal disability and has not demonstrated benefits in the chronic progressive form of multiple sclerosis

**Usual Dosage** Adults: S.C.: 20 mg daily

**Mechanism of Action** Glatiramer is a mixture of random polymers of four amino acids; L-alanine, L-glutamic acid, L-lysine and L-tyrosine, the resulting mixture is antigenically similar to myelin basic protein, which is an important component of the myelin sheath of nerves; glatiramer is thought to suppress T-lymphocytes specific for a myelin antigen, it is also proposed that glatiramer interferes with the antigen-presenting function of certain immune cells opposing pathogenic T-cell function

**Local Anesthetic/Vasoconstrictor Precautions** No information available to require special precautions

**Effects on Dental Treatment** No effects or complications reported

**Other Adverse Effects**

>10%:

- Dermatologic: Erythema
- Local: Pain

1% to 10%:

- Cardiovascular: Chest pain or tightness, flushing
- Central nervous system: Anxiety
- Hematologic: Transient eosinophilia
- Respiratory: Dyspnea
- Miscellaneous: Diaphoresis

**Contraindications** Previous hypersensitivity to any component of the copolymer formulation

**Pregnancy Risk Factor** B

**Dosage Forms** Injection: Single-use vials containing 20 mg of glatiramer and 40 mg mannitol; packaged in 2 mL vials along with 1 mL vial of diluent (sterile water for injection)


- **GlaucTabs®** *see* Methazolamide *on page 646*


## Glimepiride (GLYE me pye ride)

**Related Information**

Endocrine Disorders & Pregnancy *on page 1082*

**U.S. Brand Names** Amaryl®

**Therapeutic Category** Antidiabetic Agent; Hypoglycemic Agent, Oral; Sulfonylurea Agent

**Use**

Management of noninsulin-dependent diabetes mellitus (type II) as an adjunct to diet and exercise to lower blood glucose

Use in combination with insulin to lower blood glucose in patients whose hyperglycemia cannot be controlled by diet and exercise in conjunction with an oral hypoglycemic agent

**Usual Dosage** Oral (allow several days between dose titrations):

Adults: Initial: 1-2 mg once daily, administered with breakfast or the first main meal; usual maintenance dose: 1-4 mg once daily; after a dose of 2 mg once daily, increase in increments of 2 mg at 1- to 2-week intervals based upon the patient's blood glucose response to a maximum of 8 mg once daily

Elderly: Initial: 1 mg/day

Combination with insulin therapy (fasting glucose level for instituting combination therapy is in the range of >150 mg/dL in plasma or serum depending on the patient): 8 mg once daily with the first main meal

After starting with low-dose insulin, upward adjustments of insulin can be done approximately weekly as guided by frequent measurements of fasting blood glucose. Once stable, combination-therapy patients should monitor their capillary blood glucose on an ongoing basis, preferably daily.

**Mechanism of Action** Stimulates insulin release from the pancreatic beta cells; reduces glucose output from the liver; insulin sensitivity is increased at peripheral target sites

**Local Anesthetic/Vasoconstrictor Precautions** No information available to require special precautions

**Effects on Dental Treatment** Glipizide-dependent diabetics (noninsulin dependent, Type II) should be appointed for dental treatment in morning in order to minimize chance of stress-induced hypoglycemia

**Contraindications** Hypersensitivity to glimepiride or any component, other sulfonamides; diabetic ketoacidosis (with or without coma)

**Warnings/Precautions**

The administration of oral hypoglycemic drugs (ie, tolbutamide) has been reported to be associated with increased cardiovascular mortality as compared to treatment with diet alone or diet plus insulin

All sulfonylurea drugs are capable of producing severe hypoglycemia. Hypoglycemia is more likely to occur when caloric intake is deficient, after severe or prolonged exercise, when alcohol is ingested, or when more than one glucose-lowering drug is used.

**Drug Interactions**

Decreased effects: Beta-blockers, cholestyramine, hydantoins, rifampin, thiazide diuretics, urinary alkalines, charcoal

Increased effects: $H_2$ antagonists, anticoagulants, androgens, fluconazole, salicylates, gemfibrozil, sulfonamides, tricyclic antidepressants, probenecid, MAO inhibitors, methyldopa, digitalis glycosides, urinary acidifiers

Increased toxicity: Cimetidine → ↑ hypoglycemic effects

**Drug Uptake**

Duration of action: 24 hours

Peak blood glucose reductions: Within 2-3 hours

Absorption: 100% absorbed; delayed when given with food

Serum half-life: 5-9 hours

**Pregnancy Risk Factor** C

**Generic Available** No

## Glipizide (GLIP i zide)

**Related Information**

Endocrine Disorders & Pregnancy *on page 1082*

**U.S. Brand Names** Glucotrol®; Glucotrol® XL

**Therapeutic Category** Antidiabetic Agent; Hypoglycemic Agent, Oral; Sulfonylurea Agent

**Use** Management of noninsulin-dependent diabetes mellitus (type II)

**Usual Dosage** Oral (allow several days between dose titrations):

Adults: 2.5-40 mg/day; doses >15-20 mg/day should be divided and given twice daily

Elderly: Initial: 2.5-5 mg/day; increase by 2.5-5 mg/day at 1- to 2-week intervals

**Mechanism of Action** Stimulates insulin release from the pancreatic beta cells; reduces glucose output from the liver; insulin sensitivity is increased at peripheral target sites

**Local Anesthetic/Vasoconstrictor Precautions** No information available to require special precautions

**Effects on Dental Treatment** Glipizide-dependent diabetics (noninsulin dependent, Type II) should be appointed for dental treatment in morning in order to minimize chance of stress-induced hypoglycemia

**Other Adverse Effects**

>10%:

Central nervous system: Headache

Gastrointestinal: Anorexia, nausea, vomiting, diarrhea, epigastric fullness, constipation, heartburn

1% to 10%: Dermatologic: Rash, urticaria, photosensitivity

<1%:

Cardiovascular: Edema

Endocrine & metabolic: Hypoglycemia, hyponatremia

Hematologic: Blood dyscrasias, aplastic anemia, hemolytic anemia, bone marrow suppression, thrombocytopenia, agranulocytosis

Hepatic: Cholestatic jaundice

Renal: Diuretic effect

**Drug Interactions**

Salicylates may enhance the hypoglycemic response to glipizide due to increased plasma levels of glipizide by displacing from plasma proteins

(Continued)

## Glipizide *(Continued)*

Thiazide diuretics will increase blood glucose leading to increased requirements of glipizide

**Drug Uptake**

Duration of action: 12-24 hours
Peak blood glucose reductions: Within 1.5-2 hours
Absorption: Delayed when given with food
Serum half-life: 2-4 hours

**Pregnancy Risk Factor** C

**Generic Available** Yes

♦ **GlucaGen®** *see* Glucagon *on this page*

## Glucagon (GLOO ka gon)

**U.S. Brand Names** GlucaGen®

**Therapeutic Category** Antihypoglycemic Agent

**Use** Hypoglycemia; diagnostic aid in the radiologic examination of GI tract when a hypotonic state is needed; used with some success as a cardiac stimulant in management of severe cases of beta-adrenergic blocking agent overdosage

**Usual Dosage**

Hypoglycemia or insulin shock therapy: I.M., I.V., S.C.:
- Children: 0.025-0.1 mg/kg/dose, not to exceed 1 mg/dose, repeated in 20 minutes as needed
- Adults: 0.5-1 mg, may repeat in 20 minutes as needed

**If patient fails to respond to glucagon, I.V. dextrose must be given**

Diagnostic aid: Adults: I.M., I.V.: 0.25-2 mg 10 minutes prior to procedure

**Mechanism of Action** Stimulates adenylate cyclase to produce increased cyclic AMP, which promotes hepatic glycogenolysis and gluconeogenesis, causing a raise in blood glucose levels

**Local Anesthetic/Vasoconstrictor Precautions** No information available to require special precautions

**Effects on Dental Treatment** No effects or complications reported

**Other Adverse Effects** 1% to 10%:

Cardiovascular: Hypotension
Dermatologic: Urticaria
Gastrointestinal: Nausea, vomiting
Respiratory: Respiratory distress

**Drug Uptake**

Peak effect on blood glucose levels: Parenteral: Within 5-20 minutes
Duration of action: 60-90 minutes
Serum half-life, plasma: 3-10 minutes

**Pregnancy Risk Factor** B

**Generic Available** No

**Comments** 1 unit = 1 mg

♦ **Glucocerebrosidase** *see* Alglucerase *on page 47*

♦ **Glucophage®** *see* Metformin *on page 643*

## Glucose (GLOO kose, IN stant)

**U.S. Brand Names** B-D Glucose® [OTC]; Glutose® [OTC]; Insta-Glucose® [OTC]

**Therapeutic Category** Antihypoglycemic Agent

**Use** Management of hypoglycemia

**Usual Dosage** Adults: Oral: 10-20 g

**Local Anesthetic/Vasoconstrictor Precautions** No information available to require special precautions

**Effects on Dental Treatment** No effects or complications reported

**Other Adverse Effects** 1% to 10%:

Cardiovascular: Syncope
Gastrointestinal: Nausea, vomiting, diarrhea

**Pregnancy Risk Factor** A

**Generic Available** Yes

**Comments** 4 calories/g

## Glucose Polymers (GLOO kose POL i merz)

**U.S. Brand Names** Moducal® [OTC]; Polycose® [OTC]; Sumacal® [OTC]

**Therapeutic Category** Nutritional Supplement

**Use** Supplies calories for those persons not able to meet the caloric requirement with usual food intake

**Local Anesthetic/Vasoconstrictor Precautions** No information available to require special precautions

**Effects on Dental Treatment** No effects or complications reported

**Generic Available** Yes

- **Glucotrol®** *see* Glipizide *on page 469*
- **Glucotrol® XL** *see* Glipizide *on page 469*

## Glutamic Acid (gloo TAM ik AS id)

**Therapeutic Category** Gastrointestinal Agent, Miscellaneous
**Use** Treatment of hypochlorhydria and achlorhydria
**Usual Dosage** Adults: Oral:
Tablet/powder: 500-1000 mg/day before meals or food
Capsule: 1-3 capsules 3 times/day before meals
**Local Anesthetic/Vasoconstrictor Precautions** No information available to require special precautions
**Effects on Dental Treatment** No effects or complications reported
**Other Adverse Effects** Systemic acidosis may occur with massive overdosage
**Pregnancy Risk Factor** C
**Generic Available** Yes

## Glutethimide (gloo TETH i mide)

**Therapeutic Category** Hypnotic; Sedative
**Use** Short-term treatment of insomnia
**Usual Dosage** Oral:
Adults: 250-500 mg at bedtime, dose may be repeated but not less than 4 hours before intended awakening; maximum: 1 g/day
Elderly/debilitated patients: Total daily dose should not exceed 500 mg
**Local Anesthetic/Vasoconstrictor Precautions** No information available to require special precautions
**Effects on Dental Treatment** No effects or complications reported
**Other Adverse Effects**
>10%: Central nervous system: Daytime drowsiness
1% to 10%:
Central nervous system: Confusion, headache
Dermatologic: Skin rash
Gastrointestinal: Nausea, vomiting
Ocular: Blurred vision
<1%:
Hematologic: Blood dyscrasias
Cardiovascular: Bradycardia
Central nervous system: Paradoxical reaction, convulsions, fever
**Pregnancy Risk Factor** C
**Generic Available** Yes

- **Glutose® [OTC]** *see* Glucose *on previous page*
- **Glyate® [OTC]** *see* Guaifenesin *on page 478*

## Glyburide (GLYE byoor ide)

**Related Information**
Endocrine Disorders & Pregnancy *on page 1082*
**U.S. Brand Names** Diaβeta®; Glynase™ PresTab™; Micronase®
**Canadian Brand Names** Albert® Glyburide; Apo®-Glyburide; Euglucon®; Gen-Glybe; Novo-Glyburide; Nu-Glyburide
**Therapeutic Category** Antidiabetic Agent; Hypoglycemic Agent, Oral; Sulfonylurea Agent
**Use** Management of noninsulin-dependent diabetes mellitus (type II)
**Usual Dosage** Oral:
Adults: 1.25-5 mg to start then increase at weekly intervals to 1.25-20 mg maintenance dose/day divided in 1-2 doses
Elderly: Initial: 1.25-2.5 mg/day, increase by 1.25-2.5 mg/day every 1-3 weeks
PresTab™: Initial: 0.75-3 mg/day, increase by 1.5 mg/day in weekly intervals, maximum: 12 mg/day
**Mechanism of Action** Stimulates insulin release from the pancreatic beta cells; reduces glucose output from the liver; insulin sensitivity is increased at peripheral target sites
**Local Anesthetic/Vasoconstrictor Precautions** No information available to require special precautions
**Effects on Dental Treatment** Glyburide-dependent diabetics (noninsulin dependent, Type II) should be appointed for dental treatment in morning in order to minimize chance of stress-induced hypoglycemia
**Other Adverse Effects**
>10%:
Central nervous system: Headache, dizziness
(Continued)

## Glyburide *(Continued)*

Gastrointestinal: Nausea, epigastric fullness, heartburn, constipation, diarrhea, anorexia

1% to 10%: Dermatologic: Pruritus, rash, urticaria, photosensitivity reaction

<1%:

Endocrine & metabolic: Hypoglycemia

Genitourinary: Nocturia

Hematologic: Leukopenia, thrombocytopenia, hemolytic anemia, aplastic anemia, bone marrow suppression, agranulocytosis

Hepatic: Cholestatic jaundice

Neuromuscular & skeletal: arthralgia, paresthesia

Renal: Diuretic effect

**Drug Interactions**

Salicylates may enhance the hypoglycemic response to glyburide due to increased plasma levels of glyburide by displacing from plasma proteins

Thiazide diuretics will increase blood glucose leading to increased requirements of glyburide

**Drug Uptake**

Onset of action: Oral: Insulin levels in the serum begin to increase within 15-60 minutes after a single dose

Duration: Up to 24 hours

Serum half-life: 5-16 hours; may be prolonged with renal insufficiency or hepatic insufficiency

Time to peak serum concentration: Adults: Within 2-4 hours

**Pregnancy Risk Factor** C

**Generic Available** yes

## Glycerin (GLIS er in)

**U.S. Brand Names** Fleet® Babylax® Rectal [OTC]; Ophthalgan® Ophthalmic; Osmoglyn®; Sani-Supp® Suppository [OTC]

**Therapeutic Category** Laxative, Hyperosmolar

**Synonyms** Glycerol

**Use** Constipation; reduction of intraocular pressure; reduction of corneal edema; glycerin has been administered orally to reduce intracranial pressure

**Usual Dosage**

Constipation: Rectal:

Children <6 years: 1 infant suppository 1-2 times/day as needed or 2-5 mL as an enema

Children >6 years and Adults: 1 adult suppository 1-2 times/day as needed or 5-15 mL as an enema

Children and Adults:

Reduction of intraocular pressure: Oral: 1-1.8 g/kg 1-1½ hours preoperatively; additional doses may be administered at 5-hour intervals

Reduction of intracranial pressure: Oral: 1.5 g/kg/day divided every 4 hours; 1 g/kg/dose every 6 hours has also been used

Reduction of corneal edema: Ophthalmic solution: Instill 1-2 drops in eye(s) prior to examination OR for lubricant effect, instill 1-2 drops in eye(s) every 3-4 hours

**Mechanism of Action** Osmotic dehydrating agent which increases osmotic pressure; draws fluid into colon and thus stimulates evacuation

**Local Anesthetic/Vasoconstrictor Precautions** No information available to require special precautions

**Effects on Dental Treatment** No effects or complications reported

**Other Adverse Effects**

>10%:

Central nervous system: Headache

Gastrointestinal: Nausea, vomiting

1% to 10%:

Central nervous system: Confusion, dizziness

Endocrine: Polydipsia

Gastrointestinal: Diarrhea, dry mouth

<1%:

Cardiovascular: Arrhythmias

Endocrine & metabolic: Hyperglycemia

Gastrointestinal: Tenesmus, rectal irritation, cramping pain

**Drug Uptake**

Absorption:

Oral: Well absorbed

Rectal: Poorly absorbed

Decrease in intraocular pressure: Oral:

Onset of action: Within 10-30 minutes

Peak effect: Within 60-90 minutes
Duration: 4-8 hours
Reduction of intracranial pressure: Oral:
Onset of action: Within 10-60 minutes
Peak effect: Within 60-90 minutes
Duration: ~2-3 hours
Constipation: Suppository: Onset of action: 15-30 minutes
Serum half-life: 30-45 minutes

**Pregnancy Risk Factor** C

**Generic Available** Yes

## Glycerin, Lanolin, and Peanut Oil

(GLIS er in, LAN oh lin, & PEE nut oyl)

**U.S. Brand Names** Massé® Breast Cream [OTC]

**Therapeutic Category** Topical Skin Product

**Use** Nipple care of pregnant and nursing women

**Usual Dosage** Apply as often as needed

**Local Anesthetic/Vasoconstrictor Precautions** No information available to require special precautions

**Effects on Dental Treatment** No effects or complications reported

**Generic Available** Yes

- **Glycerol** *see* Glycerin *on previous page*
- **Glycerol-T®** *see* Theophylline and Guaifenesin *on page 973*
- **Glycerol Triacetate** *see* Triacetin *on page 1009*
- **Glycofed®** *see* Guaifenesin and Pseudoephedrine *on page 481*

## Glycopyrrolate (glye koe PYE roe late)

**U.S. Brand Names** Robinul®; Robinul® Forte

**Therapeutic Category** Anticholinergic Agent; Antispasmodic Agent, Gastrointestinal

**Use** Adjunct in treatment of peptic ulcer disease; inhibit salivation and excessive secretions of the respiratory tract preoperatively; reversal of neuromuscular blockade; control of upper airway secretions

**Usual Dosage**

Children:
Control of secretions:
Oral: 40-100 mcg/kg/dose 3-4 times/day
I.M., I.V.: 4-10 mcg/kg/dose every 3-4 hours; maximum: 0.2 mg/dose or 0.8 mg/24 hours
Intraoperative: I.V.: 4 mcg/kg not to exceed 0.1 mg; repeat at 2- to 3-minute intervals as needed
Preoperative: I.M.:
<2 years: 4.4-8.8 mcg/kg 30-60 minutes before procedure
>2 years: 4.4 mcg/kg 30-60 minutes before procedure

Children and Adults: Reverse neuromuscular blockade: I.V.: 0.2 mg for each 1 mg of neostigmine or 5 mg of pyridostigmine administered

Adults:
Intraoperative: I.V.: 0.1 mg repeated as needed at 2- to 3-minute intervals
Preoperative: I.M.: 4.4 mcg/kg 30-60 minutes before procedure
Peptic ulcer:
Oral: 1-2 mg 2-3 times/day
I.M., I.V.: 0.1-0.2 mg 3-4 times/day

**Mechanism of Action** Blocks the action of acetylcholine at parasympathetic sites in smooth muscle, secretory glands, and the CNS

**Local Anesthetic/Vasoconstrictor Precautions** No information available to require special precautions

**Effects on Dental Treatment** >10% of patients will experience significant dry mouth (reversible with cessation of drug therapy)

**Other Adverse Effects**

>10%:
Dermatologic: Dry skin
Gastrointestinal: Constipation
Local: Irritation at injection site
Respiratory: Dry nose, throat
Miscellaneous: Decreased sweating

1% to 10%:
Dermatologic: Photosensitivity
Endocrine & metabolic: Decreased flow of breast milk
Gastrointestinal: Dysphagia

(Continued)

## Glycopyrrolate *(Continued)*

<1%:
- Cardiovascular: Orthostatic hypotension, ventricular fibrillation, tachycardia, palpitations
- Central nervous system: Confusion, drowsiness, headache, loss of memory, fatigue, ataxia
- Dermatologic: Skin rash
- Gastrointestinal: Bloated feeling, nausea, vomiting
- Genitourinary: Dysuria
- Neuromuscular & skeletal: Weakness
- Ocular: Increased intraocular pain, blurred vision

**Drug Interactions**

Decreased effect of levodopa
Increased toxicity with amantadine

**Drug Uptake**

Oral: Onset of action: Within 50 minutes
I.M.: Onset of action: 20-40 minutes
I.V.: Onset of action: 10-15 minutes
Absorption: Oral: Poor and erratic

**Pregnancy Risk Factor** B

**Generic Available** Yes

- ♦ **Glycotuss® [OTC]** *see* Guaifenesin *on page 478*
- ♦ **Glycotuss-dM® [OTC]** *see* Guaifenesin and Dextromethorphan *on page 479*
- ♦ **Glynase™ PresTab™** *see* Glyburide *on page 471*
- ♦ **Gly-Oxide® Oral [OTC]** *see* Carbamide Peroxide *on page 186*
- ♦ **Glyset®** *see* Miglitol *on page 676*
- ♦ **Glytuss® [OTC]** *see* Guaifenesin *on page 478*
- ♦ **GM-CSF** *see* Sargramostim *on page 904*

## Gold Sodium Thiomalate (gold SOW dee um thye oh MAL ate)

**U.S. Brand Names** Aurolate®

**Therapeutic Category** Gold Compound

**Use** Treatment of progressive rheumatoid arthritis

**Usual Dosage** I.M.:

Children: Initial: Test dose of 10 mg is recommended, followed by 1 mg/kg/week for 20 weeks; maintenance: 1 mg/kg/dose at 2- to 4-week intervals thereafter for as long as therapy is clinically beneficial and toxicity does not develop. Administration for 2-4 months is usually required before clinical improvement is observed.

Adults: 10 mg first week; 25 mg second week; then 25-50 mg/week until 1 g cumulative dose has been given; if improvement occurs without adverse reactions, give 25-50 mg every 2-3 weeks for 2-20 weeks, then every 3-4 weeks indefinitely

**Mechanism of Action** Unknown, may decrease prostaglandin synthesis or may alter cellular mechanisms by inhibiting sulfhydryl systems

**Local Anesthetic/Vasoconstrictor Precautions** No information available to require special precautions

**Effects on Dental Treatment** No effects or complications reported

**Other Adverse Effects**

>10%:
- Dermatologic: Itching, skin rash
- Gastrointestinal: Stomatitis, gingivitis, glossitis
- Ocular: Conjunctivitis

1% to 10%:
- Dermatologic: Urticaria, alopecia
- Hematologic: Eosinophilia, leukopenia, thrombocytopenia
- Renal: Hematuria, proteinuria

<1%:
- Dermatologic: Angioedema, gray-to-blue pigmentation
- Gastrointestinal: Dysphagia, ulcerative enterocolitis, GI hemorrhage, metallic taste
- Hematologic: Agranulocytosis, anemia, aplastic anemia
- Hepatic: Hepatotoxicity
- Neuromuscular & skeletal: Peripheral neuropathy
- Respiratory: Interstitial pneumonitis

**Drug Uptake**

Serum half-life: 5 days; may lengthen with multiple doses
Time to peak serum concentration: Within 4-6 hours

**Pregnancy Risk Factor** C

**Generic Available** Yes

**Comments** Approximately 50% gold

- **GoLYTELY®** *see* Polyethylene Glycol-Electrolyte Solution *on page 815*
- **Gonak™ [OTC]** *see* Hydroxypropyl Methylcellulose *on page 517*
- **Gonal-F®** *see* Follitropin Alpha *on page 453*
- **Gonic®** *see* Chorionic Gonadotropin *on page 246*
- **Gonioscopic Ophthalmic Solution** *see* Hydroxypropyl Methylcellulose *on page 517*
- **Goniosol® [OTC]** *see* Hydroxypropyl Methylcellulose *on page 517*
- **Goody's® Headache Powders** *see* Acetaminophen, Aspirin, and Caffeine *on page 31*
- **Gordofilm® Liquid** *see* Salicylic Acid *on page 900*

## Goserelin (GOE se rel in)

**U.S. Brand Names** Zoladex® Implant

**Therapeutic Category** Gonadotropin Releasing Hormone Analog

**Use** Palliative treatment of advanced prostate cancer; in combination with flutamide for the management of locally confined stage T2b-T4 (stage B2-C) carcinoma of the prostate

**Usual Dosage**

Adults: S.C.: 3.6 mg injected into upper abdomen every 28 days; do not try to aspirate with the goserelin syringe, if the needle is in a large vessel, blood will immediately appear in syringe chamber

Prostate carcinoma: Intended for long-term administration

Endometriosis: Recommended duration is 6 months; retreatment is not recommended since safety data is not available

**Mechanism of Action** LHRH synthetic analog of luteinizing hormone-releasing hormone also known as gonadotropin-releasing hormone (GnRH) incorporated into a biodegradable depot material which allows for continuous slow release over 28 days; mechanism of action is similar to leuprolide

**Local Anesthetic/Vasoconstrictor Precautions** No information available to require special precautions

**Effects on Dental Treatment** No effects or complications reported

**Other Adverse Effects**

General: Worsening of signs and symptoms may occur during the first few weeks of therapy and are usually manifested by an increase in bone pain, increased difficulty in urinating, hot flashes, injection site irritation, and weakness; this will subside, but patients should be aware

>10%:

Endocrine & metabolic: Gynecomastia, postmenopausal symptoms, sexual dysfunction, loss of libido, hot flashes

Genitourinary: Impotence, decreased erection

1% to 10%:

Cardiovascular: Edema

Central nervous system: Headache, spinal cord compression (possible result of tumor flare), lethargy, dizziness, insomnia

Dermatologic: Rash

Endocrine & metabolic: Breast tenderness/enlargement, vaginal spotting and breakthrough bleeding

Gastrointestinal: Nausea and vomiting, anorexia, diarrhea, weight gain

Local: Pain on injection

Neuromuscular & skeletal: Bone loss, increased bone pain

Miscellaneous: Sweating

**Drug Uptake**

Absorption:

Oral: Inactive when administered orally

S.C.: Rapid and can be detected in the serum in 10 minutes

Time to peak serum concentration: S.C.: 12-15 days

Serum half-life: Following a bolus S.C. dose: 5 hours

**Pregnancy Risk Factor** X

**Generic Available** No

## Granisetron (gra NI se tron)

**U.S. Brand Names** Kytril®

**Therapeutic Category** Antiemetic; Selective 5-$HT_3$ Receptor Antagonist

**Use** Prophylaxis and treatment of chemotherapy-related emesis; may be prescribed for patients who are refractory to or have severe adverse reactions to standard antiemetic therapy. Granisetron may be prescribed for young patients (ie, <45 years of age who are more likely to develop extrapyramidal reactions to high-dose metoclopramide) who are to receive highly emetogenic chemotherapeutic agents as listed:

(Continued)

## Granisetron *(Continued)*

Agents with high emetogenic potential (>90%) (dose/m²):

- Carmustine ≥200 mg
- Cisplatin ≥75 mg
- Cyclophosphamide ≥1000 mg
- Cytarabine ≥1000 mg
- Dacarbazine ≥500 mg
- Ifosfamide ≥1000 mg
- Lomustine ≥60 mg
- Mechlorethamine
- Pentostatin
- Streptozocin

**or** two agents classified as having high or moderately high emetogenic potential as listed:

Agents with moderately high emetogenic potential (60% to 90%) (dose/m²):

- Carmustine <200 mg
- Cisplatin <75 mg
- Cyclophosphamide 1000 mg
- Cytarabine 250-1000 mg
- Dacarbazine <500 mg
- Doxorubicin ≥75 mg
- Ifosfamide
- Lomustine <60 mg
- Methotrexate ≥250 mg
- Mitomycin
- Mitoxantrone
- Procarbazine

Granisetron should not be prescribed for chemotherapeutic agents with a low emetogenic potential (eg, bleomycin, busulfan, cyclophosphamide <1000 mg, etoposide, 5-fluorouracil, vinblastine, vincristine)

**Usual Dosage**

I.V.: Children and Adults: 10 mcg/kg for 1-3 doses. Doses should be administered as a single IVPB over 5 minutes to 1 hour, given just prior to chemotherapy (15-60 minutes before); as intervention therapy for breakthrough nausea and vomiting, during the first 24 hours following chemotherapy, 2 or 3 repeat infusions (same dose) have been administered, separated by at least 10 minutes

Oral: Adults: 1 mg twice daily; the first 1 mg dose should be given up to 1 hour before chemotherapy, and the second tablet, 12 hours after the first

**Note: Granisetron should only be given on the day(s) of chemotherapy**

**Mechanism of Action** Selective 5-HT$_3$ receptor antagonist, blocking serotonin, both peripherally on vagal nerve terminals and centrally in the chemoreceptor trigger zone

**Local Anesthetic/Vasoconstrictor Precautions** No information available to require special precautions

**Effects on Dental Treatment** No effects or complications reported

**Other Adverse Effects**

>10%: Central nervous system: Headache

1% to 10%:

- Cardiovascular: Transient blood pressure changes
- Central nervous system: Dizziness, insomnia, anxiety
- Gastrointestinal: Constipation, abdominal pain, diarrhea
- Neuromuscular & skeletal: Weakness

<1%:

- Cardiovascular: Arrhythmias
- Central nervous system: Somnolence, agitation
- Endocrine & metabolic: Hot flashes
- Hepatic: Liver enzyme elevations

**Drug Interactions** No data reported

**Drug Uptake**

Onset of action: Commonly controls emesis within 1-3 minutes of administration

Duration: Effects generally last no more than 24 hours maximum

Serum half-life:

- Cancer patients: 10-12 hours
- Healthy volunteers: 3-4 hours

**Pregnancy Risk Factor** B

**Generic Available** No

♦ **Granulex** *see* Trypsin, Balsam Peru, and Castor Oil *on page 1030*

♦ **Granulocyte Colony Stimulating Factor** *see* Filgrastim *on page 430*

- **Granulocyte-Macrophage Colony Stimulating Factor** *see* Sargramostim *on page 904*

## Grepafloxacin (grep a FLOX a sin)

**U.S. Brand Names** Raxar®

**Therapeutic Category** Antibiotic, Quinolone

**Use** Treatment of acute bacterial exacerbations of chronic bronchitis caused by *Haemophilus influenzae, Streptococcus pneumoniae*, or *Moxaxella catarrhalis*; community-acquired pneumonia caused by *Mycoplasma pneumoniae* or the organisms previously mentioned; uncomplicated gonorrhea caused by *Neisseria gonorrhoeae*, and nongonococcal cervicitis and urethritis caused by *Chlamydia trachomatis*

**Usual Dosage** Adults: Oral: 400-600 mg every 24 hours (given in a single dose)

**Mechanism of Action** Inhibits DNA-gyrase in susceptible organisms; inhibits relaxation of supercoiled DNA and promotes breakage of double-stranded DNA

**Local Anesthetic/Vasoconstrictor Precautions** No information available to require special precautions

**Effects on Dental Treatment** No effects or complications reported

**Contraindications** In patients with hepatic failure; given concomitantly with class I and III antiarrhythmics or bepridil due to the potential risk of cardiac arrhythmias (including torsade de pointes)

**Drug Uptake**

Duration of action: 12 hours after dosing (400 mg), plasma levels were <0.5 mcg/mL

Absorption: Peak plasma levels at 2-5 hours

Half-life: 5-12 hours

- **Grifulvin® V** *see* Griseofulvin *on this page*
- **Grisactin®** *see* Griseofulvin *on this page*
- **Grisactin® Ultra** *see* Griseofulvin *on this page*

## Griseofulvin (gri see oh FUL vin)

**U.S. Brand Names** Fulvicin® P/G; Fulvicin-U/F®; Grifulvin® V; Grisactin®; Grisactin® Ultra; Gris-PEG®

**Canadian Brand Names** Grisovin®-FP

**Therapeutic Category** Antifungal Agent, Systemic

**Use** Treatment of susceptible tinea infections of the skin, hair, and nails

**Usual Dosage** Oral:

Children:

Microsize: 10-15 mg/kg/day in single or divided doses

Ultramicrosize: >2 months: 5.5-7.3 mg/kg/day in single or divided doses

Adults:

Microsize: 500-1000 mg/day in single or divided doses

Ultramicrosize: 330-375 mg/day in single or divided doses; doses up to 750 mg/day have been used for infections more difficult to eradicate such as tinea unguium and tinea pedis

Duration of therapy depends on the site of infection:

Tinea corporis: 2-4 weeks

Tinea capitis: 4-6 weeks or longer

Tinea pedis: 4-8 weeks

Tinea unguium: 4-6 months

**Mechanism of Action** Inhibits fungal cell mitosis at metaphase; binds to human keratin making it resistant to fungal invasion

**Local Anesthetic/Vasoconstrictor Precautions** No information available to require special precautions

**Effects on Dental Treatment** Griseofulvin may cause soreness or irritation of mouth or tongue

**Other Adverse Effects**

>10%: Dermatologic: Skin rash, urticaria

1% to 10%:

Central nervous system: Headache, fatigue, dizziness, insomnia, mental confusion

Dermatologic: Photosensitivity

Gastrointestinal: Nausea, vomiting, epigastric distress, diarrhea

Miscellaneous: Oral thrush

<1%:

Dermatologic: Angioneurotic edema

Endocrine & metabolic: Menstrual toxicity

Gastrointestinal: GI bleeding

Hematologic: Leukopenia

Hepatic: Hepatic toxicity

Renal: Proteinuria, nephrosis

(Continued)

## Griseofulvin *(Continued)*

**Drug Interactions**
Decreased effect:
Barbiturates leads to decreased levels of griseofulvin
Decreased warfarin activity
Decreased oral contraceptive effectiveness
Increased toxicity: With alcohol causes tachycardia and flushing

**Drug Uptake**
Absorption: Ultramicrosize griseofulvin absorption is almost complete; absorption of microsize griseofulvin is variable (25% to 70% of an oral dose); absorption is enhanced by ingestion of a fatty meal
Serum half-life: 9-22 hours

**Pregnancy Risk Factor** C
**Generic Available** Yes

- **Gris-PEG®** *see* Griseofulvin *on previous page*
- **Guaifed® [OTC]** *see* Guaifenesin and Pseudoephedrine *on page 481*
- **Guaifed-PD®** *see* Guaifenesin and Pseudoephedrine *on page 481*

## Guaifenesin (gwye FEN e sin)

**Related Information**
Guaifenesin and Phenylephrine *on page 480*
Guaifenesin, Pseudoephedrine, and Dextromethorphan *on page 482*

**U.S. Brand Names** Anti-Tuss® Expectorant [OTC]; Breonesin® [OTC]; Diabetic Tussin® EX [OTC]; Duratuss-G®; Fenesin™; Gee Gee® [OTC]; Genatuss® [OTC]; GG-Cen® [OTC]; Glyate® [OTC]; Glycotuss® [OTC]; Glytuss® [OTC]; Guaifenex® LA; GuiaCough® Expectorant [OTC]; Guiatuss® [OTC]; Halotussin® [OTC]; Humibid® L.A.; Humibid® Sprinkle; Hytuss® [OTC]; Hytuss-2X® [OTC]; Liquibid®; Medi-Tuss® [OTC]; Monafed®; Muco-Fen-LA®; Mytussin® [OTC]; Naldecon® Senior EX [OTC]; Organidin® NR; Pneumomist®; Respa-GF®; Robitussin® [OTC]; Scot-Tussin® [OTC]; Siltussin® [OTC]; Sinumist®-SR Capsulets®; Touro Ex®; Tusibron® [OTC]; Uni-tussin® [OTC]

**Canadian Brand Names** Balminil® Expectorant; Calmylin Expectorant

**Therapeutic Category** Expectorant

**Use** Temporary control of cough due to minor throat and bronchial irritation

**Usual Dosage** Oral:
Children:
<2 years: 12 mg/kg/day in 6 divided doses
2-5 years: 50-100 mg every 4 hours, not to exceed 600 mg/day
6-11 years: 100-200 mg every 4 hours, not to exceed 1.2 g/day
Children >12 years and Adults: 200-400 mg every 4 hours to a maximum of 2.4 g/day

**Mechanism of Action** Thought to act as an expectorant by irritating the gastric mucosa and stimulating respiratory tract secretions, thereby increasing respiratory fluid volumes and decreasing phlegm viscosity

**Local Anesthetic/Vasoconstrictor Precautions** No information available to require special precautions

**Effects on Dental Treatment** No effects or complications reported

**Other Adverse Effects** 1% to 10%:
Central nervous system: Drowsiness, headache
Dermatologic: Rash
Gastrointestinal: Nausea, vomiting, stomach pain

**Drug Interactions** No data reported

**Drug Uptake** Absorption: Well absorbed from GI tract

**Pregnancy Risk Factor** C

**Generic Available** Yes

## Guaifenesin and Codeine (gwye FEN e sin & KOE deen)

**U.S. Brand Names** Brontex® Liquid; Brontex® Tablet; Cheracol®; Guaituss AC®; Guiatussin® with Codeine; Mytussin® AC; Robafen® AC; Robitussin® A-C; Tussi-Organidin® NR

**Therapeutic Category** Antitussive; Cough Preparation; Expectorant

**Use** Temporary control of cough due to minor throat and bronchial irritation

**Usual Dosage** Oral:
Children:
2-6 years: 1-1.5 mg/kg codeine/day divided into 4 doses administered every 4-6 hours (maximum: 30 mg/24 hours)
6-12 years: 5 mL every 4 hours, not to exceed 30 mL/24 hours
Children >12 years and Adults: 5-10 mL every 4-8 hours not to exceed 60 mL/24 hours

**Mechanism of Action**
Guaifenesin is thought to act as an expectorant by irritating the gastric mucosa and stimulating respiratory tract secretions, thereby increasing respiratory fluid volumes and decreasing phlegm viscosity
Codeine is an antitussive that controls cough by depressing the medullary cough center

**Local Anesthetic/Vasoconstrictor Precautions** No information available to require special precautions

**Effects on Dental Treatment** No effects or complications reported

**Other Adverse Effects**
Codeine:
>10%:
Central nervous system: Drowsiness
Gastrointestinal: Constipation
1% to 10%:
Cardiovascular: Hypotension, palpitations, tachycardia or bradycardia, peripheral vasodilation
Central nervous system: CNS depression, sedation, confusion, headache, increased intracranial pressure, dizziness, lightheadedness, false feeling of well being, restlessness, paradoxical CNS stimulation, malaise
Dermatologic: Skin rash, urticaria
Endocrine & metabolic: Antidiuretic hormone release
Gastrointestinal: Nausea, vomiting, anorexia, dry mouth, biliary spasm
Genitourinary: Decreased urination, urinary tract spasm
Neuromuscular & skeletal: Weakness
Ocular: Miosis, blurred vision
Respiratory: Respiratory depression, dyspnea
Miscellaneous: Histamine release, physical and psychological dependence with prolonged use
<1%:
Central nervous system: Convulsions, hallucinations, mental depression, nightmares, insomnia
Gastrointestinal: Stomach cramps, paralytic ileus
Neuromuscular & skeletal: Trembling, muscle rigidity
Guaifenesin: 1% to 10%:
Central nervous system: Drowsiness, headache
Dermatologic: Rash
Gastrointestinal: Nausea, vomiting, stomach pain

**Drug Interactions** Increased toxicity: CNS depressant medications produce additive sedative properties

**Pregnancy Risk Factor** C

**Generic Available** Yes

## Guaifenesin and Dextromethorphan

(gwye FEN e sin & deks troe meth OR fan)

**U.S. Brand Names** Benylin® Expectorant [OTC]; Cheracol® D [OTC]; Clear Tussin® 30; Contac® Cough Formula Liquid [OTC]; Diabetic Tussin DM® [OTC]; Extra Action Cough Syrup [OTC]; Fenesin DM®; Genatuss DM® [OTC]; Glyco-tuss-dM® [OTC]; Guaifenex® DM; GuiaCough® [OTC]; Guiatuss-DM® [OTC]; Halotussin® DM [OTC]; Humibid® DM [OTC]; Iobid DM®; Kolephrin® GG/DM [OTC]; Monafed® DM; Muco-Fen-DM®; Mytussin® DM [OTC]; Naldecon® Senior DX [OTC]; Phanatuss® Cough Syrup [OTC]; Phenadex® Senior [OTC]; Respa-DM®; Rhinosyn-DMX® [OTC]; Robafen DM® [OTC]; Robitussin®-DM [OTC]; Safe Tussin® 30 [OTC]; Scot-Tussin® Senior Clear [OTC]; Siltussin DM® [OTC]; Synacol® CF [OTC]; Syracol-CF® [OTC]; Tolu-Sed® DM [OTC]; Tusibron-DM® [OTC]; Tuss-DM® [OTC]; Tussi-Organidin® DM NR; Uni-tussin® DM [OTC]; Vicks® 44E [OTC]; Vicks® Pediatric Formula 44E [OTC]

**Therapeutic Category** Antitussive; Cough Preparation; Expectorant

**Use** Temporary control of cough due to minor throat and bronchial irritation

**Usual Dosage** Oral:
Children: Dextromethorphan: 1-2 mg/kg/24 hours divided 3-4 times/day
Children >12 years and Adults: 5 mL every 4 hours or 10 mL every 6-8 hours not to exceed 40 mL/24 hours

**Mechanism of Action**
Guaifenesin is thought to act as an expectorant by irritating the gastric mucosa and stimulating respiratory tract secretions, thereby increasing respiratory fluid volumes and decreasing phlegm viscosity
Dextromethorphan is a chemical relative of morphine lacking narcotic properties except in overdose; controls cough by depressing the medullary cough center

**Local Anesthetic/Vasoconstrictor Precautions** No information available to require special precautions

**Effects on Dental Treatment** No effects or complications reported

(Continued)

## Guaifenesin and Dextromethorphan *(Continued)*

**Other Adverse Effects** 1% to 10%:

Central nervous system: Drowsiness, headache

Dermatologic: Rash

Gastrointestinal: Nausea, vomiting

**Warnings/Precautions** Research on chicken embryos exposed to concentrations of dextromethorphan relative to those typically taken by humans has shown to cause birth defects and fetal death; more study is needed, but it is suggested that pregnant women should be advised not to use dextromethorphan-containing medications

**Drug Interactions** No data reported

**Drug Uptake** Onset of action: Exerts its antitussive effect in 15-30 minutes after oral administration

**Pregnancy Risk Factor** C (see Warnings)

**Generic Available** Yes

♦ **Guaifenesin and Hydrocodone** *see* Hydrocodone and Guaifenesin *on page 508*

## Guaifenesin and Phenylephrine (gwye FEN e sin & fen il EF rin)

**U.S. Brand Names** Deconsal® Sprinkle®; Endal®; Sinupan®

**Therapeutic Category** Cold Preparation

**Synonyms** Phenylephrine and Guaifenesin

**Usual Dosage** Oral: Adults: 1 or 2 every 12 hours

**Mechanism of Action** See individual agents

**Local Anesthetic/Vasoconstrictor Precautions** Use with caution since phenylephrine is a sympathomimetic amine which could interact with epinephrine to cause a pressor response

**Effects on Dental Treatment**

Guaifenesin: No effects or complications reported

Phenylephrine: Up to 10% of patients could experience tachycardia, palpitations, and dry mouth; use vasoconstrictor with caution

**Other Adverse Effects** See individual agents

**Drug Interactions** See individual agents

**Dosage Forms**

Capsule, sustained release:

Deconsal® Sprinkle®: Guaifenesin 300 mg and phenylephrine hydrochloride 10 mg

Sinupan®: Guaifenesin 200 mg and phenylephrine hydrochloride 40 mg

Tablet, timed release (Endal®): Guaifenesin 300 mg and phenylephrine hydrochloride 20 mg

**Generic Available** No

## Guaifenesin and Phenylpropanolamine

(gwye FEN e sin & fen il proe pa NOLE a meen)

**U.S. Brand Names** Ami-Tex LA®; Coldlac-LA®; Conex® [OTC]; Contuss® XT; Dura-Vent®; Entex® LA; Genagesic®; Genamin® Expectorant [OTC]; Guaifenex® PPA 75; Guaipax®; Myminic® Expectorant [OTC]; Naldecon-EX® Children's Syrup [OTC]; Nolex® LA; Partuss® LA; Phenylfenesin® L.A.; Profen II®; Profen LA®; Rymed-TR®; Silaminic® Expectorant [OTC]; Sildicon-E® [OTC]; Snaplets-EX® [OTC]; Theramin® Expectorant [OTC]; Triaminic® Expectorant [OTC]; Tri-Clear® Expectorant [OTC]; Triphenyl® Expectorant [OTC]; ULR-LA®; Vicks® DayQuil® Sinus Pressure & Congestion Relief [OTC]

**Therapeutic Category** Decongestant; Expectorant

**Synonyms** Phenylpropanolamine and Guaifenesin

**Use** Symptomatic relief of those respiratory conditions where tenacious mucous plugs and congestion complicate the problem such as sinusitis, pharyngitis, bronchitis, asthma, and as an adjunctive therapy in serous otitis media

**Usual Dosage** Oral:

Children:

2-6 years: 2.5 mL every 4 hours

6-12 years: ½ tablet every 12 hours or 5 mL every 4 hours

Children >12 years and Adults: 1 tablet every 12 hours or 10 mL every 4 hours

**Local Anesthetic/Vasoconstrictor Precautions** Use with caution since phenylpropanolamine is a sympathomimetic amine which could interact with epinephrine to cause a pressor response

**Effects on Dental Treatment**

Guaifenesin: No effects or complications reported

Phenylpropanolamine: Up to 10% of patients could experience tachycardia, palpitations, and dry mouth; use vasoconstrictor with caution

**Pregnancy Risk Factor** C

**Generic Available** Yes

## Guaifenesin and Pseudoephedrine

(gwye FEN e sin & soo doe e FED rin)

**U.S. Brand Names** Congess® Jr; Congess® Sr; Congestac®; Deconsal® II; Defen-LA®; Entex® PSE; Eudal-SR®; Fedahist® Expectorant [OTC]; Fedahist® Expectorant Pediatric [OTC]; Glycofed®; Guaifed® [OTC]; Guaifed-PD®; Guaifenex® PSE; GuaiMAX-D®; Guaitab®; Guaivent®; Guai-Vent/PSE®; Guiatuss PE® [OTC]; Halotussin® PE [OTC]; Histalet® X; Nasabid™; Respa-1st®; Respaire®-60 SR; Respaire®-120 SR; Robitussin-PE® [OTC]; Robitussin® Severe Congestion Liqui-Gels® [OTC]; Ru-Tuss® DE; Rymed®; Sinufed® Timecelles®; Touro LA®; Tuss-LA®; V-Dec-M®; Versacaps®; Zephrex®; Zephrex LA®

**Therapeutic Category** Decongestant; Expectorant

**Synonyms** Pseudoephedrine and Guaifenesin

**Use** Enhance the output of respiratory tract fluid and reduce mucosal congestion and edema in the nasal passage

**Usual Dosage** Oral:

Children:

2-6 years: 2.5 mL every 4 hours not to exceed 15 mL/24 hours

6-12 years: 5 mL every 4 hours not to exceed 30 mL/24 hours

Children >12 years and Adults: 10 mL every 4 hours not to exceed 60 mL/24 hours

**Local Anesthetic/Vasoconstrictor Precautions** Use with caution since pseudoephedrine is a sympathomimetic amine which could interact with epinephrine to cause a pressor response

**Effects on Dental Treatment**

Guaifenesin: No effects or complications reported

Pseudoephedrine: Up to 10% of patients could experience tachycardia, palpitations, and dry mouth; use vasoconstrictor with caution

**Pregnancy Risk Factor** C

**Generic Available** Yes

## Guaifenesin, Phenylpropanolamine, and Dextromethorphan

(gwye FEN e sin, fen il proe pa NOLE a meen, & deks troe meth OR fan)

**U.S. Brand Names** Anatuss® [OTC]; Guiatuss CF® [OTC]; Naldecon® DX Adult Liquid [OTC]; Robafen® CF [OTC]; Robitussin-CF® [OTC]; Siltussin-CF® [OTC]

**Therapeutic Category** Cough Preparation; Decongestant; Expectorant

**Use** Temporarily relieves nasal congestion and controls cough due to minor throat and bronchial irritation; helps loosen phlegm and thin bronchial secretions to make coughs more productive

**Usual Dosage** Oral:

Children:

2-6 years: 2.5 mL every 4 hours not to exceed 15 mL/24 hours

6-12 years: 5 mL every 4 hours not to exceed 30 mL/24 hours

Children >12 years and Adults: 10 mL every 4 hours not to exceed 60 mL/24 hours

**Local Anesthetic/Vasoconstrictor Precautions** Use with caution since phenylpropanolamine is a sympathomimetic amine which could interact with epinephrine to cause a pressor response

**Effects on Dental Treatment**

Dextromethorphan, Guaifenesin: No effects or complications reported

Phenylpropanolamine: Up to 10% of patients could experience tachycardia, palpitations, and dry mouth; use vasoconstrictor with caution

**Warnings/Precautions** Research on chicken embryos exposed to concentrations of dextromethorphan relative to those typically taken by humans has shown to cause birth defects and fetal death; more study is needed, but it is suggested that pregnant women should be advised not to use dextromethorphan-containing medications

**Pregnancy Risk Factor** C (see Warnings)

**Generic Available** Yes

## Guaifenesin, Phenylpropanolamine, and Phenylephrine

(gwye FEN e sin, fen il proe pa NOLE a meen, & fen il EF rin)

**U.S. Brand Names** Coldloc®; Contuss®; Dura-Gest®; Enomine®; Entex®; Guaifenex®; Guiatex®

**Therapeutic Category** Decongestant; Expectorant

**Use** Temporary relief of nasal congestion, running nose, sneezing, itching of nose and throat, and itchy, watery eyes due to common cold, hay fever, or other upper respiratory allergies

(Continued)

## Guaifenesin, Phenylpropanolamine, and Phenylephrine *(Continued)*

**Usual Dosage** Children >12 years and Adults: 1 capsule/tablet or 10 mL 4 times/day (every 6 hours) with food or fluid

**Local Anesthetic/Vasoconstrictor Precautions** Use with caution since phenylpropanolamine and phenylephrine are sympathomimetic amines which could interact with epinephrine to cause a pressor response

**Effects on Dental Treatment**

Guaifenesin: No effects or complications reported

Phenylephrine, Phenylpropanolamine: Up to 10% of patients could experience tachycardia, palpitations, and dry mouth; use vasoconstrictor with caution

**Pregnancy Risk Factor** C

**Generic Available** Yes

## Guaifenesin, Pseudoephedrine, and Codeine

(gwye FEN e sin, soo doe e FED rin, & KOE deen)

**U.S. Brand Names** Codafed® Expectorant; Cycofed® Pediatric; Decohistine® Expectorant; Deproist® Expectorant with Codeine; Dihistine® Expectorant; Guiatuss DAC®; Guiatussin® DAC; Halotussin® DAC; Isoclor® Expectorant; Mytussin® DAC; Nucofed®; Nucofed® Pediatric Expectorant; Nucotuss®; Phenhist® Expectorant; Robitussin®-DAC; Ryna-CX®; Tussar® SF Syrup

**Therapeutic Category** Cough Preparation; Decongestant; Expectorant

**Use** Temporarily relieves nasal congestion and controls cough due to minor throat and bronchial irritation; helps loosen phlegm and thin bronchial secretions to make coughs more productive

**Usual Dosage** Oral:

Children 6-12 years: 5 mL every 4 hours, not to exceed 40 mL/24 hours

Children >12 years and Adults: 10 mL every 4 hours, not to exceed 40 mL/24 hours

**Local Anesthetic/Vasoconstrictor Precautions** Use with caution since pseudoephedrine is a sympathomimetic amine which could interact with epinephrine to cause a pressor response

**Effects on Dental Treatment**

Codeine: <1%: Dry mouth

Guaifenesin: No effects or complications reported

Pseudoephedrine: Up to 10% of patients could experience tachycardia, palpitations, and dry mouth; use vasoconstrictor with caution

**Pregnancy Risk Factor** C

**Generic Available** Yes

## Guaifenesin, Pseudoephedrine, and Dextromethorphan

(gwye FEN e sin, soo doe e FED rin, & deks troe meth OR fan)

**U.S. Brand Names** Anatuss® DM [OTC]; Dimacol® Caplets [OTC]; Novahistine® DMX Liquid [OTC]; Rhinosyn-X® Liquid [OTC]; Ru-Tuss® Expectorant [OTC]; Sudafed® Cold & Cough Liquid Caps [OTC]

**Therapeutic Category** Cold Preparation

**Synonyms** Dextromethorphan, Guaifenesin, and Pseudoephedrine; Pseudoephedrine, Dextromethorphan, and Guaifenesin

**Use** Temporarily relieves nasal congestion and controls cough due to minor throat and bronchial irritation; helps loosen phlegm and thin bronchial secretions to make coughs more productive

**Usual Dosage** Adults: Oral: 2 capsules (caplets) or 10 mL every 4 hours

**Mechanism of Action** See individual agents

**Local Anesthetic/Vasoconstrictor Precautions** Use with caution since pseudoephedrine is a sympathomimetic amine which could interact with epinephrine to cause a pressor response

**Effects on Dental Treatment**

Guaifenesin: No effects or complications reported

Pseudoephedrine: Up to 10% of patients could experience tachycardia, palpitations, and dry mouth; use vasoconstrictor with caution

Dextromethorphan: No effects or complications reported

**Other Adverse Effects** See individual agents

**Warnings/Precautions** Research on chicken embryos exposed to concentrations of dextromethorphan relative to those typically taken by humans has shown to cause birth defects and fetal death; more study is needed, but it is suggested that pregnant women should be advised not to use dextromethorphan-containing medications

**Drug Interactions** See individual agents

**Dosage Forms**

Caplets (Dimacol®): Guaifenesin 100 mg, pseudoephedrine hydrochloride 30 mg, and dextromethorphan hydrobromide 10 mg

Capsule (Sudafed® Cold & Cough Liquid Caps): Guaifenesin 100 mg, pseudoephedrine hydrochloride 30 mg, and dextromethorphan hydrobromide 10 mg

Liquid (Anatuss® DM, Novahistine® DMX Liquid, Rhinosyn-X® Liquid, Ru-Tuss® Expectorant): Guaifenesin 100 mg, pseudoephedrine hydrochloride 30 mg, and dextromethorphan hydrobromide 10 mg per 5 mL

**Generic Available** Yes

- **Guaifenex®** *see* Guaifenesin, Phenylpropanolamine, and Phenylephrine *on page 481*
- **Guaifenex® DM** *see* Guaifenesin and Dextromethorphan *on page 479*
- **Guaifenex® LA** *see* Guaifenesin *on page 478*
- **Guaifenex® PPA 75** *see* Guaifenesin and Phenylpropanolamine *on page 480*
- **Guaifenex® PSE** *see* Guaifenesin and Pseudoephedrine *on page 481*
- **GuaiMAX-D®** *see* Guaifenesin and Pseudoephedrine *on page 481*
- **Guaipax®** *see* Guaifenesin and Phenylpropanolamine *on page 480*
- **Guaitab®** *see* Guaifenesin and Pseudoephedrine *on page 481*
- **Guaituss AC®** *see* Guaifenesin and Codeine *on page 478*
- **Guaivent®** *see* Guaifenesin and Pseudoephedrine *on page 481*
- **Guai-Vent/PSE®** *see* Guaifenesin and Pseudoephedrine *on page 481*

## Guanabenz (GWAHN a benz)

**Related Information**

Cardiovascular Diseases *on page 1066*

**U.S. Brand Names** Wytensin®

**Therapeutic Category** Alpha-Adrenergic Blockers - Peripheral-Acting (Alpha$_1$-Blockers)

**Use** Management of hypertension

**Usual Dosage** Adults: Oral: Initial: 4 mg twice daily, increase in increments of 4-8 mg/day every 1-2 weeks to a maximum of 32 mg twice daily

**Mechanism of Action** Stimulates alpha$_2$-adrenoreceptors in the brain stem, thus activating an inhibitory neuron, resulting in reduced sympathetic outflow, producing a decrease in vasomotor tone and heart rate

**Local Anesthetic/Vasoconstrictor Precautions** No information available to require special precautions

**Effects on Dental Treatment** >10% of patients will experience significant dry mouth; normal salivation occurs with cessation of drug therapy

**Other Adverse Effects**

>10%:
- Central nervous system: Drowsiness, sedation, dizziness
- Neuromuscular & skeletal: Weakness

1% to 10%:
- Cardiovascular: Chest pain, edema
- Central nervous system: Headache
- Endocrine & metabolic: Decreased sexual ability
- Gastrointestinal: Nausea

<1%:
- Cardiovascular: Arrhythmias, palpitations
- Central nervous system: Anxiety, ataxia, depression, sleep disturbances
- Dermatologic: Rash, pruritus
- Endocrine & metabolic: Sexual dysfunction, gynecomastia
- Gastrointestinal: Diarrhea, vomiting, constipation, taste disorders
- Neuromuscular & skeletal: Myalgia
- Ocular: Blurring of vision
- Renal: Polyuria
- Respiratory: Nasal congestion, dyspnea

**Drug Interactions**

Decreased hypotensive effect of guanabenz with tricyclic antidepressants

Increased effect: Other hypotensive agents

**Drug Uptake**

Onset of antihypertensive effect: Within 1 hour

Absorption: ~75%

Serum half-life: 7-10 hours

**Pregnancy Risk Factor** C

**Generic Available** Yes

## Guanadrel (GWAHN a drel)

**Related Information**

Cardiovascular Diseases *on page 1066*

(Continued)

## Guanadrel *(Continued)*

**U.S. Brand Names** Hylorel®

**Therapeutic Category** Alpha-Adrenergic Blockers - Peripheral-Acting (Alpha$_1$-Blockers)

**Use** Considered a second line agent in the treatment of hypertension, usually with a diuretic

**Usual Dosage**

Adults: Oral: Initial: 10 mg/day (5 mg twice daily); adjust dosage until blood pressure is controlled, usual dosage: 20-75 mg/day, given twice daily

Elderly: Initial: 5 mg once daily

**Mechanism of Action** Acts as a false neurotransmitter that blocks the adrenergic actions of norepinephrine; it displaces norepinephrine from its presynaptic storage granules and thus exposes it to degradation; it thereby produces a reduction in total peripheral resistance and, therefore, blood pressure

**Local Anesthetic/Vasoconstrictor Precautions**

Manufacturer's information states that guanadrel may block vasopressor activity of epinephrine. This has not been observed during use of epinephrine as a vasoconstrictor in local anesthesia.

**Effects on Dental Treatment** No effects or complications reported

**Other Adverse Effects**

>10%:

- Cardiovascular: Palpitations, chest pain, peripheral edema, faintness
- Central nervous system: Fatigue, headache, drowsiness, confusion
- Gastrointestinal: Increased bowel movements, gas pain, constipation, anorexia, weight gain/loss
- Genitourinary: Nocturia, ejaculation disturbances
- Neuromuscular & skeletal: Paresthesia, aching limbs, leg cramps, backache, arthralgia
- Ocular: Visual disturbances
- Renal: Polyuria
- Respiratory: Dyspnea, coughing

1% to 10%:

- Cardiovascular: Orthostatic hypotension
- Central nervous system: Psychological problems, depression, sleep disorders
- Gastrointestinal: Glossitis, nausea, vomiting, dry mouth
- Genitourinary: Impotence
- Renal: Hematuria

<1%: Cardiovascular: Angina

**Drug Interactions**

Decreased effect with tricyclic antidepressants, indirect-acting amines (ephedrine, phenylpropanolamine), phenothiazines

Increased toxicity of direct-acting amines (epinephrine, norepinephrine)

Increased effect of beta-blockers, vasodilators

**Drug Uptake**

Peak effect: Within 4-6 hours

Duration: 4-14 hours

Absorption: Oral: Rapid

Serum half-life, biphasic:

- Initial: 1-4 hours
- Terminal: 5-45 hours

Time to peak serum concentration: Within 1.5-2 hour

**Pregnancy Risk Factor** B

**Generic Available** No

## Guanethidine (gwahn ETH i deen)

**Related Information**

Cardiovascular Diseases *on page 1066*

**U.S. Brand Names** Ismelin®

**Canadian Brand Names** Apo®-Guanethidine

**Therapeutic Category** Alpha-Adrenergic Blockers - Peripheral-Acting (Alpha$_1$-Blockers)

**Use** Treatment of moderate to severe hypertension

**Usual Dosage** Oral:

Children: Initial: 0.2 mg/kg/day, increase by 0.2 mg/kg/day at 7- to 10-day intervals to a maximum of 3 mg/kg/day

Adults:

- Ambulatory patients: Initial: 10 mg/day, increase at 5- to 7-day intervals to a maximum of 25-50 mg/day
- Hospitalized patients: Initial: 25-50 mg/day, increase by 25-50 mg/day or every other day to desired therapeutic response

Elderly: Initial: 5 mg once daily

**Mechanism of Action** Acts as a false neurotransmitter that blocks the adrenergic actions of norepinephrine; it displaces norepinephrine from its presynaptic storage granules and thus exposes it to degradation; it thereby produces a reduction in total peripheral resistance and, therefore, blood pressure

**Local Anesthetic/Vasoconstrictor Precautions** Manufacturer's information states that haloperidol may block vasopressor activity of epinephrine. This has not been observed during use of epinephrine as a vasoconstrictor in local anesthesia.

**Effects on Dental Treatment** No effects or complications reported

**Other Adverse Effects**

>10%:

- Cardiovascular: Palpitations, chest pain, peripheral edema, faintness
- Central nervous system: Fatigue, headache, drowsiness, confusion
- Gastrointestinal: Increased bowel movements, gas pain, constipation, anorexia, weight gain/loss
- Genitourinary: Nocturia, impotence, ejaculation disturbances
- Neuromuscular & skeletal: Paresthesia, aching limbs, leg cramps, backache, arthralgia
- Ocular: Visual disturbances
- Renal: Polyuria
- Respiratory: Dyspnea, coughing

1% to 10%:

- Cardiovascular: Orthostatic hypotension
- Central nervous system: Psychological problems, depression, sleep disorders
- Gastrointestinal: Glossitis, nausea, vomiting, dry mouth
- Renal: Hematuria

<1%: Cardiovascular: Angina

**Drug Interactions**

Decreased effect with tricyclic antidepressants, indirect-acting amines (ephedrine, phenylpropanolamine)

Increased toxicity of direct-acting amines (epinephrine, norepinephrine)

**Drug Uptake**

Onset of effect: Within 0.5-2 hours
Peak antihypertensive effect: Within 6-8 hours
Duration: 24-48 hours
Absorption: Irregular (3% to 55%)
Serum half-life: 5-10 days

**Pregnancy Risk Factor** C

**Generic Available** Yes

## Guanfacine (GWAHN fa seen)

**Related Information**

Cardiovascular Diseases *on page 1066*

**U.S. Brand Names** Tenex®

**Therapeutic Category** Alpha-Adrenergic Blockers - Peripheral-Acting (Alpha$_1$-Blockers)

**Use** Management of hypertension

**Usual Dosage** Adults: Oral: 1 mg usually at bedtime, may increase if needed at 3- to 4-week intervals to a maximum of 3 mg/day; 1 mg/day is most common dose

**Mechanism of Action** Stimulates alpha$_2$-adrenoreceptors in the brain stem, thus activating an inhibitory neuron, resulting in reduced sympathetic outflow, producing a decrease in vasomotor tone and heart rate

**Local Anesthetic/Vasoconstrictor Precautions** No information available to require special precautions

**Effects on Dental Treatment** >10% of patients experience dry mouth

**Other Adverse Effects**

>10%:

- Central nervous system: Somnolence, dizziness
- Gastrointestinal: Constipation

1% to 10%:

- Central nervous system: Fatigue, headache, insomnia
- Endocrine & metabolic: Decreased sexual ability
- Gastrointestinal: Nausea, vomiting
- Ocular: Conjunctivitis

<1%:

- Cardiovascular: Bradycardia, palpitations, substernal pain
- Central nervous system: Amnesia, confusion, depression, malaise
- Dermatologic: Dermatitis, pruritus, purpura
- Gastrointestinal: Abdominal pain, diarrhea, dyspepsia, dysphagia, taste perversion
- Genitourinary: Testicular disorder, urinary incontinence

(Continued)

## Guanfacine *(Continued)*

Neuromuscular & skeletal: Leg cramps, hypokinesia, paresthesia
Otic: Tinnitus
Respiratory: Rhinitis, dyspnea
Miscellaneous: Sweating

**Drug Interactions**
Decreased hypotensive effect of guanfacine with tricyclic antidepressants
Increased effect: Other hypotensive agents

**Drug Uptake**
Peak effect: Within 8-11 hours
Duration: 24 hours following a single dose
Serum half-life: 17 hours
Time to peak serum concentration: Within 1-4 hours

**Pregnancy Risk Factor** B
**Generic Available** No

- **GuiaCough® [OTC]** *see* Guaifenesin and Dextromethorphan *on page 479*
- **GuiaCough® Expectorant [OTC]** *see* Guaifenesin *on page 478*
- **Guiatex®** *see* Guaifenesin, Phenylpropanolamine, and Phenylephrine *on page 481*
- **Guiatuss® [OTC]** *see* Guaifenesin *on page 478*
- **Guiatuss CF® [OTC]** *see* Guaifenesin, Phenylpropanolamine, and Dextromethorphan *on page 481*
- **Guiatuss DAC®** *see* Guaifenesin, Pseudoephedrine, and Codeine *on page 482*
- **Guiatuss-DM® [OTC]** *see* Guaifenesin and Dextromethorphan *on page 479*
- **Guiatussin® DAC** *see* Guaifenesin, Pseudoephedrine, and Codeine *on page 482*
- **Guiatussin® with Codeine** *see* Guaifenesin and Codeine *on page 478*
- **Guiatuss PE® [OTC]** *see* Guaifenesin and Pseudoephedrine *on page 481*
- **Gum Benjamin** *see* Benzoin *on page 130*
- **G-well®** *see* Lindane *on page 592*
- **Gyne-Lotrimin® 3** *see* Clotrimazole *on page 267*
- **Gyne-Sulf®** *see* Sulfabenzamide, Sulfacetamide, and Sulfathiazole *on page 939*
- **Gynogen L.A.® Injection** *see* Estradiol *on page 387*
- **Gynol II® [OTC]** *see* Nonoxynol 9 *on page 728*
- **Habitrol™** *see* Nicotine *on page 718*

## *Haemophilus* b Conjugate Vaccine

(hem OF fi lus bee KON joo gate vak SEEN)

**U.S. Brand Names** HibTITER®; OmniHIB™; PedvaxHIB™; ProHIBiT®

**Therapeutic Category** Vaccine, Inactivated Bacteria

**Synonyms** Diphtheria $CRM_{197}$ Protein Conjugate; Diphtheria Toxoid Conjugate; *Haemophilus* b Oligosaccharide Conjugate Vaccine; *Haemophilus* b Polysaccharide Vaccine; HbCV; Hib Polysaccharide Conjugate; PRP-D

**Use** Immunization of children 24 months to 6 years of age against diseases caused by *H. influenzae* type b

**Usual Dosage** Children: I.M.: 0.5 mL as a single dose should be administered according to one of the following "brand-specific" schedules; do not inject I.V.

**Vaccination Schedule for Haemophilus b Conjugate Vaccines**

| Age at 1st Dose (mo) | HibTITER® | | PedvaxHIB® | | ProHIBiT® | |
|---|---|---|---|---|---|---|
| | Primary Series | Booster | Primary Series | Booster | Primary Series | Booster |
| 2-6* | 3 doses, 2 months apart | 15 mo† | 2 doses, 2 months apart | 12 mo† | | |
| 7-11 | 2 doses, 2 months apart | 15 mo† | 2 doses, 2 months apart | 15 mo† | | |
| 12-14 | 1 dose | 15 mo† | 1 dose | 15 mo† | | |
| 15-60 | 1 dose | — | 1 dose | — | 1 dose | — |

*It is not currently recommended that the various Haemophilus b conjugate vaccines be interchanged (ie, the same brand should be used throughout the entire vaccination series). If the health care provider does not know which vaccine was previously used, it is prudent that an infant, 2-6 months of age, be given a primary series of three doses.

†At least 2 months after previous dose.

**Mechanism of Action** Stimulates production of anticapsular antibodies and provides active immunity to *Haemophilus influenzae*; Hib conjugate vaccines use covalent binding of capsular polysaccharide of *Haemophilus influenzae* type b to diphtheria CRM 197 (HibTITER®) to produce an antigen which is postulated to convert a T-independent antigen into a T-dependent antigen to result in enhanced antibody response and on immunologic memory

**Local Anesthetic/Vasoconstrictor Precautions** No information available to require special precautions

**Effects on Dental Treatment** No effects or complications reported

**Other Adverse Effects** When administered during the same visit that DTP vaccine is given, the rates of systemic reactions do not differ from those observed only when DTP vaccine is administered

25%:
- Cardiovascular: Swelling
- Dermatologic: Local erythema
- Local: Increased risk of *Haemophilus* b infections in the week after vaccination
- Miscellaneous: Warmth

>10%: Acute febrile reactions

1% to 10%:
- Central nervous system: Fever (up to 102.2°F), irritability, lethargy
- Gastrointestinal: Anorexia, diarrhea
- Local: Irritation at injection site

<1%:
- Cardiovascular: Edema of face, eyes
- Central nervous system: Convulsions, fever >102.2°F, unusual fatigue
- Dermatologic: Urticaria, itching
- Gastrointestinal: Vomiting
- Neuromuscular & skeletal: Weakness
- Respiratory: Dyspnea
- Miscellaneous: Allergic or anaphylactic reactions

**Drug Uptake**

The seroconversion following one dose of Hib vaccine for children 18 months or 24 months of age or older is 75% to 90% respectively

Onset of serum antibody responses: 1-2 weeks after vaccination

Duration: Immunity appears to last 1.5 years

**Pregnancy Risk Factor** C

**Generic Available** No

**Comments** Federal law requires that the date of administration, the vaccine manufacturer, lot number of vaccine, and the administering person's name, title and address be entered into the patient's permanent medical record

- ***Haemophilus* b Oligosaccharide Conjugate Vaccine** *see Haemophilus* b Conjugate Vaccine *on previous page*
- ***Haemophilus* b Polysaccharide Vaccine** *see Haemophilus* b Conjugate Vaccine *on previous page*

## Halazepam (hal AZ e pam)

**U.S. Brand Names** Paxipam®

**Therapeutic Category** Benzodiazepine

**Use** Management of anxiety disorders; short-term relief of the symptoms of anxiety

**Usual Dosage** Adults: Oral: 20-40 mg 3-4 times/day

**Mechanism of Action** Benzodiazepines appear to potentiate the effects of GABA and other inhibitory neurotransmitters by binding to specific benzodiazepine-receptor sites in various areas of the CNS

**Local Anesthetic/Vasoconstrictor Precautions** No information available to require special precautions

**Effects on Dental Treatment** >10% of patients experience significant dry mouth; normal salivary flow occurs with cessation of drug therapy

**Other Adverse Effects**

>10%:
- Cardiovascular: Chest pain
- Central nervous system: Drowsiness, fatigue, lightheadedness, memory impairment, insomnia, anxiety, depression, headache, ataxia
- Dermatologic: Rash
- Endocrine & metabolic: Decreased libido
- Gastrointestinal: Constipation, diarrhea, decreased salivation, nausea, vomiting, increased or decreased appetite
- Neuromuscular & skeletal: Dysarthria
- Miscellaneous: Sweating

1% to 10%:
- Cardiovascular: Syncope, tachycardia, hypotension
- Central nervous system: Confusion, nervousness, dizziness, akathisia
- Dermatologic: Dermatitis
- Gastrointestinal: Weight gain or loss, increased salivation
- Neuromuscular & skeletal: Rigidity, tremor, muscle cramps

(Continued)

## Halazepam *(Continued)*

Ocular: Blurred vision
Otic: Tinnitus
Respiratory: Nasal congestion, hyperventilation

<1%:

Endocrine & metabolic: Menstrual irregularities
Hematologic: Blood dyscrasias
Neuromuscular & skeletal: Reflex slowing
Miscellaneous: Drug dependence

**Drug Uptake**

Half-life:

Parent: 14 hours
Active metabolite (desmethyldiazepam): 50-100 hours

Peak level: 1-3 hours

**Pregnancy Risk Factor** D

**Generic Available** No

**Comments** Halazepam offers no significant advantage over other benzodiazepines

## Halcinonide (hal SIN oh nide)

**Related Information**

Corticosteroids, Topical Comparison *on page 1222*

**U.S. Brand Names** Halog®; Halog®-E

**Therapeutic Category** Corticosteroid, Topical (High Potency)

**Use** Inflammation of corticosteroid-responsive dermatoses [high potency topical corticosteroid]

**Usual Dosage** Children and Adults: Topical: Apply sparingly 1-3 times/day, occlusive dressing may be used for severe or resistant dermatoses; a thin film of cream or ointment is effective; do not overuse

**Mechanism of Action** Decreases inflammation by suppression of migration of polymorphonuclear leukocytes and reversal of increased capillary permeability

**Local Anesthetic/Vasoconstrictor Precautions** No information available to require special precautions

**Effects on Dental Treatment** No effects or complications reported

**Other Adverse Effects** <1%:

Dermatologic: Itching, dry skin, folliculitis, hypertrichosis, acneiform eruptions, hypopigmentation, perioral dermatitis, allergic contact dermatitis, skin maceration, skin atrophy, striae
Local: Burning, irritation, miliaria
Miscellaneous: Secondary infection

**Drug Interactions** No data reported

**Drug Uptake** Absorption: Percutaneous absorption varies by location of topical application and the use of occlusive dressings

**Pregnancy Risk Factor** C

**Dosage Forms**

Cream (Halog®): 0.025% (15 g, 60 g, 240 g); 0.1% (15 g, 30 g, 60 g, 240 g)
Cream, emollient base (Halog®-E) : 0.1% (15 g, 30 g, 60 g)
Ointment, topical (Halog®): 0.1% (15 g, 30 g, 60 g, 240 g)
Solution (Halog®): 0.1% (20 mL, 60 mL)

**Generic Available** No

- **Halcion®** *see* Triazolam *on page 1013*
- **Haldol®** *see* Haloperidol *on next page*
- **Haldol® Decanoate** *see* Haloperidol *on next page*
- **Haldrone®** *see* Paramethasone Acetate *on page 765*
- **Halenol® Childrens [OTC]** *see* Acetaminophen *on page 27*
- **Haley's M-O® [OTC]** *see* Magnesium Hydroxide and Mineral Oil Emulsion *on page 612*
- **Halfan®** *see* Halofantrine *on next page*
- **Halfprin® 81® [OTC]** *see* Aspirin *on page 100*

## Halobetasol (hal oh BAY ta sol)

**U.S. Brand Names** Ultravate™

**Therapeutic Category** Corticosteroid, Topical (Very High Potency)

**Use** Relief of inflammatory and pruritic manifestations of corticosteroid-response dermatoses [very high potency topical corticosteroid]

**Usual Dosage** Children and Adults: Topical: Apply sparingly to skin twice daily, rub in gently and completely; treatment should not exceed 2 consecutive weeks and total dosage should not exceed 50 g/week

**Mechanism of Action** Corticosteroids inhibit the initial manifestations of the inflammatory process (ie, capillary dilation and edema, fibrin deposition, and migration and diapedesis of leukocytes into the inflamed site) as well as later sequelae (angiogenesis, fibroblast proliferation)

**Local Anesthetic/Vasoconstrictor Precautions** No information available to require special precautions

**Effects on Dental Treatment** No effects or complications reported

**Other Adverse Effects** <1%: Topical: Burning, itching, irritation, dryness, folliculitis, hypertrichosis, acneiform eruptions, hypopigmentation, perioral dermatitis, allergic contact dermatitis, skin maceration, secondary infection, skin atrophy, striae, miliaria

**Drug Interactions** No data reported

**Drug Uptake** Absorption: Percutaneous absorption varies by location of topical application and the use of occlusive dressings; ~3% of a topically applied dose of ointment enters the circulation within 96 hours

**Pregnancy Risk Factor** C

**Dosage Forms**

Cream, as propionate: 0.05% (15 g, 45 g)

Ointment, topical, as propionate: 0.05% (15 g, 45 g)

**Generic Available** No

## Halofantrine (ha loe FAN trin)

**U.S. Brand Names** Halfan®

**Therapeutic Category** Antimalarial Agent

**Use** Treatment of mild to moderate acute malaria caused by susceptible strains of *Plasmodium falciparum* and *Plasmodium vivax*

**Usual Dosage** Oral:

Children <40 kg: 8 mg/kg every 6 hours for 3 doses

Adults: 500 mg every 6 hours for 3 doses

**Mechanism of Action** Similar to mefloquine; destruction of asexual blood forms, possible inhibition of proton pump

**Local Anesthetic/Vasoconstrictor Precautions** No information available to require special precautions

**Effects on Dental Treatment** No effects or complications reported

**Other Adverse Effects**

>10%: Dermatologic: Pruritus

1% to 10%:

- Cardiovascular: Edema
- Central nervous system: Malaise, headache
- Gastrointestinal: Nausea, vomiting
- Hematologic: Leukocytosis
- Hepatic: Elevated LFTs
- Local: Tenderness
- Neuromuscular & skeletal: Myalgia
- Respiratory: Cough
- Miscellaneous: Lymphadenopathy

<1%:

- Cardiovascular: Tachycardia, hypotension
- Dermatologic: Urticaria
- Endocrine & metabolic: Hypoglycemia
- Local: Sterile abscesses
- Respiratory: Asthma
- Miscellaneous: Anaphylactic shock

**Drug Interactions** No data reported

**Drug Uptake**

Mean time to parasite clearance: 40-84 hours

Absorption: Erratic and variable; serum levels are proportional to dose up to 1000 mg; doses greater than this should be divided; may be increased 60% with high fat meals

Serum half-life: 23 hours; metabolite: 82 hours; may be increased in active disease

**Pregnancy Risk Factor** X

**Generic Available** No

♦ **Halog®** *see* Halcinonide *on previous page*

♦ **Halog®-E** *see* Halcinonide *on previous page*

## Haloperidol (ha loe PER i dole)

**U.S. Brand Names** Haldol®; Haldol® Decanoate

**Therapeutic Category** Antipsychotic Agent

(Continued)

## Haloperidol *(Continued)*

**Use** Treatment of psychoses, Tourette's disorder, and severe behavioral problems in children; may be used for the emergency sedation of severely agitated or delirious patients

**Usual Dosage**

Children: 3-12 years (15-40 kg): Oral:

Initial: 0.05 mg/kg/day or 0.25-0.5 mg/day given in 2-3 divided doses; increase by 0.25-0.5 mg every 5-7 days; maximum: 0.15 mg/kg/day

Usual maintenance:

Agitation or hyperkinesia: 0.01-0.03 mg/kg/day once daily

Nonpsychotic disorders: 0.05-0.075 mg/kg/day in 2-3 divided doses

Psychotic disorders: 0.05-0.15 mg/kg/day in 2-3 divided doses

Children 6-12 years: I.M. (as lactate): 1-3 mg/dose every 4-8 hours to a maximum of 0.15 mg/kg/day; change over to oral therapy as soon as able

Adults:

Oral: 0.5-5 mg 2-3 times/day; usual maximum: 30 mg/day; some patients may require up to 100 mg/day

I.M. (as lactate): 2-5 mg every 4-8 hours as needed

I.M. (as decanoate): Initial: 10-15 times the daily oral dose administered at 3- to 4-week intervals

Sedation in the Intensive Care Unit:

I.M./IVP/IVPB: May repeat bolus doses after 30 minutes until calm achieved then administer 50% of the maximum dose every 6 hours

Mild agitation: 0.5-2 mg

Moderate agitation: 2-5 mg

Severe agitation: 10-20 mg

Continuous intravenous infusion (100 mg/100 mL $D_5W$): Rates of 1-40 mg/hour have been used

Elderly (nonpsychotic patients, dementia behavior):

Initial: Oral: 0.25-0.5 mg 1-2 times/day; increase dose at 4- to 7-day intervals by 0.25-0.5 mg/day; increase dosing intervals (twice daily, 3 times/day, etc) as necessary to control response or side effects

Maximum daily dose: 50 mg; gradual increases (titration) may prevent side effects or decrease their severity

**Mechanism of Action** Blocks postsynaptic mesolimbic dopaminergic $D_1$ and $D_2$ receptors in the brain; exhibits a strong alpha-adrenergic blocking and anticholinergic effect, depresses the release of hypothalamic and hypophyseal hormones; believed to depress the reticular activating system thus affecting basal metabolism, body temperature, wakefulness, vasomotor tone, and emesis

**Local Anesthetic/Vasoconstrictor Precautions** Manufacturer's information states that haloperidol may block vasopressor activity of epinephrine. This has not been observed during use of epinephrine as a vasoconstrictor in local anesthesia.

**Effects on Dental Treatment** Orthostatic hypotension and nasal congestion possible in dental patients. Since the drug is a dopamine antagonist, extrapyramidal symptoms of the TMJ a possibility.

**Other Adverse Effects** Sedation and anticholinergic effects are more pronounced than extrapyramidal effects; EKG changes, retinal pigmentation are more common than with chlorpromazine

>10%:

Central nervous system: Sedation, drowsiness, restlessness, anxiety, extrapyramidal reactions, dystonic reactions, pseudoparkinsonian signs and symptoms, tardive dyskinesia, neuroleptic malignant syndrome, seizures, altered central temperature regulation, akathisia

Endocrine & metabolic: Swelling of breasts

Gastrointestinal: Weight gain, constipation

1% to 10%:

Cardiovascular: Hypotension (especially orthostatic), tachycardia, arrhythmias, abnormal T waves with prolonged ventricular repolarization

Central nervous system: Hallucinations, drowsiness

Gastrointestinal: Nausea, vomiting

Genitourinary: Dysuria

<1%:

Central nervous system: Tardive dystonia, heat stroke, altered central temperature regulation

Dermatologic: Hyperpigmentation, pruritus, rash, contact dermatitis, alopecia, photosensitivity (rare)

Endocrine & metabolic: Amenorrhea, galactorrhea, gynecomastia, sexual dysfunction

Gastrointestinal: Adynamic ileus, dry mouth (problem for denture user)

Genitourinary: Urinary retention, overflow incontinence, priapism

Hematologic: Agranulocytosis, leukopenia (usually inpatients with large doses for prolonged periods)
Hepatic: Cholestatic jaundice, obstructive jaundice
Ocular: Blurred vision, retinal pigmentation, decreased visual acuity (may be irreversible)
Respiratory: Laryngospasm, respiratory depression

**Drug Interactions** Cytochrome P-450 IID6 enzyme inhibitor
Decreased effect: Carbamazepine and phenobarbital may increase metabolism and decreased effectiveness of haloperidol
Increased toxicity: CNS depressants may increase adverse effects; epinephrine may cause hypotension; haloperidol and anticholinergic agents cause increased intraocular pressure; concurrent use with lithium has occasionally caused acute encephalopathy-like syndrome

**Drug Uptake**
Onset of sedation: I.V.: Within 1 hour
Duration of action: ~3 weeks for decanoate form
Serum half-life: 20 hours
Time to peak serum concentration: 20 minutes

**Pregnancy Risk Factor** C
**Generic Available** Yes

## Haloprogin (ha loe PROE jin)

**U.S. Brand Names** Halotex®
**Therapeutic Category** Antifungal Agent, Topical
**Use** Topical treatment of tinea pedis (athlete's foot), tinea cruris (jock itch), tinea corporis (ring worm), tinea manuum caused by *Trichophyton rubrum*, *Trichophyton tonsurans*, *Trichophyton mentagrophytes*, *Microsporum canis*, or *Epidermophyton floccosum*. Topical treatment of *Malassezia furfur*.
**Usual Dosage** Children and Adults: Topical: Apply liberally twice daily for 2-3 weeks; intertriginous areas may require up to 4 weeks of treatment
**Mechanism of Action** Interferes with fungal DNA replication to inhibit yeast cell respiration and disrupt its cell membrane
**Local Anesthetic/Vasoconstrictor Precautions** No information available to require special precautions
**Effects on Dental Treatment** No effects or complications reported
**Other Adverse Effects** <1%: Topical: Pruritus, folliculitis, irritation, burning sensation, vesicle formation, erythema
**Drug Interactions** No data reported
**Drug Uptake** Absorption: Poorly through the skin (~11%)
**Pregnancy Risk Factor** B
**Generic Available** No

- **Halotestin®** *see* Fluoxymesterone *on page 445*
- **Halotex®** *see* Haloprogin *on this page*
- **Halotussin® [OTC]** *see* Guaifenesin *on page 478*
- **Halotussin® DAC** *see* Guaifenesin, Pseudoephedrine, and Codeine *on page 482*
- **Halotussin® DM [OTC]** *see* Guaifenesin and Dextromethorphan *on page 479*
- **Halotussin® PE [OTC]** *see* Guaifenesin and Pseudoephedrine *on page 481*
- **Haltran® [OTC]** *see* Ibuprofen *on page 522*
- **Havrix®** *see* Hepatitis A Vaccine *on page 494*
- **Hayfebrol® Liquid [OTC]** *see* Chlorpheniramine and Pseudoephedrine *on page 233*
- **HbCV** *see Haemophilus* b Conjugate Vaccine *on page 486*
- **H-BIG®** *see* Hepatitis B Immune Globulin *on page 494*
- **Head & Shoulders® [OTC]** *see* Pyrithione Zinc *on page 869*
- **Healon®** *see* Sodium Hyaluronate *on page 922*
- **Healon® GV** *see* Sodium Hyaluronate *on page 922*
- **Helidac™** *see* Bismuth Subsalicylate, Metronidazole, and Tetracycline *on page 142*
- **Helidac™ Combination** *see* Metronidazole *on page 667*
- **Helistat®** *see* Microfibrillar Collagen Hemostat *on page 673*
- **Helixate®** *see* Antihemophilic Factor (Recombinant) *on page 90*
- **Hemabate™** *see* Carboprost Tromethamine *on page 190*
- **Hemiacidrin** *see* Citric Acid Bladder Mixture *on page 255*

## Hemin (HEE min)

**U.S. Brand Names** Panhematin®
**Therapeutic Category** Blood Modifiers
(Continued)

## Hemin *(Continued)*

**Use** Treatment of recurrent attacks of acute intermittent porphyria (AIP) only after an appropriate period of alternate therapy has been tried

**Usual Dosage** I.V.: 1-4 mg/kg/day administered over 10-15 minutes for 3-14 days; may be repeated no earlier than every 12 hours; not to exceed 6 mg/kg in any 24-hour period

**Local Anesthetic/Vasoconstrictor Precautions** No information available to require special precautions

**Effects on Dental Treatment** No effects or complications reported

**Other Adverse Effects** 1% to 10%:

Central nervous system: Mild pyrexia
Hematologic: Leukocytosis
Local: Phlebitis

**Generic Available** No

- **Hemocyte® [OTC]** *see* Ferrous Fumarate *on page 426*
- **Hemodent® Gingival Retraction Cord** *see* Aluminum Chloride *on page 54*
- **Hemofil® M** *see* Antihemophilic Factor (Human) *on page 89*
- **Hemotene®** *see* Microfibrillar Collagen Hemostat *on page 673*

## Heparin (HEP a rin)

**U.S. Brand Names** Hep-Lock®

**Therapeutic Category** Anticoagulant (Other)

**Synonyms** Heparin Lock Flush; Heparin Sodium, Heparin Calcium

**Use** Prophylaxis and treatment of thromboembolic disorders

**Usual Dosage**

Line flushing: When using daily flushes of heparin to maintain patency of single and double lumen central catheters, 10 units/mL is commonly used for younger infants (eg, <10 kg) while 100 units/mL is used for older infants, children, and adults. Capped PVC catheters and peripheral heparin locks require flushing more frequently (eg, every 6-8 hours). Volume of heparin flush is usually similar to volume of catheter (or slightly greater). Additional flushes should be given when stagnant blood is observed in catheter, after catheter is used for drug or blood administration, and after blood withdrawal from catheter.

Addition of heparin (0.5-1 unit/mL) to peripheral and central TPN has been shown to increase duration of line patency. The final concentration of heparin used for TPN solutions may need to be decreased to 0.5 units/mL in small infants receiving larger amounts of volume in order to avoid approaching therapeutic amounts. Arterial lines are heparinized with a final concentration of 1 unit/mL.

Children:

Intermittent I.V.: Initial: 50-100 units/kg, then 50-100 units/kg every 4 hours
I.V. infusion: Initial: 50 units/kg, then 15-25 units/kg/hour; increase dose by 2-4 units/kg/hour every 6-8 hours as required

**Standard Heparin Solution**
**(25,000 units/500 mL $D_5W$)**

| To Administer a Dose of | Set Infusion Rate at |
|---|---|
| 400 units/h | 8 mL/h |
| 500 units/h | 10 mL/h |
| 600 units/h | 12 mL/h |
| 700 units/h | 14 mL/h |
| 800 units/h | 16 mL/h |
| 900 units/h | 18 mL/h |
| 1000 units/h | 20 mL/h |
| 1100 units/h | 22 mL/h |
| 1200 units/h | 24 mL/h |
| 1300 units/h | 26 mL/h |
| 1400 units/h | 28 mL/h |
| 1500 units/h | 30 mL/h |
| 1600 units/h | 32 mL/h |
| 1700 units/h | 34 mL/h |
| 1800 units/h | 36 mL/h |
| 1900 units/h | 38 mL/h |
| 2000 units/h | 40 mL/h |

Adults:

Prophylaxis (low-dose heparin): S.C.: 5000 units every 8-12 hours

Intermittent I.V.: Initial: 10,000 units, then 50-70 units/kg (5000-10,000 units) every 4-6 hours

I.V. infusion: 50 units/kg to start, then 15-25 units/kg/hour as continuous infusion; increase dose by 5 units/kg/hour every 4 hours as required according to PTT results, usual range: 10-30 units/hour

Weight-based protocol: 80 units/kg I.V. push followed by continuous infusion of 18 units/kg/hour. See table.

**Mechanism of Action** Potentiates the action of antithrombin III and thereby inactivates thrombin (as well as activated coagulation factors IX, X, XI, XII, and plasmin) and prevents the conversion of fibrinogen to fibrin; heparin also stimulates release of lipoprotein lipase (lipoprotein lipase hydrolyzes triglycerides to glycerol and free fatty acids)

**Local Anesthetic/Vasoconstrictor Precautions** No information available to require special precautions

**Effects on Dental Treatment** No effects or complications reported

**Other Adverse Effects**

>10%:

Dermatologic: Unexplained bruising

Gastrointestinal: Constipation, vomiting of blood, bleeding from gums

Hematologic: Hemorrhage, blood in urine

1% to 10%:

Cardiovascular: Chest pain

Genitourinary: Frequent or persistent erection

Neuromuscular & skeletal: Peripheral neuropathy

Miscellaneous: Allergic reactions

<1%:

Central nervous system: Fever, headache, chills

Dermatologic: Urticaria

Gastrointestinal: Nausea, vomiting

Hematologic: Thrombocytopenia (heparin-associated thrombocytopenia occurs in <1% of patients, immune thrombocytopenia occurs with progressive fall in platelet counts and, in some cases, thromboembolic complications; daily platelet counts for 5-7 days at initiation of therapy may help detect the onset of this complication)

Hepatic: Elevated liver enzymes

Local: Irritation, ulceration, cutaneous necrosis have been rarely reported with deep S.C. injections

Neuromuscular & skeletal: Osteoporosis (chronic therapy effect)

**Drug Uptake**

Onset of anticoagulation:

I.V.: Immediate with use

S.C.: Within 20-30 minutes

Absorption: Oral, rectal, sublingual, I.M.: Erratic

Serum half-life:

Mean: 1.5 hours

Range: 1-2 hours; affected by obesity, renal function, hepatic function, malignancy, presence of pulmonary embolism, and infections

**Pregnancy Risk Factor** C

**Generic Available** Yes

**Comments** Heparin does not possess fibrinolytic activity and, therefore, cannot lyse established thrombi; discontinue heparin if hemorrhage occurs; severe hemorrhage or overdosage may require protamine; monitor platelet counts, signs of bleeding, PTT.

When using daily flushes of heparin to maintain patency of single and double lumen central catheters, 10 units/mL is commonly used for younger infants (eg, <10 kg) while 100 units/mL is used for older infants and children (eg, ≥10 kg). Capped PVC catheters and peripheral heparin locks require flushing more frequently (eg, every 6-8 hours). Volume of heparin flush is usually similar to volume of catheter (or slightly greater) or may be standardized according to specific hospital's policy (eg, 2-5 mL/flush). Dose of heparin flush used should not approach therapeutic per kg dose. Additional flushes should be given when stagnant blood is observed in catheter, after catheter is used for drug or blood administration, and after blood withdrawal from catheter.

Heparin 1 unit/mL (final concentration) may be added to TPN solutions, both central and peripheral. (Addition of heparin to peripheral TPN has been shown to increase duration of line patency.) The final concentration of heparin used for TPN solutions may need to be decreased to 0.5 units/mL in small infants receiving larger amounts of volume in order to avoid approaching therapeutic amounts.

(Continued)

## Heparin *(Continued)*

Arterial lines are heparinized with a final concentration of 1 unit/mL.

- **Heparin Cofactor I** *see* Antithrombin III *on page 92*
- **Heparin Lock Flush** *see* Heparin *on page 492*
- **Heparin Sodium, Heparin Calcium** *see* Heparin *on page 492*

## Hepatitis A Vaccine (hep a TYE tis aye vak SEEN)

**Related Information**

Systemic Viral Diseases *on page 1115*

**U.S. Brand Names** Havrix®

**Therapeutic Category** Vaccine, Inactivated Virus

**Use** For populations desiring protection against hepatitis A or for populations at high risk of exposure to hepatitis A virus (travelers to developing countries, household and sexual contacts of persons infected with hepatitis A), child day care employees, illicit drug users, male homosexuals, institutional workers (eg, institutions for the mentally and physically handicapped persons, prisons, etc), and healthcare workers who may be exposed to hepatitis A virus (eg, laboratory employees)

**Usual Dosage** I.M.:

Children: 0.5 mL (360 units) on days 1 and 30, with a booster dose 6-12 months later (completion of the first 2 doses [ie, the primary series] should be accomplished at least 2 weeks before anticipated exposure to hepatitis A)

Adults: 1 mL (1440 units), with a booster dose at 6-12 months

**Mechanism of Action** As an inactivated virus vaccine, hepatitis A vaccine offers active immunization against hepatitis A virus infection at an effective immune response rate in up to 99% of subjects

**Local Anesthetic/Vasoconstrictor Precautions** No information available to require special precautions

**Effects on Dental Treatment** No effects or complications reported

**Other Adverse Effects**

Central nervous system: Headache, fatigue, fever (rare)

Hepatic: Transient liver function test abnormalities

Local: Cutaneous reactions at the injection site (pain, soreness, tenderness, swelling, warmth, and redness)

**Drug Interactions** No interference of immunogenicity was reported when mixed with hepatitis B vaccine

**Drug Uptake**

Onset of action (protection): 3 weeks after a single dose

Duration: Neutralizing antibodies have persisted for >3 years; unconfirmed evidence indicates that antibody levels may persist for 5-10 years

**Pregnancy Risk Factor** C

**Generic Available** No

## Hepatitis B Immune Globulin

(hep a TYE tis bee i MYUN GLOB yoo lin)

**Related Information**

Occupational Exposure to Bloodborne Pathogens (Universal Precautions) *on page 1232*

Systemic Viral Diseases *on page 1115*

**U.S. Brand Names** H-BIG®; HyperHep®

**Therapeutic Category** Immune Globulin

**Use** Provide prophylactic passive immunity to hepatitis B infection to those individuals exposed; newborns of mothers known to be hepatitis B surface antigen positive; hepatitis B immune globulin is not indicated for treatment of active hepatitis B infections and is ineffective in the treatment of chronic active hepatitis B infection

**Usual Dosage** I.M.:

Newborns: Hepatitis B: 0.5 mL as soon after birth as possible (within 12 hours)

Adults: Postexposure prophylaxis: 0.06 mL/kg; usual dose: 3-5 mL; repeat at 28-30 days after exposure

**Mechanism of Action** Hepatitis B immune globulin (HBIG) is a nonpyrogenic sterile solution containing 10% to 18% protein of which at least 80% is monomeric immunoglobulin G (IgG). HBIG differs from immune globulin in the amount of anti-HBs. Immune globulin is prepared from plasma that is not preselected for anti-HBs content. HBIG is prepared from plasma preselected for high titer anti-HBs. In the U.S., HBIG has an anti-HBs high titer of higher than 1:100,000 by IRA. There is no evidence that the causative agent of AIDS (HTLV-III/LAV) is transmitted by HBIG.

**Local Anesthetic/Vasoconstrictor Precautions** No information available to require special precautions

**Effects on Dental Treatment** No effects or complications reported

**Other Adverse Effects**

1% to 10%:

Central nervous system: Dizziness, malaise

Dermatologic: Urticaria, angioedema, rash, erythema

Local: Pain and tenderness at injection site

Neuromuscular & skeletal: Arthralgia

<1%: Miscellaneous: Anaphylaxis

**Drug Interactions** Increased toxicity: Live virus vaccines

**Drug Uptake**

Absorption: Slow

Time to peak serum concentration: 1-6 days

**Pregnancy Risk Factor** C

**Generic Available** No

## Hepatitis B Vaccine (hep a TYE tis bee vak SEEN)

**Related Information**

Systemic Viral Diseases *on page 1115*

**U.S. Brand Names** Engerix-B®; Recombivax HB®

**Therapeutic Category** Vaccine, Inactivated Virus

**Use** Immunization against infection caused by all known subtypes of hepatitis B virus in individuals considered at high risk of potential exposure to hepatitis B virus or $HB_sAg$-positive materials

**Usual Dosage** See tables.

**Immunization Regimen of Three I.M. Hepatitis B Vaccine Doses**

| Age | Initial | | 1 mo | | 6 mo | |
|---|---|---|---|---|---|---|
| | Recombivax HB® (mL) | Engerix-B® (mL) | Recombivax HB® (mL) | Engerix-B® (mL) | Recombivax HB® (mL) | Engerix-B® (mL) |
| Birth* - 10 y | 0.25 | 0.5 | 0.25 | 0.5 | 0.25 | 0.5 |
| 11-19 y | 0.5 | 1 | 0.5 | 1 | 0.5 | 1 |
| ≥20 y | 1 | 1 | 1 | 1 | 1 | 1 |
| Dialysis or immunocompromised patients | | 2† | | 2† | | 2† |

*Infants born of $HB_s$ Ag negative mothers.

†Two 1 mL doses given at different sites.

**Recommended Dosage for Infants Born to $HB_sAg$ Positive Mothers**

| Treatment | Birth | Within 7 d | 1 mo | 6 mo |
|---|---|---|---|---|
| Engerix-B® (pediatric dose 10 mcg/0.5 mL) | * | 0.5 mL* | 0.5 mL | 0.5 mL |
| Recombivax HB® (pediatric dose 5 mcg/0.5 mL) | * | 0.5 mL* | 0.5 mL | 0.5 mL |
| Hepatitis B immune globulin | 0.5 mL | — | — | — |

*The first dose may be given at birth at the same time as HBIG, but give in the opposite anterolateral thigh. This may better ensure vaccine absorption.

**Mechanism of Action** Recombinant hepatitis B vaccine is a noninfectious subunit viral vaccine. The vaccine is derived from hepatitis B surface antigen ($HB_sAg$) produced through recombinant DNA techniques from yeast cells. The portion of the hepatitis B gene which codes for $HB_sAg$ is cloned into yeast which is then cultured to produce hepatitis B vaccine.

**Local Anesthetic/Vasoconstrictor Precautions** No information available to require special precautions

**Effects on Dental Treatment** No effects or complications reported

**Other Adverse Effects**

>10%:

Central nervous system: Fever, malaise, fatigue, headache

Local: Mild local tenderness, local inflammatory reaction

1% to 10%:

Gastrointestinal: Nausea, diarrhea

Respiratory: Pharyngitis

<1%:

Cardiovascular: Tachycardia, hypotension, flushing

Central nervous system: Lightheadedness, chills, somnolence, insomnia, irritability, agitation

Dermatologic: Pruritus, rash, erythema, urticaria

(Continued)

## Hepatitis B Vaccine *(Continued)*

Gastrointestinal: Vomiting, GI disturbances, constipation, abdominal cramps, dyspepsia, anorexia
Genitourinary: Dysuria
Neuromuscular & skeletal: Arthralgia, myalgia, stiffness in back/neck/arm or shoulder
Otic: Earache
Respiratory: Rhinitis, cough, epistaxis
Miscellaneous: Sweating, sensation of warmth

**Drug Interactions** Decreased effect: Immunosuppressive agents

**Drug Uptake** Duration of action: Following all 3 doses of hepatitis B vaccine, immunity will last approximately 5-7 years

**Pregnancy Risk Factor** C

**Generic Available** No


- **Hep-Lock®** *see* Heparin *on page 492*
- **Heptalac®** *see* Lactulose *on page 571*
- **Herceptin®** *see* Trastuzumab *on page 1006*
- **Herplex®** *see* Idoxuridine ***Withdrawn from Market 9/98*** *on page 525*
- **HES** *see* Hetastarch *on this page*
- **Hespan®** *see* Hetastarch *on this page*


## Hetastarch (HET a starch)

**U.S. Brand Names** Hespan®

**Therapeutic Category** Plasma Volume Expander

**Synonyms** HES; Hydroxyethyl Starch

**Use** Blood volume expander used in treatment of shock or impending shock when blood or blood products are not available; does not have oxygen-carrying capacity and is not a substitute for blood or plasma; an adjunct in leukapheresis to enhance the yield of granulocytes by centrifugal means

**Usual Dosage** I.V. infusion (requires an infusion pump):
Children: Safety and efficacy have not been established
Adults: 500-1000 mL (up to 1500 mL/day) or 20 mL/kg/day (up to 1500 mL/day); larger volumes (15,000 mL/24 hours) have been used safely in small numbers of patients

**Mechanism of Action** Produces plasma volume expansion by virtue of its highly colloidal starch structure, similar to albumin

**Local Anesthetic/Vasoconstrictor Precautions** No information available to require special precautions

**Effects on Dental Treatment** No effects or complications reported

**Other Adverse Effects** <1%:
Cardiovascular: Peripheral edema, heart failure, circulatory overload
Central nervous system: Fever, chills, headaches
Dermatologic: Itching, pruritus
Gastrointestinal: Vomiting
Hematologic: Bleeding, prolongation of PT, PTT, clotting time, and bleeding time
Neuromuscular & skeletal: Myalgia
Miscellaneous: Hypersensitivity

**Drug Uptake**
Onset of volume expansion: I.V.: Within 30 minutes
Duration: 24-36 hours

**Pregnancy Risk Factor** C

**Generic Available** No

**Comments** Does not have oxygen-carrying capacity and is not a substitute for blood or plasma; large volumes may interfere with platelet function and prolong PT and PTT times; safety and efficacy in children have not been established; hetastarch is a synthetic polymer derived from a waxy starch composed of amylopectin; average molecular weight = 450,000

## Hexachlorophene (heks a KLOR oh feen)

**U.S. Brand Names** pHisoHex®; pHiso® Scrub; Septisol®

**Therapeutic Category** Antibacterial, Topical; Soap

**Use** Surgical scrub and as a bacteriostatic skin cleanser; control an outbreak of gram-positive infection when other procedures have been unsuccessful

**Usual Dosage** Children and Adults: Topical: Apply 5 mL cleanser and water to area to be cleansed; lather and rinse thoroughly under running water

**Mechanism of Action** Bacteriostatic polychlorinated biphenyl which inhibits membrane-bound enzymes and disrupts the cell membrane

**Local Anesthetic/Vasoconstrictor Precautions** No information available to require special precautions

**Effects on Dental Treatment** No effects or complications reported

**Other Adverse Effects** <1%:
Central nervous system: CNS injury, seizures, irritability
Dermatologic: Photosensitivity, dermatitis, redness, dry skin

**Drug Interactions** No data reported

**Drug Uptake**
Absorption: Percutaneously through inflamed, excoriated, and intact skin
Serum half-life: Infants: 6.1-44.2 hours

**Pregnancy Risk Factor** C

**Dosage Forms**
Foam (Septisol®): 0.23% with alcohol 56% (180 mL, 600 mL)
Liquid, topical (pHisoHex®): 3% (8 mL, 150 mL, 500 mL, 3840 mL)

**Generic Available** Yes

- **Hexadrol®** *see* Dexamethasone *on page 308*
- **Hexalen®** *see* Altretamine *on page 53*
- **Hexavitamin** *see* Vitamins, Multiple *on page 1051*

## Hexobarbital (hex oh BAR bi tal)

**U.S. Brand Names** Pre-Sed®

**Therapeutic Category** Sedative

**Use** Preoperative medication; short-term sedation for diagnostic and minor surgical procedures; potentiating agent for analgesic; postoperative medication; patients suffering from mental and emotional stress that cannot fall asleep

**Restrictions** C-III

**Usual Dosage** Oral:
Children 6-12 years: One-fourth ($^1/_4$) to one-half ($^1/_2$) tablet ~15 minutes before procedure
Children >12 years: One-half (<12)[ to 1 tablet ~15 minutes before procedure
Adults: 1-2 tablets ~15 minutes before procedure

**Mechanism of Action** Interferes with transmission of impulses from the thalamus to the cortex of the brain resulting in an imbalance in central inhibitory and facilitatory mechanisms

**Local Anesthetic/Vasoconstrictor Precautions** No information available to require special precautions

**Effects on Dental Treatment** No effects or complications reported

**Contraindications** Hypersensitivity to hexobarbital or any component; pre-existing CNS depression, severe uncontrolled pain, porphyria, severe respiratory disease with dyspnea or obstruction; patients with impairment of renal function

**Warnings/Precautions** May be habit forming; untoward response attributable to barbiturates are particularly likely to occur in patients with fever, hyperthyroidism, diabetes mellitus, severe anemia, latent or manifest porphyria and congestive heart failure. Use with caution in patients with respiratory disease associated with dyspnea or obstruction; in patients with impaired hepatic function, the dose should be reduced.

**Drug Interactions** Caution should be observed when barbiturates and tranquilizers or antihistamines are administered simultaneously, as there may be a synergistic effect; smaller doses than the usual are then indicated. Barbiturate pretreatment of patients being induced with oral coumarin-type anticoagulants may prevent anticoagulation.

**Drug Uptake** Duration of action: ~1 hour

**Dosage Forms** Tablet, scored: 260 mg

**Comments** This tranquilizer has a rapid 10-minute onset time and ultra-short duration of 1 hour; developed exclusively for the dental industry to help reduce chair time. A comfortable patient will return and talk about the ease of his appointment.

## Hexylresorcinol (heks il re ZOR si nole)

**U.S. Brand Names** Sucrets® Sore Throat [OTC]

**Therapeutic Category** Local Anesthetic

**Use** Minor antiseptic and local anesthetic for sore throat

**Usual Dosage** May be used as needed, allow to dissolve slowly in mouth

**Local Anesthetic/Vasoconstrictor Precautions** No information available to require special precautions

**Effects on Dental Treatment** No effects or complications reported

**Dosage Forms** Lozenge: 2.4 mg

**Generic Available** Yes

- **Hibiclens® Topical [OTC]** *see* Chlorhexidine Gluconate *on page 225*
- **Hibistat® Topical [OTC]** *see* Chlorhexidine Gluconate *on page 225*
- **Hib Polysaccharide Conjugate** *see* *Haemophilus* b Conjugate Vaccine *on page 486*
- **HibTITER®** *see* *Haemophilus* b Conjugate Vaccine *on page 486*

- **Hiprex®** *see* Methenamine *on page 647*
- **Hismanal®** *see* Astemizole *on page 104*
- **Histalet Forte® Tablet** *see* Chlorpheniramine, Pyrilamine, Phenylephrine, and Phenylpropanolamine *on page 238*
- **Histalet® Syrup [OTC]** *see* Chlorpheniramine and Pseudoephedrine *on page 233*
- **Histalet® X** *see* Guaifenesin and Pseudoephedrine *on page 481*
- **Histatab® Plus Tablet [OTC]** *see* Chlorpheniramine and Phenylephrine *on page 232*
- **Hista-Vadrin® Tablet** *see* Chlorpheniramine, Phenylephrine, and Phenylpropanolamine *on page 235*
- **Histerone® Injection** *see* Testosterone *on page 961*
- **Histolyn-CYL® Injection** *see* Histoplasmin *on this page*

## Histoplasmin (his toe PLAZ min)

**U.S. Brand Names** Histolyn-CYL® Injection

**Therapeutic Category** Diagnostic Agent, Skin Test

**Synonyms** Histoplasmosis Skin Test Antigen

**Use** Diagnosing histoplasmosis; to assess cell-mediated immunity

**Usual Dosage** Adults: Intradermally: 0.1 mL of 1:100 dilution into volar surface of forearm; induration of ≥5 mm in diameter indicates a positive reaction

**Local Anesthetic/Vasoconstrictor Precautions** No information available to require special precautions

**Effects on Dental Treatment** No effects or complications reported

**Other Adverse Effects** 1% to 10%:

Dermatologic: Pruritus, urticaria
Local: Ulceration or necrosis may occur at test site
Respiratory: Dyspnea

**Pregnancy Risk Factor** C

**Generic Available** No

- **Histoplasmosis Skin Test Antigen** *see* Histoplasmin *on this page*
- **Histor-D® Syrup** *see* Chlorpheniramine and Phenylephrine *on page 232*
- **Histor-D® Timecelles®** *see* Chlorpheniramine, Phenylephrine, and Methscopolamine *on page 235*

## Histrelin (his TREL in)

**U.S. Brand Names** Supprelin™

**Therapeutic Category** Gonadotropin Releasing Hormone Analog

**Use** Treatment of central idiopathic precocious puberty; treatment of estrogen-associated gynecological disorders such as acute intermittent porphyria, endometriosis, leiomyomata uteri, and premenstrual syndrome

**Usual Dosage**

Central idiopathic precocious puberty: S.C.: Usual dose is 10 mcg/kg/day given as a single daily dose at the same time each day
Acute intermittent porphyria in women: S.C.: 5 mcg/day
Endometriosis: S.C.: 100 mcg/day
Leiomyomata uteri: S.C.: 20-50 mcg/day or 4 mcg/kg/day

**Mechanism of Action** Histrelin is a synthetic long-acting gonadotropin-releasing hormone analog; with daily administration, it desensitizes the pituitary to endogenous gonadotropin-releasing hormone (ie, suppresses gonadotropin release by causing down regulation of the pituitary); this results in a decrease in gonadal sex steroid production which stops the secondary sexual development

**Local Anesthetic/Vasoconstrictor Precautions** No information available to require special precautions

**Effects on Dental Treatment** No effects or complications reported

**Other Adverse Effects**

>10%:
Cardiovascular: Vasodilation
Central nervous system: Headache
Gastrointestinal: Abdominal pain
Genitourinary: Vaginal bleeding, vaginal dryness
Local: Skin reaction at injection site

1% to 10%:
Central nervous system: Mood swings
Dermatologic: Skin rashes, urticaria
Endocrine & metabolic: Breast tenderness, hot flashes
Gastrointestinal: Nausea, vomiting
Neuromuscular & skeletal: Joint stiffness, pain
Renal: Increased urinary calcium excretion

**Drug Interactions** No data reported

**Drug Uptake**

Precocious puberty: Onset of hormonal responses: Within 3 months of initiation of therapy

Acute intermittent porphyria associated with menses: Amelioration of symptoms: After 1-2 months of therapy

Treatment of endometriosis or leiomyomata uteri: Onset of responses: After 3-6 months of treatment

**Pregnancy Risk Factor** X

**Generic Available** No

- **Hi-Vegi-Lip®** *see* Pancreatin *on page 763*
- **Hivid®** *see* Zalcitabine *on page 1057*
- **HIV Infection and AIDS** *see page 1085*
- **HMS Liquifilm®** *see* Medrysone *on page 624*
- **Hold® DM [OTC]** *see* Dextromethorphan *on page 314*

## Homatropine (hoe MA troe peen)

**U.S. Brand Names** AK-Homatropine® Ophthalmic; Isopto® Homatropine Ophthalmic

**Therapeutic Category** Anticholinergic Agent, Ophthalmic; Ophthalmic Agent, Mydriatic

**Use** Producing cycloplegia and mydriasis for refraction; treatment of acute inflammatory conditions of the uveal tract

**Usual Dosage**

Children:

Mydriasis and cycloplegia for refraction: Instill 1 drop of 2% solution immediately before the procedure; repeat at 10-minute intervals as needed

Uveitis: Instill 1 drop of 2% solution 2-3 times/day

Adults:

Mydriasis and cycloplegia for refraction: Instill 1-2 drops of 2% solution or 1 drop of 5% solution before the procedure; repeat at 5- to 10-minute intervals as needed

Uveitis: Instill 1-2 drops of 2% or 5% 2-3 times/day up to every 3-4 hours as needed

**Mechanism of Action** Blocks response of iris sphincter muscle and the accommodative muscle of the ciliary body to cholinergic stimulation resulting in dilation and loss of accommodation

**Local Anesthetic/Vasoconstrictor Precautions** No information available to require special precautions

**Effects on Dental Treatment** No effects or complications reported

**Other Adverse Effects**

>10%: Ocular: Blurred vision, photophobia

1% to 10%:

Local: Stinging, local irritation

Ocular: Increased intraocular pressure

Respiratory: Congestion

<1%:

Cardiovascular: Vascular congestion, edema

Central nervous system: Drowsiness

Dermatologic: Exudate, eczematoid dermatitis

Ocular: Follicular conjunctivitis

**Drug Uptake**

Onset of accommodation and pupil effect: Ophthalmic:

Maximum mydriatic effect: Within 10-30 minutes

Maximum cycloplegic effect: Within 30-90 minutes

Duration:

Mydriasis: 6 hours to 4 days

Cycloplegia: 10-48 hours

**Pregnancy Risk Factor** C

**Generic Available** Yes

- **Homatropine and Hydrocodone** *see* Hydrocodone and Homatropine *on page 508*
- **Horse Anti-human Thymocyte Gamma Globulin** *see* Lymphocyte Immune Globulin *on page 608*
- **H.P. Acthar® Gel** *see* Corticotropin *on page 278*
- **Humalog®** *see* Insulin Preparations *on page 537*

## Human Growth Hormone (HYU man grothe HOR mone)

**U.S. Brand Names** Genotropin® Injection; Humatrope® Injection; Norditropin® Injection; Nutropin® AQ Injection; Nutropin® Injection; Protropin® Injection; Saizen® Injection; Serostim® Injection

(Continued)

## Human Growth Hormone *(Continued)*

**Therapeutic Category** Growth Hormone

**Use**

Long-term treatment of growth failure from lack of adequate endogenous growth hormone secretion

Nutropin®: Treatment of children who have growth failure associated with chronic renal insufficiency up until the time of renal transplantation

**Usual Dosage** Children (individualize dose):

Somatrem (Protropin®): I.M., S.C.: Up to 0.1 mg (0.26 units)/kg/dose 3 times/week

Somatropin (Humatrope®): I.M., S.C.: Up to 0.06 mg (0.16 units)/kg/dose 3 times/week

Somatropin (Nutropin®): S.C.:

Growth hormone inadequacy: Weekly dosage of 0.3 mg/kg (0.78 units/kg) administered daily

Chronic renal insufficiency: Weekly dosage of 0.35 mg/kg (0.91 units/kg) administered daily

Therapy should be discontinued when patient has reached satisfactory adult height, when epiphyses have fused, or when the patient ceases to respond

Growth of 5 cm/year or more is expected, if growth rate does not exceed 2.5 cm in a 6-month period, double the dose for the next 6 months, if there is still no satisfactory response, discontinue therapy

**Mechanism of Action** Somatrem and somatropin are purified polypeptide hormones of recombinant DNA origin; somatrem contains the identical sequence of amino acids found in human growth hormone while somatropin's amino acid sequence is identical plus an additional amino acid, methionine; human growth hormone stimulates growth of linear bone, skeletal muscle, and organs; stimulates erythropoietin which increases red blood cell mass; exerts both insulin-like and diabetogenic effects

**Local Anesthetic/Vasoconstrictor Precautions** No information available to require special precautions

**Effects on Dental Treatment** No effects or complications reported

**Other Adverse Effects** S.C. administration can cause local lipoatrophy or lipodystrophy and may enhance the development of neutralizing antibodies

1% to 10%: Endocrine & metabolism: Hypothyroidism

<1%:

Dermatologic: Skin rash, itching

Endocrine & metabolic: Hypoglycemia

Local: Pain at injection site

Neuromuscular & skeletal: Pain in hip/knee

Miscellaneous: Small risk for developing leukemia

**Drug Interactions** Decreased effect: Glucocorticoid therapy may inhibit growth-promoting effects.

**Drug Uptake** Somatrem and somatropin have equivalent pharmacokinetic properties

Duration of action: Maintains supraphysiologic levels for 18-20 hours

Absorption: I.M.: Well absorbed

Serum half-life: 15-50 minutes

**Pregnancy Risk Factor** C

**Generic Available** No

- **Humate-P®** *see* Antihemophilic Factor (Human) *on page 89*
- **Humatin®** *see* Paromomycin *on page 767*
- **Humatrope® Injection** *see* Human Growth Hormone *on previous page*
- **Humegon™** *see* Menotropins *on page 628*
- **Humibid® DM [OTC]** *see* Guaifenesin and Dextromethorphan *on page 479*
- **Humibid® L.A.** *see* Guaifenesin *on page 478*
- **Humibid® Sprinkle** *see* Guaifenesin *on page 478*
- **HuMist® Nasal Mist [OTC]** *see* Sodium Chloride *on page 920*
- **Humorsol®** *see* Demecarium *on page 302*
- **Humulin® 50/50** *see* Insulin Preparations *on page 537*
- **Humulin® 70/30** *see* Insulin Preparations *on page 537*
- **Humulin® L** *see* Insulin Preparations *on page 537*
- **Humulin® N** *see* Insulin Preparations *on page 537*
- **Humulin® R** *see* Insulin Preparations *on page 537*
- **Humulin® U** *see* Insulin Preparations *on page 537*
- **Hurricaine®** *see* Benzocaine *on page 128*
- **Hyaluronic Acid** *see* Sodium Hyaluronate *on page 922*

## Hyaluronidase (hye al yoor ON i dase)

**U.S. Brand Names** Wydase® Injection

**Therapeutic Category** Antidote, Extravasation

**Use** Increase the dispersion and absorption of other drugs; increase rate of absorption of parenteral fluids administered by hypodermoclysis; management of I.V. extravasations

**Usual Dosage**

Children:

Management of I.V. extravasation: Reconstitute the 150 unit vial of lyophilized powder with 1 mL normal saline; take 0.1 mL of this solution and dilute with 0.9 mL normal saline to yield 15 units/mL; using a 25- or 26-gauge needle, five 0.2 mL injections are made subcutaneously or intradermally into the extravasation site at the leading edge, changing the needle after each injection

Hypodermoclysis:

S.C.: 1 mL (150 units) is added to 1000 mL of infusion fluid and 0.5 mL (75 units) in injected into each clysis site at the initiation of the infusion

I.V.: 15 units is added to each 100 mL of I.V. fluid to be administered

Adults: Absorption and dispersion of drugs: 150 units are added to the vehicle containing the drug

**Mechanism of Action** Modifies the permeability of connective tissue through hydrolysis of hyaluronic acid, one of the chief ingredients of tissue cement which offers resistance to diffusion of liquids through tissues

**Local Anesthetic/Vasoconstrictor Precautions** No information available to require special precautions

**Effects on Dental Treatment** No effects or complications reported

**Other Adverse Effects** <1%:

Cardiovascular: Tachycardia, hypotension

Central nervous system: Dizziness, chills

Dermatologic: Urticaria, erythema

Gastrointestinal: Nausea, vomiting

**Drug Uptake**

Onset of action: Immediate by the subcutaneous or intradermal routes for the treatment of extravasation

Duration: 24-48 hours

**Pregnancy Risk Factor** C

**Generic Available** No

**Comments** The USP hyaluronidase unit is equivalent to the turbidity-reducing (TR) unit and the International Unit; each unit is defined as being the activity contained in 100 mcg of the International Standard Preparation


- **Hyate®:C** *see* Antihemophilic Factor (Porcine) *on page 89*
- **Hybolin™ Decanoate Injection** *see* Nandrolone *on page 703*
- **Hybolin™ Improved Injection** *see* Nandrolone *on page 703*
- **Hycamptamine** *see* Topotecan *on page 999*
- **Hycamtin™** *see* Topotecan *on page 999*
- **HycoClear Tuss®** *see* Hydrocodone and Guaifenesin *on page 508*
- **Hycodan®** *see* Hydrocodone and Homatropine *on page 508*
- **Hycomine®** *see* Hydrocodone and Phenylpropanolamine *on page 510*
- **Hycomine® Compound** *see* Hydrocodone, Chlorpheniramine, Phenylephrine, Acetaminophen and Caffeine *on page 510*
- **Hycomine® Pediatric** *see* Hydrocodone and Phenylpropanolamine *on page 510*
- **Hycotuss® Expectorant Liquid** *see* Hydrocodone and Guaifenesin *on page 508*
- **Hydergine®** *see* Ergoloid Mesylates *on page 380*
- **Hydergine® LC** *see* Ergoloid Mesylates *on page 380*


## Hydralazine (hye DRAL a zeen)

**Related Information**

Cardiovascular Diseases *on page 1066*

**U.S. Brand Names** Apresoline®

**Canadian Brand Names** Apo®-Hydralazine; Novo-Hylazin; Nu-Hydral

**Therapeutic Category** Vasodilator

**Use** Management of moderate to severe hypertension, congestive heart failure, hypertension secondary to pre-eclampsia/eclampsia; also used to treat primary pulmonary hypertension

(Continued)

## Hydralazine *(Continued)*

**Usual Dosage**

Children:

Oral: Initial: 0.75-1 mg/kg/day in 2-4 divided doses, not to exceed 25 mg/dose; increase over 3-4 weeks to maximum of 7.5 mg/kg/day in 2-4 divided doses; maximum daily dose: 200 mg/day

I.M., I.V.: 0.1-0.2 mg/kg/dose (not to exceed 20 mg) every 4-6 hours as needed, up to 1.7-3.5 mg/kg/day in 4-6 divided doses

Adults:

Oral: Hypertension:

Initial dose: 10 mg 4 times/day

Increase by 10-25 mg/dose every 2-5 days

Maximum dose: 300 mg/day

Oral: Congestive heart failure:

Initial dose: 10-25 mg TID

Target dose: 75 mg TID

Maximum dose: 100 mg TID

I.M., I.V.:

Hypertensive Initial: 10-20 mg/dose every 4-6 hours as needed, may increase to 40 mg/dose; change to oral therapy as soon as possible

Pre-eclampsia/eclampsia: 5 mg/dose then 5-10 mg every 20-30 minutes as needed

Elderly: Oral: Initial: 10 mg 2-3 times/day; increase by 10-25 mg/day every 2-5 days

**Mechanism of Action** Direct vasodilation of arterioles (with little effect on veins) with decreased systemic resistance

**Local Anesthetic/Vasoconstrictor Precautions** No information available to require special precautions

**Effects on Dental Treatment** No effects or complications reported

**Other Adverse Effects**

>10%:

Cardiovascular: Palpitations, flushing, tachycardia, angina pectoris

Central nervous system: Headache

Gastrointestinal: Nausea, vomiting, diarrhea, anorexia

1% to 10%:

Cardiovascular: Hypotension, redness or flushing of face

Gastrointestinal: Constipation

Ocular: Lacrimation

Respiratory: Dyspnea, nasal congestion

<1%:

Cardiovascular: Edema

Central nervous system: Malaise, fever, dizziness

Dermatologic: Rash

Neuromuscular & skeletal: Arthralgias, peripheral neuritis, weakness

**Drug Interactions** Increased toxicity: Concomitant administration of MAO inhibitors causes significant decrease in blood pressure; indomethacin leads to decreased hypotensive effects

**Drug Uptake**

Onset of action:

Oral: 20-30 minutes

I.V.: 5-20 minutes

Duration:

Oral: 2-4 hours

I.V.: 2-6 hours

Serum half-life:

Normal renal function: 2-8 hours

End-stage renal disease: 7-16 hours

**Pregnancy Risk Factor** C

**Generic Available** Yes

## Hydralazine and Hydrochlorothiazide

(hye DRAL a zeen & hye droe klor oh THYE a zide)

**U.S. Brand Names** Apresazide®

**Therapeutic Category** Antihypertensive Agent, Combination

**Synonyms** Hydrochlorothiazide and Hydralazine

**Use** Management of moderate to severe hypertension and treatment of congestive heart failure

**Usual Dosage** Adults: Oral: 1 capsule twice daily

**Local Anesthetic/Vasoconstrictor Precautions** No information available to require special precautions

**Effects on Dental Treatment** No effects or complications reported

**Pregnancy Risk Factor** C
**Generic Available** Yes

## Hydralazine, Hydrochlorothiazide, and Reserpine

(hye DRAL a zeen, hye droe klor oh THYE a zide, & re SER peen)

**U.S. Brand Names** Hydrap-ES®; Marpres®; Ser-Ap-Es®
**Therapeutic Category** Antihypertensive Agent, Combination
**Use** Hypertensive disorders
**Usual Dosage** Adults: Oral: 1-2 tablets 3 times/day
**Local Anesthetic/Vasoconstrictor Precautions** No information available to require special precautions
**Effects on Dental Treatment** No effects or complications reported
**Pregnancy Risk Factor** C
**Generic Available** Yes

- ♦ **Hydramyn® Syrup [OTC]** *see* Diphenhydramine *on page 338*
- ♦ **Hydrap-ES®** *see* Hydralazine, Hydrochlorothiazide, and Reserpine *on this page*
- ♦ **Hydrate® Injection** *see* Dimenhydrinate *on page 335*
- ♦ **Hydrea®** *see* Hydroxyurea *on page 517*
- ♦ **Hydrocet® [5/500]** *see* Hydrocodone and Acetaminophen *on page 505*

## Hydrochlorothiazide (hye droe klor oh THYE a zide)

**Related Information**
Cardiovascular Diseases *on page 1066*
Moexipril and Hydrochlorothiazide *on page 685*

**U.S. Brand Names** Esidrix®; Ezide®; HydroDIURIL®; Hydro-Par®; Oretic®
**Canadian Brand Names** Apo®-Hydro; Diuchlor®; Neo-Codema®; Novo-Hydrazide; Urozide®
**Therapeutic Category** Diuretic, Thiazide
**Use** Management of mild to moderate hypertension; treatment of edema in congestive heart failure and nephrotic syndrome
**Usual Dosage** Oral (effect of drug may be decreased when used every day):
Children (In pediatric patients, chlorothiazide may be preferred over hydrochlorothiazide as there are more dosage formulations (eg, suspension) available):
<6 months: 2-3 mg/kg/day in 2 divided doses
>6 months: 2 mg/kg/day in 2 divided doses
Adults: 25-100 mg/day in 1-2 doses
Maximum: 200 mg/day
Elderly: 12.5-25 mg once daily
Minimal increase in response and more electrolyte disturbances are seen with doses >50 mg/day
**Mechanism of Action** Inhibits sodium reabsorption in the distal tubules causing increased excretion of sodium and water as well as potassium and hydrogen ions
**Local Anesthetic/Vasoconstrictor Precautions** No information available to require special precautions
**Effects on Dental Treatment** No effects or complications reported
**Other Adverse Effects**
1% to 10%: Endocrine & metabolic: Hypokalemia
<1%:
Cardiovascular: Hypotension
Dermatologic: Photosensitivity
Endocrine & metabolic: Fluid and electrolyte imbalances (hypocalcemia, hypomagnesemia, hyponatremia), hyperglycemia
Hematologic: Rarely blood dyscrasias
Renal: Prerenal azotemia
**Drug Interactions**
Decreased effect: Decreased antidiabetic drug efficacy
Increased toxicity:
Hypotensive agents cause increased hypotensive potential
Increased digoxin related arrhythmias when given with digoxin
Increased lithium levels due to reduced lithium clearance
**Drug Uptake**
Onset of diuretic action: Oral: Within 2 hours
Peak effect: 4 hours
Duration: 6-12 hours
Absorption: Oral: ~60% to 80%
**Pregnancy Risk Factor** D
**Generic Available** Yes: Tablet

- ♦ **Hydrochlorothiazide and Amiloride** *see* Amiloride and Hydrochlorothiazide *on page 61*

- **Hydrochlorothiazide and Hydralazine** *see* Hydralazine and Hydrochlorothiazide *on page 502*
- **Hydrochlorothiazide and Methyldopa** *see* Methyldopa and Hydrochlorothiazide *on page 659*

## Hydrochlorothiazide and Reserpine

(hye droe klor oh THYE a zide & re SER peen)

**U.S. Brand Names** Hydropres®; Hydro-Serp®; Hydroserpine®

**Therapeutic Category** Antihypertensive Agent, Combination

**Synonyms** Reserpine and Hydrochlorothiazide

**Use** Management of mild to moderate hypertension; treatment of edema in congestive heart failure and nephrotic syndrome

**Usual Dosage** Adults: Oral: 1-2 tablets once or twice daily

**Local Anesthetic/Vasoconstrictor Precautions** No information available to require special precautions

**Effects on Dental Treatment** No effects or complications reported

**Pregnancy Risk Factor** C

**Generic Available** Yes

## Hydrochlorothiazide and Spironolactone

(hye droe klor oh THYE a zide & speer on oh LAK tone)

**Related Information**

Cardiovascular Diseases *on page 1066*

**U.S. Brand Names** Alazide®; Aldactazide®; Spironazide®; Spirozide®

**Canadian Brand Names** Apo®-Spirozide; Novo-Spirozine

**Therapeutic Category** Antihypertensive Agent, Combination; Diuretic, Combination

**Synonyms** Spironolactone and Hydrochlorothiazide

**Use** Management of mild to moderate hypertension; treatment of edema in congestive heart failure and nephrotic syndrome

**Usual Dosage** Oral:

Children: 1.66-3.3 mg/kg/day (of spironolactone) in 2-4 divided doses

Adults: 1-8 tablets in 1-2 divided doses

**Local Anesthetic/Vasoconstrictor Precautions** No information available to require special precautions

**Effects on Dental Treatment** No effects or complications reported

**Other Adverse Effects** 1% to 10%:

Central nervous system: Headache, lethargy

Dermatology: Rash

Endocrine & metabolic: Hyperkalemia, gynecomastia, hyperchloremic metabolic acidosis (in decompensated hepatic cirrhosis), dehydration, hyponatremia

Gastrointestinal: Anorexia, nausea, vomiting, diarrhea

**Contraindications** Anuria, hyperkalemia, renal or hepatic failure, hypersensitivity to hydrochlorothiazide, spironolactone, or any component

**Pregnancy Risk Factor** C

**Dosage Forms** Tablet:

25/25: Hydrochlorothiazide 25 mg and spironolactone 25 mg

50/50: Hydrochlorothiazide 50 mg and spironolactone 50 mg

**Generic Available** Yes

## Hydrochlorothiazide and Triamterene

(hye droe klor oh THYE a zide & trye AM ter een)

**Related Information**

Cardiovascular Diseases *on page 1066*

**U.S. Brand Names** Dyazide®; Maxzide®

**Canadian Brand Names** Apo®-Triazide; Novo-Triamzide; Nu-Triazide

**Therapeutic Category** Diuretic, Combination

**Use** Management of mild to moderate hypertension; treatment of edema in congestive heart failure and nephrotic syndrome

**Usual Dosage** Oral:

Adults: 1-2 capsules twice daily after meals

Elderly: Initial: 1 capsule/day or every other day

**Mechanism of Action** Competes with aldosterone for receptor sites in the distal renal tubules, increasing sodium, chloride, and water excretion while conserving potassium and hydrogen ions; may block the effect of aldosterone on arteriolar smooth muscle as well

Inhibits sodium reabsorption in the distal tubules causing increased excretion of sodium and water as well as potassium and hydrogen ions

**Local Anesthetic/Vasoconstrictor Precautions** No information available to require special precautions

**Effects on Dental Treatment** No effects or complications reported

**Other Adverse Effects**

1% to 10%: Gastrointestinal: Loss of appetite, nausea, vomiting, stomach cramps, diarrhea, upset stomach

<1%:

Central nervous system: Dizziness, fatigue

Dermatologic: Purpura, cracked corners of mouth

Endocrine & metabolic: Electrolyte disturbances

Gastrointestinal: Bright orange tongue, burning of tongue

Hematologic: Aplastic anemia, agranulocytosis, hemolytic anemia, leukopenia, thrombocytopenia, megaloblastic anemia

Neuromuscular & skeletal: Muscle cramps

Ocular: Xanthopsia, transient blurred vision

Respiratory: Allergic pneumonitis, pulmonary edema, respiratory distress

**Drug Interactions**

Hydrochlorothiazide:

Decreased effect of oral hypoglycemics; decreased absorption with cholestyramine and colestipol

Increased effect with furosemide and other loop diuretics

Increased toxicity/levels of lithium

Triamterene:

Increased risk of hyperkalemia if given together with amiloride, spironolactone, angiotensin-converting enzyme (ACE) inhibitors

Increased toxicity of amantadine (possibly by decreasing its renal excretion)

**Pregnancy Risk Factor** C

**Generic Available** Yes (Dyazide® strength only)

♦ **Hydrocil® [OTC]** *see* Psyllium *on page 865*

♦ **Hydro Cobex®** *see* Hydroxocobalamin *on page 515*

# Hydrocodone and Acetaminophen

(hye droe KOE done & a seet a MIN oh fen)

**Related Information**

Acetaminophen *on page 27*

Dental Drug Interactions: Update on Drug Combinations Requiring Special Considerations *on page 1225*

Narcotic Agonists *on page 1223*

Oral Pain *on page 1122*

**U.S. Brand Names** Anexsia® 5/500; Anexsia® 7.5/650; Anexsia® 10/660; Anodynos-DHC® [5/500]; Bancap HC® [5/500]; Co-Gesic® [5/500]; Dolacet® [5/500]; DuoCet™ [5/500]; Duradyne DHC® [5/500]; Hydrocet® [5/500]; Hydrogesic® [5/500]; Hy-Phen® [5/500]; Lorcet® [5/500]; Lorcet®-HD [5/500]; Lorcet® Plus [7.5/650]; Lortab® 2.5/500; Lortab® 5/500; Lortab® 7.5/500; Lortab® 10/500; Lortab® 10/650; Lortab® Elixir; Lortab® Solution; Margesic® H [5/500]; Stagesic® [5/500]; T-Gesic® [5/500]; Vicodin® [5/500]; Vicodin® ES [7.5/750]; Vicodin® HP; Zydone® [5/500]

**Canadian Brand Names** Vapocet®

**Therapeutic Category** Analgesic, Narcotic

**Use**

Dental: Treatment of postoperative pain

Medical: Relief of pain

**Restrictions** C-III; Refillable up to 5 times in 6 months

**Usual Dosage** Oral:

Children: Not recommended in pediatric dental patients

Adults: Analgesic: 1-2 tablets or capsules every 4-6 hours or 5-10 mL solution every 4-6 hours as needed for pain; maximum dose: 12 tablets or capsules/day

**Mechanism of Action**

Hydrocodone, as with other narcotic (opiate) analgesics, blocks pain perception in the cerebral cortex by binding to specific receptor molecules (opiate receptors) within the neuronal membranes of synapses. This binding results in a decreased synaptic chemical transmission throughout the CNS thus inhibiting the flow of pain sensations into the higher centers. Mu and kappa are the two subtypes of the opiate receptor which hydrocodone binds to to cause analgesia.

Acetaminophen inhibits the synthesis of prostaglandins in the CNS and peripherally blocks pain impulse generation; produces antipyresis from inhibition of hypothalamic heat-regulating center.

**Local Anesthetic/Vasoconstrictor Precautions** No information available to require special precautions

**Effects on Dental Treatment** <1% of patients experience dry mouth

**Other Adverse Effects**

>10%:

Cardiovascular: Hypotension

(Continued)

## Hydrocodone and Acetaminophen *(Continued)*

Central nervous system: Lightheadedness, dizziness, sedation

1% to 10%: Gastrointestinal: Nausea

**Contraindications** Patients with known G-6-PD deficiency; hypersensitivity to acetaminophen; hypersensitivity to hydrocodone

**Warnings/Precautions** Use with caution in patients with hypersensitivity reactions to other phenanthrene derivative opioid agonists (morphine, codeine, levorphanol, oxycodone, oxymorphone); respiratory diseases including asthma, emphysema, COPD, or severe liver or renal insufficiency; some preparations contain sulfites which may cause allergic reactions; may be habit-forming

**Drug Interactions** The use of MAO inhibitors or tricyclic antidepressants with hydrocodone may **increase** the effect of either the antidepressant or hydrocodone; concurrent use of hydrocodone with anticholinergics may cause paralytic ileus; patients taking other narcotic agents, antipsychotics, antianxiety agents or other CNS depressants (including alcohol) with hydrocodone may experience an additive CNS depression; with acetaminophen component, refer to Acetaminophen monograph

**Drug Uptake**

Onset of effect: Narcotic analgesia: Within 10-20 minutes

Duration of effect: 3-6 hours

Serum half-life: 3.8 hours

**Pregnancy Risk Factor** C

**Breast-feeding Considerations**

Hydrocodone: No data reported

Acetaminophen: May be taken while breast-feeding

**Dosage Forms**

Capsule:

Bancap HC®, Dolacet®, Hydrocet®, Hydrogesic®, Lorcet®-HD, Margesic® H, Medipain 5®, Stagesic®, T-Gesic®, Zydone®: Hydrocodone bitartrate 5 mg and acetaminophen 500 mg

Elixir (tropical fruit punch flavor) (Lortab®): Hydrocodone bitartrate 2.5 mg and acetaminophen 167 mg per 5 mL with alcohol 7% (480 mL)

Solution, oral (tropical fruit punch flavor) (Lortab®): Hydrocodone bitartrate 2.5 mg and acetaminophen 167 mg per 5 mL with alcohol 7% (480 mL)

Tablet: Hydrocodone bitartrate 5 mg and acetaminophen 400 mg; hydrocodone bitartrate 7.5 mg and acetaminophen 400 mg; hydrocodone bitartrate 10 mg and acetaminophen 400 mg; hydrocodone bitartrate 5 mg and acetaminophen 500 mg; hydrocodone bitartrate 7.5 mg and acetaminophen 750 mg; hydrocodone bitartrate 7.5 mg and acetaminophen 500 mg; hydrocodone bitartrate 7.5 mg and acetaminophen 650 mg; hydrocodone bitartrate 10 mg and acetaminophen 650 mg

Lortab® 2.5/500: Hydrocodone bitartrate 2.5 mg and acetaminophen 500 mg

Anexsia® 5/500, Anodynos-DHC®, Co-Gesic®, DuoCet™, DHC®; Hy-Phen®, Lorcet®, Lortab®® 5/500, Vicodin®: Hydrocodone bitartrate 5 mg and acetaminophen 500 mg

Lortab® 7.5/500: Hydrocodone bitartrate 7.5 mg and acetaminophen 500 mg

Anexsia® 7.5/650, Lorcet® Plus: Hydrocodone bitartrate 7.5 mg and acetaminophen 650 mg

Vicodin® ES: Hydrocodone bitartrate 7.5 mg and acetaminophen 750 mg

Norco®: Hydrocodone bitartrate 10 mg and acetaminophen 325 mg

Lortab® 10/500: Hydrocodone bitartrate 10 mg and acetaminophen 500 mg

Lorcet® 10/650: Hydrocodone bitartrate 10 mg and acetaminophen 650 mg

Vicodin® HP: Hydrocodone bitartrate 10 mg and acetaminophen 660 mg

**Dietary Considerations** No data reported

**Generic Available** Yes

**Comments** Neither hydrocodone nor acetaminophen elicit anti-inflammatory effects. Because of addiction liability of opiate analgesics, the use of hydrocodone should be limited to 2-3 days postoperatively for treatment of dental pain. Nausea is the most common adverse effect seen after use in dental patients; sedation and constipation are second. Nausea elicited by narcotic analgesics is centrally mediated and the presence or absence of food will not affect the degree nor incidence of nausea.

Acetaminophen:

A study by Hylek, et al, suggested that the combination of acetaminophen with warfarin (Coumadin®) may cause enhanced anticoagulation. The following recommendations have been made by Hylek, et al, and supported by an editorial in *JAMA* by Bell.

Dose and duration of acetaminophen should be as low as possible, individualized and monitored

The study by Hylek reported the following:

For patients who reported taking the equivalent of at least 4 regular strength (325 mg) tablets for longer than a week, the odds of having an INR >6.0 were increased 10-fold above those not taking acetaminophen. Risk decreased with lower intakes of acetaminophen reaching a background level of risk at a dose of 6 or fewer 325 mg tablets per week.

**Selected Readings**

Bell WR, "Acetaminophen and Warfarin: Undesirable Synergy," *JAMA*, Factors for Excessive Warfarin Anticoagulation," *JAMA*, 1998, 279:657-62.

Dionne RA, "New Approaches to Preventing and Treating Postoperative Pain," *J Am Dent Assoc*, 1992, 123(6):26-34.

Gobetti JP, "Controlling Dental Pain," *J Am Dent Assoc*, 1992, 123(6):47-52.

Hylek EM, Heiman H, Skates SJ, et al, "Acetaminophen and Other Risk 1998, 279:702-3.

## Hydrocodone and Aspirin (hye droe KOE done & AS pir in)

**Related Information**

Dental Drug Interactions: Update on Drug Combinations Requiring Special Considerations *on page 1225*

Narcotic Agonists *on page 1223*

**U.S. Brand Names** Alor® 5/500; Azdone®; Damason-P®; Lortab® ASA; Panasal® 5/500

**Therapeutic Category** Analgesic, Narcotic

**Use**

Dental: Treatment of postoperative pain

Medical: Relief of pain

**Restrictions** C-III; Refillable up to 5 times in 6 months

**Usual Dosage** Oral:

Children: Not recommended in pediatric dental patients

Adults: 1-2 tablets every 4-6 hours as needed for pain

**Mechanism of Action** Hydrocodone, as with other narcotic (opiate) analgesics, blocks pain perception in the cerebral cortex by binding to specific receptor molecules (opiate receptors) within the neuronal membranes of synapsis. This binding results in a decreased synaptic chemical transmission throughout the CNS thus inhibiting the flow of pain sensations into the higher centers. Mu and kappa are the two subtypes of the opiate receptor which hydrocodone binds to to cause analgesia.

Aspirin inhibits prostaglandin synthesis by decreasing the activity of the enzyme, cyclo-oxygenase, which results in decreased formation of prostaglandin precursors, acts on the hypothalamic heat-regulating center to reduce fever, blocks thromboxane synthetase action which prevents formation of the platelet-aggregating substance thromboxane $A_2$

**Local Anesthetic/Vasoconstrictor Precautions** No information available to require special precautions

**Effects on Dental Treatment** <1% of patients experience dry mouth; use with caution in patients with platelet and bleeding disorders, renal dysfunction, erosive gastritis, or peptic ulcer disease, previous nonreaction does not guarantee future safe taking of medication; do not use aspirin in children <16 years of age for chickenpox or flu symptoms due to the association with Reye's syndrome

Avoid aspirin if possible, for 1 week prior to surgery because of the possibility of postoperative bleeding; use with caution in impaired hepatic function

Elderly are a high-risk population for adverse effects from nonsteroidal anti-inflammatory agents. As much as 60% of elderly with GI complications to NSAIDs can develop peptic ulceration and/or hemorrhage asymptomatically. Also, concomitant disease and drug use contribute to the risk for GI adverse effects. Use lowest effective dose for shortest period possible. Consider renal function decline with age. Use with caution in patients with history of asthma.

**Other Adverse Effects**

>10%:

- Central nervous system: Lightheadedness, dizziness, sedation
- Gastrointestinal: Nausea, heartburn, stomach pains, dyspepsia

1% to 10%: Gastrointestinal: Gastrointestinal ulceration

**Warnings/Precautions** Because of aspirin component, use with caution in patients with impaired renal function, erosive gastritis, or peptic ulcer disease; children and teenagers should not use for chickenpox or flu symptoms before a physician is consulted about Reye's syndrome

**Drug Interactions** The use of MAO inhibitors or tricyclic antidepressants with hydrocodone may **increase** the effect of either the antidepressant or hydrocodone; concurrent use of hydrocodone with anticholinergics may cause paralytic ileus; patients taking other narcotic agents, antipsychotic, antianxiety agents or other CNS depressants (including alcohol) with hydrocodone and aspirin may experience an additive CNS depression; aspirin interacts with warfarin to cause bleeding

(Continued)

## Hydrocodone and Aspirin *(Continued)*

**Drug Uptake**

Onset of effect: Onset of narcotic analgesia: Within 10-20 minutes
Duration of effect: 3-6 hours
Serum half-life: 3.8 hours

**Pregnancy Risk Factor** D

**Breast-feeding Considerations**

Hydrocodone: No data reported
Aspirin: Cautious use due to potential adverse effects in nursing infants

**Dosage Forms** Tablet: Hydrocodone bitartrate 5 mg and aspirin 500 mg

**Dietary Considerations** May be taken with food or milk to minimize GI distress

**Generic Available** Yes

**Comments** Because of addiction liability of opiate analgesics, the use of hydrocodone should be limited to 2-3 days postoperatively for treatment of dental pain; nausea is the most common adverse effect seen after use in dental patients; sedation and constipation are second; aspirin component affects bleeding times and could influence time of wound healing

**Selected Readings**

Dionne RA, "New Approaches to Preventing and Treating Postoperative Pain," *J Am Dent Assoc*, 1992, 123(6):26-34.
Gobetti JP, "Controlling Dental Pain," *J Am Dent Assoc*, 1992, 123(6):47-52.

## Hydrocodone and Chlorpheniramine

(hye droe KOE done & klor fen IR a meen)

**U.S. Brand Names** Tussionex®

**Therapeutic Category** Antitussive; Cough Preparation

**Use** Symptomatic relief of cough

**Usual Dosage** Oral:

Children 6-12 years: 2.5 mL every 12 hours; do not exceed 5 mL/24 hours
Adults: 5 mL every 12 hours; do not exceed 10 mL/24 hours

**Local Anesthetic/Vasoconstrictor Precautions** No information available to require special precautions

**Effects on Dental Treatment** Prolonged use will cause significant xerostomia

**Pregnancy Risk Factor** C

**Generic Available** Yes

## Hydrocodone and Guaifenesin

(hye droe KOE done & gwye FEN e sin)

**U.S. Brand Names** Codiclear® DH; HycoClear Tuss®; Hycotuss® Expectorant Liquid; Kwelcof®

**Therapeutic Category** Antitussive; Cough Preparation

**Synonyms** Guaifenesin and Hydrocodone

**Use** Symptomatic relief of nonproductive coughs associated with upper and lower respiratory tract congestion

**Usual Dosage** Oral:

Children:
- <2 years: 0.3 mg/kg/day (hydrocodone) in 4 divided doses
- 2-12 years: 2.5 mL every 4 hours, after meals and at bedtime
- >12 years: 5 mL every 4 hours, after meals and at bedtime

Adults: 5 mL every 4 hours, after meals and at bedtime, not to exceed 30 mL in a 24-hour period

**Local Anesthetic/Vasoconstrictor Precautions** No information available to require special precautions

**Effects on Dental Treatment** No effects or complications reported

**Pregnancy Risk Factor** C

**Generic Available** Yes

## Hydrocodone and Homatropine

(hye droe KOE done & hoe MA troe peen)

**U.S. Brand Names** Hycodan®; Hydromet®; Oncet®; Tussigon®

**Therapeutic Category** Antitussive; Cough Preparation

**Synonyms** Homatropine and Hydrocodone

**Use** Symptomatic relief of cough

**Usual Dosage** Oral (based on hydrocodone component):

Children: 0.6 mg/kg/day in 3-4 divided doses; do not administer more frequently than every 4 hours

A single dose should not exceed 1.25 mg in children <2 years of age, 5 mg in children 2-12 years, and 10 mg in children >12 years

Adults: 5-10 mg every 4-6 hours, a single dose should not exceed 15 mg; do not administer more frequently than every 4 hours

**Local Anesthetic/Vasoconstrictor Precautions** No information available to require special precautions

**Effects on Dental Treatment** Dry mouth

**Other Adverse Effects**

>10%:
- Cardiovascular: Hypotension
- Central nervous system: Lightheadedness, dizziness, sedation, drowsiness, fatigue
- Neuromuscular & skeletal: Weakness

1% to 10%:
- Cardiovascular: Bradycardia, tachycardia
- Central nervous system: Confusion
- Gastrointestinal: Nausea, vomiting
- Renal: Decreased urination
- Respiratory: Dyspnea

<1%:
- Cardiovascular: Hypertension
- Central nervous system: Hallucinations
- Dermatologic: Dry hot skin
- Gastrointestinal: Dry mouth, anorexia, biliary spasm, impaired GI motility
- Genitourinary: Urinary tract spasm
- Ocular: Miosis, mydriasis, blurred vision, diplopia
- Miscellaneous: Histamine release, physical and psychological dependence with prolonged use

**Pregnancy Risk Factor** C

**Generic Available** Yes

## Hydrocodone and Ibuprofen

(hye droe KOE done & eye byoo PROE fen)

**U.S. Brand Names** Vicoprofen®

**Therapeutic Category** Analgesic, Narcotic

**Use** Relief of moderate to moderately severe pain

**Usual Dosage** Adults: Oral: 1-2 tablets every 4-6 hours as needed for pain

**Mechanism of Action** Refer to individual agents

**Local Anesthetic/Vasoconstrictor Precautions** No information available to require special precautions

**Effects on Dental Treatment** Use with caution in patients taking anticoagulants (ibuprofen)

**Other Adverse Effects**

>10%:
- Cardiovascular: Hypotension
- Central nervous system: Lightheadedness, dizziness, sedation, drowsiness, fatigue
- Dermatologic: Rash, urticaria
- Gastrointestinal: Abdominal cramps, heartburn, indigestion, nausea
- Neuromuscular & skeletal: Weakness

1% to 10%:
- Cardiovascular: Bradycardia
- Central nervous system: Headache, nervousness, confusion
- Dermatologic: Itching
- Endocrine & metabolic: Fluid retention
- Gastrointestinal: Dyspepsia, vomiting, abdominal pain, peptic ulcer, GI bleed, GI perforation, nausea
- Genitourinary: Decreased urination
- Otic: Tinnitus
- Respiratory: Shortness of breath, dyspnea

<1%:
- Cardiovascular: Edema, congestive heart failure, arrhythmias, tachycardia, hypertension
- Central nervous system: Confusion, hallucinations, mental depression, drowsiness, insomnia, aseptic meningitis
- Dermatologic: Urticaria, erythema multiforme, toxic epidermal necrolysis, Stevens-Johnson syndrome
- Endocrine & metabolic: Polydipsia, hot flashes
- Gastrointestinal: Gastritis, GI ulceration, xerostomia, anorexia, biliary tract spasm
- Genitourinary: Cystitis, urinary tract spasm
- Hematologic: Neutropenia, anemia, agranulocytosis, inhibition of platelet aggregation, hemolytic anemia, bone marrow suppression, leukopenia, thrombocytopenia
- Hepatic: Hepatitis
- Neuromuscular & skeletal: Peripheral neuropathy

(Continued)

## Hydrocodone and Ibuprofen *(Continued)*

Ocular: Vision changes, blurred vision, conjunctivitis, dry eyes, toxic amblyopia, diplopia, miosis

Otic: Decreased hearing

Renal: Acute renal failure, polyuria

Respiratory: Allergic rhinitis, shortness of breath, epistaxis

Miscellaneous: Histamine release, physical and psychological dependence with prolonged use

**Dosage Forms** Tablet: Hydrocodone bitartrate 7.5 mg and ibuprofen 200 mg

**Generic Available** No

**Comments** The combination of 15 mg hydrocodone bitartrate with 400 mg ibuprofen was compared to 400 mg ibuprofen alone and placebo for the ability to diminish postoperative pain (pain after cesarean section or gynecologic surgery, 120 patients). Analgesia was measured during a 6-hour period after dosing based on onset of relief, hourly and summary variables, and duration of effect. A significantly greater proportion of patients treated with the hydrocodone/ibuprofen combination reported onset of relief compared with ibuprofen or placebo. Time to onset of relief did not differ among treatments. Hydrocodone with ibuprofen and ibuprofen alone were significantly more effective than placebo for all measures. The combination of hydrocodone with ibuprofen was significantly superior to ibuprofen for all hourly analgesic evaluations, weighted sum of pain intensity differences, total pain relief, and global rating of study medications. This report demonstrated an analgesic superiority of 15 mg hydrocodone bitartrate combined with 400 mg ibuprofen compared to 400 mg ibuprofen alone.

**Selected Readings**

Dionne R, "To Tame the Pain?" *Compend Contin Educ Dent*, 1998, 19(4):426-8, 430-1.

Hargreaves KM, "Management of Pain in Endodontic Patients," *Tex Dent J*, 1997, 114(10):27-31.

Sunshine A, Olson NZ, O'Neill E, et al, "Analgesic Efficacy of a Hydrocodone With Ibuprofen Combination Compared With Ibuprofen Alone for the Treatment of Acute Postoperative Pain," *J Clin Pharmacol*, 1997, 37:908-15.

## Hydrocodone and Phenylpropanolamine

(hye droe KOE done & fen il proe pa NOLE a meen)

**U.S. Brand Names** Codamine®; Codamine® Pediatric; Hycomine®; Hycomine® Pediatric; Hydrocodone PA® Syrup

**Therapeutic Category** Cough Preparation; Decongestant

**Synonyms** Phenylpropanolamine and Hydrocodone

**Use** Symptomatic relief of cough and nasal congestion

**Usual Dosage** Oral:

Children 6-12 years: 2.5 mL every 4 hours, up to 6 doses/24 hours

Adults: 5 mL every 4 hours, up to 6 doses/24 hours

**Local Anesthetic/Vasoconstrictor Precautions** Use with caution since phenylpropanolamine is a sympathomimetic amine which could interact with epinephrine to cause a pressor response

**Effects on Dental Treatment** Up to 10% of patients could experience tachycardia, palpitations, and dry mouth; use vasoconstrictor with caution

**Pregnancy Risk Factor** C

**Generic Available** Yes

## Hydrocodone, Chlorpheniramine, Phenylephrine, Acetaminophen and Caffeine

(hye droe KOE done, klor fen IR a meen, fen il EF rin, a seet a MIN oh fen, & KAF een)

**U.S. Brand Names** Hycomine® Compound

**Therapeutic Category** Antitussive; Cough Preparation

**Use** Symptomatic relief of cough and symptoms of upper respiratory infections

**Usual Dosage** Adults: Oral: 1 tablet every 4 hours, up to 4 times/day

**Local Anesthetic/Vasoconstrictor Precautions** Use with caution since phenylephrine is a sympathomimetic amine which could interact with epinephrine to cause a pressor response

**Effects on Dental Treatment**

Acetaminophen: No effects or complications reported

Chlorpheniramine: Prolonged use will cause significant xerostomia

Phenylephrine: Up to 10% of patients could experience tachycardia, palpitations, and dry mouth; use vasoconstrictor with caution

**Pregnancy Risk Factor** C

**Generic Available** Yes

**Selected Readings**

Barker JD Jr, de Carle DJ, and Anuras S, "Chronic Excessive Acetaminophen Use in Liver Damage," *Ann Intern Med*, 1977, 87(3):299-301.

Dionne RA, Campbell RA, Cooper SA, et al, "Suppression of Postoperative Pain by Preoperative Administration of Ibuprofen in Comparison to Placebo, Acetaminophen, and Acetaminophen Plus Codeine," *J Clin Pharmacol*, 1983, 23(1):37-43.

Licht H, Seeff LB, and Zimmerman HJ, "Apparent Potentiation of Acetaminophen Hepatotoxicity by Alcohol," *Ann Intern Med*, 1980, 92(4):511.

♦ **Hydrocodone PA® Syrup** *see* Hydrocodone and Phenylpropanolamine *on previous page*

## Hydrocodone, Phenylephrine, Pyrilamine, Phenindamine, Chlorpheniramine, and Ammonium Chloride

(hye droe KOE done, fen il EF rin, peer IL a meen, fen IN da meen, klor fen IR a meen, & a MOE nee um KLOR ide)

**U.S. Brand Names** P-V-Tussin®

**Therapeutic Category** Antihistamine/Decongestant Combination; Cough Preparation

**Use** Symptomatic relief of cough and nasal congestion

**Usual Dosage** Adults: Oral: 10 mL every 4-6 hours, up to 40 mL/day

**Local Anesthetic/Vasoconstrictor Precautions** Use with caution since phenylephrine is a sympathomimetic amine which could interact with epinephrine to cause a pressor response

**Effects on Dental Treatment**

Chlorpheniramine: Prolonged use will cause significant xerostomia

Phenylephrine: Up to 10% of patients could experience tachycardia, palpitations, and dry mouth; use vasoconstrictor with caution

**Generic Available** Yes

## Hydrocodone, Pseudoephedrine, and Guaifenesin

(hye droe KOE done, soo doe e FED rin & gwye FEN e sin)

**U.S. Brand Names** Cophene XP®; Detussin® Expectorant; SRC® Expectorant; Tussafin® Expectorant

**Therapeutic Category** Cough Preparation; Decongestant; Expectorant

**Use** Symptomatic relief of irritating, nonproductive cough associated with respiratory conditions such as bronchitis, bronchial asthma, tracheobronchitis, and the common cold

**Local Anesthetic/Vasoconstrictor Precautions** Use with caution since pseudoephedrine is a sympathomimetic amine which could interact with epinephrine to cause a pressor response

**Effects on Dental Treatment**

Guaifenesin: No effects or complications reported

Pseudoephedrine: Up to 10% of patients could experience tachycardia, palpitations, and dry mouth; use vasoconstrictor with caution

**Generic Available** Yes

## Hydrocortisone (hye droe KOR ti sone)

**Related Information**

Corticosteroid Equivalencies Comparison *on page 1221*

Corticosteroids, Topical Comparison *on page 1222*

**U.S. Brand Names** Cortef®; Hydrocortone® Acetate; Hydrocortone® Phosphate; Orabase® HCA; Solu-Cortef®

**Therapeutic Category** Anti-inflammatory Agent; Corticosteroid, Systemic; Corticosteroid, Topical (Low Potency)

**Use**

Dental: Treatment of a variety of oral diseases of allergic, inflammatory or autoimmune origin

Medical: Management of adrenocortical insufficiency; relief of inflammation of corticosteroid-responsive dermatoses (low and medium potency topical corticosteroid); adjunctive treatment of ulcerative colitis

**Usual Dosage** Adults: Anti-inflammatory or immunosuppressive:

Oral: 20-240 mg/day in 2-4 divided doses;

I.M., I.V.: Succinate: 100-500 mg every 2-10 hours

I.M., I.V., S.C.: Sodium phosphate: Initially 15-240 mg/day (approximately $^1/_3$ to $^1/_2$ of the oral dose) in divided doses every 12 hours. In acute diseases, doses higher than 240 mg may be required.

**Mechanism of Action** Decreases inflammation by suppression of migration of polymorphonuclear leukocytes and reversal of increased capillary permeability

**Local Anesthetic/Vasoconstrictor Precautions** No information available to require special precautions

**Effects on Dental Treatment** No effects or complications reported

**Other Adverse Effects** >10%:

Central nervous system: Insomnia, nervousness

(Continued)

## Hydrocortisone *(Continued)*

Gastrointestinal: Increased appetite, indigestion

**Contraindications** Serious infections, except septic shock or tuberculous meningitis; known hypersensitivity to hydrocortisone; viral, fungal, or tubercular skin lesions

**Warnings/Precautions** Use with caution in patients with hyperthyroidism, cirrhosis, nonspecific ulcerative colitis, hypertension, osteoporosis, thromboembolic tendencies, CHF, convulsive disorders, myasthenia gravis, thrombophlebitis, peptic ulcer, diabetes

Acute adrenal insufficiency may occur with abrupt withdrawal after long-term therapy or with stress; young pediatric patients may be more susceptible to adrenal axis suppression from topical therapy

Because of the risk of adverse effects, systemic corticosteroids should be used cautiously in the elderly, in the smallest possible dose, and for the shortest possible time

**Drug Interactions** Insulin decreases hypoglycemic effect; phenytoin, phenobarbital, ephedrine, and rifampin have caused increased metabolism of hydrocortisone and decreased steroid blood level; oral anticoagulants change prothrombin time; potassium- depleting diuretics increase risk of hypokalemia; cardiac glucosides increase risk of arrhythmias or digitalis toxicity secondary to hypokalemia

**Drug Uptake**

Hydrocortisone acetate salt has a slow onset but long duration of action when compared with more soluble preparations

Hydrocortisone sodium phosphate salt is a water soluble salt with a rapid onset but short duration of action

Hydrocortisone sodium succinate salt is a water soluble salt with is rapidly active

Absorption: Rapid by all routes, except rectally

Serum half-life, biologic: 8-12 hours

**Pregnancy Risk Factor** C

**Breast-feeding Considerations** No data reported

**Dosage Forms**

**Hydrocortisone acetate:** Injection, suspension: 25 mg/mL (5 mL, 10 mL); 50 mg/mL (5 mL, 10 mL)

**Hydrocortisone base:** Tablet, oral: 5 mg, 10 mg, 20 mg

**Hydrocortisone cypionate:** Suspension, oral: 10 mg/5 mL (120 mL)

**Hydrocortisone sodium phosphate:** Injection, IM/IV/SC: 50 mg/mL (2 mL, 10 mL)

**Hydrocortisone sodium succinate:** Injection, IM/IV: 100 mg, 250 mg, 500 mg, 1000 mg

**Dietary Considerations** May be taken with meals to decrease GI upset; limit caffeine; need diet rich in pyridoxine, vitamin C, vitamin D, folate, calcium, and phosphorus

**Generic Available** Yes

- **Hydrocortisone and Clioquinol** *see* Clioquinol and Hydrocortisone *on page 260*
- **Hydrocortisone and Dibucaine** *see* Dibucaine and Hydrocortisone *on page 318*
- **Hydrocortisone and Pramoxine** *see* Pramoxine and Hydrocortisone *on page 828*
- **Hydrocortisone and Urea** *see* Urea and Hydrocortisone *on page 1034*
- **Hydrocortone® Acetate** *see* Hydrocortisone *on previous page*
- **Hydrocortone® Phosphate** *see* Hydrocortisone *on previous page*
- **Hydro-Crysti-12®** *see* Hydroxocobalamin *on page 515*
- **HydroDIURIL®** *see* Hydrochlorothiazide *on page 503*

## Hydroflumethiazide (hye droe floo meth EYE a zide)

**Related Information**

Cardiovascular Diseases *on page 1066*

**U.S. Brand Names** Diucardin®; Saluron®

**Therapeutic Category** Diuretic, Thiazide

**Use** Management of mild to moderate hypertension; treatment of edema in congestive heart failure and nephrotic syndrome

**Usual Dosage** Oral:

Children: 1 mg/kg/24 hours

Adults: 50-200 mg/day

**Mechanism of Action** The diuretic mechanism of action is primarily inhibition of sodium, chloride, and water reabsorption in the renal distal tubules, thereby producing diuresis with a resultant reduction in plasma volume

**Local Anesthetic/Vasoconstrictor Precautions** No information available to require special precautions

**Effects on Dental Treatment** No effects or complications reported

**Other Adverse Effects**

1% to 10%: Endocrine & metabolic: Hypokalemia

<1%:

Cardiovascular: Hypotension

Central nervous system: Drowsiness

Dermatologic: Photosensitivity, rash

Endocrine & metabolic: Fluid and electrolyte imbalances (hypocalcemia, hypomagnesemia, hyponatremia), hyperglycemia

Gastrointestinal: Anorexia

Hematologic: Aplastic anemia, hemolytic anemia, leukopenia, agranulocytosis, thrombocytopenia, rarely blood dyscrasias

Hepatic: Hepatitis

Neuromuscular & skeletal: Paresthesia

Renal: Polyuria, prerenal azotemia, uremia

**Drug Interactions**

Decreased effect of oral hypoglycemics; decreased absorption with cholestyramine and colestipol

Increased effect with furosemide and other loop diuretics

Increased toxicity/levels of lithium

**Drug Uptake**

Onset of diuretic effect: Within ~2 hours

Peak effect: Within ~4 hours

Duration of action: 12-24 hours

**Pregnancy Risk Factor** D

**Generic Available** Yes

## Hydroflumethiazide and Reserpine

(hye droe floo meth EYE a zide & re SER peen)

**U.S. Brand Names** Salutensin®

**Therapeutic Category** Antihypertensive Agent, Combination

**Use** Management of hypertension

**Usual Dosage** As determined by individual titration, usually 1 tablet once or twice daily

**Local Anesthetic/Vasoconstrictor Precautions** No information available to require special precautions

**Effects on Dental Treatment** No effects or complications reported

**Pregnancy Risk Factor** C

**Generic Available** Yes

♦ **Hydrogesic® [5/500]** *see* Hydrocodone and Acetaminophen *on page 505*

♦ **Hydromagnesium Aluminate** *see* Magaldrate *on page 610*

♦ **Hydromet®** *see* Hydrocodone and Homatropine *on page 508*

## Hydromorphone (hye droe MOR fone)

**Related Information**

Narcotic Agonists *on page 1223*

**U.S. Brand Names** Dilaudid®; Dilaudid-5®; Dilaudid-HP®; HydroStat IR®

**Canadian Brand Names** Hydromorph Contin®; PMS-Hydromorphone

**Therapeutic Category** Analgesic, Narcotic; Antitussive

**Use** Management of moderate to severe pain; antitussive at lower doses

**Usual Dosage** Doses should be titrated to appropriate analgesic effects; when changing routes of administration, note that oral doses are less than half as effective as parenteral doses (may be only one-fifth as effective)

Pain: Older Children and Adults:

Oral, I.M., I.V., S.C.: 1-4 mg/dose every 4-6 hours as needed; usual adult dose: 2 mg/dose

Rectal: 3 mg every 6-8 hours

Antitussive: Oral:

Children 6-12 years: 0.5 mg every 3-4 hours as needed

Children >12 years and Adults: 1 mg every 3-4 hours as needed

**Mechanism of Action** Binds to opiate receptors in the CNS, causing inhibition of ascending pain pathways, altering the perception of and response to pain; causes cough supression by direct central action in the medulla; produces generalized CNS depression

**Local Anesthetic/Vasoconstrictor Precautions** No information available to require special precautions

**Effects on Dental Treatment** Dry mouth and nausea in 10% of patients

(Continued)

## Hydromorphone *(Continued)*

**Other Adverse Effects**

Endocrine & metabolic: Antidiuretic hormone release
Gastrointestinal: Biliary spasm
Genitourinary: Urinary tract spasm
Ocular: Miosis
Miscellaneous: Physical and psychological dependence, histamine release

>10%:

Cardiovascular: Palpitations, hypotension, peripheral vasodilation
Central nervous system: Dizziness, lightheadedness, drowsiness
Gastrointestinal: Anorexia

1% to 10%:

Cardiovascular: Tachycardia, bradycardia, flushing of face
Central nervous system: CNS depression, increased intracranial pressure, fatigue, headache, nervousness, restlessness
Gastrointestinal: Nausea, vomiting, constipation, stomach cramps, dry mouth
Genitourinary: Ureteral spasm
Neuromuscular & skeletal: Trembling, weakness
Renal: Decreased urination
Respiratory: Respiratory depression, dyspnea

<1%:

Central nervous system: Hallucinations, mental depression, paralytic ileus
Dermatologic: Pruritus, skin rash, urticaria

**Drug Interactions** Increased toxicity: CNS depressants, phenothiazines, tricyclic antidepressants may potentiate the adverse effects of hydromorphone

**Drug Uptake**

Onset of analgesic effect: Within 15-30 minutes
Duration: 4-5 hours
Serum half-life: 1-3 hours

**Pregnancy Risk Factor** B (D if used for prolonged periods or in high doses at term)

**Generic Available** Yes

♦ **Hydromox®** *see* Quinethazone *on page 872*
♦ **Hydro-Par®** *see* Hydrochlorothiazide *on page 503*
♦ **Hydrophed®** *see* Theophylline, Ephedrine, and Hydroxyzine *on page 974*
♦ **Hydropres®** *see* Hydrochlorothiazide and Reserpine *on page 504*

## Hydroquinone (HYE droe kwin one)

**U.S. Brand Names** Ambi® Skin Tone [OTC]; Eldopaque® [OTC]; Eldopaque Forte®; Eldoquin® [OTC]; Eldoquin® Forte®; Esoterica® Facial [OTC]; Esoterica® Regular [OTC]; Esoterica® Sensitive Skin Formula [OTC]; Esoterica® Sunscreen [OTC]; Melanex®; Porcelana® [OTC]; Porcelana® Sunscreen [OTC]; Solaquin® [OTC]; Solaquin Forte®

**Canadian Brand Names** Neostrata™ HQ; Ultraquin™

**Therapeutic Category** Depigmenting Agent

**Use** Gradual bleaching of hyperpigmented skin conditions

**Usual Dosage** Children >12 years and Adults: Topical: Apply thin layer and rub in twice daily

**Mechanism of Action** Produces reversible depigmentation of the skin by suppression of melanocyte metabolic processes, in particular the inhibition of the enzymatic oxidation of tyrosine to DOPA (3,4-dihydroxyphenylalanine); sun exposure reverses this effect and will cause repigmentation.

**Local Anesthetic/Vasoconstrictor Precautions** No information available to require special precautions

**Effects on Dental Treatment** No effects or complications reported

**Other Adverse Effects** 1% to 10%: Dermatologic: Dermatitis, dryness, erythema, stinging, irritation, inflammatory reaction, sensitization

**Drug Interactions** No data reported

**Drug Uptake** Onset and duration of depigmentation produced by hydroquinone varies among individuals

**Pregnancy Risk Factor** C

**Generic Available** No

♦ **Hydro-Serp®** *see* Hydrochlorothiazide and Reserpine *on page 504*
♦ **Hydroserpine®** *see* Hydrochlorothiazide and Reserpine *on page 504*
♦ **HydroStat IR®** *see* Hydromorphone *on previous page*
♦ **Hydroxacen®** *see* Hydroxyzine *on page 518*

## Hydroxocobalamin (hye droks oh koe BAL a min)

**U.S. Brand Names** Hydro Cobex®; Hydro-Crysti-12®; LA-12®

**Canadian Brand Names** Acti-$B_{12}$®

**Therapeutic Category** Vitamin, Water Soluble

**Use** Treatment of pernicious anemia, vitamin $B_{12}$ deficiency, increased $B_{12}$ requirements due to pregnancy, thyrotoxicosis, hemorrhage, malignancy, liver or kidney disease

**Usual Dosage** Vitamin $B_{12}$ deficiency: I.M.:

Children: 1-5 mg given in single doses of 100 mcg over 2 or more weeks, followed by 30-50 mcg/month

Adults: 30 mcg/day for 5-10 days, followed by 100-200 mcg/month

**Mechanism of Action** Coenzyme for various metabolic functions, including fat and carbohydrate metabolism and protein synthesis, used in cell replication and hematopoiesis

**Local Anesthetic/Vasoconstrictor Precautions** No information available to require special precautions

**Effects on Dental Treatment** No effects or complications reported

**Other Adverse Effects**

1% to 10%:

- Dermatologic: Itching
- Gastrointestinal: Diarrhea

<1%:

- Cardiovascular: Peripheral vascular thrombosis
- Dermatologic: Urticaria
- Miscellaneous: Anaphylaxis

**Drug Interactions** No data reported

**Pregnancy Risk Factor** C

**Generic Available** Yes

## Hydroxyamphetamine (hye droks ee am FET a meen)

**U.S. Brand Names** Paredrine®

**Therapeutic Category** Ophthalmic Agent, Mydriatic

**Use** Produce mydriasis in diagnostic eye examination

**Usual Dosage** Instill 1-2 drops into conjunctival sac

**Local Anesthetic/Vasoconstrictor Precautions** No information available to require special precautions

**Effects on Dental Treatment** No effects or complications reported

**Generic Available** No

## Hydroxyamphetamine and Tropicamide

(hye droks ee am FET a meen & troe PIK a mide)

**U.S. Brand Names** Paremyd® Ophthalmic

**Therapeutic Category** Ophthalmic Agent, Mydriatic

**Use** Mydriasis with cycloplegia

**Usual Dosage** Ophthalmic: Adults: Instill 1-2 drops into conjunctival sac(s)

**Local Anesthetic/Vasoconstrictor Precautions** No information available to require special precautions

**Effects on Dental Treatment** No effects or complications reported

**Generic Available** No

♦ **Hydroxycarbamide** *see* Hydroxyurea *on page 517*

## Hydroxychloroquine (hye droks ee KLOR oh kwin)

**Related Information**

Rheumatoid Arthritis and Osteoarthritis *on page 1092*

**U.S. Brand Names** Plaquenil®

**Therapeutic Category** Antimalarial Agent

**Use** Suppresses and treats acute attacks of malaria; treatment of systemic lupus erythematosus and rheumatoid arthritis

**Usual Dosage** Oral:

Children:

Chemoprophylaxis of malaria: 5 mg/kg (base) once weekly; should not exceed the recommended adult dose; begin 2 weeks before exposure; continue for 4-6 weeks after leaving endemic area

Acute attack: 10 mg/kg (base) initial dose; followed by 5 mg/kg at 6, 24, and 48 hours

JRA or SLE: 3-5 mg/kg/day divided 1-2 times/day to a maximum of 400 mg/day; not to exceed 7 mg/kg/day

Adults:

Chemoprophylaxis of malaria: 2 tablets weekly on same day each week; begin 2 weeks before exposure; continue for 4-6 weeks after leaving endemic area

(Continued)

## Hydroxychloroquine *(Continued)*

Acute attack: 4 tablets first dose day 1; 2 tablets in 6 hours day 1; 2 tablets in 1 dose day 2; and 2 tablets in 1 dose on day 3

Rheumatoid arthritis: 2-3 tablets/day to start taken with food or milk; increase dose until optimum response level is reached; usually after 4-12 weeks dose should be reduced by 1/2 and a maintenance dose of 1-2 tablets/day given

Lupus erythematosus: 2 tablets every day or twice daily for several weeks depending on response; 1-2 tablets/day for prolonged maintenance therapy

**Mechanism of Action** Interferes with digestive vacuole function within sensitive malarial parasites by increasing the pH and interfering with lysosomal degradation of hemoglobin; inhibits locomotion of neutrophils and chemotaxis of eosinophils; impairs complement-dependent antigen-antibody reactions

**Local Anesthetic/Vasoconstrictor Precautions** No information available to require special precautions

**Effects on Dental Treatment** No effects or complications reported

**Other Adverse Effects**

>10%:

Central nervous system: Headache

Dermatologic: Itching

Gastrointestinal: Diarrhea, loss of appetite, nausea, stomach cramps, vomiting

Ocular: Ciliary muscle dysfunction

1% to 10%:

Central nervous system: Dizziness, lightheadedness, nervousness, restlessness

Dermatologic: Bleaching of hair, skin rash blue-black discoloration of skin

Ocular: Ocular toxicity, keratopathy, retinopathy

<1%:

Central nervous system: Emotional changes, seizures

Hematologic: Agranulocytosis, aplastic anemia, neutropenia, thrombocytopenia

Neuromuscular & skeletal: Neuromyopathy

Otic: Ototoxicity

**Drug Interactions** No data reported

**Drug Uptake** Absorption: Oral: Complete

**Pregnancy Risk Factor** C

**Generic Available** Yes

♦ **Hydroxydaunomycin Hydrochloride** *see* Doxorubicin *on page 353*

♦ **Hydroxyethylcellulose** *see* Artificial Tears *on page 97*

♦ **Hydroxyethyl Starch** *see* Hetastarch *on page 496*

## Hydroxyprogesterone Caproate

(hye droks ee proe JES te rone KAP roe ate)

**U.S. Brand Names** Hylutin® Injection; Hyprogest® 250 Injection

**Therapeutic Category** Progestin

**Use** Treatment of amenorrhea, abnormal uterine bleeding, endometriosis, uterine carcinoma

**Usual Dosage** Adults: Female: I.M.:

Amenorrhea: 375 mg; if no bleeding, begin cyclic treatment with estradiol valerate

Production of secretory endometrium and desquamation: (Medical D and C): 125-250 mg administered on day 10 of cycle; repeat every 7 days until supression is no longer desired.

Uterine carcinoma: 1 g one or more times/day (1-7 g/week) for up to 12 weeks

**Mechanism of Action** Natural steroid hormone that induces secretory changes in the endometrium, promotes mammary gland development, relaxes uterine smooth muscle, blocks follicular maturation and ovulation and maintains pregnancy

**Local Anesthetic/Vasoconstrictor Precautions** No information available to require special precautions

**Effects on Dental Treatment** No effects or complications reported

**Other Adverse Effects**

>10%:

Cardiovascular: Edema

Endocrine & metabolic: Breakthrough bleeding, spotting, changes in menstrual flow, amenorrhea

Gastrointestinal: Anorexia

Local: Pain at injection site

Neuromuscular & skeletal: Weakness

1% to 10%:

Central nervous system: Mental depression, insomnia, fever

Dermatologic: Melasma or chloasma, allergic rash with or without pruritus
Gastrointestinal: Weight gain or loss
Genitourinary: Changes in cervical erosion and secretions, increased breast tenderness
Hepatic: Cholestatic jaundice

**Drug Interactions** Decreased effect: Rifampin causes an increased clearance of hydroxyprogesterone

**Drug Uptake** Peak serum concentration: I.M.: 3-7 days; concentrations are measurable for 3-4 weeks after injection

**Pregnancy Risk Factor** D

**Generic Available** Yes

## Hydroxypropyl Cellulose (hye droks ee PROE pil SEL yoo lose)

**U.S. Brand Names** Lacrisert®

**Therapeutic Category** Ophthalmic Agent, Miscellaneous

**Use** Dry eyes

**Local Anesthetic/Vasoconstrictor Precautions** No information available to require special precautions

**Effects on Dental Treatment** No effects or complications reported

**Other Adverse Effects** 1% to 10%: Local irritation

**Generic Available** Yes

## Hydroxypropyl Methylcellulose

(hye droks ee PROE pil meth il SEL yoo lose)

**U.S. Brand Names** Gonak™ [OTC]; Goniosol® [OTC]

**Therapeutic Category** Ophthalmic Agent, Miscellaneous

**Synonyms** Gonioscopic Ophthalmic Solution

**Use** Ophthalmic surgical aid in cataract extraction and intraocular implantation; gonioscopic examinations

**Usual Dosage** Introduced into anterior chamber of eye with 20-gauge or larger cannula

**Local Anesthetic/Vasoconstrictor Precautions** No information available to require special precautions

**Effects on Dental Treatment** No effects or complications reported

**Other Adverse Effects** 1% to 10%: Local irritation

**Pregnancy Risk Factor** C

**Generic Available** No

## Hydroxyurea (hye droks ee yoor EE a)

**U.S. Brand Names** Droxia®; Hydrea®

**Therapeutic Category** Antineoplastic Agent, Miscellaneous

**Synonyms** Hydroxycarbamide

**Use** CML in chronic phase; radiosensitizing agent in the treatment of primary brain tumors; head and neck tumors; uterine cervix and nonsmall cell lung cancer; psoriasis; sickle cell anemia and other hemoglobinopathies; resistant chronic myelocytic leukemia; hematologic conditions such as essential thrombocythemia, polycythemia vera, hypereosinophilia, and hyperleukocytosis due to acute leukemia. Has shown activity against renal cell cancer; malignant melanoma; metastatic or inoperable carcinoma of the ovary; head, neck, and lip cancer; and prostate cancer.

Droxia™: Approved - specifically for patients >18 years of age who have had at least three "painful crises" in the previous year - to reduce frequency of these crises and the need for blood transfusions; Droxia™ is not a cure for sickle cell disease, but it may help control the symptoms of the disease.

**Unlabeled use:** Thrombocythemia

**Usual Dosage** Adults: Oral (refer to individual protocols): Dosage based on patient's actual or ideal weight, whichever is less

Solid tumors: Intermittent therapy: 80 mg/kg as a single dose every third day; continuous therapy: 20-30 mg/kg/day given as a single dose/day

Concomitant therapy with irradiation: 80 mg/kg as a single dose every third day starting at least 7 days before initiation of irradiation

Resistant chronic myelocytic leukemia: 20-30 mg/kg/day divided daily

Sickle cell anemia: Droxia™: Initial: 15 mg/kg as a single daily dose (dose based on IBW or actual body weight whichever is less); dose may be increased by 5 mg/kg every 12 weeks to highest dose which does not produce toxic blood counts over 24 weeks, or a maximum of 35 mg/kg

Do not increase dose if counts are between acceptable and toxic; if counts are considered toxic, discontinue hydroxyurea until hematologic recovery; resume dosing at a dose which is 2.5 mg/kg/day less than the dose which

(Continued)

## Hydroxyurea *(Continued)*

resulted in toxicity; further titration should proceed at 2.5 mg/kg/day increments, adjusted every 12 weeks as above; do not attempt any dosage which results in toxicity on two occasions

Acceptable: Neutrophils ≥2500 cells/mm³, platelets ≥95,000/mm³, hemoglobin >5.3 g/dL and reticulocytes ≥95,000/mm³ if the hemoglobin concentration is <9 g/dL

Toxic: Neutrophils <2000 cells/mm³, platelets <80,000/mm³, hemoglobin <4.5 g/dL and reticulocytes ≥80,000/mm³ if the hemoglobin concentration is <9 g/dL

**Mechanism of Action** Interferes with synthesis of DNA, during the S phase of cell division, without interfering with RNA synthesis; inhibits ribonucleoside diphosphate reductase preventing conversion of ribonucleotides to deoxyribonucleotides; mechanism by which hydroxyurea produces beneficial effects in sickle cell anemia is uncertain; proposed contributions include increased concentration of hemoglobin F, increased deformability of sickled cells, and reductions in neutrophils

**Local Anesthetic/Vasoconstrictor Precautions** No information available to require special precautions

**Effects on Dental Treatment** No effects or complications reported

**Other Adverse Effects**

>10%:

Central nervous system: Drowsiness

Gastrointestinal: Mild to moderate nausea and vomiting may occur, as well as diarrhea, constipation, mucositis, ulceration of the GI tract, anorexia, and stomatitis

Hematologic: Myelosuppression: Dose-limiting toxicity, causes a rapid drop in leukocyte count (seen in 4-5 days in nonhematologic malignancy and more rapidly in leukemia). Thrombocytopenia and anemia occur less often; reversal of WBC count occurs rapidly, but the platelet count may take 7-10 days to recover.

1% to 10%:

Dermatologic: Dermatologic changes (hyperpigmentation, erythema of the hands and face, maculopapular rash, or dry skin), alopecia

Hepatic: Abnormal LFTs and hepatitis

Renal: Elevated BUN/creatinine

Miscellaneous: Carcinogenic potential

<1%:

Central nervous system: Neurotoxicity, renal tubular function impairment, dizziness, disorientation, hallucination, seizures, headache

Endocrine & metabolic: Hyperuricemia

Genitourinary: Dysuria

Hepatic: Elevation of hepatic enzymes

**Drug Interactions**

Increased effect: Zidovudine, zalcitabine, didanosine: Synergy

Increased toxicity:

Fluorouracil: The potential for neurotoxicity may increase with concomitant administration

Cytarabine: Modulation of its metabolism and cytotoxicity → reduction of cytarabine dose is recommended

**Drug Uptake**

Absorption: Readily absorbed from GI tract (≥80%)

Serum half-life: 3-4 hours

Time to peak serum concentration: Within 2 hours

**Pregnancy Risk Factor** D

**Dosage Forms**

Capsule: 500 mg

Capsule (Droxia™): 200 mg, 300 mg, 400 mg

**Generic Available** Yes

## Hydroxyzine (hye DROKS i zeen)

**Related Information**

Patients Requiring Sedation *on page 1152*

**U.S. Brand Names** Anxanil®; Atarax®; Hydroxacen®; Hyzine-50®; QYS®; Vistacon®; Vistaject-25®; Vistaject-50®; Vistaquel®; Vistaril®; Vistazine®

**Canadian Brand Names** Apo®-Hydroxyzine; Multipax®; Novo-Hydroxyzin; PMS-Hydroxyzine

**Therapeutic Category** Antianxiety Agent; Antiemetic; Antihistamine; Sedative; Tranquilizer, Minor

**Use**

Dental: Treatment of anxiety, as a preoperative sedative in pediatric dentistry

Medical: Antipruritic, antiemetic, and in alcohol withdrawal symptoms

**Usual Dosage**

Children:

>6 years:

Oral: 25-50 mg 1 hour before procedure or 0.6 mg/kg/dose every 6 hours

I.M.: 0.5-1 mg/kg/dose every 4-6 hours as needed

<6 years: Oral: 12.5-25 mg 1 hours before procedure

Adults: Very rarely used in adults as preoperative sedative

Oral: 50-100 mg 1 hour before procedure

I.M.: 25-100 mg 1 hour before procedure

**Mechanism of Action** Competes with histamine for $H_1$-receptor sites on effector cells in the gastrointestinal tract, blood vessels, and respiratory tract

**Local Anesthetic/Vasoconstrictor Precautions** No information available to require special precautions

**Effects on Dental Treatment** 1% to 10% of patients experience dry mouth

**Other Adverse Effects**

>10%:

Central nervous system: Slight to moderate drowsiness

Respiratory: Thickening of bronchial secretions

1% to 10%:

Central nervous system: Headache, fatigue, nervousness, dizziness

Gastrointestinal: Appetite increase, weight gain, nausea, diarrhea, abdominal pain

Neuromuscular & skeletal: Arthralgia

Respiratory: Pharyngitis

**Contraindications** Hypersensitivity to hydroxyzine or any component

**Warnings/Precautions** S.C., intra-arterial and I.V. administration **not** recommended since thrombosis and digital gangrene can occur; extravasation can result in sterile abscess and marked tissue induration; should be used with caution in patients with narrow-angle glaucoma, prostatic hypertrophy, and bladder neck obstruction; should also be used with caution in patients with asthma or COPD

Anticholinergic effects are not well tolerated in the elderly. Hydroxyzine may be useful as a short-term antipruritic, but it is not recommended for use as a sedative or anxiolytic in the elderly.

**Drug Interactions** Increased toxicity with CNS depressants, anticholinergics

**Drug Uptake**

Absorption: Oral: Rapid

Onset of effect: Within 15-30 minutes

Duration: 4-6 hours

Serum half-life: 3-7 hours

**Pregnancy Risk Factor** C

**Breast-feeding Considerations** No data reported

**Dosage Forms**

Hydroxyzine hydrochloride:

Injection: 25 mg/mL (1 mL, 2 mL, 10 mL); 50 mg/mL (1 mL, 2 mL, 10 mL)

Syrup: 10 mg/5 mL (120 mL, 480 mL, 4000 mL)

Tablet: 10 mg, 25 mg, 50 mg, 100 mg

Hydroxyzine pamoate:

Capsule: 25 mg, 50 mg, 100 mg

Suspension, oral: 25 mg/5 mL (120 mL, 480 mL)

**Dietary Considerations** No data reported

**Generic Available** Yes

♦ **Hygroton®** *see* Chlorthalidone *on page 242*

♦ **Hylorel®** *see* Guanadrel *on page 483*

♦ **Hylutin® Injection** *see* Hydroxyprogesterone Caproate *on page 516*

## Hyoscyamine (hye oh SYE a meen)

**U.S. Brand Names** Anaspaz®; A-Spas® S/L; Cystospaz®; Cystospaz-M®; Donnamar®; ED-SPAZ®; Gastrosed™; Levbid®; Levsin®; Levsinex®; Levsin/SL®

**Therapeutic Category** Anticholinergic Agent; Antispasmodic Agent, Gastrointestinal

**Use** Treatment of GI tract disorders caused by spasm, adjunctive therapy for peptic ulcers

**Usual Dosage**

Children: Oral, S.L.: Dose as per table repeated every 4 hours as needed

Adults:

Oral or S.L.: 0.125-0.25 mg 3-4 times/day before meals or food and at bedtime

Oral: 0.375-0.75 mg (timed release) every 12 hours

I.M., I.V., S.C.: 0.25-0.5 mg every 6 hours

(Continued)

## Hyoscyamine *(Continued)*

**Hyoscyamine**

| Weight (kg) | Dose (mcg) | Maximum 24-Hour Dose (mcg) |
|---|---|---|
| **Children <2 y** | | |
| 2.3 | 12.5 | 75 |
| 3.4 | 16.7 | 100 |
| 5 | 20.8 | 125 |
| 7 | 25 | 150 |
| 10 | 31.3-33.3 | 200 |
| 15 | 45.8 | 275 |
| **Children 2-10 y** | | |
| 10 | 31.3-33.3 | Do not exceed 0.75 mg |
| 20 | 62.5 | |
| 40 | 93.8 | |
| 50 | 125 | |

**Mechanism of Action** Blocks the action of acetylcholine at parasympathetic sites in smooth muscle, secretory glands and the CNS; increases cardiac output, dries secretions, antagonizes histamine and serotonin

**Local Anesthetic/Vasoconstrictor Precautions** No information available to require special precautions

**Effects on Dental Treatment** >10% of patients experience dry mouth (normal salivary flow returns with cessation of drug therapy)

**Other Adverse Effects**

>10%:
- Dermatologic: Dry skin
- Local: Irritation at injection site
- Respiratory: Dry nose, throat
- Miscellaneous: Decreased sweating

1% to 10%:
- Dermatologic: Photosensitivity
- Gastrointestinal: Constipation, dysphagia
- Ocular: Blurred vision, mydriasis

<1%:
- Cardiovascular: Palpitations, orthostatic hypotension
- Central nervous system: Headache, lightheadedness, memory loss, fatigue, delirium, restlessness, ataxia
- Dermatologic: Skin rash
- Genitourinary: Dysuria
- Neuromuscular & skeletal: Tremor
- Ocular: Increased intraocular pressure

**Drug Interactions**

Decreased effect with antacids

Increased toxicity with amantadine, antimuscarinics, haloperidol, phenothiazines, TCAs, MAO inhibitors

**Drug Uptake**

Onset of effect: 2-3 minutes

Duration: 4-6 hours

Absorption: Oral: Absorbed well

Serum half-life: 13% to 38%

**Pregnancy Risk Factor** C

**Generic Available** Yes

## Hyoscyamine, Atropine, Scopolamine, and Phenobarbital

(hye oh SYE a meen, A troe peen, skoe POL a meen & fee noe BAR bi tal)

**U.S. Brand Names** Barbidonna®; Donnatal®; Hyosophen®; Malatal®; Spasmolin®

**Therapeutic Category** Anticholinergic Agent; Antispasmodic Agent, Gastrointestinal

**Use** Adjunct in treatment of peptic ulcer disease, irritable bowel, spastic colitis, spastic bladder, and renal colic

**Usual Dosage** Oral:

Children 2-12 years: Kinesed® dose: ½ to 1 tablet 3-4 times/day

Children: Donnatal® elixir: 0.1 mL/kg/dose every 4 hours; maximum dose: 5 mL **or** see table for alternative.

| Weight (kg) | Dose (mL) | |
|---|---|---|
| | q4h | q6h |
| 4.5 | 0.5 | 0.75 |
| 10 | 1 | 1.5 |
| 14 | 1.5 | 2 |
| 23 | 2.5 | 3.8 |
| 34 | 3.8 | 5 |
| ≥45 | 5 | 7.5 |

Adults: 1-2 capsules or tablets 3-4 times/day; or 1 Donnatal® Extentab® in sustained release form every 12 hours; or 5-10 mL elixir 3-4 times/day or every 8 hours

**Mechanism of Action** Refer to individual agents

**Local Anesthetic/Vasoconstrictor Precautions** No information available to require special precautions

**Effects on Dental Treatment** >10% of patients experience dry mouth (normal salivary flow returns with cessation of drug therapy)

**Other Adverse Effects**

>10%:
- Dermatologic: Dry skin
- Gastrointestinal: Constipation
- Local: Irritation at injection site
- Respiratory: Dry nose, throat
- Miscellaneous: Decreased sweating

1% to 10%:
- Dermatologic: Photosensitivity
- Endocrine & metabolic: Decreased flow of breast milk
- Gastrointestinal: Dysphagia

<1%:
- Cardiovascular: Orthostatic hypotension, ventricular fibrillation, tachycardia, palpitations
- Central nervous system: Confusion, drowsiness, headache, loss of memory, fatigue, ataxia
- Dermatologic: Skin rash
- Gastrointestinal: Bloated feeling, nausea, vomiting
- Genitourinary: Dysuria
- Ocular: Increased intraocular pain, blurred vision

**Drug Interactions** The following drugs may cause enhanced effects of this preparation: CNS depressants, amantadine, antihistamine, phenothiazines, corticosteroids, digitalis, griseofulvin, anticonvulsants, MAO inhibitors, tricyclic antidepressants

**Drug Uptake** Absorption: Well absorbed from GI tract

**Pregnancy Risk Factor** C

**Generic Available** Yes

## Hyoscyamine, Atropine, Scopolamine, Kaolin, and Pectin

(hye oh SYE a meen, A troe peen, skoe POL a meen, KAY oh lin & PEK tin)

**Therapeutic Category** Antidiarrheal

**Use** Antidiarrheal; also used in gastritis, enteritis, colitis, and acute gastrointestinal upsets, and nausea which may accompany any of these conditions

**Usual Dosage** Oral:

Children:
- 10-20 lb: 2.5 mL
- 20-30 lb: 5 mL
- >30 lb: 5-10 mL

Adults:
- Diarrhea: 30 mL at once and 15-30 mL with each loose stool
- Other conditions: 15 mL every 3 hours as needed

**Local Anesthetic/Vasoconstrictor Precautions** No information available to require special precautions

**Effects on Dental Treatment** Dry mouth in >10% of patients (normal salivary flow returns with cessation of drug therapy)

**Pregnancy Risk Factor** C

**Generic Available** Yes

## Hyoscyamine, Atropine, Scopolamine, Kaolin, Pectin, and Opium

(hye oh SYE a meen, A troe peen, skoe POL a meen, KAY oh lin, PEK tin, & OH pee um)

**U.S. Brand Names** Donnapectolin-PG®; Kapectolin PG®

**Therapeutic Category** Antidiarrheal

**Use** Treatment of diarrhea

**Usual Dosage**

Children 6-12 years: Initial: 10 mL, then, 5-10 mL every 3 hours thereafter

Alternate children's dosing recommendations based on body weight:

10 lb: 2.5 mL

20 lb: 5 mL

≥ 30 lb: 5-10 mL

Do not administer more than 4 doses in any 24-hour period

Children >12 years and Adults: Initial: 30 mL (1 fluid oz) followed by 15 mL every 3 hours

**Local Anesthetic/Vasoconstrictor Precautions** No information available to require special precautions

**Effects on Dental Treatment** Dry mouth in >10% of patients (normal salivary flow returns with cessation of drug therapy)

**Pregnancy Risk Factor** C

**Generic Available** Yes

**Comments** Hyoscyamine is dialyzable

- **Hyosophen®** *see* Hyoscyamine, Atropine, Scopolamine, and Phenobarbital *on page 520*
- **Hyperab®** *see* Rabies Immune Globulin (Human) *on page 875*
- **HyperHep®** *see* Hepatitis B Immune Globulin *on page 494*
- **Hyperstat® I.V.** *see* Diazoxide *on page 317*
- **Hyper-Tet®** *see* Tetanus Immune Globulin (Human) *on page 962*
- **Hy-Phen® [5/500]** *see* Hydrocodone and Acetaminophen *on page 505*
- **HypoTears PF Solution [OTC]** *see* Artificial Tears *on page 97*
- **HypoTears Solution [OTC]** *see* Artificial Tears *on page 97*
- **HypRho®-D** *see* $Rh_o$(D) Immune Globulin *on page 884*
- **HypRho®-D Mini-Dose** *see* $Rh_o$(D) Immune Globulin *on page 884*
- **Hyprogest® 250 Injection** *see* Hydroxyprogesterone Caproate *on page 516*
- **Hyrexin-50® Injection** *see* Diphenhydramine *on page 338*
- **Hytakerol®** *see* Dihydrotachysterol *on page 333*
- **Hytinic® [OTC]** *see* Polysaccharide-Iron Complex *on page 816*
- **Hytrin®** *see* Terazosin *on page 957*
- **Hytuss® [OTC]** *see* Guaifenesin *on page 478*
- **Hytuss-2X® [OTC]** *see* Guaifenesin *on page 478*
- **Hyzaar®** *see* Losartan and Hydrochlorothiazide *on page 604*
- **Hyzine-50®** *see* Hydroxyzine *on page 518*
- **Iberet-Folic-500®** *see* Ferrous Sulfate, Ascorbic Acid, Vitamin B-Complex, and Folic Acid *on page 429*
- **Iberet®-Liquid [OTC]** *see* Ferrous Sulfate, Ascorbic Acid, and Vitamin B-Complex *on page 428*
- **IBU®** *see* Ibuprofen *on this page*
- **Ibuprin® [OTC]** *see* Ibuprofen *on this page*

## Ibuprofen (eye byoo PROE fen)

**Related Information**

Dental Drug Interactions: Update on Drug Combinations Requiring Special Considerations *on page 1225*

Oral Pain *on page 1122*

Rheumatoid Arthritis and Osteoarthritis *on page 1092*

Temporomandibular Dysfunction (TMD) *on page 1149*

**U.S. Brand Names** Advil® [OTC]; Bayer® Select® Pain Relief Formula [OTC]; Children's Advil® Oral Suspension [OTC]; Children's Motrin® Oral Suspension [OTC]; Genpril® [OTC]; Haltran® [OTC]; IBU®; Ibuprin® [OTC]; Ibuprohm® [OTC]; Junior Strength Motrin® [OTC]; Menadol® [OTC]; Midol® IB [OTC]; Motrin®; Motrin® IB [OTC]; Nuprin® [OTC]; Pediatric Advil® [OTC]; Saleto-200® [OTC]; Saleto-400®; Saleto-600®; Saleto-800®

**Canadian Brand Names** Actiprofen®; Apo®-Ibuprofen; Novo-Profen®; Nu-Ibuprofen

**Therapeutic Category** Analgesic, Non-narcotic; Anti-inflammatory Agent; Nonsteroidal Anti-inflammatory Drug (NSAID), Oral

**Use**

Dental: Management of pain and swelling

Medical: Inflammatory diseases and rheumatoid disorders including juvenile rheumatoid arthritis, mild to moderate pain, fever, dysmenorrhea, gout, ankylosing spondylitis, acute migraine headache

**Usual Dosage** Oral:

Children: Analgesic: 4-10 mg/kg/dose every 6-8 hours

Adults: 400-800 mg/dose 3-4 times/day; maximum daily dose: 3.2 (3200 mg) g/day

**Mechanism of Action** Inhibits prostaglandin synthesis by decreasing the activity of the enzyme, cyclo-oxygenase, which results in decreased formation of prostaglandin precursors

**Local Anesthetic/Vasoconstrictor Precautions** No information available to require special precautions

**Effects on Dental Treatment** <1% of patients experience dry mouth; NSAID formulations are known to reversibly decrease platelet aggregation via mechanisms different than observed with aspirin. The dentist should be aware of the potential of abnormal coagulation. Caution should also be exercised in the use of NSAIDs in patients already on anticoagulant therapy with drugs such as warfarin (Coumadin®).

**Other Adverse Effects**

>10%: Gastrointestinal: Indigestion, nausea

1% to 10%: Gastrointestinal: Abdominal pain

**Contraindications** Hypersensitivity to ibuprofen, any component, aspirin, or other nonsteroidal anti-inflammatory drugs (NSAIDs)

**Warnings/Precautions** Do not exceed 3200 mg/day; use with caution in patients with congestive heart failure, hypertension, decreased renal or hepatic function, history of GI disease (bleeding or ulcers), or those receiving anticoagulants; safety and efficacy in children <6 months of age have not yet been established; elderly are a high-risk population for adverse effects from nonsteroidal anti-inflammatory agents. As much as 60% of elderly can develop peptic ulceration and/or hemorrhage asymptomatically.

Use lowest effective dose for shortest period possible. CNS adverse effects such as confusion, agitation, and hallucination are generally seen in overdose or high dose situations; but elderly may demonstrate these adverse effects at lower doses than younger adults.

**Drug Interactions**

Warfarin (Coumadin®): Ibuprofen can cause a decrease in platelet aggregation which may result in enhancement of the anticoagulant effect of coumarins

Lithium: Ibuprofen may inhibit prostaglandin-induced renal secretion of lithium, which increases lithium plasma levels and produces symptoms of lithium toxicity

Methotrexate: Ibuprofen has been reported to increase the serum levels of methotrexate resulting in possible methotrexate toxicity

Aspirin: Aspirin may decrease ibuprofen serum levels thereby reducing the effectiveness of ibuprofen

Raloxifen (Evista®): Manufacturer's information states that caution should be used when raloxifen is coadministered with other highly protein-bound drugs such as ibuprofen. Raloxifen could displace the ibuprofen and vice versa leading to increased free active form of the target drug.

**Drug Uptake**

Absorption: Rapid

Onset of effect: 30-60 minutes

Time to peak serum concentration: Within 1-2 hours

Duration of effect: 4-6 hours

Serum half-life: 2-4 hours

**Pregnancy Risk Factor** B (D if used in the 3rd trimester)

**Breast-feeding Considerations** May be taken while breast-feeding

**Dosage Forms**

Caplet: 100 mg

Drops, oral (berry flavor): 40 mg/mL (15 mL)

Suspension, oral: 100 mg/5 mL [OTC] (60 mL, 120 mL, 480 mL)

Suspension, oral, drops: 40 mg/mL [OTC]

Tablet: 100 mg [OTC], 200 mg [OTC], 300 mg, 400 mg, 600 mg, 800 mg

Tablet, chewable: 50 mg, 100 mg

**Dietary Considerations** May be taken with food or milk to decrease GI adverse effects; food decreases rate of absorption but extent remains the same

**Generic Available** Yes: Tablet

**Comments** Preoperative use of ibuprofen at a dose of 400-600 mg every 6 hours 24 hours before the appointment decreases postoperative edema and hastens healing time

(Continued)

## Ibuprofen *(Continued)*

**Selected Readings**

Brooks PM and Day RO, "Nonsteroidal Anti-inflammatory Drugs - Differences and Similarities," *N Engl J Med*, 1991, 324(24):1716-25.

Dionne RA, "New Approaches to Preventing and Treating Postoperative Pain," *J Am Dent Assoc*, 1992, 123(6):26-34.

Gobetti JP, "Controlling Dental Pain," *J Am Dent Assoc*, 1992, 123(6):47-52.

Pearlman B, Boyatzis S, Daly C, et al, "The Analgesic Efficacy of Ibuprofen in Periodontal Surgery: A Multicentre Study," *Aust Dent J*, 1997, 42(5):328-34.

Winter L Jr, Bass E, Recant B, et al, "Analgesic Activity of Ibuprofen (Motrin®) in Postoperative Oral Surgical Pain," *Oral Surg Oral Med Oral Pathol*, 1978, 45(2):159-66.

◆ **Ibuprohm® [OTC]** *see* Ibuprofen *on page 522*

## Ibutilide (i BYOO ti lide)

**U.S. Brand Names** Corvert®

**Therapeutic Category** Antiarrhythmic Agent, Class III

**Synonyms** Ibutilide Fumarate

**Use** Acute termination of atrial fibrillation or flutter of recent onset; the effectiveness of ibutilide has not been determined in patients with arrhythmias of >90 days in duration

**Usual Dosage** I.V.: Initial:

<60 kg: 0.01 mg/kg over 10 minutes

≥60 kg: 1 mg over 10 minutes

If the arrhythmia does not terminate within 10 minutes after the end of the initial infusion, a second infusion of equal strength may be infused over a 10-minute period

**Mechanism of Action** Exact mechanism of action is unknown; prolongs the action potential in cardiac tissue

**Local Anesthetic/Vasoconstrictor Precautions** No information available to require special precautions

**Effects on Dental Treatment** No effects or complications reported

**Other Adverse Effects**

1% to 10%:

Cardiovascular: Sustained polymorphic ventricular tachycardia (ie, torsade de pointes) (1.7%), often requiring cardioversion, nonsustained polymorphic ventricular tachycardia (2.7%), nonsustained monomorphic ventricular extrasystoles (5.1%), nonsustained monomorphic VT (4.9%), tachycardia/supraventricular tachycardia, hypotension (2%), bundle branch block (1.9%), A-V block (1.5%), bradycardia, Q-T segment prolongation, hypertension (1.2%), palpitations (1%)

Central nervous system: Headache (3.6%)

Gastrointestinal: Nausea (>1%)

<1%:

Cardiovascular: Supraventricular extrasystoles (0.9%), nodal arrhythmia (0.7%), congestive heart failure (0.5%), syncope, idioventricular rhythm, sustained monomorphic VT (0.2%)

Renal: Renal failure: (0.3%)

**Warnings/Precautions** Potentially fatal arrhythmias (eg, polymorphic ventricular tachycardia) can occur with ibutilide, **usually** in association with torsade de pointes (Q-T prolongation). Studies indicate a 1.7% incidence of arrhythmias in treated patients. The drug should be given in a setting of continuous EKG monitoring and by personnel trained in treating arrhythmias particularly polymorphic ventricular tachycardia. Patients with chronic atrial fibrillation may not be the best candidates for ibutilide since they often revert after conversion and the risks of treatment may not be justified when compared to alternative management. Dosing adjustments in patients with renal or hepatic dysfunction since a maximum of only two 10-minute infusions are indicated and drug distribution is one of the primary mechanisms responsible for termination of the pharmacologic effect; safety and efficacy in children have not been established.

**Drug Interactions** Increased toxicity: Class Ia antiarrhythmic drugs (disopyramide, quinidine, and procainamide) and other class III drugs such as amiodarone and sotalol, should not be given concomitantly with ibutilide due to their potential to prolong refractoriness; the potential for prolongation of the Q-T interval may occur if ibutilide is given concurrently with phenothiazines, tricyclic and tetracyclic antidepressants, and the nonsedating antihistamines (terfenadine and astemizole); signs of digoxin toxicity may be masked when coadministered with ibutilide

**Drug Uptake**

Absorption: Onset: Within 90 minutes after start of infusion (½ of conversions to sinus rhythm occur during infusion)

Serum half-life: 2-12 hours (average: 6 hours)

**Pregnancy Risk Factor** C

**Generic Available** No

♦ **Ibutilide Fumarate** *see* Ibutilide *on previous page*
♦ **Idamycin®** *see* Idarubicin *on this page*

## Idarubicin (eye da ROO bi sin)

**U.S. Brand Names** Idamycin®

**Therapeutic Category** Antineoplastic Agent, Antibiotic

**Synonyms** 4-demethoxydaunorubicin; IDR

**Use** In combination with other antineoplastic agents for treatment of acute myelogenous leukemia (AML) in adults and acute lymphocytic leukemia (ALL) in children

**Usual Dosage** I.V.:

Children:

Leukemia: 10-12 mg/$m^2$ once daily for 3 days and repeat every 3 weeks

Solid tumors: 5 mg/$m^2$ once daily for 3 days and repeat every 3 weeks

Adults: 12 mg/$m^2$/day for 3 days by slow I.V. injection (10-15 minutes) in combination with Ara-C. The Ara-C may be given as 100 mg/$m^2$/day by continuous infusion for 7 days or 25 mg/$m^2$ bolus followed by Ara-C 200 mg/$m^2$/day for 5 days continuous infusion.

**Mechanism of Action** Similar to daunorubicin, idarubicin exhibits inhibitory effects on DNA and RNA polymerase *in vitro*. Idarubicin has an affinity for DNA similar to daunorubicin and somewhat higher efficacy in stabilizing the DNA double helix against heat denaturation. Idarubicin has been as active or more active than daunorubicin in inhibiting 3H-TdR uptake by DNA or RNA of mouse embryo fibroblasts.

**Local Anesthetic/Vasoconstrictor Precautions** No information available to require special precautions

**Effects on Dental Treatment** No effects or complications reported

**Other Adverse Effects**

>10%:

Central nervous system: Headache, fever

Dermatologic: Alopecia, rash, urticaria

Gastrointestinal: Mucositis, nausea, vomiting, diarrhea, stomatitis

Genitourinary: Discoloration of urine (red)

Hematologic: Hemorrhage, anemia

Leukopenia (nadir: 8-29 days)

Thrombocytopenia (nadir: 10-15 days)

Local: Tissue necrosis upon extravasation, erythematous streaking

**Vesicant chemotherapy**

Miscellaneous: Infection

1% to 10%:

Central nervous system: Seizures

Neuromuscular & skeletal: Peripheral neuropathy

Respiratory: Pulmonary allergy

<1%:

Cardiovascular: Arrhythmias, EKG changes, cardiomyopathy, congestive heart failure, myocardial toxicity, acute life-threatening arrhythmias

Endocrine & metabolic: Hyperuricemia

Hepatic: Elevations in liver enzymes or bilirubin

**Drug Uptake**

Absorption: Oral: Rapid but erratic (20% to 30%) from GI tract

Serum half-life, elimination:

Oral: 14-35 hours

I.V.: 12-27 hours

Time to peak serum concentration: Within 2-4 hours and varies considerably

**Pregnancy Risk Factor** D

**Generic Available** No

**Comments** Discoloration of urine may persist for 48 hours

## Idoxuridine *Withdrawn from Market 9/98*

(eye doks YOOR i deen)

**U.S. Brand Names** Herplex®

**Therapeutic Category** Antiviral Agent, Ophthalmic

**Use** Treatment of herpes simplex keratitis

**Usual Dosage** Adults: Ophthalmic:

Ointment: Instill 5 times/day (every 4 hours) in the conjunctival sac with last dose at bedtime; continue therapy for 5-7 days after healing appears complete

Solution: Instill 1 drop in eye(s) every hour during day and every 2 hours at night, continue until definite improvement is noted, then reduce daytime dose to 1 drop every 2 hours and every 4 hours at night; continue for 5-7 days after healing appears complete

Alternative dosing schedule: Instill 1 drop every minute for 5 minutes; repeat every 4 hours day and night

(Continued)

## Idoxuridine *Withdrawn from Market 9/98* *(Continued)*

**Mechanism of Action** Incorporated into viral DNA in place of thymidine resulting in mutations and inhibition of viral replication

**Local Anesthetic/Vasoconstrictor Precautions** No information available to require special precautions

**Effects on Dental Treatment** No effects or complications reported

**Other Adverse Effects**

1% to 10%:

Dermatologic: Pruritus, follicular conjunctivitis

Local: Irritation, pain, inflammation, mild edema of the eyelids and cornea

Ocular: Visual haze, corneal clouding, photophobia, small punctate defects on the corneal epithelium

<1%: Ocular: Small punctate defects on the corneal epithelium

**Drug Interactions** Increased toxicity: Do not coadminister with boric acid containing solutions

**Drug Uptake** Absorption: Ophthalmic: Poorly absorbed following instillation; tissue uptake is a function of cellular metabolism, which is inhibited by high concentrations of the drug (absorption decreases as the concentration of drug increases)

**Pregnancy Risk Factor** C

**Generic Available** No

- **IDR** *see* Idarubicin *on previous page*
- **Ifex® Injection** *see* Ifosfamide *on this page*

## Ifosfamide (eye FOSS fa mide)

**U.S. Brand Names** Ifex® Injection

**Therapeutic Category** Antineoplastic Agent, Alkylating Agent

**Use** In combination with other antineoplastics in treatment of lung cancer, Hodgkin's and non-Hodgkin's lymphoma, breast cancer, acute and chronic lymphocytic leukemia, ovarian cancer, testicular cancer, and sarcomas

**Usual Dosage** I.V. **(refer to individual protocols)**:

Children: 1200-1800 mg/m²/day for 3-5 days every 21-28 days **or** 5 g/m² as a single 24-hour infusion **or** 3 g/m²/day for 2 days

Adults:

Doses may be given as 50 mg/kg/day **or** 700-2000 mg/m²/day for 5 days

Alternatives include 2400 mg/m²/day for 3 days **or** 5000 mg/m² as a single dose

Doses of 700-900 mg/m²/day for 5 days may be given IVP; courses may be repeated every 3-4 weeks

To prevent bladder toxicity, ifosfamide should be given with extensive hydration consisting of at least 2 L of oral or I.V. fluid per day. A protector, such as mesna, should also be used to prevent hemorrhagic cystitis. The dose-limiting toxicity is hemorrhagic cystitis and ifosfamide should be used in conjunction with a uroprotective agent.

**Mechanism of Action** Causes cross-linking of strands of DNA by binding with nucleic acids and other intracellular structures; inhibits protein synthesis and DNA synthesis; an analogue of cyclophosphamide, and like cyclophosphamide, it undergoes activation by microsomal enzymes in the liver. Ifosfamide is metabolized to active compounds, ifosfamide mustard, and acrolein

**Local Anesthetic/Vasoconstrictor Precautions** No information available to require special precautions

**Effects on Dental Treatment** No effects or complications reported

**Other Adverse Effects**

>10%:

Dermatologic: Alopecia occurs in 50% to 83% of patients 2-4 weeks after initiation of therapy; may be as high as 100% in combination therapy patients.

Endocrine & metabolic: Metabolic acidosis may occur in up to 31% of

Gastrointestinal: Nausea and vomiting in 58% of patients is dose and schedule related (more common with higher doses and after bolus regimens); nausea and vomiting can persist up to 3 days after therapy; also anorexia, diarrhea, constipation, and stomatitis noted.

Emetic potential: Moderate (58%)

Genitourinary toxicity: Hemorrhagic cystitis has been frequently associated with the use of ifosfamide. A urinalysis prior to each dose should be obtained. **Ifosfamide should never be administered without a uroprotective agent (MESNA).**

Hepatic: Transient elevation in LFTS

Renal: Hematuria has been reported in 6% to 92% of patients. Renal toxicity occurs in 6% of patients and is manifested as an elevation in BUN or serum creatinine and is most likely related to tubular damage.

1% to 10%:

Cardiovascular: Cardiotoxicity

Central nervous system: Polyneuropathy, somnolence, confusion, hallucinations in 12% and coma (rare) have occurred and are usually reversible; usually occur with higher doses; depressive psychoses

Dermatologic: Skin hyperpigmentation, dermatitis

Endocrine & metabolic: SIADH

Gastrointestinal: Stomatitis

Hematologic: Leukopenia is mild to moderate, thrombocytopenia and anemia are rare

Myelosuppression: Less of a problem than with cyclophosphamide if used alone. However, myelosuppression can be severe when used with other chemotherapeutic agents. Be cautious with patients with compromised bone marrow reserve. WBC: Moderate; Platelets: Mild; Onset (days): 7; Nadir (days): 10-14; Recovery (days): 21

Hepatic: Elevated liver enzymes

Local: Phlebitis

Respiratory: Nasal congestion, pulmonary fibrosis

Miscellaneous: Immunosuppression, sterility, nail ridging, possible secondary malignancy, impaired wound healing, and allergic reactions

**Drug Uptake** Pharmacokinetics are dose-dependent

Absorption: Oral: Peak plasma levels occur within 1 hour

Serum half-life: Beta phase: 11-15 hours with high-dose (3800-5000 mg/m$^2$) or 4-7 hours with lower doses (1800 mg/m$^2$)

**Pregnancy Risk Factor** D

**Generic Available** No

**Comments** Usually used in combination with mesna, a prophylactic agent for hemorrhagic cystitis


- **IL-2** *see* Aldesleukin *on page 44*
- **IL-11** *see* Oprelvekin *on page 743*
- **Ilopan®** *see* Dexpanthenol *on page 310*
- **Ilopan-Choline®** *see* Dexpanthenol *on page 310*
- **Ilosone® Oral** *see* Erythromycin *on page 383*
- **Ilotycin® Ophthalmic** *see* Erythromycin, Topical *on page 386*
- **Ilozyme®** *see* Pancrelipase *on page 763*
- **Imdur™** *see* Isosorbide Mononitrate *on page 556*
- **I-Methasone®** *see* Dexamethasone *on page 308*
- **Imidazole Carboxamide** *see* Dacarbazine *on page 292*


## Imiglucerase (imi GLOO ser ase)

**U.S. Brand Names** Cerezyme®

**Therapeutic Category** Enzyme, Glucocerebrosidase

**Use** Long-term enzyme replacement therapy for patients with Type 1 Gaucher's disease

**Usual Dosage** I.V.: 2.5 units/kg 3 times a week up to as much as 60 units/kg administered as frequently as once a week or as infrequently as every 4 weeks; 60 units/kg administered every 2 weeks is the most common dose

**Local Anesthetic/Vasoconstrictor Precautions** No information available to require special precautions

**Effects on Dental Treatment** No effects or complications reported

**Pregnancy Risk Factor** C

**Generic Available** No

## Imipenem and Cilastatin (i mi PEN em & sye la STAT in)

**Related Information**

Animal and Human Bites Guidelines *on page 1164*

**U.S. Brand Names** Primaxin®

**Therapeutic Category** Antibiotic, Miscellaneous

**Use** Treatment of documented multidrug resistant gram-negative infection due to organisms proven or suspected to be susceptible to imipenem/cilastatin; treatment of multiple organism infection in which other agents have an insufficient spectrum of activity or are contraindicated due to toxic potential; Antibacterial activity includes resistant gram-negative bacilli (*Pseudomonas aeruginosa* and *Enterobacter* sp.), gram-positive bacteria (methicillin-sensitive *Staphylococcus aureus* and *Enterococcus* sp.) and anaerobes

**Usual Dosage** I.M. and I.V. (dosing based on imipenem component):

Children: I.V.: 60-100 mg/kg/24 hours divided every 6 hours (maximum: 4 g/day)

(Continued)

## Imipenem and Cilastatin *(Continued)*

Adults: I.V.: 500 mg every 6-8 hours (1 g every 6-8 hours for severe *Pseudomonas* infection); infuse each 250-500 mg dose over 20-30 minutes; infuse each 1 g dose over 40-60 minutes

Mild to moderate infection **only**: I.M.: 500-750 mg every 12 hours (**Note:** 750 mg is recommended for intra-abdominal and more severe respiratory, dermatologic, or gynecologic infections; total daily I.M. dosages >1500 mg are not recommended; deep I.M. injection should be carefully made into a large muscle mass only)

**Mechanism of Action**

A carbapenem with broad-spectrum antibacterial activity including resistant gram-negative bacilli (*Pseudomonas aeruginosa* and *Enterococcus* sp.), gram-positive bacteria (methicillin-sensitive *Staphylococcus aureus* and *Enterococcus* sp.) and anaerobes

Inhibits cell wall synthesis by binding to penicillin-binding proteins on the bacterial outer membrane; cilastatin prevents renal metabolism of imipenem by competitive inhibition of dehydropeptidase along the brush border of the proximal renal tubules

**Local Anesthetic/Vasoconstrictor Precautions** No information available to require special precautions

**Effects on Dental Treatment** No effects or complications reported

**Other Adverse Effects**

1% to 10%:

Gastrointestinal: Nausea, diarrhea, vomiting

Local: Phlebitis

<1%:

Cardiovascular: Hypotension, palpitations

Central nervous system: Seizures

Dermatologic: Rash

Gastrointestinal: Pseudomembranous colitis

Hematologic: Neutropenia, eosinophilia

Local: Pain at injection site

Miscellaneous: Emergence of resistant strains of *P. aeruginosa*

**Drug Interactions** Increased toxicity: Probenecid causes increased toxic potential

**Drug Uptake** Serum half-life:

Imipenem: 1 hour, extended with renal insufficiency

Cilastatin: 1 hour, extended with renal insufficiency

**Pregnancy Risk Factor** C

**Generic Available** No

## Imipramine (im IP ra meen)

**U.S. Brand Names** Tofranil®; Tofranil-PM®

**Canadian Brand Names** Apo®-Imipramine; Novo-Pramine; PMS-Imipramine

**Therapeutic Category** Antidepressant, Tricyclic

**Use** Treatment of various forms of depression, often in conjunction with psychotherapy; enuresis in children; analgesic for certain chronic and neuropathic pain

**Usual Dosage** Maximum antidepressant effect may not be seen for 2 or more weeks after initiation of therapy.

Children: Oral:

Depression: 1.5 mg/kg/day with dosage increments of 1 mg/kg every 3-4 days to a maximum dose of 5 mg/kg/day in 1-4 divided doses; monitor carefully especially with doses ≥3.5 mg/kg/day

Enuresis: ≥6 years: Initial: 10-25 mg at bedtime, if inadequate response still seen after 1 week of therapy, increase by 25 mg/day; dose should not exceed 2.5 mg/kg/day or 50 mg at bedtime if 6-12 years of age or 75 mg at bedtime if ≥12 years of age

Adjunct in the treatment of cancer pain: Initial: 0.2-0.4 mg/kg at bedtime; dose may be increased by 50% every 2-3 days up to 1-3 mg/kg/dose at bedtime

Adolescents: Oral: Initial: 25-50 mg/day; increase gradually; maximum: 100 mg/day in single or divided doses

Adults:

Oral: Initial: 25 mg 3-4 times/day, increase dose gradually, total dose may be given at bedtime; maximum: 300 mg/day

I.M.: Initial: Up to 100 mg/day in divided doses; change to oral as soon as possible

Elderly: Initial: 10-25 mg at bedtime; increase by 10-25 mg every 3 days for inpatients and weekly for outpatients if tolerated; average daily dose to achieve a therapeutic concentration: 100 mg/day; range: 50-150 mg/day

**Mechanism of Action** Traditionally believed to increase the synaptic concentration of serotonin and/or norepinephrine in the central nervous system by inhibition of their reuptake by the presynaptic neuronal membrane. However, additional receptor effects have been found including desensitization of adenyl cyclase, down regulation of beta-adrenergic receptors, and down regulation of serotonin receptors.

**Local Anesthetic/Vasoconstrictor Precautions** Use with caution; epinephrine, norepinephrine and levonordefrin have been shown to have an increased pressor response in combination with TCAs

**Effects on Dental Treatment** >10% of patients experience dry mouth; long-term treatment with TCAs such as imipramine increases the risk of caries by reducing salivation and salivary buffer capacity. In a study by Rundergren, et al, pathological alterations were observed in the oral mucosa of 72% of 58 patients; 55% had new carious lesions after taking TCAs for a median of 5½ years. Current research is investigating the use of the salivary stimulant pilocarpine to overcome the xerostomia from imipramine.

**Other Adverse Effects** Less sedation and anticholinergic effects than amitriptyline

>10%:

- Central nervous system: Dizziness, drowsiness, headache
- Gastrointestinal: Increased appetite, nausea, unpleasant taste, weight gain, constipation
- Genitourinary: Urinary retention
- Neuromuscular & skeletal: Weakness

1% to 10%:

- Cardiovascular: Postural hypotension, arrhythmias, tachycardia, sudden death
- Central nervous system: Confusion, delirium, hallucinations, nervousness, restlessness, parkinsonian syndrome, insomnia
- Endocrine & metabolic: Sexual dysfunction
- Gastrointestinal: Diarrhea, heartburn
- Genitourinary: Dysuria
- Neuromuscular & skeletal: Fine muscle tremors
- Ocular: Blurred vision, eye pain
- Miscellaneous: Excessive sweating

<1%:

- Central nervous system: Anxiety, seizures
- Dermatologic: Alopecia, photosensitivity
- Endocrine & metabolic: Breast enlargement, galactorrhea, SIADH
- Genitourinary: Testicular swelling
- Hematologic: Leukopenia, eosinophilia, rarely agranulocytosis
- Hepatic: Elevated liver enzymes, cholestatic jaundice
- Ocular: Increased intraocular pressure
- Otic: Tinnitus
- Miscellaneous: Allergic reactions, trouble with gums, decreased lower esophageal sphincter tone may cause GE reflux, allergic reactions, has been associated with falls

**Drug Interactions**

Decreased effect: Phenobarbital may increase the metabolism of imipramine; imipramine blocks the uptake of guanethidine and thus prevents the hypotensive effect of guanethidine

Increased toxicity: Clonidine may increase hypertensive crisis; imipramine may be additive with or may potentiate the action of other CNS depressants such as sedatives or hypnotics; with MAO inhibitors, hyperpyrexia, hypertension, tachycardia, confusion, and seizures. Imipramine may increase the prothrombin time in patients stabilized on warfarin; imipramine potentiates the pressor and cardiac effects of sympathomimetic agents such as isoproterenol, epinephrine, etc; cimetidine and methylphenidate may decrease the metabolism of imipramine

Additive anticholinergic effects seen with other anticholinergic agents

**Drug Uptake**

Peak antidepressant effect: Usually after ≥2 weeks

Absorption: Oral: Well absorbed

Serum half-life: 6-18 hours

**Pregnancy Risk Factor** D

**Generic Available** Yes: Tablet

**Selected Readings**

Boakes AJ, Laurence DR, Teoh PC, et al, "Interactions Between Sympathomimetic Amines and Antidepressant Agents in Man," *Br Med J*, 1973, 1(849):311-5.

Jastak JT and Yagiela JA, "Vasoconstrictors and Local Anesthesia: A Review and Rationale for Use," *J Am Dent Assoc*, 1983, 107(4):623-30.

Larochelle P, Hamet P, and Enjalbert M, "Responses to Tyramine and Norepinephrine After Imipramine and Trazodone," *Clin Pharmacol Ther*, 1979, 26(1):24-30.

(Continued)

## Imipramine *(Continued)*

Mitchell JR, "Guanethidine and Related Agents. III Antagonism by Drugs Which Inhibit the Norepinephrine Pump in Man," *J Clin Invest*, 1970, 49(8):1596-604.
Rundegren J, van Dijken J, Mörnstad H, et al, "Oral Conditions in Patients Receiving Long-Term Treatment With Cyclic Antidepressant Drugs," *Swed Dent J*, 1985, 9(2):55-64.
Svedmyr N, "The Influence of a Tricyclic Antidepressive Agent (Protriptyline) on Some of the Circulatory Effects of Noradrenaline and Adrenalin in Man," *Life Sci*, 1968, 7(1):77-84.
Wynn RL, "New Antidepressant Medications," *Gen Dent*, 1997, 45(1):24-8.

## Imiquimod (i mi KWI mod)

**U.S. Brand Names** Aldara™

**Therapeutic Category** Immune Response Modifier

**Use** Genital and perianal warts (condyloma acuminata)

**Usual Dosage** Adults: Topical: Apply three times/week, prior to bedtime, leave on for 6-10 hours, remove cream by washing area with mild soap and water

**Mechanism of Action** Mechanism of action is unknown; however, induces cytokines, including interferon-alpha and others

**Local Anesthetic/Vasoconstrictor Precautions** No information available to require special precautions

**Effects on Dental Treatment** No effects or complications reported

**Drug Uptake** Absorption: Minimal

**Pregnancy Risk Factor** B

♦ **Imitrex®** *see* Sumatriptan Succinate *on page 949*

## Immune Globulin, Intramuscular

(i MYUN GLOB yoo lin, IN tra MUS kyoo ler)

**Related Information**

Systemic Viral Diseases *on page 1115*

**U.S. Brand Names** Gamastan®; Gammar®

**Therapeutic Category** Immune Globulin

**Use** Household and sexual contacts of persons with hepatitis A, measles, varicella, and possibly rubella; travelers to high-risk areas outside tourist routes; staff, attendees, and parents of diapered attendees in day-care center outbreaks

For travelers, IG is not an alternative to careful selection of foods and water; immune globulin can interfere with the antibody response to parenterally administered live virus vaccines. Frequent travelers should be tested for hepatitis A antibody, immune hemolytic anemia, and neutropenia (with ITP, I.V. route is usually used).

**Usual Dosage** I.M.:

Hepatitis A:

- Pre-exposure prophylaxis upon travel into endemic areas:
  - 0.02 mL/kg for anticipated risk 1-3 months
  - 0.06 mL/kg for anticipated risk >3 months
  - Repeat approximate dose every 4-6 months if exposure continues
- Postexposure prophylaxis: 0.02 mL/kg given within 2 weeks of exposure

Measles:

- Prophylaxis: 0.25 mL/kg/dose (maximum dose: 15 mL) given within 6 days of exposure followed by live attenuated measles vaccine in 3 months or at 15 months of age (whichever is later)
- For patients with leukemia, lymphoma, immunodeficiency disorders, generalized malignancy, or receiving immunosuppressive therapy: 0.5 mL/kg (maximum dose: 15 mL)

Poliomyelitis: Prophylaxis: 0.3 mL/kg/dose as a single dose

Rubella: Prophylaxis: 0.55 mL/kg/dose within 72 hours of exposure

Varicella:: Prophylaxis: 0.6-1.2 mL/kg (varicella zoster immune globulin preferred) within 72 hours of exposure

IgG deficiency: 1.3 mL/kg, then 0.66 mL/kg in 3-4 weeks

Hepatitis B: Prophylaxis: 0.06 mL/kg/dose (HBIG preferred)

**Mechanism of Action** Provides passive immunity by increasing the antibody titer and antigen-antibody reaction potential

**Local Anesthetic/Vasoconstrictor Precautions** No information available to require special precautions

**Effects on Dental Treatment** No effects or complications reported

**Other Adverse Effects**

>10%: Local: Pain, tenderness, muscle stiffness at I.M. site

1% to 10%:

- Cardiovascular: Flushing
- Central nervous system: Chills
- Gastrointestinal: Nausea

<1%:

- Central nervous system: Lethargy, fever

Dermatologic: Urticaria, angioedema, erythema
Gastrointestinal: Vomiting
Neuromuscular & skeletal: Myalgia
Miscellaneous: Hypersensitivity reactions

**Drug Interactions** Increased toxicity: Live virus, vaccines (measles, mumps, rubella); do not administer within 3 months after administration of these vaccines

**Drug Uptake**
Duration of immune effect: Usually 3-4 weeks
Serum half-life: 23 days
Time to peak serum concentration: I.M.: Within 24-48 hours

**Pregnancy Risk Factor** C

**Generic Available** Yes

## Immune Globulin, Intravenous

(i MYUN GLOB yoo lin, IN tra VEE nus)

**Related Information**
Systemic Viral Diseases *on page 1115*

**U.S. Brand Names** Gamimune® N; Gammagard®; Gammagard® S/D; Gammar®-P I.V.; Polygam®; Polygam® S/D; Sandoglobulin®; Venoglobulin®-I; Venoglobulin®-S

**Therapeutic Category** Immune Globulin

**Synonyms** IVIG

**Use** Immunodeficiency syndrome, idiopathic thrombocytopenic purpura (ITP) and B-cell chronic lymphocytic leukemia (CLL); used in conjunction with appropriate anti-infective therapy to prevent or modify acute bacterial or viral infections in patients with iatrogenically-induced or disease-associated immunodepression; autoimmune neutropenia, bone marrow transplantation patients, Kawasaki disease, Guillain-Barré syndrome, demyelinating polyneuropathies

**Usual Dosage** Children and Adults: I.V.:

**Dosages should be based on ideal body weight** and not actual body weight in morbidly obese patients

Primary immunodeficiency disorders: 200-400 mg/kg every 4 weeks or as per monitored serum IgG concentrations

Chronic lymphocytic leukemia (CLL): 400 mg/kg/dose every 3 weeks

Idiopathic thrombocytopenic purpura (ITP): Maintenance dose:
400 mg/kg/day for 5 consecutive days
800 mg/kg/day for 2 consecutive days

Chronic ITP: 400-1000 mg/kg/dose every 7 or 14 days

Kawasaki disease:
400 mg/kg/day for 4 days within 10 days of onset of fever
800 mg/kg/day for 1-2 days within 10 days of onset of fever
2 g/kg for one dose only

Acquired immunodeficiency syndrome (patients must be symptomatic):
200-250 mg/kg/dose every 2 weeks
400-500 mg/kg/dose every month or every 4 weeks

Autoimmune hemolytic anemia and neutropenia: 1000 mg/kg/dose for 2-3 days

Autoimmune diseases: 400 mg/kg/day for 4 days

Post allogeneic bone marrow transplant: 500 mg/kg/week for 4 months post-transplant

Adjuvant to severe cytomegalovirus infections: 500 mg/kg/dose every other day for 7 doses

Severe systemic viral and bacterial infections:
Children: 500-1000 mg/kg/week

Prevention of gastroenteritis: Children: Oral: 50 mg/kg/day divided every 6 hours

Guillain-Barré syndrome:
400 mg/kg/day for 4 days
1000 mg/kg/day for 2 days
2000 mg/kg/day for one day

Refractory dermatomyositis: 2 g/kg/dose every month x 3-4 doses

Refractory polymyositis: 1 g/kg/day x 2 days every month x 4 doses

Chronic inflammatory demyelinating polyneuropathy:
400 mg/kg/day for 5 doses once each month
800 mg/kg/day for 3 doses once each month
1000 mg/kg/day for 2 days once each month

**Mechanism of Action** Replacement therapy for primary and secondary immunodeficiencies; interference with $F_c$ receptors on the cells of the reticuloendothelial system for autoimmune cytopenias and ITP; possible role of contained antiviral-type antibodies

**Local Anesthetic/Vasoconstrictor Precautions** No information available to require special precautions

**Effects on Dental Treatment** No effects or complications reported

(Continued)

## Immune Globulin, Intravenous *(Continued)*

**Other Adverse Effects**

1% to 10%:

Cardiovascular: Flushing of the face, tachycardia
Central nervous system: Chills
Gastrointestinal: Nausea
Respiratory: Dyspnea

<1%:

Cardiovascular: Hypotension, tightness in the chest
Central nervous system: Dizziness, fever, headache
Miscellaneous: Sweating, hypersensitivity reactions

**Drug Uptake** I.V. provides immediate antibody levels

Half-life: 21-24 days

**Pregnancy Risk Factor** C

**Generic Available** No

**Comments** Gammagard®, Polygam®, or Iveegam® have low titers of IgA and may be used in patients with IgA deficiency

- **Imodium®** *see* Loperamide *on page 599*
- **Imodium® A-D [OTC]** *see* Loperamide *on page 599*
- **Imogam®** *see* Rabies Immune Globulin (Human) *on page 875*
- **Imovax® Rabies I.D. Vaccine** *see* Rabies Virus Vaccine *on page 876*
- **Imovax® Rabies Vaccine** *see* Rabies Virus Vaccine *on page 876*
- **Imuran®** *see* Azathioprine *on page 112*
- **I-Naphline® Ophthalmic** *see* Naphazoline *on page 703*
- **Inapsine®** *see* Droperidol *on page 358*

## Indapamide (in DAP a mide)

**Related Information**

Cardiovascular Diseases *on page 1066*

**U.S. Brand Names** Lozol®

**Canadian Brand Names** Apo®-Indapadmide; Lozide®

**Therapeutic Category** Diuretic, Thiazide

**Use** Management of mild to moderate hypertension; treatment of edema in congestive heart failure and nephrotic syndrome

**Usual Dosage** Adults: Oral: 2.5-5 mg/day. **Note:** There is little therapeutic benefit to increasing the dose >5 mg/day; there is, however, an increased risk of electrolyte disturbances.

**Mechanism of Action** Diuretic effect is localized at the proximal segment of the distal tubule of the nephron; it does not appear to have significant effect on glomerular filtration rate nor renal blood flow; like other diuretics, it enhances sodium, chloride, and water excretion by interfering with the transport of sodium ions across the renal tubular epithelium

**Local Anesthetic/Vasoconstrictor Precautions** No information available to require special precautions

**Effects on Dental Treatment** No effects or complications reported

**Other Adverse Effects**

1% to 10%: Endocrine & metabolic: Hypokalemia

<1%:

Cardiovascular: Arrhythmia, weak pulse, hypotension
Central nervous system: Mood changes
Dermatologic: Photosensitivity
Endocrine & metabolic: Fluid and electrolyte imbalances (hypocalcemia, hypomagnesemia, hyponatremia), hyperglycemia
Gastrointestinal: Dry mouth, increased thirst
Hematologic: Rarely blood dyscrasias
Neuromuscular & skeletal: Numbness in hands, feet, or lips; paresthesia, muscle cramps or pain, weakness (unusual)
Renal: Prerenal azotemia
Respiratory: Dyspnea

**Drug Interactions**

Decreased effect of oral hypoglycemics; decreased absorption with cholestyramine and colestipol
Increased effect with furosemide and other loop diuretics
Increased toxicity/levels of lithium; when given with digoxin, diuretic-induced hypokalemia increases the risk of digoxin toxicity

**Drug Uptake**

Absorption: Completely from GI tract
Serum half-life: 14-18 hours
Time to peak serum concentration: 2-2.5 hours

**Pregnancy Risk Factor** D

**Generic Available** Yes

- **Inderal®** *see* Propranolol *on page 857*
- **Inderal® LA** *see* Propranolol *on page 857*
- **Inderide®** *see* Propranolol and Hydrochlorothiazide *on page 859*

## Indinavir (in DIN a veer)

**Related Information**

HIV Infection and AIDS *on page 1085*
Systemic Viral Diseases *on page 1115*

**U.S. Brand Names** Crixivan®

**Therapeutic Category** Antiviral Agent, Oral; Protease Inhibitor

**Use** Treatment of HIV infection, especially advanced disease; usually administered as part of a three-drug regimen (two nucleosides plus a protease inhibitor) or double therapy (one nucleoside plus a protease inhibitor)

**Usual Dosage** Adults: Oral: 800 mg every 8 hours

**Mechanism of Action** Indinavir is a protease inhibitor which prevents cleavage of protein precursors essential for HIV infection of new cells and viral replication. Some patients with advanced HIV infection have significantly improved clinically with the use of a protease inhibitor; resistant strains are cross-resistant to ritonavir and saquinavir.

**Local Anesthetic/Vasoconstrictor Precautions** No information available to require special precautions

**Effects on Dental Treatment** No effects or complications reported

**Other Adverse Effects** 1% to 10%:

Hepatic: Mild elevation of indirect bilirubin (10%)
Renal: Kidney stones (2% to 3%)

**Contraindications** Hypersensitivity to the drug or its components; avoid use with terfenadine, astemizole, cisapride, or benzodiazepines

**Warnings/Precautions** Use caution in patients with hepatic insufficiency; dosage reduction may be needed; nephrolithiasis may occur with use; if signs and symptoms of nephrolithiasis occur, interrupt therapy for 1-3 days; ensure adequate hydration

**Drug Interactions**

Decreased effect: Concurrent use of rifampin and rifabutin may decrease the effectiveness of indinavir; dosage decreases of rifampin/rifabutin is recommended

Increased toxicity: Gastric pH is lowered and absorption may be decreased when didanosine and indinavir are taken <1 hour apart; a reduction of dose is often required when coadministered with ketoconazole; astemizole, cisapride, and benzodiazepines should be avoided with indinavir due to a potentially serious toxicity. Clarithromycin can increase indinavir serum concentration resulting in toxicity. Indinavir increases clarithromycin blood levels; it is not known what effect this has. Erythromycin is likely also to increase indinavir serum concentrations. Azithromycin and dirithromycin are unlikely to affect indinavir.

**Drug Uptake**

Bioavailability: Oral: Good; $T_{max}$: 0.8 ± 0.3 hour
Half-life: 1.8 ± 0.4 hour

**Pregnancy Risk Factor** C

**Dosage Forms** Capsule: 400 mg

**Generic Available** No

**Comments** One study of previously untreated patients with a mean CD4-cell count of 250 cell/$mm^3$ found that indinavir plus zidovudine lowered serum HIV below detectable levels in 56% of 52 patients treated for 24 weeks. Other studies show similar results. Indinavir alone has suppressed serum HIV below detectable levels in 40% to 60% of patients treated up to 48 weeks.

- **Indochron E-R®** *see* Indomethacin *on next page*
- **Indocin®** *see* Indomethacin *on next page*
- **Indocin® I.V.** *see* Indomethacin *on next page*
- **Indocin® SR** *see* Indomethacin *on next page*

## Indocyanine Green (in doe SYE a neen green)

**U.S. Brand Names** Cardio-Green®

**Therapeutic Category** Diagnostic Agent, Cardiac Function

**Use** Determining hepatic function, cardiac output and liver blood flow and for ophthalmic angiography

**Usual Dosage**

Angiography: Use 40 mg of dye in 2 mL of aqueous solvent, in some patients, half the volume (1 mL) has been found to produce angiograms of comparable resolution; immediately following the bolus dose of dye, a bolus of sodium

(Continued)

## Indocyanine Green *(Continued)*

chloride 0.9% is given; this regimen will deliver a spatially limited dye bolus of optimal concentration to the choroidal vasculature following I.V. injection

Determination of cardiac output: Dye is injected as rapidly as possible into the right atrium, right ventricle, or pulmonary artery through a cardiac catheter; the usual dose is 1.25 mg for infants, 2.5 mg for children, and 5 mg for adults; total dose should not exceed 2 mg/kg; the dye is diluted with sterile water for injection or sodium chloride 0.9% to make a final volume of 1 mL; doses are repeated periodically to obtain several dilution curves; the dye should be flushed from the catheter with sodium chloride 0.9% to prevent hemolysis

**Local Anesthetic/Vasoconstrictor Precautions** No information available to require special precautions

**Effects on Dental Treatment** No effects or complications reported

**Other Adverse Effects** 1% to 10%:

Central nervous system: Headache

Dermatologic: Pruritus, skin discoloration

Miscellaneous: Sweating, anaphylactoid reactions

**Pregnancy Risk Factor** C

**Generic Available** Yes

## Indomethacin (in doe METH a sin)

**Related Information**

Rheumatoid Arthritis and Osteoarthritis *on page 1092*

**U.S. Brand Names** Indochron E-R®; Indocin®; Indocin® I.V.; Indocin® SR

**Canadian Brand Names** Apo®-Indomethacin; Indocid®; Indocid® SR; Novo-Methacin; Nu-Indo; Pro-Indo®

**Therapeutic Category** Analgesic, Non-narcotic; Anti-inflammatory Agent; Nonsteroidal Anti-inflammatory Drug (NSAID), Oral; Nonsteroidal Anti-inflammatory Drug (NSAID), Parenteral

**Use** Management of inflammatory diseases and rheumatoid disorders; moderate pain; acute gouty arthritis; I.V. form used as alternative to surgery for closure of patent ductus arteriosus in neonates

**Usual Dosage**

Patent ductus arteriosus:

Neonates: I.V.: Initial: 0.2 mg/kg; followed with: 2 doses of 0.1 mg/kg at 12- to 24-hour intervals if age <48 hours at time of first dose; 0.2 mg/kg 2 times if 2-7 days old at time of first dose; or 0.25 mg/kg 2 times if over 7 days at time of first dose; discontinue if significant adverse effects occur. Dose should be withheld if patient has anuria or oliguria.

Analgesia:

Children: Oral: Initial: 1-2 mg/kg/day in 2-4 divided doses; maximum: 4 mg/kg/day; not to exceed 150-200 mg/day

Adults: Oral, rectal: 25-50 mg/dose 2-3 times/day; maximum dose: 200 mg/day; extended release capsule should be given on a 1-2 times/day schedule

**Mechanism of Action** Inhibits prostaglandin synthesis by decreasing the activity of the enzyme, cyclo-oxygenase, which results in decreased formation of prostaglandin precursors

**Local Anesthetic/Vasoconstrictor Precautions** No information available to require special precautions

**Effects on Dental Treatment** NSAID formulations are known to reversibly decrease platelet aggregation via mechanisms different than observed with aspirin. The dentist should be aware of the potential of abnormal coagulation. Caution should also be exercised in the use of NSAIDs in patients already on anticoagulant therapy with drugs such as warfarin (Coumadin®).

**Other Adverse Effects**

>10%:

Central nervous system: Dizziness

Dermatologic: Rash

Gastrointestinal: Nausea, epigastric pain, abdominal pain, anorexia, GI bleeding, ulcers, perforation, abdominal cramps, heartburn, indigestion

1% to 10%:

Central nervous system: Headache, nervousness

Dermatologic: Itching

Endocrine & metabolic: Fluid retention

Gastrointestinal: Vomiting

Otic: Tinnitus

<1%:

Cardiovascular: Hypertension, congestive heart failure, arrhythmias, tachycardia

Central nervous system: Somnolence, fatigue, depression, confusion, hallucinations

Dermatologic: Urticaria, erythema multiforme, toxic epidermal necrolysis, Stevens-Johnson syndrome, angioedema
Endocrine & metabolic: Hyperkalemia, dilutional hyponatremia (I.V.), oliguria, hypoglycemia (I.V.), hot flashes, polydipsia
Gastrointestinal: Gastritis
Genitourinary: Cystitis
Hematologic: Hemolytic anemia, bone marrow suppression, agranulocytosis, thrombocytopenia, inhibition of platelet aggregation, anemia, leukopenia
Hepatic: Hepatitis
Neuromuscular & skeletal: Peripheral neuropathy
Ocular: Corneal opacities, blurred vision, conjunctivitis, dry eyes, toxic amblyopia
Otic: Decreased hearing
Renal: Polyuria, renal failure
Respiratory: Dyspnea, allergic rhinitis, epistaxis
Miscellaneous: Aseptic meningitis, hypersensitivity reactions

**Drug Interactions**
Decreased effect: May decrease antihypertensive effects of beta-blockers, hydralazine and captopril
Increased toxicity: May increase serum potassium with potassium-sparing diuretics; probenecid may increase indomethacin serum concentrations; other NSAIDs may increase GI adverse effects; may increase nephrotoxicity of cyclosporin
Indomethacin may increase serum concentrations of digoxin, methotrexate, lithium, and aminoglycosides (reported with I.V. use in neonates)

**Drug Uptake**
Onset of action: Within 30 minutes
Duration: 4-6 hours
Absorption: Prompt and extensive
Serum half-life: 4.5 hours
Time to peak serum concentration: Oral: Within 3-4 hours

**Pregnancy Risk Factor** B (D if used longer than 48 hours or after 34-week gestation)

**Generic Available** Yes (capsule and oral suspension)

- **Infants Feverall™ [OTC]** *see* Acetaminophen *on page 27*
- **Infants' Silapap® [OTC]** *see* Acetaminophen *on page 27*
- **Infasurf®** *see* Calfactant *on page 178*
- **InFed™ Injection** *see* Iron Dextran Complex *on page 550*
- **Inflamase®** *see* Prednisolone *on page 832*
- **Inflamase® Mild** *see* Prednisolone *on page 832*

## Infliximab

**U.S. Brand Names** Remicade™

**Therapeutic Category** Gastrointestinal Agent, Miscellaneous; Monoclonal Antibody

**Use** Treatment of moderately to severely active Crohn's disease for the reduction of the signs and symptoms in patients who have an inadequate response to conventional therapy or for the treatment of patients with fistulizing Crohn's disease for the reduction in the number of draining enterocutaneous fistula(s)

**Usual Dosage**
Moderately to severely active Crohn's disease: Adults: I.V.: 5 mg/kg as a single infusion over a minimum of 2 hours
Fistulizing Crohn's disease: 5 mg/kg as an infusion over a minimum of 2 hours, dose repeated at 2 and 6 weeks after the initial infusion

**Local Anesthetic/Vasoconstrictor Precautions** No information available to require special precautions

**Effects on Dental Treatment** Candidiasis reported in ~5% of patients

**Other Adverse Effects**
>10%:
Central nervous system: Headache (22.6%), fatigue (10.6%), fever (10.1%)
Gastrointestinal: Nausea (16.6%), abdominal pain (12.1%)
Local: Infusion reactions (16%)
Respiratory: Upper respiratory tract infection (16.1%)
Miscellaneous: Infections (21%)
1% to 10%:
Cardiovascular: Chest pain (5.5%)
Central nervous system: Pain (8.5%), dizziness (8%)
Dermatologic: Rash (6%), pruritus (5%)
Gastrointestinal: Vomiting (8.5%)
Neuromuscular & skeletal: Myalgia (5%), back pain (5%)
(Continued)

## Infliximab *(Continued)*

Respiratory: Pharyngitis (8.5%), bronchitis (7%), rhinitis (6%), cough (5%), sinusitis (5%)

Miscellaneous: Development of antibodies to double-stranded DNA (9%), candidiasis (5%), serious infection (3%)

<1%: Lupus-like syndrome (2 patients); a proportion of patients (12%) with fistulizing disease developed new abscess 8-16 weeks after the last infusion of infliximab

**Drug Interactions** Specific drug interaction studies have not been conducted

**Drug Uptake** Serum half-life: 9.5 days

**Pregnancy Risk Factor** C

**Dosage Forms** Powder for injection: 100 mg

## Influenza Virus Vaccine (in floo EN za VYE rus vak SEEN)

**U.S. Brand Names** Fluogen®; Fluzone®

**Therapeutic Category** Vaccine, Inactivated Virus

**Use** Provide active immunity to influenza virus strains contained in the vaccine; for high risk persons, previous year vaccines should not be to prevent present year influenza

Those at risk for influenza injection:

Persons ≥65 years of age

Institutionalized patients

Persons of any age with chronic disorders of pulmonary and/or cardiovascular system

Persons who have required medical follow-up following hospitalization for other chronic diseases such as diabetes, renal disease, immunodepressive disorders, etc

Travelers, especially those at risk (above)

**Usual Dosage** Adults: I.M.: 0.5 mL each year of appropriate vaccine for the year, one dose is all that is necessary; administer in late fall to allow maximum titers to develop by peak epidemic periods usually occurring in early December

**Local Anesthetic/Vasoconstrictor Precautions** No information available to require special precautions

**Effects on Dental Treatment** No effects or complications reported

**Other Adverse Effects**

1% to 10%:

Central nervous system: Fever, malaise

Local: Tenderness, redness, or induration at the site of injection

<1%:

Central nervous system: Guillain-Barré syndrome

Dermatologic: Urticaria, angioedema

Neuromuscular & skeletal: Myalgia

Respiratory: Asthma

Miscellaneous: Anaphylactoid reactions (most likely to residual egg protein), allergic reactions

**Drug Interactions**

Decreased effect with immunosuppressive agents; do not administer within 7 days after administration of diphtheria and tetanus toxoids and pertussis vaccine adsorbed (DTP)

Increased effect/toxicity of theophylline and warfarin

**Pregnancy Risk Factor** C

**Generic Available** No

♦ **Infumorph™ Injection** *see* Morphine Sulfate *on page 688*

♦ **INH™** *see* Isoniazid *on page 552*

♦ **Inocor®** *see* Amrinone *on page 84*

## Insect Sting Kit (IN sekt sting kit)

**U.S. Brand Names** Ana-Kit®

**Therapeutic Category** Antidote, Insect Sting

**Use** Anaphylaxis emergency treatment of insect bites or stings by the sensitive patient that may occur within minutes of insect sting or exposure to an allergic substance

**Usual Dosage** Children and Adults:

Epinephrine:

<2 years: 0.05-0.1 mL

2-6 years: 0.15 mL

6-12 years: 0.2 mL

>12 years : 0.3 mL

Chlorpheniramine:

<6 years: 1 tablet

6-12 years: 2 tablets
>12 years: 4 tablets

**Local Anesthetic/Vasoconstrictor Precautions** No information available to require special precautions

**Effects on Dental Treatment** No effects or complications reported

**Generic Available** No

**Comments** Not intended for I.V. use (I.M. or S.C. only)

◆ **Insta-Char® [OTC]** *see* Charcoal *on page 219*

◆ **Insta-Glucose® [OTC]** *see* Glucose *on page 470*

## Insulin Preparations (IN su lin prep a RAY shuns)

**Related Information**

Endocrine Disorders & Pregnancy *on page 1082*

**U.S. Brand Names** Humalog®; Humulin® 50/50; Humulin® 70/30; Humulin® L; Humulin® N; Humulin® R; Humulin® U; Lente® Iletin® I; Lente® Iletin® II; Lente® Insulin; Lente® L; Novolin® 70/30; Novolin® L; Novolin® N; Novolin® R; NPH Iletin® I; NPH Insulin; NPH-N; Pork NPH Iletin® II; Pork Regular Iletin® II; Regular (Concentrated) Iletin® II U-500; Regular Iletin® I; Regular Insulin; Regular Purified Pork Insulin; Velosulin® Human

**Therapeutic Category** Antidiabetic Agent

**Use** Treatment of insulin-dependent diabetes mellitus, also noninsulin-dependent diabetes mellitus unresponsive to treatment with diet and/or oral hypoglycemics; to assure proper utilization of glucose and reduce glucosuria in nondiabetic patients receiving parenteral nutrition whose glucosuria cannot be adequately controlled with infusion rate adjustments or those who require assistance in achieving optimal caloric intakes; hyperkalemia (use with glucose to shift potassium into cells to lower serum potassium levels)

**Usual Dosage** Dose requires continuous medical supervision; may administer I.V. (regular), I.M., S.C.

Diabetes mellitus:

Children and Adults: 0.5-1 unit/kg/day in divided doses

Adolescents (growth spurts): 0.8-1.2 units/kg/day in divided doses

Adjust dose to maintain premeal and bedtime blood glucose of 80-140 mg/dL (children <5 years: 100-200 mg/dL)

Hyperkalemia: Give calcium gluconate and $NaHCO_3$ first then 50% dextrose at 0.5-1 mL/kg and insulin 1 unit for every 4-5 g dextrose given

Diabetic ketoacidosis: Children and Adults: I.V. loading dose: 0.1 unit/kg, then maintenance continuous infusion: 0.1 unit/kg/hour (range: 0.05-0.2 units/kg/hour depending upon the rate of decrease of serum glucose - too rapid decrease of serum glucose may lead to cerebral edema).

Optimum rate of decrease (serum glucose): 80-100 mg/dL/hour

**Note:** Newly diagnosed patients with IDDM presenting in DKA and patients with blood sugars <800 mg/dL may be relatively "sensitive" to insulin and should receive loading and initial maintenance doses approximately ½ of those indicated above.

**Mechanism of Action** Replacement therapy for persons unable to produce the hormone naturally or in insufficient amounts to maintain glycemic control

**Drug Interactions With Insulin Injection**

| Decrease Hypoglycemic Effect of Insulin | Increase Hypoglycemic Effect of Insulin |
|---|---|
| Contraceptives, oral | Alcohol |
| Corticosteroids | Alpha blockers |
| Dextrothyroxine | Anabolic steroids |
| Diltiazem | Beta-blockers* |
| Dobutamine | Clofibrate |
| Epinephrine | Fenfluramine |
| Smoking | Guanethidine |
| Thiazide diuretics | MAO inhibitors |
| Thyroid hormone | Pentamidine |
| Niacin | Phenylbutazone |
| | Salicylates |
| | Sulfinpyrazone |
| | Tetracyclines |

*Nonselective beta-blockers may delay recovery from hypoglycemic episodes and mask signs/symptoms of hypoglycemia. Cardioselective agents may be alternatives.

(Continued)

## Insulin Preparations *(Continued)*

**Local Anesthetic/Vasoconstrictor Precautions** No information available to require special precautions

**Effects on Dental Treatment** Insulin-dependent diabetics (juvenile onset, type I) should be appointed for dental treatment in the morning in order to minimize chance of stress-induced hypoglycemia

**Other Adverse Effects** 1% to 10%:

Cardiovascular: Palpitation, tachycardia, pallor

Central nervous system: Fatigue, mental confusion, loss of consciousness, headache, hypothermia

Dermatologic: Urticaria

Endocrine & metabolic: Hypoglycemia

Gastrointestinal: Hunger, nausea, numbness of mouth

Local: Itching, redness, swelling, stinging, or warmth at injection site, atrophy or hypertrophy of S.C. fat tissue

Neuromuscular & skeletal: Muscle weakness, tremor, paresthesia

Ocular: Transient presbyopia, blurred vision

Miscellaneous: Perspiration, anaphylaxis

**Drug Interactions** See table on previous page.

**Drug Uptake**

Onset and duration of hypoglycemic effects depend upon preparation administered. See table.

**Pharmacokinetics/Pharmacodynamics: Onset and Duration of Hypoglycemic Effects Depend Upon Preparation Administered**

| | Onset (h) | Peak (h) | Duration (h) |
|---|---|---|---|
| Insulin, regular (Novolin® R) | 0.5–1 | 2-3 | 5–7 |
| Prompt insulin zinc suspension (Semilente®) | 0.5–1 | 4–7 | 18–24 |
| Insulin zinc suspension (NPH) (Novolin® N) | 1–1.5 | 4–12 | 18–24 |
| Isophane insulin suspension (Lente®) | 1–2.5 | 8–12 | 18–24 |
| Isophane insulin suspension and regular insulin injection (Novolin® 70/30) | 0.5 | 4-8 | 24 |
| Prompt zinc insulin suspension (PZI) | 4-8 | 14-24 | 36 |
| Extended insulin zinc suspension (Ultralente®) | 4-8 | 16–18 | >36 |

Onset and duration: Biosynthetic NPH human insulin shows a more rapid onset and shorter duration of action than corresponding porcine insulins; human insulin and purified porcine regular insulin are similarly efficacious following S.C. administration. The duration of action of highly purified porcine insulins is shorter than that of conventional insulin equivalents. Duration depends on type of preparation and route of administration as well as patient related variables. In general, the larger the dose of insulin, the longer the duration of activity.

Absorption: Biosynthetic regular human insulin is absorbed from the S.C. injection site more rapidly than insulins of animal origin (60-90 minutes peak vs 120-150 minutes peak respectively) and lowers the initial blood glucose much faster. Human Ultralente® insulin is absorbed about twice as quickly as its bovine equivalent, and bioavailability is also improved. Human Lente® insulin preparations are also absorbed more quickly than their animal equivalents.

**Pregnancy Risk Factor** B

**Generic Available** Yes

- **Intal®** *see* Cromolyn Sodium *on page 281*
- **Integrilin®** *see* Eptifibatide *on page 379*

## Interferon Alfa-2a (in ter FEER on AL fa too aye)

**Related Information**

Systemic Viral Diseases *on page 1115*

**U.S. Brand Names** Roferon-A®

**Therapeutic Category** Antineoplastic Agent, Miscellaneous; Interferon

**Use** FDA approved: Patients >18 years of age: Hairy cell leukemia, AIDS related Kaposi's sarcoma; multiple **unlabeled uses**; indications and dosage regimens are specific for a particular brand of interferon

**Usual Dosage** Refer to individual protocols

Children: Hemangiomas of infancy, pulmonary hemangiomatosis: S.C.: 1-3 million units/$m^2$/day once daily

Adults >18 years: I.M., S.C.:

Hairy cell leukemia:

Induction: 3 million units/day for 16-24 weeks.

Maintenance: 3 million units 3 times/week (may be treated for up to 20 consecutive weeks)

AIDS-related Kaposi's sarcoma:

Induction: 36 million units/day for 10-12 weeks

Maintenance: 36 million units 3 times/week (may begin with dose escalation from 3-9-18 million units each day over 3 consecutive days followed by 36 million units/day for the remainder of the 10-12 weeks of induction)

If severe adverse reactions occur, modify dosage (50% reduction) or temporarily discontinue therapy until adverse reactions abate

**Mechanism of Action** Inhibits cellular growth, alters the state of cellular differentiation, interferes with oncogene expression, alters cell surface antigen expression, increases phagocytic activity of macrophages and augments cytotoxicity of lymphocytes for target cells

**Local Anesthetic/Vasoconstrictor Precautions** No information available to require special precautions

**Effects on Dental Treatment** >10% of patients experience significant dry mouth and metallic taste

**Other Adverse Effects**

>10%:

Central nervous system: Dizziness, fatigue, malaise, fever (usually within 4-6 hours), chills

Dermatologic: Skin rash

Gastrointestinal: Nausea, vomiting, diarrhea, abdominal cramps, weight loss

Hematologic: Mildly myelosuppressive and well tolerated if used without adjunct antineoplastic agents; thrombocytosis has been reported, leukopenia (mainly neutropenia), anemia, thrombocytopenia, decreased hemoglobin, hematocrit, platelets

Neuromuscular & skeletal: Rigors, arthralgia

Miscellaneous: Flu-like syndrome, sweating

1% to 10%:

Central nervous system: Headache, delirium, somnolence, neurotoxicity

Dermatologic: alopecia, dry skin

Gastrointestinal: Anorexia, stomatitis

Hepatic: Hepatotoxicity

Neuromuscular & skeletal: Peripheral neuropathy, leg cramps

Ocular: Blurred vision

<1%:

Cardiovascular: Tachycardia, arrhythmias, chest pain, hypotension, SVT, edema

Central nervous system: Confusion, sensory neuropathy, psychiatric effects, EEG abnormalities, depression

Dermatologic: Partial alopecia

Endocrine & metabolic: Hypothyroidism, hyperuricemia

Gastrointestinal: Change in taste

Hepatic: Elevated hepatic transaminase

Local: Sensitivity to injection

Neuromuscular & skeletal: Myalgia

Ocular: Visual disturbances

Renal: Proteinuria, elevated Cr, elevated BUN

Respiratory: Coughing, chest pain, dyspnea, nasal congestion

Miscellaneous: Neutralizing antibodies; usually patient can build up a tolerance to side effects

**Drug Interactions**

Increased effect:

Cimetidine: May augment the antitumor effects of interferon in melanoma

Theophylline: Clearance has been reported to be decreased in hepatitis patients receiving interferon

Increased toxicity: Vinblastine: Enhances interferon toxicity in several patients; increased incidence of paresthesia has also been noted

**Drug Uptake**

Absorption: Filtered and absorbed at the renal tubule

Serum half-life: Elimination:

I.M., I.V.: 2 hours after administration

S.C.: 3 hours

Time to peak serum concentration: I.M., S.C.: ~6-8 hours

**Pregnancy Risk Factor** C

**Generic Available** No

## Interferon Alfa-2b (in ter FEER on AL fa too bee)

**Related Information**

Systemic Viral Diseases *on page 1115*

**U.S. Brand Names** Intron® A

**Therapeutic Category** Antineoplastic Agent, Miscellaneous; Biological Response Modulator; Interferon

**Use** FDA approved: Patients >18 years of age: Hairy cell leukemia, condylomata acuminata, AIDS-related Kaposi's sarcoma, chronic hepatitis non-A, non-B(C), chronic hepatitis B; indications and dosage regimens are specific for a particular brand of interferon

**Usual Dosage** Adults (**refer to individual protocols**):

Hairy cell leukemia: I.M., S.C.: 2 million units/m$^2$ 3 times/week for 2 to ≥6 months of therapy

AIDS-related Kaposi's sarcoma: I.M., S.C. (use 50 million unit vial): 30 million units/m$^2$ 3 times/week

Condylomata acuminata: Intralesionally (use 10 million unit vial): 1 million units/lesion 3 times/week for 4-8 weeks; not to exceed 5 million units per treatment (maximum: 5 lesions at one time)

Chronic hepatitis C (non-A/non-B): I.M., S.C.: 3 million units 3 times/week for approximately a 6-month course

Chronic hepatitis B: I.M., S.C.: 5 million units/day or 10 million units 3 times/week for 16 weeks; if severe adverse reactions occur, reduce dosage 50% or temporarily discontinue therapy until adverse reactions abate; when platelet/granulocyte count returns to normal, reinstitute therapy

**Mechanism of Action** Alpha interferons are a family of proteins, produced by nucleated cells, that have antiviral, antiproliferative, and immune-regulating activity. There are 16 known subtypes of alpha interferons. Interferons interact with cells through high affinity cell surface receptors. Following activation, multiple effects can be detected including induction of gene transcription. Inhibits cellular growth, alters the state of cellular differentiation, interferes with oncogene expression, alters cell surface antigen expression, increases phagocytic activity of macrophages, and augments cytotoxicity of lymphocytes for target cells

**Local Anesthetic/Vasoconstrictor Precautions** No information available to require special precautions

**Effects on Dental Treatment** >10% of patients experience dry mouth and metallic taste

**Other Adverse Effects**

>10%:

- Central nervous system: Dizziness, fatigue, malaise, fever (usually within 4-6 hours)
- Dermatologic: Skin rash
- Gastrointestinal: Nausea, vomiting, diarrhea, abdominal cramps, weight loss, anorexia
- Hematologic: Mildly myelosuppressive and well tolerated if used without adjunct antineoplastic agents; thrombocytosis has been reported, leukopenia (mainly neutropenia), anemia, thrombocytopenia, decreased hemoglobin, hematocrit, platelets
- Neuromuscular & skeletal: Rigors, arthralgia
- Miscellaneous: Flu-like syndrome, sweating

1% to 10%:

- Central nervous system: Neurotoxicity
- Dermatologic: Dry skin, alopecia
- Gastrointestinal: Stomatitis
- Hepatic: Hepatotoxicity
- Neuromuscular & skeletal: Peripheral neuropathy, leg cramps
- Ocular: Blurred vision

<1%:

- Cardiovascular: Cardiotoxicity, tachycardia, arrhythmias, hypotension, SVT, arrhythmias, chest pain, edema
- Central nervous system: EEG abnormalities, confusion, sensory neuropathy, headache, psychiatric effects, delirium, somnolence
- Dermatologic: Partial alopecia
- Endocrine & metabolic: Hypothyroidism, hyperuricemia
- Gastrointestinal: Change in taste
- Hepatic: Elevated hepatic transaminase, elevated ALT and AST
- Local: Sensitivity to injection
- Neuromuscular & skeletal: Myalgia
- Ocular: Visual disturbances
- Renal: Proteinuria, elevated creatinine, elevated BUN
- Respiratory: Coughing, dyspnea, nasal congestion
- Miscellaneous: Neutralizing antibodies; usually patient can build up a tolerance to side effects

**Drug Interactions**

Increased effect: Cimetidine: May augment the antitumor effects of interferon in melanoma

Increased toxicity:

Theophylline: Clearance has been reported to be decreased in hepatitis patients receiving interferon

Vinblastine: Enhances interferon toxicity in several patients; increased incidence of paresthesia has also been noted

**Drug Uptake**

Absorption: Filtered and absorbed at the renal tubule

Serum half-life: Elimination:

I.M., I.V.: 2 hours

S.C.: 3 hours

Time to peak serum concentration: I.M., S.C.: ~6-8 hours

**Pregnancy Risk Factor** C

**Generic Available** No

## Interferon Alfa-2b and Ribavirin Combination Pack

(in ter FEER on AL fa too bee)

**U.S. Brand Names** Rebetron™

**Therapeutic Category** Antineoplastic Agent, Miscellaneous; Antiviral Agent, Inhalation Therapy; Biological Response Modulator; Interferon

**Use** The combination therapy is indicated for the treatment of chronic hepatitis C in patients with compensated liver disease who have relapsed following alpha interferon therapy

**Usual Dosage** The recommended dosage of combination therapy is 3 million int. units of Intron® A injected subcutaneously 3 times/week and 1000-1200 mg of Rebetol® capsules administered orally in a divided daily (morning and evening) dose for 24 weeks; patients weighing 75 kg (165 pounds) or less should receive 1000 mg of Rebetol® daily, while patients weighing more than 75 kg should receive 1200 mg of Rebetol® daily

**Mechanism of Action**

Interferon Alfa-2b: Alpha interferons are a family of proteins, produced by nucleated cells, that have antiviral, antiproliferative, and immune-regulating activity. There are 16 known subtypes of alpha interferons. Interferons interact with cells through high affinity cell surface receptors. Following activation, multiple effects can be detected including induction of gene transcription. Inhibits cellular growth, alters the state of cellular differentiation, interferes with oncogene expression, alters cell surface antigen expression, increases phagocytic activity of macrophages, and augments cytotoxicity of lymphocytes for target cells

Ribavirin: Inhibits replication of RNA and DNA viruses; inhibits influenza virus RNA polymerase activity and inhibits the initiation and elongation of RNA fragments resulting in inhibition of viral protein synthesis

**Local Anesthetic/Vasoconstrictor Precautions** No information available to require special precautions

**Effects on Dental Treatment** >10% of patients experience dry mouth and metallic taste

**Other Adverse Effects**

Interferon Alfa-2b

>10%:

Central nervous system: Dizziness, fatigue, malaise, fever (usually within 4-6 hours), chills

Dermatologic: Skin rash

Gastrointestinal: Xerostomia, nausea, vomiting, diarrhea, dizziness, abdominal cramps, weight loss, metallic taste, anorexia

Hematologic: Mildly myelosuppressive and well tolerated if used without adjunct antineoplastic agents; thrombocytosis has been reported, leukopenia (mainly neutropenia), anemia, thrombocytopenia, decreased hemoglobin, hematocrit, platelets

Myelosuppressive:

WBC: Mild

Platelets: Mild

Onset (days): 7-10

Nadir (days): 14

Recovery (days): 21

Neuromuscular & skeletal: Rigors, arthralgia

Miscellaneous: Flu-like syndrome, diaphoresis

1% to 10%:

Central nervous system: Neurotoxicity

Dermatologic: Dry skin, alopecia

Gastrointestinal: Stomatitis

(Continued)

# Interferon Alfa-2b and Ribavirin Combination Pack *(Continued)*

Hepatic: Hepatotoxicity
Neuromuscular & skeletal: Peripheral neuropathy, leg cramps
Ocular: Blurred vision

<1%:

Cardiovascular: Cardiotoxicity, tachycardia, arrhythmias, hypotension, SVT, arrhythmias, chest pain, edema
Central nervous system: EEG abnormalities, confusion, sensory neuropathy, fever, headache, psychiatric effects, delirium, somnolence, chills
Dermatologic: Partial alopecia, rash
Endocrine & metabolic: Increased uric acid level, hypothyroidism
Gastrointestinal: Weight loss, change in taste
Hematologic: Decreased hemoglobin, hematocrit, platelets
Hepatic: Increased hepatic transaminase, increased ALT and AST
Local: Sensitivity to injection
Neuromuscular & skeletal: Myalgia, arthralgia, rigors
Ocular: Visual disturbances, blurred vision
Renal: Proteinuria, increased creatinine, increased BUN
Respiratory: Coughing, dyspnea, nasal congestion
Miscellaneous: Neutralizing antibodies; usually patient can build up a tolerance to side effects

Ribavirin

1% to 10%:

Central nervous system: Fatigue, headache, insomnia
Gastrointestinal: Nausea, anorexia
Hematologic: Anemia

<1%:

Cardiovascular: Hypotension, cardiac arrest, digitalis toxicity
Dermatologic: Rash, skin irritation
Ocular: Conjunctivitis
Respiratory: Mild bronchospasm, worsening of respiratory function, apnea

**Contraindications** Known hypersensitivity to interferon alfa-2b or any component; females of childbearing age

**Warnings/Precautions**

Interferon Alfa-2b: The U.S. Food and Drug Administration (FDA) currently recommends that procedures for proper handling and disposal of antineoplastic agents be considered. Use with caution in patients with seizure disorders, brain metastases, compromised CNS, multiple sclerosis, and patients with pre-existing cardiac disease, severe renal or hepatic impairment, or myelosuppression; safety and efficacy in children <18 years of age have not been established. Higher doses in the elderly or in malignancies other than hairy cell leukemia may result in severe obtundation.

Ribavirin: Use with caution in patients requiring assisted ventilation because precipitation of the drug in the respiratory equipment may interfere with safe and effective patient ventilation; monitor carefully in patients with COPD and asthma for deterioration of respiratory function. Ribavirin is potentially mutagenic, tumor-promoting, and gonadotoxic.

Anemia (hemoglobin <10 g/dL) was observed in 10% of treated patients in clinical trials; anemia occurred within 1-2 weeks of initiation of therapy; because of this initial acute drop in hemoglobin, it is advised that complete blood counts (CBC) should be obtained pretreatment and at week 2 and week 4 of therapy or more frequently if clinically indicated; patients should then be followed as clinically appropriate

**Drug Interactions**

Interferon Alfa-2b:

Increased effect: Cimetidine: May augment the antitumor effects of interferon in melanoma

Increased toxicity:

Theophylline: Clearance has been reported to be decreased in hepatitis patients receiving interferon
Vinblastine: Enhances interferon toxicity in several patients; increased incidence of paresthesia has also been noted

Ribavirin: Decreased effect of zidovudine

**Drug Uptake**

Absorption: Filtered and absorbed at the renal tubule
Distribution: The $V_d$ of interferon is 31 L; but has been noted to be much greater (370-720 L) in leukemia patients receiving continuous infusion IFN; IFN does not penetrate the CSF
Metabolism: Majority of dose thought to be metabolized in the kidney

Bioavailability:
- I.M.: 83%
- S.C.: 90%

Half-life: Elimination:
- I.M., I.V.: 2 hours
- S.C.: 3 hours

Time to peak serum concentration: I.M., S.C.: ~6-8 hours

**Pregnancy Risk Factor** X

**Generic Available** No

**Comments** Myelosuppressive effects:
- WBC: Mild
- Platelets: Mild
- Onset (days): 7-10
- Nadir (days): 14
- Recovery (days): 21

## Interferon Alfa-n3 (in ter FEER on AL fa en three)

**Related Information**

Systemic Viral Diseases *on page 1115*

**U.S. Brand Names** Alferon® N

**Therapeutic Category** Antineoplastic Agent, Miscellaneous; Interferon

**Use** FDA approved: Patients ≥18 years of age: Condylomata acuminata, intralesional treatment of refractory or recurring genital or venereal warts; useful in patients who do not respond or are not candidates for usual treatments; indications and dosage regimens are specific for a particular brand of interferon

**Usual Dosage** Adults: Inject 250,000 units (0.05 mL) in each wart twice weekly for a maximum of 8 weeks; therapy should not be repeated for at least 3 months after the initial 8-week course of therapy

**Mechanism of Action** Interferons interact with cells through high affinity cell surface receptors. Following activation, multiple effects can be detected including induction of gene transcription. Inhibits cellular growth, alters the state of cellular differentiation, interferes with oncogene expression, alters cell surface antigen expression, increases phagocytic activity of macrophages, and augments cytotoxicity of lymphocytes for target cells

**Local Anesthetic/Vasoconstrictor Precautions** No information available to require special precautions

**Effects on Dental Treatment** >10% of patients experience dry mouth and metallic taste

**Other Adverse Effects**

>10%:
- Central nervous system: Fatigue, malaise, fever (usually within 4-6 hours), chills, dizziness
- Dermatologic: Skin rash
- Gastrointestinal: Nausea, vomiting, diarrhea, abdominal cramps, weight loss, anorexia
- Hematologic: Mildly myelosuppressive and well tolerated if used without adjunct antineoplastic agents; thrombocytosis has been reported, leukopenia (mainly neutropenia), anemia, thrombocytopenia, decreased hemoglobin, hematocrit, platelets
- Neuromuscular & skeletal: Arthralgia, rigors
- Miscellaneous: Flu-like syndrome, sweating

1% to 10%:
- Central nervous system: Headache, delirium, somnolence, neurotoxicity
- Dermatologic: Alopecia, dry skin
- Gastrointestinal: Stomatitis
- Hepatic: Hepatotoxicity
- Neuromuscular & skeletal: Peripheral neuropathy, leg cramps
- Ocular: Blurred vision

<1%:
- Cardiovascular: Tachycardia, arrhythmias, chest pain, hypotension, SVT, edema
- Central nervous system: EEG abnormalities, confusion, sensory neuropathy, confusion, psychiatric effects, depression
- Dermatologic: Rash, partial alopecia, local sensitivity to injection
- Endocrine & metabolic: Hypothyroidism, hyperuricemia
- Gastrointestinal: Change in taste
- Hepatic: Elevated hepatic transaminase, elevated ALT and AST
- Neuromuscular & skeletal: Myalgia
- Ocular: Visual disturbances
- Renal: Proteinuria, elevated Cr, elevated BUN
- Respiratory: Coughing, chest pain, dyspnea, cough, nasal congestion

(Continued)

## Interferon Alfa-n3 *(Continued)*

Miscellaneous: Neutralizing antibodies, usually patient can build up a tolerance to side effects

**Drug Interactions**

Increased effect: Cimetidine: May augment the antitumor effects of interferon in melanoma

Increased toxicity:

Vinblastine: Enhances interferon toxicity in several patients; increased incidence of paresthesia has also been noted

Theophylline: Clearance has been reported to be decreased in hepatitis patients receiving interferon

**Pregnancy Risk Factor** C

**Generic Available** No

## Interferon Beta-1a (in ter FEER on BAY ta won aye)

**U.S. Brand Names** Avonex™

**Therapeutic Category** Biological Response Modulator

**Use** Treatment of relapsing forms of multiple sclerosis (MS); to slow the accumulation of physical disability and decrease the frequency of clinical exacerbations

**Usual Dosage** Adults >18 years: I.M.: 30 mcg once weekly

**Mechanism of Action** Interferon beta differs from naturally occurring human protein by a single amino acid substitution and the lack of carbohydrate side chains; alters the expression and response to surface antigens and can enhance immune cell activities. Properties of interferon beta that modify biologic responses are mediated by cell surface receptor interactions; mechanism in the treatment of MS is unknown.

**Local Anesthetic/Vasoconstrictor Precautions** No information available to require special precautions

**Effects on Dental Treatment** No effects or complications reported

**Other Adverse Effects** 1% to 10%:

Cardiovascular: CHF (rare), tachycardia, syncope

Central nervous system: Headache, lethargy, depression, emotional lability, anxiety, suicidal ideations, somnolence, agitation, confusion

Dermatologic: Alopecia (rare)

Endocrine & metabolic: Hypocalcemia

Gastrointestinal: Nausea, anorexia, vomiting, diarrhea, chronic weight loss

Hematologic: Leukopenia, thrombocytopenia, anemia (frequent, dose-related, but not usually severe)

Hepatic: Elevated liver enzymes (mild, transient)

Local: Pain/redness at injection site (80%)

Neuromuscular & skeletal: Weakness

Ocular: Retinal toxicity/visual changes

Renal: Elevated BUN and $S_{cr}$

Miscellaneous: Flu-like syndrome (fever, nausea, malaise, myalgia) occurs in most patients, but is usually controlled by acetaminophen or NSAIDs; dose related abortifacient activity was reported in rhesus monkeys

**Warnings/Precautions** Interferon beta-1a should be used with caution in patients with a history of depression, seizures, or cardiac disease; because its use has not been evaluated during lactation, its use in breast-feeding mothers may not be safe and should be warned against

**Drug Interactions** Decreases clearance of zidovudine thus increasing zidovudine toxicity

**Drug Uptake** Limited data due to small doses used

Serum half-life: 10 hours

Time to peak serum concentration: 3-15 hours

**Pregnancy Risk Factor** C

**Generic Available** No

## Interferon Beta-1b (in ter FEER on BAY ta won bee)

**U.S. Brand Names** Betaseron®

**Therapeutic Category** Interferon

**Use** Reduces the frequency of clinical exacerbations in ambulatory patients with relapsing-remitting multiple sclerosis (MS)

**Usual Dosage** S.C.:

Children <18 years: Not recommended

Adults >18 years: 0.25 mg (8 million units) every other day

**Mechanism of Action** Interferon beta-1b differs from naturally occurring human protein by a single amino acid substitution and the lack of carbohydrate side chains; alters the expression and response to surface antigens and can enhance immune cell activities. Properties of interferon beta-1b that modify biologic responses are mediated by cell surface receptor interactions; mechanism in the treatment of MS is unknown.

**Local Anesthetic/Vasoconstrictor Precautions** No information available to require special precautions

**Effects on Dental Treatment** No effects or complications reported

**Other Adverse Effects** Due to the pivotal position of interferon in the immune system, toxicities can affect nearly every organ system. Injection site reactions, injection site necrosis, flu-like symptoms, menstrual disorders, depression (with suicidal ideations), somnolence, palpitations, peripheral vascular disorders, hypertension, blood dyscrasias, dyspnea, laryngitis, cystitis, gastrointestinal complaints.

**Drug Interactions** No data reported

**Drug Uptake** Limited data due to small doses used

Half-life: 8 minutes to 4.3 hours

Time to peak serum concentration: 1-8 hours

**Pregnancy Risk Factor** C

**Generic Available** No

## Interferon Gamma-1b (in ter FEER on GAM ah won bee)

**U.S. Brand Names** Actimmune®

**Therapeutic Category** Biological Response Modulator; Interferon

**Use** Reduce the frequency and severity of serious infections associated with chronic granulomatous disease

**Usual Dosage** Children >1 year and Adults: S.C.:

BSA ≤0.5 $m^2$: 1.5 mcg/kg/dose

BSA >0.5 $m^2$: 50 mcg/$m^2$ (1.5 million units/$m^2$) 3 times/week

**Local Anesthetic/Vasoconstrictor Precautions** No information available to require special precautions

**Effects on Dental Treatment** No effects or complications reported

**Other Adverse Effects**

>10%:

- Central nervous system: Fever, headache, chills, fatigue
- Dermatologic: Rash
- Gastrointestinal: Diarrhea, vomiting, nausea

1% to 10%:

- Central nervous system: Depression
- Gastrointestinal: Abdominal pain, weight loss, anorexia
- Neuromuscular & skeletal: Arthralgia, back pain, myalgia

**Drug Uptake**

Absorption: Slowly absorbed from I.M. and S.C. injection

Half-life: Elimination:

- I.V.: 38 minutes
- I.M., S.C.: 3-6 hours

Time to peak plasma concentration:

- I.M.: 4 hours (1.5 ng/mL)
- S.C.: 7 hours (0.6 ng/mL)

**Pregnancy Risk Factor** C

**Generic Available** No

**Comments** More heat- and acid-labile than alfa interferons


- ♦ **Interleukin-2** *see* Aldesleukin *on page 44*
- ♦ **Interleukin-11** *see* Oprelvekin *on page 743*
- ♦ **Intralipid®** *see* Fat Emulsion *on page 419*
- ♦ **Intravenous Fat Emulsion** *see* Fat Emulsion *on page 419*
- ♦ **Intron® A** *see* Interferon Alfa-2b *on page 540*
- ♦ **Inversine®** *see* Mecamylamine *on page 620*
- ♦ **Invirase®** *see* Saquinavir *on page 903*
- ♦ **Iobid DM®** *see* Guaifenesin and Dextromethorphan *on page 479*
- ♦ **Iodex® Regular** *see* Povidone-Iodine *on page 827*


## Iodinated Glycerol (EYE oh di nay ted GLI ser ole)

**U.S. Brand Names** Iophen®; Organidin®; Par Glycerol®; R-Gen®

**Therapeutic Category** Expectorant

**Use** Mucolytic expectorant in adjunctive treatment of bronchitis, bronchial asthma, pulmonary emphysema, cystic fibrosis, or chronic sinusitis

**Usual Dosage** Oral:

Children: Up to 30 mg 4 times/day

Adults: 60 mg 4 times/day

**Mechanism of Action** Increases respiratory tract secretions by decreasing surface tension and thereby decreases the viscosity of mucus, which aids in removal of the mucus

(Continued)

## Iodinated Glycerol *(Continued)*

**Local Anesthetic/Vasoconstrictor Precautions** No information available to require special precautions

**Effects on Dental Treatment** No effects or complications reported

**Other Adverse Effects**

1% to 10%: Gastrointestinal: Diarrhea, nausea, vomiting

<1%:

Central nervous system: Headache
Dermatologic: Acne, dermatitis
Endocrine & metabolic: Acute parotitis, thyroid gland enlargement
Gastrointestinal: GI irritation
Ocular: Swelling of the eyelids
Respiratory: Pulmonary edema
Miscellaneous: Hypersensitivity

**Drug Interactions** Increased toxicity: Disulfiram, metronidazole, procarbazine, MAO inhibitors, CNS depressants, lithium

**Drug Uptake** Absorption: From GI tract

**Pregnancy Risk Factor** X

**Dosage Forms** Organically bound iodine in brackets

Elixir: 60 mg/5 mL [30 mg/5 mL] (120 mL, 480 mL)
Solution: 50 mg/mL [25 mg/mL] (30 mL)
Tablet: 30 mg [15 mg]

## Iodine (EYE oh dyne)

**Therapeutic Category** Topical Skin Product

**Use** Used topically as an antiseptic in the management of minor, superficial skin wounds and has been used to disinfect the skin preoperatively

**Usual Dosage** Apply topically as necessary to affected areas of skin

**Local Anesthetic/Vasoconstrictor Precautions** No information available to require special precautions

**Effects on Dental Treatment** No effects or complications reported

**Other Adverse Effects** 1% to 10%:

Central nervous system: Fever, headache
Dermatologic: Skin rash, angioedema, urticaria, acne
Gastrointestinal: Metallic taste, diarrhea
Endocrine & metabolic: Hypothyroidism
Hematologic: Eosinophilia, hemorrhage (mucosal)
Neuromuscular & skeletal: Arthralgia
Ocular: Swelling of eyelids
Respiratory: Pulmonary edema
Miscellaneous: Lymph node enlargement

**Pregnancy Risk Factor** D

**Generic Available** Yes

**Comments** Sodium thiosulfate inactivates iodine and is an effective chemical antidote for codeine poisoning; solutions of sodium thiosulfate may be used to remove iodine stains from skin and clothing

♦ **Iodine** *see* Trace Metals *on page 1001*
♦ **Iodochlorhydroxyquin and Hydrocortisone** *see* Clioquinol and Hydrocortisone *on page 260*
♦ **Iodopen®** *see* Trace Metals *on page 1001*

## Iodoquinol (eye oh doe KWIN ole)

**U.S. Brand Names** Yodoxin®

**Canadian Brand Names** Diodoquin®

**Therapeutic Category** Amebicide

**Use** Treatment of acute and chronic intestinal amebiasis; asymptomatic cyst passers; *Blastocystis hominis* infections; ineffective for amebic hepatitis or hepatic abscess

**Usual Dosage** Oral:

Children: 30-40 mg/kg/day (maximum: 650 mg/dose) in 3 divided doses for 20 days; not to exceed 1.95 g/day
Adults: 650 mg 3 times/day after meals for 20 days; not to exceed 2 g/day

**Mechanism of Action** Contact amebicide that works in the lumen of the intestine by an unknown mechanism

**Local Anesthetic/Vasoconstrictor Precautions** No information available to require special precautions

**Effects on Dental Treatment** No effects or complications reported

**Other Adverse Effects**

>10%: Gastrointestinal: Diarrhea, nausea, vomiting, stomach pain

1% to 10%:
  Central nervous system: Fever, chills, agitation, retrograde amnesia, headache
  Dermatologic: Skin rash, urticaria
  Endocrine & metabolic: Thyroid gland enlargement
  Gastrointestinal: Itching of rectal area
  Neuromuscular & skeletal: Peripheral neuropathy, weakness
  Ocular: Optic neuritis, optic atrophy, visual impairment

**Drug Interactions** No data reported

**Drug Uptake**
Absorption: Oral: Poor and irregular

**Pregnancy Risk Factor** C

**Generic Available** No

## Iodoquinol and Hydrocortisone

(eye oh doe KWIN ole & hye droe KOR ti sone)

**U.S. Brand Names** Vytone® Topical

**Therapeutic Category** Antifungal Agent, Topical; Corticosteroid, Topical (Low Potency)

**Use** Treatment of eczema; infectious dermatitis; chronic eczematoid otitis externa; mycotic dermatoses

**Usual Dosage** Apply 3-4 times/day

**Local Anesthetic/Vasoconstrictor Precautions** No information available to require special precautions

**Effects on Dental Treatment** No effects or complications reported

**Pregnancy Risk Factor** C

**Generic Available** No


- **Iofed®** *see* Brompheniramine and Pseudoephedrine *on page 154*
- **Iofed® PD** *see* Brompheniramine and Pseudoephedrine *on page 154*
- **Ionamin®** *see* Phentermine *on page 793*
- **Iophen®** *see* Iodinated Glycerol *on page 545*
- **Iopidine®** *see* Apraclonidine *on page 93*
- **I-Paracaine®** *see* Proparacaine *on page 852*


## Ipecac Syrup (IP e kak SIR up)

**Therapeutic Category** Antidote, Emetic

**Use** Treatment of acute oral drug overdosage and certain poisonings

**Usual Dosage** Oral:
Children:
  6-12 months: 5-10 mL followed by 10-20 mL/kg of water; repeat dose one time if vomiting does not occur within 20 minutes
  1-12 years: 15 mL followed by 10-20 mL/kg of water; repeat dose one time if vomiting does not occur within 20 minutes
  If emesis does not occur within 30 minutes after second dose, ipecac must be removed from stomach by gastric lavage
Adults: 15-30 mL followed by 200-300 mL of water; repeat dose one time if vomiting does not occur within 20 minutes

**Mechanism of Action** Irritates the gastric mucosa and stimulates the medullary chemoreceptor trigger zone to induce vomiting

**Local Anesthetic/Vasoconstrictor Precautions** No information available to require special precautions

**Effects on Dental Treatment** No effects or complications reported

**Other Adverse Effects** 1% to 10%:
  Cardiovascular: Cardiotoxicity
  Central nervous system: Lethargy
  Gastrointestinal: Protracted vomiting, diarrhea
  Ocular: Myopathy

**Drug Uptake**
Onset of action: Within 15-30 minutes
Duration: 20-25 minutes; can last longer, 60 minutes in some cases
Absorption: Significant amounts, mainly when it does not produce emesis

**Pregnancy Risk Factor** C

**Generic Available** Yes


- **I-Pentolate®** *see* Cyclopentolate *on page 285*
- **I-Phrine® Ophthalmic Solution** *see* Phenylephrine *on page 795*
- **IPOL™** *see* Poliovirus Vaccine, Inactivated *on page 813*


## Ipratropium (i pra TROE pee um)

**Related Information**
Ipratropium and Albuterol *on next page*
Respiratory Diseases *on page 1079*
(Continued)

## Ipratropium *(Continued)*

**U.S. Brand Names** Atrovent®

**Therapeutic Category** Anticholinergic Agent; Bronchodilator

**Use** Anticholinergic bronchodilator in bronchospasm associated with COPD, bronchitis, and emphysema; symptomatic relief of rhinorrhea associated with the common cold in children ages 5-11 years

**Usual Dosage**

Children:

- <2 years: Nebulization: 250 mcg 3 times/day
- 3-14 years: Metered dose inhaler: 1-2 inhalations 3 times/day, up to 6 inhalations/24 hours

Children >12 years and Adults: Nebulization: 500 mcg (1 unit-dose vial) administered 3-4 times/day by oral nebulization, with doses 6-8 hours apart

Children >14 years and Adults: Metered dose inhaler: 2 inhalations 4 times/day every 4-6 hours up to 12 inhalations in 24 hours

**Mechanism of Action** Blocks the action of acetylcholine at parasympathetic sites in bronchial smooth muscle causing bronchodilation

**Local Anesthetic/Vasoconstrictor Precautions** No information available to require special precautions

**Effects on Dental Treatment** >10% of patients experience dry mouth

**Other Adverse Effects Note:** Ipratropium is poorly absorbed from the lung, so systemic effects are rare

>10%:

- Central nervous system: Nervousness, dizziness, fatigue, headache
- Gastrointestinal: Nausea, stomach upset
- Respiratory: Cough

1% to 10%:

- Cardiovascular: Palpitations, hypotension
- Central nervous system: Insomnia
- Genitourinary: Urinary retention
- Neuromuscular & skeletal: Trembling
- Ocular: Blurred vision
- Respiratory: Nasal congestion

<1%:

- Dermatologic: Skin rash, urticaria
- Gastrointestinal: Stomatitis

**Drug Interactions**

Increased effect with albuterol

Increased toxicity with anticholinergics or drugs with anticholinergic properties, dronabinol

**Drug Uptake**

Onset of bronchodilation: 1-3 minutes after administration

Duration: Up to 4-6 hours

Absorption: Not readily absorbed into the systemic circulation from the surface of the lung or from the GI tract

**Pregnancy Risk Factor** B

**Generic Available** Yes

## Ipratropium and Albuterol (i pra TROE pee um & al BYOO ter ole)

**U.S. Brand Names** Combivent®

**Therapeutic Category** Bronchodilator

**Use** Treatment of chronic obstructive pulmonary disease (COPD) in those patients that are currently on a regular bronchodilator who continue to have bronchospasms and require a second bronchodilator

**Usual Dosage** Adults: 2 inhalations 4 times/day, maximum of 12 inhalations/24 hours

**Mechanism of Action** See individual agents

**Local Anesthetic/Vasoconstrictor Precautions** No information available to require special precautions

**Effects on Dental Treatment** >10% of patients experience dry mouth

**Other Adverse Effects** See individual agents

**Drug Interactions** See individual agents

**Dosage Forms** Aerosol: Ipratropium bromide 21 mcg and albuterol sulfate 120 mcg per actuation [200 doses] (14.7 g)

**Generic Available** No

♦ **IPV** *see* Poliovirus Vaccine, Inactivated *on page 813*

## Irbesartan (ir be SAR tan)

**U.S. Brand Names** Avapro®

**Therapeutic Category** Angiotensin II Antagonist

**Use** Treatment of hypertension alone or in combination with other antihypertensives

**Usual Dosage** Adults: Oral: 150 mg once daily with or without food; patients may be titrated to 300 mg once daily

**Mechanism of Action** Irbesartan is an angiotensin receptor antagonist. Angiotensin II acts as a vasoconstrictor. In addition to causing direct vasoconstriction, angiotensin II also stimulates the release of aldosterone. Once aldosterone is released, sodium as well as water are reabsorbed. The end result is an elevation in blood pressure. Irbesartan binds to the AT1 angiotensin II receptor. This binding prevents angiotensin II from binding to the receptor thereby blocking the vasoconstriction and the aldosterone secreting effects of angiotensin II.

**Local Anesthetic/Vasoconstrictor Precautions** No information available to require special precautions

**Effects on Dental Treatment** No effects or complications reported

**Drug Interactions** CYP2C9 enzyme substrate; hydrochlorothiazide has an added effect

**Drug Uptake**

Serum half-life: Terminal: 11-15 hours

Time to peak serum concentration: 1.5-2 hours

**Dosage Forms** Tablet: 75 mg, 150 mg, 300 mg

♦ **Ircon® [OTC]** *see* Ferrous Fumarate *on page 426*

## Irinotecan (eye rye no TEE kan)

**U.S. Brand Names** Camptosar®

**Therapeutic Category** Antineoplastic Agent, Miscellaneous

**Use** Treatment of metastatic carcinoma of the colon or rectum which has recurred or progressed following 5-FU fluorouracil-based therapy

**Usual Dosage** Adults: I.V.: The recommended starting dose is 125 mg/m$^2$ (I.V. infusion over 90 minutes) once a week for 4 weeks, followed by a 2-week rest period; additional 6-week cycles of treatment (4 weeks on therapy, followed by 2 weeks off therapy) may be repeated in patients who remain stable or do not develop intolerable toxicities

**Mechanism of Action** Irinotecan and its active metabolite (SN-38) bind reversibly to topoisomerase I and stabilize the cleavable complex so that religation of the cleaved DNA strand cannot occur. This results in the accumulation of cleavable complexes and single-strand DNA breaks. This interaction results in double-stranded DNA breaks and cell death consistent with S-phase cell cycle specificity.

**Local Anesthetic/Vasoconstrictor Precautions** No information available to require special precautions

**Effects on Dental Treatment** No effects or complications reported

**Other Adverse Effects**

>10%:

Cardiovascular: Vasodilation

Central nervous system: Insomnia, dizziness, fever (45.4%)

Dermatologic: Alopecia (60.5%), rash

Gastrointestinal: Irinotecan therapy may induce two different forms of diarrhea. Onset, symptoms, proposed mechanisms and treatment are different. Overall, 56.9% of patients treated experience abdominal pain and/or cramping during therapy. Anorexia, constipation, flatulence, stomatitis, and dyspepsia have also been reported.

Diarrhea: Dose-limiting toxicity with weekly dosing regimen

Early diarrhea (50.7% incidence) usually occurs during or within 24 hours of administration. May be accompanied by symptoms of cramping, vomiting, flushing, and diaphoresis. It is thought to be mediated by cholinergic effects which can be successfully managed with atropine (refer to Warnings/Precautions).

Late diarrhea (87.8% incidence) usually occurs >24 hours after treatment. National Cancer Institute (NCI) grade 3 or 4 diarrhea occurs in 30.6% of patients. Late diarrhea generally occurs with a median of 11 days after therapy and lasts approximately 3 days. Patients experiencing grade 3 or 4 diarrhea were noted to have symptoms a total of 7 days. Correlated with irinotecan or SN-38 levels in plasma and bile. Due to the duration, dehydration and electrolyte imbalances are significant clinical concerns. Loperamide therapy is recommended. The incidence of grade 3 or 4 late diarrhea is significantly higher in patients ≥ 65 years of age: close monitoring and prompt initiation of high-dose loperamide therapy is prudent (refer to Warnings/Precautions).

Emetic potential: Moderately high (86.2% incidence, however, only 12.5% grade 3 or 4 vomiting)

(Continued)

## Irinotecan *(Continued)*

Hematologic: Myelosuppressive: Dose-limiting toxicity with 3 week dosing regimen

Grade 1-4 neutropenia occurred in 53.9% of patients. Patients who had previously received pelvic or abdominal radiation therapy were noted to have a significantly increased incidence of grade 3 or 4 neutropenia. White blood cell count nadir is 15 days after administration and is more frequent than thrombocytopenia. Recovery is usually within 24-28 days and cumulative toxicity has not been observed.

WBC: Mild to severe
Platelets: Mild
Onset (days): 10
Nadir (days): 14-16
Recovery (days): 21-28

Neuromuscular & skeletal: Weakness (75.7%)
Respiratory: Dyspnea (22%), coughing, rhinitis
Miscellaneous: Diaphoresis

1% to 10%: Irritant chemotherapy; thrombophlebitis has been reported

**Drug Interactions** Increased toxicity: Prochlorperazine: Increased incidence of akathisia

**Drug Uptake** Serum half-life: Terminal: Irinotecan = 10 hours; SN-38 = 10 hours

**Pregnancy Risk Factor** D

**Dosage Forms** Injection: 20 mg/mL (5 mL)

**Generic Available** No

## Iron Dextran Complex (EYE ern DEKS tran KOM pleks)

**U.S. Brand Names** Dexferrum® Injection; InFed™ Injection

**Canadian Brand Names** Infufer®

**Therapeutic Category** Iron Salt

**Use** Treatment of microcytic, hypochromic anemia resulting from iron deficiency when oral iron administration is infeasible or ineffective

**Usual Dosage** I.M. (Z-track method should be used for I.M. injection), I.V.:

A 0.5 mL test dose (0.25 mL in infants) should be given prior to starting iron dextran therapy; total dose should be divided into a daily schedule for I.M., total dose may be given as a single continuous infusion

Iron deficiency anemia: Dose (mL) = 0.0476 x wt (kg) x (normal hemoglobin - observed hemoglobin) + (1 mL/5 kg) to maximum of 14 mL for iron stores

Iron replacement therapy for blood loss: Replacement iron (mg) = blood loss (mL) x hematocrit

Maximum daily dose (can give total dose at one time I.V.):

Children:
5-10 kg: 50 mg iron (1 mL)
10-50 kg: 100 mg iron (2 mL)

Adults >50 kg: 100 mg iron (2 mL)

**Mechanism of Action** The released iron, from the plasma, eventually replenishes the depleted iron stores in the bone marrow where it is incorporated into hemoglobin

**Local Anesthetic/Vasoconstrictor Precautions** No information available to require special precautions

**Effects on Dental Treatment** No effects or complications reported

**Other Adverse Effects**

>10%:
Central nervous system: Chills, fever, headache
Gastrointestinal: Metallic taste, nausea, vomiting
Local: Pain at injection site, staining of skin at the site of I.M. injection
Miscellaneous: Sweating

1% to 10%:
Gastrointestinal: Diarrhea
Genitourinary: Discolored urine

<1%:
Cardiovascular: Flushing
Local: Phlebitis
Neuromuscular & skeletal: Arthralgia
Respiratory: Respiratory difficulty
Miscellaneous: Lymphadenopathy

**Drug Uptake** Absorption:

I.M.: 50% to 90% is promptly absorbed, the balance is slowly absorbed over month

I.V.: Uptake of iron by the reticuloendothelial system appears to be constant at about 10-20 mg/hour

**Pregnancy Risk Factor** C

**Generic Available** Yes

**Comments** 2 mL of undiluted iron dextran is the maximum recommended daily dose; epinephrine should be immediately available in the event of acute hypersensitivity reaction

- **Ismelin®** *see* Guanethidine *on page 484*
- **Ismo®** *see* Isosorbide Mononitrate *on page 556*
- **Ismotic®** *see* Isosorbide *on page 555*
- **Isobamate** *see* Carisoprodol, Aspirin, and Codeine *on page 192*
- **Isocaine® HCl** *see* Mepivacaine *on page 632*
- **Isocaine® HCl 2%** *see* Mepivacaine and Levonordefrin *on page 632*
- **Isocaine® HCl 3%** *see* Mepivacaine Dental Anesthetic *on page 634*
- **Isocal® [OTC]** *see* Enteral Nutritional Products *on page 371*

## Isocarboxazid (eye soe kar BOKS a zid)

**U.S. Brand Names** Marplan®

**Therapeutic Category** Antidepressant, Monoamine Oxidase Inhibitor

**Use** Symptomatic treatment of atypical, nonendogenous or neurotic depression

**Usual Dosage** Adults: Oral: 10 mg 3 times/day; reduce to 10-20 mg/day in divided doses when condition improves

**Mechanism of Action** Thought to act by increasing endogenous concentrations of epinephrine, norepinephrine, dopamine, and serotonin through inhibition of the enzyme (monoamine oxidase) responsible for the breakdown of these neurotransmitters

**Local Anesthetic/Vasoconstrictor Precautions** Attempts should be made to avoid use of vasoconstrictor due to possibility of hypertensive episodes with monoamine oxidase inhibitors

**Effects on Dental Treatment** Orthostatic hypotension in >10% of patients; meperidine should be avoided as an analgesic due to toxic reactions with MAO inhibitors

**Other Adverse Effects**

>10%:
- Cardiovascular: Orthostatic hypotension
- Central nervous system: Drowsiness
- Endocrine & metabolic: Decreased sexual ability
- Neuromuscular & skeletal: Trembling, weakness
- Ocular: Blurred vision

1% to 10%:
- Cardiovascular: Tachycardia, peripheral edema
- Central nervous system: Nervousness, chills
- Gastrointestinal: Diarrhea, anorexia, dry mouth, constipation

<1%:
- Central nervous system: Parkinsonian syndrome
- Hematologic: Leukopenia
- Hepatic: Hepatitis

**Drug Interactions**

Decreased effect of antihypertensives

Increased toxicity with disulfiram (possible seizures), fluoxetine (and other serotonin active agents), TCAs (cardiovascular instability), meperidine (cardiovascular instability), phenothiazines (hyperpyretic crisis), levodopa, sympathomimetics (hypertensive crisis), barbiturates, rauwolfia alkaloids (eg, reserpine), dextroamphetamine (psychoses), foods containing tyramine

**Pregnancy Risk Factor** C

**Generic Available** No

- **Isoclor® Expectorant** *see* Guaifenesin, Pseudoephedrine, and Codeine *on page 482*
- **Isocom®** *see* Acetaminophen, Isometheptene, and Dichloralphenazone *on page 32*
- **Isodine® [OTC]** *see* Povidone-Iodine *on page 827*

## Isoetharine (eye soe ETH a reen)

**Related Information**

Respiratory Diseases *on page 1079*

**U.S. Brand Names** Arm-a-Med® Isoetharine; Beta-2®; Bronkometer®; Bronkosol®; Dey-Lute® Isoetharine

**Therapeutic Category** Adrenergic Agonist Agent; Antiasthmatic; Bronchodilator

**Use** Bronchodilator in bronchial asthma and for reversible bronchospasm occurring with bronchitis and emphysema

(Continued)

## Isoetharine *(Continued)*

**Usual Dosage** Treatments are usually not repeated more often than every 4 hours, except in severe cases

Nebulizer: Children: 0.01 mL/kg; minimum dose 0.1 mL; maximum dose: 0.5 mL diluted in 2-3 mL normal saline

Inhalation: Oral: Adults: 1-2 inhalations every 4 hours as needed

**Mechanism of Action** Relaxes bronchial smooth muscle by action on $beta_2$-receptors with very little effect on heart rate

**Local Anesthetic/Vasoconstrictor Precautions** Isoetharine is selective for beta-adrenergic receptors and not alpha receptors; therefore, there is no precaution in the use of vasoconstrictor

**Effects on Dental Treatment** Dry mouth in 1% to 10% of patients

**Other Adverse Effects**

1% to 10%:

Cardiovascular: Tachycardia, hypertension, pounding heartbeat

Central nervous system: Dizziness, lightheadedness, headache, nervousness, insomnia

Gastrointestinal: Dry mouth, nausea, vomiting

Neuromuscular & skeletal: Trembling, weakness

<1%: Respiratory: Paradoxical bronchospasm

**Drug Interactions**

Decreased effect with beta-blockers

Increased toxicity with other sympathomimetics (eg, epinephrine)

**Drug Uptake** Duration: 1-4 hours

**Pregnancy Risk Factor** C

**Generic Available** Yes

## Isoflurophate (eye soe FLURE oh fate)

**U.S. Brand Names** Floropryl®

**Therapeutic Category** Antiglaucoma Agent; Cholinergic Agent, Ophthalmic; Ophthalmic Agent, Miotic

**Use** Treat primary open-angle glaucoma and conditions that obstruct aqueous outflow and to treat accommodative convergent strabismus

**Usual Dosage** Adults: Ophthalmic:

Glaucoma: Instill 0.25" strip in eye every 8-72 hours

Strabismus: Instill 0.25" strip to each eye every night for 2 weeks then reduce to 0.25" every other night to once weekly for 2 months

**Mechanism of Action** Cholinesterase inhibitor that causes contraction of the iris and ciliary muscles producing miosis, reduced intraocular pressure, and increased aqueous humor outflow

**Local Anesthetic/Vasoconstrictor Precautions** No information available to require special precautions

**Effects on Dental Treatment** No effects or complications reported

**Other Adverse Effects**

1% to 10%: Ocular: Stinging, burning, myopia, visual blurring

<1%:

Cardiovascular: Bradycardia, hypotension, flushing

Gastrointestinal: Nausea, vomiting, diarrhea

Neuromuscular & skeletal: Muscle weakness

Ocular: Retinal detachment, browache, miosis, twitching eyelids, watering eyes

Respiratory: Dyspnea

Miscellaneous: Sweating

**Drug Interactions** Increased toxicity: Succinylcholine, systemic anticholinesterases, carbamate or organic phosphate insecticides, cause decrease in cholinesterase levels

**Drug Uptake**

Peak IOP reduction: 24 hours

Duration: 1 week

Onset of miosis: Within 5-10 minutes

Duration: Up to 4 weeks

**Pregnancy Risk Factor** X

**Generic Available** No

♦ **Isollyl Improved®** *see* Butalbital Compound *on page 163*
♦ **Isollyl® Improved** *see* Butalbital Compound and Aspirin *on page 165*
♦ **Isomeprobamate** *see* Carisoprodol *on page 191*

## Isoniazid (eye soe NYE a zid)

**Related Information**

Nonviral Infectious Diseases *on page 1095*

**U.S. Brand Names** INH™; Laniazid® Oral; Nydrazid® Injection

**Canadian Brand Names** PMS-Isoniazid

**Therapeutic Category** Antitubercular Agent

**Use** Treatment of susceptible tuberculosis infections and prophylactically to those individuals exposed to tuberculosis

**Usual Dosage** Oral, I.M. (recommendations often change due to resistant strains and newly developed information; consult *MMWR* for current CDC recommendations):

Children: 10-20 mg/kg/day in 1-2 divided doses (maximum: 300 mg total dose)
Prophylaxis: 10 mg/kg/day given daily (up to 300 mg total dose) for 6 months

Adults: 5 mg/kg/day given daily (usual dose is 300 mg)
Disseminated disease: 10 mg/kg/day in 1-2 divided doses
Treatment should be continued for 9 months with rifampin or for 6 months with rifampin and pyrazinamide
Prophylaxis: 300 mg/day given daily for 6 months

American Thoracic Society and CDC currently recommend twice weekly therapy as part of a short-course regimen which follows 1-2 months of daily treatment for uncomplicated pulmonary tuberculosis in compliant patients
Children: 20-40 mg/kg/dose (up to 900 mg) twice weekly
Adults: 15 mg/kg/dose (up to 900 mg) twice weekly

**Mechanism of Action** Unknown, but may include the inhibition of myocolic acid synthesis resulting in disruption of the bacterial cell wall

**Local Anesthetic/Vasoconstrictor Precautions** No information available to require special precautions

**Effects on Dental Treatment** No effects or complications reported

**Other Adverse Effects**

>10%:
Gastrointestinal: Loss of appetite, nausea, vomiting, stomach pain
Hepatic: Hepatitis
Neuromuscular & skeletal: Peripheral neuritis, weakness

1% to 10%:
Central nervous system: Dizziness, slurred speech, lethargy
Neuromuscular & skeletal: Hyper-reflexia

<1%:
Central nervous system: Fever, seizures, mental depression, psychosis
Dermatologic: Skin rash
Hematologic: Blood dyscrasias
Neuromuscular & skeletal: Arthralgia
Ocular: Blurred vision, loss of vision

**Drug Interactions**

Decreased effect/levels of isoniazid with aluminum salts

Increased toxicity/levels of oral anticoagulants, carbamazepines, cycloserine, hydantoins, hepatically metabolized benzodiazepines; reaction with disulfiram

**Drug Uptake**

Absorption: Oral, I.M.: Rapid and complete; rate can be slowed when orally administered with food

Serum half-life:
Fast acetylators: 30-100 minutes
Slow acetylators: 2-5 hours; half-life may be prolonged in patients with impaired hepatic function or severe renal impairment

Time to peak serum concentration: Within 1-2 hours

**Pregnancy Risk Factor** C

**Generic Available** Yes

♦ **Isonipecaine** *see* Meperidine *on page 629*

♦ **Isopap®** *see* Acetaminophen, Isometheptene, and Dichloralphenazone *on page 32*

## Isoproterenol (eye soe proe TER e nole)

**Related Information**

Cardiovascular Diseases *on page 1066*

**U.S. Brand Names** Arm-a-Med® Isoproterenol; Dey-Dose® Isoproterenol; Isuprel®; Medihaler-Iso®

**Therapeutic Category** Adrenergic Agonist Agent; Bronchodilator

**Use** Treatment of reversible airway obstruction as in asthma or COPD; used parenterally in ventricular arrhythmias due to A-V nodal block; hemodynamically compromised bradyarrhythmias or atropine-resistant bradyarrhythmias; temporary use in third degree A-V block until pacemaker insertion; low cardiac output; vasoconstrictive shock states

(Continued)

## Isoproterenol *(Continued)*

**Usual Dosage**

Children:

Bronchodilation: Inhalation: Metered dose inhaler: 1-2 metered doses up to 5 times/day

Bronchodilation (using 1:200 inhalation solution) 0.01 mL/kg/dose every 4 hours as needed (maximum: 0.05 mL/dose) diluted with NS to 2 mL

Sublingual: 5-10 mg every 3-4 hours, not to exceed 30 mg/day

Cardiac arrhythmias: I.V.: Start 0.1 mcg/kg/minute (usual effective dose 0.2-2 mcg/kg/minute)

Adults:

Bronchodilation: Inhalation: Metered dose inhaler: 1-2 metered doses 4-6 times/day

Bronchodilation: 1-2 inhalations of a 0.25% solution, no more than 2 inhalations at any one time (1-5 minutes between inhalations); no more than 6 inhalations in any hour during a 24-hour period; maintenance therapy: 1-2 inhalations 4-6 times/day. Alternatively: 0.5% solution via hand bulb nebulizer is 5-15 deep inhalations repeated once in 5-10 minutes if necessary; treatments may be repeated up to 5 times/day.

Sublingual: 10-20 mg every 3-4 hours; not to exceed 60 mg/day

Cardiac arrhythmias: I.V.: 5 mcg/minute initially, titrate to patient response (2-20 mcg/minute)

Shock: I.V.: 0.5-5 mcg/minute; adjust according to response

**Mechanism of Action** Stimulates $beta_1$- and $beta_2$-receptors resulting in relaxation of bronchial, GI, and uterine smooth muscle, increased heart rate and contractility, vasodilation of peripheral vasculature

**Local Anesthetic/Vasoconstrictor Precautions** Isoproterenol is selective for beta-adrenergic receptors and not alpha receptors; therefore, there is no precaution in the use of vasoconstrictor such as epinephrine

**Effects on Dental Treatment** >10% of patients experience dry mouth

**Other Adverse Effects**

>10%:

Central nervous system: Insomnia, restlessness

Gastrointestinal: Dry throat, discoloration of saliva (pinkish-red)

1% to 10%:

Cardiovascular: Flushing of the face or skin, ventricular arrhythmias, tachycardias, profound hypotension, hypertension

Central nervous system: Nervousness, anxiety, dizziness, headache, lightheadedness

Gastrointestinal: Vomiting, nausea

Neuromuscular & skeletal: Trembling, tremor, weakness

Miscellaneous: Sweating

<1%:

Cardiovascular: Arrhythmias, chest pain

Respiratory: Paradoxical bronchospasm

**Drug Interactions** Increased toxicity: Sympathomimetic agents lead to headaches; general anesthetics lead to arrhythmias

**Drug Uptake**

Onset of bronchodilation: Oral inhalation: Immediately

Duration:

Oral inhalation: 1 hour

S.C.: Up to 2 hours

Serum half-life: 2.5-5 minutes

Time to peak serum concentration: Oral: Within 1-2 hours

**Pregnancy Risk Factor** C

**Generic Available** Yes

## Isoproterenol and Phenylephrine

(eye soe proe TER e nole & fen il EF rin)

**U.S. Brand Names** Duo-Medihaler® Aerosol

**Therapeutic Category** Adrenergic Agonist Agent

**Use** Treatment of bronchospasm associated with acute and chronic bronchial asthma, bronchitis, pulmonary emphysema, and bronchiectasis

**Usual Dosage** Daily maintenance: 1-2 inhalations 4-6 times/day, no more than 2 inhalations at any one time or more than 6 in any 1 hour within 24 hours

**Local Anesthetic/Vasoconstrictor Precautions** No information available to require special precautions

**Effects on Dental Treatment** No effects or complications reported

**Generic Available** No

♦ **Isoptin®** *see* Verapamil *on page 1043*

♦ **Isoptin® SR** *see* Verapamil *on page 1043*

- ♦ **Isopto® Atropine** *see* Atropine *on page 108*
- ♦ **Isopto® Carbachol Ophthalmic** *see* Carbachol *on page 185*
- ♦ **Isopto® Carpine®** *see* Pilocarpine *on page 802*
- ♦ **Isopto® Cetamide® Ophthalmic** *see* Sulfacetamide Sodium *on page 939*
- ♦ **Isopto® Cetapred® Ophthalmic** *see* Sulfacetamide Sodium and Prednisolone *on page 940*
- ♦ **Isopto® Eserine®** *see* Physostigmine *on page 801*
- ♦ **Isopto® Homatropine Ophthalmic** *see* Homatropine *on page 499*
- ♦ **Isopto® Hyoscine Ophthalmic** *see* Scopolamine *on page 905*
- ♦ **Isopto® Plain Solution [OTC]** *see* Artificial Tears *on page 97*
- ♦ **Isopto® Tears Solution [OTC]** *see* Artificial Tears *on page 97*
- ♦ **Isordil®** *see* Isosorbide Dinitrate *on this page*


## Isosorbide (eye soe SOR bide)

**U.S. Brand Names** Ismotic®

**Therapeutic Category** Antiglaucoma Agent; Diuretic, Osmotic; Ophthalmic Agent, Osmotic

**Use** Short-term emergency treatment of acute angle-closure glaucoma and short-term reduction of intraocular pressure prior to and following intraocular surgery; may be used to interrupt an acute glaucoma attack; preferred agent when need to avoid nausea and vomiting

**Usual Dosage** Adults: Oral: Initial: 1.5 g/kg with a usual range of 1-3 g/kg 2-4 times/day as needed

**Mechanism of Action** Elevates osmolarity of glomerular filtrate to hinder the tubular resorption of water and increase excretion of sodium and chloride to result in diuresis; creates an osmotic gradient between plasma and ocular fluids

**Local Anesthetic/Vasoconstrictor Precautions** No information available to require special precautions

**Effects on Dental Treatment** No effects or complications reported

**Other Adverse Effects**

1% to 10%:

Central nervous system: Headache, confusion, disorientation

Gastrointestinal: Vomiting

<1%:

Cardiovascular: Syncope

Central nervous system: Lethargy, vertigo, dizziness, lightheadedness, irritability

Dermatologic: Rash

Endocrine & metabolic: Hypernatremia, hyperosmolarity

Gastrointestinal: Nausea, abdominal/gastric discomfort (infrequently), anorexia, thirst

Miscellaneous: Hiccups

**Drug Interactions** No data reported

**Drug Uptake**

Onset of action: Within 10-30 minutes

Peak action: 1-1.5 hours

Duration: 5-6 hours

Serum half-life: 5-9.5 hours

**Pregnancy Risk Factor** B

**Generic Available** No

## Isosorbide Dinitrate (eye soe SOR bide dye NYE trate)

**Related Information**

Cardiovascular Diseases *on page 1066*

**U.S. Brand Names** Dilatrate®-SR; Isordil®; Sorbitrate®

**Canadian Brand Names** Apo®-ISDN; Cedocard®-SR; Coradur®

**Therapeutic Category** Antianginal Agent; Nitrate; Vasodilator, Coronary

**Use** Prevention and treatment of angina pectoris; for congestive heart failure; to relieve pain, dysphagia, and spasm in esophageal spasm with GE reflux

**Usual Dosage** Adults (elderly should be given lowest recommended daily doses initially and titrate upward):

Oral: Angina: 5-40 mg 4 times/day or 40 mg every 8-12 hours in sustained released dosage form

Oral: Congestive heart failure:

Initial dose: 10 mg 3 times/day

Target dose: 40 mg 3 times/day

Maximum dose: 80 mg 3 times/day

Sublingual: 2.5-10 mg every 4-6 hours

Chew: 5-10 mg every 2-3 hours

Tolerance to nitrate effects develops with chronic exposure

(Continued)

## Isosorbide Dinitrate *(Continued)*

Dose escalation does not overcome this effect. Tolerance can only be overcome by short periods of nitrate absence from the body. Short periods (10-12 hours) or nitrate withdrawal help minimize tolerance.

**Mechanism of Action** Stimulation of intracellular cyclic-GMP results in vascular smooth muscle relaxation of both arterial and venous vasculature. Increased venous pooling decreases left ventricular pressure (preload) and arterial dilatation decreases arterial resistance (afterload). Therefore, this reduces cardiac oxygen demand by decreasing left ventricular pressure and systemic vascular resistance by dilating arteries. Additionally, coronary artery dilation improves collateral flow to ischemic regions; esophageal smooth muscle is relaxed via the same mechanism.

**Local Anesthetic/Vasoconstrictor Precautions** No information available to require special precautions

**Effects on Dental Treatment** No effects or complications reported

**Other Adverse Effects**

>10%:

Cardiovascular: Flushing, postural hypotension

Central nervous system: Headache, lightheadedness, dizziness

Neuromuscular & skeletal: Weakness

1% to 10%: Dermatologic: Drug rash, exfoliative dermatitis

<1%:

Gastrointestinal: Nausea, vomiting

Hematologic: Methemoglobinemia (overdose)

**Drug Interactions** No data reported

**Drug Uptake** Serum half-life:

Parent drug: 1-4 hours

Metabolite (5-mononitrate): 4 hours

**Pregnancy Risk Factor** C

**Generic Available** Yes

## Isosorbide Mononitrate (eye soe SOR bide mon oh NYE trate)

**Related Information**

Cardiovascular Diseases *on page 1066*

**U.S. Brand Names** Imdur™; Ismo®; Monoket®

**Therapeutic Category** Antianginal Agent; Vasodilator, Coronary

**Use** Long-acting metabolite of the vasodilator isosorbide dinitrate used for the prophylactic treatment of angina pectoris

**Usual Dosage** Adults: Oral:

Regular tablet: 20 mg twice daily separated by 7 hours

Extended release tablet (Imdur™): Initial: 30-60 mg once daily; after several days the dosage may be increased to 120 mg/day (given as two 60 mg tablets); daily dose should be taken in the morning upon arising; maximum: 240 mg/day

Asymmetrical dosing regimen of 7 AM and 3 PM or 9 AM and 5 PM to allow for a nitrate-free dosing interval to minimize nitrate tolerance

**Mechanism of Action** Prevailing mechanism of action for nitroglycerin (and other nitrates) is systemic venodilation, decreasing preload as measured by pulmonary capillary wedge pressure and left ventricular end diastolic volume and pressure; the average reduction in LVEDV is 25% at rest, with a corresponding increase in ejection fractions of 50% to 60%. This effect improves congestive symptoms in heart failure and improves the myocardial perfusion gradient in patients with coronary artery disease.

**Local Anesthetic/Vasoconstrictor Precautions** No information available to require special precautions

**Effects on Dental Treatment** No effects or complications reported

**Other Adverse Effects**

>10%: Central nervous system: Headache, dizziness

1% to 10%: Gastrointestinal: Nausea, vomiting

<1%:

Cardiovascular: Angina pectoris, arrhythmias, atrial fibrillation, hypotension, palpitations, postural hypotension, premature ventricular contractions, supraventricular tachycardia, syncope, edema

Central nervous system: Malaise, agitation, anxiety, confusion, hypoesthesia, insomnia, nervousness, nightmares

Dermatologic: Pruritus, rash

Gastrointestinal: Abdominal pain, diarrhea, dyspepsia, tenesmus, increased appetite

Genitourinary: Impotence, dysuria

Hematologic: Methemoglobinemia (rarely)

Neuromuscular & skeletal: Neck stiffness, rigors, arthralgia, dyscoordination, weakness

Ocular: Blurred vision, diplopia
Renal: Polyuria
Respiratory: Bronchitis, pneumonia, upper respiratory tract infection
Miscellaneous: Tooth disorder, cold sweat

**Drug Interactions** No data reported

**Drug Uptake** Absorption: Oral: Nearly complete and low intersubject variability in its pharmacokinetic parameters and plasma concentrations

**Pregnancy Risk Factor** C

**Generic Available** No

## Isotretinoin (eye soe TRET i noyn)

**U.S. Brand Names** Accutane®

**Canadian Brand Names** Isotrex®

**Therapeutic Category** Acne Products; Retinoic Acid Derivative; Vitamin A Derivative

**Use** Treatment of severe recalcitrant cystic and/or conglobate acne unresponsive to conventional therapy; used investigationally for the treatment of children with metastatic neuroblastoma or leukemia that does not respond to conventional therapy

**Usual Dosage** Oral:

Children: Maintenance therapy for neuroblastoma: 100-250 mg/m$^2$/day in 2 divided doses has been used investigationally

Children and Adults: 0.5-2 mg/kg/day in 2 divided doses (dosages as low as 0.05 mg/kg/day have been reported to be beneficial) for 15-20 weeks or until the total cyst count decreases by 70%, whichever is sooner

**Mechanism of Action** Reduces sebaceous gland size and reduces sebum production; regulates cell proliferation and differentiation

**Local Anesthetic/Vasoconstrictor Precautions** No information available to require special precautions

**Effects on Dental Treatment** >10% of patients experience dry mouth

**Other Adverse Effects**

>10%:
Dermatologic: Cheilitis, inflammation of lips, dry skin, pruritus, photosensitivity
Endocrine/metabolic: Elevated serum concentration of triglycerides
Local: Burning, redness
Neuromuscular & skeletal: Bone pain, arthralgia, myalgia
Ocular: Itching of eye
Respiratory: Dry nose, epistaxis

1% to 10%:
Central nervous system: Fatigue, headache, mental depression
Dermatologic: Skin peeling on hands or soles of feet, skin rash
Gastrointestinal: Stomach upset
Ocular: Dry eyes, photophobia

<1%:
Central nervous system: Mood changes, pseudomotor cerebri
Dermatologic: Alopecia
Endocrine & metabolic: Hyperuricemia
Gastrointestinal: Anorexia, nausea, vomiting, inflammatory bowel syndrome, bleeding of gums
Hematologic: Elevated erythrocyte sedimentation rate, decrease in hemoglobin and hematocrit
Hepatic: Hepatitis
Ocular: Conjunctivitis, corneal opacities, optic neuritis, cataracts

**Note:** Not to be used in women of childbearing potential unless woman is capable of complying with effective contraceptive measures; therapy is normally begun on the second or third day of next normal menstrual period; effective contraception must be used for at least 1 month before beginning therapy, during therapy, and for 1 month after discontinuation of therapy. Because of the high likelihood of teratogenic effects (~20%), physicians do not prescribe isotretinoin for women who are or who are likely to become pregnant while using the drug.

**Drug Interactions**

Increased effect: Increased clearance of carbamazepine
Increased toxicity: Avoid other vitamin A products; may interfere with medications used to treat hypertriglyceridemia

**Drug Uptake**

Absorption: Oral: Demonstrates biphasic absorption
Serum half-life, terminal:
Parent drug: 10-20 hours
Time to peak serum concentration: Within 3 hours

**Pregnancy Risk Factor** X

**Generic Available** No

♦ **Isovex®** *see* Ethaverine *on page 398*

## Isoxsuprine (eye SOKS syoo preen)

**U.S. Brand Names** Vasodilan®

**Therapeutic Category** Vasodilator

**Use** Treatment of peripheral vascular diseases, such as arteriosclerosis obliterans and Raynaud's disease

**Usual Dosage** Adults: 10-20 mg 3-4 times/day; start with lower dose in elderly due to potential hypotension

**Mechanism of Action** In studies on normal human subjects, isoxsuprine increases muscle blood flow, but skin blood flow is usually unaffected. Rather than increasing muscle blood flow by beta-receptor stimulation, isoxsuprine probably has a direct action on vascular smooth muscle. The generally accepted mechanism of action of isoxsuprine on the uterus is beta-adrenergic stimulation. Isoxsuprine was shown to inhibit prostaglandin synthetase at high serum concentrations, with low concentrations there was an increase in the P-G synthesis.

**Local Anesthetic/Vasoconstrictor Precautions** No information available to require special precautions

**Effects on Dental Treatment** No effects or complications reported

**Other Adverse Effects**

1% to 10%: Gastrointestinal: Nausea, vomiting

<1%:

- Cardiovascular: Chest pain, hypotension
- Dermatologic: Rash
- Respiratory: Pulmonary edema

**Drug Interactions** No data reported

**Drug Uptake**

Absorption: Nearly complete

Serum half-life, serum: 1.25 hours mean

Time to peak serum concentration: Oral, I.M.: Within 1 hour

**Pregnancy Risk Factor** C

**Generic Available** Yes

## Isradipine (iz RA di peen)

**Related Information**

Calcium Channel Blockers & Gingival Hyperplasia *on page 1204*

Cardiovascular Diseases *on page 1066*

**U.S. Brand Names** DynaCirc®

**Therapeutic Category** Calcium Channel Blocker

**Use** Treatment of hypertension, congestive heart failure, migraine prophylaxis

**Usual Dosage** Adults: 2.5 mg twice daily; antihypertensive response seen in 2-3 hours; maximal response in 2-4 weeks; increase dose at 2- to 4-week intervals at 2.5-5 mg increments; usual dose range: 5-20 mg/day. **Note**: Most patients show no improvement with doses >10 mg/day except adverse reaction rate increases; therefore, maximal dose in elderly should be 10 mg/day.

**Mechanism of Action** Inhibits calcium ion from entering the "slow channels" or select voltage-sensitive areas of vascular smooth muscle and myocardium during depolarization, producing a relaxation of coronary vascular smooth muscle and coronary vasodilation; increases myocardial oxygen delivery in patients with vasospastic angina

**Local Anesthetic/Vasoconstrictor Precautions** No information available to require special precautions

**Effects on Dental Treatment** Other drugs of this class can cause gingival hyperplasia (ie, nifedipine) but there have been no reports for isradipine

**Other Adverse Effects**

>10%: Central nervous system: Headache

1% to 10%:

- Cardiovascular: Edema, palpitations, flushing, chest pain, tachycardia, hypotension
- Central nervous system: Dizziness, fatigue
- Dermatologic: Rash
- Gastrointestinal: Nausea, abdominal discomfort, vomiting, diarrhea
- Neuromuscular & skeletal: Weakness
- Respiratory: Dyspnea

<1%:

- Cardiovascular: Heart failure, atrial and ventricular fibrillation, TIAs, A-V block, myocardial infarction, abnormal EKG
- Central nervous system: Disturbed sleep
- Dermatologic: Pruritus, urticaria
- Gastrointestinal: Dry mouth
- Genitourinary: Nocturia

Hematologic: Leukopenia
Neuromuscular & skeletal: Foot cramps, paresthesia
Ocular: Visual disturbance
Respiratory: Cough

**Drug Interactions** Increased toxicity/effect/levels: $H_2$-blockers cause increased bioavailability of isradipine

Severe hypotension has been reported during fentanyl anesthesia with concomitant use of beta-blockers and calcium channel blockers; even though such interactions have not been seen specifically with isradipine, caution is suggested in using isradipine with fentanyl

**Drug Uptake**

Absorption: Oral: 90% to 95%
Serum half-life: 8 hours
Time to peak: Serum concentration: 1-1.5 hours

**Pregnancy Risk Factor** C

**Generic Available** No

**Selected Readings**

Westbrook P, Bednarczyk EM, Carlson M, et al, "Regression of Nifedipine-Induced Gingival Hyperplasia Following Switch to a Same Class Calcium Channel Blocker, Isradipine," *J Periodontol*, 1997, 68(7):645-50.

♦ **Isuprel®** *see* Isoproterenol *on page 553*
♦ **Itch-X® [OTC]** *see* Pramoxine *on page 828*

## Itraconazole (i tra KOE na zole)

**Related Information**

Oral Fungal Infections *on page 1134*

**U.S. Brand Names** Sporanox®

**Therapeutic Category** Antifungal Agent, Systemic

**Use**

Dental: Treatment of susceptible fungal infections in immunocompromised and immunocompetent patients including blastomycosis and histoplasmosis; also has activity against *Aspergillus, Candida, Coccidioides, Cryptococcus, Sporothrix* and chromomycosis

Medical: Treatment of susceptible fungal infection as described for dental use

**Usual Dosage** Oral (absorption is best if taken with food, therefore, it is best to administer itraconazole after meals):

Children: Efficacy and safety have not been established; a small number of patients 3-16 years of age have been treated with 100 mg/day for systemic fungal infections with no serious adverse effects reported

Adults: 200 mg once daily, if obvious improvement or there is evidence of progressive fungal disease, increase the dose in 100 mg increments to a maximum of 400 mg/day; doses >200 mg/day are given in 2 divided doses

**Mechanism of Action** Inhibits fungal cytochrome P-450-dependent enzymes (cytochrome P-450 3A4 and cytochrome P-450 2C); this blocks the synthesis of ergosterol which is the vital component in the fungal cell membrane. Triazoles contain three nitrogen atoms in the five-membered azole ring; the triazole ring increases tissue penetration, prolongs half-life, and enhances efficacy while decreasing toxicity compared with the imidazoles.

**Local Anesthetic/Vasoconstrictor Precautions** No information available to require special precautions

**Effects on Dental Treatment** No effects or complications reported

**Other Adverse Effects**

>10%: Gastrointestinal: Nausea

1% to 10%:
Central nervous system: Headache
Dermatologic: Rash
Gastrointestinal: Abdominal pain, vomiting

**Contraindications** Known hypersensitivity to itraconazole or other azoles; terfenadine

**Warnings/Precautions** Rare cases of serious cardiovascular adverse event, including death, ventricular tachycardia and torsade de pointes have been observed due to increased terfenadine concentrations induced by itraconazole; patients who develop abnormal liver function tests during fluconazole therapy should be monitored and therapy discontinued if symptoms of liver disease develop

**Drug Interactions** Decreased serum levels with isoniazid and phenytoin; decreased/undetectable serum levels with rifampin - **should not be administered concomitantly with rifampin**; absorption requires gastric acidity, therefore, antacids, $H_2$ antagonists (cimetidine and ranitidine), omeprazole, and sucralfate significantly reduce bioavailability resulting in treatment failures and should not be administered concomitantly; amphotericin B or fluconazole should be used instead. May increase cyclosporine levels (by 50%) when high doses

(Continued)

## Itraconazole *(Continued)*

are used; may increase phenytoin serum concentration; may inhibit warfarins metabolism; may increase digoxin serum levels; may increase terfenadine levels - **concomitant administration is not recommended.** If used concomitantly with an HMG-CoA reductase inhibitor (atorvastatin, lovastatin, pravastatin, simvastatin) itraconazole can increase HMG-CoA levels significantly (possibly 20-fold). This is probably due to hepatic enzyme inhibition or competition. In order to decrease the risk of myositis or myopathy, it may be necessary to temporarily stop HMG-CoA reductase inhibitors if systemic azole antifungals are needed. Coadministration with cisapride may cause toxic increases in cisapride blood levels.

**Drug Uptake**

Absorption: Oral: ~55%

Serum half-life: After single 200 mg dose: 21±5 hours

Time to peak serum concentration: 1-2 hours

**Pregnancy Risk Factor** C

**Breast-feeding Considerations** No data reported

**Dosage Forms**

Capsule: 100 mg

Solution, oral: 100 mg/10 mL (150 mL)

**Dietary Considerations** Absorption enhanced by food and requires gastric acidity

**Generic Available** No

♦ **I-Tropine®** *see* Atropine *on page 108*

## Ivermectin (eye ver MEK tin)

**U.S. Brand Names** Stromectol®

**Therapeutic Category** Antibiotic, Miscellaneous

**Use** Treatment of the following infections: Strongyloidiasis of the intestinal tract due the nematode parasite *Strongyloides stercoralis.* Onchocerciasis due to the nematode parasite *Onchocerca volvulus.* Note: Ivermectin is ineffective against adult *Onchocerca volvulus* parasites because they reside in subcutaneous nodules which are infrequently palpable. Surgical excision of these nodules may be considered in the management of patients with onchocerciasis.

**Usual Dosage** Oral:

Children >5 years: 150 mcg/kg as a single dose once every 12 months

Adults: 150 mcg/kg as a single dose; may be repeated every 6-12 **months**

**Local Anesthetic/Vasoconstrictor Precautions** No information available to require special precautions

**Effects on Dental Treatment** No effects or complications reported

**Drug Uptake** Half life: 22-28 hours

**Pregnancy Risk Factor** C

**Dosage Forms** Tablet: 6 mg

**Generic Available** No

♦ **IVIG** *see* Immune Globulin, Intravenous *on page 531*

♦ **IvyBlock®** *see* Bentoquatam *on page 127*

## Japanese Encephalitis Virus Vaccine, Inactivated

(jap a NEESE en sef a LYE tis VYE rus vak SEEN, in ak ti VAY ted)

**U.S. Brand Names** JE-VAX®

**Therapeutic Category** Vaccine, Live Virus

**Use** Active immunization against Japanese encephalitis for persons spending a month or longer in endemic areas, especially if travel will include rural areas

**Usual Dosage** US recommended primary immunization schedule:

Children >3 years and Adults: S.C.: Three 1 mL doses given on days 0, 7, and 30. Give third dose on day 14 when time does not permit waiting; 2 doses a week apart produce immunity in about 80% of vaccines; the longest regimen yields highest titers after 6 months

Children 1-3 years: S.C.: Three 0.5 mL doses given on days 0, 7, and 30; abbreviated schedules should be used only when necessary due to time constraints

Booster dose: Give after 2 years, or according to current recommendation

**Note:** Travel should not commence for at least 10 days after the last dose of vaccine, to allow adequate antibody formation and recognition of any delayed adverse reaction

Advise concurrent use of other means to reduce the risk of mosquito exposure when possible, including bed nets, insect repellents, protective clothing, avoidance of travel in endemic areas, and avoidance of outdoor activity during twilight and evening periods

**Local Anesthetic/Vasoconstrictor Precautions** No information available to require special precautions

**Effects on Dental Treatment** No effects or complications reported

**Other Adverse Effects**

1% to 10%:

Cardiovascular: Hypotension
Central nervous system: Fever, headache, malaise, chills, dizziness
Dermatologic: Rash, urticaria, itching with or without accompanying rash
Gastrointestinal: Nausea, vomiting, abdominal pain
Local: Tenderness, redness, and swelling at injection site
Neuromuscular & skeletal: Myalgia

<1%:

Central nervous system: Encephalitis, encephalopathy, seizure
Dermatologic: Erythema multiforme, erythema nodosum, angioedema
Neuromuscular & skeletal: Peripheral neuropathy, joint swelling
Respiratory: Dyspnea
Miscellaneous: Anaphylactic reaction

Report allergic or unusual adverse reactions to the Vaccine Adverse Event Reporting System (VAERS 1-800-822-7967)

**Pregnancy Risk Factor** C

**Generic Available** No

**Comments** Japanese encephalitis vaccine is currently available only from the Centers for Disease Control. Contact Centers for Disease Control at (404) 639-6370 (Mon-Fri) or (404) 639-2888 (nights, weekends, or holidays).

- **Jenest-28™** *see* Ethinyl Estradiol and Norethindrone *on page 404*
- **JE-VAX®** *see* Japanese Encephalitis Virus Vaccine, Inactivated *on previous page*
- **Junior Strength Motrin® [OTC]** *see* Ibuprofen *on page 522*
- **Junior Strength Panadol® [OTC]** *see* Acetaminophen *on page 27*
- **Just Tears® Solution [OTC]** *see* Artificial Tears *on page 97*
- **K+ 10®** *see* Potassium Chloride *on page 822*
- **Kabikinase®** *see* Streptokinase *on page 933*
- **Kadian™ Capsule** *see* Morphine Sulfate *on page 688*
- **Kalcinate®** *see* Calcium Gluconate *on page 175*

## Kanamycin (kan a MYE sin)

**Related Information**

Nonviral Infectious Diseases *on page 1095*

**U.S. Brand Names** Kantrex®

**Therapeutic Category** Antibiotic, Aminoglycoside

**Use**

Oral: Preoperative bowel preparation in the prophylaxis of infections and adjunctive treatment of hepatic coma (oral kanamycin is not indicated in the treatment of systemic infections); treatment of susceptible bacterial infection including gram-negative aerobes, gram-positive *Bacillus* as well as some mycobacteria
Parenteral: Rarely used in antibiotic irrigations during surgery

**Usual Dosage**

Children:

Infections: I.M., I.V.: 15-30 mg/kg/day in divided doses every 8 hours
Suppression of bowel flora: Oral: 150-250 mg/kg/day in divided doses administered every 1-6 hours

Adults:

Infections: I.M., I.V.: 5-7.5 mg/kg/dose in divided doses every 8-12 hours
Preoperative intestinal antisepsis: Oral: 1 g every 4-6 hours for 36-72 hours
Hepatic coma: Oral: 8-12 g/day in divided doses

**Mechanism of Action** Interferes with protein synthesis in bacterial cell by binding to ribosomal subunit

**Local Anesthetic/Vasoconstrictor Precautions** No information available to require special precautions

**Effects on Dental Treatment** No effects or complications reported

**Other Adverse Effects**

>10%: Renal: Nephrotoxicity

1% to 10%:

Cardiovascular: Swelling
Central nervous system: Neurotoxicity
Dermatologic: Skin itching, redness, rash
Otic: Ototoxicity (auditory), ototoxicity (vestibular)

<1%:

Central nervous system: Drowsiness, headache, pseudomotor cerebri
Dermatologic: Photosensitivity, erythema

(Continued)

## Kanamycin *(Continued)*

Gastrointestinal: Anorexia, nausea, vomiting, weight loss, increased salivation, enterocolitis
Hematologic: Granulocytopenia, agranulocytosis, thrombocytopenia
Local: Burning, stinging
Neuromuscular & skeletal: Tremors, muscle cramps, weakness
Respiratory: Dyspnea

**Drug Interactions** Increased toxicity:
Penicillins, cephalosporins, amphotericin B, diuretics cause increased nephrotoxicity of kanamycin
Neuromuscular blocking agents cause increased neuromuscular blockade of kanamycin

**Drug Uptake**
Absorption: Oral: Not absorbed following administration
Serum half-life: 2-4 hours, increases in anuria to 80 hours
End-stage renal disease: 40-96 hours
Time to peak serum concentration: I.M.: 1-2 hours

**Pregnancy Risk Factor** D
**Generic Available** Yes


- ♦ **Kantrex®** *see* Kanamycin *on previous page*
- ♦ **Kaochlor®** *see* Potassium Chloride *on page 822*
- ♦ **Kaochlor-Eff®** *see* Potassium Bicarbonate, Potassium Chloride, and Potassium Citrate *on page 821*
- ♦ **Kaochlor® SF** *see* Potassium Chloride *on page 822*
- ♦ **Kaodene® [OTC]** *see* Kaolin and Pectin *on this page*


## Kaolin and Pectin (KAY oh lin & PEK tin)

**U.S. Brand Names** Kaodene® [OTC]; Kao-Spen® [OTC]; Kapectolin® [OTC]
**Therapeutic Category** Antidiarrheal
**Synonyms** Pectin and Kaolin
**Use** Treatment of uncomplicated diarrhea
**Usual Dosage** Oral:
Children:
<6 years: Do not use
6-12 years: 30-60 mL after each loose stool
Adults: 60-120 mL after each loose stool

**Local Anesthetic/Vasoconstrictor Precautions** No information available to require special precautions
**Effects on Dental Treatment** No effects or complications reported
**Other Adverse Effects** 1% to 10%: Gastrointestinal: Constipation, fecal impaction
**Pregnancy Risk Factor** C
**Generic Available** Yes

## Kaolin and Pectin With Opium
(KAY oh lin & PEK tin with OH pee um)

**U.S. Brand Names** Parepectolin®
**Canadian Brand Names** Donnagel®-PG Capsule; Donnagel®-PG Suspension
**Therapeutic Category** Antidiarrheal
**Use** Symptomatic relief of diarrhea
**Usual Dosage** Oral:
Children:
3-6 years: 7.5 mL with each loose bowel movement, not to exceed 30 mL in 12 hours
6-12 years: 5-10 mL with each loose bowel movement, not to exceed 40 mL in 12 hours
Children >12 years and Adults: 15-30 mL with each loose bowel movement, not to exceed 120 mL in 12 hours

**Local Anesthetic/Vasoconstrictor Precautions** No information available to require special precautions
**Effects on Dental Treatment** No effects or complications reported
**Pregnancy Risk Factor** C
**Generic Available** Yes


- ♦ **Kaon®** *see* Potassium Gluconate *on page 824*
- ♦ **Kaon-Cl®** *see* Potassium Chloride *on page 822*
- ♦ **Kaon-Cl-10®** *see* Potassium Chloride *on page 822*
- ♦ **Kaopectate® Advanced Formula [OTC]** *see* Attapulgite *on page 109*
- ♦ **Kaopectate® II [OTC]** *see* Loperamide *on page 599*
- ♦ **Kaopectate® Maximum Strength Caplets** *see* Attapulgite *on page 109*

- ♦ **Kao-Spen® [OTC]** *see* Kaolin and Pectin *on previous page*
- ♦ **Kapectolin® [OTC]** *see* Kaolin and Pectin *on previous page*
- ♦ **Kapectolin PG®** *see* Hyoscyamine, Atropine, Scopolamine, Kaolin, Pectin, and Opium *on page 522*
- ♦ **Karidium®** *see* Fluoride *on page 441*
- ♦ **Karigel®** *see* Fluoride *on page 441*
- ♦ **Karigel®-N** *see* Fluoride *on page 441*
- ♦ **Kasof® [OTC]** *see* Docusate *on page 346*
- ♦ **Kay Ciel®** *see* Potassium Chloride *on page 822*
- ♦ **K+ Care®** *see* Potassium Chloride *on page 822*
- ♦ **K+ Care® Effervescent** *see* Potassium Bicarbonate *on page 820*
- ♦ **K-Dur® 10** *see* Potassium Chloride *on page 822*
- ♦ **K-Dur® 20** *see* Potassium Chloride *on page 822*
- ♦ **Keflex®** *see* Cephalexin *on page 214*
- ♦ **Keflin®** *see* Cephalothin *on page 216*
- ♦ **Keftab®** *see* Cephalexin *on page 214*
- ♦ **Kefurox®** *see* Cefuroxime *on page 210*
- ♦ **Kefzol®** *see* Cefazolin *on page 199*
- ♦ **K-Electrolyte® Effervescent** *see* Potassium Bicarbonate *on page 820*
- ♦ **Kemadrin®** *see* Procyclidine *on page 845*
- ♦ **Kenacort®** *see* Triamcinolone *on page 1010*
- ♦ **Kenaject-40®** *see* Triamcinolone *on page 1010*
- ♦ **Kenalog®** *see* Triamcinolone *on page 1010*
- ♦ **Kenalog-10®** *see* Triamcinolone *on page 1010*
- ♦ **Kenalog-40®** *see* Triamcinolone *on page 1010*
- ♦ **Kenalog® H** *see* Triamcinolone *on page 1010*
- ♦ **Kenalog® in Orabase®** *see* Triamcinolone *on page 1010*
- ♦ **Kenalog® in Orabase®** *see* Triamcinolone Acetonide Dental Paste *on page 1011*
- ♦ **Kenonel®** *see* Triamcinolone *on page 1010*
- ♦ **Keoxifene Hydrochloride** *see* Raloxifene *on page 876*
- ♦ **Keralyt® Gel** *see* Salicylic Acid and Propylene Glycol *on page 901*
- ♦ **Kerlone®** *see* Betaxolol *on page 138*
- ♦ **Kestrone®** *see* Estrone *on page 393*
- ♦ **Ketalar®** *see* Ketamine *on this page*


## Ketamine (KEET a meen)

**U.S. Brand Names** Ketalar®

**Therapeutic Category** General Anesthetic, Intravenous

**Use** Induction of anesthesia; short surgical procedures; dressing changes

**Usual Dosage** Used in combination with anticholinergic agents to ↓ hypersalivation

Children: Initial induction:

- Oral: 6-10 mg/kg for 1 dose (mixed in 0.2-0.3 mL/kg of cola or other beverage) given 30 minutes before the procedure
- I.M.: 3-7 mg/kg
- I.V.: Range: 0.5-2 mg/kg, use smaller doses (0.5-1 mg/kg) for sedation for minor procedures; usual induction dosage: 1-2 mg/kg

Continuous I.V. infusion: Sedation: 5-20 mcg/kg/minute

Adults: Initial induction:

- I.M.: 3-8 mg/kg
- I.V.: Range: 1-4.5 mg/kg; usual induction dosage: 1-2 mg/kg

Children and Adults: Maintenance: Supplemental doses of $1/2$ to the full induction dose; repeat as needed

**Mechanism of Action** Produces dissociative anesthesia by direct action on the cortex and limbic system

**Local Anesthetic/Vasoconstrictor Precautions** No information available to require special precautions

**Effects on Dental Treatment** No effects or complications reported

**Other Adverse Effects**

>10%:

- Cardiovascular: Hypertension, tachycardia, increased cardiac output, paradoxical direct myocardial depression
- Central nervous system: Increased intracranial pressure, vivid dreams, visual hallucinations
- Neuromuscular & skeletal: Tonic-clonic movements, tremors
- Miscellaneous: Emergence reactions, vocalization

(Continued)

## Ketamine *(Continued)*

1% to 10%:
- Cardiovascular: Bradycardia, hypotension
- Dermatologic: Skin rash
- Gastrointestinal: Vomiting, anorexia, nausea
- Local: Pain at injection site
- Ocular: Nystagmus, diplopia
- Respiratory: Respiratory depression

<1%:
- Cardiovascular: Cardiac arrhythmias, myocardial depression, increases in cerebral blood
- Endocrine & metabolic: Increased metabolic rate
- Gastrointestinal: Hypersalivation
- Neuromuscular & skeletal: Increased skeletal muscle tone, fasciculations
- Ocular: Increased intraocular pressure
- Respiratory: Increased airway resistance, cough reflex may be depressed, decreased bronchospasm, respiratory depression or apnea with large doses or rapid infusions, laryngospasm

**Drug Interactions** Increased toxicity:
- Barbiturates, narcotics, hydroxyzine increase prolonged recovery from ketamine
- Muscle relaxants, thyroid hormones cause increased blood pressure and heart rate in combination with ketamine
- Halothane causes decreased blood pressure in combination with ketamine

**Drug Uptake** Duration of action (following a single dose):
- Unconsciousness: 10-15 minutes
- Analgesia: 30-40 minutes
- Amnesia: May persist for 1-2 hours

**Pregnancy Risk Factor** D

**Generic Available** No

## Ketoconazole (kee toe KOE na zole)

**Related Information**

Dental Drug Interactions: Update on Drug Combinations Requiring Special Considerations *on page 1225*
Oral Fungal Infections *on page 1134*
Respiratory Diseases *on page 1079*

**U.S. Brand Names** Nizoral®

**Therapeutic Category** Antifungal Agent, Systemic; Antifungal Agent, Topical

**Use**
- Dental: Treatment of susceptible fungal infections in the oral cavity including candidiasis, oral thrush, and chronic mucocutaneous candidiasis
- Medical: Treatment of susceptible fungal infections including blastomycosis, histoplasmosis, paracoccidioidomycosis, as well as certain recalcitrant cutaneous dermatophytosis; used topically for treatment of tinea corporis, tinea cruris, tinea versicolor, and cutaneous candidiasis, seborrheic dermatitis

**Usual Dosage**

Children >2 years:
- Oral: 5-10 mg/kg/day divided every 12-24 hours for 2-4 weeks
- Topical: Rub gently to affected area 1-2 times/day

Adults:
- Oral: 200-400 mg/day as a single daily dose
- Topical: Rub gently to affected area 1-2 times/day

**Mechanism of Action** Alters the permeability of the cell wall; inhibits biosynthesis of triglycerides and phospholipids by fungi; inhibits several fungal enzymes that results in a build-up of toxic concentrations of hydrogen peroxide

**Local Anesthetic/Vasoconstrictor Precautions** No information available to require special precautions

**Effects on Dental Treatment** No effects or complications reported

**Other Adverse Effects**

Oral: 1% to 10%:
- Dermatologic: Pruritus
- Gastrointestinal: Nausea, vomiting, abdominal pain, diarrhea

Cream: Dermatologic: Severe irritation, pruritus, stinging (~5%)

Shampoo: Increases in normal hair loss, irritation (<1%), abnormal hair texture, scalp pustules, mild dryness of skin, itching, oiliness/dryness of hair

**Contraindications** Hypersensitivity to ketoconazole or any component; CNS fungal infections (due to poor CNS penetration); coadministration with terfenadine is contraindicated

**Warnings/Precautions** Use with caution in patients with impaired hepatic function; has been associated with hepatotoxicity, including some fatalities; perform periodic liver function tests; high doses of ketoconazole may depress adrenocortical function.

**Drug Interactions** Decreased serum levels with isoniazid and phenytoin; decreased/undetectable serum levels with rifampin - **should not be administered concomitantly with rifampin**; absorption requires gastric acidity, therefore, antacids, $H_2$ antagonists (cimetidine and ranitidine), omeprazole, and sucralfate significantly reduce bioavailability resulting in treatment failures and should not be administered concomitantly; amphotericin B or fluconazole should be used instead. May increase cyclosporine levels (by 50%) when high doses are used; may increase phenytoin serum concentration; may inhibit warfarins metabolism; may increase digoxin serum levels. Coadministration with astemizole could result in cardiotoxicity. Concomitant use of cisapride and ketoconazole may cause toxic increases in cisapride blood levels.

**Drug Uptake**

Serum half-life: Biphasic: Initial: 2 hours; terminal: 8 hours

Time to peak serum concentration: 1-2 hours

**Pregnancy Risk Factor** C

**Breast-feeding Considerations** No data reported

**Dosage Forms**

Cream: 2% (15 g, 30 g, 60 g)

Shampoo: 2% (120 mL)

Tablet: 200 mg

**Dietary Considerations** May be taken with food or milk to decrease GI adverse effects

**Generic Available** No

## Ketoprofen (kee toe PROE fen)

**Related Information**

Oral Pain *on page 1122*

Rheumatoid Arthritis and Osteoarthritis *on page 1092*

**U.S. Brand Names** Actron® [OTC]; Orudis®; Orudis® KT [OTC]; Oruvail®

**Canadian Brand Names** Apo®-Keto; Apo®-Keto-E; Novo-Keto-EC; Nu-Ketoprofen; Nu-Ketoprofen-E; Orafen; PMS-Ketoprofen; Rhodis™; Rhodis-EC™

**Therapeutic Category** Analgesic, Non-narcotic; Anti-inflammatory Agent; Nonsteroidal Anti-inflammatory Drug (NSAID), Oral

**Use**

Dental: Management of pain and swelling

Medical: Acute and long-term treatment of rheumatoid arthritis and osteoarthritis; primary dysmenorrhea; mild to moderate pain

**Usual Dosage** Oral:

Children: Not recommended

Adults: 25-50 mg every 6-8 hours as necessary; daily doses >300 mg are not recommended

**Mechanism of Action** Inhibits prostaglandin synthesis by decreasing the activity of the enzyme, cyclo-oxygenase, which results in decreased formation of prostaglandin precursors

**Local Anesthetic/Vasoconstrictor Precautions** No information available to require special precautions

**Effects on Dental Treatment** NSAID formulations are known to reversibly decrease platelet aggregation via mechanisms different than observed with aspirin. The dentist should be aware of the potential of abnormal coagulation. Caution should also be exercised in the use of NSAIDs in patients already on anticoagulant therapy with drugs such as warfarin (Coumadin®).

**Other Adverse Effects** >10%:

Central nervous system: Dizziness

Dermatologic: Skin rash

Gastrointestinal: Cramps, heartburn, nausea

**Contraindications** Ketoprofen is contraindicated in patients who have known hypersensitivity to it; should not be given to patients in whom aspirin or other nonsteroidal anti-inflammatory drugs induce asthma, urticaria, or other allergic-type reactions because severe, rarely fatal, anaphylactic reactions to ketoprofen have been reported in such patients

**Warnings/Precautions** Use lowest effective dose for shortest period possible; use with caution in patients with a history of GI disease (bleeding or ulcers)

**Drug Interactions** Probenecid increases both free and bound ketoprofen by reducing the plasma clearance of ketoprofen to about one-third, as well as decreasing its protein-binding; the combination of ketoprofen and probenecid is not recommended; coadministration of ketoprofen and methotrexate should be avoided because increased toxicity due to displacement of protein-bound methotrexate has been reported to occur

(Continued)

## Ketoprofen *(Continued)*

**Drug Uptake**
Absorption: Rapid and complete
Onset of effect: 30-60 minutes
Serum half-life: 2-4 hours
Time to peak serum concentration: 0.5-2 hours

**Pregnancy Risk Factor** B (D if used in the 3rd trimester or near delivery)

**Breast-feeding Considerations** May be taken while breast-feeding

**Dosage Forms**
Capsule (Orudis®): 25 mg, 50 mg, 75 mg
Actron®, Orudis® KT [OTC]: 12.5 mg
Capsule, extended release (Oruvail®): 100 mg, 200 mg

**Dietary Considerations** In order to minimize gastrointestinal effects, ketoprofen can be prescribed to be taken with food or milk; although food affects the bioavailability of ketoprofen, analgesic efficacy is not significantly diminished; food slows rate of absorption resulting in delayed and reduced peak serum concentrations

**Generic Available** Yes

**Selected Readings**

Balevi B, "Ketorolac Versus Ibuprofen: A Simple Cost-Efficacy Comparison for Dental Use," *J Can Dent Assoc*, 1994, 60(1):31-2.
Brooks PM and Day RO, "Nonsteroidal Anti-Inflammatory Drugs - Differences and Similarities," *N Engl J Med*, 1991, 324(24):1716-25.
Cooper SA, "Ketoprofen in Oral Surgery Pain: A Review," *J Clin Pharmacol*, 1988, 28(12 Suppl):S40-6.
Hersh EV, "The Efficacy and Safety of Ketoprofen in Postsurgical Dental Pain," *Compendium*, 1991, 12(4):234.


## Ketorolac Tromethamine (KEE toe role ak troe METH a meen)

**Related Information**
Dental Drug Interactions: Update on Drug Combinations Requiring Special Considerations *on page 1225*

**U.S. Brand Names** Acular® Ophthalmic; Toradol® Injection; Toradol® Oral

**Therapeutic Category** Analgesic, Non-narcotic; Anti-inflammatory Agent; Nonsteroidal Anti-inflammatory Drug (NSAID), Oral

**Use**
Dental: Short-term (<5 days) management of pain
Medical: First parenteral NSAID for analgesia; 30 mg I.M. provides the analgesia comparable to 12 mg of morphine or 100 mg of meperidine

**Usual Dosage** Adults: Treatment of acute postsurgical pain:
Manufacturer recommendation: I.M.: 30 mg followed by an oral dose (10 mg) as needed, then 10 mg every 4-6 hours as needed thereafter; total time for drug administration should be no longer than 5 days; maximum oral daily dose: 40 mg (or 120 mg combined oral and I.M.)
I.M.: Initial: 30-60 mg, then 15-30 mg every 6 hours as needed for up to 5 days maximum; maximum dose in the first 24 hours: 150 mg with 120 mg/24 hours for up to 5 days total

**Mechanism of Action** Inhibits prostaglandin synthesis by decreasing the activity of the enzyme, cyclo-oxygenase, which results in decreased formation of prostaglandin precursors

**Local Anesthetic/Vasoconstrictor Precautions** No information available to require special precautions

**Effects on Dental Treatment** NSAID formulations are known to reversibly decrease platelet aggregation via mechanisms different than observed with aspirin. The dentist should be aware of the potential of abnormal coagulation. Caution should also be exercised in the use of NSAIDs in patients already on anticoagulant therapy with drugs such as warfarin (Coumadin®).

**Other Adverse Effects** 1% to 10%: Gastrointestinal: Abdominal pain, nausea, gastric ulcers

**Contraindications** In patients who have developed nasal polyps, angioedema, or bronchospastic reactions to other NSAIDs, active peptic ulcer disease, recent GI bleeding or perforation, patients with advanced renal disease or risk of renal failure, labor and delivery, nursing mothers, patients with hypersensitivity to ketorolac, aspirin, or other NSAIDs, **prophylaxis before major surgery**, suspected or confirmed cerebrovascular bleeding, hemorrhagic diathesis, concurrent aspirin or other NSAIDs, epidural or intrathecal administration, concomitant probenecid

**Warnings/Precautions** Use extra caution and reduce dosages in the elderly because it is cleared renally somewhat slower, and the elderly are also more sensitive to the renal effects of NSAIDs; use with caution in patients with congestive heart failure, hypertension, decreased renal or hepatic function, history of GI disease (bleeding or ulcers), or those receiving anticoagulants

**Drug Interactions** High dose salicylates may increase plasma levels of ketorolac by displacing from plasma proteins; coadministration with probenecid reduces renal excretion of ketorolac causing increased plasma levels; ketorolac reduces diuretic effect of furosemide; some NSAIDs may prevent renal excretion of lithium; effect of ketorolac on lithium is unknown

**Drug Uptake**

Absorption: Oral: Rapid and complete
Onset of effect: I.M.: Within 10 minutes
Duration of effect: 6-8 hours
Serum half-life: 2-8 hours
Time to peak serum concentration: I.M.: 30-60 minutes

**Pregnancy Risk Factor** B (D if used in the 3rd trimester)

**Breast-feeding Considerations** No data reported

**Dosage Forms**

Injection: 15 mg/mL (1 mL); 30 mg/mL (1 mL, 2 mL)
Solution, ophthalmic: 0.5% (5 mL)
Tablet: 10 mg

**Dietary Considerations** May be taken with food to decrease GI distress; food decreases rate of absorption but extent remains the same

**Generic Available** Yes (tablet)

**Comments** According to the manufacturer, ketorolac has been used inappropriately by physicians in the past. The drug had been prescribed to NSAID-sensitive patients, patients with GI bleeding, and for long-term use; a warning has been issued regarding increased incidence and severity of GI complications with increasing doses and duration of use. Labeling now includes the statement that ketorolac inhibits platelet function and is indicated for up to 5 days use only.

**Selected Readings**


Ahmad N, Grad HA, Haas DA, et al, "The Efficacy of Nonopioid Analgesics for Postoperative Dental Pain: A Meta-Analysis," *Anesth Prog*, 1997, 44(4):119-26.

Balevi B, "Ketorolac Versus Ibuprofen: A Simple Cost-Efficacy Comparison for Dental Use," *J Can Dent Assoc*, 1994, 60(1):31-2.

Brown CR, Moodie JE, Evans SE, et al, "Efficacy of Intramuscular (I.M.) Ketorolac and Meperidine in Pain Following Major Oral Surgery," *Clin Pharmacol Ther*, 1988, 43:161 (abstract).

Forbes JA, Butterworth GA, Burchfield WH, et al, "Evaluation of Ketorolac, Aspirin, and an Acetaminophen-Codeine Combination in Postoperative Oral Surgery Pain," *Pharmacotherapy*, 1990, 10(6 Pt 2): 77S-93S.

Forbes JA, Kehm CJ, Grodin CD, et al, "Evaluation of Ketorolac, Ibuprofen, Acetaminophen, and an Acetaminophen-Codeine Combination in Postoperative Oral Surgery Pain," *Pharmacotherapy*, 1990, 10(6 Pt 2):94S-105S.

Fricke JR Jr, Angelocci D, Fox K, et al, "Comparison of the Efficacy and Safety of Ketorolac and Meperidine in the Relief of Dental Pain," *J Clin Pharmacol*, 1992, 32(4):376-84.

Fricke J, Halladay SC, Bynum L, et al, "Pain Relief After Dental Impaction Surgery Using Ketorolac, Hydrocodone Plus Acetaminophen, or Placebo," *Clin Ther*, 1993, 15(3):500-9.

Gannon R, "Focus on Ketorolac: A Nonsteroidal, Anti-inflammatory Agent for the Treatment of Moderate to Severe Pain," *Hosp Formul*, 1989, 24:695-702.

Pendeville PE, Van Boven MJ, Contreras V, et al, "Ketorolac Tromethamine for Postoperative Analgesia in Oral Surgery," *Acta Anaesthesiol Belg*, 1995, 46(1):25-30.

Swift JQ, Roszkowski MT, Alton T, "Effect of Intra-articular Versus Systemic Anti-inflammatory Drugs in a Rabbit Model of Temporomandibular Joint Inflammation," *J Oral Maxillofac Surg*, 1998, 56(11):1288-95 (discussion 1295-6).

Walton GM, Rood JP, Snowdon AT, et al, "Ketorolac and Diclofenac for Postoperative Pain Relief Following Oral Surgery," *Br J Oral Maxillofac Surg*, 1993, 31(3):158-60.

Wynn RL, "Ketorolac (Toradol®) for Dental Pain," *Gen Dent*, 1992, 40(6):476-9.


- **Key-Pred®** *see* Prednisolone *on page 832*
- **Key-Pred-SP®** *see* Prednisolone *on page 832*
- **K-G®** *see* Potassium Gluconate *on page 824*
- **K-Gen® Effervescent** *see* Potassium Bicarbonate *on page 820*
- **K-Ide®** *see* Potassium Bicarbonate and Potassium Citrate, Effervescent *on page 821*
- **Kinevac®** *see* Sincalide *on page 916*
- **Klaron® Lotion** *see* Sulfacetamide Sodium *on page 939*
- **K-Lease®** *see* Potassium Chloride *on page 822*
- **Klerist-D® Tablet [OTC]** *see* Chlorpheniramine and Pseudoephedrine *on page 233*
- **Klonopin™** *see* Clonazepam *on page 264*
- **K-Lor™** *see* Potassium Chloride *on page 822*
- **Klor-Con®** *see* Potassium Chloride *on page 822*
- **Klor-Con® 8** *see* Potassium Chloride *on page 822*
- **Klor-Con® 10** *see* Potassium Chloride *on page 822*
- **Klor-Con/25®** *see* Potassium Chloride *on page 822*
- **Klor-Con®/EF** *see* Potassium Bicarbonate and Potassium Citrate, Effervescent *on page 821*
- **Klor-Con M20®** *see* Potassium Chloride *on page 822*
- **Klorvess®** *see* Potassium Chloride *on page 822*

- **Klorvess® Effervescent** *see* Potassium Bicarbonate and Potassium Chloride, Effervescent *on page 820*
- **Klotrix®** *see* Potassium Chloride *on page 822*
- **K-Lyte®** *see* Potassium Bicarbonate and Potassium Citrate, Effervescent *on page 821*
- **K/Lyte/CL®** *see* Potassium Bicarbonate and Potassium Chloride, Effervescent *on page 820*
- **K-Lyte®/Cl** *see* Potassium Chloride *on page 822*
- **K-Lyte® Effervescent** *see* Potassium Bicarbonate *on page 820*
- **K-Norm®** *see* Potassium Chloride *on page 822*
- **Koāte®-HP** *see* Antihemophilic Factor (Human) *on page 89*
- **Koāte®-HS** *see* Antihemophilic Factor (Human) *on page 89*
- **Kogenate®** *see* Antihemophilic Factor (Recombinant) *on page 90*
- **Kolephrin® GG/DM [OTC]** *see* Guaifenesin and Dextromethorphan *on page 479*
- **Kolyum®** *see* Potassium Chloride and Potassium Gluconate *on page 823*
- **Konakion®** *see* Phytonadione *on page 801*
- **Kondon's Nasal® [OTC]** *see* Ephedrine *on page 371*
- **Konsyl® [OTC]** *see* Psyllium *on page 865*
- **Konsyl-D® [OTC]** *see* Psyllium *on page 865*
- **Konȳne® 80** *see* Factor IX Complex (Human) *on page 417*
- **Koromex® [OTC]** *see* Nonoxynol 9 *on page 728*
- **K-Phos® Neutral** *see* Potassium Phosphate and Sodium Phosphate *on page 826*
- **K-Phos® Original** *see* Potassium Acid Phosphate *on page 820*
- **K-Tab®** *see* Potassium Chloride *on page 822*
- **Ku-Zyme® HP** *see* Pancrelipase *on page 763*
- **K-Vescent®** *see* Potassium Bicarbonate and Potassium Citrate, Effervescent *on page 821*
- **Kwelcof®** *see* Hydrocodone and Guaifenesin *on page 508*
- **Kytril®** *see* Granisetron *on page 475*
- **LA-12®** *see* Hydroxocobalamin *on page 515*

## Labetalol (la BET a lole)

**Related Information**

Cardiovascular Diseases *on page 1066*

**U.S. Brand Names** Normodyne®; Trandate®

**Therapeutic Category** Alpha-/Beta- Adrenergic Blocker

**Use** Treatment of mild to severe hypertension; I.V. for hypertensive emergencies

**Usual Dosage** Due to limited documentation of its use, labetalol should be initiated cautiously in pediatric patients with careful dosage adjustment and blood pressure monitoring

Children:

Oral: Limited information regarding labetalol use in pediatric patients is currently available in literature. Some centers recommend initial oral doses of 4 mg/kg/day in 2 divided doses. Reported oral doses have started at 3 mg/kg/day and 20 mg/kg/day and have increased up to 40 mg/kg/day.

I.V., intermittent bolus doses of 0.3-1 mg/kg/dose have been reported

For treatment of pediatric hypertensive emergencies, initial continuous infusions of 0.4-1 mg/kg/hour with a maximum of 3 mg/kg/hour have been used; administration requires the use of an infusion pump

Adults:

Oral: Initial: 100 mg twice daily, may increase as needed every 2-3 days by 100 mg until desired response is obtained; usual dose: 200-400 mg twice daily; not to exceed 2.4 g/day

I.V.: 20 mg or 1-2 mg/kg whichever is lower, IVP over 2 minutes, may give 40-80 mg at 10-minute intervals, up to 300 mg total dose

I.V. infusion: Initial: 2 mg/minute; titrate to response up to 300 mg total dose; administration requires the use of an infusion pump

**I.V. infusion (500 mg/250 mL $D_5$)** rates:

1 mg/minute: 30 mL/hour
2 mg/minute: 60 mL/hour
3 mg/minute: 90 mL/hour
4 mg/minute: 120 mL/hour
5 mg/minute: 150 mL/hour
6 mg/minute: 180 mL/hour

**Mechanism of Action** Blocks alpha-, $beta_1$-, and $beta_2$-adrenergic receptor sites; elevated renins are reduced

**Local Anesthetic/Vasoconstrictor Precautions** Use with caution; epinephrine has interacted with nonselective beta-blockers to result in initial hypertensive episode followed by bradycardia

**Effects on Dental Treatment** Noncardioselective beta-blockers (ie, propranolol, nadolol) enhance the pressor response to epinephrine, resulting in hypertension and bradycardia. Many nonsteroidal anti-inflammatory drugs such as ibuprofen and indomethacin can reduce the hypotensive effect of beta-blockers after 3 or more weeks of therapy with the NSAID. Short-term NSAID use (ie, 3 days) requires no special precautions in patients taking beta-blockers.

**Other Adverse Effects**

1% to 10%:

- Cardiovascular: Congestive heart failure, arrhythmia, reduced peripheral circulation, orthostatic hypotension
- Central nervous system: Mental depression, dizziness, drowsiness
- Dermatologic: Itching, numbness of skin
- Endocrine & metabolic: Decreased sexual ability
- Gastrointestinal: Nausea, vomiting, stomach discomfort, changes in taste
- Neuromuscular & skeletal: Weakness
- Respiratory: Dyspnea, nasal congestion

<1%:

- Cardiovascular: Bradycardia, chest pain
- Dermatologic: Skin rash
- Gastrointestinal: Diarrhea
- Hepatic: Hepatotoxicity
- Neuromuscular & skeletal: Arthralgia
- Ocular: Dry eyes

**Drug Interactions**

Decreased effect of beta-blockers:

- Barbiturates (increased liver metabolism of beta-blockers to result in lower serum levels)
- NSAIDs (attenuate the hypotensive therapeutic effects of beta-blockers)
- Rifampin (increased liver metabolism of beta-blockers to result in lower serum levels)

Increased effects of beta-blockers:

- Calcium channel blockers (increase serum levels of beta-blockers by unknown mechanism to enhance hypotension)

Beta-blockers increase the effects of:

- Epinephrine (vasoconstrictor; initial hypertensive episode followed by bradycardia) only from noncardioselective type beta-blockers
- Phenylephrine (Neosynephrine®; enhanced pressor response)
- Theophylline (inhibit theophylline metabolism causing increase in serum concentrations)

**Drug Uptake**

Onset of action:

- Oral: 20 minutes to 2 hours
- I.V.: 2-5 minutes

Peak effect:

- Oral: 1-4 hours
- I.V.: 5-15 minutes

Duration:

- Oral: 8-24 hours (dose-dependent)
- I.V.: 2-4 hours

Serum half-life, normal renal function: 6-8 hours

**Pregnancy Risk Factor** C

**Generic Available** No

- ♦ **Lac-Hydrin®** *see* Lactic Acid With Ammonium Hydroxide *on next page*
- ♦ **Lacril® Ophthalmic Solution [OTC]** *see* Artificial Tears *on page 97*
- ♦ **Lacrisert®** *see* Hydroxypropyl Cellulose *on page 517*
- ♦ **LactAid® [OTC]** *see* Lactase *on this page*

## Lactase (LAK tase)

**U.S. Brand Names** Dairy Ease® [OTC]; LactAid® [OTC]; Lactrase® [OTC]

**Therapeutic Category** Nutritional Supplement

**Use** Help digest lactose in milk for patients with lactose intolerance

**Usual Dosage**

Capsule: 1-2 capsules taken with milk or meal; pretreat milk with 1-2 capsules/quart of milk

Liquid: 5-15 drops/quart of milk

Tablet: 1-3 tablets with meals

**Local Anesthetic/Vasoconstrictor Precautions** No information available to require special precautions

(Continued)

## Lactase *(Continued)*

**Effects on Dental Treatment** No effects or complications reported

**Generic Available** No

- **Lactic Acid and Salicylic Acid** *see* Salicylic Acid and Lactic Acid *on page 900*

## Lactic Acid and Sodium-PCA

(LAK tik AS id & SOW dee um-pee see aye)

**U.S. Brand Names** LactiCare® [OTC]

**Therapeutic Category** Topical Skin Product

**Synonyms** Sodium-PCA and Lactic Acid

**Use** Lubricate and moisturize the skin counteracting dryness and itching

**Usual Dosage** Apply as needed

**Local Anesthetic/Vasoconstrictor Precautions** No information available to require special precautions

**Effects on Dental Treatment** No effects or complications reported

**Generic Available** No

## Lactic Acid With Ammonium Hydroxide

(LAK tik AS id with a MOE nee um hye DROKS ide)

**U.S. Brand Names** Lac-Hydrin®

**Therapeutic Category** Topical Skin Product

**Synonyms** Ammonium Lactate

**Use** Treatment of moderate to severe xerosis and ichthyosis vulgaris

**Usual Dosage** Shake well; apply to affected areas, use twice daily, rub in well

**Local Anesthetic/Vasoconstrictor Precautions** No information available to require special precautions

**Effects on Dental Treatment** No effects or complications reported

**Generic Available** No

- **LactiCare® [OTC]** *see* Lactic Acid and Sodium-PCA *on this page*
- **Lactinex® [OTC]** *see Lactobacillus acidophilus* and *Lactobacillus bulgaricus* *on this page*

## *Lactobacillus acidophilus* and *Lactobacillus bulgaricus*

(lak toe ba SIL us as i DOF fil us & lak toe ba SIL us bul GAR i cus)

**Related Information**

Oral Nonviral Soft Tissue Ulcerations or Erosions *on page 1141*

**U.S. Brand Names** Bacid® [OTC]; Lactinex® [OTC]; More-Dophilus® [OTC]

**Canadian Brand Names** Fermalac®

**Therapeutic Category** Antidiarrheal

**Use** Treatment of uncomplicated diarrhea particularly that caused by antibiotic therapy; re-establish normal physiologic and bacterial flora of the intestinal tract

**Usual Dosage** Children >3 years and Adults: Oral:

Capsules: 2 capsules 2-4 times/day

Granules: 1 packet added to or taken with cereal, food, milk, fruit juice, or water, 3-4 times/day

Powder: 1 teaspoonful daily with liquid

Tablet, chewable: 4 tablets 3-4 times/day; may follow each dose with a small amount of milk, fruit juice, or water

**Mechanism of Action** Creates an environment unfavorable to potentially pathogenic fungi or bacteria through the production of lactic acid, and favors establishment of an aciduric flora, thereby suppressing the growth of pathogenic microorganisms; helps re-establish normal intestinal flora

**Local Anesthetic/Vasoconstrictor Precautions** No information available to require special precautions

**Effects on Dental Treatment** No effects or complications reported

**Other Adverse Effects** 1% to 10%: Gastrointestinal: Flatulence

**Drug Interactions** No data reported

**Drug Uptake** Absorption: Oral: Not absorbed

**Pregnancy Risk Factor** No rating

**Dosage Forms**

Capsule: 50s, 100s

Granules: 1 g/packet (12 packets/box)

Powder: 12 oz

Tablet, chewable: 50s

**Generic Available** No

- **Lactrase® [OTC]** *see* Lactase *on previous page*

## Lactulose (LAK tyoo lose)

**U.S. Brand Names** Cephulac®; Cholac®; Chronulac®; Constilac®; Constulose®; Duphalac®; Enulose®; Evalose®; Heptalac®; Lactulose PSE®

**Therapeutic Category** Ammonium Detoxicant; Laxative, Miscellaneous

**Use** Adjunct in the prevention and treatment of portal-systemic encephalopathy (PSE); treatment of chronic constipation

**Usual Dosage** Diarrhea may indicate overdosage and responds to dose reduction

Prevention of portal systemic encephalopathy (PSE): Oral:

Older Children: Daily dose of 40-90 mL divided 3-4 times/day; if initial dose causes diarrhea, then reduce it immediately; adjust dosage to produce 2-3 stools/day

Constipation: Children: 5 g/day (7.5 mL) after breakfast

Adults:

Acute PSE:

Oral: 20-30 g (30-45 mL) every 1-2 hours to induce rapid laxation; adjust dosage daily to produce 2-3 soft stools; doses of 30-45 mL may be given hourly to cause rapid laxation, then reduce to recommended dose; usual daily dose: 60-100 g or 20-30 g (30-45 mL), 3-4 times/day

Rectal administration: 200 g (300 mL) diluted with 700 mL of $H_20$ or NS; administer rectally via rectal balloon catheter and retain 30-60 minutes every 4-6 hours

Constipation: Oral: 15-30 mL/day increased to 60 mL/day if necessary

**Mechanism of Action** The bacterial degradation of lactulose resulting in an acidic pH inhibits the diffusion of $NH_3$ into the blood by causing the conversion of $NH_3$ to $NH_4+$; also enhances the diffusion of $NH_3$ from the blood into the gut where conversion to $NH_4+$ occurs; produces an osmotic effect in the colon with resultant distention promoting peristalsis

**Local Anesthetic/Vasoconstrictor Precautions** No information available to require special precautions

**Effects on Dental Treatment** No effects or complications reported

**Other Adverse Effects**

>10%: Gastrointestinal: Flatulence, diarrhea (excessive dose)

1% to 10%: Gastrointestinal: Abdominal discomfort, nausea, vomiting

**Drug Uptake** Absorption: Oral: Not absorbed appreciably following administration; this is desirable since the intended site of action is within the colon

**Pregnancy Risk Factor** B

**Generic Available** Yes


- **Lactulose PSE®** *see* Lactulose *on this page*
- **Ladakamycin** *see* Azacitidine *on page 111*
- **Lamictal®** *see* Lamotrigine *on next page*
- **Lamisil®** *see* Terbinafine *on page 958*
- **Lamisil® Oral** *see* Terbinafine, Oral *on page 958*


## Lamivudine (la MI vyoo deen)

**Related Information**


HIV Infection and AIDS *on page 1085*

Systemic Viral Diseases *on page 1115*

Zidovudine and Lamivudine *on page 1059*


**U.S. Brand Names** Epivir®; Epivir®-HBV™

**Therapeutic Category** Antiviral Agent, Oral

**Synonyms** 3TC

**Use**

Epivir®: In combination with zidovudine (or other nucleoside) and often a protease inhibitor for treatment of HIV infection when therapy is warranted based on clinical and/or immunological evidence of disease progression; recommended with zidovudine for prophylaxis of HIV following needle sticks

Epivir®-HBV™: Treatment of chronic hepatitis B associated with evidence of hepatitis B viral replication and active liver inflammation

**Usual Dosage** Oral:

Hepatitis B virus (HBV): 100 mg once daily

HIV:

Children 3 months to 12 years: 4 mg/kg twice daily (maximum: 150 mg twice daily) with zidovudine

Adolescents 12-16 years and Adults: 150 mg twice daily with zidovudine

Adults <50 kg: 2 mg/kg twice daily with zidovudine

**Mechanism of Action** *In vitro*, lamivudine is phosphorylated to its active 5′-triphosphate metabolite (L-TP), which inhibits HIV reverse transcription via viral DNA chain termination; L-TP also inhibits the RNA- and DNA-dependent DNA polymerase activities of reverse transcriptase

(Continued)

## Lamivudine *(Continued)*

**Local Anesthetic/Vasoconstrictor Precautions** No information available to require special precautions

**Effects on Dental Treatment** No effects or complications reported

**Other Adverse Effects**

>10%:

- Central nervous system: Headache, insomnia, malaise, fatigue, pain
- Gastrointestinal: Nausea, diarrhea, vomiting
- Neuromuscular & skeletal: Peripheral neuropathy, paresthesia
- Respiratory: Nasal signs and symptoms, cough

1% to 10%:

- Central nervous system: Dizziness, depression, fever, chills
- Dermatologic: Rashes
- Gastrointestinal: Anorexia, abdominal pain, dyspepsia, elevated amylase
- Hematologic: Neutropenia, anemia
- Hepatic: Elevated AST, ALT
- Neuromuscular & skeletal: Myalgia, arthralgia

<1%:

- Gastrointestinal: Pancreatitis
- Hematologic: Thrombocytopenia
- Hepatic: Hyperbilirubinemia

**Drug Interactions** Increased effect: Zidovudine concentrations increase significantly (~39%) with coadministration with lamivudine; trimethoprim/sulfamethoxazole increases lamivudine's AUC and decreases its renal clearance by 44% and 29%, respectively; although the AUC was not significantly affected, absorption of lamivudine was slowed and $C_{max}$ was 40% lower when administered to patients in the fed versus the fasted state

**Drug Uptake**

Absorption: Oral: Rapid in HIV-infected patients

Serum half-life:

- Children: 2 hours
- Adults: 5-7 hours

**Pregnancy Risk Factor** C

**Dosage Forms**

Solution, oral:

- Epivir®: 10 mg/mL (240 mL)
- Epivir®-HBV™: 5 mg/mL (240 mL)

Tablet:

- Epivir®: 150 mg
- Epivir®-HBV™: 100 mg

**Generic Available** No

## Lamotrigine (la MOE tri jeen)

**U.S. Brand Names** Lamictal®

**Therapeutic Category** Anticonvulsant, Miscellaneous

**Use** Partial/secondary generalized seizures in adults; childhood epilepsy (not approved for use in children <16 years of age); adjunctive treatment of Lennox-Gastaut syndrome in pediatric and adult patients; conversion to monotherapy in adults with partial seizures who are receiving treatment with a single enzyme-inducing antiepileptic drug

**Usual Dosage** Oral:

Children: 2-15 mg/kg/day in 2 divided doses

Adults: Initial dose: 50-100 mg/day then titrate to daily maintenance dose of 100-400 mg/day in 1-2 divided daily doses

With concomitant valproic acid therapy: Initial dose: 25 mg/day then titrate to maintenance dose of 50-200 mg/day in 1-2 divided daily doses

**Mechanism of Action** A triazine derivative which inhibits release of glutamate (an excitatory amino acid) and inhibits voltage-sensitive sodium channels, which stabilizes neuronal membranes

**Local Anesthetic/Vasoconstrictor Precautions** No information available to require special precautions

**Effects on Dental Treatment** No effects or complications reported

**Other Adverse Effects** 1% to 10%:

- Central nervous system: Dizziness, sedation, ataxia
- Dermatologic: Hypersensitivity rash, Stevens-Johnson syndrome, angioedema
- Ocular: Nystagmus, diplopia
- Renal: Hematuria

**Drug Interactions**

Decreased effect: Acetaminophen (increases renal clearance); carbamazepine, phenobarbital, and phenytoin (increases metabolic clearance)

Increased effect: Valproic acid increases half-life of lamotrigine (decreased metabolic clearance)

**Drug Uptake** Serum half-life: 24 hours; increases to 59 hours with concomitant valproic acid therapy; decreases with concomitant phenytoin or carbamazepine therapy to 15 hours

**Pregnancy Risk Factor** C

**Generic Available** No

- **Lamprene®** *see* Clofazimine *on page 261*
- **Lanacane® [OTC]** *see* Benzocaine *on page 128*
- **Laniazid® Oral** *see* Isoniazid *on page 552*

## Lanolin, Cetyl Alcohol, Glycerin, and Petrolatum

(LAN oh lin, SEE til AL koe hol, GLIS er in, & pe troe LAY tum)

**U.S. Brand Names** Lubriderm® [OTC]

**Therapeutic Category** Topical Skin Product

**Use** Treatment of dry skin

**Usual Dosage** Topical: Apply to skin as necessary

**Local Anesthetic/Vasoconstrictor Precautions** No information available to require special precautions

**Effects on Dental Treatment** No effects or complications reported

**Other Adverse Effects** 1% to 10%: Local irritation

**Pregnancy Risk Factor** C

**Generic Available** Yes

- **Lanorinal®** *see* Butalbital Compound *on page 163*
- **Lanorinal®** *see* Butalbital Compound and Aspirin *on page 165*
- **Lanoxicaps®** *see* Digoxin *on page 329*
- **Lanoxin®** *see* Digoxin *on page 329*

## Lansoprazole (lan SOE pra zole)

**U.S. Brand Names** Prevacid®

**Therapeutic Category** Gastric Acid Secretion Inhibitor

**Use** Short-term treatment (up to 4 weeks) for healing and symptom relief of active duodenal ulcers (should not be used for maintenance therapy of duodenal ulcers); up to 8 weeks of treatment for all grades of erosive esophagitis (8 additional weeks can be given for incompletely healed esophageal erosions or for recurrence); and long-term treatment of pathological hypersecretory conditions, including Zollinger-Ellison syndrome

**Usual Dosage**

Duodenal or gastric ulcer: 30 mg once daily for 4-8 weeks

Erosive esophagitis: 30 mg once daily for 4-8 weeks

Hypersecretory conditions: 30-180 mg once daily, titrated to reduce acid secretion to <10 mEq/hour (5 mEq/hour in patients with prior gastric surgery)

**Mechanism of Action** Similar to omeprazole; a proton pump inhibitor which decreases acid secretion in gastric parietal cells

**Local Anesthetic/Vasoconstrictor Precautions** No information available to require special precautions

**Effects on Dental Treatment** No effects or complications reported

**Other Adverse Effects**

1% to 10%:

Central nervous system: Fatigue, dizziness, headache

Gastrointestinal: Abdominal pain, diarrhea, nausea, increased appetite, hypergastrinoma

<1%:

Dermatologic: Rash

Otic: Tinnitus

Renal: Proteinuria

**Drug Uptake**

Duration of effect: 1 day

Absorption: Food decreases absorption by 50%

Half-life:

Healthy patients: 1.5 hours

Elderly: 2.9 hours

Cirrhosis: 7 hours

**Pregnancy Risk Factor** B

**Dosage Forms** Capsule, delayed release: 15 mg, 30 mg

**Generic Available** No

- **Lariam®** *see* Mefloquine *on page 625*
- **Larodopa®** *see* Levodopa *on page 581*
- **Larotid®** *see* Amoxicillin *on page 76*

♦ **Lasix®** *see* Furosemide *on page 460*
♦ **L-asparaginase** *see* Asparaginase *on page 98*
♦ **Lassar's Zinc Paste** *see* Zinc Oxide *on page 1061*

## Latanoprost (la TAN oh prost)

**U.S. Brand Names** Xalatan®

**Therapeutic Category** Ophthalmic Agent, Miscellaneous

**Use** Reduction of elevated intraocular pressure in patients with open-angle glaucoma and ocular hypertension who are intolerant of the other IOP lowering medications or insufficiently responsive (failed to achieve target IOP determined after multiple measurements over time) to another IOP lowering medication

**Usual Dosage** Ophthalmic: Recommended dosage is one drop (1.5 g) in the affected eye(s) once daily in the evening. Dosage should not exceed once daily.

**Mechanism of Action** Latanoprost is a prostaglandin $F_2$-alpha analog believed to reduce intraocular pressure by increasing the outflow of the aqueous humor

**Local Anesthetic/Vasoconstrictor Precautions** No information available to require special precautions

**Effects on Dental Treatment** No effects or complications reported

**Other Adverse Effects**

>10%: Ocular: Blurred vision, burning and stinging, conjunctival hyperemia, foreign body sensation, itching, increased pigmentation of the iris, and punctate epithelial keratopathy

1% to 10%:

Cardiovascular: Chest pain, angina pectoris

Dermatologic: Rash, allergic skin reaction

Neuromuscular & skeletal: Myalgia, arthralgia, back pain

Ocular: Dry eye, excessive tearing, eye pain, lid crusting, lid edema, lid erythema, lid discomfort/pain, photophobia

Respiratory: Upper respiratory tract infection, cold, flu

<1%: Ocular: Conjunctivitis, diplopia, discharge from the eye, retinal artery embolus, retinal detachment, vitreous hemorrhage from diabetic retinopathy

**Drug Interactions** Decreased effect: *In vitro* studies have shown that precipitation occurs when eye drops containing thimerosal are mixed with latanoprost. If such drugs are used, administer with an interval of at least 5 minutes between applications

**Drug Uptake**

Onset of effect: 3-4 hours

Maximum effect: 8-12 hours

Absorption: Through the cornea where the isopropyl ester prodrug is hydrolyzed by esterases to the biologically active acid. Peak concentration is reached in 2 hours after topical administration in the aqueous humor.

Serum half-life: 17 minutes

**Pregnancy Risk Factor** C

**Dosage Forms** Solution, ophthalmic: 0.005% (2.5 mL)

**Generic Available** No

♦ **L-Carnitine** *see* Levocarnitine *on page 580*
♦ **LCD** *see* Coal Tar *on page 270*
♦ **LCR** *see* Vincristine *on page 1046*
♦ **Lederplex® [OTC]** *see* Vitamin B Complex *on page 1050*

## Leflunomide

**Related Information**

Rheumatoid Arthritis and Osteoarthritis *on page 1092*

**U.S. Brand Names** Arava™

**Therapeutic Category** Antimetabolite

**Use** Treatment of active rheumatoid arthritis to reduce signs and symptoms and to retard structural damage as evidenced by x-ray erosions and joint space narrowing

**Usual Dosage**

Adults: Oral: Initial: 100 mg/day for 3 days, followed by 20 mg/day; dosage may be decreased to 10 mg/day in patients who have difficulty tolerating the 20 mg dose. Due to the long half-life of the active metabolite, plasma levels may require a prolonged period to decline after dosage reduction.

Guidelines for dosage adjustment or discontinuation based on the severity and persistence of ALT elevation have been developed. For ALT elevations >2 times the upper limit of normal, dosage reduction to 10 mg/day may allow continued administration. Cholestyramine 8 g 3 times/day for 1-3 days may be administered to decrease plasma levels. If elevations >2 times but ≤3 times the upper limit of normal persist, liver biopsy is recommended. If elevations >3 times the upper limit of normal persist despite cholestyramine administration and dosage reduction, leflunomide should be discontinued and drug elimination should be enhanced with additional cholestyramine as indicated.

Elderly: Although hepatic function may decline with age, no specific dosage adjustment is recommended. Patients should be monitored closely for adverse effects which may require dosage adjustment.

**Mechanism of Action** Inhibits pyrimidine synthesis, resulting in antiproliferative and anti-inflammatory effects

**Local Anesthetic/Vasoconstrictor Precautions** No information available to require special precautions

**Effects on Dental Treatment** 1% to 10% of patients may experience stomatitis (3%), gingivitis, candidiasis (oral), enlarged salivary gland, tooth disorder, dry mouth, and taste disturbance

**Other Adverse Effects**

>10%:

Gastrointestinal: Diarrhea (17%)

Respiratory: Respiratory tract infection (15%)

1% to 10%:

Cardiovascular: Hypertension (10%), chest pain (2%), palpitation, tachycardia, vasculitis, vasodilation, varicose vein, edema (peripheral)

Central nervous system: Headache (7%), dizziness (4%), pain (2%), fever, malaise, migraine, anxiety, depression, insomnia, sleep disorder

Dermatologic: Alopecia (10%), rash (10%), pruritus (4%), dry skin (2%), eczema (2%), acne, dermatitis, hair discoloration, hematoma, herpes infection, nail disorder, subcutaneous nodule, skin disorder/discoloration, skin ulcer, bruising

Endocrine & metabolic: Hypokalemia (1%), diabetes mellitus, hyperglycemia, hyperlipidemia, hyperthyroidism, menstrual disorder

Gastrointestinal: Nausea (9%), abdominal pain (5%), dyspepsia (5%), weight loss (4%), anorexia (3%), gastroenteritis (3%), vomiting (3%), cholelithiasis, colitis, constipation, esophagitis, flatulence, gastritis, melena

Genitourinary: Urinary tract infection (5%), albuminuria, cystitis, dysuria, hematuria, vaginal candidiasis, prostate disorder, urinary frequency

Hematologic: Anemia

Hepatic: Abnormal liver function tests (5%)

Neuromuscular & skeletal: Back pain (5%), joint disorder (4%), weakness (3%), tenosynovitis (3%), synovitis (2%), arthralgia (1%), paresthesia (2%), muscle cramps (1%), neck pain, pelvic pain, increased CPK, arthrosis, bursitis, myalgia, bone necrosis, bone pain, tendon rupture, neuralgia, neuritis

Ocular: Blurred vision, cataract, conjunctivitis, eye disorder

Respiratory: Bronchitis (7%), cough (3%), pharyngitis (3%), pneumonia (2%), rhinitis (2%), sinusitis (2%), asthma, dyspnea, epistaxis, lung disorder

Miscellaneous: Infection (4%), accidental injury (5%), allergic reactions (2%), diaphoresis

<1%: Anaphylaxis, urticaria, eosinophilia, thrombocytopenia, leukopenia

**Drug Interactions** Cytochrome P-450 2C9 enzyme inhibitor

Increased effect: Theoretically, the concomitant use of drugs metabolized by this enzyme, which includes many NSAIDs, may result in increased serum concentrations and possible toxic effects. Coadministration with methotrexate increases the risk of hepatotoxicity. Leflunomide may also enhance the hepatotoxicity of other drugs. Tolbutamide free fraction may be increased. Rifampin may increase the serum concentrations of leflunomide. Leflunomide has uricosuric activity and may enhance activity of other uricosuric agents.

Decreased effect: Administration of cholestyramine and activated charcoal enhance the elimination of leflunomide's active metabolite

**Drug Uptake**

Serum half-life: Mean 14-15 days; enterohepatic recycling appears to contribute to the long half-life of this agent, since activated charcoal and cholestyramine substantially reduce plasma half-life

Time to peak: 6-12 hours

**Pregnancy Risk Factor** X

- **Legatrin® [OTC]** *see* Quinine *on page 874*
- **Lente® Iletin® I** *see* Insulin Preparations *on page 537*
- **Lente® Iletin® II** *see* Insulin Preparations *on page 537*
- **Lente® Insulin** *see* Insulin Preparations *on page 537*
- **Lente® L** *see* Insulin Preparations *on page 537*

## Lepirudin (leh puh ROO din)

**Related Information**

Cardiovascular Diseases *on page 1066*

**U.S. Brand Names** Refludan®

**Therapeutic Category** Anticoagulant (Other)

(Continued)

## Lepirudin *(Continued)*

**Synonyms** Lepirudin (rDNA); Recombinant Hirudin

**Use** Indicated for anticoagulation in patient with heparin-induced thrombocytopenia (HIT) and associated thromboembolic disease in order to prevent further thromboembolic complications

Investigational: Prevention or reduction of ischemic complications associated with unstable angina

**Usual Dosage** Maximum dose: Do not exceed 0.21 mg/kg/hour unless an evaluation of coagulation abnormalities limiting response has been completed. Dosing is weight-based, however, patients weighing >110 kg should not receive doses greater than the recommended dose for a patient weighing 110 kg (44 mg bolus and initial maximal infusion rate of 16.5 mg/hour).

Patients with heparin-induced thrombocytopenia: Bolus dose: 0.4 mg/kg IVP (over 15-20 seconds), followed by continuous infusion at 0.15 mg/kg/hour; bolus and infusion must be reduced in renal insufficiency

Concomitant use with thrombolytic therapy: Bolus dose: 0.2 mg/kg IVP (over 15-20 seconds), followed by continuous infusion at 0.1 mg/kg/hour

Dosing adjustments during infusions: Monitor first APTT 4 hours after the start of the infusion. Subsequent determinations of APTT should be obtained at least once daily during treatment. More frequent monitoring is recommended in renally impaired patients. Any APTT ratio measurement out of range (1.5-2.5) should be confirmed prior to adjusting dose, unless a clinical need for immediate reaction exists. If the APTT is below target range, increase infusion by 20%. If the APTT is in excess of the target range, decrease infusion rate by 50%. A repeat APTT should be obtained 4 hours after any dosing change.

Use in patients scheduled for switch to oral anticoagulants: Reduce lepirudin dose gradually to reach APTT ratio just above 1.5 before starting warfarin therapy; as soon as INR reaches 2.0, lepirudin therapy should be discontinued

**Mechanism of Action** Lepirudin is a highly specific direct thrombin inhibitor. Each molecule is capable of binding one molecule of thrombin and inhibiting its thrombogenic activity.

**Local Anesthetic/Vasoconstrictor Precautions** No information available to require special precautions

**Effects on Dental Treatment** Mouth bleeding, tongue edema has been reported

**Other Adverse Effects**

**HIT patients:**

>10%: Hematologic: Anemia (12.4%), bleeding from puncture sites (10.6%), hematoma 10.8%

1% to 10%:

Gastrointestinal: GI bleeding/rectal bleeding (5.3%)
Genitourinary: Vaginal bleeding (1.8%)
Renal: Hematuria (4.4%)
Respiratory: Epistaxis (4.4%)

<1%:

Gastrointestinal: Hemoptysis, mouth bleeding
Hepatic: Liver bleeding
Respiratory: Pulmonary bleeding
Miscellaneous: Hemoperitoneum, retroperitoneal bleeding

**Non-HIT populations** (including those receiving thrombolytics and/or contrast media):

1% to 10%: Respiratory: Bronchospasm/stridor/dyspnea/cough

<1%:

Dermatologic: Edema, angioedema, laryngeal edema, tongue edema
Hematologic: Intracranial bleeding (0.6%)
Miscellaneous: Allergic reactions (unspecified), skin reactions, anaphylactoid reactions, anaphylaxis

**Drug Interactions** Thrombolytics may enhance anticoagulant properties of lepirudin on APTT and can increase the risk of bleeding complications. Bleeding risk may also be increased by oral anticoagulants (Coumadin®) and platelet function inhibitors (nonsteroidal anti-inflammatory drugs, dipyridamole, ticlopidine, clopidogrel, IIb/IIIa antagonists, and aspirin).

**Drug Uptake** Serum half-life: Variable, 1.3 hours in healthy volunteers; up to 2 days in marked renal insufficiency ($Cl_{cr}$ <15 mL/minute)

**Pregnancy Risk Factor** B

**Dosage Forms** Injection: 50 mg

♦ **Lepirudin (rDNA)** *see* Lepirudin *on previous page*

♦ **Lescol®** *see* Fluvastatin *on page 451*

## Letrozole (LET roe zole)

**U.S. Brand Names** Femara™

**Therapeutic Category** Antineoplastic Agent, Hormone (Antiestrogen)

**Use** Treatment of advanced breast cancer in postmenopausal women with disease progression following tamoxifen therapy. Patients with ER-negative disease and patients who did not respond to tamoxifen therapy rarely responded to anastrozole.

**Usual Dosage** Adults: Oral: 2.5 mg once/day, without regard to meals

**Mechanism of Action** Letrozole inhibits the aromatase enzyme responsible for conversion of androstenedione to estrone and testosterone to estradiol; resulting in reduction of plasma estrogen levels

**Local Anesthetic/Vasoconstrictor Precautions** No information available to require special precautions

**Effects on Dental Treatment** No effects or complications reported

**Drug Uptake**

Absorption: Nearly 100%

Half-life: Terminal: 2 days

**Dosage Forms** Tablet: 2.5 mg

## Leucovorin (loo koe VOR in)

**U.S. Brand Names** Wellcovorin®

**Therapeutic Category** Antidote, Methotrexate; Folic Acid Derivative

**Synonyms** Calcium Leucovorin; Citrovorum Factor; Folinic Acid; 5-Formyl Tetrahydrofolate; Leucovorin Calcium

**Use** Antidote for folic acid antagonists; treatment of folate deficient megaloblastic anemias of infancy, sprue, pregnancy; nutritional deficiency when oral folate therapy is not possible

**Usual Dosage** Children and Adults:

Treatment of folic acid antagonist overdosage (eg, pyrimethamine or trimethoprim): Oral: 2-15 mg/day for 3 days or until blood counts are normal or 5 mg every 3 days; doses of 6 mg/day are needed for patients with platelet counts <100,000/mm³

Folate-deficient megaloblastic anemia: I.M.: 1 mg/day

Megaloblastic anemia secondary to congenital deficiency of dihydrofolate reductase: I.M.: 3-6 mg/day

Rescue dose (rescue therapy should start within 24 hours of MTX therapy): I.V.: 10 mg/m² to start, then 10 mg/m² every 6 hours orally for 72 hours until serum MTX concentration is $<10^{-8}$ molar; if serum creatinine 24 hours after methotrexate is elevated 50% or more above the pre-MTX serum creatinine **or** the serum MTX concentration is $>5 \times 10^{-6}$ molar (see graph), increase dose to 100 mg/m²/dose every 3 hours until serum methotrexate level is $<1 \times 10^{-8}$ molar

Investigational: Post I.T. methotrexate: Oral, I.V.: 12 mg/m² as a single dose; post high-dose methotrexate: 100-1000 mg/m²/dose until the serum methotrexate level is less than $1 \times 10^{-7}$ molar

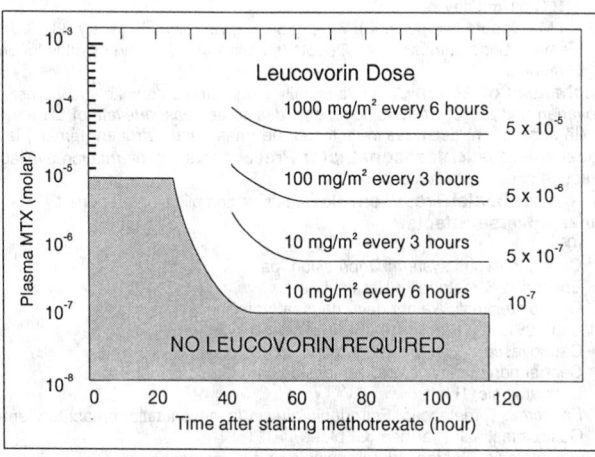

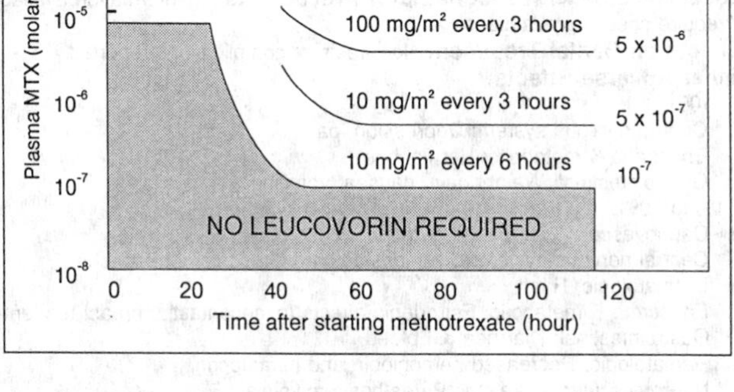


(Continued)

## Leucovorin *(Continued)*

**The drug should be given parenterally instead of orally in patients with GI toxicity, nausea, vomiting, and when individual doses are >25 mg**

**Mechanism of Action** A reduced form of folic acid, but does not require a reduction reaction by an enzyme for activation, allows for purine and thymidine synthesis, a necessity for normal erythropoiesis; leucovorin supplies the necessary cofactor blocked by MTX, enters the cells via the same active transport system as MTX

**Local Anesthetic/Vasoconstrictor Precautions** No information available to require special precautions

**Effects on Dental Treatment** No effects or complications reported

**Other Adverse Effects** <1%:
- Dermatologic: Rash, pruritus, erythema, urticaria
- Hematologic: Thrombocytosis
- Respiratory: Wheezing

**Drug Uptake**
- Onset of activity:
  - Oral: Within 30 minutes
  - I.V.: Within 5 minutes
- Absorption: Oral, I.M.: Rapid
- Serum half-life:
  - Leucovorin: 15 minutes
  - 5MTHF: 33-35 minutes

**Pregnancy Risk Factor** C

**Generic Available** Yes

**Comments** Drug should be given parenterally instead of orally in patients with GI toxicity, nausea, vomiting, and when individual doses are >25 mg

- ♦ **Leucovorin Calcium** *see* Leucovorin *on previous page*
- ♦ **Leukeran®** *see* Chlorambucil *on page 221*
- ♦ **Leukine™** *see* Sargramostim *on page 904*

## Leuprolide Acetate (loo PROE lide AS e tate)

**U.S. Brand Names** Lupron®; Lupron® Depot; Lupron® Depot-Ped

**Therapeutic Category** Antineoplastic Agent, Hormone (Gonadotropin Hormone-Releasing Antigen); Gonadotropin Releasing Hormone Analog

**Synonyms** Leuprorelin Acetate

**Use** Treatment of precocious puberty; palliative treatment of advanced prostate carcinoma

**Usual Dosage** Requires parenteral administration
- Children: Precocious puberty:
  - S.C.: 20-45 mcg/kg/day
  - I.M. (Depot®) formulation: 0.3 mg/kg/dose given every 28 days
    - ≤25 kg: 7.5 mg
    - >25-37.5 kg: 11.25 mg
    - >37.5 kg: 15 mg
- Adults:
  - Male: Advanced prostatic carcinoma:
    - S.C.: 1 mg/day **or**
    - I.M., Depot® (suspension): 7.5 mg/dose given monthly (every 28-33 days)
  - Female: Endometriosis: I.M., Depot® (suspension): 3.75 mg monthly for up to 6 months

**Mechanism of Action** Continuous daily administration results in suppression of ovarian and testicular steroidogenesis due to decreased levels of LH and FSH with subsequent decrease in testosterone (male) and estrogen (female) levels

**Local Anesthetic/Vasoconstrictor Precautions** No information available to require special precautions

**Effects on Dental Treatment** No effects or complications reported

**Other Adverse Effects**
- >10%:
  - Central nervous system: Depression, pain
  - Endocrine & metabolic: Hot flashes
  - Gastrointestinal: Weight gain, nausea, vomiting
- 1% to 10%:
  - Cardiovascular: Cardiac arrhythmias, edema
  - Central nervous system: Dizziness, lethargy, insomnia, headache
  - Dermatologic: Rash
  - Endocrine & metabolic: Estrogenic effects (gynecomastia, breast tenderness)
  - Gastrointestinal: Diarrhea, GI bleed
  - Hematologic: Decreased hemoglobin and hematocrit
  - Neuromuscular & skeletal: Paresthesia, myalgia

Ocular: Blurred vision
<1%:
Cardiovascular: Myocardial infarction
Local: Thrombophlebitis
Respiratory: Pulmonary embolism

**Drug Uptake**
Onset of action: Serum testosterone levels first increase within 3 days of therapy
Duration: Levels decrease after 2-4 weeks with continued therapy
Serum half-life: 3-4.25 hours

**Pregnancy Risk Factor** X

**Generic Available** No

**Comments** Has the advantage of not increasing risk of atherosclerotic vascular disease, causing swelling of breasts, fluid retention, and thromboembolism as compared to estrogen therapy

- **Leuprorelin Acetate** *see* Leuprolide Acetate *on previous page*
- **Leurocristine** *see* Vincristine *on page 1046*
- **Leustatín™** *see* Cladribine *on page 255*

## Levamisole (lee VAM i sole)

**U.S. Brand Names** Ergamisol®

**Therapeutic Category** Immune Modulator

**Use** Adjuvant treatment with fluorouracil in Dukes stage C colon cancer

**Usual Dosage** Adults: Oral: Initial: 50 mg every 8 hours for 3 days, then 50 mg every 8 hours for 3 days every 2 weeks (fluorouracil is always given concomitantly)

**Mechanism of Action** Clinically, combined therapy with levamisole and 5-fluorouracil has been effective in treating colon cancer patients, whereas demonstrable activity has been. Due to the broad range of pharmacologic activities of levamisole, it has been suggested that the drug may act as a biochemical modulator (of fluorouracil, for example, in colon cancer), an effect entirely independent of immune modulation. Further studies are needed to evaluate the mechanisms of action of the drug in cancer patients.

**Local Anesthetic/Vasoconstrictor Precautions** No information available to require special precautions

**Effects on Dental Treatment** No effects or complications reported

**Other Adverse Effects**
>10%: Gastrointestinal: Nausea, diarrhea
1% to 10%:
Cardiovascular: Edema
Central nervous system: Fatigue, fever, dizziness, headache, somnolence, depression, nervousness, insomnia
Dermatologic: Dermatitis, alopecia
Gastrointestinal: Stomatitis, vomiting, anorexia, abdominal pain, constipation, taste perversion
Hematologic: Leukopenia
Neuromuscular & skeletal: Rigors, arthralgia, myalgia, paresthesia
Miscellaneous: Infection
<1%:
Cardiovascular: Chest pain
Central nervous system: Anxiety
Dermatologic: Pruritus, urticaria
Gastrointestinal: Flatulence, dyspepsia
Hematologic: Thrombocytopenia, anemia, granulocytopenia
Ocular: Abnormal tearing, blurred vision, conjunctivitis
Respiratory: Epistaxis
Miscellaneous: Altered sense of smell

**Drug Uptake**
Absorption: Well absorbed
Half-life, elimination: 2-6 hours
Time to peak serum concentration: 1-2 hours

**Pregnancy Risk Factor** C

**Generic Available** No

**Comments** Should not be used at dose exceeding the recommended dose or frequency due to increasing adverse reactions

- **Levaquin™** *see* Levofloxacin *on page 583*
- **Levarterenol Bitartrate** *see* Norepinephrine *on page 729*
- **Levatol®** *see* Penbutolol *on page 771*
- **Levbid®** *see* Hyoscyamine *on page 519*
- **Levlen®** *see* Ethinyl Estradiol and Levonorgestrel *on page 402*
- **Levlite®** *see* Ethinyl Estradiol and Levonorgestrel *on page 402*

## Levobunolol (lee voe BYOO noe lole)

**U.S. Brand Names** AKBeta®; Betagan®

**Therapeutic Category** Antiglaucoma Agent; Beta-Adrenergic Blocker, Ophthalmic

**Use** To lower intraocular pressure in chronic open-angle glaucoma or ocular hypertension

**Usual Dosage** Adults: Instill 1 drop in the affected eye(s) 1-2 times/day

**Mechanism of Action** A nonselective beta-adrenergic blocking agent that lowers intraocular pressure by reducing aqueous humor production and possibly increases the outflow of aqueous humor

**Local Anesthetic/Vasoconstrictor Precautions** No information available to require special precautions

**Effects on Dental Treatment** No effects or complications reported

**Other Adverse Effects**

>10%: Ocular: Stinging/burning of eye

1% to 10%:

- Cardiovascular: Bradycardia, arrhythmia, hypotension
- Central nervous system: Dizziness, headache
- Dermatologic: Alopecia, erythema
- Local: Stinging, burning
- Ocular: Blepharoconjunctivitis, conjunctivitis
- Respiratory: Bronchospasm

<1%:

- Dermatologic: Skin rash
- Local: Itching
- Ocular: Visual disturbances, keratitis, decreased visual acuity

**Drug Interactions** Increased toxicity:

- Systemic beta-adrenergic blocking agents
- Ophthalmic epinephrine (increased blood pressure/loss of IOP effect)
- Quinidine (sinus bradycardia)
- Verapamil (bradycardia and asystole have been reported)

**Drug Uptake**

- Onset of action: Decreases in intraocular pressure (IOP) can be noted within 1 hour
- Peak effect: 2-6 hours
- Duration: 1-7 days

**Pregnancy Risk Factor** C

**Generic Available** Yes

## Levocabastine (LEE voe kab as teen)

**U.S. Brand Names** Livostin®

**Therapeutic Category** Ophthalmic Agent, Miscellaneous

**Use** Treatment of allergic conjunctivitis

**Usual Dosage** Children >12 years and Adults: Instill 1 drop in affected eye(s) 4 times/day for up to 2 weeks

**Mechanism of Action** Potent, selective histamine $H_1$-receptor antagonist for topical ophthalmic use

**Local Anesthetic/Vasoconstrictor Precautions** No information available to require special precautions

**Effects on Dental Treatment** No effects or complications reported

**Other Adverse Effects**

>10%: Local: Transient burning, stinging, discomfort

1% to 10%:

- Central nervous system: Headache, somnolence, fatigue
- Dermatologic: Rash
- Gastrointestinal: Dry mouth
- Ocular: Blurred vision, eye pain, red eyes, eyelid edema
- Respiratory: Dyspnea

**Drug Interactions** No data reported

**Drug Uptake** Absorption: Topical: Systemically absorbed

**Pregnancy Risk Factor** B

**Dosage Forms** Suspension, ophthalmic, as hydrochloride: 0.05% (2.5 mL, 5 mL, 10 mL)

**Generic Available** No

## Levocarnitine (lee voe KAR ni teen)

**U.S. Brand Names** Carnitor® Injection; Carnitor® Oral; VitaCarn® Oral

**Therapeutic Category** Dietary Supplement

**Synonyms** L-Carnitine

**Use** Treatment of primary or secondary carnitine deficiency

**Usual Dosage**
Oral:
Children: 50-100 mg/kg/day divided 2-3 times/day, maximum: 3 g/day; dosage must be individualized based upon patient response; higher dosages have been used
Adults: 1-3 g/day for 50 kg subject; start at 1 g/day, increase slowly assessing tolerance and response
I.V.: Children and Adults: 50 mg/kg as a loading dose, followed (in severe cases) by 50 mg/kg/day infusion; maintenance: 50 mg/kg/day given every 4-6 hours, increase as needed to a maximum of 300 mg/kg/day

**Local Anesthetic/Vasoconstrictor Precautions** No information available to require special precautions

**Effects on Dental Treatment** No effects or complications reported

**Pregnancy Risk Factor** B

**Generic Available** Yes

**Comments** Tolerance may be improved by mixing the product with liquids or food and spacing doses evenly throughout the day with meals

## Levodopa (lee voe DOE pa)

**U.S. Brand Names** Dopar®; Larodopa®

**Therapeutic Category** Anti-Parkinson's Agent

**Use** Treatment of Parkinson's disease; used as a diagnostic agent for growth hormone deficiency

**Usual Dosage** Oral:
Children (give as a single dose to evaluate growth hormone deficiency):
$0.5\ g/m^2$ **or**
<30 lb: 125 mg
30-70 lb: 250 mg
>70 lb: 500 mg
Adults: 500-1000 mg/day in divided doses every 6-12 hours; increase by 100-750 mg/day every 3-7 days until response or total dose of 8,000 mg is reached
A significant therapeutic response may not be obtained for 6 months

**Mechanism of Action** Increases dopamine levels in the brain, then stimulates dopaminergic receptors in the basal ganglia to improve the balance between cholinergic and dopaminergic activity

**Local Anesthetic/Vasoconstrictor Precautions** No information available to require special precautions

**Effects on Dental Treatment** Dopaminergic therapy in Parkinson's disease (ie, treatment with levodopa) is associated with orthostatic hypotension. Patients medicated with levodopa should be carefully assisted from the chair and observed for signs of orthostatic hypotension.

**Other Adverse Effects**
>10%:
Cardiovascular: Orthostatic hypotension, arrhythmias
Central nervous system: Dizziness, anxiety, confusion, nightmares
Gastrointestinal: Anorexia, nausea, vomiting, constipation
Genitourinary: Dysuria
Neuromuscular & skeletal: Choreiform and involuntary movements
Ocular: Blepharospasm
1% to 10%:
Central nervous system: Headache
Gastrointestinal: Diarrhea, dry mouth
Genitourinary: Discoloration of urine
Neuromuscular & skeletal: Muscle twitching
Ocular: Eyelid spasms
Miscellaneous: Discoloration of sweat
<1%:
Cardiovascular: Hypertension
Gastrointestinal: Duodenal ulcer, GI bleeding
Hematologic: Hemolytic anemia
Ocular: Blurred vision

**Drug Interactions**
Decreased effect:
Hydantoins cause decreased effectiveness of levodopa
Phenothiazines and hypotensive agents cause decreased effect of levodopa
Pyridoxine causes increased peripheral conversion, causing decreased levodopa effectiveness
Increased toxicity:
Monoamine oxidase inhibitors may increase hypertensive reactions
Antacids cause increased levodopa

**Drug Uptake**
Time to peak serum concentration: Oral: 1-2 hours
(Continued)

## Levodopa *(Continued)*

Serum half-life: 1.2-2.3 hours

**Pregnancy Risk Factor** C

**Generic Available** No

## Levodopa and Carbidopa (lee voe DOE pa & kar bi DOE pa)

**U.S. Brand Names** Sinemet®

**Therapeutic Category** Anti-Parkinson's Agent

**Use** Treatment of parkinsonian syndrome; 50-100 mg/day of carbidopa is needed to block the peripheral conversion of levodopa to dopamine. "On-off" can be managed by giving smaller, more frequent doses of Sinemet® or adding a dopamine agonist or selegiline; when adding a new agent, doses of Sinemet® should usually be decreased.

**Usual Dosage** Oral:

Adults: Initial: 25/100 2-4 times/day, increase as necessary to a maximum of 200/2000 mg/day

Elderly: Initial: 25/100 twice daily, increase as necessary

**Conversion from Sinemet® to Sinemet® CR (50/200):** (Sinemet® [total daily dose of levodopa] / Sinemet® CR)

300-400 mg / 1 tablet twice daily

500-600 mg / 1½ tablets twice daily or one 3 times/day

700-800 mg / 4 tablets in 3 or more divided doses

900-1000 mg / 5 tablets in 3 or more divided doses

Intervals between doses of Sinemet® CR should be 4-8 hours while awake

**Mechanism of Action** Parkinson's symptoms are due to a lack of striatal dopamine; levodopa circulates in the plasma to the blood-brain-barrier (BBB), where it crosses, to be converted by striatal enzymes to dopamine; carbidopa inhibits the peripheral plasma breakdown of levodopa by inhibiting its decarboxylation, and thereby increases available levodopa at the BBB

**Local Anesthetic/Vasoconstrictor Precautions** No information available to require special precautions

**Effects on Dental Treatment** Dopaminergic therapy in Parkinson disease (ie, treatment with levodopa and carbidopa combination) is associated with orthostatic hypotension. Patients medicated with this drug combination should be carefully assisted from the chair and observed for signs of orthostatic hypotension.

**Other Adverse Effects**

>10%:

Cardiovascular: Orthostatic hypotension, palpitations, cardiac arrhythmias

Central nervous system: Confusion, nightmares, dizziness, anxiety

Gastrointestinal: Nausea, vomiting, anorexia, constipation

Genitourinary: Dysuria

Neuromuscular & skeletal: Dystonic movements, "on-off", choreiform and involuntary movements

Ocular: Blepharospasm

1% to 10%:

Central nervous system: Headache

Gastrointestinal: Diarrhea, dry mouth

Genitourinary: Discoloration of urine

Neuromuscular & skeletal: Muscle twitching

Ocular: Eyelid spasms

Miscellaneous: Discoloration of sweat

<1%:

Cardiovascular: Hypertension

Central nervous system: Memory loss, nervousness, insomnia, fatigue, hallucinations, ataxia

Gastrointestinal: Duodenal ulcer, GI bleeding

Hematologic: Hemolytic anemia

Ocular: Blurred vision

**Drug Interactions**

Decreased effect:

Hydantoins cause decreased effectiveness

Phenothiazines and hypotensive agents cause decreased effect of levodopa

Increased toxicity: Monoamine oxidase inhibitors may increase hypertensive reactions

**Drug Uptake**

Carbidopa:

Absorption: Oral: 40% to 70%

Serum half-life: 1-2 hours

Levodopa:

Absorption: May be decreased if given with a high protein meal

Serum half-life: 1.2-2.3 hours

**Pregnancy Risk Factor** C

**Generic Available** Yes

♦ **Levo-Dromoran®** *see* Levorphanol *on page 585*

## Levofloxacin (lee voe FLOKS a sin)

**U.S. Brand Names** Levaquin™

**Therapeutic Category** Antibiotic, Quinolone

**Use** Treatment of bacterial respiratory tract infections; uncomplicated urinary tract infection (UTI)

**Usual Dosage** Adults: Oral, I.V. (infuse I.V. solution over 60 minutes):

Acute bacterial exacerbation of chronic bronchitis: 500 mg every 24 hours for at least 7 days

Community acquired pneumonia: 500 mg every 24 hours for 7-14 days

Acute maxillary sinusitis: 500 mg every 24 hours for 10-14 days

Uncomplicated skin infections: 500 mg every 24 hours for 7-10 days

Complicated urinary tract infections include acute pyelonephritis: 250 mg every 24 hours for 10 days

**Mechanism of Action** As the S (-) enantiomer of the fluoroquinolone, ofloxacin, levofloxacin, inhibits DNA-gyrase in susceptible organisms; inhibits relaxation of supercoiled DNA and promotes breakage of double-stranded DNA

**Local Anesthetic/Vasoconstrictor Precautions** No information available to require special precautions

**Effects on Dental Treatment** No effects or complications reported

**Other Adverse Effects**

>1%:

Central nervous system: Dizziness, headache, insomnia

Dermatologic: Rash

Gastrointestinal: Nausea, vomiting, increased transaminases

Hematologic: Leukopenia, thrombocytopenia

Neuromuscular & skeletal: Tremor, arthralgia

**Warnings/Precautions** Not recommended in children <18 years of age; other quinolones have caused transient arthropathy in children; CNS stimulation may occur (tremor, restlessness, confusion, and very rarely hallucinations or seizures); use with caution in patients with known or suspected CNS disorders or renal dysfunction; prolonged use may result in superinfection; if an allergic reaction (itching, urticaria, dyspnea, pharyngeal or facial edema, loss of consciousness, tingling, cardiovascular collapse) occurs, discontinue the drug immediately; use caution to avoid possible photosensitivity reactions during and for several days following fluoroquinolone therapy; pseudomembranous colitis may occur and should be considered in patients who present with diarrhea

**Drug Interactions**

Decreased effect: Decreased absorption with antacids containing aluminum, magnesium, and/or calcium (by up to 98% if given at the same time); phenytoin serum levels may be reduced by quinolones; antineoplastic agents may also decrease serum levels of fluoroquinolones

Increased toxicity/serum levels: Quinolones cause increased levels of caffeine, warfarin, azlocillin, cyclosporine, and theophylline (one study indicates no effect on theophylline metabolism); azlocillin, cimetidine, and probenecid increases quinolone levels; an increased incidence of seizures may occur with foscarnet

**Drug Uptake**

Absorption: Well absorbed

Serum half-life: 6 hours

Time to peak serum concentration: 1 hour

**Pregnancy Risk Factor** C

**Generic Available** No

♦ **Levomepromazine** *see* Methotrimeprazine *on page 654*

## Levomethadyl Acetate Hydrochloride

(lee voe METH a dil AS e tate hye droe KLOR ide)

**U.S. Brand Names** ORLAAM®

**Therapeutic Category** Analgesic, Narcotic

**Use** Management of opiate dependence

**Usual Dosage** Adults: Oral: 20-40 mg 3 times/week, with ranges of 10 mg to as high as 140 mg 3 times/week; always dilute before administration and mix with diluent prior to dispensing

**Local Anesthetic/Vasoconstrictor Precautions** No information available to require special precautions

**Effects on Dental Treatment** No effects or complications reported

(Continued)

## Levomethadyl Acetate Hydrochloride *(Continued)*

**Other Adverse Effects**

>10%:

Cardiovascular: Bradycardia, hypotension

Central nervous system: Drowsiness

Gastrointestinal: Nausea, vomiting

Respiratory: Respiratory depression

1% to 10%:

Cardiovascular: Peripheral vasodilation, orthostatic hypotension

Central nervous system: Dizziness/vertigo, CNS depression, confusion, sedation, increased intracranial pressure

Endocrine & metabolic: Antidiuretic hormone release

Gastrointestinal: Constipation, biliary spasm

Genitourinary: Urinary tract spasm

Ocular: Miosis, blurred vision

**Drug Interactions** Decreased effect/levels with phenobarbital

**Pregnancy Risk Factor** C

**Dosage Forms** Solution, oral: 10 mg/mL (474 mL)

**Generic Available** No

## Levonorgestrel (LEE voe nor jes trel)

**Related Information**

Endocrine Disorders & Pregnancy *on page 1082*

**U.S. Brand Names** Norplant® Implant

**Therapeutic Category** Contraceptive, Implant (Progestin); Contraceptive, Progestin Only; Progestin

**Use** Prevention of pregnancy. The net cumulative 5 year pregnancy rate for levonorgestrel implant use has been reported to be from 1.5-3.9 pregnancies/100 users. Norplant® is a very efficient, yet reversible, method of contraception. The long duration of action may be particularly advantageous in women who desire an extended period of contraceptive protection without sacrificing the possibility of future fertility.

**Usual Dosage** Total administration doses (implanted): 216 mg in 6 capsules which should be implanted during the first 7 days of onset of menses subdermally in the upper arm; each Norplant® silastic capsule releases 80 mcg of drug/day for 6-18 months, following which a rate of release of 25-30 mcg/day is maintained for ≤5 years; capsules should be removed by end of 5th year

**Mechanism of Action** Ovulation is inhibited in about 50% to 60% of implant users from a negative feedback mechanism on the hypothalamus, leading to reduced secretion of follicle stimulating hormone (FSH) and luteinizing hormone (LH). An insufficient luteal phase has also been demonstrated with levonorgestrel administration and may result from defective gonadotropin stimulation of the ovary or from a direct effect of the drug on progesterone synthesis by the corpora lutea.

**Local Anesthetic/Vasoconstrictor Precautions** No information available to require special precautions

**Effects on Dental Treatment** Progestins may predispose the patient to gingival bleeding

**Other Adverse Effects**

>10%: Endocrine & metabolic: Prolonged menstrual flow, spotting

1% to 10%:

Central nervous system: Headache, nervousness, dizziness

Dermatologic: Dermatitis, acne

Endocrine & metabolic: Amenorrhea, irregular menstrual cycles, scanty bleeding, breast discharge

Gastrointestinal: Nausea, change in appetite, weight gain

Genitourinary: Vaginitis, leukorrhea

Local: Pain or itching at implant site

Neuromuscular & skeletal: Myalgia

<1%: Miscellaneous: Infection at implant site

**Drug Interactions** Decreased effect: Carbamazepine/phenytoin

**Drug Uptake** Serum half-life, terminal: 11-45 hours

**Pregnancy Risk Factor** X

**Generic Available** No


- **Levophed® Injection** *see* Norepinephrine *on page 729*
- **Levoprome®** *see* Methotrimeprazine *on page 654*
- **Levora®** *see* Ethinyl Estradiol and Levonorgestrel *on page 402*

## Levorphanol (lee VOR fa nole)

**Related Information**

Narcotic Agonists *on page 1223*

**U.S. Brand Names** Levo-Dromoran®

**Therapeutic Category** Analgesic, Narcotic

**Use** Relief of moderate to severe pain; also used parenterally for preoperative sedation and an adjunct to nitrous oxide/oxygen anesthesia; 2 mg levorphanol produces analgesia comparable to that produced by 10 mg of morphine

**Usual Dosage** Adults:

Oral: 2 mg every 6-24 hours as needed

S.C.: 2 mg, up to 3 mg if necessary, every 6-8 hours

**Mechanism of Action** Levorphanol tartrate is a synthetic opioid agonist that is classified as a morphinan derivative. Opioids interact with stereospecific opioid receptors in various parts of the central nervous system and other tissues. Analgesic potency parallels the affinity for these binding sites. These drugs do not alter the threshold or responsiveness to pain, but the perception of pain.

**Local Anesthetic/Vasoconstrictor Precautions** No information available to require special precautions

**Effects on Dental Treatment** ~10% of patients experience dry mouth (will disappear with cessation of therapy)

**Other Adverse Effects**

>10%:

- Cardiovascular: Palpitations, hypotension, bradycardia, peripheral vasodilation
- Central nervous system: CNS depression, fatigue, drowsiness, dizziness
- Dermatologic: Pruritus
- Gastrointestinal: Nausea, vomiting
- Neuromuscular & skeletal: Weakness

1% to 10%:

- Central nervous system: Nervousness, headache, restlessness, anorexia, malaise, confusion
- Endocrine & metabolic: Antidiuretic hormone release
- Gastrointestinal: Stomach cramps, constipation, biliary spasm
- Genitourinary: Decreased urination, urinary tract spasm
- Local: Pain at injection site
- Ocular: Miosis
- Respiratory: Respiratory depression

<1%:

- Central nervous system: Mental depression, hallucinations, paradoxical CNS stimulation, increased intracranial pressure
- Dermatologic: Skin rash, urticaria
- Gastrointestinal: Paralytic ileus
- Miscellaneous: Physical and psychological dependence, histamine release

**Drug Interactions** Increased toxicity: CNS depressants increased CNS depression

**Pregnancy Risk Factor** B (D if used for prolonged periods or in high doses at term)

**Generic Available** No

♦ **Levo-T™** *see* Levothyroxine *on this page*

♦ **Levothroid®** *see* Levothyroxine *on this page*

## Levothyroxine (lee voe thye ROKS een)

**Related Information**

Endocrine Disorders & Pregnancy *on page 1082*

**U.S. Brand Names** Eltroxin™; Levo-T™; Levothroid®; Levoxyl®; Synthroid®

**Canadian Brand Names** Eltroxin®; PMS-Levothyroxine Sodium

**Therapeutic Category** Thyroid Product

**Use** Replacement or supplemental therapy in hypothyroidism; some clinicians suggest levothyroxine is the drug of choice for replacement therapy

**Usual Dosage**

Children:

Oral:

- 0-6 months: 8-10 mcg/kg/day **or** 25-50 mcg/day
- 6-12 months: 6-8 mcg/kg/day **or** 50-75 mcg/day
- 1-5 years: 5-6 mcg/kg/day **or** 75-100 mcg/day
- 6-12 years: 4-5 mcg/kg/day **or** 100-150 mcg/day
- >12 years: 2-3 mcg/kg/day **or** ≥150 mcg/day

I.M., I.V.: 50% to 75% of the oral dose

Adults:

Oral: 12.5-50 mcg/day to start, then increase by 25-50 mcg/day at intervals of 2-4 weeks; average adult dose: 100-200 mcg/day

I.M., I.V.: 50% of the oral dose

(Continued)

## Levothyroxine *(Continued)*

Myxedema coma or stupor: I.V.: 200-500 mcg one time, then 100-300 mcg the next day if necessary

Thyroid suppression therapy: Oral: 2-6 mcg/kg/day for 7-10 days

**Mechanism of Action** Exact mechanism of action is unknown; however, it is believed the thyroid hormone exerts its many metabolic effects through control of DNA transcription and protein synthesis; involved in normal metabolism, growth, and development; promotes gluconeogenesis, increases utilization and mobilization of glycogen stores, and stimulates protein synthesis, increases basal metabolic rate

**Local Anesthetic/Vasoconstrictor Precautions** No precautions with vasoconstrictor are necessary if patient is well controlled with levothyroxine

**Effects on Dental Treatment** No effects or complications reported

**Other Adverse Effects** <1%:

Cardiovascular: Palpitations, cardiac arrhythmias, tachycardia, chest pain

Central nervous system: Nervousness, headache, insomnia, fever, clumsiness

Dermatologic: Alopecia

Endocrine: Changes in menstrual cycle

Gastrointestinal: Weight loss, increased appetite, diarrhea, abdominal cramps, constipation

Neuromuscular & skeletal: Myalgia, hand tremors, tremor

Respiratory: Dyspnea

Miscellaneous: Sweating

**Drug Interactions**

Decreased effect:

Phenytoin may decreased levothyroxine levels

Cholestyramine may decreased absorption of levothyroxine

Increases oral hypoglycemic requirements

Increased effect: Increased effects of oral anticoagulants

Increased toxicity: Tricyclic antidepressants cause increased toxic potential of both drugs

**Drug Uptake**

Onset of therapeutic effect:

Oral: 3-5 days

I.V. Within 6-8 hours

Peak effect: I.V.: Within 24 hours

Absorption: Oral: Erratic

Time to peak serum concentration: 2-4 hours

**Pregnancy Risk Factor** A

**Generic Available** Yes


♦ **Levoxyl®** *see* Levothyroxine *on previous page*

♦ **Levsin®** *see* Hyoscyamine *on page 519*

♦ **Levsinex®** *see* Hyoscyamine *on page 519*

♦ **Levsin/SL®** *see* Hyoscyamine *on page 519*

♦ **Levulose, Dextrose and Phosphoric Acid** *see* Phosphorated Carbohydrate Solution *on page 800*

♦ **Lexxel™** *see* Enalapril and Felodipine *on page 368*

♦ **Librax®** *see* Clidinium and Chlordiazepoxide *on page 258*

♦ **Libritabs®** *see* Chlordiazepoxide *on page 224*

♦ **Librium®** *see* Chlordiazepoxide *on page 224*

♦ **Lice-Enz® Shampoo [OTC]** *see* Pyrethrins *on page 867*

♦ **Lida-Mantle HC® Topical** *see* Lidocaine and Hydrocortisone *on page 589*

♦ **Lidex®** *see* Fluocinonide *on page 440*

♦ **Lidex-E®** *see* Fluocinonide *on page 440*


## Lidocaine (LYE doe kane)

**Related Information**


Cardiovascular Diseases *on page 1066*

Oral Pain *on page 1122*

Oral Viral Infections *on page 1137*

Patients Undergoing Cancer Therapy *on page 1154*


**U.S. Brand Names** Dilocaine®; Duo-Trach®; Nervocaine®; Octocaine®; Xylocaine®

**Canadian Brand Names** PMS-Lidocaine Viscous; Xylocard®

**Therapeutic Category** Antiarrhythmic Agent (Supraventricular & Ventricular); Dental/Local Anesthetics; Local Anesthetic, Injectable

**Use**

Dental: Amide-type injectable local anesthetic and topical local anesthetic; Patch: Production of mild topical anesthesia of accessible mucous membranes of the mouth prior to superficial dental procedures

Medical: Drug of choice for ventricular ectopy, ventricular tachycardia, ventricular fibrillation; for pulseless VT or VF preferably give **after** defibrillation and epinephrine; control of premature ventricular contractions, wide-complex PSVT

**Usual Dosage** Dental anesthetic, infiltration, or conduction block: Do not exceed 6.6 mg/kg of body weight or 300 mg/dental appointment. A 2% solution of lidocaine hydrochloride provides 20 mg of anesthetic per mL. The effective anesthetic dose varies with procedure, intensity of anesthesia needed, duration of anesthesia required, and physical condition of the patient. Always use the lowest effective dose along with careful aspiration.

**Note:** Maximum dose for lidocaine hydrochloride cited from USP Dispensing Information (USP DI) 17th ed, The United Pharmacopeial Convention, Inc, Rockville, MD, 1997, 137.

**Mechanism of Action** Class IB antiarrhythmic; local anesthetics bind selectively to the intracellular surface of sodium channels to block influx of sodium into the axon. As a result, depolarization necessary for action potential propagation and subsequent nerve function is prevented. The block at the sodium channel is reversible. When drug diffuses away from the axon, sodium channel function is restored and nerve propagation returns.

**Local Anesthetic/Vasoconstrictor Precautions** No information available to require special precautions

**Effects on Dental Treatment** No effects or complications reported

**Other Adverse Effects** No data reported

**Contraindications** Known hypersensitivity to amide-type local anesthetics; patients with Adams-Stokes syndrome or with severe degree of S-A, A-V, or intraventricular heart block (without a pacemaker)

**Drug Interactions** No data reported

**Drug Uptake**

Onset of action (single bolus dose): 45-90 seconds

Duration: 10-20 minutes

Half-life (biphasic): Increased with CHF, liver disease, shock, severe renal disease

Initial: 7-30 minutes

Terminal:

Infants, premature: 3.2 hours

Adults: 1.5-2 hours

**Pregnancy Risk Factor** C

**Breast-feeding Considerations** May be taken while breast-feeding

**Dosage Forms**

Injection: 0.5% [5 mg/mL] (50 mL); 1% [10 mg/mL] (2 mL, 5 mL, 10 mL, 20 mL, 30 mL, 50 mL); 1.5% [15 mg/mL] (20 mL); 2% [20 mg/mL] (2 mL, 5 mL, 10 mL, 20 mL, 30 mL, 50 mL); 4% [40 mg/mL] (5 mL)

Liquid, viscous: 2% (20 mL, 100 mL)

**Generic Available** Yes

**Comments** Lidocaine without epinephrine is not marketed as a dental 1.8 mL carpule and as such is not used as a dental local anesthetic

## Lidocaine and Epinephrine (LYE doe kane & ep i NEF rin)

**Related Information**

Oral Pain *on page 1122*

**U.S. Brand Names** Octocaine® 50; Octocaine® 100; Xylocaine® With Epinephrine

**Therapeutic Category** Dental/Local Anesthetics; Local Anesthetic, Injectable

**Use** Dental: Amide-type anesthetic used for local infiltration anesthesia; injection near nerve trunks to produce nerve block

**Usual Dosage**

Children <10 years: Dental anesthesia, infiltration, or conduction block: 20-30 mg (1-1.5 mL) of lidocaine hydrochloride as a 2% solution with epinephrine 1:100,000; maximum: 4-5 mg of lidocaine hydrochloride/kg of body weight or 100-150 mg as a single dose

Children >10 years and Adults: Dental anesthesia, infiltration, or conduction block: Do not exceed 6.6 mg/kg body weight or 300 mg of lidocaine hydrochloride and 3 mcg (0.003 mg) of epinephrine/kg of body weight or 0.2 mg epinephrine per dental appointment. The effective anesthetic dose varies with procedure, intensity of anesthesia needed, duration of anesthesia required, and physical condition of the patient. Always use the lowest effective dose along with careful aspiration. The following numbers of dental carpules (1.8

(Continued)

## Lidocaine and Epinephrine *(Continued)*

mL) provide the indicated amounts of lidocaine hydrochloride 2% and epinephrine 1:100,000.

| # of Cartridges | Mg Lidocaine (2%) | Mg Vasoconstrictor (Epinephrine 1:100,000) |
|---|---|---|
| 1 | 36 | 0.018 |
| 2 | 72 | 0.036 |
| 3 | 108 | 0.054 |
| 4 | 144 | 0.072 |
| 5 | 180 | 0.090 |
| 6 | 216 | 0.108 |
| 7 | 252 | 0.126 |
| 8 | 288 | 0.144 |
| 9 | 324 | 0.162 |
| 10 | 360 | 0.180 |

For most routine dental procedures, lidocaine hydrochloride 2% with epinephrine 1:100,000 is preferred. When a more pronounced hemostasis is required, a 1:50,000 epinephrine concentration should be used. The following numbers of dental carpules (1.8 mL) provide the indicated amounts of lidocaine hydrochloride 2% and epinephrine 1:50,000.

| # of Cartridges | Mg Lidocaine (2%) | Mg Vasoconstrictor (Epinephrine 1:50,000) |
|---|---|---|
| 1 | 36 | 0.036 |
| 2 | 72 | 0.072 |
| 3 | 108 | 0.108 |
| 4 | 144 | 0.144 |
| 5 | 180 | 0.180 |
| 6 | 216 | 0.216 |

**Note:** Adult and children doses of lidocaine hydrochloride and epinephrine cited from USP Dispensing Information (USP DI) 17th ed, The United States Pharmacopeial Convention, Inc, Rockville, MD, 1997, 138-9.

**Mechanism of Action** Local anesthetics bind selectively to the intracellular surface of sodium channels to block influx of sodium into the axon. As a result, depolarization necessary for action potential propagation and subsequent nerve function is prevented. The block at the sodium channel is reversible. When drug diffuses away from the axon, sodium channel function is restored and nerve propagation returns.

Epinephrine prolongs the duration of the anesthetic actions of lidocaine by causing vasoconstriction (alpha adrenergic receptor agonist) of the vasculature surrounding the nerve axons. This prevents the diffusion of lidocaine away from the nerves resulting in a longer retention in the axon.

**Local Anesthetic/Vasoconstrictor Precautions** No information available to require special precautions

**Effects on Dental Treatment** No effects or complications reported

**Other Adverse Effects** Degree of adverse effects in the central nervous system and cardiovascular system are directly related to the blood levels of lidocaine. The effects below are more likely to occur after systemic administration rather than infiltration.

Cardiovascular: Myocardial effects include a decrease in contraction force as well as a decrease in electrical excitability and myocardial conduction rate resulting in bradycardia and reduction in cardiac output.

Central nervous system: High blood levels result in anxiety, restlessness, disorientation, confusion, dizziness, tremors and seizures. This is followed by depression of CNS resulting in somnolence, unconsciousness and possible respiratory arrest. In some cases, symptoms of CNS stimulation may be absent and the primary CNS effects are somnolence and unconsciousness.

Gastrointestinal: Nausea and vomiting may occur

Hypersensitivity reactions: Extremely rare, but may be manifest as dermatologic reactions and edema at injection site. Asthmatic syndromes have occurred. Patients may exhibit hypersensitivity to bisulfites contained in local anesthetic solution to prevent oxidation of epinephrine. In general, patients reacting to bisulfites have a history of asthma and their airways are hyper-reactive to asthmatic syndrome.

Psychogenic reactions: It is common to misinterpret psychogenic responses to local anesthetic injection as an allergic reaction. Intraoral injections are perceived by many patients as a stressful procedure in dentistry. Common symptoms to this stress are sweating, palpitations, hyperventilation, generalized pallor and a fainting feeling

**Contraindications** Hypersensitivity to local anesthetics of the amide-type

**Warnings/Precautions** Should be avoided in patients with uncontrolled hyperthyroidism. Should be used in minimal amounts in patients with significant cardiovascular problems (because of epinephrine component). Aspirate the syringe after tissue penetration and before injection to minimize chance of direct vascular injection.

**Drug Interactions** Due to epinephrine component, use with tricyclic antidepressants or MAO inhibitors could result in increased pressor response; use with nonselective beta-blockers (ie, propranolol) could result in serious hypertension and reflex bradycardia

**Drug Uptake**

Onset of action: Infiltration less than 2 minutes; nerve block 2-4 minutes

Duration after infiltration: Soft tissue anesthesia ~2.5 hours; pulp anesthesia <60 minutes

Duration after nerve block: Soft tissue anesthesia ~3.25 hours; pulp anesthesia at least 90 minutes

**Pregnancy Risk Factor** B

**Breast-feeding Considerations** Usual infiltration doses of lidocaine with epinephrine given to nursing mothers has not been shown to affect the health of the nursing infant

**Dosage Forms** Injection:

Lidocaine Hydrochloride 2% with epinephrine 1:100,000 (Octocaine® 100, Xylocaine®): (1.8 mL dental cartridges)

Lidocaine Hydrochloride 2% with epinephrine 1:50,000 (Octocaine® 50, Xylocaine®): (1.8 mL dental cartridges)

**Dietary Considerations** No data reported

**Generic Available** Yes

**Selected Readings**

Ayoub ST and Coleman AE, "A Review of Local Anesthetics," *Gen Dent*, 1992, 40(4):285-7, 289-90.

Jastak JT and Yagiela JA, "Vasoconstrictors and Local Anesthesia: A Review and Rationale for Use," *J Am Dent Assoc*, 1983, 107(4):623-30.

MacKenzie TA and Young ER, "Local Anesthetic Update," *Anesth Prog*, 1993, 40(2):29-34.

Wynn RL, "Epinephrine Interactions With Beta-Blockers," *Gen Dent*, 1994, 42(1):16, 18.

Wynn RL, "Recent Research on Mechanisms of Local Anesthetics," *Gen Dent*, 1995, 43(4):316-8.

Yagiela JA, "Local Anesthetics," *Anesth Prog*, 1991, 38(4-5):128-41.

## Lidocaine and Hydrocortisone

(LYE doe kane & hye droe KOR ti sone)

**U.S. Brand Names** Lida-Mantle HC® Topical

**Therapeutic Category** Corticosteroid, Topical (Low Potency); Local Anesthetic, Topical

**Use** Topical anti-inflammatory and anesthetic for skin disorders

**Usual Dosage** Topical: Apply 2-4 times/day

**Local Anesthetic/Vasoconstrictor Precautions** No information available to require special precautions

**Effects on Dental Treatment** No effects or complications reported

**Generic Available** No

## Lidocaine and Prilocaine (LYE doe kane & PRIL oh kane)

**U.S. Brand Names** EMLA® Cream; EMLA® Disc

**Therapeutic Category** Analgesic, Topical; Antipruritic, Topical; Local Anesthetic, Topical

**Use**

Dental: Amide-type topical anesthetic for use on normal intact skin to provide local analgesia for minor procedures such as I.V. cannulation or venipuncture

Medical: Has also been used for painful procedures such as lumbar puncture and skin graft harvesting; topical anesthetic for local anesthesia on normal skin

**Usual Dosage** Children and Adults:

**EMLA® cream should not be used in infants under the age of 1 month or in infants, under the age of 12 months, who are receiving treatment with methemoglobin-inducing agents**

Choose 2 application sites available for intravenous access

Apply a thick layer (2.5 g/site - 1/2 of a 5 g tube) of cream to each designated site of intact skin

Cover each site with the occlusive dressing (Tegaderm®)

Mark the time on the dressing

(Continued)

## Lidocaine and Prilocaine *(Continued)*

**Allow at least 1 hour for optimum therapeutic effect.** Remove the dressing and wipe off excess EMLA® cream (gloves should be worn).

**EMLA® Cream Maximum Recommended Application Area* for Infants and Children Based on Application to Intact Skin**

| Body Weight (kg) | Maximum Application Area ($cm^2$)† |
|---|---|
| <10 | 100 |
| 10-20 | 600 |
| >20 | 2000 |

*These are broad guidelines for avoiding systemic toxicity in applying EMLA® to patients with normal intact skin and with normal renal and hepatic function.

†For more individualized calculation of how much lidocaine and prilocaine may be absorbed, use the following estimates of lidocaine and prilocaine absorption for children and adults:

Estimated mean (±SD) absorption of lidocaine: 0.045 (±0.016) $mg/cm^2/h$.

Estimated mean (±SD) absorption of prilocaine: 0.077 (±0.036) $mg/cm^2/h$.

**Debilitated patients, small children or patients with impaired elimination (ie, hepatic or renal dysfunction):** Smaller areas of treatment are recommended

**Mechanism of Action** Local anesthetics bind selectively to the intracellular surface of sodium channels to block influx of sodium into the axon. As a result, depolarization necessary for action potential propagation and subsequent nerve function is prevented. The block at the sodium channel is reversible. When drug diffuses away from the axon, sodium channel function is restored and nerve propagation returns.

**Local Anesthetic/Vasoconstrictor Precautions** No information available to require special precautions

**Effects on Dental Treatment** No effects or complications reported

**Other Adverse Effects** 1% to 10%:

Dermatologic: Angioedema, contact dermatitis

Local: Burning, stinging

**Contraindications** Known hypersensitivity to lidocaine, prilocaine, any component or local anesthetics of the amide type; patients with congenital or idiopathic methemoglobinemia, infants <1 month of age, infants <12 months of age who are receiving concurrent treatment with methemoglobin-inducing agents (ie, sulfas, acetaminophen, benzocaine, chloroquine, dapsone, nitrofurantoin, nitroglycerin, nitroprusside, phenobarbital, phenytoin)

**Warnings/Precautions** Use with caution in patients receiving class I antiarrhythmic drugs, since systemic absorption occurs and synergistic toxicity is possible

**Drug Interactions** Increased toxicity with Class I antiarrhythmic drugs (tocainide, mexiletine) - effects are additive and potentially synergistic and with drugs known to induce methemoglobinemia

**Drug Uptake**

Absorption: Related to the duration of application and to the area over which it is applied

3-hour application: 3.6% lidocaine and 6.1% prilocaine were absorbed

24-hour application: 16.2% lidocaine and 33.5% prilocaine were absorbed

Onset of action: 1 hour for sufficient dermal analgesia

Peak effect: 2-3 hours

Duration: 1-2 hours after removal of the cream

Serum half-life:

Lidocaine: 65-150 minutes, prolonged with cardiac or hepatic dysfunction

Prilocaine: 10-150 minutes, prolonged in hepatic or renal dysfunction

**Pregnancy Risk Factor** B

**Breast-feeding Considerations** Usual infiltration doses of lidocaine and prilocaine given to nursing mothers has not been shown to affect the health of the nursing infant

**Dosage Forms**

Cream: Lidocaine 2.5% and prilocaine 2.5% [2 Tegaderm® dressings] (5 g, 30 g)

Disc:

**Generic Available** No

**Selected Readings**

Vickers ER, Mazbani N, Gerzina TM, et al, "Pharmacokinetics of EMLA Cream 5% Application to Oral Mucosa," *Anesth Prog*, 1997, 44:32-7.

## Lidocaine Transoral (LYE doe kane)

**Related Information**

Oral Pain *on page 1122*

**U.S. Brand Names** Dentipatch®

**Therapeutic Category** Local Anesthetic, Transoral

**Use** Local anesthesia of the oral mucosa prior to oral injections and soft-tissue dental procedures

**Usual Dosage** One patch on selected area of oral mucosa

**Mechanism of Action** Blocks both the initiation and conduction of nerve impulses by decreasing the neuronal membrane's permeability to sodium ions, which results in inhibition of depolarization with resultant blockade of conduction

**Local Anesthetic/Vasoconstrictor Precautions** No information available to require special precautions

**Effects on Dental Treatment** No effects or complications reported

**Other Adverse Effects** No data reported

**Contraindications** Known hypersensitivity to any of its components

**Drug Uptake**

Onset of action: 2 minutes

Duration of anesthesia after patch application: Based on 15-minute wear period, effect is present for at least 40 minutes

**Dosage Forms** Patch: 23 mg/2 $cm^2$, 46.1 mg/2 $cm^2$ (50s, 100s)

**Generic Available** No

**Comments** The manufacturer claims Dentipatch® is safe, with "negligible systemic absorption" of lidocaine. The agent is "clinically proven to prevent injection pain from 25-gauge needles that are inserted to the level of the bone." Data from controlled studies (235 patients) have shown no serious adverse effects with the application of lidocaine patch to the oral mucosa for 15 minutes. Peak plasma levels were 10% of those seen following local infiltration anesthesia with 1.8 mL lidocaine and 1:100,000 epinephrine. According to the manufacturer, tips for applying lidocaine patch are the following:

- Cotton roll isolation for all procedures except palatal application
- Air dry with syringe on dental unit for 30 seconds
- Apply patch to gingiva or mucosa
- Apply firm finger pressure to patch for 30 seconds

Leave patch in place during scaling and root planing procedure; remove after 15 minutes. Patch should be removed after 5-10 minutes prior to giving injection.

**Selected Readings**

Hersh EV, Houpt MI, Cooper SA, et al, "Analgesic Efficacy and Safety of an Intraoral Lidocaine Patch," *J Am Dent Assoc*, 1996, 127(11):1626-34.

Houpt MI, Heins P, Lamster I, et al, "An Evaluation of Intraoral Lidocaine Patches in Reducing Needle-Insertion Pain," *Compendium*, 1997, 4:309-16.

"The Lidocaine Patch: A New Delivery System," *Biological Therapies in Dentistry*, Sept 1997, vol 13.

◆ **Limbitrol® DS 10-25** *see* Amitriptyline and Chlordiazepoxide *on page 68*

◆ **Lincocin®** *see* Lincomycin *on this page*

## Lincomycin (lin koe MYE sin)

**U.S. Brand Names** Lincocin®

**Therapeutic Category** Antibiotic, Macrolide

**Use** Treatment of susceptible bacterial infections, mainly those caused by streptococci and staphylococci resistant to other agents

**Usual Dosage**

Children >1 month:

- Oral: 30-60 mg/kg/day in divided doses every 8 hours
- I.M.: 10 mg/kg every 8-12 hours
- I.V.: 10-20 mg/kg/day in divided doses every 8-12 hours

Adults:

- Oral: 500 mg every 6-8 hours
- I.M.: 600 mg every 12-24 hours
- I.V.: 600-1 g every 8-12 hours up to 8 g/day

**Mechanism of Action** Lincosamide antibiotic which was isolated from a strain of *Streptomyces lincolnensis*; lincomycin, like clindamycin, inhibits bacterial protein synthesis by specifically binding on the 50S subunit and affecting the process of peptide chain initiation. Other macrolide antibiotics (erythromycin) also bind to the 50S subunit. Since only one molecule of antibiotic can bind to a single ribosome, the concomitant use of erythromycin and lincomycin is not recommended.

**Local Anesthetic/Vasoconstrictor Precautions** No information available to require special precautions

**Effects on Dental Treatment** No effects or complications reported

**Other Adverse Effects**

1% to 10%: Gastrointestinal: Nausea, vomiting, diarrhea

<1%:

- Cardiovascular: Hypotension
- Central nervous system: Vertigo

(Continued)

## Lincomycin *(Continued)*

Dermatologic: Urticaria, rash, Stevens-Johnson syndrome
Gastrointestinal: Pseudomembranous colitis, glossitis, stomatitis, pruritus ani
Genitourinary: Vaginitis
Hematologic: Granulocytopenia, thrombocytopenia, pancytopenia
Hepatic: Elevation of liver enzymes
Local: Sterile abscess at I.M. injection site, thrombophlebitis
Otic: Tinnitus

**Drug Interactions**
Decreased effect with erythromycin
Increased activity/toxicity of neuromuscular blocking agents

**Drug Uptake**
Absorption: Oral: ~20% to 30%
Serum half-life, elimination: 2-11.5 hours
Time to peak serum concentration:
Oral: 2-4 hours
I.M.: 1 hour

**Pregnancy Risk Factor** B
**Generic Available** No

## Lindane (LIN dane)

**U.S. Brand Names** G-well®; Scabene®
**Canadian Brand Names** Hexit®; Kwellada™; PMS-Lindane
**Therapeutic Category** Antiparasitic Agent, Topical; Pediculocide; Scabicidal Agent; Shampoos
**Use** Treatment of scabies (*Sarcoptes scabiei*), *Pediculus capitis* (head lice), and *Pediculus pubis* (crab lice)
**Usual Dosage** Children and Adults: Topical:
Scabies: Apply a thin layer of lotion or cream and massage it on skin from the neck to the toes (head to toe in infants). For adults, bathe and remove the drug after 8-12 hours; for children, wash off 6-8 hours after application (for infants, wash off 6 hours after application); repeat treatment in 7 days if lice or nits are still present
Pediculosis, capitis and pubis: 15-30 mL of shampoo is applied and lathered for 4-5 minutes; rinse hair thoroughly and comb with a fine tooth comb to remove nits; repeat treatment in 7 days if lice or nits are still present
**Mechanism of Action** Directly absorbed by parasites and ova through the exoskeleton; stimulates the nervous system resulting in seizures and death of parasitic arthropods
**Local Anesthetic/Vasoconstrictor Precautions** No information available to require special precautions
**Effects on Dental Treatment** No effects or complications reported
**Other Adverse Effects** <1%:
Cardiovascular: Cardiac arrhythmia
Central nervous system: Dizziness, restlessness, seizures, headache, ataxia
Dermatologic: Eczematous eruptions, contact dermatitis, skin and adipose tissue may act as repositories
Gastrointestinal: Nausea, vomiting
Hematologic: Aplastic anemia
Hepatic: Hepatitis
Local: Burning and stinging
Renal: Hematuria
Respiratory: Pulmonary edema
**Drug Interactions** Increased toxicity: Oil-based hair dressing may increase toxic potential
**Drug Uptake**
Absorption: Systemic absorption of up to 13% may occur
Serum half-life: Children: 17-22 hours
Time to peak serum concentration: Topical: Children: 6 hours
**Pregnancy Risk Factor** B
**Generic Available** Yes

♦ **Lioresal®** *see* Baclofen *on page 118*

## Liothyronine (lye oh THYE roe neen)

**Related Information**
Endocrine Disorders & Pregnancy *on page 1082*
**U.S. Brand Names** Cytomel®; Triostat™
**Therapeutic Category** Thyroid Product

**Use** Replacement or supplemental therapy in hypothyroidism, management of nontoxic goiter, chronic lymphocytic thyroiditis, as an adjunct in thyrotoxicosis and as a diagnostic aid; **levothyroxine is recommended for chronic therapy**

**Usual Dosage**

Congenital hypothyroidism: Children: Oral: 5 mcg/day increase by 5 mcg every 3 days to 20 mcg/day for infants, 50 mcg/day for children 1-3 years of age, and give adult dose for children >3 years.

Hypothyroidism: Oral:

Adults: 25 mcg/day increase by 12.5-25 mcg/day every 1-2 weeks to a maximum of 100 mcg/day

Elderly: Initial: 5 mcg/day, increase by 5 mcg/day every 1-2 weeks; usual maintenance dose: 25-75 mcg/day

$T_3$ suppression test: Oral: 75-100 mcg/day for 7 days; use lowest dose for elderly

Myxedema coma: I.V.: 25-50 mcg

Patients with known or suspected cardiovascular disease: 10-20 mcg

**Note:** Normally, at least 4 hours should be allowed between doses to adequately assess therapeutic response and no more than 12 hours should elapse between doses to avoid fluctuations in hormone levels. Oral therapy should be resumed as soon as the clinical situation has been stabilized and the patient is able to take oral medication. If levothyroxine rather than liothyronine sodium is used in initiating oral therapy, the physician should bear in mind that there is a delay of several days in the onset of levothyroxine activity and that I.V. therapy should be discontinued gradually.

**Mechanism of Action** Primary active compound is $T_3$ (triiodothyronine), which may be converted from $T_4$ (thyroxine) and then circulates throughout the body to influence growth and maturation of various tissues; exact mechanism of action is unknown; however, it is believed the thyroid hormone exerts its many metabolic effects through control of DNA transcription and protein synthesis; involved in normal metabolism, growth, and development; promotes gluconeogenesis, increases utilization and mobilization of glycogen stores, and stimulates protein synthesis, increases basal metabolic rate

**Local Anesthetic/Vasoconstrictor Precautions** No precautions with vasoconstrictor are necessary if patient is well controlled with liothyronine

**Effects on Dental Treatment** No effects or complications reported

**Other Adverse Effects** <1%:

Cardiovascular: Palpitations, tachycardia, cardiac arrhythmias, chest pain

Central nervous system: Nervousness, fever, headache, insomnia, clumsiness

Dermatologic: Alopecia

Endocrine & metabolic: Changes in menstrual cycle

Gastrointestinal: Weight loss, increased appetite, diarrhea, abdominal cramps, constipation

Neuromuscular & skeletal: Myalgia, hand tremors, tremor

Respiratory: Dyspnea

Miscellaneous: Sweating

**Drug Interactions**

Decreased effect:

Cholestyramine resin causes decreased absorption of liothyronine

Antidiabetic drug requirements are increased

Estrogens cause increased thyroid requirements

Increased effect: Increased oral anticoagulant effects

**Drug Uptake**

Onset of effect: Within 24-72 hours

Duration: Up to 72 hours

Absorption: Oral: Well absorbed (~85% to 90%)

Serum half-life: 16-49 hours

**Pregnancy Risk Factor** A

**Generic Available** Yes

## Liotrix (LYE oh triks)

**Related Information**

Endocrine Disorders & Pregnancy *on page 1082*

**U.S. Brand Names** Thyrolar®

**Therapeutic Category** Thyroid Product

**Use** Replacement or supplemental therapy in hypothyroidism (uniform mixture of $T_4$:$T_3$ in 4:1 ratio by weight); little advantage to this product exists and cost is not justified

**Usual Dosage** Oral:

Congenital hypothyroidism:

Children (dose of $T_4$ or levothyroxine/day):

0-6 months: 8-10 mcg/kg or 25-50 mcg/day

6-12 months: 6-8 mcg/kg or 50-75 mcg/day

(Continued)

## Liotrix *(Continued)*

1-5 years: 5-6 mcg/kg or 75-100 mcg/day
6-12 years: 4-5 mcg/kg or 100-150 mcg/day
>12 years: 2-3 mcg/kg or >150 mcg/day

Hypothyroidism (dose of thyroid equivalent):
Adults: 30 mg/day, increasing by 15 mg/day at 2- to 3-week intervals to a maximum of 180 mg/day (usual maintenance dose: 60-120 mg/day)
Elderly: Initial: 15 mg, adjust dose at 2- to 4-week intervals by increments of 15 mg

**Mechanism of Action** The primary active compound is $T_3$ (triiodothyronine), which may be converted from $T_4$ (thyroxine) and then circulates throughout the body to influence growth and maturation of various tissues. Liotrix is uniform mixture of synthetic $T_4$ and $T_3$ in 4:1 ratio; exact mechanism of action is unknown; however, it is believed the thyroid hormone exerts its many metabolic effects through control of DNA transcription and protein synthesis; involved in normal metabolism, growth, and development; promotes gluconeogenesis, increases utilization and mobilization of glycogen stores and stimulates protein synthesis, increases basal metabolic rate

**Local Anesthetic/Vasoconstrictor Precautions** No precautions with vasoconstrictor are necessary if patient is well controlled with liotrix

**Effects on Dental Treatment** No effects or complications reported

**Other Adverse Effects** <1%:
Cardiovascular: Palpitations, tachycardia, cardiac arrhythmias, chest pain
Central nervous system: Nervousness, headache, insomnia, fever, clumsiness
Dermatologic: Alopecia
Endocrine & metabolic: Excessive bone loss with overtreatment (excess thyroid replacement), heat intolerance, changes in menstrual cycle
Gastrointestinal: Weight loss, increased appetite, diarrhea, abdominal cramps, vomiting, constipation
Neuromuscular & skeletal: Tremor, myalgia, hand tremors
Respiratory: Dyspnea
Miscellaneous: Sweating

**Drug Interactions**
Decreased effect:
Thyroid hormones increase hypoglycemic drug requirements
Phenytoin may decrease clinical lymphothyroidism
Cholestyramine causes decreased drug absorption of liotrix
Increased effect: Increased oral anticoagulant effect
Increased toxicity: Tricyclic antidepressants cause increased potential of both drugs

**Drug Uptake**
Absorption: 50% to 95% from GI tract
Serum half-life: 6-7 days
Time to peak serum concentration: 12-48 hours

**Pregnancy Risk Factor** A
**Generic Available** No

- **Lipancreatin** *see* Pancrelipase *on page 763*
- **Lipidil®** *see* Fenofibrate *on page 422*
- **Lipitor®** *see* Atorvastatin *on page 106*
- **Liposyn®** *see* Fat Emulsion *on page 419*
- **Lipovite® [OTC]** *see* Vitamin B Complex *on page 1050*
- **Liquibid®** *see* Guaifenesin *on page 478*
- **Liqui-Char® [OTC]** *see* Charcoal *on page 219*
- **Liquid Pred®** *see* Prednisone *on page 833*
- **Liqui-E®** *see* Tocophersolan *on page 992*
- **Liquifilm® Forte Solution [OTC]** *see* Artificial Tears *on page 97*
- **Liquifilm® Tears Solution [OTC]** *see* Artificial Tears *on page 97*
- **Liquiprin® [OTC]** *see* Acetaminophen *on page 27*

## Lisinopril (lyse IN oh pril)

**Related Information**
Cardiovascular Diseases *on page 1066*

**U.S. Brand Names** Prinivil®; Zestril®

**Canadian Brand Names** Apo®-Lisinopril

**Therapeutic Category** Angiotensin-Converting Enzyme (ACE) Inhibitor

**Use** Treatment of hypertension, either alone or in combination with other antihypertensive agents; adjunctive therapy in treatment of CHF (afterload reduction)

**Usual Dosage**

Adults: Initial: 10 mg/day; increase doses 5-10 mg/day at 1- to 2-week intervals; maximum daily dose: 40 mg

Elderly: Initial: 2.5-5 mg/day; increase doses 2.5-5 mg/day at 1- to 2-week intervals; maximum daily dose: 40 mg

Patients taking diuretics should have them discontinued 2-3 days prior to initiating lisinopril if possible; restart diuretic after blood pressure is stable if needed; in patients with hyponatremia (<130 mEq/L), start dose at 2.5 mg/day

Acute myocardial infarction (within 24 hours in hemodynamically stable patients): Oral: 5 mg immediately, then 5 mg at 24 hours, 10 mg at 48 hours, and 10 mg every day thereafter for 6 weeks; patients should continue to receive standard treatments such as thrombolytics, aspirin, and beta-blockers

**Mechanism of Action** Competitive inhibitor of angiotensin-converting enzyme (ACE); prevents conversion of angiotensin I to angiotensin II, a potent vasoconstrictor; results in lower levels of angiotensin II which causes an increase in plasma renin activity and a reduction in aldosterone secretion; a CNS mechanism may also be involved in hypotensive effect as angiotensin II increases adrenergic outflow from CNS; vasoactive kallikreins may be decreased in conversion to active hormones by ACE inhibitors, thus reducing blood pressure

**Local Anesthetic/Vasoconstrictor Precautions** No information available to require special precautions

**Effects on Dental Treatment** No effects or complications reported

**Other Adverse Effects**

1% to 10%:

- Cardiovascular: Hypotension
- Central nervous system: Dizziness, headache, fatigue
- Gastrointestinal: Diarrhea
- Renal: Elevated BUN and serum creatinine
- Respiratory: Upper respiratory symptoms, cough

<1%:

- Cardiovascular: Chest discomfort, flushing, myocardial infarction, angina pectoris, orthostatic hypotension, rhythm disturbances, tachycardia, peripheral edema, vasculitis, palpitations, syncope
- Central nervous system: Fever, malaise, depression, somnolence, insomnia
- Dermatologic: Urticaria, pruritus, angioedema
- Endocrine & metabolic: Gout
- Gastrointestinal: Pancreatitis, abdominal pain, anorexia, constipation, flatulence, dry mouth
- Hematologic: Neutropenia, bone marrow suppression
- Hepatic: Hepatitis
- Neuromuscular & skeletal: Arthralgia, shoulder pain
- Ocular: Blurred vision
- Respiratory: Bronchitis, sinusitis, pharyngeal pain
- Miscellaneous: Sweating

**Drug Interactions** See table.

**Drug-Drug Interactions With ACEIs**

| Precipitant Drug | Drug (Category) and Effect | Description |
|---|---|---|
| Antacids | ACE Inhibitors: decreased | Decreased bioavailability of ACEIs. May be more likely with captopril. Separate administration times by 1-2 hours. |
| NSAIDs (indomethacin) | ACEIs: decreased | Reduced hypotensive effects of ACEIs. More prominent in low renin or volume dependent hypertensive patients. |
| Phenothiazines | ACEIs: increased | Pharmacologic effects of ACEIs may be increased. |
| ACEIs | Allopurinol: increased | Higher risk of hypersensitivity reaction possible when given concurrently. Three case reports of Stevens-Johnson syndrome with captopril. |
| ACEIs | Digoxin: increased | Increased plasma digoxin levels. |
| ACEIs | Lithium: increased | Increased serum lithium levels and symptoms of toxicity may occur. |
| ACEIs | Potassium preps/ potassium sparing diuretics increased | Coadministration may result in elevated potassium levels. |

Increased toxicity: Lisinopril and diuretics have additive hypotensive effects

**Drug Uptake**

Peak hypotensive effect: Oral: Within 6 hours

(Continued)

## Lisinopril *(Continued)*

Absorption: Well absorbed; unaffected by food
Serum half-life: 11-12 hours

**Pregnancy Risk Factor** C (first trimester); D (second and third trimesters)

**Generic Available** No

## Lisinopril and Hydrochlorothiazide

(lyse IN oh pril & hye droe klor oh THYE a zide)

**Related Information**

Cardiovascular Diseases *on page 1066*

**U.S. Brand Names** Prinzide®; Zestoretic®

**Therapeutic Category** Antihypertensive Agent, Combination

**Use** Treatment of hypertension

**Local Anesthetic/Vasoconstrictor Precautions** No information available to require special precautions

**Effects on Dental Treatment** No effects or complications reported

**Generic Available** No

- **Listerine® Antiseptic [OTC]** *see* Mouthwash, Antiseptic *on page 690*
- **Listermint® with Fluoride [OTC]** *see* Fluoride *on page 441*

## Lithium (LITH ee um)

**Related Information**

Dental Drug Interactions: Update on Drug Combinations Requiring Special Considerations *on page 1225*

**U.S. Brand Names** Eskalith®; Lithobid®; Lithonate®; Lithotabs®

**Therapeutic Category** Antimanic Agent

**Use** Management of acute manic episodes, bipolar disorders, and depression

**Usual Dosage** Oral: Monitor serum concentrations and clinical response (efficacy and toxicity) to determine proper dose

Children 6-12 years: 15-60 mg/kg/day in 3-4 divided doses; dose not to exceed usual adult dosage

Adults: 300-600 mg 3-4 times/day; usual maximum maintenance dose: 2.4 g/day or 450-900 mg of sustained release twice daily

Elderly: Initial dose: 300 mg twice daily; increase weekly in increments of 300 mg/day, monitoring levels; rarely need to go >900-1200 mg/day

**Mechanism of Action** Alters cation transport across cell membrane in nerve and muscle cells and influences reuptake of serotonin and/or norepinephrine

**Local Anesthetic/Vasoconstrictor Precautions** No information available to require special precautions

**Effects on Dental Treatment** Avoid NSAIDs if analgesics are required since lithium toxicity has been reported with concomitant administration; acetaminophen products (ie, singly or with narcotics) are recommended

**Other Adverse Effects**

>10%:
- Endocrine & metabolic: Polydipsia, stress
- Gastrointestinal: Nausea, diarrhea, impaired taste
- Neuromuscular & skeletal: Trembling

1% to 10%:
- Central nervous system: Fatigue
- Dermatologic: Skin rash
- Gastrointestinal: Bloated feeling, weight gain
- Neuromuscular: Muscle twitching, weakness

<1%:
- Central nervous system: Lethargy, dizziness, vertigo, pseudotumor cerebri
- Dermatologic: Eruptions, discoloration of fingers and toes
- Endocrine & metabolic: Hypothyroidism, goiter, acneiform, diabetes insipidus
- Gastrointestinal: Anorexia, dry mouth
- Hematologic: Leukocytosis
- Neuromuscular & skeletal: Muscle weakness, cogwheel rigidity, chronic movements of the limbs, tremor
- Ocular: Vision problems
- Renal: Nonspecific nephron atrophy, renal tubular acidosis

**Drug Interactions**

Decreased effect with xanthines (eg, theophylline, caffeine)

Increased effect/toxicity of CNS depressants, alfentanil, iodide salts increased hypothyroid effect

Increased toxicity with thiazide diuretics (dose may need to be reduced by 30%), NSAIDs, haloperidol, phenothiazines (neurotoxicity), neuromuscular blockers, carbamazepine, fluoxetine, ACE inhibitors

**Drug Uptake**

Serum half-life: 18-24 hours; can increase to more than 36 hours in elderly or patients with renal impairment

Time to peak serum concentration (nonsustained release product): Within 0.5-2 hours following oral absorption

**Pregnancy Risk Factor** D

**Generic Available** Yes

- ♦ **Lithobid®** *see* Lithium *on previous page*
- ♦ **Lithonate®** *see* Lithium *on previous page*
- ♦ **Lithostat®** *see* Acetohydroxamic Acid *on page 35*
- ♦ **Lithotabs®** *see* Lithium *on previous page*
- ♦ **Livostin®** *see* Levocabastine *on page 580*
- ♦ **LKV-Drops® [OTC]** *see* Vitamins, Multiple *on page 1051*

## L-Lysine (el LYE seen)

**U.S. Brand Names** Enisyl® [OTC]; Lycolan® Elixir [OTC]

**Therapeutic Category** Dietary Supplement

**Use** Improves utilization of vegetable proteins

**Usual Dosage** Adults: Oral: 334-1500 mg/day

**Local Anesthetic/Vasoconstrictor Precautions** No information available to require special precautions

**Effects on Dental Treatment** No effects or complications reported

**Pregnancy Risk Factor** C

**Generic Available** Yes

- ♦ **LMD®** *see* Dextran *on page 311*
- ♦ **Lodine®** *see* Etodolac *on page 413*
- ♦ **Lodine® XL** *see* Etodolac *on page 413*
- ♦ **Lodosyn®** *see* Carbidopa *on page 188*

## Lodoxamide Tromethamine (loe DOKS a mide troe METH a meen)

**U.S. Brand Names** Alomide®

**Therapeutic Category** Ophthalmic Agent, Miscellaneous

**Use** Treatment of vernal keratoconjunctivitis, vernal conjunctivitis, and vernal keratitis

**Usual Dosage** Children >2 years and Adults: Instill 1-2 drops in eye(s) 4 times/day for up to 3 months

**Mechanism of Action** Mast cell stabilizer that inhibits the *in vivo* type I immediate hypersensitivity reaction to increase cutaneous vascular permeability associated with IgE and antigen-mediated reactions

**Local Anesthetic/Vasoconstrictor Precautions** No information available to require special precautions

**Effects on Dental Treatment** No effects or complications reported

**Other Adverse Effects**

>10%: Local: Transient burning, stinging, discomfort

1% to 10%:

Central nervous system: Headache

Ocular: Blurred vision, corneal erosion/ulcer, eye pain, corneal abrasion, blepharitis

<1%:

Central nervous system: Dizziness, somnolence

Dermatologic: Rash

Gastrointestinal: Nausea, stomach discomfort

Ocular: Blepharitis

Respiratory: Sneezing, dry nose

**Drug Interactions** No data reported

**Drug Uptake** Absorption: Topical: Very small and undetectable

**Pregnancy Risk Factor** B

**Dosage Forms** Solution, ophthalmic: 0.1% (10 mL)

**Generic Available** No

- ♦ **Loestrin®** *see* Ethinyl Estradiol and Norethindrone *on page 404*
- ♦ **Logen®** *see* Diphenoxylate and Atropine *on page 340*
- ♦ **Lomanate®** *see* Diphenoxylate and Atropine *on page 340*

## Lomefloxacin (loe me FLOKS a sin)

**U.S. Brand Names** Maxaquin®

**Therapeutic Category** Antibiotic, Quinolone

**Use** Quinolone antibiotic for skin and skin structure, lower respiratory and urinary tract infections, and sexually transmitted diseases

**Usual Dosage** Adults: Oral: 400 mg once daily for 10-14 days

(Continued)

## Lomefloxacin *(Continued)*

**Mechanism of Action** Inhibits DNA-gyrase in susceptible organisms thereby inhibits relaxation of supercoiled DNA and promotes breakage of DNA strands. DNA gyrase (topoisomerase II), is an essential bacterial enzyme that maintains the superhelical structure of DNA and is required for DNA replication and transcription, DNA repair, recombination, and transposition.

**Local Anesthetic/Vasoconstrictor Precautions** No information available to require special precautions

**Effects on Dental Treatment** No effects or complications reported

**Other Adverse Effects**

1% to 10%:

- Central nervous system: Headache, dizziness
- Dermatologic: Photosensitivity
- Gastrointestinal: Nausea

<1%:

- Cardiovascular: Flushing, chest pain, hypotension, hypertension, edema, syncope, tachycardia, bradycardia, arrhythmia, extrasystoles, cyanosis, cardiac failure, angina pectoris, myocardial infarction, face edema
- Central nervous system: Fatigue, malaise, chills, convulsions, vertigo, coma
- Dermatologic: Purpura, rash
- Endocrine & metabolic: Gout, hypoglycemia
- Gastrointestinal: Abdominal pain, vomiting, flatulence, constipation, dry mouth, thirst, taste perversion, tongue discoloration
- Genitourinary: Micturition disorder, dysuria
- Hematologic: Thrombocytopenia
- Neuromuscular & skeletal: Back pain, hyperkinesia, tremor, paresthesias, leg cramps, myalgia, weakness
- Otic: Earache
- Renal: Hematuria, anuria
- Respiratory: Dyspnea, cough, epistaxis
- Miscellaneous: Increased sweating, allergic reaction, flu-like symptoms, decreased heat tolerance, increased fibrinolysis

**Drug Interactions**

Decreased effect: Decreased absorption with antacids containing aluminum, magnesium, and/or calcium (by up to 98% if given at the same time)

Increased toxicity/serum levels: Quinolones cause increased levels of caffeine, warfarin, cyclosporine, and theophylline; azlocillin, cimetidine, probenecid increase quinolone levels

**Drug Uptake**

Absorption: Well absorbed

Serum half-life, elimination: 5-7.5 hours

**Pregnancy Risk Factor** C

**Generic Available** No

♦ **Lomotil®** *see* Diphenoxylate and Atropine *on page 340*

## Lomustine (loe MUS teen)

**U.S. Brand Names** CeeNU® Oral

**Therapeutic Category** Antineoplastic Agent, Alkylating Agent (Nitrosourea)

**Synonyms** CCNU

**Use** Treatment of brain tumors, Hodgkin's and non-Hodgkin's lymphomas, melanoma, renal carcinoma, lung cancer, colon cancer

**Usual Dosage** Oral (**refer to individual protocols**):

Children: 75-150 mg/m$^2$ as a single dose every 6 weeks. Subsequent doses are readjusted after initial treatment according to platelet and leukocyte counts.

Adults: 100-130 mg/m$^2$ as a single dose every 6 weeks; readjust after initial treatment according to platelet and leukocyte counts

With compromised marrow function: Initial dose: 100 mg/m$^2$ as a single dose every 6 weeks

**Subsequent dosing adjustment based on nadir:**

Leukocytes 2000-2900/mm$^3$, platelets 25,000-74,999/mm$^3$: Administer 70% of prior dose

Leukocytes <2000/mm$^3$, platelets <25,000/mm$^3$: Administer 50% of prior dose

**Mechanism of Action** Inhibits DNA and RNA synthesis via carbamylation of DNA polymerase, alkylation of DNA, and alteration of RNA, proteins, and enzymes

**Local Anesthetic/Vasoconstrictor Precautions** No information available to require special precautions

**Effects on Dental Treatment** No effects or complications reported

**Other Adverse Effects**

>10%:

Gastrointestinal: Nausea and vomiting occur 3-6 hours after oral administration; this is due to a centrally mediated mechanism, not a direct effect on the GI lining; if vomiting occurs, it is not necessary to replace the dose unless it occurs immediately after drug administration

Hematologic: Anemia; myelosuppressive effects occur 4-6 weeks after a dose and may persist for 1-2 weeks

1% to 10%:

Central nervous system: Neurotoxicity

Dermatologic: Rash

Gastrointestinal: Stomatitis, diarrhea

Hematologic: Anemia

<1%:

Central nervous system: Disorientation, lethargy, ataxia

Dermatologic: Alopecia

Hepatic: Hepatotoxicity

Neuromuscular & skeletal: Dysarthria

Renal: Renal failure

Respiratory: Pulmonary fibrosis with cumulative doses >600 mg

**Drug Uptake**

Absorption: Complete from GI tract; appears in plasma within 3 minutes after administration

Serum half-life: Parent drug: 16-72 hours

Active metabolite: Terminal half-life: 1.3-2 days

Time to peak serum concentration: Active metabolite: Within 3 hours

**Pregnancy Risk Factor** D

**Generic Available** No

**Comments** Myelosuppression is delayed about 4-6 weeks after a dose

♦ **Loniten®** *see* Minoxidil *on page 678*

♦ **Lonox®** *see* Diphenoxylate and Atropine *on page 340*

♦ **Lo/Ovral®** *see* Ethinyl Estradiol and Norgestrel *on page 407*

## Loperamide (loe PER a mide)

**U.S. Brand Names** Diar-aid® [OTC]; Imodium®; Imodium® A-D [OTC]; Kaopectate® II [OTC]; Pepto® Diarrhea Control [OTC]

**Canadian Brand Names** PMS-Loperamine

**Therapeutic Category** Antidiarrheal

**Use** Treatment of acute diarrhea and chronic diarrhea associated with inflammatory bowel disease; chronic functional diarrhea (idiopathic), chronic diarrhea caused by bowel resection or organic lesions; to decrease the volume of ileostomy discharge

**Unlabeled use:** Treatment of traveler's diarrhea in combination with trimethoprim-sulfamethoxazole (co-trimoxazole) (3 days therapy)

**Usual Dosage** Oral:

Children:

Acute diarrhea: Initial doses (in first 24 hours):

2-6 years: 1 mg three times/day

6-8 years: 2 mg twice daily

8-12 years: 2 mg three times/day

Maintenance: After initial dosing, 0.1 mg/kg doses after each loose stool, but not exceeding initial dosage

Chronic diarrhea: 0.08-0.24 mg/kg/day divided 2-3 times/day, maximum: 2 mg/dose

Adults: Initial: 4 mg (2 capsules), followed by 2 mg after each loose stool, up to 16 mg/day (8 capsules)

**Mechanism of Action** Acts directly on intestinal muscles to inhibit peristalsis and prolongs transit time enhancing fluid and electrolyte movement through intestinal mucosa; reduces fecal volume, increases viscosity, and diminishes fluid and electrolyte loss; demonstrates antisecretory activity; exhibits peripheral action

**Local Anesthetic/Vasoconstrictor Precautions** No information available to require special precautions

**Effects on Dental Treatment** No effects or complications reported

**Other Adverse Effects**

Central nervous system: Sedation, fatigue, dizziness, drowsiness

Dermatologic: Rash

Gastrointestinal: Nausea, vomiting, constipation, abdominal cramping, dry mouth, abdominal distention

**Drug Interactions** Increased toxicity: CNS depressants, phenothiazines, tricyclic antidepressants may potentiate the adverse effects of loperamide

(Continued)

## Loperamide *(Continued)*

**Drug Uptake**
Onset of action: Oral: Within 0.5-1 hour
Absorption: Oral: <40%; levels in breast milk expected to be very low
Serum half-life: 7-14 hours

**Pregnancy Risk Factor** B

**Generic Available** Yes

- **Lopid®** *see* Gemfibrozil *on page 465*
- **Lopremone** *see* Protirelin *on page 861*
- **Lopressor® [Tartrate]** *see* Metoprolol *on page 666*
- **Loprox®** *see* Ciclopirox *on page 247*
- **Lorabid™** *see* Loracarbef *on this page*

## Loracarbef (lor a KAR bef)

**U.S. Brand Names** Lorabid™

**Therapeutic Category** Antibiotic, Carbacephem

**Use** Infections caused by susceptible organisms involving the respiratory tract, acute otitis media, sinusitis, skin and skin structure, bone and joint, and urinary tract and gynecologic

**Usual Dosage** Oral:
Children:
Acute otitis media: 15 mg/kg twice daily for 10 days
Pharyngitis: 7.5-15 mg/kg twice daily for 10 days
Adults: Women:
Uncomplicated urinary tract infections: 200 mg once daily for 7 days
Skin and soft tissue: 200-400 mg every 12-24 hours
Uncomplicated pyelonephritis: 400 mg every 12 hours for 14 days

**Mechanism of Action** Inhibits bacterial cell wall synthesis by binding to one or more of the penicillin binding proteins (PBPs); inhibits the final transpeptidation step of peptidoglycan synthesis in bacterial cell walls, thus inhibiting cell wall biosynthesis. It is thought that beta-lactam antibiotics inactivate transpeptidase via acylation of the enzyme with cleavage of the CO-N bond of the beta-lactam ring. Upon exposure to beta-lactam antibiotics, bacteria eventually lyse due to ongoing activity of cell wall autolytic enzymes (autolysins and murein hydrolases) while cell wall assembly is arrested.

**Local Anesthetic/Vasoconstrictor Precautions** No information available to require special precautions

**Effects on Dental Treatment** No effects or complications reported

**Other Adverse Effects**
1% to 10%:
Central nervous system: Headache
Dermatologic: Skin rashes
Gastrointestinal: Diarrhea, nausea, vomiting, abdominal pain, anorexia
Genitourinary: Vaginitis, vaginal moniliasis
<1%:
Cardiovascular: Vasodilation
Central nervous system: Somnolence, nervousness, dizziness
Hematologic: Transient thrombocytopenia, leukopenia, and eosinophilia
Hepatic: Transient elevations of ALT, AST, alkaline phosphatase
Renal: Transient elevations of BUN and creatinine

**Drug Interactions** Increased serum levels with probenecid

**Drug Uptake**
Absorption: Oral: Rapid
Serum half-life, elimination: ~1 hour
Time to peak serum concentration: Oral: Within 1 hour

**Pregnancy Risk Factor** B

**Generic Available** No

## Loratadine (lor AT a deen)

**U.S. Brand Names** Claritin®

**Therapeutic Category** Antihistamine

**Use** Relief of nasal and non-nasal symptoms of seasonal allergic rhinitis

**Usual Dosage** Children >12 years and Adults: Oral: 10 mg/day on an empty stomach

**Mechanism of Action** Long-acting tricyclic antihistamine with selective peripheral histamine $H_1$ receptor antagonistic properties

**Local Anesthetic/Vasoconstrictor Precautions** No information available to require special precautions

**Effects on Dental Treatment** >10% of patients experience dry mouth which will disappear with cessation of drug therapy

**Other Adverse Effects**

>10%: Central nervous system: Headache, somnolence, fatigue

1% to 10%:

Cardiovascular: Hypotension, hypertension, palpitations, tachycardia

Central nervous system: Anxiety, depression

Endocrine & metabolic: Breast pain

Neuromuscular & skeletal: Hyperkinesia, arthralgias

Respiratory: Nasal dryness, pharyngitis, dyspnea

Miscellaneous: Sweating

**Drug Interactions**

Increased plasma concentrations of loratadine and its active metabolite with ketoconazole; erythromycin increases the AUC of loratadine and its active metabolite; no change in QTc interval was seen

Increased toxicity: Procarbazine, other antihistamines, alcohol

**Drug Uptake**

Onset of action: Within 1-3 hours

Peak effect: 8-12 hours

Duration: >24 hours

Absorption: Rapid

Serum half-life: 12-15 hours

**Pregnancy Risk Factor** B

**Dosage Forms**

Syrup: 1 mg/mL (480 mL)

Tablet: 10 mg

Rapid-disintegrating tablets: 10 mg (RediTabs®)

**Generic Available** No

## Loratadine and Pseudoephedrine

(lor AT a deen & soo doe e FED rin)

**Related Information**

Oral Bacterial Infections *on page 1128*

**U.S. Brand Names** Claritin-D®; Claritin-D 24-Hour®

**Canadian Brand Names** Chlor-Tripolon® N.D.; Claritin® Extra

**Therapeutic Category** Antihistamine/Decongestant Combination

**Use** Temporary relief of symptoms of seasonal and perennial allergic rhinitis, and vasomotor rhinitis, including nasal obstruction

**Usual Dosage** Adults: Oral: 1 tablet every 12 hours

**Local Anesthetic/Vasoconstrictor Precautions** Use with caution since pseudoephedrine is a sympathomimetic amine which could interact with epinephrine to cause a pressor response

**Effects on Dental Treatment** Up to 10% of patients could experience tachycardia, palpitations, and dry mouth; use vasoconstrictor with caution; over 10% of patients may experience dry mouth which will disappear with cessation of drug therapy

**Other Adverse Effects**

>10%:

Cardiovascular: Tachycardia

Central nervous system: Slight to moderate drowsiness, nervousness, transient stimulation, insomnia

Respiratory: Thickening of bronchial secretions

1% to 10%:

Central nervous system: Headache, fatigue, dizziness

Gastrointestinal: Appetite increase, weight gain, nausea, diarrhea, abdominal pain, dry mouth

Genitourinary: Dysuria

Neuromuscular & skeletal: Arthralgia, weakness

Respiratory: Pharyngitis

Miscellaneous: Sweating

<1%:

Cardiovascular: Edema, palpitations, hypotension

Central nervous system: Depression, sedation, paradoxical excitement, convulsions, hallucinations

Dermatologic: Angioedema, rash, photosensitivity

Genitourinary: Urinary retention

Hepatic: Hepatitis

Neuromuscular & skeletal: Myalgia, paresthesia, tremor

Ocular: Blurred vision

Respiratory: Bronchospasm, epistaxis, dyspnea

**Generic Available** No

## Lorazepam (lor A ze pam)

**Related Information**

Patients Requiring Sedation *on page 1152*
Temporomandibular Dysfunction (TMD) *on page 1149*

**U.S. Brand Names** Ativan®

**Canadian Brand Names** Apo®-Lorazepam; Novo-Lorazepam; Nu-Loraz; PMS-Lorazepam; Pro-Lorazepam®

**Therapeutic Category** Antianxiety Agent; Benzodiazepine; Hypnotic; Sedative; Tranquilizer, Minor

**Use** Management of anxiety, status epilepticus, preoperative sedation, for desired amnesia, and as an antiemetic adjunct

**Unapproved uses:** Alcohol detoxification, insomnia, psychogenic catatonia, partial complex seizures

**Usual Dosage**

Antiemetic:
- Children 2-15 years: I.V.: 0.05 mg/kg (up to 2 mg/dose) prior to chemotherapy
- Adults: Oral, I.V.: 0.5-2 mg every 4-6 hours as needed

Anxiety and sedation:
- Children: Oral, I.V.: Usual: 0.05 mg/kg/dose (range: 0.02-0.09 mg/kg) every 4-8 hours
- Adults: Oral: 1-10 mg/day in 2-3 divided doses; usual dose: 2-6 mg/day in divided doses

Insomnia: Adults: Oral: 2-4 mg at bedtime

Preoperative: Adults:
- I.M.: 0.05 mg/kg administered 2 hours before surgery; maximum: 4 mg/dose
- I.V.: 0.044 mg/kg 15-20 minutes before surgery; usual maximum: 2 mg/dose

Operative amnesia: Adults: I.V.: up to 0.05 mg/kg; maximum: 4 mg/dose

Status epilepticus: I.V.:
- Children: 0.1 mg/kg slow I.V. over 2-5 minutes, do not exceed 4 mg/single dose; may repeat second dose of 0.05 mg/kg slow I.V. in 10-15 minutes if needed
- Adolescents: 0.07 mg/kg slow I.V. over 2-5 minutes; maximum: 4 mg/dose; may repeat in 10-15 minutes
- Adults: 4 mg/dose given slowly over 2-5 minutes; may repeat in 10-15 minutes; usual maximum dose: 8 mg

**Mechanism of Action** Depresses all levels of the CNS, including the limbic and reticular formation, probably through the increased action of gamma-aminobutyric acid (GABA), which is a major inhibitory neurotransmitter in the brain.

**Local Anesthetic/Vasoconstrictor Precautions** No information available to require special precautions

**Effects on Dental Treatment** >10% of patients experience dry mouth; normal salivary flow occurs with cessation of drug therapy

**Other Adverse Effects**

>10%: Central nervous system: Sedation

1% to 10%:
- Central nervous system: Dizziness, unsteadiness
- Neuromuscular & skeletal: Weakness

<1%:
- Cardiovascular: Hypotension
- Central nervous system: Disorientation, fatigue, depression, headache, sleep disturbance
- Gastrointestinal: Nausea, appetite changes

**Drug Interactions**

Decreased effect with oral contraceptives (combination products), cigarette smoking; decreased effect of levodopa
Increased effect with morphine
Increased toxicity with alcohol, CNS depressants, MAO inhibitors, loxapine, tricyclic antidepressants

**Drug Uptake**

Onset of hypnosis: I.M.: 20-30 minutes
Duration: 6-8 hours
Absorption: Oral, I.M.: Prompt following administration
Serum half-life:
- Older Children: 10.5 hours
- Adults: 12.9 hours
- Elderly: 15.9 hours
- End-stage renal disease: 32-70 hours

**Pregnancy Risk Factor** D

**Dosage Forms**
Injection: 2 mg/mL (1 mL, 10 mL); 4 mg/mL (1 mL, 10 mL)
Solution, oral concentrated, alcohol and dye free: 2 mg/mL (30 mL)
Tablet: 0.5 mg, 1 mg, 2 mg

**Generic Available** Yes


- ♦ **Lorcet® [5/500]** *see* Hydrocodone and Acetaminophen *on page 505*
- ♦ **Lorcet®-HD [5/500]** *see* Hydrocodone and Acetaminophen *on page 505*
- ♦ **Lorcet® Plus [7.5/650]** *see* Hydrocodone and Acetaminophen *on page 505*
- ♦ **Lorelco®** *see* Probucol *on page 840*
- ♦ **Loroxide® [OTC]** *see* Benzoyl Peroxide *on page 130*
- ♦ **Lortab® 2.5/500** *see* Hydrocodone and Acetaminophen *on page 505*
- ♦ **Lortab® 5/500** *see* Hydrocodone and Acetaminophen *on page 505*
- ♦ **Lortab® 7.5/500** *see* Hydrocodone and Acetaminophen *on page 505*
- ♦ **Lortab® 10/500** *see* Hydrocodone and Acetaminophen *on page 505*
- ♦ **Lortab® 10/650** *see* Hydrocodone and Acetaminophen *on page 505*
- ♦ **Lortab® ASA** *see* Hydrocodone and Aspirin *on page 507*
- ♦ **Lortab® Elixir** *see* Hydrocodone and Acetaminophen *on page 505*
- ♦ **Lortab® Solution** *see* Hydrocodone and Acetaminophen *on page 505*


## Losartan (loe SAR tan)

**Related Information**
Cardiovascular Diseases *on page 1066*

**U.S. Brand Names** Cozaar®

**Therapeutic Category** Angiotensin II Antagonist

**Synonyms** DuP 753; Losartan Potassium; MK594

**Use** Treatment of hypertension alone or in combination with other antihypertensives; in considering the use of monotherapy with Cozaar®, it should be noted that in controlled trials Cozaar® had an effect on blood pressure that was notably less in black patients than in nonblacks, a finding similar to the small effect of ACE inhibitors in blacks

**Usual Dosage** Oral: The usual starting dose is 50 mg once daily; can be administered once or twice daily with total daily doses ranging from 25 mg to 100 mg
Usual initial doses in patients receiving diuretics or those with intravascular volume depletion: 25 mg
Patients not receiving diuretics: 50 mg

**Mechanism of Action** As a selective and competitive, nonpeptide angiotensin II receptor antagonist, losartan blocks the vasoconstrictor and aldosterone-secreting effects of angiotensin II; losartan interacts reversibly at the AT1 and AT2 receptors of many tissues and has slow dissociation kinetics; its affinity for the AT1 receptor is 1000 times greater than the AT2 receptor. Angiotensin II receptor antagonists may induce a more complete inhibition of the renin-angiotensin system than ACE inhibitors, they do not affect the response to bradykinin, and are less likely to be associated with nonrenin-angiotensin effects (eg, cough and angioedema). Losartan increases urinary flow rate and in addition to being natriuretic and kaliuretic, increases excretion of chloride, magnesium, uric acid, calcium, and phosphate.

**Local Anesthetic/Vasoconstrictor Precautions** No information available to require special precautions

**Effects on Dental Treatment** No effects or complications reported

**Other Adverse Effects**
1% to 10%:
Cardiovascular: Hypotension without reflex tachycardia
Central nervous system: Dizziness, insomnia
Endocrine & metabolic: Hyperkalemia
Gastrointestinal: Diarrhea, dyspepsia
Hematologic: Slight decreases in hemoglobin and hematocrit
Neuromuscular & skeletal: Back and leg pain, myalgia
Renal: Hypouricemia (with large doses)
Respiratory: Cough (less than ACE inhibitors), nasal congestion, sinus disorders, sinusitis

<1%:
Cardiovascular: Orthostatic effects, angina, second degree A-V block, CVA, palpitations, sinus bradycardia, tachycardia, flushing, facial edema
Central nervous system: Anxiety, ataxia, confusion, depression, dream abnormality, migraine headache, sleep disorders, vertigo, fever
Dermatologic: Alopecia, dermatitis, dry skin, bruising, erythema, photosensitivity, pruritus, rash, urticaria
Endocrine & metabolic: Gout, decreased libido
Gastrointestinal: Anorexia, constipation, flatulence, vomiting, taste alteration, gastritis

(Continued)

## Losartan *(Continued)*

Genitourinary: Impotence, nocturia, urinary tract infection
Hepatic: Slight elevations of LFTs and bilirubin
Neuromuscular & skeletal: Paresthesia; tremor; arm, hip, shoulder, and knee pain; joint swelling; fibromyalgia; muscle weakness
Ocular: Blurred vision, burning and stinging eyes, conjunctivitis, decreased visual acuity
Otic: Tinnitus
Renal: Mild elevation in BUN/creatinine, polyuria
Respiratory: Dyspnea, bronchitis, pharyngeal discomfort, epistaxis, rhinitis, respiratory congestion
Miscellaneous: Sweating

**Drug Uptake**
Onset of effect: 6 hours
Serum half-life:
Losartan: 1.5-2 hours
E-3174: 6-9 hours
Time to peak: Peak serum levels of losartan: 1 hour; metabolite, E-3174: 3-4 hours

**Pregnancy Risk Factor** C (first trimester); D (second & third trimester)
**Generic Available** No
**Comments** Cozaar® may be administered with other antihypertensive agents

## Losartan and Hydrochlorothiazide

(loe SAR tan & hye droe klor oh THYE a zide)
**U.S. Brand Names** Hyzaar®
**Therapeutic Category** Angiotensin II Antagonist; Diuretic, Thiazide
**Use** Treatment of hypertension
**Usual Dosage** Adults: Oral: 1 tablet daily
**Local Anesthetic/Vasoconstrictor Precautions** No information available to require special precautions
**Effects on Dental Treatment** No effects or complications reported
**Pregnancy Risk Factor** C (1st trimester); D (2nd and 3rd trimesters)
**Generic Available** No

♦ **Losartan Potassium** *see* Losartan *on previous page*
♦ **Lotemax®** *see* Loteprednol *on this page*
♦ **Lotensin®** *see* Benazepril *on page 125*
♦ **Lotensin HCT®** *see* Benazepril and Hydrochlorothiazide *on page 126*

## Loteprednol (loe te PRED nol)

**U.S. Brand Names** Alrex™; Lotemax®
**Therapeutic Category** Corticosteroid, Ophthalmic
**Synonyms** Loteprednol Etabonate
**Use**
0.2% suspension (Alrex™): Temporary relief of signs and symptoms of seasonal allergic conjunctivitis
0.5% suspension (Lotemax®): Inflammatory conditions (treatment of steroid-responsive inflammatory conditions of the palpebral and bulbar conjunctiva, cornea, and anterior segment of the globe such as allergic conjunctivitis, acne rosacea, superficial punctate keratitis, herpes zoster keratitis, iritis, cyclitis, selected infective conjunctivitis, when the inherent hazard of steroid use is accepted to obtain an advisable diminution in edema and inflammation) and treatment of postoperative inflammation following ocular surgery

**Usual Dosage** Adults: Ophthalmic:
0.2% suspension (Alrex™): Instill 1 drop into affected eye(s) 4 times/day
0.5% suspension (Lotemax®):
Inflammatory conditions: Apply 1-2 drops into the conjunctival sac of the affected eye(s) 4 times/day. During the initial treatment within the first week, the dosing may be increased up to 1 drop every hour. Advise patients not to discontinue therapy prematurely. If signs and symptoms fail to improve after 2 days, re-evaluate the patient.
Postoperative inflammation: Apply 1-2 drops into the conjunctival sac of the operated eye(s) 4 times/day beginning 24 hours after surgery and continuing throughout the first 2 weeks of the postoperative period

**Mechanism of Action** Corticosteroids inhibit the inflammatory response including edema, capillary dilation, leukocyte migration, and scar formation. Loteprednol is highly lipid soluble and penetrates cells readily to induce the production of lipocortins. These proteins modulate the activity of prostaglandins and leukotrienes.

**Local Anesthetic/Vasoconstrictor Precautions** No information available to require special precautions

**Effects on Dental Treatment** No effects or complications reported

**Other Adverse Effects**

Ocular: Increased intraocular pressure, changes in visual acuity and/or field defects, cataract formation, secondary ocular infection, globe perforation in disease which thins cornea or sclera

10% to 15%:

Central nervous system: Headache

Respiratory: Rhinitis, pharyngitis

5% to 10%: Ocular: Abnormal vision/blurring, burning on instillation, chemosis, dry eyes, itching, injection

<5%: Ocular: Conjunctivitis/irritation, corneal abnormalities, eyelid erythema, papillae uveitis

**Drug Uptake** Plasma levels following intraocular administration were not detectable

**Pregnancy Risk Factor** C

**Dosage Forms** Suspension, ophthalmic, as etabonate:

0.2% (Alrex™): 5 mL, 10 mL

0.5% (Lotemax®): 2.5 mL, 5 mL, 10 mL, 15 mL

**Generic Available** No

- **Loteprednol Etabonate** *see* Loteprednol *on previous page*
- **Lotrel®** *see* Amlodipine and Benazepril *on page 72*
- **Lotrimin® AF Powder [OTC]** *see* Miconazole *on page 672*
- **Lotrimin® AF Spray Liquid [OTC]** *see* Miconazole *on page 672*
- **Lotrimin® AF Spray Powder [OTC]** *see* Miconazole *on page 672*
- **Lotrisone®** *see* Betamethasone and Clotrimazole *on page 137*

## Lovastatin (LOE va sta tin)

**Related Information**

Cardiovascular Diseases *on page 1066*

**U.S. Brand Names** Mevacor®

**Canadian Brand Names** Apo®-Lovastatin

**Therapeutic Category** HMG-CoA Reductase Inhibitor; Lipid Lowering Drugs

**Use** Adjunct to dietary therapy to decrease elevated serum total and LDL cholesterol concentrations in primary hypercholesterolemia

**Usual Dosage** Adults: Oral: Initial: 20 mg with evening meal, then adjust at 4-week intervals; maximum dose: 80 mg/day; before initiation of therapy, patients should be placed on a standard cholesterol-lowering diet for 3-6 months and the diet should be continued during drug therapy

**Mechanism of Action** Lovastatin acts by competitively inhibiting 3-hydroxyl-3-methylglutaryl-coenzyme A (HMG-CoA) reductase, the enzyme that catalyzes the rate-limiting step in cholesterol biosynthesis

**Local Anesthetic/Vasoconstrictor Precautions** No information available to require special precautions

**Effects on Dental Treatment** No effects or complications reported

**Other Adverse Effects** Endocrine & metabolic: Gynecomastia

1% to 10%: Elevated creatine phosphokinase (CPK)

Central nervous system: Headache, dizziness

Dermatologic: Rash, pruritus

Gastrointestinal: Flatulence, abdominal pain, cramps, diarrhea, pancreatitis, constipation, nausea, dyspepsia, heartburn

Neuromuscular & skeletal: Myalgia

<1%:

Gastrointestinal: Dysgeusia

Ocular: Blurred vision, myositis, lenticular opacities

**Drug Interactions**

Increased toxicity: Gemfibrozil (musculoskeletal effects such as myopathy, myalgia and/or muscle weakness accompanied by markedly elevated CK concentrations, rash and/or pruritus); clofibrate, niacin (myopathy), erythromycin, cyclosporine, oral anticoagulants (elevated PT)

Increased effect/toxicity of levothyroxine

Concurrent use of erythromycin and lovastatin may result in rhabdomyolysis

**Drug Uptake**

Onset of effect: 3 days of therapy required for LDL cholesterol concentration reductions

Absorption: Oral: 30%

Serum half-life: 1.1-1.7 hours

Time to peak serum concentration: Oral: 2-4 hours

**Pregnancy Risk Factor** X

(Continued)

## Lovastatin *(Continued)*

**Generic Available** No

♦ **Lovenox®** *see* Enoxaparin *on page 370*

## Loxapine (LOKS a peen)

**U.S. Brand Names** Loxitane®

**Canadian Brand Names** Loxapac®

**Therapeutic Category** Antiemetic; Antipsychotic Agent; Phenothiazine Derivative

**Use** Treatment of psychoses, nausea and vomiting; Tourette's syndrome; mania; intractable hiccups (adults); behavioral problems (children)

**Usual Dosage** Adults:

Oral: 10 mg twice daily, increase dose until psychotic symptoms are controlled; usual dose range: 60-100 mg/day in divided doses 2-4 times/day; dosages >250 mg/day are not recommended

I.M.: 12.5-50 mg every 4-6 hours or longer as needed and change to oral therapy as soon as possible

**Mechanism of Action** Blocks postsynaptic mesolimbic dopaminergic receptors in the brain; exhibits a strong alpha-adrenergic blocking effect and depresses the release of hypothalamic and hypophyseal hormones; believed to depress the reticular-activating system, thus affecting basal metabolism, body temperatures, wakefulness, vasomotor tone, and emesis

**Local Anesthetic/Vasoconstrictor Precautions** Most pharmacology textbooks state that in presence of phenothiazines, systemic doses of epinephrine paradoxically decrease the blood pressure. This is the so called "epinephrine reversal" phenomenon. This has never been observed when epinephrine is given by infiltration as part of the anesthesia procedure.

**Effects on Dental Treatment** >10% of patients experience dry mouth. Significant hypotension may occur, especially when the drug is administered parenterally; orthostatic hypotension is due to alpha-receptor blockade, the elderly are at greater risk for orthostatic hypotension

Tardive dyskinesia: Prevalence rate may be 40% in elderly; development of the syndrome and the irreversible nature are proportional to duration and total cumulative dose over time

Extrapyramidal reactions are more common in elderly with up to 50% developing these reactions after 60 years of age; drug-induced **Parkinson's syndrome** occurs often; **Akathisia** is the most common extrapyramidal reaction in elderly

Increased confusion, memory loss, psychotic behavior, and agitation frequently occur as a consequence of anticholinergic effects

Antipsychotic associated sedation in nonpsychotic patients is extremely unpleasant due to feelings of depersonalization, derealization, and dysphoria

**Other Adverse Effects**

>10%:
- Cardiovascular: Orthostatic hypotension
- Central nervous system: Drowsiness, extrapyramidal effects (parkinsonian), confusion, persistent tardive dyskinesia
- Ocular: Blurred vision

1% to 10%:
- Dermatologic: Skin rash
- Endocrine & metabolic: Enlargement of breasts
- Gastrointestinal: Constipation, nausea, vomiting

<1%:
- Cardiovascular: Tachycardia, arrhythmias, abnormal T-waves with prolonged ventricular repolarization
- Central nervous system: Neuroleptic malignant syndrome (NMS), sedation, restlessness, anxiety, seizures, altered central temperature regulation
- Dermatologic: Hyperpigmentation, pruritus, rash, photosensitivity
- Endocrine & metabolic: Galactorrhea, amenorrhea, gynecomastia, sexual dysfunction
- Gastrointestinal: Weight gain, adynamic ileus
- Genitourinary: Urinary retention, overflow incontinence, priapism
- Hematologic: Agranulocytosis (more often in women between fourth and tenth week of therapy), leukopenia (usually in patients with large doses for prolonged periods)
- Hepatic: Cholestatic jaundice
- Ocular: Retinal pigmentation

**Drug Interactions**

Decreased effect of guanethidine, phenytoin

Increased toxicity with CNS depressants, metrizamide (increased seizure potential), guanabenz, MAO inhibitors

**Drug Uptake**

Onset of neuroleptic effect: Oral: Within 20-30 minutes

Peak effect: 1.5-3 hours

Duration: ~12 hours

Serum half-life, biphasic:

Initial: 5 hours

Terminal: 12-19 hours

**Pregnancy Risk Factor** C

**Generic Available** Yes

- **Loxitane®** *see* Loxapine *on previous page*
- **Lozol®** *see* Indapamide *on page 532*
- **L-PAM** *see* Melphalan *on page 626*
- **L-Sarcolysin** *see* Melphalan *on page 626*
- **Lubriderm® [OTC]** *see* Lanolin, Cetyl Alcohol, Glycerin, and Petrolatum *on page 573*
- **LubriTears® Solution [OTC]** *see* Artificial Tears *on page 97*
- **Ludiomil®** *see* Maprotiline *on page 615*
- **Lufyllin®** *see* Dyphylline *on page 361*
- **Luminal®** *see* Phenobarbital *on page 790*
- **Lupron®** *see* Leuprolide Acetate *on page 578*
- **Lupron® Depot** *see* Leuprolide Acetate *on page 578*
- **Lupron® Depot-Ped** *see* Leuprolide Acetate *on page 578*
- **Luride®** *see* Fluoride *on page 441*
- **Luride® Lozi-Tab®** *see* Fluoride *on page 441*
- **Luride®-SF Lozi-Tab®** *see* Fluoride *on page 441*
- **Luvox®** *see* Fluvoxamine *on page 451*
- **Lycolan® Elixir [OTC]** *see* L-Lysine *on page 597*

# Lyme Disease Vaccine

**U.S. Brand Names** LYMErix®

**Therapeutic Category** Vaccine

**Synonyms** Lyme Disease Vaccine (Recombinant OspA)

**Use** Active immunization against Lyme disease in individuals between 15-70 years of age

**Usual Dosage** Adults: I.M.: Vaccination with 3 doses of 30 mcg (0.5 mL), administered at 0, 1 and 12 months, is recommended for optimal protection

**Mechanism of Action** Lyme disease vaccine is a recombinant, noninfectious lipoprotein (OspA) derived from the outer surface of *Borrelia burgdorfi*, the causative agent of Lyme disease. Vaccination stimulates production of antibodies directed against this organism, including antibodies against the LA-2 epitope, which have bactericidal activity. Since OspA expression is down-regulated after inoculation into the human host, at least part of the vaccine's efficacy may be related to neutralization of bacteria within the midgut of the tick vector, preventing transmission to the human host.

**Local Anesthetic/Vasoconstrictor Precautions** No information available to require special precautions

**Effects on Dental Treatment** No effects or complications reported

**Other Adverse Effects** (Limited to overall self-reported events occurring within 30 days following a dose)

>10%: Local: Injection site pain (21.9%)

1% to 10%:

Central nervous system: Headache (5.6%), fatigue (3.9%), fever (2.6%), chills (2%), dizziness (1%)

Dermatologic: Rash (1.4%)

Gastrointestinal: Nausea (1.1%)

Neuromuscular & skeletal: Arthralgia (6.8%), myalgia (4.8%), muscle aches (2.8%), back pain (1.9%), stiffness (1%)

Respiratory: Upper respiratory tract infection (4.4%), sinusitis (3.2%), pharyngitis (2.5%), rhinitis (2.4%), cough (1.5%), bronchitis (1.1%)

Miscellaneous: Viral infection (2.8%), flu-like syndrome (2.5%)

Solicited adverse event rates were higher than unsolicited event rates (above). These included local reactions of soreness (93.5%), redness (41.8%), and swelling (29.9%). In addition, general systemic symptoms included fatigue (40.8%), headache (38.6%), arthralgia (25.6%), rash (11.7%) and fever (3.5%)

Patients with a history of Lyme disease were noted to experience a higher frequency of early musculoskeletal reactions. Other differences in the observed

(Continued)

## Lyme Disease Vaccine *(Continued)*

rate of adverse reactions were not significantly different between vaccine and placebo recipients.

**Drug Interactions** No data available

**Pregnancy Risk Factor** C

**Dosage Forms** Injection:

Vial: 30 mcg/0.5 mL

Prefilled syringe (Tip-Lok™): 30 mcg/0.5 mL

- ♦ **Lyme Disease Vaccine (Recombinant OspA)** *see* Lyme Disease Vaccine *on previous page*
- ♦ **LYMErix®** *see* Lyme Disease Vaccine *on previous page*

## Lymphocyte Immune Globulin (LIM foe site i MYUN GLOB yoo lin)

**U.S. Brand Names** Atgam®

**Therapeutic Category** Immunosuppressant Agent

**Synonyms** Antithymocyte Globulin (Equine); Antithymocyte Immunoglobulin; ATG; Horse Anti-human Thymocyte Gamma Globulin

**Use** Prevention and treatment of acute allograft rejection; treatment of moderate to severe aplastic anemia in patients not considered suitable candidates for bone marrow transplantation; prevention of graft-vs-host disease following bone marrow transplantation

**Usual Dosage** An intradermal skin test is recommended prior to administration of the initial dose of ATG; use 0.1 mL of a 1:1000 dilution of ATG in normal saline

Children: I.V.:

Aplastic anemia protocol: 10-20 mg/kg/day for 8-14 days, then give every other day for 7 more doses

Cardiac allograft: 10 mg/kg/day for 7 days

Renal allograft: 5-25 mg/kg/day

Adults: I.V.:

Aplastic anemia protocol: 10-20 mg/kg/day for 8-14 days, then give every other day for 7 more doses **or** 40 mg/kg/day for 4 days

Rejection prevention: 15 mg/kg/day for 14 days, then give every other day for 7 more doses for a total of 21 doses in 28 days; initial dose should be administered within 24 hours before or after transplantation

Rejection treatment: 10-15 mg/kg/day for 14 days, then give every other day for 7 more doses

**Mechanism of Action** May involve elimination of antigen-reactive T-lymphocytes (killer cells) in peripheral blood or alteration of T-cell function

**Local Anesthetic/Vasoconstrictor Precautions** No information available to require special precautions

**Effects on Dental Treatment** No effects or complications reported

**Other Adverse Effects**

>10%:

Central nervous system: Fever, chills

Dermatologic: Rash

Hematologic: Leukopenia, thrombocytopenia

Miscellaneous: Systemic infection

1% to 10%:

Cardiovascular: Hypotension, hypertension, tachycardia, edema, chest pain

Central nervous system: Headache, malaise

Gastrointestinal: Diarrhea, nausea, stomatitis, GI bleeding

Respiratory: Dyspnea

Local: Pain, swelling or redness at injection site, thrombophlebitis

Neuromuscular & skeletal: Myalgia, back pain

Renal: Abnormal renal function tests

Miscellaneous: Viral infection, anaphylaxis may be indicated by hypotension, respiratory distress, serum sickness

<1%:

Central nervous system: Seizures

Dermatologic: Pruritus, urticaria

Hematologic: Hemolysis, anemia

Neuromuscular & skeletal: Arthralgia, weakness

Renal: Acute renal failure

Miscellaneous: Lymphadenopathy

**Drug Uptake** Serum half-life: 1.5-12 days

**Pregnancy Risk Factor** C

**Generic Available** No

**Comments** Do not dilute with $D_5W$ (may cause precipitation). The use of highly acidic infusion solutions is not recommended because of possible physical instability. When the dose of corticosteroids and other immunosuppressants is being reduced, some previously masked reaction to Atgam® may appear.

- ♦ **Lyphocin®** *see* Vancomycin *on page 1039*

## Lypressin (lye PRES in)

**U.S. Brand Names** Diapid®

**Therapeutic Category** Antidiuretic Hormone Analog

**Use** Controls or prevents signs and complications of neurogenic diabetes insipidus

**Usual Dosage** Children and Adults: Instill 1-2 sprays into one or both nostrils whenever frequency of urination increases or significant thirst develops; usual dosage is 1-2 sprays 4 times/day; range: 1 spray/day at bedtime to 10 sprays each nostril every 3-4 hours

**Mechanism of Action** Increases cyclic adenosine monophosphate (cAMP) which increases water permeability at the renal tubule resulting in decreased urine volume and increased osmolality; causes peristalsis by directly stimulating the smooth muscle in the GI tract

**Local Anesthetic/Vasoconstrictor Precautions** No information available to require special precautions

**Effects on Dental Treatment** No effects or complications reported

**Other Adverse Effects**

1% to 10%:

Central nervous system: Dizziness, headache

Gastrointestinal: Abdominal cramping, increased bowel movements

Respiratory: Chest tightness, coughing, dyspnea, rhinorrhea, nasal congestion, irritation or burning

<1%:

Endocrine & metabolic: Water intoxication

Respiratory: Inadvertent inhalation

**Drug Interactions** Increased effect: Chlorpropamide, clofibrate, carbamazepine causes prolongation of antidiuretic effects

**Drug Uptake**

Onset of antidiuretic effect: Intranasal spray: Within 0.5-2 hours

Duration: 3-8 hours

Serum half-life: 15-20 minutes

**Pregnancy Risk Factor** C

**Generic Available** No

- ♦ **Lysodren®** *see* Mitotane *on page 681*
- ♦ **Maalox® [OTC]** *see* Aluminum Hydroxide and Magnesium Hydroxide *on page 56*
- ♦ **Maalox® Anti-Gas® [OTC]** *see* Simethicone *on page 915*
- ♦ **Maalox® Plus [OTC]** *see* Aluminum Hydroxide, Magnesium Hydroxide, and Simethicone *on page 56*
- ♦ **Maalox® Therapeutic Concentrate [OTC]** *see* Aluminum Hydroxide and Magnesium Hydroxide *on page 56*
- ♦ **Macrobid®** *see* Nitrofurantoin *on page 724*
- ♦ **Macrodantin®** *see* Nitrofurantoin *on page 724*
- ♦ **Macrodex®** *see* Dextran *on page 311*

## Mafenide (MA fe nide)

**U.S. Brand Names** Sulfamylon®

**Therapeutic Category** Antibacterial, Topical; Antibiotic, Topical

**Use** Adjunct in the treatment of second and third degree burns to prevent septicemia caused by susceptible organisms such as *Pseudomonas aeruginosa*; prevention of graft loss of meshed autografts on excised burn wounds

**Usual Dosage** Children and Adults: Topical: Apply once or twice daily with a sterile gloved hand; apply to a thickness of approximately 16 mm; the burned area should be covered with cream at all times

**Mechanism of Action** Interferes with bacterial folic acid synthesis through competitive inhibition of para-aminobenzoic acid

**Local Anesthetic/Vasoconstrictor Precautions** No information available to require special precautions

**Effects on Dental Treatment** No effects or complications reported

**Other Adverse Effects**

>10%: Local: Burning sensation, excoriation, pain

1% to 10%:

Cardiovascular: Swelling of face

Dermatologic: Skin rash

Respiratory: Dyspnea

(Continued)

## Mafenide *(Continued)*

<1%:

Dermatologic: Erythema

Endocrine & metabolic: Hyperchloremia, metabolic acidosis

Hematologic: Bone marrow suppression, hemolytic anemia, bleeding, porphyria

Respiratory: Hyperventilation, tachypnea

Miscellaneous: Hypersensitivity

**Drug Interactions** No data reported

**Drug Uptake**

Absorption: Diffuses through devascularized areas and is rapidly absorbed from burned surface

Time to peak serum concentration: Topical: 2-4 hours

**Pregnancy Risk Factor** C

**Generic Available** No

## Magaldrate (MAG al drate)

**U.S. Brand Names** Riopan® [OTC]

**Therapeutic Category** Antacid

**Synonyms** Hydromagnesium Aluminate

**Use** Symptomatic relief of hyperacidity associated with peptic ulcer, gastritis, peptic esophagitis and hiatal hernia

**Usual Dosage** Adults: Oral: 540-1080 mg between meals and at bedtime

**Local Anesthetic/Vasoconstrictor Precautions** No information available to require special precautions

**Effects on Dental Treatment** No effects or complications reported

**Other Adverse Effects**

>10%: Gastrointestinal: Constipation, chalky taste, stomach cramps, fecal impaction

1% to 10%: Gastrointestinal: Nausea, vomiting, discoloration of feces (white speckles)

<1%: Endocrine & metabolic: Hypophosphatemia, hypomagnesemia

**Pregnancy Risk Factor** C

**Generic Available** Yes

**Comments** Chemical entity known as hydroxy magnesium aluminate equivalent to magnesium oxide and aluminum oxide; unlike other magnesium-containing antacids, Riopan® is safe to use in renal patients

## Magaldrate and Simethicone (MAG al drate & sye METH i kone)

**U.S. Brand Names** Riopan Plus® [OTC]

**Canadian Brand Names** Riopan® Plus Extra Strength

**Therapeutic Category** Antacid; Antiflatulent

**Synonyms** Simethicone and Magaldrate

**Use** Relief of hyperacidity associated with peptic ulcer, gastritis, peptic esophagitis and hiatal hernia which are accompanied by symptoms of gas

**Usual Dosage** Adults: Oral: 5-10 mL between meals and at bedtime

**Local Anesthetic/Vasoconstrictor Precautions** No information available to require special precautions

**Effects on Dental Treatment** No effects or complications reported

**Pregnancy Risk Factor** C

**Generic Available** Yes

**Comments** Chemical entity known as hydroxy magnesium aluminate equivalent to magnesium oxide and aluminum oxide; unlike other magnesium containing antacids, Riopan® is safe to use in renal patients if used cautiously

♦ **Magalox Plus® [OTC]** *see* Aluminum Hydroxide, Magnesium Hydroxide, and Simethicone *on page 56*

♦ **Magan®** *see* Magnesium Salicylate *on page 613*

♦ **Magnacal® [OTC]** *see* Enteral Nutritional Products *on page 371*

## Magnesium Chloride (mag NEE zhum KLOR ide)

**U.S. Brand Names** Slow-Mag® [OTC]

**Therapeutic Category** Magnesium Salt

**Use** Correct or prevent hypomagnesemia

**Usual Dosage**

Oral: Adults: Dietary supplement: 54-283 mg/day in divided doses

I.V. in TPN:

Children: 2-10 mEq/day

The usual recommended pediatric maintenance intake of magnesium ranges from 0.2-0.6 mEq/kg/day. The dose of magnesium may also be based on the caloric intake; on that basis, 3-10 mEq/day of magnesium are needed; maximum maintenance dose: 8-16 mEq/day

Adults: 8-24 mEq/day

**Local Anesthetic/Vasoconstrictor Precautions** No information available to require special precautions

**Effects on Dental Treatment** Magnesium products may prevent gastrointestinal absorption of tetracyclines by forming a large ionized chelated molecule with the tetracyclines in the stomach. Tetracyclines should be given at least 1 hour before magnesium.

**Other Adverse Effects** 1% to 10%:

Cardiovascular: Flushing

Central nervous system: Depressed CNS, somnolence

Gastrointestinal: Diarrhea

Neuromuscular & skeletal: Blocked peripheral neuromuscular transmission, deep tendon reflexes

Respiratory: Respiratory paralysis

**Pregnancy Risk Factor** D

**Generic Available** Yes

## Magnesium Citrate (mag NEE zhum SIT rate)

**U.S. Brand Names** Evac-Q-Mag® [OTC]

**Therapeutic Category** Laxative, Saline

**Synonyms** Citrate of Magnesia

**Use** To evacuate bowel prior to certain surgical and diagnostic procedures

**Usual Dosage** Cathartic: Oral:

Children:

<6 years: 0.5 mL/kg up to a maximum of 200 mL repeated every 4-6 hours until stools are clear

6-12 years: 100-150 mL

Children ≥12 years and Adults: ½ to 1 full bottle (120-300 mL)

**Mechanism of Action** Promotes bowel evacuation by causing osmotic retention of fluid which distends the colon with increased peristaltic activity

**Local Anesthetic/Vasoconstrictor Precautions** No information available to require special precautions

**Effects on Dental Treatment** Magnesium products may prevent gastrointestinal absorption of tetracyclines by forming a large ionized chelated molecule with the tetracyclines in the stomach. Tetracyclines should be given at least 1 hour before magnesium.

**Other Adverse Effects** 1% to 10%:

Cardiovascular: Hypotension

Endocrine & metabolic: Hypermagnesemia

Gastrointestinal: Abdominal cramps, diarrhea, gas formation

Respiratory: Respiratory depression

**Drug Uptake** Absorption: Oral: 15% to 30%

**Pregnancy Risk Factor** B

**Generic Available** Yes

**Comments** Magnesium content of 5 mL: 3.85-4.71 mEq

## Magnesium Gluconate (mag NEE zhum GLOO koe nate)

**U.S. Brand Names** Magonate® [OTC]

**Therapeutic Category** Magnesium Salt

**Use** Dietary supplement for treatment of magnesium deficiencies

**Usual Dosage** The recommended dietary allowance (RDA) of magnesium is 4.5 mg/kg which is a total daily allowance of 350-400 mg for adult men and 280-300 mg for adult women. During pregnancy the RDA is 300 mg and during lactation the RDA is 355 mg. Average daily intakes of dietary magnesium have declined in recent years due to processing of food. The latest estimate of the average American dietary intake was 349 mg/day.

Dietary supplement: Oral:

Children: 3-6 mg/kg/day in divided doses 3-4 times/day; maximum: 400 mg/day

Adults: 27-54 mg 2-3 times/day or 100 mg 4 times/day

**Mechanism of Action** Magnesium is important as a cofactor in many enzymatic reactions in the body involving protein synthesis and carbohydrate metabolism, (at least 300 enzymatic reactions require magnesium). Actions on lipoprotein lipase have been found to be important in reducing serum cholesterol and on sodium/potassium ATPase in promoting polarization (ie, neuromuscular functioning).

**Local Anesthetic/Vasoconstrictor Precautions** No information available to require special precautions

**Effects on Dental Treatment** Magnesium products may prevent gastrointestinal absorption of tetracyclines by forming a large ionized chelated molecule with

(Continued)

## Magnesium Gluconate *(Continued)*

the tetracyclines in the stomach. Tetracyclines should be given at least 1 hour before magnesium.

**Other Adverse Effects**

1% to 10%: Gastrointestinal: Diarrhea (excessive dose)

<1%:

Endocrine & metabolic: Hypotension, hypermagnesemia
Gastrointestinal: Abdominal cramps
Neuromuscular & skeletal: Muscle weakness
Respiratory: Respiratory depression

**Drug Uptake** Absorption: Oral: 15% to 30%

**Generic Available** Yes

**Comments** Magnesium content of 500 mg: 27 mg

## Magnesium Hydroxide (mag NEE zhum hye DROKS ide)

**U.S. Brand Names** Phillips'® Milk of Magnesia [OTC]

**Therapeutic Category** Antacid; Laxative, Saline; Magnesium Salt

**Use** Short-term treatment of occasional constipation and symptoms of hyperacidity, magnesium replacement therapy

**Usual Dosage** Oral:

Laxative:

<2 years: 0.5 mL/kg/dose
2-5 years: 5-15 mL/day or in divided doses
6-12 years: 15-30 mL/day or in divided doses
≥12 years: 30-60 mL/day or in divided doses

Antacid:

Children: 2.5-5 mL as needed up to 4 times/day
Adults: 5-15 mL or 650 mg to 1.3 g tablets up to 4 times/day as needed

**Mechanism of Action** Promotes bowel evacuation by causing osmotic retention of fluid which distends the colon with increased peristaltic activity; reacts with hydrochloric acid in stomach to form magnesium chloride

**Local Anesthetic/Vasoconstrictor Precautions** No information available to require special precautions

**Effects on Dental Treatment** Magnesium products may prevent gastrointestinal absorption of tetracyclines by forming a large ionized chelated molecule with the tetracyclines in the stomach. Tetracyclines should be given at least 1 hour before magnesium.

**Other Adverse Effects**

>10%: Diarrhea

1% to 10%:

Cardiovascular: Hypotension
Endocrine & metabolic: Hypermagnesemia
Gastrointestinal: Abdominal cramps
Neuromuscular & skeletal: Muscle weakness
Respiratory: Respiratory depression

**Drug Interactions** Decreased effect: Decreased absorption of tetracyclines, digoxin, indomethacin, or iron salts

**Drug Uptake** Onset of laxative action: 4-8 hours

**Pregnancy Risk Factor** B

**Generic Available** Yes

♦ **Magnesium Hydroxide and Aluminum Hydroxide** *see* Aluminum Hydroxide and Magnesium Hydroxide *on page 56*

## Magnesium Hydroxide and Mineral Oil Emulsion

(mag NEE zhum hye DROKS ide & MIN er al oyl e MUL shun)

**U.S. Brand Names** Haley's M-O® [OTC]

**Therapeutic Category** Laxative, Lubricant; Laxative, Saline

**Synonyms** MOM/Mineral Oil Emulsion

**Use** Short-term treatment of occasional constipation

**Usual Dosage** Adults: Oral: 5-45 mL at bedtime

**Local Anesthetic/Vasoconstrictor Precautions** No information available to require special precautions

**Effects on Dental Treatment** Magnesium products may prevent gastrointestinal absorption of tetracyclines by forming a large ionized chelated molecule with the tetracyclines in the stomach. Tetracyclines should be given at least 1 hour before magnesium.

**Pregnancy Risk Factor** B

**Generic Available** Yes

## Magnesium Oxide (mag NEE zhum OKS ide)

**U.S. Brand Names** Maox®

**Therapeutic Category** Antacid

**Use** Short-term treatment of occasional constipation and symptoms of hyperacidity

**Usual Dosage** Magnesium RDA: 4.5 mg/kg, which is a total daily allowance of 350 mg for adult men and 280-300 mg for adult women. During pregnancy, the RDA is 200 mg and during lactation it is 355 mg. Average daily intakes of dietary magnesium have declined in recent years due to processing of food. The latest estimate of the average American dietary intake was 349 mg/day.

Adults: Oral:

Dietary supplement: 27-54 mEq (1-2 tablets) 2-3 times/day

Antacid: $^1/_2$ to 3 tablets (0.21-1.68 g) with water or milk 4 times/day after meals and at bedtime

Laxative: 2-4 g at bedtime with full glass of water

**Mechanism of Action** Promotes bowel evacuation by causing osmotic retention of fluid which distends the colon with increased peristaltic activity

**Local Anesthetic/Vasoconstrictor Precautions** No information available to require special precautions

**Effects on Dental Treatment** Magnesium products may prevent gastrointestinal absorption of tetracyclines by forming a large ionized chelated molecule with the tetracyclines in the stomach. Tetracyclines should be given at least 1 hour before magnesium.

**Other Adverse Effects**

>10%: Diarrhea

1% to 10%:

Cardiovascular: Hypotension, EKG changes

Central nervous system: Mental depression, coma

Gastrointestinal: Nausea, vomiting

Respiratory: Respiratory depression

**Drug Interactions** Decreased effect: Tetracyclines, digoxin, indomethacin, iron salts, isoniazid, quinolones

**Drug Uptake** Onset of laxative action: 4-8 hours

**Pregnancy Risk Factor** B

**Generic Available** Yes

## Magnesium Salicylate (mag NEE zhum sa LIS i late)

**U.S. Brand Names** Doan's®, Original [OTC]; Extra Strength Doan's® [OTC]; Magan®; Mobidin®

**Therapeutic Category** Nonsteroidal Anti-inflammatory Drug (NSAID), Oral

**Use** Mild to moderate pain, fever, various inflammatory conditions

**Usual Dosage** Oral: Adults: 650 mg 4 times daily or 1090 mg 3 times daily; may increase to 3.6-4.8 mg/day in 3 or 4 divided doses

**Local Anesthetic/Vasoconstrictor Precautions** No information available to require special precautions

**Effects on Dental Treatment** NSAID formulations are known to reversibly decrease platelet aggregation via mechanisms different than observed with aspirin. The dentist should be aware of the potential of abnormal coagulation. Caution should also be exercised in the use of NSAIDs in patients already on anticoagulant therapy with drugs such as warfarin (Coumadin®).

**Dosage Forms**

Caplet:

Doan's®, Original: 325 mg

Extra Strength Doan's®: 500 mg

Tablet:

Magan®: 545 mg

Mobidin®: 600 mg

**Generic Available** Yes

## Magnesium Sulfate (mag NEE zhum SUL fate)

**Therapeutic Category** Anticonvulsant, Miscellaneous; Electrolyte Supplement, Parenteral; Laxative, Saline; Magnesium Salt

**Synonyms** Epsom Salts

**Use** Treatment and prevention of hypomagnesemia; hypertension; encephalopathy and seizures associated with acute nephritis in children; also used as a cathartic

**Usual Dosage** The recommended dietary allowance (RDA) of magnesium is 4.5 mg/kg which is a total daily allowance of 350-400 mg for adult men and 280-300 mg for adult women. During pregnancy the RDA is 300 mg and during lactation the RDA is 355 mg. Average daily intakes of dietary magnesium have declined in recent years due to processing of food. The latest estimate of the average

(Continued)

## Magnesium Sulfate *(Continued)*

American dietary intake was 349 mg/day. Dose represented as $MgSO_4$ unless stated otherwise.

**Note:** Serum magnesium is poor reflection of repletional status as the majority of magnesium is intracellular; serum levels may be transiently normal for a few hours after a dose is given, therefore, aim for consistently high normal serum levels in patients with normal renal function for most efficient repletion

Hypomagnesemia:

Children: I.M., I.V.: 25-50 mg/kg/dose (0.2-0.4 mEq/kg/dose) every 4-6 hours for 3-4 doses, maximum single dose: 2000 mg (16 mEq), may repeat if hypomagnesemia persists (higher dosage up to 100 mg/kg/dose $MgSO_4$ I.V. has been used); maintenance: I.V.: 30-60 mg/kg/day (0.25-0.5 mEq/kg/day)

Management of seizures and hypertension:

Children:

Oral: 100-200 mg/kg/dose 4 times/day

I.M., I.V.: 20-100 mg/kg/dose every 4-6 hours as needed; in severe cases doses as high as 200 mg/kg/dose have been used

Adults:

Oral: 3 g every 6 hours for 4 doses as needed

I.M., I.V.: 1 g every 6 hours for 4 doses; for severe hypomagnesemia: 8-12 g $MgSO_4$/day in divided doses has been used

Eclampsia, pre-eclampsia: Adults:

I.M.: 1-4 g every 4 hours

I.V.: Initial: 4 g, then switch to I.M. or 1-4 g/hour by continuous infusion

Maximum dose should not exceed 30-40 g/day; maximum rate of infusion: 1-2 g/hour

Maintenance electrolyte requirements:

Daily requirements: 0.2-0.5 mEq/kg/24 hours or 3-10 mEq/1000 kcal/24 hours

Maximum: 8-16 mEq/24 hours

Cathartic: Oral:

Children: 0.25 g/kg every 4-6 hours

Adults: 10-15 g in a glass of water

**Mechanism of Action** Promotes bowel evacuation by causing osmotic retention of fluid which distends the colon with increased peristaltic activity when taken orally; parenterally, decreases acetylcholine in motor nerve terminals and acts on myocardium by slowing rate of S-A node impulse formation and prolonging conduction time

**Local Anesthetic/Vasoconstrictor Precautions** No information available to require special precautions

**Effects on Dental Treatment** Magnesium products may prevent gastrointestinal absorption of tetracyclines by forming a large ionized chelated molecule with the tetracyclines in the stomach. Tetracyclines should be given at least 1 hour before magnesium.

**Other Adverse Effects**

1% to 10%:

Serum magnesium levels >3 mg/dL:

Central nervous system: Depressed CNS

Gastrointestinal: Diarrhea

Neuromuscular & skeletal: Blocked peripheral neuromuscular transmission leading to anticonvulsant effects

Serum magnesium levels >5 mg/dL:

Cardiovascular: Flushing

Central nervous system: Somnolence

Serum magnesium levels >12.5 mg/dL:

Cardiovascular: Complete heart block

Respiratory: Respiratory paralysis

**Drug Uptake**

Oral: Onset of cathartic action: Within 1-2 hours

I.M.:

Onset of action: 1 hour

Duration: 3-4 hours

I.V.:

Onset of action: Immediate

Duration: 30 minutes

**Pregnancy Risk Factor** B

**Generic Available** Yes

**Comments** $MgSO_4$ 500 mg = magnesium 4.06 mEq = elemental magnesium 49.3 mg

- **Magonate® [OTC]** *see* Magnesium Gluconate *on page 611*
- **Malatal®** *see* Hyoscyamine, Atropine, Scopolamine, and Phenobarbital *on page 520*
- **Mallamint® [OTC]** *see* Calcium Carbonate *on page 172*
- **Mallazine® Eye Drops [OTC]** *see* Tetrahydrozoline *on page 967*

## Malt Soup Extract (malt soop EKS trakt)

**U.S. Brand Names** Maltsupex® [OTC]

**Therapeutic Category** Laxative, Bulk-Producing

**Use** Short-term treatment of constipation

**Usual Dosage** Oral:

Infants >1 month:

Breast fed: 1-2 teaspoonfuls in 2-4 oz of water or fruit juice 1-2 times/day

Bottle fed: 1/2 to 2 tablespoonfuls/day in formula for 3-4 days, then 1-2 teaspoonfuls/day

Children 2-11 years: 1-2 tablespoonfuls 1-2 times/day

Children ≥12 years and Adults:

Liquid: 2 tablespoonfuls twice daily for 3-4 days, then 1-2 tablespoonfuls every evening

Tablet: 4 tablets 4 times/day

**Local Anesthetic/Vasoconstrictor Precautions** No information available to require special precautions

**Effects on Dental Treatment** No effects or complications reported

**Other Adverse Effects** 1% to 10%: Gastrointestinal: Abdominal cramps, diarrhea, rectal obstruction

**Generic Available** No

- **Maltsupex® [OTC]** *see* Malt Soup Extract *on this page*
- **Mandelamine®** *see* Methenamine *on page 647*
- **Mandol®** *see* Cefamandole *on page 199*
- **Manganese** *see* Trace Metals *on page 1001*
- **Mantoux** *see* Tuberculin Purified Protein Derivative *on page 1031*
- **Maolate®** *see* Chlorphenesin *on page 231*
- **Maox®** *see* Magnesium Oxide *on page 613*
- **Mapap® [OTC]** *see* Acetaminophen *on page 27*

## Maprotiline (ma PROE ti leen)

**Related Information**

Vasoconstrictor Interactions With Antidepressants *on page 1277*

**U.S. Brand Names** Ludiomil®

**Therapeutic Category** Antidepressant, Tetracyclic

**Use** Treatment of depression and anxiety associated with depression

**Usual Dosage** Oral:

Children 6-14 years: 10 mg/day, increase to a maximum daily dose of 75 mg

Adults: 75 mg/day to start, increase by 25 mg every 2 weeks up to 150-225 mg/day; given in 3 divided doses or in a single daily dose

Elderly: Initial: 25 mg at bedtime, increase by 25 mg every 3 days for inpatients and weekly for outpatients if tolerated; usual maintenance dose: 50-75 mg/day, higher doses may be necessary in nonresponders

**Mechanism of Action** Traditionally believed to increase the synaptic concentration of norepinephrine in the central nervous system by inhibition of their reuptake by the presynaptic neuronal membrane. However, additional receptor effects have been found including desensitization of adenyl cyclase, down regulation of beta-adrenergic receptors, and down regulation of serotonin receptors.

**Local Anesthetic/Vasoconstrictor Precautions** Use with caution; epinephrine, norepinephrine and levonordefrin have been shown to have an increased pressor response in combination with TCAs

**Effects on Dental Treatment** >10% of patients experience dry mouth; long-term treatment with TCAs such as amoxapine increases the risk of caries by reducing salivation and salivary buffer capacity

**Other Adverse Effects**

>10%:

Cardiovascular: Orthostatic hypotension

Central nervous system: Drowsiness

Dermatologic: Skin rash

Genitourinary: Urinary retention

Neuromuscular & skeletal: Weakness

1% to 10%:

Central nervous system: Insomnia

Gastrointestinal: Constipation, nausea, vomiting, increased appetite and weight gain, weight loss

(Continued)

## Maprotiline *(Continued)*

Neuromuscular & skeletal: Trembling

<1%:

Central nervous system: Confusion
Endocrine & metabolic: Breast enlargement
Genitourinary: Swelling of testicles
Hepatic: Cholestatic hepatitis
Ocular: Blurred vision, increased intraocular pressure
Otic: Tinnitus

**Drug Interactions**

Decreased effect: Phenobarbital may increase the metabolism of maprotiline; maprotiline blocks the uptake of guanethidine and thus prevents the hypotensive effect of guanethidine

Increased toxicity: Clonidine causes hypertensive crisis; maprotiline may be additive with or may potentiate the action of other CNS depressants such as sedatives or hypnotics; with MAO inhibitors, hyperpyrexia, hypertension, tachycardia, confusion, and seizures. Maprotiline may increase the prothrombin time in patients stabilized on warfarin; maprotiline potentiate the pressor and cardiac effects of sympathomimetic agents such as isoproterenol, epinephrine, etc; cimetidine and methylphenidate may decrease the metabolism of maprotiline

Additive anticholinergic effects seen with other anticholinergic agents

**Drug Uptake**

Absorption: Slow
Serum half-life: 27-58 hours (mean, 43 hours)
Time to peak serum concentration: Within 12 hours

**Pregnancy Risk Factor** B

**Generic Available** Yes

**Selected Readings**

Boakes AJ, Laurence DR, Teoh PC, et al, "Interactions Between Sympathomimetic Amines and Antidepressant Agents in Man," *Br Med J*, 1973, 1(849):311-5.

Jastak JT and Yagiela JA, "Vasoconstrictors and Local Anesthesia: A Review and Rationale for Use," *J Am Dent Assoc*, 1983, 107(4):623-30.

Larochelle P, Hamet P, and Enjalbert M, "Responses to Tyramine and Norepinephrine After Imipramine and Trazodone," *Clin Pharmacol Ther*, 1979, 26(1):24-30.

Mitchell JR, "Guanethidine and Related Agents. III Antagonism by Drugs Which Inhibit the Norepinephrine Pump in Man," *J Clin Invest*, 1970, 49(8):1596-604.

Rundegren J, van Dijken J, Mörnstad H, et al, "Oral Conditions in Patients Receiving Long-Term Treatment With Cyclic Antidepressant Drugs," *Swed Dent J*, 1985, 9(2):55-64.

Svedmyr N, "The Influence of a Tricyclic Antidepressive Agent (Protriptyline) on Some of the Circulatory Effects of Noradrenaline and Adrenalin in Man," *Life Sci*, 1968, 7(1):77-84.

Wynn RL, "New Antidepressant Medications," *Gen Dent*, 1997, 45(1):24-8.


- ♦ **Maranox® [OTC]** *see* Acetaminophen *on page 27*
- ♦ **Marax®** *see* Theophylline, Ephedrine, and Hydroxyzine *on page 974*
- ♦ **Marcaine®** *see* Bupivacaine *on page 157*
- ♦ **Marcaine® With Epinephrine** *see* Bupivacaine and Epinephrine *on page 158*
- ♦ **Marcillin®** *see* Ampicillin *on page 81*
- ♦ **Marezine® [OTC]** *see* Cyclizine *on page 283*
- ♦ **Margesic® H [5/500]** *see* Hydrocodone and Acetaminophen *on page 505*
- ♦ **Marinol®** *see* Dronabinol *on page 358*
- ♦ **Marnal®** *see* Butalbital Compound *on page 163*
- ♦ **Marplan®** *see* Isocarboxazid *on page 551*
- ♦ **Marpres®** *see* Hydralazine, Hydrochlorothiazide, and Reserpine *on page 503*
- ♦ **Marthritic®** *see* Salsalate *on page 902*


## Masoprocol (ma SOE pro kole)

**U.S. Brand Names** Actinex®

**Therapeutic Category** Topical Skin Product

**Use** Treatment of actinic keratosis

**Usual Dosage** Adults: Topical: Wash and dry area; gently massage into affected area every morning and evening for 28 days

**Mechanism of Action** Antiproliferative activity against keratinocytes

**Local Anesthetic/Vasoconstrictor Precautions** No information available to require special precautions

**Effects on Dental Treatment** No effects or complications reported

**Other Adverse Effects**

>10%:

Dermatologic: Erythema, flaking, dryness, itching
Local: Burning

1% to 10%:

Dermatologic: Soreness, rash
Neuromuscular & skeletal: Paresthesia

Ocular: Eye irritation

<1%: Dermatologic: Blistering, excoriation, skin roughness, wrinkling

**Drug Interactions** No data reported

**Drug Uptake** Absorption: Topical: <1% to 2%

**Pregnancy Risk Factor** B

**Dosage Forms** Cream: 10% (30 g)

**Generic Available** Yes

- **Massé® Breast Cream [OTC]** *see* Glycerin, Lanolin, and Peanut Oil *on page 473*
- **Matulane®** *see* Procarbazine *on page 842*
- **Mavik®** *see* Trandolapril *on page 1003*
- **Maxair™** *see* Pirbuterol *on page 809*
- **Maxalt®** *see* Rizatriptan *on page 894*
- **Maxalt-MLT™** *see* Rizatriptan *on page 894*
- **Maxaquin®** *see* Lomefloxacin *on page 597*
- **Max-Caro® [OTC]** *see* Beta-Carotene *on page 135*
- **Maxiflor®** *see* Diflorasone *on page 327*
- **Maximum Strength Anbesol® [OTC]** *see* Benzocaine *on page 128*
- **Maximum Strength Desenex® Antifungal Cream [OTC]** *see* Miconazole *on page 672*
- **Maximum Strength Dex-A-Diet® [OTC]** *see* Phenylpropanolamine *on page 797*
- **Maximum Strength Dexatrim® [OTC]** *see* Phenylpropanolamine *on page 797*
- **Maximum Strength Nytol® [OTC]** *see* Diphenhydramine *on page 338*
- **Maximum Strength Orajel® [OTC]** *see* Benzocaine *on page 128*
- **Maxipime®** *see* Cefepime *on page 201*
- **Maxitrol®** *see* Neomycin, Polymyxin B, and Dexamethasone *on page 711*
- **Maxivate®** *see* Betamethasone *on page 136*
- **Maxolon®** *see* Metoclopramide *on page 664*
- **Maxzide®** *see* Hydrochlorothiazide and Triamterene *on page 504*
- **Mazanor®** *see* Mazindol *on this page*

## Mazindol (MAY zin dole)

**U.S. Brand Names** Mazanor®; Sanorex®

**Therapeutic Category** Anorexiant

**Use** Short-term adjunct in exogenous obesity

**Usual Dosage** Adults: Oral: Initial: 1 mg once daily and adjust to patient response; usual dose is 1 mg 3 times daily, 1 hour before meals, or 2 mg once daily, 1 hour before lunch; take with meals to avoid GI discomfort

**Local Anesthetic/Vasoconstrictor Precautions** No information available to require special precautions

**Effects on Dental Treatment** No effects or complications reported

**Other Adverse Effects**

>10%:

Cardiovascular: Hypertension

Central nervous system: Euphoria, nervousness, insomnia

1% to 10%:

Central nervous system: Confusion, mental depression, restlessness

Endocrine & metabolic: Changes in libido

Gastrointestinal: Nausea, vomiting, constipation

Hematologic: Blood dyscrasias

Neuromuscular & skeletal: Tremor

Ocular: Blurred vision

<1%:

Cardiovascular: Tachycardia, arrhythmias

Central nervous system: Headache

Dermatologic: Alopecia

Gastrointestinal: Diarrhea, abdominal cramps

Genitourinary: Dysuria, testicular pain

Neuromuscular & skeletal: Myalgia

Renal: Polyuria

Respiratory: Dyspnea

Miscellaneous: Increased sweating

**Pregnancy Risk Factor** C

**Generic Available** No

## m-Cresyl Acetate (em-KREE sil AS e tate)

**U.S. Brand Names** Cresylate®

**Therapeutic Category** Otic Agent, Anti-infective

**Use** Provides an acid medium; for external otitis infections caused by susceptible bacteria or fungus

**Usual Dosage** Instill 2-4 drops as required

**Local Anesthetic/Vasoconstrictor Precautions** No information available to require special precautions

**Effects on Dental Treatment** No effects or complications reported

**Generic Available** No

♦ **MCT Oil® [OTC]** *see* Medium Chain Triglycerides *on page 622*

## Measles and Rubella Vaccines, Combined

(MEE zels & roo BEL a vak SEENS, kom BINED)

**U.S. Brand Names** M-R-VAX® II

**Therapeutic Category** Vaccine, Live Virus

**Synonyms** Rubella and Measles Vaccines, Combined

**Use** Simultaneous immunization against measles and rubella

**Usual Dosage** Children at 15 months and Adults: S.C.: Inject 0.5 mL into outer aspect of upper arm; no routine booster for rubella

**Local Anesthetic/Vasoconstrictor Precautions** No information available to require special precautions

**Effects on Dental Treatment** No effects or complications reported

**Other Adverse Effects** All serious adverse reactions must be reported to the FDA

>10%:
- Central nervous system: Fever <100°F
- Dermatologic: Urticaria, rash, local erythema
- Local: Burning at injection site, local tenderness
- Neuromuscular & skeletal: Arthralgias

1% to 10%:
- Central nervous system: Fever between 100°F and 103°F, malaise, headache
- Gastrointestinal: Sore throat
- Miscellaneous: Allergic reaction (delayed type), lymphadenopathy

<1%:
- Central nervous system: Fatigue, convulsions, encephalitis, confusion, severe headache, fever >103°F (prolonged)
- Dermatologic: Itching, reddening of skin (especially around ears and eyes)
- Gastrointestinal: Vomiting
- Hematologic: Thrombocytopenic purpura
- Neuromuscular & skeletal: Stiff neck
- Ocular: Diplopia, optic neuritis
- Respiratory: Dyspnea
- Miscellaneous: Hypersensitivity

The chance of a child having a convulsion after receiving the measles vaccine is small. The risk is up to 5 times greater if the child has ever had a convulsion before or if the child's brother, sister, or parent has ever had a convulsion.

**Pregnancy Risk Factor** X

**Generic Available** No

**Comments** Federal law requires that the date of administration, the vaccine manufacturer, lot number of vaccine, and the administering person's name, title and address be entered into the patient's permanent medical record

## Measles, Mumps, and Rubella Vaccines, Combined

(MEE zels, mumpz & roo BEL a vak SEENS, kom BINED)

**U.S. Brand Names** M-M-R® II

**Therapeutic Category** Vaccine, Live Virus

**Synonyms** MMR; Mumps, Measles and Rubella Vaccines, Combined; Rubella, Measles and Mumps Vaccines, Combined

**Use** Measles, mumps, and rubella prophylaxis

**Usual Dosage**

Infants <12 months: If there is risk of exposure to measles, single-antigen measles vaccine should be administered at 6-11 months of age with a second dose (of MMR) at >12 months of age

Give S.C. in outer aspect of the upper arm to children ≥15 months of age:
- 0.5 mL at 15 months of age and then repeated at 4-6 years* of age
- In some areas, MMR vaccine may be given at 12 months
- *Many experts recommend that this dose of MMR be given at entry to middle school or junior high school

**Local Anesthetic/Vasoconstrictor Precautions** No information available to require special precautions

**Effects on Dental Treatment** No effects or complications reported

**Other Adverse Effects** All serious adverse reactions must be reported to the FDA

1% to 10%:

Dermatologic: Transient rash, tenderness erythema and swelling

Gastrointestinal: Sore throat

Miscellaneous: Allergic reactions

<1%: Central nervous system: Seizures, malaise, fever

The chance of a child having a convulsion after receiving the measles vaccine is small. The risk is up to 5 times greater if the child has ever had a convulsion before or if the child's brother, sister, or parent has ever had a convulsion.

**Pregnancy Risk Factor** X

**Generic Available** No

**Comments** Federal law requires that the date of administration, the vaccine manufacturer, lot number of vaccine, and the administering person's name, title and address be entered into the patient's permanent medical record

## Measles Virus Vaccine, Live (MEE zels VYE rus vak SEEN, live)

**U.S. Brand Names** Attenuvax®

**Therapeutic Category** Vaccine, Live Virus

**Synonyms** More Attenuated Enders Strain; Rubeola Vaccine

**Use** Immunization against measles (rubeola) in persons ≥15 months of age

**Usual Dosage** Children >15 months and Adults: S.C.: 0.5 mL in outer aspect of the upper arm, no routine boosters

**Local Anesthetic/Vasoconstrictor Precautions** No information available to require special precautions

**Effects on Dental Treatment** No effects or complications reported

**Other Adverse Effects** All serious adverse reactions must be reported to the FDA

Dermatologic: Rarely urticaria, erythema

>10%:

Cardiovascular: Swelling

Central nervous system: Fever <100°F

Local: Burning or stinging, induration

1% to 10%:

Central nervous system: Fever between 100°F and 103°F

Miscellaneous: Allergic reaction (delayed type)

<1%:

Central nervous system: Fatigue, convulsions, confusion, severe headache, fever >103°F (prolonged)

Dermatologic: Itching, reddening of skin (especially around ears and eyes)

Gastrointestinal: Vomiting, sore throat

Hematologic: Thrombocytopenic purpura

Ocular: Diplopia

Neuromuscular & skeletal: Stiff neck

Respiratory: Dyspnea, coryza

Miscellaneous: Lymphadenopathy

**Pregnancy Risk Factor** X

**Generic Available** No

**Comments** Federal law requires that the date of administration, the vaccine manufacturer, lot number of vaccine, and the administering person's name, title and address be entered into the patient's permanent medical record

♦ **Mebaral®** *see* Mephobarbital *on page 631*

## Mebendazole (me BEN da zole)

**U.S. Brand Names** Vermox®

**Therapeutic Category** Anthelmintic

**Use** Treatment of pinworms, whipworms, roundworms, and hookworms

**Usual Dosage** Children and Adults: Oral:

Pinworms: 100 mg as a single dose; may need to repeat after 2 weeks; treatment should include family members in close contact with patient

Whipworms, roundworms, hookworms: One tablet twice daily, morning and evening on 3 consecutive days; if patient is not cured within 3-4 weeks, a second course of treatment may be administered

Capillariasis: 200 mg twice daily for 20 days

**Mechanism of Action** Selectively and irreversibly blocks glucose uptake and other nutrients in susceptible adult intestine-dwelling helminths

**Local Anesthetic/Vasoconstrictor Precautions** No information available to require special precautions

(Continued)

## Mebendazole *(Continued)*

**Effects on Dental Treatment** No effects or complications reported

**Other Adverse Effects**

1% to 10%: Gastrointestinal: Abdominal pain, diarrhea, nausea, vomiting

<1%:

- Central nervous system: Fever, dizziness, headache, fatigue
- Dermatologic: Skin rash, itching, alopecia (with high dose)
- Gastrointestinal: Sore throat
- Hematologic: Neutropenia
- Neuromuscular & skeletal: Weakness

**Drug Interactions** Decreased effect: Anticonvulsants such as carbamazepine and phenytoin may increase metabolism of mebendazole

**Drug Uptake**

Absorption: Only 2% to 10%

Serum half-life: 1-11.5 hours

Time to peak serum concentration: Within 2-4 hours

**Pregnancy Risk Factor** C

**Generic Available** Yes

## Mecamylamine (mek a MIL a meen)

**U.S. Brand Names** Inversine®

**Therapeutic Category** Ganglionic Blocking Agent

**Use** Treatment of moderately severe to severe hypertension and in uncomplicated malignant hypertension

**Usual Dosage** Adults: Oral: 2.5 mg twice daily after meals for 2 days; increased by increments of 2.5 mg at intervals ≥2 days until desired blood pressure response is achieved; average daily dose: 25 mg

**Mechanism of Action** Mecamylamine is a ganglionic blocker. This agent inhibits acetylcholine at the autonomic ganglia, causing a decrease in blood pressure. Mecamylamine also blocks central nicotinic cholinergic receptors, which inhibits the effects of nicotine and may suppress the desire to smoke.

**Local Anesthetic/Vasoconstrictor Precautions** No information available to require special precautions

**Effects on Dental Treatment** >10% of patients experience dry mouth

**Other Adverse Effects**

>10%:

- Cardiovascular: Postural hypotension
- Central nervous system: Drowsiness
- Endocrine & metabolic: Decreased sexual ability
- Ocular: Blurred vision, enlarged pupils

1% to 10%:

- Gastrointestinal: Loss of appetite, nausea, vomiting
- Genitourinary: Dysuria

<1%:

- Central nervous system: Convulsions, confusion, mental depression
- Gastrointestinal: Bloating, frequent stools, followed by severe constipation
- Neuromuscular & skeletal: Uncontrolled movements of hands, arms, legs, or face, trembling
- Respiratory: Dyspnea

**Pregnancy Risk Factor** C

**Generic Available** No

♦ **Meclan®** *see* Meclocycline *on next page*

## Meclizine (MEK li zeen)

**U.S. Brand Names** Antivert®; Antrizine®; Bonine® [OTC]; Dizmiss® [OTC]; Dramamine® II [OTC]; Meni-D®; Ru-Vert-M®; Vergon® [OTC]

**Therapeutic Category** Antiemetic; Antihistamine

**Use** Prevention and treatment of symptoms of motion sickness; management of vertigo with diseases affecting the vestibular system

**Usual Dosage** Children >12 years and Adults: Oral:

Motion sickness: 12.5-25 mg 1 hour before travel, repeat dose every 12-24 hours if needed; doses up to 50 mg may be needed

Vertigo: 25-100 mg/day in divided doses

**Mechanism of Action** Has central anticholinergic action by blocking chemoreceptor trigger zone; decreases excitability of the middle ear labyrinth and blocks conduction in the middle ear vestibular-cerebellar pathways

**Local Anesthetic/Vasoconstrictor Precautions** No information available to require special precautions

**Effects on Dental Treatment** Up to 10% of patients will have significant dry mouth which will disappear with cessation of drug therapy

**Other Adverse Effects**

>10%:

Central nervous system: Slight to moderate drowsiness

Respiratory: Thickening of bronchial secretions

1% to 10%:

Central nervous system: Headache, fatigue, nervousness, dizziness

Gastrointestinal: Appetite increase, weight gain, nausea, diarrhea, abdominal pain, dry mouth

Neuromuscular & skeletal: Arthralgia

Respiratory: Pharyngitis

<1%:

Cardiovascular: Palpitations, hypotension

Central nervous system: Depression, sedation

Dermatologic: Photosensitivity, rash, angioedema

Genitourinary: Urinary retention

Hepatic: Hepatitis

Neuromuscular & skeletal: Myalgia, tremor, paresthesia

Ocular: Blurred vision

Respiratory: Bronchospasm, epistaxis

**Drug Interactions** Increased toxicity: CNS depressants, neuroleptics, anticholinergics

**Drug Uptake**

Onset of action: Oral: Within 1 hour

Duration: 8-24 hours

Serum half-life: 6 hours

**Pregnancy Risk Factor** B

**Generic Available** Yes

## Meclocycline (me kloe SYE kleen)

**U.S. Brand Names** Meclan®

**Therapeutic Category** Antibiotic, Topical; Topical Skin Product, Acne

**Use** Topical treatment of inflammatory acne vulgaris

**Usual Dosage** Children >11 years and Adults: Topical: Apply generously to affected areas twice daily

**Mechanism of Action** Inhibits bacterial protein synthesis by binding with the 30S and possibly the 50S ribosomal subunit(s) of susceptible bacteria; may also cause alterations in the cytoplasmic membrane

**Local Anesthetic/Vasoconstrictor Precautions** No information available to require special precautions

**Effects on Dental Treatment** No effects or complications reported

**Other Adverse Effects**

>10%: Topical: Follicular staining, yellowing of the skin, burning/stinging feeling

1% to 10%: Topical: Pain, redness, skin irritation, dermatitis

**Drug Interactions** No data reported

**Drug Uptake** Absorption: Topical: Very little

**Pregnancy Risk Factor** B

**Dosage Forms** Cream, topical, as sulfosalicylate: 1% (20 g, 45 g)

**Generic Available** No

## Meclofenamate (me kloe fen AM ate)

**Related Information**

Rheumatoid Arthritis and Osteoarthritis *on page 1092*

**U.S. Brand Names** Meclomen®

**Therapeutic Category** Analgesic, Non-narcotic; Anti-inflammatory Agent; Nonsteroidal Anti-inflammatory Drug (NSAID), Oral

**Use** Treatment of inflammatory disorders

**Usual Dosage** Children >14 years and Adults: Oral:

Mild to moderate pain: 50 mg every 4-6 hours, not to exceed 400 mg/day

Rheumatoid arthritis/osteoarthritis: 200-400 mg/day in 3-4 equal doses

**Mechanism of Action** Inhibits prostaglandin synthesis by decreasing the activity of the enzyme, cyclo-oxygenase, which results in decreased formation of prostaglandin precursors

**Local Anesthetic/Vasoconstrictor Precautions** No information available to require special precautions

**Effects on Dental Treatment** NSAID formulations are known to reversibly decrease platelet aggregation via mechanisms different than observed with aspirin. The dentist should be aware of the potential of abnormal coagulation. Caution should also be exercised in the use of NSAIDs in patients already on anticoagulant therapy with drugs such as warfarin (Coumadin®). Recovery of platelet function usually occurs 1-2 days after discontinuation of NSAIDs.

(Continued)

## Meclofenamate *(Continued)*

**Other Adverse Effects**

>10%:

Central nervous system: Dizziness
Dermatologic: Skin rash
Gastrointestinal: Abdominal cramps, heartburn, indigestion, nausea

1% to 10%:

Cardiovascular: Fluid retention
Central nervous system: Headache, nervousness
Dermatologic: Itching
Gastrointestinal: Vomiting
Otic: Tinnitus

<1%:

Cardiovascular: Congestive heart failure, hypertension, arrhythmia, tachycardia
Central nervous system: Confusion, hallucinations, aseptic meningitis, mental depression, drowsiness, insomnia
Dermatologic: Urticaria, erythema multiforme, toxic epidermal necrolysis, Stevens-Johnson syndrome, angioedema
Endocrine & metabolic: Polydipsia, hot flashes
Gastrointestinal: Gastritis, GI ulceration
Genitourinary: Cystitis
Hematologic: Agranulocytosis, anemia, hemolytic anemia, bone marrow suppression, leukopenia, thrombocytopenia
Hepatic: Hepatitis
Neuromuscular & skeletal: Peripheral neuropathy
Ocular: Toxic amblyopia, blurred vision, conjunctivitis, dry eyes
Otic: Decreased hearing
Renal: Polyuria, acute renal failure
Respiratory: Allergic rhinitis, dyspnea, epistaxis

**Drug Interactions**

Decreased effect with aspirin; decreased effect of diuretics, antihypertensives
Increased effect/toxicity of warfarin, methotrexate

**Drug Uptake**

Duration of action: 2-4 hours
Serum half-life: 2-3.3 hours
Time to peak serum concentration: Within 0.5-1.5 hours

**Pregnancy Risk Factor** B (D if used in the 3rd trimester)

**Generic Available** Yes


- **Meclomen®** *see* Meclofenamate *on previous page*
- **Medigesic®** *see* Butalbital Compound *on page 163*
- **Medigesic®** *see* Butalbital Compound and Acetaminophen *on page 164*
- **Medihaler-Iso®** *see* Isoproterenol *on page 553*
- **Mediplast® Plaster [OTC]** *see* Salicylic Acid *on page 900*
- **Medi-Quick® Topical Ointment [OTC]** *see* Bacitracin, Neomycin, and Polymyxin B *on page 118*
- **Medi-Tuss® [OTC]** *see* Guaifenesin *on page 478*


## Medium Chain Triglycerides

(mee DEE um chane trye GLIS er ides)

**U.S. Brand Names** MCT Oil® [OTC]

**Therapeutic Category** Nutritional Supplement

**Synonyms** Triglycerides, Medium Chain

**Use** Dietary supplement for those who cannot digest long chain fats; malabsorption associated with disorders such as pancreatic insufficiency, bile salt deficiency, and bacterial overgrowth of the small bowel; induce ketosis as a prevention for seizures (akinetic, clonic, and petit mal)

**Usual Dosage** Oral:

Infants: Initial: 0.5 mL every other feeding, then advance to every feeding, then increase in increments of 0.25-0.5 mL/feeding at intervals of 2-3 days as tolerated

Seizures: About 39 mL with each meal or 50% to 70% (800-1120 kcal) of total calories (1600 kcal) as the oil will induce ketosis necessary for seizure control

Cystic fibrosis: 3 tablespoons/day is tolerated without adverse symptoms by most children

Adults: 15 mL 3-4 times/day

**Local Anesthetic/Vasoconstrictor Precautions** No information available to require special precautions

**Effects on Dental Treatment** No effects or complications reported

**Other Adverse Effects**

Central nervous system: May result in **narcosis** and **coma** in cirrhotic patients due to high levels of medium chain fatty acids in the serum which then enter the cerebral spinal fluid; electroencephalogram effects include slowing of the alpha wave (can occur during infusion of fatty acids of 2-6 carbon lengths)

Endocrine & metabolic:

MCT therapy does not produce recognized metabolic side effects of any clinical importance, nor do they interfere with the metabolism of other food stuffs or with the absorption of drugs; when administered in the form of a mixed diet with carbohydrates and protein, there is no clinical evidence of **hyperketonemia**; hyperketonemia may occur in normal or diabetic subjects in the absence of carbohydrates; has been reported that MCT may increase hepatic free fatty acid synthesis and reduce ketone clearance

Fecal water, sodium and potassium excretion are decreased in patients with steatorrhea who are treated with MCT; enhanced calcium absorption has been demonstrated in patients with steatorrhea who are given MCT

Gastrointestinal: Nausea, occasional vomiting, gastritis and distention, diarrhea, and borborygmi are common adverse reactions occurring in about 10% of the patients receiving supplements or diets containing MCT; these symptoms may be related to rapid hydrolysis of MCT, high concentrations of free fatty acids in the stomach and small intestine, hyperosmolarity causing influx of large amounts of fluid, and lactose intolerance; abdominal cramps, nausea and vomiting occurred despite cautionary administration of MCT in small sips throughout meals, but subsided with continued administration

**Pregnancy Risk Factor** C

**Generic Available** No

**Comments** Does not provide any essential fatty acids; only saturated fats are contained; supplementation with safflower, corn oil, or other polyunsaturated vegetable oil must be given to provide the patient with the essential fatty acids. The minimum daily requirement has not been established for oral intake, but 10-15 mL of safflower oil (60% to 70% linoleic acid) appears to be satisfactory. Contains 7.7 kcal/mL

♦ **Medralone**® *see* Methylprednisolone *on page 661*

♦ **Medrol**® *see* Methylprednisolone *on page 661*

## Medroxyprogesterone Acetate

(me DROKS ee proe JES te rone AS e tate)

**Related Information**

Endocrine Disorders & Pregnancy *on page 1082*

**U.S. Brand Names** Amen®; Curretab®; Cycrin®; Depo-Provera®; Provera®

**Canadian Brand Names** Novo-Medrone

**Therapeutic Category** Contraceptive, Progestin Only; Progestin

**Use** Endometrial carcinoma or renal carcinoma as well as secondary amenorrhea or abnormal uterine bleeding due to hormonal imbalance; prevention of pregnancy; reduction of endometrial hyperplasia in postmenopausal women conjugated estrogens (0.625 mg) for 12-14 consecutive days per month, either beginning on the first day of the cycle or the sixteenth day of cycle

**Usual Dosage**

Adolescents and Adults: Oral:

Amenorrhea: 5-10 mg/day for 5-10 days or 2.5 mg/day

Abnormal uterine bleeding: 5-10 mg for 5-10 days starting on day 16 or 21 of cycle

Accompanying cyclic estrogen therapy, postmenopausal: 2.5-10 mg the last 10-13 days of estrogen dosing each month

Adults: I.M.:

Endometrial or renal carcinoma: 400-1000 mg/week

Contraception: 150 mg every 3 months or 450 mg every 6 months

**Mechanism of Action** Inhibits secretion of pituitary gonadotropins, which prevents follicular maturation and ovulation, stimulates growth of mammary tissue

**Local Anesthetic/Vasoconstrictor Precautions** No information available to require special precautions

**Effects on Dental Treatment** Progestins may predispose the patient to gingival bleeding

**Other Adverse Effects**

>10%:

Cardiovascular: Edema

Endocrine & metabolic: Breakthrough bleeding, spotting, changes in menstrual flow, amenorrhea

Gastrointestinal: Anorexia

Local: Pain at injection site

(Continued)

## Medroxyprogesterone Acetate *(Continued)*

Neuromuscular & skeletal: Weakness

1% to 10%:

Cardiovascular: Embolism, central thrombosis

Central nervous system: Mental depression, fever, insomnia

Dermatologic: Melasma or chloasma, allergic rash with or without pruritus

Endocrine & metabolic: Changes in cervical erosion and secretions, increased breast tenderness

Gastrointestinal: Weight gain or loss

Hepatic: Cholestatic jaundice

Local: Thrombophlebitis

**Drug Interactions** Decreased effect: Aminoglutethimide may decrease effects by increasing hepatic metabolism

**Drug Uptake** Absorption: I.M.: Slow

**Pregnancy Risk Factor** X

**Generic Available** Yes

## Medrysone (ME dri sone)

**U.S. Brand Names** HMS Liquifilm®

**Therapeutic Category** Anti-inflammatory Agent, Ophthalmic; Corticosteroid, Ophthalmic

**Use** Treatment of allergic conjunctivitis, vernal conjunctivitis, episcleritis, ophthalmic epinephrine sensitivity reaction

**Usual Dosage** Children and Adults: Ophthalmic: Instill 1 drop in conjunctival sac 2-4 times/day up to every 4 hours; may use every 1-2 hours during first 1-2 days

**Mechanism of Action** Decreases inflammation by suppression of migration of polymorphonuclear leukocytes and reversal of increased capillary permeability

**Local Anesthetic/Vasoconstrictor Precautions** No information available to require special precautions

**Effects on Dental Treatment** No effects or complications reported

**Other Adverse Effects**

1% to 10%: Ocular: Temporary mild blurred vision

<1%: Ocular: Stinging, burning eyes, corneal thinning, increased intraocular pressure, glaucoma, damage to the optic nerve, defects in visual activity, cataracts, secondary ocular infection

**Drug Uptake** Absorption: Through aqueous humor

**Pregnancy Risk Factor** C

**Dosage Forms** Solution, ophthalmic: 1% (5 mL, 10 mL)

**Generic Available** No

**Comments** Medrysone is a synthetic corticosteroid; structurally related to progesterone; if no improvement after several days of treatment, discontinue medrysone and institute other therapy; duration of therapy: 3-4 days to several weeks dependent on type and severity of disease; taper dose to avoid disease exacerbation

## Mefenamic Acid (me fe NAM ik AS id)

**U.S. Brand Names** Ponstel®

**Canadian Brand Names** Apo®-Mefenamic; Ponstan®

**Therapeutic Category** Analgesic, Non-narcotic; Nonsteroidal Anti-inflammatory Drug (NSAID), Oral

**Use** Short-term relief of mild to moderate pain including primary dysmenorrhea

**Usual Dosage** Children >14 years and Adults: Oral: 500 mg to start then 250 mg every 4 hours as needed; maximum therapy: 1 week

**Mechanism of Action** Inhibits prostaglandin synthesis by decreasing the activity of the enzyme, cyclo-oxygenase, which results in decreased formation of prostaglandin precursors

**Local Anesthetic/Vasoconstrictor Precautions** No information available to require special precautions

**Effects on Dental Treatment** NSAID formulations are known to reversibly decrease platelet aggregation via mechanisms different than observed with aspirin. The dentist should be aware of the potential of abnormal coagulation. Caution should also be exercised in the use of NSAIDs in patients already on anticoagulant therapy with drugs such as warfarin (Coumadin®). Recovery of platelet function usually occurs 1-2 days after discontinuation of NSAIDs.

**Other Adverse Effects**

>10%:

Central nervous system: Dizziness

Dermatologic: Skin rash

Gastrointestinal: Abdominal cramps, heartburn, indigestion, nausea

1% to 10%:
- Central nervous system: Headache, nervousness
- Dermatologic: Itching
- Endocrine & metabolic: Fluid retention
- Gastrointestinal: Vomiting
- Otic: Tinnitus

<1%:
- Cardiovascular: Congestive heart failure, hypertension, arrhythmias, tachycardia
- Central nervous system: Confusion, hallucinations, aseptic meningitis, mental depression, drowsiness, insomnia
- Dermatologic: Urticaria, erythema multiforme, toxic epidermal necrolysis, Stevens-Johnson syndrome, angioedema
- Endocrine & metabolic: Polydipsia, hot flashes
- Gastrointestinal: Gastritis, GI ulceration
- Genitourinary: Cystitis
- Hematologic: Agranulocytosis, anemia, hemolytic anemia, bone marrow suppression, leukopenia, thrombocytopenia
- Hepatic: Hepatitis
- Neuromuscular & skeletal: Peripheral neuropathy
- Ocular: Toxic amblyopia, blurred vision, conjunctivitis, dry eyes
- Otic: Decreased hearing
- Renal: Polyuria, acute renal failure
- Respiratory: Dyspnea, allergic rhinitis, epistaxis

**Drug Interactions**

Decreased effect of diuretics, antihypertensives; decreased effect with aspirin
Increased effect/toxicity with oral anticoagulants, methotrexate

**Drug Uptake**

Duration of action: Up to 6 hours
Serum half-life: 3.5 hours

**Pregnancy Risk Factor** C

**Generic Available** No

## Mefloquine (ME floe kwin)

**U.S. Brand Names** Lariam®

**Therapeutic Category** Antimalarial Agent

**Use** Treatment of acute malarial infections and prevention of malaria

**Usual Dosage** Oral:

Children: Malaria prophylaxis:
- 15-19 kg: 1/4 tablet
- 20-30 kg: 1/2 tablet
- 31-45 kg: 3/4 tablet
- >45 kg: 1 tablet
- Administer weekly starting 1 week before travel, continuing weekly during travel and for 4 weeks after leaving endemic area

Adults:
- Treatment of mild to moderate malaria infection: 5 tablets (1250 mg) as a single dose with at least 8 oz of water
- Malaria prophylaxis: 1 tablet (250 mg) weekly starting 1 week before travel, continuing weekly during travel and for 4 weeks after leaving endemic area

**Mechanism of Action** Mefloquine is a quinoline-methanol compound structurally similar to quinine; mefloquine's effectiveness in the treatment and prophylaxis of malaria is due to the destruction of the asexual blood forms of the malarial pathogens that affect humans, *Plasmodium falciparum, P. vivax, P. malariae, P. ovale*

**Local Anesthetic/Vasoconstrictor Precautions** No information available to require special precautions

**Effects on Dental Treatment** No effects or complications reported

**Other Adverse Effects**

1% to 10%:
- Central nervous system: Difficulty concentrating, headache, insomnia, lightheadedness, vertigo
- Gastrointestinal: Vomiting, diarrhea, stomach pain, nausea
- Ocular: Visual disturbances
- Otic: Tinnitus

<1%:
- Cardiovascular: Bradycardia, extrasystoles, syncope
- Central nervous system: Anxiety, dizziness, confusion, seizures, hallucinations, mental depression, psychosis

**Drug Uptake**

Absorption: Oral: Well absorbed
Serum half-life: 21-22 days

(Continued)

## Mefloquine *(Continued)*

**Pregnancy Risk Factor** C

**Generic Available** No

**Comments** To avoid relapse after initial treatment with mefloquine, patients should subsequently be treated with an 8-aminoquinolone (eg, primaquine)

- **Mefoxin®** *see* Cefoxitin *on page 205*
- **Mega B® [OTC]** *see* Vitamin B Complex *on page 1050*
- **Megace®** *see* Megestrol Acetate *on this page*
- **Megaton™ [OTC]** *see* Vitamin B Complex *on page 1050*

## Megestrol Acetate (me JES trole AS e tate)

**U.S. Brand Names** Megace®

**Therapeutic Category** Antineoplastic Agent, Hormone; Progestin

**Use** Palliative treatment of breast and endometrial carcinomas, appetite stimulation, and promotion of weight gain in cachexia

**Usual Dosage** Adults: Oral (**refer to individual protocols**):

Female:

Breast carcinoma: 40 mg 4 times/day

Endometrial: 40-320 mg/day in divided doses; use for 2 months to determine efficacy; maximum doses used have been up to 800 mg/day

Uterine bleeding: 40 mg 2-4 times/day

Male and Female: HIV-related cachexia: Initial dose: 800 mg/day; daily doses of 400 and 800 mg/day were found to be clinically effective

**Mechanism of Action** Megestrol is an antineoplastic progestin thought to act through an antileutenizing effect mediated via the pituitary

**Local Anesthetic/Vasoconstrictor Precautions** No information available to require special precautions

**Effects on Dental Treatment** No effects or complications reported

**Other Adverse Effects**

>10%:

Cardiovascular: Edema

Endocrine & metabolic: Breakthrough bleeding and amenorrhea, spotting, changes in menstrual flow

Neuromuscular & skeletal: Weakness

1% to 10%:

Central nervous system: Insomnia, depression, fever, headache

Dermatologic: Allergic rash with or without pruritus, melasma or chloasma, skin rash, and rarely alopecia

Endocrine & metabolic: Changes in cervical erosion and secretions, increased breast tenderness, changes in vaginal bleeding pattern, fluid retention, hyperglycemia

Gastrointestinal: Weight gain (not attributed to edema or fluid retention), nausea, vomiting, stomach cramps

Hepatic: Cholestatic jaundice, hepatotoxicity

Hematologic: Myelosuppressive: WBC: None; Platelets: None

Local: Thrombophlebitis

Neuromuscular & skeletal: Carpal tunnel syndrome

Respiratory: Hyperpnea

**Drug Interactions** No data reported

**Drug Uptake**

Onset of action: At least 2 months of continuous therapy is necessary

Absorption: Oral: Well absorbed

Serum half-life, elimination: 15-20 hours

Time to peak serum concentration: Oral: Within 1-3 hours

**Pregnancy Risk Factor** X

**Generic Available** Yes

- **Melanex®** *see* Hydroquinone *on page 514*
- **Melfiat-105® Unicelles®** *see* Phendimetrazine *on page 788*
- **Mellaril®** *see* Thioridazine *on page 978*
- **Mellaril-S®** *see* Thioridazine *on page 978*

## Melphalan (MEL fa lan)

**U.S. Brand Names** Alkeran®

**Therapeutic Category** Antineoplastic Agent, Alkylating Agent (Nitrogen Mustard)

**Synonyms** L-PAM; L-Sarcolysin; Phenylalanine Mustard

**Use** Palliative treatment of multiple myeloma and nonresectable epithelial ovarian carcinoma; neuroblastoma, rhabdomyosarcoma, breast cancer, sarcoma; I.V. formulation: Use in patients in whom oral therapy is not appropriate

**Usual Dosage**

Oral (refer to individual protocols); dose should always be adjusted to patient response and weekly blood counts:

Children: 4-20 mg/m²/day for 1-21 days

Adults:

Multiple myeloma: 6 mg/day initially adjusted as indicated **or** 0.15 mg/kg/day for 7 days **or** 0.25 mg/kg/day for 4 days; repeat at 4- to 6-week intervals

Ovarian carcinoma: 0.2 mg/kg/day for 5 days, repeat every 4-5 weeks

I.V. (refer to individual protocols):

Children:

Pediatric rhabdomyosarcoma: 10-35 mg/m²/dose every 21-28 days

High-dose melphalan with bone marrow transplantation for neuroblastoma: 70-100 mg/m²/day on day 7 and 6 before BMT; **or** 140-220 mg/m² single dose before BMT **or** 50 mg/m²/day for 4 days; **or** 70 mg/m²/day for 3 days

Adults: Multiple myeloma: 16 mg/m² administered at 2-week intervals for 4 doses, then repeat monthly as per protocol for multiple myeloma

**Mechanism of Action** Alkylating agent which is a derivative of mechlorethamine that inhibits DNA and RNA synthesis via formation of carbonium ions; cross-links strands of DNA

**Local Anesthetic/Vasoconstrictor Precautions** No information available to require special precautions

**Effects on Dental Treatment** No effects or complications reported

**Other Adverse Effects**

>10%:

Dermatologic: Alopecia, pruritus, rash

Endocrine & metabolic: SIADH, amenorrhea

Hematologic: Leukopenia and thrombocytopenia are the most common effects of melphalan; anemia, agranulocytosis, hemolytic anemia; irreversible bone marrow failure has been reported

Myelosuppression: WBC: Moderate; Platelets: Moderate; Onset (days): 7; Nadir (days): 8-10 and 27-32; Recovery (days): 42-50

Second malignancies: Reported are melphalan more frequently

Respiratory: Pulmonary fibrosis, interstitial pneumonitis

Miscellaneous: Sterility, hypersensitivity

1% to 10%:

Cardiovascular: Vasculitis

Dermatologic: Vesiculation of skin

Gastrointestinal: Nausea and vomiting are mild; stomatitis and diarrhea are infrequent

Genitourinary: Bladder irritation, hemorrhagic cystitis

**Drug Uptake**

Absorption: Oral: Variable and incomplete from the GI tract; food interferes with absorption

Serum half-life, terminal: 1.5 hours

Time to peak serum concentration: Reportedly within 2 hours

**Pregnancy Risk Factor** D

**Generic Available** No

- **Menadol® [OTC]** *see* Ibuprofen *on page 522*
- **Menest®** *see* Estrogens, Esterified *on page 392*
- **Meni-D®** *see* Meclizine *on page 620*

## Meningococcal Polysaccharide Vaccine, Groups A, C, Y, and W-135

(me NIN joe kok al pol i SAK a ride vak SEEN groops aye, see, why & dubl yoo won thur tee fyve)

**U.S. Brand Names** Menomune®-A/C/Y/W-135

**Therapeutic Category** Vaccine, Live Bacteria

**Use** Immunization against infection caused by *Neisseria meningitidis* groups A,C,Y, and W-135 in persons ≥2 years

**Usual Dosage** One dose I.M. (0.5 mL); the need for booster is unknown

**Mechanism of Action** Induces the formation of bactericidal antibodies to meningococcal antigens; the presence of these antibodies is strongly correlated with immunity to meningococcal disease caused by *Neisseria meningitidis* groups A, C, Y and W-135.

**Local Anesthetic/Vasoconstrictor Precautions** No information available to require special precautions

**Effects on Dental Treatment** No effects or complications reported

**Other Adverse Effects**

>10%:

Central nervous system: Pain

(Continued)

## Meningococcal Polysaccharide Vaccine, Groups A, C, Y, and W-135 *(Continued)*

Dermatologic: Erythema and induration
Local: Tenderness
1% to 10%: Central nervous system: Headache, malaise, fever, chills

**Drug Uptake**
Onset: Antibody levels are achieved within 10-14 days after administration
Duration: Antibodies against group A and C polysaccharides decline markedly (to prevaccination levels) over the first 3 years following a single dose of vaccine, especially in children <4 years of age

**Pregnancy Risk Factor** C

**Generic Available** No

♦ **Menomune®-A/C/Y/W-135** *see* Meningococcal Polysaccharide Vaccine, Groups A, C, Y, and W-135 *on previous page*

## Menotropins (men oh TROE pins)

**U.S. Brand Names** Humegon™; Pergonal®

**Therapeutic Category** Gonadotropin; Ovulation Stimulator

**Use** Sequentially with hCG to induce ovulation and pregnancy in the infertile woman with functional anovulation; used with hCG in men to stimulate spermatogenesis in those with primary hypogonadotropic hypogonadism

**Usual Dosage** Adults: I.M.:
Male: Following pretreatment with hCG, 1 ampul 3 times/week and hCG 2000 units twice weekly until sperm is detected in the ejaculate (4-6 months) then may be increased to 2 ampuls of menotropins (150 units FSH/150 units LH) 3 times/week
Female: 1 ampul/day (75 units of FSH and LH) for 9-12 days followed by 10,000 units hCG 1 day after the last dose; repeated at least twice at same level before increasing dosage to 2 ampuls (150 units FSH/150 units LH)

**Mechanism of Action** Actions occur as a result of both follicle stimulating hormone (FSH) effects and luteinizing hormone (LH) effects; menotropins stimulate the development and maturation of the ovarian follicle (FSH), cause ovulation (LH), and stimulate the development of the corpus luteum (LH); in males it stimulates spermatogenesis (LH)

**Local Anesthetic/Vasoconstrictor Precautions** No information available to require special precautions

**Effects on Dental Treatment** No effects or complications reported

**Other Adverse Effects**
Male:
>10%: Endocrine & metabolic: Gynecomastia
1% to 10%: Erythrocytosis (shortness of breath, dizziness, anorexia, syncope, epistaxis)
Female:
>10%:
Endocrine & metabolic: Ovarian enlargement
Gastrointestinal: Abdominal distention
Local: Pain/rash at injection site
1% to 10%: Ovarian hyperstimulation syndrome
<1%:
Cardiovascular: Thromboembolism,
Central nervous system: Pain, febrile reactions

**Drug Interactions** No data reported

**Pregnancy Risk Factor** X

**Dosage Forms** Injection:
Follicle stimulating hormone activity 75 units and luteinizing hormone activity 75 units per 2 mL ampul
Follicle stimulating hormone activity 150 units and luteinizing hormone activity 150 units per 2 mL ampul

**Generic Available** Yes

♦ **Mentax®** *see* Butenafine *on page 166*

## Mepenzolate Bromide (me PEN zoe late)

**U.S. Brand Names** Cantil®

**Therapeutic Category** Anticholinergic Agent; Antispasmodic Agent, Gastrointestinal

**Use** Management of peptic ulcer disease; inhibit salivation and excessive secretions in respiratory tract preoperatively

**Usual Dosage** Adults: Oral: 25-50 mg 4 times/day with meal and at bedtime

**Local Anesthetic/Vasoconstrictor Precautions** No information available to require special precautions

**Effects on Dental Treatment** >10% of patients experience dry mouth

**Other Adverse Effects**

>10%:
- Dermatologic: Dry skin
- Gastrointestinal: Constipation
- Respiratory: Dry nose, throat
- Miscellaneous: Decreased sweating

1% to 10%: Gastrointestinal: Dysphagia

<1%:
- Cardiovascular: Tachycardia
- Central nervous system: Confusion, headache, loss of memory, fatigue, drowsiness, nervousness, insomnia
- Dermatologic: Rash
- Gastrointestinal: Bloated feeling, nausea, vomiting
- Genitourinary: Urinary retention
- Neuromuscular & skeletal: Weakness
- Ocular: Increased intraocular pressure, blurred vision

**Pregnancy Risk Factor** C

**Generic Available** No

◆ **Mepergan**® *see* Meperidine and Promethazine *on next page*

## Meperidine (me PER i deen)

**Related Information**

Dental Drug Interactions: Update on Drug Combinations Requiring Special Considerations *on page 1225*
Narcotic Agonists *on page 1223*
Oral Pain *on page 1122*

**U.S. Brand Names** Demerol®

**Therapeutic Category** Analgesic, Narcotic

**Synonyms** Isonipecaine; Pethidine Hydrochloride

**Use**

Dental: Adjunct in preoperative intravenous conscious sedation in patients undergoing dental surgery; alternate oral narcotic in patients allergic to codeine to treat moderate to moderate-severe pain

Medical: Management of moderate to severe pain

**Restrictions** C-II; Nonrefillable

**Usual Dosage**

Children: Oral: 25-50 mg every 4-6 hours as needed for pain

Adults:
- I.V.: 50-100 mg titrated as a single dose to produce sedation
- Oral: 50-100 mg every 4-6 hours as needed for pain

**Mechanism of Action** Binds to opiate receptors in the CNS, causing inhibition of ascending pain pathways, altering the perception of and response to pain; produces generalized CNS depression

**Local Anesthetic/Vasoconstrictor Precautions** No information available to require special precautions

**Effects on Dental Treatment** 1% to 10% of patients experience dry mouth

**Other Adverse Effects** >10%:
- Cardiovascular: Hypotension
- Central nervous system: Fatigue, drowsiness, dizziness
- Gastrointestinal: Nausea, vomiting, constipation
- Neuromuscular & skeletal: Weakness
- Miscellaneous: Histamine release

**Contraindications** Hypersensitivity to meperidine or any component; patients receiving MAO inhibitors presently or in the past 14 days

**Warnings/Precautions** Use with caution in patients with pulmonary, hepatic, renal disorders, or increased intracranial pressure; use with caution in patients with renal failure or seizure disorders or those receiving high-dose meperidine; normeperidine (an active metabolite and CNS stimulant) may accumulate and precipitate twitches, tremors, or seizures; some preparations contain sulfites which may cause allergic reaction

Enhanced analgesia has been seen in elderly patients on therapeutic doses of narcotics; duration of action may be increased in the elderly; the elderly may be particularly susceptible to the CNS depressant and constipating effects of narcotics

**Drug Interactions** Phenytoin may decrease the analgesic effects of meperidine; meperidine may aggravate the adverse effects of isoniazid; MAO inhibitors, fluoxetine, and other serotonin uptake inhibitors greatly potentiate the effects of meperidine; acute opioid overdosage symptoms can be seen, including severe toxic reactions; CNS depressants, tricyclic antidepressants, and phenothiazines may potentiate the effects of meperidine; concurrent use with sibutramine may

(Continued)

## Meperidine *(Continued)*

increase the risk of serotonin syndrome (serotonin syndrome includes fever, sweating, agitation, and restlessness)

**Drug Uptake**

Onset of effect: I.V.: Within 5 minutes

Duration: 4-6 hours

Serum half-life:

Parent drug, terminal phase:

Adults: 2.5-4 hours

Adults with liver disease: 7-11 hours

Normeperidine (active metabolite): 15-30 hours; dependent on renal function and can accumulate with higher doses or in patients with decreased renal function

Time to peak serum concentration: Oral: 90-120 minutes

**Pregnancy Risk Factor** B (D if used for prolonged periods or in high doses at term)

**Breast-feeding Considerations** Considered compatible by AAO in 1983 statement; however, not included in the 1989 statement

**Dosage Forms**

Syrup: 50 mg/5 mL (500 mL)

Tablet: 50 mg, 100 mg

**Dietary Considerations** No data reported

**Generic Available** Yes

**Comments** Meperidine is not to be used as the narcotic drug of first choice. It is recommended only to be used in codeine-allergic patients when a narcotic analgesic is indicated. Meperidine is not an anti-inflammatory agent. Meperidine, as with other narcotic analgesics, is recommended only for limited acute dosing (ie, 3 days or less); common adverse effects in the dental patient are nausea, sedation, and constipation. Meperidine has a significant addiction liability, especially when given long term.

## Meperidine and Promethazine

(me PER i deen & proe METH a zeen)

**U.S. Brand Names** Mepergan®

**Therapeutic Category** Analgesic, Narcotic

**Use** Management of moderate to severe pain

**Usual Dosage** Adults:

Oral: One (1) capsule every 4-6 hours

I.M.: Inject 1-2 mL every 3-4 hours

**Local Anesthetic/Vasoconstrictor Precautions** No information available to require special precautions

**Effects on Dental Treatment** 1% to 10% of patients experience dry mouth

**Pregnancy Risk Factor** B

**Generic Available** No

## Mephenytoin (me FEN i toyn)

**U.S. Brand Names** Mesantoin®

**Therapeutic Category** Anticonvulsant, Hydantoin

**Use** Treatment of tonic-clonic and partial seizures in patients who are uncontrolled with less toxic anticonvulsants

**Usual Dosage** Oral:

Children: 3-15 mg/kg/day in 3 divided doses; usual maintenance dose: 100-400 mg/day in 3 divided doses

Adults: Initial dose: 50-100 mg/day given daily; increase by 50-100 mg at weekly intervals; usual maintenance dose: 200-600 mg/day in 3 divided doses; maximum: 800 mg/day

**Mechanism of Action** Stabilizes neuronal membranes and decreases seizure activity by increasing efflux or decreasing influx of sodium ions across cell membranes in the motor cortex during generation of nerve impulses; prolongs effective refractory period and suppresses ventricular pacemaker automaticity, shortens action potential in the heart

**Local Anesthetic/Vasoconstrictor Precautions** No information available to require special precautions

**Effects on Dental Treatment** Mephenytoin, like phenytoin, causes gingival hyperplasia. Usually starts during the first 6 months of dental treatment as gingivitis. The incidence is higher in patients under 20 years of age. To minimize severity and growth rate of gingival tissue begin a program of professional cleaning and patient plaque control within 10 days of starting anticonvulsant therapy. GH induced by mephenytoin disappears with cessation of drug therapy.

**Other Adverse Effects**

>10%:

Central nervous system: Psychiatric changes, slurred speech, dizziness, somnolence

Gastrointestinal: Constipation, nausea, vomiting

Neuromuscular & skeletal: Trembling

1% to 10%:

Central nervous system: Headache, insomnia

Dermatologic: Skin rash

Gastrointestinal: Anorexia, weight loss

Hematologic: Leukopenia

Hepatic: Hepatitis

Renal: Elevated serum creatinine

<1%:

Cardiovascular: Hypotension, bradycardia, cardiac arrhythmias, cardiovascular collapse

Central nervous system: Confusion, fever, ataxia

Dermatologic: Stevens-Johnson syndrome or SLE-like syndrome

Gastrointestinal: Gingival hyperplasia

Hematologic: Blood dyscrasias, Hodgkin's disease-like syndrome

Local: Venous irritation and pain, thrombophlebitis

Neuromuscular & skeletal: Paresthesia, peripheral neuropathy

Ocular: Diplopia, nystagmus, blurred vision, photophobia

Miscellaneous: Lymphadenopathy, serum sickness

**Drug Interactions**

Decreased effect with carbamazepine, TCAs, calcium antacids; decreased effect of oral anticoagulants, oral contraceptives, steroids, quinidine, vitamin D, vitamin K, doxycycline, furosemide, TCAs

Increased effect/toxicity with alcohol, sulfonamides, chloramphenicol, cimetidine, isoniazid, disulfiram, phenothiazines, benzodiazepines

**Pregnancy Risk Factor** C

**Generic Available** No

## Mephobarbital (me foe BAR bi tal)

**U.S. Brand Names** Mebaral®

**Therapeutic Category** Anticonvulsant, Barbiturate

**Use** Sedative; treatment of grand mal and petit mal epilepsy

**Usual Dosage** Oral:

Epilepsy:

Children: 6-12 mg/kg/day in 2-4 divided doses

Adults: 200-600 mg/day in 2-4 divided doses

Sedation:

Children:

<5 years: 16-32 mg 3-4 times/day

>5 years: 32-64 mg 3-4 times/day

Adults: 32-100 mg 3-4 times/day

**Mechanism of Action** Increases seizure threshold in the motor cortex; depresses monosynaptic and polysynaptic transmission in the CNS

**Local Anesthetic/Vasoconstrictor Precautions** No information available to require special precautions

**Effects on Dental Treatment** No effects or complications reported

**Other Adverse Effects**

>10%: Central nervous system: Dizziness, lightheadedness, drowsiness, "hang-over" effect

1% to 10%:

Central nervous system: Confusion, mental depression, unusual excitement, nervousness, faint feeling, headache, insomnia, nightmares

Gastrointestinal: Constipation, nausea, vomiting

<1%:

Cardiovascular: Hypotension

Central nervous system: Hallucinations

Dermatologic: Skin rash, exfoliative dermatitis, Stevens-Johnson syndrome, angioedema

Hematologic: Agranulocytosis, megaloblastic anemia, thrombocytopenia

Local: Thrombophlebitis

Respiratory: Respiratory depression

Miscellaneous: Dependence

**Drug Interactions**

Mephobarbital causes decreased effects of the following drugs: Phenothiazines, haloperidol, quinidine, cyclosporine, TCAs, corticosteroids, theophylline, ethosuximide, warfarin, oral contraceptives, chloramphenicol, griseofulvin, doxycycline, beta-blockers

(Continued)

## Mephobarbital *(Continued)*

The following drugs enhance the CNS effects of mephobarbital: Propoxyphene, benzodiazepines, CNS depressants, valproic acid, methylphenidate, chloramphenicol

**Drug Uptake**

Onset of action: 20-60 minutes
Duration: 6-8 hours
Absorption: Oral: ~50%
Serum half-life: 34 hours

**Pregnancy Risk Factor** D

**Generic Available** No

♦ **Mephyton®** *see* Phytonadione *on page 801*

## Mepivacaine (me PIV a kane)

**U.S. Brand Names** Carbocaine®; Isocaine® HCl; Polocaine®

**Therapeutic Category** Local Anesthetic

**Synonyms** Mepivacaine Hydrochloride

**Use** Local anesthesia by nerve block; infiltration in dental procedures

**Usual Dosage** Children and Adults: Injectable local anesthetic: Varies with procedure, degree of anesthesia needed, vascularity of tissue, duration of anesthesia required, and physical condition of patient

**Mechanism of Action** Mepivacaine is an amino amide local anesthetic similar to lidocaine; like all local anesthetics, mepivacaine acts by preventing the generation and conduction of nerve impulses

**Local Anesthetic/Vasoconstrictor Precautions** No information available to require special precautions

**Effects on Dental Treatment** No effects or complications reported

**Other Adverse Effects**

<1%:

Cardiovascular: Bradycardia, myocardial depression, hypotension, cardiovascular collapse, edema
Central nervous system: Anxiety, restlessness, disorientation, confusion, seizures, drowsiness, unconsciousness, chills
Dermatologic: Urticaria
Gastrointestinal: Nausea, vomiting
Local: Transient stinging or burning at injection site
Neuromuscular & skeletal: Tremors
Ocular: Blurred vision
Otic: Tinnitus
Respiratory: Respiratory arrest
Miscellaneous: Anaphylactoid reactions, shivering

**Warnings/Precautions** Use with caution in patients with cardiac disease, renal disease, and hyperthyroidism; convulsions due to systemic toxicity leading to cardiac arrest have been reported presumably due to intravascular injection

**Drug Uptake**

Onset of action: Epidural: Within 7-15 minutes
Duration: 2-2.5 hours; similar onset and duration is seen following infiltration
Protein binding: 70% to 85%
Metabolism: Chiefly in the liver by N-demethylation, hydroxylation, and glucuronidation
Half-life: 1.9 hours
Elimination: Urinary excretion (95% as metabolites)

**Pregnancy Risk Factor** C

**Dosage Forms** Injection, as hydrochloride: 1% [10 mg/mL] (30 mL, 50 mL); 1.5% [15 mg/mL] (30 mL); 2% [20 mg/mL] (20 mL, 50 mL); 3% [30 mg/mL] (1.8 mL)

**Generic Available** Yes

**Selected Readings**

Dodson WE, Hillman RE, and Hillman LS, "Brain Tissue Levels in a Fatal Case of Neonatal Mepivacaine (Carbocaine®) Poisoning," *J Pediatr*, 1975, 86(4):624-7.

Torres MJ, Garcia JJ, del Cano Moratinos AM, et al, "Fixed Drug Eruption Induced by Mepivacaine," *J Allergy Clin Immunol*, 1995, 96(1):130-1.

## Mepivacaine and Levonordefrin

(me PIV a kane & lee voe nor DEF rin)

**Related Information**

Oral Pain *on page 1122*

**U.S. Brand Names** Carbocaine® 2% With Neo-Cobefrin®; Isocaine® HCl 2%; Polocaine® 2%

**Canadian Brand Names** Polocaine® and Levonordefrin

**Therapeutic Category** Dental/Local Anesthetics; Local Anesthetic, Injectable

**Use** Dental: Amide-type anesthetic used for local infiltration anesthesia; injection near nerve trunks to produce nerve block

**Usual Dosage**

Children <10 years: Maximum pediatric dosage must be carefully calculated on the basis of patient's weight but should not exceed 6.6 mg/kg of body weight or 180 mg of mepivacaine hydrochloride as a 2% solution with levonordefrin 1:20,000

Children >10 years and Adults:

Dental infiltration and nerve block, single site: 36 mg (1.8 mL) of mepivacaine hydrochloride as a 2% solution with levonordefrin 1:20,000

Entire oral cavity: 180 mg (9 mL) of mepivacaine hydrochloride as a 2% solution with levonordefrin 1:20,000; up to a maximum of 6.6 mg/kg of body weight but not to exceed 400 mg of mepivacaine hydrochloride per appointment. The effective anesthetic dose varies with procedure, intensity of anesthesia needed, duration of anesthesia required, and physical condition of the patient. Always use the lowest effective dose along with careful aspiration.

The following numbers of dental carpules (1.8 mL) provide the indicated amounts of mepivacaine hydrochloride 2% and levonordefrin 1:20,000.

| # of Cartridges | Mg Mepivacaine (2%) | Mg Vasoconstrictor (Levonordefrin 1:20,000) |
|---|---|---|
| 1 | 36 | 0.090 |
| 2 | 72 | 0.180 |
| 3 | 108 | 0.270 |
| 4 | 144 | 0.360 |
| 5 | 180 | 0.450 |
| 6 | 216 | 0.540 |
| 7 | 252 | 0.630 |
| 8 | 288 | 0.720 |
| 9 | 324 | 0.810 |
| 10 | 360 | 0.900 |

**Note:** Adult and children doses of mepivacaine hydrochloride with levonordefrin cited from USP Dispensing Information (USP DI), 17th ed, The United States Pharmacopeial Convention, Inc, Rockville, MD, 1997, 139.

**Mechanism of Action** Local anesthetics bind selectively to the intracellular surface of sodium channels to block influx of sodium into the axon. As a result, depolarization necessary for action potential propagation and subsequent nerve function is prevented. The block at the sodium channel is reversible. When drug diffuses away from the axon, sodium channel function is restored and nerve propagation returns.

Levonordefrin prolongs the duration of the anesthetic actions of mepivacaine by causing vasoconstriction (alpha adrenergic receptor agonist) of the vasculature surrounding the nerve axons. This prevents the diffusion of mepivacaine away from the nerves resulting in a longer retention in the axon.

**Local Anesthetic/Vasoconstrictor Precautions** No information available to require special precautions

**Effects on Dental Treatment** No effects or complications reported

**Other Adverse Effects** Degree of adverse effects in the CNS and cardiovascular system are directly related to the blood levels of mepivacaine. The effects below are more likely to occur after systemic administration rather than infiltration.

Central nervous system: High blood levels result in anxiety, restlessness, disorientation, confusion, dizziness, and seizures. This is followed by depression of CNS resulting in somnolence, unconsciousness and possible respiratory arrest. In some cases, symptoms of CNS stimulation may be absent and the primary CNS effects are somnolence and unconsciousness.

Cardiovascular: Myocardial effects include a decrease in contraction force as well as a decrease in electrical excitability and myocardial conduction rate resulting in bradycardia and reduction in cardiac output.

Gastrointestinal: Nausea and vomiting may occur

Hypersensitivity reactions: Extremely rare, but may be manifest as dermatologic reactions and edema at injection site. Asthmatic syndromes have occurred. Patients may exhibit hypersensitivity to bisulfites contained in local anesthetic solution to prevent oxidation of levonordefrin. In general, patients reacting to bisulfites have a history of asthma and their airways are hyper-reactive to asthmatic syndrome.

Neuromuscular & skeletal: Tremors

(Continued)

## Mepivacaine and Levonordefrin *(Continued)*

Psychogenic reactions: It is common to misinterpret psychogenic responses to local anesthetic injection as an allergic reaction. Intraoral injections are perceived by many patients as a stressful procedure in dentistry. Common symptoms to this stress are sweating, palpitations, hyperventilation, generalized pallor and a fainting feeling.

**Contraindications** Hypersensitivity to local anesthetics of the amide-type

**Warnings/Precautions** Should be avoided in patients with uncontrolled hyperthyroidism. Should be used in minimal amounts in patients with significant cardiovascular problems (because of levonordefrin component). Aspirate the syringe after tissue penetration and before injection to minimize chance of direct vascular injection.

**Drug Interactions** Due to levonordefrin component, use with tricyclic antidepressants or MAO inhibitors could result in increased pressor response; use with nonselective beta-blockers (ie, propranolol) could result in serious hypertension and reflex bradycardia

**Drug Uptake**

Duration: 1-2.5 hours in upper jaw and 2.5-5.5 hours in lower jaw

Infiltration: 50 minutes

Inferior alveolar block: 60-75 minutes

**Pregnancy Risk Factor** C

**Breast-feeding Considerations** Usual infiltration doses of mepivacaine with levonordefrin given to nursing mothers has not been shown to affect the health of the nursing infant

**Dosage Forms** Injection: Mepivacaine hydrochloride 2% with levonordefrin 1:20,000 (1.8 mL dental cartridges)

**Dietary Considerations** No data reported

**Generic Available** No

**Selected Readings**

Ayoub ST and Coleman AE, "A Review of Local Anesthetics," *Gen Dent*, 1992, 40(4):285-7, 289-90.

Jastak JT and Yagiela JA, "Vasoconstrictors and Local Anesthesia: A Review and Rationale for Use," *J Am Dent Assoc*, 1983, 107(4):623-30.

MacKenzie TA and Young ER, "Local Anesthetic Update," *Anesth Prog*, 1993, 40(2):29-34.

Wynn RL, "Epinephrine Interactions With Beta-Blockers," *Gen Dent*, 1994, 42(1):16, 18.

Wynn RL, "Recent Research on Mechanisms of Local Anesthetics," *Gen Dent*, 1995, 43(4):316-8.

Yagiela JA, "Local Anesthetics," *Anesth Prog*, 1991, 38(4-5):128-41.

## Mepivacaine Dental Anesthetic

(me PIV a kane DEN tal an es THE tik)

**Related Information**

Oral Pain *on page 1122*

**U.S. Brand Names** Carbocaine® 3%; Isocaine® HCl 3%; Polocaine® 3%

**Canadian Brand Names** Polocaine®

**Therapeutic Category** Dental/Local Anesthetics; Local Anesthetic, Injectable

**Use** Dental: Amide-type anesthetic used for local infiltration anesthesia; injection near nerve trunks to produce nerve block

**Usual Dosage**

Children <10 years: Up to 5-6 mg/kg of body weight; maximum pediatric dosage must be carefully calculated on the basis of patient's weight but must not exceed 270 mg (9 mL) of the 3% solution

Children >10 years and Adults:

Dental anesthesia, single site in upper or lower jaw: 54 mg (1.8 mL) as a 3% solution

Infiltration and nerve block of entire oral cavity: 270 mg (9 mL) as a 3% solution; up to a maximum of 6.6 mg/kg of body weight but not to exceed 300 mg per appointment. Manufacturer's maximum recommended dose is not more than 400 mg to normal healthy adults. The effective anesthetic dose varies with procedure, intensity of anesthesia needed, duration of anesthesia required, and physical condition of the patient. Always use the lowest effective dose along with careful aspiration.

The following number of dental carpules (1.8 mL) provide the indicated amounts of mepivacaine dental anesthetic 3%.

| # of Cartridges | Mg Mepivacaine (3%) |
|---|---|
| 1 | 54 |
| 2 | 108 |
| 3 | 162 |
| 4 | 216 |
| 5 | 270 |
| 6 | 324 |
| 7 | 378 |
| 8 | 432 |

**Note:** Adult and children doses of mepivacaine dental anesthetic cited from USP Dispensing Information (USP DI), 17th ed, The United States Pharmacopeial Convention, Inc, Rockville, MD, 1997, 138-9.

**Mechanism of Action** Local anesthetics bind selectively to the intracellular surface of sodium channels to block influx of sodium into the axon. As a result, depolarization necessary for action potential propagation and subsequent nerve function is prevented. The block at the sodium channel is reversible. When drug diffuses away from the axon, sodium channel function is restored and nerve propagation returns.

**Local Anesthetic/Vasoconstrictor Precautions** No information available to require special precautions

**Effects on Dental Treatment** No effects or complications reported

**Other Adverse Effects** Degree of adverse effects in the CNS and cardiovascular system are directly related to the blood levels of local anesthetic.

Cardiovascular: Myocardial effects include a decrease in contraction force as well as a decrease in electrical excitability and myocardial conduction rate resulting in bradycardia and reduction in cardiac output

Central nervous system: High blood levels result in anxiety, restlessness, disorientation, confusion, dizziness, and seizures. This is followed by depression of CNS resulting in somnolence, unconsciousness and possible respiratory arrest. In some cases, symptoms of CNS stimulation may be absent and the primary CNS effects are somnolence and unconsciousness.

Gastrointestinal: Nausea and vomiting may occur

Hypersensitivity reactions: May manifest as dermatologic reactions and edema at injection site. Asthmatic syndromes have occurred.

Neuromuscular & skeletal: Tremors

Psychogenic reactions: It is common to misinterpret psychogenic responses to local anesthetic injection as an allergic reaction. Intraoral injections is perceived by many patients as a stressful procedure in dentistry. Common symptoms to this stress are sweating, palpitations, hyperventilation, generalized pallor and a fainting feeling.

**Contraindications** Hypersensitivity to local anesthetics of the amide type

**Warnings/Precautions** Aspirate the syringe after tissue penetration and before injection to minimize chance of direct vascular injection

**Drug Interactions** No data reported

**Drug Uptake**

Onset of action: 30-120 seconds in upper jaw; 1-4 minutes in lower jaw

Duration: 20 minutes in upper jaw; 40 minutes in lower jaw

Serum half-life: 1.9 hours

**Pregnancy Risk Factor** C

**Breast-feeding Considerations** Usual infiltration doses of mepivacaine dental anesthetic given to nursing mothers has not been shown to affect the health of the nursing infant

**Dosage Forms** Injection: Mepivacaine hydrochloride 3% (1.8 mL dental cartridges)

**Dietary Considerations** No data reported

**Generic Available** Yes

**Selected Readings**

Ayoub ST and Coleman AE, "A Review of Local Anesthetics," *Gen Dent*, 1992, 40(4):285-7, 289-90.

Wynn RL, "Recent Research on Mechanisms of Local Anesthetics," *Gen Dent*, 1995, 43(4):316-8.

♦ **Mepivacaine Hydrochloride** *see* Mepivacaine *on page 632*

## Meprobamate (me proe BA mate)

**U.S. Brand Names** Equanil®; Miltown®; Neuramate®

**Canadian Brand Names** Apo®-Meprobamate; Meditran®; Novo-Mepro

**Therapeutic Category** Antianxiety Agent; Muscle Relaxant; Skeletal Muscle Relaxant; Tranquilizer, Minor

**Use**

Dental: Treatment of muscle spasm associated with acute temporomandibular joint pain; management of dental anxiety disorders

Medical: Management of anxiety disorders

**Unlabeled use:** Demonstrated value for muscle contraction, headache, premenstrual tension, external sphincter spasticity, muscle rigidity, opisthotonos-associated with tetanus

**Restrictions** C-IV; Refillable up to 5 times in 6 months

(Continued)

## Meprobamate *(Continued)*

**Usual Dosage** Oral:

Children 6-12 years: 100-200 mg 2-3 times/day

Sustained release: 200 mg twice daily

Adults: 400 mg 3-4 times/day, up to 2400 mg/day

Sustained release: 400-800 mg twice daily

**Mechanism of Action** Precise mechanism is not yet clear, but many effects have been ascribed to its central depressant actions

**Local Anesthetic/Vasoconstrictor Precautions** No information available to require special precautions

**Effects on Dental Treatment** <1% of patients experience stomatitis

**Other Adverse Effects**

>10%: Central nervous system: Drowsiness, clumsiness, ataxia, loss of motor coordination

1% to 10%: Central nervous system: Dizziness

**Contraindications** Acute intermittent porphyria; hypersensitivity to meprobamate or any component; do not use in patients with pre-existing CNS depression, narrow-angle glaucoma, or severe uncontrolled pain

**Warnings/Precautions** Physical and psychological dependence and abuse may occur; not recommended in children <6 years of age; allergic reaction may occur in patients with history of dermatological condition (usually by fourth dose); use with caution in patients with renal or hepatic impairment, or with a history of seizures

**Drug Interactions** CNS depressants cause increased CNS depression

**Drug Uptake**

Absorption: Oral: Rapid and nearly complete

Onset of sedation: Oral: Within 1 hour

Serum half-life: 10 hours

**Pregnancy Risk Factor** D

**Breast-feeding Considerations** Milk concentrations are higher then plasma; effects unknown; not recommended

**Dosage Forms**

Capsule, sustained release: 200 mg, 400 mg

Tablet: 200 mg, 400 mg, 600 mg

**Dietary Considerations** No data reported

**Generic Available** Yes

♦ **Meprobamate and Aspirin** *see* Aspirin and Meprobamate *on page 103*

♦ **Mepron™** *see* Atovaquone *on page 107*

## Merbromin (mer BROE min)

**U.S. Brand Names** Mercurochrome®

**Therapeutic Category** Topical Skin Product

**Use** Topical antiseptic

**Usual Dosage** Apply freely, until injury has healed

**Local Anesthetic/Vasoconstrictor Precautions** No information available to require special precautions

**Effects on Dental Treatment** No effects or complications reported

**Generic Available** Yes

## Mercaptopurine (mer kap toe PYOOR een)

**U.S. Brand Names** Purinethol®

**Therapeutic Category** Antineoplastic Agent, Antimetabolite; Antineoplastic Agent, Purine

**Synonyms** 6-Mercaptopurine; 6-MP

**Use** Treatment of acute leukemias (ALL, CML)

**Usual Dosage** Oral (**refer to individual protocols**):

Children:

Induction: 2.5-5 mg/kg/day given once daily

Maintenance: 1.5-2.5 mg/kg/day given once daily **or** 70-100 $mg/m^2$/day once daily

Adults:

Induction: 2.5-5 mg/kg/day (100-200 mg)

Maintenance: 1.5-2.5 mg/kg/day **or** 80-100 $mg/m^2$/day given once daily

Elderly: Due to renal decline with age, start with lower recommended doses for adults

**Mechanism of Action** Purine antagonist which inhibits DNA and RNA synthesis; acts as false metabolite and is incorporated into DNA and RNA, eventually inhibiting their synthesis. 6-MP is substituted for hypoxanthine; must be metabolized to active nucleotides once inside the cell.

**Local Anesthetic/Vasoconstrictor Precautions** No information available to require special precautions

**Effects on Dental Treatment** No effects or complications reported

**Other Adverse Effects**

>10%: Hepatic: 6-MP can cause an intrahepatic cholestasis and focal centralobular necrosis manifested as hyperbilirubinemia, elevated alkaline phosphatase, and elevated AST. This may be dose related, occurring more frequently at doses >2.5 mg/kg/day; jaundice is noted 1-2 months into therapy, but has ranged from 1 week to 8 years.

1% to 10%:

Central nervous system: Drug fever
Dermatologic: Hyperpigmentation, rash
Endocrine & metabolic: Hyperuricemia
Gastrointestinal: Nausea, vomiting, diarrhea, stomatitis, anorexia, stomach pain, and mucositis may require parenteral nutrition and dose reduction; 6-TG is less GI toxic than 6-MP
Hematologic: Leukopenia, thrombocytopenia, anemia may occur at high doses
Myelosuppressive: WBC: Moderate; Platelets: Moderate; Onset (days): 7-10; Nadir (days): 14; Recovery (days): 21
Neuromuscular & skeletal: Weakness
Renal: Renal toxicity

<1%:

Dermatologic: Dry, scaling rash
Gastrointestinal: Glossitis, tarry stools
Hematologic: Eosinophilia

**Drug Uptake**

Absorption: Variable and incomplete (16% to 50%)
Serum half-life (age-dependent):
Children: 21 minutes
Adults: 47 minutes
Time to peak serum concentration: Within 2 hours

**Pregnancy Risk Factor** D

**Generic Available** No

♦ **6-Mercaptopurine** *see* Mercaptopurine *on previous page*

## Mercuric Oxide (mer KYOOR ik OKS ide)

**Therapeutic Category** Antibiotic, Ophthalmic

**Synonyms** Yellow Mercuric Oxide

**Use** Treatment of irritation and minor infections of the eyelids

**Usual Dosage** Apply small amount to inner surface of lower eyelid once or twice daily

**Local Anesthetic/Vasoconstrictor Precautions** No information available to require special precautions

**Effects on Dental Treatment** No effects or complications reported

**Generic Available** Yes

♦ **Mercurochrome®** *see* Merbromin *on previous page*

♦ **Meridia™** *see* Sibutramine *on page 912*

## Meropenem (mer oh PEN em)

**U.S. Brand Names** Merrem® I.V.

**Therapeutic Category** Antibiotic, Carbacephem

**Use** Meropenem is indicated as single agent therapy for the treatment of intra-abdominal infections including complicated appendicitis and peritonitis in adults and bacterial meningitis in pediatric patients >3 months of age caused by *S. pneumoniae*, *H. influenzae*, and *N. meningitidis* (penicillin-resistant pneumococci have not been studied in clinical trials); it is better tolerated than imipenem and highly effective against a broad range of bacteria

**Usual Dosage**

Children:
Intra-abdominal infections: 20 mg/kg every 8 hours (maximum dose: 1 g every 8 hours)
Meningitis: 40 mg/kg every 8 hours (maximum dose: 2 g every 8 hours)
Adults: 1 g every 8 hours (see Administration)

**Mechanism of Action** Inhibits bacterial cell wall synthesis by binding to several of the penicillin-binding proteins, which in turn inhibit the final transpeptidation step of peptidoglycan synthesis in bacterial cell walls, thus inhibiting cell wall biosynthesis; bacteria eventually lyse due to ongoing activity of cell wall autolytic enzymes (autolysins and murein hydrolases) while cell wall assembly is arrested

**Local Anesthetic/Vasoconstrictor Precautions** No information available to require special precautions

(Continued)

## Meropenem *(Continued)*

**Effects on Dental Treatment** 1% to 10% of patients will experience oral moniliasis and glossitis

**Other Adverse Effects**

1% to 10%:
- Central nervous system: Headache
- Dermatologic: Rash, pruritus
- Gastrointestinal: Diarrhea, nausea/vomiting, constipation, glossitis
- Local: Injection site reaction/thrombophlebitis
- Respiratory: Apnea
- Miscellaneous: Oral moniliasis

<1%:
- Cardiovascular: Heart failure, other cardiac symptoms including myocardial infarction and arrhythmias, edema
- Central nervous system: Pain, fever, agitation/delirium, dizziness, seizure, hallucinations
- Dermatologic: Urticaria
- Gastrointestinal: Anorexia, flatulence
- Hematologic: Bleeding event, anemia, hematologic effects both increase and decrease in cell counts
- Hepatic: Hepatic failure, hepatic effects, elevated LFTs
- Renal: Kidney failure
- Respiratory: Dyspnea
- Miscellaneous: Sweating

**Warnings/Precautions** Do not administer to patients with serious hypersensitivity reactions to beta-lactam agents. Seizures and other CNS events have been reported during treatment with meropenem; these experiences have occurred most commonly in patients with pre-existing CNS disorders, with bacterial meningitis, and/or decreased renal function; may cause pseudomembranous colitis

**Drug Interactions** Probenecid interferes with renal excretion of meropenem

**Drug Uptake** Serum half-life: ~1 hours

**Pregnancy Risk Factor** B

**Generic Available** No

**Comments** 1 g of meropenem contains 90.2 mg of sodium as sodium carbonate (3.92 mEq)

**Selected Readings**

Wiseman LR, Wagstaff AJ, Brogden RN, et al, "Meropenem. A Review of Its Antibacterial Activity, Pharmacokinetic Properties, and Clinical Efficacy," *Drugs*, 1995, 50(1):73-101.


- **Merrem® I.V.** *see* Meropenem *on previous page*
- **Mersol® [OTC]** *see* Thimerosal *on page 976*
- **Merthiolate® [OTC]** *see* Thimerosal *on page 976*
- **Meruvax® II** *see* Rubella Virus Vaccine, Live *on page 899*


## Mesalamine (me SAL a meen)

**U.S. Brand Names** Asacol®; Pentasa®; Rowasa®

**Therapeutic Category** 5-Aminosalicylic Acid Derivative; Anti-inflammatory Agent, Rectal

**Use** Treatment of ulcerative colitis, proctosigmoiditis, and proctitis

**Usual Dosage** Adults (usual course of therapy is 3-6 weeks):

Oral:
- Capsule: 1 g 4 times/day
- Tablet: 800 mg 3 times/day

Retention enema: 60 mL (4 g) at bedtime, retained overnight, approximately 8 hours

Rectal suppository: Insert 1 suppository in rectum twice daily

Some patients may require rectal and oral therapy concurrently

**Mechanism of Action** Mesalamine (5-aminosalicylic acid) is the active component of sulfasalazine; the specific mechanism of action of mesalamine is unknown; however, it is thought that it modulates local chemical mediators of the inflammatory response, especially leukotrienes; action appears topical rather than systemic

**Local Anesthetic/Vasoconstrictor Precautions** No information available to require special precautions

**Effects on Dental Treatment** No effects or complications reported

**Other Adverse Effects**

>10%:
- Central nervous system: Headache, malaise
- Gastrointestinal: Abdominal pain, cramps, flatulence, gas

1% to 10%: Dermatologic: Alopecia, rash

<1%: Anal irritation, acute intolerance syndrome (bloody diarrhea, severe abdominal cramps, severe headache)

**Drug Interactions** Decreased effect: Decreased digoxin bioavailability

**Drug Uptake**

Absorption: Rectal: ~15%; variable and dependent upon retention time, underlying GI disease, and colonic pH

Serum half-life:

5-ASA: 0.5-1.5 hours

Acetyl 5-ASA: 5-10 hours

Time to peak serum concentration: Within 4-7 hours

**Pregnancy Risk Factor** B

**Generic Available** No

♦ **Mesantoin®** *see* Mephenytoin *on page 630*

## Mesoridazine (mez oh RID a zeen)

**U.S. Brand Names** Serentil®

**Therapeutic Category** Antipsychotic Agent; Phenothiazine Derivative

**Use** Symptomatic management of psychotic disorders, including schizophrenia, behavioral problems, alcoholism as well as reducing anxiety and tension occurring in neurosis

**Usual Dosage** Concentrate may be diluted just prior to administration with distilled water, acidified tap water, orange or grape juice; do not prepare and store bulk dilutions

Adults:

Oral: 25-50 mg 3 times/day; maximum: 100-400 mg/day

I.M.: 25 mg initially, repeat in 30-60 minutes as needed; optimal dosage range: 25-200 mg/day

**Mechanism of Action** Blockade of postsynaptic CNS dopamine receptors

**Local Anesthetic/Vasoconstrictor Precautions** No information available to require special precautions

**Effects on Dental Treatment** No effects or complications reported

**Other Adverse Effects**

>10%:

Cardiovascular: Hypotension, orthostatic hypotension

Central nervous system: Pseudoparkinsonism, akathisia, dystonias, tardive dyskinesia (persistent), dizziness

Gastrointestinal: Constipation

Ocular: Pigmentary retinopathy

Respiratory: Nasal congestion

Miscellaneous: Decreased sweating

1% to 10%:

Dermatologic: Photosensitivity, skin rash

Endocrine & metabolic: Changes in menstrual cycle, changes in libido, pain in breasts

Gastrointestinal: Weight gain, nausea, vomiting, stomach pain

Genitourinary: Dysuria, ejaculatory disturbances

Neuromuscular & skeletal: Trembling of fingers

<1%:

Central nervous system: Neuroleptic malignant syndrome (NMS), impairment of temperature regulation, lowering of seizures threshold

Dermatologic: Discoloration of skin (blue-gray)

Endocrine & metabolic: Galactorrhea

Genitourinary: Priapism

Hematologic: Agranulocytosis, leukopenia

Hepatic: Cholestatic jaundice, hepatotoxicity

Ocular: Cornea and lens changes, pigmentary retinopathy

**Drug Interactions**

Decreased effect with anticonvulsants, anticholinergics

Increased toxicity with CNS depressants, metrizamide (increased seizures), propranolol

**Drug Uptake**

Duration of action: 4-6 hours

Absorption: Very erratic with oral tablet; oral liquids much more dependable

Serum half-life: 24-48 hours

Time to peak serum concentration: 2-4 hours

**Pregnancy Risk Factor** C

**Generic Available** No

## Mestranol and Norethindrone (MES tra nole & nor eth IN drone)

**Related Information**

Endocrine Disorders & Pregnancy *on page 1082*

**U.S. Brand Names** Genora® 1/50; Nelova™ 1/50M; Norethin™ 1/50M; Norinyl® 1+50; Ortho-Novum™ 1/50

(Continued)

## Mestranol and Norethindrone *(Continued)*

**Therapeutic Category** Contraceptive, Oral; Progestin

**Use** Prevention of pregnancy; treatment of hypermenorrhea, endometriosis, female hypogonadism [monophasic oral contraceptive]

**Usual Dosage** Adults: Female: Oral:

Contraception: 1 tablet daily, beginning on day 5 of menstrual cycle (first day of menstrual flow is day 1). With 20-tablet and 21-tablet packages, new dosing cycle begins 7 days after last tablet taken. With 28-tablet packages, dosage is 1 tablet daily without interruption; extra tablets are placebos or contain iron. If next menstrual period does not begin on schedule, rule out pregnancy before starting new dosing cycle. If menstrual period begins, start new dosing cycle 7 days after last tablet was taken. If all doses have been taken on schedule and one menstrual period is missed, continue dosing cycle. If two consecutive menstrual periods are missed, pregnancy test is required before new dosing cycle is started.

One dose missed: Take as soon as remembered or take 2 tablets next day

Two doses missed: Take 2 tablets as soon as remembered or 2 tablets next 2 days

Three doses missed: Begin new compact of tablets starting on day 1 of next cycle

**Mechanism of Action** Inhibits ovulation via a negative feedback mechanism on the hypothalamus, which alters the normal pattern of gonadotropin secretion of a follicle-stimulating hormone (FSH) and luteinizing hormone by the anterior pituitary. Follicular phase FSH and midcycle surge of gonadotropins are inhibited. Produces alterations in the genital tract, including changes in the cervical mucus, rendering it unfavorable for sperm penetration even if ovulation occurs. Changes in the endometrium may also occur, producing an unfavorable environment for nidation. May alter the tubal transport of the ova through the fallopian tubes. Progestational agents may also alter sperm fertility.

**Local Anesthetic/Vasoconstrictor Precautions** No information available to require special precautions

**Effects on Dental Treatment** When prescribing antibiotics, patients must be advised to use additional methods of birth control when taking oral contraceptives

**Other Adverse Effects**

>10%:
- Cardiovascular: Peripheral edema
- Central nervous system: Headache
- Endocrine: Enlargement of breasts, breast tenderness, increased libido
- Gastrointestinal: Nausea, anorexia, bloating

1% to 10%: Gastrointestinal: Vomiting, diarrhea

<1%:
- Cardiovascular: Hypertension, thromboembolism, edema, myocardial infarction
- Central nervous system: Depression, dizziness, anxiety, stroke
- Dermatologic: Chloasma, melasma, rash
- Endocrine: Decreased glucose tolerance, breast tumors, amenorrhea, alterations in frequency and flow of menses, elevated triglycerides and LDL
- Gastrointestinal: GI distress
- Hepatic: Cholestatic jaundice
- Ocular: Intolerance to contact lenses
- Miscellaneous: Increased susceptibility to *Candida* infection

See tables.

### Achieving Proper Hormonal Balance in an Oral Contraceptive

| Estrogen | | Progestin | |
|---|---|---|---|
| **Excess** | **Deficiency** | **Excess** | **Deficiency** |
| Nausea, bloating | Early or midcycle breakthrough bleeding | Increased appetite | Late breakthrough bleeding |
| Cervical mucorrhea, polyposis | Increased spotting | Weight gain | Amenorrhea |
| Melasma | Hypomenorrhea | Tiredness, fatigue | Hypermenorrhea |
| Migraine headache | | Hypomenorrhea | |
| Breast fullness or tenderness | | Acne, oily scalp* | |
| Edema | | Hair loss, hirsutism* | |
| Hypertension | | Depression | |
| | | Monilial vaginitis | |
| | | Breast regression | |

*Result of androgenic activity of progestins.

**Pharmacological Effects of Progestins Used in Oral Contraceptives**

| | Progestin | Estrogen | Antiestrogen | Androgen |
|---|---|---|---|---|
| Norgestrel/levonorgestrel | +++ | 0 | ++ | +++ |
| Ethynodiol diacetate | ++ | +* | +* | + |
| Norethindrone acetate | + | + | +++ | + |
| Norethindrone | + | +* | +* | + |
| Norethynodrel | + | +++ | 0 | 0 |

*Has estrogenic effect at low doses; may have antiestrogenic effect at higher doses.

+++ = pronounced effect

++ = moderate effect

+ = slight effect

0 = no effect

**Drug Interactions**

Decreased effect of oral contraceptives with barbiturates, hydantoins - phenytoin, rifampin, antibiotics - penicillins, tetracyclines, erythromycins, clindamycin, griseofulvin

Increased toxicity of acetaminophen, anticoagulants, benzodiazepines, caffeine, corticosteroids, metoprolol, theophylline, tricyclic antidepressants

**Pregnancy Risk Factor** X

**Generic Available** Yes

# Mestranol and Norethynodrel

(MES tra nole & nor e THYE noe drel)

**Related Information**

Endocrine Disorders & Pregnancy *on page 1082*

**U.S. Brand Names** Enovid®

**Therapeutic Category** Contraceptive, Oral

**Use** Treatment of hypermenorrhea, endometriosis, female hypogonadism

**Usual Dosage** Adults: Female: Oral:

Endometriosis: 5-10 mg/day for 2 weeks beginning on day 5 of menstrual cycle; increase by 5-10 mg increments at 2-week intervals up to 20 mg/day for 6-9 months

Hypermenorrhea: 20-30 mg/day until bleeding is controlled, then reduce to 10 mg/day and continue through day 24 of cycle; administer 5-10 mg/day from day 5 through day 24 of next 2-3 cycles

**Mechanism of Action** Inhibits ovulation via a negative feedback mechanism on the hypothalamus, which alters the normal pattern of gonadotropin secretion of a follicle-stimulating hormone (FSH) and luteinizing hormone by the anterior pituitary. The follicular phase FSH and midcycle surge of gonadotropins are inhibited. Oral contraceptives produce alterations in the genital tract, including changes in the cervical mucus, rendering it unfavorable for sperm penetration even if ovulation occurs. Changes in the endometrium may also occur, producing an unfavorable environment for nidation. May alter the tubal transport of the ova through the fallopian tubes. Progestational agents may also alter sperm fertility.

**Local Anesthetic/Vasoconstrictor Precautions** No information available to require special precautions

**Effects on Dental Treatment** When prescribing antibiotics, patients must be advised to use additional methods of birth control when taking oral contraceptives

**Other Adverse Effects**

>10%:

- Cardiovascular: Peripheral edema
- Endocrine & metabolic: Enlargement of breasts, breast tenderness
- Gastrointestinal: Nausea, anorexia, bloating

1% to 10%:

- Central nervous system: Headache
- Endocrine & metabolic: Increased libido
- Gastrointestinal: Vomiting, diarrhea

<1%:

- Cardiovascular: Hypertension, thromboembolism, myocardial infarction, edema
- Central nervous system: Depression, dizziness, anxiety, stroke
- Dermatologic: Chloasma, melasma, rash
- Endocrine & metabolic: Decreased glucose tolerance, breast tumors, amenorrhea, alterations in frequency and flow of menses, elevated triglycerides and LDL
- Gastrointestinal: GI distress
- Hepatic: Cholestatic jaundice

(Continued)

## Mestranol and Norethynodrel *(Continued)*

Ocular: Intolerance to contact lenses
Miscellaneous: Increased susceptibility to *Candida* infection

**Drug Interactions**
Decreased effect with barbiturates, hydantoins - phenytoin, rifampin, antibiotics - penicillins, tetracyclines, erythromycins, clindamycin, griseofulvin
Increased toxicity of acetaminophen, anticoagulants, benzodiazepines, caffeine, corticosteroids, metoprolol, theophylline, tricyclic antidepressants

**Drug Uptake**
Mestranol:
Demethylated to ethinyl estradiol
Serum half-life: 6-20 hours
Norethynodrel: Serum half-life, terminal: 5-14 hours

**Pregnancy Risk Factor** X
**Generic Available** Yes

- **Metahydrin®** *see* Trichlormethiazide *on page 1014*
- **Metamucil® [OTC]** *see* Psyllium *on page 865*
- **Metamucil® Instant Mix [OTC]** *see* Psyllium *on page 865*
- **Metaprel®** *see* Metaproterenol *on this page*

## Metaproterenol (met a proe TER e nol)

**Related Information**
Respiratory Diseases *on page 1079*

**U.S. Brand Names** Alupent®; Arm-a-Med® Metaproterenol; Dey-Dose® Metaproterenol; Metaprel®; Prometa®

**Therapeutic Category** Adrenergic Agonist Agent; Antiasthmatic; Beta$_2$-Adrenergic Agonist Agent; Bronchodilator

**Use** Bronchodilator in reversible airway obstruction due to asthma or COPD; because of its delayed onset of action (one hour) and prolonged effect (4 or more hours), this may not be the drug of choice for assessing response to a bronchodilator

**Usual Dosage**
Oral:
Children:
<2 years: 0.4 mg/kg/dose given 3-4 times/day; in infants, the dose can be given every 8-12 hours
2-6 years: 1-2.6 mg/kg/day divided every 6 hours
6-9 years: 10 mg/dose 3-4 times/day
Children >9 years and Adults: 20 mg 3-4 times/day
Elderly: Initial: 10 mg 3-4 times/day, increasing as necessary up to 20 mg 3-4 times/day
Inhalation: Children >12 years and Adults: 2-3 inhalations every 3-4 hours, up to 12 inhalations in 24 hours
Nebulizer:
Children: 0.01-0.02 mL/kg of 5% solution; minimum dose: 0.1 mL; maximum dose: 0.3 mL diluted in 2-3 mL normal saline every 4-6 hours (may be given more frequently according to need)
Adolescents and Adults: 5-20 breaths of full strength 5% metaproterenol **or** 0.2 to 0.3 mL 5% metaproterenol in 2.5-3 mL normal saline until nebulized every 4-6 hours (can be given more frequently according to need)

**Mechanism of Action** Relaxes bronchial smooth muscle by action on beta$_2$-receptors with very little effect on heart rate

**Local Anesthetic/Vasoconstrictor Precautions** No information available to require special precautions

**Effects on Dental Treatment** No effects or complications reported

**Other Adverse Effects**
>10%:
Central nervous system: Nervousness
Neuromuscular & skeletal: Tremor
1% to 10%:
Cardiovascular: Tachycardia, palpitations, hypertension
Central nervous system: Headache, dizziness
Gastrointestinal: Nausea, vomiting, bad taste
Neuromuscular & skeletal: Trembling, muscle cramps, weakness
Respiratory: Coughing
Miscellaneous: Increased sweating
<1%: Respiratory: Paradoxical bronchospasm

**Drug Interactions**
Decreased effect: Beta-blockers
Increased toxicity: Sympathomimetics, TCAs, MAO inhibitors

**Drug Uptake**
Oral:
Onset of bronchodilation: Within 15 minutes
Peak effect: Within 1 hour
Duration of action: ~1-5 hours
Inhalation:
Onset of effects: Within 60 seconds
Duration of action: Similar (~1-5 hours) regardless of route administered
**Pregnancy Risk Factor** C
**Generic Available** Yes (except inhaler)

♦ **Metasep® [OTC]** *see* Parachlorometaxylenol *on page 765*

## Metaxalone (me TAKS a lone)

**U.S. Brand Names** Skelaxin®
**Therapeutic Category** Muscle Relaxant; Skeletal Muscle Relaxant
**Use** Relief of discomfort associated with acute, painful musculoskeletal conditions
**Usual Dosage** Children >12 years and Adults: Oral: 800 mg 3-4 times/day
**Mechanism of Action** Does not have a direct effect on skeletal muscle; most of its therapeutic effect comes from actions on the central nervous system
**Local Anesthetic/Vasoconstrictor Precautions** No information available to require special precautions
**Effects on Dental Treatment** No effects or complications reported
**Other Adverse Effects**
>10%:
Central nervous system: Paradoxical stimulation, headache, somnolence, dizziness
Gastrointestinal: Nausea, vomiting, stomach cramps
<1%:
Dermatologic: Allergic dermatitis
Hematologic: Leukopenia, hemolytic anemia
Hepatic: Hepatotoxicity
Miscellaneous: Anaphylaxis
**Drug Interactions** Increased effect of alcohol, CNS depressants
**Drug Uptake**
Onset of action: ~1 hour
Duration: ~4-6 hours
Serum half-life: 2-3 hours
**Pregnancy Risk Factor** C
**Generic Available** No

## Metformin (met FOR min)

**Related Information**
Endocrine Disorders & Pregnancy *on page 1082*
**U.S. Brand Names** Glucophage®
**Canadian Brand Names** Novo-Metformin
**Therapeutic Category** Hypoglycemic Agent, Oral
**Use** Management of noninsulin-dependent diabetes mellitus [NIDDM] (type II) as monotherapy when hyperglycemia cannot be managed on diet alone. May be used concomitantly with a sulfonylurea when diet and metformin or sulfonylurea alone do not result in adequate glycemic control. May also be used with metformin and insulin in NIDDM.
**Usual Dosage** Oral (allow 1-2 weeks between dose titrations):
Adults:
500 mg tablets: Initial: 500 mg twice daily (given with the morning and evening meals). Dosage increases should be made in increments of one tablet every week, given in divided doses, up to a maximum of 2,500 mg/day. Doses of up to 2000 mg/day may be given twice daily. If a dose of 2,500 mg/day is required, it may be better tolerated 3 times/day (with meals).
850 mg tablets: Initial: 850 mg once daily (given with the morning meal). Dosage increases should be made in increments of one tablet every OTHER week, given in divided doses, up to a maximum of 2550 mg/day. The usual maintenance dose is 850 mg twice daily (with the morning and evening meals). Some patients may be given 850 mg 3 times/day (with meals).
Elderly patients: The initial and maintenance dosing should be conservative, due to the potential for decreased renal function. Generally, elderly patients should not be titrated to the maximum dose of metformin.

**Transfer from other antidiabetic agents:** No transition period is generally necessary except when transferring from chlorpropamide. When transferring from chlorpropamide, care should be exercised during the first 2 weeks because of the prolonged retention of chlorpropamide in the body, leading to overlapping drug effects and possible hypoglycemia.
(Continued)

## Metformin *(Continued)*

**Concomitant metformin and oral sulfonylurea therapy:** If patients have not responded to 4 weeks of the maximum dose of metformin monotherapy, consideration to a gradually addition of an oral sulfonylurea while continuing metformin at the maximum dose, even if prior primary or secondary failure to a sulfonylurea has occurred.

**Mechanism of Action** Decreases hepatic glucose production, decreasing intestinal absorption of glucose and improves insulin sensitivity (increases peripheral glucose uptake and utilization)

**Local Anesthetic/Vasoconstrictor Precautions** No information available to require special precautions

**Effects on Dental Treatment** Metformin-dependent diabetics (noninsulin dependent, Type II) should be appointed for dental treatment in morning in order to minimize chance of stress-induced hypoglycemia

**Other Adverse Effects**

>10%: Gastrointestinal: Anorexia, nausea, vomiting, diarrhea, epigastric fullness, constipation, heartburn

1% to 10%:

- Dermatologic: Rash, urticaria, photosensitivity
- Endocrine & metabolic: Decreased vitamin $B_{12}$ levels

<1%: Hematologic: Blood dyscrasias, aplastic anemia, hemolytic anemia, bone marrow suppression, thrombocytopenia, agranulocytosis

**Drug Interactions**

Decreased effects: Drugs which tend to produce hyperglycemia (eg, diuretics, corticosteroids, phenothiazines, thyroid products, estrogens, oral contraceptives, phenytoin, nicotinic acid, sympathomimetics, calcium channel blocking drugs, isoniazid) may lead to a loss of glycemic control

Increased toxicity:

- Cationic drugs (eg, amiloride, digoxin, morphine, procainamide, quinidine, quinine, ranitidine, triamterene, trimethoprim, and vancomycin) which are eliminated by renal tubular secretion could have the potential for interaction with metformin by competing for common renal tubular transport systems
- Cimetidine increases (by 60%) peak metformin plasma and whole blood concentrations

**Drug Uptake** Serum half-life, plasma elimination: 6.2 hours

**Pregnancy Risk Factor** B

**Generic Available** No

## Methadone (METH a done)

**Related Information**

Narcotic Agonists *on page 1223*

**U.S. Brand Names** Dolophine®

**Canadian Brand Names** Methadose®

**Therapeutic Category** Analgesic, Narcotic

**Use** Management of severe pain, used in narcotic detoxification maintenance programs

**Usual Dosage** Doses should be titrated to appropriate effects

Children: Analgesia:

- Oral, I.M., S.C.: 0.7 mg/kg/24 hours divided every 4-6 hours as needed or 0.1-0.2 mg/kg every 4-12 hours as needed; maximum: 10 mg/dose
- I.V.: 0.1 mg/kg every 4 hours initially for 2-3 doses, then every 6-12 hours as needed; maximum: 10 mg/dose

Adults:

- Analgesia: Oral, I.M., I.V., S.C.: 2.5-10 mg every 3-8 hours as needed, up to 5-20 mg every 6-8 hours
- Detoxification: Oral: 15-40 mg/day; should not exceed 21 days and may not be repeated earlier than 4 weeks after completion of preceding course
- Maintenance of opiate dependence: Oral: 20-120 mg/day

**Mechanism of Action** Binds to opiate receptors in the CNS, causing inhibition of ascending pain pathways, altering the perception of and response to pain; produces generalized CNS depression

**Local Anesthetic/Vasoconstrictor Precautions** No information available to require special precautions

**Effects on Dental Treatment** 1% to 10% of patients experience significant dry mouth which will disappear with cessation of drug therapy

**Other Adverse Effects**

- Central nervous system: CNS depression
- Endocrine & metabolic: Antidiuretic hormone release
- Ocular: Miosis
- Respiratory: Respiratory depression

>10%:
- Cardiovascular: Palpitations, hypotension, bradycardia, peripheral vasodilation
- Central nervous system: Fatigue, drowsiness, dizziness
- Gastrointestinal: Nausea, vomiting, constipation
- Neuromuscular & skeletal: Weakness
- Miscellaneous: Histamine release

1% to 10%:
- Central nervous system: Nervousness, headache, restlessness, anorexia, malaise, confusion, increased intracranial pressure
- Gastrointestinal: Stomach cramps, dry mouth, biliary spasm
- Genitourinary: Decreased urination, urinary tract spasm
- Local: Pain at injection site
- Respiratory: Dyspnea

<1%:
- Central nervous system: Mental depression, hallucinations, paradoxical CNS stimulation
- Dermatologic: Pruritus, skin rash, urticaria
- Gastrointestinal: Paralytic ileus
- Miscellaneous: Physical and psychological dependence

**Drug Interactions**

Decreased effect: Phenytoin, pentazocine and rifampin may increase the metabolism of methadone and may precipitate withdrawal

Increased toxicity: CNS depressants, phenothiazines, tricyclic antidepressants, MAO inhibitors may potentiate the adverse effects of methadone

**Drug Uptake**

Oral:
- Onset of analgesia: Within 0.5-1 hour
- Duration: 6-8 hours, increases to 22-48 hours with repeated doses

Parenteral:
- Onset of effect: Within 10-20 minutes
- Peak effect: Within 1-2 hours

Serum half-life: 15-29 hours, may be prolonged with alkaline pH

**Pregnancy Risk Factor** B (D if used for prolonged periods or in high doses at term)

**Generic Available** Yes

## Methamphetamine (meth am FET a meen)

**U.S. Brand Names** Desoxyn®

**Therapeutic Category** Amphetamine; Central Nervous System Stimulant, Amphetamine

**Use** Treatment of narcolepsy, exogenous obesity, abnormal behavioral syndrome in children (minimal brain dysfunction)

**Usual Dosage**

Attention deficit disorder: Children >6 years: 2.5-5 mg 1-2 times/day, may increase by 5 mg increments weekly until optimum response is achieved, usually 20-25 mg/day

Exogenous obesity: Children >12 years and Adults: 5 mg, 30 minutes before each meal; long-acting formulation: 10-15 mg in morning; treatment duration should not exceed a few weeks

**Local Anesthetic/Vasoconstrictor Precautions** Use vasoconstriction with caution in patients taking methamphetamine. Amphetamines enhance the sympathomimetic response of epinephrine and norepinephrine leading to potential hypertension and cardiotoxicity.

**Effects on Dental Treatment** Up to 10% of patients taking dextroamphetamines may present with hypertension. The use of local anesthetic without vasoconstrictor is recommended in these patients.

**Other Adverse Effects**

>10%:
- Cardiovascular: Arrhythmia
- Central nervous system: False feeling of well being, nervousness, restlessness, insomnia

1% to 10%:
- Cardiovascular: Hypertension
- Central nervous system: Mood or mental changes, dizziness, lightheadedness, headache
- Endocrine & metabolic: Changes in libido
- Gastrointestinal: Diarrhea, nausea, vomiting, stomach cramps, constipation, anorexia, weight loss, dry mouth
- Ocular: Blurred vision
- Miscellaneous: Increased sweating

<1%:
- Cardiovascular: Chest pain

(Continued)

## Methamphetamine *(Continued)*

Central nervous system: CNS stimulation (severe), Tourette's syndrome, hyperthermia, seizures, paranoia
Dermatologic: Skin rash, urticaria
Miscellaneous: Tolerance and withdrawal with prolonged use

**Drug Interactions** Increased toxicity with MAO inhibitors (hypertensive crisis)
**Pregnancy Risk Factor** C
**Generic Available** No

## Methantheline (meth AN tha leen)

**U.S. Brand Names** Banthine®
**Therapeutic Category** Anticholinergic Agent; Antispasmodic Agent, Gastrointestinal
**Synonyms** Methanthelinium Bromide
**Use** Adjunctive treatment of peptic ulcer, irritable bowel syndrome, pancreatitis, ureteral and urinary bladder spasm; to reduce duodenal motility during diagnostic radiologic procedures and treatment of an uninhibited neurogenic bladder
**Usual Dosage** Oral:
Neonates: 12.5 mg twice daily then 3 times/day
Children:
<1 year: 12.5-25 mg 4 times/day
>1 year: 12.5-50 mg 4 times/day
Adults: 50-100 mg every 6 hours
**Local Anesthetic/Vasoconstrictor Precautions** No information available to require special precautions
**Effects on Dental Treatment** >10% of patients experience dry mouth
**Other Adverse Effects**
>10%:
Dermatologic: Dry skin
Gastrointestinal: Constipation
Respiratory: Dry nose, throat
Miscellaneous: Decreased sweating
1% to 10%: Gastrointestinal: Dysphagia
<1%:
Cardiovascular: Tachycardia
Central nervous system: Confusion, headache, loss of memory, fatigue, drowsiness, nervousness, insomnia
Dermatologic: Rash
Gastrointestinal: Bloated feeling, nausea, vomiting
Genitourinary: Urinary retention
Neuromuscular & skeletal: Weakness
Ocular: Increased intraocular pressure, blurred vision
**Pregnancy Risk Factor** C
**Generic Available** No

♦ **Methanthelinium Bromide** *see* Methantheline *on this page*

## Methazolamide (meth a ZOE la mide)

**U.S. Brand Names** GlaucTabs®; Neptazane®
**Therapeutic Category** Antiglaucoma Agent; Carbonic Anhydrase Inhibitor; Diuretic, Carbonic Anhydrase Inhibitor
**Use** Adjunctive treatment of open-angle or secondary glaucoma; short-term therapy of narrow-angle glaucoma when delay of surgery is desired
**Usual Dosage** Adults: Oral: 50-100 mg 2-3 times/day
**Mechanism of Action** Noncompetitive inhibition of the enzyme carbonic anhydrase; thought that carbonic anhydrase is located at the luminal border of cells of the proximal tubule. When the enzyme is inhibited, there is an increase in urine volume and a change to an alkaline pH with a subsequent decrease in the excretion of titratable acid and ammonia.
**Local Anesthetic/Vasoconstrictor Precautions** No information available to require special precautions
**Effects on Dental Treatment** No effects or complications reported
**Other Adverse Effects**
>10%:
Central nervous system: Malaise
Gastrointestinal: Metallic taste, anorexia
Neuromuscular & skeletal: Weakness
Renal: Polyuria
1% to 10%:
Central nervous system: Mental depression, drowsiness, dizziness
Renal: Crystalluria

<1%:

Central nervous system: Fever, headache, seizures, unsteadiness, fatigue
Dermatologic: Rash, sulfonamide rash, Stevens-Johnson syndrome
Endocrine & metabolic: Hyperchloremic metabolic acidosis, hypokalemia, hyperglycemia
Gastrointestinal: GI irritation, constipation, anorexia, dry mouth, black tarry stools
Genitourinary: Dysuria
Hematologic: Bone marrow suppression
Neuromuscular & skeletal: Paresthesia, trembling
Ocular: Myopia
Otic: Tinnitus
Miscellaneous: Loss of smell, hypersensitivity

**Drug Interactions**

Increased toxicity:

May induce hypokalemia which would sensitize a patient to digitalis toxicity
May increase the potential for salicylate toxicity
Hypokalemia may be compounded with concurrent diuretic use or steroids
Primidone absorption may be delayed

Decreased effect: Increased lithium excretion and altered excretion of other drugs by alkalinization of the urine, such as amphetamines, quinidine, procainamide, methenamine, phenobarbital, salicylates

**Drug Uptake**

Onset of action: Slow in comparison with acetazolamide (2-4 hours)
Peak effect: 6-8 hours
Duration: 10-18 hours
Absorption: Slowly from GI tract
Serum half-life: ~14 hours

**Pregnancy Risk Factor** C

**Generic Available** Yes

## Methenamine (meth EN a meen)

**U.S. Brand Names** Hiprex®; Mandelamine®; Urex®; Urised®

**Canadian Brand Names** Dehydral™; Hip-Rex™; Urasal®

**Therapeutic Category** Antibiotic, Miscellaneous

**Use** Prophylaxis or suppression of recurrent urinary tract infections; urinary tract discomfort secondary to hypermotility; should not be used to treat infections outside of urinary tract

**Usual Dosage** Oral:

Children: 6-12 years:

Hippurate: 25-50 mg/kg/day divided every 12 hours
Mandelate: 50-75 mg/kg/day divided every 6 hours

Children >12 years and Adults:

Hippurate: 1 g twice daily
Mandelate: 1 g 4 times/day after meals and at bedtime

**Mechanism of Action** Methenamine is hydrolyzed to formaldehyde and ammonia in acidic urine; formaldehyde has nonspecific bactericidal action

**Local Anesthetic/Vasoconstrictor Precautions** No information available to require special precautions

**Effects on Dental Treatment** No effects or complications reported

**Other Adverse Effects**

1% to 10%:

Dermatologic: Skin rash
Gastrointestinal: Nausea, vomiting, diarrhea, anorexia, abdominal cramping

<1%:

Central nervous system: Headache
Genitourinary: Bladder irritation, dysuria
Hepatic: Elevation in AST and ALT
Renal: Hematuria, crystalluria

**Drug Interactions**

Decreased effect: Sodium bicarbonate and acetazolamide will decrease effect secondary to alkalinization of urine

Increased toxicity: Sulfonamides (may precipitate)

**Drug Uptake**

Absorption: Readily absorbed from GI tract
Serum half-life: 3-6 hours

**Pregnancy Risk Factor** C

**Generic Available** Yes

♦ **Methergine®** *see* Methylergonovine *on page 659*

## Methicillin (meth i SIL in)

**U.S. Brand Names** Staphcillin®

**Therapeutic Category** Antibiotic, Penicillin

**Use** Treatment of susceptible bacterial infections such as osteomyelitis, septicemia, endocarditis, and CNS infections due to penicillinase-producing strains of *Staphylococcus*; other antistaphylococcal penicillins are usually preferred

**Usual Dosage** I.M., I.V.:

Children: 150-200 mg/kg/day divided every 6 hours; 200-400 mg/kg/day divided every 4-6 hours has been used for treatment of severe infections; maximum dose: 12 g/day

Adults: 4-12 g/day in divided doses every 4-6 hours

**Mechanism of Action** Inhibits bacterial cell wall synthesis by binding to one or more of the penicillin binding proteins (PBPs); which in turn inhibits the final transpeptidation step of peptidoglycan synthesis in bacterial cell walls, thus inhibiting cell wall biosynthesis. Bacteria eventually lyse due to ongoing activity of cell wall autolytic enzymes (autolysins and murein hydrolases) while cell wall assembly is arrested.

**Local Anesthetic/Vasoconstrictor Precautions** No information available to require special precautions

**Effects on Dental Treatment** Prolonged use of penicillins may lead to development of oral candidiasis

**Other Adverse Effects**

1% to 10%:

- Dermatologic: Skin rash
- Renal: Acute interstitial nephritis

<1%:

- Central nervous system: Fever
- Dermatologic: Rash
- Genitourinary: Hemorrhagic cystitis
- Hematologic: Eosinophilia, anemia, leukopenia, neutropenia, thrombocytopenia
- Local: Phlebitis
- Miscellaneous: Serum sickness-like reactions

**Drug Interactions**

Decreased effect: Efficacy of oral contraceptives may be reduced

Increased effect: Disulfiram, probenecid may increase penicillin levels, increased effect of anticoagulants

**Drug Uptake**

Serum half-life (with normal renal function):

- Children 2-16 years: 0.8 hour
- Adults: 0.4-0.5 hour

Time to peak serum concentration:

- I.M.: 0.5-1 hour
- I.V. infusion: Within 5 minutes

**Pregnancy Risk Factor** B

**Generic Available** No

## Methimazole (meth IM a zole)

**Related Information**

Endocrine Disorders & Pregnancy *on page 1082*

**U.S. Brand Names** Tapazole®

**Therapeutic Category** Antithyroid Agent

**Use** Palliative treatment of hyperthyroidism, return the hyperthyroid patient to a normal metabolic state prior to thyroidectomy, and to control thyrotoxic crisis that may accompany thyroidectomy. The use of antithyroid thioamides is as effective in elderly as they are in younger adults; however, the expense, potential adverse effects, and inconvenience (compliance, monitoring) make them undesirable. The use of radioiodine due to ease of administration and less concern for long-term side effects and reproduction problems (some older males) makes it a more appropriate therapy.

**Usual Dosage** Oral: Administer in 3 equally divided doses at approximately 8-hour intervals

Children: Initial: 0.4 mg/kg/day in 3 divided doses; maintenance: 0.2 mg/kg/day in 3 divided doses up to 30 mg/24 hours maximum

Adults: Initial: 5 mg every 8 hours; maintenance dose: 5-15 mg/day up to 60 mg/day for severe hyperthyroidism

Adjust dosage as required to achieve and maintain serum $T_3$, $T_4$, and TSH levels in the normal range. An elevated $T_3$ may be the sole indicator of inadequate treatment. An elevated TSH indicates excessive antithyroid treatment.

**Mechanism of Action** Inhibits the synthesis of thyroid hormones by blocking the oxidation of iodine in the thyroid gland, blocking iodine's ability to combine with tyrosine to form thyroxine and triiodothyronine ($T_3$), does not inactivate circulating $T_4$ and $T_3$

**Local Anesthetic/Vasoconstrictor Precautions** No information available to require special precautions

**Effects on Dental Treatment** No effects or complications reported

**Other Adverse Effects**

>10%:
- Central nervous system: Fever
- Dermatologic: Skin rash
- Hematologic: Leukopenia

1% to 10%:
- Central nervous system: Dizziness
- Gastrointestinal: Nausea, vomiting, stomach pain, dysgeusia
- Hematologic: Agranulocytosis
- Miscellaneous: SLE-like syndrome

<1%:
- Cardiovascular: Edema
- Central nervous system: Drowsiness, vertigo, headache
- Dermatologic: Rash, urticaria, pruritus, alopecia
- Endocrine & metabolic: Goiter
- Gastrointestinal: Constipation, weight gain, swollen salivary glands
- Hematologic: Thrombocytopenia, aplastic anemia
- Hepatic: Cholestatic jaundice
- Neuromuscular & skeletal: Arthralgia, paresthesia
- Renal: Nephrotic syndrome

**Drug Interactions** Increased toxicity: Iodinated glycerol, lithium, potassium iodide; anticoagulant activity increased

**Drug Uptake**

Onset of antithyroid effect: Oral: Within 30-40 minutes

Duration: 2-4 hours

Serum half-life: 4-13 hours

**Pregnancy Risk Factor** D

**Generic Available** No

## Methionine (me THYE oh neen)

**U.S. Brand Names** Pedameth®

**Therapeutic Category** Dietary Supplement

**Use** Treatment of diaper rash and control of odor, dermatitis and ulceration caused by ammoniacal urine

**Usual Dosage** Oral:

Children: Control of diaper rash: 75 mg in formula or other liquid 3-4 times/day for 3-5 days

Adults:

Control of odor in incontinent adults: 200-400 mg 3-4 times/day

Dietary supplement: 500 mg/day

**Local Anesthetic/Vasoconstrictor Precautions** No information available to require special precautions

**Effects on Dental Treatment** No effects or complications reported

**Generic Available** Yes

## Methocarbamol (meth oh KAR ba mole)

**Related Information**

Temporomandibular Dysfunction (TMD) *on page 1149*

**U.S. Brand Names** Robaxin®

**Therapeutic Category** Muscle Relaxant; Skeletal Muscle Relaxant

**Use**

Dental: Treatment of muscle spasm associated with acute temporomandibular joint pain

Medical: Treatment of muscle spasm associated with acute painful musculoskeletal conditions, supportive therapy in tetanus

**Usual Dosage** Adults: Muscle spasm: Oral: 1.5 g 4 times/day for 2-3 days, then decrease to 4-4.5 g/day in 3-6 divided doses

**Mechanism of Action** Causes skeletal muscle relaxation by reducing the transmission of impulses from the spinal cord to skeletal muscle

**Local Anesthetic/Vasoconstrictor Precautions** No information available to require special precautions

**Effects on Dental Treatment** No effects or complications reported

**Other Adverse Effects** >10%: Central nervous system: Drowsiness, dizziness, lightheadedness

(Continued)

## Methocarbamol *(Continued)*

**Contraindications** Renal impairment, hypersensitivity to methocarbamol or any component

**Warnings/Precautions** Rate of injection should not exceed 3 mL/minute; solution is hypertonic; avoid extravasation; use with caution in patients with a history of seizures

**Drug Interactions** Increased effect/toxicity with CNS depressants

**Drug Uptake**

Absorption: Rapid

Onset of muscle relaxation: Oral: Within 30 minutes

Serum half-life: 1-2 hours

Time to peak serum concentration: Oral: ~2 hours

**Pregnancy Risk Factor** C

**Breast-feeding Considerations** May be taken while breast-feeding

**Dosage Forms**

Injection: 100 mg/mL in polyethylene glycol 50% (10 mL)

Tablet: 500 mg, 750 mg

**Dietary Considerations** Tablets may be crushed and mixed with food or liquid if needed

**Generic Available** Yes

## Methocarbamol and Aspirin (meth oh KAR ba mole & AS pir in)

**U.S. Brand Names** Robaxisal®

**Therapeutic Category** Muscle Relaxant; Skeletal Muscle Relaxant

**Use**

Dental: Treatment of muscle spasm associated with acute temporomandibular joint pain

Medical: Treatment of muscle spasm associated with acute painful musculoskeletal conditions, supportive therapy in tetanus

**Usual Dosage** Children >12 years and Adults: Oral: 2 tablets 4 times/day

**Mechanism of Action** Causes skeletal muscle relaxation by reducing the transmission of impulses from the spinal cord to skeletal muscle

**Local Anesthetic/Vasoconstrictor Precautions** No information available to require special precautions

**Effects on Dental Treatment** Use with caution in patients with platelet and bleeding disorders, renal dysfunction, erosive gastritis, or peptic ulcer disease, previous nonreaction does not guarantee future safe taking of medication; do not use aspirin in children <16 years of age for chickenpox or flu symptoms due to the association with Reye's syndrome

Avoid aspirin if possible, for 1 week prior to surgery because of the possibility of postoperative bleeding; use with caution in impaired hepatic function

Elderly are a high-risk population for adverse effects from nonsteroidal anti-inflammatory agents. As much as 60% of elderly with GI complications to NSAIDs can develop peptic ulceration and/or hemorrhage asymptomatically. Also, concomitant disease and drug use contribute to the risk for GI adverse effects. Use lowest effective dose for shortest period possible. Consider renal function decline with age. Use with caution in patients with history of asthma

**Other Adverse Effects**

Methocarbamol: >10%: Central nervous system: Drowsiness, dizziness, lightheadedness

Aspirin:

>10%: Gastrointestinal: Nausea, vomiting, dyspepsia, epigastric discomfort, heartburn, stomach pains

1% to 10%: Gastrointestinal: Ulceration

**Contraindications**

Methocarbamol: Renal impairment, hypersensitivity to methocarbamol or any component

Aspirin: Bleeding disorders (factor VII or IX deficiencies), hypersensitivity to salicylates or other NSAIDs, tartrazine dye and asthma

**Warnings/Precautions** Use aspirin with caution in patients with platelet and bleeding disorders, renal dysfunction, erosive gastritis, or peptic ulcer disease, previous nonreaction does not guarantee future safe taking of medication; do not use aspirin in children <16 years of age for chickenpox or flu symptoms due to the association with Reye's syndrome

Avoid aspirin if possible, for 1 week prior to surgery because of the possibility of postoperative bleeding; use with caution in impaired hepatic function

Elderly are a high-risk population for adverse effects from nonsteroidal anti-inflammatory agents. As much as 60% of elderly with GI complications to NSAIDs can develop peptic ulceration and/or hemorrhage asymptomatically.

Also, concomitant disease and drug use contribute to the risk for GI adverse effects. Use lowest effective dose for shortest period possible. Consider renal function decline with age. Use with caution in patients with history of asthma

**Drug Interactions**

Methocarbamol: Increased effect/toxicity with CNS depressants

Aspirin: Concomitant use of aspirin may result in possible decreased serum concentration of NSAIDs; aspirin may antagonize effects of probenecid; aspirin may increase methotrexate serum levels. Aspirin may displace valproic acid from binding sites which can result in toxicity; warfarin and aspirin result in increased bleeding; NSAIDs and aspirin result in increased GI adverse effects.

**Drug Uptake**

Methocarbamol:

- Absorption: Rapid
- Onset of muscle relaxation: Oral: Within 30 minutes
- Time to peak serum concentration: Oral: ~2 hours
- Serum half-life: 1-2 hours

Aspirin:

- Absorption: Rapid
- Time to peak serum concentration: ~1-2 hours
- Serum half-life:
  - Parent drug: 15-20 minutes
  - Salicylates (dose-dependent): From 3 hours at lower doses (300-600 mg), to 5-6 hours (after 1 g) to 10 hours with higher doses

**Pregnancy Risk Factor** C (D if full-dose aspirin in 3rd trimester)

**Breast-feeding Considerations** Use cautiously due to potential adverse effects in nursing infants

**Dosage Forms** Tablet: Methocarbamol 400 mg and aspirin 325 mg

**Dietary Considerations** Food decreases rate but not extent of absorption (oral)

**Generic Available** Yes

## Methohexital (meth oh HEKS i tal)

**U.S. Brand Names** Brevital® Sodium

**Canadian Brand Names** Brietal Sodium®

**Therapeutic Category** Barbiturate; General Anesthetic, Intravenous; Sedative

**Use**

Dental: I.V. induction and maintenance of general anesthesia for short periods

Medical: None

**Restrictions** C-IV

**Usual Dosage** I.V.:

Children: 1-2 mg/kg/dose

Adults: 50-120 mg to start; 20-40 mg every 4-7 minutes

**Mechanism of Action** Ultrashort-acting I.V. barbiturate anesthetic; acts as agonist within the multisubunit $GABA_A$ receptor ion chloride-channel complex in central nervous system neurons; this leads to inhibition of many brain functions resulting in loss of consciousness. May also dissolve in neuronal membranes to cause stabilization and eventual loss of action potentials which also leads to inhibition of brain function.

**Local Anesthetic/Vasoconstrictor Precautions** No information available to require special precautions

**Effects on Dental Treatment** No effects or complications reported

**Other Adverse Effects** >10%: Local: Pain on I.M. injection

**Contraindications** Porphyria, hypersensitivity to methohexital or any component

**Warnings/Precautions** Use with extreme caution in patients with liver impairment, asthma, cardiovascular instability

**Drug Interactions** CNS depressants worsen CNS depression

**Drug Uptake**

Onset of effect: Immediately after I.V. injection

Duration: 10-20 minutes after a single dose

**Pregnancy Risk Factor** C

**Breast-feeding Considerations** No data reported

**Dosage Forms** Injection, as sodium: 500 mg, 2.5 g, 5 g

**Dietary Considerations** Should not be given to patients with food in stomach because of danger of vomiting during anesthesia

**Generic Available** No

## Methotrexate (meth oh TREKS ate)

**Related Information**

Rheumatoid Arthritis and Osteoarthritis *on page 1092*

**U.S. Brand Names** Folex® PFS; Rheumatrex®

**Therapeutic Category** Antineoplastic Agent, Antimetabolite

(Continued)

## Methotrexate *(Continued)*

**Use** Treatment of trophoblastic neoplasms; leukemias; psoriasis; rheumatoid arthritis; breast, head, and lung carcinomas; osteosarcoma; sarcomas; carcinoma of gastric, esophagus, testes; lymphomas

**Usual Dosage** Refer to individual protocols. May be administered orally, I.M., intra-arterially, intrathecally, I.V., or S.C.

Leucovorin may be administered concomitantly or within 24 hours of methotrexate

Children:

Juvenile rheumatoid arthritis: Oral, I.M.: 5-15 mg/m²/week as a single dose **or** as 3 divided doses given 12 hours apart

Antineoplastic dosage range:

Oral, I.M.: 7.5-30 mg/m²/week **or** every 2 weeks

I.V.: 10-12,000 mg/m² bolus dosing **or** continuous infusion over 6-42 hours

**Methotrexate Dosing Schedules**

| | Dose | Route | Frequency |
|---|---|---|---|
| Conventional dose | 15-20 mg/m²<br>30-50 mg/m²<br>15 mg/day for 5 days | Oral<br>Oral, I.V.<br>Oral, I.M. | Twice weekly<br>Weekly<br>Every 2-3 weeks |
| Intermediate dose | 50-150 mg/m²<br>240 mg/m²*<br>0.5-1 g/m²* | I.V. push<br>I.V. infusion<br>I.V. infusion | Every 2-3 weeks<br>Every 4-7 days<br>Every 2-3 weeks |
| High dose | 1-12 g/m²* | I.V. infusion | Every 1-3 weeks |

Pediatric solid tumors: I.V.:

<12 years: 12 g/m² (dosage range: 12-18 g)

≥ 12 years: 8 g/m² (maximum: 18 g)

Meningeal leukemia: I.V.: Loading dose: 6 g/m² followed by I.V. continuous infusion of 1.2 g/m²/hour for 23 hours

Acute lymphocytic leukemia (high dose): I.V.: Loading: 200 mg/m² followed by a 24-hour infusion of 1200 mg/m²/day

ANLL: I.V.: 7.5 mg/m²/day on days 1-5

Resistant ANLL: I.V.: 100 mg/m²/dose on day 1

Hodgkin's lymphoma: I.V.: 200-500 mg/m²; repeat every 28 days

Induction of remission in acute lymphoblastic leukemias: Oral: 3.3 mg/m²/day for 4-6 weeks; remission maintenance: Oral, I.M.: 20-30 mg/m² twice weekly

Meningeal leukemia: I.T.: 10-15 mg/m² (maximum dose: 15 mg)

**or**

≤3 months: 3 mg/dose

4-11 months: 6 mg/dose

1 year: 8 mg/dose

2 years: 10 mg/dose

≥3 years: 12 mg/dose

I.T. doses are prepared with preservative-free MTX **only**. Hydrocortisone may be added to the I.T. preparation; total volume should range from 3-6 mL. Doses should be repeated at 2- to 5-day intervals until CSF counts return to normal followed by a dose once weekly for 2 weeks then monthly thereafter.

Adults: I.V.: Range is wide from 30-40 mg/m²/week to 100-7500 mg/m² with leucovorin rescue

Doses not requiring leucovorin rescue range from 30-40 mg/m² I.V. or I.M. repeated weekly, or oral regimens of 10 mg/m² twice weekly

**High-dose MTX is considered to be >100 mg/m² and can be as high as 1500-7500 mg/m²**. These doses require leucovorin rescue. Patients receiving doses ≥1000 mg/m² should have their urine alkalinized with bicarbonate or Bicitra® prior to and following MTX therapy.

Trophoblastic neoplasms: Oral, I.M.: 15-30 mg/day for 5 days; repeat in 7 days for 3-5 courses

Head and neck cancer: Oral, I.M., I.V.: 25-50 mg/m² once weekly

Rheumatoid arthritis: Oral: 7.5 mg once weekly **or** 2.5 mg every 12 hours for 3 doses/week; not to exceed 20 mg/week

Psoriasis: Oral: 2.5-5 mg/dose every 12 hours for 3 doses given once weekly

**or**

Oral, I.M.: 10-25 mg/dose given once weekly

Elderly: Rheumatoid arthritis/psoriasis: Oral:

Initial: 5 mg once weekly

If nausea occurs, split dose to 2.5 mg every 12 hours for the day of administration

Dose may be increased to 7.5 mg/week based on response, not to exceed 20 mg/week

Ectopic pregnancy: I.M./I.V.: 50 mg/m$^2$ single-dose without leucovorin rescue

**Mechanism of Action** Antimetabolite that inhibits DNA synthesis and cell reproduction in cancerous cells

Folates must be in the reduced form ($FH_4$) to be active

Folates are activated by dihydrofolate reductase (DHFR)

DHFR is inhibited by MTX (by binding irreversibly), causing an increase in the intracellular dihydrofolate pool (the inactive cofactor) and inhibition of both purine and thymidylate synthesis (TS)

MTX enters the cell through an energy-dependent and temperature-dependent process which is mediated by an intramembrane protein; this carrier mechanism is also used by naturally occurring reduced folates, including folinic acid (leucovorin), making this a competitive process

At high drug concentrations (>20 µM), MTX enters the cell by a second mechanism which is not shared by reduced folates; the process may be passive diffusion or a specific, saturable process, and provides a rationale for high-dose MTX

A small fraction of MTX is converted intracellularly to polyglutamates, which leads to a prolonged inhibition of DHFR

**Local Anesthetic/Vasoconstrictor Precautions** No information available to require special precautions

**Effects on Dental Treatment** Methotrexate commonly causes ulceration stomatitis, gingivitis, and pharyngitis associated with oral discomfort

**Other Adverse Effects**

>10%:

Gastrointestinal: Mucositis is dose-dependent; appears in 3-7 days after therapy, resolving within 2 weeks

Cardiovascular: Vasculitis

Central nervous system (with I.T. administration only):

Arachnoiditis: Acute reaction manifested as severe headache, nuchal rigidity, vomiting, and fever; may be alleviated by reducing the dose

Subacute toxicity: 10% of patients treated with 12-15 mg/m$^2$ of I.T. MTX may develop this in the second or third week of therapy; consists of motor paralysis of extremities, cranial nerve palsy, seizures, or coma. This has also been seen in pediatric cases receiving very high-dose MTX (when enough MTX can get across into the CSF).

Demyelinating encephalopathy: Seen months or years after receiving MTX; usually in association with cranial irradiation or other systemic chemotherapy

Dermatologic: Reddening of skin

Gastrointestinal: Ulcerative stomatitis, pharyngitis, glossitis, gingivitis, nausea, vomiting, diarrhea, anorexia, intestinal perforation

Emetic potential: <100 mg: Moderately low (10% to 30%); ≥100 mg or <250 mg: Moderate (30% to 60%); ≥250 mg: Moderately high (60% to 90%)

Endocrine & metabolic: Hyperuricemia

Hematologic: Leukopenia, thrombocytopenia

Renal: Renal failure, azotemia, nephropathy

1% to 10%:

Central nervous system: Dizziness, malaise, encephalopathy, seizures, fever, chills

Dermatologic: Alopecia, rash, photosensitivity, depigmentation or hyperpigmentation of skin

Endocrine & metabolic: Diabetes

Genitourinary: Cystitis

Hematologic: Hemorrhage

Myelosuppressive: This is the primary dose-limiting factor (along with mucositis) of MTX; occurs about 5-7 days after MTX therapy, and should resolve within 2 weeks; WBC: Mild; Platelets: Moderate; Onset (days): 7; Nadir (days): 10; Recovery (days): 21

Hepatic abnormalities: Cirrhosis and portal fibrosis have been associated with chronic MTX therapy; acute elevation of liver enzymes are common after high-dose MTX, and usually resolve within 10 days

Neuromuscular & skeletal: Arthralgia

Ocular: Blurred vision

Respiratory: Pneumonitis associated with fever, cough, and interstitial pulmonary infiltrates; treatment is to withhold MTX during the acute reaction

Renal dysfunction: Manifested by an abrupt rise in serum creatinine and BUN and a fall in urine output; more common with high-dose MTX, and may be due to precipitation of the drug. The best treatment is prevention: Aggressively hydrate with 3 L/m$^2$/day starting 12 hours before therapy and continue

(Continued)

## Methotrexate *(Continued)*

for 24-36 hours; alkalinize the urine by adding 50 mEq of bicarbonate to each liter of fluid; keep urine flow >100 mL/hour and urine pH >7.

Renal: Vasculitis

Miscellaneous: Anaphylaxis, decreased resistance to infection

**Drug Interactions**

Decreased effect: Decreased phenytoin, 5-FU, nonsteroidal anti-inflammatory drugs (NSAIDs)

Corticosteroids: Reported to decrease uptake of MTX into leukemia cells. Administration of these drugs should be separated by 12 hours. Dexamethasone has been reported to not affect methotrexate influx into cells.

Increased toxicity:

Live virus vaccines cause vaccinia infections

Vincristine: Inhibits MTX efflux from the cell, leading to increased and prolonged MTX levels in the cell; the dose of VCR needed to produce this effect is not achieved clinically

Organic acids: Salicylates, sulfonamides, probenecid, and high doses of penicillins compete with MTX for transport and reduce renal tubular secretion. Salicylates and sulfonamides may also displace MTX from plasma proteins, increasing MTX levels.

Ara-C: Increased formation of the Ara-C nucleotide can occur when MTX precedes Ara-C, thus promoting the action of Ara-C

Cyclosporine: CSA and MTX interfere with each others renal elimination, which may result in increased toxicity

**Drug Uptake**

Absorption:

Oral: Rapid; well absorbed orally at low doses (<30 mg/m$^2$), incomplete absorption after large doses

I.M. injection: Completely absorbed

Serum half-life: 8-12 hours with high doses and 3-10 hours with low doses

Time to peak serum concentration:

Oral: 1-2 hours

Parenteral: 30-60 minutes

**Pregnancy Risk Factor** D

**Generic Available** Yes

## Methotrimeprazine (meth oh trye MEP ra zeen)

**U.S. Brand Names** Levoprome®

**Canadian Brand Names** Nozinan®

**Therapeutic Category** Analgesic, Non-narcotic; Phenothiazine Derivative; Sedative

**Synonyms** Levomepromazine; Methotrimeprazine Hydrochloride

**Use** Relief of moderate to severe pain in nonambulatory patients; for analgesia and sedation when respiratory depression is to be avoided, as in obstetrics; preanesthetic for producing sedation, somnolence and relief of apprehension and anxiety

**Usual Dosage** Adults: I.M.:

Sedation analgesia: 10-20 mg every 4-6 hours as needed

Preoperative medication: 2-20 mg, 45 minutes to 3 hours before surgery

Postoperative analgesia: 2.5-7.5 mg every 4-6 hours is suggested as necessary since residual effects of anesthetic may be present

Pre- and postoperative hypotension: I.M.: 5-10 mg

**Mechanism of Action** Methotrimeprazine is a phenothiazine with sites of action thought to be in the thalamus, hypothalamus, reticular and limbic systems, producing suppression of sensory impulses. This results with sedation, an elevated pain threshold, and induction of amnesia. The analgesic effect of methotrimeprazine is comparable to meperidine and morphine without the respiratory suppression. This agent also has antihistamine, anticholinergic, and antiepinephrine effects.

**Local Anesthetic/Vasoconstrictor Precautions** No information available to require special precautions

**Effects on Dental Treatment** Anticholinergic side effects can cause a reduction of saliva production or secretion contributes to discomfort and dental disease (ie, caries, oral candidiasis and periodontal disease); phenothiazines can cause extrapyramidal reactions which may appear as muscle twitching or increased motor activity of the face, neck or head

**Other Adverse Effects**

>10%:

Cardiovascular: Hypotension, orthostatic hypotension

Central nervous system: Pseudoparkinsonism, akathisia, dystonias, tardive dyskinesia (persistent), dizziness

Gastrointestinal: Constipation
Ocular: Pigmentary retinopathy
Respiratory: Nasal congestion
Miscellaneous: Decreased sweating

1% to 10%:
Dermatologic: Photosensitivity, skin rash
Endocrine & metabolic: Changes in menstrual cycle, changes in libido, pain in breasts
Gastrointestinal: Weight gain, nausea, vomiting, stomach pain
Genitourinary: Dysuria, ejaculatory disturbances
Neuromuscular & skeletal: Trembling of fingers

<1%:
Central nervous system: Neuroleptic malignant syndrome (NMS), impairment of temperature regulation, lowering of seizures threshold
Dermatologic: Discoloration of skin (blue-gray)
Endocrine & metabolic: Galactorrhea
Genitourinary: Priapism
Hematologic: Agranulocytosis, leukopenia
Hepatic: Cholestatic jaundice, hepatotoxicity
Ocular: Cornea and lens changes, pigmentary retinopathy

**Drug Interactions** Increased toxicity: Additive effects with other CNS-depressants

**Drug Uptake**
Peak effect: Within 20-40 minutes
Duration: 4 hours
Serum half-life, elimination: 20 hours
Time to peak serum concentration: Within 0.5-1.5 hours

**Pregnancy Risk Factor** C

**Generic Available** No

♦ **Methotrimeprazine Hydrochloride** *see* Methotrimeprazine *on previous page*

## Methoxsalen (meth OKS a len)

**U.S. Brand Names** Oxsoralen® Topical; Oxsoralen-Ultra® Oral

**Canadian Brand Names** Ultramop™

**Therapeutic Category** Psoralen

**Synonyms** Methoxypsoralen; 8-Methoxypsoralen; 8-MOP

**Use** Symptomatic control of severe, recalcitrant, disabling psoriasis in conjunction with long wave ultraviolet radiation; induce repigmentation in vitiligo topical repigmenting agent in conjunction with controlled doses of ultraviolet A (UVA) or sunlight

**Usual Dosage**
Psoriasis: Adults: Oral: 10-70 mg 1½-2 hours before exposure to ultraviolet light, 2-3 times at least 48 hours apart; dosage is based upon patient's body weight and skin type
Vitiligo: Children >12 years and Adults:
Oral: 20 mg 2-4 hours before exposure to UVA light or sunlight; limit exposure to 15-40 minutes based on skin basic color and exposure
Topical: Apply lotion 1-2 hours before exposure to UVA light, no more than once weekly

**Mechanism of Action** Bonds covalently to pyrimidine bases in DNA, inhibits the synthesis of DNA, and suppresses cell division. The augmented sunburn reaction involves excitation of the methoxsalen molecule by radiation in the long-wave ultraviolet light (UVA), resulting in transference of energy to the methoxsalen molecule producing an excited state ("triplet electronic state"). The molecule, in this "triplet state", then reacts with cutaneous DNA.

**Local Anesthetic/Vasoconstrictor Precautions** No information available to require special precautions

**Effects on Dental Treatment** No effects or complications reported

**Other Adverse Effects**
>10%:
Dermatologic: Itching
Gastrointestinal: Nausea

1% to 10%:
Cardiovascular: Severe edema, hypotension
Central nervous system: Nervousness, vertigo, depression
Dermatologic: Pruritus, freckling, hypopigmentation, rash, cheilitis, erythema; painful blistering, burning, and peeling of skin
Neuromuscular & skeletal: Loss of muscle coordination

**Drug Uptake** Time to peak serum concentration: Oral: 2-4 hours

**Pregnancy Risk Factor** C

**Generic Available** No

(Continued)

## Methoxsalen *(Continued)*

**Comments** Absorption is increased with food; peak levels occur in 30 minutes to 1 hour after ingestion; plasma half-life is approximately 2 hours

## Methoxycinnamate and Oxybenzone

(meth OKS ee SIN a mate & oks i BEN zone)

**U.S. Brand Names** PreSun® 29 [OTC]; Ti-Screen® [OTC]

**Therapeutic Category** Sunscreen

**Synonyms** Sunscreen, PABA-Free

**Use** Reduce the chance of premature aging of the skin and skin cancer from overexposure to the sun

**Local Anesthetic/Vasoconstrictor Precautions** No information available to require special precautions

**Effects on Dental Treatment** No effects or complications reported

**Generic Available** Yes

♦ **Methoxypsoralen** *see* Methoxsalen *on previous page*

♦ **8-Methoxypsoralen** *see* Methoxsalen *on previous page*

## Methscopolamine (meth skoe POL a meen)

**U.S. Brand Names** Pamine®

**Therapeutic Category** Anticholinergic Agent; Antispasmodic Agent, Gastrointestinal

**Use** Adjunctive therapy in the treatment of peptic ulcer

**Usual Dosage** Adults: Oral: 2.5 mg 30 minutes before meals or food and 2.5-5 mg at bedtime

**Mechanism of Action** Methscopolamine is a peripheral anticholinergic agent that does not cross the blood-brain barrier and provides a peripheral blockade of muscarinic receptors. This agent reduces the volume and the total acid content of gastric secretions, inhibits salivation, and reduces gastrointestinal motility.

**Local Anesthetic/Vasoconstrictor Precautions** No information available to require special precautions

**Effects on Dental Treatment** >10% of patients experience dry mouth; anticholinergic side effects can cause a reduction of saliva production or secretion contributes to discomfort and dental disease (ie, caries, oral candidiasis and periodontal disease)

**Other Adverse Effects**

>10%:

- Dermatologic: Dry skin
- Gastrointestinal: Constipation
- Respiratory: Dry nose, throat
- Miscellaneous: Decreased sweating

1% to 10%: Gastrointestinal: Dysphagia

<1%:

- Cardiovascular: Tachycardia
- Central nervous system: Confusion, drowsiness, nervousness, insomnia, headache, loss of memory, fatigue
- Dermatologic: Rash
- Gastrointestinal: Bloated feeling, nausea, vomiting
- Genitourinary: Urinary retention
- Neuromuscular & skeletal: Weakness
- Ocular: Increased intraocular pressure, blurred vision

**Drug Interactions** No data reported

**Pregnancy Risk Factor** C

**Generic Available** No

## Methsuximide (meth SUKS i mide)

**U.S. Brand Names** Celontin®

**Canadian Brand Names** Celontin®

**Therapeutic Category** Anticonvulsant, Succinimide

**Use** Control of absence (petit mal) seizures; useful adjunct in refractory, partial complex (psychomotor) seizures

**Usual Dosage** Oral:

- Children: Initial: 10-15 mg/kg/day in 3-4 divided doses; increase weekly up to maximum of 30 mg/kg/day
- Adults: 300 mg/day for the first week; may increase by 300 mg/day at weekly intervals up to 1.2 g/day in 2-4 divided doses/day

**Mechanism of Action** Increases the seizure threshold and suppresses paroxysmal spike-and-wave pattern in absence seizures; depresses nerve transmission in the motor cortex

**Local Anesthetic/Vasoconstrictor Precautions** No information available to require special precautions

**Effects on Dental Treatment** No effects or complications reported

**Other Adverse Effects**

>10%:

Central nervous system: Ataxia, dizziness, drowsiness, headache
Dermatologic: Stevens-Johnson syndrome
Gastrointestinal: Anorexia, nausea, vomiting, weight loss
Miscellaneous: Hiccups, SLE

1% to 10%:

Central nervous system: Aggressiveness, mental depression, nightmares, fatigue
Neuromuscular & skeletal: Weakness

<1%:

Central nervous system: Paranoid psychosis
Dermatologic: Urticaria, exfoliative dermatitis
Hematologic: Agranulocytosis, leukopenia, aplastic anemia, thrombocytopenia, pancytopenia

**Drug Interactions** No data reported

**Drug Uptake**

Serum half-life: 2-4 hours
Time to peak serum concentration: Oral: Within 1-3 hours

**Pregnancy Risk Factor** C

**Generic Available** No

## Methyclothiazide (meth i kloe THYE a zide)

**Related Information**

Cardiovascular Diseases *on page 1066*

**U.S. Brand Names** Aquatensen®; Enduron®

**Therapeutic Category** Diuretic, Thiazide

**Use** Management of mild to moderate hypertension; treatment of edema in congestive heart failure and nephrotic syndrome

**Usual Dosage** Oral:

Children: 0.05-0.2 mg/kg/day
Adults:
Edema: 2.5-10 mg/day
Hypertension: 2.5-5 mg/day

**Mechanism of Action** Inhibits sodium reabsorption in the distal tubules causing increased excretion of sodium and water, as well as, potassium and hydrogen ions

**Local Anesthetic/Vasoconstrictor Precautions** No information available to require special precautions

**Effects on Dental Treatment** No effects or complications reported

**Other Adverse Effects**

1% to 10%: Endocrine & metabolic: Hypokalemia

<1%:

Cardiovascular: Hypotension
Central nervous system: Drowsiness
Dermatologic: Photosensitivity, rash
Endocrine & metabolic: Fluid and electrolyte imbalances (hypocalcemia, hypomagnesemia, hyponatremia), hyperglycemia
Gastrointestinal: Nausea, vomiting, anorexia
Hematologic: Rarely blood dyscrasias, aplastic anemia, hemolytic anemia, leukopenia, agranulocytosis, thrombocytopenia
Hepatic: Hepatitis
Neuromuscular & skeletal: Paresthesia
Renal: Polyuria, prerenal azotemia, uremia

**Drug Interactions** Increased toxicity/levels of lithium

**Drug Uptake**

Onset of diuresis: Oral: 2 hours
Peak effect: 6 hours
Duration: ~1 day

**Pregnancy Risk Factor** D

**Generic Available** Yes

## Methyclothiazide and Deserpidine

(meth i kloe THYE a zide & de SER pi deen)

**U.S. Brand Names** Enduronyl®; Enduronyl® Forte

**Therapeutic Category** Antihypertensive Agent, Combination

**Use** Management of mild to moderately severe hypertension

**Usual Dosage** Oral: Individualized, normally 1-4 tablets/day

(Continued)

## Methyclothiazide and Deserpidine *(Continued)*

**Local Anesthetic/Vasoconstrictor Precautions** No information available to require special precautions
**Effects on Dental Treatment** No effects or complications reported
**Pregnancy Risk Factor** C
**Generic Available** No

## Methyclothiazide and Pargyline

(meth i kloe THYE a zide & PAR gi leen)
**U.S. Brand Names** Eutron®
**Therapeutic Category** Antihypertensive Agent, Combination
**Synonyms** Pargyline and Methyclothiazide
**Use** Management of hypertension
**Usual Dosage** Oral: Individualized, normally 1-4 tablets/day
**Local Anesthetic/Vasoconstrictor Precautions** No information available to require special precautions
**Effects on Dental Treatment** No effects or complications reported
**Pregnancy Risk Factor** C
**Generic Available** No

## Methylbenzethonium Chloride

(meth il ben ze THOE nee um KLOR ide)
**U.S. Brand Names** Diaparene® [OTC]; Puri-Clens™ [OTC]; Sween® Cream [OTC]
**Therapeutic Category** Topical Skin Product
**Use** Diaper rash and ammonia dermatitis
**Usual Dosage** Apply topically to area as needed
**Local Anesthetic/Vasoconstrictor Precautions** No information available to require special precautions
**Effects on Dental Treatment** No effects or complications reported
**Generic Available** No

## Methylcellulose (meth il SEL yoo lose)

**U.S. Brand Names** Citrucel® [OTC]
**Canadian Brand Names** Murocel™
**Therapeutic Category** Ophthalmic Agent, Miscellaneous
**Use** Adjunct in treatment of constipation
**Usual Dosage** Oral:
Children ≤12 years: Half the adult dose in 4 oz of cold water, 1-3 times/day
Children ≥12 years and Adults: 1 heaping tablespoon (19 g) in 8 oz of cold water, 1-3 times/day
**Local Anesthetic/Vasoconstrictor Precautions** No information available to require special precautions
**Effects on Dental Treatment** No effects or complications reported
**Pregnancy Risk Factor** C
**Generic Available** Yes
**Comments** Each dose contains sodium 3 mg, potassium 105 mg, and 60 calories from sucrose

## Methyldopa (meth il DOE pa)

**Related Information**
Cardiovascular Diseases *on page 1066*
**U.S. Brand Names** Aldomet®
**Canadian Brand Names** Apo®-Methyldopa; Dopamet®; Medimet®; Novo-Medopa®; Nu-Medopa
**Therapeutic Category** Alpha-Adrenergic Blockers - Peripheral-Acting (Alpha$_1$-Blockers)
**Use** Management of moderate to severe hypertension
**Usual Dosage**
Children:
Oral: Initial: 10 mg/kg/day in 2-4 divided doses; increase every 2 days as needed to maximum dose of 65 mg/kg/day; do not exceed 3 g/day
I.V.: 5-10 mg/kg/dose every 6-8 hours up to a total dose of 65 mg/kg/24 hours or 3 g/24 hours
Adults:
Oral: Initial: 250 mg 2-3 times/day; increase every 2 days as needed; usual dose 1-1.5 g/day in 2-4 divided doses; maximum dose: 3 g/day
I.V.: 250-1000 mg every 6-8 hours; maximum dose: 1 g every 6 hours

**Mechanism of Action** Stimulation of central alpha-adrenergic receptors by a false transmitter that results in a decreased sympathetic outflow to the heart, kidneys, and peripheral vasculature

**Local Anesthetic/Vasoconstrictor Precautions** No information available to require special precautions

**Effects on Dental Treatment** Anticholinergic side effects can cause a reduction of saliva production or secretion. This may result in discomfort and dental disease (ie, caries, oral candidiasis and periodontal disease)

**Other Adverse Effects**

>10%: Cardiovascular: Peripheral edema

1% to 10%:

Central nervous system: Drug fever, mental depression, anxiety, nightmares, drowsiness, headache

Gastrointestinal: Dry mouth

<1%:

Cardiovascular: Orthostatic hypotension, bradycardia (sinus)

Central nervous system: Fever, chills, sedation, vertigo, depression, memory lapse

Dermatologic: Rash

Endocrine & metabolic: Sodium retention, sexual dysfunction, gynecomastia, hyperprolactinemia

Gastrointestinal: Colitis, pancreatitis, diarrhea, nausea, vomiting, "black" tongue

Genitourinary: Decreased libido

Hematologic: Thrombocytopenia, hemolytic anemia, positive Coombs' test, leukopenia, transient leukopenia or granulocytopenia

Hepatic: Cholestasis or hepatitis and heptocellular injury, elevated liver enzymes, jaundice, cirrhosis

Neuromuscular & skeletal: Paresthesias, weakness

Respiratory: Dyspnea

Miscellaneous: SLE-like syndrome

**Drug Interactions**

Decreased effect: Iron supplements can interact and cause a significant **increase** in blood pressure

Increased toxicity: Lithium causes increased lithium toxicity; tolbutamide and levodopa effects/toxicity increased

**Drug Uptake**

Peak hypotensive effect: Oral, parenteral: Within 3-6 hours

Duration: 12-24 hours

Serum half-life: 75-80 minutes

End-stage renal disease: 6-16 hours

**Pregnancy Risk Factor** C

**Generic Available** Yes

♦ **Methyldopa and Chlorothiazide** *see* Chlorothiazide and Methyldopa *on page 229*

## Methyldopa and Hydrochlorothiazide

(meth il DOE pa & hye droe klor oh THYE a zide)

**U.S. Brand Names** Aldoril®

**Canadian Brand Names** Aldoril®-15; Aldoril®-25; Apo®-Methazide; Novo-Doparil; PMS-Dopazide

**Therapeutic Category** Antihypertensive Agent, Combination

**Synonyms** Hydrochlorothiazide and Methyldopa

**Use** Management of moderate to severe hypertension

**Usual Dosage** Oral: 1 tablet 2-3 times/day for first 48 hours, then decrease or increase at intervals of not less than 2 days until an adequate response is achieved

**Local Anesthetic/Vasoconstrictor Precautions** No information available to require special precautions

**Effects on Dental Treatment** Anticholinergic side effects can cause a reduction of saliva production or secretion. This may result in discomfort and dental disease (ie, caries, oral candidiasis and periodontal disease)

**Pregnancy Risk Factor** C

**Generic Available** Yes

## Methylergonovine (meth il er goe NOE veen)

**U.S. Brand Names** Methergine®

**Therapeutic Category** Ergot Alkaloid and Derivative

**Use** Prevention and treatment of postpartum and postabortion hemorrhage caused by uterine atony or subinvolution

(Continued)

## Methylergonovine *(Continued)*

**Usual Dosage** Adults:

Oral: 0.2 mg 3-4 times/day for 2-7 days

I.M.: 0.2 mg after delivery of anterior shoulder, after delivery of placenta, or during puerperium; may be repeated as required at intervals of 2-4 hours

I.V.: Same dose as I.M., but should not be routinely administered I.V. because of possibility of inducing sudden hypertension and cerebrovascular accident

**Mechanism of Action** Similar smooth muscle actions as seen with ergotamine; however, it affects primarily uterine smooth muscles producing sustained contractions and thereby shortens the third stage of labor

**Local Anesthetic/Vasoconstrictor Precautions** No information available to require special precautions

**Effects on Dental Treatment** No effects or complications reported

**Other Adverse Effects**

>10%:

- Cardiovascular: Hypertension
- Central nervous system: Headache, seizures

1% to 10%: Gastrointestinal: Nausea, vomiting

<1%:

- Cardiovascular: Temporary chest pain, palpitations
- Central nervous system: Hallucinations, dizziness
- Endocrine & metabolic: Water intoxication
- Gastrointestinal: Diarrhea, foul taste
- Local: Thrombophlebitis
- Neuromuscular & skeletal: Leg cramps
- Otic: Tinnitus
- Renal: Hematuria
- Respiratory: Dyspnea, nasal congestion
- Miscellaneous: Sweating

**Drug Interactions** No data reported

**Drug Uptake**

Onset of oxytocic effect:

- Oral: 5-10 minutes
- I.M.: 2-5 minutes
- I.V.: Immediately

Duration of action:

- Oral: ~3 hours
- I.M.: ~3 hours
- I.V.: 45 minutes

Absorption: Rapid

Serum half-life (biphasic):

- Initial: 1-5 minutes
- Terminal: 30 minutes to 2 hours

Time to peak serum concentration: Within 30 minutes to 3 hours

**Pregnancy Risk Factor** C

**Generic Available** No

♦ **Methylmorphine** *see* Codeine *on page 272*

♦ **Methylone®** *see* Methylprednisolone *on next page*

## Methylphenidate (meth il FEN i date)

**U.S. Brand Names** Ritalin®; Ritalin-SR®

**Canadian Brand Names** PMS-Methylphenidate; Riphenidate

**Therapeutic Category** Central Nervous System Stimulant, Nonamphetamine

**Use** Treatment of attention deficit disorder and symptomatic management of narcolepsy; many **unlabeled uses**

**Usual Dosage** Oral: (Discontinue periodically to re-evaluate or if no improvement occurs within 1 month)

Children ≥6 years: Attention deficit disorder: Initial: 0.3 mg/kg/dose or 2.5-5 mg/dose given before breakfast and lunch; increase by 0.1 mg/kg/dose or by 5-10 mg/day at weekly intervals; usual dose: 0.5-1 mg/kg/day; maximum dose: 2 mg/kg/day or 60 mg/day

Adults:

- Narcolepsy: 10 mg 2-3 times/day, up to 60 mg/day
- Depression: Initial: 2.5 mg every morning before 9 AM; dosage may be increased by 2.5-5 mg every 2-3 days as tolerated to a maximum of 20 mg/day; may be divided (ie, 7 AM and 12 noon), but should not be given after noon; do not use sustained release product

**Mechanism of Action** Blocks the reuptake mechanism of dopaminergic neurons; appears to stimulate the cerebral cortex and subcortical structures similar to amphetamines

**Local Anesthetic/Vasoconstrictor Precautions** No information available to require special precautions

**Effects on Dental Treatment** Up to 10% of patients taking dextroamphetamines or amphetamine-like drugs may present with hypertension. The use of local anesthetic without vasoconstrictor is recommended in these patients.

**Other Adverse Effects**

>10%:

Cardiovascular: Tachycardia

Central nervous system: Nervousness, insomnia

Gastrointestinal: Anorexia

1% to 10%:

Central nervous system: Dizziness, drowsiness

Gastrointestinal: Stomach pain

Miscellaneous: Hypersensitivity reactions

<1%:

Cardiovascular: Hypertension, hypotension, palpitations, cardiac arrhythmias

Central nervous system: Movement disorders, precipitation of Tourette's syndrome, and toxic psychosis (rare), fever, headache, convulsions

Dermatologic: Rash

Gastrointestinal: Nausea, weight loss, vomiting

Endocrine & metabolic: Growth retardation

Hematologic: Thrombocytopenia, anemia, leukopenia

Ocular: Blurred vision

**Drug Interactions**

Decreased effect: Effects of guanethidine, bretylium may be antagonized by methylphenidate

Increased toxicity: May increase serum concentrations of tricyclic antidepressants, warfarin, phenytoin, phenobarbital, and primidone; MAO inhibitors may potentiate effects of methylphenidate

**Drug Uptake**

Immediate release tablet:

Duration: 3-6 hours

Sustained release tablet:

Peak effect: Within 4-7 hours

Duration: 8 hours

Absorption: Slow and incomplete from GI tract

Serum half-life: 2-4 hours

**Pregnancy Risk Factor** C

**Generic Available** Yes

## Methylprednisolone (meth il pred NIS oh lone)

**Related Information**

Corticosteroid Equivalencies Comparison *on page 1221*

Corticosteroids, Topical Comparison *on page 1222*

Respiratory Diseases *on page 1079*

**U.S. Brand Names** Adlone®; A-methaPred®; depMedalone®; Depoject®; Depo-Medrol®; Depopred®; Duralone®; Medralone®; Medrol®; Methylone®; Solu-Medrol®

**Canadian Brand Names** Medrol® Veriderm® Cream

**Therapeutic Category** Adrenal Corticosteroid; Anti-inflammatory Agent; Corticosteroid, Systemic; Corticosteroid, Topical (Low Potency)

**Use**

Dental: Treatment of a variety of oral diseases of allergic, inflammatory or autoimmune origin

Medical: Primarily as an anti-inflammatory or immunosuppressant agent in the treatment of a variety of diseases including those of hematologic, allergic, inflammatory, neoplastic, and autoimmune origin

**Usual Dosage Only sodium succinate salt may be given I.V.**. Methylprednisolone sodium succinate is highly soluble and has a rapid effect by I.M. and I.V. routes. Methylprednisolone acetate has a low solubility and has a sustained I.M. effect.

Children:

Anti-inflammatory or immunosuppressive: Oral, I.M., I.V. (sodium succinate): 0.12-1.7 mg/kg/day or 5-25 mg/m²/day in divided doses every 6-12 hours

Adults:

Anti-inflammatory or immunosuppressive: Oral: 2-60 mg/day in 1-4 divided doses to start, followed by gradual reduction in dosage to the lowest possible level consistent with maintaining an adequate clinical response

I.M. (sodium succinate): 10-80 mg/day once daily

I.M. (acetate): 40-120 mg every 1-2 weeks

(Continued)

## Methylprednisolone *(Continued)*

I.V. (sodium succinate): 10-40 mg over a period of several minutes and repeated I.V. or I.M. at intervals depending on clinical response; when high dosages are needed, give 30 mg/kg over a period of 10-20 minutes and may be repeated every 4-6 hours for 48 hours

**Mechanism of Action** Decreases inflammation by suppression of migration of polymorphonuclear leukocytes and reversal of increased capillary permeability

**Local Anesthetic/Vasoconstrictor Precautions** No information available to require special precautions

**Effects on Dental Treatment** No effects or complications reported

**Other Adverse Effects** >10%:

Central nervous system: Insomnia, nervousness

Gastrointestinal: Increased appetite, indigestion

**Contraindications** Serious infections, except septic shock or tuberculous meningitis; known hypersensitivity to methylprednisolone; viral, fungal, or tubercular skin lesions; administration of live virus vaccines

**Warnings/Precautions**

Use with caution in patients with hyperthyroidism, cirrhosis, nonspecific ulcerative colitis, hypertension, osteoporosis, thromboembolic tendencies, CHF, convulsive disorders, myasthenia gravis, thrombophlebitis, peptic ulcer, diabetes

Acute adrenal insufficiency may occur with abrupt withdrawal after long-term therapy or with stress; young pediatric patients may be more susceptible to adrenal axis suppression from topical therapy

Because of the risk of adverse effects, systemic corticosteroids should be used cautiously in the elderly, in the smallest possible dose, and for the shortest possible time.

**Drug Interactions** Phenytoin, phenobarbital, rifampin increases clearance of methylprednisolone; potassium depleting diuretics enhance potassium depletion; skin test antigens, immunizations increase response and increase potential infections; methylprednisolone may increase circulating glucose levels → may need adjustments of insulin or oral hypoglycemics

**Drug Uptake** Methylprednisolone sodium succinate is highly soluble and has a rapid effect by I.M. and I.V. routes; methylprednisolone acetate has a low solubility and has a sustained I.M. effect

Serum half-life: 3-3.5 hours

Time to obtain peak effect and the duration of these effects is dependent upon the route of administration. See table.

| Route | Peak Effect | Duration |
|---|---|---|
| Oral | 1-2 h | 30-36 h |
| I.M. | 4-8 d | 1-4 wk |
| Intra-articular | 1 wk | 1-5 wk |

**Pregnancy Risk Factor** C

**Breast-feeding Considerations** No data reported

**Dosage Forms**

Injection, as sodium succinate: 40 mg (1 mL, 3 mL); 125 mg (2 mL, 5 mL); 500 mg (1 mL, 4 mL, 8 mL, 20 mL); 1,000 mg (1 mL, 8 mL, 50 mL); 2,000 mg (30.6 mL)

Injection, as acetate: 20 mg/mL (5 mL, 10 mL); 40 mg/mL (1 mL, 5 mL, 10 mL); 80 mg/mL (1 mL, 5 mL)

Tablet: 2 mg, 4 mg, 8 mg, 16 mg, 24 mg, 32 mg

Tablet, dose pack: 4 mg (21s)

**Dietary Considerations** Should be taken after meals or with food or milk; limit caffeine; need diet rich in pyridoxine, vitamin C, vitamin D, folate, calcium, phosphorus, and protein

**Generic Available** Yes

♦ **4-Methylpyrazole** *see* Fomepizole *on page 453*

## Methyltestosterone (meth il tes TOS te rone)

**U.S. Brand Names** Android-25®; Oreton® Methyl; Testred®; Virilon®

**Therapeutic Category** Androgen

**Use**

Male: Hypogonadism; delayed puberty; impotence and climacteric symptoms

Female: Palliative treatment of metastatic breast cancer; postpartum breast pain and/or engorgement

**Usual Dosage** Adults (buccal absorption produces twice the androgenic activity of oral tablets):

Male:
  Oral: 10-40 mg/day
  Buccal: 5-25 mg/day
Female:
  Breast pain/engorgement:
    Oral: 80 mg/day for 3-5 days
    Buccal: 40 mg/day for 3-5 days
  Breast cancer:
    Oral: 50-200 mg/day
    Buccal: 25-100 mg/day

**Mechanism of Action** Stimulates receptors in organs and tissues to promote growth and development of male sex organs and maintains secondary sex characteristics in androgen-deficient males

**Local Anesthetic/Vasoconstrictor Precautions** No information available to require special precautions

**Effects on Dental Treatment** No effects or complications reported

**Other Adverse Effects**

>10%:
  Male: Virilism, priapism
  Female: Virilism, menstrual problems (amenorrhea), breast soreness
  Cardiovascular: Edema
  Dermatologic: Acne

1% to 10%:
  Females: Hirsutism (increase in pubic hair growth)
  Men: Prostatic hypertrophy, prostatic carcinoma, impotence, testicular atrophy
  Gastrointestinal: GI irritation, nausea, vomiting
  Hepatic: Hepatic dysfunction

<1%:
  Endocrine & metabolic: Gynecomastia, amenorrhea, hypercalcemia
  Hematologic: Leukopenia, polycythemia
  Hepatic: Hepatic necrosis, cholestatic hepatitis
  Miscellaneous: Hypersensitivity reactions

**Drug Interactions** Decreased effect: Oral anticoagulant effect or insulin requirements may be increased

**Drug Uptake**

Absorption: From GI tract and oral mucosa

**Pregnancy Risk Factor** X

**Generic Available** Yes

## Methysergide (meth i SER jide)

**U.S. Brand Names** Sansert®

**Therapeutic Category** Ergot Alkaloid and Derivative

**Use** Prophylaxis of vascular headache

**Usual Dosage** Adults: Oral: 4-8 mg/day with meals; if no improvement is noted after 3 weeks, drug is unlikely to be beneficial; must not be given continuously for longer than 6 months, and a drug-free interval of 3-4 weeks must follow each 6-month course

**Mechanism of Action** Ergotamine congener, however actions appear to differ; methysergide has minimal ergotamine-like oxytocic or vasoconstrictive properties, and has significantly greater serotonin-like properties

**Local Anesthetic/Vasoconstrictor Precautions** No information available to require special precautions

**Effects on Dental Treatment** No effects or complications reported

**Other Adverse Effects**

>10%:
  Cardiovascular: Postural hypotension, peripheral ischemia
  Central nervous system: Insomnia
  Gastrointestinal: Nausea, vomiting, abdominal pain, diarrhea

1% to 10%:
  Cardiovascular: Peripheral edema, tachycardia, bradycardia
  Dermatologic: Skin rash
  Gastrointestinal: Heartburn

<1%:
  Central nervous system: Overstimulation, drowsiness, mild euphoria, lethargy, mental depression, vertigo, unsteadiness, confusion, hyperesthesia; rebound headache may occur if methysergide is discontinued abruptly
  Ocular: Visual disturbances
  Respiratory: Fibrosis

**Drug Interactions** No data reported

**Drug Uptake**

Serum half-life, plasma elimination: ~10 hours

(Continued)

## Methysergide *(Continued)*

**Pregnancy Risk Factor** X
**Generic Available** No

- **Meticorten®** *see* Prednisone *on page 833*
- **Metimyd® Ophthalmic** *see* Sulfacetamide Sodium and Prednisolone *on page 940*

## Metipranolol (met i PRAN oh lol)

**U.S. Brand Names** OptiPranolol®

**Therapeutic Category** Antiglaucoma Agent; Beta-Adrenergic Blocker, Ophthalmic

**Use** Agent for lowering intraocular pressure in patients with chronic open-angle glaucoma

**Usual Dosage** Ophthalmic: Adults: Instill 1 drop in the affected eye(s) twice daily

**Mechanism of Action** Beta-adrenoceptor-blocking agent; lacks intrinsic sympathomimetic activity and membrane-stabilizing effects and possesses only slight local anesthetic activity; mechanism of action of metipranolol in reducing intraocular pressure appears to be via reduced production of aqueous humor. This effect may be related to a reduction in blood flow to the iris root-ciliary body. It remains unclear if the reduction in intraocular pressure observed with beta-blockers is actually secondary to beta-adrenoceptor blockade.

**Local Anesthetic/Vasoconstrictor Precautions** No information available to require special precautions

**Effects on Dental Treatment** No effects or complications reported

**Other Adverse Effects**

>10%: Ocular: Mild ocular stinging and discomfort, eye irritation
1% to 10%: Ocular: Blurred vision, browache
<1%:
- Cardiovascular: Bradycardia, A-V block, congestive heart failure
- Neuromuscular & skeletal: Weakness
- Ocular: Conjunctivitis, blepharitis, tearing, erythema, itching, keratitis, photophobia, decreased corneal sensitivity
- Respiratory: Bronchospasm

**Drug Interactions** No data reported

**Drug Uptake**

Onset of action: ≤30 minutes
Maximum effects: ~2 hours
Duration of action: Intraocular pressure reduction has persisted for 24 hours following ocular instillation
Serum half-life, elimination: ~3 hours

**Pregnancy Risk Factor** C
**Generic Available** No

## Metoclopramide (met oh kloe PRA mide)

**Related Information**

Endocrine Disorders & Pregnancy *on page 1082*

**U.S. Brand Names** Maxolon®; Octamide® PFS; Reglan®

**Canadian Brand Names** Apo®-Metoclop; Maxeran®

**Therapeutic Category** Antiemetic

**Use** Symptomatic treatment of diabetic gastric stasis, gastroesophageal reflux; prevention of nausea associated with chemotherapy or postsurgery and facilitates intubation of the small intestine

**Usual Dosage**

Children:
- Gastroesophageal reflux: Oral: 0.1-0.2 mg/kg/dose up to 4 times/day; efficacy of continuing metoclopramide beyond 12 weeks in reflux has not been determined; total daily dose should not exceed 0.5 mg/kg/day
- Gastrointestinal hypomotility (gastroparesis): Oral, I.M., I.V.: 0.1 mg/kg/dose up to 4 times/day, not to exceed 0.5 mg/kg/day
- Antiemetic (chemotherapy-induced emesis): I.V.: 1-2 mg/kg 30 minutes before chemotherapy and every 2-4 hours
- Facilitate intubation: I.V.:
  - <6 years: 0.1 mg/kg
  - 6-14 years: 2.5-5 mg

Adults:
- Gastroesophageal reflux: Oral: 10-15 mg/dose up to 4 times/day 30 minutes before meals or food and at bedtime; single doses of 20 mg are occasionally needed for provoking situations; efficacy of continuing metoclopramide beyond 12 weeks in reflux has not been determined
- Gastrointestinal hypomotility (gastroparesis):
  - Oral: 10 mg 30 minutes before each meal and at bedtime for 2-8 weeks

I.V. (for severe symptoms): 10 mg over 1-2 minutes; 10 days of I.V. therapy may be necessary for best response

Antiemetic (chemotherapy-induced emesis): I.V.: 1-2 mg/kg 30 minutes before chemotherapy and every 2-4 hours to every 4-6 hours (and usually given with diphenhydramine 25-50 mg I.V./oral)

Postoperative nausea and vomiting: I.M.: 10 mg near end of surgery; 20 mg doses may be used

Facilitate intubation: I.V.: 10 mg

Elderly:

Gastroesophageal reflux: Oral: 5 mg 4 times/day (30 minutes before meals and at bedtime); increase dose to 10 mg 4 times/day if no response at lower dose

Gastrointestinal hypomotility:

Oral: Initial: 5 mg 30 minutes before meals and at bedtime for 2-8 weeks; increase if necessary to 10 mg doses

I.V.: Initiate at 5 mg over 1-2 minutes; increase to 10 mg if necessary

Postoperative nausea and vomiting: I.M.: 5 mg near end of surgery; may repeat dose if necessary

**Mechanism of Action** Blocks dopamine receptors in chemoreceptor trigger zone of the CNS; enhances the response to acetylcholine of tissue in upper GI tract causing enhanced motility and accelerated gastric emptying without stimulating gastric, biliary, or pancreatic secretions

**Local Anesthetic/Vasoconstrictor Precautions** No information available to require special precautions

**Effects on Dental Treatment** No effects or complications reported

**Other Adverse Effects**

>10%:

Central nervous system: Restlessness, drowsiness

Gastrointestinal: Diarrhea

Neuromuscular & skeletal: Weakness

1% to 10%:

Central nervous system: Insomnia, depression

Dermatologic: Skin rash

Endocrine & metabolic: Breast tenderness, prolactin stimulation

Gastrointestinal: Nausea, dry mouth

<1%:

Cardiovascular: Tachycardia, hypertension or hypotension

Central nervous system: Extrapyramidal reactions*, tardive dyskinesia, fatigue, anxiety, agitation

Gastrointestinal: Constipation

Hematologic: Methemoglobinemia

***Note:** A recent study suggests the incidence of extrapyramidal reactions due to metoclopramide may be as high as 34% and the incidence appears more often in the elderly

**Drug Interactions**

Decreased effect: Anticholinergic agents antagonize metoclopramide's actions

Increased toxicity: Opiate analgesics causes increased CNS depression

**Drug Uptake**

Onset of effect:

Oral: Within 0.5-1 hour

I.V.: Within 1-3 minutes

Duration of therapeutic effect: 1-2 hours, regardless of route administered

Serum half-life, normal renal function: 4-7 hours (may be dose-dependent)

**Pregnancy Risk Factor** B

**Generic Available** Yes

## Metolazone (me TOLE a zone)

**Related Information**

Cardiovascular Diseases *on page 1066*

**U.S. Brand Names** Mykrox®; Zaroxolyn®

**Therapeutic Category** Diuretic, Thiazide

**Use** Management of mild to moderate hypertension; treatment of edema in congestive heart failure and nephrotic syndrome, impaired renal function

**Usual Dosage** Oral:

Children: 0.2-0.4 mg/kg/day divided every 12-24 hours

Adults:

Edema: 5-20 mg/dose every 24 hours

Hypertension: 2.5-5 mg/dose every 24 hours

Hypertension (Mykrox®): 0.5 mg/day; if response is not adequate, increase dose to maximum of 1 mg/day

(Continued)

## Metolazone *(Continued)*

**Mechanism of Action** Inhibits sodium reabsorption in the distal tubules causing increased excretion of sodium and water, as well as, potassium and hydrogen ions

**Local Anesthetic/Vasoconstrictor Precautions** No information available to require special precautions

**Effects on Dental Treatment** No effects or complications reported

**Other Adverse Effects**

1% to 10%: Endocrine & metabolic: Hypokalemia

<1%:

- Cardiovascular: Hypotension
- Central nervous system: Drowsiness
- Dermatologic: Photosensitivity, rash
- Endocrine & metabolic: Fluid and electrolyte imbalances (hypocalcemia, hypomagnesemia, hyponatremia), hyperglycemia
- Gastrointestinal: Nausea, vomiting, anorexia
- Hematologic: Rarely blood dyscrasias, aplastic anemia, hemolytic anemia, leukopenia, agranulocytosis, thrombocytopenia
- Hepatic: Hepatitis
- Neuromuscular & skeletal: Paresthesia
- Renal: Prerenal azotemia, polyuria, uremia

**Drug Interactions** Increased toxicity:

Concurrent administration with furosemide may cause excessive volume and electrolyte depletion

Increased digitalis glycosides toxicity

Increased lithium toxicity

**Drug Uptake** Same for all routes:

Onset of diuresis: Within 60 minutes

Duration: 12-24 hours

Absorption: Oral: Incomplete

Serum half-life: 6-20 hours, renal function dependent

**Pregnancy Risk Factor** D

**Generic Available** No

## Metoprolol (me toe PROE lole)

**Related Information**

Cardiovascular Diseases *on page 1066*

**U.S. Brand Names** Lopressor® [Tartrate]; Toprol XL® [Succinate]

**Canadian Brand Names** Apo®-Metoprolol (Type L); Betaloc®; Betaloc® Durules®; Novo-Metoprolol; Nu-Metop

**Therapeutic Category** Beta-adrenergic Blocker, Cardioselective

**Use** Treatment of hypertension and angina pectoris; prevention of myocardial infarction, atrial fibrillation, flutter, symptomatic treatment of hypertrophic subaortic stenosis

**Unlabeled use:** Treatment of ventricular arrhythmias, atrial ectopy, migraine prophylaxis, essential tremor, aggressive behavior

**Usual Dosage**

Children: Oral: 1-5 mg/kg/24 hours divided twice daily; allow 3 days between dose adjustments

Adults:

- Oral: 100-450 mg/day in 2-3 divided doses, begin with 50 mg twice daily and increase doses at weekly intervals to desired effect
- I.V.: 5 mg every 2 minutes for 3 doses in early treatment of myocardial infarction; thereafter give 50 mg orally every 6 hours 15 minutes after last I.V. dose and continue for 48 hours; then administer a maintenance dose of 100 mg twice daily

Elderly: Oral: Initial: 25 mg/day; usual range: 25-300 mg/day

**Mechanism of Action** Selective inhibitor of $beta_1$-adrenergic receptors; competitively blocks $beta_1$-receptors, with little or no effect on $beta_2$-receptors at doses <100 mg; does not exhibit any membrane stabilizing or intrinsic sympathomimetic activity

**Local Anesthetic/Vasoconstrictor Precautions** No information available to require special precautions

**Effects on Dental Treatment** Noncardioselective beta-blockers (ie, propranolol, nadolol) enhance the pressor response to epinephrine, resulting in hypertension and bradycardia. This has not been reported for metoprolol, a cardioselective beta-blocker. Therefore, local anesthetic with vasoconstrictor can be safely used in patients medicated with metoprolol. Many nonsteroidal anti-inflammatory drugs such as ibuprofen and indomethacin can reduce the hypotensive effect of beta-blockers after 3 or more weeks of therapy with the NSAID. Short-term

NSAID use (ie, 3 days) requires no special precautions in patients taking beta-blockers.

**Other Adverse Effects**

>10%:

Central nervous system: Mental depression, fatigue, dizziness

Neuromuscular & skeletal: Weakness

1% to 10%:

Cardiovascular: Bradycardia, arrhythmia, reduced peripheral circulation

Gastrointestinal: Heartburn

Respiratory: Wheezing

<1%:

Cardiovascular: Chest pain, heart failure, Raynaud's phenomenon

Central nervous system: Insomnia, nightmares, confusion, headache

Dermatologic: Rash, itching

Endocrine & metabolic: Decreased sexual activity

Gastrointestinal: Constipation, nausea, vomiting, stomach discomfort

Genitourinary: Impotence

Miscellaneous: Cold extremities

**Drug Interactions**

Decreased effect of beta-blockers:

Barbiturates (increased liver metabolism of beta-blockers to result in lower serum levels)

NSAIDs (attenuate the hypotensive therapeutic effects of beta-blockers)

Rifampin (increased liver metabolism of beta-blockers to result in lower serum levels)

Increased effects of beta-blockers:

Calcium channel blockers (increase serum levels of beta-blockers by unknown mechanism to enhance hypotension)

Beta-blockers increase the effects of:

Epinephrine (vasoconstrictor; initial hypertensive episode followed by bradycardia) only from noncardioselective type beta-blockers

Phenylephrine (Neosynephrine®; enhanced pressor response)

Theophylline (inhibit theophylline metabolism causing increase in serum concentrations)

**Drug Uptake**

Peak antihypertensive effect: Oral: Within 1.5-4 hours

Duration: 10-20 hours

Absorption: 95%

Serum half-life: 3-4 hours

End-stage renal disease: 2.5-4.5 hours

**Pregnancy Risk Factor** B

**Generic Available** Yes

**Selected Readings**

Foster CA and Aston SJ, "Propranolol-Epinephrine Interaction: A Potential Disaster," *Plast Reconstr Surg*, 1983, 72(1):74-8.

Wong DG, Spence JD, Lamki L, et al, "Effect of Nonsteroidal Anti-inflammatory Drugs on Control of Hypertension of Beta-Blockers and Diuretics," *Lancet*, 1986, 1(8488):997-1001.

Wynn RL, "Dental Nonsteroidal Anti-inflammatory Drugs and Prostaglandin-Based Drug Interactions, Part Two," *Gen Dent*, 1992, 40(2):104, 106, 108.

Wynn RL, "Epinephrine Interactions With Beta-Blockers," *Gen Dent*, 1994, 42(1):16, 18.

♦ **Metreton®** *see* Prednisolone *on page 832*

♦ **Metrodin® Injection** *see* Urofollitropin *on page 1034*

♦ **MetroGel®** *see* Metronidazole *on this page*

♦ **Metro I.V.®** *see* Metronidazole *on this page*

## Metronidazole (me troe NI da zole)

**Related Information**

Oral Bacterial Infections *on page 1128*

Oral Nonviral Soft Tissue Ulcerations or Erosions *on page 1141*

Periodontal Diseases *on page 1132*

**U.S. Brand Names** Flagyl®; Helidac™ Combination; MetroGel®; Metro I.V.®; Noritate® Cream; Protostat®

**Canadian Brand Names** Apo®-Metronidazole; Novo-Nidazol

**Therapeutic Category** Amebicide; Antibiotic, Anaerobic; Antibiotic, Topical; Antiprotozoal

**Use**

Dental: Treatment of oral soft tissue infections due to anaerobic bacteria including all anaerobic cocci, anaerobic gram-negative bacilli (*Bacteroides*), and gram-positive spore-forming bacilli (*Clostridium*). Useful as single agent or in combination with amoxicillin, Augmentin®, or ciprofloxacin in the treatment of periodontitis associated with the presence of *Actinobacillus actinomycetemcomitans*, (AA).

(Continued)

## Metronidazole *(Continued)*

Medical: Treatment of susceptible anaerobic bacterial and protozoal infections in the following conditions: amebiasis, symptomatic and asymptomatic trichomoniasis; skin and skin structure infections; CNS infections; intra-abdominal infections; systemic anaerobic infections; topically for the treatment of acne rosacea; treatment of antibiotic-associated pseudomembranous colitis (AAPC); Helidac™ in combination with an $H_2$ antagonist for the treatment active duodenal ulcer associated with *H. pylori* infection; topical cream is indicated for topical application in the treatment of inflammatory papules, pustules and erythema of rosacea

**Usual Dosage** Adults: Oral:

Anaerobic infections: 500 mg every 6-8 hours, not to exceed 4 g/day

Treatment of periodontitis associated with AA:

Oral, singly: 200-400 mg 3 times/day for 7-10 days;

In combination: Metronidazole plus Augmentin® 250 mg 3 times/day each for 7 days; metronidazole 250 mg plus amoxicillin 250 mg each 3 times/day for 7 days; metronidazole plus ciprofloxacin 500 mg each twice daily for 8 days

Helidac™: Take metronidazole 250 mg tablet, bismuth subsalicylate 262.4 mg tablet twice daily, and tetracycline 500 mg capsule plus an $H_2$ antagonist 4 times/day at meals and bedtime for 14 days; chew and swallow the bismuth subsalicylate tablets, swallow the metronidazole tablet and tetracycline capsule with a full glass of water

**Mechanism of Action** Reduced to a product which interacts with DNA to cause a loss of helical DNA structure and strand breakage resulting in inhibition of protein synthesis and cell death in susceptible organisms

**Local Anesthetic/Vasoconstrictor Precautions** No information available to require special precautions

**Effects on Dental Treatment** <1% of patients may experience dry mouth and metallic taste

**Other Adverse Effects**

>10%:

Central nervous system: Dizziness, headache

Gastrointestinal: Nausea, diarrhea, loss of appetite, vomiting

<1%: Endocrine & metabolic: Disulfiram-type reaction with alcohol

**Contraindications** Hypersensitivity to metronidazole or any component, 1st trimester of pregnancy

**Warnings/Precautions** Use with caution in patients with liver impairment, blood dyscrasias; history of seizures, congestive heart failure, or other sodium retaining states; reduce dosage in patients with severe liver impairment, CNS disease, and severe renal failure. Has been shown to be carcinogenic in rodents.

**Drug Interactions** Phenytoin, phenobarbital cause decreased metronidazole half-life; alcohol, disulfiram cause disulfiram-like reactions which includes flushing, headache, nausea, and in some patients, vomiting and chest and/or abdominal pain, therefore, absolutely contraindicated with alcohol; warfarin increases PT prolongation

**Drug Uptake**

Absorption: Oral: ~80%

Serum half-life: 6-8 hours, increases with hepatic impairment

Time to peak serum concentration: Within 1-2 hours

**Pregnancy Risk Factor** B

**Breast-feeding Considerations** Not compatible; resume breast-feeding 12-24 hours after last dose

**Dosage Forms**

Gel, topical: 0.75% [7.5 mg/mL] (30 g)

Injection, ready to use: 5 mg/mL (100 mL)

Powder for injection, as hydrochloride: 500 mg

Tablet: 250 mg, 500 mg

Helidac™ (one-day supply): Contains metronidazole 250 mg tablet (#4), bismuth subsalicylate 262.4 mg tablet [Pepto-Bismol®] (#8), and tetracycline 500 mg capsule (#4)

**Dietary Considerations** Food has no effect on extent of absorption, but delays rate and decreases maximum concentration; however, may be taken with food if gastric irritation

**Generic Available** Yes

**Selected Readings**

Eisenberg L, Suchow R, Coles RS, et al, "The Effects of Metronidazole Administration on Clinical and Microbiologic Parameters of Periodontal Disease," *Clin Prev Dent*, 1991, 13(1):28-34.

Jenkins WM, MacFarlane TW, Gilmour WH, et al, "Systemic Metronidazole in the Treatment of Periodontitis," *J Clin Periodontol*, 1989, 16(7):433-50.

Loesche WJ, Giordano JR, Hujoel P, et al, "Metronidazole in Periodontitis: Reduced Need for Surgery," *J Clin Periodontol*, 1992, 19(2):103-12.

Loesche WJ, Schmidt E, Smith BA, et al, "Effects of Metronidazole on Periodontal Treatment Needs," *J Periodontol*, 1991, 62(4):247-57.

Soder PO, Frithiof L, Wikner S, et al, "The Effect of Systemic Metronidazole After Nonsurgical Treatment in Moderate and Advanced Periodontitis in Young Adults," *J Periodontol*, 1990, 61(5):281-8.

## Metyrosine (me TYE roe seen)

**U.S. Brand Names** Demser®

**Therapeutic Category** Tyrosine Hydroxylase Inhibitor

**Synonyms** AMPT; OGMT

**Use** Short-term management of pheochromocytoma before surgery, long-term management when surgery is contraindicated or when malignant

**Usual Dosage** Children >12 years and Adults: Oral: Initial: 250 mg 4 times/day, increased by 250-500 mg/day up to 4 g/day; maintenance: 2-3 g/day in 4 divided doses; for preoperative preparation, administer optimum effective dosage for 5-7 days

**Mechanism of Action** Blocks the rate-limiting step in the biosynthetic pathway of catecholamines. It is a tyrosine hydroxylase inhibitor, blocking the conversion of tyrosine to dihydroxyphenylalanine. This inhibition results in decreased levels of endogenous catecholamines. Catecholamine biosynthesis is reduced by 35% to 80% in patients treated with metyrosine 1-4 g/day.

**Local Anesthetic/Vasoconstrictor Precautions** No information available to require special precautions

**Effects on Dental Treatment** No effects or complications reported

**Other Adverse Effects**

>10%:
- Central nervous system: Drowsiness, extrapyramidal symptoms
- Gastrointestinal: Diarrhea

1% to 10%:
- Endocrine & metabolic: Galactorrhea, edema of the breasts
- Gastrointestinal: Nausea, vomiting, xerostomia
- Genitourinary: Impotence
- Respiratory: Nasal congestion

<1%:
- Cardiovascular: Lower extremity edema
- Central nervous system: Depression, hallucinations, disorientation, parkinsonism
- Dermatologic: Urticaria
- Genitourinary: Urinary problems
- Hematologic: Anemia, eosinophilia
- Renal: Hematuria
- Miscellaneous: Hyperstimulation after withdrawal

**Contraindications** Hypertension of unknown etiology, known hypersensitivity to metyrosine

**Warnings/Precautions** Maintain fluid volume during and after surgery; use with caution in patients with impaired renal or hepatic function

**Drug Uptake** Serum half-life: 7.2 hours

**Pregnancy Risk Factor** C

**Dosage Forms** Capsule: 250 mg

**Dietary Considerations** Alcohol: Additive CNS effect, avoid use

**Generic Available** No

♦ **Mevacor®** *see* Lovastatin *on page 605*

## Mexiletine (MEKS i le teen)

**Related Information**

Cardiovascular Diseases *on page 1066*

**U.S. Brand Names** Mexitil®

**Therapeutic Category** Antiarrhythmic Agent, Class I-B; Antiarrhythmic Agent (Supraventricular & Ventricular)

**Use** Management of serious ventricular arrhythmias; suppression of PVCs

**Unlabeled use:** Diabetic neuropathy

**Usual Dosage** Adults: Oral: Initial: 200 mg every 8 hours (may load with 400 mg if necessary); adjust dose every 2-3 days; usual dose: 200-300 mg every 8 hours; maximum dose: 1.2 g/day (some patients respond to every 12-hour dosing); patients with hepatic impairment or CHF may require dose reduction; when switching from another antiarrhythmic, initiate a 200 mg dose 6-12 hours after stopping former agents, 3-6 hours after stopping procainamide

**Mechanism of Action** Class IB antiarrhythmic, structurally related to lidocaine, which may cause increase in systemic vascular resistance and decrease in cardiac output; no significant negative inotropic effect; inhibits inward sodium

(Continued)

## Mexiletine *(Continued)*

current, decreases rate of rise of phase 0, increases effective refractory period/action potential duration ratio

**Local Anesthetic/Vasoconstrictor Precautions** No information available to require special precautions

**Effects on Dental Treatment** No effects or complications reported

**Other Adverse Effects**

>10%:

- Central nervous system: Lightheadedness, dizziness, nervousness
- Neuromuscular & skeletal: Trembling, unsteady gait

1% to 10%:

- Cardiovascular: Chest pain, premature ventricular contractions
- Central nervous system: Confusion, headache, insomnia
- Dermatologic: Rash
- Gastrointestinal: Constipation or diarrhea
- Hepatic: Elevated LFTs
- Neuromuscular & skeletal: Numbness of fingers/toes, weakness
- Ocular: Blurred vision
- Otic: Tinnitus
- Respiratory: Dyspnea

<1%:

- Hematologic: Leukopenia, agranulocytosis, thrombocytopenia, positive antinuclear antibody
- Ocular: Diplopia

**Drug Interactions**

Decreased plasma levels: Phenobarbital, phenytoin, rifampin, and other hepatic enzyme inducers, cimetidine and drugs which make the urine acidic

Increased effect: Allopurinol

Increased toxicity/levels of caffeine and theophylline

**Drug Uptake**

Absorption: Elderly have a slightly slower rate of absorption but extent of absorption is the same as young adults

Serum half-life: Adults: 10-14 hours (average: 14.4 hours elderly, 12 hours in younger adults); increase in half-life with hepatic or heart failure

Time to peak: Peak levels attained in 2-3 hours

**Pregnancy Risk Factor** C

**Generic Available** Yes

♦ **Mexitil®** *see* Mexiletine *on previous page*

♦ **Mezlin®** *see* Mezlocillin *on this page*

## Mezlocillin (mez loe SIL in)

**U.S. Brand Names** Mezlin®

**Therapeutic Category** Antibiotic, Penicillin

**Use** Treatment of infections caused by susceptible gram-negative aerobic bacilli (*Klebsiella, Proteus, Escherichia coli, Enterobacter, Pseudomonas aeruginosa, Serratia*) involving the skin and skin structure, bone and joint, respiratory tract, urinary tract, gastrointestinal tract, as well as, septicemia

**Usual Dosage** I.M., I.V.:

Children: 200-300 mg/kg/day divided every 4-6 hours; maximum: 24 g/day

Adults:

- Uncomplicated urinary tract infection: 1.5-2 g every 6 hours
- Serious infections: 3-4 g every 4-6 hours

**Mechanism of Action** Interferes with bacterial cell wall synthesis during active multiplication causing cell death and resultant bactericidal activity against susceptible bacteria

**Local Anesthetic/Vasoconstrictor Precautions** No information available to require special precautions

**Effects on Dental Treatment** Prolonged use of penicillins may lead to development of oral candidiasis

**Other Adverse Effects**

1% to 10%: Gastrointestinal: Nausea, diarrhea

<1%:

- Central nervous system: Fever, seizures, dizziness, headache
- Dermatologic: Rash, exfoliative dermatitis
- Endocrine & metabolic: Hypokalemia, hypernatremia
- Gastrointestinal: Vomiting
- Hematologic: Eosinophilia, leukopenia, neutropenia, thrombocytopenia, agranulocytosis, hemolytic anemia, prolonged bleeding time, positive Coombs' [direct]
- Hepatic: Hepatotoxicity, elevated liver enzymes
- Renal: Hematuria, elevated serum creatinine and BUN, interstitial nephritis

Miscellaneous: Serum sickness-like reactions

**Drug Interactions** Aminoglycosides (synergy), probenecid (decreased clearance), vecuronium (increased duration of neuromuscular blockade), heparin (increased risk of bleeding)

**Drug Uptake**

Absorption: I.M.: 63%

Serum half-life: Dose dependent:

Children 2-19 years: 0.9 hour

Adults: 50-70 minutes, increased in renal impairment

Time to peak serum concentration:

I.M.: 45-90 minutes after administration

I.V. infusion: Within 5 minutes

**Pregnancy Risk Factor** B

**Generic Available** No

- **Miacalcin® Injection** *see* Calcitonin *on page 169*
- **Miacalcin® Nasal Spray** *see* Calcitonin *on page 169*
- **Mibefradil Dihydrochloride** *see* Mibefradil ***Withdrawn from Market 6/8/98*** *on this page*
- **Mibefradilum** *see* Mibefradil ***Withdrawn from Market 6/8/98*** *on this page*

## Mibefradil *Withdrawn from Market 6/8/98* (mi be FRA dil)

**U.S. Brand Names** Posicor®

**Therapeutic Category** Calcium Channel Blocker; Vasodilator

**Synonyms** Mibefradil Dihydrochloride; Mibefradilum

**Mechanism of Action** Blocks low-voltage (T type) and high voltage (L type) calcium channels, with greater selectivity for T-type channels, in contrast to benzothiazepine, dihydropyridine, and phenyalkylamine calcium antagonists, which at therapeutic concentrations block only the L-type channels. Does not induce reflex tachycardia but rather causes a slight reduction in heart rate and acts directly on vascular smooth muscle to cause a reduction in peripheral vascular resistance. In chronic stable angina pectoris, mibefradil causes a decreased cardiac workload and oxygen demand by inducing a reduction in heart rate, total peripheral resistance (afterload), and double product (heart rate times systolic blood pressure).

**Warnings/Precautions**

Roche Laboratories has announced that it is voluntarily withdrawing this drug from the market as a result of new information about potentially harmful interactions with other drugs. In many cases, drug interactions can be addressed by appropriate labeling changes and public education, but due to the complexity of the prescribing information needed in this case, and seriousness of side effects, FDA and Roche agreed that it would be difficult to administer it safely.

When it entered the market in August of 1997, its enzyme-inhibiting properties were described in the labeling. The labeling specifically listed three drugs (astemizole, cisapride, and terfenadine) that could be expected to accumulate to dangerous levels if mibefradil is coadministered. In December, after learning of several cases in which patients suffered serious adverse reactions after taking mibefradil with one or more of the other drugs, FDA strengthened the labeling. and two more drugs (lovastatin and simvastatin) were added to the label's list of those that should never be coadministered with mibefradil, FDA also issued a public warning about this problem and the company issued a "Dear Doctor" letter to physicians.

From spontaneous reports and ongoing trials, FDA and Roche have continued to learn of adverse reactions related to coadministration of mibefradil with several other drugs. At present, more than 25 drugs are known to be potentially dangerous if used with mibefradil -- a number and diversity of drugs that cannot be practically addressed by standard label warnings.

Patients now taking mibefradil should not simply discontinue treatment because stopping medications can be risky. Instead, patients should promptly consult with their physicians about appropriate alternative therapy. In addition, patients now taking mibefradil should not add any new medication to their current treatment without consulting their physicians.

The following is the text of the letter that was sent out on June 8, 1998:

Dear Doctor:

Roche Laboratories announced today the voluntary market withdrawal of the antihypertensive and antianginal medication Posicor® (mibefradil dihydrochloride).

The company is taking this action based on evolving information concerning the potential for drug interactions, some of them serious, that may occur when Posicor® is taken together with some other medications. The decision follows the analysis of the preliminary results of a 3-year long-term study of Posicor® in congestive heart failure. The study demonstrated no overall

(Continued)

## Mibefradil *Withdrawn from Market 6/8/98 (Continued)*

difference between Posicor® or placebo when added to standard therapy in this patient population, but it provided further information on drug interactions.

In both hypertension and chronic angina pectoris, Posicor® has consistently proved to be effective and well tolerated, when used appropriately; however, the combination of Posicor® and some other commonly used drugs, among them cardiovascular agents, may increase the frequency of the side-effects of these other medications. In principle, drug interactions can be addressed by appropriate labeling; however, with respect to Posicor®, Roche Laboratories believes that the complexity of such prescribing information would make it too difficult to implement. As patient well-being is of highest priority to Roche, the company has decided to voluntarily withdraw the compound from the market.

The company is working closely with the Food and Drug Administration to inform physicians and other healthcare professionals of its decision.

Please immediately discontinue prescribing and dispensing Posicor®, and immediately contact your patients who are currently prescribed Posicor® so that they can discontinue treatment and receive appropriate alternative therapy.

Roche Laboratories provided this information in a "Dear Doctor" letter to physicians, pharmacists, nurse practitioners, and other healthcare professionals. Questions about the withdrawal of Posicor® can be addressed to Roche's 24-hour hotline at 1-800-205-4611.

**Drug Interactions**

**The following is a list of drugs that depend on the same liver enzyme as Posicor® (mibefradil). Use of them in combination with Posicor® could be dangerous.**

Generic Name (Trade Name)
Amiodarone (Cordarone®)
Astemizole (Hismanal®)
Bepridil (Vascor®)
Cisapride (Propulsid®)
Cyclosporine (Neoral®, Sandimmune®)
Cyclophosphamide (Cytoxan®)
Desipramine (Norpramin®)
Erythromycin (Erythrocin®, Ilosone®, others)
Etoposide (VePesid®)
Flecainide (Tambocor®)
Flutamide (Eulexin®)
Halofantrine (Halfan®)
Ifosfamide (Ifex®)
Imipramine (Tofranil®)
Lovastatin (Mevacor®)
Mexiletine (Mexitil®)
Pimozide (Orap®)
Propafenone (Rythmol®)
Quinidine (Cardioquin®, Quinaglute®, Quinidex®, others)
Simvastatin (Zocor™)
Tacrolimus (Prograf®)
Tamoxifen (Nolvadex®)
Terfenadine (Seldane®)
Thioridazine (Mellaril®)
Vinblastine (Velban®)
Vincristine (Oncovin®)

**Dosage Forms** Tablet, as dihydrochloride: 50 mg, 100 mg

♦ **Micanol® Cream** *see* Anthralin *on page 88*
♦ **Micardis®** *see* Telmisartan *on page 955*
♦ **Micatin® Topical [OTC]** *see* Miconazole *on this page*

## Miconazole (mi KON a zole)

**U.S. Brand Names** Absorbine® Antifungal Foot Powder [OTC]; Breezee® Mist Antifungal [OTC]; Femizol-M® [OTC]; Fungoid® Creme; Fungoid® Tincture; Lotrimin® AF Powder [OTC]; Lotrimin® AF Spray Liquid [OTC]; Lotrimin® AF Spray Powder [OTC]; Maximum Strength Desenex® Antifungal Cream [OTC]; Micatin® Topical [OTC]; Monistat-Derm™ Topical; Monistat i.v.™ Injection; Monistat™ Vaginal; Ony-Clear® Spray; Prescription Strength Desenex® [OTC]; Zeasorb-AF® Powder [OTC]

**Canadian Brand Names** Monazole-7®

**Therapeutic Category** Antifungal Agent, Topical; Antifungal Agent, Vaginal

**Use**

I.V.: Treatment of severe systemic fungal infections and fungal meningitis that are refractory to standard treatment

Topical: Treatment of vulvovaginal candidiasis and a variety of skin and mucous membrane fungal infections

**Usual Dosage**

Children:

I.V.: 20-40 mg/kg/day divided every 8 hours

Topical: Apply twice daily for up to 1 month

Adults:

Topical: Apply twice daily for up to 1 month

I.T.: 20 mg every 1-2 days

I.V.: Initial: 200 mg, then 1.2-3.6 g/day divided every 8 hours for up to 20 weeks

Bladder candidal infections: 200 mg diluted solution instilled in the bladder

Vaginal: Insert contents of 1 applicator of vaginal cream (100 mg) or 100 mg suppository at bedtime for 7 days, or 200 mg suppository at bedtime for 3 days

**Mechanism of Action** Inhibits biosynthesis of ergosterol, damaging the fungal cell wall membrane, which increases permeability causing leaking of nutrients

**Local Anesthetic/Vasoconstrictor Precautions** No information available to require special precautions

**Effects on Dental Treatment** No effects or complications reported

**Other Adverse Effects**

>10%:

Central nervous system: Fever, chills

Dermatologic: Skin rash, itching

Local: Pain at injection site

Gastrointestinal: Anorexia, diarrhea, nausea, vomiting

1% to 10%: Hematologic: Anemia, thrombocytopenia

<1%:

Cardiovascular: Flushing of face or skin

Central nervous system: Drowsiness

**Drug Interactions** Warfarin (increased anticoagulant effect), oral sulfonylureas, amphotericin B (decreased antifungal effect of both agents), phenytoin (levels may be increased); coadministration with astemizole could result in cardiotoxicity

**Drug Uptake** Serum half-life, multiphasic:

Initial: 40 minutes

Secondary: 126 minutes

Terminal phase: 24 hours

**Pregnancy Risk Factor** C

**Dosage Forms**

Cream:

Topical, as nitrate: 2% (15 g, 30 g, 56.7 g, 85 g)

Vaginal, as nitrate: 2% (45 g is equivalent to 7 doses)

Injection: 1% [10 mg/mL] (20 mL)

Lotion, as nitrate: 2% (30 mL, 60 mL)

Powder, topical: 2% (45 g, 90 g, 113 g)

Spray, topical: 2% (105 mL)

Suppository, vaginal, as nitrate: 100 mg (7s); 200 mg (3s)

Tincture: 2% with alcohol (7.39 mL, 29.57 mL)

**Generic Available** Yes

♦ **MICRhoGAM™** *see* $Rh_o$(D) Immune Globulin *on page 884*

## Microfibrillar Collagen Hemostat

(mye kro FI bri lar KOL la jen HEE moe stat)

**U.S. Brand Names** Avitene®; Helistat®; Hemotene®

**Therapeutic Category** Hemostatic Agent

**Use** Dental & Medical: Adjunct to hemostasis when control of bleeding by ligature is ineffective or impractical

**Usual Dosage** Apply dry directly to source of bleeding

**Mechanism of Action** Microfibrillar collagen hemostat (MCH) is an absorbable topical hemostatic agent prepared from purified bovine corium collagen and shredded into fibrils. Physically, microfibrillar collagen hemostat yields a large surface area. Chemically, it is collagen with hydrochloric acid noncovalently bound to some of the available amino groups in the collagen molecules. When in contact with a bleeding surface, microfibrillar collagen hemostat attracts platelets which adhere to its fibrils and undergo the release phenomenon. This triggers aggregation of the platelets into thrombi in the interstices of the fibrous mass, initiating the formation of a physiologic platelet plug.

**Local Anesthetic/Vasoconstrictor Precautions** No information available to require special precautions

(Continued)

## Microfibrillar Collagen Hemostat *(Continued)*

**Effects on Dental Treatment** No effects or complications reported

**Other Adverse Effects** 1% to 10%:

Local: Adhesion formation

Miscellaneous: Potentiation of infection, allergic reaction

**Contraindications** Closure of skin incisions, contaminated wounds

**Warnings/Precautions** Fragments of MCH may pass through filters of blood scavenging systems, avoid reintroduction of blood from operative sites treated with MCH; after several minutes remove excess material

**Drug Interactions** No data reported

**Drug Uptake** Resorption: By animal tissue in 3 months

**Pregnancy Risk Factor** C

**Breast-feeding Considerations** No data reported

**Dosage Forms**

Fibrous: 1 g, 5 g

Nonwoven web: 70 mm x 70 mm x 1 mm; 70 mm x 35 mm x 1 mm

**Generic Available** No


- **Micro-K® 10** *see* Potassium Chloride *on page 822*
- **Micro-K® Extencaps®** *see* Potassium Chloride *on page 822*
- **Micro-K® LS** *see* Potassium Chloride *on page 822*
- **Microlipid™ [OTC]** *see* Enteral Nutritional Products *on page 371*
- **Micronase®** *see* Glyburide *on page 471*
- **microNefrin®** *see* Epinephrine, Racemic *on page 375*
- **Micronor®** *see* Norethindrone *on page 730*
- **Microsulfon®** *see* Sulfadiazine *on page 941*
- **Midamor®** *see* Amiloride *on page 61*


## Midazolam (MID aye zoe lam)

**U.S. Brand Names** Versed® Injection; Versed® Syrup

**Therapeutic Category** Benzodiazepine; Hypnotic; Sedative

**Use**

Dental: Sedation component in I.V. conscious sedation in oral surgery patients; syrup formulation is used for children to help alleviate anxiety before a dental procedure

Medical: In medicine, preoperative sedation and provides conscious sedation prior to diagnostic or radiographic procedures

**Restrictions** C-IV

**Usual Dosage**

Preoperative sedation: Children:

Oral:

<5 years: 0.5 mg/kg;

>5 years: 0.4-0.5 mg/kg; doses as high as 0.5-0.75 mg/kg have provided effective preanesthetic sedation

I.M.: 0.07-0.08 mg/kg 30 minutes to 1 hour before surgery; range: 0.05-0.1 mg/kg

I.V.: 0.035 mg/kg/dose, repeat over several minutes as required to achieve the desired sedative effect up to a total dose of 0.1-0.2 mg/kg or 5 mg total

Conscious sedation during mechanical ventilation:

Neonates: I.V. continuous infusion: 0.15-1 mcg/kg/minute

Children:

I.V.: 0.1-0.2 mg/kg; follow loading dose with a 1-2 mcg/kg/minute continuous infusion; titrate to the desired effect; range: 0.4-6 mcg/kg/minute

I.V. intermittent infusion: 0.05-0.2 mg/kg every 1-2 hours as needed

Conscious sedation for procedures:

Children:

Oral: 0.2-0.4 mg/kg; dose as high as 1 mg/kg have been used in younger (6 months to <6 years of age) and less cooperative patients; (maximum: 20 mg) 30-45 minutes before the procedure

Intranasal: 0.2-0.4 mg/kg (use undiluted 5 mg/mL injectable drug for intranasal administration)

I.V.: 0.05-0.1 mg/kg 3 minutes before procedure

Adolescents >12 years:

Sedation for procedure: I.V.: 0.5 mg every 3-4 minutes until effect achieved

Preoperative sedation: I.M.: 0.07-0.08 mg/kg 30-60 minutes before surgery; usual dose: 5 mg

Adults: Conscious sedation: I.V.: Initial: 0.5-2 mg slow I.V. over at least 2 minutes; slowly titrate to effect by repeating doses every 2-3 minutes if needed; usual total dose: 2.5-5 mg; use decreased doses in elderly

Healthy Adults <60 years: I.V.: Some patients respond to doses as low as 1 mg; no more than 2.5 mg should be administered over a period of 2 minutes. Additional doses of midazolam may be administered after a 2-minute waiting period and evaluation of sedation after each dose increment. A total dose >5 mg is generally not needed. If narcotics or other CNS depressants are administered concomitantly, the midazolam dose should be reduced by 30%.

**Mechanism of Action** Depresses all levels of the CNS, including the limbic and reticular formation, probably through the increased action of gamma-aminobutyric acid (GABA), which is a major inhibitory neurotransmitter in the brain

**Local Anesthetic/Vasoconstrictor Precautions** No information available to require special precautions

**Effects on Dental Treatment** No effects or complications reported

**Other Adverse Effects**

>10%: Miscellaneous: Hiccups

1% to 10%:

Central nervous system: Drowsiness, ataxia, amnesia, dizziness, sedation

Respiratory: Respiratory depression and arrest, apnea, laryngospasm, bronchospasm

**Contraindications** Hypersensitivity to midazolam or any component (cross-sensitivity with other benzodiazepines may occur); uncontrolled pain; existing CNS depression; shock; narrow-angle glaucoma

**Warnings/Precautions** Use with caution in patients with congestive heart failure, renal impairment, pulmonary disease, hepatic dysfunction, the elderly, and those receiving concomitant narcotics; midazolam may cause respiratory depression/arrest; deaths and hypoxic encephalopathy have resulted when these were not promptly recognized and treated appropriately

**Drug Interactions** Theophylline may antagonize the sedative effects of midazolam; CNS depressants cause increased sedation and respiratory depression; doses of general anesthetic agents should be reduced when used in conjunction with midazolam; cimetidine may increase midazolam serum concentrations

**Note:** If narcotics or other CNS depressants are administered concomitantly, the midazolam dose should be reduced by 30% if <65 years of age or by at least 50% if >65 years of age.

**Drug Uptake**

Onset of sedation:

Oral: Within 20-30 minutes

I.M.: Within 5-15 minutes

I.V.: Within 1-5 minutes

Intranasal: Within 8-12 minutes

Peak sedation:

I.M.: Within 30-60 minutes

Intranasal: 10 minutes

Duration:

I.M. mean: 2 hours, up to 6 hours; prolonged effect with hepatic/renal dysfunction

Intranasal: 30-60 minutes

Protein binding: 95%

Metabolism: In the liver via hydroxylation then glucuronide conjugation; active hydroxy metabolite may accumulate with prolonged infusion

Bioavailability: Oral: 15% to 45%

Half-life:

Neonates: 4-12 hours

Children: 1-2 hours

Adults: 3 hours (may be increased with obesity, age, and reduced hepatic or cardiac function)

Elimination: Excreted as conjugated metabolites in urine; ~2% to 10% excreted in feces after oral dose; <1% eliminated as unchanged drug in the urine

**Pregnancy Risk Factor** D

**Breast-feeding Considerations** No data reported

**Dosage Forms**

Injection, as hydrochloride: 1 mg/mL (2 mL, 5 mL, 10 mL); 5 mg/mL (1 mL, 2 mL, 5 mL, 10 mL)

Syrup, as hydrochloride: 2 mg/mL (118 mL)

**Dietary Considerations** No data reported

**Generic Available** No

♦ **Midchlor®** *see* Acetaminophen, Isometheptene, and Dichloralphenazone *on page 32*

## Midodrine (MI doe dreen)

**U.S. Brand Names** ProAmatine®

**Therapeutic Category** Alpha-Adrenergic Agonist

(Continued)

## Midodrine *(Continued)*

**Synonyms** Midodrine Hydrochloride

**Use** Treatment of symptomatic orthostatic hypotension in patients whose lives are considerably impaired despite standard clinical care.

**Usual Dosage** Adults: Oral: 10 mg 3 times/day during daytime hours (every 3-4 hours) when patient is upright (maximum: 40 mg/day)

**Mechanism of Action** Midodrine forms an active metabolite, desglymidodrine, that is an $alpha_1$-agonist. This agent increases arteriolar and venous tone resulting in a rise in standing, sitting, and supine systolic and diastolic blood pressure in patients with orthostatic hypotension.

**Local Anesthetic/Vasoconstrictor Precautions** No information available to require special precautions

**Effects on Dental Treatment** 1% to 10% of patients experience significant dry mouth

**Other Adverse Effects**

>10%:
- Dermatologic: Piloerection, pruritus
- Genitourinary: Urinary urgency, retention, or polyuria
- Neuromuscular & skeletal: Paresthesia

1% to 10%:
- Cardiovascular: Supine hypertension, facial flushing
- Central nervous system: Confusion, anxiety, dizziness, chills
- Dermatologic: Rash, dry skin
- Gastrointestinal: Xerostomia, nausea, abdominal pain
- Genitourinary: Dysuria
- Neuromuscular & skeletal: Pain

<1%:
- Cardiovascular: Flushing
- Central nervous system: Headache, insomnia
- Gastrointestinal: Flatulence
- Neuromuscular & skeletal: Leg cramps
- Ocular: Visual changes

**Warnings/Precautions** Only indicated for patients for whom orthostatic hypotension significantly impairs their daily life. Use is not recommended with supine hypertension and caution should be exercised in patients with diabetes, visual problems, urinary retention (reduce initial dose) or hepatic dysfunction; monitor renal and hepatic function prior to and periodically during therapy; safety and efficacy has not been established in children; discontinue and re-evaluate therapy if signs of bradycardia occur.

**Drug Interactions** Increased effect: Concomitant fludrocortisone results in hypernatremia or an increase in intraocular pressure and glaucoma; bradycardia may be accentuated with concomitant administration of cardiac glycosides, psychotherapeutics, and beta-blockers; alpha-agonists may increase the pressure effects and alpha-antagonists may negate the effects of midodrine

**Drug Uptake**

Absorption: Rapid

Serum half-life: ~3-4 hours (active drug); 25 minutes (prodrug)

Time to peak serum concentration: 1-2 hours (active drug); 30 minutes (prodrug)

**Pregnancy Risk Factor** C

**Generic Available** No

- ♦ **Midodrine Hydrochloride** *see* Midodrine *on previous page*
- ♦ **Midol® IB [OTC]** *see* Ibuprofen *on page 522*
- ♦ **Midol® PM [OTC]** *see* Acetaminophen and Diphenhydramine *on page 30*
- ♦ **Midrin®** *see* Acetaminophen, Isometheptene, and Dichloralphenazone *on page 32*

## Miglitol

**U.S. Brand Names** Glyset®

**Therapeutic Category** Antidiabetic Agent; Hypoglycemic Agent, Oral

**Use** As an adjunct to diet to lower blood glucose in patients with noninsulin-dependent diabetes mellitus (NIDDM)

**Usual Dosage** Oral: Adults: 25 mg three times/day with the first bite of food at each meal; the dose may be increased to 50 mg three times/day after 4-8 weeks; maximum recommended dose is 100 mg three times/day

**Mechanism of Action** In contrast to sulfonylureas, miglitol does not enhance insulin secretion; the antihyperglycemic action of miglitol results from a reversible inhibition of membrane-bound intestinal a-glucosidases which hydrolyze oligosaccharides and disaccharides to glucose and other monosaccharides in the brush border of the small intestine; in diabetic patients, this enzyme inhibition results in delayed glucose absorption and lowering of postprandial hyperglycemia

**Local Anesthetic/Vasoconstrictor Precautions** No information available to require special precautions

**Effects on Dental Treatment** No effects or complications reported

**Dosage Forms** Tablet: 25 mg, 50 mg, 100 mg

- ♦ **Migranal® Nasal Spray** *see* Dihydroergotamine *on page 332*
- ♦ **Migratine®** *see* Acetaminophen, Isometheptene, and Dichloralphenazone *on page 32*
- ♦ **Miles Nervine® Caplets [OTC]** *see* Diphenhydramine *on page 338*
- ♦ **Milontin®** *see* Phensuximide *on page 793*
- ♦ **Milophene®** *see* Clomiphene *on page 263*

## Milrinone (MIL ri none)

**U.S. Brand Names** Primacor®

**Therapeutic Category** Cardiovascular Agent, Other

**Use** Short-term I.V. therapy of congestive heart failure; used for calcium antagonist intoxication

**Usual Dosage** Adults: I.V.: Loading dose: 50 mcg/kg administered over 10 minutes followed by a maintenance dose titrated according to the hemodynamic and clinical response

**Mechanism of Action** Phosphodiesterase inhibitor resulting in vasodilation

**Local Anesthetic/Vasoconstrictor Precautions** No information available to require special precautions

**Effects on Dental Treatment** No effects or complications reported

**Other Adverse Effects**

>10%: Cardiovascular: Ventricular arrhythmias

1% to 10%:

Cardiovascular: Supraventricular arrhythmias, hypotension, angina, chest pain
Central nervous system: Headache

<1%:

Cardiovascular: Ventricular fibrillation
Endocrine & metabolic: Hypokalemia
Hematologic: Thrombocytopenia
Neuromuscular & skeletal: Tremor

**Drug Interactions** No data reported

**Drug Uptake**

Serum level: I.V.: Following a 125 mcg/kg dose, peak plasma concentrations of ~1000 ng/mL were observed at 2 minutes postinjection, decreasing to <100 ng/mL in 2 hours

Therapeutic effect: Oral: Following doses of 7.5-15 mg, peak hemodynamic effects occurred at 90 minutes

Serum half-life, elimination: I.V.: 136 minutes in patients with CHF; patients with severe CHF have a more prolonged half-life, with values ranging from 1.7-2.7 hours. Patients with CHF have a reduction in the systemic clearance of milrinone, resulting in a prolonged elimination half-life. Alternatively, one study reported that 1 month of therapy with milrinone did not change the pharmacokinetic parameters for patients with CHF despite improvement in cardiac function.

**Pregnancy Risk Factor** C

**Generic Available** No

- ♦ **Miltown®** *see* Meprobamate *on page 635*
- ♦ **Mini-Gamulin® Rh** *see* $Rh_o$(D) Immune Globulin *on page 884*
- ♦ **Minipress®** *see* Prazosin *on page 830*
- ♦ **Minitran®** *see* Nitroglycerin *on page 725*
- ♦ **Minizide®** *see* Prazosin and Polythiazide *on page 831*
- ♦ **Minocin® IV Injection** *see* Minocycline *on this page*
- ♦ **Minocin® Oral** *see* Minocycline *on this page*

## Minocycline (mi noe SYE kleen)

**U.S. Brand Names** Dynacin® Oral; Minocin® IV Injection; Minocin® Oral

**Canadian Brand Names** Apo®-Minocycline; Syn-Minocycline

**Therapeutic Category** Antibiotic, Tetracycline Derivative

**Use**

Dental: Treatment of periodontitis associated with presence of *Actinobacillus actinomycetemocomitams* (AA); as adjunctive therapy in recurrent aphthous ulcers

Medical: Treatment of susceptible bacterial infections of both gram-negative and gram-positive organisms; acne, meningococcal carrier state

**Usual Dosage** Infection: Oral, I.V.:

(Continued)

## Minocycline *(Continued)*

Children >8 years: Initial: 4 mg/kg followed by 2 mg/kg/dose every 12 hours
Adults: 200 mg stat, 100 mg every 12 hours not to exceed 400 mg/24 hours

**Mechanism of Action** Inhibits bacterial protein synthesis by binding with the 30S and possibly the 50S ribosomal subunit(s) of susceptible bacteria; cell wall synthesis is not affected

**Local Anesthetic/Vasoconstrictor Precautions** No information available to require special precautions

**Effects on Dental Treatment** Opportunistic "superinfection" with *Candida albicans*; tetracycline's are not recommended for use during pregnancy or in children ≤8 years of age since they have been reported to cause enamel hypoplasia and permanent teeth discoloration. The use of tetracycline's should only be used in these patients if other agents are contraindicated or alternative antimicrobials will not eradicate the organism. Long-term use associated with oral candidiasis.

**Other Adverse Effects**

>10%: Miscellaneous: Discoloration of teeth in children

1% to 10%:
- Dermatologic: Photosensitivity
- Gastrointestinal: Nausea, diarrhea

**Warnings/Precautions** Use of tetracyclines during tooth development may cause permanent discoloration of the teeth and enamel, hypoplasia and retardation of skeletal development and bone growth with risk being the greatest for children <4 years of age and those receiving high doses; use with caution in patients with renal or hepatic impairment and in pregnancy; dosage modification required in patients with renal impairment; pseudotumor cerebri has been reported with tetracycline use; outdated drug can cause nephropathy.

**Drug Interactions** Decreased effect with antacids (aluminum, calcium, zinc, or magnesium), bismuth salts, barbiturates, carbamazepine, hydantoins; decreased effect of oral contraceptives; increased effect of warfarin

**Drug Uptake** Serum half-life: 15 hours

**Pregnancy Risk Factor** D

**Breast-feeding Considerations** No data reported

**Dosage Forms**

Capsule, as hydrochloride: 50 mg, 100 mg
Capsule, as hydrochloride (Dynacin®): 50 mg, 100 mg
Capsule, pellet-filled, as hydrochloride (Minocin®): 50 mg, 100 mg
Injection, as hydrochloride (Minocin® IV): 100 mg
Suspension, oral, as hydrochloride (Minocin®)50 mg/5 mL (60 mL)

**Dietary Considerations** No data reported

**Generic Available** Yes

## Minoxidil (mi NOKS i dil)

**Related Information**

Cardiovascular Diseases *on page 1066*

**U.S. Brand Names** Loniten®; Rogaine® Extra Strength for Men [OTC]; Rogaine® for Men [OTC]; Rogaine® for Women [OTC]

**Canadian Brand Names** Apo®-Gain; Gen-Minoxidil®

**Therapeutic Category** Vasodilator

**Use** Management of severe hypertension (usually in combination with a diuretic and beta-blocker); treatment of male pattern baldness (alopecia androgenetica)

**Usual Dosage**

Children <12 years: Hypertension: Oral: Initial: 0.1-0.2 mg/kg once daily; maximum: 5 mg/day; increase gradually every 3 days; usual dosage: 0.25-1 mg/kg/day in 1-2 divided doses; maximum: 50 mg/day

Children >12 years and Adults:
- Hypertension: Oral: Initial: 5 mg once daily, increase gradually every 3 days; usual dose: 10-40 mg/day in 1-2 divided doses; maximum: 100 mg/day
- Alopecia: Topical: Apply twice daily; 4 months of therapy may be necessary for hair growth

Elderly: Initial: 2.5 mg once daily; increase gradually

**Mechanism of Action** Produces vasodilation by directly relaxing arteriolar smooth muscle, with little effect on veins; effects may be mediated by cyclic AMP; stimulation of hair growth is secondary to vasodilation, increased cutaneous blood flow and stimulation of resting hair follicles

**Local Anesthetic/Vasoconstrictor Precautions** No information available to require special precautions

**Effects on Dental Treatment** No effects or complications reported

**Other Adverse Effects**

>10%:
- Cardiovascular: EKG changes, tachycardia, congestive heart failure, edema
- Dermatologic: Hypertrichosis (commonly occurs within 1-2 months of therapy)

1% to 10%: Endocrine & metabolic: Fluid and electrolyte imbalance

<1%:

Cardiovascular: Angina, pericardial effusion tamponade

Central nervous system: Dizziness, headache

Dermatologic: Rashes, coarsening facial features, dermatologic reactions, Stevens-Johnson syndrome, sunburn

Endocrine & metabolic: Breast tenderness

Gastrointestinal: Weight gain

Hematologic: Thrombocytopenia, leukopenia

**Drug Interactions** Increased toxicity:

Concurrent administration with guanethidine may cause profound orthostatic hypotensive effects

Additive hypotensive effects with other hypotensive agents or diuretics

**Drug Uptake**

Onset of hypotensive effect: Oral: Within 30 minutes

Duration: Up to 2-5 days

Serum half-life: Adults: 3.5-4.2 hours

Peak effect: Within 2-8 hours

**Pregnancy Risk Factor** C

**Generic Available** Yes

- **Mintezol®** *see* Thiabendazole *on page 975*
- **Minute-Gel®** *see* Fluoride *on page 441*
- **Miochol-E®** *see* Acetylcholine *on page 36*
- **Miostat® Intraocular** *see* Carbachol *on page 185*
- **Mirapex®** *see* Pramipexole *on page 828*
- **Mircette®** *see* Ethinyl Estradiol and Desogestrel *on page 399*

## Mirtazapine (mir TAZ a peen)

**U.S. Brand Names** Remeron®

**Therapeutic Category** Antidepressant, Tetracyclic

**Use** Treatment of depression

**Usual Dosage** Adults: Oral: Initial: 15 mg nightly, titrate up to 15-45 mg/day with dose increases made no more frequently than every 1-2 weeks; there is an inverse relationship between dose and sedation

**Mechanism of Action** Mirtazapine is a tetracyclic antidepressant that works by its central presynaptic alpha$_2$-adrenergic antagonist effects, which results in increased release of norepinephrine and serotonin. It is also a potent antagonist of 5HT2 and 5HT3 serotonin receptors and H1 histamine receptors and a moderate peripheral alpha$_1$-adrenergic and muscarinic antagonist; it does not inhibit the reuptake of norepinephrine or serotonin.

**Local Anesthetic/Vasoconstrictor Precautions** No information available to require special precautions

**Effects on Dental Treatment** Significant xerostomia occurs in up to 25% of patients

**Other Adverse Effects**

>10%:

Central nervous system: Somnolence

Endocrine & metabolic: Increased cholesterol

Gastrointestinal: Constipation, increased appetite, weight gain

1% to 10%:

Cardiovascular: Hypertension, vasodilatation, peripheral edema, edema

Central nervous system: Dizziness, abnormal dreams, abnormal thoughts, confusion, malaise

Endocrine & metabolic: Increased triglycerides

Gastrointestinal: Vomiting, anorexia, eructation, glossitis, cholecystitis

Genitourinary: Polyuria

Neuromuscular & skeletal: Myalgia, back pain, arthralgias, tremor, weakness

Respiratory: Dyspnea

Miscellaneous: Flu-like symptoms, thirst

<1%:

Cardiovascular: Orthostatic hypotension

Central nervous system: Seizures (1 case reported)

Endocrine & metabolic: Dehydration

Gastrointestinal: Weight loss

Hematologic: Agranulocytosis, neutropenia, lymphadenopathy

Hepatic: Liver function test increases

**Warnings/Precautions** Use with caution in patients with cardiac conduction disturbances, history of hyperthyroid, renal, or hepatic dysfunction; safe use of tricyclic antidepressants in children <12 years of age has not been established; to avoid cholinergic crisis do not discontinue abruptly in patients receiving high doses chronically

(Continued)

## Mirtazapine *(Continued)*

**Drug Interactions** CYP1A2, 2C9, 2D6, and 3A3/4 enzyme substrate

Increased toxicity: Impairment of cognitive and motor skills are additive with those produced by alcohol, benzodiazepines, and other CNS depressants; possibly serious or fatal reactions can occur when given with or when given within 14 days of a monoamine oxidase inhibitor

**Drug Uptake**

Serum half-life: 20-40 hours

Time to peak serum concentration: 2 hours

**Pregnancy Risk Factor** C

**Dosage Forms** Tablet: 15 mg, 30 mg

**Generic Available** No

## Misoprostol (mye soe PROST ole)

**U.S. Brand Names** Cytotec®

**Therapeutic Category** Prostaglandin

**Use** Prevention of NSAID-induced gastric ulcers

**Usual Dosage** Adults: Oral: 200 mcg 4 times/day with food; if not tolerated, may decrease dose to 100 mcg 4 times/day with food or 200 mcg twice daily with food

**Mechanism of Action** Misoprostol is a synthetic prostaglandin $E_1$ analog that replaces the protective prostaglandins consumed with prostaglandin-inhibiting therapies eg, nonsteroidal anti-inflammatory drugs

**Local Anesthetic/Vasoconstrictor Precautions** No information available to require special precautions

**Effects on Dental Treatment** No effects or complications reported

**Other Adverse Effects**

>10%: Gastrointestinal: Diarrhea, abdominal pain

1% to 10%:

- Central nervous system: Headache
- Gastrointestinal: Constipation, flatulence

<1%:

- Gastrointestinal: Nausea, vomiting
- Genitourinary: Uterine stimulation, vaginal bleeding

**Drug Interactions** No data reported

**Drug Uptake**

Absorption: Oral: Rapid

Serum half-life (parent and metabolite combined): 1.5 hours

Time to peak serum concentration (active metabolite): Within 15-30 minutes

**Pregnancy Risk Factor** X

**Dosage Forms** Tablet: 100 mcg, 200 mcg

**Generic Available** No

♦ **Mithracin®** *see* Plicamycin *on page 811*

## Mitomycin (mye toe MYE sin)

**U.S. Brand Names** Mutamycin®

**Therapeutic Category** Antineoplastic Agent, Antibiotic

**Synonyms** Mitomycin-C; MTC

**Use** Therapy of disseminated adenocarcinoma of stomach, colon, or pancreas in combination with other approved chemotherapeutic agents; bladder cancer, breast cancer

**Usual Dosage Refer to individual protocols.**

Children and Adults: I.V.:

- Single agent therapy: 20 mg/m² every 6-8 weeks
- Combination therapy: 10 mg/m² every 6-8 weeks
- Bone marrow transplant:
  - 40-50 mg/m²
  - 2-40 mg/m²/day for 3 days
- Total cumulative dose should not exceed 50 mg/m²; see table.

| Nadir After Prior Dose/mm³ | | % of Prior Dose to Be Given |
|---|---|---|
| Leukocytes | Platelets | |
| 4000 | >100,000 | 100 |
| 3000-3999 | 75,000-99,999 | 100 |
| 2000-2999 | 25,000-74,999 | 70 |
| 2000 | <25,000 | 50 |

**Mechanism of Action** Isolated from *Streptomyces caespitosus*; acts primarily as an alkylating agent and produces DNA cross-linking (primarily with guanine and cytosine pairs); cell-cycle nonspecific; inhibits DNA and RNA synthesis by alkylation and cross-linking the strands of DNA

**Local Anesthetic/Vasoconstrictor Precautions** No information available to require special precautions

**Effects on Dental Treatment** No effects or complications reported

**Other Adverse Effects**

>10%:

Extravasation: May cause severe tissue irritation if infiltrated; can progress to cellulitis, ulceration, and sloughing of tissue

Gastrointestinal: Emetic potential: Moderately high (60% to 90%); **nausea and vomiting (mild to moderate) seen in almost 100% of patients**; usually begins 1-2 hours after treatment and persists for 3 hours to 4 days; other toxicities include stomatitis, hepatic toxicity, diarrhea, anorexia

Hematologic: Myelosuppressive: Dose-related toxicity and may be cumulative; related to both total dose (incidence higher at doses >50 mg) and schedule

1% to 10%:

Dermatologic: Discolored fingernails (violet), alopecia

Gastrointestinal: Mouth ulcers

Neuromuscular & skeletal: Paresthesia

Respiratory: Interstitial pneumonitis or pulmonary fibrosis have been noticed in 7% of patients, and it occurs independent of dosing. Manifested as dry cough and progressive dyspnea; usually is responsive to steroid therapy.

Renal: Elevation of creatinine seen in 2% of patients; hemolytic uremic syndrome observed in <10% of patients and is dose-dependent (doses >30 mg have higher risk)

<1%:

Cardiovascular: Cardiac failure (in patients treated with doses >30 mg)

Central nervous system: Malaise, fever

Dermatologic: Pruritus, rash

Hematologic: Bone marrow suppression (leukopenia, thrombocytopenia), microangiopathic hemolytic anemia

Local: Thrombophlebitis

Neuromuscular & skeletal: Weakness

**Drug Uptake**

Absorption: Fairly well from the GI tract

Serum half-life: 23-78 minutes

Terminal: 50 minutes

**Pregnancy Risk Factor** C

**Generic Available** No

♦ **Mitomycin-C** *see* Mitomycin *on previous page*

## Mitotane (MYE toe tane)

**U.S. Brand Names** Lysodren®

**Therapeutic Category** Antiadrenal Agent; Antineoplastic Agent, Miscellaneous

**Synonyms** o,p'-DDD

**Use** Treatment of inoperable adrenal cortical carcinoma

**Usual Dosage** Oral:

Children: 0.1-0.5 mg/kg or 1-2 g/day in divided doses increasing gradually to a maximum of 5-7 g/day

Adults: Start at 1-6 g/day in divided doses, then increase incrementally to 8-10 g/day in 3-4 divided doses; dose is changed on basis of side effect with aim of giving as high a dose as tolerated; maximum daily dose: 18 g

**Mechanism of Action** Causes adrenal cortical atrophy; drug affects mitochondria in adrenal cortical cells and decreases production of cortisol; also alters the peripheral metabolism of steroids

**Local Anesthetic/Vasoconstrictor Precautions** No information available to require special precautions

**Effects on Dental Treatment** No effects or complications reported

**Other Adverse Effects**

>10%:

Central nervous system: Vertigo, mental depression, dizziness; all are reversible with discontinuation of the drug and can occur in 15% to 26% of patients

Dermatologic: Rash (15%) which may subside without discontinuation of therapy, hyperpigmentation

Gastrointestinal: 75% to 80% will experience nausea, vomiting, and anorexia; diarrhea can occur in 20% of patients

Ocular: Visual disturbances, diplopia, blurred vision; all are reversible with discontinuation of drug

1% to 10%:

Cardiovascular: Orthostatic hypotension, flushing of skin

Central nervous system: Fever

(Continued)

## Mitotane *(Continued)*

Genitourinary: Hemorrhagic cystitis
Neuromuscular & skeletal: Myalgia

<1%:

Cardiovascular: Hypertension
Central nervous system: Lethargy, somnolence, mental depression, irritability, confusion, fatigue, headache
Endocrine & metabolic: Hypercholesterolemia, adrenal insufficiency may develop and may require steroid replacement
Genitourinary: Hemorrhagic cystitis, hypouricemia
Hematologic: Myelosuppressive: WBC: None; Platelets: None
Neuromuscular & skeletal: Tremor, weakness
Ocular: Lens opacities, toxic retinopathy
Renal: Hematuria, albuminuria
Respiratory: Dyspnea, wheezing

**Drug Uptake**

Absorption: Oral: ~35% to 40%
Serum half-life: 18-159 days
Time to peak serum concentration: Within 3-5 hours

**Pregnancy Risk Factor** C

**Generic Available** No

**Comments** Myelosuppressive effects:
WBC: None
Platelets: None

## Mitoxantrone (mye toe ZAN trone)

**U.S. Brand Names** Novantrone®

**Therapeutic Category** Antineoplastic Agent, Anthracycline; Antineoplastic Agent, Antibiotic

**Synonyms** DHAD; Mitoxantrone Hydrochloride

**Use** FDA approved for remission-induction therapy of acute nonlymphocytic leukemia (ANLL); mitoxantrone is also active against other various leukemias, lymphoma, and breast cancer, and moderately active against pediatric sarcoma

**Usual Dosage Refer to individual protocols.** I.V. (may dilute in $D_5W$ or NS):

ANLL leukemias:

Children ≤2 years: 0.4 mg/kg/day once daily for 3-5 days
Children >2 years and Adults: 12 $mg/m^2$/day once daily for 3 days; acute leukemia in relapse: 8-12 $mg/m^2$/day once daily for 4-5 days

Solid tumors:

Children: 18-20 $mg/m^2$ every 3-4 weeks **OR** 5-8 $mg/m^2$ every week
Adults: 12-14 $mg/m^2$ every 3-4 weeks **OR** 2-4 $mg/m^2$/day for 5 days
Maximum total dose: 80-120 $mg/m^2$ in patients with predisposing factor and <160 mg in patients with no predisposing factor

**Mechanism of Action** Analogue of the anthracyclines, but different in mechanism of action, cardiac toxicity, and potential for tissue necrosis; mitoxantrone does intercalate DNA; binds to nucleic acids and inhibits DNA and RNA synthesis by template disordering and steric obstruction; replication is decreased by binding to DNA topoisomerase II (enzyme responsible for DNA helix supercoiling); active throughout entire cell cycle; does not appear to produce free radicals

**Local Anesthetic/Vasoconstrictor Precautions** No information available to require special precautions

**Effects on Dental Treatment** No effects or complications reported

**Other Adverse Effects**

>10%:

Central nervous system: Headache
Dermatologic: Alopecia
Gastrointestinal: Nausea, vomiting, diarrhea, abdominal pain, mucositis, stomatitis, GI bleeding
Emetic potential: Moderate (31% to 72%)
Genitourinary: Discoloration of urine (blue-green)
Hepatic: Abnormal LFTs
Respiratory: Coughing, dyspnea

1% to 10%:

Cardiac toxicity: Much reduced compared to doxorubicin and has been reported primarily in patients who have received prior anthracycline therapy, congestive heart failure, hypotension
Central nervous system: Seizures, fever
Dermatologic: Pruritus, skin desquamation
Hepatic: Transient elevation of liver enzymes, jaundice
Ocular: Conjunctivitis

Renal: Renal failure
<1%: Local: Pain or redness at injection site

**Drug Uptake**
Absorption: Oral: Poor
Serum half-life: Terminal: 37 hours; may be prolonged with liver impairment

**Pregnancy Risk Factor** D

**Generic Available** No

- **Mitoxantrone Hydrochloride** *see* Mitoxantrone *on previous page*
- **Mitran®** *see* Chlordiazepoxide *on page 224*
- **Mitrolan® Chewable Tablet [OTC]** *see* Calcium Polycarbophil *on page 177*
- **MK594** *see* Losartan *on page 603*
- **M-KYA® [OTC]** *see* Quinine *on page 874*
- **MMR** *see* Measles, Mumps, and Rubella Vaccines, Combined *on page 618*
- **M-M-R® II** *see* Measles, Mumps, and Rubella Vaccines, Combined *on page 618*
- **Moban®** *see* Molindone *on page 685*
- **Mobidin®** *see* Magnesium Salicylate *on page 613*

## Modafinil

**U.S. Brand Names** Provigil®

**Therapeutic Category** Central Nervous System Stimulant, Nonamphetamine

**Use** Improve wakefulness in patients with excessive daytime sleepiness associated with narcolepsy

**Restrictions** C-IV

**Usual Dosage** Adults: Oral: Initial: 200 mg as a single daily dose

**Mechanism of Action** The mechanism(s) of action for modafinil have not been defined. It does not appear to stimulate receptors commonly associated with sleep/wake regulation (including norepinephrine, serotonin, melatonin, GABA, dopamine, adenosine, and histamine-3 receptors).

**Local Anesthetic/Vasoconstrictor Precautions** No information available to require special precautions

**Effects on Dental Treatment** Dry mouth, mouth ulceration, and gingivitis have been reported

**Other Adverse Effects** Limited to events which were equal to or greater than placebo:

1% to 10%:

Cardiovascular: Chest pain (2%), hypertension (2%), hypotension (2%), vasodilation (1%), arrhythmia (1%), syncope (1%)

Central nervous system: Nervousness (8%), dizziness (5%), depression (4%), anxiety (4%), cataplexy (3%), insomnia (3%), dyskinesia (2%), chills (2%), fever (1%), confusion (1%), amnesia (1%), emotional lability (1%), ataxia (1%)

Dermatologic: Dry skin (1%)

Endocrine & metabolic: Hyperglycemia (1%), albuminuria (1%)

Gastrointestinal: Diarrhea (8%), dry mouth (5%), anorexia (5%), vomiting (1%), mouth ulceration (1%), gingivitis (1%)

Genitourinary: Abnormal urine (1%), urinary retention (1%), ejaculatory disturbance (1%)

Hematologic: Eosinophilia (1%)

Hepatic: Abnormal liver function (3%), elevated GGT

Neuromuscular & skeletal: Neck pain (2%), hypertonia (2%), neck rigidity (1%), joint disorder (1%), tremor (1%), paresthesia (3%)

Ocular: Amblyopia (2%), abnormal vision (2%)

Respiratory: Pharyngitis (6%), lung disorder (4%), dyspnea (2%), asthma (1%), epistaxis (1%)

**Warnings/Precautions** Caution when operating machinery or driving. Although functional impairment has not been demonstrated for modafinil, any agent affecting the CNS may alter judgment, thinking, or motor skills. Use with caution in patients with a recent history of myocardial infarction, unstable angina, hypertension, or history of psychosis. Efficacy of oral contraceptives may be reduced - use alternative contraceptive measures. Prolonged administration may lead to drug dependence.

**Drug Interactions**

Decreased effects/toxicity: Modafinil is a cytochrome P-450 isoenzyme 3A4 substrate and induces CYP 1A2, 2B6, and 3A4. Modafinil may induce its own metabolism. Coadministration with other substrates of CYP3A4 such as oral contraceptives, cyclosporine, and (to a limited degree) theophylline may result in decreased serum concentrations/efficacy of these agents. Agents which induce CYP3A4, including phenobarbital, carbamazepine, and rifampin, may result in decreased concentrations of modafinil.

(Continued)

## Modafinil *(Continued)*

Increased effects/toxicity:

Modafinil is a cytochrome P-450 isoenzyme 2C19 inhibitor. Coadministration with drugs metabolized by CYP2C19, including diazepam, phenytoin, and propranolol, may result in increased serum concentrations/toxicity from these agents. In populations deficient in CYP2D6, where CYP2C19 acts as a secondary metabolic pathway, concentrations of agents such as tricyclic antidepressants and SSRI's may be increased during coadministration. Clomipramine concentrations may be increased.

Modafinil may suppress CYP2C9, potentially increasing the concentrations/toxicity of agents metabolized by this isoenzyme, including warfarin and phenytoin.

Agents which inhibit CYP3A4, including ketoconazole and itraconazole, may result in increased concentrations/toxicity of modafinil.

**Drug Uptake**

Serum half-life: 15 hours

Time to peak: 2-4 hours

**Pregnancy Risk Factor** C

**Dosage Forms** Tablet: 100 mg, 200 mg

- **Modane® Bulk [OTC]** *see* Psyllium *on page 865*
- **Modane® Soft [OTC]** *see* Docusate *on page 346*
- **Modicon™** *see* Ethinyl Estradiol and Norethindrone *on page 404*
- **Modified Dakin's Solution** *see* Sodium Hypochlorite Solution *on page 922*
- **Modified Shohl's Solution** *see* Sodium Citrate and Citric Acid *on page 921*
- **Moducal® [OTC]** *see* Glucose Polymers *on page 470*
- **Moduretic®** *see* Amiloride and Hydrochlorothiazide *on page 61*

## Moexipril (mo EKS i pril)

**Related Information**

Cardiovascular Diseases *on page 1066*

Moexipril and Hydrochlorothiazide *on next page*

**U.S. Brand Names** Univasc®

**Therapeutic Category** Angiotensin-Converting Enzyme (ACE) Inhibitor

**Use** Treatment of hypertension, alone or in combination with thiazide diuretics

**Usual Dosage** Adults: Oral: Initial: 7.5 mg once daily (in patients **not** receiving diuretics), one hour prior to a meal **or** 3.75 mg once daily (when combined with thiazide diuretics); maintenance dose: 7.5-30 mg/day in 1 or 2 divided doses one hour before meals

**Mechanism of Action** Competitive inhibitor of angiotensin-converting enzyme (ACE); prevents conversion of angiotensin I to angiotensin II, a potent vasoconstrictor; results in lower levels of angiotensin II which causes an increase in plasma renin activity and a reduction in aldosterone secretion

**Local Anesthetic/Vasoconstrictor Precautions** No information available to require special precautions

**Effects on Dental Treatment** No effects or complications reported

**Other Adverse Effects**

1% to 10%:

Cardiovascular: Flushing

Central nervous system: Headache, dizziness, fatigue

Dermatologic: Rash, pruritus, alopecia, rash

Endocrine & metabolic: Hyperkalemia

Gastrointestinal: Diarrhea

Renal: Oliguria, reversible elevations in creatinine or BUN, polyuria

Respiratory: Nonproductive cough (6%), pharyngitis, upper respiratory infections, rhinitis

Miscellaneous: Flu-like symptoms

<1%:

Cardiovascular: Symptomatic hypotension, chest pain, angina, peripheral edema, myocardial infarction, palpitations, arrhythmias

Central nervous system: Sleep disturbances, anxiety, mood changes

Dermatologic: Angioedema, photosensitivity, pemphigus

Endocrine & metabolic: Hypercholesterolemia

Gastrointestinal: Abdominal pain, taste disturbance, constipation, vomiting, changes in appetite, pancreatitis, dysgeusia

Hematologic: Neutropenia

Hepatic: Elevated LFTs

Neuromuscular & skeletal: Myalgia, arthralgia

Renal: Proteinuria

Respiratory: Bronchospasm, dyspnea

**Drug Uptake**
Absorption: Food decreases bioavailability (AUC decreased by ~40%)
Serum half-life:
Moexipril: 1 hour
Moexiprilat: 2-10 hours
Time to peak: 1.5 hours
**Pregnancy Risk Factor** D
**Generic Available** No

## Moexipril and Hydrochlorothiazide

(mo EKS i pril & hye droe klor oh THYE a zide)
**U.S. Brand Names** Uniretic™
**Therapeutic Category** Angiotensin-Converting Enzyme (ACE) Inhibitor; Diuretic, Thiazide
**Use** Treatment of hypertension
**Usual Dosage** Adults: Oral: 7.5-30 mg of moexipril, taken either in a single or divided dose one hour before meals
**Mechanism of Action** See individual agents
**Local Anesthetic/Vasoconstrictor Precautions** No information available to require special precautions
**Effects on Dental Treatment** No effects or complications reported
**Other Adverse Effects** See individual agents
**Drug Interactions** See individual agents
**Dosage Forms** Tablet: Moexipril hydrochloride 7.5 mg and hydrochlorothiazide 12.5 mg; moexipril hydrochloride 15 mg and hydrochlorothiazide 25 mg
**Generic Available** No

♦ **Moi-Stir® Solution [OTC]** *see* Saliva Substitute *on page 901*
♦ **Moi-Stir® Swabsticks [OTC]** *see* Saliva Substitute *on page 901*
♦ **Moisture® Ophthalmic Drops [OTC]** *see* Artificial Tears *on page 97*

## Molindone (moe LIN done)

**U.S. Brand Names** Moban®
**Therapeutic Category** Antipsychotic Agent
**Use** Management of psychotic disorder
**Usual Dosage** Oral:
Children:
3-5 years: 1-2.5 mg/day divided into 4 doses
5-12 years: 0.5-1 mg/kg/day in 4 divided doses
Adults: 50-75 mg/day increase at 3- to 4-day intervals up to 225 mg/day
**Mechanism of Action** Mechanism of action mimics that of chlorpromazine; however, it produces more extrapyramidal effects and less sedation than chlorpromazine
**Local Anesthetic/Vasoconstrictor Precautions** No information available to require special precautions
**Effects on Dental Treatment** >10% of patients experience dry mouth; anticholinergic side effects can cause a reduction of saliva production or secretion. This may result in discomfort and dental disease (ie, caries, oral candidiasis and periodontal disease); molindone can cause extrapyramidal reactions which may appear as muscle twitching or increased motor activity of the face, neck or head
**Other Adverse Effects**
>10%:
Cardiovascular: Orthostatic hypotension
Central nervous system: Akathisia, extrapyramidal effects, persistent tardive dyskinesia
Gastrointestinal: Constipation
Ocular: Blurred vision
Miscellaneous: Decreased sweating
1% to 10%:
Central nervous system: Mental depression
Endocrine & metabolic: Change in menstrual periods, swelling of breasts
<1%:
Cardiovascular: Tachycardia, arrhythmias
Central nervous system: Sedation, drowsiness, restlessness, anxiety, seizures, neuroleptic malignant syndrome (NMS), altered central temperature regulation
Dermatologic: Hyperpigmentation, pruritus, rash, photosensitivity
Endocrine & metabolic: Galactorrhea, gynecomastia
Gastrointestinal: Weight gain
Genitourinary: Urinary retention
(Continued)

## Molindone *(Continued)*

Hematologic: Agranulocytosis (more often in women between fourth and tenth weeks of therapy), leukopenia (usually in patients with large doses for prolonged periods)

Ocular: Retinal pigmentation

**Drug Interactions** Increased toxicity: CNS depressants, antihypertensives, anticonvulsants

**Drug Uptake**

Serum half-life: 1.5 hours

Time to peak serum concentration: Oral: Within 1.5 hours

**Pregnancy Risk Factor** C

**Generic Available** No

- **Mol-Iron® [OTC]** *see* Ferrous Sulfate *on page 427*
- **Mollifene® Ear Wax Removing Formula [OTC]** *see* Carbamide Peroxide *on page 186*
- **Molybdenum** *see* Trace Metals *on page 1001*
- **Molypen®** *see* Trace Metals *on page 1001*

## Mometasone Furoate (moe MET a sone FYOOR oh ate)

**U.S. Brand Names** Elocon®; Nasonex®

**Canadian Brand Names** Elocom

**Therapeutic Category** Corticosteroid, Topical (Medium Potency)

**Use** Topical forms for the relief of the inflammatory and pruritic manifestations of corticosteroid-responsive dermatoses (medium potency topical corticosteroid); nasal spray used for the prophylaxis and treatment of nasal symptoms of seasonal allergic rhinitis and the treatment of nasal symptoms of perennial allergic rhinitis in adults and children 12 years of age and older

**Usual Dosage** Adults: Topical: Apply sparingly to area once daily, do not use occlusive dressings

**Mechanism of Action** May depress the formation, release, and activity of endogenous chemical mediators of inflammation (kinins, histamine, liposomal enzymes, prostaglandins). Leukocytes and macrophages may have to be present for the initiation of responses mediated by the above substances. Inhibits the margination and subsequent cell migration to the area of injury, and also reverses the dilatation and increased vessel permeability in the area resulting in decreased access of cells to the sites of injury.

**Local Anesthetic/Vasoconstrictor Precautions** No information available to require special precautions

**Effects on Dental Treatment** No effects or complications reported

**Other Adverse Effects** <1%:

Dermatologic: Acne, hypopigmentation, allergic dermatitis, maceration of the skin, skin atrophy, striae, miliaria, folliculitis, hypertrichosis

Endocrine & metabolic: HPA suppression, Cushing's syndrome, growth retardation

Local: Burning, itching, irritation, dryness

Miscellaneous: Secondary infection

**Drug Interactions** No data reported

**Pregnancy Risk Factor** C

**Generic Available** No

- **MOM/Mineral Oil Emulsion** *see* Magnesium Hydroxide and Mineral Oil Emulsion *on page 612*
- **Monafed®** *see* Guaifenesin *on page 478*
- **Monafed® DM** *see* Guaifenesin and Dextromethorphan *on page 479*
- **Monistat-Derm™ Topical** *see* Miconazole *on page 672*
- **Monistat i.v.™ Injection** *see* Miconazole *on page 672*
- **Monistat™ Vaginal** *see* Miconazole *on page 672*

## Monobenzone (mon oh BEN zone)

**U.S. Brand Names** Benoquin®

**Therapeutic Category** Topical Skin Product

**Use** Final depigmentation in extensive vitiligo

**Usual Dosage** Adults: Topical: Apply 2-3 times daily

**Local Anesthetic/Vasoconstrictor Precautions** No information available to require special precautions

**Effects on Dental Treatment** No effects or complications reported

**Other Adverse Effects** 1% to 10%: Irritation, burning sensation, dermatitis

**Pregnancy Risk Factor** C

**Generic Available** No

- **Monocid®** *see* Cefonicid *on page 202*

- **Monoclate-P®** *see* Antihemophilic Factor (Human) *on page 89*
- **Monoclonal Antibody** *see* Muromonab-CD3 *on page 692*
- **Monoethanolamine** *see* Ethanolamine Oleate *on page 397*
- **Mono-Gesic®** *see* Salsalate *on page 902*
- **Monoket®** *see* Isosorbide Mononitrate *on page 556*
- **Mononine®** *see* Factor IX Complex (Human) *on page 417*
- **Monopril®** *see* Fosinopril *on page 457*


## Montelukast (mon te LOO kast)

**Related Information**

Respiratory Diseases *on page 1079*

**U.S. Brand Names** Singulair®

**Therapeutic Category** Leukotriene Receptor Antagonist

**Synonyms** Montelukast Sodium

**Use** Prophylaxis and chronic treatment of asthma in adults and children ≥6 years of age

**Usual Dosage** Oral:

Children 6-14 years: 5 mg once daily

Children >14 years and Adults: 10 mg once daily

**Mechanism of Action** Selective leukotriene receptor antagonist that blocks leukotriene $D_4$ receptor ($LTD_4$), thereby decreasing migration, mucous production, and airway wall edema

**Local Anesthetic/Vasoconstrictor Precautions** No information available to require special precautions

**Effects on Dental Treatment** No effects or complications reported

**Drug Uptake**

Absorption: Rapid

Half-life, plasma: Mean: 2.7-5.5 hours

Time to peak serum concentration: 3-4 hours for 10 mg tablet and 2-2.5 hours for 5 mg tablet

**Dosage Forms**

Tablet, as sodium: 10 mg

Tablet, chewable (cherry), as sodium: 5 mg


- **Montelukast Sodium** *see* Montelukast *on this page*
- **Monurol™** *see* Fosfomycin *on page 456*
- **8-MOP** *see* Methoxsalen *on page 655*
- **More Attenuated Enders Strain** *see* Measles Virus Vaccine, Live *on page 619*
- **More-Dophilus® [OTC]** *see Lactobacillus acidophilus* and *Lactobacillus bulgaricus on page 570*


## Moricizine (mor I siz een)

**Related Information**

Cardiovascular Diseases *on page 1066*

**U.S. Brand Names** Ethmozine®

**Therapeutic Category** Antiarrhythmic Agent, Class I; Antiarrhythmic Agent (Supraventricular & Ventricular)

**Use** For treatment of ventricular tachycardia and life-threatening ventricular arrhythmias

**Unlabeled use:** PVCs, complete and nonsustained ventricular tachycardia

**Usual Dosage** Adults: Oral: 200-300 mg every 8 hours, adjust dosage at 150 mg/day at 3-day intervals. See table for dosage recommendations of transferring from other antiarrhythmic agents to Ethmozine®.

**Moricizine**

| Transferred From | Start Ethmozine® |
|---|---|
| Encainide, propafenone, tocainide, or mexiletine | 8-12 hours after last dose |
| Flecainide | 12-24 hours after last dose |
| Procainamide | 3-6 hours after last dose |
| Quinidine, disopyramide | 6-12 hours after last dose |

**Mechanism of Action** Class I antiarrhythmic agent; reduces the fast inward current carried by sodium ions, shortens Phase I and Phase II repolarization, resulting in decreased action potential duration and effective refractory period

**Local Anesthetic/Vasoconstrictor Precautions** No information available to require special precautions

**Effects on Dental Treatment** No effects or complications reported

(Continued)

## Moricizine *(Continued)*

**Other Adverse Effects**

>10%: Central nervous system: Dizziness

1% to 10%:

Cardiovascular: Proarrhythmia, palpitations, cardiac death, EKG abnormalities, congestive heart failure

Central nervous system: Headache, fatigue, insomnia

Endocrine & metabolic: Decreased libido

Gastrointestinal: Nausea, diarrhea, ileus

Ocular: Blurred vision, periorbital edema

Respiratory: Dyspnea

<1%:

Cardiovascular: Ventricular tachycardia, cardiac chest pain, hypotension or hypertension, syncope, supraventricular arrhythmias, myocardial infarction

Central nervous system: Anxiety, drug fever, confusion, loss of memory, vertigo, anorexia

Dermatologic: Rash, dry skin

Gastrointestinal: GI upset, vomiting, dyspepsia, flatulence, bitter taste

Genitourinary: Urinary retention, urinary incontinence, impotence

Neuromuscular & skeletal: Tremor

Otic: Tinnitus

Respiratory: Apnea

Miscellaneous: Sweating

**Drug Interactions**

Decreased levels of theophylline (50%)

Increased levels with cimetidine (50%)

**Drug Uptake** Serum half-life:

Normal patients: 3-4 hours

Cardiac disease patients: 6-13 hours

**Pregnancy Risk Factor** B

**Generic Available** No

## Morphine Sulfate (MOR feen SUL fate)

**Related Information**

Narcotic Agonists *on page 1223*

**U.S. Brand Names** Astramorph™ PF Injection; Duramorph® Injection; Infumorph™ Injection; Kadian™ Capsule; MS Contin® Oral; MSIR® Oral; MS/L®; MS/S®; OMS® Oral; Oramorph SR™ Oral; RMS® Rectal; Roxanol™ Oral; Roxanol Rescudose®; Roxanol SR™ Oral

**Canadian Brand Names** Epimorph®; M-Eslon®; Morphine-HP®; MS-IR®; MST Continus; Statex®

**Therapeutic Category** Analgesic, Narcotic

**Use** Relief of moderate to severe acute and chronic pain; pain of myocardial infarction; relieves dyspnea of acute left ventricular failure and pulmonary edema; preanesthetic medication

**Usual Dosage** Doses should be titrated to appropriate effect; when changing routes of administration in chronically treated patients, please note that oral doses are approximately one-half as effective as parenteral dose

Children:

Oral: Tablet and solution (prompt release): 0.2-0.5 mg/kg/dose every 4-6 hours as needed; tablet (controlled release): 0.3-0.6 mg/kg/dose every 12 hours

I.M., I.V., S.C.: 0.1-0.2 mg/kg/dose every 2-4 hours as needed; usual maximum: 15 mg/dose; may initiate at 0.05 mg/kg/dose

I.V., S.C. continuous infusion: Sickle cell or cancer pain: 0.025-2 mg/kg/hour; postoperative pain: 0.01-0.04 mg/kg/hour

Sedation/analgesia for procedures: I.V.: 0.05-0.1 mg/kg 5 minutes before the procedure

Adolescents >12 years: Sedation/analgesia for procedures: I.V.: 3-4 mg and repeat in 5 minutes if necessary

Adults:

Oral: Prompt release: 10-30 mg every 4 hours as needed; controlled release: 15-30 mg every 8-12 hours

I.M., I.V., S.C.: 2.5-20 mg/dose every 2-6 hours as needed; usual: 10 mg/dose every 4 hours as needed

I.V., S.C. continuous infusion: 0.8-10 mg/hour; may increase depending on pain relief/adverse effects; usual range: up to 80 mg/hour

Epidural: Initial: 5 mg in lumbar region; if inadequate pain relief within 1 hour, give 1-2 mg, maximum dose: 10 mg/24 hours

Intrathecal ($^1/_{10}$ of epidural dose): 0.2-1 mg/dose; repeat doses **not** recommended

Rectal: 10-20 mg every 4 hours

**Mechanism of Action** Binds to opiate receptors in the CNS, causing inhibition of ascending pain pathways, altering the perception of and response to pain; produces generalized CNS depression

**Local Anesthetic/Vasoconstrictor Precautions** No information available to require special precautions

**Effects on Dental Treatment** >10% of patients experience dry mouth; anticholinergic side effects can cause a reduction of saliva production or secretion contributes to discomfort and dental disease (ie, caries, oral candidiasis and periodontal disease)

**Other Adverse Effects**

Cardiovascular: Flushing
Central nervous system: CNS depression, drowsiness, sedation
Endocrine & metabolic: Antidiuretic hormone release
Miscellaneous: Physical and psychological dependence

>10%:
- Cardiovascular: Palpitations, hypotension, bradycardia
- Central nervous system: Dizziness
- Gastrointestinal: Nausea, vomiting, constipation
- Local: Pain at injection site
- Neuromuscular & skeletal: Weakness
- Miscellaneous: Histamine release, sweating

1% to 10%:
- Central nervous system: Restlessness, headache, false feeling of well being, confusion
- Gastrointestinal: Anorexia, GI irritation, dry mouth, paralytic ileus
- Genitourinary: Decreased urination
- Neuromuscular & skeletal: Trembling
- Ocular: Vision problems
- Respiratory: Respiratory depression, dyspnea

<1%:
- Cardiovascular: Peripheral vasodilation
- Central nervous system: Insomnia, mental depression, hallucinations, paradoxical CNS stimulation
- Dermatologic: Pruritus
- Gastrointestinal: Biliary spasm
- Genitourinary: Urinary tract spasm
- Neuromuscular & skeletal: Muscle rigidity
- Ocular: Miosis

**Drug Interactions**

Decreased effect: Phenothiazines may antagonize the analgesic effect of morphine and other opiate agonists

Increased toxicity: CNS depressants, tricyclic antidepressants may potentiate the effects of morphine and other opiate agonists; dextroamphetamine may enhance the analgesic effect of morphine and other opiate agonists

**Drug Uptake**

Absorption: Oral: Variable
Serum half-life: Adults: 2-4 hours

**Pregnancy Risk Factor** B (D if used for prolonged periods or in high doses at term)

**Generic Available** Yes

## Morrhuate Sodium (MOR yoo ate SOW dee um)

**U.S. Brand Names** Scleromate™

**Therapeutic Category** Sclerosing Agent

**Use** Treatment of small, uncomplicated varicose veins of the lower extremities

**Usual Dosage** I.V.:

Children 1-18 years: Esophageal hemorrhage: 2, 3, or 4 mL of 5% repeated every 3-4 days until bleeding is controlled, then every 6 weeks until varices obliterated

Adults: 50-250 mg, repeated at 5- to 7-day intervals (50-100 mg for small veins, 150-250 mg for large veins)

**Mechanism of Action** Both varicose veins and esophageal varices are treated by the thrombotic action of morrhuate sodium. By causing inflammation of the vein's intima, a thrombus is formed. Occlusion secondary to the fibrous tissue and the thrombus results in the obliteration of the vein.

**Local Anesthetic/Vasoconstrictor Precautions** No information available to require special precautions

**Effects on Dental Treatment** No effects or complications reported

**Other Adverse Effects**

>10%:
- Cardiovascular: Thrombosis, valvular incompetency

(Continued)

## Morrhuate Sodium *(Continued)*

Dermatologic: Urticaria
Local: Burning at the site of injection, severe extravasation effects

<1%:

Cardiovascular: Vascular collapse
Central nervous system: Drowsiness, headache, dizziness
Gastrointestinal: Nausea, vomiting
Neuromuscular & skeletal: Weakness
Respiratory: Asthma
Miscellaneous: Anaphylaxis

**Drug Interactions** No data reported

**Drug Uptake**

Onset of action: ~5 minutes
Absorption: Most of the dose stays at the site of injection

**Pregnancy Risk Factor** C

**Generic Available** No

♦ **Mosco® Liquid [OTC]** *see* Salicylic Acid *on page 900*
♦ **Motofen®** *see* Difenoxin and Atropine *on page 326*
♦ **Motrin®** *see* Ibuprofen *on page 522*
♦ **Motrin® IB [OTC]** *see* Ibuprofen *on page 522*
♦ **Motrin® IB Sinus [OTC]** *see* Pseudoephedrine and Ibuprofen *on page 864*
♦ **Mouthkote® Solution [OTC]** *see* Saliva Substitute *on page 901*
♦ **Mouth Pain, Cold Sore, Canker Sore Products** *see page 1253*

## Mouthwash, Antiseptic

**Related Information**

Oral Bacterial Infections *on page 1128*
Oral Nonviral Soft Tissue Ulcerations or Erosions *on page 1141*
Oral Rinse Products *on page 1257*
Periodontal Diseases *on page 1132*

**U.S. Brand Names** Cool Mint Listerine® Antiseptic [OTC]; Fresh Burst Listerine® Antiseptic [OTC]; Listerine® Antiseptic [OTC]

**Therapeutic Category** Antimicrobial Mouth Rinse; Antiplaque Agent; Mouthwash

**Use** Help prevent and reduce plaque and gingivitis; bad breath

**Usual Dosage** Rinse full strength for 30 seconds with 20 mL ($^2/_3$ fluid ounce or 4 teaspoonfuls) morning and night

**Local Anesthetic/Vasoconstrictor Precautions** No information available to require special precautions

**Effects on Dental Treatment** No effects or complications reported

**Other Adverse Effects** No data reported

**Contraindications** Known hypersensitivity to any of its components

**Dosage Forms** Rinse: 250 mL, 500 mL, 1000 mL

**Comments**

Active ingredients:

Listerine® Antiseptic: Thymol 0.064%, eucalyptus 0.092%, methyl salicylate 0.060%, menthol 0.042%, alcohol 26.9%, water, benzoic acid, poloxamer 407, sodium benzoate, caramel

Fresh Burst Listerine® Antiseptic: Thymol 0.064%, eucalyptus 0.092%, methyl salicylate 0.060%, menthol 0.042%, alcohol 26.9%, water, benzoic acid, poloxamer 407, sodium benzoate, flavoring, sodium, saccharin, sodium citrate, citric acid, D&C yellow #10, FD&C green #3

Cool Mint Listerine® Antiseptic: Thymol 0.064%, eucalyptus 0.092%, methyl salicylate 0.060%, menthol 0.042%, alcohol 26.9%, water, benzoic acid, poloxamer 407, sodium benzoate, flavoring, sodium, saccharin, sodium citrate, citric acid, FD&C green #3

The following information is endorsed on the label of the Listerine® products by the Council on Scientific Affairs, American Dental Association: "Listerine® Antiseptic has been shown to help prevent and reduce supragingival plaque accumulation and gingivitis when used in a conscientiously applied program of oral hygiene and regular professional care. Its effect on periodontitis has not been determined."

♦ **4-MP** *see* Fomepizole *on page 453*
♦ **6-MP** *see* Mercaptopurine *on page 636*
♦ **M-R-VAX® II** *see* Measles and Rubella Vaccines, Combined *on page 618*
♦ **MS Contin® Oral** *see* Morphine Sulfate *on page 688*
♦ **MSIR® Oral** *see* Morphine Sulfate *on page 688*
♦ **MS/L®** *see* Morphine Sulfate *on page 688*
♦ **MS/S®** *see* Morphine Sulfate *on page 688*

- **MTC** *see* Mitomycin *on page 680*
- **M.T.E.-4®** *see* Trace Metals *on page 1001*
- **M.T.E.-5®** *see* Trace Metals *on page 1001*
- **M.T.E.-6®** *see* Trace Metals *on page 1001*
- **Muco-Fen-DM®** *see* Guaifenesin and Dextromethorphan *on page 479*
- **Muco-Fen-LA®** *see* Guaifenesin *on page 478*
- **Mucomyst®** *see* Acetylcysteine *on page 36*
- **Mucoplex® [OTC]** *see* Vitamin B Complex *on page 1050*
- **Mucosil™** *see* Acetylcysteine *on page 36*
- **Multe-pak-4®** *see* Trace Metals *on page 1001*
- **Multe-pak-5®** *see* Trace Metals *on page 1001*
- **Multiple Sulfonamides** *see* Sulfadiazine, Sulfamethazine, and Sulfamerazine *on page 942*
- **Multiple Vitamins** *see* Vitamins, Multiple *on page 1051*
- **Multitest CMI®** *see* Skin Test Antigens, Multiple *on page 917*
- **Multivitamins/Fluoride** *see* Vitamins, Multiple *on page 1051*
- **Multi Vit® Drops [OTC]** *see* Vitamins, Multiple *on page 1051*
- **Mumps, Measles and Rubella Vaccines, Combined** *see* Measles, Mumps, and Rubella Vaccines, Combined *on page 618*
- **Mumpsvax®** *see* Mumps Virus Vaccine, Live, Attenuated *on this page*

## Mumps Virus Vaccine, Live, Attenuated

(mumpz VYE rus vak SEEN, live, a ten YOO ate ed)

**U.S. Brand Names** Mumpsvax®

**Therapeutic Category** Vaccine, Live Virus

**Use** Mumps prophylaxis by promoting active immunity

**Usual Dosage** 1 vial (5000 units) S.C. in outer aspect of the upper arm, no booster

**Local Anesthetic/Vasoconstrictor Precautions** No information available to require special precautions

**Effects on Dental Treatment** No effects or complications reported

**Other Adverse Effects**

>10%: Local: Burning or stinging at injection site

1% to 10%:

Central nervous system: Fever ≤100°F

Dermatologic: Rash

Endocrine & metabolic: Parotitis

<1%:

Central nervous system: Convulsions, confusion, severe or continuing headache, fever >103°F

Genitourinary: Orchitis in postpubescent and adult males

Hematologic: Thrombocytopenic purpura

Miscellaneous: Anaphylactic reactions

**Drug Interactions** Decreased effect with concurrent infection, immunoglobulin with in 1 month, other live vaccines with the exception of attenuated measles, rubella, or polio

**Pregnancy Risk Factor** X

**Dosage Forms** Injection: Single dose

**Generic Available** No

**Comments** Federal law requires that the date of administration, the vaccine manufacturer, lot number of vaccine, and the administering person's name, title and address be entered into the patient's permanent medical record

## Mupirocin (myoo PEER oh sin)

**U.S. Brand Names** Bactroban®; Bactroban® Nasal

**Therapeutic Category** Antibiotic, Topical

**Use** Topical treatment of impetigo due to *Staphylococcus aureus*, beta-hemolytic *Streptococcus* and *S. pyogenes*; intranasally for the eradication of nasal colonization with methicillin-resistant *Streptococcus aureus* in adult patients and healthcare workers during institutional outbreaks; eradication of nasal colonization with methicillin-resistant *Staphylococcus aureus* in adult patients and health care workers; use as part of a comprehensive infection control program to reduce the risk of infection among patients at high risk of methicillin-resistant *S. aureus* infection during institutional outbreaks of infections with this pathogen

**Usual Dosage** Children and Adults: Topical: Apply small amount to affected area 2-5 times/day for 5-14 days

**Mechanism of Action** Binds to bacterial isoleucyl transfer-RNA synthetase resulting in the inhibition of protein and RNA synthesis

**Local Anesthetic/Vasoconstrictor Precautions** No information available to require special precautions

(Continued)

## Mupirocin *(Continued)*

**Effects on Dental Treatment** No effects or complications reported

**Other Adverse Effects** 1% to 10%:

Dermatologic: Pruritus, rash, erythema, dry skin

Local: Burning, stinging, pain, tenderness, swelling

**Drug Interactions** No data reported

**Drug Uptake**

Absorption: Topical: Penetrates the outer layers of the skin; systemic absorption minimal through intact skin

Serum half-life: 17-36 minutes

**Pregnancy Risk Factor** B

**Generic Available** No

- **Murine® Ear Drops [OTC]** *see* Carbamide Peroxide *on page 186*
- **Murine® Plus Ophthalmic [OTC]** *see* Tetrahydrozoline *on page 967*
- **Murine® Solution [OTC]** *see* Artificial Tears *on page 97*
- **Muro 128® Ophthalmic [OTC]** *see* Sodium Chloride *on page 920*
- **Murocel® Ophthalmic Solution [OTC]** *see* Artificial Tears *on page 97*
- **Murocoll-2® Ophthalmic** *see* Phenylephrine and Scopolamine *on page 796*

## Muromonab-CD3 (myoo roe MOE nab see dee three)

**U.S. Brand Names** Orthoclone® OKT3

**Therapeutic Category** Immunosuppressant Agent

**Synonyms** Monoclonal Antibody; OKT3

**Use** Treatment of acute allograft rejection in renal transplant patients; effective in reversing acute hepatic, cardiac, and bone marrow transplant rejection episodes resistant to conventional treatment

**Usual Dosage** I.V. (**refer to individual protocols**):

Children <30 kg: 2.5 mg/day once daily for 7-14 days

Children >30 kg: 5 mg/day once daily for 7-14 days

**or**

Children <12 years: 0.1 mg/kg/day once daily for 10-14 days

Children ≥12 years and Adults: 5 mg/day once daily for 10-14 days

**Mechanism of Action** Reverses graft rejection by binding to T cells and interfering with their function

**Local Anesthetic/Vasoconstrictor Precautions** No information available to require special precautions

**Effects on Dental Treatment** No effects or complications reported

**Other Adverse Effects**

1% to 10%:

- Central nervous system: Headache
- Neuromuscular & skeletal: Stiff neck
- Ocular: Photophobia
- Respiratory: Pulmonary edema

<1%:

- Cardiovascular: Hypertension, hypotension, chest pain, tightness in chest
- Central nervous system: Aseptic meningitis, seizures, fatigue, confusion, coma, hallucinations, pyrexia
- Dermatologic: Pruritus, rash
- Neuromuscular & skeletal: Arthralgia, tremor
- Renal: Elevated BUN/creatinine
- Respiratory: Wheezing
- Miscellaneous: Flu-like symptoms (ie, fever, chills), infection, anaphylactic-type reactions

**Drug Uptake**

Absorption: I.V.: Immediate

Time to steady-state: Trough level: 3-14 days; pretreatment levels are restored within 7 days after treatment is terminated

**Pregnancy Risk Factor** C

**Generic Available** No

**Comments** Recommend decreasing dose of prednisone to 0.5 mg/kg, azathioprine to 0.5 mg/kg (approximate 50% decrease in dose), and discontinuing cyclosporine while patient is receiving OKT3

- **Muroptic-5® [OTC]** *see* Sodium Chloride *on page 920*
- **Muse® Pellet** *see* Alprostadil *on page 51*
- **Mutamycin®** *see* Mitomycin *on page 680*
- **M.V.I.®** *see* Vitamins, Multiple *on page 1051*
- **M.V.I.®-12** *see* Vitamins, Multiple *on page 1051*
- **M.V.I.® Concentrate** *see* Vitamins, Multiple *on page 1051*
- **M.V.I.® Pediatric** *see* Vitamins, Multiple *on page 1051*

- **Myambutol®** *see* Ethambutol *on page 396*
- **Mycelex® Troche** *see* Clotrimazole *on page 267*
- **Mycifradin® Sulfate** *see* Neomycin *on page 709*
- **Mycinettes® [OTC]** *see* Benzocaine *on page 128*
- **Mycobutin®** *see* Rifabutin *on page 885*
- **Mycogen II Topical** *see* Nystatin and Triamcinolone *on page 735*
- **Mycolog®-II Topical** *see* Nystatin and Triamcinolone *on page 735*
- **Myconel® Topical** *see* Nystatin and Triamcinolone *on page 735*


**Adverse Reactions Reported in >10%**

| Adverse Reaction | MM 2 g/day | MM 3 g/day |
|---|---|---|
| **Body as a Whole** | | |
| Pain | 33 | 31.2 |
| Abdominal pain | 12.1-24.7 | 11.9-27.6 |
| Fever | 20.4 | 23.3 |
| Headache | 20.1 | 16.1 |
| Infection | 12.7-18.2 | 15.6-20.9 |
| Sepsis | 17.6-20.8 | 17.5-19.7 |
| Asthenia | 13.7 | 16.1 |
| Chest pain | 13.4 | 13.3 |
| Back pain | 11.6 | 12.1 |
| Hypertension | 17.6-32.4 | 16.9-28.2 |
| **Central Nervous System** | | |
| Tremor | 11 | 11.8 |
| Insomnia | 8.9 | 11.8 |
| Dizziness | 5.7 | 11.2 |
| **Dermatologic** | | |
| Acne | 10.1 | 9.7 |
| Rash | 7.7 | 6.4 |
| **Gastrointestinal** | | |
| Diarrhea | 16.4-31 | 18.8-36.1 |
| Constipation | 21.9 | 18.5 |
| Nausea | 19.9 | 23.6 |
| Dyspepsia | 17.6 | 13.6 |
| Vomiting | 12.5 | 13.6 |
| Nausea & vomiting | 10.4 | 9.7 |
| Oral monoliasis | 10.1 | 12.1 |
| **Hemic/Lymphatic** | | |
| Anemia | 25.6 | 25.8 |
| Leukopenia | 11.5-23.2 | 16.3-34.5 |
| Thrombocytopenia | 10.1 | 8.2 |
| Hypochromic anemia | 7.4 | 11.5 |
| Leukocytosis | 7.1 | 10.9 |
| **Metabolic/Nutritional** | | |
| Peripheral edema | 28.6 | 27 |
| Hypercholesterolemia | 12.8 | 8.5 |
| Hypophosphatemia | 12.5 | 15.8 |
| Edema | 12.2 | 11.8 |
| Hypokalemia | 10.1 | 10 |
| Hyperkalemia | 8.9 | 10.3 |
| Hyperglycemia | 8.6 | 12.4 |
| **Respiratory** | | |
| Infection | 15.8-21 | 13.1-23.9 |
| Dyspnea | 15.5 | 17.3 |
| Cough increase | 15.5 | 13.3 |
| Pharyngitis | 9.5 | 11.2 |
| Bronchitis | 8.5 | 11.9 |
| Pneumonia | 3.6 | 10.6 |
| **Urogenital** | | |
| UTI | 37.2-45.5 | 37-44.4 |
| Hematuria | 14 | 12.1 |
| Kidney tubular necrosis | 6.3 | 10 |
| Urinary tract disorder | 6.7 | 10.6 |

## Mycophenolate (mye koe FEN oh late)

**U.S. Brand Names** CellCept®

**Therapeutic Category** Immunosuppressant Agent

**Use** Immunosuppressant used with corticosteroids and cyclosporine to prevent organ rejection in patients receiving allogenic renal transplants

**Usual Dosage** Adults: I.V./Oral: 1 g twice daily (2 g daily dose), administered within 72 hours of transplantation, when administered in combination with corticosteroids and cyclosporine

**Mechanism of Action** Inhibition of purine synthesis of human lymphocytes and proliferation of human lymphocytes

**Local Anesthetic/Vasoconstrictor Precautions** No information available to require special precautions

**Effects on Dental Treatment** No effects or complications reported

**Other Adverse Effects** See table on previous page.

**Drug Interactions**

Decreased effect: Antacids and cholestyramine decrease serum levels of mycophenolate

Increased toxicity: Acyclovir and ganciclovir levels may elevate due to competition for tubular secretion of these drugs; probenecid may elevate mycophenolate levels due to inhibition of tubular secretion; salicylates: high doses may increase free fraction of mycophenolic acid

**Drug Uptake**

Absorption: Mycophenolate mofetil is hydrolyzed to mycophenolic acid in the liver and gastrointestinal tract; food does not alter the extent of absorption, but the maximum concentration is decreased

Serum half-life: 18 hours

Serum concentrations: Correlation of toxicity or efficacy is still being developed, however, one study indicated that 12-hour AUCs of >40 mcg/mL/hour were correlated with efficacy and decreased episodes of rejection

**Pregnancy Risk Factor** C

**Dosage Forms**

Capsule, as mofetil: 250 mg

Powder for injection, as hydrochloride: 500 mg

Tablet, as mofetil: 500 mg

**Generic Available** No


- **Mycostatin®** *see* Nystatin *on page 734*
- **Myco-Triacet® II** *see* Nystatin and Triamcinolone *on page 735*
- **Mydfrin® Ophthalmic Solution** *see* Phenylephrine *on page 795*
- **Mydriacyl®** *see* Tropicamide *on page 1029*
- **Mykrox®** *see* Metolazone *on page 665*
- **Mylanta® [OTC]** *see* Aluminum Hydroxide, Magnesium Hydroxide, and Simethicone *on page 56*
- **Mylanta® Gas® [OTC]** *see* Simethicone *on page 915*
- **Mylanta® Gelcaps®** *see* Calcium Carbonate and Magnesium Carbonate *on page 172*
- **Mylanta®-II [OTC]** *see* Aluminum Hydroxide, Magnesium Hydroxide, and Simethicone *on page 56*
- **Myleran®** *see* Busulfan *on page 161*
- **Mylicon® [OTC]** *see* Simethicone *on page 915*
- **Mylosar®** *see* Azacitidine *on page 111*
- **Myminic® Expectorant [OTC]** *see* Guaifenesin and Phenylpropanolamine *on page 480*
- **Myoflex® [OTC]** *see* Triethanolamine Salicylate *on page 1016*
- **Myotonachol™** *see* Bethanechol *on page 139*
- **Myphetane DC®** *see* Brompheniramine, Phenylpropanolamine, and Codeine *on page 155*
- **Mysoline®** *see* Primidone *on page 838*
- **Mytelase® Caplets®** *see* Ambenonium *on page 58*
- **Mytrex® F Topical** *see* Nystatin and Triamcinolone *on page 735*
- **Mytussin® [OTC]** *see* Guaifenesin *on page 478*
- **Mytussin® AC** *see* Guaifenesin and Codeine *on page 478*
- **Mytussin® DAC** *see* Guaifenesin, Pseudoephedrine, and Codeine *on page 482*
- **Mytussin® DM [OTC]** *see* Guaifenesin and Dextromethorphan *on page 479*

## Nabilone (NA bi lone)

**U.S. Brand Names** Cesamet®

**Therapeutic Category** Antiemetic

**Use** Treatment of nausea and vomiting associated with cancer chemotherapy

**Usual Dosage** Oral:

Children >4 years:

<18 kg: 0.5 mg twice daily

18-30 kg: 1 mg twice daily

>30 kg: 1 mg 3 times/day

Adults: 1-2 mg twice daily beginning 1-3 hours before chemotherapy is administered and continuing around-the-clock until 1 dose after chemotherapy is completed; maximum daily dose: 6 mg divided in 3 doses

**Mechanism of Action** Nabilone is a synthetic cannabinoid utilized as an antiemetic drug in the control of nausea and vomiting in patients receiving cancer chemotherapy; like delta-9-tetrahydrocannabinol (the active principal of marijuana), nabilone is a dibenzo(b,d)pyrans

**Local Anesthetic/Vasoconstrictor Precautions** No information available to require special precautions

**Effects on Dental Treatment** >10% of patients experience dry mouth

**Other Adverse Effects**

>10%: Central nervous system: Dizziness, drowsiness, vertigo, euphoria, clumsiness

1% to 10%:

Cardiovascular: Orthostatic hypotension

Central nervous system: Depression

Ocular: Blurred vision

<1%:

Central nervous system: Changes of mood, confusion, hallucinations, headache

Gastrointestinal: Loss of appetite

Respiratory: Dyspnea

**Drug Interactions** No data reported

**Drug Uptake**

Absorption: Rapid

Serum half-life: 35 hours

**Pregnancy Risk Factor** C

**Generic Available** No

## Nabumetone (na BYOO me tone)

**Related Information**

Rheumatoid Arthritis and Osteoarthritis *on page 1092*

**U.S. Brand Names** Relafen®

**Therapeutic Category** Nonsteroidal Anti-inflammatory Drug (NSAID), Oral

**Use** Management of osteoarthritis and rheumatoid arthritis

**Unlabeled use**: Sunburn, mild to moderate pain

**Usual Dosage** Adults: Oral: 1000 mg/day; an additional 500-1000 mg may be needed in some patients to obtain more symptomatic relief; may be administered once or twice daily

**Mechanism of Action** Nabumetone is a nonacidic, nonsteroidal anti-inflammatory drug that is rapidly metabolized after absorption to a major active metabolite, 6-methoxy-2-naphthylacetic acid. As found with previous nonsteroidal anti-inflammatory drugs, nabumetone's active metabolite inhibits the cyclo-oxygenase enzyme which is indirectly responsible for the production of inflammation and pain during arthritis by way of enhancing the production of endoperoxides and prostaglandins $E_2$ and $I_2$ (prostacyclin). The active metabolite of nabumetone is felt to be the compound primarily responsible for therapeutic effect. Comparatively, the parent drug is a poor inhibitor of prostaglandin synthesis.

**Local Anesthetic/Vasoconstrictor Precautions** No information available to require special precautions

**Effects on Dental Treatment** NSAID formulations are known to reversibly decrease platelet aggregation via mechanisms different than observed with aspirin. The dentist should be aware of the potential of abnormal coagulation. Caution should also be exercised in the use of NSAIDs in patients already on anticoagulant therapy with drugs such as warfarin (Coumadin®).

**Other Adverse Effects**

>10%:

Central nervous system: Dizziness

Dermatologic: Skin rash

Gastrointestinal: Abdominal cramps, heartburn, indigestion, nausea

(Continued)

## Nabumetone *(Continued)*

1% to 10%:
- Central nervous system: Headache, nervousness
- Dermatologic: Itching
- Endocrine & metabolic: Fluid retention
- Gastrointestinal: Vomiting
- Otic: Tinnitus

<1%:
- Cardiovascular: Congestive heart failure, hypertension, arrhythmia, tachycardia
- Central nervous system: Confusion, hallucinations, aseptic meningitis, mental depression, drowsiness, insomnia
- Dermatologic: Angioedema, urticaria, erythema multiforme, toxic epidermal necrolysis, Stevens-Johnson syndrome
- Endocrine & metabolic: Polydipsia, hot flashes
- Gastrointestinal: Gastritis, GI ulceration
- Genitourinary: Cystitis
- Hematologic: Agranulocytosis, anemia, hemolytic anemia, bone marrow suppression, leukopenia, thrombocytopenia
- Hepatic: Hepatitis
- Neuromuscular & skeletal: Peripheral neuropathy
- Ocular: Toxic amblyopia, blurred vision, conjunctivitis, dry eyes
- Otic: Decreased hearing
- Renal: Polyuria, acute renal failure
- Respiratory: Allergic rhinitis, dyspnea, epistaxis

**Drug Interactions** No data reported

**Drug Uptake**

Serum half-life, elimination: Major metabolite: 24 hours

Time to peak serum concentration: Metabolite: Oral: Within 3-6 hours

**Pregnancy Risk Factor** C

**Generic Available** No

♦ **NaCl** *see* Sodium Chloride *on page 920*

## Nadolol (nay DOE lole)

**Related Information**

Cardiovascular Diseases *on page 1066*

**U.S. Brand Names** Corgard®

**Canadian Brand Names** Apo®-Nadol; Syn-Nadolol

**Therapeutic Category** Antianginal Agent; Beta-adrenergic Blocker, Noncardioselective

**Use** Treatment of hypertension and angina pectoris; prevention of myocardial infarction; prophylaxis of migraine headaches

**Usual Dosage** Oral:

Children: No information regarding pediatric dosage is currently available in the literature

Adults: Initial: 40-80 mg/day, increase dosage gradually by 40-80 mg increments at 3- to 7-day intervals until optimum clinical response is obtained with profound slowing of heart rate; doses up to 160-240 mg/day in angina and 240-320 mg/day in hypertension may be necessary; doses as high as 640 mg/day have been used

Elderly: Initial: 20 mg/day; increase doses by 20 mg increments at 3- to 7-day intervals; usual dosage range: 20-240 mg/day

**Mechanism of Action** Competitively blocks response to $beta_1$- and $beta_2$-adrenergic stimulation; does not exhibit any membrane stabilizing or intrinsic sympathomimetic activity

**Local Anesthetic/Vasoconstrictor Precautions** Use with caution; epinephrine has interacted with nonselective beta-blockers to result in initial hypertensive episode followed by bradycardia

**Effects on Dental Treatment** Noncardioselective beta-blockers (ie, propranolol, nadolol) may enhance the pressor response to epinephrine, resulting in hypertension and bradycardia. Many nonsteroidal anti-inflammatory drugs such as ibuprofen and indomethacin can reduce the hypotensive effect of beta-blockers after 3 or more weeks of therapy with the NSAID. Short-term NSAID use (ie, 3 days) requires no special precautions in patients taking beta-blockers.

**Other Adverse Effects**

>10%: Cardiovascular: Bradycardia

1% to 10%:
- Cardiovascular: Reduced peripheral circulation
- Central nervous system: Mental depression, dizziness
- Endocrine & metabolic: Decreased sexual ability
- Gastrointestinal: Constipation

Neuromuscular & skeletal: Weakness
Respiratory: Dyspnea, wheezing

<1%:

Cardiovascular: Congestive heart failure, chest pain, orthostatic hypotension, edema, Raynaud's phenomenon
Central nervous system: Drowsiness, nightmares, vivid dreams, insomnia, lethargy, fatigue, confusion, headache
Dermatologic: Itching, rash
Gastrointestinal: Vomiting, stomach discomfort, diarrhea, nausea
Genitourinary: Impotence
Hematologic: Thrombocytopenia
Neuromuscular & skeletal: Paresthesia
Ocular: Dry eyes
Respiratory: Nasal congestion
Miscellaneous: Cold extremities

**Drug Interactions**

Decreased effect of beta-blockers:

Barbiturates (increased liver metabolism of beta-blockers to result in lower serum levels)
NSAIDs (attenuate the hypotensive therapeutic effects of beta-blockers)
Rifampin (increased liver metabolism of beta-blockers to result in lower serum levels)

Increased effects of beta-blockers:

Calcium channel blockers (increase serum levels of beta-blockers by unknown mechanism to enhance hypotension)

Beta-blockers increase the effects of:

Epinephrine (vasoconstrictor; initial hypertensive episode followed by bradycardia) only from noncardioselective type beta-blockers
Phenylephrine (Neosynephrine®; enhanced pressor response)
Theophylline (inhibit theophylline metabolism causing increase in serum concentrations)

**Drug Uptake**

Duration of effect: 24 hours
Absorption: Oral: 30% to 40%
Time to peak serum concentration: Within 2-4 hours persisting for 17-24 hours
Serum half-life: Adults: 10-24 hours; increased half-life with decreased renal function
End-stage renal disease: 45 hours

**Pregnancy Risk Factor** C

**Generic Available** Yes

**Selected Readings**

Foster CA and Aston SJ, "Propranolol-Epinephrine Interaction: A Potential Disaster," *Plast Reconstr Surg*, 1983, 72(1):74-8.
Wong DG, Spence JD, Lamki L, et al, "Effect of Nonsteroidal Anti-inflammatory Drugs on Control of Hypertension of Beta-Blockers and Diuretics," *Lancet*, 1986, 1(8488):997-1001.
Wynn RL, "Dental Nonsteroidal Anti-inflammatory Drugs and Prostaglandin-Based Drug Interactions, Part Two," *Gen Dent*, 1992, 40(2):104, 106, 108.
Wynn RL, "Epinephrine Interactions With Beta-Blockers," *Gen Dent*, 1994, 42(1):16, 18.

## Nafarelin (NAF a re lin)

**U.S. Brand Names** Synarel®

**Therapeutic Category** Hormone, Posterior Pituitary; Luteinizing Hormone-Releasing Hormone Analog

**Use** Treatment of endometriosis, including pain and reduction of lesions; treatment of central precocious puberty (gonadotropin-dependent precocious puberty) in children of both sexes

**Usual Dosage**

Endometriosis: Adults: Female: 1 spray (200 mcg) in 1 nostril each morning and the other nostril each evening starting on days 2-4 of menstrual cycle for 6 months
Central precocious puberty: Children: Male/Female: 2 sprays (400 mcg) into each nostril in the morning 2 sprays (400 mcg) into each nostril in the evening. If inadequate suppression, may increase dose to 3 sprays (600 mcg) into alternating nostrils 3 times/day.

**Mechanism of Action** Potent synthetic decapeptide analogue of gonadotropin-releasing hormone (GnRH; LHRH) which is approximately 200 times more potent than GnRH in terms of pituitary release of luteinizing hormone (LH) and follicle-stimulating hormone (FSH). Effects on the pituitary gland and sex hormones are dependent upon its length of administration. After acute administration, an initial stimulation of the release of LH and FSH from the pituitary is observed; an

(Continued)

## Nafarelin *(Continued)*

increase in androgens and estrogens subsequently follows. Continued administration of nafarelin, however, suppresses gonadotrope responsiveness to endogenous GnRH resulting in reduced secretion of LH and FSH and, secondarily, decreased ovarian and testicular steroid production.

**Local Anesthetic/Vasoconstrictor Precautions** No information available to require special precautions

**Effects on Dental Treatment** No effects or complications reported

**Other Adverse Effects**

>10%:

Central nervous system: Headache, emotional lability
Dermatologic: Acne
Endocrine & metabolic: Hot flashes, decreased libido, decreased breast size
Genitourinary: Vaginal dryness
Neuromuscular & skeletal: Myalgia
Respiratory: Nasal irritation

1% to 10%:

Cardiovascular: Edema
Central nervous system: Insomnia
Dermatologic: Urticaria, rash, pruritus, seborrhea
Respiratory: Dyspnea, chest pain

<1%:

Endocrine & metabolic: Increased libido
Gastrointestinal: Weight loss

**Drug Interactions** No data reported

**Drug Uptake**

Absorption: Not absorbed from GI tract
Maximum serum concentration: 10-45 minutes

**Pregnancy Risk Factor** X

**Generic Available** No

♦ **Nafazair® Ophthalmic** *see* Naphazoline *on page 703*
♦ **Nafcil™** *see* Nafcillin *on this page*

## Nafcillin (naf SIL in)

**U.S. Brand Names** Nafcil™; Nallpen®; Unipen®

**Therapeutic Category** Antibiotic, Penicillin

**Use** Treatment of susceptible bacterial infections such as osteomyelitis, septicemia, endocarditis, and CNS infections due to penicillinase-producing strains of *Staphylococcus*

**Usual Dosage**

Children: I.M., I.V.:

Mild to moderate infections: 50-100 mg/kg/day in divided doses every 6 hours
Severe infections: 100-200 mg/kg/day in divided doses every 4-6 hours
Maximum dose: 12 g/day

Adults:

I.M.: 500 mg every 4-6 hours
I.V.: 500-2000 mg every 4-6 hours

**Mechanism of Action** Interferes with bacterial cell wall synthesis during active multiplication, causing cell wall death and resultant bactericidal activity against susceptible bacteria

**Local Anesthetic/Vasoconstrictor Precautions** No information available to require special precautions

**Effects on Dental Treatment** Prolonged use of penicillins may lead to the development of oral candidiasis

**Other Adverse Effects** <1%:

Central nervous system: Fever, pain
Dermatologic: Skin rash
Gastrointestinal: Nausea, diarrhea
Hematologic: Neutropenia
Local: Thrombophlebitis; oxacillin (less likely to cause phlebitis) is often preferred in pediatric patients
Renal: Acute interstitial nephritis
Miscellaneous: Hypersensitivity reactions

**Drug Interactions**

Decreased effect: Chloramphenicol may decrease nafcillin levels; oral contraceptive may have a decreased effectiveness
Increased effect: Probenecid may increase nafcillin levels
Increased toxicity: Oral anticoagulants, heparin increase risk of bleeding

**Drug Uptake**

Absorption: Oral: Poor and erratic

Serum half-life:
Adults: 0.5-1.5 hours, with normal hepatic function
End-stage renal disease: 1.2 hours
Time to peak serum concentration:
Oral: Within 2 hours
I.M.: Within 0.5-1 hour
**Pregnancy Risk Factor** B
**Generic Available** Yes

## Naftifine (NAF ti feen)

**U.S. Brand Names** Naftin®
**Therapeutic Category** Antifungal Agent, Topical
**Use** Topical treatment of tinea cruris (jock itch), tinea corporis (ring worm), and tinea pedis (athlete's foot)
**Usual Dosage** Adults: Topical: Apply cream once daily and gel twice daily (morning and evening) for up to 4 weeks
**Mechanism of Action** Synthetic, broad-spectrum antifungal agent in the allylamine class; appears to have both fungistatic and fungicidal activity. Exhibits antifungal activity by selectively inhibiting the enzyme squalene epoxidase in a dose-dependent manner which results in the primary sterol, ergosterol, within the fungal membrane not being synthesized.
**Local Anesthetic/Vasoconstrictor Precautions** No information available to require special precautions
**Effects on Dental Treatment** No effects or complications reported
**Other Adverse Effects**
>10%: Local: Burning, stinging
1% to 10%: Local: Dryness, erythema, itching, irritation
**Drug Interactions** No data reported
**Drug Uptake**
Absorption: Systemic, 6% for cream, ≤4% for gel
Serum half-life: 2-3 days
**Pregnancy Risk Factor** B
**Generic Available** No

◆ **Naftin®** *see* Naftifine *on this page*
◆ **$NaHCO_3$** *see* Sodium Bicarbonate *on page 918*

## Nalbuphine (NAL byoo feen)

**Related Information**
Narcotic Agonists *on page 1223*
**U.S. Brand Names** Nubain®
**Therapeutic Category** Analgesic, Narcotic
**Use** Relief of moderate to severe pain; preoperative analgesia, postoperative and surgical anesthesia, and obstetrical analgesia during labor and delivery
**Usual Dosage** I.M., I.V., S.C.:
Children 10 months to 14 years: Premedication: 0.2 mg/kg; maximum: 20 mg/dose
Adults: 10 mg/70 kg every 3-6 hours; maximum single dose: 20 mg; maximum daily dose: 160 mg
**Mechanism of Action** Binds to opiate receptors in the CNS, causing inhibition of ascending pain pathways, altering the perception of and response to pain; produces generalized CNS depression
**Local Anesthetic/Vasoconstrictor Precautions** No information available to require special precautions
**Effects on Dental Treatment** Anticholinergic side effects can cause a reduction of saliva production or secretion contributes to discomfort and dental disease (ie, caries, oral candidiasis and periodontal disease)
**Other Adverse Effects**
>10%:
Central nervous system: Drowsiness, CNS depression
Miscellaneous: Histamine release, narcotic withdrawal
1% to 10%:
Cardiovascular: Hypotension, flushing
Central nervous system: Dry mouth, dizziness, headache
Dermatologic: Urticaria, skin rash
Gastrointestinal: Nausea, vomiting, anorexia
Local: Pain at injection site
Neuromuscular & skeletal: Weakness
Respiratory: Pulmonary edema
<1%:
Cardiovascular: Hypertension, tachycardia
(Continued)

## Nalbuphine *(Continued)*

Central nervous system: Mental depression, hallucinations, confusion, paradoxical CNS stimulation, nervousness, restlessness, nightmares, insomnia
Gastrointestinal: GI irritation, ureteral spasm, biliary spasm, toxic megacolon
Genitourinary: Decreased urination
Ocular: Blurred vision
Respiratory: Dyspnea, respiratory depression

**Drug Interactions** Increased toxicity: Barbiturate anesthetics cause increased CNS depression

**Drug Uptake** Serum half-life: 3.5-5 hours

**Pregnancy Risk Factor** B (D if used for prolonged periods or in high doses at term)

**Generic Available** Yes

- ♦ **Naldecon®** *see* Chlorpheniramine, Phenyltoloxamine, Phenylpropanolamine, and Phenylephrine *on page 237*
- ♦ **Naldecon® DX Adult Liquid [OTC]** *see* Guaifenesin, Phenylpropanolamine, and Dextromethorphan *on page 481*
- ♦ **Naldecon-EX® Children's Syrup [OTC]** *see* Guaifenesin and Phenylpropanolamine *on page 480*
- ♦ **Naldecon® Senior DX [OTC]** *see* Guaifenesin and Dextromethorphan *on page 479*
- ♦ **Naldecon® Senior EX [OTC]** *see* Guaifenesin *on page 478*
- ♦ **Naldelate®** *see* Chlorpheniramine, Phenyltoloxamine, Phenylpropanolamine, and Phenylephrine *on page 237*
- ♦ **Nalfon®** *see* Fenoprofen *on page 424*
- ♦ **Nalgest®** *see* Chlorpheniramine, Phenyltoloxamine, Phenylpropanolamine, and Phenylephrine *on page 237*

## Nalidixic Acid (nal i DIKS ik AS id)

**U.S. Brand Names** NegGram®

**Therapeutic Category** Antibiotic, Quinolone

**Use** Treatment of urinary tract infections

**Usual Dosage** Oral:

Children 3 months to 12 years: 55 mg/kg/day divided every 6 hours; suppressive therapy is 33 mg/kg/day divided every 6 hours

Adults: 1 g 4 times/day for 2 weeks; then suppressive therapy of 500 mg 4 times/day

**Mechanism of Action** Inhibits DNA polymerization in late stages of chromosomal replication

**Local Anesthetic/Vasoconstrictor Precautions** No information available to require special precautions

**Effects on Dental Treatment** No effects or complications reported

**Other Adverse Effects**

>10%: Central nervous system: Dizziness, drowsiness, headache

1% to 10%: Gastrointestinal: Nausea, vomiting

<1%:

Central nervous system: Increased intracranial pressure, malaise, vertigo, confusion, toxic psychosis, convulsions, fever, chills
Dermatologic: Rash, urticaria, photosensitivity reactions
Endocrine & metabolic: Metabolic acidosis
Hematologic: Leukopenia, thrombocytopenia
Hepatic: Hepatotoxicity
Ocular: Visual disturbances

**Drug Interactions**

Decreased effect with antacids
Increased effect of warfarin

**Drug Uptake**

Serum half-life: 6-7 hours; increases significantly with renal impairment
Time to peak serum concentration: Oral: Within 1-2 hours

**Pregnancy Risk Factor** B

**Generic Available** Yes

- ♦ **Nallpen®** *see* Nafcillin *on page 698*

## Nalmefene (NAL me feen)

**U.S. Brand Names** Revex®

**Therapeutic Category** Antidote for Narcotic Agonists

**Use** Complete or partial of opioid drug effects; management of known or suspected opioid overdose

**Usual Dosage**

Reversal of postoperative opioid depression: Blue labeled product (100 mcg/mL): Titrate to reverse the undesired effects of opioids; initial dose for nonopioid dependent patients: 0.25 mcg/kg followed by 0.25 mcg/kg incremental doses at 2- to 5-minute intervals; after a total dose of >1 mcg/kg, further therapeutic response is unlikely

Management of known/suspected opioid overdose: Green labeled product (1000 mcg/mL): Initial dose: 0.5 mg/70 kg; may repeat with 1 mg/70 kg in 2-5 minutes; further increase beyond a total dose of 1.5 mg/70 kg will not likely result in improved response and may result in cardiovascular stress and precipitated withdrawal syndrome. (If opioid dependency is suspected, administer a challenge dose of 0.1 mg/70 kg; if no withdrawal symptoms are observed in 2 minutes, the recommended doses can be administered.)

**Mechanism of Action** As a 6-methylene analog of naltrexone, nalmefene acts as a competitive antagonist at opioid receptor sites, preventing or reversing the respiratory depression, sedation, and hypotension induced by opiates; no pharmacologic activity of its own (eg, opioid agonist activity) has been demonstrated

**Local Anesthetic/Vasoconstrictor Precautions** No information available to require special precautions

**Effects on Dental Treatment** No effects or complications reported

**Other Adverse Effects**

>10%: Gastrointestinal: Nausea

1% to 10%:
- Cardiovascular: Tachycardia, hypertension
- Central nervous system: Postoperative pain, fever, dizziness
- Gastrointestinal: Vomiting

<1%:
- Cardiovascular: Hypotension, vasodilation, arrhythmia
- Central nervous system: Headache, chills, nervousness, confusion
- Gastrointestinal: Diarrhea, dry mouth
- Genitourinary: Urinary retention
- Neuromuscular & skeletal: Tremor
- Miscellaneous: Withdrawal syndrome

**Drug Uptake**

Onset of action: I.M., S.C.: 5-15 minutes
Serum half-life: 10.8 hours
Time to peak serum concentration: 2.3 hours

**Pregnancy Risk Factor** B

**Generic Available** No

**Comments** Nalmefene is supplied in two concentrations 100 mcg/mL has a blue label, 1000 mcg/mL has a green label; proper steps should be used to prevent use of the incorrect dosage strength; duration of action of nalmefene is as long as most opioid analgesics; may cause acute withdrawal symptoms in individuals who have some degree of tolerance to and dependence on opioids

## Naloxone (nal OKS one)

**Related Information**

Narcotic Agonists *on page 1223*

**U.S. Brand Names** Narcan®

**Therapeutic Category** Narcotic Antagonist

**Use**

Dental: Reverses CNS and respiratory depressant effects of fentanyl and meperidine during I.V. conscious state

Medical: Reverses CNS and respiratory depression in suspected narcotic overdose; neonatal opiate depression; coma of unknown etiology

**Usual Dosage** Adults: Narcotic overdose: I.V.: 0.4-2 mg every 2-3 minutes as needed; may need to repeat doses every 20-60 minutes, if no response is observed after 10 mg, question the diagnosis. **Note:** Use 0.1-0.2 mg increments in patients who are opioid-dependent and in postoperative patients to avoid large cardiovascular changes.

**Mechanism of Action** Competes and displaces narcotics at narcotic receptor sites (mu, kappa, delta, and sigma subtypes)

**Local Anesthetic/Vasoconstrictor Precautions** No information available to require special precautions

**Effects on Dental Treatment** No effects or complications reported

**Other Adverse Effects** 1% to 10%:
- Cardiovascular: Hypertension, hypotension, tachycardia, ventricular arrhythmias
- Central nervous system: Insomnia, irritability, anxiety
- Dermatologic: Rash
- Gastrointestinal: Nausea, vomiting
- Ocular: Blurred vision
- Miscellaneous: Narcotic withdrawal, sweating

(Continued)

## Naloxone *(Continued)*

**Contraindications** Hypersensitivity to naloxone or any component

**Warnings/Precautions** Use with caution in patients with cardiovascular disease; excessive dosages should be avoided after use of opiates in surgery, because naloxone may cause an increase in blood pressure and reversal of anesthesia; may precipitate withdrawal symptoms in patients addicted to opiates, including pain, hypertension, sweating, agitation, irritability, shrill cry, failure to feed

**Drug Interactions** Decreased effect of narcotic analgesics

**Drug Uptake**

Onset of effect: I.V.: Within 2 minutes

Duration of effect: 20-60 minutes; since shorter than that of most opioids, repeated doses are usually needed

Time to peak serum concentration: 5-15 minutes

Serum half-life: 1-1.5 hours

**Pregnancy Risk Factor** B

**Breast-feeding Considerations** No data reported

**Dosage Forms** Injection: 0.02 mg/mL (2 mL); 0.4 mg/mL (1 mL, 2 mL, 10 mL); 1 mg/mL (2 mL, 10 mL)

**Dietary Considerations** No data reported

**Generic Available** Yes

**Comments** Naloxone is an antagonist to all narcotic analgesics. Its use in dental practice is to reverse overdose effects of the two narcotic agents fentanyl and meperidine, used in the technique of I.V. conscious sedation.

♦ **Nalspan®** *see* Chlorpheniramine, Phenyltoloxamine, Phenylpropanolamine, and Phenylephrine *on page 237*

## Naltrexone (nal TREKS one)

**U.S. Brand Names** ReVia® Oral

**Therapeutic Category** Narcotic Antagonist

**Use** Adjunct to the maintenance of an opioid-free state in detoxified individual

**Usual Dosage** Do not give until patient is opioid-free for 7-10 days as required by urine analysis

Adults: Oral: 25 mg; if no withdrawal signs within 1 hour give another 25 mg; maintenance regimen is flexible, variable and individualized (50 mg/day to 100-150 mg 3 times/week)

**Mechanism of Action** Naltrexone is a cyclopropyl derivative of oxymorphone similar in structure to naloxone and nalorphine (a morphine derivative); it acts as a competitive antagonist at opioid receptor sites

**Local Anesthetic/Vasoconstrictor Precautions** No information available to require special precautions

**Effects on Dental Treatment** No effects or complications reported

**Other Adverse Effects**

>10%:
- Central nervous system: Insomnia, nervousness, headache
- Gastrointestinal: Abdominal cramping, nausea, vomiting
- Neuromuscular & skeletal: Arthralgia

1% to 10%:
- Central nervous system: Dizziness
- Dermatologic: Skin rash
- Gastrointestinal: Anorexia
- Endocrine & metabolic: Polydipsia
- Respiratory: Sneezing

<1%:
- Central nervous system: Irritability, anxiety
- Hematologic: Thrombocytopenia, agranulocytosis, hemolytic anemia
- Ocular: Blurred vision
- Miscellaneous: Narcotic withdrawal

**Drug Interactions** No data reported

**Drug Uptake**

Duration of action:
- 50 mg: 24 hours
- 100 mg: 48 hours
- 150 mg: 72 hours

Absorption: Oral: Almost completely

Serum half-life: 4 hours; 6-β-naltrexol: 13 hours

Time to peak serum concentration: Within 60 minutes

**Pregnancy Risk Factor** C

**Generic Available** No

## Nandrolone (NAN droe lone)

**U.S. Brand Names** Anabolin® Injection; Androlone®-D Injection; Androlone® Injection; Deca-Durabolin® Injection; Hybolin™ Decanoate Injection; Hybolin™ Improved Injection; Neo-Durabolic Injection

**Therapeutic Category** Androgen

**Use** Control of metastatic breast cancer; management of anemia of renal insufficiency

**Usual Dosage** Deep I.M. (into gluteal muscle):

Children 2-13 years: (decanoate): 25-50 mg every 3-4 weeks
Adults:
Male:
Breast cancer (phenpropionate): 50-100 mg/week
Anemia of renal insufficiency (decanoate): 100-200 mg/week
Female: 50-100 mg/week
Breast cancer (phenproprionate): 50-100 mg/week
Anemia of renal insufficiency (decanoate): 50-100 mg/week

**Mechanism of Action** Promotes tissue-building processes, increases production of erythropoietin, causes protein anabolism; increases hemoglobin and red blood cell volume

**Local Anesthetic/Vasoconstrictor Precautions** No information available to require special precautions

**Effects on Dental Treatment** No effects or complications reported

**Other Adverse Effects**

**Male:**
Postpubertal:
>10%:
Dermatologic: Acne
Endocrine & metabolic: Gynecomastia
Genitourinary: Bladder irritability, priapism
1% to 10%:
Central nervous system: Insomnia, chills
Endocrine & metabolic: Decreased libido
Gastrointestinal: Nausea, diarrhea
Genitourinary: Prostatic hypertrophy (elderly)
Hematologic: Iron deficiency anemia, suppression of clotting factors
Hepatic: Hepatic dysfunction
<1%:
Hepatic: Hepatic necrosis, hepatocellular carcinoma
Prepubertal:
>10%:
Dermatologic: Acne
Endocrine & metabolic: Virilism
1% to 10%:
Central nervous system: Chills, insomnia
Dermatologic: Hyperpigmentation
Gastrointestinal: Diarrhea, nausea
Hematologic: Iron deficiency anemia, suppression of clotting
<1%: Hepatic: necrosis, hepatocellular carcinoma

**Female:**
>10%: Endocrine & metabolic: Virilism
1% to 10%:
Central nervous system: Chills, insomnia
Endocrine & metabolic: Hypercalcemia
Gastrointestinal: Nausea, diarrhea
Hematologic: Iron deficiency anemia, suppression of clotting factors
Hepatic: Hepatic dysfunction
<1%: Hepatic: Hepatic necrosis, hepatocellular carcinoma

**Drug Interactions** Increased toxicity: Oral anticoagulants, insulin, oral hypoglycemic agents, adrenal steroids, ACTH

**Pregnancy Risk Factor** X

**Generic Available** Yes

## Naphazoline (naf AZ oh leen)

**U.S. Brand Names** AK-Con® Ophthalmic; Albalon® Liquifilm® Ophthalmic; Allerest® Eye Drops [OTC]; Clear Eyes® [OTC]; Comfort® Ophthalmic [OTC]; Degest® 2 Ophthalmic [OTC]; Estivin® II Ophthalmic [OTC]; I-Naphline® Ophthalmic; Nafazair® Ophthalmic; Naphcon Forte® Ophthalmic; Naphcon® Ophthalmic [OTC]; Opcon® Ophthalmic; Privine® Nasal [OTC]; VasoClear® Ophthalmic [OTC]; Vasocon Regular® Ophthalmic

**Therapeutic Category** Adrenergic Agonist Agent, Ophthalmic; Decongestant, Nasal; Nasal Agent, Vasoconstrictor; Ophthalmic Agent, Vasoconstrictor

(Continued)

## Naphazoline *(Continued)*

**Use** Topical ocular vasoconstrictor; will temporarily relieve congestion, itching, and minor irritation, and to control hyperemia in patients with superficial corneal vascularity

**Usual Dosage**

Nasal:

Children:

<6 years: Intranasal: Not recommended (especially infants) due to CNS depression

6-12 years: 1 spray of 0.05% into each nostril every 6 hours if necessary; therapy should not exceed 3-5 days

Children >12 years and Adults: 0.05%, instill 1-2 drops or sprays every 6 hours if needed; therapy should not exceed 3-5 days

Ophthalmic:

Children <6 years: Not recommended for use due to CNS depression (especially in infants)

Children >6 years and Adults: Instill 1-2 drops into conjunctival sac of affected eye(s) every 3-4 hours; therapy generally should not exceed 3-4 days

**Mechanism of Action** Stimulates alpha-adrenergic receptors in the arterioles of the conjunctiva and the nasal mucosa to produce vasoconstriction

**Local Anesthetic/Vasoconstrictor Precautions** No information available to require special precautions

**Effects on Dental Treatment** No effects or complications reported

**Other Adverse Effects** 1% to 10%:

Cardiovascular: Systemic cardiovascular stimulation

Central nervous system: Dizziness, headache, nervousness

Gastrointestinal: Nausea

Local: Transient stinging, nasal mucosa irritation, dryness

Ocular: Mydriasis, increased intraocular pressure, blurring of vision

Respiratory: Sneezing, rebound congestion

**Drug Interactions** Increased toxicity: Anesthetics (discontinue mydriatic prior to use of anesthetics that sensitize the myocardium to sympathomimetics, ie, cyclopropane, halothane), MAO inhibitors, tricyclic antidepressants causes hypertensive reactions

**Drug Uptake**

Onset of decongestant action: Topical: Within 10 minutes

Duration: 2-6 hours

**Pregnancy Risk Factor** C

**Generic Available** Yes

## Naphazoline and Antazoline (naf AZ oh leen & an TAZ oh leen)

**U.S. Brand Names** Albalon-A® Ophthalmic; Antazoline-V® Ophthalmic; Vasocon-A® [OTC] Ophthalmic

**Therapeutic Category** Ophthalmic Agent, Vasoconstrictor

**Use** Topical ocular congestion, irritation and itching

**Usual Dosage** 1-2 drops every 3-4 hours

**Local Anesthetic/Vasoconstrictor Precautions** No information available to require special precautions

**Effects on Dental Treatment** No effects or complications reported

**Other Adverse Effects** 1% to 10%:

Cardiovascular: Systemic cardiovascular stimulation, hypertension

Central nervous system: Nervousness, dizziness, headache

Gastrointestinal: Nausea

Local: Transient stinging

Neuromuscular & skeletal: Weakness

Ocular: Mydriasis, increased intraocular pressure, blurring of vision

Respiratory: Nasal mucosa irritation, dryness, rebound congestion

Miscellaneous: Sweating

**Pregnancy Risk Factor** C

**Generic Available** No

**Comments** Discontinue drug and consult physician if ocular pain or visual changes occur, ocular redness or irritation, or condition worsens or persists for more than 72 hours

## Naphazoline and Pheniramine (naf AZ oh leen & fen NIR a meen)

**U.S. Brand Names** Naphcon-A® Ophthalmic [OTC]

**Therapeutic Category** Ophthalmic Agent, Vasoconstrictor

**Synonyms** Pheniramine and Naphazoline

**Use** Topical ocular vasoconstrictor

**Usual Dosage** 1-2 drops every 3-4 hours

**Local Anesthetic/Vasoconstrictor Precautions** No information available to require special precautions

**Effects on Dental Treatment** No effects or complications reported

**Other Adverse Effects** 1% to 10%:

Cardiovascular: Systemic effects due to absorption (hypertension, cardiac irregularities, hyperglycemia)

Ocular: Pupillary dilation, increase in intraocular pressure

**Pregnancy Risk Factor** C

**Generic Available** No

- **Naphcon-A® Ophthalmic [OTC]** *see* Naphazoline and Pheniramine *on previous page*
- **Naphcon Forte® Ophthalmic** *see* Naphazoline *on page 703*
- **Naphcon® Ophthalmic [OTC]** *see* Naphazoline *on page 703*
- **Naprosyn® (Naproxen Base)** *see* Naproxen *on this page*

## Naproxen (na PROKS en)

**Related Information**

Dental Drug Interactions: Update on Drug Combinations Requiring Special Considerations *on page 1225*

Oral Pain *on page 1122*

Rheumatoid Arthritis and Osteoarthritis *on page 1092*

Temporomandibular Dysfunction (TMD) *on page 1149*

**U.S. Brand Names** Aleve® (Naproxen Sodium) (OTC); Anaprox® (Naproxen Sodium); Naprosyn® (Naproxen Base)

**Canadian Brand Names** Apo®-Naproxen; Naxen®; Novo-Naprox; Nu-Naprox

**Therapeutic Category** Analgesic, Non-narcotic; Anti-inflammatory Agent; Nonsteroidal Anti-inflammatory Drug (NSAID), Oral

**Use**

Dental: Management of pain and swelling

Medical: Management of inflammatory disease and rheumatoid disorders (including juvenile rheumatoid arthritis); acute gout; mild to moderate pain; dysmenorrhea; fever, migraine headache

**Usual Dosage** Adults: Oral:

Naproxen base: Initial: 500 mg, then 250 mg every 6-8 hours

Naproxen sodium: Initial: 550 mg, then 275 mg every 6-8 hours

Maximum daily dose: 1250 mg/day naproxen base and 1375 mg naproxen sodium

**Mechanism of Action** Inhibits prostaglandin synthesis by decreasing the activity of the enzyme, cyclo-oxygenase, which results in decreased formation of prostaglandin precursors

**Local Anesthetic/Vasoconstrictor Precautions** No information available to require special precautions

**Effects on Dental Treatment** NSAID formulations are known to reversibly decrease platelet aggregation via mechanisms different than observed with aspirin. The dentist should be aware of the potential of abnormal coagulation. Caution should also be exercised in the use of NSAIDs in patients already on anticoagulant therapy with drugs such as warfarin (Coumadin®).

**Other Adverse Effects** >10%: Gastrointestinal: Nausea, heartburn, ulcers, indigestion

**Contraindications** Hypersensitivity to naproxen, aspirin, or other nonsteroidal anti-inflammatory drugs (NSAIDs)

**Warnings/Precautions** Use with caution in patients with GI disease (bleeding or ulcers), cardiovascular disease (CHF, hypertension), renal or hepatic impairment, and patients receiving anticoagulants; perform ophthalmologic evaluation for those who develop eye complaints during therapy (blurred vision, diminished vision, changes in color vision, retinal changes); NSAIDs may mask signs/symptoms of infections; photosensitivity reported; elderly are at especially high-risk for adverse effects

**Drug Interactions** Decreased effect of furosemide; naproxen could displace other highly protein bound drugs, such as oral anticoagulants, hydantoins, salicylates, sulfonamides, and sulfonylureas; naproxen and warfarin may result in slight increase in free warfarin; naproxen and probenecid may result in increased plasma half-life of naproxen; naproxen and methotrexate may result in significantly increased and prolonged blood methotrexate concentration, which may be severe or fatal. Manufacturer's information for raloxifen (Evista®) states that caution should be used when raloxifen is coadministered with other highly protein-bound drugs such as naproxen. Raloxifen could displace the naproxen and vice versa leading to increased free active form of the target drug. In healthy volunteers receiving naproxen, concomitant administration of clopidogrel was associated with increased occult gastrointestinal blood loss.

(Continued)

## Naproxen *(Continued)*

**Drug Uptake**
Onset of effect: 1 hour
Duration of effect: Up to 7 hours
Serum half-life: 12-15 hours
Time to peak serum concentration: Within 1-2 hours and persisting for up to 12 hours

**Pregnancy Risk Factor** B (D if used in the 3rd trimester or near delivery)

**Breast-feeding Considerations** May be taken while breast-feeding

**Dosage Forms**
Suspension, oral: 125 mg/5 mL (15 mL, 30 mL, 480 mL)
Tablet, as sodium:
220 mg (200 mg base)
Anaprox®: 220 mg (200 mg base); 275 mg (250 mg base); 550 mg (500 mg base)
Tablet:
Aleve®: 200 mg
Naprosyn®: 250 mg, 375 mg, 500 mg
Tablet, controlled release (Naprelan®): 375 mg, 500 mg

**Dietary Considerations** May be taken with food, milk, or antacids to decrease GI adverse effects

**Generic Available** Yes

**Comments** The sodium salt of naproxen provides better effects because of better oral absorption; the sodium salt also provides a faster onset and a longer duration of action

**Selected Readings**

Brooks PM and Day RO, "Nonsteroidal Anti-inflammatory Drugs - Differences and Similarities," *N Engl J Med*, 1991, 324(24):1716-25.
Forbes JA, Keller CK, Smith JW, et al, "Analgesic Effect of Naproxen Sodium, Codeine, a Naproxen-Codeine Combination and Aspirin on the Postoperative Pain of Oral Surgery," *Pharmacotherapy*, 1986, 6(5):211-8.

- **Naqua®** *see* Trichlormethiazide *on page 1014*

## Naratriptan (NAR a trip tan)

**U.S. Brand Names** Amerge®

**Therapeutic Category** Antimigraine Agent; Serotonin Agonist

**Synonyms** Naratriptan Hydrochloride

**Use** Acute treatment of migraine with or without aura

**Usual Dosage** Oral: Adults: 1 mg or 2.5 mg (maximum dose: 5 mg); if no response, dose may be repeated in 4 hours

**Mechanism of Action** Potent $5HT_{1B}$ and $5HT_{1D}$ agonist

**Local Anesthetic/Vasoconstrictor Precautions** No information available to require special precautions

**Effects on Dental Treatment** No effects or complications reported

**Drug Uptake** Half-life: 5-6 hours

**Dosage Forms** Tablet: 1 mg, 2.5 mg

- **Naratriptan Hydrochloride** *see* Naratriptan *on this page*
- **Narcan®** *see* Naloxone *on page 701*
- **Narcotic Agonists** *see page 1223*
- **Nardil®** *see* Phenelzine *on page 789*
- **Naropin™** *see* Ropivacaine *on page 896*
- **Nasabid™** *see* Guaifenesin and Pseudoephedrine *on page 481*
- **Nasacort®** *see* Triamcinolone *on page 1010*
- **Nasacort® AQ** *see* Triamcinolone *on page 1010*
- **Nasahist B®** *see* Brompheniramine *on page 151*
- **NāSal™ [OTC]** *see* Sodium Chloride *on page 920*
- **Nasalcrom®** *see* Cromolyn Sodium *on page 281*
- **Nasalide® Nasal Aerosol** *see* Flunisolide *on page 439*
- **Nasal Moist® [OTC]** *see* Sodium Chloride *on page 920*
- **Nasarel® Nasal Spray** *see* Flunisolide *on page 439*
- **Nasonex®** *see* Mometasone Furoate *on page 686*
- **Natabec® [OTC]** *see* Vitamins, Multiple *on page 1051*
- **Natabec® FA [OTC]** *see* Vitamins, Multiple *on page 1051*
- **Natabec® Rx** *see* Vitamins, Multiple *on page 1051*
- **Natacyn®** *see* Natamycin *on next page*
- **Natalins® [OTC]** *see* Vitamins, Multiple *on page 1051*
- **Natalins® Rx** *see* Vitamins, Multiple *on page 1051*

## Natamycin (na ta MYE sin)

**U.S. Brand Names** Natacyn®

**Therapeutic Category** Antifungal Agent, Ophthalmic

**Use** Treatment of blepharitis, conjunctivitis, and keratitis caused by susceptible fungi (*Aspergillus, Candida*), *Cephalosporium, Curvularia, Fusarium, Penicillium, Microsporum, Epidermophyton, Blastomyces dermatitidis, Coccidioides immitis, Cryptococcus neoformans, Histoplasma capsulatum, Sporothrix schenckii, Trichomonas vaginalis*

**Usual Dosage** Adults: Ophthalmic: Instill 1 drop in conjunctival sac every 1-2 hours, after 3-4 days reduce to 1 drop 6-8 times/day; usual course of therapy is 2-3 weeks

**Mechanism of Action** Increases cell membrane permeability in susceptible fungi

**Local Anesthetic/Vasoconstrictor Precautions** No information available to require special precautions

**Effects on Dental Treatment** No effects or complications reported

**Other Adverse Effects** <1%: Ocular: Blurred vision, photophobia, eye pain, eye irritation not present before therapy

**Drug Interactions** Increased toxicity: Topical corticosteroids (concomitant use contraindicated)

**Drug Uptake** Absorption: Ophthalmic: <2% systemically absorbed

**Pregnancy Risk Factor** C

**Dosage Forms** Suspension, ophthalmic: 5% (15 mL)

**Generic Available** No

- **Natural Products, Herbals, and Dietary Supplements** *see page 1167*
- **Nature's Tears® Solution [OTC]** *see* Artificial Tears *on page 97*
- **Naturetin®** *see* Bendroflumethiazide *on page 127*
- **Naus-A-Way® [OTC]** *see* Phosphorated Carbohydrate Solution *on page 800*
- **Nausetrol® [OTC]** *see* Phosphorated Carbohydrate Solution *on page 800*
- **Navane®** *see* Thiothixene *on page 980*
- **Navelbine®** *see* Vinorelbine *on page 1047*
- **ND-Stat®** *see* Brompheniramine *on page 151*
- **Nebcin® Injection** *see* Tobramycin *on page 990*
- **NebuPent™ Inhalation** *see* Pentamidine *on page 778*

## Nedocromil Sodium (ne doe KROE mil SOW dee um)

**Related Information**

Respiratory Diseases *on page 1079*

**U.S. Brand Names** Tilade® Inhalation Aerosol

**Canadian Brand Names** Mireze®

**Therapeutic Category** Antiasthmatic; Antihistamine, Inhalation

**Use** Maintenance therapy in patients with mild to moderate bronchial asthma

**Usual Dosage** Children >12 years and Adults: Inhalation: 2 inhalations 4 times/day; may reduce dosage to 2-3 times/day once desired clinical response to initial dose is observed

**Local Anesthetic/Vasoconstrictor Precautions** No information available to require special precautions

**Effects on Dental Treatment** No effects or complications reported

**Other Adverse Effects** 1% to 10%:

Cardiovascular: Chest pain
Central nervous system: Dizziness, headache, fatigue
Gastrointestinal: Nausea, vomiting, dry mouth, diarrhea, unpleasant taste
Respiratory: Coughing, pharyngitis, rhinitis, bronchitis, dyspnea, bronchospasm

**Drug Uptake**

Duration of therapeutic effect: 2 hours
Serum half-life: 1.5-2 hours

**Pregnancy Risk Factor** B

**Generic Available** No

**Comments Not** a bronchodilator and, therefore, should not be used for reversal of acute bronchospasm; has no known therapeutic systemic activity when delivered by inhalation

- **N.E.E.® 1/35** *see* Ethinyl Estradiol and Norethindrone *on page 404*

## Nefazodone (nef AY zoe done)

**U.S. Brand Names** Serzone®

**Therapeutic Category** Antidepressant, Miscellaneous

**Use** Treatment of depression

**Usual Dosage** Oral: Adults: 200 mg/day, administered in two divided doses initially, with a range of 300-600 mg/day in two divided doses thereafter

(Continued)

## Nefazodone *(Continued)*

**Mechanism of Action** Inhibits reuptake of serotonin and norepinephrine by the presynaptic neuronal membrane and desensitization of adenyl cyclase, down regulation of beta-adrenergic receptors, and down regulation of serotonin receptors

**Local Anesthetic/Vasoconstrictor Precautions** No information available to require special precautions

**Effects on Dental Treatment** >10% of patients experience significant dry mouth which will disappear with cessation of drug therapy

**Other Adverse Effects**

>10%:

Central nervous system: Headache, drowsiness, insomnia, agitation, dizziness, confusion

Gastrointestinal: Nausea

Neuromuscular & skeletal: Tremor

1% to 10%:

Cardiovascular: Postural hypotension

Gastrointestinal: Constipation, vomiting

Neuromuscular & skeletal: Weakness

Ocular: Blurred vision, amblyopia

<1%:

Gastrointestinal: Diarrhea

Genitourinary: Prolonged priapism

**Drug Interactions**

Alprazolam and triazolam: Coadministration with nefazodone has resulted in significant increased blood levels of these two benzodiazepines. A 50% reduction in alprazolam dosage is recommended; a 75% reduction in triazolam dosage is recommended

Digoxin: Coadministration with nefazodone has resulted in increased blood levels of digoxin; because of the narrow margin of safety of digoxin, caution is advised in administration with nefazodone

Monoamine oxidase inhibitors: In patients taking antidepressants similar to nefazodone, concomitant administration of monoamine oxidase inhibitors has resulted in serious, sometimes fatal, reactions. It is recommended that nefazodone not be given in combination with monoamine oxidase inhibitors.

**Drug Uptake**

Onset of action: Therapeutic effects take at least 2 weeks to appear

Serum half-life: 2-4 hours (parent compound), active metabolites persist longer

Time to peak serum concentration: 30 minutes, prolonged in presence of food

**Pregnancy Risk Factor** C

**Generic Available** No

♦ **NegGram®** *see* Nalidixic Acid *on page 700*

## Nelfinavir (nel FIN a veer)

**Related Information**

HIV Infection and AIDS *on page 1085*

**U.S. Brand Names** Viracept®

**Therapeutic Category** Protease Inhibitor

**Use** As monotherapy or preferably in combination with nucleoside analogs in the treatment of HIV infection when antiretroviral therapy is warranted

**Usual Dosage** Oral:

Children 2-13 years: 20-30 mg/kg 3 times/day with a meal or light snack; if tablets are unable to be taken, use oral powder in small amount of water, milk, formula, or dietary supplements; do not use acidic food/juice or store for >6 hours

Adults: 750 mg 3 times/day with meals

**Mechanism of Action** Inhibits the HIV-1 protease; inhibition of the viral protease prevents cleavage of the gag-pol polyprotein resulting in the production of immature, noninfectious virus; cross-resistance with other protease inhibitors is possible although, as yet, unknown

**Local Anesthetic/Vasoconstrictor Precautions** No information available to require special precautions

**Effects on Dental Treatment** <1% of patients experience mouth ulcers

**Other Adverse Effects**

>10%: Gastrointestinal: Diarrhea

1% to 10%:

Central nervous system: Decreased concentration

Dermatologic: Rash

Gastrointestinal: Nausea, flatulence, abdominal pain

Neuromuscular & skeletal: Weakness

<1%:

Central nervous system: Anxiety, depression, dizziness, emotional lability, hyperkinesia, insomnia, migraine, seizures, sleep disorder, somnolence, suicide ideation, fever, headache, malaise

Dermatologic: Dermatitis, pruritus, urticaria

Endocrine & metabolic: Increased LFTs, hyperlipemia, hyperuricemia, hypoglycemia

Gastrointestinal: Anorexia, dyspepsia, epigastric pain, mouth ulceration, GI bleeding, pancreatitis, vomiting

Genitourinary: Kidney calculus, sexual dysfunction

Hematologic: Anemia, leukopenia, thrombocytopenia

Hepatic: Hepatitis

Neuromuscular & skeletal: Arthralgia, arthritis, cramps, myalgia, myasthenia, myopathy, paresthesia, back pain

Respiratory: Dyspnea, pharyngitis, rhinitis, sinusitis

Miscellaneous: Diaphoresis, allergy

**Warnings/Precautions** Avoid use of powder in phenylketonurics since contains phenylalanine; use extreme caution when administered to patients with hepatic insufficiency since nelfinavir is metabolized in the liver and excreted predominantly in the feces; avoid use, if possible, with terfenadine, astemizole, cisapride, triazolam, or midazolam. Concurrent use with some anticonvulsants may significantly limit nelfinavir's effectiveness.

**Drug Interactions** Unlike other protease inhibitors, nelfinavir may be administered with dapsone, trimethoprim/sulfamethoxazole, clarithromycin, azithromycin, erythromycin, itraconazole, and fluconazole

Increased effect: Nelfinavir inhibits the metabolism of cisapride and astemizole and should, therefore, not be administered concurrently due to risk of cardiac arrhythmias. A 20% increase in rifabutin plasma AUC has been observed when coadministered with nelfinavir (decrease rifabutin's dose by 50%). An increase in midazolam and triazolam serum levels may occur resulting in significant oversedation when administered with nelfinavir. These drugs should not be administered together. Indinavir and ritonavir may increase nelfinavir plasma concentrations resulting in potential increases in side effects (the safety of these combinations have not been established).

Decreased effect: Rifampin decreases nelfinavir's plasma AUC by ~82%; the two drugs should not be administered together. Serum levels of the hormones in oral contraceptives may decrease significantly with administration of nelfinavir. Patients should use alternative methods of contraceptives during nelfinavir therapy. Phenobarbital, phenytoin, and carbamazepine may decrease serum levels and consequently effectiveness of nelfinavir.

**Drug Uptake**

Serum half-life: 3.5-5 hours

Time to peak serum concentration: 2-4 hours

**Pregnancy Risk Factor** B

- **Nelova™ 0.5/35E** *see* Ethinyl Estradiol and Norethindrone *on page 404*
- **Nelova™ 1/50M** *see* Mestranol and Norethindrone *on page 639*
- **Nelova™ 10/11** *see* Ethinyl Estradiol and Norethindrone *on page 404*
- **Nembutal®** *see* Pentobarbital *on page 780*
- **Neo-Calglucon® [OTC]** *see* Calcium Glubionate *on page 174*
- **Neo-Cortef®** *see* Neomycin and Hydrocortisone *on page 711*
- **NeoDecadron® Ophthalmic** *see* Neomycin and Dexamethasone *on next page*
- **NeoDecadron® Topical** *see* Neomycin and Dexamethasone *on next page*
- **Neo-Dexameth® Ophthalmic** *see* Neomycin and Dexamethasone *on next page*
- **Neo-Durabolic Injection** *see* Nandrolone *on page 703*
- **Neo-fradin®** *see* Neomycin *on this page*
- **Neoloid® [OTC]** *see* Castor Oil *on page 196*
- **Neomixin® Topical [OTC]** *see* Bacitracin, Neomycin, and Polymyxin B *on page 118*

## Neomycin (nee oh MYE sin)

**Related Information**

Neomycin and Polymyxin B *on page 711*

Neomycin, Polymyxin B, and Dexamethasone *on page 711*

Neomycin, Polymyxin B, and Prednisolone *on page 713*

**U.S. Brand Names** Mycifradin® Sulfate; Neo-fradin®; Neo-Tabs®

**Therapeutic Category** Ammonium Detoxicant; Antibiotic, Aminoglycoside; Antibiotic, Topical

(Continued)

## Neomycin *(Continued)*

**Use** Prepares GI tract for surgery; treat minor skin infections; treat diarrhea caused by *E. coli*; adjunct in the treatment of hepatic encephalopathy, as irrigant during surgery

**Usual Dosage**

Children: Oral:

Preoperative intestinal antisepsis: 90 mg/kg/day divided every 4 hours for 2 days; or 25 mg/kg at 1 PM, 2 PM, and 11 PM on the day preceding surgery as an adjunct to mechanical cleansing of the intestine and in combination with erythromycin base

Hepatic coma: 50-100 mg/kg/day in divided doses every 6-8 hours or 2.5-7 g/$m^2$/day divided every 4-6 hours for 5-6 days not to exceed 12 g/day

Children and Adults: Topical: Apply ointment 1-4 times/day; topical solutions containing 0.1% to 1% neomycin have been used for irrigation

Adults: Oral:

Preoperative intestinal antisepsis: 1 g each hour for 4 doses then 1 g every 4 hours for 5 doses; or 1 g at 1 PM, 2 PM, and 11 PM on day preceding surgery as an adjunct to mechanical cleansing of the bowel and oral erythromycin; or 6 g/day divided every 4 hours for 2-3 days

Hepatic coma: 500-2000 mg every 6-8 hours or 4-12 g/day divided every 4-6 hours for 5-6 days

Chronic hepatic insufficiency: 4 g/day for an indefinite period

**Mechanism of Action** Interferes with bacterial protein synthesis by binding to 30S ribosomal subunits

**Local Anesthetic/Vasoconstrictor Precautions** No information available to require special precautions

**Effects on Dental Treatment** No effects or complications reported

**Other Adverse Effects**

1% to 10%:

Dermatologic: Dermatitis, rash, urticaria, erythema

Local: Burning

Ocular: Contact conjunctivitis

<1%:

Gastrointestinal: Nausea, vomiting, diarrhea

Neuromuscular & skeletal: Neuromuscular blockade

Otic: Ototoxicity

Renal: Nephrotoxicity

**Drug Interactions**

Decreased effect: May decrease GI absorption of digoxin and methotrexate

Increased effect: Synergistic effects with penicillins

Increased toxicity:

Oral neomycin may potentiate the effects of oral anticoagulants

Increased adverse effects with other neurotoxic, ototoxic, or nephrotoxic drugs

**Drug Uptake**

Absorption: Oral, percutaneous: Poor (3%)

Serum half-life: 3 hours (age and renal function dependent)

Time to peak serum concentration:

Oral: 1-4 hours

I.M.: Within 2 hours

**Pregnancy Risk Factor** C

**Generic Available** Yes

## Neomycin and Dexamethasone

(nee oh MYE sin & deks a METH a sone)

**U.S. Brand Names** AK-Neo-Dex® Ophthalmic; NeoDecadron® Ophthalmic; NeoDecadron® Topical; Neo-Dexameth® Ophthalmic

**Therapeutic Category** Antibiotic, Ophthalmic; Corticosteroid, Ophthalmic

**Synonyms** Dexamethasone and Neomycin

**Use** Treatment of steroid responsive inflammatory conditions of the palpebral and bulbar conjunctiva, lid, cornea, and anterior segment of the globe

**Usual Dosage**

Ophthalmic: Instill 1-2 drops in eye(s) every 3-4 hours

Topical: Apply thin coat 3-4 times/day until favorable response is observed, then reduce dose to one application/day

**Local Anesthetic/Vasoconstrictor Precautions** No information available to require special precautions

**Effects on Dental Treatment** No effects or complications reported

**Other Adverse Effects** <1%:

Local: Transient stinging, burning, or local irritation

Ocular: Increased intraocular pressure, mydriasis, ptosis, epithelial punctate keratitis, and possible corneal or scleral malacia can occur

**Pregnancy Risk Factor** C

**Generic Available** No

## Neomycin and Hydrocortisone

(nee oh MYE sin & hye droe KOR ti sone)

**U.S. Brand Names** Neo-Cortef®

**Therapeutic Category** Antibiotic, Topical; Corticosteroid, Topical (Low Potency)

**Use** Treatment of susceptible topical bacterial infections with associated swelling

**Usual Dosage** Topical: Apply to area in a thin film 2-4 times/day

**Local Anesthetic/Vasoconstrictor Precautions** No information available to require special precautions

**Effects on Dental Treatment** No effects or complications reported

**Generic Available** No

## Neomycin and Polymyxin B (nee oh MYE sin & pol i MIKS in bee)

**U.S. Brand Names** Neosporin® Cream [OTC]; Neosporin® G.U. Irrigant

**Therapeutic Category** Antibiotic, Topical; Antibiotic, Urinary Irrigation

**Use** Short-term as a continuous irrigant or rinse in the urinary bladder to prevent bacteriuria and gram-negative rod septicemia associated with the use of indwelling catheters; to help prevent infection in minor cuts, scrapes, and burns; treatment of superficial ocular infections involving the conjunctiva or cornea

**Usual Dosage** Children and Adults:

Bladder irrigation: **Not for injection**; add 1 mL irrigant to 1 liter isotonic saline solution and connect container to the inflow of lumen of 3-way catheter. Continuous irrigant or rinse in the urinary bladder for up to a maximum of 10 days with administration rate adjusted to patient's urine output; usually no more than 1 L of irrigant is used per day.

Ophthalmic:

Ointment: Instill ½" ribbon into the conjunctival sac every 3-4 hours for acute infections or 2-3 times/day for mild to moderate infections for 7-10 days

Solution: Instill 1-2 drops every 15-30 minutes for acute infections; 1-2 drops every 3-6 hours for mild-moderate infections.

Topical: Apply cream 1-4 times/day to affected area

**Mechanism of Action** Refer to individual monographs

**Local Anesthetic/Vasoconstrictor Precautions** No information available to require special precautions

**Effects on Dental Treatment** No effects or complications reported

**Other Adverse Effects** 1% to 10%:

Dermatologic: Contact dermatitis, erythema, rash, urticaria

Genitourinary: Bladder irritation

Local: Burning

Neuromuscular & skeletal: Neuromuscular blockade

Otic: Ototoxicity

Renal: Nephrotoxicity

**Drug Interactions** No data reported

**Drug Uptake** Absorption: Topical: Not absorbed following application to intact skin; absorbed through denuded or abraded skin, peritoneum, wounds, or ulcers

**Pregnancy Risk Factor** C (D - G.U. irrigant)

**Dosage Forms**

Cream: Neomycin sulfate 3.5 mg and polymyxin B sulfate 10,000 units per g (0.94 g, 15 g)

Solution, irrigant: Neomycin sulfate 40 mg and polymyxin B sulfate 200,000 units per mL (1 mL, 20 mL)

**Generic Available** Yes

## Neomycin, Polymyxin B, and Dexamethasone

(nee oh MYE sin, pol i MIKS in bee, & deks a METH a sone)

**U.S. Brand Names** AK-Trol®; Dexacidin®; Dexasporin®; Maxitrol®

**Therapeutic Category** Antibiotic, Ophthalmic

**Use** Steroid-responsive inflammatory ocular conditions in which a corticosteroid is indicated and where bacterial infection or a risk of bacterial infection exists

**Usual Dosage** Children and Adults: Ophthalmic:

Ointment: Place a small amount (~½") in the affected eye 3-4 times/day or apply at bedtime as an adjunct with drops

Solution: Instill 1-2 drops into affected eye(s) every 3-4 hours; in severe disease, drops may be used hourly and tapered to discontinuation

**Mechanism of Action** Refer to individual monographs

(Continued)

## Neomycin, Polymyxin B, and Dexamethasone *(Continued)*

**Local Anesthetic/Vasoconstrictor Precautions** No information available to require special precautions

**Effects on Dental Treatment** No effects or complications reported

**Other Adverse Effects** 1% to 10%:

Dermatologic: Contact dermatitis, delayed wound healing

Ocular: Cutaneous sensitization, eye pain, development of glaucoma, cataract, increased intraocular pressure, optic nerve damage

**Drug Interactions** No data reported

**Drug Uptake** Refer to individual monographs

**Pregnancy Risk Factor** C

**Generic Available** Yes

## Neomycin, Polymyxin B, and Gramicidin

(nee oh MYE sin, pol i MIKS in bee, & gram i SYE din)

**U.S. Brand Names** AK-Spore® Ophthalmic Solution; Neosporin® Ophthalmic Solution

**Therapeutic Category** Antibiotic, Ophthalmic

**Use** Treatment of superficial ocular infection, infection prophylaxis in minor skin abrasions

**Usual Dosage** Children and Adults: Ophthalmic: Instill 1-2 drops 4-6 times/day or more frequently as required for severe infections

**Mechanism of Action** Interferes with bacterial protein synthesis by binding to 30S ribosomal subunits; binds to phospholipids, alters permeability, and damages the bacterial cytoplasmic membrane permitting leakage of intracellular constituents

**Local Anesthetic/Vasoconstrictor Precautions** No information available to require special precautions

**Effects on Dental Treatment** No effects or complications reported

**Other Adverse Effects** 1% to 10%:

Cardiovascular: Edema

Dermatologic: Itching

Local: Reddening, failure to heal

Ocular: Low grade conjunctivitis

**Drug Interactions** No data reported

**Pregnancy Risk Factor** C

**Generic Available** Yes

## Neomycin, Polymyxin B, and Hydrocortisone

(nee oh MYE sin, pol i MIKS in bee, & hye droe KOR ti sone)

**U.S. Brand Names** AK-Spore H.C.® Ophthalmic Suspension; AK-Spore H.C.® Otic; AntibiOtic® Otic; Cortatrigen® Otic; Cortisporin® Ophthalmic Suspension; Cortisporin® Otic; Cortisporin® Topical Cream; Octicair® Otic; Otic-Care® Otic; Otocort® Otic; Otosporin® Otic; Pediotic® Otic; UAD Otic®

**Therapeutic Category** Antibiotic, Ophthalmic; Antibiotic, Otic; Antibiotic, Topical; Corticosteroid, Ophthalmic; Corticosteroid, Otic; Corticosteroid, Topical (Low Potency)

**Use** Steroid-responsive inflammatory condition for which a corticosteroid is indicated and where bacterial infection or a risk of bacterial infection exists

**Usual Dosage** Duration of use should be limited to 10 days unless otherwise directed by the physician

Otic solution is used **only** for swimmer's ear (infections of external auditory canal)

Otic:

- Children: Instill 3 drops into affected ear 3-4 times/day
- Adults: Instill 4 drops 3-4 times/day; otic suspension is the preferred otic preparation

Children and Adults:

- Ophthalmic: Drops: Instill 1-2 drops 2-4 times/day, or more frequently as required for severe infections; in acute infections, instill 1-2 drops every 15-30 minutes gradually reducing the frequency of administration as the infection is controlled
- Topical: Apply a thin layer 1-4 times/day

**Mechanism of Action** Refer to individual monographs for neomycin, Polymyxin B, and Hydrocortisone

**Local Anesthetic/Vasoconstrictor Precautions** No information available to require special precautions

**Effects on Dental Treatment** No effects or complications reported

**Other Adverse Effects**
>10%: Miscellaneous: Hypersensitivity
1% to 10%:
Dermatologic: Contact dermatitis, erythema, rash, urticaria
Genitourinary: Bladder irritation
Local: Burning, itching, swelling, pain, stinging
Neuromuscular & skeletal: Neuromuscular blockade
Ocular: Increased intraocular pressure, glaucoma, cataracts, conjunctival erythema
Otic: Ototoxicity
Renal: Nephrotoxicity
Miscellaneous: Sensitization to neomycin, secondary infections

**Drug Interactions** No data reported
**Pregnancy Risk Factor** C
**Generic Available** Yes

## Neomycin, Polymyxin B, and Prednisolone

(nee oh MYE sin, pol i MIKS in bee, & pred NIS oh lone)

**U.S. Brand Names** Poly-Pred®
**Therapeutic Category** Antibiotic, Ophthalmic; Corticosteroid, Ophthalmic
**Use** Steroid-responsive inflammatory ocular condition in which bacterial infection or a risk of bacterial ocular infection exists
**Usual Dosage** Children and Adults: Ophthalmic: Instill 1-2 drops every 3-4 hours; acute infections may require every 30-minute instillation initially with frequency of administration reduced as the infection is brought under control. To treat the lids: Instill 1-2 drops every 3-4 hours, close the eye and rub the excess on the lids and lid margins.
**Mechanism of Action** Refer to individual monographs
**Local Anesthetic/Vasoconstrictor Precautions** No information available to require special precautions
**Effects on Dental Treatment** No effects or complications reported
**Other Adverse Effects** 1% to 10%:
Dermatologic: Cutaneous sensitization, skin rash, delayed wound healing
Ocular: Increased intraocular pressure, glaucoma, optic nerve damage, cataracts, conjunctival sensitization

**Drug Interactions** No data reported
**Drug Uptake** Refer to individual monographs
**Pregnancy Risk Factor** C
**Generic Available** Yes

- **Neonatal Trace Metals** *see* Trace Metals *on page 1001*
- **Neopap® [OTC]** *see* Acetaminophen *on page 27*
- **Neoral® Oral** *see* Cyclosporine *on page 288*
- **Neosar®** *see* Cyclophosphamide *on page 285*
- **Neosporin® Cream [OTC]** *see* Neomycin and Polymyxin B *on page 711*
- **Neosporin® G.U. Irrigant** *see* Neomycin and Polymyxin B *on page 711*
- **Neosporin® Ophthalmic Ointment** *see* Bacitracin, Neomycin, and Polymyxin B *on page 118*
- **Neosporin® Ophthalmic Solution** *see* Neomycin, Polymyxin B, and Gramicidin *on previous page*
- **Neosporin® Topical Ointment [OTC]** *see* Bacitracin, Neomycin, and Polymyxin B *on page 118*
- **Neo-Synephrine® 12 Hour Nasal Solution [OTC]** *see* Oxymetazoline *on page 755*
- **Neo-Synephrine® Nasal Solution [OTC]** *see* Phenylephrine *on page 795*
- **Neo-Synephrine® Ophthalmic Solution** *see* Phenylephrine *on page 795*
- **Neo-Tabs®** *see* Neomycin *on page 709*
- **Neotrace-4®** *see* Trace Metals *on page 1001*
- **Neotricin HC® Ophthalmic Ointment** *see* Bacitracin, Neomycin, Polymyxin B, and Hydrocortisone *on page 118*
- **NeoVadrin® [OTC]** *see* Vitamins, Multiple *on page 1051*
- **NeoVadrin® B Complex [OTC]** *see* Vitamin B Complex *on page 1050*
- **Nephro-Calci® [OTC]** *see* Calcium Carbonate *on page 172*
- **Nephrocaps® [OTC]** *see* Vitamin B Complex With Vitamin C and Folic Acid *on page 1050*
- **Nephro-Fer™ [OTC]** *see* Ferrous Fumarate *on page 426*
- **Nephron®** *see* Epinephrine, Racemic *on page 375*
- **Nephrox Suspension [OTC]** *see* Aluminum Hydroxide *on page 55*
- **Neptazane®** *see* Methazolamide *on page 646*
- **Nervocaine®** *see* Lidocaine *on page 586*

- ♦ **Nesacaine®** *see* Chloroprocaine *on page 226*
- ♦ **Nesacaine®-MPF** *see* Chloroprocaine *on page 226*
- ♦ **Nestrex®** *see* Pyridoxine *on page 867*



## Netilmicin (ne til MYE sin)

**U.S. Brand Names** Netromycin®

**Therapeutic Category** Antibiotic, Aminoglycoside

**Use** Short-term treatment of serious or life-threatening infections including septicemia, peritonitis, intra-abdominal abscess, lower respiratory tract infections, urinary tract infections; skin, bone, and joint infections caused by sensitive *Pseudomonas aeruginosa, Escherichia coli, Proteus, Klebsiella, Serratia, Enterobacter, Citrobacter,* and *Staphylococcus*

**Usual Dosage** Individualization is critical because of the low therapeutic index. Use of ideal body weight (IBW) for determining the mg/kg/dose appears to be more accurate than dosing on the basis of total body weight (TBW). In morbid obesity, dosage requirement may best be estimated using a dosing weight of IBW + 0.4 (TBW - IBW). Peak and trough plasma drug levels should be determined, particularly in critically ill patients with serious infections or in disease states known to significantly alter aminoglycoside pharmacokinetics (eg, cystic fibrosis, burns, or major surgery).

Once daily dosing: Higher peak serum drug concentration to MIC ratios, demonstrated aminoglycoside postantibiotic effect, decreased renal cortex drug uptake, and improved cost-time efficiency are supportive reasons for the use of once daily dosing regimens for aminoglycosides. Current research indicates these regimens to be as effective for nonlife-threatening infections, with no higher incidence of nephrotoxicity, than those requiring multiple daily doses. Doses are determined by calculating the entire day's dose via usual multiple dose calculation techniques and administering this quantity as a single dose. Doses are then adjusted to maintain mean serum concentrations above the MIC(s) of the causative organism(s). (Example: 4.5-6.5 mg/kg as a single dose; expected $Cp_{max}$: 10-20 mcg/mL, and $Cp_{min}$: <1 mcg/mL). Further research is needed for universal recommendation in all patient populations and gram-negative disease; exceptions may include those with known high clearance (eg, children, patients with cystic fibrosis, or burns who may require shorter dosage intervals) and patients with renal function impairment for whom longer than conventional dosage intervals are usually required.

I.M., I.V.:
- Children 6 weeks to 12 years: 1-2.5 mg/kg/dose every 8 hours
- Children >12 years and Adults: 1.5-2 mg/kg/dose every 8-12 hours
- Some clinicians suggest a daily dose of 4-7 mg/kg for all patients with normal renal function. This dose is at least as efficacious with similar, if not less, toxicity than conventional dosing.

**Mechanism of Action** Interferes with protein synthesis in bacterial cell by binding to ribosomal subunit

**Local Anesthetic/Vasoconstrictor Precautions** No information available to require special precautions

**Effects on Dental Treatment** No effects or complications reported

**Other Adverse Effects**

>10%:
- Central nervous system: Neurotoxicity
- Otic: Ototoxicity (auditory), ototoxicity (vestibular)
- Renal: Decreased creatinine clearance, nephrotoxicity

1% to 10%:
- Cardiovascular: Swelling
- Dermatologic: Skin itching, redness, rash

<1%:
- Central nervous system: Drowsiness, headache, pseudomotor cerebri
- Dermatologic: Photosensitivity, erythema
- Gastrointestinal: Anorexia, nausea, vomiting, weight loss, increased salivation, enterocolitis
- Hematologic: Granulocytopenia, agranulocytosis, thrombocytopenia
- Local: Burning, stinging
- Neuromuscular & skeletal: Tremors, muscle cramps, weakness
- Respiratory: Dyspnea

**Drug Interactions** Increased toxicity:

Penicillins, cephalosporins, amphotericin B, loop diuretics, vancomycin cause increased nephrotoxic potential

Neuromuscular blocking agents cause increased neuromuscular blockade

**Drug Uptake**

Absorption: I.M.: Well absorbed

Serum half-life: 2-3 hours (age and renal function dependent)

Time to peak serum concentration: I.M.: Within 0.5-1 hour

**Pregnancy Risk Factor** D

**Generic Available** No

- **Netromycin®** *see* Netilmicin *on previous page*
- **Neumega®** *see* Oprelvekin *on page 743*
- **Neupogen® Injection** *see* Filgrastim *on page 430*
- **Neuramate®** *see* Meprobamate *on page 635*
- **Neurontin®** *see* Gabapentin *on page 461*
- **Neut® Injection** *see* Sodium Bicarbonate *on page 918*
- **Neutra-Phos®** *see* Potassium Phosphate and Sodium Phosphate *on page 826*
- **Neutra-Phos®-K** *see* Potassium Phosphate *on page 825*
- **Neutrexin®** *see* Trimetrexate Glucuronate *on page 1023*
- **Neutrogena® Acne Mask [OTC]** *see* Benzoyl Peroxide *on page 130*
- **Neutrogena® T/Derm** *see* Coal Tar *on page 270*

## Nevirapine (ne VYE ra peen)

**U.S. Brand Names** Viramune®

**Therapeutic Category** Antiviral Agent, Parenteral

**Use** In combination therapy with nucleoside antiretroviral agents in HIV-1 infected adults previously treated for whom current therapy is deemed inadequate

**Usual Dosage** Adults: Oral: 200 mg once daily for 2 weeks followed by 200 mg twice daily

**Mechanism of Action** Nevirapine is a non-nucleoside reverse transcriptase inhibitor specific for HIV-1; nevirapine does not require intracellular phosphorylation for antiviral activity

**Local Anesthetic/Vasoconstrictor Precautions** No information available to require special precautions

**Effects on Dental Treatment** No effects or complications reported

**Other Adverse Effects** >10%:

Central nervous system: Headache, drowsiness, drug fever

Dermatologic: Rash

Gastrointestinal: Diarrhea, nausea

Hepatic: LFTs (elevated)

**Contraindications** Previous hypersensitivity to nevirapine

**Drug Interactions** Decreased effect: Rifampin and rifabutin may decrease nevirapine trough concentrations due to induction of CYP3A; since nevirapine may decrease concentrations of protease inhibitors, they should not be administered concomitantly; nevirapine may decrease the effectiveness of oral contraceptives - suggest alternate method of birth control

**Drug Uptake**

Absorption: Rapidly absorbed with peak levels occurring within 2 hours of administration

Serum half-life: 22-84 hours

**Pregnancy Risk Factor** C

**Generic Available** No

- **New Decongestant®** *see* Chlorpheniramine, Phenyltoloxamine, Phenylpropanolamine, and Phenylephrine *on page 237*
- **N.G.T.® Topical** *see* Nystatin and Triamcinolone *on page 735*

## Niacin (NYE a sin)

**Related Information**

Cardiovascular Diseases *on page 1066*

**U.S. Brand Names** Nicobid® [OTC]; Nicolar® [OTC]; Nicotinex [OTC]; Slo-Niacin® [OTC]

**Therapeutic Category** Lipid Lowering Drugs; Vitamin, Water Soluble

**Use** Adjunctive treatment of hyperlipidemias; peripheral vascular disease and circulatory disorders; treatment of pellagra; dietary supplement

**Usual Dosage** Give I.M., I.V., or S.C. only if oral route is unavailable and use only for vitamin deficiencies (not for hyperlipidemia)

Children: Pellagra: Oral: 50-100 mg/dose 3 times/day

Oral: Recommended daily allowances:

0-0.5 years: 5 mg/day

0.5-1 year: 6 mg/day

1-3 years: 9 mg/day

4-6 years: 12 mg/day

7-10 years: 13 mg/day

Males:

11-14 years: 17 mg/day

15-18 years: 20 mg/day

(Continued)

## Niacin *(Continued)*

19-24 years: 19 mg/day
Females: 11-24 years: 15 mg/day

Adults: Oral:
Recommended daily allowances:
Males: 25-50 years: 19 mg/day; >51 years: 15 mg/day
Females: 25-50 years: 15 mg/day; >51 years: 13 mg/day
Hyperlipidemia: 1.5-6 g/day in 3 divided doses with or after meals
Pellagra: 50-100 mg 3-4 times/day, maximum: 500 mg/day
Niacin deficiency: 10-20 mg/day, maximum: 100 mg/day

**Mechanism of Action** Component of two coenzymes which is necessary for tissue respiration, lipid metabolism, and glycogenolysis; inhibits the synthesis of very low density lipoproteins

**Local Anesthetic/Vasoconstrictor Precautions** No information available to require special precautions

**Effects on Dental Treatment** No effects or complications reported

**Other Adverse Effects**

1% to 10%:
Cardiovascular: Generalized flushing with sensation of warmth
Central nervous system: Headache
Gastrointestinal: Bloating, flatulence, nausea
Hepatic: Abnormalities of hepatic function tests, jaundice
Neuromuscular & skeletal: Paresthesia
Miscellaneous: Increased sebaceous gland activity

<1%:
Cardiovascular: Tachycardia, syncope, vasovagal attacks
Central nervous system: Dizziness
Dermatologic: Skin rash
Hepatic: Chronic liver damage
Ocular: Blurred vision
Respiratory: Wheezing

**Drug Interactions**

Decreased effect of oral hypoglycemics; may inhibit uricosuric effects of sulfinpyrazone and probenecid
Decreased toxicity (flush) with aspirin
Increased toxicity with lovastatin (myopathy) and possibly with other HMG-CoA reductase inhibitors; adrenergic blocking agents → additive vasodilating effect and postural hypotension

**Drug Uptake**

Serum half-life: 45 minutes
Peak serum concentrations: Oral: Within 45 minutes

**Pregnancy Risk Factor** A (C if used in doses greater than RDA suggested doses)

**Generic Available** Yes

## Niacinamide (nye a SIN a mide)

**Therapeutic Category** Vitamin, Water Soluble

**Use** Prophylaxis and treatment of pellagra

**Usual Dosage** Oral:

Children: Pellagra: 100-300 mg/day in divided doses
Adults: 50 mg 3-10 times/day
Pellagra: 300-500 mg/day
Recommended daily allowance: 13-19 mg/day

**Mechanism of Action** Used by the body as a source of niacin; is a component of two coenzymes which is necessary for tissue respiration, lipid metabolism, and glycogenolysis; inhibits the synthesis of very low density lipoproteins

**Local Anesthetic/Vasoconstrictor Precautions** No information available to require special precautions

**Effects on Dental Treatment** No effects or complications reported

**Other Adverse Effects**

1% to 10%:
Gastrointestinal: Bloating, flatulence, nausea
Neuromuscular & skeletal: Paresthesia
Miscellaneous: Increased sebaceous gland activity

<1%:
Cardiovascular: Tachycardia
Dermatologic: Skin rash
Ocular: Blurred vision
Respiratory: Wheezing

**Drug Interactions** No data reported

**Drug Uptake**

Absorption: Rapid from GI tract

Serum half-life: 45 minutes

Time to peak serum concentration: 20-70 minutes

**Pregnancy Risk Factor** A (C if used in doses greater than RDA suggested doses)

**Generic Available** Yes

## Nicardipine (nye KAR de peen)

**Related Information**

Calcium Channel Blockers & Gingival Hyperplasia *on page 1204*

Cardiovascular Diseases *on page 1066*

**U.S. Brand Names** Cardene®; Cardene® SR

**Canadian Brand Names** Ridene

**Therapeutic Category** Antianginal Agent; Calcium Channel Blocker

**Use** Chronic stable angina; management of essential hypertension, migraine prophylaxis

**Unlabeled use:** CHF

**Usual Dosage** Adults:

Oral: 40 mg 3 times/day (allow 3 days between dose increases)

Oral, sustained release: Initial: 30 mg twice daily, titrate up to 60 mg twice daily

I.V. (dilute to 0.1 mg/mL): Initial: 5 mg/hour increased by 2.5 mg/hour every 15 minutes to a maximum of 15 mg/hour

**Mechanism of Action** Inhibits calcium ion from entering the "slow channels" or select voltage-sensitive areas of vascular smooth muscle and myocardium during depolarization, producing a relaxation of coronary vascular smooth muscle and coronary vasodilation; increases myocardial oxygen delivery in patients with vasospastic angina

**Local Anesthetic/Vasoconstrictor Precautions** No information available to require special precautions

**Effects on Dental Treatment** Other drugs of this class can cause gingival hyperplasia (ie, nifedipine). The first case of nicardipine-induced gingival hyperplasia has been reported in a child taking 40-50 mg daily for 20 months

**Other Adverse Effects**

1% to 10%:

- Cardiovascular: Flushing, palpitations, tachycardia, pedal edema
- Central nervous system: Headache, dizziness, somnolence
- Gastrointestinal: Nausea
- Neuromuscular & skeletal: Weakness

<1%:

- Cardiovascular: Edema, syncope, abnormal EKG
- Central nervous system: Insomnia, malaise, abnormal dreams
- Dermatologic: Rash
- Gastrointestinal: Vomiting, constipation, dyspepsia, dry mouth
- Genitourinary: Nocturia
- Neuromuscular & skeletal: Tremor

**Drug Interactions**

Increased toxicity/effect/levels:

- Calcium channel blockers (CCB) and $H_2$-blockers cause increased bioavailability CCB
- CCB and beta-blockers cause increased cardiac depressant effects on A-V conduction
- $H_2$-blockers cause increased bioavailability of nicardipine

Severe hypotension has been reported during fentanyl anesthesia with concomitant use of beta-blockers and calcium channel blockers; even though such interactions have not been seen specifically with nicardipine, caution is suggested in using nicardipine with fentanyl

**Drug Uptake**

Absorption: Oral: Well absorbed, ~100%

Serum half-life: 2-4 hours

Time to peak: Peak serum levels occur within 20-120 minutes and an onset of hypotension occurs within 20 minutes

**Pregnancy Risk Factor** C

**Generic Available** Yes: Capsule

**Selected Readings**

Pascual-Castroviejo I and Pascual Pascual SI, "Nicardipine-Induced Gingival Hyperplasia," *Neurologia*, 1997, 12(1):37-9.

- **N'ice® Vitamin C Drops [OTC]** *see* Ascorbic Acid *on page 97*
- **Niclocide®** *see* Niclosamide *on next page*

## Niclosamide (ni KLOE sa mide)

**U.S. Brand Names** Niclocide®

**Therapeutic Category** Anthelmintic

**Use** Treatment of intestinal beef and fish tapeworm infections and dwarf tapeworm infections

**Usual Dosage** Oral:

Beef and fish tapeworm:
- Children:
  - 11-34 kg: 1 g (2 tablets) as a single dose
  - >34 kg: 1.5 g (3 tablets) as a single dose
- Adults: 2 g (4 tablets) in a single dose
- May require a second course of treatment 7 days later

Dwarf tapeworm:
- Children:
  - 11-34 g: 1 g (2 tablets) chewed thoroughly in a single dose the first day, then 500 mg/day (1 tablet) for next 6 days
  - >34 g: 1.5 g (3 tablets) in a single dose the first day, then 1 g/day for 6 days
- Adults: 2 g (4 tablets) in a single daily dose for 7 days

**Mechanism of Action** Inhibits the synthesis of ATP through inhibition of oxidative phosphorylation in the mitochondria of cestodes

**Local Anesthetic/Vasoconstrictor Precautions** No information available to require special precautions

**Effects on Dental Treatment** No effects or complications reported

**Other Adverse Effects**

1% to 10%:
- Central nervous system: Drowsiness, dizziness, headache
- Gastrointestinal: Nausea, vomiting, loss of appetite, diarrhea

<1%:
- Cardiovascular: Palpitations, edema in the arm
- Central nervous system: Fever
- Dermatologic: Rash, pruritus ani, alopecia
- Gastrointestinal: Constipation, oral irritation, bad taste in mouth, rectal bleeding
- Neuromuscular & skeletal: Backache, weakness
- Miscellaneous: Sweating

**Drug Interactions** No data reported

**Drug Uptake** Absorption: Oral: Not significant

**Pregnancy Risk Factor** B

**Generic Available** No

♦ **Nicobid® [OTC]** *see* Niacin *on page 715*

♦ **Nicoderm®** *see* Nicotine *on this page*

♦ **Nicolar® [OTC]** *see* Niacin *on page 715*

♦ **Nicorette®** *see* Nicotine *on this page*

## Nicotine (nik oh TEEN)

**U.S. Brand Names** Habitrol™; Nicoderm®; Nicorette®; Nicotrol®; Nicotrol® NS; ProStep®

**Canadian Brand Names** Nicorette®; Nicorette® Plus

**Therapeutic Category** Smoking Deterrent

**Use**

Dental: Treatment aid to smoking cessation while participating in a behavioral modification program under dental or medical supervision

Medical: None

**Usual Dosage**

Gum: Chew 1 piece of gum when urge to smoke, up to 30 pieces/day; most patients require 10-12 pieces of gum/day

Inhaler: Usually 6 to 16 cartridges per day; best effect was achieved by frequent continuous puffing (20 minutes); recommended duration of treatment is 3 months, after which patients may be weaned from the inhaler by gradual reduction of the daily dose over 6-12 weeks

Transdermal patch (patients should be advised to completely stop smoking upon initiation of therapy): Apply new patch every 24 hours to nonhairy, clean, dry skin on the upper body or upper outer arm; each patch should be applied to a different site
- Initial starting dose: 21 mg/day for 4-8 weeks for most patients
- First weaning dose: 14 mg/day for 2-4 weeks
- Second weaning dose: 7 mg/day for 2-4 weeks
- Initial starting dose for patients <100 pounds, smoke <10 cigarettes/day, have a history of cardiovascular disease: 14 mg/day for 4-8 weeks followed by 7 mg/day for 2-4 weeks

In patients who are receiving >600 mg/day of cimetidine: Decrease to the next lower patch size

Benefits of use of nicotine transdermal patches beyond 3 months have not been demonstrated

Spray: 1-2 sprays/hour; do not exceed more than 5 doses (10 sprays) per hour; each dose (2 sprays) contains 1 mg of nicotine. **Warning:** A dose of 40 mg can cause fatalities.

**Mechanism of Action** Nicotine is one of two naturally-occurring alkaloids which exhibit their primary effects via autonomic ganglia stimulation. The other alkaloid is lobeline which has many actions similar to those of nicotine but is less potent. Nicotine is a potent ganglionic and central nervous system stimulant, the actions of which are mediated via nicotine-specific receptors. Biphasic actions are observed depending upon the dose administered. The main effect of nicotine in small doses is stimulation of all autonomic ganglia; with larger doses, initial stimulation is followed by blockade of transmission. Biphasic effects are also evident in the adrenal medulla; discharge of catecholamines occurs with small doses, whereas prevention of catecholamines release is seen with higher doses as a response to splanchnic nerve stimulation. Stimulation of the central nervous system (CNS) is characterized by tremors and respiratory excitation. However, convulsions may occur with higher doses, along with respiratory failure secondary to both central paralysis and peripheral blockade to respiratory muscles.

**Local Anesthetic/Vasoconstrictor Precautions** No information available to require special precautions

**Effects on Dental Treatment** >10% of patients using chewing gum form of product experience excessive salivation, mouth, or throat soreness

**Other Adverse Effects**

Chewing gum:

>10%:

Cardiovascular: Tachycardia

Central nervous system: Headache (mild)

Gastrointestinal: Nausea, vomiting, indigestion, excessive salivation, belching, increased appetite, mouth or throat soreness

Neuromuscular & skeletal: Jaw muscle ache

Miscellaneous: Hiccups

1% to 10%:

Central nervous system: Insomnia, dizziness, nervousness

Endocrine & metabolic: Dysmenorrhea

Gastrointestinal: GI distress, eructation

Neuromuscular & skeletal: Myalgia

Respiratory: Hoarseness

Miscellaneous: Hiccups

<1%:

Cardiovascular: Atrial fibrillation

Dermatologic: Erythema, itching, hypersensitivity reactions

Transdermal systems:

>10%:

Cardiovascular: Tachycardia

Central nervous system: Headache (mild)

Dermatologic: Pruritus, erythema

Gastrointestinal: Increased appetite

1% to 10%:

Central nervous system: Insomnia, nervousness

Endocrine & metabolic: Dysmenorrhea

<1%:

Cardiovascular: Atrial fibrillation

Dermatologic: Itching

Miscellaneous: Hypersensitivity reactions

**Contraindications** Nonsmokers, patients with a history of hypersensitivity or allergy to nicotine or any components used in the transdermal system, pregnant or nursing women, patients who are smoking during the postmyocardial infarction period, patients with life-threatening arrhythmias, or severe or worsening angina pectoris, active temporomandibular joint disease (gum)

**Warnings/Precautions** Use with caution in oropharyngeal inflammation and in patients with history of esophagitis, peptic ulcer, coronary artery disease, vasospastic disease, angina, hypertension, hyperthyroidism, diabetes, and hepatic dysfunction; nicotine is known to be one of the most toxic of all poisons; while the gum is being used to help the patient overcome a health hazard, it also must be considered a hazardous drug vehicle

Nicotine nasal spray: Fatal dose: 40 mg

(Continued)

## Nicotine *(Continued)*

**Drug Interactions**

Smoking cessation may alter response to concomitant medications:

Decreased effect of caffeine, imipramine, oxazepam, pentazocine, propranolol, theophylline, glutethimide

Increased effect of furosemide, insulin, propoxyphene

Smoking and nicotine can increase circulating cortisol and catecholamines; therapy with adrenergic agonists or adrenergic blockers may need to be adjusted

Decrease dose of patch in patients taking lithium

**Drug Uptake** Intranasal nicotine may more closely approximate the time course of plasma nicotine levels observed after cigarette smoking than other dosage forms

Duration of action: Transdermal: 24 hours

Absorption: Transdermal: Slow

Serum half-life, elimination: 4 hours

Time to peak serum concentration: Transdermal: 8-9 hours

**Pregnancy Risk Factor** D (transdermal)/X (chewing gum)

**Breast-feeding Considerations** No data reported

**Dosage Forms**

Inhaler, oral (cartridge): 10 mg [delivering 4 mg] (42s); each unit consists of one mouthpiece, 7 storage trays each containing 6 cartridges and one storage case

Patch, transdermal:

Habitrol™: 21 mg/day; 14 mg/day; 7 mg/day (30 systems/box)

Nicoderm®: 21 mg/day; 14 mg/day; 7 mg/day (14 systems/box)

Nicotrol® [OTC]: 15 mg/day (gradually released over 16 hours)

ProStep®: 22 mg/day; 11 mg/day (7 systems/box)

Pieces, chewing gum, as polacrilex: 2 mg/square [OTC] (96 pieces/box); 4 mg/square (96 pieces/box)

Spray, nasal: 0.5 mg/actuation [10 mg/mL-200 actuations] (10 mL)

**Dietary Considerations** No data reported

**Generic Available** No

**Comments** At least 10 reported studies have documented the effectiveness of nicotine patches in smoking cessation. Approximately 45% of treated patients quit smoking after 6 weeks of patch therapy. Control patients given placebo patches accounted for about a 20% success rate. At 52 weeks, approximately 1/2 of the 45% 6-week successful patients continued to abstain. Control placebo patients accounted for an approximate 11% success rate after 52 weeks.

**Selected Readings**

Christen AG and Christen JA, "The Prescription of Transdermal Nicotine Patches for Tobacco-Using Dental Patients: Current Status in Indiana," *J Indiana Dent Assoc*, 1992, 71(6):12-8.

Li Wan Po A, "Transdermal Nicotine in Smoking Cessation. A Meta-Analysis," *Eur J Clin Pharmacol*, 1993, 45(6):519-28.

Stafne EE, "The Nicotine Transdermal Patch: Use in the Dental Office Tobacco Cessation Program," *Northwest Dent*, 1994, 73(3):19-22.

Transdermal Nicotine Study Group, "Transdermal Nicotine for Smoking Cessation. Six-month Results from Two Multicenter Controlled Clinical Trials," *JAMA*, 1991, 266(22):3133-8.

Westman EC, Levin ED, and Rose JE, "The Nicotine Patch in Smoking Cessation," *Arch Intern Med*, 1993, 153(16):1917-23.

Wynn RL, "Nicotine Patches in Smoking Cessation," *AGD Impact*, 1994, 22:14.

♦ **Nicotinex [OTC]** *see* Niacin *on page 715*

♦ **Nicotrol®** *see* Nicotine *on page 718*

♦ **Nicotrol® NS** *see* Nicotine *on page 718*

## Nifedipine (nye FED i peen)

**Related Information**

Calcium Channel Blockers & Gingival Hyperplasia *on page 1204*

Cardiovascular Diseases *on page 1066*

**U.S. Brand Names** Adalat®; Adalat® CC; Procardia®; Procardia XL®

**Canadian Brand Names** Adalat PA®; Apo®-Nifed; Gen-Nifedipine; Novo-Nifedin; Nu-Nifedin

**Therapeutic Category** Antianginal Agent; Calcium Channel Blocker

**Use** Angina, hypertrophic cardiomyopathy, hypertension (sustained release only), pulmonary hypertension

**Usual Dosage** Capsule may be punctured and drug solution administered sublingually to reduce blood pressure

Children: Oral, S.L.:

Hypertensive emergencies: 0.25-0.5 mg/kg/dose

Hypertrophic cardiomyopathy: 0.6-0.9 mg/kg/24 hours in 3-4 divided doses

Adults:

Initial: 10 mg 3 times/day as capsules or 30 mg once daily as sustained release

Usual dose: 10-30 mg 3 times/day as capsules or 30-60 mg once daily as sustained release

Maximum dose: 120-180 mg/day

*Increase sustained release at 7- to 14-day intervals*

**Mechanism of Action** Inhibits calcium ion from entering the "slow channels" or select voltage-sensitive areas of vascular smooth muscle and myocardium during depolarization, producing a relaxation of coronary vascular smooth muscle and coronary vasodilation; increases myocardial oxygen delivery in patients with vasospastic angina

**Local Anesthetic/Vasoconstrictor Precautions** No information available to require special precautions

**Effects on Dental Treatment** Nifedipine has the greatest incidence in causing gingival hyperplasia than any other calcium channel blocker. Effects from the use of nifedipine (30-100 mg/day) have appeared after 1-9 months. Discontinuance of the drug results in complete disappearance or marked regression of symptoms; symptoms will reappear upon remedication. Marked regression occurs after 1 week and complete disappearance of symptoms has occurred within 15 days. If a gingivectomy is performed and use of the drug is continued or resumed, hyperplasia usually will reoccur. The success of the gingivectomy usually requires that the medication be discontinued or that a switch to a noncalcium channel blocker be made. If for some reason, nifedipine cannot be discontinued, hyperplasia has not reoccurred after gingivectomy when extensive plaque control was performed. If nifedipine is changed to another class of cardiovascular agent, the gingival hyperplasia will probably regress and disappear. A switch to another calcium channel blocker probably may result in continued hyperplasia.

**Other Adverse Effects**

>10%:

- Cardiovascular: Flushing
- Central nervous system: Dizziness, lightheadedness, giddiness, headache
- Gastrointestinal: Nausea, heartburn
- Neuromuscular & skeletal: Weakness
- Miscellaneous: Heat sensation

1% to 10%:

- Cardiovascular: Peripheral edema, palpitations, hypotension
- Central nervous system: Nervousness, mood changes
- Gastrointestinal: Sore throat
- Neuromuscular & skeletal: Muscle cramps, tremor
- Respiratory: Dyspnea, cough, nasal congestion

<1%:

- Cardiovascular: Tachycardia, syncope
- Central nervous system: Fever, chills
- Dermatologic: Dermatitis, urticaria, purpura
- Gastrointestinal: Diarrhea, constipation, gingival hyperplasia
- Hematologic: Thrombocytopenia, leukopenia, anemia
- Neuromuscular & skeletal: Joint stiffness, arthritis with increased ANA
- Ocular: Blurred vision, transient blindness
- Miscellaneous: Sweating

**Drug Interactions**

Increased toxicity/effect/levels:

- $H_2$-blockers cause increased bioavailability of nifedipine
- Beta-blockers cause increased cardiac depressant effects on A-V conduction

Severe hypotension has been reported during fentanyl anesthesia with concomitant use of beta-blockers and calcium channel blockers; even though such interactions have not been seen specifically with nifedipine, caution is suggested in using nifedipine with fentanyl

**Drug Uptake**

Onset of action:

- Oral: Within 20 minutes
- S.L.: Within 1-5 minutes

Serum half-life:

- Adults, normal: 2-5 hours
- Adults with cirrhosis: 7 hours

**Pregnancy Risk Factor** C

**Generic Available** Yes: Capsule

**Selected Readings**

Deen-Duggins L, Fry HR, Clay JR, et al, "Nifedipine-Associated Gingival Overgrowth: A Survey of the Literature and Report of Four Cases," *Quintessence Int*, 1996, 27(3):163-70.

Desai P and Silver JG, "Drug-Induced Gingival Enlargements," *J Can Dent Assoc*, 1998, 64(4):263-8.

Harel-Raviv M, Eckler M, Lalani K, et al, "Nifedipine-Induced Gingival Hyperplasia. A Comprehensive Review and Analysis," *Oral Surg Oral Med Oral Pathol Oral Radiol Endod*, 1995, 79(6):715-22.

Lederman D, Lumerman H, Reuben S, et al, "Gingival Hyperplasia Associated With Nifedipine Therapy," *Oral Surg Oral Med Oral Pathol*, 1984, 57(6):620-2.

(Continued)

## Nifedipine *(Continued)*

Lucas RM, Howell LP, and Wall BA, "Nifedipine-Induced Gingival Hyperplasia: A Histochemical and Ultrastructural Study," *J Periodontol*, 1985, 56(4):211-5.

Nery EB, Edson RG, Lee KK, et al, "Prevalence of Nifedipine-Induced Gingival Hyperplasia," *J Periodontol*, 1995, 66(7):572-8.

Nishikawa SJ, Tada H, Hamasaki A, et al, "Nifedipine-Induced Gingival Hyperplasia: A Clinical and In Vitro Study," *J Periodontol*, 1991, 62(1):30-5.

Pilloni A, Camargo PM, Carere M, et al, "Surgical Treatment of Cyclosporine A- and Nifedipine-Induced Gingival Enlargements: Gingivectomy Versus Periodontal Flap," *J Periodontol*, 1998, 69(7):791-7.

Saito K, Mori S, Iwakura M, et al, "Immunohistochemical Localization of Transforming Growth Factor Beta, Basic Fibroblast Growth Factor and Heparin Sulphate Glycosaminoglycan in Gingival Hyperplasia Induced by Nifedipine and Phenytoin," *J Periodontal Res*, 1996, 31(8):545-5.

Silverstein LH, Koch JP, Lefkove MD, et al, "Nifedipine-Induced Gingival Enlargement Around Dental Implants: A Clinical Report," *J Oral Implantol*, 1995, 21(2):116-20.

Westbrook P, Bednarczyk EM, Carlson M, et al, "Regression of Nifedipine-Induced Gingival Hyperplasia Following Switch to a Same Class Calcium Channel Blocker, Isradipine," *J Periodontol*, 1997, 68(7):645-50.

Wynn RL, "Calcium Channel Blockers and Gingival Hyperplasia," *Gen Dent*, 1991, 39(4):240-3.

Wynn RL, "Update on Calcium Channel Blocker-Induced Gingival Hyperplasia," *Gen Dent*, 1995, 43(3):218-22.

- **Niferex® [OTC]** *see* Polysaccharide-Iron Complex *on page 816*
- **Niferex®-PN** *see* Vitamins, Multiple *on page 1051*
- **Nilandron™** *see* Nilutamide *on this page*
- **Nilstat®** *see* Nystatin *on page 734*

## Nilutamide (ni LU ta mide)

**U.S. Brand Names** Nilandron™

**Canadian Brand Names** Anandron®

**Therapeutic Category** Antineoplastic Agent, Miscellaneous

**Use** In combination with surgical castration in treatment of metastatic prostatic carcinoma (Stage $D_2$); for maximum benefit, nilutamide treatment must begin on the same day as or on the day after surgical castration

**Usual Dosage** Adults: Oral: 300 mg (6-50 mg tablets) once daily for 30 days, then 150 mg (3-50 mg tablets) once daily; starting on the same day or day after surgical castration

**Mechanism of Action** Nonsteroidal antiandrogen that inhibits androgen uptake or inhibits binding of androgen in target tissues

**Local Anesthetic/Vasoconstrictor Precautions** No information available to require special precautions

**Effects on Dental Treatment** No effects or complications reported

**Other Adverse Effects**

>10%:

Central nervous system: Pain, headache, insomnia
Gastrointestinal: Nausea, constipation, anorexia
Genitourinary: Impotence, testicular atrophy, gynecomastia
Endocrine & metabolic: Loss of libido, hot flashes
Neuromuscular & skeletal: Weakness
Ocular: Impaired adaption to dark

1% to 10%:

Cardiovascular: Hypertension
Central nervous system: Flu syndrome, fever, dizziness, depression, hypesthesia
Dermatologic: Alopecia, dry skin, rash
Gastrointestinal: Dyspepsia, vomiting, abdominal pain
Genitourinary: Urinary tract infection, hematuria, urinary tract disorder, nocturia
Respiratory: Dyspnea, upper respiratory infection, pneumonia
Ocular: Chromatopsia, impaired adaption to light, abnormal vision
Miscellaneous: Diaphoresis

**Drug Uptake**

Absorption: Rapid and complete
Serum half-life: 38-59 hours

**Pregnancy Risk Factor** C

**Dosage Forms** Tablet: 50 mg

- **NIM** *see* Bleomycin *on page 145*

## Nimodipine (nye MOE di peen)

**Related Information**

Calcium Channel Blockers & Gingival Hyperplasia *on page 1204*
Cardiovascular Diseases *on page 1066*

**U.S. Brand Names** Nimotop®

**Therapeutic Category** Calcium Channel Blocker

**Use** Improvement of neurological deficits due to spasm following subarachnoid hemorrhage from ruptured congenital intracranial aneurysms in patients who are in good neurological condition postictus

**Usual Dosage** Adults: Oral: 60 mg every 4 hours for 21 days, start therapy within 96 hours after subarachnoid hemorrhage

**Mechanism of Action** Nimodipine shares the pharmacology of other calcium channel blockers; animal studies indicate that nimodipine has a greater effect on cerebral arterials than other arterials; this increased specificity may be due to the drug's increased lipophilicity and cerebral distribution as compared to nifedipine; inhibits calcium ion from entering the "slow channels" or select voltage sensitive areas of vascular smooth muscle and myocardium during depolarization

**Local Anesthetic/Vasoconstrictor Precautions** No information available to require special precautions

**Effects on Dental Treatment** Other drugs of this class can cause gingival hyperplasia (ie, nifedipine) but there have been no reports for nimodipine

**Other Adverse Effects**

1% to 10%: Cardiovascular: Reductions in systemic blood pressure

<1%:

- Cardiovascular: Edema, EKG abnormalities, tachycardia, bradycardia
- Central nervous system: Headache, depression
- Dermatologic: Rash, acne
- Gastrointestinal: Diarrhea, nausea
- Hematologic: Hemorrhage
- Hepatic: Hepatitis
- Neuromuscular & skeletal: Muscle cramps
- Respiratory: Dyspnea

**Drug Interactions**

Increased toxicity/effect/levels:

- $H_2$ blockers cause increased bioavailability of nimodipine
- Beta-blockers cause increased cardiac depressant effects on A-V conduction

Severe hypotension has been reported during fentanyl anesthesia with concomitant use of beta-blockers and calcium channel blockers; even though such interactions have not been seen specifically with nimodipine, caution is suggested in using nimodipine with fentanyl

**Drug Uptake**

Serum half-life: 3 hours, increases with reduced renal function

Time to peak serum concentration: Oral: Within 1 hour

**Pregnancy Risk Factor** C

**Generic Available** No

♦ **Nimotop®** *see* Nimodipine *on previous page*

♦ **Nipent™ Injection** *see* Pentostatin *on page 782*

♦ **Nipride®** *see* Nitroprusside *on page 726*

## Nisoldipine (NYE sole di peen)

**Related Information**

Cardiovascular Diseases *on page 1066*

**U.S. Brand Names** Sular®

**Therapeutic Category** Calcium Channel Blocker

**Use** Management of hypertension, may be used alone or in combination with other antihypertensive agents

**Usual Dosage** Adults: Oral: Initial: 20 mg once daily, then increase by 10 mg/week (or longer intervals) to attain adequate control of blood pressure; doses >60 mg once daily are not recommended. A starting dose not exceeding 10 mg/day is recommended for the elderly and those with hepatic impairment.

**Mechanism of Action** As a dihydropyridine calcium channel blocker, structurally similar to nifedipine, nisoldipine impedes the movement of calcium ions into vascular smooth muscle and cardiac muscle. Dihydropyridines are potent vasodilators and are not as likely to suppress cardiac contractility and slow cardiac conduction as other calcium antagonists such as verapamil and diltiazem; nisoldipine is 5-10 times as potent a vasodilator as nifedipine.

**Local Anesthetic/Vasoconstrictor Precautions** No information available to require special precautions

**Effects on Dental Treatment** Other drugs in this class can cause gingival hyperplasia, but there have been no reports for nisoldipine

**Other Adverse Effects**

Cardiovascular: Peripheral edema, tachycardia

Central nervous system: Dizziness, headache

**Warnings/Precautions** Increased angina and/or myocardial infarction in patients with coronary artery disease

**Drug Interactions** Increased toxicity:

Nisoldipine and digoxin may increase digoxin effect

(Continued)

## Nisoldipine *(Continued)*

Nisoldipine and propranolol may increase cardiovascular adverse effects
Nisoldipine and $H_2$-antagonists increase bioavailability and may increase nisoldipine serum concentration
Nisoldipine and omeprazole increase bioavailability and may increase nisoldipine serum concentration

**Drug Uptake**
Absorption: Well absorbed
Serum half-life: 7-12 hours

**Pregnancy Risk Factor** C

**Dosage Forms** Tablet, extended release: 10 mg, 20 mg, 30 mg, 40 mg

**Generic Available** No

- ♦ **Nitalapram** *see* Citalopram *on page 254*
- ♦ **Nitro-Bid®** *see* Nitroglycerin *on next page*
- ♦ **Nitrocine®** *see* Nitroglycerin *on next page*
- ♦ **Nitrodisc®** *see* Nitroglycerin *on next page*
- ♦ **Nitro-Dur®** *see* Nitroglycerin *on next page*

## Nitrofurantoin (nye troe fyoor AN toyn)

**U.S. Brand Names** Furadantin®; Macrobid®; Macrodantin®

**Canadian Brand Names** Apo®-Nitrofurantoin; Nephronex®; Novo-Furan

**Therapeutic Category** Antibiotic, Miscellaneous

**Use** Prevention and treatment of urinary tract infections caused by susceptible gram-negative and some gram-positive organisms; *Pseudomonas, Serratia*, and most species of *Proteus* are generally resistant to nitrofurantoin

**Usual Dosage** Oral:
Children >1 month: 5-7 mg/kg/day in divided doses every 6 hours; maximum: 400 mg/day
Chronic therapy: 1-2 mg/kg/day in divided doses every 24 hours; maximum dose: 400 mg/day
Adults: 50-100 mg/dose every 6 hours (not to exceed 400 mg/24 hours)
Prophylaxis: 50-100 mg/dose at at bedtime

**Mechanism of Action** Inhibits several bacterial enzyme systems including acetyl coenzyme A interfering with metabolism and possibly cell wall synthesis

**Local Anesthetic/Vasoconstrictor Precautions** No information available to require special precautions

**Effects on Dental Treatment** No effects or complications reported

**Other Adverse Effects**
>10%:
Cardiovascular: Chest pains
Central nervous system: Chills, fever
Gastrointestinal: Stomach upset, diarrhea, loss of appetite, vomiting
Respiratory: Cough, dyspnea
1% to 10%:
Central nervous system: Fatigue, drowsiness, headache, dizziness
Gastrointestinal: Sore throat
Neuromuscular & skeletal: Paresthesia, weakness
<1%:
Dermatologic: Skin rash, itching
Hematologic: Hemolytic anemia
Hepatic: Hepatitis
Neuromuscular & skeletal: Arthralgia

**Drug Interactions**
Decreased effect: Antacids (decreases absorption of nitrofurantoin)
Increased toxicity: Probenecid (decreases renal excretion of nitrofurantoin)

**Drug Uptake**
Absorption: Well absorbed from GI tract; the macrocrystalline form is absorbed more slowly due to slower dissolution, but causes less GI distress
Serum half-life: 20-60 minutes; prolonged with renal impairment

**Pregnancy Risk Factor** B

**Generic Available** Yes: Tablet and suspension

## Nitrofurazone (nye troe FYOOR a zone)

**U.S. Brand Names** Furacin®

**Therapeutic Category** Antibacterial, Topical

**Use** Antibacterial agent in second and third degree burns and skin grafting

**Usual Dosage** Children and Adults: Topical: Apply once daily or every few days to lesion or place on gauze

**Mechanism of Action** A broad antibacterial spectrum; it acts by inhibiting bacterial enzymes involved in carbohydrate metabolism; effective against a wide range of gram-negative and gram-positive organisms; bactericidal against most bacteria commonly causing surface infections including *Staphylococcus aureus*, *Streptococcus*, *Escherichia coli*, *Enterobacter cloacae*, *Clostridium perfringens*, *Aerobacter aerogenes*, and *Proteus* sp; not particularly active against most *Pseudomonas aeruginosa* strains and does not inhibit viruses or fungi. Topical preparations of nitrofurazone are readily soluble in blood, pus, and serum and are nonmacerating.

**Local Anesthetic/Vasoconstrictor Precautions** No information available to require special precautions

**Effects on Dental Treatment** No effects or complications reported

**Other Adverse Effects** Women should inform their physicians if signs or symptoms of any of the following occur thromboembolic or thrombotic disorders including sudden severe headache or vomiting, disturbance of vision or speech, loss of vision, numbness or weakness in an extremity, sharp or crushing chest pain, calf pain, dyspnea, severe abdominal pain or mass, mental depression or unusual bleeding

Women should discontinue taking the medication if they suspect they are pregnant or become pregnant. Notify physician if area under dermal patch becomes irritated or a rash develops.

**Drug Interactions** Decreased effect: Sutilains decrease activity of nitrofurazone

**Pregnancy Risk Factor** C

**Generic Available** Yes

♦ **Nitrogard**® *see* Nitroglycerin *on this page*

## Nitroglycerin (nye troe GLI ser in)

**Related Information**

Cardiovascular Diseases *on page 1066*

**U.S. Brand Names** Deponit®; Minitran®; Nitro-Bid®; Nitrocine®; Nitrodisc®; Nitro-Dur®; Nitrogard®; Nitroglyn®; Nitrol®; Nitrolingual®; Nitrong®; Nitrostat®; Transdermal-NTG®; Transderm-Nitro®; Tridil®

**Therapeutic Category** Antianginal Agent; Nitrate; Vasodilator, Coronary

**Use** Treatment of angina pectoris; I.V. for congestive heart failure (especially when associated with acute myocardial infarction); pulmonary hypertension; hypertensive emergencies occurring perioperatively (especially during cardiovascular surgery)

**Usual Dosage Note:** Hemodynamic and antianginal tolerance often develop within 24-48 hours of continuous nitrate administration

Children: Pulmonary hypertension: Continuous infusion: Start 0.25-0.5 mcg/kg/minute and titrate by 1 mcg/kg/minute at 20- to 60-minute intervals to desired effect; usual dose: 1-3 mcg/kg/minute; maximum: 5 mcg/kg/minute

Adults:

- Buccal: Initial: 1 mg every 3-5 hours while awake (3 times/day); titrate dosage upward if angina occurs with tablet in place
- Oral: 2.5-9 mg 2-4 times/day (up to 26 mg 4 times/day)
- I.V.: 5 mcg/minute, increase by 5 mcg/minute every 3-5 minutes to 20 mcg/minute; if no response at 20 mcg/minute increase by 10 mcg/minute every 3-5 minutes, up to 200 mcg/minute
- Ointment: 1" to 2" every 8 hours up to 4" to 5" every 4 hours
- Patch, transdermal: 0.2-0.4 mg/hour initially and titrate to doses of 0.4-0.8 mg/hour; tolerance is minimized by using a patch-on period of 12-14 hours and patch-off period of 10-12 hours
- Sublingual: 0.2-0.6 mg every 5 minutes for maximum of 3 doses in 15 minutes; may also use prophylactically 5-10 minutes prior to activities which may provoke an attack
- Translingual: 1-2 sprays into mouth under tongue every 3-5 minutes for maximum of 3 doses in 15 minutes, may also be used 5-10 minutes prior to activities which may provoke an attack prophylactically

May need to use nitrate-free interval (10-12 hours/day) to avoid tolerance development; tolerance may possibly be reversed with acetylcysteine; gradually decrease dose in patients receiving NTG for prolonged period to avoid withdrawal reaction

**Mechanism of Action** Reduces cardiac oxygen demand by decreasing left ventricular pressure and systemic vascular resistance; dilates coronary arteries and improves collateral flow to ischemic regions

**Local Anesthetic/Vasoconstrictor Precautions** No information available to require special precautions

**Effects on Dental Treatment** No effects or complications reported

**Other Adverse Effects**

>10%:

Cardiovascular: Postural hypotension, flushing

(Continued)

## Nitroglycerin *(Continued)*

Central nervous system: Headache, lightheadedness, dizziness
Neuromuscular & skeletal: Weakness

1% to 10%: Dermatologic: Drug rash, exfoliative dermatitis

<1%:

Cardiovascular: Reflex tachycardia, bradycardia, coronary vascular insufficiency, arrhythmias
Dermatologic: Allergic contact dermatitis, exfoliative dermatitis
Gastrointestinal: Nausea, vomiting
Hematologic: Methemoglobinemia (overdose)
Miscellaneous: Perspiration, collapse, alcohol intoxication

**Drug Interactions**

Decreased effect: I.V. nitroglycerin may antagonize the anticoagulant effect of heparin, monitor closely; may need to decrease heparin dosage when nitroglycerin is discontinued

Increased toxicity: Alcohol, beta-blockers, calcium channel blockers may enhance nitroglycerin's hypotensive effect

**Drug Uptake**

Onset and duration of action is dependent upon dosage form administered
Serum half-life: 1-4 minutes

**Pregnancy Risk Factor** C

**Generic Available** Yes

- **Nitroglyn®** *see* Nitroglycerin *on previous page*
- **Nitrol®** *see* Nitroglycerin *on previous page*
- **Nitrolingual®** *see* Nitroglycerin *on previous page*
- **Nitrong®** *see* Nitroglycerin *on previous page*
- **Nitropress®** *see* Nitroprusside *on this page*

## Nitroprusside (nye troe PRUS ide)

**U.S. Brand Names** Nipride®; Nitropress®

**Therapeutic Category** Vasodilator

**Use** Management of hypertensive crises; congestive heart failure; used for controlled hypotension to reduce bleeding during surgery

**Usual Dosage** Administration requires the use of an infusion pump. Average dose: 5 mcg/kg/minute

Children: Pulmonary hypertension: I.V.: Initial: 1 mcg/kg/minute by continuous I.V. infusion; increase in increments of 1 mcg/kg/minute at intervals of 20-60 minutes; titrating to the desired response; usual dose: 3 mcg/kg/minute, rarely need >4 mcg/kg/minute; maximum: 5 mcg/kg/minute.

Adults: I.V. Initial: 0.3-0.5 mcg/kg/minute; increase in increments of 0.5 mcg/kg/minute, titrating to the desired hemodynamic effect or the appearance of headache or nausea; usual dose: 3 mcg/kg/minute; rarely need >4 mcg/kg/minute; maximum: 10 mcg/kg/minute. When >500 mcg/kg is administered by prolonged infusion of faster than 2 mcg/kg/minute, cyanide is generated faster than an unaided patient can handle.

**Mechanism of Action** Causes peripheral vasodilation by direct action on venous and arteriolar smooth muscle, thus reducing peripheral resistance; will increase cardiac output by decreasing afterload; reduces aortal and left ventricular impedance

**Local Anesthetic/Vasoconstrictor Precautions** No information available to require special precautions

**Effects on Dental Treatment** No effects or complications reported

**Other Adverse Effects** 1% to 10%:

Cardiovascular: Excessive hypotensive response, palpitations, substernal distress
Central nervous system: Disorientation, psychosis, headache, restlessness
Endocrine & metabolic: Thyroid suppression
Gastrointestinal: Nausea, vomiting
Neuromuscular & skeletal: Muscle spasm, weakness
Otic: Tinnitus
Respiratory: Hypoxia
Miscellaneous: Sweating, thiocyanate toxicity

**Drug Interactions** No data reported

**Drug Uptake**

Onset of hypotensive effect: <2 minutes
Duration: Within 1-10 minutes following discontinuation of therapy, effects cease
Serum half-life:

Parent drug: <10 minutes
Thiocyanate: 2.7-7 days

**Pregnancy Risk Factor** C
**Generic Available** Yes

♦ **Nitrostat®** *see* Nitroglycerin *on page 725*

## Nitrous Oxide (NYE trus OKS ide)

**Related Information**

Patients Requiring Sedation *on page 1152*

**Therapeutic Category** Dental Gases

**Use**

Dental: To induce sedation and analgesia in anxious dental patients

Medical: A principal adjunct to inhalation and intravenous general anesthesia in medical patients undergoing surgery; prehospital relief of pain of differing etiologies (ie, burns, fractures, back injury, abrasions, lacerations)

**Usual Dosage** Children and Adults: For sedation and analgesia: Concentrations of 25% to 50% nitrous oxide with oxygen inhaled through the nose via a nasal mask

**Mechanism of Action** General CNS depressant action; may act similarly as inhalant general anesthetics by mildly stabilizing axonal membranes to partially inhibit action potentials leading to sedation; may partially act on opiate receptor systems to cause mild analgesia

**Local Anesthetic/Vasoconstrictor Precautions** No information available to require special precautions

**Effects on Dental Treatment** No effects or complications reported

**Other Adverse Effects**

An increased risk of renal and hepatic diseases and peripheral neuropathy similar to that of vitamin $B_{12}$ deficiency have been reported in dental personnel who work in areas where nitrous oxide is used

Methionine synthase, a vitamin $B_{12}$ dependent enzyme, is inactivated following very prolonged administration of nitrous oxide, and the subsequent interference with DNA synthesis prevents production of both leukocytes and red blood cells by bone marrow. These effects do not occur within the time frame of clinical sedation.

Female dental personnel who were exposed to unscavenged nitrous oxide for more than 5 hours/week were significantly less fertile than women who were not exposed, or who were exposed to lower levels of scavenged or unscavenged nitrous oxide. Fertility was measured by the number of menstrual cycles, without use of contraception, required to become pregnant. Women who were exposed to nitrous oxide for more than 5 hours/week were only 41% as likely as unexposed women to conceive during each monthly cycle.

**Contraindications** Nitrous oxide should not be administered without oxygen. Nitrous oxide should not be given to patients after a full meal

**Warnings/Precautions** Nausea and vomiting occurs postoperatively in ~15% of patients. Prolonged use may produce bone marrow suppression and/or neurologic dysfunction. Oxygen should be briefly administered during emergence from prolonged anesthesia with nitrous oxide to prevent diffusion hypoxia. Patients with vitamin $B_{12}$ deficiency (pernicious anemia) and those with other nutritional deficiencies (alcoholics) are at increased risk of developing neurologic disease and bone marrow suppression with exposure to nitrous oxide. May be addictive

**Drug Interactions** No data reported

**Drug Uptake** Nitrous oxide is rapidly absorbed via inhalation. The blood/gas partition coefficient is 0.5. The gas is rapidly eliminated via the lungs, with minimal amounts eliminated through the skin.

Onset time: Inhalation: 5-10 minutes

**Pregnancy Risk Factor** No data reported

**Breast-feeding Considerations** No data reported

**Dosage Forms** Supplied in blue cylinders

**Dietary Considerations** No data reported

**Generic Available** Yes

**Comments** Results of a mail survey of more than 30,000 dentists and 30,000 chairside assistants, who were exposed to trace anesthetics in dental operatories were published in 1980 (Cohen et al, 1980). This study suggested that long-term exposure to nitrous oxide and to nitrous oxide/halogenated anesthetics was associated with an increase in general health problems and reproductive difficulties in these dental personnel. Schuyt et al (1986) observed that 4 female dental personnel who were exposed to inhalation sedation with 35% nitrous oxide reported 6 spontaneous abortions among 7 pregnancies over 17 months

**Selected Readings**

Babich S and Burakoff RP, "Occupational Hazards of Dentistry. A Review of Literature From 1990," *N Y State Dent J*, 1997, 63(8):26-31.

Baird PA, "Occupational Exposure to Nitrous Oxide - Not a Laughing Matter," *N Engl J Med*, 1992, 327(14):1026-7.

(Continued)

## Nitrous Oxide *(Continued)*

Cohen EN, Gift HC, Brown BW, et al, "Occupational Disease in Dentistry and Chronic Exposure to Trace Anesthetic Gases," *J Am Dent Assoc*, 1980, 101(1):21-31.
Dunning DG, McFarland K, and Safarik M, "Nitrous-Oxide Use. II. Risks, Compliance, and Exposure Levels Among Nebraska Dentists and Dental Assistants," *Gen Dent*, 1997, 45(1):82-6.
Howard WR, "Nitrous Oxide in the Dental Environment: Assessing the Risk, Reducing the Exposure," *J Am Dent Assoc*, 1997, 128(3):356-60.
Johnsen KG, "Nitrous Oxide Safety," *J Am Dent Assoc*, 1997, 128(8):1066-7.
"Nitrous Oxide in the Dental Office. ADA Council on Scientific Affairs; ADA Council on Dental Practice," *J Am Dent Assoc*, 1997, 128(3):364-5.
Petersen JK, "Nitrous Oxide Analgesia in Dental Practice," *Acta Anaesthesiol Scand*, 1994, 38(8):773-4.
Quarnstrom F, "Nitrous Oxide," *J Am Dent Assoc*, 1997, 128(6):690, 692.
Rowland AS, Baird DD, Weinberg CR, et al, "Reduced Fertility Among Women Employed as Female Dental Assistants Exposed to High Levels of Nitrous Oxide," *N Engl J Med*, 1992, 327(14):993-7.
Schuyt HC, Brakel K, Oostendorp SG, et al, "Abortions Among Dental Personnel Exposed to Nitrous Oxide," *Anaesthesia*, 1986, 41(1):82-3.
Wynn RL, "Nitrous Oxide and Fertility, Part I," *Gen Dent*, 1993, 41(2):122-3.
Wynn RL, "Nitrous Oxide and Fertility, Part II," *Gen Dent*, 1993, 41(3):212, 214.

♦ **Nix™ [OTC]** *see* Permethrin *on page 785*

## Nizatidine (ni ZA ti deen)

**U.S. Brand Names** Axid®; Axid® AR [OTC]
**Canadian Brand Names** Apo®-Nizatidine
**Therapeutic Category** Histamine $H_2$ Antagonist
**Use** Treatment and maintenance of duodenal ulcer; treatment of gastroesophageal reflux disease (GERD)
**Usual Dosage** Adults: Active duodenal ulcer: Oral:
Treatment: 300 mg at bedtime or 150 mg twice daily
Maintenance: 150 mg/day
**Mechanism of Action** Nizatidine is an $H_2$-receptor antagonist. In healthy volunteers, nizatidine has been effective in suppressing gastric acid secretion induced by pentagastrin infusion or food. Nizatidine reduces gastric acid secretion by 29.4% to 78.4%. This compares with a 60.3% reduction by cimetidine. Nizatidine 100 mg is reported to provide equivalent acid suppression as cimetidine 300 mg.
**Local Anesthetic/Vasoconstrictor Precautions** No information available to require special precautions
**Effects on Dental Treatment** No effects or complications reported
**Other Adverse Effects**
1% to 10%:
Central nervous system: Dizziness, headache
Gastrointestinal: Constipation, diarrhea
<1%:
Cardiovascular: Bradycardia, tachycardia, palpitations, hypertension
Central nervous system: Fever, fatigue, seizures, insomnia, drowsiness
Dermatologic: Acne, pruritus, urticaria, dry skin
Gastrointestinal: Abdominal discomfort, flatulence, belching, anorexia
Hematologic: Agranulocytosis, neutropenia, thrombocytopenia
Hepatic: Elevated AST, ALT
Neuromuscular & skeletal: Paresthesia, weakness
Renal: Elevated BUN and creatinine, proteinuria
Respiratory: Bronchospasm
Miscellaneous: Allergic reaction
**Drug Interactions** No data reported
**Pregnancy Risk Factor** C
**Generic Available** No

♦ **Nizoral®** *see* Ketoconazole *on page 564*
♦ **N-Methylhydrazine** *see* Procarbazine *on page 842*
♦ **Nolahist® [OTC]** *see* Phenindamine *on page 790*
♦ **Nolamine®** *see* Chlorpheniramine, Phenindamine, and Phenylpropanolamine *on page 234*
♦ **Nolex® LA** *see* Guaifenesin and Phenylpropanolamine *on page 480*
♦ **Nolvadex®** *see* Tamoxifen *on page 952*

## Nonoxynol 9 (non OKS i nole nine)

**U.S. Brand Names** Because® [OTC]; Delfen® [OTC]; Emko® [OTC]; Encare® [OTC]; Gynol II® [OTC]; Koromex® [OTC]; Ramses® [OTC]; Semicid® [OTC]; Shur-Seal® [OTC]
**Therapeutic Category** Spermicide
**Use** Spermatocide in contraception
**Usual Dosage** Insert into vagina at least 15 minutes before intercourse
**Local Anesthetic/Vasoconstrictor Precautions** No information available to require special precautions

**Effects on Dental Treatment** No effects or complications reported

**Pregnancy Risk Factor** C

**Generic Available** Yes

- ♦ **Nonviral Infectious Diseases** *see page 1095*
- ♦ **No Pain-HP® [OTC]** *see* Capsaicin *on page 181*
- ♦ **Noradrenaline** *see* Norepinephrine *on this page*
- ♦ **Noradrenaline Acid Tartrate** *see* Norepinephrine *on this page*
- ♦ **Nordette®** *see* Ethinyl Estradiol and Levonorgestrel *on page 402*
- ♦ **Norditropin® Injection** *see* Human Growth Hormone *on page 499*

## Norepinephrine (nor ep i NEF rin)

**U.S. Brand Names** Levophed® Injection

**Therapeutic Category** Adrenergic Agonist Agent

**Synonyms** Levarterenol Bitartrate; Noradrenaline; Noradrenaline Acid Tartrate; Norepinephrine Bitartrate

**Use** Treatment of shock which persists after adequate fluid volume replacement; severe hypotension; cardiogenic shock

**Usual Dosage Note:** Norepinephrine dosage is stated in terms of norepinephrine base and intravenous formulation is norepinephrine bitartrate

**Norepinephrine bitartrate 2 mg = norepinephrine base 1 mg**

Continuous I.V. infusion:

Children:

Initial: 0.05-0.1 mcg/kg/minute; titrate to desired effect

Maximum dose: 1-2 mcg/kg/minute

Adults: Initiate at 4 mcg/minute and titrate to desired response; 8-12 mcg/minute is usual range

ACLS dosing range: 0.5-30 mcg/minute

**Rate of infusion**: 4 mg in 500 mL $D_5W$

2 mcg/minute = 15 mL/hour
4 mcg/minute = 30 mL/hour
6 mcg/minute = 45 mL/hour
8 mcg/minute = 60 mL/hour
10 mcg/minute = 75 mL/hour
12 mcg/minute = 90 mL/hour
14 mcg/minute = 105 mL/hour
16 mcg/minute = 120 mL/hour
18 mcg/minute = 135 mL/hour
20 mcg/minute = 150 mL/hour

**Mechanism of Action** Stimulates $beta_1$-adrenergic receptors and alpha-adrenergic receptors causing increased contractility and heart rate as well as vasoconstriction, thereby increasing systemic blood pressure and coronary blood flow; clinically alpha effects (vasoconstriction) are greater than beta effects (inotropic and chronotropic effects)

**Local Anesthetic/Vasoconstrictor Precautions** No information available to require special precautions

**Effects on Dental Treatment** No effects or complications reported

**Other Adverse Effects**

1% to 10%:

Central nervous system: Dizziness, anxiety, headache, insomnia

Endocrine & metabolic: Thyroid gland enlargement

Neuromuscular & skeletal: Trembling

<1%:

Cardiovascular: Cardiac arrhythmias, palpitations, bradycardia, tachycardia, hypertension, chest pain, pallor, gangrene of extremities

Gastrointestinal: Vomiting

Genitourinary: Uterine contractions

Local: Sloughing at the infusion site

Ocular: Photophobia

Respiratory: Respiratory distress

Miscellaneous: Diaphoresis

**Warnings/Precautions** Blood/volume depletion should be corrected, if possible, before norepinephrine therapy; extravasation may cause severe tissue necrosis, administer into a large vein. The drug should not be given to patients with peripheral or mesenteric vascular thrombosis because ischemia may be increased and the area of infarct extended; use with caution during cyclopropane and halothane anesthesia; use with caution in patients with occlusive vascular disease; some products may contain sulfites

(Continued)

## Norepinephrine *(Continued)*

**Drug Interactions**

Increased effect with tricyclic antidepressants, MAO inhibitors, antihistamines (diphenhydramine, tripelennamine), guanethidine, ergot alkaloids, and methyldopa

Atropine sulfate may block the reflex bradycardia caused by norepinephrine and enhances the pressor response

**Drug Uptake**

Onset of action: I.V.: Very rapid-acting

Duration: Limited

Metabolism: By catechol-o-methyltransferase (COMT) and monoamine oxidase (MAO)

Elimination: In urine (84% to 96% as inactive metabolites)

**Pregnancy Risk Factor** D

**Dosage Forms** Injection, as bitartrate: 1 mg/mL (4 mL)

**Generic Available** No

**Selected Readings**

Martin C, Papazian L, Perrin G, et al, "Norepinephrine or Dopamine for the Treatment of Hyperdynamic Septic Shock?" *Chest*, 1993, 103(6):1826-31.

- **Norepinephrine Bitartrate** *see* Norepinephrine *on previous page*
- **Norethin™ 1/35E** *see* Ethinyl Estradiol and Norethindrone *on page 404*
- **Norethin™ 1/50M** *see* Mestranol and Norethindrone *on page 639*

## Norethindrone (nor eth IN drone)

**Related Information**

Endocrine Disorders & Pregnancy *on page 1082*

**U.S. Brand Names** Aygestin®; Micronor®; Nor-QD®

**Therapeutic Category** Contraceptive, Oral; Contraceptive, Progestin Only; Progestin

**Use** Treatment of amenorrhea; abnormal uterine bleeding; endometriosis, oral contraceptive; **higher rate of failure with progestin only contraceptives**

**Usual Dosage** Adolescents and Adults: Female: Oral:

Contraception: Progesterone only: Norethindrone 0.35 mg every day of the year starting on first day of menstruation; if one dose is missed take as soon as remembered; then next tablet at regular time; if two doses are missed, take one of the missed doses, discard the other, and take daily dose at usual time; if three doses are missed, use another form of birth control until menses appear or pregnancy is ruled out

Amenorrhea and abnormal uterine bleeding:

Norethindrone: 5-20 mg/day on days 5-25 of menstrual cycle

Acetate salt: 2.5-10 mg on days 5-25 of menstrual cycle

Endometriosis:

Norethindrone: 10 mg/day for 2 weeks; increase at increments of 5 mg/day every 2 weeks until 30 mg/day; continue for 6-9 months or until breakthrough bleeding demands temporary termination

Acetate salt: 5 mg/day for 14 days; increase at increments of 2.5 mg/day every 2 weeks up to 15 mg/day; continue for 6-9 months or until breakthrough bleeding demands temporary termination

**Mechanism of Action** Inhibits secretion of pituitary gonadotropin (LH) which prevents follicular maturation and ovulation

**Local Anesthetic/Vasoconstrictor Precautions** No information available to require special precautions

**Effects on Dental Treatment** Until we know more about the mechanism of interaction, caution is required in prescribing antibiotics to female dental patients taking progestin-only oral contraceptives

**Other Adverse Effects**

>10%:

Cardiovascular: Edema

Endocrine & metabolic: Breakthrough bleeding, spotting, changes in menstrual flow, amenorrhea

Gastrointestinal: Anorexia

Neuromuscular & skeletal: Weakness

1% to 10%:

Cardiovascular: Embolism, central thrombosis

Central nervous system: Mental depression, fever, insomnia

Dermatologic: Melasma or chloasma, allergic rash with or without pruritus

Endocrine & metabolic: Changes in cervical erosion and secretions, weight gain or loss, increased breast tenderness

Hepatic: Cholestatic jaundice

Local: Thrombophlebitis

**Drug Interactions** Decreased effect: Aminoglutethimide may decrease effects by increasing hepatic metabolism

**Pregnancy Risk Factor** X

**Generic Available** No

♦ **Norflex™** *see* Orphenadrine *on page 744*

## Norfloxacin (nor FLOKS a sin)

**U.S. Brand Names** Chibroxin™; Noroxin®

**Therapeutic Category** Antibiotic, Quinolone

**Use** Complicated and uncomplicated urinary tract infections caused by susceptible gram-negative and gram-positive bacteria; ophthalmic solution for conjunctivitis

**Usual Dosage**

Ophthalmic: Children >1 year and Adults: Instill 1-2 drops in affected eye(s) 4 times/day for up to 7 days

Oral: Adults:

Urinary tract infections: 400 mg twice daily for 3-21 days depending on severity of infection or organism sensitivity; maximum: 800 mg/day

Uncomplicated gonorrhea: 800 mg as a single dose (CDC recommends as an alternative regimen to ciprofloxacin or ofloxacin)

Prostatitis: 400 mg every 12 hours for 4 weeks

**Mechanism of Action** Norfloxacin is a DNA gyrase inhibitor. DNA gyrase is an essential bacterial enzyme that maintains the superhelical structure of DNA. DNA gyrase is required for DNA replication and transcription, DNA repair, recombination, and transposition; bactericidal

**Local Anesthetic/Vasoconstrictor Precautions** No information available to require special precautions

**Effects on Dental Treatment** No effects or complications reported

**Other Adverse Effects**

1% to 10%:

Central nervous system: Headache, dizziness, fatigue

Gastrointestinal: Nausea

<1%:

Central nervous system: Somnolence, depression, insomnia, fever

Dermatologic: Pruritus, hyperhidrosis, erythema, rash

Gastrointestinal: Abdominal pain, dyspepsia, constipation, flatulence, heartburn, dry mouth, diarrhea, vomiting, loose stools, anorexia, bitter taste, GI bleeding

Hepatic: Elevated liver enzymes

Neuromuscular & skeletal: Back pain, weakness

Renal: Elevated serum creatinine and BUN, acute renal failure

**Drug Interactions**

Decreased effect: Decreased absorption with antacids containing aluminum, magnesium, and/or calcium (by up to 98% if given at the same time)

Increased toxicity/serum levels: Quinolones cause increased levels of caffeine, warfarin, cyclosporine, and theophylline; azlocillin, cimetidine, probenecid increase quinolone levels

**Drug Uptake**

Absorption: Oral: Rapid, up to 40%

Serum half-life: 4.8 hours (can be higher with reduced glomerular filtration rates)

Time to peak serum concentration: Within 1-2 hours

**Pregnancy Risk Factor** C

**Generic Available** No

♦ **Norgesic™** *see* Orphenadrine, Aspirin, and Caffeine *on page 745*

♦ **Norgesic™ Forte** *see* Orphenadrine, Aspirin, and Caffeine *on page 745*

♦ **Norgestimate and Ethinyl Estradiol** *see* Ethinyl Estradiol and Norgestimate *on page 406*

## Norgestrel (nor JES trel)

**Related Information**

Endocrine Disorders & Pregnancy *on page 1082*

**U.S. Brand Names** Ovrette®

**Therapeutic Category** Contraceptive, Oral; Progestin

**Use** Prevention of pregnancy; **progestin only products have higher risk of failure in contraceptive use**

**Usual Dosage** Administer daily, starting the first day of menstruation, take 1 tablet at the same time each day, every day of the year. If 1 dose is missed, take as soon as remembered, then next tablet at regular time; if 2 doses are missed, take 1 tablet and discard the other, then take daily at usual time; if 3 doses are missed, use an additional form of birth control until menses or pregnancy is ruled out.

(Continued)

## Norgestrel *(Continued)*

**Mechanism of Action** Inhibits secretion of pituitary gonadotropin (LH) which prevents follicular maturation and ovulation

**Local Anesthetic/Vasoconstrictor Precautions** No information available to require special precautions

**Effects on Dental Treatment** Until we know more about the mechanism of interaction, caution is required in prescribing antibiotics to female dental patients taking progestin-only oral contraceptives

**Other Adverse Effects**

>10%:
- Cardiovascular: Edema
- Endocrine & metabolic: Breakthrough bleeding, spotting, changes in menstrual flow, amenorrhea
- Gastrointestinal: Anorexia
- Neuromuscular & skeletal: Weakness

1% to 10%:
- Cardiovascular: Embolism, central thrombosis
- Central nervous system: Mental depression, fever, insomnia
- Dermatologic: Melasma or chloasma, allergic rash with or without pruritus
- Endocrine & metabolic: Changes in cervical erosion and secretions, weight gain or loss, increased breast tenderness
- Hepatic: Cholestatic jaundice
- Local: Thrombophlebitis

**Drug Interactions** Decreased effect: Aminoglutethimide may decrease effects by increasing hepatic metabolism

**Pregnancy Risk Factor** X

**Generic Available** No

- ♦ **Norinyl® 1+35** *see* Ethinyl Estradiol and Norethindrone *on page 404*
- ♦ **Norinyl® 1+50** *see* Mestranol and Norethindrone *on page 639*
- ♦ **Noritate® Cream** *see* Metronidazole *on page 667*
- ♦ **Normal Saline** *see* Sodium Chloride *on page 920*
- ♦ **Normiflo®** *see* Ardeparin *on page 94*
- ♦ **Normodyne®** *see* Labetalol *on page 568*
- ♦ **Noroxin®** *see* Norfloxacin *on previous page*
- ♦ **Norpace®** *see* Disopyramide *on page 343*
- ♦ **Norplant® Implant** *see* Levonorgestrel *on page 584*
- ♦ **Norpramin®** *see* Desipramine *on page 304*
- ♦ **Nor-QD®** *see* Norethindrone *on page 730*

## Nortriptyline (nor TRIP ti leen)

**U.S. Brand Names** Aventyl® Hydrochloride; Pamelor®

**Canadian Brand Names** Apo®-Nortriptyline

**Therapeutic Category** Antidepressant, Tricyclic

**Use** Treatment of various forms of depression, often in conjunction with psychotherapy. Maximum antidepressant effect may not be seen for 2 or more weeks after initiation of therapy; has also demonstrated effectiveness for chronic pain.

**Usual Dosage** Oral:

Nocturnal enuresis:
- Children:
  - 6-7 years (20-25 kg): 10 mg/day
  - 8-11 years (25-35 kg): 10-20 mg/day
  - >11 years (35-54 kg): 25-35 mg/day

Depression:
- Adolescents: 30-50 mg/day in divided doses
- Adults: 25 mg 3-4 times/day up to 150 mg/day
- Elderly:
  - Initial: 10-25 mg at bedtime
  - Dosage can be increased by 25 mg every 3 days for inpatients and weekly for outpatients if tolerated
  - Usual maintenance dose: 75 mg as a single bedtime dose, however, lower or higher doses may be required to stay within the therapeutic window

**Mechanism of Action** Traditionally believed to increase the synaptic concentration of serotonin and/or norepinephrine in the central nervous system by inhibition of their reuptake by the presynaptic neuronal membrane. However, additional receptor effects have been found including desensitization of adenyl cyclase, down regulation of beta-adrenergic receptors, and down regulation of serotonin receptors.

**Local Anesthetic/Vasoconstrictor Precautions** Use with caution; epinephrine, norepinephrine and levonordefrin have been shown to have an increased pressor response in combination with TCAs

**Effects on Dental Treatment** >10% of patients experience dry mouth; long-term treatment with TCAs such as nortriptyline increases the risk of caries by reducing salivation and salivary buffer capacity

**Other Adverse Effects**

>10%:

Central nervous system: Dizziness, drowsiness, headache

Gastrointestinal: Constipation, increased appetite, nausea, unpleasant taste, weight gain

Neuromuscular & skeletal: Weakness

1% to 10%:

Cardiovascular: Postural hypotension, arrhythmias, tachycardia, sudden death

Central nervous system: Confusion, delirium, hallucinations, nervousness, restlessness, parkinsonian syndrome, insomnia

Endocrine & metabolic: Sexual dysfunction

Gastrointestinal: Diarrhea, heartburn

Genitourinary: Dysuria

Ocular: Blurred vision, eye pain

Neuromuscular & skeletal: Fine muscle tremors

Miscellaneous: Excessive sweating

<1%:

Central nervous system: Anxiety, seizures

Dermatologic: Alopecia, photosensitivity

Endocrine & metabolic: Breast enlargement, galactorrhea, SIADH

Gastrointestinal: Trouble with gums, decreased lower esophageal sphincter tone may cause GE reflux

Genitourinary: Testicular swelling

Hematologic: Leukopenia, rarely agranulocytosis, eosinophilia

Hepatic: Elevated liver enzymes, cholestatic jaundice

Otic: Tinnitus

Miscellaneous: Allergic reactions

**Drug Interactions** Blocks the uptake of guanethidine and thus prevents the hypotensive effect of guanethidine; may be additive with or may potentiate the action of other CNS depressants such as sedatives or hypnotics; potentiates the pressor and cardiac effects of sympathomimetic agents such as isoproterenol, epinephrine, etc; with MAO inhibitors, hyperpyrexia, hypertension, tachycardia, confusion, seizures, and death have been reported; anticholinergic effect seen with other anticholinergic agents; cimetidine reduces the metabolism of nortriptyline; may increase the prothrombin time in patients stabilized on warfarin

**Drug Uptake**

Onset of action: 1-3 weeks before therapeutic effects are seen

Serum half-life: 28-31 hours

Time to peak serum concentration: Oral: Within 7-8.5 hours

**Pregnancy Risk Factor** D

**Generic Available** Yes

**Selected Readings**

Boakes AJ, Laurence DR, Teoh PC, et al, "Interactions Between Sympathomimetic Amines and Antidepressant Agents in Man," *Br Med J*, 1973, 1(849):311-5.

Jastak JT and Yagiela JA, "Vasoconstrictors and Local Anesthesia: A Review and Rationale for Use," *J Am Dent Assoc*, 1983, 107(4):623-30.

Larochelle P, Hamet P, and Enjalbert M, "Responses to Tyramine and Norepinephrine After Imipramine and Trazodone," *Clin Pharmacol Ther*, 1979, 26(1):24-30.

Mitchell JR, "Guanethidine and Related Agents. III Antagonism by Drugs Which Inhibit the Norepinephrine Pump in Man," *J Clin Invest*, 1970, 49(8):1596-604.

Rundegren J, van Dijken J, Mörnstad H, et al, "Oral Conditions in Patients Receiving Long-Term Treatment With Cyclic Antidepressant Drugs," *Swed Dent J*, 1985, 9(2):55-64.

Svedmyr N, "The Influence of a Tricyclic Antidepressive Agent (Protriptyline) on Some of the Circulatory Effects of Noradrenaline and Adrenalin in Man," *Life Sci*, 1968, 7(1):77-84.

- **Norvasc®** *see* Amlodipine *on page 71*
- **Norvir®** *see* Ritonavir *on page 892*
- **Norzine®** *see* Thiethylperazine *on page 976*
- **Nōstrilla® [OTC]** *see* Oxymetazoline *on page 755*
- **Nostril® Nasal Solution [OTC]** *see* Phenylephrine *on page 795*
- **Novacet® Topical** *see* Sulfur and Sulfacetamide Sodium *on page 947*
- **Novahistine® DMX Liquid [OTC]** *see* Guaifenesin, Pseudoephedrine, and Dextromethorphan *on page 482*
- **Novantrone®** *see* Mitoxantrone *on page 682*
- **Novocain®** *see* Procaine *on page 842*
- **Novolin® 70/30** *see* Insulin Preparations *on page 537*
- **Novolin® L** *see* Insulin Preparations *on page 537*
- **Novolin® N** *see* Insulin Preparations *on page 537*
- **Novolin® R** *see* Insulin Preparations *on page 537*
- **NP-27® [OTC]** *see* Tolnaftate *on page 997*

- **NPH Iletin® I** *see* Insulin Preparations *on page 537*
- **NPH Insulin** *see* Insulin Preparations *on page 537*
- **NPH-N** *see* Insulin Preparations *on page 537*
- **NSC-102816** *see* Azacitidine *on page 111*
- **NSC-106977** *see* Erwinia Asparaginase *on page 382*
- **NTZ® Long Acting Nasal Solution [OTC]** *see* Oxymetazoline *on page 755*
- **Nubain®** *see* Nalbuphine *on page 699*
- **Nucofed®** *see* Guaifenesin, Pseudoephedrine, and Codeine *on page 482*
- **Nucofed® Pediatric Expectorant** *see* Guaifenesin, Pseudoephedrine, and Codeine *on page 482*
- **Nucotuss®** *see* Guaifenesin, Pseudoephedrine, and Codeine *on page 482*
- **Nu-Iron® [OTC]** *see* Polysaccharide-Iron Complex *on page 816*
- **Nullo® [OTC]** *see* Chlorophyll *on page 226*
- **NuLytely®** *see* Polyethylene Glycol-Electrolyte Solution *on page 815*
- **Numorphan®** *see* Oxymorphone *on page 756*
- **Numzitdent® [OTC]** *see* Benzocaine *on page 128*
- **Numzit Teething® [OTC]** *see* Benzocaine *on page 128*
- **Nupercainal® [OTC]** *see* Dibucaine *on page 318*
- **Nuprin® [OTC]** *see* Ibuprofen *on page 522*
- **Nu-Tears® II Solution [OTC]** *see* Artificial Tears *on page 97*
- **Nu-Tears® Solution [OTC]** *see* Artificial Tears *on page 97*
- **Nutraplus® [OTC]** *see* Urea *on page 1034*
- **Nutrilipid®** *see* Fat Emulsion *on page 419*
- **Nutropin® AQ Injection** *see* Human Growth Hormone *on page 499*
- **Nutropin® Injection** *see* Human Growth Hormone *on page 499*
- **Nydrazid® Injection** *see* Isoniazid *on page 552*

## Nylidrin (NYE li drin)

**U.S. Brand Names** Arlidin®

**Canadian Brand Names** PMS-Nylidrin®

**Therapeutic Category** Vasodilator, Peripheral

**Use** Considered "possibly effective" for increasing blood supply to treat peripheral disease (arteriosclerosis obliterans, diabetic vascular disease, nocturnal leg cramps, Raynaud's disease, frost bite, ischemic ulcer, thrombophlebitis) and circulatory disturbances of the inner ear (cochlear ischemia, macular or ampullar ischemia, etc)

**Usual Dosage** Adults: Oral: 3-12 mg 3-4 times/day

**Mechanism of Action** Nylidrin is a peripheral vasodilator; this results from direct relaxation of vascular smooth muscle and beta agonist action. Nylidrin does not appear to affect cutaneous blood flow; it reportedly increases heart rate and cardiac output; cutaneous blood flow is not enhanced to any appreciable extent.

**Local Anesthetic/Vasoconstrictor Precautions** No information available to require special precautions

**Effects on Dental Treatment** No effects or complications reported

**Other Adverse Effects**

1% to 10%:
- Central nervous system: Nervousness
- Neuromuscular & skeletal: Trembling

<1%:
- Cardiovascular: Palpitations, postural hypotension
- Central nervous system: Dizziness
- Gastrointestinal: Nausea, vomiting
- Neuromuscular & skeletal: Weakness

**Drug Interactions** No data reported

**Pregnancy Risk Factor** C

## Nystatin (nye STAT in)

**Related Information**

Oral Fungal Infections *on page 1134*

Patients Undergoing Cancer Therapy *on page 1154*

**U.S. Brand Names** Mycostatin®; Nilstat®; Nystex®

**Canadian Brand Names** Mestatin®; Nadostine®; Nyaderm; PMS-Nystatin

**Therapeutic Category** Antifungal Agent, Oral Nonabsorbed; Antifungal Agent, Topical; Antifungal Agent, Vaginal

**Use**

Dental: Treatment of susceptible cutaneous, mucocutaneous, and oral cavity fungal infections normally caused by the *Candida* species

Medical: None

**Usual Dosage** Oral candidiasis: Suspension (swish and swallow orally):

Children and Adults: 400,000-600,000 units 4 times/day; troche: 200,000-400,000 units 4-5 times/day

Adults: 400,000-600,000 units 4 times/day; pastilles: 200,000-400,000 units 4-5 times/day

**Mechanism of Action** Binds to sterols in fungal cell membrane, changing the cell wall permeability allowing for leakage of cellular contents

**Local Anesthetic/Vasoconstrictor Precautions** No information available to require special precautions

**Effects on Dental Treatment** No effects or complications reported

**Other Adverse Effects**

1% to 10%: Gastrointestinal: Nausea, vomiting, diarrhea, abdominal pain

<1%:

Dermatologic: Contact dermatitis, Stevens-Johnson syndrome

Miscellaneous: Hypersensitivity reactions

**Contraindications** Hypersensitivity to nystatin or any component

**Drug Interactions** No data reported

**Drug Uptake**

Onset of symptomatic relief from candidiasis: Within 24-72 hours

Absorption: Not absorbed through mucous membranes or intact skin; poorly absorbed from GI tract

**Pregnancy Risk Factor** B/C (oral)

**Breast-feeding Considerations** Compatible (not absorbed orally)

**Dosage Forms**

Cream: 100,000 units/g (15 g, 30 g)

Ointment, topical: 100,000 units/g (15 g, 30 g)

Powder, for preparation of oral suspension: 50 million units, 1 billion units, 2 billion units, 5 billion units

Powder, topical: 100,000 units/g (15 g)

Suspension, oral: 100,000 units/mL (5 mL, 60 mL, 480 mL)

Tablet:

Oral: 500,000 units

Vaginal: 100,000 units (15 and 30/box with applicator)

Troche: 200,000 units

**Dietary Considerations** No data reported

**Generic Available** Yes

## Nystatin and Triamcinolone (nye STAT in & trye am SIN oh lone)

**Related Information**

Oral Fungal Infections *on page 1134*

**U.S. Brand Names** Mycogen II Topical; Mycolog®-II Topical; Myconel® Topical; Myco-Triacet® II; Mytrex® F Topical; N.G.T.® Topical; Tri-Statin® II Topical

**Therapeutic Category** Antifungal Agent, Topical; Corticosteroid, Topical (Medium Potency)

**Use** Treatment of cutaneous candidiasis

**Usual Dosage** Children and Adults: Topical: Apply sparingly 2-4 times/day

**Mechanism of Action** Nystatin is an antifungal agent that binds to sterols in fungal cell membrane, changing the cell wall permeability allowing for leakage of cellular contents. Triamcinolone is a synthetic corticosteroid; it decreases inflammation by suppression of migration of polymorphonuclear leukocytes and reversal of increased capillary permeability. It suppresses the immune system reducing activity and volume of the lymphatic system. It suppresses adrenal function at high doses.

**Local Anesthetic/Vasoconstrictor Precautions** No information available to require special precautions

**Effects on Dental Treatment** No effects or complications reported

**Other Adverse Effects** 1% to 10%:

Dermatologic: Dryness, folliculitis, hypertrichosis, acne, hypopigmentation, allergic dermatitis, maceration of the skin, skin atrophy

Local: Burning, itching, irritation

Miscellaneous: Increased incidence of secondary infection

**Contraindications** Known hypersensitivity to nystatin or triamcinolone

**Warnings/Precautions** Avoid use of occlusive dressings; limit therapy to least amount necessary for effective therapy, pediatric patients may be more susceptible to HPA axis suppression due to larger BSA to weight ratio

**Drug Interactions** No data reported

**Pregnancy Risk Factor** C

**Breast-feeding Considerations**

Nystatin: Compatible

Triamcinolone: No data reported

(Continued)

## Nystatin and Triamcinolone *(Continued)*

**Dosage Forms**

Cream: Nystatin 100,000 units and triamcinolone acetonide 0.1% (15 g, 30 g, 45 g, 60 g, 240 g)

Ointment, topical: Nystatin 100,000 units and triamcinolone acetonide 0.1% (15 g, 30 g, 60 g, 120 g)

**Generic Available** Yes


- **Nystex®** *see* Nystatin *on page 734*
- **Nytol® Oral [OTC]** *see* Diphenhydramine *on page 338*
- **Occlusal®-HP Liquid** *see* Salicylic Acid *on page 900*
- **Occupational Exposure to Bloodborne Pathogens (Universal Precautions)** *see page 1232*
- **Ocean Nasal Mist [OTC]** *see* Sodium Chloride *on page 920*
- **OCL®** *see* Polyethylene Glycol-Electrolyte Solution *on page 815*
- **Octamide® PFS** *see* Metoclopramide *on page 664*
- **Octicair® Otic** *see* Neomycin, Polymyxin B, and Hydrocortisone *on page 712*
- **Octocaine®** *see* Lidocaine *on page 586*
- **Octocaine® 50** *see* Lidocaine and Epinephrine *on page 587*
- **Octocaine® 100** *see* Lidocaine and Epinephrine *on page 587*


## Octreotide Acetate (ok TREE oh tide AS e tate)

**U.S. Brand Names** Sandostatin®; Sandostatin LAR®

**Therapeutic Category** Antisecretory Agent; Somatostatin Analog

**Use** Control of symptoms in patients with metastatic carcinoid and vasoactive intestinal peptide-secreting tumors (VIPomas); acromegaly, insulinomas, Zollinger-Ellison syndrome, pancreatic tumors, gastrinoma, postgastrectomy dumping syndrome, bleeding esophageal varices, small bowel fistulas, AIDS-associated secretory diarrhea, chemotherapy-induced diarrhea, GVHD-induced diarrhea, control of bleeding of esophageal varices; depot suspension is indicated for long term maintenance therapy in acromegalic patients for whom medical treatment is appropriate and who have been shown to respond to and can tolerate the injection; reduction of growth hormone and IGF-1 in acromegaly, suppression of severe diarrhea and flushing associated with malignant carcinoid syndrome, and for the treatment of profuse water diarrhea associated with VIPoma (vasoactive intestinal peptide tumor).

**Usual Dosage** Adults: S.C.:

Acromegaly: Patients not currently receiving octreotide acetate should begin therapy with the regular injection given subcutaneously in an initial dose of 50 mcg 3 times/day. Beginning with this low dose may permit adaptation adverse gastrointestinal effects for patients who require higher doses. Multiple growth hormone (GH) determinations at 0-8 hours after a subcutaneous injection will guide dosage titration. The goal is to attempt to normalize GH and IGF-I (somatomedin C) levels. Most patients require doses of 100-200 mcg 3 times/day for maximum effect but some patients require up to 500 mcg 3 times/day; injection sites should be rotated in a systematic manner to avoid irritation patients currently receiving the regular injection can be switched directly to the depot in a dose of 20 mg given I.M. intragluteally at 4-week intervals for 3 months. (Deltoid injections are to be avoided because of significant discomfort at the injection site when given in that area. Gluteal injection sites should be alternated to avoid irritation.)

Carcinoid: S.C.:100-600 mcg/day in 2-4 divided doses

VIPomas: S.C.: 200-300 mcg/day in 2-4 divided doses

Diarrhea: Initial: I.V.: 50-100 mcg every 8 hours; increase by 100 mcg/dose at 48-hour intervals; maximum dose: 500 mcg every 8 hours

Esophageal varices bleeding: I.V. bolus: 25-50 mcg followed by continuous I.V. infusion of 25-50 mcg/hour

**Mechanism of Action** Mimics natural somatostatin by inhibiting serotonin release, and the secretion of gastrin, VIP, insulin, glucagon, secretin, motilin, and pancreatic polypeptide

**Local Anesthetic/Vasoconstrictor Precautions** No information available to require special precautions

**Effects on Dental Treatment** No effects or complications reported

**Other Adverse Effects**

1% to 10%:

Cardiovascular: Flushing, edema

Central nervous system: Headache, dizziness, fatigue

Endocrine & metabolic: Hyperglycemia, hypoglycemia

Gastrointestinal: Nausea, diarrhea, abdominal pain, vomiting, fat malabsorption

Local: Pain at injection site

Neuromuscular & skeletal: Weakness
<1%:
Cardiovascular: Chest pain
Central nervous system: Anxiety, fever
Dermatologic: Erythema, alopecia, rash
Endocrine & metabolic: Galactorrhea
Gastrointestinal: Constipation, flatulence, throat discomfort
Hepatic: Hepatitis
Respiratory: Dyspnea, rhinorrhea
Ocular: Burning eyes
Neuromuscular & skeletal: Leg cramps, Bell's palsy

**Drug Uptake**
Duration of action: 6-12 hours
Absorption:
Oral: Absorbed but still under study
S.C.: Rapid
Serum half-life: 60-110 minutes

**Pregnancy Risk Factor** B

**Generic Available** No

**Comments** Doses of 1-10 mcg/kg every 12 hours have been used in children beginning at the low end of the range and increasing by 0.3 mcg/kg/dose at 3-day intervals; suppression of growth hormone (animal data) is of concern when used as long-term therapy

- **Ocu-Carpine®** *see* Pilocarpine *on page 802*
- **OcuClear® Ophthalmic [OTC]** *see* Oxymetazoline *on page 755*
- **OcuCoat® Ophthalmic Solution [OTC]** *see* Artificial Tears *on page 97*
- **OcuCoat® PF Ophthalmic Solution [OTC]** *see* Artificial Tears *on page 97*
- **Ocuflox™** *see* Ofloxacin *on this page*
- **Ocupress®** *see* Carteolol *on page 194*
- **Ocusert® Pilo** *see* Pilocarpine *on page 802*
- **Ocusert Pilo-20®** *see* Pilocarpine *on page 802*
- **Ocusert Pilo-40®** *see* Pilocarpine *on page 802*
- **Ocusulf-10® Ophthalmic** *see* Sulfacetamide Sodium *on page 939*
- **Ocutricin® Topical Ointment** *see* Bacitracin, Neomycin, and Polymyxin B *on page 118*
- **Off-Ezy® Wart Remover [OTC]** *see* Salicylic Acid *on page 900*

## Ofloxacin (oh FLOKS a sin)

**Related Information**
Nonviral Infectious Diseases *on page 1095*

**U.S. Brand Names** Floxin® Oral; Floxin® Otic; Ocuflox™

**Therapeutic Category** Antibiotic, Quinolone

**Use** Quinolone antibiotic for skin and skin structure, lower respiratory and urinary tract infections, and sexually transmitted diseases, bacterial conjunctivitis caused by susceptible organisms; for the ear, otitis externa; acute otitis media in children 1-12 years of age with tympanostomy tubes; chronic suppurative otitis media in children ≥12 years of age with perforated tympanic membranes

**Usual Dosage**
Children >1 year and Adults: Ophthalmic: Instill 1-2 drops in affected eye(s) every 2-4 hours for the first 2 days, then use 4 times/day for an additional 5 days
Adults: Oral, I.V.: 200-400 mg every 12 hours for 7-10 days for most infections or for 6 weeks for prostatitis
Children >1 year and Adults: Otic: 5 or 10 drops, respectively, twice daily

**Mechanism of Action** Ofloxacin, a fluorinated quinolone, is a pyridine carboxylic acid derivative which exerts a broad spectrum bactericidal effect. It inhibits DNA gyrase, an essential bacterial enzyme that maintains the superhelical structure of DNA. DNA gyrase is required for DNA replication and transcription, DNA repair, recombination, and transposition within the bacteria.

**Local Anesthetic/Vasoconstrictor Precautions** No information available to require special precautions

**Effects on Dental Treatment** No effects or complications reported

**Other Adverse Effects**
>10%: Gastrointestinal: Nausea
1% to 10%:
Cardiovascular: Chest pain
Central nervous system: Headache, insomnia, dizziness, fatigue, somnolence, sleep disorders, nervousness, pyrexia
Dermatologic: External genital pruritus in women, rash, pruritus
Gastrointestinal: Diarrhea, vomiting, GI distress, pain and cramps, flatulence, dysgeusia, dry mouth, decreased appetite
(Continued)

## Ofloxacin *(Continued)*

Genitourinary: Vaginitis
Neuromuscular & skeletal: Trunk pain
Ocular: Superinfection (ophthalmic), photophobia, lacrimation, dry eyes, stinging, visual disturbances

<1%:

Cardiovascular: Syncope, edema, hypertension, palpitations, vasodilation
Central nervous system: Anxiety, cognitive change, depression, dream abnormality, euphoria, hallucinations, vertigo, chills, malaise, extremity pain
Gastrointestinal: Thirst, weight loss
Neuromuscular & skeletal: Paresthesia, weakness
Ocular: Photophobia
Otic: Decreased hearing acuity, tinnitus
Respiratory: Cough

**Drug Interactions**

Decreased effect: decreased absorption with antacids containing aluminum, magnesium, and/or calcium (by up to 98% if given at the same time)

Increased toxicity/serum levels: Quinolones cause increased caffeine, warfarin, cyclosporine, and theophylline levels; azlocillin, cimetidine, probenecid increase quinolone levels

**Drug Uptake**

Absorption: Well absorbed; administration with food causes only minor alterations in absorption

Serum half-life, elimination 5-7.5 hours

**Pregnancy Risk Factor** C

**Generic Available** No

- **Ogen®** *see* Estropipate *on page 394*
- **OGMT** *see* Metyrosine *on page 669*
- **OKT3** *see* Muromonab-CD3 *on page 692*

## Olanzapine (oh LAN za peen)

**U.S. Brand Names** Zyprexa™

**Therapeutic Category** Antipsychotic Agent

**Use** Treatment of manifestations of psychotic disorders

**Usual Dosage** Adults: Oral: Usual starting dose: 5-10 mg/day, given in a once-a-day dosing schedule; up to a maximum of 20 mg/day

**Mechanism of Action** Olanzapine is a thienobenzodiazepine neuroleptic; thought to work by antagonizing dopamine and serotonin activities. It is a selective monoaminergic antagonist with high affinity binding to serotonin $5HT2_A$ and $5HT2_C$, dopamine $D_{1-4}$, muscarinic $M_{1-5}$, histamine $H_1$ and alpha$_1$-adrenergic receptor sites.

**Local Anesthetic/Vasoconstrictor Precautions** No information available to require special precautions

**Effects on Dental Treatment** No effects or complications reported

**Other Adverse Effects**

>10%: Central nervous system: Headache, somnolence, insomnia, agitation, nervousness, hostility, dizziness

1% to 10%:

Central nervous system: Dystonic reactions, Parkinsonian events, akathisia, anxiety, personality changes, fever
Gastrointestinal: Xerostomia, constipation, abdominal pain, weight gain
Neuromuscular & skeletal: Arthralgia
Ocular: Amblyopia
Respiratory: Rhinitis, cough, pharyngitis

<1%:

Cardiovascular: Peripheral edema
Central nervous system: Tardive dyskinesia, neuroleptic malignant syndrome

**Drug Interactions**

Decreased effect: Cigarette smoking, levodopa, pergolide, bromocriptine, charcoal, and reduction of effects may be seen with cytochrome P-450 enzyme inducers such as rifampin, omeprazole, carbamazepine

Increased effect: Effects may be potentiated with cytochrome P-450 $1A_2$ inhibitors such as fluvoxamine

Increased toxicity: Increased sedation with alcohol or other CNS depressants, increased risk of hypotension and orthostatic hypotension with antihypertensives

**Drug Uptake**

Absorption: Well absorbed; not affected by food

Peak concentrations: ~6 hours

Half-life: 21-54 hours; approximately 1.5 times greater in elderly

**Pregnancy Risk Factor** C

**Dosage Forms** Tablet: 5 mg, 7.5 mg, 10 mg

**Comments** Olanzapine (Zyprexa™) is chemically similar to clozapine (Clozaril®), but without as many side effects. Also, olanzapine (Zyprexa™) does not produce side effects such as Parkinson's disease-like tremors which are associated with other antipsychotics such as haloperidol.

## Olopatadine (oh LOP ah tah deen)

**U.S. Brand Names** Patanol®

**Therapeutic Category** Antihistamine

**Use** Allergic conjunctivitis

**Usual Dosage** Adults: Ophthalmic: One drop in affected eye(s) every 6-8 hours (2 times daily)

**Local Anesthetic/Vasoconstrictor Precautions** No information available to require special precautions

**Effects on Dental Treatment** No effects or complications reported

**Pregnancy Risk Factor** C

**Dosage Forms** Solution, ophthalmic: 0.1% (5 mL)

## Olsalazine (ole SAL a zeen)

**U.S. Brand Names** Dipentum®

**Therapeutic Category** 5-Aminosalicylic Acid Derivative; Anti-inflammatory Agent

**Use** Maintenance of remission of ulcerative colitis in patients intolerant to sulfasalazine

**Usual Dosage** Adults: Oral: 1 g/day in 2 divided doses

**Mechanism of Action** The mechanism of action appears to be topical rather than systemic

**Local Anesthetic/Vasoconstrictor Precautions** No information available to require special precautions

**Effects on Dental Treatment** No effects or complications reported

**Other Adverse Effects**

>10%: Gastrointestinal: Diarrhea, cramps, abdominal pain

1% to 10%:

- Central nervous system: Headache, fatigue, depression
- Dermatologic: Rash, itching
- Gastrointestinal: Nausea, dyspepsia, bloating, anorexia
- Neuromuscular & skeletal: Arthralgia

<1%:

- Central nervous system: Fever
- Gastrointestinal: Bloody diarrhea
- Hematologic: Blood dyscrasias
- Hepatic: Hepatitis

**Drug Interactions** No data reported

**Drug Uptake**

Absorption: <3%; very little intact olsalazine is systemically absorbed

Serum half-life, elimination: 56 minutes or 55 hours depending on the analysis used

**Pregnancy Risk Factor** C

**Dosage Forms** Capsule, as sodium: 250 mg

**Generic Available** No

## Omeprazole (oh ME pray zol)

**U.S. Brand Names** Prilosec™

**Canadian Brand Names** Losec®

**Therapeutic Category** Gastric Acid Secretion Inhibitor

**Use** Short-term (4-8 weeks) treatment of severe erosive esophagitis (grade 2 or above), diagnosed by endoscopy and short-term treatment of symptomatic gastroesophageal reflux disease (GERD) poorly responsive to customary medical treatment; pathological hypersecretory conditions; peptic ulcer disease; eradication of *H. pylori* in patients with duodenal ulcer disease

**Unlabeled use:** Gastric ulcer therapy and healing NSAID-induced ulcers

**Usual Dosage** Adults: Oral:

Active duodenal ulcer: 20 mg/day for 4-8 weeks

GERD or severe erosive esophagitis: 20 mg/day for 4-8 weeks

Pathological hypersecretory conditions: 60 mg once daily to start; doses up to 120 mg 3 times/day have been administered; administer daily doses >80 mg in divided doses

(Continued)

## Omeprazole *(Continued)*

*Helicobacter pylori*: Combination therapy with bismuth subsalicylate, tetracycline, clarithromycin, and $H_2$ antagonist; or clarithromycin and omeprazole. Adult dose: Oral: 20 mg twice daily

Gastric ulcers: 40 mg/day for 4-8 weeks

**Mechanism of Action** Suppresses gastric acid secretion by inhibiting the parietal cell H+/K+ ATP pump

**Local Anesthetic/Vasoconstrictor Precautions** No information available to require special precautions

**Effects on Dental Treatment** No effects or complications reported

**Other Adverse Effects**

1% to 10%:

Cardiovascular: Angina, tachycardia, bradycardia, edema
Central nervous system: Headache (7%), dizziness
Dermatologic: Rash, urticaria, pruritus, dry skin
Gastrointestinal: Diarrhea, nausea, abdominal pain, vomiting, constipation, anorexia, irritable colon, fecal discoloration, esophageal candidiasis, dry mouth, taste alterations
Genitourinary: Testicular pain, urinary tract infection
Neuromuscular & skeletal: Back pain, muscle cramps, myalgia, arthralgia, leg pain, weakness
Renal: Pyuria, proteinuria, hematuria, glycosuria, polyuria
Respiratory: Cough

<1%:

Cardiovascular: Chest pain
Central nervous system: Fever, fatigue, malaise, apathy, somnolence, nervousness, anxiety, pain
Gastrointestinal: Abdominal swelling

**Drug Interactions**

Cytochrome P-450 1A2 enzyme inducer and cytochrome P-450 IIC enzyme inhibitor

Decreased effect: Decreased ketoconazole; decreased itraconazole because of reduced absorption from gastrointestinal tract

Increased toxicity: Diazepam causes increased half-life; increased digoxin, increased phenytoin, increased warfarin

**Drug Uptake**

Onset of antisecretory action: Oral: Within 1 hour
Duration: 72 hours
Serum half-life: 30-90 minutes

**Pregnancy Risk Factor** C

**Dosage Forms** Capsule, delayed release: 10 mg, 20 mg, 40 mg

**Generic Available** No


- **Omnicef**® *see* Cefdinir *on page 200*
- **OmniHIB**™ *see Haemophilus* b Conjugate Vaccine *on page 486*
- **Omnipen**® *see* Ampicillin *on page 81*
- **Omnipen®-N** *see* Ampicillin *on page 81*
- **OMS® Oral** *see* Morphine Sulfate *on page 688*
- **Oncaspar**® *see* Pegaspargase *on page 769*
- **Oncet**® *see* Hydrocodone and Homatropine *on page 508*
- **Oncovin® Injection** *see* Vincristine *on page 1046*


## Ondansetron (on DAN se tron)

**U.S. Brand Names** Zofran®

**Therapeutic Category** Antiemetic; Selective 5-$HT_3$ Receptor Antagonist

**Use** May be prescribed for patients who are refractory to or have severe adverse reactions to standard antiemetic therapy. Ondansetron may be prescribed for young patients (ie, <45 years of age who are more likely to develop extrapyramidal reactions to high-dose metoclopramide) who are to receive highly emetogenic chemotherapeutic agents as listed:

Agents with high emetogenic potential (>90%) (dose/$m^2$):

Carmustine ≥200 mg
Cisplatin ≥75 mg
Cyclophosphamide ≥1000 mg
Cytarabine ≥1000 mg
Dacarbazine ≥500 mg
Ifosfamide ≥1000 mg
Lomustine ≥60 mg
Mechlorethamine
Pentostatin

Streptozocin

**or** two agents classified as having high or moderately high emetogenic potential as listed:

Agents with moderately high emetogenic potential (60% to 90%) (dose/$m^2$):
- Carmustine <200 mg
- Cisplatin <75 mg
- Cyclophosphamide 1000 mg
- Cytarabine 250-1000 mg
- Dacarbazine <500 mg
- Doxorubicin ≥75 mg
- Ifosfamide
- Lomustine <60 mg
- Methotrexate ≥250 mg
- Mitomycin
- Mitoxantrone
- Procarbazine

Ondansetron should not be prescribed for chemotherapeutic agents with a low emetogenic potential (eg, bleomycin, busulfan, cyclophosphamide <1000 mg, etoposide, 5-fluorouracil, vinblastine, vincristine)

**Usual Dosage**

Oral:
- Children 4-11 years: 4 mg 30 minutes before chemotherapy; repeat 4 and 8 hours after initial dose
- Children >11 years and Adults: 8 mg 30 minutes before chemotherapy; repeat 4 and 8 hours after initial dose or every 8 hours for a maximum of 48 hours

I.V.: Administer either three 0.15 mg/kg doses or a single 32 mg dose; with the 3-dose regimen, the initial dose is given 30 minutes prior to chemotherapy with subsequent doses administered 4 and 8 hours after the first dose. With the single-dose regimen 32 mg is infused over 15 minutes beginning 30 minutes before the start of emetogenic chemotherapy. Dosage should be calculated based on weight:
- Children: Pediatric dosing should follow the manufacturer's guidelines for 0.15 mg/kg/dose administered 30 minutes prior to chemotherapy, 4 and 8 hours after the first dose. While not as yet FDA-approved, literature supports the day's total dose administered as a single dose 30 minutes prior to chemotherapy.
- Adults:
  - >80 kg: 12 mg IVPB
  - 45-80 kg: 8 mg IVPB
  - <45 kg: 0.15 mg/kg/dose IVPB

**Mechanism of Action** Selective 5-$HT_3$ receptor antagonist, blocking serotonin, both peripherally on vagal nerve terminals and centrally in the chemoreceptor trigger zone

**Local Anesthetic/Vasoconstrictor Precautions** No information available to require special precautions

**Effects on Dental Treatment** No effects or complications reported

**Other Adverse Effects**

>10%:
- Central nervous system: Headache, fever
- Gastrointestinal: Constipation, diarrhea

1% to 10%:
- Central nervous system: Dizziness
- Gastrointestinal: Abdominal cramps, dry mouth
- Neuromuscular & skeletal: Weakness

<1%:
- Cardiovascular: Tachycardia
- Central nervous system: Lightheadedness, seizures
- Dermatologic: Rash
- Endocrine & metabolic: Hypokalemia
- Hepatic: Transient elevations in serum levels of aminotransferases and bilirubin
- Respiratory: Bronchospasm, dyspnea, wheezing

**Drug Interactions**

Decreased effect: Metabolized by the hepatic cytochrome P-450 enzymes; therefore, the drug's clearance and half-life may be changed with concomitant use of cytochrome P-450 inducers (eg, barbiturates, carbamazepine, rifampin, phenytoin, and phenylbutazone)

Increased toxicity: Inhibitors (eg, cimetidine, allopurinol, and disulfiram)

**Drug Uptake** Serum half-life:
- Children <15 years: 2-3 hours
- Adults: 4 hours

(Continued)

## Ondansetron *(Continued)*

**Pregnancy Risk Factor** B

**Generic Available** No

- **Ony-Clear® Nail** *see* Triacetin *on page 1009*
- **Ony-Clear® Spray** *see* Miconazole *on page 672*
- **OP-CCK** *see* Sincalide *on page 916*
- **Opcon® Ophthalmic** *see* Naphazoline *on page 703*
- **o,p'-DDD** *see* Mitotane *on page 681*
- **Ophthalgan® Ophthalmic** *see* Glycerin *on page 472*
- **Ophthetic®** *see* Proparacaine *on page 852*
- **Ophthochlor®** *see* Chloramphenicol *on page 222*
- **Ophthocort® Ophthalmic** *see* Chloramphenicol, Polymyxin B, and Hydrocortisone *on page 223*

## Opium Alkaloids (OH pee um AL ka loyds)

**U.S. Brand Names** Pantopon®

**Therapeutic Category** Analgesic, Narcotic

**Use** For relief of severe pain

**Usual Dosage** Adults: I.M., S.C.: 5-20 mg every 4-5 hours

**Local Anesthetic/Vasoconstrictor Precautions** No information available to require special precautions

**Effects on Dental Treatment** 1% to 10% of patients will experience significant dry mouth

**Other Adverse Effects**

>10%:

Cardiovascular: Hypotension
Central nervous system: Fatigue, drowsiness, dizziness
Gastrointestinal: Nausea, vomiting
Neuromuscular & skeletal: Weakness

1% to 10%:

Central nervous system: Nervousness, headache, confusion restlessness, malaise
Gastrointestinal: Anorexia, stomach cramps, dry mouth, constipation, biliary tract spasm
Genitourinary: Ureteral spasms, decreased urination
Local: Pain at injection site
Respiratory: Dyspnea

<1%:

Central nervous system: Mental depression, paradoxical CNS stimulation, hallucinations, increased intracranial pressure
Dermatologic: Skin rash, urticaria
Gastrointestinal: Paralytic ileus
Miscellaneous: Histamine release, physical and psychological dependence

**Pregnancy Risk Factor** B (D if used for prolonged periods or in high doses at term)

**Generic Available** Yes

**Comments** Abrupt discontinuation after sustained use (generally >10 days) may cause withdrawal symptoms

## Opium Tincture (OH pee um TING chur)

**Therapeutic Category** Analgesic, Narcotic; Antidiarrheal

**Use** Treatment of diarrhea or relief of pain

**Usual Dosage** Oral:

Children:

Diarrhea: 0.005-0.01 mL/kg/dose every 3-4 hours for a maximum of 6 doses/24 hours
Analgesia: 0.01-0.02 mL/kg/dose every 3-4 hours

Adults:

Diarrhea: 0.3-1 mL/dose every 2-6 hours to maximum of 6 mL/24 hours
Analgesia: 0.6-1.5 mL/dose every 3-4 hours

**Mechanism of Action** Contains many narcotic alkaloids including morphine; its mechanism for gastric motility inhibition is primarily due to this morphine content; it results in a decrease in digestive secretions, an increase in GI muscle tone, and therefore a reduction in GI propulsion

**Local Anesthetic/Vasoconstrictor Precautions** No information available to require special precautions

**Effects on Dental Treatment** No effects or complications reported

**Other Adverse Effects**

>10%:

Cardiovascular: Palpitations, hypotension, bradycardia

Central nervous system: Drowsiness, dizziness
Neuromuscular & skeletal: Weakness

1% to 10%:

Central nervous system: Restlessness, headache, malaise
Genitourinary: Decreased urination
Miscellaneous: Histamine release

<1%:

Cardiovascular: Peripheral vasodilation
Central nervous system: CNS depression, increased intracranial pressure, insomnia, mental depression
Gastrointestinal: Nausea, vomiting, constipation, anorexia, stomach cramps, biliary spasm
Genitourinary: Urinary tract spasm
Ocular: Miosis
Respiratory: Respiratory depression
Miscellaneous: Physical and psychological dependence

**Drug Interactions**

Decreased effect: Phenothiazines may antagonize the analgesic effect of opiate agonists

Increased toxicity: CNS depressants, MAO inhibitors, tricyclic antidepressants may potentiate the effects of opiate agonists; dextroamphetamine may enhance the analgesic effect of opiate agonists

**Drug Uptake**

Duration of effect: 4-5 hours
Absorption: Variable from GI tract

**Pregnancy Risk Factor** B (D if used for prolonged periods or in high doses at term)

**Generic Available** No

## Oprelvekin (oh PREL ve kin)

**U.S. Brand Names** Neumega®

**Therapeutic Category** Hematopoietic Growth Factor

**Synonyms** IL-11; Interleukin-11; Recombinant Human Interleukin-11; Recombinant Interleukin-11; rhIL-11; rIL-11

**Use** Prevention and treatment of severe thrombocytopenia following myelosuppressive chemotherapy

**Usual Dosage** Refer to individual protocols

Children: 75-100 mcg/kg/day for 10-21 days (until platelet count >50,000/mm$^3$)
Adults: 50 mcg/kg/day for 10-21 days (until platelet count >50,000/mm$^3$)

**Mechanism of Action** Oprelvekin stimulates multiple stages of megakaryocytopoiesis and thrombopoiesis, resulting in proliferation of megakaryocyte progenitors and megakaryocyte maturation

**Local Anesthetic/Vasoconstrictor Precautions** No information available to require special precautions

**Effects on Dental Treatment** No effects or complications reported

**Other Adverse Effects**

>10%:

Cardiovascular: Tachycardia (19% to 30%), palpitations (14% to 24%), atrial arrhythmias (12%), peripheral edema (60% to 75%)
Central nervous system: Headache (41%), dizziness (38%), insomnia (33%), fatigue (30%), fever, (36%)
Dermatologic: Rash (25%)
Endocrine & metabolic: Fluid retention
Gastrointestinal: Nausea (50% to 77%), vomiting, anorexia
Hematologic: Anemia (100%), probably a dilutional phenomena; appears within 3 days of initiation of therapy, resolves in about 2 weeks after cessation of oprelvekin
Neuromuscular & skeletal: Arthralgia, myalgias
Respiratory: Dyspnea (48%), pleural effusions (10%)

1% to 10%:

Cardiovascular: Syncope (6% to 13%)
Gastrointestinal: Weight gain (5%)

**Drug Uptake**

Half-life: Terminal: 5-8 hours
Time to peak serum concentration: 1-6 hours

**Generic Available** No

♦ **Opticyl®** *see* Tropicamide *on page 1029*
♦ **Optigene® Ophthalmic [OTC]** *see* Tetrahydrozoline *on page 967*
♦ **Optimine®** *see* Azatadine *on page 111*
♦ **Optimoist® Solution [OTC]** *see* Saliva Substitute *on page 901*
♦ **OptiPranolol®** *see* Metipranolol *on page 664*

- ♦ **OPV** *see* Poliovirus Vaccine, Live, Trivalent, Oral *on page 813*
- ♦ **Orabase®-B [OTC]** *see* Benzocaine *on page 128*
- ♦ **Orabase® HCA** *see* Hydrocortisone *on page 511*
- ♦ **Orabase®-O [OTC]** *see* Benzocaine *on page 128*
- ♦ **Orabase® Plain [OTC]** *see* Gelatin, Pectin, and Methylcellulose *on page 464*
- ♦ **Orabase® With Benzocaine [OTC]** *see* Benzocaine, Gelatin, Pectin, and Sodium Carboxymethylcellulose *on page 129*
- ♦ **Oracit®** *see* Sodium Citrate and Citric Acid *on page 921*
- ♦ **Orajel® Brace-Aid Oral Anesthetic [OTC]** *see* Benzocaine *on page 128*
- ♦ **Orajel® Maximum Strength [OTC]** *see* Benzocaine *on page 128*
- ♦ **Orajel® Mouth-Aid [OTC]** *see* Benzocaine *on page 128*
- ♦ **Orajel® Perioseptic® [OTC]** *see* Carbamide Peroxide *on page 186*
- ♦ **Oral Bacterial Infections** *see page 1128*
- ♦ **Oral Fungal Infections** *see page 1134*
- ♦ **Oral Nonviral Soft Tissue Ulcerations or Erosions** *see page 1141*
- ♦ **Oral Pain** *see page 1122*
- ♦ **Oral Rinse Products** *see page 1257*
- ♦ **Oral Viral Infections** *see page 1137*
- ♦ **Oramorph SR™ Oral** *see* Morphine Sulfate *on page 688*
- ♦ **Orap™** *see* Pimozide *on page 805*
- ♦ **Orasept® [OTC]** *see* Benzocaine *on page 128*
- ♦ **Orasol® [OTC]** *see* Benzocaine *on page 128*
- ♦ **Orasone®** *see* Prednisone *on page 833*
- ♦ **Orazinc® [OTC]** *see* Zinc Supplements *on page 1062*
- ♦ **Orazinc® Oral [OTC]** *see* Zinc Sulfate *on page 1062*
- ♦ **Ordrine AT® Extended Release Capsule** *see* Caramiphen and Phenylpropanolamine *on page 184*
- ♦ **Oretic®** *see* Hydrochlorothiazide *on page 503*
- ♦ **Oreton® Methyl** *see* Methyltestosterone *on page 662*
- ♦ **Orexin® [OTC]** *see* Vitamin B Complex *on page 1050*
- ♦ **Organidin®** *see* Iodinated Glycerol *on page 545*
- ♦ **Organidin® NR** *see* Guaifenesin *on page 478*
- ♦ **Orgaran®** *see* Danaparoid *on page 295*
- ♦ **Orimune®** *see* Poliovirus Vaccine, Live, Trivalent, Oral *on page 813*
- ♦ **Orinase®** *see* Tolbutamide *on page 994*
- ♦ **ORLAAM®** *see* Levomethadyl Acetate Hydrochloride *on page 583*
- ♦ **Ormazine** *see* Chlorpromazine *on page 238*
- ♦ **Ornade® Spansule®** *see* Chlorpheniramine and Phenylpropanolamine *on page 233*
- ♦ **Ornex® No Drowsiness [OTC]** *see* Acetaminophen and Pseudoephedrine *on page 31*
- ♦ **Ornidyl® Injection** *see* Eflornithine *on page 365*

## Orphenadrine (or FEN a dreen)

**Related Information**

Temporomandibular Dysfunction (TMD) *on page 1149*

**U.S. Brand Names** Norflex™

**Therapeutic Category** Muscle Relaxant; Skeletal Muscle Relaxant

**Use** Treatment of muscle spasm associated with acute painful musculoskeletal conditions; supportive therapy in tetanus

**Usual Dosage** Adults:

Oral: 100 mg twice daily

I.M., I.V.: 60 mg every 12 hours

**Mechanism of Action** Indirect skeletal muscle relaxant thought to work by central atropine-like effects; has some euphorgenic and analgesic properties

**Local Anesthetic/Vasoconstrictor Precautions** No information available to require special precautions

**Effects on Dental Treatment** The peripheral anticholinergic effects of orphenadrine may decrease or inhibit salivary flow; normal salivation will return with cessation of drug therapy

**Other Adverse Effects**

>10%:

Central nervous system: Drowsiness, dizziness

Ocular: Blurred vision

1% to 10%:

Cardiovascular: Flushing of face, tachycardia, syncope

Dermatologic: Skin rash

Gastrointestinal: Nausea, vomiting, constipation

Genitourinary: Decreased urination
Neuromuscular & skeletal: Weakness
Ocular: Nystagmus, increased intraocular pressure
Respiratory: Nasal congestion

<1%:

Central nervous system: Hallucinations
Hematologic: Aplastic anemia

**Drug Interactions** No data reported

**Drug Uptake**

Duration: 4-6 hours
Serum half-life: 14-16 hours

**Pregnancy Risk Factor** C

**Generic Available** Yes

## Orphenadrine, Aspirin, and Caffeine

(or FEN a dreen, AS pir in, & KAF een)

**U.S. Brand Names** Norgesic™; Norgesic™ Forte

**Therapeutic Category** Analgesic, Non-narcotic; Muscle Relaxant; Skeletal Muscle Relaxant

**Use** Relief of discomfort associated with skeletal muscular conditions

**Usual Dosage** Oral: 1-2 tablets 3-4 times/day

**Local Anesthetic/Vasoconstrictor Precautions** No information available to require special precautions

**Effects on Dental Treatment** The peripheral anticholinergic effects of orphenadrine may decrease or inhibit salivary flow; normal salivation will return with cessation of drug therapy

**Pregnancy Risk Factor** D

**Generic Available** Yes

- **Ortho-Cept®** *see* Ethinyl Estradiol and Desogestrel *on page 399*
- **Orthoclone® OKT3** *see* Muromonab-CD3 *on page 692*
- **Ortho-Cyclen®** *see* Ethinyl Estradiol and Norgestimate *on page 406*
- **Ortho®-Dienestrol Vaginal** *see* Dienestrol *on page 324*
- **Ortho-Est®** *see* Estropipate *on page 394*
- **Ortho-Novum® 1/35** *see* Ethinyl Estradiol and Norethindrone *on page 404*
- **Ortho-Novum™ 1/50** *see* Mestranol and Norethindrone *on page 639*
- **Ortho-Novum® 7/7/7** *see* Ethinyl Estradiol and Norethindrone *on page 404*
- **Ortho-Novum® 10/11** *see* Ethinyl Estradiol and Norethindrone *on page 404*
- **Ortho Tri-Cyclen®** *see* Ethinyl Estradiol and Norgestimate *on page 406*
- **Or-Tyl® Injection** *see* Dicyclomine *on page 322*
- **Orudis®** *see* Ketoprofen *on page 565*
- **Orudis® KT [OTC]** *see* Ketoprofen *on page 565*
- **Oruvail®** *see* Ketoprofen *on page 565*
- **Os-Cal® 500 [OTC]** *see* Calcium Carbonate *on page 172*
- **Osmoglyn®** *see* Glycerin *on page 472*
- **Osmolite® HN [OTC]** *see* Enteral Nutritional Products *on page 371*
- **Osteocalcin® Injection** *see* Calcitonin *on page 169*
- **Otic-Care® Otic** *see* Neomycin, Polymyxin B, and Hydrocortisone *on page 712*
- **Otic Domeboro®** *see* Aluminum Acetate and Acetic Acid *on page 54*
- **Otobiotic® Otic** *see* Polymyxin B and Hydrocortisone *on page 816*
- **Otocalm® Ear** *see* Antipyrine and Benzocaine *on page 91*
- **Otocort® Otic** *see* Neomycin, Polymyxin B, and Hydrocortisone *on page 712*
- **Otosporin® Otic** *see* Neomycin, Polymyxin B, and Hydrocortisone *on page 712*
- **Otrivin® [OTC]** *see* Xylometazoline *on page 1055*
- **Ovcon® 35** *see* Ethinyl Estradiol and Norethindrone *on page 404*
- **Ovcon® 50** *see* Ethinyl Estradiol and Norethindrone *on page 404*
- **Ovral®** *see* Ethinyl Estradiol and Norgestrel *on page 407*
- **Ovrette®** *see* Norgestrel *on page 731*

## Oxacillin (oks a SIL in)

**U.S. Brand Names** Bactocill®

**Therapeutic Category** Antibiotic, Penicillin

**Use** Treatment of susceptible bacterial infections such as osteomyelitis, septicemia, endocarditis, and CNS infections due to penicillinase-producing strains of *Staphylococcus*

**Usual Dosage**

Children:

Oral: 50-100 mg/kg/day divided every 6 hours

(Continued)

## Oxacillin *(Continued)*

I.M., I.V.: 150-200 mg/kg/day in divided doses every 6 hours; maximum dose: 12 g/day

Adults:

Oral: 500-1000 mg every 4-6 hours for at least 5 days

I.M., I.V.: 250 mg to 2 g/dose every 4-6 hours

**Mechanism of Action** Inhibits bacterial cell wall synthesis by binding to one or more of the penicillin binding proteins (PBPs); which in turn inhibits the final transpeptidation step of peptidoglycan synthesis in bacterial cell walls, thus inhibiting cell wall biosynthesis. Bacteria eventually lyse due to ongoing activity of cell wall autolytic enzymes (autolysins and murein hydrolases) while cell wall assembly is arrested.

**Local Anesthetic/Vasoconstrictor Precautions** No information available to require special precautions

**Effects on Dental Treatment** Prolonged use of penicillins may lead to development of oral candidiasis

**Other Adverse Effects**

1% to 10%: Gastrointestinal: Nausea, diarrhea

<1%:

Central nervous system: Fever

Dermatologic: Rash

Gastrointestinal: Vomiting

Hematologic: Eosinophilia, leukopenia, neutropenia, thrombocytopenia, agranulocytosis

Hepatic: Hepatotoxicity, elevated AST

Renal: Hematuria, acute interstitial nephritis

Miscellaneous: Serum sickness-like reactions

**Drug Interactions**

Decreased effect: Efficacy of oral contraceptives may be reduced

Increased effect: Disulfiram, probenecid causes increased penicillin levels

**Drug Uptake**

Absorption: Oral: 35% to 67%

Serum half-life:

Children 1 week to 2 years: 0.9-1.8 hours

Adults: 23-60 minutes (prolonged with reduced renal function and in neonates)

Time to peak serum concentration:

Oral: Within 2 hours

I.M.: Within 30-60 minutes

**Pregnancy Risk Factor** B

**Generic Available** Yes

## Oxamniquine (oks AM ni kwin)

**U.S. Brand Names** Vansil™

**Therapeutic Category** Anthelmintic

**Use** Treat all stages of *Schistosoma mansoni* infection

**Usual Dosage** Oral:

Children <30 kg: 20 mg/kg in 2 divided doses of 10 mg/kg at 2- to 8-hour intervals

Adults: 12-15 mg/kg as a single dose

**Local Anesthetic/Vasoconstrictor Precautions** No information available to require special precautions

**Effects on Dental Treatment** No effects or complications reported

**Other Adverse Effects**

>10%: Central nervous system: Dizziness, drowsiness, headache

<10%:

Central nervous system: Insomnia, malaise, hallucinations, behavior changes

Dermatologic: Rash, urticaria, pruritus

Gastrointestinal: GI effects

Genitourinary: Urine discoloration (orange/red)

Hepatic: Elevated LFTs

Renal: Proteinuria

**Pregnancy Risk Factor** C

**Generic Available** No

**Comments** Strains other than from the western hemisphere may require higher doses

♦ **Oxandrin®** *see* Oxandrolone *on this page*

## Oxandrolone (oks AN droe lone)

**U.S. Brand Names** Oxandrin®

**Therapeutic Category** Androgen

**Use** Treatment of catabolic or tissue-depleting processes

**Usual Dosage** Adults: Oral: 2.5 mg 2-4 times daily

**Local Anesthetic/Vasoconstrictor Precautions** No information available to require special precautions

**Effects on Dental Treatment** No effects or complications reported

**Other Adverse Effects**

Male:

Postpubertal:

>10%: Bladder irritability, priapism, gynecomastia, acne

1% to 10%: Decreased libido, hepatic dysfunction, chills, nausea, diarrhea, insomnia, iron deficiency anemia, suppression of clotting factors, prostatic hypertrophy (geriatric)

<1%: Hepatic necrosis, hepatocellular carcinoma

Prepubertal: Virilism

>10%: Acne, virilism

1% to 10%: Hyperpigmentation, chills, diarrhea, nausea, insomnia, iron deficiency anemia, suppression of clotting factors

<1%: Hepatic necrosis, hepatocellular carcinoma

Female:

>10%: Virilism

1% to 10%: Hypercalcemia, hepatic dysfunction, nausea, chills, diarrhea, insomnia, iron deficiency anemia, suppression of clotting factors

<1%: Hepatic necrosis, hepatocellular carcinoma

**Pregnancy Risk Factor** X

**Generic Available** No

**Comments** This medication is currently on the market as an Orphan Drug. It is distributed by Gynex Pharmaceuticals, Inc. to physicians who document their expertise in endocrinology and agree to participate in a study to gather data for the FDA.

## Oxaprozin (oks a PROE zin)

**Related Information**

Rheumatoid Arthritis and Osteoarthritis *on page 1092*

**U.S. Brand Names** Daypro™

**Therapeutic Category** Nonsteroidal Anti-inflammatory Drug (NSAID), Oral

**Use** Acute and long-term use in the management of signs and symptoms of osteoarthritis and rheumatoid arthritis

**Usual Dosage** Adults: Oral (individualize dosage to lowest effective dose to minimize adverse effects):

Osteoarthritis: 600-1200 mg once daily

Rheumatoid arthritis: 1200 mg once daily

Maximum dose: 1800 mg/day or 26 mg/kg (whichever is lower) in divided doses

**Mechanism of Action** Inhibits prostaglandin synthesis by decreasing the activity of the enzyme, cyclo-oxygenase, which results in decreased formation of prostaglandin precursors

**Local Anesthetic/Vasoconstrictor Precautions** No information available to require special precautions

**Effects on Dental Treatment** NSAID formulations are known to reversibly decrease platelet aggregation via mechanisms different than observed with aspirin. The dentist should be aware of the potential of abnormal coagulation. Caution should also be exercised in the use of NSAIDs in patients already on anticoagulant therapy with drugs such as warfarin (Coumadin®).

**Other Adverse Effects**

>10%:

Central nervous system: Dizziness

Dermatologic: Skin rash

Gastrointestinal: Abdominal cramps, heartburn, indigestion, nausea

1% to 10%:

Cardiovascular: Angina pectoris, arrhythmia

Central nervous system: Nervousness

Dermatologic: Itching

Gastrointestinal: GI ulceration, vomiting

Genitourinary: Vaginal bleeding

Otic: Tinnitus

<1%:

Cardiovascular: Chest pain, congestive heart failure, hypertension, tachycardia

Central nervous system: Convulsions, forgetfulness, mental depression, drowsiness, insomnia

Dermatologic: Urticaria, exfoliative dermatitis, erythema multiforme, Stevens-Johnson syndrome, angioedema

Gastrointestinal: Stomatitis

Genitourinary: Cystitis

(Continued)

## Oxaprozin *(Continued)*

Hematologic: Agranulocytosis, anemia, pancytopenia, leukopenia, thrombocytopenia
Hepatic: Hepatitis
Neuromuscular & skeletal: Peripheral neuropathy, trembling, weakness
Ocular: Blurred vision, change in vision
Otic: Decreased hearing
Renal: Interstitial nephritis, nephrotic syndrome, renal impairment
Respiratory: Dyspnea, wheezing, laryngeal edema, epistaxis
Miscellaneous: Anaphylaxis, increased sweating

**Drug Interactions** Oxaprozin, like other NSAIDs, may cause increased toxicity of aspirin, oral anticoagulants, diuretics

**Drug Uptake**
Absorption: Almost completely
Serum half-life: 40-50 hours
Time to peak: 2-4 hours

**Pregnancy Risk Factor** C

**Generic Available** No

## Oxazepam (oks A ze pam)

**Related Information**
Patients Requiring Sedation *on page 1152*

**U.S. Brand Names** Serax®

**Canadian Brand Names** Apo®-Oxazepam; Novo-Oxazepam; Oxpam®; PMS-Oxazepam; Zapex®

**Therapeutic Category** Benzodiazepine

**Use** Treatment of anxiety and management of alcohol withdrawal; may also be used as an anticonvulsant in management of simple partial seizures

**Usual Dosage** Oral:
Children: 1 mg/kg/day has been administered
Adults:
Anxiety: 10-30 mg 3-4 times/day
Alcohol withdrawal: 15-30 mg 3-4 times/day
Hypnotic: 15-30 mg

**Mechanism of Action** Benzodiazepine anxiolytic sedative that produces CNS depression at the subcortical level, except at high doses, whereby it works at the cortical level

**Local Anesthetic/Vasoconstrictor Precautions** No information available to require special precautions

**Effects on Dental Treatment** >10% of patients experience dry mouth which disappears with cessation of drug therapy

**Other Adverse Effects**
>10%: Central nervous system: Drowsiness
1% to 10%: Central nervous system: Dizziness, vertigo, headache
<1%:
Cardiovascular: Syncope
Central nervous system: Slurred speech, lethargy, ataxia
Dermatologic: Rash
Endocrine & metabolic: Altered libido
Gastrointestinal: Nausea
Hematologic: Leukopenia
Hepatic: Jaundice
Neuromuscular & skeletal: Tremor

**Drug Interactions** Increased toxicity (CNS depression): Alcohol, tricyclic antidepressants, sedative-hypnotics, MAO inhibitors

**Drug Uptake**
Absorption: Oral: Almost completely
Serum half-life: 2.8-5.7 hours
Time to peak serum concentration: Within 2-4 hours

**Pregnancy Risk Factor** D

**Generic Available** Yes

## Oxiconazole (oks i KON a zole)

**U.S. Brand Names** Oxistat®

**Therapeutic Category** Antifungal Agent, Topical

**Use** Treatment of tinea pedis (athlete's foot), tinea cruris (jock itch), and tinea corporis (ring worm)

**Usual Dosage** Children and Adults: Topical: Apply once to twice daily to affected areas for 2 weeks (tinea corporis/tinea cruris) to 1 month (tinea pedis)

**Mechanism of Action** Inhibition of ergosterol synthesis. Effective for treatment of tinea pedis, tinea cruris, and tinea corporis. Active against *Trichophyton*

*rubrum, Trichophyton mentagrophytes, Trichophyton violaceum, Microsporum canis, Microsporum audouini, Microsporum gypseum, Epidermophyton floccosum, Candida albicans,* and *Malassezia furfur.*

**Local Anesthetic/Vasoconstrictor Precautions** No information available to require special precautions

**Effects on Dental Treatment** No effects or complications reported

**Other Adverse Effects** 1% to 10%: Local: Itching, transient burning, local irritation, stinging, erythema, dryness

**Drug Interactions** No data reported

**Drug Uptake**

Absorption: In each layer of the dermis; very little is absorbed systemically after one topical dose

**Pregnancy Risk Factor** B

**Generic Available** No

- **Oxipor® VHC [OTC]** *see* Coal Tar *on page 270*
- **Oxistat®** *see* Oxiconazole *on previous page*
- **Oxsoralen® Topical** *see* Methoxsalen *on page 655*
- **Oxsoralen-Ultra® Oral** *see* Methoxsalen *on page 655*

## Oxtriphylline (oks TRYE fi lin)

**Related Information**

Respiratory Diseases *on page 1079*

**U.S. Brand Names** Choledyl®

**Therapeutic Category** Antiasthmatic; Bronchodilator; Theophylline Derivative

**Synonyms** Choline Theophyllinate

**Use** Bronchodilator in symptomatic treatment of asthma and reversible bronchospasm

**Usual Dosage** Oral:

Children: 1-9 years: 6.2 mg/kg/dose every 6 hours

Children 9-16 years and Adult smokers: 4.7 mg/kg/dose every 6 hours

Adults: 4.7 mg/kg every 8 hours; sustained release: administer every 12 hours

**Local Anesthetic/Vasoconstrictor Precautions** No information available to require special precautions

**Effects on Dental Treatment** Do not prescribe any erythromycin product to patients taking theophylline products. Erythromycin will delay the normal metabolic inactivation of theophyllines leading to increased blood levels; this has resulted in nausea, vomiting and CNS restlessness

**Other Adverse Effects** Uncommon with theophylline levels <20 mcg/mL

1% to 10%:

Cardiovascular: Tachycardia

Central nervous system: Nervousness, restlessness

Gastrointestinal: Nausea, vomiting

<1%:

Central nervous system: Insomnia, irritability, seizures

Dermatologic: Skin rash

Gastrointestinal: Gastric irritation

Neuromuscular & skeletal: Tremor

Miscellaneous: Allergic reactions

**Pregnancy Risk Factor** C

**Generic Available** Yes

**Comments** Oxtriphylline is 64% theophylline

- **Oxy-5® Advanced Formula for Sensitive Skin [OTC]** *see* Benzoyl Peroxide *on page 130*
- **Oxy-5® Tinted [OTC]** *see* Benzoyl Peroxide *on page 130*
- **Oxy-10® Advanced Formula for Sensitive Skin [OTC]** *see* Benzoyl Peroxide *on page 130*
- **Oxy 10® Wash [OTC]** *see* Benzoyl Peroxide *on page 130*

## Oxybutynin (oks i BYOO ti nin)

**U.S. Brand Names** Ditropan®; Ditropan® XL

**Canadian Brand Names** Albert® Oxybutynin

**Therapeutic Category** Antispasmodic Agent, Urinary

**Use** Antispasmodic for neurogenic bladder (urgency, frequency, urge incontinence) and uninhibited bladder

**Usual Dosage** Oral:

Children:

1-5 years: 0.2 mg/kg/dose 2-4 times/day

>5 years: 5 mg twice daily, up to 5 mg 4 times/day maximum

Adults: 5 mg 2-3 times/day up to 5 mg 4 times/day maximum

Elderly: 2.5-5 mg twice daily; increase by 2.5 mg increments every 1-2 days

(Continued)

## Oxybutynin *(Continued)*

Ditropan® XL (extended release): 5 mg or 10 mg once daily

**Note:** Should be discontinued periodically to determine whether the patient can manage without the drug and to minimize resistance to the drug

**Mechanism of Action** Direct antispasmodic effect on smooth muscle, also inhibits the action of acetylcholine on smooth muscle (exhibits ¹/₅ the anticholinergic activity of atropine, but is 4-10 times the antispasmodic activity); does not block effects at skeletal muscle or at autonomic ganglia; increases bladder capacity, decreases uninhibited contractions, and delays desire to void; therefore, decreases urgency and frequency

**Local Anesthetic/Vasoconstrictor Precautions** No information available to require special precautions

**Effects on Dental Treatment** >10% of patients experience dry mouth; prolonged use of oxybutynin may decrease or inhibit salivary flow; normal salivation returns with cessation of drug therapy

**Other Adverse Effects**

>10%:

Central nervous system: Drowsiness
Gastrointestinal: Constipation
Miscellaneous: Decreased sweating

1% to 10%:

Cardiovascular: Tachycardia, palpitations
Central nervous system: Dizziness, insomnia, fever, headache
Dermatologic: Rash
Endocrine & metabolic: Hot flashes, decreased flow of breast milk
Gastrointestinal: Nausea, vomiting
Genitourinary: Urinary hesitancy or retention, decreased sexual ability
Neuromuscular & skeletal: Weakness
Ocular: Blurred vision, mydriatic effect

<1%:

Ocular: Increased intraocular pressure
Miscellaneous: Allergic reaction

**Drug Interactions**

Increased toxicity:
Additive sedation with CNS depressants and alcohol
Additive anticholinergic effects with antihistamines and anticholinergic agents

**Drug Uptake**

Onset of effect: Oral: 30-60 minutes
Peak effect: 3-6 hours
Duration: 6-10 hours
Absorption: Oral: Rapid and well absorbed
Serum half-life: 1-2.3 hours
Time to peak serum concentration: Within 60 minutes

**Pregnancy Risk Factor** B

**Generic Available** Yes

♦ **Oxycel®** *see* Cellulose, Oxidized *on page 213*

## Oxychlorosene (oks i KLOR oh seen)

**U.S. Brand Names** Clorpactin® WCS-90

**Therapeutic Category** Antibiotic, Topical

**Use** Treating localized infections

**Usual Dosage** Topical (0.1% to 0.5% solutions): Apply by irrigation, instillation, spray, soaks, or wet compresses

**Local Anesthetic/Vasoconstrictor Precautions** No information available to require special precautions

**Effects on Dental Treatment** No effects or complications reported

**Generic Available** No

**Comments** Product is available as powder which must be diluted with sterile water or isotonic saline

## Oxycodone (oks i KOE done)

**U.S. Brand Names** OxyContin®; OxyIR™; Percolone™; Roxicodone™

**Canadian Brand Names** Supeudol®

**Therapeutic Category** Analgesic, Narcotic

**Synonyms** Dihydrohydroxycodeinone; Oxycodone Hydrochloride

**Use**

Dental: Treatment of postoperative pain

Medical: Management of moderate to severe pain, normally used in combination with non-narcotic analgesics; management of moderate to severe pain where use of an opioid analgesic is appropriate for more than a few days

**Restrictions** C-II

**Usual Dosage** Oral:

Immediate release:

Children:

6-12 years: 1.25 mg every 6 hours as needed

>12 years: 2.5 mg every 6 hours as needed

Adults: 5 mg every 6 hours as needed

Controlled release: Adults: 10 mg every 12 hours around-the-clock

**Mechanism of Action** Oxycodone, as with other narcotic (opiate) analgesics, blocks pain perception in the cerebral cortex by binding to specific receptor molecules (opiate receptors) within the neuronal membranes of synapses. This binding results in a decreased synaptic chemical transmission throughout the CNS thus inhibiting the flow of pain sensations into the higher centers. Mu and kappa are the two subtypes of the opiate receptor which oxycodone binds to to cause analgesia.

**Local Anesthetic/Vasoconstrictor Precautions** No information available to require special precautions

**Effects on Dental Treatment** 1% to 10% of patients experience dry mouth

**Other Adverse Effects**

>10%:

Central nervous system: Fatigue, drowsiness, dizziness

Gastrointestinal: Nausea, vomiting

1% to 10%: Gastrointestinal: Anorexia, stomach cramps, xerostomia, constipation, biliary spasm

**Contraindications** Patients with known hypersensitivity to oxycodone

**Warnings/Precautions** Use with caution in patients with hypersensitivity reactions to other phenanthrene derivative opioid agonists (morphine, hydrocodone, hydromorphone, levorphanol, oxycodone, oxymorphone); respiratory diseases including asthma, emphysema, COPD, or severe liver or renal insufficiency; some preparations contain sulfites which may cause allergic reactions; may be habit-forming

**Drug Interactions** The use of MAO inhibitors or tricyclic antidepressants with oxycodone may **increase** the effect of either the antidepressant or oxycodone; concurrent use of oxycodone with anticholinergics may cause paralytic ileus; patients taking other narcotic agents, antipsychotics, antianxiety agents or other CNS depressants (including alcohol) with oxycodone may experience an additive CNS depression

**Drug Uptake**

Onset of effect: Narcotic analgesia: 0.5-1 hour

Duration of effect: 4-6 hours

Serum half-life: 2-3 hours

**Pregnancy Risk Factor** B (D if used for prolonged periods or in high doses at term)

**Dosage Forms**

Capsule, as hydrochloride, immediate release (OxyIR™): 5 mg

Liquid, oral, as hydrochloride: 5 mg/5 mL (500 mL)

Solution, oral concentrate, as hydrochloride: 20 mg/mL (30 mL)

Tablet, as hydrochloride: 5 mg

Percolone™: 5 mg

Tablet, controlled release, as hydrochloride (OxyContin®): 10 mg, 20 mg, 40 mg, 80 mg

Tablet, sustained release, as hydrochloride (Roxicodone™): 10 mg, 30 mg

**Dietary Considerations** No data reported

**Generic Available** No

**Comments** Prophylactic use of a laxative should be considered; oxycodone, as with other narcotic analgesics, is recommended only for limited acute dosing (ie, 3 days or less). The most common adverse effect is nausea, followed by sedation and constipation. Oxycodone has an addictive liability, especially when given long term.

## Oxycodone and Acetaminophen

(oks i KOE done & a seet a MIN oh fen)

**Related Information**

Acetaminophen *on page 27*

Dental Drug Interactions: Update on Drug Combinations Requiring Special Considerations *on page 1225*

Narcotic Agonists *on page 1223*

Oral Pain *on page 1122*

**U.S. Brand Names** Percocet®; Roxicet® 5/500; Roxilox®; Tylox®

**Canadian Brand Names** Endocet®; Oxycocet; Percocet®-Demi

**Therapeutic Category** Analgesic, Narcotic

(Continued)

## Oxycodone and Acetaminophen *(Continued)*

**Use**

Dental: Treatment of postoperative pain
Medical: Relief of pain

**Restrictions** C-II; Nonrefillable

**Usual Dosage** Oral:

Children: Not recommended in pediatric dental patients
Adults: 1-2 tablets every 4-6 hours as needed for pain; maximum dose: 12 tablets/day

**Mechanism of Action**

Oxycodone, as with other narcotic (opiate) analgesics, blocks pain perception in the cerebral cortex by binding to specific receptor molecules (opiate receptors) within the neuronal membranes of synapses. This binding results in a decreased synaptic chemical transmission throughout the CNS thus inhibiting the flow of pain sensations into the higher centers. Mu and kappa are the two subtypes of the opiate receptor which oxycodone binds to to cause analgesia.

Acetaminophen inhibits the synthesis of prostaglandins in the CNS and peripherally blocks pain impulse generation; produces antipyresis from inhibition of hypothalamic heat-regulating center

**Local Anesthetic/Vasoconstrictor Precautions** No information available to require special precautions

**Effects on Dental Treatment** 1% to 10% of patients experience dry mouth

**Other Adverse Effects**

>10%:

Central nervous system: Drowsiness, dizziness, sedation
Gastrointestinal: Nausea

1% to 10%: Gastrointestinal: Constipation

**Contraindications** Patients with known G-6-PD deficiency; hypersensitivity to acetaminophen; hypersensitivity to oxycodone

**Warnings/Precautions** Use with caution in patients with hypersensitivity reactions to other phenanthrene derivative opioid agonists (morphine, codeine, hydrocodone, hydromorphone, levorphanol, oxymorphone); respiratory diseases including asthma, emphysema, COPD, or severe liver or renal insufficiency; some preparations contain sulfites which may cause allergic reactions; may be habit-forming

Enhanced analgesia has been seen in elderly patients on therapeutic doses of narcotics; duration of action may be increased in the elderly; the elderly may be particularly susceptible to the CNS depressant and constipating effects of narcotics

**Drug Interactions** The use of MAO inhibitors or tricyclic antidepressants with oxycodone may **increase** the effect of either the antidepressant or oxycodone; concurrent use of oxycodone with anticholinergics may cause paralytic ileus; patients taking other narcotic agents, antipsychotics, antianxiety agents or other CNS depressants (including alcohol) with oxycodone may experience an additive CNS depression; with acetaminophen component, refer to Acetaminophen monograph

**Drug Uptake**

Onset of effect: Narcotic analgesia: 0.5-1 hour
Duration of effect: 4-6 hours
Serum half-life: Oxycodone: 2-3 hours

**Pregnancy Risk Factor** C

**Breast-feeding Considerations**

Oxycodone: No data reported
Acetaminophen: May be taken while breast-feeding

**Dosage Forms**

Caplet: Oxycodone hydrochloride 5 mg and acetaminophen 500 mg
Capsule: Oxycodone hydrochloride 5 mg and acetaminophen 500 mg
Solution, oral: Oxycodone hydrochloride 5 mg and acetaminophen 325 mg per 5 mL (5 mL, 500 mL)
Tablet: Oxycodone hydrochloride 5 mg and acetaminophen 325 mg

**Dietary Considerations** No data reported

**Generic Available** Yes

**Comments** Oxycodone, as with other narcotic analgesics, is recommended only for limited acute dosing (ie, 3 days or less). The most common adverse effect is nausea, followed by sedation and constipation. Oxycodone has an addictive liability, especially when given long term. The acetaminophen component requires use with caution in patients with alcoholic liver disease.

Acetaminophen:

A study by Hylek, et al, suggested that the combination of acetaminophen with warfarin (Coumadin®) may cause enhanced anticoagulation. The following recommendations have been made by Hylek, et al, and supported by an editorial in *JAMA* by Bell.

Dose and duration of acetaminophen should be as low as possible, individualized and monitored

The study by Hylek reported the following:

For patients who reported taking the equivalent of at least 4 regular strength (325 mg) tablets for longer than a week, the odds of having an INR >6.0 were increased 10-fold above those not taking acetaminophen. Risk decreased with lower intakes of acetaminophen reaching a background level of risk at a dose of 6 or fewer 325 mg tablets per week.

**Selected Readings**


Bell WR, "Acetaminophen and Warfarin: Undesirable Synergy," *JAMA*, Factors for Excessive Warfarin Anticoagulation," *JAMA*, 1998, 279:657-62.

Cooper SA, Precheur H, Rauch D, et al, "Evaluation of Oxycodone and Acetaminophen in Treatment of Postoperative Pain," *Oral Surg Oral Med Oral Pathol*, 1980, 50(6):496-501.

Dionne RA, "New Approaches to Preventing and Treating Postoperative Pain," *J Am Dent Assoc*, 1992, 123(6):26-34.

Gobetti JP, "Controlling Dental Pain," *J Am Dent Assoc*, 1992, 123(6):47-52.

Hylek EM, Heiman H, Skates SJ, et al, "Acetaminophen and Other Risk 1998, 279:702-3.


## Oxycodone and Aspirin (oks i KOE done & AS pir in)

**Related Information**


Dental Drug Interactions: Update on Drug Combinations Requiring Special Considerations *on page 1225*

Narcotic Agonists *on page 1223*

Oral Pain *on page 1122*


**U.S. Brand Names** Codoxy®; Percodan®; Percodan®-Demi; Roxiprin®

**Canadian Brand Names** Endodan®; Oxycodan

**Therapeutic Category** Analgesic, Narcotic

**Use**

Dental: Treatment of postoperative pain

Medical: Relief of pain

**Restrictions** C-II; Nonrefillable

**Usual Dosage** Oral:

Children: Not recommended in pediatric dental patients

Adults: Percodan®: 1 tablet every 6 hours as needed for pain or Percodan®-Demi: 1-2 tablets every 6 hours as needed for pain

**Mechanism of Action**

Oxycodone, as with other narcotic (opiate) analgesics, blocks pain perception in the cerebral cortex by binding to specific receptor molecules (opiate receptors) within the neuronal membranes of synapses. This binding results in a decreased synaptic chemical transmission throughout the CNS thus inhibiting the flow of pain sensations into the higher centers. Mu and kappa are the two subtypes of the opiate receptor which oxycodone binds to to cause analgesia.

Aspirin inhibits prostaglandin synthesis by decreasing the activity of the enzyme, cyclo-oxygenase, which results in decreased formation of prostaglandin precursors, acts on the hypothalamic heat-regulating center to reduce fever, blocks thromboxane synthetase action which prevents formation of the platelet-aggregating substance thromboxane $A_2$

**Local Anesthetic/Vasoconstrictor Precautions** No information available to require special precautions

**Effects on Dental Treatment** 1% to 10% of patients experience dry mouth; use with caution in patients with platelet and bleeding disorders, renal dysfunction, erosive gastritis, or peptic ulcer disease, previous nonreaction does not guarantee future safe taking of medication; do not use aspirin in children <16 years of age for chickenpox or flu symptoms due to the association with Reye's syndrome

Avoid aspirin if possible, for 1 week prior to surgery because of the possibility of postoperative bleeding; use with caution in impaired hepatic function

Elderly are a high-risk population for adverse effects from nonsteroidal anti-inflammatory agents. As much as 60% of elderly with GI complications to NSAIDs can develop peptic ulceration and/or hemorrhage asymptomatically. Also, concomitant disease and drug use contribute to the risk for GI adverse effects. Use lowest effective dose for shortest period possible. Consider renal function decline with age. Use with caution in patients with history of asthma.

**Other Adverse Effects**

>10%:

Central nervous system: Drowsiness, dizziness, sedation

Gastrointestinal: Nausea, heartburn, stomach pains, dyspepsia

1% to 10%: Gastrointestinal: Constipation

**Contraindications** Known hypersensitivity to oxycodone or aspirin; severe respiratory depression

(Continued)

## Oxycodone and Aspirin *(Continued)*

**Warnings/Precautions** Use with caution in patients with hypersensitivity to other phenanthrene derivative opioid agonists (morphine, codeine, hydrocodone, hydromorphone, oxymorphone, levorphanol); children and teenagers should not be given aspirin products if chickenpox or flu symptoms are present; aspirin use has been associated with Reye's syndrome; severe liver or renal insufficiency, pre-existing CNS and depression

Enhanced analgesia has been seen in elderly patients on therapeutic doses of narcotics; duration of action may be increased in the elderly; the elderly may be particularly susceptible to the CNS depressant and constipating effects of narcotics

**Drug Interactions** The use of MAO inhibitors or tricyclic antidepressants with oxycodone may **increase** effect of either the antidepressant or oxycodone; concurrent use of oxycodone with anticholinergics may cause paralytic ileus; patients taking other narcotic agents, antipsychotics, antianxiety agents or other CNS depressants (including alcohol) with oxycodone and aspirin may experience an additive CNS depression; aspirin interacts with warfarin to cause bleeding

**Drug Uptake**

Onset of effect: Narcotic analgesia: 0.5-1 hour

Duration of effect 4-6 hours

Serum half-life: Oxycodone: 2-3 hours

**Pregnancy Risk Factor** D

**Breast-feeding Considerations**

Aspirin: Caution is suggested due to potential adverse effects in nursing infants

Oxycodone: No data reported

**Dosage Forms** Tablet:

Percodan®: Oxycodone hydrochloride 4.5 mg, oxycodone terephthalate 0.38 mg, and aspirin 325 mg

Percodan®-Demi: Oxycodone hydrochloride 2.25 mg, oxycodone terephthalate 0.19 mg, and aspirin 325 mg

**Dietary Considerations** May be taken with food or water

**Generic Available** Yes

**Comments** Oxycodone, as with other narcotic analgesics, is recommended only for limited acute dosing (ie, 3 days or less). The most common adverse effect is nausea, followed by sedation and constipation. Oxycodone has an addictive liability, especially when given long term. The oxycodone with aspirin could have anticoagulant effects and could possibly affect bleeding times.

**Selected Readings**

Dionne RA, "New Approaches to Preventing and Treating Postoperative Pain," *J Am Dent Assoc*, 1992, 123(6):26-34.

Gobetti JP, "Controlling Dental Pain," *J Am Dent Assoc*, 1992, 123(6):47-52.

♦ **Oxycodone Hydrochloride** *see* Oxycodone *on page 750*

♦ **OxyContin®** *see* Oxycodone *on page 750*

## Oxygen (OKS i jen)

**Therapeutic Category** Dental Gases

**Use**

Dental: Administered as a supplement with nitrous oxide to ensure adequate ventilation during sedation; a resuscitative agent for medical emergencies in dental office

Medical: To treat various clinical disorders, both respiratory and nonrespiratory; relief of arterial hypoxia and secondary complications; treatment of pulmonary hypertension, polycythemia secondary to hypoxemia, chronic disease states complicated by anemia, cancer, migraine headaches, coronary artery disease, seizure disorders, sickle-cell crisis and sleep apnea

**Usual Dosage** Children and Adults: Average rate of 2 L/minute

**Mechanism of Action** Increased oxygen in tidal volume and oxygenation of tissues at molecular level

**Local Anesthetic/Vasoconstrictor Precautions** No information available to require special precautions

**Effects on Dental Treatment** No effects or complications reported

**Other Adverse Effects** No data reported

**Contraindications** No data reported

**Warnings/Precautions** Oxygen-induced hypoventilation is the greatest potential hazard of oxygen therapy. In patients with severe chronic obstructive pulmonary disease (COPD), the respiratory drive results from hypoxic stimulation of the carotid chemoreceptors. If this hypoxic drive is diminished by excessive oxygen therapy, hypoventilation may occur and further carbon dioxide retention with possible cessation of ventilation could result.

**Drug Interactions** No data reported

**Pregnancy Risk Factor** No data reported
**Breast-feeding Considerations** No data reported
**Dosage Forms** Liquid system with large reservoir holding 75-100 lb of liquid oxygen; compressed gas system consisting of high-pressure tank; tank sizes are "H" (6900 L of oxygen), "E" (622 L of oxygen) and "D" (356 L of oxygen)
**Dietary Considerations** No data reported
**Generic Available** Yes

♦ **OxyIR™** *see* Oxycodone *on page 750*

## Oxymetazoline (oks i met AZ oh leen)

**Related Information**

Oral Bacterial Infections *on page 1128*

**U.S. Brand Names** Afrin® Children's Nose Drops [OTC]; Afrin® Sinus [OTC]; Allerest® 12 Hour Nasal Solution [OTC]; Chlorphed®-LA Nasal Solution [OTC]; Dristan® Long Lasting Nasal Solution [OTC]; Duramist® Plus [OTC]; Duration® Nasal Solution [OTC]; Neo-Synephrine® 12 Hour Nasal Solution [OTC]; Nōstrilla® [OTC]; NTZ® Long Acting Nasal Solution [OTC]; OcuClear® Ophthalmic [OTC]; Sinarest® 12 Hour Nasal Solution; Sinex® Long-Acting [OTC]; Twice-A-Day® Nasal [OTC]; Visine® L.R. Ophthalmic [OTC]; 4-Way® Long Acting Nasal Solution [OTC]
**Canadian Brand Names** Drixoral® Nasal
**Therapeutic Category** Adrenergic Agonist Agent; Decongestant, Nasal; Nasal Agent, Vasoconstrictor
**Use**

Dental: Symptomatic relief of nasal mucosal congestion

Medical:

Adjunctive therapy of middle ear infections, associated with acute or chronic rhinitis, the common cold, sinusitis, hay fever, or other allergies

Ophthalmic: Relief of redness of eye due to minor eye irritations

**Usual Dosage** Intranasal (therapy should not exceed 3-5 days):

Children 2-5 years: 0.025% solution: Instill 2-3 drops in each nostril twice daily

Children ≥6 years and Adults: 0.05% solution: Instill 2-3 drops or 2-3 sprays into each nostril twice daily

**Mechanism of Action** Stimulates alpha-adrenergic receptors in the arterioles of the nasal mucosa to produce vasoconstriction
**Local Anesthetic/Vasoconstrictor Precautions** No information available to require special precautions
**Effects on Dental Treatment** No effects or complications reported
**Other Adverse Effects**

>10%:

Local: Transient burning, stinging

Respiratory: Dryness of the nasal mucosa, sneezing

1% to 10%:

Cardiovascular: Hypertension, palpitations

Respiratory: Rebound congestion with prolonged use

**Contraindications** Hypersensitivity to oxymetazoline or any component
**Warnings/Precautions** Rebound congestion may occur with extended use (>3 days); use with caution in the presence of hypertension, diabetes, hyperthyroidism, heart disease, coronary artery disease, cerebral arteriosclerosis, or long-standing bronchial asthma
**Drug Interactions** Increased toxicity with MAO inhibitors
**Drug Uptake**

Onset of effect: Intranasal: Within 5-10 minutes

Duration: 5-6 hours

**Pregnancy Risk Factor** C
**Breast-feeding Considerations** No data reported
**Dosage Forms** Solution, nasal:

Drops: 0.05% drops (15 mL, 20 mL)

Drops, pediatric: 0.025% (20 mL)

Spray: 0.05% (15 mL, 30 mL)

**Dietary Considerations** No data reported
**Generic Available** Yes

## Oxymetholone (oks i METH oh lone)

**U.S. Brand Names** Anadrol®
**Canadian Brand Names** Anapolon®
**Therapeutic Category** Anabolic Steroid
**Use** Anemias caused by the administration of myelotoxic drugs
**Usual Dosage** Adults: Erythropoietic effects: Oral: 1-5 mg/kg/day in 1 daily dose; maximum: 100 mg/day; give for a minimum trial of 3-6 months because response may be delayed

(Continued)

## Oxymetholone *(Continued)*

**Mechanism of Action** Stimulates receptors in organs and tissues to promote growth and development of male sex organs and maintains secondary sex characteristics in androgen-deficient males

**Local Anesthetic/Vasoconstrictor Precautions** No information available to require special precautions

**Effects on Dental Treatment** No effects or complications reported

**Other Adverse Effects**

**Male:**

Postpubertal:

>10%:

Dermatologic: Acne

Endocrine & metabolic: Gynecomastia

Genitourinary: Bladder irritability, priapism

1% to 10%:

Central nervous system: Insomnia, chills

Endocrine & metabolic: Decreased libido

Gastrointestinal: Nausea, diarrhea

Genitourinary: Prostatic hypertrophy (elderly)

Hematologic: Iron deficiency anemia, suppression of clotting factors

Hepatic: Hepatic dysfunction

<1%:

Hepatic: Hepatic necrosis, hepatocellular carcinoma

Prepubertal:

>10%:

Dermatologic: Acne

Endocrine & metabolic: Virilism

1% to 10%:

Central nervous system: Chills, insomnia

Dermatologic: Hyperpigmentation

Gastrointestinal: Diarrhea, nausea

Hematologic: Iron deficiency anemia, suppression of clotting factors

<1%: Hepatic: Hepatic necrosis, hepatocellular carcinoma

**Female:**

>10%: Endocrine & metabolic: Virilism

1% to 10%:

Central nervous system: Chills, insomnia

Endocrine & metabolic: Hypercalcemia

Gastrointestinal: Nausea, diarrhea

Hematologic: Iron deficiency anemia, suppression of clotting factors

Hepatic: Hepatic dysfunction

<1%: Hepatic: Hepatic necrosis, hepatocellular carcinoma

**Drug Interactions** Increased toxicity: Increased oral anticoagulants, insulin requirements may be decreased

**Drug Uptake** Serum half-life: 9 hours

**Pregnancy Risk Factor** X

**Generic Available** No

## Oxymorphone (oks i MOR fone)

**Related Information**

Narcotic Agonists *on page 1223*

**U.S. Brand Names** Numorphan®

**Therapeutic Category** Analgesic, Narcotic

**Use** Management of moderate to severe pain and preoperatively as a sedative and a supplement to anesthesia

**Usual Dosage** Adults:

I.M., S.C.: 0.5 mg initially, 1-1.5 mg every 4-6 hours as needed

I.V.: 0.5 mg initially

Rectal: 5 mg every 4-6 hours

**Mechanism of Action** Oxymorphone hydrochloride (Numorphan®) is a potent narcotic analgesic with uses similar to those of morphine. The drug is a semisynthetic derivative of morphine (phenanthrene derivative) and is closely related to hydromorphone chemically (Dilaudid®).

**Local Anesthetic/Vasoconstrictor Precautions** No information available to require special precautions

**Effects on Dental Treatment** Anticholinergic side effects can cause a reduction of saliva production or secretion contributes to discomfort and dental disease (ie, caries, oral candidiasis and periodontal disease)

**Other Adverse Effects**

>10%:

Cardiovascular: Hypotension

Central nervous system: Fatigue, drowsiness, dizziness
Gastrointestinal: Nausea, vomiting, constipation
Neuromuscular & skeletal: Weakness
Miscellaneous: Histamine release

1% to 10%:
Central nervous system: Nervousness, headache, restlessness, malaise, confusion
Gastrointestinal: Anorexia, stomach cramps, dry mouth, biliary spasm
Genitourinary: Decreased urination, ureteral spasms
Local: Pain at injection site
Respiratory: Dyspnea

<1%:
Central nervous system: Mental depression, hallucinations, paradoxical CNS stimulation, increased intracranial pressure
Dermatologic: Skin rash, urticaria
Gastrointestinal: Paralytic ileus
Miscellaneous: Histamine release, physical and psychological dependence

**Drug Interactions**
Decreased effect with phenothiazines
Increased effect/toxicity with CNS depressants, TCAs, dextroamphetamine

**Drug Uptake**
Onset of analgesia:
I.V., I.M., S.C.: Within 5-10 minutes
Rectal: Within 15-30 minutes
Duration of analgesia: Parenteral, rectal: 3-4 hours

**Pregnancy Risk Factor** B (D if used for prolonged periods or in high doses at term)

**Generic Available** No

## Oxyphenbutazone (oks i fen BYOO ta zone)

**Therapeutic Category** Analgesic, Non-narcotic; Nonsteroidal Anti-inflammatory Drug (NSAID), Oral

**Use** Management of inflammatory disorders, as an analgesic in the treatment of mild to moderate pain and as an antipyretic; I.V. form used as an alternate to surgery in management of patent ductus arteriosus in premature neonates; acute gouty arthritis

**Usual Dosage** Adults: Oral:
Rheumatoid arthritis: 100-200 mg 3-4 times/day until desired effect, then reduce dose to not exceeding 400 mg/day
Acute gouty arthritis: Initial: 400 mg then 100 mg every 4 hours until acute attack subsides, not longer than 1 week

**Local Anesthetic/Vasoconstrictor Precautions** No information available to require special precautions

**Effects on Dental Treatment** NSAID formulations are known to reversibly decrease platelet aggregation via mechanisms different than observed with aspirin. The dentist should be aware of the potential of abnormal coagulation. Caution should also be exercised in the use of NSAIDs in patients already on anticoagulant therapy with drugs such as warfarin (Coumadin®).

**Other Adverse Effects**
>10%:
Central nervous system: Dizziness
Dermatologic: Skin rash
Gastrointestinal: Abdominal cramps, heartburn, indigestion, nausea

1% to 10%:
Central nervous system: Headache, nervousness
Dermatologic: Itching
Endocrine & metabolic: Fluid retention
Gastrointestinal: Vomiting
Otic: Tinnitus

<1%:
Cardiovascular: Congestive heart failure, hypertension, arrhythmia, tachycardia
Central nervous system: Confusion, hallucinations, aseptic meningitis, mental depression, drowsiness, insomnia
Dermatologic: Urticaria, erythema multiforme, toxic epidermal necrolysis, Stevens-Johnson syndrome, angioedema
Endocrine & metabolic: Polydipsia, hot flashes
Gastrointestinal: Gastritis, GI ulceration
Genitourinary: Cystitis
Hematologic: Agranulocytosis, anemia, hemolytic anemia, bone marrow suppression, leukopenia, thrombocytopenia
Hepatic: Hepatitis

(Continued)

## Oxyphenbutazone *(Continued)*

Neuromuscular & skeletal: Peripheral neuropathy
Ocular: Toxic amblyopia, blurred vision, conjunctivitis, dry eyes
Otic: Decreased hearing
Renal: Polyuria, acute renal failure
Respiratory: Allergic rhinitis, dyspnea, epistaxis

**Pregnancy Risk Factor** D

**Generic Available** Yes

## Oxyphencyclimine (oks i fen SYE kli meen)

**U.S. Brand Names** Daricon®

**Therapeutic Category** Anticholinergic Agent; Antispasmodic Agent, Gastrointestinal

**Use** Adjunctive treatment of peptic ulcer

**Usual Dosage** Children >12 years and Adults: Oral: 10 mg twice daily or 5 mg 3 times/day

**Local Anesthetic/Vasoconstrictor Precautions** No information available to require special precautions

**Effects on Dental Treatment** >10% of patients experience dry mouth

**Other Adverse Effects**

>10%:
- Dermatologic: Dry skin
- Gastrointestinal: Constipation, dry throat
- Respiratory: Dry nose
- Miscellaneous: Decreased sweating

1% to 10%:
- Gastrointestinal: Dysphagia
- Ocular: Photosensitivity

<1%:
- Cardiovascular: Tachycardia
- Central nervous system: Confusion, headache, loss of memory, fatigue, drowsiness, nervousness, insomnia
- Dermatologic: Rash
- Gastrointestinal: Bloated feeling, nausea, vomiting
- Genitourinary: Urinary retention
- Neuromuscular & skeletal: Weakness
- Ocular: Increased intraocular pressure, blurred vision

**Pregnancy Risk Factor** C

**Generic Available** No

## Oxytetracycline (oks i tet ra SYE kleen)

**U.S. Brand Names** Terramycin® I.M. Injection; Terramycin® Oral

**Therapeutic Category** Antibiotic, Tetracycline Derivative

**Use** Treatment of susceptible bacterial infections; both gram-positive and gram-negative, as well as, *Rickettsia* and *Mycoplasma* organisms

**Usual Dosage**

Oral:
- Children: 40-50 mg/kg/day in divided doses every 6 hours (maximum: 2 g/24 hours)
- Adults: 250-500 mg/dose every 6 hours

I.M.:
- Children >8 years: 15-25 mg/kg/day (maximum: 250 mg/dose) in divided doses every 8-12 hours
- Adults: 250-500 mg every 24 hours or 300 mg/day divided every 8-12 hours

**Mechanism of Action** Inhibits bacterial protein synthesis by binding with the 30S and possibly the 50S ribosomal subunit(s) of susceptible bacteria, cell wall synthesis is not affected

**Local Anesthetic/Vasoconstrictor Precautions** No information available to require special precautions

**Effects on Dental Treatment** Tetracycline's are not recommended for use during pregnancy or in children ≤8 years of age since they have been reported to cause enamel hypoplasia and permanent teeth discoloration. The use of tetracycline's should only be used in these patients if other agents are contraindicated or alternative antimicrobials will not eradicate the organism. Long-term use associated with oral candidiasis.

**Other Adverse Effects**

>10%: Miscellaneous: Discoloration of teeth and enamel hypoplasia (infants)

1% to 10%:
- Dermatologic: Photosensitivity
- Gastrointestinal: Nausea, diarrhea

<1%:

Cardiovascular: Pericarditis

Central nervous system: Increased intracranial pressure, bulging fontanels in infants, pseudotumor cerebri

Dermatologic: Pruritus, exfoliative dermatitis, dermatologic effects

Endocrine & metabolic: Diabetes insipidus syndrome

Gastrointestinal: Vomiting, esophagitis, anorexia, abdominal cramps, antibiotic-associated pseudomembranous colitis, staphylococcal enterocolitis

Hepatic: Hepatotoxicity

Local: Thrombophlebitis,

Neuromuscular & skeletal: Paresthesia

Renal: Renal damage, acute renal failure, azotemia

Miscellaneous: Superinfections, anaphylaxis, pigmentation of nails, hypersensitivity reactions, candidal superinfection

**Drug Interactions**

Decreased effect with antacids containing aluminum, calcium or magnesium

Iron and bismuth subsalicylate may decrease oxytetracycline bioavailability

Barbiturates, phenytoin, and carbamazepine decrease oxytetracycline's half-life

Increased effect of warfarin

**Drug Uptake**

Absorption:

Oral: Adequate (~75%)

I.M.: Poor

Serum half-life: 8.5-9.6 hours (increases with renal impairment)

Time to peak serum concentration: Within 2-4 hours

**Pregnancy Risk Factor** D

**Dosage Forms**

Capsule, as hydrochloride: 250 mg

Injection, as hydrochloride, with lidocaine 2%: 5% [50 mg/mL] (2 mL, 10 mL); 12.5% [125 mg/mL] (2 mL)

**Generic Available** Yes

## Oxytetracycline and Hydrocortisone

(oks i tet ra SYE kleen & hye droe KOR ti sone)

**U.S. Brand Names** Terra-Cortril® Ophthalmic Suspension

**Therapeutic Category** Antibiotic, Ophthalmic

**Use** Treatment of susceptible ophthalmic bacterial infections with associated swelling

**Local Anesthetic/Vasoconstrictor Precautions** No information available to require special precautions

**Effects on Dental Treatment** No effects or complications reported

**Pregnancy Risk Factor** C

**Generic Available** Yes

## Oxytetracycline and Polymyxin B

(oks i tet ra SYE kleen & pol i MIKS in bee)

**U.S. Brand Names** Terak® Ophthalmic Ointment; Terramycin® Ophthalmic Ointment; Terramycin® w/Polymyxin B Ophthalmic Ointment

**Therapeutic Category** Antibiotic, Ophthalmic

**Synonyms** Polymyxin B and Oxytetracycline

**Use** Treatment of superficial ocular infections involving the conjunctiva and/or cornea

**Usual Dosage** Topical: Apply ½" of ointment onto the lower lid of affected eye 2-4 times/day

**Local Anesthetic/Vasoconstrictor Precautions** No information available to require special precautions

**Effects on Dental Treatment** No effects or complications reported

**Pregnancy Risk Factor** D

**Generic Available** No

## Oxytocin (oks i TOE sin)

**U.S. Brand Names** Pitocin®; Syntocinon®

**Canadian Brand Names** Toesen®

**Therapeutic Category** Oxytocic Agent

**Use** Induces labor at term; controls postpartum bleeding; nasal preparation used to promote milk letdown in lactating females

**Usual Dosage** I.V. administration requires the use of an infusion pump

(Continued)

## Oxytocin *(Continued)*

Adults:

Induction of labor: I.V.: 0.001-0.002 units/minute; increase by 0.001-0.002 units every 15-30 minutes until contraction pattern has been established; maximum dose should not exceed 20 milliunits/minute

Postpartum bleeding:

I.M.: Total dose of 10 units after delivery

I.V.: 10-40 units by I.V. infusion in 1000 mL of intravenous fluid at a rate sufficient to control uterine atony

Promotion of milk letdown: Intranasal: 1 spray or 3 drops in one or both nostrils 2-3 minutes before breast-feeding

**Mechanism of Action** Produces the rhythmic uterine contractions characteristic to delivery and stimulates breast milk flow during nursing

**Local Anesthetic/Vasoconstrictor Precautions** No information available to require special precautions

**Effects on Dental Treatment** No effects or complications reported

**Other Adverse Effects**

Fetal: <1%:

Cardiovascular: Bradycardia, arrhythmias

Central nervous system: Brain damage, intracranial hemorrhage

Hepatic: Neonatal jaundice

Respiratory: Hypoxia

Miscellaneous: Death

Maternal: <1%:

Cardiovascular: Cardiac arrhythmias, premature ventricular contractions, hypotension, tachycardia, arrhythmias

Central nervous system: Seizures, coma

Endocrine & metabolic: SIADH with hyponatremia

Gastrointestinal: Nausea, vomiting

Genitourinary: Increased uterine motility, pelvic hematoma

Hematologic: Postpartum hemorrhage, fatal afibrinogenemia, increased blood loss

Miscellaneous: Death, anaphylactic reactions

**Drug Interactions** No data reported

**Drug Uptake**

Onset of uterine contractions: I.V.: Within 1 minute

Duration: <30 minutes

Serum half-life: 1-5 minutes

**Pregnancy Risk Factor** X (nasal solution)

**Generic Available** Yes

- **Oyst-Cal 500 [OTC]** *see* Calcium Carbonate *on page 172*
- **Oystercal® 500** *see* Calcium Carbonate *on page 172*
- **P-071** *see* Cetirizine *on page 218*

## Paclitaxel (PAK li taks el)

**U.S. Brand Names** Taxol®

**Therapeutic Category** Antineoplastic Agent, Antimicrotubular

**Use** Treatment of metastatic carcinoma of the ovary after failure of first-line or subsequent chemotherapy; treatment of metastatic breast cancer; in combination with cisplatin for the first-line treatment of nonsmall cell lung cancer in patients who are not candidates for potentially curative surgery and/or radiation therapy

**Usual Dosage** Corticosteroids (dexamethasone), $H_1$ antagonists (diphenhydramine), and $H_2$ antagonists (cimetidine or ranitidine), should be administered prior to paclitaxel administration to minimize potential for anaphylaxis

Adults: I.V. infusion: **Refer to individual protocol**

Ovarian carcinoma: 135-175 mg/m$^2$ over 1-24 hours administered every 3 weeks

Metastatic breast cancer: Treatment is still undergoing investigation; most protocols have used doses of 175-250 mg/m$^2$ over 1-24 hours every 3 weeks

**Mechanism of Action** In the cell, paclitaxel causes formation of stable microtubule bundles, interfering with the late G-2 mitotic phase of the cell cycle and inhibiting cell replication

**Local Anesthetic/Vasoconstrictor Precautions** No information available to require special precautions

**Effects on Dental Treatment** No effects or complications reported

**Other Adverse Effects**

>10%:

Bone marrow suppression: Major dose-limiting (ie, more severe at doses of 200-250 mg/m$^2$) toxicity

Dermatologic: Alopecia has been observed in almost all patients; loss of scalp hair occurs suddenly between day 14 and 21 and is reversible. Some patients experience a loss of all body hair. Local venous effects include erythema, tenderness, and discomfort during infusion and areas of extravasation include erythema, swelling, and induration. Necrotic changes and ulcers have not been reported even after extravasation of large volumes of infusate.

Hypersensitivity: Based on observations during early clinical trials, reactions were principally nonimmunologically mediated by the direct release of histamine or other vasoactive substances from mast cells and basophils

Neurotoxicity: Typically cumulative, with symptoms progressing after each treatment at both high and low doses. Patients with pre-existing neuropathies due to previous chemotherapy or coexisting medical illness (diabetes mellitus, alcoholism) appear to be predisposed to neurotoxicity. Neurotoxic effects such as sensory neuropathy, motor neuropathy, autonomic neuropathy, myopathy or myopathic effects, and central nervous system toxicity have been reported. Sensory neuropathy occurs invariably when the paclitaxel dose approaches 250 $mg/m^2$. Symptoms include numbness, tingling, and/or burning pain in the distal lower extremities, toes and/or fingers and begin as early as 24-72 hours after treatment with high single doses. Motor neuropathy occurs primarily at relatively high doses (250-275 $mg/m^2$) and in those patients with diabetes mellitus who may be more predisposed to toxic neuropathies. Myopathy effects are commonly observed after treatment with moderate to high doses (ie, >200 $mg/m^2$) administered over 6-24 hours. These symptoms generally occur 2-3 days after treatment and resolve within 5-6 days.

Miscellaneous: Hypersensitivity reactions, myalgia, abnormal liver function tests

1% to 10%:

Cardiovascular: Bradycardia, severe cardiovascular events

Gastrointestinal: Nausea and vomiting are not severe at any dose level

Irritant chemotherapy

**Drug Interactions** Increased toxicity:

In phase I trials, myelosuppression was more profound when given after cisplatin than with alternative sequence; pharmacokinetic data demonstrates a decrease in clearance of -33% when administered following cisplatin

Possibility of an inhibition of metabolism in patients treated with ketoconazole

**Drug Uptake** Administered by I.V. infusion and exhibits a biphasic decline in plasma concentrations

Serum half-life, mean, terminal: 5.3-17.4 hours after 1- and 6-hour infusions at dosing levels of 15-275 $mg/m^2$

**Pregnancy Risk Factor** D

**Generic Available** No

## Palivizumab (pah li VIZ u mab)

**U.S. Brand Names** Synagis®

**Therapeutic Category** Monoclonal Antibody

**Use** Prevention of serious lower respiratory tract disease caused by respiratory syncytial virus (RSV) in pediatric patients at high risk of RSV disease; safety and efficacy were established in infants with bronchopulmonary dysplasia (BPD) and infants with a history of prematurity ≤35 weeks gestational age

**Usual Dosage** Children: I.M.: 15 mg/kg of body weight, monthly throughout RSV season (First dose administered prior to commencement of RSV season)

**Mechanism of Action** Exhibits neutralizing and fusion-inhibitory activity against RSV; these activities inhibit RSV replication in laboratory and clinical studies

**Local Anesthetic/Vasoconstrictor Precautions** No information available to require special precautions

**Effects on Dental Treatment** No effects or complications reported

**Other Adverse Effects** The incidence of adverse events was similar between the palivizumab and placebo groups

>1%:

Central nervous system: Nervousness

Dermatologic: Oral *Monilia*, fungal dermatitis, eczema, seborrhea

Gastrointestinal: Diarrhea, vomiting, gastroenteritis

Hematologic: Anemia

Hepatic: ALT increase, liver function abnormality

Local: Injection site reaction

Ocular: Conjunctivitis

Respiratory: Cough, wheeze, bronchiolitis, pneumonia, bronchitis, asthma, croup, dyspnea, sinusitis, apnea

Miscellaneous: Failure to thrive, viral infection, flu syndrome

**Drug Interactions** No formal drug interaction studies have been conducted

(Continued)

## Palivizumab *(Continued)*

**Drug Uptake** Serum half-life: ~18 days

**Pregnancy Risk Factor** C

**Dosage Forms** Injection, lyophilized: 100 mg

**Selected Readings**


Johnson S, Oliver C, Prince GA, et al, "Development of a Humanized Monoclonal Antibody (MEDI-493) With Potent *In Vitro* Activity Against Respiratory Syncytial Virus," *J Infect Dis*, 1997, 176:1215-24.

Subramanian KN, Weisman, LE, Rhodes T, et al, "Safety, Tolerance and Pharmacokinetics of a Humanized Monoclonal Antibody to Respiratory Syncytial Virus in Premature Infants With Bronchopulmonary Dysplasia. MEDI-493 Study Group," *Pediatr Infect Dis J*, 1998, 17:110-5.

Welliver RC, "Respiratory Syncytial Virus Immunoglobulin and Monoclonal Antibodies in the Prevention and Treatment of Respiratory Syncytial Virus Infection," *Semin Perinatol*, 1998, 22:87-95.



♦ **PALS® [OTC]** *see* Chlorophyll *on page 226*

♦ **Pamelor®** *see* Nortriptyline *on page 732*


## Pamidronate (pa mi DROE nate)

**U.S. Brand Names** Aredia™

**Therapeutic Category** Antidote, Hypercalcemia; Bisphosphonate Derivative

**Use** FDA-approved: Treatment of hypercalcemia associated with malignancy; treatment of osteolytic bone lesions associated with multiple myeloma; treatment of osteolytic bone metastases of breast cancer; moderate to severe Paget's disease of bone

**Usual Dosage** Drug must be diluted properly before administration and infused slowly (over at least 1 hour)

Adults: I.V.:

- Moderate cancer-related hypercalcemia (corrected serum calcium: 12-13 mg/dL): 60-90 mg given as a slow infusion over 2-24 hours
- Severe cancer-related hypercalcemia (corrected serum calcium: >13.5 mg/dL): 90 mg as a slow infusion over 2-24 hours
  - A period of 7 days should elapse before the use of second course; repeat infusions every 2-3 weeks have been suggested, however, could be administered every 2-3 months according to the degree and of severity of hypercalcemia and/or the type of malignancy

Osteolytic bone lesions with multiple myeloma: 90 mg in 500 mL $D_5W$, 0.45% NaCl or 0.9% NaCl administered over 4 hours on a monthly basis

Paget's disease: 30 mg in 500 mL 0.45% NaCl, 0.9% NaCl or $D_5W$ administered over 4 hours for 3 consecutive days

**Mechanism of Action** A biphosphonate which inhibits bone resorption via actions on osteoclasts or on osteoclast precursors. Does not appear to produce any significant effects on renal tubular calcium handling and is poorly absorbed following oral administration (high oral doses have been reported effective); therefore, I.V. therapy is preferred.

**Local Anesthetic/Vasoconstrictor Precautions** No information available to require special precautions

**Effects on Dental Treatment** No effects or complications reported

**Other Adverse Effects**

1% to 10%:

- Central nervous system: Malaise, fever, convulsions
- Endocrine & metabolic: Hypomagnesemia, hypocalcemia, hypokalemia, hypophosphatemia, fluid overload
- Gastrointestinal: GI symptoms, nausea, diarrhea, constipation, anorexia
- Hepatic: Abnormal hepatic function
- Neuromuscular & skeletal: Bone pain
- Respiratory: Dyspnea

<1%:

- Central nervous system: Pain
- Dermatologic: Skin rash, angioedema
- Gastrointestinal: Dysgeusia, occult blood in stools
- Hematologic: Leukopenia
- Neuromuscular & skeletal: Increased risk of fractures
- Renal: Nephrotoxicity
- Miscellaneous: Hypersensitivity reactions

**Drug Interactions** No data reported

**Drug Uptake**

Onset of effect: 24-48 hours

Maximum effect: 5-7 days

Absorption: Poorly from the GI tract; pharmacokinetic studies are lacking

Serum half-life, unmetabolized: 2.5 hours

**Pregnancy Risk Factor** C

**Generic Available** No

- ♦ **Pamine®** *see* Methscopolamine *on page 656*
- ♦ **p-Aminoclonidine** *see* Apraclonidine *on page 93*
- ♦ **Panadol® [OTC]** *see* Acetaminophen *on page 27*
- ♦ **Panasal® 5/500** *see* Hydrocodone and Aspirin *on page 507*
- ♦ **Pancrease®** *see* Pancrelipase *on this page*
- ♦ **Pancrease® MT 4** *see* Pancrelipase *on this page*
- ♦ **Pancrease® MT 10** *see* Pancrelipase *on this page*
- ♦ **Pancrease® MT 16** *see* Pancrelipase *on this page*
- ♦ **Pancrease® MT 20** *see* Pancrelipase *on this page*


## Pancreatin (PAN kree a tin)

**U.S. Brand Names** Creon®; Digepepsin®; Donnazyme®; Hi-Vegi-Lip®

**Therapeutic Category** Pancreatic Enzyme

**Use** Replacement therapy in symptomatic treatment of malabsorption syndrome caused by pancreatic insufficiency

**Usual Dosage** The following dosage recommendations are only an approximation for initial dosages. The actual dosage will depend on the digestive requirements of the individual patient.

Children:
- <1 year: 2000 units of lipase with meals/feedings
- 1-6 years: 4000-8000 units of lipase with meals and 4,000 units with snacks
- 7-12 years: 4000-12,000 units of lipase with meals and snacks

Adults: 4000-16,000 units of lipase with meals and with snacks

**Local Anesthetic/Vasoconstrictor Precautions** No information available to require special precautions

**Effects on Dental Treatment** No effects or complications reported

**Other Adverse Effects**

1% to 10%: High doses:
- Endocrine & metabolic: Hyperuricemia
- Gastrointestinal: Nausea, cramps, constipation, diarrhea
- Ocular: Lacrimation
- Renal: Hyperuricosuria
- Respiratory: Sneezing

<1%:
- Dermatologic: Rash
- Gastrointestinal: Irritation of the mouth
- Respiratory: Dyspnea, bronchospasm

**Pregnancy Risk Factor** C

**Generic Available** No

**Comments** On a weight basis, pancreatin has 1/12 the lipolytic activity of pancrelipase

## Pancrelipase (pan kre LI pase)

**U.S. Brand Names** Cotazym®; Cotazym-S®; Creon® 10; Creon® 20; Ilozyme®; Ku-Zyme® HP; Pancrease®; Pancrease® MT 4; Pancrease® MT 10; Pancrease® MT 16; Pancrease® MT 20; Protilase®; Ultrase® MT12; Ultrase® MT20; Viokase®; Zymase®

**Therapeutic Category** Pancreatic Enzyme

**Synonyms** Lipancreatin

**Use** Replacement therapy in symptomatic treatment of malabsorption syndrome caused by pancreatic insufficiency

**Usual Dosage** Oral:

Powder: Actual dose depends on the digestive requirements of the patient
- Children <1 year: Start with 1/8 teaspoonful with feedings
- Adults: 0.7 g with meals

Enteric coated microspheres and microtablets: The following dosage recommendations are only an approximation for initial dosages. The actual dosage will depend on the digestive requirements of the individual patient.
- Children:
  - <1 year: 2000 units of lipase with meals
  - 1-6 years: 4000-8000 units of lipase with meals and 4000 units with snacks
  - 7-12 years: 4000-12,000 units of lipase with meals and snacks
- Adults: 4000-16,000 units of lipase with meals and with snacks or 1-3 tablets/capsules before or with meals and snacks; in severe deficiencies, dose may be increased to 8 tablets/capsules

Occluded feeding tubes: One tablet of Viokase® crushed with one 325 mg tablet of sodium bicarbonate (to activate the Viokase®) in 5 mL of water can be instilled into the nasogastric tube and clamped for 5 minutes; then, flushed with 50 mL of tap water

(Continued)

## Pancrelipase *(Continued)*

**Mechanism of Action** Replaces endogenous pancreatic enzymes to assist in digestion of protein, starch and fats

**Local Anesthetic/Vasoconstrictor Precautions** No information available to require special precautions

**Effects on Dental Treatment** No effects or complications reported

**Other Adverse Effects**

1% to 10%: High doses:
- Endocrine & metabolic: Hyperuricemia
- Gastrointestinal: Nausea, cramps, constipation, diarrhea
- Ocular: Lacrimation
- Renal: Hyperuricosuria
- Respiratory: Sneezing

<1%:
- Dermatologic: Rash
- Gastrointestinal: Irritation of the mouth
- Respiratory: Dyspnea, bronchospasm

**Drug Uptake** Absorption: Not absorbed, acts locally in GI tract

**Pregnancy Risk Factor** C

**Generic Available** Yes

**Comments** Concomitant administration of conventional pancreatin enzymes with an $H_2$-receptor antagonist has been used to decrease the inactivation of enzyme activity


- ♦ **Panhematin®** *see* Hemin *on page 491*
- ♦ **PanOxyl®-AQ** *see* Benzoyl Peroxide *on page 130*
- ♦ **PanOxyl® Bar [OTC]** *see* Benzoyl Peroxide *on page 130*
- ♦ **Panscol® [OTC]** *see* Salicylic Acid *on page 900*
- ♦ **Panthoderm® [OTC]** *see* Dexpanthenol *on page 310*
- ♦ **Pantopon®** *see* Opium Alkaloids *on page 742*


## Pantothenic Acid (pan toe THEN ik AS id)

**Therapeutic Category** Vitamin, Water Soluble

**Synonyms** Calcium Pantothenate; Vitamin $B_5$

**Use** Pantothenic acid deficiency

**Usual Dosage** Adults: Oral: Recommended daily dose 4-7 mg/day

**Local Anesthetic/Vasoconstrictor Precautions** No information available to require special precautions

**Effects on Dental Treatment** No effects or complications reported

**Pregnancy Risk Factor** A (C if used in doses above RDA recommendations)

**Generic Available** Yes

## Papaverine (pa PAV er een)

**U.S. Brand Names** Genabid®; Pavabid®; Pavatine®

**Therapeutic Category** Vasodilator

**Use**

Oral: Relief of peripheral and cerebral ischemia associated with arterial spasm; smooth muscle relaxant

Parenteral: Various vascular spasms associated with muscle spasms as in myocardial infarction, angina, peripheral and pulmonary embolism, peripheral vascular disease, angiospastic states, and visceral spasm (ureteral, biliary, and GI colic); testing for impotence

**Usual Dosage**

Children: I.M., I.V.: 1.5 mg/kg 4 times/day

Adults:
- Oral: 100-300 mg 3-5 times/day
- Oral, sustained release: 150-300 mg every 12 hours
- I.M., I.V.: 30-120 mg every 3 hours as needed; for cardiac extrasystoles, give 2 doses 10 minutes apart I.V. or I.M.

**Mechanism of Action** Smooth muscle spasmolytic producing a generalized smooth muscle relaxation including: vasodilatation, gastrointestinal sphincter relaxation, bronchiolar muscle relaxation, and potentially a depressed myocardium (with large doses); muscle relaxation may occur due to inhibition or cyclic nucleotide phosphodiesterase, increasing cyclic AMP; muscle relaxation is unrelated to nerve innervation; papaverine increases cerebral blood flow in normal subjects; oxygen uptake is unaltered

**Local Anesthetic/Vasoconstrictor Precautions** No information available to require special precautions

**Effects on Dental Treatment** No effects or complications reported

**Other Adverse Effects** <1%:
Cardiovascular: Flushing of the face, tachycardia, hypotension, arrhythmias with rapid I.V. use
Central nervous system: Depression, dizziness, vertigo, drowsiness, sedation, lethargy, headache
Dermatologic: Pruritus
Gastrointestinal: Dry mouth, nausea, constipation
Hepatic: Hepatic hypersensitivity
Local: Thrombosis at the I.V. administration site
Respiratory: Apnea with rapid I.V. use
Miscellaneous: Sweating

**Drug Interactions**
Decreased effect: Papaverine decreases the effects of levodopa
Increased toxicity: Additive effects with CNS depressants or morphine

**Drug Uptake**
Onset of action: Oral: Rapid
Serum half-life: 0.5-1.5 hours

**Pregnancy Risk Factor** C

**Generic Available** Yes

## Para-Aminosalicylate Sodium

(PAIR a-a MEE noe sa LIS i late SOW dee um)

**Related Information**
Nonviral Infectious Diseases *on page 1095*

**Therapeutic Category** Analgesic, Non-narcotic; Salicylate

**Synonyms** Aminosalicylate Sodium; PAS

**Use** Adjunctive treatment of tuberculosis

**Usual Dosage** Oral:
Children: 240-360 mg/kg/day in 3-4 divided doses
Adults: 12-15 g/day in 3-4 divided doses

**Local Anesthetic/Vasoconstrictor Precautions** No information available to require special precautions

**Effects on Dental Treatment** No effects or complications reported

**Other Adverse Effects** 1% to 10%:
Endocrine & metabolic: Hypokalemia
Gastrointestinal: Nausea, vomiting, diarrhea
Hepatic: Hepatitis, jaundice
Miscellaneous: Allergy reactions

**Pregnancy Risk Factor** C

**Generic Available** No

**Comments** Capsules contain bentonite which may decrease absorption of concomitantly ingested drugs

## Parachlorometaxylenol (PAIR a klor oh met a ZYE le nol)

**U.S. Brand Names** Metasep® [OTC]

**Therapeutic Category** Antiseborrheic Agent, Topical

**Synonyms** PCMX

**Use** Aid in relief of dandruff and associated conditions

**Usual Dosage** Massage to a foamy lather, allow to remain on hair for 5 minutes, rinse thoroughly and repeat

**Local Anesthetic/Vasoconstrictor Precautions** No information available to require special precautions

**Effects on Dental Treatment** No effects or complications reported

**Generic Available** No

♦ **Paraflex®** *see* Chlorzoxazone *on page 242*
♦ **Parafon Forte™ DSC** *see* Chlorzoxazone *on page 242*
♦ **Para-Hist AT®** *see* Promethazine, Phenylephrine, and Codeine *on page 850*

## Paramethasone Acetate (par a METH a sone AS e tate)

**U.S. Brand Names** Haldrone®; Stemex®

**Therapeutic Category** Adrenal Corticosteroid

**Use** Treatment of variety of diseases including those of hematologic, allergic, inflammatory, neoplastic, and autoimmune in origin

**Usual Dosage** Oral: 2-24 mg/day

**Local Anesthetic/Vasoconstrictor Precautions** No information available to require special precautions

**Effects on Dental Treatment** No effects or complications reported

**Pregnancy Risk Factor** C

**Generic Available** No

(Continued)

## Paramethasone Acetate *(Continued)*

**Comments** Likely to inhibit maturation and growth in adolescents; at high doses (>15 mg/d) increased urinary excretion of nitrogen and calcium will occur

- ♦ **Paraplatin®** *see* Carboplatin *on page 190*
- ♦ **Par Decon®** *see* Chlorpheniramine, Phenyltoloxamine, Phenylpropanolamine, and Phenylephrine *on page 237*
- ♦ **Paredrine®** *see* Hydroxyamphetamine *on page 515*

## Paregoric (par e GOR ik)

**Therapeutic Category** Analgesic, Narcotic; Antidiarrheal

**Use** Treatment of diarrhea or relief of pain; neonatal opiate withdrawal

**Usual Dosage** Oral:

Neonatal opiate withdrawal: Instill 3-6 drops every 3-6 hours as needed, or initially 0.2 mL every 3 hours; increase dosage by approximately 0.05 mL every 3 hours until withdrawal symptoms are controlled; it is rare to exceed 0.7 mL/dose. Stabilize withdrawal symptoms for 3-5 days, then gradually decrease dosage over a 2- to 4-week period.

Children: 0.25-0.5 mL/kg 1-4 times/day

Adults: 5-10 mL 1-4 times/day

**Mechanism of Action** Increases smooth muscle tone in GI tract, decreases motility and peristalsis, diminishes digestive secretions

**Local Anesthetic/Vasoconstrictor Precautions** No information available to require special precautions

**Effects on Dental Treatment** No effects or complications reported

**Other Adverse Effects**

>10%:

Cardiovascular: Hypotension
Central nervous system: Drowsiness, dizziness
Gastrointestinal: Constipation
Neuromuscular & skeletal: Weakness

1% to 10%:

Central nervous system: Restlessness, headache, malaise
Genitourinary: Ureteral spasms, decreased urination
Miscellaneous: Histamine release

<1%:

Cardiovascular: Peripheral vasodilation
Central nervous system: Insomnia, CNS depression, mental depression, increased intracranial pressure
Gastrointestinal: Anorexia, stomach cramps, nausea, vomiting, biliary spasm
Genitourinary: Urinary tract spasm
Ocular: Miosis
Respiratory: Respiratory depression
Miscellaneous: Physical and psychological dependence

**Drug Interactions** Increased effect/toxicity with CNS depressants (eg, alcohol, narcotics, benzodiazepines, TCAs, MAO inhibitors, phenothiazine)

**Pregnancy Risk Factor** B (D when used long-term or in high doses)

**Generic Available** Yes

- ♦ **Paremyd® Ophthalmic** *see* Hydroxyamphetamine and Tropicamide *on page 515*
- ♦ **Parenteral Multiple Vitamin** *see* Vitamins, Multiple *on page 1051*
- ♦ **Parepectolin®** *see* Kaolin and Pectin With Opium *on page 562*
- ♦ **Par Glycerol®** *see* Iodinated Glycerol *on page 545*
- ♦ **Pargyline and Methyclothiazide** *see* Methyclothiazide and Pargyline *on page 658*

## Paricalcitol (par eh CAL ci tol)

**U.S. Brand Names** Zemplar™

**Therapeutic Category** Vitamin D Analog

**Use** Prevention and treatment of secondary hyperparathyroidism associated with chronic renal failure

**Usual Dosage** Adults: I.V.: 0.04-0.1 mcg/kg (2.8-7 mcg) given as a bolus dose no more frequently than every other day at any time during dialysis; dose as high as 0.24 mcg/kg (16.8 mcg) have been administered safely

**Mechanism of Action** Synthetic vitamin D analog which has been shown to reduce PTH serum concentrations

**Local Anesthetic/Vasoconstrictor Precautions** No information available to require special precautions

**Effects on Dental Treatment** No effects or complications reported

**Other Adverse Effects** The three most frequently reported events in the clinical studies were nausea, vomiting and edema, which are commonly seen in hemodialysis patients.

>10%: Gastrointestinal: Nausea (13%)

<10%:

Cardiovascular: Palpitations, peripheral edema (7%)
Central nervous system: Chills, malaise, fever, lightheadedness (5%)
Gastrointestinal: Vomiting (8%), GI bleeding (5%), xerostomia (3%)
Respiratory: Pneumonia (5%)
Miscellaneous: Flu-like symptoms, sepsis

**Drug Interactions** Phosphate or vitamin D-related compounds should not be taken concurrently; digitalis toxicity is potentiated by hypercalcemia

**Pregnancy Risk Factor** C

**Generic Available** No

♦ **Parlodel®** *see* Bromocriptine *on page 150*

♦ **Parnate®** *see* Tranylcypromine *on page 1005*

## Paromomycin (par oh moe MYE sin)

**U.S. Brand Names** Humatin®

**Therapeutic Category** Amebicide

**Use** Treatment of acute and chronic intestinal amebiasis due to susceptible *Entamoeba histolytica* (not effective in the treatment of extraintestinal amebiasis); tapeworm infestations; adjunctive management of hepatic coma; treatment of cryptosporidial diarrhea

**Usual Dosage** Oral:

Intestinal amebiasis: Children and Adults: 25-35 mg/kg/day in 3 divided doses for 5-10 days

*Dientamoeba fragilis*: Children and Adults: 25-30 mg/kg/day in 3 divided doses for 7 days

*Cryptosporidium*: Adults with AIDS: 1.5-2.25 g/day in 3-6 divided doses for 10-14 days (occasionally courses of up to 4-8 weeks may be needed)

Tapeworm (fish, dog, bovine, porcine):
Children: 11 mg/kg every 15 minutes for 4 doses
Adults: 1 g every 15 minutes for 4 doses

Hepatic coma: Adults: 4 g/day in 2-4 divided doses for 5-6 days

Dwarf tapeworm: Children and Adults: 45 mg/kg/dose every day for 5-7 days

**Mechanism of Action** Acts directly on ameba; has antibacterial activity against normal and pathogenic organisms in the GI tract; interferes with bacterial protein synthesis by binding to 30S ribosomal subunits

**Local Anesthetic/Vasoconstrictor Precautions** No information available to require special precautions

**Effects on Dental Treatment** No effects or complications reported

**Other Adverse Effects**

1% to 10%: Gastrointestinal: Diarrhea, abdominal cramps, nausea, vomiting, heartburn

<1%:

Central nervous system: Headache, vertigo
Dermatologic: Rash, pruritus, exanthema
Gastrointestinal: Steatorrhea, secondary enterocolitis
Hematologic: Eosinophilia
Otic: Ototoxicity

**Drug Uptake**

Absorption: Not absorbed via oral route

**Pregnancy Risk Factor** C

**Generic Available** No

## Paroxetine (pa ROKS e teen)

**Related Information**

Vasoconstrictor Interactions With Antidepressants *on page 1277*

**U.S. Brand Names** Paxil™

**Therapeutic Category** Antidepressant, Selective Serotonin Reuptake Inhibitor

**Use** Treatment of depression; indicated for treatment of obsessions and compulsions in patients with obsessive-compulsive disorder (OCD) as defined in the DSM-IV

**Usual Dosage** Adults: Oral:

Depression: 20 mg once daily (maximum: 60 mg/day), preferably in the morning; in elderly, debilitated, or patients with hepatic or renal impairment, start with 10 mg/day (maximum: 40 mg/day); adjust doses at 7-day intervals

Panic disorder and obsessive compulsive disorder: Recommended average daily dose: 40 mg, this dosage should be given after an adequate trial on 20 mg/day and then titrating upward

(Continued)

## Paroxetine *(Continued)*

**Mechanism of Action** Paroxetine is a selective serotonin reuptake inhibitor, chemically unrelated to tricyclic, tetracyclic, or other antidepressants; presumably, the inhibition of serotonin reuptake from brain synapse stimulated serotonin activity in the brain

**Local Anesthetic/Vasoconstrictor Precautions** Although caution should be used in patients taking tricyclic antidepressants, no interactions have been reported with vasoconstrictor and paroxetine, a nontricyclic antidepressant which acts to increase serotonin

**Effects on Dental Treatment** >10% of patients experience dry mouth; prolonged use of paroxetine may decrease or inhibit salivary flow; normal salivary flow will resume with cessation of drug therapy

**Other Adverse Effects**

>10%:

- Central nervous system: Headache, somnolence, dizziness, insomnia
- Gastrointestinal: Nausea, constipation, diarrhea
- Genitourinary: Ejaculatory disturbances
- Neuromuscular & skeletal: Weakness
- Miscellaneous: Sweating

1% to 10%:

- Cardiovascular: Palpitations, vasodilation, postural hypotension
- Central nervous system: Nervousness, anxiety
- Endocrine & metabolic: Decreased libido
- Gastrointestinal: Anorexia, flatulence, vomiting
- Neuromuscular & skeletal: Tremor, paresthesia

<1%:

- Cardiovascular: Bradycardia, hypotension
- Central nervous system: Migraine, akinesia
- Dermatologic: Alopecia
- Endocrine & metabolic: Amenorrhea
- Gastrointestinal: Gastritis, thirst
- Hematologic: Anemia, leukopenia
- Neuromuscular & skeletal: Arthritis
- Otic: Ear pain
- Ocular: Eye pain
- Respiratory: Asthma
- Miscellaneous: Bruxism

**Drug Interactions**

Decreased effect of paroxetine when taken with phenobarbital, phenytoin

Increased toxicity: Alcohol, cimetidine, MAO inhibitors (hyperpyrexic crisis); increased effect/toxicity of tricyclic antidepressants, fluoxetine, sertraline, phenothiazines, class 1C antiarrhythmics, warfarin

**Drug Uptake** Serum half-life: 21 hours

**Pregnancy Risk Factor** B

**Generic Available** No


- ♦ **Partuss® LA** *see* Guaifenesin and Phenylpropanolamine *on page 480*
- ♦ **PAS** *see* Para-Aminosalicylate Sodium *on page 765*
- ♦ **Patanol®** *see* Olopatadine *on page 739*
- ♦ **Pathilon®** *see* Tridihexethyl *on page 1015*
- ♦ **Pathocil®** *see* Dicloxacillin *on page 321*
- ♦ **Patients Requiring Sedation** *see page 1152*
- ♦ **Patients Undergoing Cancer Therapy** *see page 1154*
- ♦ **Pavabid®** *see* Papaverine *on page 764*
- ♦ **Pavatine®** *see* Papaverine *on page 764*
- ♦ **Paxil™** *see* Paroxetine *on previous page*
- ♦ **Paxipam®** *see* Halazepam *on page 487*
- ♦ **PBZ®** *see* Tripelennamine *on page 1025*
- ♦ **PBZ-SR®** *see* Tripelennamine *on page 1025*
- ♦ **PCE® Oral** *see* Erythromycin *on page 383*
- ♦ **PCMX** *see* Parachlorometaxylenol *on page 765*
- ♦ **Pectin and Kaolin** *see* Kaolin and Pectin *on page 562*
- ♦ **Pedameth®** *see* Methionine *on page 649*
- ♦ **Pedia Care® Oral** *see* Pseudoephedrine *on page 863*
- ♦ **Pediacof®** *see* Chlorpheniramine, Phenylephrine, and Codeine *on page 234*
- ♦ **Pediaflor®** *see* Fluoride *on page 441*
- ♦ **Pedialyte® [OTC]** *see* Enteral Nutritional Products *on page 371*
- ♦ **Pediapred®** *see* Prednisolone *on page 832*
- ♦ **Pediatric Advil® [OTC]** *see* Ibuprofen *on page 522*

- **Pediatric Triban®** *see* Trimethobenzamide *on page 1020*
- **Pediazole®** *see* Erythromycin and Sulfisoxazole *on page 385*
- **Pedi-Boro® [OTC]** *see* Aluminum Sulfate and Calcium Acetate *on page 57*
- **Pedi-Cort V® Creme** *see* Clioquinol and Hydrocortisone *on page 260*
- **Pediotic® Otic** *see* Neomycin, Polymyxin B, and Hydrocortisone *on page 712*
- **Pedi-Pro Topical [OTC]** *see* Undecylenic Acid and Derivatives *on page 1033*
- **Pedituss®** *see* Chlorpheniramine, Phenylephrine, and Codeine *on page 234*
- **PedtE-PAK-4®** *see* Trace Metals *on page 1001*
- **Pedtrace-4®** *see* Trace Metals *on page 1001*
- **PedvaxHIB™** *see Haemophilus* b Conjugate Vaccine *on page 486*

## Pegademase Bovine (peg A de mase BOE vine)

**U.S. Brand Names** Adagen™

**Therapeutic Category** Enzyme, Replacement Therapy

**Use** Enzyme replacement therapy for adenosine deaminase (ADA) deficiency in patients with severe combined immunodeficiency disease (SCID) who cannot benefit from bone marrow transplant; not a cure for SCID, unlike bone marrow transplants, injections must be used the rest of the child's life, therefore, is not really an alternative

**Usual Dosage** Children: I.M.: Dose given every 7 days, 10 units/kg the first dose, 15 units/kg the second dose, and 20 units/kg the third dose; maintenance dose: 20 units/kg/week is recommended depending on patient's ADA level; maximum single dose: 30 units/kg

**Mechanism of Action** Adenosine deaminase is an enzyme that catalyzes the deamination of both adenosine and deoxyadenosine. Hereditary lack of adenosine deaminase activity results in severe combined immunodeficiency disease, a fatal disorder of infancy characterized by profound defects of both cellular and humoral immunity. It is estimated that 25% of patients with the autosomal recessive form of severe combined immunodeficiency lack adenosine deaminase.

**Local Anesthetic/Vasoconstrictor Precautions** No information available to require special precautions

**Effects on Dental Treatment** No effects or complications reported

**Other Adverse Effects** <1%:

Central nervous system: Headache

Local: Pain at injection site

**Drug Interactions** Decreased effect: Vidarabine

**Drug Uptake**

Plasma adenosine deaminase activity generally normalizes after 2-3 weeks of weekly I.M. injections

Absorption: Rapid

Serum half-life: 48-72 hours

**Pregnancy Risk Factor** C

**Generic Available** No

- **Peganone®** *see* Ethotoin *on page 409*

## Pegaspargase (peg AS par jase)

**U.S. Brand Names** Oncaspar®

**Therapeutic Category** Antineoplastic Agent, Miscellaneous

**Synonyms** PEG-L-asparaginase

**Use** Induction treatment of acute lymphoblastic leukemia in combination with other chemotherapeutic agents in patients who have developed hypersensitivity to native forms of asparaginase derived from *E. coli* and/or *Erwinia chrysanthemia*, treatment of lymphoma

**Usual Dosage**

Dose must be individualized based upon clinical response and tolerance of the patient (refer to individual protocols)

I.M. administration is **preferred** over I.V. administration; I.M. administration may decrease the incidence of hepatotoxicity, coagulopathy, and GI and renal disorders

Children: I.M., I.V.:

Body surface area ≤0.6 $m^2$: 82.5 units/kg every 14 days

Body surface area ≥0.6 $m^2$: 2500 units/$m^2$ every 14 days

Adults: I.M., I.V.: 2,500 units/$m^2$ every 14 days

**Mechanism of Action**

Pegaspargase is a modified version of the enzyme asparaginase. The asparaginase used in the manufacture of pegaspargase is derived from *Escherichia coli*.

Some malignant cells (ie, lymphoblastic leukemia cells and those of lymphocyte derivation) must acquire the amino acid asparagine from surrounding fluid such

(Continued)

## Pegaspargase *(Continued)*

as blood, whereas normal cells can synthesize their own asparagine. asparaginase is an enzyme that deaminates asparagine to aspartic acid and ammonia in the plasma and extracellular fluid and therefore deprives tumor cells of the amino acid for protein synthesis.

**Local Anesthetic/Vasoconstrictor Precautions** No information available to require special precautions

**Effects on Dental Treatment** No effects or complications reported

**Other Adverse Effects** Overall, the adult patients had a somewhat higher incidence of asparaginase toxicities, except for hypersensitivity reactions, than the pediatric patients

>10%:
- Cardiovascular: Edema
- Central nervous system: Pain
- Dermatologic: Urticaria, erythema
- Gastrointestinal: Pancreatitis, (sometimes fulminant and fatal); elevated serum amylase and lipase, swelling lip
- Hepatic: Elevations of AST, ALT, and bilirubin (direct and indirect); jaundice, ascites and hypoalbuminemia, fatty changes in the liver; liver failure
- Local: Induration, tenderness
- Neuromuscular: Arthralgia
- Respiratory: Bronchospasm, dyspnea
- Miscellaneous: Hypersensitivity (acute or delayed), acute anaphylaxis,

>5%:
- Allergic reactions: Rash, erythema, edema, pain, fever, chills, dyspnea or bronchospasm
- Central nervous system: Malaise
- Gastrointestinal: Emetic potential: Mild (>5%)

1% to 5%:
- Cardiovascular: Hypotension, tachycardia, thrombosis
- Central nervous system: Chills
- Dermatologic: Lip edema
- Gastrointestinal: Abdominal pain
- Hematologic: Decreased anticoagulant effect, disseminated intravascular coagulation, decreased fibrinogen, hemolytic anemia, leukopenia, pancytopenia, thrombocytopenia, increased thromboplastin.
  - Myelosuppressive effects: WBC: Mild; Platelets: Mild; Onset (days): 7; Nadir (days): 14; Recovery (days): 21
- Local: Injection site hypersensitivity
- Respiratory: Dyspnea

**Drug Uptake**
Serum half-life: 5.73 days

**Pregnancy Risk Factor** C

**Generic Available** No

♦ **PEG-L-asparaginase** *see* Pegaspargase *on previous page*

## Pemoline (PEM oh leen)

**U.S. Brand Names** Cylert®

**Therapeutic Category** Central Nervous System Stimulant, Nonamphetamine

**Use** Treatment of attention deficit disorder with hyperactivity (ADDH); narcolepsy

**Usual Dosage** Children ≥6 years: Oral: Initial: 37.5 mg given once daily in the morning, increase by 18.75 mg/day at weekly intervals; usual effective dose range: 56.25-75 mg/day; maximum: 112.5 mg/day; dosage range: 0.5-3 mg/kg/24 hours; significant benefit may not be evident until third or fourth week of administration

**Mechanism of Action** Blocks the reuptake mechanism of dopaminergic neurons, appears to act at the cerebral cortex and subcortical structures; CNS and respiratory stimulant with weak sympathomimetic effects; actions may be mediated via increase in CNS dopamine

**Local Anesthetic/Vasoconstrictor Precautions** Pemoline has minimal sympathomimetic effects; there are no precautions in using vasoconstrictors

**Effects on Dental Treatment** No effects or complications reported

**Other Adverse Effects**

>10%:
- Central nervous system: Insomnia
- Gastrointestinal: Anorexia, weight loss

1% to 10%:
- Central nervous system: Dizziness, drowsiness, mental depression
- Dermatologic: Skin rash
- Gastrointestinal: Stomach pain, nausea

<1%:

Central nervous system: Seizures, precipitation of Tourette's syndrome, hallucination, headache, movement disorders

Endocrine & metabolic: Growth reaction

Gastrointestinal: Diarrhea

Hepatic: Elevated liver enzymes (usually reversible upon discontinuation), hepatitis, jaundice

**Drug Interactions** Decreased effect of insulin

**Drug Uptake**

Duration: 8 hours

Serum half-life:

Children: 7-8.6 hours

Adults: 12 hours

Time to peak serum concentration: Oral: Within 2-4 hours

**Pregnancy Risk Factor** B

**Generic Available** No

## Penbutolol (pen BYOO toe lole)

**Related Information**

Cardiovascular Diseases *on page 1066*

**U.S. Brand Names** Levatol®

**Therapeutic Category** Beta-adrenergic Blocker, Noncardioselective

**Use** Treatment of mild to moderate arterial hypertension

**Usual Dosage** Adults: Oral: Initial: 20 mg once daily, full effect of a 20 or 40 mg dose is seen by the end of a 2-week period, doses of 40-80 mg have been tolerated but have shown little additional antihypertensive effects

**Mechanism of Action** Blocks both $beta_1$- and $beta_2$-receptors and has mild intrinsic sympathomimetic activity; has negative inotropic and chronotropic effects and can significantly slow A-V nodal conduction

**Local Anesthetic/Vasoconstrictor Precautions** No information available to require special precautions

**Effects on Dental Treatment** No effects or complications reported

**Other Adverse Effects**

1% to 10%:

Cardiovascular: Congestive heart failure, arrhythmia

Central nervous system: Mental depression, headache, dizziness

Neuromuscular & skeletal: Back pain, arthralgia

<1%:

Cardiovascular: Bradycardia, chest pain, mesenteric arterial thrombosis, A-V block, persistent bradycardia, hypotension, chest pain, edema, Raynaud's phenomenon

Central nervous system: Fatigue, insomnia, lethargy, nightmares, depression, confusion

Dermatologic: Purpura

Endocrine & metabolic: Hyperglycemia

Gastrointestinal: Ischemic colitis, constipation, nausea, diarrhea

Genitourinary: Impotence

Hematologic: Thrombocytopenia

Respiratory: Bronchospasm

Miscellaneous: Cold extremities

**Drug Uptake**

Absorption: Well absorbed, ~100%

Half-life: 5 hours

**Pregnancy Risk Factor** C

**Generic Available** No

## Penciclovir (pen SYE kloe veer)

**Related Information**

Oral Viral Infections *on page 1137*

**U.S. Brand Names** Denavir™

**Therapeutic Category** Antiviral Agent, Topical

**Use** Antiviral cream for the treatment of recurrent herpes labialis (cold sores) in adults

**Usual Dosage** Apply cream at the first sign or symptom of cold sore (eg, tingling, swelling); apply every 2 hours during waking hours for 4 days

**Mechanism of Action** In cells infected with HSV-1 or HSV-2, viral thymidine kinase phosphorylates penciclovir to a monophosphate form which, in turn, is converted to penciclovir triphosphate by cellular kinases. Penciclovir triphosphate inhibits HSV polymerase competitively with deoxyguanosine triphosphate. Consequently, herpes viral DNA synthesis and, therefore, replication are selectively inhibited

(Continued)

## Penciclovir *(Continued)*

**Local Anesthetic/Vasoconstrictor Precautions** No information available to require special precautions

**Effects on Dental Treatment** No effects or complications reported

**Other Adverse Effects** 1% to 10%:

Central nervous system: Headache

Local: Application site reaction

**Contraindications** Patients with known hypersensitivity to the product or any of its components

**Warnings/Precautions** Penciclovir should only be used on herpes labialis on the lips and face; because no data are available, application to mucous membranes is not recommended. Avoid application in or near eyes since it may cause irritation. The effect of penciclovir has not been established in immunocompromised patients.

**Drug Interactions** No data reported

**Drug Uptake** Measurable penciclovir concentrations were not detected in plasma or urine of health male volunteers following single or repeat application of the 1% cream at a dose of 180 mg penciclovir daily (approximately 67 times the usual clinical dose)

**Pregnancy Risk Factor** B

**Dosage Forms** Cream: 1% [10 mg/g] (2 g)

**Generic Available** No

♦ **Penetrex™** *see* Enoxacin *on page 369*

## Penicillamine (pen i SIL a meen)

**U.S. Brand Names** Cuprimine®; Depen®

**Therapeutic Category** Chelating Agent

**Synonyms** D-3-Mercaptovaline; β,β-Dimethylcysteine; D-Penicillamine

**Use** Treatment of Wilson's disease, cystinuria, adjunct in the treatment of severe rheumatoid arthritis; lead poisoning, primary biliary cirrhosis

**Usual Dosage** Oral:

Rheumatoid arthritis:

- Children: Initial: 3 mg/kg/day (≤250 mg/day) for 3 months, then 6 mg/kg/day (≤500 mg/day) in divided doses twice daily for 3 months to a maximum of 10 mg/kg/day in 3-4 divided doses
- Adults: 125-250 mg/day, may increase dose at 1- to 3-month intervals up to 1-1.5 g/day

Wilson's disease (doses titrated to maintain urinary copper excretion >1 mg/day):

- Infants <6 months: 250 mg/dose once daily
- Children <12 years: 250 mg/dose 2-3 times/day
- Adults: 250 mg 4 times/day

Cystinuria:

- Children: 30 mg/kg/day in 4 divided doses
- Adults: 1-4 g/day in divided doses every 6 hours

Lead poisoning (continue until blood lead level is <60 μg/dL): Children and Adults: 25-35 mg/kg/d, administered in 3-4 divided doses; initiating treatment at 25% of this dose and gradually increasing to the full dose over 2-3 weeks may minimize adverse reactions

Primary biliary cirrhosis: 250 mg/day to start, increase by 250 mg every 2 weeks up to a maintenance dose of 1 g/day, usually given 250 mg 4 times/day

Arsenic poisoning: Children: 100 mg/kg/day in divided doses every 6 hours for 5 days; maximum: 1 g/day

**Mechanism of Action** Chelates with lead, copper, mercury and other heavy metals to form stable, soluble complexes that are excreted in urine; depresses circulating IgM rheumatoid factor, depresses T-cell but not B-cell activity; combines with cystine to form a compound which is more soluble, thus cystine calculi are prevented

**Local Anesthetic/Vasoconstrictor Precautions** No information available to require special precautions

**Effects on Dental Treatment** No effects or complications reported

**Other Adverse Effects**

>10%:

- Central nervous system: Fever
- Dermatologic: Rash, urticaria, itching
- Gastrointestinal: Hypogeusia
- Neuromuscular & skeletal: Arthralgia

1% to 10%:

- Cardiovascular: Edema of the face, feet, or lower legs
- Central nervous system: Fever, chills

Gastrointestinal: Weight gain, sore throat
Genitourinary: Bloody or cloudy urine
Hematologic: Aplastic or hemolytic anemia, leukopenia, thrombocytopenia
Miscellaneous: White spots on lips or mouth

<1%:

Central nervous system: Fatigue
Dermatologic: Toxic epidermal necrolysis, pemphigus, increased friability of the skin
Endocrine & metabolic: Iron deficiency
Gastrointestinal: Nausea, vomiting, anorexia, pancreatitis
Hepatic: Cholestatic jaundice, hepatitis
Neuromuscular & skeletal: Myasthenia gravis syndrome, weakness
Ocular: Optic neuritis
Otic: Tinnitus
Renal: Nephrotic syndrome
Respiratory: Coughing, wheezing
Miscellaneous: SLE-like syndrome, spitting of blood allergic reactions, lymphadenopathy

**Warnings/Precautions** Cross-sensitivity with penicillin is possible; therefore, should be used cautiously in patients with a history of penicillin allergy. Patients on penicillamine for Wilson's disease or cystinuria should receive pyridoxine supplementation 25 mg/day; once instituted for Wilson's disease or cystinuria, continue treatment on a daily basis; interruptions of even a few days have been followed by hypersensitivity with reinstitution of therapy. Penicillamine has been associated with fatalities due to agranulocytosis, aplastic anemia, thrombocytopenia, Goodpasture's syndrome, and myasthenia gravis; patients should be warned to report promptly any symptoms suggesting toxicity; approximately 33% of patients will experience an allergic reaction; since toxicity may be dose related, it is recommended not to exceed 750 mg/day in elderly.

**Drug Interactions**

Decreased effect with iron and zinc salts, antacids (magnesium, calcium, aluminum) and food
Decreased effect/levels of digoxin
Increased effect of gold, antimalarials, immunosuppressants, phenylbutazone (hematologic, renal toxicity)

**Drug Uptake**

Absorption: Oral: 40% to 70%
Serum half-life: 1.7-3.2 hours
Time to peak serum concentration: Within 2 hours

**Pregnancy Risk Factor** D

**Dosage Forms**

Capsule: 125 mg, 250 mg
Tablet: 250 mg

**Dietary Considerations** Should be administered at least 1 hour before a meal on an empty stomach; do not administer with milk; iron and zinc may decrease drug action; increase dietary intake of pyridoxine; for Wilson's disease, decrease copper in diet and omit chocolate, nuts, shellfish, mushrooms, liver, raisins, broccoli, and molasses; for lead poisoning, decrease calcium in diet

Patients unable to swallow capsules may mix contents of capsule with fruit juice or chilled pureed fruit; limit alcohol

**Generic Available** No

**Selected Readings**

Aronow R and Fleschmann LE, "Mercury Poisoning in Children," *Clin Pediatr (Phila)*, 1976, 15(10):936-45.
Hryhorczuk DO, Meyers L, and Chen G, "Treatment of Mercury Intoxication in a Dentist With N-Acetyl-D,L-Penicillamine," *J Toxicol Clin Toxicol*, 1982, 19(4):401-8.
Lyle WH, "Penicillamine in Metal Poisoning," *J Rheumatol Suppl*, 1981, 7:96-9.
Rosa FW, "Teratogen Update. Penicillamine," *Teratology*, 1986, 33(1):127-31.

## Penicillin G Benzathine (pen i SIL in jee BENZ a theen)

**Related Information**

Dental Drug Interactions: Update on Drug Combinations Requiring Special Considerations *on page 1225*
Nonviral Infectious Diseases *on page 1095*

**U.S. Brand Names** Bicillin® L-A; Permapen®

**Canadian Brand Names** Megacillin® Susp

**Therapeutic Category** Antibiotic, Penicillin

**Use** Active against some gram-positive organisms, few gram-negative organisms such as *Neisseria gonorrhoeae*, and some anaerobes and spirochetes; used only for the treatment of mild to moderately severe infections caused by organisms susceptible to low concentrations of penicillin G or for prophylaxis of infections caused by these organisms; used when patient cannot be kept in a hospital environment and neurosyphilis has been ruled out

(Continued)

## Penicillin G Benzathine *(Continued)*

The CDC and AAP do not currently recommend the use of penicillin G benzathine to treat congenital syphilis or neurosyphilis due to reported treatment failures and lack of published clinical data on its efficacy

**Usual Dosage** I.M.: Give undiluted injection; higher doses result in more sustained rather than higher levels. Use a penicillin G benzathine-penicillin G procaine combination to achieve early peak levels in acute infections.

Children:

- Group A streptococcal upper respiratory infection: 25,000-50,000 units/kg as a single dose; maximum: 1.2 million units
- Prophylaxis of recurrent rheumatic fever: 25,000-50,000 units/kg every 3-4 weeks; maximum: 1.2 million units/dose
- Early syphilis: 50,000 units/kg as a single injection; maximum: 2.4 million units
- Syphilis of more than 1-year duration: 50,000 units/kg every week for 3 doses; maximum: 2.4 million units/dose

Adults:

- Group A streptococcal upper respiratory infection: 1.2 million units as a single dose
- Prophylaxis of recurrent rheumatic fever: 1.2 million units every 3-4 weeks or 600,000 units twice monthly
- Early syphilis: 2.4 million units as a single dose in 2 injection sites
- Syphilis of more than 1-year duration: 2.4 million units in 2 injection sites once weekly for 3 doses
- Not indicated as single drug therapy for neurosyphilis, but may be given 1 time/week for 3 weeks following I.V. treatment (refer to Penicillin G monograph for dosing)

**Mechanism of Action** Interferes with bacterial cell wall synthesis during active multiplication, causing cell wall death and resultant bactericidal activity against susceptible bacteria

**Local Anesthetic/Vasoconstrictor Precautions** No information available to require special precautions

**Effects on Dental Treatment** No effects or complications reported

**Other Adverse Effects**

1% to 10%: Local: Pain

<1%:

- Central nervous system: Convulsions, confusion, drowsiness, fever
- Dermatologic: Rash
- Endocrine & metabolic: Electrolyte imbalance
- Hematologic: Hemolytic anemia, positive Coombs' reaction
- Local: Thrombophlebitis
- Neuromuscular & skeletal: Myoclonus
- Renal: Acute interstitial nephritis
- Miscellaneous: Hypersensitivity reactions, anaphylaxis, Jarisch-Herxheimer reaction

**Drug Interactions**

Decreased effect: Tetracyclines cause decreased penicillin effectiveness

Increased effect: Probenecid causes increased penicillin levels

**Drug Uptake**

Absorption: I.M.: Slow

Time to peak serum concentration: Within 12-24 hours; serum levels are usually detectable for 1-4 weeks depending on the dose; larger doses result in more sustained levels rather than higher levels

**Pregnancy Risk Factor** B

**Generic Available** No

## Penicillin G Benzathine and Procaine Combined

(pen i SIL in jee BENZ a theen & PROE kane KOM bined)

**U.S. Brand Names** Bicillin® C-R 900/300 Injection; Bicillin® C-R Injection

**Therapeutic Category** Antibiotic, Penicillin

**Synonyms** Penicillin G Procaine and Benzathine Combined

**Use** Active against most gram-positive organisms, mostly streptococcal and pneumococcal

**Usual Dosage** I.M.:

Children:

- <30 lb: 600,000 units in a single dose
- 30-60 lb: 900,000 units to 1.2 million units in a single dose

Children >60 lb and Adults: 2.4 million units in a single dose

**Local Anesthetic/Vasoconstrictor Precautions** No information available to require special precautions

**Effects on Dental Treatment** No effects or complications reported

**Other Adverse Effects** 1% to 10%:
Central nervous system: CNS toxicity (convulsions, confusion, drowsiness, myoclonus)
Hematologic: Positive Coombs' reaction, hemolytic anemia
Renal: Interstitial nephritis
Miscellaneous: Hypersensitivity reactions, Jarisch-Herxheimer reaction
**Pregnancy Risk Factor** B
**Generic Available** No

## Penicillin G, Parenteral, Aqueous

(pen i SIL in jee, pa REN ter al, AYE kwee us)

**Related Information**
Dental Drug Interactions: Update on Drug Combinations Requiring Special Considerations *on page 1225*
Nonviral Infectious Diseases *on page 1095*
**U.S. Brand Names** Pfizerpen®
**Therapeutic Category** Antibiotic, Penicillin
**Use** Active against some gram-positive organisms, generally not *Staphylococcus aureus*; some gram-negative such as *Neisseria gonorrhoeae*, and some anaerobes and spirochetes; although ceftriaxone is now the drug of choice for Lyme disease and gonorrhea
**Usual Dosage** I.M., I.V.:
Children (sodium salt is preferred in children): 100,000-250,000 units/kg/day in divided doses every 4 hours; maximum: 4.8 million units/24 hours
Severe infections: Up to 400,000 units/kg/day in divided doses every 4 hours; maximum dose: 24 million units/day
Adults: 2-24 million units/day in divided doses every 4 hours

Disseminated gonococcal infections or gonococcus ophthalmia (if organism proven sensitive): 100,000 units/kg/day in 2 equal doses (4 equal doses/day for infants >1 week)

Gonococcal meningitis: 150,000 units/kg in 2 equal doses (4 doses/day for infants >1 week)
**Mechanism of Action** Interferes with bacterial cell wall synthesis during active multiplication, causing cell wall death and resultant bactericidal activity against susceptible bacteria
**Local Anesthetic/Vasoconstrictor Precautions** No information available to require special precautions
**Effects on Dental Treatment** No effects or complications reported
**Other Adverse Effects** <1%:
Central nervous system: Convulsions, confusion, drowsiness, fever
Dermatologic: Rash
Endocrine & metabolic: Electrolyte imbalance
Hematologic: Hemolytic anemia, positive Coombs' reaction
Local: Thrombophlebitis
Neuromuscular & skeletal: Myoclonus
Renal: Acute interstitial nephritis
Miscellaneous: Hypersensitivity reactions, anaphylaxis, Jarisch-Herxheimer reaction
**Drug Interactions**
Decreased effect: Tetracyclines cause decreased penicillin effectiveness
Increased effect: Probenecid causes increased penicillin levels
**Drug Uptake**
Serum half-life:
Children and adults with normal renal function: 20-50 minutes
End-stage renal disease: 3.3-5.1 hours
Time to peak serum concentration:
I.M.: Within 30 minutes
I.V. Within 1 hour
**Pregnancy Risk Factor** B
**Generic Available** Yes

## Penicillin G Procaine (pen i SIL in jee PROE kane)

**Related Information**
Dental Drug Interactions: Update on Drug Combinations Requiring Special Considerations *on page 1225*
**U.S. Brand Names** Crysticillin® A.S.; Pfizerpen®-AS; Wycillin®
**Canadian Brand Names** Ayercillin®
**Therapeutic Category** Antibiotic, Penicillin
**Use** Moderately severe infections due to *Neisseria gonorrhoeae*, *Treponema pallidum* and other penicillin G-sensitive microorganisms that are susceptible to low but prolonged serum penicillin concentrations
(Continued)

## Penicillin G Procaine *(Continued)*

**Usual Dosage** I.M.:

Children: 25,000-50,000 units/kg/day in divided doses 1-2 times/day; not to exceed 4.8 million units/24 hours

Gonorrhea: 100,000 units/kg (maximum 4.8 million units) one time (in 2 injection sites) along with probenecid 25 mg/kg (maximum: 1 g orally) 30 minutes prior to procaine penicillin

Congenital syphilis: 50,000 units/kg/day for 10-14 days

Adults: 0.6-4.8 million units/day in divided doses every 12-24 hours

Uncomplicated gonorrhea: 1 g probenecid orally, then 4.8 million units procaine penicillin divided into 2 injection sites 30 minutes later

Endocarditis caused by susceptible viridans *Streptococcus* (when used in conjunction with an aminoglycoside): 1.2 million units every 6 hours for 2-4 weeks

Neurosyphilis: I.M.: 2-4 million units/day with 500 mg probenecid by mouth 4 times/day for 10-14 days; **penicillin G aqueous I.V. is the preferred agent**

**Mechanism of Action** Inhibits bacterial cell wall synthesis by binding to one or more of the penicillin binding proteins (PBPs); which in turn inhibits the final transpeptidation step of peptidoglycan synthesis in bacterial cell walls, thus inhibiting cell wall biosynthesis. Bacteria eventually lyse due to ongoing activity of cell wall autolytic enzymes (autolysins and murein hydrolases) while cell wall assembly is arrested.

**Local Anesthetic/Vasoconstrictor Precautions** No information available to require special precautions

**Effects on Dental Treatment** No effects or complications reported

**Other Adverse Effects**

>10%: Local: Pain at injection site

<1%:

Cardiovascular: Myocardial depression, vasodilation, conduction disturbances

Central nervous system: CNS stimulation, seizures, confusion, drowsiness

Hematologic: Hemolytic anemia, positive Coombs' reaction

Local: Sterile abscess at injection site

Neuromuscular & skeletal: Myoclonus

Renal: Interstitial nephritis

Miscellaneous: Pseudoanaphylactic reactions, hypersensitivity reactions, Jarisch-Herxheimer reaction

**Drug Interactions**

Decreased effect: Tetracyclines cause decreased penicillin effectiveness

Increased effect: Probenecid causes increased penicillin levels

**Drug Uptake**

Absorption: I.M.: Slowly absorbed

Time to peak serum concentration: Within 1-4 hours; can persist within the therapeutic range for 15-24 hours

**Pregnancy Risk Factor** B

**Generic Available** Yes

♦ **Penicillin G Procaine and Benzathine Combined** *see* Penicillin G Benzathine and Procaine Combined *on page 774*

## Penicillin V Potassium (pen i SIL in vee poe TASS ee um)

**Related Information**

Dental Drug Interactions: Update on Drug Combinations Requiring Special Considerations *on page 1225*

Oral Bacterial Infections *on page 1128*

Oral Viral Infections *on page 1137*

**U.S. Brand Names** Beepen-VK®; Betapen®-VK; Pen.Vee® K; Robicillin® VK; V-Cillin K®; Veetids®

**Canadian Brand Names** Apo®-Pen VK; Nadopen-V®; Novo-Pen-VK®; Nu-Pen-VK; PVF® K

**Therapeutic Category** Antibiotic, Penicillin

**Use**

Dental: Antibiotic of first choice in treating common orofacial infections caused by aerobic gram-positive cocci and anaerobes. These orofacial infections include cellulitis, periapical abscess, periodontal abscess, acute suppurative pulpitis, oronasal fistula, pericoronitis, osteitis, osteomyelitis, postsurgical and post-traumatic infection. It is no longer recommended for dental procedure prophylaxis.

Medical: Treatment of moderate to severe susceptible bacterial infections involving the respiratory tract, otitis media, sinusitis, skin, and and urinary tract

**Usual Dosage**

Children <12 years: Daily dose: 25-50 mg/kg in divided doses every 6-8 hours for 7 days; maximum daily dose: 3 g

Children >12 years and Adults: 250-500 mg every 6 hours for at least 7 days

**Mechanism of Action** Inhibits bacterial cell wall synthesis by binding to one or more of the penicillin binding proteins (PBPs); which in turn inhibits the final transpeptidation step of peptidoglycan synthesis in bacterial cell walls, thus inhibiting cell wall biosynthesis. Bacteria eventually lyse due to ongoing activity of cell wall autolytic enzymes (autolysins and murein hydrolases) while cell wall assembly is arrested.

**Local Anesthetic/Vasoconstrictor Precautions** No information available to require special precautions

**Effects on Dental Treatment** Prolonged use of penicillins may lead to development of oral candidiasis

**Other Adverse Effects**

>10%: Gastrointestinal: Mild diarrhea, vomiting, nausea

1% to 10%: Miscellaneous: Hypersensitivity reactions

**Contraindications** Known hypersensitivity to penicillin or any component

**Warnings/Precautions** Use with caution in patients with severe renal impairment (modify dosage) or hypersensitivity to cephalosporins

**Drug Interactions** Tetracyclines may decrease penicillin effectiveness; probenecid may increase penicillin levels; aminoglycosides cause synergistic efficacy

**Drug Uptake**

Absorption: Oral: 60% to 73% from GI tract

Time to peak serum concentration: Oral: Within 0.5-1 hour

Serum half-life: 0.5 hours

**Pregnancy Risk Factor** B

**Breast-feeding Considerations** No data reported; however, other penicillins may be taken while breast-feeding

**Dosage Forms**

Powder for oral solution: 125 mg/5 mL (3 mL, 100 mL, 150 mL, 200 mL); 250 mg/5 mL (100 mL, 150 mL, 200 mL)

Tablet: 125 mg, 250 mg, 500 mg

**Dietary Considerations** Peak concentration may be delayed with food; may be taken with water on an empty stomach 1 hour before or 2 hours after meals or may be taken with food

**Generic Available** Yes

**Selected Readings**

Wynn RL and Bergman SA, "Antibiotics and Their Use in the Treatment of Orofacial Infections, Part I and Part II," *Gen Dent*, 1994, 42(5):398-402, 498-502.

♦ **Pentacarinat® Injection** *see* Pentamidine *on next page*

## Pentaerythritol Tetranitrate (pen ta er ITH ri tole te tra NYE trate)

**Related Information**

Cardiovascular Diseases *on page 1066*

**U.S. Brand Names** Duotrate®; Peritrate®; Peritrate® SA

**Therapeutic Category** Antianginal Agent; Nitrate; Vasodilator, Coronary

**Use** Possibly effective for the prophylactic long-term management of angina pectoris. **Note:** Not indicated to abort acute anginal episodes

**Usual Dosage** Adults: Oral: 10-20 mg 4 times/day up to 40 mg 4 times/day before or after meals and at bedtime; sustained release preparation 80 mg twice daily; use lowest recommended doses in elderly initially; titrations up to 240 mg/day are tolerated, however, headache may occur with increasing doses (reduce dose for a few days; if headache returns or is persistent, an analgesic can be used to treat symptoms)

**Mechanism of Action** Stimulation of intracellular cyclic-GMP results in vascular smooth muscle relaxation of both arterial and venous vasculature. Increased venous pooling decreases left ventricular pressure (preload) and arterial dilatation decreases arterial resistance (afterload). Therefore, this reduces cardiac oxygen demand by decreasing left ventricular pressure and systemic vascular resistance by dilating arteries. Additionally, coronary artery dilation improves collateral flow to ischemic regions; esophageal smooth muscle is relaxed via the same mechanism.

**Local Anesthetic/Vasoconstrictor Precautions** No information available to require special precautions

**Effects on Dental Treatment** No effects or complications reported

**Other Adverse Effects**

>10%:

Cardiovascular: Flushing, postural hypotension

Central nervous system: Headache, lightheadedness, dizziness

Neuromuscular & skeletal: Weakness

1% to 10%: Dermatologic: Drug rash, exfoliative dermatitis

<1%:

Gastrointestinal: Nausea, vomiting

(Continued)

## Pentaerythritol Tetranitrate *(Continued)*

Hematologic: Methemoglobinemia (overdose)

**Drug Interactions** No data reported

**Drug Uptake**

Onset of hemodynamic effect: Oral: Within 20-60 minutes

Duration: 4-5 hours, or up to 12 hours with the sustained release formulations

Serum half-life: 10 minutes

**Pregnancy Risk Factor** C

**Generic Available** Yes

## Pentagastrin (pen ta GAS trin)

**U.S. Brand Names** Peptavlon®

**Therapeutic Category** Diagnostic Agent, Gastric Acid Secretory Function

**Use** Evaluate gastric acid secretory function in pernicious anemia, gastric carcinoma; in suspected duodenal ulcer or Zollinger-Ellison tumor

**Usual Dosage** Adults:

I.M., S.C.: 6 mcg/kg

I.V. infusion: 0.1-12 mcg/kg/hour in 0.9% sodium chloride

**Mechanism of Action** Excites the oxyntic cells of the stomach to secrete to their maximum capacity similar to the naturally occurring hormone, gastrin

**Local Anesthetic/Vasoconstrictor Precautions** No information available to require special precautions

**Effects on Dental Treatment** No effects or complications reported

**Other Adverse Effects**

>10%: Gastrointestinal: Abdominal pain, desire to defecate, nausea, vomiting

1% to 10%:

- Cardiovascular: Flushing, tachycardia, palpitations, hypotension, faintness
- Central nervous system: Dizziness, headache
- Respiratory: Dyspnea

<1%: Miscellaneous: Allergic reactions

**Drug Uptake**

Absorption: I.M., S.C.: Well absorbed

Serum half-life: 1 minute

**Pregnancy Risk Factor** C

**Generic Available** No

♦ **Pentam-300® Injection** *see* Pentamidine *on this page*

## Pentamidine (pen TAM i deen)

**U.S. Brand Names** NebuPent™ Inhalation; Pentacarinat® Injection; Pentam-300® Injection

**Therapeutic Category** Antibiotic, Miscellaneous

**Use** Treatment and prevention of pneumonia caused by *Pneumocystis carinii*; treatment of trypanosomiasis

**Usual Dosage**

Children:

- Treatment: I.M., I.V. (I.V. preferred): 4 mg/kg/day once daily for 10-14 days
- Prevention:
  - I.M., I.V.: 4 mg/kg monthly or every 2 weeks
  - Inhalation (aerosolized pentamidine in children ≥5 years): 300 mg/dose given every 3-4 weeks via Respirgard® II inhaler (8 mg/kg dose has also been used in children <5 years)
- Treatment of trypanosomiasis: I.V.: 4 mg/kg/day once daily for 10 days

Adults:

- Treatment: I.M., I.V. (I.V. preferred): 4 mg/kg/day once daily for 14 days
- Prevention: Inhalation: 300 mg every 4 weeks via Respirgard® II nebulizer

**Mechanism of Action** Interferes with RNA/DNA, phospholipids and protein synthesis, through inhibition of oxidative phosphorylation and/or interference with incorporation of nucleotides and nucleic acids into RNA and DNA, in protozoa

**Local Anesthetic/Vasoconstrictor Precautions** No information available to require special precautions

**Effects on Dental Treatment** No effects or complications reported

**Other Adverse Effects**

>10%:

- Cardiovascular: Chest pain
- Dermatologic: Skin rash
- Endocrine & metabolic: Hyperkalemia
- Local: Local reactions at injection site
- Respiratory: Wheezing, dyspnea, coughing, pharyngitis

1% to 10%: Gastrointestinal: Bitter or metallic taste

<1%:
- Cardiovascular: Hypotension, tachycardia
- Central nervous system: Dizziness, fever, fatigue
- Endocrine & metabolic: Hyperglycemia or hypoglycemia, hypocalcemia
- Gastrointestinal: Pancreatitis, vomiting
- Hematologic: Megaloblastic anemia, granulocytopenia, leukopenia, thrombocytopenia
- Hepatic: Mild hepatic injury
- Renal: Renal insufficiency, mild renal injury
- Respiratory: Extrapulmonary pneumocystosis, irritation of the airway, pneumothorax
- Miscellaneous: Jarisch-Herxheimer-like reaction

**Drug Interactions** No data reported

**Drug Uptake**

Absorption: I.M.: Well absorbed

Serum half-life, terminal: 6.4-9.4 hours; may be prolonged in patients with severe renal impairment

**Pregnancy Risk Factor** C

**Generic Available** Yes

- ♦ **Pentasa®** *see* Mesalamine *on page 638*
- ♦ **Pentaspan®** *see* Pentastarch *on this page*

## Pentastarch (PEN ta starch)

**U.S. Brand Names** Pentaspan®

**Therapeutic Category** Blood Modifiers

**Use** Adjunct in leukapheresis to improve the harvesting and increase the yield of leukocytes by centrifugal means

**Usual Dosage** 250-700 mL to which citrate anticoagulant has been added is administered by adding to the input line of the centrifugation apparatus at a ratio of 1:8-1:13 to venous whole blood

**Local Anesthetic/Vasoconstrictor Precautions** No information available to require special precautions

**Effects on Dental Treatment** No effects or complications reported

**Generic Available** No

## Pentazocine (pen TAZ oh seen)

**Related Information**

Narcotic Agonists *on page 1223*

**U.S. Brand Names** Talwin®; Talwin® NX

**Therapeutic Category** Analgesic, Narcotic

**Use** Relief of moderate to severe pain; has also been used as a sedative prior to surgery and as a supplement to surgical anesthesia

**Usual Dosage**

Children: I.M., S.C.:
- 5-8 years: 15 mg
- 8-14 years: 30 mg

Children >12 years and Adults: Oral: 50 mg every 3-4 hours; may increase to 100 mg/dose if needed, but should not exceed 600 mg/day

Adults:
- I.M., S.C.: 30-60 mg every 3-4 hours, not to exceed total daily dose of 360 mg
- I.V.: 30 mg every 3-4 hours

**Mechanism of Action** Binds to opiate receptors in the CNS, causing inhibition of ascending pain pathways, altering the perception of and response to pain; produces generalized CNS depression; partial agonist-antagonist

**Local Anesthetic/Vasoconstrictor Precautions** No information available to require special precautions

**Effects on Dental Treatment** No effects or complications reported

**Other Adverse Effects**

>10%:
- Central nervous system: Euphoria, drowsiness
- Gastrointestinal: Nausea, vomiting
- Neuromuscular & skeletal: Weakness

1% to 10%:
- Cardiovascular: Hypotension
- Central nervous system: Malaise, headache, restlessness, nightmares
- Dermatologic: Skin rash
- Gastrointestinal: Dry mouth
- Genitourinary: Ureteral spasm
- Ocular: Blurred vision
- Respiratory: Dyspnea

(Continued)

## Pentazocine *(Continued)*

<1%:

Cardiovascular: Palpitations, bradycardia, peripheral vasodilation

Central nervous system: Insomnia, CNS depression, sedation, hallucinations, confusion, disorientation, seizures may occur in seizure-prone patients, increased intracranial pressure

Dermatologic: Pruritus

Endocrine & metabolic: Antidiuretic hormone release

Gastrointestinal: GI irritation, constipation, biliary spasm

Genitourinary: Urinary tract spasm

Local: Tissue damage and irritation with I.M./S.C. use

Ocular: Miosis

Miscellaneous: Histamine release physical and psychological dependence

**Drug Interactions** May potentiate or reduce analgesic effect of opiate agonist, (eg, morphine) depending on patients tolerance to opiates can precipitate withdrawal in narcotic addicts

Increased effect/toxicity with tripelennamine (can be lethal), CNS depressants (phenothiazines, tranquilizers, anxiolytics, sedatives, hypnotics, or alcohol)

**Drug Uptake**

Onset of action:

Oral, I.M., S.C.: Within 15-30 minutes

I.V.: Within 2-3 minutes

Duration:

Oral: 4-5 hours

Parenteral: 2-3 hours

Serum half-life: 2-3 hours; increased with decreased hepatic function

**Pregnancy Risk Factor** B (D if used for prolonged periods or in high doses at term)

**Dosage Forms**

Injection, as lactate: 30 mg/mL (1 mL, 1.5 mL, 2 mL, 10 mL)

Tablet: Pentazocine hydrochloride 50 mg and naloxone hydrochloride 0.5 mg

**Generic Available** Yes

## Pentazocine Compound (pen TAZ oh seen KOM pownd)

**U.S. Brand Names** Talacen®; Talwin® Compound

**Therapeutic Category** Analgesic, Narcotic

**Use** Relief of moderate to severe pain; has also been used as a sedative prior to surgery and as a supplement to surgical anesthesia

**Usual Dosage** Adults: Oral: 2 tablets 3-4 times/day

**Local Anesthetic/Vasoconstrictor Precautions** No information available to require special precautions

**Effects on Dental Treatment** No effects or complications reported

**Pregnancy Risk Factor** D

**Generic Available** No

**Comments** Abrupt discontinuation after sustained use (generally >10 days) may cause withdrawal symptoms

## Pentobarbital (pen toe BAR bi tal)

**U.S. Brand Names** Nembutal®

**Therapeutic Category** Barbiturate; Sedative

**Use** Short-term treatment of insomnia; preoperative sedation; high-dose barbiturate coma for treatment of increased intracranial pressure or status epilepticus unresponsive to other therapy

**Usual Dosage**

Children:

Sedative: Oral: 2-6 mg/kg/day divided in 3 doses; maximum: 100 mg/day

Hypnotic: I.M.: 2-6 mg/kg; maximum: 100 mg/dose

Rectal:

2 months to 1 year (10-20 lb): 30 mg

1-4 years (20-40 lb): 30-60 mg

5-12 years (40-80 lb): 60 mg

12-14 years (80-110 lb): 60-120 mg

**or**

<4 years: 3-6 mg/kg/dose

>4 years: 1.5-3 mg/kg/dose

Preoperative/preprocedure sedation: ≥6 months:

Oral, I.M., rectal: 2-6 mg/kg; maximum: 100 mg/dose

I.V.: 1-3 mg/kg to a maximum of 100 mg until asleep

Children 5-12 years: Conscious sedation prior to a procedure: I.V.: 2 mg/kg 5-10 minutes before procedures, may repeat one time

Adolescents: Conscious sedation: Oral, I.V.: 100 mg prior to a procedure

Adults:
- Hypnotic:
  - Oral: 100-200 mg at bedtime or 20 mg 3-4 times/day for daytime sedation
  - I.M.: 150-200 mg
  - I.V.: Initial: 100 mg, may repeat every 1-3 minutes up to 200-500 mg total dose
- Rectal: 120-200 mg at bedtime
- Preoperative sedation: I.M.: 150-200 mg

Children and Adults: Barbiturate coma in head injury patients: I.V.: Loading dose: 5-10 mg/kg given slowly over 1-2 hours; monitor blood pressure and respiratory rate; Maintenance infusion: Initial: 1 mg/kg/hour; may increase to 2-3 mg/kg/hour; maintain burst suppression on EEG

**Mechanism of Action** Short-acting barbiturate with sedative, hypnotic, and anticonvulsant properties

**Local Anesthetic/Vasoconstrictor Precautions** No information available to require special precautions

**Effects on Dental Treatment** No effects or complications reported

**Other Adverse Effects**

Renal: Oliguria

>10%:
- Cardiovascular: Cardiac arrhythmias, bradycardia, hypotension, arterial spasm, and gangrene with inadvertent intra-arterial injection
- Central nervous system: Drowsiness, lethargy, CNS excitation or depression, impaired judgment, "hangover" effect
- Local: Pain at injection site, thrombophlebitis with I.V. use

1% to 10%:
- Central nervous system: Confusion, mental depression, unusual excitement, nervousness, faint feeling, headache, insomnia, nightmares
- Gastrointestinal: Nausea, vomiting, constipation

<1%:
- Cardiovascular: Hypotension
- Central nervous system: Hallucinations, hypothermia
- Dermatologic: Rash, exfoliative dermatitis, Stevens-Johnson syndrome
- Hematologic: Agranulocytosis, thrombocytopenia, megaloblastic anemia
- Local: Thrombophlebitis
- Respiratory: Laryngospasm, respiratory depression, apnea (especially with rapid I.V. use)

**Drug Interactions**

Decreased effect: Decreased chloramphenicol; decreased doxycycline effects

Increased toxicity: Increased CNS depressants, cimetidine; causes increase effect of pentobarbital

**Drug Uptake**

Onset of action:
- Oral, rectal: 15-60 minutes
- I.M.: Within 10-15 minutes
- I.V.: Within 1 minute

Duration:
- Oral, rectal: 1-4 hours
- I.V.: 15 minutes

Serum half-life, terminal:
- Children: 25 hours
- Adults, normal: 22 hours; range: 35-50 hours

**Pregnancy Risk Factor** D

**Generic Available** Yes

## Pentosan Polysulfate Sodium

(PEN toe san pol i SUL fate SOW dee um)

**U.S. Brand Names** Elmiron®

**Therapeutic Category** Analgesic, Urinary

**Synonyms** PPS

**Use** Bladder pain relief or discomfort associated with interstitial cystitis

**Usual Dosage** Adults: Oral: 100 mg 3 times/day taken with water 1 hour before or 2 hours after meals

Patients should be evaluated at 3 months and may be continued an additional 3 months if there has been no improvement and if there are no therapy-limiting side effects. **The risks and benefits of continued use beyond 6 months in patients who have not responded is not yet known.**

**Mechanism of Action** Although pentosan polysulfate sodium is a low-molecular weight heparinoid, it is not known whether these properties play a role in its mechanism of action in treating interstitial cystitis; the drug appears to adhere to

(Continued)

## Pentosan Polysulfate Sodium *(Continued)*

the bladder wall mucosa where it may act as a buffer to protect the tissues from irritating substances in the urine.

**Local Anesthetic/Vasoconstrictor Precautions** No information available to require special precautions

**Effects on Dental Treatment** <1% of patients experience gum bleeding, mouth ulcers

**Other Adverse Effects**

1% to 10%:

Central nervous system: Headache, dizziness
Dermatologic: Alopecia, rash
Gastrointestinal: Diarrhea, nausea, dyspepsia, abdominal pain
Hepatic: Liver function test abnormalities

<1%:

Dermatologic: Pruritus, urticaria, photosensitivity, bruising
Gastrointestinal: Vomiting, mouth ulcer, colitis, esophagitis, gastritis, flatulence, constipation, anorexia, gum bleeding
Hematologic: Anemia, increased prothrombin time, increased partial thromboplastin time, leukopenia, thrombocytopenia
Ocular: Conjunctivitis, optic neuritis, amblyopia, retinal hemorrhage
Otic: Tinnitus
Respiratory: Pharyngitis, rhinitis, epistaxis, dyspnea
Miscellaneous: Allergic reactions

**Warnings/Precautions** Pentosan polysulfate is a low-molecular weight heparin-like compound with anticoagulant and fibrinolytic effects, therefore, bleeding complications such as ecchymosis, epistaxis and gum bleeding, may occur; patients with the following diseases should be carefully evaluated before initiating therapy: aneurysm, thrombocytopenia, hemophilia, gastrointestinal ulcerations, polyps, diverticula, or hepatic insufficiency; patients undergoing invasive procedures or having signs or symptoms of underlying coagulopathies or other increased risk of bleeding (eg, receiving heparin, warfarin, thrombolytics, or high dose aspirin) should be evaluated for hemorrhage; elevations in transaminases and alopecia can occur

**Drug Interactions** Although there is no information about potential drug interactions, it is expected that pentosan polysulfate sodium would have at least additive anticoagulant effects when administered with anticoagulant drugs such as warfarin or heparin, and possible similar effects when administered with aspirin or thrombolytics

**Drug Uptake**

Absorption: ~3%
Serum half-life: 4-8 hours

**Pregnancy Risk Factor** B

**Generic Available** No

## Pentostatin (PEN toe stat in)

**U.S. Brand Names** Nipent™ Injection

**Therapeutic Category** Antineoplastic Agent, Antimetabolite; Antineoplastic Agent, Nonirritant

**Synonyms** DCF; Deoxycoformycin; 2′-deoxycoformycin

**Use** Treatment of adult patients with alpha-interferon-refractory hairy cell leukemia; significant antitumor activity in various lymphoid neoplasms has been demonstrated; pentostatin also is known as 2'-deoxycoformycin; it is a purine analogue capable of inhibiting adenosine deaminase

**Usual Dosage** Refractory hairy cell leukemia: Adults (refer to individual protocols): 4 $mg/m^2$ every other week; I.V. bolus over ≥3-5 minutes in $D_5W$ or NS at concentrations ≥2 mg/mL

**Mechanism of Action** An antimetabolite inhibiting adenosine deaminase (ADA), prevents ADA from controlling intracellular adenosine levels through the irreversible deamination of adenosine and deoxyadenosine. ADA is found to exhibit the highest activity in lymphoid tissue. Patients receiving pentostatin accumulate deoxyadenosine (dAdo) and deoxyadenosine 5′-triphosphate (dATP); accumulation of dATP results in cell death, probably through inhibiting DNA or RNA synthesis. Following a single dose, pentostatin has the ability to inhibit ADA for periods exceeding 1 week.

**Local Anesthetic/Vasoconstrictor Precautions** No information available to require special precautions

**Effects on Dental Treatment** No effects or complications reported

**Other Adverse Effects**

>10%:

Central nervous system: Headache, neurologic disorder, fever, fatigue, chills, pain

Dermatologic: Rash
Gastrointestinal: Vomiting, nausea, anorexia, diarrhea
Hematologic: Leukopenia, anemia, thrombocytopenia
Hepatic: Hepatic disorder, liver function tests (abnormal)
Neuromuscular & skeletal: Myalgia
Respiratory: Coughing
Miscellaneous: Allergic reaction

1% to 10%:
Cardiovascular: Chest pain, arrhythmia, peripheral edema
Central nervous system: Anxiety, confusion, depression, dizziness, insomnia, lethargy, coma, seizures, malaise
Dermatologic: Dry skin, eczema, pruritus
Gastrointestinal: Constipation, flatulence, stomatitis, weight loss
Genitourinary: Dysuria
Hematologic: Myelosuppression
Hepatic: Liver dysfunction
Local: Thrombophlebitis
Neuromuscular & skeletal: Arthralgia, paresthesia, back pain, weakness
Ocular: Abnormal vision, eye pain, keratoconjunctivitis
Otic: Ear pain
Renal: Renal failure, hematuria
Respiratory: Bronchitis, dyspnea, lung edema, pneumonia
Miscellaneous: Death, opportunistic infections, sweating

**Drug Uptake** Serum half-life, terminal: 5-15 hours
**Pregnancy Risk Factor** D
**Generic Available** No

♦ **Pentothal® Sodium** *see* Thiopental *on page 977*

## Pentoxifylline (pen toks I fi leen)

**U.S. Brand Names** Trental®
**Canadian Brand Names** Albert® Pentoxifylline; Apo®-Pentoxifylline SR
**Therapeutic Category** Blood Viscosity Reducer Agent
**Use** Symptomatic management of peripheral vascular disease, mainly intermittent claudication

**Unapproved use:** AIDS patients with increased TNF, CVA, cerebrovascular diseases, diabetic atherosclerosis, diabetic neuropathy, gangrene, hemodialysis shunt thrombosis, vascular impotence, cerebral malaria, septic shock, sickle cell syndromes, and vasculitis

**Usual Dosage** Adults: Oral: 400 mg 3 times/day with meals; may reduce to 400 mg twice daily if GI or CNS side effects occur
**Mechanism of Action** Mechanism of action remains unclear; is thought to reduce blood viscosity and improve blood flow by altering the rheology of red blood cells
**Local Anesthetic/Vasoconstrictor Precautions** No information available to require special precautions
**Effects on Dental Treatment** No effects or complications reported
**Other Adverse Effects**

1% to 10%:
Central nervous system: Dizziness, headache
Gastrointestinal: Dyspepsia, nausea, vomiting

<1%:
Cardiovascular: Mild hypotension, angina
Central nervous system: Agitation
Ocular: Blurred vision
Otic: Earache

**Drug Interactions** Increased effect/toxic potential with cimetidine (increased levels) and other $H_2$ antagonists, warfarin; increased effect of antihypertensives
**Drug Uptake**
Absorption: Oral: Well absorbed
Serum half-life:
Parent drug: 24-48 minutes
Metabolites: 60-96 minutes
Time to peak serum concentration: Within 2-4 hours
**Pregnancy Risk Factor** C
**Generic Available** Yes

♦ **Pentrax® [OTC]** *see* Coal Tar *on page 270*
♦ **Pen.Vee® K** *see* Penicillin V Potassium *on page 776*
♦ **Pepcid®** *see* Famotidine *on page 419*
♦ **Pepcid® AC Acid Controller [OTC]** *see* Famotidine *on page 419*
♦ **Peptavlon®** *see* Pentagastrin *on page 778*

♦ **Pepto-Bismol® (subsalicylate) [OTC]** *see* Bismuth *on page 142*
♦ **Pepto® Diarrhea Control [OTC]** *see* Loperamide *on page 599*
♦ **Percocet®** *see* Oxycodone and Acetaminophen *on page 751*
♦ **Percodan®** *see* Oxycodone and Aspirin *on page 753*
♦ **Percodan®-Demi** *see* Oxycodone and Aspirin *on page 753*
♦ **Percogesic® [OTC]** *see* Acetaminophen and Phenyltoloxamine *on page 30*
♦ **Percolone™** *see* Oxycodone *on page 750*
♦ **Perdiem® Plain [OTC]** *see* Psyllium *on page 865*
♦ **Perfectoderm® Gel [OTC]** *see* Benzoyl Peroxide *on page 130*

## Pergolide Mesylate (PER go lide)

**U.S. Brand Names** Permax®

**Therapeutic Category** Anti-Parkinson's Agent; Ergot Alkaloid and Derivative

**Use** Adjunctive treatment to levodopa/carbidopa in the management of Parkinson's Disease

**Usual Dosage** When adding pergolide to levodopa/carbidopa, the dose of the latter can usually and should be decreased. Patients no longer responsive to bromocriptine may benefit by being switched to pergolide.

Adults: Oral: Start with 0.05 mg/day for 2 days, then increase dosage by 0.1 or 0.15 mg/day every 3 days over next 12 days, increase dose by 0.25 mg/day every 3 days until optimal therapeutic dose is achieved, up to 5 mg/day maximum; usual dosage range: 2-3 mg/day in 3 divided doses

**Mechanism of Action** Pergolide is a semisynthetic ergot alkaloid similar to bromocriptine but stated to be more potent and longer acting; it is a centrally-active dopamine agonist stimulating both $D_1$ and $D_2$ receptors

**Local Anesthetic/Vasoconstrictor Precautions** No information available to require special precautions

**Effects on Dental Treatment** Pergolide may decrease or inhibit salivary flow; normal salivary flow will resume with cessation of drug therapy; prolonged salivary reduction could enhance development of periodontal disease, oral candidiasis and discomfort

**Other Adverse Effects**

>10%:

- Central nervous system: Dizziness, somnolence, insomnia, confusion, hallucinations, anxiety, dystonia
- Gastrointestinal: Nausea, constipation
- Neuromuscular & skeletal: Dyskinesias
- Respiratory: Rhinitis

1% to 10%:

- Cardiovascular: Myocardial infarction, postural hypotension, syncope, arrhythmias, peripheral edema, vasodilation, palpitations, chest pain
- Central nervous system: Chills
- Gastrointestinal: Diarrhea, abdominal pain, vomiting, dry mouth, anorexia, weight gain
- Neuromuscular & skeletal: Weakness
- Ocular: Abnormal vision
- Respiratory: Dyspnea
- Miscellaneous: Flu syndrome

**Drug Interactions** Decreased effect: Dopamine antagonists, metoclopramide

**Drug Uptake** Absorption: Oral: Well absorbed

**Pregnancy Risk Factor** B

**Generic Available** No

♦ **Pergonal®** *see* Menotropins *on page 628*
♦ **Periactin®** *see* Cyproheptadine *on page 289*
♦ **Peri-Colace® [OTC]** *see* Docusate and Casanthranol *on page 347*
♦ **Peridex® Oral Rinse** *see* Chlorhexidine Gluconate *on page 225*

## Perindopril Erbumine (per IN doe pril er BYOO meen)

**U.S. Brand Names** Aceon®

**Therapeutic Category** Antihypertensive Agent

**Use** Treatment of stage I or II hypertension and congestive heart failure

**Usual Dosage** Adults: Oral:

- Congestive heart failure: 4 mg once daily
- Hypertension: Initial: 4 mg/day but may be titrated to response; usual range: 4-8 mg/day, maximum: 16 mg/day

**Mechanism of Action** Competitive inhibitor of angiotensin-converting enzyme (ACE); prevents conversion of angiotensin I to angiotensin II, a potent vasoconstrictor; results in lower levels of angiotensin II which, in turn, causes an increase in plasma renin activity and a reduction in aldosterone secretion

**Local Anesthetic/Vasoconstrictor Precautions** No information available to require special precautions

**Effects on Dental Treatment** <1%: Taste disturbances

**Other Adverse Effects**

1% to 10%

Central nervous system: Headache, dizziness, mood and sleep disorders, fatigue

Dermatologic: Rash, pruritus

Gastrointestinal: Nausea, epigastric pain, diarrhea, vomiting

Neuromuscular & skeletal: Muscle cramps

Respiratory: Cough (incidence is greater in women, 3:1)

<1%:

Cardiovascular: Hypotension

Dermatologic: Angioedema, psoriasis

Endocrine & metabolic: Hyperkalemia

Genitourinary: Impotence

Hematologic: Agranulocytosis for all ACE inhibitors (especially in patients with renal impairment or collagen vascular disease), possibly neutropenia

Ocular: Dry eyes, blurred vision, optic phosphenes

Renal: Decreases in creatinine clearance in some elderly hypertensive patients or those with chronic renal failure, worsening of renal function in patients with bilateral renal artery stenosis, or furosemide therapy; proteinuria

**Drug Interactions** See table.

**Drug-Drug Interactions With ACEIs**

| Precipitant Drug | Drug (Category) and Effect | Description |
|---|---|---|
| Antacids | ACE Inhibitors: decreased | Decreased bioavailability of ACEIs. May be more likely with captopril. Separate administration times by 1-2 hours. |
| NSAIDs (indomethacin) | ACEIs: decreased | Reduced hypotensive effects of ACEIs. More prominent in low renin or volume dependent hypertensive patients. |
| Phenothiazines | ACEIs: increased | Pharmacologic effects of ACEIs may be increased. |
| ACEIs | Allopurinol: increased | Higher risk of hypersensitivity reaction possible when given concurrently. Three case reports of Stevens-Johnson syndrome with captopril. |
| ACEIs | Digoxin: increased | Increased plasma digoxin levels. |
| ACEIs | Lithium: increased | Increased serum lithium levels and symptoms of toxicity may occur. |
| ACEIs | Potassium preps/ potassium sparing diuretics increased | Coadministration may result in elevated potassium levels. |

**Drug Uptake**

Serum half-life:

Parent drug: 1.5-3 hours

Metabolite: 25-30 hours

Time to peak: Occurs in 1 and 3-4 hours for perindopril and perindoprilat, respectively after chronic therapy; (maximum perindoprilat serum levels are 2-3 times higher and $T_{max}$ is shorter following chronic therapy); in CHF, the peak of perindoprilat is prolonged to 6 hours

**Pregnancy Risk Factor** D (especially during 2nd and 3rd trimester)

**Generic Available** No

- **Periochip®** *see* Chlorhexidine Gluconate *on page 225*
- **Periodontal Diseases** *see page 1132*
- **PerioGard®** *see* Chlorhexidine Gluconate *on page 225*
- **Periostat™** *see* Doxycycline *on page 355*
- **Peritrate®** *see* Pentaerythritol Tetranitrate *on page 777*
- **Peritrate® SA** *see* Pentaerythritol Tetranitrate *on page 777*
- **Permapen®** *see* Penicillin G Benzathine *on page 773*
- **Permax®** *see* Pergolide Mesylate *on previous page*

## Permethrin (per METH rin)

**U.S. Brand Names** Elimite™; Nix™ [OTC]

**Therapeutic Category** Antiparasitic Agent, Topical; Scabicidal Agent

**Use** Single application treatment of infestation with *Pediculus humanus capitis* (head louse) and its nits or *Sarcoptes scabiei* (scabies)

(Continued)

## Permethrin *(Continued)*

**Usual Dosage** Topical: Children >2 months and Adults:

Head lice: After hair has been washed with shampoo, rinsed with water, and towel dried, apply a sufficient volume of topical liquid to saturate the hair and scalp. Leave on hair for 10 minutes before rinsing off with water; remove remaining nits; may repeat in 1 week if lice or nits still present.

Scabies: Apply cream from head to toe; leave on for 8-14 hours before washing off with water; for infants, also apply on the hairline, neck, scalp, temple, and forehead; may reapply in 1 week if live mites appear

Permethrin 5% cream was shown to be safe and effective when applied to an infant <1 month of age with neonatal scabies; time of application was limited to 6 hours before rinsing with soap and water

**Mechanism of Action** Inhibits sodium ion influx through nerve cell membrane channels in parasites resulting in delayed repolarization and thus paralysis and death of the pest

**Local Anesthetic/Vasoconstrictor Precautions** No information available to require special precautions

**Effects on Dental Treatment** No effects or complications reported

**Other Adverse Effects** 1% to 10%:

Cardiovascular: Local edema

Dermatologic: Pruritus, erythema, rash of the scalp, numbness or scalp discomfort

Local: Burning, stinging, tingling

**Drug Interactions** No data reported

**Drug Uptake** Absorption: Topical: Minimal (<2%)

**Pregnancy Risk Factor** B

**Generic Available** No

♦ **Permitil®** *see* Fluphenazine *on page 446*
♦ **Pernox® [OTC]** *see* Sulfur and Salicylic Acid *on page 947*
♦ **Peroxin A5®** *see* Benzoyl Peroxide *on page 130*
♦ **Peroxin A10®** *see* Benzoyl Peroxide *on page 130*

## Perphenazine (per FEN a zeen)

**U.S. Brand Names** Trilafon®

**Canadian Brand Names** Apo®-Perphenazine; PMS-Perphenazine

**Therapeutic Category** Antiemetic; Antipsychotic Agent; Phenothiazine Derivative

**Use** Management of manifestations of psychotic disorders, depressive neurosis, alcohol withdrawal, nausea and vomiting, nonpsychotic symptoms associated with dementia in elderly, Tourette's syndrome, Huntington's chorea, spasmodic torticollis and Reye's syndrome

**Usual Dosage**

Children:
- Psychoses: Oral:
  - 1-6 years: 4-6 mg/day in divided doses
  - 6-12 years: 6 mg/day in divided doses
  - >12 years: 4-16 mg 2-4 times/day
  - I.M.: 5 mg every 6 hours
- Nausea/vomiting: I.M.: 5 mg every 6 hours

Adults:
- Psychoses:
  - Oral: 4-16 mg 2-4 times/day not to exceed 64 mg/day
  - I.M.: 5 mg every 6 hours up to 15 mg/day in ambulatory patients and 30 mg/day in hospitalized patients
- Nausea/vomiting:
  - Oral: 8-16 mg/day in divided doses up to 24 mg/day
  - I.M.: 5-10 mg every 6 hours as necessary up to 15 mg/day in ambulatory patients and 30 mg/day in hospitalized patients
  - I.V. (severe): 1 mg at 1- to 2-minute intervals up to a total of 5 mg

**Mechanism of Action** Blocks postsynaptic mesolimbic dopaminergic receptors in the brain; exhibits a strong alpha-adrenergic blocking effect and depresses the release of hypothalamic and hypophyseal hormones

**Local Anesthetic/Vasoconstrictor Precautions** Most pharmacology textbooks state that in presence of phenothiazines, systemic doses of epinephrine paradoxically decrease the blood pressure. This is the so called "epinephrine reversal" phenomenon. This has never been observed when epinephrine is given by infiltration as part of the anesthesia procedure.

**Effects on Dental Treatment** Significant hypotension may occur, especially when the drug is administered parenterally; orthostatic hypotension is due to alpha-receptor blockade, the elderly are at greater risk for orthostatic hypotension

Tardive dyskinesia: Prevalence rate may be 40% in elderly; development of the syndrome and the irreversible nature are proportional to duration and total cumulative dose over time

Extrapyramidal reactions are more common in elderly with up to 50% developing these reactions after 60 years of age; drug-induced **Parkinson's syndrome** occurs often; **Akathisia** is the most common extrapyramidal reaction in elderly

Increased confusion, memory loss, psychotic behavior, and agitation frequently occur as a consequence of anticholinergic effects

Antipsychotic associated sedation in nonpsychotic patients is extremely unpleasant due to feelings of depersonalization, derealization, and dysphoria

**Other Adverse Effects**

>10%:
- Cardiovascular: Hypotension, orthostatic hypotension
- Central nervous system: Pseudoparkinsonism, akathisia, dystonias, tardive dyskinesia (persistent), dizziness
- Gastrointestinal: Constipation
- Ocular: Pigmentary retinopathy
- Respiratory: Nasal congestion
- Miscellaneous: Decreased sweating

1% to 10%:
- Dermatologic: Photosensitivity, skin rash
- Endocrine & metabolic: Changes in menstrual cycle, changes in libido, pain in breasts
- Gastrointestinal: Weight gain, vomiting, stomach pain, nausea
- Genitourinary: Dysuria, ejaculatory disturbances
- Neuromuscular & skeletal: Trembling of fingers

<1%:
- Central nervous system: Neuroleptic malignant syndrome (NMS), impairment of temperature regulation, lowering of seizures threshold
- Dermatologic: Discoloration of skin (blue-gray)
- Endocrine & metabolic: Galactorrhea
- Genitourinary: Priapism
- Hematologic: Agranulocytosis, leukopenia
- Hepatic: Cholestatic jaundice, hepatotoxicity
- Ocular: Cornea and lens changes, pigmentary retinopathy

**Drug Interactions** Increased toxicity: Additive effects with other CNS depressants

**Drug Uptake**
- Absorption: Oral: Well absorbed
- Serum half-life: 9 hours
- Time to peak serum concentration: Within 4-8 hours

**Pregnancy Risk Factor** C

**Generic Available** Yes

- ♦ **Perphenazine and Amitriptyline** *see* Amitriptyline and Perphenazine *on page 69*
- ♦ **Persa-Gel®** *see* Benzoyl Peroxide *on page 130*
- ♦ **Persantine®** *see* Dipyridamole *on page 342*
- ♦ **Pertofrane®** *see* Desipramine *on page 304*
- ♦ **Pertussin® CS [OTC]** *see* Dextromethorphan *on page 314*
- ♦ **Pertussin® ES [OTC]** *see* Dextromethorphan *on page 314*
- ♦ **Pethidine Hydrochloride** *see* Meperidine *on page 629*
- ♦ **Pfizerpen®** *see* Penicillin G, Parenteral, Aqueous *on page 775*
- ♦ **Pfizerpen®-AS** *see* Penicillin G Procaine *on page 775*
- ♦ **$PGE_1$** *see* Alprostadil *on page 51*
- ♦ **$PGE_2$** *see* Dinoprostone *on page 337*
- ♦ **$PGF_{2\alpha}$** *see* Dinoprost Tromethamine *on page 338*
- ♦ **Phanatuss® Cough Syrup [OTC]** *see* Guaifenesin and Dextromethorphan *on page 479*
- ♦ **Pharmacology of Drug Metabolism and Interactions** *see page 12*
- ♦ **Pharmaflur®** *see* Fluoride *on page 441*
- ♦ **Phazyme® [OTC]** *see* Simethicone *on page 915*
- ♦ **Phenadex® Senior [OTC]** *see* Guaifenesin and Dextromethorphan *on page 479*
- ♦ **Phenahist-TR®** *see* Chlorpheniramine, Phenylephrine, Phenylpropanolamine, and Belladonna Alkaloids *on page 236*
- ♦ **Phenameth® DM** *see* Promethazine and Dextromethorphan *on page 849*

♦ **Phenaphen® With Codeine** *see* Acetaminophen and Codeine *on page 28*

♦ **Phenazine®** *see* Promethazine *on page 847*

## Phenazopyridine (fen az oh PEER i deen)

**U.S. Brand Names** Azo-Standard® [OTC]; Baridium® [OTC]; Prodium® [OTC]; Pyridiate®; Pyridium®; Urodine®; Urogesic®

**Canadian Brand Names** Phenazo; Pyronium®; Vito Reins®

**Therapeutic Category** Analgesic, Urinary; Local Anesthetic, Urinary

**Use** Symptomatic relief of urinary burning, itching, frequency and urgency in association with urinary tract infection or following urologic procedures

**Usual Dosage** Oral:

Children: 12 mg/kg/day in 3 divided doses administered after meals for 2 days

Adults: 100-200 mg 3 times/day after meals for 2 days when used concomitantly with an antibacterial agent

**Mechanism of Action** An azo dye which exerts local anesthetic or analgesic action on urinary tract mucosa through an unknown mechanism

**Local Anesthetic/Vasoconstrictor Precautions** No information available to require special precautions

**Effects on Dental Treatment** No effects or complications reported

**Other Adverse Effects**

1% to 10%:

- Central nervous system: Headache, dizziness
- Gastrointestinal: Stomach cramps

<1%:

- Central nervous system: Vertigo
- Dermatologic: Skin pigmentation, rash
- Hematologic: Methemoglobinemia, hemolytic anemia
- Hepatic: Hepatitis
- Renal: Acute renal failure

**Drug Interactions** No data reported

**Pregnancy Risk Factor** B

**Generic Available** Yes

♦ **Phenchlor® S.H.A.** *see* Chlorpheniramine, Phenylephrine, Phenylpropanolamine, and Belladonna Alkaloids *on page 236*

## Phendimetrazine (fen dye ME tra zeen)

**U.S. Brand Names** Bontril PDM®; Bontril® Slow-Release; Dital®; Dyrexan-OD®; Melfiat-105® Unicelles®; Plegine®; Prelu-2®; Rexigen Forte®

**Therapeutic Category** Anorexiant

**Synonyms** Phendimetrazine Tartrate

**Use** An appetite suppressant during the first few weeks of dieting to help establish new eating habits; its effectiveness lasts only for short periods (3-12 weeks)

**Restrictions** C-III

**Usual Dosage** Adults: Oral:

Regular capsule or tablet: 35 mg 2 or 3 times daily, 1 hour before meals

Sustained release: 105 mg once daily in the morning before breakfast

**Local Anesthetic/Vasoconstrictor Precautions** Use vasoconstrictor with caution in patients taking phendimetrazine. Phendimetrazine can enhance the sympathomimetic response to epinephrine leading to potential hypertension and cardiotoxicity.

**Effects on Dental Treatment** Patients taking phendimetrazine may present with hypertension; monitor blood pressure

**Other Adverse Effects**

>10%:

- Cardiovascular: Hypertension
- Central nervous system: Euphoria, nervousness, insomnia

1% to 10%:

- Central nervous system: Confusion, mental depression, restlessness
- Gastrointestinal: Nausea, vomiting, constipation
- Endocrine & metabolic: Changes in libido
- Hematologic: Blood dyscrasias
- Neuromuscular & skeletal: Tremor
- Ocular: Blurred vision

<1%:

- Cardiovascular: Tachycardia, arrhythmias
- Central nervous system: Restlessness, headache
- Dermatologic: Alopecia
- Gastrointestinal: Diarrhea, abdominal cramps
- Genitourinary: Dysuria
- Neuromuscular & skeletal: Myalgia
- Renal: Polyuria

Respiratory: Dyspnea
Miscellaneous: Diaphoresis (increased)

**Contraindications** Known hypersensitivity to phendimetrazine

**Warnings/Precautions** Anorexigens have been reported to be associated with the occurrence of serious regurgitant cardiac valvular disease, including disease of the mitral, aortic, and/or tricuspid valves. Primary pulmonary hypertension (PPH) - a rare, frequently fatal disease of the lungs - has been found to occur with increased frequency in patients receiving anorexigens. There have been reports of PPH and valvular irregularities in users of phendimetrazine tartrate tablets. The safety and effectiveness of the combined use of phendimetrazine with other anorexigens in the treatment of obesity have not been established, and there is no approved use of these products together in the treatment of obesity. Phendimetrazine is approved only as a single agent for short-term use (ie, a few weeks).

**Generic Available** Yes

- **Phendimetrazine Tartrate** *see* Phendimetrazine *on previous page*
- **Phendry® Oral [OTC]** *see* Diphenhydramine *on page 338*

## Phenelzine (FEN el zeen)

**U.S. Brand Names** Nardil®

**Therapeutic Category** Antidepressant, Monoamine Oxidase Inhibitor

**Use** Symptomatic treatment of atypical, nonendogenous or neurotic depression

The MAO inhibitors are usually reserved for patients who do not tolerate or respond to the traditional "cyclic" or "second generation" antidepressants. The brain activity of monoamine oxidase increases with age and even more so in patients with Alzheimer's disease. Therefore, the MAO inhibitors may have an increased role in patients with Alzheimer's disease who are depressed. Phenelzine is less stimulating than tranylcypromine.

**Usual Dosage** Oral:

Adults: 15 mg 3 times/day; may increase to 60-90 mg/day during early phase of treatment, then reduce to dose for maintenance therapy slowly after maximum benefit is obtained; takes 2-4 weeks for a significant response to occur

Elderly: Initial: 7.5 mg/day; increase by 7.5-15 mg/day every 3-4 days as tolerated; usual therapeutic dose: 15-60 mg/day in 3-4 divided doses

**Mechanism of Action** Thought to act by increasing endogenous concentrations of epinephrine, norepinephrine, dopamine and serotonin through inhibition of the enzyme (monoamine oxidase) responsible for the breakdown of these neurotransmitters

**Local Anesthetic/Vasoconstrictor Precautions** Attempts should be made to avoid use of vasoconstrictor due to possibility of hypertensive episodes with monoamine oxidase inhibitors

**Effects on Dental Treatment** Orthostatic hypotension in >10% of patients; meperidine should be avoided as an analgesic due to toxic reactions with MAO inhibitors

**Other Adverse Effects**

>10%:
Cardiovascular: Orthostatic hypotension
Central nervous system: Drowsiness
Endocrine & metabolic: Decreased sexual ability
Neuromuscular & skeletal: Trembling, weakness
Ocular: Blurred vision

1% to 10%:
Cardiovascular; Tachycardia, peripheral edema
Central nervous system: Nervousness, chills
Gastrointestinal: Diarrhea, anorexia, dry mouth, constipation

<1%:
Central nervous system: Parkinsonism syndrome
Hematologic: Leukopenia
Hepatic: Hepatitis

**Drug Interactions**

Decreased effect of antihypertensives

Increased toxicity with disulfiram (possible seizures), fluoxetine (and other serotonin active agents), tricyclic antidepressants (cardiovascular instability), meperidine (cardiovascular instability),. phenothiazines (hyperpyretic crisis), levodopa, sympathomimetics (hypertensive crisis), barbiturates, rauwolfia alkaloids (eg, reserpine), dextroamphetamine (psychoses), foods containing tyramine

**Drug Uptake**

Onset of action: Within 2-4 weeks

Duration: May continue to have a therapeutic effect and interactions 2 weeks after discontinuing therapy

(Continued)

## Phenelzine *(Continued)*

Absorption: Oral: Well absorbed

**Pregnancy Risk Factor** C

**Generic Available** No

- **Phenerbel-S®** *see* Belladonna, Phenobarbital, and Ergotamine Tartrate *on page 125*
- **Phenergan®** *see* Promethazine *on page 847*
- **Phenergan® VC Syrup** *see* Promethazine and Phenylephrine *on page 849*
- **Phenergan® VC With Codeine** *see* Promethazine, Phenylephrine, and Codeine *on page 850*
- **Phenergan® With Codeine** *see* Promethazine and Codeine *on page 848*
- **Phenergan® with Dextromethorphan** *see* Promethazine and Dextromethorphan *on page 849*
- **Phenetron®** *see* Chlorpheniramine *on page 231*
- **Phenhist® Expectorant** *see* Guaifenesin, Pseudoephedrine, and Codeine *on page 482*

## Phenindamine (fen IN dah meen)

**U.S. Brand Names** Nolahist® [OTC]

**Therapeutic Category** Decongestant, Nasal

**Use** Treatment of perennial and seasonal allergic rhinitis and chronic urticaria

**Usual Dosage** Oral:

Children <6 years: As directed by physician

Children 6 to <12 years: 12.5 mg every 4-6 hours, up to 75 mg/24 hours

Adults: 25 mg every 4-6 hours, up to 150 mg/24 hours

**Local Anesthetic/Vasoconstrictor Precautions** No information available to require special precautions

**Effects on Dental Treatment** No effects or complications reported

**Generic Available** Yes

- **Pheniramine and Naphazoline** *see* Naphazoline and Pheniramine *on page 704*

## Pheniramine, Phenylpropanolamine, and Pyrilamine

(fen EER a meen, fen il proe pa NOLE a meen, & peer IL a meen)

**U.S. Brand Names** Triaminic® Oral Infant Drops

**Therapeutic Category** Antihistamine/Decongestant Combination

**Use** Symptomatic relief of nasal congestion and postnasal drip as well as allergic rhinitis

**Usual Dosage**

Infants <1 year: Drops: 0.05 mL/kg/dose 4 times/day

Children: Syrup:

<1 year: 0.4 mL/kg/dose 4 times/day

1-6 years: 2.5 mL/dose every 4 hours

6-12 years: 5 mL dose every 4 hours

**Local Anesthetic/Vasoconstrictor Precautions** No information available to require special precautions

**Effects on Dental Treatment** No effects or complications reported

**Pregnancy Risk Factor** C

**Generic Available** Yes

## Phenobarbital (fee noe BAR bi tal)

**U.S. Brand Names** Barbita®; Luminal®; Solfoton®

**Canadian Brand Names** Barbilixir®

**Therapeutic Category** Anticonvulsant, Barbiturate; Barbiturate; Hypnotic; Sedative

**Use** Management of generalized tonic-clonic (grand mal) and partial seizures; neonatal seizures; febrile seizures in children; sedation; may also be used for prevention and treatment of neonatal hyperbilirubinemia and lowering of bilirubin in chronic cholestasis

**Usual Dosage**

Children:

Sedation: Oral: 2 mg/kg 3 times/day

Hypnotic: I.M., I.V., S.C.: 3-5 mg/kg at bedtime

Preoperative sedation: Oral, I.M., I.V.: 1-3 mg/kg 1-1.5 hours before procedure

Anticonvulsant: Status epilepticus: **Loading dose:** I.V.:

Children: 10-20 mg/kg in a single or divided dose; in select patients may give additional 5 mg/kg/dose every 15-30 minutes until seizure is controlled or a total dose of 40 mg/kg is reached

Adults: 300-800 mg initially followed by 120-240 mg/dose at 20-minute intervals until seizures are controlled or a total dose of 1-2 g

Anticonvulsant maintenance dose: Oral, I.V.:

Children:

1-5 years: 6-8 mg/kg/day in 1-2 divided doses

5-12 years: 4-6 mg/kg/day in 1-2 divided doses

Children >12 years and Adults: 1-3 mg/kg/day in divided doses or 50-100 mg 2-3 times/day

Adults:

Sedation: Oral, I.M.: 30-120 mg/day in 2-3 divided doses

Hypnotic: Oral, I.M., I.V., S.C.: 100-320 mg at bedtime

Preoperative sedation: I.M.: 100-200 mg 1-1.5 hours before procedure

**Mechanism of Action** Interferes with transmission of impulses from the thalamus to the cortex of the brain resulting in an imbalance in central inhibitory and facilitatory mechanisms

**Local Anesthetic/Vasoconstrictor Precautions** No information available to require special precautions

**Effects on Dental Treatment** No effects or complications reported

**Other Adverse Effects**

>10%:

Cardiovascular: Hypotension, cardiac arrhythmias, bradycardia, arterial spasm, and gangrene with inadvertent intra-arterial injection

Central nervous system: Dizziness, lightheadedness, "hangover" effect, drowsiness, lethargy, CNS excitation or depression, impaired judgment

Local: Pain at injection site, thrombophlebitis with I.V. use

1% to 10%:

Central nervous system: Confusion, mental depression, unusual excitement, nervousness, faint feeling, headache, insomnia, nightmares

Gastrointestinal: Nausea, vomiting, constipation

<1%:

Central nervous system: Hallucinations, hypothermia

Dermatologic: Exfoliative dermatitis, Stevens-Johnson syndrome, rash

Hematologic: Agranulocytosis, megaloblastic anemia, thrombocytopenia

Respiratory: Laryngospasm, respiratory depression, apnea (especially with rapid I.V. use)

**Drug Interactions**

Decreased effect: Phenobarbital appears to increase the metabolism of the following drugs to cause a decrease in their actions: Phenothiazines, haloperidol, quinidine, cyclosporine, tricyclic antidepressants, corticosteroids, theophylline, ethosuximide, warfarin, oral contraceptives, chloramphenicol, griseofulvin, doxycycline, beta-blockers

Increased toxicity: Phenobarbital enhances the sedative effects of propoxyphene, benzodiazepines, CNS depressants, valproic acid, methylphenidate, chloramphenicol

**Drug Uptake**

Oral:

Onset of hypnosis: Within 20-60 minutes

Duration: 6-10 hours

I.V.:

Onset of action: Within 5 minutes

Duration: 4-10 hours

Absorption: Oral: 70% to 90%

Serum half-life:

Children: 37-73 hours

Adults: 53-140 hours

Time to peak serum concentration: Oral: Within 1-6 hours

**Pregnancy Risk Factor** D

**Generic Available** Yes

## Phenol (FEE nol)

**Related Information**

Mouth Pain, Cold Sore, Canker Sore Products *on page 1253*

**U.S. Brand Names** Baker's P&S Topical [OTC]; Cēpastat® [OTC]; Chloraseptic® Oral [OTC]

**Therapeutic Category** Pharmaceutical Aid

**Synonyms** Carbolic Acid

**Use** Relief of sore throat pain, mouth, gum, and throat irritations

**Usual Dosage**

Allow to dissolve slowly in mouth; may be repeated every 2 hours as needed

For each neurolysis procedure: 0.5-2 mL (up to 7.5 mL may be needed)

(Continued)

## Phenol *(Continued)*

**Local Anesthetic/Vasoconstrictor Precautions** No information available to require special precautions

**Effects on Dental Treatment** No effects or complications reported

**Other Adverse Effects** In overdose situation:

1% to 10%:

- Cardiovascular: Hypotension, cardiovascular collapse, tachycardia, atrial and ventricular arrhythmias, edema
- Central nervous system: slurred speech, CNS depression, agitation, confusion, seizures, coma
- Dermatologic: White, red, or brown skin discoloration
- Gastrointestinal: Nausea, vomiting, oral burns GI ulceration, GI bleeding
- Genitourinary: Urine discoloration (green)
- Hematologic: Hemorrhage
- Local: Irritation, burns
- Renal: Nephritis
- Respiratory: Bronchospasm/wheezing, coughing, dyspnea, pneumonia, pulmonary

When used for spinal neurolysis/motor point blocks: 1% to 10%:

- Cardiovascular: Dysrhythmias
- Central nervous system: Headache, hyperesthesia, dysesthesia
- Gastrointestinal: Bowel incontinence
- Genitourinary: Urinary incontinence
- Local: Tissue necrosis, pain at injection site
- Neuromuscular & skeletal: Motor weakness, nerve damage
- Respiratory: Pleural irritation

**Pregnancy Risk Factor** C

**Generic Available** Yes

**Comments** Cepastat® contains 8 calories/lozenge (2 g sorbitol)

♦ **Phenoxine® [OTC]** *see* Phenylpropanolamine *on page 797*

## Phenoxybenzamine (fen oks ee BEN za meen)

**U.S. Brand Names** Dibenzyline®

**Therapeutic Category** Alpha-Adrenergic Blocking Agent, Oral; Antihypertensive Agent; Vasodilator, Coronary

**Use** Symptomatic management of pheochromocytoma; treatment of hypertensive crisis caused by sympathomimetic amines

**Unlabeled use:** Micturition problems associated with neurogenic bladder, functional outlet obstruction, and partial prostate obstruction

**Usual Dosage** Oral:

Children: Initial: 0.2 mg/kg (maximum: 10 mg) once daily, increase by 0.2 mg/kg increments; usual maintenance dose: 0.4-1.2 mg/kg/day every 6-8 hours, higher doses may be necessary

Adults: Initial: 10 mg twice daily, increase by 10 mg every other day until optimum dose is achieved; usual range: 20-40 mg 2-3 times/day

**Mechanism of Action** Produces long-lasting noncompetitive alpha-adrenergic blockade of postganglionic synapses in exocrine glands and smooth muscle; relaxes urethra and increases opening of the bladder

**Local Anesthetic/Vasoconstrictor Precautions** No information available to require special precautions

**Effects on Dental Treatment** No effects or complications reported

**Other Adverse Effects**

>10%:

- Cardiovascular: Postural hypotension, tachycardia, syncope
- Ocular: Miosis
- Respiratory: Nasal congestion

1% to 10%:

- Cardiovascular: Shock
- Central nervous system: Lethargy, headache, confusion, fatigue
- Gastrointestinal: Vomiting, nausea, diarrhea, dry mouth
- Genitourinary: Inhibition of ejaculation
- Neuromuscular & skeletal: Weakness

**Drug Interactions**

Decreased effect: Alpha agonists

Increased toxicity: Beta-blockers (hypotension, tachycardia)

**Drug Uptake**

Onset of action: Oral: Within 2 hours

Duration: Can continue for 4 or more days

Serum half-life: 24 hours

**Pregnancy Risk Factor** C

**Generic Available** No

## Phensuximide (fen SUKS i mide)

**U.S. Brand Names** Milontin®

**Therapeutic Category** Anticonvulsant, Succinimide

**Use** Control of absence (petit mal) seizures

**Usual Dosage** Children and Adults: Oral: 0.5-1 g 2-3 times/day

**Local Anesthetic/Vasoconstrictor Precautions** No information available to require special precautions

**Effects on Dental Treatment** No effects or complications reported

**Other Adverse Effects**

>10%:

- Central nervous system: Ataxia, dizziness, drowsiness, headache
- Dermatologic: Stevens-Johnson syndrome
- Gastrointestinal: Anorexia, nausea, vomiting, weight loss
- Miscellaneous: Systemic lupus erythematosus (SLE), hiccups

1% to 10%:

- Central nervous system: Mental depression, nightmares, fatigue, aggressiveness
- Neuromuscular & skeletal: Weakness

<1%:

- Central nervous system: Paranoid psychosis
- Dermatologic: Urticaria, exfoliative dermatitis
- Hematologic: Agranulocytosis, leukopenia, aplastic anemia, thrombocytopenia, pancytopenia

**Pregnancy Risk Factor** D

**Generic Available** No

## Phentermine (FEN ter meen)

**U.S. Brand Names** Adipex-P®; Fastin®; Ionamin®; Zantryl®

**Therapeutic Category** Anorexiant

**Use** Short-term adjunct in exogenous obesity

**Usual Dosage** Oral:

Children 3-15 years: 5-15 mg/day for 4 weeks

Adults: 8 mg 3 times/day 30 minutes before meals or food or 15-37.5 mg/day before breakfast or 10-14 hours before retiring

**Mechanism of Action** Phentermine is structurally similar to dextroamphetamine and is comparable to dextroamphetamine as an appetite suppressant, but is generally associated with a lower incidence and severity of CNS side effects. Phentermine, like other anorexiants, stimulates the hypothalamus to result in decreased appetite; anorexiant effects are most likely mediated via norepinephrine and dopamine metabolism. However, other CNS effects or metabolic effects may be involved.

**Local Anesthetic/Vasoconstrictor Precautions** Use vasoconstriction with caution in patients taking phentermine. Amphetamines enhance the sympathomimetic response of epinephrine and norepinephrine leading to potential hypertension and cardiotoxicity.

**Effects on Dental Treatment** Up to 10% of patients may present with hypertension. The use of local anesthetic without vasoconstrictor is recommended in these patients.

**Other Adverse Effects**

>10%:

- Cardiovascular: Hypertension
- Central nervous system: Euphoria, nervousness, insomnia

1% to 10%:

- Central nervous system: Confusion, mental depression, restlessness
- Gastrointestinal: Nausea, vomiting, constipation
- Endocrine & metabolic: Changes in libido
- Hematologic: Blood dyscrasias
- Neuromuscular & skeletal: Tremor
- Ocular: Blurred vision

<1%:

- Cardiovascular: Tachycardia, arrhythmias
- Central nervous system: Headache
- Dermatologic: Alopecia
- Gastrointestinal: Diarrhea, abdominal cramps
- Genitourinary: Dysuria
- Neuromuscular & skeletal: Myalgia
- Renal: Polyuria
- Respiratory: Dyspnea
- Miscellaneous: Increased sweating

(Continued)

## Phentermine *(Continued)*

**Drug Interactions**

Adrenergic blockers are inhibited by amphetamines

Amphetamines enhance the activity of tricyclic or sympathomimetic agents

MAO inhibitors slow the metabolism of amphetamines

Amphetamines will counteract the sedative effects of antihistamines

Amphetamines potentiate the analgesic effects of meperidine

**Drug Uptake**

Absorption: Well absorbed; resin absorbed slower and produces more prolonged clinical effects

Serum half-life: 20 hours

**Pregnancy Risk Factor** C

**Generic Available** Yes

**Comments** Many diet doctors have prescribed fenfluramine ("fen") and phentermine ("phen"). When taken together the combination is known as "fen-phen". The diet drug dexfenfluramine (Redux®) is chemically similar to fenfluramine (Pondimin®) and was also used in combination with phentermine called "Redux-phen". While each of the three drugs alone had approval from the FDA for sale in the treatment of obesity, neither combination had an official approval. The use of the combinations in the treatment of obesity was considered an "off-label" use. Reports in medical literature have been accumulating for some years about significant side effects associated with fenfluramine and dexfenfluramine. In 1997, the manufacturers, at the urging of the FDA, agreed to voluntarily withdraw the drugs from the market. The action was based on findings from physicians who evaluated patients taking fenfluramine and dexfenfluramine with echocardiograms. The findings indicated that approximately 30% of patients had abnormal echocardiograms, even though they had no symptoms. This was a much higher than expected percentage of abnormal test results. This conclusion was based on a sample of 291 patients examined by five different physicians. Under normal conditions, fewer than 1% of patients would be expected to show signs of heart valve disease. The findings suggested that fenfluramine and dexfenfluramine were the likely cause of heart valve problems of the type that promoted FDA's earlier warnings concerning "fen-phen". The earlier warning included the following: The mitral valve and other valves in the heart are damaged by a strange white coating and allow blood to flow back, causing heart muscle damage. In several cases, valve replacement surgery has been done. As a rule, the person must, thereafter for life, be on a blood thinner to prevent clots from the mechanical valve. This type of valve damage had only been seen before in persons who were exposed to large amounts of serotonin. The fenfluramine increases the availability of serotonin.

## Phentolamine (fen TOLE a meen)

**U.S. Brand Names** Regitine®

**Canadian Brand Names** Rogitine®

**Therapeutic Category** Alpha-Adrenergic Blocking Agent, Parenteral; Alpha-Adrenergic Inhibitors, Central; Antidote, Extravasation; Antihypertensive Agent; Diagnostic Agent, Pheochromocytoma; Vasodilator, Coronary

**Use** Diagnosis of pheochromocytoma and treatment of hypertension associated with pheochromocytoma or other caused by excess sympathomimetic amines; as treatment of dermal necrosis after extravasation of drugs with alpha-adrenergic effects (norepinephrine, dopamine, epinephrine, dobutamine)

**Usual Dosage**

Treatment of alpha-adrenergic drug extravasation: S.C.:

Children: 0.1-0.2 mg/kg diluted in 10 mL 0.9% sodium chloride infiltrated into area of extravasation within 12 hours

Adults: Infiltrate area with small amount of solution made by diluting 5-10 mg in 10 mL 0.9% sodium chloride within 12 hours of extravasation

If dose is effective, normal skin color should return to the blanched area within 1 hour

Diagnosis of pheochromocytoma: I.M., I.V.:

Children: 0.05-0.1 mg/kg/dose, maximum single dose: 5 mg

Adults: 5 mg

Surgery for pheochromocytoma: Hypertension: I.M., I.V.:

Children: 0.05-0.1 mg/kg/dose given 1-2 hours before procedure; repeat as needed every 2-4 hours until hypertension is controlled; maximum single dose: 5 mg

Adults: 5 mg given 1-2 hours before procedure and repeated as needed every 2-4 hours

Hypertensive crisis: Adults: 5-20 mg

**Mechanism of Action** Competitively blocks alpha-adrenergic receptors to produce brief antagonism of circulating epinephrine and norepinephrine to reduce hypertension caused by alpha effects of these catecholamines; also has a positive inotropic and chronotropic effect on the heart

**Local Anesthetic/Vasoconstrictor Precautions** Although the alpha-adrenergic blocking effects could antagonize epinephrine, there is no information available to require special precautions

**Effects on Dental Treatment** No effects or complications reported

**Other Adverse Effects**

>10%:

Cardiovascular: Hypotension, tachycardia, arrhythmias, reflex tachycardia, anginal pain, orthostatic hypotension

Gastrointestinal: Nausea, vomiting, diarrhea, exacerbation of peptic ulcer, abdominal pain

Respiratory: Nasal congestion

1% to 10%:

Cardiovascular: Flushing of face, syncope

Central nervous system: Dizziness

Neuromuscular & skeletal: Weakness

<1%:

Cardiovascular: Myocardial infarction

Central nervous system: Severe headache

**Drug Interactions**

Decreased effect: Epinephrine, ephedrine

Increased toxicity: Ethanol (disulfiram reaction)

**Drug Uptake**

Onset of action:

I.M.: Within 15-20 minutes

I.V.: Immediate

Duration:

I.M.: 30-45 minutes

I.V.: 15-30 minutes

Serum half-life: 19 minutes

**Pregnancy Risk Factor** C

**Generic Available** No

♦ **Phenylalanine Mustard** *see* Melphalan *on page 626*

♦ **Phenyldrine® [OTC]** *see* Phenylpropanolamine *on page 797*

## Phenylephrine (fen il EF rin)

**Related Information**

Dentin Hypersensitivity; High Caries Index; Xerostomia *on page 1145*

Guaifenesin and Phenylephrine *on page 480*

**U.S. Brand Names** AK-Dilate® Ophthalmic Solution; AK-Nefrin® Ophthalmic Solution; Alconefrin® Nasal Solution [OTC]; I-Phrine® Ophthalmic Solution; Mydfrin® Ophthalmic Solution; Neo-Synephrine® Nasal Solution [OTC]; Neo-Synephrine® Ophthalmic Solution; Nostril® Nasal Solution [OTC]; Prefrin™ Ophthalmic Solution; Relief® Ophthalmic Solution; Rhinall® Nasal Solution [OTC]; Sinarest® Nasal Solution [OTC]; St. Joseph® Measured Dose Nasal Solution [OTC]; Vicks Sinex® Nasal Solution [OTC]

**Canadian Brand Names** Dionephrine; Novahistine® Decongestant; Prefrin™ Liquifilm®

**Therapeutic Category** Adrenergic Agonist Agent; Adrenergic Agonist Agent, Ophthalmic; Antiglaucoma Agent; Nasal Agent, Vasoconstrictor; Ophthalmic Agent, Mydriatic

**Use** Treatment of hypotension, vascular failure in shock; as a vasoconstrictor in regional analgesia; symptomatic relief of nasal and nasopharyngeal mucosal congestion; as a mydriatic in ophthalmic procedures and treatment of wide-angle glaucoma; supraventricular tachycardia

**Usual Dosage**

Ophthalmic procedures:

Children and Adults: Instill 1 drop of 2.5% or 10% solution, may repeat in 10-60 minutes as needed

Nasal decongestant: (therapy should not exceed 5 continuous days)

Children:

2-6 years: Instill 1 drop every 2-4 hours of 0.125% solution as needed

6-12 years: Instill 1-2 sprays or instill 1-2 drops every 4 hours of 0.25% solution as needed

Children >12 years and Adults: Instill 1-2 sprays or instill 1-2 drops every 4 hours of 0.25% to 0.5% solution as needed; 1% solution may be used in adult in cases of extreme nasal congestion; do not use nasal solutions more than 3 days

(Continued)

## Phenylephrine *(Continued)*

Hypotension/shock:
Children:
I.M., S.C.: 0.1 mg/kg/dose every 1-2 hours as needed (maximum: 5 mg)
I.V. bolus: 5-20 mcg/kg/dose every 10-15 minutes as needed
I.V. infusion: 0.1-0.5 mcg/kg/minute
Adults:
I.M., S.C.: 2-5 mg/dose every 1-2 hours as needed (initial dose should not exceed 5 mg)
I.V. bolus: 0.1-0.5 mg/dose every 10-15 minutes as needed (initial dose should not exceed 0.5 mg)
I.V. infusion: 10 mg in 250 mL $D_5W$ or NS (1:25,000 dilution) (40 mcg/mL); start at 100-180 mcg/minute (2-5 mL/minute; 50-90 drops/minute) initially; when blood pressure is stabilized, maintenance rate: 40-60 mcg/minute (20-30 drops/minute)
Paroxysmal supraventricular tachycardia: I.V.:
Children: 5-10 mcg/kg/dose over 20-30 seconds
Adults: 0.25-0.5 mg/dose over 20-30 seconds

**Mechanism of Action** Potent, direct-acting alpha-adrenergic stimulator with weak beta-adrenergic activity; causes vasoconstriction of the arterioles of the nasal mucosa and conjunctiva; activates the dilator muscle of the pupil to cause contraction; produces vasoconstriction of arterioles in the body; produces systemic arterial vasoconstriction

**Local Anesthetic/Vasoconstrictor Precautions** Use with caution since phenylephrine is a sympathomimetic amine which could interact with epinephrine to cause a pressor response

**Effects on Dental Treatment** Up to 10% of patients could experience tachycardia, palpitations, and dry mouth; use vasoconstrictor with caution

**Other Adverse Effects**
Nasal:
>10%: Respiratory: Burning, rebound congestion, sneezing
1% to 10%: Respiratory: Stinging, dryness
Ophthalmic:
>10%: Ocular: Transient stinging
1% to 10%:
Central nervous system: Headache, browache
Ocular: Blurred vision, photophobia, lacrimation
Systemic:
>10%: Neuromuscular & skeletal: Tremor
1% to 10%:
Cardiovascular: Peripheral vasoconstriction hypertension, angina, reflex bradycardia, arrhythmias
Central nervous system: Restlessness, excitability

**Drug Interactions**
Decreased effect of phenylephrine with alpha- and beta-adrenergic blocking agents
Increased effect of phenylephrine with oxytocic drugs
Increased toxicity: With sympathomimetics, tachycardia or arrhythmias may occur; with MAO inhibitors, actions may be potentiated

**Drug Uptake**
Onset of effect:
I.M., S.C.: Within 10-15 minutes
I.V.: Immediate
Duration:
I.M.: 30 minutes to 2 hours
I.V.: 15-30 minutes
S.C.: 1 hour
Serum half-life: 2.5 hours

**Pregnancy Risk Factor** C
**Generic Available** Yes

- ♦ **Phenylephrine and Chlorpheniramine** *see* Chlorpheniramine and Phenylephrine *on page 232*
- ♦ **Phenylephrine and Cyclopentolate** *see* Cyclopentolate and Phenylephrine *on page 285*
- ♦ **Phenylephrine and Guaifenesin** *see* Guaifenesin and Phenylephrine *on page 480*

## Phenylephrine and Scopolamine

(fen il EF rin & skoe POL a meen)

**U.S. Brand Names** Murocoll-2® Ophthalmic
**Therapeutic Category** Ophthalmic Agent, Mydriatic

**Synonyms** Scopolamine and Phenylephrine
**Use** Mydriasis, cycloplegia, and to break posterior synechiae in iritis
**Usual Dosage** Instill 1-2 drops into eye(s); repeat in 5 minutes
**Local Anesthetic/Vasoconstrictor Precautions** Use with caution since phenylephrine is a sympathomimetic amine which could interact with epinephrine to cause a pressor response
**Effects on Dental Treatment** This form of phenylephrine will have no effect on dental treatment when given as eye drops
**Pregnancy Risk Factor** C
**Generic Available** Yes

## Phenylephrine and Zinc Sulfate (fen il EF rin & zingk SUL fate)

**U.S. Brand Names** Zincfrin® Ophthalmic [OTC]
**Therapeutic Category** Ophthalmic Agent, Miscellaneous
**Use** Soothe, moisturize, and remove redness due to minor eye irritation
**Usual Dosage** Instill 1-2 drops in eye(s) 2-4 times/day as needed
**Local Anesthetic/Vasoconstrictor Precautions** No information available to require special precautions
**Effects on Dental Treatment** No effects or complications reported
**Generic Available** Yes

- ♦ **Phenylephrine, Chlorpheniramine, Phenylpropanolamine, and Belladonna Alkaloids** *see* Chlorpheniramine, Phenylephrine, Phenylpropanolamine, and Belladonna Alkaloids *on page 236*
- ♦ **Phenylfenesin® L.A.** *see* Guaifenesin and Phenylpropanolamine *on page 480*

## Phenylpropanolamine (fen il proe pa NOLE a meen)

**Related Information**
Phenyltoloxamine, Phenylpropanolamine, Pyrilamine, and Pheniramine *on next page*
**U.S. Brand Names** Acutrim® 16 Hours [OTC]; Acutrim® II, Maximum Strength [OTC]; Acutrim® Late Day [OTC]; Control® [OTC]; Dexatrim® Pre-Meal [OTC]; Maximum Strength Dex-A-Diet® [OTC]; Maximum Strength Dexatrim® [OTC]; Phenoxine® [OTC]; Phenyldrine® [OTC]; Propagest® [OTC]; Rhindecon®; Unitrol® [OTC]
**Therapeutic Category** Adrenergic Agonist Agent; Anorexiant; Decongestant; Nasal Agent, Vasoconstrictor
**Use** Anorexiant; nasal decongestant
**Usual Dosage** Oral:
Children: Decongestant:
2-6 years: 6.25 mg every 4 hours
6-12 years: 12.5 mg every 4 hours not to exceed 75 mg/day
Adults:
Decongestant: 25 mg every 4 hours or 50 mg every 8 hours, not to exceed 150 mg/day
Anorexic: 25 mg 3 times/day 30 minutes before meals or 75 mg (timed release) once daily in the morning
Precision release: 75 mg after breakfast
**Mechanism of Action** Releases tissue stores of epinephrine and thereby produces an alpha- and beta-adrenergic stimulation; this causes vasoconstriction and nasal mucosa blanching; also appears to depress central appetite centers
**Local Anesthetic/Vasoconstrictor Precautions** Use with caution since phenylpropanolamine is a sympathomimetic amine which could interact with epinephrine to cause a pressor response
**Effects on Dental Treatment** Up to 10% of patients could experience tachycardia, palpitations, and dry mouth; use vasoconstrictor with caution
**Other Adverse Effects**
>10%: Cardiovascular: Hypertension, palpitations
1% to 10%:
Central nervous system: Insomnia, restlessness, dizziness
Gastrointestinal: Dry mouth, nausea
<1%:
Cardiovascular: Tightness in chest, bradycardia, arrhythmias, angina
Central nervous system: Severe headache, anxiety, nervousness
Genitourinary: Dysuria
**Drug Interactions**
Decreased effect of antihypertensives
Increased effect/toxicity with MAO inhibitors (hypertensive crisis), beta-blockers (increased pressor effects)
**Drug Uptake**
Absorption: Oral: Well absorbed
Serum half-life: 4.6-6.6 hours
(Continued)

## Phenylpropanolamine *(Continued)*

**Pregnancy Risk Factor** C

**Generic Available** Yes

- **Phenylpropanolamine and Brompheniramine** *see* Brompheniramine and Phenylpropanolamine *on page 153*
- **Phenylpropanolamine and Caramiphen** *see* Caramiphen and Phenylpropanolamine *on page 184*
- **Phenylpropanolamine and Chlorpheniramine** *see* Chlorpheniramine and Phenylpropanolamine *on page 233*
- **Phenylpropanolamine and Guaifenesin** *see* Guaifenesin and Phenylpropanolamine *on page 480*
- **Phenylpropanolamine and Hydrocodone** *see* Hydrocodone and Phenylpropanolamine *on page 510*
- **Phenylpropanolamine, Chlorpheniramine, Phenylephrine, and Belladonna Alkaloids** *see* Chlorpheniramine, Phenylephrine, Phenylpropanolamine, and Belladonna Alkaloids *on page 236*

## Phenyltoloxamine, Phenylpropanolamine, and Acetaminophen

(fen il tol OKS a meen, fen il proe pa NOLE a meen, & a seet a MIN oh fen)

**U.S. Brand Names** Sinubid®

**Therapeutic Category** Analgesic, Non-narcotic; Antihistamine/Decongestant Combination

**Use** Intermittent symptomatic treatment of nasal congestion in sinus or other frontal headache; allergic rhinitis, vasomotor rhinitis, coryza; facial pain and pressure of acute and chronic sinusitis

**Usual Dosage** Oral:

Children 6-12 years: 1/2 tablet every 12 hours (twice daily)

Adults: 1 tablet every 12 hours (twice daily)

**Local Anesthetic/Vasoconstrictor Precautions** Use with caution since phenylpropanolamine is a sympathomimetic amine which could interact with epinephrine to cause a pressor response

**Effects on Dental Treatment**

Acetaminophen: No effects or complications reported

Phenylpropanolamine: Up to 10% of patients could experience tachycardia, palpitations, and dry mouth; use vasoconstrictor with caution

**Pregnancy Risk Factor** C

**Generic Available** Yes

**Selected Readings**

Barker JD Jr, de Carle DJ, and Anuras S, "Chronic Excessive Acetaminophen Use in Liver Damage," *Ann Intern Med*, 1977, 87(3):299-301.

Dionne RA, Campbell RA, Cooper SA, et al, "Suppression of Postoperative Pain by Preoperative Administration of Ibuprofen in Comparison to Placebo, Acetaminophen, and Acetaminophen Plus Codeine," *J Clin Pharmacol*, 1983, 23(1):37-43.

Licht H, Seeff LB, and Zimmerman HJ, "Apparent Potentiation of Acetaminophen Hepatotoxicity by Alcohol," *Ann Intern Med*, 1980, 92(4):511.

## Phenyltoloxamine, Phenylpropanolamine, Pyrilamine, and Pheniramine

(fen il tol OKS a meen, fen il proe pa NOLE a meen, peer IL a meen, & fen IR a meen)

**U.S. Brand Names** Poly-Histine-D® Capsule

**Therapeutic Category** Cold Preparation

**Use** Treatment of nasal congestion

**Usual Dosage** Oral: Adults: One capsule every 8-12 hours

**Local Anesthetic/Vasoconstrictor Precautions** Use with caution since phenylpropanolamine is a sympathomimetic amine which could interact with epinephrine to cause a pressor response

**Effects on Dental Treatment**

Phenylpropanolamine: Up to 10% of patients could experience tachycardia, palpitations, and dry mouth; use vasoconstrictor with caution

Pyrilamine: No effects or complications reported

Pheniramine: No effects or complications reported

**Other Adverse Effects** See individual agents

**Drug Interactions** See individual agents

**Dosage Forms** Capsule: Phenyltoloxamine citrate 16 mg, phenylpropanolamine hydrochloride 50 mg, pyrilamine maleate 16 mg, and pheniramine maleate 16 mg

**Generic Available** Yes

## Phenytoin (FEN i toyn)

**Related Information**

Cardiovascular Diseases *on page 1066*

**U.S. Brand Names** Dilantin®; Diphenylan Sodium®

**Canadian Brand Names** Tremytoine®

**Therapeutic Category** Antiarrhythmic Agent, Class I-B; Antiarrhythmic Agent (Supraventricular & Ventricular); Anticonvulsant, Hydantoin

**Use** Management of generalized tonic-clonic (grand mal), simple partial and complex partial seizures; prevention of seizures following head trauma/neurosurgery; ventricular arrhythmias, including those associated with digitalis intoxication, prolonged Q-T interval and surgical repair of congenital heart diseases in children; also used for epidermolysis bullosa

**Usual Dosage**

Status epilepticus: I.V.:

- Children: Loading dose: 15-20 mg/kg in a single or divided dose; maintenance dose: Initial: 5 mg/kg/day in 2 divided doses, usual doses:
  - 6 months to 3 years: 8-10 mg/kg/day
  - 4-6 years: 7.5-9 mg/kg/day
  - 7-9 years: 7-8 mg/kg/day
  - 10-16 years: 6-7 mg/kg/day, some patients may require every 8 hours dosing
- Adults: Loading dose: 15-20 mg/kg in a single or divided dose, followed by 100-150 mg/dose at 30-minute intervals up to a maximum of 1500 mg/24 hours; maintenance dose: 300 mg/day or 5-6 mg/kg/day in 3 divided doses or 1-2 divided doses using extended release

Anticonvulsant: Children and Adults: Oral:

- Loading dose: 15-20 mg/kg; based on phenytoin serum concentrations and recent dosing history; administer oral loading dose in 3 divided doses given every 2-4 hours to decrease GI adverse effects and to ensure complete oral absorption; maintenance dose: same as I.V.

**Mechanism of Action** Stabilizes neuronal membranes and decreases seizure activity by increasing efflux or decreasing influx of sodium ions across cell membranes in the motor cortex during generation of nerve impulses; prolongs effective refractory period and suppresses ventricular pacemaker automaticity, shortens action potential in the heart

**Local Anesthetic/Vasoconstrictor Precautions** No information available to require special precautions

**Effects on Dental Treatment** Gingival hyperplasia is a common problem observed during the first 6 months of phenytoin therapy appearing as gingivitis or gum inflammation. To minimize severity and growth rate of gingival tissue begin a program of professional cleaning and patient plaque control within 10 days of starting anticonvulsant therapy.

**Other Adverse Effects**

>10%:

- Central nervous system: Psychiatric changes, slurred speech, dizziness, drowsiness
- Gastrointestinal: Constipation, nausea, vomiting, gingival hyperplasia
- Neuromuscular & skeletal: Trembling

1% to 10%:

- Central nervous system: Headache, insomnia
- Dermatologic: Skin rash
- Gastrointestinal: Anorexia, weight loss
- Hematologic: Leukopenia, elevated serum creatinine
- Hepatic: Hepatitis

<1%:

- Cardiovascular: Hypotension, bradycardia, cardiac arrhythmias, cardiovascular collapse
- Central nervous system: Confusion, fever, ataxia
- Local: Thrombophlebitis, venous irritation and pain
- Neuromuscular & skeletal: Peripheral neuropathy, paresthesia
- Ocular: Diplopia, nystagmus, blurred vision

Rarely seen effects: SLE-like syndrome, lymphadenopathy, hepatitis, Stevens-Johnson syndrome, blood dyscrasias, dyskinesias, pseudolymphoma, lymphoma

**Drug Interactions** Phenytoin is an inducer of cytochrome P-450 IIIA enzymes and is associated with many drug interactions

Decreased effect: Rifampin, cisplatin, vinblastine, bleomycin, folic acid, continuous NG feedings

Increased toxicity: Amiodarone decreases metabolism of phenytoin; disulfiram decreases metabolism of phenytoin; fluconazole, itraconazole decreases phenytoin serum concentrations; isoniazid may increase phenytoin serum concentrations

(Continued)

## Phenytoin *(Continued)*

Increased effect/toxicity of valproic acid, ethosuximide, primidone, warfarin, oral contraceptives, corticosteroids, cyclosporine, theophylline, chloramphenicol, rifampin, doxycycline, quinidine, mexiletine, disopyramide, dopamine, nondepolarizing skeletal muscle relaxants

**Drug Uptake**

Absorption: Oral: Slow

Time to peak serum concentration (dependent upon formulation administered): Oral:

Extended-release capsule: Within 4-12 hours

Immediate release preparation: Within 2-3 hours

**Pregnancy Risk Factor** D

**Generic Available** Yes

**Selected Readings**

Dooley G and Vasan N, "Dilantin® Hyperplasia: A Review of the Literature," *J N Z Soc Periodontol*, 1989, 68:19-22.

Iacopino AM, Doxey D, Cutler CW, et al, "Phenytoin and Cyclosporine A Specifically Regulate Macrophage Phenotype and Expression of Platelet-Derived Growth Factor and Interleukin-1 In Vitro and In Vivo: Possible Molecular Mechanism of Drug-Induced Gingival Hyperplasia," *J Periodontol*, 1997, 68(1):73-83.

Pihlstrom BL, "Prevention and Treatment of Dilantin®-Associated Gingival Enlargement," *Compendium*, 1990, 14:S506-10.

Saito K, Mori S, Iwakura M, et al, "Immunohistochemical Localization of Transforming Growth Factor Beta, Basic Fibroblast Growth Factor and Heparin Sulphate Glycosaminoglycan in Gingival Hyperplasia Induced by Nifedipine and Phenytoin," *J Periodontal Res*, 1996, 31(8):545-5.

Zhou LX, Pihlstrom B, Hardwick JP, et al, "Metabolism of Phenytoin by the Gingiva of Normal Humans: The Possible Role of Reactive Metabolites of Phenytoin in the Initiation of Gingival Hyperplasia," *Clin Pharmacol Ther*, 1996, 60(2):191-8.

## Phenytoin With Phenobarbital (FEN i toyn with fee noe BAR bi tal)

**U.S. Brand Names** Dilantin® With Phenobarbital

**Therapeutic Category** Anticonvulsant, Barbiturate; Anticonvulsant, Hydantoin

**Use** Management of generalized tonic-clonic (grand mal), simple partial and complex partial seizures

**Usual Dosage** Adults: Oral: Initial:

Rheumatoid arthritis: 100-200 mg 3-4 times/day until desired effect, then reduce dose to not exceeding 400 mg/day

Acute gouty arthritis: 400 mg, 100 mg every 4 hours until acute attack subsides, not to continue longer than 1 week

**Local Anesthetic/Vasoconstrictor Precautions** No information available to require special precautions

**Effects on Dental Treatment** Gingival hyperplasia is a common problem observed during the first 6 months of phenytoin therapy appearing as gingivitis or gum inflammation. To minimize severity and growth rate of gingival tissue begin a program of professional cleaning and patient plaque control within 10 days of starting anticonvulsant therapy.

**Pregnancy Risk Factor** D

**Generic Available** No

- **Pherazine® VC w/ Codeine** *see* Promethazine, Phenylephrine, and Codeine *on page 850*
- **Pherazine® w/DM** *see* Promethazine and Dextromethorphan *on page 849*
- **Pherazine® With Codeine** *see* Promethazine and Codeine *on page 848*
- **Phicon® [OTC]** *see* Pramoxine *on page 828*
- **Phillips'® Milk of Magnesia [OTC]** *see* Magnesium Hydroxide *on page 612*
- **pHisoHex®** *see* Hexachlorophene *on page 496*
- **pHiso® Scrub** *see* Hexachlorophene *on page 496*
- **Phos-Flur®** *see* Fluoride *on page 441*
- **PhosLo®** *see* Calcium Acetate *on page 171*
- **Phospholine Iodide®** *see* Echothiophate Iodide *on page 361*

## Phosphorated Carbohydrate Solution

(FOS for ate ed kar boe HYE drate soe LOO shun)

**U.S. Brand Names** Emecheck® [OTC]; Emetrol® [OTC]; Naus-A-Way® [OTC]; Nausetrol® [OTC]

**Therapeutic Category** Antiemetic

**Synonyms** Dextrose, Levulose and Phosphoric Acid; Levulose, Dextrose and Phosphoric Acid; Phosphoric Acid, Levulose and Dextrose

**Use** Relief of nausea associated with upset stomach that occurs with intestinal flu, pregnancy, food indiscretions, and emotional upsets

**Usual Dosage**

Morning sickness: 15-30 mL on arising; repeat every 3 hours or when nausea threatens

Motion sickness and vomiting due to drug therapy: 5 mL doses for young children; 15 mL doses for older children and adults

Regurgitation in infants: 5 or 10 mL, 10-15 minutes before each feeding; in refractory cases: 10-15 mL, 30 minutes before each feeding

Vomiting due to psychogenic factors:

Children: 5-10 mL; repeat dose every 15 minutes until distress subsides; do not take for more than 1 hour

Adults: 15-30 mL; repeat dose every 15 minutes until distress subsides; do not take for more than 1 hour

**Local Anesthetic/Vasoconstrictor Precautions** No information available to require special precautions

**Effects on Dental Treatment** No effects or complications reported

**Other Adverse Effects** 1% to 10%: Gastrointestinal: Abdominal pain, diarrhea

**Generic Available** Yes

- **Phosphoric Acid, Levulose and Dextrose** *see* Phosphorated Carbohydrate Solution *on previous page*
- **Photofrin®** *see* Porfimer *on page 817*
- **Phrenilin®** *see* Butalbital Compound *on page 163*
- **Phrenilin®** *see* Butalbital Compound and Acetaminophen *on page 164*
- **Phrenilin® Forte®** *see* Butalbital Compound *on page 163*
- **Phrenilin® Forte®** *see* Butalbital Compound and Acetaminophen *on page 164*
- **Phyllocontin®** *see* Aminophylline *on page 63*
- **Phylloquinone** *see* Phytonadione *on this page*

## Physostigmine (fye zoe STIG meen)

**U.S. Brand Names** Antilirium®; Isopto® Eserine®

**Therapeutic Category** Antidote, Anticholinergic Agent; Antiglaucoma Agent; Cholinergic Agent; Cholinergic Agent, Ophthalmic

**Use** Reverse toxic CNS effects caused by anticholinergic drugs; used as miotic in treatment of glaucoma

**Usual Dosage**

Children: Anticholinergic drug overdose: Reserve for life-threatening situations only: I.V.: 0.01-0.03 mg/kg/dose, (maximum: 0.5 mg/minute); may repeat after 5-10 minutes to a maximum total dose of 2 mg or until response occurs or adverse cholinergic effects occur

Adults: Anticholinergic drug overdose:

I.M., I.V., S.C.: 0.5-2 mg to start, repeat every 20 minutes until response occurs or adverse effect occurs

Repeat 1-4 mg every 30-60 minutes as life-threatening signs (arrhythmias, seizures, deep coma) recur; maximum I.V. rate: 1 mg/minute

Ophthalmic:

Ointment: Instill a small quantity to lower fornix up to 3 times/day

Solution: Instill 1-2 drops into eye(s) up to 4 times/day

**Mechanism of Action** Inhibits destruction of acetylcholine by acetylcholinesterase which facilitates transmission of impulses across myoneural junction and prolongs the central and peripheral effects of acetylcholine

**Local Anesthetic/Vasoconstrictor Precautions** No information available to require special precautions

**Effects on Dental Treatment** No effects or complications reported

**Other Adverse Effects** Ophthalmic:

>10%:

Ocular: Lacrimation, marked miosis, blurred vision, eye pain

Miscellaneous: Sweating

1% to 10%:

Central nervous system: Headache, browache

Dermatologic: Burning, redness

**Drug Interactions** No data reported with ophthalmic use

**Drug Uptake**

Onset of action:

Ophthalmic instillation: Within 2 minutes

Parenteral: Within 5 minutes

Absorption: I.M., ophthalmic, S.C.: Readily absorbed

Serum half-life: 15-40 minutes

**Pregnancy Risk Factor** C

**Generic Available** Yes: Ophthalmic

- **Phytomenadione** *see* Phytonadione *on this page*

## Phytonadione (fye toe na DYE one)

**U.S. Brand Names** AquaMEPHYTON®; Konakion®; Mephyton®

**Therapeutic Category** Vitamin, Fat Soluble

(Continued)

## Phytonadione *(Continued)*

**Synonyms** Phylloquinone; Phytomenadione

**Use** Prevention and treatment of hypoprothrombinemia caused by drug-induced or anticoagulant-induced vitamin K deficiency, hemorrhagic disease of the newborn; phytonadione is more effective and is preferred to other vitamin K preparations in the presence of impending hemorrhage; oral absorption depends on the presence of bile salts

**Usual Dosage** I.V. route should be restricted for emergency use only

Minimum daily requirement: Not well established

Adults: 0.03 mcg/kg/day

Hemorrhagic disease of the newborn:

Prophylaxis: I.M., S.C.: 0.5-1 mg within 1 hour of birth

Treatment: I.M., S.C.: 1-2 mg/dose/day

Oral anticoagulant overdose:

Children and Adults: Oral, I.M., I.V., S.C.: 2.5-10 mg/dose; rarely up to 25-50 mg has been used; may repeat in 6-8 hours if given by I.M., I.V., S.C. route; may repeat 12-48 hours after oral route

Vitamin K deficiency: Due to drugs, malabsorption or decreased synthesis of vitamin K

Children:

Oral: 2.5-5 mg/24 hours

I.M., I.V.: 1-2 mg/dose as a single dose

Adults:

Oral: 5-25 mg/24 hours

I.M., I.V.: 10 mg

**Mechanism of Action** Promotes liver synthesis of clotting factors (II, VII, IX, X); however, the exact mechanism as to this stimulation is unknown. Menadiol is a water soluble form of vitamin K; phytonadione has a more rapid and prolonged effect than menadione; menadiol sodium diphosphate ($K_4$) is half as potent as menadione ($K_3$).

**Local Anesthetic/Vasoconstrictor Precautions** No information available to require special precautions

**Effects on Dental Treatment** No effects or complications reported

**Other Adverse Effects** <1%:

Cardiovascular: Transient flushing reaction, rarely hypotension, cyanosis

Central nervous system: Rarely dizziness, pain

Gastrointestinal: Dysgeusia, GI upset (oral)

Hematologic: Hemolysis in neonates and in patients with G-6-PD deficiency

Local: Tenderness at injection site

Respiratory: Dyspnea

Miscellaneous: Sweating, anaphylaxis, hypersensitivity reactions

**Drug Interactions** Warfarin sodium, dicumarol, and anisindione effects antagonized by phytonadione

**Drug Uptake**

Onset of increased coagulation factors:

Oral: Within 6-12 hours

Parenteral: Within 1-2 hours; patient may become normal after 12-14 hours

Absorption: Oral: Absorbed from the intestines in the presence of bile

**Pregnancy Risk Factor** C

**Generic Available** Yes

♦ **Pilagan®** *see* Pilocarpine *on this page*

♦ **Pilocar®** *see* Pilocarpine *on this page*

## Pilocarpine (pye loe KAR peen)

**Related Information**

Dentin Hypersensitivity; High Caries Index; Xerostomia *on page 1145*

Patients Undergoing Cancer Therapy *on page 1154*

**U.S. Brand Names** Adsorbocarpine®; Akarpine®; Isopto® Carpine®; Ocu-Carpine®; Ocusert® Pilo; Ocusert Pilo-20®; Ocusert Pilo-40®; Pilagan®; Pilocar®; Pilopine HS®; Piloptic®; Pilostat®

**Canadian Brand Names** Minims® Pilocarpine

**Therapeutic Category** Antiglaucoma Agent; Cholinergic Agent, Ophthalmic; Ophthalmic Agent, Miotic

**Use** Management of chronic simple glaucoma, chronic and acute angle-closure glaucoma; counter effects of cycloplegics

**Usual Dosage** Adults:

Ophthalmic:

Nitrate solution: Shake well before using; instill 1-2 drops 2-4 times/day

Hydrochloride solution:

Instill 1-2 drops up to 6 times/day; adjust the concentration and frequency as required to control elevated intraocular pressure

To counteract the mydriatic effects of sympathomimetic agents: Instill 1 drop of a 1% solution in the affected eye

Gel: Instill 0.5" ribbon into lower conjunctival sac once daily at bedtime

Ocular systems: Systems are labeled in terms of mean rate of release of pilocarpine over 7 days; begin with 20 mcg/hour at night and adjust based on response

Oral: 5 mg 3 times/day, titration up to 10 mg 3 times/day may be considered for patients who have not responded adequately

**Mechanism of Action** Directly stimulates cholinergic receptors in the eye causing miosis (by contraction of the iris sphincter), loss of accommodation (by constriction of ciliary muscle), and lowering of intraocular pressure (with decreased resistance to aqueous humor outflow)

**Local Anesthetic/Vasoconstrictor Precautions** No information available to require special precautions

**Effects on Dental Treatment** No effects or complications reported

**Other Adverse Effects**

>10%: Ocular: Blurred vision, miosis

1% to 10%:

Central nervous system: Headache, browache

Genitourinary: Frequent urination

Local: Stinging, burning, lacrimation

Ocular: Ciliary spasm, retinal detachment, photophobia, acute iritis, conjunctival and ciliary congestion early in therapy

Miscellaneous: Hypersensitivity reactions

<1%:

Cardiovascular: Hypertension, tachycardia

Gastrointestinal: Nausea, vomiting, diarrhea, salivation

Miscellaneous: Sweating

**Drug Interactions** Concurrent use with beta-blockers may cause conduction disturbances; pilocarpine may antagonize the effects of anticholinergic drugs

**Drug Uptake**

Ophthalmic instillation:

Miosis:

Onset of effect: Within 10-30 minutes

Duration: 4-8 hours

Intraocular pressure reduction:

Onset of effect: 1 hour required

Duration: 4-12 hours

Ocusert® Pilo application:

Miosis: Onset of effect: 1.5-2 hours

Reduced intraocular pressure:

Onset: Within 1.5-2 hours; miosis within 10-30 minutes

Duration: ~1 week

**Pregnancy Risk Factor** C

**Dosage Forms** See table.

**Pilocarpine**

| Dosage Form | Strength % | 1 mL | 2 mL | 15 mL | 30 mL | 3.5 g |
|---|---|---|---|---|---|---|
| Gel | 4 | | | | | x |
| Solution as hydrochloride | 0.25 | | | x | | |
| | 0.5 | | | x | x | |
| | 1 | x | x | x | x | |
| | 2 | x | x | x | x | |
| | 3 | | | x | x | |
| | 4 | x | x | x | x | |
| | 6 | | | x | x | |
| | 8 | | x | | | |
| | 10 | | | x | | |
| Solution as nitrate | 1 | | | x | | |
| | 2 | | | x | | |
| | 4 | | | x | | |
| Ocusert® Pilo-20: Releases 20 mcg/hour for 1 week | | | | | | |
| Ocusert® Pilo-40: Releases 40 mcg/hour for 1 week | | | | | | |

(Continued)

## Pilocarpine *(Continued)*

**Generic Available** Yes: Hydrochloride Solution

## Pilocarpine and Epinephrine (pye loe KAR peen & ep i NEF rin)

**U.S. Brand Names** E-Pilo-x® Ophthalmic; $P_xE_x$® Ophthalmic

**Canadian Brand Names** E-Pilo®

**Therapeutic Category** Antiglaucoma Agent; Ophthalmic Agent, Miotic

**Use** Treatment of glaucoma; counter effect of cycloplegics

**Usual Dosage** Instill 1-2 drops up to 6 times/day

**Local Anesthetic/Vasoconstrictor Precautions** No information available to require special precautions

**Effects on Dental Treatment** No effects or complications reported

**Other Adverse Effects** 1% to 10%:

Cardiovascular: Tachycardia, hypertension
Central nervous system: Headache
Gastrointestinal: Salivation
Ocular: Miosis, ciliary spasm, blurred vision, retinal detachment, stinging, lacrimation, itching, vitreous hemorrhages, photophobia, acute iritis
Miscellaneous: Hypersensitivity reactions

**Pregnancy Risk Factor** C

**Generic Available** No

## Pilocarpine (Dental) (pye loe KAR peen)

**U.S. Brand Names** Salagen®

**Canadian Brand Names** Minims® Pilocarpine

**Therapeutic Category** Cholinergic Agent

**Use**

Dental: Treatment of xerostomia caused by radiation therapy in patients with head and neck cancer and from Sjögren's syndrome
Medical: No data reported

**Usual Dosage** Adults: 1-2 tablets 3-4 times/day not to exceed 30 mg/day; patients should be treated for a minimum of 90 days for optimum effects

**Mechanism of Action** Pilocarpine stimulates the muscarinic-type acetylcholine receptors in the salivary glands within the parasympathetic division of the autonomic nervous system to cause an increase in serous-type saliva

**Local Anesthetic/Vasoconstrictor Precautions** No information available to require special precautions

**Effects on Dental Treatment** Salivation - therapeutic effect

**Other Adverse Effects**

>10%: Miscellaneous: Sweating
1% to 10%:
Central nervous system: Chills, headache, dizziness
Gastrointestinal: Nausea
Ocular: Lacrimation
Renal: Polyuria
Respiratory: Rhinitis, pharyngitis

**Contraindications** In patients with uncontrolled asthma, known hypersensitivity to pilocarpine and when miosis is undesirable (eg, narrow-angle glaucoma)

**Warnings/Precautions** In patients with chronic obstructive pulmonary disease, pilocarpine may stimulate the mucous cells of the respiratory tract and may increase airway resistance. Patients with cardiovascular disease may be unable to compensate for changes in heart rhythm that could be induced by pilocarpine.

**Drug Interactions** Concurrent use with anticholinergics may cause antagonism of pilocarpine's cholinergic effect; medications with cholinergic actions may result in additive cholinergic effects; beta-adrenergic receptor blocking drugs when used with pilocarpine may increase the possibility of myocardial conduction disturbances

**Drug Uptake**

Onset of action after single dose: 20 minutes
Duration: 3-5 hours
Serum half-life: 0.76 hours
Time to peak serum concentration: 1.25 hours

**Pregnancy Risk Factor** C

**Breast-feeding Considerations** May be taken while breast-feeding

**Dosage Forms** Tablet: 5 mg

**Dietary Considerations** No data reported

**Generic Available** Yes: Hydrochloride Solution

**Comments** Pilocarpine may have potential as a salivary stimulant in individuals suffering from xerostomia induced by antidepressants and other medications. At the present time however, the FDA has not approved pilocarpine for use in drug-induced xerostomia. Clinical studies are needed to evaluate pilocarpine for this type of indication. In an attempt to discern the efficacy of pilocarpine as a salivary stimulant in patients suffering from Sjögren's syndrome (SS), Rhodus and Schuh studied 9 patients with SS given daily doses of pilocarpine over a 6-week period. A dose of 5 mg daily produced a significant overall increase in both whole unstimulated salivary flow and parotid stimulated salivary flow. These results support the use of pilocarpine to increase salivary flow in patients with SS.

**Selected Readings**

Davies AN and Singer J, "A Comparison of Artificial Saliva and Pilocarpine in Radiation-Induced Xerostomia," *J Laryngol Otol*, 1994, 108(8):663-5.

Fox PC, "Management of Dry Mouth," *Dent Clin North Am*, 1997, 41(4):863-75.

Fox PC, Atkinson JC, Macynski AA, et al, " Pilocarpine Treatment of Salivary Gland Hypofunction and Dry Mouth (Xerostomia)," *Arch Intern Med*, 1991, 151(6):1149-52.

Garg AK and Malo M, "Manifestations and Treatment of Xerostomia and Associated Oral Effects Secondary to Head and Neck Radiation Therapy," *J Am Dent Assoc*, 1997, 128(8):1128-33.

Greenspan D and Daniels TE, "The Use of Pilocarpine in Postradiation Xerostomia," *J Dent Res*, 1979, 58:420.

Johnson JT, Ferretti GA, Nethery WJ, et al, "Oral Pilocarpine for Post-Irradiation Xerostomia in Patients With Head and Neck Cancer," *N Engl J Med*, 1993, 329(6):390-5.

Nagler RM and Laufer D, "Protection Against Irradiation-Induced Damage to Salivary Glands by Adrenergic Agonist Administration," *Int J Radiat Oncol Biol Phys*, 1998, 40(2):477-81.

Nelson JD, Friedlaender M, Yeatts RP, et al, "Oral Pilocarpine for Symptomatic Relief of Keratoconjunctivitis Sicca in Patients With Sjögren's Syndrome. The MGI PHARMA Sjögren's Syndrome Study Group," *Adv Exp Med Biol*, 1998, 438:979-83.

Rhodus NL and Schuh MJ, "Effects of Pilocarpine on Salivary Flow in Patients With Sjögren's Syndrome," *Oral Surg Oral Med Oral Pathol*, 1991, 72:545-9.

Rieke JW, Hafermann MD, Johnson JT, et al, "Oral Pilocarpine for Radiation-Induced Xerostomia: Integrated Efficacy and Safety Results From Two Prospective Randomized Clinical Trials," *Int J Radiat Oncol Biol Phys*, 1995, 31(3):661-9.

Rousseau P, "Pilocarpine in Radiation-Induced Xerostomia," *Am J Hosp Palliat Care*, 1995, 12(2):38-9.

Schuller DE, Stevens P, Clausen KP, et al, "Treatment of Radiation Side Effects With Pilocarpine," *J Surg Oncol*, 1989, 42(4):272-6.

Singhal S, Mehta J, Rattenbury H, et al, "Oral Pilocarpine Hydrochloride for the Treatment of Refractory Xerostomia Associated With Chronic Graft-Versus-Host Disease," *Blood*, 1995, 85(4):1147-8.

Valdez IH, Wolff A, Atkinson JC, et al, "Use of Pilocarpine During Head and Neck Radiation Therapy to Reduce Xerostomia Salivary Dysfunction," *Cancer*, 1993, 71(5):1848-51.

Wiseman LR and Faulds D, "Oral Pilocarpine: A Review of Its Pharmacological Properties and Clinical Potential in Xerostomia," *Drugs*, 1995, 49(1):143-55.

Wynn RL, "Oral Pilocarpine (Salagen®) - A Recently Approved Salivary Stimulant," *Gen Dent*, 1996, 44(1):26,29-30.

Zimmerman RP, Mark RJ, Tran LM, et al, "Concomitant Pilocarpine During Head and Neck Irradiation Is Associated With Decreased Post-Treatment Xerostomia," *Int J Radiat Oncol Biol Phys*, 1997, 37(3):571-5.

♦ **Pilopine HS®** *see* Pilocarpine *on page 802*
♦ **Piloptic®** *see* Pilocarpine *on page 802*
♦ **Pilostat®** *see* Pilocarpine *on page 802*
♦ **Pima®** *see* Potassium Iodide *on page 824*

## Pimozide (PI moe zide)

**U.S. Brand Names** Orap™

**Therapeutic Category** Neuroleptic Agent

**Use** Suppression of severe motor and phonic tics in patients with Tourette's disorder

**Usual Dosage** Children >12 years and Adults: Oral: Initial: 1-2 mg/day, then increase dosage as needed every other day; range is usually 7-16 mg/day, maximum dose: 20 mg/day or 0.3 mg/kg/day should not be exceeded

**Mechanism of Action** A potent centrally acting dopamine receptor antagonist resulting in its characteristic neuroleptic effects

**Local Anesthetic/Vasoconstrictor Precautions** No information available to require special precautions

**Effects on Dental Treatment** >10% of patients experience dry mouth

**Other Adverse Effects**

>10%:
- Cardiovascular: Tachycardia, orthostatic hypotension
- Central nervous system: Akathisia, akinesia, extrapyramidal effects, drowsiness
- Dermatologic: Skin rash
- Endocrine & metabolic: Swelling of breasts
- Gastrointestinal: Constipation

1% to 10%:
- Cardiovascular: Swelling of face
- Central nervous system: Tardive dyskinesia, mental depression
- Gastrointestinal: Diarrhea, anorexia

<1%:
- Central nervous system: Neuroleptic malignant syndrome (NMS)
- Hematologic: Blood dyscrasias
- Hepatic: Jaundice

(Continued)

## Pimozide *(Continued)*

**Contraindications** Simple tics other than Tourette's, history of cardiac dysrhythmias, known hypersensitivity to pimozide; use in patients receiving macrolide antibiotics such as clarithromycin, erythromycin, azithromycin, and dirithromycin

**Drug Interactions** Increased effect/toxicity of alfentanil, CNS depressants, guanabenz (increased sedation), MAO inhibitors

**Drug Uptake**

Absorption: Oral: 50%
Serum half-life: 50 hours
Time to peak serum concentration: Within 6-8 hours

**Pregnancy Risk Factor** C

**Generic Available** No

**Selected Readings**

"Pimozide (Orap) Contraindicated With Clarithromycin (Biaxin™) and Other Macrolide Antibiotics," *FDA Medical Bulletin*, October 1996, 3.

## Pindolol (PIN doe lole)

**Related Information**

Cardiovascular Diseases *on page 1066*

**U.S. Brand Names** Visken®

**Canadian Brand Names** Apo®-Pindol; Gen-Pindolol; Novo-Pindol; Nu-Pindol; Syn-Pindol®

**Therapeutic Category** Beta-adrenergic Blocker, Noncardioselective

**Use** Management of hypertension

**Unlabeled use:** Ventricular arrhythmias/tachycardia, antipsychotic-induced akathisia, situational anxiety; aggressive behavior associated with dementia

**Usual Dosage**

Adults: Initial: 5 mg twice daily, increase as necessary by 10 mg/day every 3-4 weeks; maximum daily dose: 60 mg

Elderly: Initial: 5 mg once daily, increase as necessary by 5 mg/day every 3-4 weeks

**Mechanism of Action** Blocks both beta$_1$- and beta$_2$-receptors and has mild intrinsic sympathomimetic activity; pindolol has negative inotropic and chronotropic effects and can significantly slow A-V nodal conduction

**Local Anesthetic/Vasoconstrictor Precautions** Use with caution; epinephrine has interacted with nonselective beta-blockers to result in initial hypertensive episode followed by bradycardia

**Effects on Dental Treatment** Noncardioselective beta-blockers (ie, propranolol, nadolol, pindolol) enhance the pressor response to epinephrine, resulting in hypertension and bradycardia. Many nonsteroidal anti-inflammatory drugs such as ibuprofen and indomethacin can reduce the hypotensive effect of beta-blockers after 3 or more weeks of therapy with the NSAID. Short-term NSAID use (ie, 3 days) requires no special precautions in patients taking beta-blockers.

**Other Adverse Effects**

>10%:
- Central nervous system: Anxiety, dizziness, insomnia, fatigue
- Endocrine & metabolic: Decreased sexual ability
- Neuromuscular & skeletal: Arthralgia, back pain, weakness

1% to 10%:
- Cardiovascular: Congestive heart failure, arrhythmia, reduced peripheral circulation
- Central nervous system: Hallucinations, nightmares, vivid dreams
- Dermatologic: Skin rash, itching
- Gastrointestinal: Diarrhea, nausea, vomiting, stomach discomfort
- Neuromuscular & skeletal: Numbness of extremities
- Respiratory: Dyspnea

<1%:
- Cardiovascular: Bradycardia, chest pain
- Central nervous system: Confusion, mental depression
- Hematologic: Thrombocytopenia
- Ocular: Dry eyes

**Drug Interactions**

Decreased effect of beta-blockers:
- Barbiturates (increased liver metabolism of beta-blockers to result in lower serum levels)
- NSAIDs (attenuate the hypotensive therapeutic effects of beta-blockers)
- Rifampin (increased liver metabolism of beta-blockers to result in lower serum levels)

Increased effects of beta-blockers:
Calcium channel blockers (increase serum levels of beta-blockers by unknown mechanism to enhance hypotension)
Beta-Blockers increase the effects of:
Epinephrine (vasoconstrictor; initial hypertensive episode followed by bradycardia) only from noncardioselective type beta-blockers

**Drug Uptake**
Absorption: Oral: Rapid, 50% to 95%
Serum half-life: 2.5-4 hours; increased with renal insufficiency, age, and cirrhosis
Time to peak serum concentration: Within 1-2 hours

**Pregnancy Risk Factor** B

**Generic Available** Yes

**Selected Readings**

Foster CA and Aston SJ, "Propranolol-Epinephrine Interaction: A Potential Disaster," *Plast Reconstr Surg*, 1983, 72(1):74-8.
Wong DG, Spence JD, Lamki L, et al, "Effect of Nonsteroidal Anti-inflammatory Drugs on Control of Hypertension of Beta-Blockers and Diuretics," *Lancet*, 1986, 1(8488):997-1001.
Wynn RL, "Dental Nonsteroidal Anti-inflammatory Drugs and Prostaglandin-Based Drug Interactions, Part Two," *Gen Dent*, 1992, 40(2):104, 106, 108.
Wynn RL, "Epinephrine Interactions With Beta-Blockers," *Gen Dent*, 1994, 42(1):16, 18.

- **Pink Bismuth® (subsalicylate) [OTC]** *see* Bismuth *on page 142*
- **Pin-Rid® [OTC]** *see* Pyrantel Pamoate *on page 865*
- **Pin-X® [OTC]** *see* Pyrantel Pamoate *on page 865*

## Piperacillin (pi PER a sil in)

**U.S. Brand Names** Pipracil®

**Therapeutic Category** Antibiotic, Penicillin

**Use** Treatment of susceptible infections such as septicemia, acute and chronic respiratory tract infections, skin and soft tissue infections, and urinary tract infections due to susceptible strains of *Pseudomonas, Proteus*, and *Escherichia coli* and *Enterobacter*, normally used with other antibiotics (ie, aminoglycosides)

**Usual Dosage**
Children: I.M., I.V.: 200-300 mg/kg/day in divided doses every 4-6 hours; maximum dose: 24 g/day
Higher doses have been used in cystic fibrosis: 350-500 mg/kg/day in divided doses every 4 hours
Adults:
I.M.: 2-3 g/dose every 6-12 hours; maximum: 24 g/24 hours
I.V.: 3-4 g/dose every 4-6 hours; maximum: 24 g/24 hours

**Mechanism of Action** Inhibits bacterial cell wall synthesis by binding to one or more of the penicillin binding proteins (PBPs); which in turn inhibits the final transpeptidation step of peptidoglycan synthesis in bacterial cell walls, thus inhibiting cell wall biosynthesis. Bacteria eventually lyse due to ongoing activity of cell wall autolytic enzymes (autolysins and murein hydrolases) while cell wall assembly is arrested.

**Local Anesthetic/Vasoconstrictor Precautions** No information available to require special precautions

**Effects on Dental Treatment** Prolonged use of penicillins may lead to development of oral candidiasis

**Other Adverse Effects** <1%:
Central nervous system: Convulsions, confusion, drowsiness, fever
Dermatologic: Rash
Endocrine & metabolic: Electrolyte imbalance
Hematologic: Hemolytic anemia, positive Coombs' reaction, abnormal platelet aggregation and prolonged prothrombin time (high doses)
Local: Thrombophlebitis
Neuromuscular: Myoclonus
Renal: Acute interstitial nephritis
Miscellaneous: Hypersensitivity reactions, anaphylaxis, Jarisch-Herxheimer reaction

**Drug Interactions**
Decreased effect: Tetracyclines cause decreased penicillin effectiveness
Increased effect: Probenecid causes increased penicillin levels

**Drug Uptake**
Absorption: I.M.: 70% to 80%
Serum half-life: Dose-dependent; prolonged with moderately severe renal or hepatic impairment:
Adults: 36-80 minutes
Time to peak serum concentration: I.M.: Within 30-50 minutes

**Pregnancy Risk Factor** B

**Generic Available** No

## Piperacillin and Tazobactam Sodium

(pi PER a sil in & ta zoe BAK tam SOW dee um)

**U.S. Brand Names** Zosyn™

**Therapeutic Category** Antibiotic, Penicillin

**Use**

Treatment of infections of lower respiratory tract, urinary tract, skin and skin structures, gynecologic, bone and joint infections, and septicemia caused by susceptible organisms. Tazobactam expands activity of piperacillin to include beta-lactamase producing strains of *S. aureus*, *H. influenzae*, *Enterobacteriaceae*, *Pseudomonas*, *Klebsiella*, *Citrobacter*, *Serratia*, *Bacteroides*, and other gram-negative anaerobes.

Application to nosocomial infections may be limited by restricted activity against gram-negative organisms producing class I beta-lactamases and inactivity against methicillin-resistant *Staphylococcus aureus*

**Usual Dosage**

Children <12 years: Not recommended due to lack of data

Children >12 years and Adults:

Severe infections: I.V.: Piperacillin/tazobactam 4/0.5 g every 8 hours or 3/0.375 g every 6 hours

Moderate infections: I.M.: Piperacillin/tazobactam 2/0.25 g every 6-1 hours; treatment should be continued for ≥7-10 days depending on severity of disease

**Mechanism of Action** Piperacillin interferes with bacterial cell wall synthesis during active multiplication, causing cell wall death and resultant bactericidal activity against susceptible bacteria; tazobactam prevents degradation of piperacillin by binding to the active side on beta-lactamase; tazobactam inhibits many beta-lactamases, including staphylococcal penicillinase and Richmond and Sykes types II, III, IV, and V, including extended spectrum enzymes; it has only limited activity against class I beta-lactamases other than class Ic types

**Local Anesthetic/Vasoconstrictor Precautions** No information available to require special precautions

**Effects on Dental Treatment** Prolonged use of penicillins may lead to development of oral candidiasis

**Other Adverse Effects**

>10%: Gastrointestinal: Diarrhea

1% to 10%:

Central nervous system: Insomnia, headache

Dermatologic: Rash, pruritus

Gastrointestinal: Constipation, nausea, vomiting, dyspepsia

Hematologic: Leukopenia

Miscellaneous: Serum sickness-like reaction

<1%:

Cardiovascular: Hypertension, hypotension, edema

Central nervous system: Dizziness, agitation, confusion

Gastrointestinal: Pseudomembranous colitis

Respiratory: Bronchospasm

Several laboratory abnormalities have rarely been associated with piperacillin/tazobactam including reversible eosinophilia, and neutropenia (associated most often with prolonged therapy), positive direct Coombs' test, prolonged PT and PTT, transient elevations of LFT, elevated creatinine

**Drug Interactions**

Decreased effect: Tetracyclines cause decreased penicillin effectiveness

Increased effect: Probenecid causes increased penicillin levels

**Drug Uptake** Both AUC and peak concentrations are dose proportional

Serum half-life:

Piperacillin: 1 hour

Metabolite: 1-1.5 hours

Tazobactam: 0.7-0.9 hour

**Pregnancy Risk Factor** B

**Generic Available** No

## Piperazine (PI per a zeen)

**U.S. Brand Names** Vermizine®

**Therapeutic Category** Anthelmintic

**Use** Treatment of pinworm and roundworm infections (used as an alternative to first-line agents, mebendazole, or pyrantel pamoate)

**Usual Dosage** Oral:

Pinworms: Children and Adults: 65 mg/kg/day (not to exceed 2.5 g/day) as a single daily dose for 7 days; in severe infections, repeat course after a 1-week interval

Roundworms:
Children: 75 mg/kg/day as a single daily dose for 2 days; maximum: 3.5 g/day
Adults: 3.5 g/day for 2 days (in severe infections, repeat course, after a 1-week interval)

**Mechanism of Action** Causes muscle paralysis of the roundworm by blocking the effects of acetylcholine at the neuromuscular junction

**Local Anesthetic/Vasoconstrictor Precautions** No information available to require special precautions

**Effects on Dental Treatment** No effects or complications reported

**Other Adverse Effects** <1%:
Central nervous system: Dizziness, seizures, EEG changes, headache, vertigo
Gastrointestinal: Nausea, vomiting, diarrhea
Hematologic: Hemolytic anemia
Neuromuscular & skeletal: Weakness
Ocular: Visual impairment
Respiratory: Bronchospasms
Miscellaneous: Hypersensitivity reactions

**Drug Interactions** None reported

**Drug Uptake**
Absorption: Well absorbed from GI tract
Time to peak serum concentration: 1 hour

**Pregnancy Risk Factor** B

**Generic Available** Yes

## Pipobroman (pi poe BROE man)

**U.S. Brand Names** Vercyte®

**Therapeutic Category** Antineoplastic Agent, Alkylating Agent

**Use** Treat polycythemia vera; chronic myelocytic leukemia

**Usual Dosage** Children >15 years and Adults: Oral:
Polycythemia: 1 mg/kg/day for 30 days; may increase to 1.5-3 mg/kg until hematocrit reduced to 50% to 55%; maintenance: 0.1-0.2 mg/kg/day
Myelocytic leukemia: 1.5-2.5 mg/kg/day until WBC drops to 10,000/$mm^3$ then start maintenance 7-175 mg/day; stop if WBC falls to <3000/$mm^3$ or platelets fall to <150,000/$mm^3$

**Mechanism of Action** An alkylating agent considered to be cell-cycle nonspecific and capable of killing tumor cells in any phase of the cell cycle. Alkylating agents form covalent cross-links with DNA thereby resulting in cytotoxic, mutagenic, and carcinogenic effects. The end result of the alkylation process results in the misreading of the DNA code and the inhibition of DNA, RNA, and protein synthesis in rapidly proliferating tumor cells.

**Local Anesthetic/Vasoconstrictor Precautions** No information available to require special precautions

**Effects on Dental Treatment** No effects or complications reported

**Other Adverse Effects** 1% to 10%:
Dermatologic: Rash
Gastrointestinal: Vomiting, diarrhea, nausea, abdominal cramps
Hematologic: Leukopenia, thrombocytopenia, anemia

**Pregnancy Risk Factor** D

**Generic Available** No

♦ **Pipracil®** *see* Piperacillin *on page 807*

## Pirbuterol (peer BYOO ter ole)

**Related Information**
Respiratory Diseases *on page 1079*

**U.S. Brand Names** Maxair™

**Therapeutic Category** Antiasthmatic; $Beta_2$-Adrenergic Agonist Agent; Bronchodilator

**Use** Prevention and treatment of reversible bronchospasm including asthma

**Usual Dosage** Children >12 years and Adults: 2 inhalations every 4-6 hours for prevention; two inhalations at an interval of at least 1-3 minutes, followed by a third inhalation in treatment of bronchospasm, not to exceed 12 inhalations/day

**Mechanism of Action** Pirbuterol is a $beta_2$-adrenergic agonist with a similar structure to albuterol, specifically a pyridine ring has been substituted for the benzene ring in albuterol. The increased $beta_2$ selectivity of pirbuterol results from the substitution of a tertiary butyl group on the nitrogen of the side chain, which additionally imparts resistance of pirbuterol to degradation by monoamine oxidase and provides a lengthened duration of action in comparison to the less selective previous beta-agonist agents.

**Local Anesthetic/Vasoconstrictor Precautions** No information available to require special precautions

**Effects on Dental Treatment** No effects or complications reported

(Continued)

## Pirbuterol *(Continued)*

**Other Adverse Effects**

>10%:

Central nervous system: Nervousness, restlessness
Neuromuscular & skeletal: Trembling

1% to 10%:

Central nervous system: Headache, dizziness
Gastrointestinal: Taste changes, vomiting, nausea

<1%:

Cardiovascular: Hypertension, arrhythmias, chest pain
Central nervous system: Insomnia
Dermatologic: Bruising
Gastrointestinal: Anorexia
Neuromuscular & skeletal: Numbness in hands, weakness
Respiratory: Paradoxical bronchospasm

**Drug Interactions** Increased toxicity: Cardiovascular effects are potentiated in patients also receiving MAO inhibitors, tricyclic antidepressants, sympathomimetic agents (eg, amphetamine, dopamine, dobutamine), inhaled anesthetics (eg, enflurane)

**Drug Uptake**

Peak therapeutic effect:

Oral: 2-3 hours with peak serum concentration of 6.2-9.8 mcg/L
Inhalation: 0.5-1 hour

Serum half-life: 2-3 hours

**Pregnancy Risk Factor** C

**Generic Available** No

## Piroxicam (peer OKS i kam)

**Related Information**

Rheumatoid Arthritis and Osteoarthritis *on page 1092*

**U.S. Brand Names** Feldene®

**Canadian Brand Names** Apo®-Piroxicam; Novo-Piroxicam; Nu-Pirox; Pro-Piroxicam®

**Therapeutic Category** Analgesic, Non-narcotic; Anti-inflammatory Agent; Nonsteroidal Anti-inflammatory Drug (NSAID), Oral

**Use** Management of inflammatory disorders; symptomatic treatment of acute and chronic rheumatoid arthritis, osteoarthritis, and ankylosing spondylitis; also used to treat sunburn

**Usual Dosage** Oral:

Children: 0.2-0.3 mg/kg/day once daily; maximum dose: 15 mg/day
Adults: 10-20 mg/day once daily; although associated with increase in GI adverse effects, doses >20 mg/day have been used (ie, 30-40 mg/day)

**Mechanism of Action** Inhibits prostaglandin synthesis, acts on the hypothalamus heat-regulating center to reduce fever, blocks prostaglandin synthetase action which prevents formation of the platelet-aggregating substance thromboxane $A_2$; decreases pain receptor sensitivity. Other proposed mechanisms of action for salicylate anti-inflammatory action are lysosomal stabilization, kinin and leukotriene production, alteration of chemotactic factors, and inhibition of neutrophil activation. This latter mechanism may be the most significant pharmacologic action to reduce inflammation.

**Local Anesthetic/Vasoconstrictor Precautions** No information available to require special precautions

**Effects on Dental Treatment** NSAID formulations are known to reversibly decrease platelet aggregation via mechanisms different than observed with aspirin. The dentist should be aware of the potential of abnormal coagulation. Caution should also be exercised in the use of NSAIDs in patients already on anticoagulant therapy with drugs such as warfarin (Coumadin®).

**Other Adverse Effects**

>10%:

Central nervous system: Dizziness
Dermatologic: Skin rash
Gastrointestinal: Abdominal cramps, heartburn, indigestion, nausea

1% to 10%:

Central nervous system: Headache, nervousness
Dermatologic: Itching
Endocrine & metabolic: Fluid retention
Gastrointestinal: Vomiting
Otic: Tinnitus

<1%:

Cardiovascular: Congestive heart failure, hypertension, arrhythmias, tachycardia

Central nervous system: Confusion, hallucinations, aseptic meningitis, mental depression, drowsiness, insomnia
Dermatologic: Urticaria, erythema multiforme, toxic epidermal necrolysis, Stevens-Johnson syndrome, angioedema
Endocrine & metabolic: Polydipsia, hot flashes
Gastrointestinal: Gastritis, GI ulceration
Genitourinary: Cystitis
Hematologic: Agranulocytosis, anemia, hemolytic anemia, bone marrow suppression, leukopenia, thrombocytopenia
Hepatic: Hepatitis
Neuromuscular & skeletal: Peripheral neuropathy
Ocular: Toxic amblyopia, blurred vision, conjunctivitis, dry eyes
Otic: Decreased hearing
Renal: Polyuria, acute renal failure
Respiratory: Allergic rhinitis, dyspnea, epistaxis

**Drug Interactions**

Decreased effect of diuretics, beta-blockers; decreased effect with aspirin, antacids, cholestyramine
Increased effect/toxicity of lithium, warfarin, methotrexate (controversial)

**Drug Uptake**

Onset of analgesia: Oral: Within 1 hour
Serum half-life: 45-50 hours

**Pregnancy Risk Factor** B (D if used in the 3rd trimester or near delivery)

**Generic Available** Yes


- **Pitocin®** *see* Oxytocin *on page 759*
- **Pitressin®** *see* Vasopressin *on page 1042*
- **Pix Carbonis** *see* Coal Tar *on page 270*
- **Placidyl®** *see* Ethchlorvynol *on page 398*
- **Plaquenil®** *see* Hydroxychloroquine *on page 515*
- **Platinol®** *see* Cisplatin *on page 252*
- **Platinol®-AQ** *see* Cisplatin *on page 252*
- **Plavix®** *see* Clopidogrel *on page 266*
- **Plegine®** *see* Phendimetrazine *on page 788*
- **Plendil®** *see* Felodipine *on page 421*


## Plicamycin (plye kay MYE sin)

**U.S. Brand Names** Mithracin®

**Therapeutic Category** Antidote, Hypercalcemia; Antineoplastic Agent, Antibiotic

**Use** Malignant testicular tumors, in the treatment of hypercalcemia and hypercalciuria of malignancy not responsive to conventional treatment; Paget's disease

**Usual Dosage Refer to individual protocols.** Dose should be diluted in 1 L of $D_5W$ or NS and administered over 4-6 hours

**Dosage should be based on the patient's body weight. If a patient has abnormal fluid retention (ie, edema, hydrothorax or ascites), the patient's ideal weight rather than actual body weight should be used to calculate the dose.**

Adults: I.V.:
Testicular cancer: 25-30 mcg/kg/day for 8-10 days
Blastic chronic granulocytic leukemia: 25 mcg/kg over 2-4 hours every other day for 3 weeks
Paget's disease: 15 mcg/kg/day once daily for 10 days
Hypercalcemia:
25 mcg/kg single dose which may be repeated in 48 hours if no response occurs
**or** 25 mcg/kg for 3-4 days
**or** 25-50 mcg/kg every other day for 3-8 doses

**Mechanism of Action** Potent osteoclast inhibitor; may inhibit parathyroid hormone effect on osteoclasts; inhibits bone resorption; forms a complex with DNA in the presence of magnesium or other divalent cations inhibiting DNA-directed RNA synthesis

**Local Anesthetic/Vasoconstrictor Precautions** No information available to require special precautions

**Effects on Dental Treatment** No effects or complications reported

**Other Adverse Effects**

>10%: Gastrointestinal: Nausea and vomiting occur in almost 100% of patients within the first 6 hours after treatment; incidence increases with rapid injection; stomatitis has also occurred; anorexia, diarrhea
1% to 10%:
Cardiovascular: Facial flushing
(Continued)

## Plicamycin *(Continued)*

Central nervous system: Headache, fever, mental depression, drowsiness
Endocrine & metabolic: Hypocalcemia
Hematologic: Hemorrhagic diathesis, mild leukopenia and thrombocytopenia
Clotting disorders: May also depress hepatic synthesis of clotting factors, leading to a form of coagulopathy; petechiae, increased prothrombin time, epistaxis, and thrombocytopenia may be seen and may require discontinuation of the drug
Hepatic: Elevation in liver enzymes, hepatotoxicity
Local: Extravasation: Irritant; may produce local tissue irritation or cellulitis if infiltrated; if extravasation occurs, follow hospital procedure, discontinue I.V., and apply ice for 24 hours
Irritant chemotherapy
Neuromuscular & skeletal: Weakness
Renal: Nephrotoxicity, azotemia

**Drug Interactions** Increased toxicity: Calcitonin, etidronate, glucagon, causes additive hypoglycemic effects

**Drug Uptake**
Decreasing calcium levels:
Onset of action: Within 24 hours
Peak effect: 48-72 hours
Duration: 5-15 days
Serum half-life, plasma: 1 hour

**Pregnancy Risk Factor** D
**Generic Available** No

♦ **Pneumomist®** *see* Guaifenesin *on page 478*
♦ **Podocon-25™** *see* Podophyllum Resin *on this page*

## Podofilox (po do FIL oks)

**U.S. Brand Names** Condylox®
**Therapeutic Category** Keratolytic Agent
**Use** Treatment of external genital warts
**Usual Dosage** Adults: Apply twice daily (morning and evening) for 3 consecutive days, then withhold use for 4 consecutive days; this cycle may be repeated up to 4 times until there is no visible wart tissue
**Local Anesthetic/Vasoconstrictor Precautions** No information available to require special precautions
**Effects on Dental Treatment** No effects or complications reported
**Pregnancy Risk Factor** C
**Generic Available** No

♦ **Podofin®** *see* Podophyllum Resin *on this page*

## Podophyllin and Salicylic Acid (po DOF fil um & sal i SIL ik AS id)

**U.S. Brand Names** Verrex-C&M®
**Therapeutic Category** Keratolytic Agent
**Synonyms** Salicylic Acid and Podophyllin
**Use** Topical treatment of benign growths including external genital and perianal warts, papillomas, fibroids
**Usual Dosage** Apply daily with applicator, allow to dry; remove necrotic tissue before each application
**Local Anesthetic/Vasoconstrictor Precautions** No information available to require special precautions
**Effects on Dental Treatment** No effects or complications reported
**Generic Available** No

## Podophyllum Resin (po DOF fil um REZ in)

**U.S. Brand Names** Podocon-25™; Podofin®
**Canadian Brand Names** Podofilm®
**Therapeutic Category** Keratolytic Agent
**Use** Topical treatment of benign growths including external genital and perianal warts, papillomas, fibroids; compound benzoin tincture generally is used as the medium for topical application
**Usual Dosage** Topical:
Children and Adults: 10% to 25% solution in compound benzoin tincture; apply drug to dry surface, use 1 drop at a time allowing drying between drops until area is covered; total volume should be limited to <0.5 mL per treatment session

Condylomata acuminatum: 25% solution is applied daily; use a 10% solution when applied to or near mucous membranes

Verrucae: 25% solution is applied 3-5 times/day directly to the wart

**Mechanism of Action** Directly affects epithelial cell metabolism by arresting mitosis through binding to a protein subunit of spindle microtubules (tubulin)

**Local Anesthetic/Vasoconstrictor Precautions** No information available to require special precautions

**Effects on Dental Treatment** No effects or complications reported

**Other Adverse Effects** Local: Pain, swelling

1% to 10%:

Dermatologic: Pruritus

Gastrointestinal: Nausea, vomiting, abdominal pain, diarrhea

<1%:

Central nervous system: Confusion, lethargy, hallucinations

Hematologic: Leukopenia, thrombocytopenia

Hepatic: Hepatotoxicity

Neuromuscular & skeletal: Peripheral neuropathy

Renal: Renal failure

**Drug Interactions** No data reported

**Pregnancy Risk Factor** X

**Generic Available** Yes

♦ **Point-Two®** *see* Fluoride *on page 441*

♦ **Poladex®** *see* Dexchlorpheniramine *on page 309*

♦ **Polaramine®** *see* Dexchlorpheniramine *on page 309*

## Poliovirus Vaccine, Inactivated

(POE lee oh VYE rus vak SEEN, in ak ti VAY ted)

**U.S. Brand Names** IPOL™

**Therapeutic Category** Vaccine, Live Virus and Inactivated Virus

**Synonyms** Enhanced-potency Inactivated Poliovirus Vaccine; IPV; Salk Vaccine

**Use** Although a protective immune response to E-IPV cannot be assured in the immunocompromised individual, E-IPV is recommended because the vaccine is safe and some protection may result from its administration.

**Usual Dosage** Subcutaneous: **Enhanced-potency inactivated poliovirus vaccine (E-IPV) is preferred for primary vaccination of adults**, 2 doses S.C. 4-8 weeks apart, a third dose 6-12 months after the second. For adults with a completed primary series and for whom a booster is indicated, either OPV or E-IPV can be given. If immediate protection is needed, either OPV or E-IPV is recommended.

**Local Anesthetic/Vasoconstrictor Precautions** No information available to require special precautions

**Effects on Dental Treatment** No effects or complications reported

**Other Adverse Effects** All serious adverse reactions must be reported to the FDA

1% to 10%:

Central nervous system: Fever >101.3°F

Dermatologic: Skin rash

Local: Tenderness or pain at injection site

<1%:

Central nervous system: Fatigue, fussiness, sleepiness, crying, Guillain-Barré

Dermatologic: Reddening of skin, erythema

Gastrointestinal: Decreased appetite

Neuromuscular & skeletal: Weakness

Respiratory: Dyspnea

**Drug Interactions** Decreased effect with immunosuppressive agents, immune globulin, other live vaccines within 1 month; may temporarily suppress tuberculin skin test sensitivity (4-6 weeks)

**Pregnancy Risk Factor** C

**Generic Available** No

## Poliovirus Vaccine, Live, Trivalent, Oral

(POE lee oh VYE rus vak SEEN, live, try VAY lent, OR al)

**U.S. Brand Names** Orimune®

**Therapeutic Category** Vaccine, Live Virus

**Synonyms** OPV; Sabin Vaccine; TOPV

**Use** Poliovirus immunization

**Usual Dosage** Oral:

Infants: 0.5 mL dose at age 2 months, 4 months, and 18 months; optional dose may be given at 6 months in areas where poliomyelitis is endemic

Older Children, Adolescents, and Adults: Two 0.5 mL doses 8 weeks apart; third dose of 0.5 mL 6-12 months after second dose; a reinforcing dose of 0.5 mL should be given before entry to school, in children who received the third primary dose before their fourth birthday

(Continued)

## Poliovirus Vaccine, Live, Trivalent, Oral *(Continued)*

**Local Anesthetic/Vasoconstrictor Precautions** No information available to require special precautions

**Effects on Dental Treatment** No effects or complications reported

**Other Adverse Effects** All serious adverse reactions must be reported to the Vaccine Adverse Event Reporting System (1-800-822-7967)

**Pregnancy Risk Factor** C

**Generic Available** No

**Comments**

Oral vaccine: Live, attenuated vaccine

Federal law requires that the date of administration, the vaccine manufacturer, lot number of vaccine, and the administering person's name, title and address be entered into the patient's permanent medical record; live virus vaccine


- ♦ **Polocaine®** *see* Mepivacaine *on page 632*
- ♦ **Polocaine® 2%** *see* Mepivacaine and Levonordefrin *on page 632*
- ♦ **Polocaine® 3%** *see* Mepivacaine Dental Anesthetic *on page 634*
- ♦ **Polycillin-N®** *see* Ampicillin *on page 81*
- ♦ **Polycillin-PRB®** *see* Ampicillin and Probenecid *on page 82*
- ♦ **Polycitra®** *see* Sodium Citrate and Potassium Citrate Mixture *on page 922*
- ♦ **Polycitra®-K** *see* Potassium Citrate and Citric Acid *on page 823*
- ♦ **Polycose® [OTC]** *see* Glucose Polymers *on page 470*
- ♦ **Polycose® [OTC]** *see* Enteral Nutritional Products *on page 371*


## Polyestradiol (pol i es tra DYE ole)

**U.S. Brand Names** Estradurin®

**Therapeutic Category** Estrogen Derivative

**Use** Palliative treatment of advanced, inoperable carcinoma of the prostate

**Usual Dosage** Adults: Deep I.M.: 40 mg every 2-4 weeks or less frequently; maximum dose: 80 mg

**Mechanism of Action** Estrogens exert their primary effects on the interphase DNA-protein complex (chromatin) by binding to a receptor (usually located in the cytoplasm of a target cell) and initiating translocation of the hormone-receptor complex to the nucleus

**Local Anesthetic/Vasoconstrictor Precautions** No information available to require special precautions

**Effects on Dental Treatment** No effects or complications reported

**Other Adverse Effects**

>10%:

- Cardiovascular: Peripheral edema
- Endocrine & metabolic: Enlargement of breasts (female and male), breast tenderness
- Gastrointestinal: Nausea, anorexia, bloating

1% to 10%:

- Central nervous system: Headache
- Endocrine & metabolic: Increased libido (female), decrease libido (male)
- Gastrointestinal: Vomiting, diarrhea

<1%:

- Cardiovascular: Hypertension, thromboembolism, myocardial infarction, edema
- Central nervous system: Depression, dizziness, anxiety, stroke
- Dermatologic: Chloasma, melasma, rash
- Endocrine & metabolic: Breast tumors, amenorrhea, alterations in frequency and flow of menses, decreased glucose tolerance, elevated triglycerides and LDL
- Gastrointestinal: GI distress
- Hepatic: Cholestatic jaundice
- Ocular: Intolerance to contact lenses
- Miscellaneous: Increased susceptibility to *Candida* infection

**Drug Interactions** No data reported

**Drug Uptake**

90% of injected dose leaves blood stream within 24 hours

Passive storage in reticuloendothelial system

Increasing the dose prolongs duration of action

**Pregnancy Risk Factor** X

**Generic Available** No

## Polyethylene Glycol-Electrolyte Solution

(pol i ETH i leen GLY kol ee LEK troe lite soe LOO shun)

**U.S. Brand Names** Colovage®; CoLyte®; GoLYTELY®; NuLytely®; OCL®

**Canadian Brand Names** Klean-Prep®; Peglyte™

**Therapeutic Category** Laxative, Bowel Evacuant

**Synonyms** Electrolyte Lavage Solution

**Use** For bowel cleansing prior to GI examination

**Usual Dosage** The recommended dose for adults is 4 L of solution prior to gastrointestinal examination, as ingestion of this dose produces a satisfactory preparation in >95% of patients. Ideally the patient should fast for approximately 3-4 hours prior to administration, but in no case should solid food be given for at least 2 hours before the solution is given. The solution is usually administered orally, but may be given via nasogastric tube to patients who are unwilling or unable to drink the solution.

Children: Oral: 25-40 mL/kg/hour for 4-10 hours

Adults:

Oral: At a rate of 240 mL (8 oz) every 10 minutes, until 4 liters are consumed or the rectal effluent is clear; rapid drinking of each portion is preferred to drinking small amounts continuously

Nasogastric tube: At a rate of 20-30 mL/minute (1.2-1.8 L/hour); the first bowel movement should occur approximately 1 hour after the start of administration

**Mechanism of Action** Induces catharsis by strong electrolyte and osmotic effects

**Local Anesthetic/Vasoconstrictor Precautions** No information available to require special precautions

**Effects on Dental Treatment** No effects or complications reported

**Other Adverse Effects** GI side effect may be reduced by premedication with single doses of simethicone and metoclopramide, given 30 minutes to 1 hour prior to beginning prep

>10%: Gastrointestinal: Nausea, abdominal fullness, bloating

1% to 10%: Gastrointestinal: Abdominal cramps, vomiting, anal irritation

<1%: Dermatologic: Skin rash

**Drug Uptake** Onset of effect: Oral: Within 1-2 hours

**Pregnancy Risk Factor** C

**Generic Available** No

**Comments** Do not add flavorings as additional ingredients before use


- **Polygam®** *see* Immune Globulin, Intravenous *on page 531*
- **Polygam® S/D** *see* Immune Globulin, Intravenous *on page 531*
- **Poly-Histine CS®** *see* Brompheniramine, Phenylpropanolamine, and Codeine *on page 155*
- **Poly-Histine-D® Capsule** *see* Phenyltoloxamine, Phenylpropanolamine, Pyrilamine, and Pheniramine *on page 798*


## Polymyxin B (pol i MIKS in bee)

**Related Information**

Neomycin and Polymyxin B *on page 711*

Neomycin, Polymyxin B, and Dexamethasone *on page 711*

Neomycin, Polymyxin B, and Prednisolone *on page 713*

**U.S. Brand Names** Aerosporin®

**Therapeutic Category** Antibiotic, Ophthalmic; Antibiotic, Topical

**Use**

Topical: Wound irrigation and bladder irrigation against *Pseudomonas aeruginosa*; used occasionally for gut decontamination

Parenteral use of polymyxin B has mainly been replaced by less toxic antibiotics; it is reserved for life-threatening infections caused by organisms resistant to the preferred drugs.

**Usual Dosage**

Otic: 1-2 drops, 3-4 times/day; should be used sparingly to avoid accumulation of excess debris

Children ≥2 years and Adults:

I.M.: 25,000-30,000 units/kg/day divided every 4-6 hours

I.V.: 15,000-25,000 units/kg/day divided every 12 hours or by continuous infusion

Intrathecal: 50,000 units/day for 3-4 days, then every other day for at least 2 weeks

Total daily dose should not exceed 2,000,000 units/day

Bladder irrigation: Continuous irrigant or rinse in the urinary bladder for up to 10 days using 20 mg (equal to 200,000 units) added to 1 L of normal saline; usually no more than 1 L of irrigant is used per day unless urine flow rate is high; administration rate is adjusted to patient's urine output

(Continued)

## Polymyxin B *(Continued)*

Topical irrigation or topical solution: 500,000 units/L of normal saline; topical irrigation should not exceed 2 million units/day in adults

Gut sterilization: Oral: 15,000-25,000 units/kg/day in divided doses every 6 hours

*Clostridium difficile* enteritis: Oral: 25,000 units every 6 hours for 10 days

Ophthalmic: A concentration of 0.1% to 0.25% is administered as 1-3 drops every hour, then increasing the interval as response indicates to 1-2 drops 4-6 times/day

**Mechanism of Action** Binds to phospholipids, alters permeability, and damages the bacterial cytoplasmic membrane permitting leakage of intracellular constituents

**Local Anesthetic/Vasoconstrictor Precautions** No information available to require special precautions

**Effects on Dental Treatment** No effects or complications reported

**Other Adverse Effects** <1%:

Cardiovascular: Facial flushing

Central nervous system: Neurotoxicity, irritability, drowsiness, ataxia, drug fever

Dermatologic: Urticarial rash

Endocrine & metabolic: Hypocalcemia, hyponatremia, hypokalemia, hypochloremia

Neuromuscular & skeletal: Neuromuscular blockade, perioral paresthesia, weakness

Ocular: Blurring of vision

Renal: Nephrotoxicity

Respiratory: Respiratory arrest

Miscellaneous: Anaphylactoid reaction, meningeal irritation with intrathecal administration

**Drug Interactions** Increased/prolonged effect of neuromuscular blocking agents

**Drug Uptake**

Absorption: Well absorbed from the peritoneum; minimal absorption from the GI tract (except in neonates) from mucous membranes or intact skin

Serum half-life: 4.5-6 hours, increased with reduced renal function

Time to peak serum concentration: I.M.: Within 2 hours

**Pregnancy Risk Factor** B

**Generic Available** Yes

## Polymyxin B and Hydrocortisone

(pol i MIKS in bee & hye droe KOR ti sone)

**U.S. Brand Names** Otobiotic® Otic

**Therapeutic Category** Antibacterial, Otic; Corticosteroid, Otic

**Use** Treatment of superficial bacterial infections of external ear canal

**Usual Dosage** Instill 4 drops 3-4 times/day

**Local Anesthetic/Vasoconstrictor Precautions** No information available to require special precautions

**Effects on Dental Treatment** No effects or complications reported

**Pregnancy Risk Factor** C

**Generic Available** No

- **Polymyxin B and Oxytetracycline** *see* Oxytetracycline and Polymyxin B *on page 759*
- **Polymyxin B and Trimethoprim** *see* Trimethoprim and Polymyxin B *on page 1021*
- **Polymyxin E** *see* Colistin *on page 275*
- **Poly-Pred®** *see* Neomycin, Polymyxin B, and Prednisolone *on page 713*

## Polysaccharide-Iron Complex

(pol i SAK a ride-EYE ern KOM pleks)

**U.S. Brand Names** Hytinic® [OTC]; Niferex® [OTC]; Nu-Iron® [OTC]

**Therapeutic Category** Iron Salt

**Use** Prevention and treatment of iron deficiency anemias

**Usual Dosage** Oral:

Children: 3 mg/kg 3 times/day

Adults: 200 mg 3-4 times/day

**Local Anesthetic/Vasoconstrictor Precautions** No information available to require special precautions

**Effects on Dental Treatment** No effects or complications reported

**Other Adverse Effects**

>10%: Gastrointestinal: Stomach cramping, constipation, nausea, vomiting, dark stools, GI irritation, epigastric pain, nausea

1% to 10%:
Gastrointestinal: Heartburn, diarrhea
Genitourinary: Discolored urine
Miscellaneous: Staining of teeth
<1%: Dermatologic: Contact irritation

**Pregnancy Risk Factor** A
**Generic Available** Yes
**Comments** 100% elemental iron

- **Polysporin® Ophthalmic** *see* Bacitracin and Polymyxin B *on page 117*
- **Polysporin® Topical** *see* Bacitracin and Polymyxin B *on page 117*
- **Polytar® [OTC]** *see* Coal Tar *on page 270*

## Polythiazide (pol i THYE a zide)

**Related Information**
Cardiovascular Diseases *on page 1066*

**U.S. Brand Names** Renese®
**Therapeutic Category** Diuretic, Thiazide
**Use** Adjunctive therapy in treatment of edema and hypertension
**Usual Dosage** Adults: Oral: 1-4 mg/day
**Mechanism of Action** The diuretic mechanism of action of the thiazides is primarily inhibition of sodium, chloride, and water reabsorption in the renal distal tubules, thereby producing diuresis with a resultant reduction in plasma volume. The antihypertensive mechanism of action of the thiazides is unknown. It is known that doses of thiazides produce greater reductions in blood pressure than equivalent diuretic doses of loop diuretics (eg, furosemide). There has been speculation that the thiazides may have some influence on vascular tone mediated through sodium depletion, but this remains to be proven.
**Local Anesthetic/Vasoconstrictor Precautions** No information available to require special precautions
**Effects on Dental Treatment** No effects or complications reported
**Other Adverse Effects**
1% to 10%: Endocrine & metabolic: Hypokalemia
<1%:
Cardiovascular: Hypotension
Central nervous system: Drowsiness
Dermatologic: Photosensitivity, rash
Endocrine & metabolic: Fluid and electrolyte imbalances (hypocalcemia, hypomagnesemia, hyponatremia), hyperglycemia
Gastrointestinal: Nausea, vomiting, anorexia
Hematologic: Rarely blood dyscrasias
Hepatic: Hepatitis
Renal: Prerenal azotemia, polyuria, uremia

**Drug Interactions** Increased toxicity/levels of lithium
**Drug Uptake**
Onset of diuretic effect: Within ~2 hours
Duration: 24-48 hours

**Pregnancy Risk Factor** D
**Generic Available** No

- **Polytrim® Ophthalmic** *see* Trimethoprim and Polymyxin B *on page 1021*
- **Poly-Vi-Flor®** *see* Vitamins, Multiple *on page 1051*
- **Polyvinyl Alcohol** *see* Artificial Tears *on page 97*
- **Poly-Vi-Sol® [OTC]** *see* Vitamins, Multiple *on page 1051*
- **Ponstel®** *see* Mefenamic Acid *on page 624*
- **Pontocaine®** *see* Tetracaine *on page 964*
- **Pontocaine® With Dextrose Injection** *see* Tetracaine and Dextrose *on page 964*
- **Porcelana® [OTC]** *see* Hydroquinone *on page 514*
- **Porcelana® Sunscreen [OTC]** *see* Hydroquinone *on page 514*

## Porfimer (POR fi mer)

**U.S. Brand Names** Photofrin®
**Therapeutic Category** Antineoplastic Agent, Miscellaneous
**Synonyms** Porfimer Sodium
**Use** Esophageal cancer: Photodynamic therapy (PDT) with porfimer for palliation of patients with completely obstructing esophageal cancer, or of patients with partially obstructing esophageal cancer who cannot be satisfactorily treated with Nd:YAG laser therapy

Photodynamic therapy for reduction of obstruction and palliation of symptoms in patients with completely or partially obstructing endobronchial nonsmall cell lung cancer (NSCLC)

(Continued)

## Porfimer *(Continued)*

**Usual Dosage** I.V. (refer to individual protocols):

Children: Safety and efficacy have not been established

Adults: I.V.: 2 mg/kg over 3-5 minutes

Photodynamic therapy is a two-stage process requiring administration of both drug and light. The first stage of PDT is the I.V. injection of porfimer. Illumination with laser light 40-50 hours following the injection with porfimer constitutes the second stage of therapy. A second laser light application may be given 90-120 hours after injection, preceded by gentle debridement of residual tumor.

Patients may receive a second course of PDT a minimum of 30 days after the initial therapy; up to three courses of PDT (each separated by a minimum of 30 days) can be given. Before each course of treatment, evaluate patients for the presence of a tracheoesophageal or bronchoesophageal fistula.

**Mechanism of Action** Photosensitizing agent used in the photodynamic therapy (PDT) of tumors: cytotoxic and antitumor actions of porfimer are light and oxygen dependent. Cellular damage caused by porfimer PDT is a consequence of the propagation of radical reactions.

**Local Anesthetic/Vasoconstrictor Precautions** No information available to require special precautions

**Effects on Dental Treatment** No effects or complications reported

**Other Adverse Effects**

>10%:

Cardiovascular: Atrial fibrillation, chest pain

Central nervous system: Fever, pain, insomnia

Dermatologic: Photosensitivity reaction

Gastrointestinal: abdominal pain, constipation, dysphagia, nausea, vomiting

Hematologic: Anemia

Neuromuscular & skeletal: Back pain

Respiratory: Dyspnea, pharyngitis, pleural effusion, pneumonia, respiratory insufficiency

1% to 10%:

Cardiovascular: Hypertension, hypotension, edema, cardiac failure, tachycardia, chest pain (substernal)

Central nervous system: Anxiety, confusion

Endocrine & metabolic: Dehydration

Gastrointestinal: Diarrhea, dyspepsia, eructation, esophageal edema, esophageal tumor bleeding, esophageal stricture, esophagitis, hematemesis, melena, weight loss, anorexia

Genitourinary: Urinary tract infection

Neuromuscular & skeletal: Weakness

Respiratory: Coughing, tracheoesophageal fistula

Miscellaneous: Moniliasis, surgical complication

**Warnings/Precautions** The U.S. Food and Drug Administration (FDA) currently recommends that procedures for proper handling and disposal of antineoplastic agents be considered. If the esophageal tumor is eroding into the trachea or bronchial tree, the likelihood of tracheoesophageal or bronchoesophageal fistula resulting from treatment is sufficiently high that PDT is not recommended. All patients who receive porfimer sodium will be photosensitive and must observe precautions to avoid exposure of skin and eyes to direct sunlight or bright indoor light for 30 days. The photosensitivity is due to residual drug which will be present in all parts of the skin. Exposure of the skin to ambient indoor light is, however, beneficial because the remaining drug will be inactivated gradually and safely through a photobleaching reaction. Patients should not stay in a darkened room during this period and should be encouraged to expose their skin to ambient indoor light. Ocular discomfort has been reported; for 30 days, when outdoors, patients should wear dark sunglasses which have an average white light transmittance of <4%.

**Drug Interactions**

Decreased effect: Compounds that quench active oxygen species or scavenge radicals (eg, dimethyl sulfoxide, beta-carotene, ethanol, mannitol) would be expected to decrease PDT activity; allopurinol, calcium channel blockers and some prostaglandin synthesis inhibitors could interfere with porfimer; drugs that decrease clotting, vasoconstriction or platelet aggregation could decrease the efficacy of PDT; glucocorticoid hormones may decrease the efficacy of the treatment

Increased toxicity: Concomitant administration of other photosensitizing agents (eg, tetracyclines, sulfonamides, phenothiazines, sulfonylureas, thiazide diuretics, griseofulvin) could increase the photosensitivity reaction

**Drug Uptake**

Serum half-life: 250 hours

Time to peak serum concentration: Within 2 hours

**Pregnancy Risk Factor** C

**Generic Available** No

- ♦ **Porfimer Sodium** *see* Porfimer *on page 817*
- ♦ **Pork NPH Iletin® II** *see* Insulin Preparations *on page 537*
- ♦ **Pork Regular Iletin® II** *see* Insulin Preparations *on page 537*
- ♦ **Portagen® [OTC]** *see* Enteral Nutritional Products *on page 371*
- ♦ **Porton Asparaginase** *see* Erwinia Asparaginase *on page 382*
- ♦ **Posicor®** *see* Mibefradil ***Withdrawn from Market 6/8/98*** *on page 671*
- ♦ **Posture® [OTC]** *see* Calcium Phosphate, Tribasic *on page 177*
- ♦ **Potasalan®** *see* Potassium Chloride *on page 822*

## Potassium Acetate (poe TASS ee um AS e tate)

**Therapeutic Category** Electrolyte Supplement, Parenteral; Potassium Salt

**Use** Potassium deficiency; to avoid chloride when high concentration of potassium is needed, source of bicarbonate

**Usual Dosage** I.V. doses should be incorporated into the patient's maintenance I.V. fluids, intermittent I.V. potassium administration should be reserved for severe depletion situations and requires EKG monitoring; doses listed as mEq of potassium

Treatment of hypokalemia: I.V.:
- Children: 2-5 mEq/kg/day
- Adults: 40-100 mEq/day

I.V. intermittent infusion (must be diluted prior to administration):
- Children: 0.5-1 mEq/kg/dose (maximum: 30 mEq) to infuse at 0.3-0.5 mEq/kg/hour (maximum: 1 mEq/kg/hour)
- Adults: 10-20 mEq/dose (maximum: 40 mEq/dose) to infuse over 2-3 hours (maximum: 40 mEq over 1 hour)

**Mechanism of Action** Potassium is the major cation of intracellular fluid and is essential for the conduction of nerve impulses in heart, brain, and skeletal muscle; contraction of cardiac, skeletal and smooth muscles; maintenance of normal renal function, acid-base balance, carbohydrate metabolism, and gastric secretion

**Local Anesthetic/Vasoconstrictor Precautions** No information available to require special precautions

**Effects on Dental Treatment** No effects or complications reported

**Other Adverse Effects**

>10%: Gastrointestinal: Diarrhea, nausea, stomach pain, flatulence, vomiting (oral)

1% to 10%:
- Cardiovascular: Bradycardia
- Endocrine & metabolic: Hyperkalemia
- Local: Local tissue necrosis with extravasation
- Neuromuscular & skeletal: Weakness
- Respiratory: Dyspnea

<1%:
- Cardiovascular: Chest pain
- Central nervous system: Mental confusion
- Endocrine & metabolic: Alkalosis
- Gastrointestinal: Abdominal pain, throat pain
- Local: Phlebitis
- Neuromuscular & skeletal: Paresthesias, paralysis

**Drug Interactions** Increased effect/levels with potassium-sparing diuretics, salt substitutes, ACE inhibitors

**Drug Uptake**

Absorption: Absorbed well from upper GI tract

**Pregnancy Risk Factor** C

**Generic Available** Yes

## Potassium Acetate, Potassium Bicarbonate, and Potassium Citrate

(poe TASS ee um AS e tate, poe TASS ee um bye KAR bun ate, & poe TASS ee um SIT rate)

**U.S. Brand Names** Tri-K®

**Therapeutic Category** Electrolyte Supplement, Oral; Potassium Salt

**Use** Treatment or prevention of hypokalemia

**Usual Dosage** Oral:

Children: 1-4 mEq/kg/24 hours in divided doses as required to maintain normal serum potassium

(Continued)

## Potassium Acetate, Potassium Bicarbonate, and Potassium Citrate *(Continued)*

Adults:
- Prevention: 16-24 mEq/day in 2-4 divided doses
- Treatment: 40-100 mEq/day in 2-4 divided doses

**Local Anesthetic/Vasoconstrictor Precautions** No information available to require special precautions

**Effects on Dental Treatment** No effects or complications reported

**Pregnancy Risk Factor** C

**Generic Available** Yes

## Potassium Acid Phosphate (poe TASS ee um AS id FOS fate)

**U.S. Brand Names** K-Phos® Original

**Therapeutic Category** Electrolyte Supplement, Oral; Potassium Salt; Urinary Acidifying Agent

**Use** Acidifies urine and lowers urinary calcium concentration; reduces odor and rash caused by ammoniacal urine; increases the antibacterial activity of methenamine

**Usual Dosage** Adults: Oral: 1000 mg dissolved in 6-8 oz of water 4 times/day with meals and at bedtime; for best results, soak tablets in water for 2-5 minutes, then stir and swallow

**Mechanism of Action** The principal intracellular cation; involved in transmission of nerve impulses, muscle contractions, enzyme activity, and glucose utilization

**Local Anesthetic/Vasoconstrictor Precautions** No information available to require special precautions

**Effects on Dental Treatment** No effects or complications reported

**Other Adverse Effects**

>10%: Gastrointestinal: Diarrhea, nausea, stomach pain, flatulence, vomiting

1% to 10%:
- Cardiovascular: Bradycardia
- Endocrine & metabolic: Hyperkalemia
- Local: Local tissue necrosis with extravasation
- Neuromuscular & skeletal: Weakness
- Respiratory: Dyspnea

<1%:
- Cardiovascular: Chest pain, arrhythmia, edema
- Central nervous system: Mental confusion, tetany
- Endocrine & metabolic: Hyperphosphatemia, hypocalcemia, alkalosis
- Gastrointestinal: Abdominal pain, weight gain, thirst, throat pain
- Genitourinary: Decreased urine output
- Local: Phlebitis
- Neuromuscular & skeletal: Paresthesias, paralysis, bone pain, arthralgia, pain/weakness of extremities

**Drug Interactions**

Increased effect/levels with potassium-sparing diuretics, salt substitutes, salicylates, ACE inhibitors

**Drug Uptake** Absorption: Absorbed well from upper GI tract

**Pregnancy Risk Factor** C

**Generic Available** No

## Potassium Bicarbonate (poe TASS ee um bye KAR bun ate)

**U.S. Brand Names** K+ Care® Effervescent; K-Electrolyte® Effervescent; K-Gen® Effervescent; K-Lyte® Effervescent

**Therapeutic Category** Electrolyte Supplement, Oral; Potassium Salt

**Use** Potassium deficiency, hypokalemia

**Usual Dosage**

Children: 1-4 mEq/kg/day

Adults: 25 mEq 2-4 times/day

**Local Anesthetic/Vasoconstrictor Precautions** No information available to require special precautions

**Effects on Dental Treatment** No effects or complications reported

**Pregnancy Risk Factor** C

**Generic Available** No

## Potassium Bicarbonate and Potassium Chloride, Effervescent

(poe TASS ee um bye KAR bun ate & poe TASS ee um KLOR ide, ef er VES ent)

**U.S. Brand Names** Klorvess® Effervescent; K/Lyte/CL®

**Therapeutic Category** Electrolyte Supplement, Oral; Potassium Salt

**Use** Treatment or prevention of hypokalemia

**Usual Dosage** Oral:

Children: 1-4 mEq/kg/24 hours in divided doses as required to maintain normal serum potassium

Adults:

Prevention: 16-24 mEq/day in 2-4 divided doses

Treatment: 40-100 mEq/day in 2-4 divided doses

**Local Anesthetic/Vasoconstrictor Precautions** No information available to require special precautions

**Effects on Dental Treatment** No effects or complications reported

**Pregnancy Risk Factor** C

**Generic Available** Yes

## Potassium Bicarbonate and Potassium Citrate, Effervescent

(poe TASS ee um bye KAR bun ate & poe TASS ee um SIT rate, ef er VES ent)

**U.S. Brand Names** Effer-K™; K-Ide®; Klor-Con®/EF; K-Lyte®; K-Vescent®

**Therapeutic Category** Electrolyte Supplement, Oral; Potassium Salt

**Use** Treatment or prevention of hypokalemia

**Usual Dosage** Oral:

Children: 1-4 mEq/kg/24 hours in divided doses as required to maintain normal serum potassium

Adults:

Prevention: 16-24 mEq/day in 2-4 divided doses

Treatment: 40-100 mEq/day in 2-4 divided doses

**Mechanism of Action** Needed for the conduction of nerve impulses in heart, brain, and skeletal muscle; contraction of cardiac, skeletal and smooth muscles; maintenance of normal renal function

**Local Anesthetic/Vasoconstrictor Precautions** No information available to require special precautions

**Effects on Dental Treatment** No effects or complications reported

**Other Adverse Effects**

>10%: Gastrointestinal: Diarrhea, nausea, stomach pain, flatulence, vomiting

1% to 10%:

Cardiovascular: Bradycardia

Endocrine & metabolic: Hyperkalemia

Local: Local tissue necrosis with extravasation

Neuromuscular & skeletal: Weakness

Respiratory: Dyspnea

<1%:

Cardiovascular: Chest pain

Central nervous system: Mental confusion

Endocrine & metabolic: Alkalosis

Gastrointestinal: Abdominal pain, throat pain

Local: Phlebitis

Neuromuscular & skeletal: Paresthesias, paralysis

**Drug Interactions** Increased effect/levels with potassium-sparing diuretics, salt substitutes, ACE inhibitors

**Drug Uptake** Absorption: Absorbed well from upper GI tract

**Pregnancy Risk Factor** C

**Generic Available** No

## Potassium Bicarbonate, Potassium Chloride, and Potassium Citrate

(poe TASS ee um bye KAR bun ate, poe TASS ee um KLOR ide & poe TASS ee um SIT rate)

**U.S. Brand Names** Kaochlor-Eff®

**Therapeutic Category** Electrolyte Supplement, Oral; Potassium Salt

**Use** Treatment or prevention of hypokalemia

**Usual Dosage** Oral:

Children: 1-4 mEq/kg/24 hours in divided doses as required to maintain normal serum potassium

Adults:

Prevention: 16-24 mEq/day in 2-4 divided doses

Treatment: 40-100 mEq/day in 2-4 divided doses

**Local Anesthetic/Vasoconstrictor Precautions** No information available to require special precautions

**Effects on Dental Treatment** No effects or complications reported

**Pregnancy Risk Factor** C

(Continued)

## Potassium Bicarbonate, Potassium Chloride, and Potassium Citrate *(Continued)*

**Generic Available** Yes

## Potassium Chloride (poe TASS ee um KLOR ide)

**U.S. Brand Names** Cena-K®; Gen-K®; K+ 10®; Kaochlor®; Kaochlor® SF; Kaon-Cl®; Kaon-Cl-10®; Kay Ciel®; K+ Care®; K-Dur® 10; K-Dur® 20; K-Lease®; K-Lor™; Klor-Con®; Klor-Con® 8; Klor-Con® 10; Klor-Con/25®; Klor-Con M20®; Klor-vess®; Klotrix®; K-Lyte®/Cl; K-Norm®; K-Tab®; Micro-K® 10; Micro-K® Extencaps®; Micro-K® LS; Potasalan®; Rum-K®; Slow-K®; Ten-K®

**Therapeutic Category** Electrolyte Supplement, Oral; Electrolyte Supplement, Parenteral; Potassium Salt

**Use** Treatment or prevention of hypokalemia

**Usual Dosage** I.V. doses should be incorporated into the patient's maintenance I.V. fluids; intermittent I.V. potassium administration should be reserved for severe depletion situations in patients undergoing EKG monitoring.

Normal daily requirements: Oral, I.V.:
- Children: 2-3 mEq/kg/day
- Adults: 40-80 mEq/day

Prevention during diuretic therapy: Oral:
- Children: 1-2 mEq/kg/day in 1-2 divided doses
- Adults: 20-40 mEq/day in 1-2 divided doses

Treatment of hypokalemia: Children:
- Oral: 1-2 mEq/kg initially, then as needed based on frequently obtained lab values. If deficits are severe or ongoing losses are great, I.V. route should be considered.
- I.V.: 1 mEq/kg over 1-2 hours initially, then repeated as needed based on frequently obtained lab values; severe depletion or ongoing losses may require >200% of normal limit needs
- I.V. intermittent infusion: Dose should not exceed 1 mEq/kg/hour, or 40 mEq/hour; if it exceeds 0.5 mEq/kg/hour, physician should be at bedside and patient should have continuous EKG monitoring

Treatment of hypokalemia: Adults:
- I.V. intermittent infusion: 10-20 mEq/hour, not to exceed 40 mEq/hour and 150 mEq/day. See table.

**Potassium Dosage/Rate of Infusion Guidelines**

| Serum Potassium* | Maximum Infusion Rate | Maximum Concentration | Maximum 24-Hour Dose |
|---|---|---|---|
| >2.5 mEq/L | 10 mEq/h | 40 mEq/L | 200 mEq |
| <2.5 mEq/L | 40 mEq/h | 80 mEq/L | 400 mEq |

Potassium >2.5 mEq/L:
- Oral: 60-80 mEq/day plus additional amounts if needed
- I.V.: 10 mEq over 1 hour with additional doses if needed

Potassium <2.5 mEq/L:
- Oral: Up to 40-60 mEq initial dose, followed by further doses based on lab values; deficits at a plasma level of 2 mEq/L may be as high as 400-800 mEq of potassium
- I.V.: Up to 40 mEq over 1 hour, with doses based on frequent lab monitoring; deficits at a plasma level of 2 mEq/L may be as high as 400-800 mEq of potassium

**Mechanism of Action** Potassium is the major cation of intracellular fluid and is essential for the conduction of nerve impulses in heart, brain, and skeletal muscle; contraction of cardiac, skeletal and smooth muscles; maintenance of normal renal function, acid-base balance, carbohydrate metabolism, and gastric secretion

**Local Anesthetic/Vasoconstrictor Precautions** No information available to require special precautions

**Effects on Dental Treatment** No effects or complications reported

**Other Adverse Effects**

>10%: Gastrointestinal: Diarrhea, nausea, stomach pain, flatulence, vomiting (oral)

1% to 10%:
- Cardiovascular: Bradycardia
- Endocrine & metabolic: Hyperkalemia
- Local: Local tissue necrosis with extravasation, pain at the site of injection
- Neuromuscular & skeletal: Weakness

Respiratory: Dyspnea
<1%:
Cardiovascular: Chest pain, arrhythmias, heart block, hypotension
Central nervous system: Mental confusion
Endocrine & metabolic: Alkalosis
Gastrointestinal: Abdominal pain, throat pain
Local: Phlebitis
Neuromuscular & skeletal: Paresthesias, paralysis

**Drug Interactions** No data reported
**Drug Uptake** Absorption: Absorbed well from upper GI tract
**Pregnancy Risk Factor** A
**Generic Available** Yes

## Potassium Chloride and Potassium Gluconate

(poe TASS ee um KLOR ide & poe TASS ee um GLOO coe nate)

**U.S. Brand Names** Kolyum®
**Therapeutic Category** Electrolyte Supplement, Oral; Potassium Salt
**Use** Treatment or prevention of hypokalemia
**Usual Dosage** Oral:
Children: 1-4 mEq/kg/24 hours in divided doses as required to maintain normal serum potassium
Adults:
Prevention: 16-24 mEq/day in 2-4 divided doses
Treatment: 40-100 mEq/day in 2-4 divided doses
**Local Anesthetic/Vasoconstrictor Precautions** No information available to require special precautions
**Effects on Dental Treatment** No effects or complications reported
**Generic Available** Yes

## Potassium Citrate (poe TASS ee um SIT rate)

**U.S. Brand Names** Urocit®-K
**Canadian Brand Names** K-Lyte®
**Therapeutic Category** Alkalinizing Agent, Oral
**Use** Prevention of uric acid nephrolithiasis; prevention of calcium renal stones in patients with hypocitraturia; urinary alkalinizer when sodium citrate is contraindicated
**Usual Dosage** Adults: Oral: 10-20 mEq 3 times/day with meals up to 100 mEq/day
**Local Anesthetic/Vasoconstrictor Precautions** No information available to require special precautions
**Effects on Dental Treatment** No effects or complications reported
**Pregnancy Risk Factor** A
**Generic Available** Yes
**Comments** Parenteral $K_3PO_4$ contains 3 mmol of phosphorous/mL and 4.4 mEq of potassium/mL. If ordering by phosphorous content, use mmol instead of mEq since the mEq value for phosphorous varies with the pH of the solution due to valence changes of the phosphorus ion. (1 mmol of phosphorous = 31 mg)

## Potassium Citrate and Citric Acid

(poe TASS ee um SIT rate & SI trik AS id)

**U.S. Brand Names** Polycitra®-K
**Therapeutic Category** Electrolyte Supplement, Oral; Potassium Salt
**Use** Treatment of metabolic acidosis; alkalinizing agent in conditions where long-term maintenance of an alkaline urine is desirable
**Usual Dosage** Oral:
Mild to moderate hypocitraturia: 10 mEq 3 times/day with meals
Severe hypocitraturia: Initial: 20 mEq 3 times/day or 15 mEq 4 times/day with meals or within 30 minutes after meals; do not exceed 100 mEq/day
**Local Anesthetic/Vasoconstrictor Precautions** No information available to require special precautions
**Effects on Dental Treatment** No effects or complications reported
**Pregnancy Risk Factor** C
**Generic Available** No
**Comments** Potassium citrate 3.4 mmol/5 mL and citric acid 1.6 mmol/5 mL = total of 5.0 mmol/5 mL citrate content

## Potassium Citrate and Potassium Gluconate

(poe TASS ee um SIT rate & poe TASS ee um GLOO coe nate)

**U.S. Brand Names** Twin-K®
**Therapeutic Category** Electrolyte Supplement, Oral; Potassium Salt

(Continued)

## Potassium Citrate and Potassium Gluconate *(Continued)*

**Use** Treatment or prevention of hypokalemia

**Usual Dosage** Oral:

Children: 1-4 mEq/kg/24 hours in divided doses as required to maintain normal serum potassium

Adults:

Prevention: 16-24 mEq/day in 2-4 divided doses

Treatment: 40-100 mEq/day in 2-4 divided doses

**Local Anesthetic/Vasoconstrictor Precautions** No information available to require special precautions

**Effects on Dental Treatment** No effects or complications reported

**Pregnancy Risk Factor** C

**Generic Available** Yes

## Potassium Gluconate (poe TASS ee um GLOO coe nate)

**U.S. Brand Names** Kaon®; K-G®

**Therapeutic Category** Electrolyte Supplement, Oral; Potassium Salt

**Use** Treatment or prevention of hypokalemia

**Usual Dosage** Oral (doses listed as mEq of potassium):

Normal daily requirement:

Children: 2-3 mEq/kg/day

Adults: 40-80 mEq/day

Prevention of hypokalemia during diuretic therapy:

Children: 1-2 mEq/kg/day in 1-2 divided doses

Adults: 16-24 mEq/day in 1-2 divided doses

Treatment of hypokalemia:

Children: 2-5 mEq/kg/day in 2-4 divided doses

Adults: 40-100 mEq/day in 2-4 divided doses

**Mechanism of Action** Potassium is the major cation of intracellular fluid and is essential for the conduction of nerve impulses in heart, brain, and skeletal muscle; contraction of cardiac, skeletal and smooth muscles; maintenance of normal renal function, acid-base balance, carbohydrate metabolism, and gastric secretion

**Local Anesthetic/Vasoconstrictor Precautions** No information available to require special precautions

**Effects on Dental Treatment** No effects or complications reported

**Other Adverse Effects**

>10%: Gastrointestinal: Diarrhea, nausea, stomach pain, flatulence, vomiting (oral)

1% to 10%:

Cardiovascular: Bradycardia

Endocrine & metabolic: Hyperkalemia

Neuromuscular & skeletal: Weakness

Respiratory: Dyspnea

<1%:

Cardiovascular: Chest pain

Central nervous system: Mental confusion

Endocrine & metabolic: Alkalosis

Gastrointestinal: Throat pain

Local: Phlebitis

Neuromuscular & skeletal: Paresthesias, paralysis

**Drug Interactions**

Increased effect/levels with potassium-sparing diuretics, salt substitutes, ACE inhibitors

Increased effect of digitalis

**Drug Uptake** Absorption: Absorbed well from upper GI tract

**Pregnancy Risk Factor** A

**Generic Available** Yes

## Potassium Iodide (poe TASS ee um EYE oh dide)

**Related Information**

Endocrine Disorders & Pregnancy *on page 1082*

**U.S. Brand Names** Pima®; SSKI®; Thyro-Block®

**Therapeutic Category** Antithyroid Agent; Expectorant

**Use** Facilitate bronchial drainage and cough; reduce thyroid vascularity prior to thyroidectomy and management of thyrotoxic crisis; block thyroidal uptake of radioactive isotopes of iodine in a radiation emergency

**Usual Dosage** Oral:

Adults: RDA: 130 mcg

Expectorant:
Children: 60-250 mg every 6-8 hours; maximum single dose: 500 mg
Adults: 300-650 mg 2-3 times/day
Preoperative thyroidectomy: Children and Adults: 50-250 mg (1-5 drops SSKI®) 3 times/day **or** 0.1-0.3 mL (3-5 drops) of strong iodine (Lugol's solution) 3 times/day; give for 10 days before surgery
Thyrotoxic crisis:
Children and Adults: 300-500 mg (6-10 drops SSKI®) 3 times/day or 1 mL strong iodine (Lugol's solution) 3 times/day
Graves' disease in neonates: 1 drop of strong iodine (Lugol's solution) 3 times/day
Sporotrichosis:
Initial:
Preschool: 50 mg/dose 3 times/day
Children: 250 mg/dose 3 times/day
Adults: 500 mg/dose 3 times/day
Oral increase 50 mg/dose daily
Maximum dose:
Preschool: 500 mg/dose 3 times/day
Children and Adults: 1-2 g/dose 3 times/day
Continue treatment for 4-6 weeks after lesions have completely healed

**Mechanism of Action** Reduces viscosity of mucus by increasing respiratory tract secretions; inhibits secretion of thyroid hormone, fosters colloid accumulation in thyroid follicles

**Local Anesthetic/Vasoconstrictor Precautions** No information available to require special precautions

**Effects on Dental Treatment** No effects or complications reported

**Other Adverse Effects** 1% to 10%:
Central nervous system: Fever, headache
Dermatologic: Urticaria, acne, angioedema
Endocrine & metabolic: Goiter with hypothyroidism
Gastrointestinal: Metallic taste, GI upset, soreness of teeth and gums
Hematologic: Cutaneous and mucosal hemorrhage, eosinophilia
Neuromuscular & skeletal: Arthralgia
Respiratory: Rhinitis
Miscellaneous: Lymph node enlargement

**Drug Interactions** Increased toxicity: Lithium causes additive hypothyroid effects

**Drug Uptake**
Onset of action: 24-48 hours
Peak effect: 10-15 days after continuous therapy

**Pregnancy Risk Factor** D

**Generic Available** Yes

## Potassium Phosphate (poe TASS ee um FOS fate)

**U.S. Brand Names** Neutra-Phos®-K

**Therapeutic Category** Electrolyte Supplement, Parenteral; Phosphate Salt; Potassium Salt

**Use** Treatment and prevention of hypophosphatemia or hypokalemia

**Usual Dosage** I.V. doses should be incorporated into the patient's maintenance I.V. fluids; intermittent I.V. infusion should be reserved for severe depletion situations in patients undergoing continuous EKG monitoring. It is difficult to determine total body phosphorus deficit; the following dosages are empiric guidelines:

Normal requirements elemental phosphorus: Oral:
0-6 months: 240 mg
6-12 months: 360 mg
1-10 years: 800 mg
>10 years: 1200 mg
Pregnancy lactation: Additional 400 mg/day

Adults RDA: 800 mg

Treatment: It is difficult to provide concrete guidelines for the treatment of severe hypophosphatemia because the extent of total body deficits and response to therapy are difficult to predict. Aggressive doses of phosphate may result in a transient serum elevation followed by redistribution into intracellular compartments or bone tissue. It is recommended that repletion of severe hypophosphatemia (<1 mg/dL in adults) be done I.V. because large doses of oral phosphate may cause diarrhea and intestinal absorption may be unreliable

**Pediatric I.V. phosphate repletion:** Children: 0.25-0.5 mmol/kg **administer over 4-6 hours and repeat if symptomatic hypophosphatemia persists;**

(Continued)

## Potassium Phosphate *(Continued)*

to assess the need for further phosphate administration, obtain serum inorganic phosphate after administration of the first dose and base further doses on serum levels and clinical status

**Adult I.V. phosphate repletion:**

Initial dose: 0.08 mmol/kg if recent uncomplicated hypophosphatemia

Initial dose: 0.16 mmol/kg if prolonged hypophosphatemia with presumed total body deficits; increase dose by 25% to 50% if patient symptomatic with severe hypophosphatemia

**Do not exceed 0.24 mmol/kg/day; administer over 6 hours by I.V. infusion**

**With orders for I.V. phosphate, there is considerable confusion associated with the use of millimoles (mmol) versus milliequivalents (mEq) to express the phosphate requirement.** Because inorganic phosphate exists as monobasic and dibasic anions, with the mixture of valences dependent on pH, ordering by mEq amounts is unreliable and may lead to large dosing errors. In addition, I.V. phosphate is available in the sodium and potassium salt; therefore, the content of these cations must be considered when ordering phosphate. The most reliable method of ordering I.V. phosphate is by millimoles, then specifying the potassium or sodium salt. For example, an order for 15 mmol of phosphate as potassium phosphate in one liter of normal saline would also provide 22 mEq of potassium.

Maintenance:

I.V. solutions:

Children: 0.5-1.5 mmol/kg/24 hours I.V. or 2-3 mmol/kg/24 hours orally in divided doses

Adults: 15-30 mmol/24 hours I.V. or 50-150 mmol/24 hours orally in divided doses

Oral:

Children <4 years: 1 capsule (250 mg phosphorus/8 mmol) 4 times/day; dilute as instructed

Children >4 years and Adults: 1-2 capsules (250-500 mg phosphorus/8-16 mmol) 4 times/day; dilute as instructed

**Local Anesthetic/Vasoconstrictor Precautions** No information available to require special precautions

**Effects on Dental Treatment** No effects or complications reported

**Other Adverse Effects**

>10%: Gastrointestinal: Diarrhea, nausea, stomach pain, flatulence, vomiting

1% to 10%:

Cardiovascular: Bradycardia
Endocrine & metabolic: Hyperkalemia
Neuromuscular & skeletal: Weakness
Respiratory: Dyspnea

<1%:

Cardiovascular: Chest pain
Central nervous system: Mental confusion
Endocrine & metabolic: Alkalosis
Gastrointestinal: Abdominal pain, throat pain
Local: Phlebitis
Neuromuscular & skeletal: Paresthesias, paralysis
Renal: Acute renal failure

**Drug Interactions**

Decreased effect/levels with aluminum and magnesium-containing antacids or sucralfate which can act as phosphate binders

Increased effect/levels with potassium-sparing diuretics, salt substitutes, or ACE-inhibitors

Increased effect of digitalis

**Pregnancy Risk Factor** C

**Generic Available** Yes

## Potassium Phosphate and Sodium Phosphate

(poe TASS ee um FOS fate & SOW dee um FOS fate)

**U.S. Brand Names** K-Phos® Neutral; Neutra-Phos®; Uro-KP-Neutral®

**Therapeutic Category** Electrolyte Supplement, Oral; Phosphate Salt; Potassium Salt

**Use** Treatment of conditions associated with excessive renal phosphate loss or inadequate GI absorption of phosphate; to acidify the urine to lower calcium concentrations; to increase the antibacterial activity of methenamine; reduce odor and rash caused by ammonia in urine

**Usual Dosage** All dosage forms to be mixed in 6-8 oz of water prior to administration

Children: 2-3 mmol phosphate/kg/24 hours given 4 times/day **or** 1 capsule 4 times/day

Adults: 1-2 capsules (250-500 mg phosphorus/8-16 mmol) 4 times/day after meals and at bedtime

**Local Anesthetic/Vasoconstrictor Precautions** No information available to require special precautions

**Effects on Dental Treatment** No effects or complications reported

**Other Adverse Effects**

>10%: Gastrointestinal: Diarrhea, nausea, stomach pain, flatulence, vomiting

1% to 10%:
- Cardiovascular: Bradycardia
- Endocrine & metabolic: Hyperkalemia
- Neuromuscular & skeletal: Weakness
- Respiratory: Dyspnea

<1%:
- Cardiovascular: Arrhythmia, chest pain, edema
- Central nervous system: Mental confusion, tetany
- Endocrine & metabolic: Alkalosis
- Gastrointestinal: Weight gain, thirst, throat pain
- Genitourinary: Decreased urine output
- Local: Phlebitis
- Neuromuscular & skeletal: Paresthesias, paralysis, pain/weakness of extremities, bone pain, arthralgia
- Renal: Acute renal failure

**Drug Interactions**

Decreased effect/levels with aluminum and magnesium-containing antacids or sucralfate which can act as phosphate binders

Increased effect/levels with potassium-sparing diuretics or ACE-inhibitors

Increased effect/levels of digitalis, salicylates

**Pregnancy Risk Factor** C

**Generic Available** Yes

## Povidone-Iodine (POE vi done EYE oh dyne)

**Related Information**

Patients Undergoing Cancer Therapy *on page 1154*

**U.S. Brand Names** Betadine® [OTC]; Efodine® [OTC]; Iodex® Regular; Isodine® [OTC]

**Therapeutic Category** Antibacterial, Topical

**Use** External antiseptic with broad microbicidal spectrum against bacteria, fungi, viruses, protozoa, and yeasts

**Usual Dosage**

Shampoo: Apply 2 tsp to hair and scalp, lather and rinse; repeat application 2 times/week until improvement is noted, then shampoo weekly

Topical: Apply as needed for treatment and prevention of susceptible microbial infections

**Mechanism of Action** Povidone-iodine is known to be a powerful broad spectrum germicidal agent effective against a wide range of bacteria, viruses, fungi, protozoa, and spores.

**Local Anesthetic/Vasoconstrictor Precautions** No information available to require special precautions

**Effects on Dental Treatment** No effects or complications reported

**Other Adverse Effects**

1% to 10%:
- Cardiovascular: Local edema
- Dermatologic: Rash, pruritus

<1%:
- Endocrine & metabolic: Metabolic acidosis
- Local: Systemic absorption in extensive burns causing iododerma
- Renal: Renal impairment

**Drug Interactions** No data reported

**Drug Uptake** Absorption: In normal individuals, topical application results in very little systemic absorption; with vaginal administration, however, absorption is rapid and serum concentrations of total iodine and inorganic iodide are increased significantly

**Pregnancy Risk Factor** D

**Generic Available** Yes


- ♦ **PPD** *see* Tuberculin Purified Protein Derivative *on page 1031*
- ♦ **PPS** *see* Pentosan Polysulfate Sodium *on page 781*
- ♦ **PrameGel® [OTC]** *see* Pramoxine *on next page*
- ♦ **Pramet® FA** *see* Vitamins, Multiple *on page 1051*
- ♦ **Pramilet® FA** *see* Vitamins, Multiple *on page 1051*

## Pramipexole (pra mi PEX ole)

**U.S. Brand Names** Mirapex®
**Therapeutic Category** Anti-Parkinson's Agent
**Use** Treatment of the signs and symptoms of idiopathic Parkinson's Disease
**Usual Dosage** Adults: Oral: Initial: 0.375 mg/day given in 3 divided doses, increase gradually by 0.125 mg/dose every 5-7 days; range: 1.5-4.5 mg/day
**Mechanism of Action** Pre- and postsynaptic D-2 receptor agonist with preferential affinity for the dopamine D-$2_3$-receptor subtypes
**Local Anesthetic/Vasoconstrictor Precautions** No information available to require special precautions
**Effects on Dental Treatment** No effects or complications reported
**Drug Uptake**
Half-life: 11-14 hours
Peak concentration: 5:44-7.17 μg/mL
**Pregnancy Risk Factor** C
**Dosage Forms** Tablet: 0.125 mg, 0.25 mg, 1 mg, 1.5 mg

♦ **Pramosone®** *see* Pramoxine and Hydrocortisone *on this page*

## Pramoxine (pra MOKS een)

**U.S. Brand Names** Anusol® Ointment [OTC]; Fleet® Pain Relief [OTC]; Itch-X® [OTC]; Phicon® [OTC]; PrameGel® [OTC]; Prax® [OTC]; ProctoFoam® NS [OTC]; Tronolane® [OTC]
**Therapeutic Category** Local Anesthetic, Topical
**Use** Temporary relief of pain and itching associated with anogenital pruritus or irritation; dermatosis, minor burns, or hemorrhoids
**Usual Dosage** Adults: Topical: Apply as directed, usually every 3-4 hours to affected area (maximum adult dose: 200 mg)
**Mechanism of Action** Pramoxine, like other anesthetics, decreases the neuronal membrane's permeability to sodium ions; both initiation and conduction of nerve impulses are blocked, thus depolarization of the neuron is inhibited
**Local Anesthetic/Vasoconstrictor Precautions** No information available to require special precautions
**Effects on Dental Treatment** No effects or complications reported
**Other Adverse Effects**
1% to 10%:
Dermatologic: Angioedema
Local: Contact dermatitis, burning, stinging
<1%:
Cardiovascular: Edema
Dermatologic: Urticaria
Genitourinary: Urethritis
Hematologic: Methemoglobinemia in infants
Local: Tenderness
**Drug Interactions** No data reported
**Drug Uptake**
Onset of therapeutic effect: Within 2-5 minutes
Peak effect: 3-5 minutes
Duration: May last for several days
**Pregnancy Risk Factor** C
**Generic Available** No

## Pramoxine and Hydrocortisone

(pra MOKS een & hye droe KOR ti sone)
**U.S. Brand Names** Enzone®; Pramosone®; Proctofoam®-HC; Zone-A Forte®
**Therapeutic Category** Anti-inflammatory Agent; Corticosteroid, Topical (Low Potency); Local Anesthetic, Topical
**Synonyms** Hydrocortisone and Pramoxine
**Use** Treatment of severe anorectal or perianal swelling
**Usual Dosage** Apply to affected areas 3-4 times/day
**Local Anesthetic/Vasoconstrictor Precautions** No information available to require special precautions
**Effects on Dental Treatment** No effects or complications reported
**Pregnancy Risk Factor** C
**Generic Available** No

♦ **Prandin™** *see* Repaglinide *on page 881*
♦ **Pravachol®** *see* Pravastatin *on this page*

## Pravastatin (PRA va stat in)

**Related Information**
Cardiovascular Diseases *on page 1066*

**U.S. Brand Names** Pravachol®

**Therapeutic Category** HMG-CoA Reductase Inhibitor; Lipid Lowering Drugs

**Use** Adjunct to diet for the reduction of elevated total and LDL cholesterol levels in patients with hypercholesterolemia (type IIa, IIb, and IIc); used in hypercholesterolemic patients without clinically evident heart disease to reduce the risk of myocardial infarction, to reduce the risk for revascularization, and reduce the risk of death due to cardiovascular causes with no increase in death from noncardiovascular diseases

**Usual Dosage** Adults: Oral: 10-20 mg once daily at bedtime, may increase to 40 mg/day at bedtime

**Mechanism of Action** Pravastatin is a competitive inhibitor of 3-hydroxy-3-methylglutaryl coenzyme A (HMG-CoA) reductase, which is the rate-limiting enzyme involved in *de novo* cholesterol synthesis.

**Local Anesthetic/Vasoconstrictor Precautions** No information available to require special precautions

**Effects on Dental Treatment** No effects of complications reported

**Other Adverse Effects**

1% to 10%:

Central nervous system: Headache, dizziness

Dermatologic: Rash

Gastrointestinal: flatulence, abdominal cramps, diarrhea, constipation, nausea, dyspepsia, heartburn

Neuromuscular & skeletal: Myalgia, elevated creatine phosphokinase (CPK)

<1%:

Gastrointestinal: Dysgeusia

Ocular: Lenticular opacities, blurred vision

**Drug Interactions**

Increased effect with cholestyramine

Increased effect/toxicity of oral anticoagulants

Increased toxicity with gemfibrozil, clofibrate

Concurrent use of erythromycin and HMG-CoA reductase inhibitors may result in rhabdomyolysis

**Drug Uptake**

Absorption: Poor

Serum half-life, elimination: ~2-3 hours

Time to peak serum concentration: 1-1.5 hours

**Pregnancy Risk Factor** X

**Generic Available** No

♦ **Prax® [OTC]** *see* Pramoxine *on previous page*

## Prazepam (PRA ze pam)

**U.S. Brand Names** Centrax®

**Therapeutic Category** Antianxiety Agent; Anticonvulsant, Benzodiazepine; Benzodiazepine; Tranquilizer, Minor

**Use** Treatment of anxiety and management of alcohol withdrawal; may also be used as an anticonvulsant in management of simple partial seizures

**Usual Dosage** Adults: Oral: 30 mg/day in divided doses, may increase gradually to a maximum of 60 mg/day

**Mechanism of Action** Benzodiazepine anxiolytic sedative that produces CNS depression at the subcortical level, except at high doses, whereby it works at the cortical level

**Local Anesthetic/Vasoconstrictor Precautions** No information available to require special precautions

**Effects on Dental Treatment** >10% of patients experience dry mouth which disappears with cessation of drug therapy

**Other Adverse Effects**

>10%:

Cardiovascular Tachycardia, chest pain

Central nervous system: Drowsiness, fatigue, lightheadedness, memory impairment, insomnia, anxiety, depression, headache, impaired coordination

Dermatologic: Rash

Endocrine & metabolic: Decreased libido

Gastrointestinal: Constipation, diarrhea, decreased salivation, nausea, vomiting, increased or decreased appetite

Neuromuscular & skeletal: Dysarthria

Ocular: Blurred vision

Miscellaneous: Sweating

1% to 10%:

Cardiovascular: Syncope, hypotension

Central nervous system: Confusion, nervousness, dizziness, akathisia

Dermatologic: Dermatitis

(Continued)

## Prazepam *(Continued)*

Gastrointestinal: Weight gain or loss, increased salivation
Neuromuscular & skeletal: Muscle cramps, rigidity, tremor
Ocular: Blurred vision
Otic: Tinnitus
Respiratory: Hyperventilation, nasal congestion

<1%:
Endocrine & metabolic: Menstrual irregularities
Hematologic: Blood dyscrasias
Neuromuscular & skeletal: Reflex slowing
Miscellaneous: Drug dependence

**Drug Interactions** Increased toxicity (CNS depression): Alcohol, tricyclic antidepressants, sedative-hypnotics, MAO inhibitors

**Drug Uptake**
Duration: 48 hours
Serum half-life:
Parent drug: 78 minutes
Desmethyldiazepam: 30-100 hours

**Pregnancy Risk Factor** D

**Generic Available** Yes

## Praziquantel (pray zi KWON tel)

**U.S. Brand Names** Biltricide®

**Therapeutic Category** Anthelmintic

**Use** Treatment of all stages of schistosomiasis caused by *Schistosoma* species pathogenic to humans; also active in the treatment of clonorchiasis, opisthorchiasis, cysticercosis, and many intestinal tapeworm infections and trematode

**Usual Dosage** Children >4 years and Adults: Oral:
Schistosomiasis: 20 mg/kg/dose 2-3 times/day for 1 day at 4- to 6-hour intervals
Flukes: 25 mg/kg/dose every 8 hours for 1-2 days
Cysticercosis: 50 mg/kg/day divided every 8 hours for 14 days
Tapeworms: 10-20 mg/kg as a single dose (25 mg/kg for *Hymenolepis nana*)

**Mechanism of Action** Increases the cell permeability to calcium in schistosomes, causing strong contractions and paralysis of worm musculature leading to detachment of suckers from the blood vessel walls and to dislodgment

**Local Anesthetic/Vasoconstrictor Precautions** No information available to require special precautions

**Effects on Dental Treatment** No effects or complications reported

**Other Adverse Effects**

1% to 10%:
Central nervous system: Dizziness, drowsiness, headache, malaise
Gastrointestinal: Abdominal pain, loss of appetite, nausea, vomiting
Miscellaneous: Sweating

<1%:
Central nervous system: Fever
Dermatologic: Skin rash, urticaria, itching
Gastrointestinal: Diarrhea
Miscellaneous: CSF reaction syndrome in patients being treated for neurocysticercosis

**Drug Uptake**
Absorption: Oral: ~80%; CSF concentration is 14% to 20% of plasma concentration
Serum half-life:
Parent drug: 0.8-1.5 hours
Metabolites: 4.5 hours
Time to peak serum concentration: Within 1-3 hours

**Pregnancy Risk Factor** B

**Generic Available** No

## Prazosin (PRA zoe sin)

**Related Information**
Cardiovascular Diseases *on page 1066*

**U.S. Brand Names** Minipress®

**Canadian Brand Names** Apo®-Prazo; Novo-Prazin; Nu-Prazo

**Therapeutic Category** Alpha-Adrenergic Blockers - Peripheral-Acting (Alpha$_1$-Blockers); Antihypertensive Agent; Vasodilator, Coronary

**Use** Treatment of hypertension, severe congestive heart failure (in conjunction with diuretics and cardiac glycosides); reduce mortality in stable postmyocardial patients with left ventricular dysfunction (ejection fraction ≤40%)

**Unlabeled use:** Symptoms of benign prostatic hypertrophy

**Usual Dosage** Oral:

Children: Initial: 5 mcg/kg/dose (to assess hypotensive effects); usual dosing interval: every 6 hours; increase dosage gradually up to maximum of 25 mcg/kg/dose every 6 hours

Adults: Initial: 1 mg/dose 2-3 times/day; usual maintenance dose: 3-15 mg/day in divided doses 2-4 times/day; maximum daily dose: 20 mg

**Mechanism of Action** Competitively inhibits postsynaptic alpha-adrenergic receptors which results in vasodilation of veins and arterioles and a decrease in total peripheral resistance and blood pressure

**Local Anesthetic/Vasoconstrictor Precautions** No information available to require special precautions

**Effects on Dental Treatment** Significant orthostatic hypotension a possibility; monitor patient when getting out of dental chair; significant dry mouth in up to 10% of patients

**Other Adverse Effects**

>10%:

Cardiovascular: Orthostatic hypotension

Central nervous system: Dizziness, lightheadedness, drowsiness, headache, malaise

1% to 10%:

Cardiovascular: Edema, palpitations

Central nervous system: Fatigue, nervousness

Gastrointestinal: Dry mouth

Genitourinary: Urinary incontinence

<1%:

Cardiovascular: Angina

Central nervous system: Nightmares, hypothermia

Dermatologic: Rash

Endocrine & metabolic: Sexual dysfunction

Gastrointestinal: Nausea

Genitourinary: Priapism

Renal: Polyuria

Respiratory: Dyspnea, nasal congestion

**Drug Interactions**

Decreased effect in combination with NSAIDs: Indomethacin pretreatment has been reported to inhibit the hypotensive effect of a single dose of prazosin. The effect of chronic therapy with both drugs is not known. It is suggested however that, as a general rule, indomethacin may inhibit the antihypertensive response to prazosin. The effect of other NSAIDs is not known and the use of NSAIDs such as ibuprofen for treatment of acute postoperative pain in patients taking prazosin is not contraindicated. Inhibition of prostaglandin synthesis by NSAIDs is probably responsible for the decreased effect of prazosin.

Increased effect (hypotensive) with diuretics and antihypertensive medications (especially beta-blockers)

**Drug Uptake**

Onset of hypotensive effect: Within 2 hours

Maximum decrease: 2-4 hours

Duration: 10-24 hours

Serum half-life: 2-4 hours; increased with congestive heart failure

**Pregnancy Risk Factor** C

**Generic Available** Yes

## Prazosin and Polythiazide (PRA zoe sin & pol i THYE a zide)

**U.S. Brand Names** Minizide®

**Therapeutic Category** Antihypertensive Agent, Combination

**Use** Management of mild to moderate hypertension

**Usual Dosage** Adults: Oral: 1 capsule 2-3 times/day

**Local Anesthetic/Vasoconstrictor Precautions** No information available to require special precautions

**Effects on Dental Treatment** No effects or complications reported

**Pregnancy Risk Factor** C

**Generic Available** No

♦ **Precose®** *see* Acarbose *on page 25*
♦ **Predair®** *see* Prednisolone *on next page*
♦ **Predaject®** *see* Prednisolone *on next page*
♦ **Predalone T.B.A.®** *see* Prednisolone *on next page*
♦ **Predcor®** *see* Prednisolone *on next page*
♦ **Predcor-TBA®** *see* Prednisolone *on next page*
♦ **Pred Forte®** *see* Prednisolone *on next page*
♦ **Pred-G® Ophthalmic** *see* Prednisolone and Gentamicin *on page 833*

♦ **Pred Mild**® *see* Prednisolone *on this page*

## Prednicarbate (PRED ni kar bate)

**U.S. Brand Names** Dermatop®

**Therapeutic Category** Corticosteroid, Topical (Medium Potency)

**Use** Relief of the inflammatory and pruritic manifestations of corticosteroid-responsive dermatoses (medium potency topical corticosteroid)

**Usual Dosage** Adults: Topical: Apply a thin film to affected area twice daily

**Mechanism of Action** Topical corticosteroids have anti-inflammatory, antipruritic, vasoconstrictive, and antiproliferative actions

**Local Anesthetic/Vasoconstrictor Precautions** No information available to require special precautions

**Effects on Dental Treatment** No effects or complications reported

**Other Adverse Effects** <10%:

Dermatologic: Acne, hypopigmentation, allergic dermatitis, maceration of the skin, skin atrophy, folliculitis, hypertrichosis

Endocrine & metabolic: HPA suppression, Cushing's syndrome, growth retardation

Local: Burning, itching, irritation, dryness

Miscellaneous: Secondary infection

**Drug Interactions** No data reported

**Pregnancy Risk Factor** C

**Dosage Forms** Cream: 0.1% (15 g, 60 g)

**Generic Available** No

♦ **Prednicen-M**® *see* Prednisone *on next page*

## Prednisolone (pred NIS oh lone)

**Related Information**

Corticosteroid Equivalencies Comparison *on page 1221*

Corticosteroids, Topical Comparison *on page 1222*

Neomycin, Polymyxin B, and Prednisolone *on page 713*

Respiratory Diseases *on page 1079*

**U.S. Brand Names** AK-Pred®; Articulose-50®; Delta-Cortef®; Econopred®; Econopred® Plus; Inflamase®; Inflamase® Mild; Key-Pred®; Key-Pred-SP®; Metreton®; Pediapred®; Predair®; Predaject®; Predalone T.B.A.®; Predcor®; Predcor-TBA®; Pred Forte®; Pred Mild®; Prelone®

**Canadian Brand Names** Novo-Prednisolone

**Therapeutic Category** Adrenal Corticosteroid; Anti-inflammatory Agent; Corticosteroid, Ophthalmic; Corticosteroid, Systemic

**Use**

Dental: Treatment of a variety of oral diseases of allergic, inflammatory or autoimmune origin

Medical: Treatment of palpebral and bulbar conjunctivitis; corneal injury from chemical, radiation, thermal burns, or foreign body penetration; endocrine disorders, rheumatic disorders, collagen diseases, dermatologic diseases, allergic states, ophthalmic diseases, respiratory diseases, hematologic disorders, neoplastic diseases, edematous states, and gastrointestinal diseases; useful in patients with inability to activate prednisone (liver disease)

**Usual Dosage** Dose depends upon condition being treated and response of patient; dosage for infants and children should be based on severity of the disease and response of the patient rather than on strict adherence to dosage indicated by age, weight, or body surface area. Consider alternate day therapy for long-term therapy. Discontinuation of long-term therapy requires gradual withdrawal by tapering the dose.

Children: Anti-inflammatory or immunosuppressive dose: Oral, I.V., I.M. (sodium phosphate salt): 0.1-2 mg/kg/day in divided doses 1-4 times/day

Adults: Oral, I.V., I.M. (sodium phosphate salt): 5-60 mg/day

Elderly: Use lowest effective adult dose

**Mechanism of Action** Decreases inflammation by suppression of migration of polymorphonuclear leukocytes and reversal of increased capillary permeability; suppresses the immune system by reducing activity and volume of the lymphatic system

**Local Anesthetic/Vasoconstrictor Precautions** No information available to require special precautions

**Effects on Dental Treatment** No effects or complications reported

**Other Adverse Effects** >10%:

Central nervous system: Insomnia, nervousness

Gastrointestinal: Increased appetite, indigestion

**Contraindications** Acute superficial herpes simplex keratitis; systemic fungal infections; varicella; hypersensitivity to prednisolone or any component

**Warnings/Precautions** Use with caution in patients with hyperthyroidism, cirrhosis, nonspecific ulcerative colitis, hypertension, osteoporosis, thromboembolic tendencies, CHF, convulsive disorders, myasthenia gravis, thrombophlebitis, peptic ulcer, diabetes; acute adrenal insufficiency may occur with abrupt withdrawal after long-term therapy or with stress; young pediatric patients may be more susceptible to adrenal axis suppression from topical therapy. Because of the risk of adverse effects, systemic corticosteroids should be used cautiously in the elderly, in the smallest possible dose, and for the shortest possible time.

**Drug Interactions** Decreased effect with barbiturates, phenytoin, rifampin; decreased effect of salicylates, vaccines, toxoids

**Drug Uptake**

Absorption: Rapid and nearly complete

Serum half-life: 3.6 hours; biological: 18-36 hours

**Pregnancy Risk Factor** C

**Breast-feeding Considerations** May be taken while breast-feeding

**Dosage Forms**

Injection, as acetate (for I.M., intralesional, intra-articular, or soft tissue administration only): 25 mg/mL (10 mL, 30 mL); 50 mg/mL (30 mL)

Injection, as sodium phosphate (for I.M., I.V., intra-articular, intralesional, or soft tissue administration): 20 mg/mL (2 mL, 5 mL, 10 mL)

Injection, as tebutate (for intra-articular, intralesional, soft tissue administration only): 20 mg/mL (1 mL, 5 mL, 10 mL)

Liquid, oral, as sodium phosphate: 5 mg/5 mL (120 mL)

Solution, ophthalmic, as sodium phosphate: 0.125% (5 mL, 10 mL, 15 mL); 1% (5 mL, 10 mL, 15 mL)

Syrup: 15 mg/5 mL (240 mL)

Tablet: 5 mg

**Dietary Considerations** Should be taken after meals or with food or milk to decrease GI effects; limit caffeine; increase dietary intake of pyridoxine, vitamin C, vitamin D, folate, calcium, and phosphorus

**Generic Available** Yes

## Prednisolone and Gentamicin (pred NIS oh lone & jen ta MYE sin)

**U.S. Brand Names** Pred-G® Ophthalmic

**Therapeutic Category** Antibiotic, Ophthalmic; Corticosteroid, Ophthalmic

**Synonyms** Gentamicin and Prednisolone

**Use** Treatment of steroid responsive inflammatory conditions and superficial ocular infections due to strains of microorganisms susceptible to gentamicin such as *Staphylococcus, E. coli, H. influenzae, Klebsiella, Neisseria, Pseudomonas, Proteus,* and *Serratia* species

**Usual Dosage** Children and Adults: Ophthalmic: 1 drop 2-4 times/day; during the initial 24-48 hours, the dosing frequency may be increased if necessary

**Local Anesthetic/Vasoconstrictor Precautions** No information available to require special precautions

**Effects on Dental Treatment** No effects or complications reported

**Other Adverse Effects** 1% to 10%:

Dermatologic: Delayed wound healing

Local: Burning, stinging

Ocular: Increased intraocular pressure, glaucoma, superficial punctate keratitis, infrequent optic nerve damage, posterior subcapsular cataract formation

Miscellaneous: Development of secondary infection, allergic sensitization

**Pregnancy Risk Factor** C

**Generic Available** Yes

## Prednisone (PRED ni sone)

**Related Information**

Corticosteroid Equivalencies Comparison *on page 1221*

Oral Nonviral Soft Tissue Ulcerations or Erosions *on page 1141*

Respiratory Diseases *on page 1079*

Rheumatoid Arthritis and Osteoarthritis *on page 1092*

**U.S. Brand Names** Deltasone®; Liquid Pred®; Meticorten®; Orasone®; Prednicen-M®; Sterapred®

**Canadian Brand Names** Apo®-Prednisone; Jaa-Prednisone®; Novo-Prednisone; Wimpred

**Therapeutic Category** Adrenal Corticosteroid; Anti-inflammatory Agent; Corticosteroid, Systemic

**Use**

Dental: Treatment of a variety of oral diseases of allergic, inflammatory or autoimmune origin

(Continued)

## Prednisone *(Continued)*

Medical: Treatment of a variety of diseases including adrenocortical insufficiency, hypercalcemia, rheumatic and collagen disorders; dermatologic, ocular, respiratory, gastrointestinal, and neoplastic diseases; organ transplantation; not available in injectable form, prednisolone must be used

**Usual Dosage** Dose depends upon condition being treated and response of patient; dosage for infants and children should be based on severity of the disease and response of the patient rather than on strict adherence to dosage indicated by age, weight, or body surface area. Consider alternate day therapy for long-term therapy. Discontinuation of long-term therapy requires gradual withdrawal by tapering the dose.

Children: Oral: Anti-inflammatory or immunosuppressive dose: 0.05-2 mg/kg/day divided 1-4 times/day

Adults: 5-60 mg/day in divided doses 1-4 times/day

Elderly: Use the lowest effective dose

**Mechanism of Action** Decreases inflammation by suppression of migration of polymorphonuclear leukocytes and reversal of increased capillary permeability; suppresses the immune system by reducing activity and volume of the lymphatic system; suppresses adrenal function at high doses

**Local Anesthetic/Vasoconstrictor Precautions** No information available to require special precautions

**Effects on Dental Treatment** No effects or complications reported

**Other Adverse Effects** >10%:

Central nervous system: Insomnia, nervousness

Gastrointestinal: Increased appetite, indigestion

**Contraindications** Serious infections, except septic shock or tuberculous meningitis; systemic fungal infections; hypersensitivity to prednisone or any component; varicella

**Warnings/Precautions** Use with caution in patients with hypothyroidism, cirrhosis, hypertension, congestive heart failure, ulcerative colitis, thromboembolic disorders, and patients with an increased risk for peptic ulcer disease; may retard bone growth; gradually taper dose to withdraw therapy. Because of the risk of adverse effects, systemic corticosteroids should be used cautiously in the elderly, in the smallest possible dose, and for the shortest possible time.

**Drug Interactions** Decreased effect with barbiturates, phenytoin, rifampin; decreased effect of salicylates, vaccines, toxoids

**Drug Uptake** Prednisone is inactive and must be metabolized to prednisolone which may be impaired in patients with impaired liver function

Absorption: Rapid and nearly complete

Serum half-life: Normal renal function: 2.5-3.5 hours

**Pregnancy Risk Factor** B

**Breast-feeding Considerations** May be taken while breast-feeding

**Dosage Forms**

Solution, oral: Concentrate (30% alcohol): 5 mg/mL (30 mL); Nonconcentrate (5% alcohol): 5 mg/5 mL (5 mL, 500 mL)

Syrup: 5 mg/5 mL (120 mL, 240 mL)

Tablet: 1 mg, 2.5 mg, 5 mg, 10 mg, 20 mg, 50 mg

**Dietary Considerations** Should be taken after meals or with food or milk; limit caffeine; increase dietary intake of pyridoxine, vitamin C, vitamin D, folate, calcium, and phosphorus

**Generic Available** Yes

- ♦ **Predominant Cultivable Microorganisms From Various Sites of the Oral Cavity** *see page 1237*
- ♦ **Prefrin™ Ophthalmic Solution** *see* Phenylephrine *on page 795*
- ♦ **Pregestimil® [OTC]** *see* Enteral Nutritional Products *on page 371*
- ♦ **Pregnyl®** *see* Chorionic Gonadotropin *on page 246*
- ♦ **Prelone®** *see* Prednisolone *on page 832*
- ♦ **Prelu-2®** *see* Phendimetrazine *on page 788*
- ♦ **Premarin®** *see* Estrogens, Conjugated *on page 391*
- ♦ **Premarin® With Methyltestosterone Oral** *see* Estrogens and Methyltestosterone *on page 391*
- ♦ **Premphase™** *see* Estrogens and Medroxyprogesterone *on page 390*
- ♦ **Prempro™** *see* Estrogens and Medroxyprogesterone *on page 390*
- ♦ **Prenatal Vitamins** *see* Vitamins, Multiple *on page 1051*
- ♦ **Prenavite® [OTC]** *see* Vitamins, Multiple *on page 1051*
- ♦ **Pre-Pen®** *see* Benzylpenicilloyl-polylysine *on page 133*
- ♦ **Prepidil® Vaginal Gel** *see* Dinoprostone *on page 337*
- ♦ **Prescription Strength Desenex® [OTC]** *see* Miconazole *on page 672*

- ♦ **Prescription Writing** *see page 1273*
- ♦ **Pre-Sed®** *see* Hexobarbital *on page 497*
- ♦ **PreSun® 29 [OTC]** *see* Methoxycinnamate and Oxybenzone *on page 656*
- ♦ **Pretz® [OTC]** *see* Sodium Chloride *on page 920*
- ♦ **Pretz-D® [OTC]** *see* Ephedrine *on page 371*
- ♦ **Prevacid®** *see* Lansoprazole *on page 573*
- ♦ **Prevalite®** *see* Cholestyramine Resin *on page 244*
- ♦ **Preven®** *see* Ethinyl Estradiol and Levonorgestrel *on page 402*
- ♦ **Preveon®** *see* Adefovir *on page 40*
- ♦ **PreviDent®** *see* Fluoride *on page 441*
- ♦ **Priftin®** *see* Rifapentine *on page 888*


## Prilocaine (PRIL oh kane)

**Related Information**

Oral Pain *on page 1122*

**U.S. Brand Names** Citanest Plain 4% Injection

**Therapeutic Category** Dental/Local Anesthetics; Local Anesthetic, Injectable

**Use** Dental: Amide-type anesthetic used for local infiltration anesthesia; injection near nerve trunks to produce nerve block

**Usual Dosage**

Children <10 years: Doses >40 mg (1 mL) as a 4% solution per procedure rarely needed

Children >10 years and Adults: Dental anesthesia, infiltration, or conduction block: Initial: 40-80 mg (1-2 mL) as a 4% solution; up to a maximum of 400 mg (10 mL) as a 4% solution within a 2-hour period. Manufacturer's maximum recommended dose is not more than 600 mg to normal healthy adults. The effective anesthetic dose varies with procedure, intensity of anesthesia needed, duration of anesthesia required and physical condition of the patient. Always use the lowest effective dose along with careful aspiration.

The following numbers of dental carpules (1.8 mL) provide the indicated amounts of prilocaine hydrochloride 4%.

| # of Cartridges | Mg Prilocaine (4%) |
|---|---|
| 1 | 72 |
| 2 | 144 |
| 3 | 216 |
| 4 | 288 |
| 5 | 360 |
| 6 | 432 |
| 7 | 504 |
| 8 | 576 |

**Note:** Adult and children doses of prilocaine hydrochloride cited from USP Dispensing Information (USP DI), 17th ed, The United States Pharmacopeial Convention, Inc, Rockville, MD, 1997, 139.

**Mechanism of Action** Local anesthetics bind selectively to the intracellular surface of sodium channels to block influx of sodium into the axon. As a result, depolarization necessary for action potential propagation and subsequent nerve function is prevented. The block at the sodium channel is reversible. When drug diffuses away from the axon, sodium channel function is restored and nerve propagation returns.

**Local Anesthetic/Vasoconstrictor Precautions** No information available to require special precautions

**Effects on Dental Treatment** No effects or complications reported

**Other Adverse Effects** Degree of adverse effects in the central nervous system and cardiovascular system are directly related to the blood levels of local anesthetic. The effects below are more likely to occur after systemic administration rather than infiltration.

Cardiovascular: Myocardial effects include a decrease in contraction force as well as a decrease in electrical excitability and myocardial conduction rate resulting in bradycardia and reduction in cardiac output.

Central nervous system: High blood levels result in anxiety, restlessness, disorientation, confusion, dizziness, tremors and seizures. This is followed by depression of CNS resulting in somnolence, unconsciousness and possible respiratory arrest. Nausea and vomiting may also occur. In some cases, symptoms of CNS stimulation may be absent and the primary CNS effects are somnolence and unconsciousness.

(Continued)

## Prilocaine *(Continued)*

Hypersensitivity reactions: May be manifest as dermatologic reactions and edema at injection site. Asthmatic syndromes have occurred.

Psychogenic reactions: It is common to misinterpret psychogenic responses to local anesthetic injection as an allergic reaction. Intraoral injections are perceived by many patients as a stressful procedure in dentistry. Common symptoms to this stress are sweating, palpitations, hyperventilation, generalized pallor and a fainting feeling

**Contraindications** Hypersensitivity to local anesthetics of the amide type

**Warnings/Precautions** Aspirate the syringe after tissue penetration and before injection to minimize chance of direct vascular injection

**Drug Interactions** No data reported

**Drug Uptake**

Infiltration:

Onset: ~2 minutes

Duration: Complete anesthesia for procedures lasting 20 minutes

Inferior alveolar nerve block:

Onset: ~3 minutes

Duration: ~2.5 hours

**Pregnancy Risk Factor** B

**Breast-feeding Considerations** Usual infiltration doses of prilocaine given to nursing mothers has not been shown to affect the health of the nursing infant

**Dosage Forms** Prilocaine hydrochloride 4%, 1.8 mL cartridges, containers of 100

**Dietary Considerations** No data reported

**Generic Available** No

**Selected Readings**

Jastak JT and Yagiela JA, "Vasoconstrictors and Local Anesthesia: A Review and Rationale for Use," *J Am Dent Assoc*, 1983, 107(4):623-30.
MacKenzie TA and Young ER, "Local Anesthetic Update," *Anesth Prog*, 1993, 40(2):29-34.
Wynn RL, "Epinephrine Interactions With Beta-Blockers," *Gen Dent*, 1994, 42(1):16, 18.
Yagiela JA, "Local Anesthetics," *Anesth Prog*, 1991, 38(4-5):128-41.

## Prilocaine With Epinephrine (PRIL oh kane with ep i NEF rin)

**Related Information**

Oral Pain *on page 1122*

**U.S. Brand Names** Citanest Forte® With Epinephrine

**Therapeutic Category** Dental/Local Anesthetics; Local Anesthetic, Injectable

**Use** Dental: Amide-type anesthetic used for local infiltration anesthesia; injection near nerve trunks to produce nerve block

**Usual Dosage**

Children <10 years: Doses >40 mg (1 mL) of prilocaine hydrochloride as a 4% solution with epinephrine 1:200,000 are rarely needed

Children >10 years and Adults: Dental anesthesia, infiltration, or conduction block: Initial: 40-80 mg (1-2 mL) of prilocaine hydrochloride as a 4% solution with epinephrine 1:200,000; up to a maximum of 400 mg (10 mL) of prilocaine hydrochloride within a 2-hour period. The effective anesthetic dose varies with procedure, intensity of anesthesia needed, duration of anesthesia required, and physical condition of the patient. Always use the lowest effective dose along with careful aspiration.

The following numbers of dental carpules (1.8 mL) provide the indicated amounts of prilocaine hydrochloride 4% and epinephrine 1:200,000.

| # of Cartridges | Mg Prilocaine (4%) | Mg Vasoconstrictor (Epinephrine 1:200,000) |
|---|---|---|
| 1 | 72 | 0.009 |
| 2 | 144 | 0.018 |
| 3 | 216 | 0.027 |
| 4 | 288 | 0.036 |
| 5 | 360 | 0.045 |
| 6 | 432 | 0.054 |
| 7 | 504 | 0.063 |
| 8 | 576 | 0.072 |

**Note:** Adult and children doses of prilocaine hydrochloride with epinephrine cited from USP Dispensing Information (USP DI), 17th ed, The United States Pharmacopeial Convention, Inc, Rockville, MD, 1997, 140.

**Mechanism of Action** Local anesthetics bind selectively to the intracellular surface of sodium channels to block influx of sodium into the axon. As a result, depolarization necessary for action potential propagation and subsequent nerve function is prevented. The block at the sodium channel is reversible. When drug diffuses away from the axon, sodium channel function is restored and nerve propagation returns.

Epinephrine prolongs the duration of the anesthetic actions of prilocaine by causing vasoconstriction (alpha adrenergic receptor agonist) of the vasculature surrounding the nerve axons. This prevents the diffusion of prilocaine away from the nerves resulting in a longer retention in the axon.

**Local Anesthetic/Vasoconstrictor Precautions** No information available to require special precautions

**Effects on Dental Treatment** No effects or complications reported

**Other Adverse Effects** Degree of adverse effects in the CNS and cardiovascular system are directly related to the blood levels of prilocaine. The effects below are more likely to occur after systemic administration rather than infiltration.

Cardiovascular: Myocardial effects include a decrease in contraction force as well as a decrease in electrical excitability and myocardial conduction rate resulting in bradycardia and reduction in cardiac output.

Central nervous system: High blood levels result in anxiety, restlessness, disorientation, confusion, dizziness, tremors and seizures. This is followed by depression of CNS resulting in somnolence, unconsciousness and possible respiratory arrest. Nausea and vomiting may also occur. In some cases, symptoms of CNS stimulation may be absent and the primary CNS effects are somnolence and unconsciousness.

Hypersensitivity reactions: Extremely rare, but may be manifest as dermatologic reactions and edema at injection site. Asthmatic syndromes have occurred. Patients may exhibit hypersensitivity to bisulfites contained in local anesthetic solution to prevent oxidation of epinephrine. In general, patients reacting to bisulfites have a history of asthma and their airways are hyper-reactive to asthmatic syndrome.

Psychogenic reactions: It is common to misinterpret psychogenic responses to local anesthetic injection as an allergic reaction. Intraoral injections are perceived by many patients as a stressful procedure in dentistry. Common symptoms to this stress are sweating, palpitations, hyperventilation, generalized pallor, and a fainting feeling.

**Contraindications** Hypersensitivity to local anesthetics of the amide-type

**Warnings/Precautions** Should be avoided in patients with uncontrolled hyperthyroidism. Should be used in minimal amounts in patients with significant cardiovascular problems (because of epinephrine component). Aspirate the syringe after tissue penetration and before injection to minimize chance of direct vascular injection

**Drug Interactions** Due to epinephrine component, use with tricyclic antidepressants or MAO inhibitors could result in increased pressor response; use with nonselective beta-blockers (ie, propranolol) could result in serious hypertension and reflex bradycardia

**Drug Uptake**

Onset of action:

Infiltration <2 minutes

Inferior alveolar nerve block: <3 minutes

Duration:

Infiltration 2.25 hours

Inferior alveolar nerve block: 3 hours

**Pregnancy Risk Factor** C

**Breast-feeding Considerations** Usual infiltration doses of prilocaine with epinephrine given to nursing mothers has not been shown to affect the health of the nursing infant

**Dosage Forms** Injection: Prilocaine hydrochloride 4% with epinephrine 1:200,000 (1.8 mL cartridges, in boxes of 100)

**Dietary Considerations** No data reported

**Generic Available** No

**Selected Readings**

Ayoub ST and Coleman AE, "A Review of Local Anesthetics," *Gen Dent*, 1992, 40(4):285-7, 289-90.

Blanton PL and Roda RS, "The Anatomy of Local Anesthesia," *J Calif Dent Assoc*, 1995, 23(4):55-65.

Jastak JT and Yagiela JA, "Vasoconstrictors and Local Anesthesia: A Review and Rationale for Use," *J Am Dent Assoc*, 1983, 107(4):623-30.

MacKenzie TA and Young ER, "Local Anesthetic Update," *Anesth Prog*, 1993, 40(2):29-34.

Wynn RL, "Epinephrine Interactions With Beta-Blockers," *Gen Dent*, 1994, 42(1):16, 18.

Yagiela JA, "Local Anesthetics," *Anesth Prog*, 1991, 38(4-5):128-41.

Yagiela JA, "Vasoconstrictor Agents for Local Anesthesia," *Anesth Prog*, 1995, 42(3-4):116-20.

- **Prilosec™** *see* Omeprazole *on page 739*
- **Primacor®** *see* Milrinone *on page 677*

## Primaquine Phosphate (PRIM a kween FOS fate)

**Therapeutic Category** Antimalarial Agent

**Use** Provides radical cure of *P. vivax* or *P. ovale* malaria after a clinical attack has been confirmed by blood smear or serologic titer and postexposure prophylaxis

**Usual Dosage** Oral:

Children: 0.3 mg base/kg/day once daily for 14 days (not to exceed 15 mg/day) or 0.9 mg base/kg once weekly for 8 weeks not to exceed 45 mg base/week

Adults: 15 mg/day (base) once daily for 14 days or 45 mg base once weekly for 8 weeks

**Mechanism of Action** Eliminates the primary tissue exoerythrocytic forms of *P. falciparum*; disrupts mitochondria and binds to DNA

**Local Anesthetic/Vasoconstrictor Precautions** No information available to require special precautions

**Effects on Dental Treatment** No effects or complications reported

**Other Adverse Effects**

>10%:

Gastrointestinal: Abdominal pain, nausea, vomiting

Hematologic: Hemolytic anemia

1% to 10%: Hematologic: Methemoglobinemia

<1%:

Cardiovascular: Arrhythmias

Central nervous system: Headache

Dermatologic: Pruritus

Hematologic: Leukopenia, agranulocytosis, leukocytosis

Ocular: Interference with visual accommodation

**Drug Interactions** Increased toxicity/levels with quinacrine

**Drug Uptake**

Absorption: Oral: Well absorbed

Serum half-life: 3.7-9.6 hours

Time to peak serum concentration: Within 1-2 hours

**Pregnancy Risk Factor** C

**Generic Available** Yes

♦ **Primaxin®** *see* Imipenem and Cilastatin *on page 527*

## Primidone (PRI mi done)

**U.S. Brand Names** Mysoline®

**Canadian Brand Names** Apo®-Primidone; Sertan®

**Therapeutic Category** Anticonvulsant, Barbiturate

**Use** Management of grand mal, complex partial, and focal seizures

**Unlabeled use:** Benign familial tremor (essential tremor)

**Usual Dosage** Oral:

Children <8 years: Initial: 50-125 mg/day given at bedtime; increase by 50-125 mg/day increments every 3-7 days; usual dose: 10-25 mg/kg/day in divided doses 3-4 times/day

Children >8 years and Adults: Initial: 125-250 mg/day at bedtime; increase by 125-250 mg/day every 3-7 days; usual dose: 750-1500 mg/day in divided doses 3-4 times/day with maximum dosage of 2 g/day

**Mechanism of Action** Decreases neuron excitability, raises seizure threshold similar to phenobarbital; primidone has two active metabolites, phenobarbital and phenylethylmalonamide (PEMA); PEMA may enhance the activity of phenobarbital

**Local Anesthetic/Vasoconstrictor Precautions** No information available to require special precautions

**Effects on Dental Treatment** No effects or complications reported

**Other Adverse Effects**

>10%: Central nervous system: Drowsiness, vertigo, ataxia, lethargy, behavior change, sedation, headache

1% to 10%:

Gastrointestinal: Nausea, vomiting, anorexia

Genitourinary: Impotence

<1%:

Dermatologic: Rash

Hematologic: Leukopenia, malignant lymphoma-like syndrome, megaloblastic anemia

Ocular: Diplopia, nystagmus

Miscellaneous: Systemic lupus-like syndrome

**Drug Interactions**

Decreased effect: Primidone may decrease serum concentrations of ethosuximide, valproic acid, griseofulvin; phenytoin may decrease primidone serum concentrations

Increased toxicity: Methylphenidate may increase primidone serum concentrations; valproic acid may increase phenobarbital concentrations derived from primidone

**Drug Uptake**

Serum half-life (age dependent):

Primidone: 10-12 hours

PEMA: 16 hours

Phenobarbital: 52-118 hours

Time to peak serum concentration: Oral: Within 4 hours

**Pregnancy Risk Factor** D

**Generic Available** Yes: Tablet

- ♦ **Principen®** *see* Ampicillin *on page 81*
- ♦ **Prinivil®** *see* Lisinopril *on page 594*
- ♦ **Prinzide®** *see* Lisinopril and Hydrochlorothiazide *on page 596*
- ♦ **Priscoline®** *see* Tolazoline *on page 993*
- ♦ **Privine® Nasal [OTC]** *see* Naphazoline *on page 703*
- ♦ **ProAmatine®** *see* Midodrine *on page 675*
- ♦ **Probalan®** *see* Probenecid *on this page*
- ♦ **Probampacin®** *see* Ampicillin and Probenecid *on page 82*
- ♦ **Pro-Banthine®** *see* Propantheline *on page 851*

## Probenecid (proe BEN e sid)

**Related Information**

Dental Drug Interactions: Update on Drug Combinations Requiring Special Considerations *on page 1225*

**U.S. Brand Names** Benemid®; Probalan®

**Canadian Brand Names** Benuryl™

**Therapeutic Category** Adjuvant Therapy, Penicillin Level Prolongation; Uric Acid Lowering Agent

**Use** Prevention of gouty arthritis; hyperuricemia; prolongation of beta-lactam effect (ie, serum levels)

**Usual Dosage** Oral:

Children:

<2 years: Not recommended

2-14 years: Prolong penicillin serum levels: 25 mg/kg starting dose, then 40 mg/kg/day given 4 times/day

Gonorrhea: <45 kg: 25 mg/kg x 1 (maximum: 1 g/dose) 30 minutes before penicillin, ampicillin or amoxicillin

Adults:

Hyperuricemia with gout: 250 mg twice daily for one week; increase to 250-500 mg/day; may increase by 500 mg/month, if needed, to maximum of 2-3 g/day (dosages may be increased by 500 mg every 6 months if serum urate concentrations are controlled)

Prolong penicillin serum levels: 500 mg 4 times/day

Gonorrhea: 1 g 30 minutes before penicillin, ampicillin or amoxicillin

**Mechanism of Action** Competitively inhibits the reabsorption of uric acid at the proximal convoluted tubule, thereby promoting its excretion and reducing serum uric acid levels; increases plasma levels of weak organic acids (penicillins, cephalosporins, or other beta-lactam antibiotics) by competitively inhibiting their renal tubular secretion

**Local Anesthetic/Vasoconstrictor Precautions** No information available to require special precautions

**Effects on Dental Treatment** No effects or complications reported

**Other Adverse Effects**

>10%:

Central nervous system: Headache

Gastrointestinal: Anorexia, nausea, vomiting

Neuromuscular & skeletal: Gouty arthritis (acute)

1% to 10%:

Central nervous system: Dizziness

Cardiovascular: Flushing of face

Dermatologic: Skin rash, itching

Gastrointestinal: Sore gums

Genitourinary: Painful urination

Renal: Renal calculi

<1%:

Hematologic: Leukopenia, hemolytic anemia, aplastic anemia

Hepatic: Hepatic necrosis

Renal: Urate nephropathy, nephrotic syndrome

Miscellaneous: Anaphylaxis

(Continued)

## Probenecid *(Continued)*

**Drug Interactions**

Decreased effect:

Salicylates (high dose) cause decreased uricosuria

Decreased urinary levels of nitrofurantoin cause decreased efficacy

Increased toxicity:

Increased methotrexate toxic potential

Increased penicillin and cephalosporin (beta-lactam) serum levels

Increased toxicity of acyclovir, thiopental, benzodiazepines, dapsone, sulfonylureas, zidovudine

**Drug Uptake**

Onset of action: Effect on penicillin levels reached in about 2 hours

Absorption: Rapid and complete from GI tract

Serum half-life: Normal renal function: 6-12 hours and is dose dependent

Time to peak serum concentration: 2-4 hours

**Pregnancy Risk Factor** B

**Generic Available** Yes

♦ **Probenecid and Colchicine** *see* Colchicine and Probenecid *on page 274*

## Probucol (PROE byoo kole)

**Related Information**

Cardiovascular Diseases *on page 1066*

**U.S. Brand Names** Lorelco®

**Therapeutic Category** Lipid Lowering Drugs

**Use** Adjunct to dietary therapy to decrease elevated serum total and LDL cholesterol concentrations in primary hypercholesterolemia

**Usual Dosage** Oral:

Children:

<27 kg: 250 mg twice daily with meals

>27 kg: 500 mg twice daily with meals

Adults: 500 mg twice daily administered with the morning and evening meals

**Mechanism of Action** Increases the fecal loss of bile acid-bound low density lipoprotein cholesterol, decreases the synthesis of cholesterol and inhibits enteral cholesterol absorption

**Local Anesthetic/Vasoconstrictor Precautions** No information available to require special precautions

**Effects on Dental Treatment** No effects or complications reported

**Other Adverse Effects**

>10%:

Cardiovascular: Q-T prolongation, serious arrhythmias

Gastrointestinal: Bloating, diarrhea, stomach pain, nausea, vomiting

1% to 10%:

Central nervous system: Dizziness, headache

Neuromuscular & skeletal: Paresthesia

<1%:

Cardiovascular: Tachycardia

Hematologic: Anemia, thrombocytopenia

**Drug Interactions** Increased toxicity: Drugs that prolong the Q-T interval (eg, tricyclic antidepressants, some antiarrhythmic agents, phenothiazines) or with drugs that affect the atrial rate (eg, beta-adrenergic blocking agents) or that can cause A-V block (eg, digoxin)

**Pregnancy Risk Factor** B

**Generic Available** No

## Procainamide (proe kane A mide)

**Related Information**

Cardiovascular Diseases *on page 1066*

**U.S. Brand Names** Procanbid™; Pronestyl®

**Canadian Brand Names** Apo®-Procainamide

**Therapeutic Category** Antiarrhythmic Agent, Class I-A; Antiarrhythmic Agent (Supraventricular & Ventricular)

**Use** Treatment of ventricular tachycardia, premature ventricular contractions, paroxysmal atrial tachycardia, and atrial fibrillation; to prevent recurrence of ventricular tachycardia, paroxysmal supraventricular tachycardia, atrial fibrillation or flutter

**Usual Dosage** Must be titrated to patient's response

Children:

Oral: 15-50 mg/kg/24 hours divided every 3-6 hours; maximum: 4 g/24 hours

I.M.: 20-30 mg/kg/24 hours divided every 4-6 hours in divided doses; maximum: 4 g/24 hours

I.V. (infusion requires use of an infusion pump):
Load: 3-6 mg/kg/dose over 5 minutes not to exceed 100 mg/dose; may repeat every 5-10 minutes to maximum of 15 mg/kg/load
Maintenance as continuous I.V. infusion: 20-80 mcg/kg/minute; maximum: 2 g/24 hours

Adults:
Oral: 250-500 mg/dose every 3-6 hours or 500 mg to 1 g every 6 hours sustained release; usual dose: 50 mg/kg/24 hours; maximum: 4 g/24 hours
I.M.: 0.5-1 g every 4-8 hours until oral therapy is possible
I.V. (infusion requires use of an infusion pump): Loading dose: 15-18 mg/kg administered as slow infusion over 25-30 minutes or 100-200 mg/dose repeated every 5 minutes as needed to a total dose of 1 g; maintenance dose: 1-6 mg/minute by continuous infusion
Infusion rate: 2 g/250 mL $D_5W$/NS (I.V. infusion requires use of an infusion pump):
1 mg/minute: 7 mL/hour
2 mg/minute: 15 mL/hour
3 mg/minute: 21 mL/hour
4 mg/minute: 30 mL/hour
5 mg/minute: 38 mL/hour
6 mg/minute: 45 mL/hour
Refractory ventricular fibrillation: 30 mg/minute, up to a total of 17 mg/kg; I.V. maintenance infusion: 1-4 mg/minute; monitor levels and do not exceed 3 mg/minute for >24 hours in adults with renal failure
ACLS guidelines: I.V.: Infuse 20 mg/minute until arrhythmia is controlled, hypotension occurs, QRS complex widens by 50% of its original width, or total of 17 mg/kg is given

**Mechanism of Action** Decreases myocardial excitability and conduction velocity and may depress myocardial contractility, by increasing the electrical stimulation threshold of ventricle, HIS-Purkinje system and through direct cardiac effects

**Local Anesthetic/Vasoconstrictor Precautions** No information available to require special precautions

**Effects on Dental Treatment** No effects or complications reported

**Other Adverse Effects**
>10%: Miscellaneous: SLE-like syndrome
1% to 10%:
Cardiovascular: Tachycardia, arrhythmias, A-V block, Q-T prolongation, widening QRS complex
Central nervous system: Dizziness, lightheadedness
Gastrointestinal: Diarrhea
<1%:
Cardiovascular: Hypotension
Central nervous system: Confusion, hallucinations, mental depression, confusion, disorientation, drug fever
Dermatologic: Rash
Gastrointestinal: Nausea, vomiting, GI complaints
Hematologic: Hemolytic anemia, agranulocytosis, neutropenia, thrombocytopenia, positive Coombs' test
Neuromuscular & skeletal: Arthralgia, myalgia
Respiratory: Pleural effusion

**Drug Interactions**
Increased plasma procainamide and procainamide metabolite concentrations with cimetidine, ranitidine, beta-blockers, and amiodarone
Increased effect of skeletal muscle relaxants, quinidine and lidocaine and neuromuscular blockers (succinylcholine)
Increased procainamide metabolite levels/toxicity with trimethoprim

**Drug Uptake**
Onset of action: I.M. 10-30 minutes
Serum half-life:
Procainamide: (Dependent upon hepatic acetylator, phenotype, cardiac function, and renal function):
Adults: 2.5-4.7 hours
Anephric: 11 hours
NAPA: (Dependent upon renal function):
Children: 6 hours
Adults: 6-8 hours
Anephric: 42 hours
Time to peak serum concentration:
Capsule: Within 45 minutes to 2.5 hours
I.M.: 15-60 minutes

**Pregnancy Risk Factor** C

**Generic Available** Yes

## Procaine (PROE kane)

**Related Information**

Oral Pain *on page 1122*

**U.S. Brand Names** Novocain®

**Therapeutic Category** Local Anesthetic, Injectable

**Use** Produces spinal anesthesia and epidural and peripheral nerve block by injection and infiltration methods

**Usual Dosage** Dose varies with procedure, desired depth, and duration of anesthesia, desired muscle relaxation, vascularity of tissues, physical condition, and age of patient

**Mechanism of Action** Blocks both the initiation and conduction of nerve impulses by decreasing the neuronal membrane's permeability to sodium ions, which results in inhibition of depolarization with resultant blockade of conduction

**Local Anesthetic/Vasoconstrictor Precautions** No information available to require special precautions

**Effects on Dental Treatment** This is no longer a useful anesthetic in dentistry because of high incidence of allergic reactions

**Other Adverse Effects**

1% to 10%: Local: Burning sensation at site of injection, pain, tissue irritation

<1%:

- Central nervous system: Aseptic meningitis resulting in paralysis can occur, CNS stimulation followed by CNS depression, chills
- Dermatologic: Skin discoloration
- Gastrointestinal: Nausea, vomiting
- Ocular: Miosis
- Otic: Tinnitus
- Miscellaneous: Anaphylactoid reaction

**Drug Interactions**

Decreased effect of sulfonamides with the PABA metabolite of procaine, chloroprocaine, and tetracaine

Decreased/increased effect of vasopressors, ergot alkaloids, and MAO inhibitors on blood pressure when using anesthetic solutions with a vasoconstrictor

**Drug Uptake**

Onset of effect: Injection: Within 2-5 minutes

Duration: 0.5-1.5 hours (dependent upon patient, type of block, concentration, and method of anesthesia)

Serum half-life: 7.7 minutes

**Pregnancy Risk Factor** C

**Dosage Forms** Injection, as hydrochloride: 1% [10 mg/mL] (2 mL, 6 mL, 30 mL, 100 mL); 2% [20 mg/mL] (30 mL, 100 mL); 10% (2 mL)

**Generic Available** Yes

♦ **Pro-Cal-Sof® [OTC]** *see* Docusate *on page 346*

♦ **Procanbid™** *see* Procainamide *on page 840*

## Procarbazine (proe KAR ba zeen)

**U.S. Brand Names** Matulane®

**Therapeutic Category** Antineoplastic Agent, Miscellaneous

**Synonyms** Benzmethyzin; N-Methylhydrazine; Procarbazine Hydrochloride

**Use** Treatment of Hodgkin's disease, non-Hodgkin's lymphoma, brain tumor, bronchogenic carcinoma

**Usual Dosage** Refer to individual protocols

Oral (dose based on patients ideal weight if the patients has abnormal fluid retention):

Children:

- BMT aplastic anemia conditioning regimen: 12.5 mg/kg/dose every other day for 4 doses
- Hodgkin's disease: MOPP/IC-MOPP regimens: 100 mg/m²/day for 14 days and repeated every 4 weeks
- Neuroblastoma and medulloblastoma: Doses as high as 100-200 mg/m²/day once daily have been used

Adults: Initial: 2-4 mg/kg/day in single or divided doses for 7 days then increase dose to 4-6 mg/kg/day until response is obtained or leukocyte count decreased <4000/mm³ or the platelet count decreased <100,000/mm³; maintenance: 1-2 mg/kg/day

In MOPP, 100 mg/m²/day on days 1-14 of a 28-day cycle

**Mechanism of Action** Mechanism of action is not clear, methylating of nucleic acids; inhibits DNA, RNA, and protein synthesis; may damage DNA directly and suppresses mitosis; metabolic activation required by host

**Local Anesthetic/Vasoconstrictor Precautions** No information available to require special precautions

**Effects on Dental Treatment** No effects or complications reported

**Other Adverse Effects**

>10%:

Central nervous system: Mental depression, manic reactions, hallucinations, dizziness, headache, nervousness, insomnia, nightmares, ataxia, foot drop, confusion, and seizures

Endocrine & metabolic: Amenorrhea

Gastrointestinal: Severe nausea and vomiting occur frequently and may be dose-limiting; anorexia, abdominal pain, stomatitis, dysphagia, diarrhea, and constipation; use a nonphenothiazine antiemetic, when possible

Emetic potential: Moderately high (60% to 90%)

Hematologic: May be dose-limiting toxicity; procarbazine should be discontinued if leukocyte count is $<4000/mm^3$ or platelet count $<100,000/mm^3$

Neuromuscular & skeletal: Paresthesia, neuropathies, disorientation, decreased reflexes, tremors

Ocular: Nystagmus

Respiratory: Pleural effusion, cough

1% to 10%:

Dermatologic: Alopecia, hyperpigmentation

Hepatic: Hepatotoxicity

<1%:

Cardiovascular: Hypotension (orthostatic), hypertensive crisis

Central nervous system: Irritability, somnolence

Dermatologic: Dermatitis, hypersensitivity rash, pruritus

Endocrine & metabolic: Cessation of menses, disulfiram-like reaction of alcohol

Hepatic: Jaundice

Neuromuscular & skeletal: Arthralgia, myalgia

Ocular: Diplopia, photophobia

Respiratory: Pneumonitis, hoarseness

Miscellaneous: Flu-like syndrome, secondary malignancy, allergic reactions

**Drug Uptake**

Absorption: Oral: Rapid and complete

Serum half-life: 1 hour

**Pregnancy Risk Factor** D

**Generic Available** No

- **Procarbazine Hydrochloride** *see* Procarbazine *on previous page*
- **Procardia®** *see* Nifedipine *on page 720*
- **Procardia XL®** *see* Nifedipine *on page 720*

## Prochlorperazine (proe klor PER a zeen)

**U.S. Brand Names** Compazine®

**Canadian Brand Names** Nu-Prochlor; PMS-Prochlorperazine; Prorazin®; Stemetil®

**Therapeutic Category** Antiemetic; Antipsychotic Agent; Phenothiazine Derivative

**Use** Management of nausea and vomiting; acute and chronic psychosis

**Usual Dosage**

Antiemetic: Children:

Oral, rectal:

>10 kg: 0.4 mg/kg/24 hours in 3-4 divided doses; **or**

9-14 kg: 2.5 mg every 12-24 hours as needed; maximum: 7.5 mg/day

14-18 kg: 2.5 mg every 8-12 hours as needed; maximum: 10 mg/day

18-39 kg: 2.5 mg every 8 hours or 5 mg every 12 hours as needed; maximum: 15 mg/day

I.M.: 0.1-0.15 mg/kg/dose; usual: 0.13 mg/kg/dose; change to oral as soon as possible

I.V.: Not recommended in children <10 kg or <2 years

Antiemetic: Adults:

Oral: 5-10 mg 3-4 times/day; usual maximum: 40 mg/day

I.M.: 5-10 mg every 3-4 hours; usual maximum: 40 mg/day

I.V.: 2.5-10 mg; maximum 10 mg/dose or 40 mg/day; may repeat dose every 3-4 hours as needed

Rectal: 25 mg twice daily

Antipsychotic:

Children 2-12 years:

Oral, rectal: 2.5 mg 2-3 times/day; increase dosage as needed to maximum daily dose of 20 mg for 2-5 years and 25 mg for 6-12 years

I.M.: 0.13 mg/kg/dose; change to oral as soon as possible

Adults:

Oral: 5-10 mg 3-4 times/day; doses up to 150 mg/day may be required in some patients for treatment of severe disturbances

(Continued)

## Prochlorperazine *(Continued)*

I.M.: 10-20 mg every 4-6 hours may be required in some patients for treatment of severe disturbances; change to oral as soon as possible

Dementia behavior (nonpsychotic): Elderly: Initial: 2.5-5 mg 1-2 times/day; increase dose at 4- to 7-day intervals by 2.5-5 mg/day; increase dosing intervals (twice daily, 3 times/day, etc) as necessary to control response or side effects; maximum daily dose should probably not exceed 75 mg in elderly; gradual increases (titration) may prevent some side effects or decrease their severity

**Mechanism of Action** Blocks postsynaptic mesolimbic dopaminergic $D_1$ and $D_2$ receptors in the brain, including the medullary chemoreceptor trigger zone; exhibits a strong alpha-adrenergic and anticholinergic blocking effect and depresses the release of hypothalamic and hypophyseal hormones; believed to depress the reticular activating system, thus affecting basal metabolism, body temperature, wakefulness, vasomotor tone and emesis

**Local Anesthetic/Vasoconstrictor Precautions** Most pharmacology textbooks state that in presence of phenothiazines, systemic doses of epinephrine paradoxically decrease the blood pressure. This is the so called "epinephrine reversal" phenomenon. This has never been observed when epinephrine is given by infiltration as part of the anesthesia procedure.

**Effects on Dental Treatment** >10% of patients experience dry mouth

Significant hypotension may occur especially when the drug is administered parenterally; orthostatic hypotension is due to alpha-receptor blockade, the elderly are at greater risk for orthostatic hypotension

Tardive dyskinesia: Prevalence rate may be 40% in elderly; development of the syndrome and the irreversible nature are proportional to duration and total cumulative dose over time

Extrapyramidal reactions are more common in elderly with up to 50% developing these reactions after 60 years of age; drug-induced **Parkinson's syndrome** occurs often; **Akathisia** is the most common extrapyramidal reaction in elderly

Increased confusion, memory loss, psychotic behavior, and agitation frequently occur as a consequence of anticholinergic effects

Antipsychotic associated sedation in nonpsychotic patients is extremely unpleasant due to feelings of depersonalization, derealization, and dysphoria

**Other Adverse Effects** Incidence of extrapyramidal reactions are higher with prochlorperazine than chlorpromazine

Central nervous system: Sedation, drowsiness, restlessness, anxiety, extrapyramidal reactions, parkinsonian signs and symptoms, seizures, altered central temperature regulation

Dermatologic: Photosensitivity, hyperpigmentation, pruritus, rash

Endocrine & metabolic: Amenorrhea, gynecomastia

Miscellaneous: Anaphylactoid reactions

>10%:

- Cardiovascular: Hypotension (especially with I.V. use), orthostatic hypotension, tachycardia, arrhythmias
- Central nervous system: Pseudoparkinsonism, akathisia, tardive dyskinesia (persistent), dizziness, dystonias
- Gastrointestinal: Constipation
- Genitourinary: Urinary retention
- Ocular: Pigmentary retinopathy, blurred vision
- Respiratory: Nasal congestion
- Miscellaneous: Decreased sweating

1% to 10%:

- Dermatologic: Skin rash
- Endocrine & metabolic: Changes in menstrual cycle pain in breasts, changes in libido
- Gastrointestinal: Weight gain, nausea, vomiting, stomach pain
- Genitourinary: Dysuria, ejaculatory disturbances
- Neuromuscular & skeletal: Trembling of fingers

<1%:

- Central nervous system: Neuroleptic malignant syndrome (NMS), impairment of temperature regulation lowering of seizures threshold
- Dermatologic: Discoloration of skin (blue-gray)
- Endocrine & metabolic: Galactorrhea
- Genitourinary: Priapism
- Hematologic: Agranulocytosis, leukopenia, thrombocytopenia
- Hepatic: Cholestatic jaundice, hepatotoxicity
- Ocular: Cornea and lens changes, pigmentary retinopathy

**Drug Interactions** Increased toxicity: Additive effects with other CNS depressants

**Drug Uptake**

Onset of effect:

Oral: Within 30-40 minutes

I.M.: Within 10-20 minutes

Rectal: Within 60 minutes

Duration: Persists longest with I.M. and oral extended-release doses (12 hours); shortest following rectal and immediate release oral administration (3-4 hours)

Serum half-life: 23 hours

**Pregnancy Risk Factor** C

**Generic Available** Yes

- **Procrit®** *see* Epoetin Alfa *on page 376*
- **Proctofoam®-HC** *see* Pramoxine and Hydrocortisone *on page 828*
- **ProctoFoam® NS [OTC]** *see* Pramoxine *on page 828*

## Procyclidine (proe SYE kli deen)

**U.S. Brand Names** Kemadrin®

**Canadian Brand Names** PMS-Procyclidine; Procyclid

**Therapeutic Category** Anticholinergic Agent; Anti-Parkinson's Agent

**Use** Relieves symptoms of parkinsonian syndrome and drug-induced extrapyramidal symptoms

**Usual Dosage** Adults: Oral: 2.5 mg 3 times/day after meals; if tolerated, gradually increase dose, maximum of 20 mg/day if necessary

**Mechanism of Action** Thought to act by blocking excess acetylcholine at cerebral synapses; many of its effects are due to its pharmacologic similarities with atropine

**Local Anesthetic/Vasoconstrictor Precautions** No information available to require special precautions

**Effects on Dental Treatment** >10% of patients experience dry mouth; prolonged use of antidyskinetics may decrease or inhibit salivary flow and could contribute to development of periodontal disease, oral candidiasis or discomfort

**Other Adverse Effects**

>10%:

Dermatologic: Dry skin

Gastrointestinal: Constipation

Respiratory: Dry nose, throat

Miscellaneous: Decreased sweating

1% to 10%:

Dermatologic: Photosensitivity

Endocrine & metabolic: Decreased flow of breast milk

Gastrointestinal: Dysphagia

<1%:

Cardiovascular: Orthostatic hypotension, ventricular fibrillation, tachycardia, palpitations

Central nervous system: Confusion, drowsiness, headache, loss of memory, fatigue, ataxia

Dermatologic: Skin rash

Gastrointestinal: Bloated feeling, nausea, vomiting

Genitourinary: Dysuria

Neuromuscular & skeletal: Weakness

Ocular: Increased intraocular pain, blurred vision

**Drug Interactions**

Decreased effect of psychotropics

Increased toxicity with phenothiazines, meperidine, TCAs

**Drug Uptake**

Onset of effect: Oral: Within 30-40 minutes

Duration: 4-6 hours

**Pregnancy Risk Factor** C

**Generic Available** No

- **Products for Xerostomia** *on page 1260*
- **Profasi® HP** *see* Chorionic Gonadotropin *on page 246*
- **Profenal®** *see* Suprofen *on page 949*
- **Profen II®** *see* Guaifenesin and Phenylpropanolamine *on page 480*
- **Profen LA®** *see* Guaifenesin and Phenylpropanolamine *on page 480*
- **Profilate® OSD** *see* Antihemophilic Factor (Human) *on page 89*
- **Profilate® SD** *see* Antihemophilic Factor (Human) *on page 89*
- **Profilnine® Heat-Treated** *see* Factor IX Complex (Human) *on page 417*
- **Progestasert®** *see* Progesterone *on next page*

## Progesterone (proe JES ter one)

**U.S. Brand Names** Crinone™ Vaginal Gel; Progestasert®; Prometrium®

**Canadian Brand Names** PMS-Progesterone; Progesterone Oil

**Therapeutic Category** Progestin

**Use** Intrauterine contraception in women who have had at least 1 child, are in a stable, mutually monogamous relationship, and have no history of pelvic inflammatory disease; amenorrhea; functional uterine bleeding; prevention of endometrial hyperplasia in nonhysterectomized postmenopausal women who are receiving conjugated estrogen tablets

**Usual Dosage** Adults: Female: Insert a single system into the uterine cavity; contraceptive effectiveness is retained for 1 year and system must be replaced 1 year after insertion

**Mechanism of Action** Natural steroid hormone that induces secretory changes in the endometrium, promotes mammary gland development, relaxes uterine smooth muscle, blocks follicular maturation and ovulation, and maintains pregnancy

**Local Anesthetic/Vasoconstrictor Precautions** No information available to require special precautions

**Effects on Dental Treatment** Progestins may predispose the patient to gingival bleeding

**Other Adverse Effects**

>10%:
- Cardiovascular: Edema
- Endocrine & metabolic: Breakthrough bleeding, spotting, changes in menstrual flow, amenorrhea
- Gastrointestinal: Anorexia
- Local: Pain at injection site
- Neuromuscular & skeletal: Weakness

1% to 10%:
- Cardiovascular: Embolism, central thrombosis
- Central nervous system: Mental depression, fever, insomnia
- Dermatologic: Melasma or chloasma, allergic rash with or without pruritus
- Endocrine: Changes in cervical erosion and secretions, increased breast tenderness
- Gastrointestinal: Weight gain or loss
- Hepatic: Cholestatic jaundice
- Local: Thrombophlebitis

**Drug Interactions** Decreased effect: Aminoglutethimide may decrease effect by increasing hepatic metabolism

**Drug Uptake**
- Duration of action: 24 hours
- Serum half-life: 5 minutes

**Pregnancy Risk Factor** X

**Generic Available** Yes


- ♦ **Proglycem®** *see* Diazoxide *on page 317*
- ♦ **Prograf®** *see* Tacrolimus *on page 951*
- ♦ **ProHIBiT®** *see Haemophilus* b Conjugate Vaccine *on page 486*
- ♦ **Prolastin® Injection** *see* Alpha$_1$-Proteinase Inhibitor *on page 49*
- ♦ **Proleukin®** *see* Aldesleukin *on page 44*
- ♦ **Prolixin®** *see* Fluphenazine *on page 446*
- ♦ **Prolixin Decanoate®** *see* Fluphenazine *on page 446*
- ♦ **Prolixin Enanthate®** *see* Fluphenazine *on page 446*
- ♦ **Proloprim®** *see* Trimethoprim *on page 1021*


## Promazine (PROE ma zeen)

**U.S. Brand Names** Sparine®

**Therapeutic Category** Antipsychotic Agent; Phenothiazine Derivative

**Use** Management of manifestations of psychotic disorders; depressive neurosis; alcohol withdrawal; nausea and vomiting; nonpsychotic symptoms associated with dementia in elderly, Tourette's syndrome; Huntington's chorea; spasmodic torticollis and Reye's syndrome

**Usual Dosage** Oral, I.M.:
- Children >12 years: Antipsychotic: 10-25 mg every 4-6 hours
- Adults:
  - Psychosis: 10-200 mg every 4-6 hours not to exceed 1000 mg/day
  - Antiemetic: 25-50 mg every 4-6 hours as needed

**Mechanism of Action** Blocks postsynaptic mesolimbic dopaminergic $D_1$ and $D_2$ receptors in the brain; exhibits a strong alpha-adrenergic blocking and anticholinergic effect, depresses the release of hypothalamic and hypophyseal hormones;

believed to depress the reticular activating system thus affecting basal metabolism, body temperature, wakefulness, vasomotor tone, and emesis

**Local Anesthetic/Vasoconstrictor Precautions** Most pharmacology textbooks state that in presence of phenothiazines, systemic doses of epinephrine paradoxically decrease the blood pressure. This is the so called "epinephrine reversal" phenomenon. This has never been observed when epinephrine is given by infiltration as part of the anesthesia procedure.

**Effects on Dental Treatment** Significant hypotension may occur, especially when the drug is administered parenterally; orthostatic hypotension is due to alpha-receptor blockade, the elderly are at greater risk for orthostatic hypotension

Tardive dyskinesia: Prevalence rate may be 40% in elderly; development of the syndrome and the irreversible nature are proportional to duration and total cumulative dose over time

Extrapyramidal reactions are more common in elderly with up to 50% developing these reactions after 60 years of age; drug-induced **Parkinson's syndrome** occurs often; **Akathisia** is the most common extrapyramidal reaction in elderly

Increased confusion, memory loss, psychotic behavior, and agitation frequently occur as a consequence of anticholinergic effects

Antipsychotic associated sedation in nonpsychotic patients is extremely unpleasant due to feelings of depersonalization, derealization, and dysphoria

**Other Adverse Effects**

>10%:

- Cardiovascular: Hypotension, orthostatic hypotension
- Central nervous system: Pseudoparkinsonism, akathisia, dystonias, tardive dyskinesia (persistent), dizziness
- Gastrointestinal: Constipation
- Ocular: Pigmentary retinopathy
- Respiratory: Nasal congestion
- Miscellaneous: Decreased sweating

1% to 10%:

- Dermatologic: Photosensitivity, skin rash
- Endocrine & metabolic: Changes in menstrual cycle, changes in libido, pain in breasts
- Gastrointestinal: Weight gain, nausea, vomiting, stomach pain
- Genitourinary: Dysuria, ejaculatory disturbances
- Neuromuscular & skeletal: Trembling of fingers

<1%:

- Central nervous system: Neuroleptic malignant syndrome (NMS), impairment of temperature regulation, lowering of seizures threshold
- Dermatologic: Discoloration of skin (blue-gray)
- Endocrine & metabolic: Galactorrhea
- Genitourinary: Priapism
- Hematologic: Agranulocytosis, leukopenia
- Hepatic: Cholestatic jaundice, hepatotoxicity
- Ocular: Cornea and lens changes

**Drug Interactions** Increased toxicity: Additive effects with other CNS depressants

**Drug Uptake** The specific pharmacokinetics of promazine are poorly established but probably resemble those of other phenothiazines.

Serum half-life: Most phenothiazines have long half-lives in the range of 24 hours or more

**Pregnancy Risk Factor** C

**Generic Available** Yes: Injection only

♦ **Prometa®** *see* Metaproterenol *on page 642*

## Promethazine (proe METH a zeen)

**U.S. Brand Names** Anergan®; Phenazine®; Phenergan®; Prorex®

**Therapeutic Category** Antiemetic; Antihistamine; Phenothiazine Derivative; Sedative

**Use** Symptomatic treatment of various allergic conditions, antiemetic, motion sickness, and as a sedative

**Usual Dosage**

Children:

- Antihistamine: Oral, rectal: 0.1 mg/kg/dose every 6 hours during the day and 0.5 mg/kg/dose at bedtime as needed
- Antiemetic: Oral, I.M., I.V., rectal: 0.25-1 mg/kg 4-6 times/day as needed
- Motion sickness: Oral, rectal: 0.5 mg/kg/dose 30 minutes to 1 hour before departure, then every 12 hours as needed
- Sedation: Oral, I.M., I.V., rectal: 0.5-1 mg/kg/dose every 6 hours as needed

(Continued)

## Promethazine *(Continued)*

Adults:
- Antihistamine (including allergic reactions to blood or plasma):
  - Oral, rectal: 12.5 mg 3 times/day and 25 mg at bedtime
  - I.M., I.V.: 25 mg, may repeat in 2 hours when necessary; switch to oral route as soon as feasible
- Antiemetic: Oral, I.M., I.V., rectal: 12.5-25 mg every 4 hours as needed
- Motion sickness: Oral, rectal: 25 mg 30-60 minutes before departure, then every 12 hours as needed
- Sedation: Oral, I.M., I.V., rectal: 25-50 mg/dose

**Mechanism of Action** Blocks postsynaptic mesolimbic dopaminergic receptors in the brain; exhibits a strong alpha-adrenergic blocking effect and depresses the release of hypothalamic and hypophyseal hormones; competes with histamine for the $H_1$-receptor; reduces stimuli to the brainstem reticular system

**Local Anesthetic/Vasoconstrictor Precautions** Most pharmacology textbooks state that in presence of phenothiazines, systemic doses of epinephrine paradoxically decrease the blood pressure. This is the so called "epinephrine reversal" phenomenon. This has never been observed when epinephrine is given by infiltration as part of the anesthesia procedure.

**Effects on Dental Treatment** Significant hypotension may occur, especially when the drug is administered parenterally; orthostatic hypotension is due to alpha-receptor blockade, the elderly are at greater risk for orthostatic hypotension

Tardive dyskinesia: Prevalence rate may be 40% in elderly; development of the syndrome and the irreversible nature are proportional to duration and total cumulative dose over time

Extrapyramidal reactions are more common in elderly with up to 50% developing these reactions after 60 years of age; drug-induced **Parkinson's syndrome** occurs often; **akathisia** is the most common extrapyramidal reaction in elderly

Increased confusion, memory loss, psychotic behavior, and agitation frequently occur as a consequence of anticholinergic effects

Antipsychotic associated sedation in nonpsychotic patients is extremely unpleasant due to feelings of depersonalization, derealization, and dysphoria

**Other Adverse Effects**
- Hematologic: Thrombocytopenia
- Hepatic: Jaundice

>10%:
- Central nervous system: Slight to moderate drowsiness
- Respiratory: Thickening of bronchial secretions

1% to 10%:
- Central nervous system: Headache, fatigue, nervousness, dizziness
- Gastrointestinal: Dry mouth, abdominal pain, nausea, diarrhea, appetite increase, weight gain
- Neuromuscular & skeletal: Arthralgia
- Respiratory: Pharyngitis

<1%:
- Cardiovascular: Tachycardia, bradycardia, palpitations, hypotension
- Central nervous system: Sedation (pronounced), confusion, excitation, extrapyramidal reactions with high doses, dystonia, faintness with I.V. administration, depression, insomnia, sedation (pronounced)
- Dermatologic: Photosensitivity, rash, angioedema
- Genitourinary: Urinary retention
- Hepatic: Hepatitis
- Neuromuscular & skeletal: Tremor, paresthesia, myalgia
- Ocular: Blurred vision
- Respiratory: Irregular respiration, bronchospasm, epistaxis
- Miscellaneous: Allergic reactions

**Drug Interactions** Increased toxicity: Additive effects with other CNS depressants

**Drug Uptake**
- Onset of effect: I.V.: Within 20 minutes (3-5 minutes with I.V. injection)
- Duration: 2-6 hours

**Pregnancy Risk Factor** C

**Generic Available** Yes

## Promethazine and Codeine (proe METH a zeen & KOE deen)

**U.S. Brand Names** Phenergan® With Codeine; Pherazine® With Codeine; Prothazine-DC®

**Therapeutic Category** Antihistamine; Antitussive; Cough Preparation

**Use** Temporary relief of coughs and upper respiratory symptoms associated with allergy or the common cold

**Usual Dosage** Oral (in terms of codeine):

Children: 1-1.5 mg/kg/day every 4 hours as needed; maximum: 30 mg/day **or**

2-6 years: 1.25-2.5 mL every 4-6 hours or 2.5-5 mg/dose every 4-6 hours as needed; maximum: 30 mg codeine/day

6-12 years: 2.5-5 mL every 4-6 hours as needed or 5-10 mg/dose every 4-6 hours as needed; maximum: 60 mg codeine/day

Adults: 10-20 mg/dose every 4-6 hours as needed; maximum: 120 mg codeine/day; or 5-10 mL every 4-6 hours as needed

**Local Anesthetic/Vasoconstrictor Precautions** No information available to require special precautions

**Effects on Dental Treatment** Although promethazine is a phenothiazine derivative, extrapyramidal reactions or tardive dyskinesias are not seen with the use of this drug.

**Pregnancy Risk Factor** C

**Generic Available** Yes

## Promethazine and Dextromethorphan

(proe METH a zeen & deks troe meth OR fan)

**U.S. Brand Names** Phenameth® DM; Phenergan® with Dextromethorphan; Pherazine® w/DM

**Therapeutic Category** Antitussive; Cough Preparation

**Use** Temporary relief of coughs and upper respiratory symptoms associated with allergy or the common cold

**Usual Dosage** Oral:

Children:

2-6 years: 1.25-2.5 mL every 4-6 hours up to 10 mL in 24 hours

6-12 years: 2.5-5 mL every 4-6 hours up to 20 mL in 24 hours

Adults: 5 mL every 4-6 hours up to 30 mL in 24 hours

**Local Anesthetic/Vasoconstrictor Precautions** No information available to require special precautions

**Effects on Dental Treatment** Although promethazine is a phenothiazine derivative, extrapyramidal reactions or tardive dyskinesias are not seen with the use of this drug.

**Warnings/Precautions** Research on chicken embryos exposed to concentrations of dextromethorphan relative to those typically taken by humans has shown to cause birth defects and fetal death; more study is needed, but it is suggested that pregnant women should be advised not to use dextromethorphan-containing medications

**Pregnancy Risk Factor** C (see Warnings)

**Generic Available** Yes

## Promethazine and Phenylephrine

(proe METH a zeen & fen il EF rin)

**U.S. Brand Names** Phenergan® VC Syrup; Promethazine VC Plain Syrup; Promethazine VC Syrup; Prometh VC Plain Liquid

**Therapeutic Category** Antihistamine/Decongestant Combination

**Use** Temporary relief of upper respiratory symptoms associated with allergy or the common cold

**Usual Dosage** Oral:

Children:

2-6 years: 1.25 mL every 4-6 hours, not to exceed 7.5 mL in 24 hours

6-12 years: 2.5 mL every 4-6 hours, not to exceed 15 mL in 24 hours

Children >12 years and Adults: 5 mL every 4-6 hours, not to exceed 30 mL in 24 hours

**Local Anesthetic/Vasoconstrictor Precautions**

Phenylephrine: Use with caution since phenylephrine is a sympathomimetic amine which could interact with epinephrine to cause a pressor response

Promethazine: No information available to require special precautions

**Effects on Dental Treatment**

Phenylephrine: Up to 10% of patients could experience tachycardia, palpitations, and dry mouth; use vasoconstrictor with caution

Although promethazine is a phenothiazine derivative, extrapyramidal reactions or tardive dyskinesias are not seen with the use of this drug.

**Pregnancy Risk Factor** C

**Generic Available** Yes

## Promethazine, Phenylephrine, and Codeine

(proe METH a zeen, fen il EF rin, & KOE deen)

**U.S. Brand Names** Para-Hist AT®; Phenergan® VC With Codeine; Pherazine® VC w/ Codeine; Promethist® with Codeine; Prometh® VC with Codeine

**Therapeutic Category** Antihistamine/Decongestant Combination; Antitussive; Cough Preparation

**Use** Temporary relief of coughs and upper respiratory symptoms including nasal congestion

**Usual Dosage** Oral:

Children (expressed in terms of codeine dosage): 1-1.5 mg/kg/day every 4 hours, maximum: 30 mg/day **or**

<2 years: Not recommended

2 to 6 years:

Weight 25 lb: 1.25-2.5 mL every 4-6 hours, not to exceed 6 mL/24 hours

Weight 30 lb: 1.25-2.5 mL every 4-6 hours, not to exceed 7 mL/24 hours

Weight 35 lb: 1.25-2.5 mL every 4-6 hours, not to exceed 8 mL/24 hours

Weight 40 lb: 1.25-2.5 mL every 4-6 hours, not to exceed 9 mL/24 hours

6 to <12 years: 2.5-5 mL every 4-6 hours, not to exceed 15 mL/24 hours

Adults: 5 mL every 4-6 hours, not to exceed 30 mL/24 hours

**Local Anesthetic/Vasoconstrictor Precautions**

Phenylephrine: Use with caution since phenylephrine is a sympathomimetic amine which could interact with epinephrine to cause a pressor response

Promethazine: No information available to require special precautions

**Effects on Dental Treatment**

Phenylephrine: Up to 10% of patients could experience tachycardia, palpitations, and dry mouth; use vasoconstrictor with caution

Although promethazine is a phenothiazine derivative, extrapyramidal reactions or tardive dyskinesias are not seen with the use of this drug.

**Pregnancy Risk Factor** C

**Generic Available** Yes

- **Promethazine VC Plain Syrup** *see* Promethazine and Phenylephrine *on previous page*
- **Promethazine VC Syrup** *see* Promethazine and Phenylephrine *on previous page*
- **Promethist® with Codeine** *see* Promethazine, Phenylephrine, and Codeine *on this page*
- **Prometh VC Plain Liquid** *see* Promethazine and Phenylephrine *on previous page*
- **Prometh® VC with Codeine** *see* Promethazine, Phenylephrine, and Codeine *on this page*
- **Prometrium®** *see* Progesterone *on page 846*
- **Promit®** *see* Dextran 1 *on page 311*
- **Pronestyl®** *see* Procainamide *on page 840*
- **Pronto® Shampoo [OTC]** *see* Pyrethrins *on page 867*
- **Propac™ [OTC]** *see* Enteral Nutritional Products *on page 371*
- **Propacet®** *see* Propoxyphene and Acetaminophen *on page 855*

## Propafenone (proe pa FEEN one)

**Related Information**

Cardiovascular Diseases *on page 1066*

**U.S. Brand Names** Rythmol®

**Therapeutic Category** Antiarrhythmic Agent, Class I-C; Antiarrhythmic Agent (Supraventricular & Ventricular)

**Use** Life-threatening ventricular arrhythmias

**Unlabeled use:** Supraventricular tachycardias, including those patients with Wolff-Parkinson-White syndrome

**Usual Dosage** Adults: Oral: 150 mg every 8 hours, increase at 3- to 4-day intervals up to 300 mg every 8 hours. **Note:** Patients who exhibit significant widening of QRS complex or second or third degree A-V block may need dose reduction.

**Mechanism of Action** Propafenone is a 1C antiarrhythmic agent which possesses local anesthetic properties, blocks the fast inward sodium current, and slows the rate of increase of the action potential. prolongs conduction and refractoriness in all areas of the myocardium, with a slightly more pronounced effect on intraventricular conduction; it prolongs effective refractory period, reduces spontaneous automaticity and exhibits some beta-blockade activity.

**Local Anesthetic/Vasoconstrictor Precautions** No information available to require special precautions

**Effects on Dental Treatment** >10% of patients experience significant dry mouth; normal salivary flow will resume with cessation of drug therapy

**Other Adverse Effects**

>10%: Central nervous system: Dizziness, drowsiness

1% to 10%:
- Cardiovascular: A-V block (first and second degree), cardiac conduction disturbances, palpitations, congestive heart failure, angina, bradycardia
- Central nervous system: Headache, anxiety, loss of balance
- Gastrointestinal: Dysgeusia, constipation, nausea, vomiting, abdominal pain, dyspepsia, anorexia, flatulence, diarrhea
- Ocular: Blurred vision
- Respiratory: Dyspnea

<1%:
- Cardiovascular: New or worsened arrhythmias (proarrhythmic effect), bundle branch block
- Central nervous system: Abnormal speech, vision, or dreams
- Hematologic: Leukopenia, thrombocytopenia, agranulocytosis
- Neuromuscular & skeletal: Paresthesia

**Drug Interactions**
- Decreased levels with rifampin
- Increased levels with cimetidine, quinidine, and beta-blockers
- Increased effect/levels of warfarin, beta-blockers metabolized by the liver, local anesthetics, cyclosporine, and digoxin (**Note:** Reduce dose of digoxin by 25%)

**Drug Uptake**
- Absorption: Well absorbed
- Serum half-life after a single dose (100-300 mg): 2-8 hours; half-life after chronic dosing ranges from 10-32 hours
- Time to peak: Peak levels occur in 2 hours with a 150 mg dose and 3 hours after a 300 mg dose; this agent exhibits nonlinear pharmacokinetics; when dose is increased from 300 mg to 900 mg/day, serum concentrations increase tenfold; this nonlinearity is thought to be due to saturable first-pass hepatic enzyme metabolism

**Pregnancy Risk Factor** C

**Generic Available** No

♦ **Propagest® [OTC]** *see* Phenylpropanolamine *on page 797*

## Propantheline (proe PAN the leen)

**U.S. Brand Names** Pro-Banthine®

**Therapeutic Category** Anticholinergic Agent; Antispasmodic Agent, Gastrointestinal

**Use**
- Dental: Induce dry field (xerostomia) in oral cavity
- Medical: Adjunctive treatment of peptic ulcer, irritable bowel syndrome, pancreatitis, ureteral and urinary bladder spasm; reduce duodenal motility during diagnostic radiologic procedures

**Usual Dosage** Adults: 15-30 mg as a single dose to induce xerostomia 1 hour before procedure

**Mechanism of Action** Competitively blocks the action of acetylcholine at postganglionic parasympathetic receptor sites

**Local Anesthetic/Vasoconstrictor Precautions** No information available to require special precautions

**Effects on Dental Treatment** Significant xerostomia in >10% of patients - (therapeutic effect)

**Other Adverse Effects**

>10%:
- Gastrointestinal: Constipation
- Miscellaneous: Decreased sweating

1% to 10%: Gastrointestinal: Dysphagia

**Contraindications** Narrow-angle glaucoma, known hypersensitivity to propantheline; ulcerative colitis; toxic megacolon; obstructive disease of the GI or urinary tract

**Warnings/Precautions** Use with caution in patients with hyperthyroidism, hepatic, cardiac, or renal disease, hypertension, GI infections, or other endocrine diseases

**Drug Interactions** Decreased effect with antacids (decreases absorption); decreased effect of sustained release dosage forms (decreases absorption); increased effect/toxicity with anticholinergics, disopyramide, narcotic analgesics, bretylium, type I antiarrhythmics, antihistamines, phenothiazines, TCAs, corticosteroids (increases intraocular pressure), CNS depressants (sedation), adenosine, amiodarone, beta-blockers, amoxapine

**Drug Uptake**
- Onset of effect: Oral: Within 30-45 minutes
- Duration: 4-6 hours
- Serum half-life: 1.6 hours (average)

**Pregnancy Risk Factor** C

(Continued)

## Propantheline *(Continued)*

**Breast-feeding Considerations** No data reported; however, atropine may be taken while breast-feeding

**Dosage Forms** Tablet, as bromide: 7.5 mg, 15 mg

**Dietary Considerations** Should be taken 30 minutes before meals so that the drug's peak effect occurs at the proper time

**Generic Available** Yes: 15 mg tablet

## Proparacaine (proe PAR a kane)

**U.S. Brand Names** AK-Taine®; Alcaine®; I-Paracaine®; Ophthetic®

**Therapeutic Category** Local Anesthetic, Ophthalmic

**Use** Anesthesia for tonometry, gonioscopy; suture removal from cornea; removal of corneal foreign body; cataract extraction, glaucoma surgery; short operative procedure involving the cornea and conjunctiva

**Usual Dosage** Children and Adults:

Ophthalmic surgery: Instill 1 drop of 0.5% solution in eye every 5-10 minutes for 5-7 doses

Tonometry, gonioscopy, suture removal: Instill 1-2 drops of 0.5% solution in eye just prior to procedure

**Mechanism of Action** Prevents initiation and transmission of impulse at the nerve cell membrane by decreasing ion permeability through stabilizing

**Local Anesthetic/Vasoconstrictor Precautions** No information available to require special precautions

**Effects on Dental Treatment** No effects or complications reported

**Other Adverse Effects**

1% to 10%: Local: Burning, stinging, redness

<1%:

- Cardiovascular: Arrhythmias
- Central nervous system: CNS depression
- Dermatologic: Allergic contact dermatitis
- Local: Irritation, sensitization
- Ocular: Lacrimation, keratitis, iritis, erosion of the corneal epithelium, conjunctival congestion and hemorrhage, corneal opacification, blurred vision
- Miscellaneous: Increased sweating

**Drug Interactions** Increased effect of phenylephrine, tropicamide

**Drug Uptake**

Onset of action: Within 20 seconds of instillation

Duration: 15-20 minutes

**Pregnancy Risk Factor** C

**Dosage Forms** Ophthalmic, solution, as hydrochloride: 0.5% (2 mL, 15 mL)

**Generic Available** Yes

## Proparacaine and Fluorescein

(proe PAR a kane & FLURE e seen)

**U.S. Brand Names** Fluoracaine® Ophthalmic

**Therapeutic Category** Diagnostic Agent, Ophthalmic Dye; Local Anesthetic, Ophthalmic

**Use** Anesthesia for tonometry, gonioscopy; suture removal from cornea; removal of corneal foreign body; cataract extraction, glaucoma surgery

**Usual Dosage**

Ophthalmic surgery: Children and Adults: Instill 1 drop in each eye every 5-10 minutes for 5-7 doses

Tonometry, gonioscopy, suture removal: Adults: Instill 1-2 drops in each eye just prior to procedure

**Mechanism of Action** Prevents initiation and transmission of impulse at the nerve cell membrane by decreasing ion permeability through stabilizing

**Local Anesthetic/Vasoconstrictor Precautions** No information available to require special precautions

**Effects on Dental Treatment** No effects or complications reported

**Other Adverse Effects**

1% to 10%: Local: Burning, stinging of eye

<1%:

- Dermatologic: Allergic contact dermatitis
- Local: Irritation, sensitization
- Ocular: Keratitis, iritis, erosion of the corneal epithelium, conjunctival congestion and hemorrhage, corneal opacification

**Drug Interactions** No data reported

**Drug Uptake**

Onset of action: Within 20 seconds of instillation

Duration: 15-20 minutes

**Pregnancy Risk Factor** C
**Generic Available** Yes

- ♦ **Propecia®** *see* Finasteride *on page 431*
- ♦ **Propine® Ophthalmic** *see* Dipivefrin *on page 341*

## Propiomazine (proe pee OH ma zeen)

**Therapeutic Category** Antianxiety Agent; Antiemetic; Phenothiazine Derivative; Sedative; Tranquilizer, Minor

**Use** Relief of restlessness, nausea, and apprehension before and during surgery or during labor

**Usual Dosage** I.M., I.V.:

Children <27 kg: 0.55-1.1 mg/kg

Adults: 10-40 mg prior to procedure, additional may be repeated at 3-hour intervals

**Local Anesthetic/Vasoconstrictor Precautions** No information available to require special precautions

**Effects on Dental Treatment** >10% of patients experience dry mouth

**Other Adverse Effects**

>10%: Central nervous system: Dizziness, drowsiness

1% to 10%:

Cardiovascular: Tachycardia
Central nervous system: Confusion
Dermatologic: Skin rash
Gastrointestinal: Diarrhea, stomach pain
Respiratory: Dyspnea

<1%: Central nervous system: Neuroleptic malignant syndrome

**Generic Available** No

**Comments** Do not use injection if cloudy or contains a precipitate

- ♦ **Proplex® SX-T** *see* Factor IX Complex (Human) *on page 417*
- ♦ **Proplex® T** *see* Factor IX Complex (Human) *on page 417*

## Propofol (PROE po fole)

**U.S. Brand Names** Diprivan® Injection

**Therapeutic Category** General Anesthetic, Intravenous

**Use** Induction or maintenance of anesthesia; sedation

Not recommended for use in children <3 years of age; not recommended for sedation of PICU patients, especially at high doses or for prolonged periods of time; metabolic acidosis with fatal cardiac failure has occurred in several children (4 weeks to 11 years of age) who received propofol infusions at average rates of infusion of 4.5-10 mg/kg/hour for 66-115 hours (maximum rates of infusion 6.2-11.5 mg/kg/hour); see Parke, 1992; Strickland, 1995; and Bray, 1995

**Usual Dosage** Dosage must be individualized based on total body weight and titrated to the desired clinical effect; however, as a general guideline:

No pediatric dose has been established; however, induction for children 1-12 years 2-2.8 mg/kg has been used

Induction: I.V.:

Adults ≤55 years, and/or ASA I or II patients: 2-2.5 mg/kg of body weight (approximately 40 mg every 10 seconds until onset of induction)

Elderly, debilitated, hypovolemic, and/or ASA III or IV patients: 1-1.5 mg/kg of body weight (approximately 20 mg every 10 seconds until onset of induction)

Maintenance: I.V. infusion:

Adults ≤55 years, and/or ASA I or II patients: 0.1-0.2 mg/kg of body weight/minute (6-12 mg/kg of body weight/hour)

Elderly, debilitated, hypovolemic, and/or ASA III or IV patients: 0.05-0.1 mg/kg of body weight/minute (3-6 mg/kg of body weight/hour)

I.V. intermittent: 25-50 mg increments, as needed

ICU sedation: Rapid bolus injection should be avoided. Bolus injection can result in hypotension, oxyhemoglobin desaturation, apnea, airway obstruction, and oxygen desaturation. The preferred route of administration is slow infusion. Doses are based on individual need and titrated to response.

Recommended starting dose: 1-3 mg/kg/hour

Adjustments in dose can occur at 3- to 5-minute intervals. An 80% reduction in dose should be considered in elderly, debilitated, and ASA II or IV patients. Once sedation is established, the dose should be decreased for the maintenance infusion period and adjusted to response. The dose required for maintenance is 1.5-4.5 mg/kg/hour or 25-75 mcg/kg/minute. An alternative, but less preferred method of administration is intermittent slow I.V. bolus injection of 10-20 mg, administered over 3-5 minutes.

(Continued)

## Propofol *(Continued)*

**Mechanism of Action** Propofol is a hindered phenolic compound with intravenous general anesthetic properties. The drug is unrelated to any of the currently used barbiturate, opioid, benzodiazepine, arylcyclohexylamine, or imidazole intravenous anesthetic agents.

**Local Anesthetic/Vasoconstrictor Precautions** No information available to require special precautions

**Effects on Dental Treatment** No effects or complications reported

**Other Adverse Effects**

>10%: Gastrointestinal: Nausea

1% to 10%:

Cardiovascular: Hypotension, bradycardia, flushing
Central nervous system: Fever
Gastrointestinal: Vomiting, abdominal cramping
Respiratory: Cough, apnea

<1%:

Cardiovascular: Chest pain, tachycardia, syncope
Central nervous system: Agitation, somnolence, confusion
Dermatologic: Pruritus
Gastrointestinal: Dry mouth, diarrhea
Neuromuscular & skeletal: Tremor, twitching
Otic: Ear pain
Respiratory: Bronchospasm, dyspnea

**Drug Uptake**

Onset of anesthesia: Within 9-51 seconds (average 30 seconds) after bolus infusion (dose dependent)
Duration: 3-10 minutes depending on the dose and the rate of administration
Serum half-life, elimination (biphasic):
Initial: 40 minutes
Terminal: 1-3 days

**Pregnancy Risk Factor** B

**Generic Available** No

**Comments** Formulated into an emulsion containing 10% w/v soybean oil, 1.2% w/v purified egg phosphatide, and 2.25% w/v glycerol; this emulsion vehicle is chemically similar to 10% Intralipid®

## Propoxyphene (proe POKS i feen)

**Related Information**

Narcotic Agonists *on page 1223*

**U.S. Brand Names** Darvon®; Darvon-N®; Dolene®

**Canadian Brand Names** Novo-Propoxyn; 624® Tablets

**Therapeutic Category** Analgesic, Narcotic

**Use** Management of mild to moderate pain

**Usual Dosage** Oral:

Children: Doses for children are not well established; doses of the hydrochloride of 2-3 mg/kg/d divided every 6 hours have been used

Adults:

Hydrochloride: 65 mg every 3-4 hours as needed for pain; maximum: 390 mg/day
Napsylate: 100 mg every 4 hours as needed for pain; maximum: 600 mg/day

**Mechanism of Action** Binds to opiate receptors in the CNS, causing inhibition of ascending pain pathways, altering the perception of and response to pain; produces generalized CNS depression

**Local Anesthetic/Vasoconstrictor Precautions** No information available to require special precautions

**Effects on Dental Treatment** No effects or complications reported

**Other Adverse Effects** Hepatic: Increased liver enzymes

>10%:

Cardiovascular: Hypotension
Central nervous system: Dizziness, lightheadedness, sedation, paradoxical excitement, insomnia, fatigue, drowsiness
Gastrointestinal: GI upset, nausea, vomiting, constipation
Neuromuscular & skeletal: Weakness
Miscellaneous: Histamine release

1% to 10%:

Central nervous system: Nervousness, headache, restlessness, malaise, confusion
Gastrointestinal: Anorexia, stomach cramps, dry mouth, biliary spasm
Genitourinary: Decreased urination, ureteral spasms
Respiratory: Dyspnea

<1%:

Central nervous system: Mental depression hallucinations, paradoxical CNS stimulation, increased intracranial pressure

Dermatologic: Rash, urticaria

Gastrointestinal: Paralytic ileus

Miscellaneous: Psychologic and physical dependence with prolonged use

**Drug Interactions**

Decreased effect with charcoal, cigarette smoking

Increased toxicity: CNS depressants may potentiate pharmacologic effects; propoxyphene may inhibit the metabolism and increase the serum concentrations of carbamazepine, phenobarbital, MAO inhibitors, tricyclic antidepressants, and warfarin

**Drug Uptake**

Onset of effect: Oral: Within 0.5-1 hour

Duration: 4-6 hours

Serum half-life: Adults:

Parent drug: 8-24 hours (mean: ~15 hours)

Norpropoxyphene: 34 hours

**Pregnancy Risk Factor** C (D if used for prolonged periods)

**Dosage Forms**

Capsule, as hydrochloride: 65 mg

Tablet, as napsylate: 100 mg

**Dietary Considerations** Should be taken with glass of water on empty stomach

**Generic Available** Yes: Capsule

## Propoxyphene and Acetaminophen

(proe POKS i feen & a seet a MIN oh fen)

**U.S. Brand Names** Darvocet-N®; Darvocet-N® 100; Propacet®; Wygesic®

**Therapeutic Category** Analgesic, Narcotic

**Use**

Dental: Management of postoperative pain

Medical: Relief of pain

**Restrictions** C-IV; Refillable up to 5 times in 6 months

**Usual Dosage**

Children: Not recommended in pediatric dental patients

Adults:

Darvocet-N®: 1-2 tablets every 4 hours as needed; maximum: 600 mg propoxyphene napsylate/day

Darvocet-N® 100: 1 tablet every 4 hours as needed; maximum: 600 mg propoxyphene napsylate/day

**Mechanism of Action**

Propoxyphene is a weak narcotic analgesic which acts through binding to opiate receptors to inhibit ascending pain pathways

Propoxyphene, as with other narcotic (opiate) analgesics, blocks pain perception in the cerebral cortex by binding to specific receptor molecules (opiate receptors) within the neuronal membranes of synapses. This binding results in a decreased synaptic chemical transmission throughout the CNS thus inhibiting the flow of pain sensations into the higher centers. Mu and kappa are the two subtypes of the opiate receptor which propoxyphene binds to to cause analgesia.

Acetaminophen inhibits the synthesis of prostaglandins in the CNS and peripherally blocks pain impulse generation; produces antipyresis from inhibition of hypothalamic heat-regulating center

**Local Anesthetic/Vasoconstrictor Precautions** No information available to require special precautions

**Effects on Dental Treatment** No effects or complications reported

**Other Adverse Effects** 1% to 10%:

Central nervous system: Dizziness, lightheadedness, headache, sedation

Gastrointestinal: Nausea, vomiting

Neuromuscular & skeletal: Weakness

Miscellaneous: Psychologic and physical dependence

**Contraindications** Hypersensitivity to propoxyphene, acetaminophen, or any component; patients with known G-6-PD deficiency

**Warnings/Precautions** When given in excessive doses, either alone or in combination with other CNS depressants, propoxyphene is a major cause of drug-related deaths; do not exceed recommended dosage; give with caution in patients dependent on opiates, substitution may result in acute opiate withdrawal symptoms

**Drug Interactions** Decreased effect with charcoal, cigarette smoking; increased toxicity with cimetidine, CNS depressants; increased toxicity/effect of carbamazepine, phenobarbital, TCAs, MAO inhibitors, benzodiazepines

(Continued)

## Propoxyphene and Acetaminophen *(Continued)*

**Drug Uptake**
Onset of action: 15-60 minutes
Time to peak serum concentration: 2-2.5 hours
Duration: 4-6 hours
Serum half-life:
Propoxyphene: 6-12 hours
Norpropoxyphene: 30-36 hours

**Pregnancy Risk Factor** C

**Breast-feeding Considerations** Both propoxyphene and acetaminophen may be taken while breast-feeding

**Dosage Forms** Tablet:
Darvocet-N®: Propoxyphene napsylate 50 mg and acetaminophen 325 mg
Darvocet-N® 100: Propoxyphene napsylate 100 mg and acetaminophen 650 mg
Genagesic®, Wygesic®: Propoxyphene hydrochloride 65 mg and acetaminophen 650 mg

**Dietary Considerations** Should be taken with water on an empty stomach

**Generic Available** Yes

**Comments** Propoxyphene is a narcotic analgesic and shares many properties including addiction liability. The acetaminophen component requires use with caution in patients with alcoholic liver disease.

## Propoxyphene and Aspirin (proe POKS i feen & AS pir in)

**Related Information**
Narcotic Agonists *on page 1223*

**U.S. Brand Names** Bexophene®; Darvon® Compound-65 Pulvules®

**Canadian Brand Names** Darvon-N® With ASA; Novo-Propoxyn Compound (contains caffeine); Darvon-N® Compound (contains caffeine)

**Therapeutic Category** Analgesic, Narcotic

**Use**
Dental: Management of postoperative pain
Medical: Relief of pain

**Restrictions** C-IV; Refillable up to 5 times in 6 months

**Usual Dosage** Oral:
Children: Not recommended
Adults: 1-2 capsules every 4 hours as needed

**Mechanism of Action**
Propoxyphene is a weak narcotic analgesic which acts through binding to opiate receptors to inhibit ascending pain pathways

Propoxyphene, as with other narcotic (opiate) analgesics, blocks pain perception in the cerebral cortex by binding to specific receptor molecules (opiate receptors) within the neuronal membranes of synapses. This binding results in a decreased synaptic chemical transmission throughout the CNS thus inhibiting the flow of pain sensations into the higher centers. Mu and kappa are the two subtypes of the opiate receptor which propoxyphene binds to to cause analgesia.

Aspirin inhibits prostaglandin synthesis by decreasing the activity of the enzyme, cyclo-oxygenase, which results in decreased formation of prostaglandin precursors, acts on the hypothalamic heat-regulating center to reduce fever, blocks thromboxane synthetase action which prevents formation of the platelet-aggregating substance thromboxane $A_2$

**Local Anesthetic/Vasoconstrictor Precautions** No effects or complications reported

**Effects on Dental Treatment** Use with caution in patients with platelet and bleeding disorders, renal dysfunction, erosive gastritis, or peptic ulcer disease, previous nonreaction does not guarantee future safe taking of medication; do not use aspirin in children <16 years of age for chickenpox or flu symptoms due to the association with Reye's syndrome

Avoid aspirin if possible, for 1 week prior to surgery because of the possibility of postoperative bleeding; use with caution in impaired hepatic function

Elderly are a high-risk population for adverse effects from nonsteroidal anti-inflammatory agents. As much as 60% of elderly with GI complications to NSAIDs can develop peptic ulceration and/or hemorrhage asymptomatically. Also, concomitant disease and drug use contribute to the risk for GI adverse effects. Use lowest effective dose for shortest period possible. Consider renal function decline with age. Use with caution in patients with history of asthma

**Other Adverse Effects** 1% to 10%:
Central nervous system: Dizziness, lightheadedness, headache, sedation
Gastrointestinal: Nausea, vomiting
Neuromuscular & skeletal: Weakness

Miscellaneous: Psychologic and physical dependence

**Contraindications** Hypersensitivity to propoxyphene, aspirin or any component

**Warnings/Precautions** When given in excessive doses, either alone or in combination with other CNS depressants, propoxyphene is a major cause of drug-related deaths; do not exceed recommended dosage; because of aspirin component, children and teenagers should not use for chickenpox or flu symptoms before a physician is consulted about Reye's syndrome

**Drug Interactions** Decreased effect with charcoal, cigarette smoking; increased toxicity with cimetidine, CNS depressants; increased toxicity/effect of carbamazepine, phenobarbital, TCAs, warfarin, MAO inhibitors, benzodiazepines, warfarin (bleeding); see Aspirin

**Drug Uptake**

Onset of action: 15-60 minutes

Time to peak serum concentration: 2-2.5 hours

Duration: 4-6 hours

Serum half-life:

Propoxyphene: 6-12 hours

Norpropoxyphene: 30-36 hours

**Pregnancy Risk Factor** D

**Breast-feeding Considerations**

Propoxyphene: May be taken while breast-feeding

Aspirin: Use cautiously due to potential adverse effects in nursing infants

**Dosage Forms**

Capsule: Propoxyphene hydrochloride 65 mg and aspirin 389 mg with caffeine 32.4 mg

Tablet (Darvon-N® with A.S.A.): Propoxyphene napsylate 100 mg and aspirin 325 mg

**Dietary Considerations** No data reported

**Generic Available** Yes

**Comments** Propoxyphene is a narcotic analgesic and shares many properties including addiction liability. The aspirin component could have anticoagulant effects and could possibly affect bleeding times.

## Propranolol (proe PRAN oh lole)

**Related Information**

Cardiovascular Diseases *on page 1066*

Endocrine Disorders & Pregnancy *on page 1082*

**U.S. Brand Names** Betachron E-R® Capsule; Inderal®; Inderal® LA

**Canadian Brand Names** Apo®-Propranolol; Detensol®; Nu-Propranolol

**Therapeutic Category** Antianginal Agent; Antiarrhythmic Agent, Class I-B; Antiarrhythmic Agent, Class II; Antiarrhythmic Agent (Supraventricular & Ventricular); Beta-adrenergic Blocker, Noncardioselective

**Use** Management of hypertension, angina pectoris, pheochromocytoma, essential tremor, tetralogy of Fallot cyanotic spells, and arrhythmias (such as atrial fibrillation and flutter, A-V nodal re-entrant tachycardias, and catecholamine-induced arrhythmias); prevention of myocardial infarction, migraine headache; symptomatic treatment of hypertrophic subaortic stenosis

**Unlabeled use:** Tremor due to Parkinson's disease, alcohol withdrawal, aggressive behavior, antipsychotic-induced akathisia, esophageal varices bleeding, anxiety, schizophrenia, acute panic, and gastric bleeding in portal hypertension

**Usual Dosage**

Tachyarrhythmias:

Oral:

Children: Initial: 0.5-1 mg/kg/day in divided doses every 6-8 hours; titrate dosage upward every 3-7 days; usual dose: 2-4 mg/kg/day; higher doses may be needed; do not exceed 16 mg/kg/day or 60 mg/day

Adults: 10-30 mg/dose every 6-8 hours

Elderly: Initial: 10 mg twice daily; increase dosage every 3-7 days; usual dosage range: 10-320 mg given in 2 divided doses

I.V.:

Children: 0.01-0.1 mg/kg slow IVP over 10 minutes; maximum dose: 1 mg

Adults: 1 mg/dose slow IVP; repeat every 5 minutes up to a total of 5 mg

Hypertension: Oral:

Children: Initial: 0.5-1 mg/kg/day in divided doses every 6-12 hours; increase gradually every 3-7 days; maximum: 2 mg/kg/24 hours

Adults: Initial: 40 mg twice daily; increase dosage every 3-7 days; usual dose: ≤320 mg divided in 2-3 doses/day; maximum daily dose: 640 mg

Migraine headache prophylaxis: Oral:

Children: 0.6-1.5 mg/kg/day **or**

≤35 kg: 10-20 mg 3 times/day

>35 kg: 20-40 mg 3 times/day

(Continued)

## Propranolol *(Continued)*

Adults: Initial: 80 mg/day divided every 6-8 hours; increase by 20-40 mg/dose every 3-4 weeks to a maximum of 160-240 mg/day given in divided doses every 6-8 hours; if satisfactory response not achieved within 6 weeks of starting therapy, drug should be withdrawn gradually over several weeks

Tetralogy spells: Children:

Oral: 1-2 mg/kg/day every 6 hours as needed, may increase by 1 mg/kg/day to a maximum of 5 mg/kg/day, or if refractory may increase slowly to a maximum of 10-15 mg/kg/day

I.V.: 0.15-0.25 mg/kg/dose slow IVP; may repeat in 15 minutes

Thyrotoxicosis:

Adolescents and Adults: Oral: 10-40 mg/dose every 6 hours

Adults: I.V.: 1-3 mg/dose slow IVP as a single dose

Adults: Oral:

Angina: 80-320 mg/day in doses divided 2-4 times/day

Pheochromocytoma: 30-60 mg/day in divided doses

Myocardial infarction prophylaxis: 180-240 mg/day in 3-4 divided doses

Hypertrophic subaortic stenosis: 20-40 mg 3-4 times/day

Essential tremor: 40 mg twice daily initially; maintenance doses: usually 120-320 mg/day

**Mechanism of Action** Nonselective beta-adrenergic blocker (class II antiarrhythmic); competitively blocks response to $beta_1$- and $beta_2$-adrenergic stimulation which results in decreases in heart rate, myocardial contractility, blood pressure, and myocardial oxygen demand

**Local Anesthetic/Vasoconstrictor Precautions** Use with caution; epinephrine has interacted with nonselective beta-blockers to result in initial hypertensive episode followed by bradycardia

**Effects on Dental Treatment** Noncardioselective beta-blockers (ie, propranolol, nadolol) enhance the pressor response to epinephrine, resulting in hypertension and bradycardia. Many nonsteroidal anti-inflammatory drugs such as ibuprofen and indomethacin can reduce the hypotensive effect of beta-blockers after 3 or more weeks of therapy with the NSAID. Short-term NSAID use (ie, 3 days) requires no special precautions in patients taking beta-blockers.

**Other Adverse Effects**

>10%:

Cardiovascular: Bradycardia

Central nervous system: Mental depression

Endocrine & metabolic: Decreased sexual ability

1% to 10%:

Cardiovascular: Congestive heart failure, reduced peripheral circulation

Central nervous system: Confusion, hallucinations, dizziness, insomnia, fatigue

Dermatologic: Skin rash

Gastrointestinal: Diarrhea, nausea, vomiting, stomach discomfort

Neuromuscular & skeletal: Weakness

Respiratory: Wheezing

<1%:

Cardiovascular: Chest pain, hypotension, impaired myocardial contractility, worsening of A-V conduction disturbances

Central nervous system: Nightmares, vivid dreams, lethargy

Dermatologic: Red, scaling, or crusted skin

Endocrine & metabolic: Hypoglycemia, hyperglycemia

Gastrointestinal: GI distress

Hematologic: Leukopenia, thrombocytopenia, agranulocytosis

Respiratory: Bronchospasm

Miscellaneous: Cold extremities

**Drug Interactions**

Decreased effect of beta-blockers with aluminum salts, barbiturates, calcium salts, cholestyramine, colestipol, NSAIDs, penicillins (ampicillin), rifampin, salicylates and sulfinpyrazone due to decreased bioavailability and plasma levels

Increased effect/toxicity of beta-blockers with calcium blockers (diltiazem, felodipine, nicardipine), contraceptives, flecainide, haloperidol (propranolol, hypotensive effects), $H_2$ antagonists (metoprolol, propranolol only by cimetidine, possibly ranitidine), hydralazine (metoprolol, propranolol), loop diuretics (propranolol, not atenolol), MAO inhibitors (metoprolol, nadolol, bradycardia), phenothiazines (propranolol), propafenone (metoprolol, propranolol), quinidine (in extensive metabolizers), ciprofloxacin, thyroid hormones (metoprolol, propranolol, when hypothyroid patient is converted to euthyroid state)

Beta-blockers may increase the effect/toxicity* of flecainide, haloperidol (hypotensive effects), hydralazine, phenothiazines, acetaminophen, anticoagulants (propranolol, warfarin), benzodiazepines (not atenolol), clonidine (hypertensive crisis after or during withdrawal of either agent), epinephrine (initial hypertensive episode followed by bradycardia), nifedipine and verapamil lidocaine*, ergots* (peripheral ischemia), prazosin (postural hypotension)

Beta-blockers may decrease the effect of sulfonylureas

Beta-blockers may also affect the action or levels of ethanol, disopyramide, nondepolarizing muscle relaxants and theophylline although the effects are difficult to predict

**Drug Uptake**

Onset of beta blockade: Oral: Within 1-2 hours

Duration: ~6 hours

Serum half-life:

Children: 3.9-6.4 hours

Adults: 4-6 hours

**Pregnancy Risk Factor** C

**Generic Available** Yes

**Selected Readings**

Foster CA and Aston SJ, "Propranolol-Epinephrine Interaction: A Potential Disaster," *Plast Reconstr Surg*, 1983, 72(1):74-8.

Wong DG, Spence JD, Lamki L, et al, "Effect of Nonsteroidal Anti-inflammatory Drugs on Control of Hypertension of Beta-Blockers and Diuretics," *Lancet*, 1986, 1(8488):997-1001.

Wynn RL, "Dental Nonsteroidal Anti-inflammatory Drugs and Prostaglandin-Based Drug Interactions, Part Two," *Gen Dent*, 1992, 40(2):104, 106, 108.

Wynn RL, "Epinephrine Interactions With Beta-Blockers," *Gen Dent*, 1994, 42(1):16, 18.

## Propranolol and Hydrochlorothiazide

(proe PRAN oh lole & hye droe klor oh THYE a zide)

**U.S. Brand Names** Inderide®

**Therapeutic Category** Antihypertensive Agent, Combination

**Use** Management of hypertension

**Usual Dosage** Dose is individualized

**Local Anesthetic/Vasoconstrictor Precautions** Use with caution; epinephrine has interacted with nonselective beta-blockers to result in initial hypertensive episode followed by bradycardia

**Effects on Dental Treatment** Noncardioselective beta-blockers (ie, propranolol, nadolol) enhance the pressor response to epinephrine, resulting in hypertension and bradycardia. Many nonsteroidal anti-inflammatory drugs such as ibuprofen and indomethacin can reduce the hypotensive effect of beta-blockers after 3 or more weeks of therapy with the NSAID. Short-term NSAID use (ie, 3 days) requires no special precautions in patients taking beta-blockers.

**Pregnancy Risk Factor** C

**Generic Available** Immediate release: Yes

♦ **Propulsid®** *see* Cisapride *on page 251*

♦ **Propylene Glycol and Salicylic Acid** *see* Salicylic Acid and Propylene Glycol *on page 901*

## Propylhexedrine (proe pil HEKS e dreen)

**U.S. Brand Names** Benzedrex® [OTC]

**Therapeutic Category** Decongestant

**Use** Topical nasal decongestant

**Usual Dosage** Inhale through each nostril while blocking the other

**Local Anesthetic/Vasoconstrictor Precautions** No information available to require special precautions

**Effects on Dental Treatment** No effects or complications reported

**Generic Available** No

**Comments** Drug has been extracted from inhaler and injected I.V. as an amphetamine substitute

## Propylthiouracil (proe pil thye oh YOOR a sil)

**Related Information**

Endocrine Disorders & Pregnancy *on page 1082*

**Canadian Brand Names** Propyl-Thyracil®

**Therapeutic Category** Antithyroid Agent

**Use** Palliative treatment of hyperthyroidism as an adjunct to ameliorate hyperthyroidism in preparation for surgical treatment or radioactive iodine therapy and in the management of thyrotoxic crisis. The use of antithyroid thioamides is as effective in elderly as they are in younger adults; however, the expense, potential adverse effects, and inconvenience (compliance, monitoring) make them undesirable. The use of radioiodine, due to ease of administration and less concern for long-term side effects and reproduction problems, makes it a more appropriate therapy.

**Usual Dosage** Oral: Administer in 3 equally divided doses at approximately 8-hour intervals. Adjust dosage to maintain $T_3$, $T_4$, and TSH levels in normal range;

(Continued)

## Propylthiouracil *(Continued)*

elevated $T_3$ may be sole indicator of inadequate treatment. Elevated TSH indicates excessive antithyroid treatment.

Children: Initial: 5-7 mg/kg/day in divided doses every 8 hours **or**
- 6-10 years: 50-150 mg/day
- >10 years: 150-300 mg/day
- Maintenance: 1/3 to 2/3 of the initial dose in divided doses every 8-12 hours. This usually begins after 2 months on an effective initial dose.

Adults: Initial: 300-450 mg/day in divided doses every 8 hours (severe hyperthyroidism may require 600-1200 mg/day); maintenance: 100-150 mg/day in divided doses every 8-12 hours

Elderly: Use lower dose recommendations; initial dose: 150-300 mg/day

**Mechanism of Action** Inhibits the synthesis of thyroid hormones by blocking the oxidation of iodine in the thyroid gland; blocks synthesis of thyroxine and triiodothyronine

**Local Anesthetic/Vasoconstrictor Precautions** No information available to require special precautions

**Effects on Dental Treatment** No effects or complications reported

**Other Adverse Effects**

>10%:
- Central nervous system: Fever
- Dermatologic: Skin rash
- Hematologic: Leukopenia

1% to 10%:
- Central nervous system: Dizziness
- Gastrointestinal: Nausea, vomiting, dysgeusia, stomach pain
- Hematologic: Agranulocytosis
- Miscellaneous: SLE-like syndrome

<1%:
- Cardiovascular: Edema, cutaneous vasculitis
- Central nervous system: Drowsiness, neuritis, vertigo, headache
- Dermatologic: Urticaria, pruritus, exfoliative dermatitis, alopecia
- Endocrine & metabolic: Goiter
- Gastrointestinal: Constipation, weight gain, swollen salivary glands
- Hematologic: Thrombocytopenia, bleeding, aplastic anemia
- Hepatic: Cholestatic jaundice, hepatitis
- Neuromuscular & skeletal: Arthralgia, paresthesia
- Renal: Nephritis

**Drug Interactions** Increased effect: Increased anticoagulant activity

**Drug Uptake**

Onset of action: For significant therapeutic effects 24-36 hours are required

Peak effect: Remissions of hyperthyroidism do not usually occur before 4 months of continued therapy

Serum half-life: 1.5-5 hours

End-stage renal disease: 8.5 hours

Time to peak serum concentration: Oral: Within 1 hour; persists for 2-3 hours

**Pregnancy Risk Factor** D

**Generic Available** Yes


- ♦ **Prorex®** *see* Promethazine *on page 847*
- ♦ **Proscar®** *see* Finasteride *on page 431*
- ♦ **Pro-Sof® Plus [OTC]** *see* Docusate and Casanthranol *on page 347*
- ♦ **ProSom™** *see* Estazolam *on page 386*
- ♦ **Prostaglandin $E_1$** *see* Alprostadil *on page 51*
- ♦ **Prostaglandin $E_2$** *see* Dinoprostone *on page 337*
- ♦ **Prostaglandin $F_2$ Alpha** *see* Dinoprost Tromethamine *on page 338*
- ♦ **ProStep®** *see* Nicotine *on page 718*
- ♦ **Prostin $E_2$® Vaginal Suppository** *see* Dinoprostone *on page 337*
- ♦ **Prostin $F_2$ Alpha®** *see* Dinoprost Tromethamine *on page 338*
- ♦ **Prostin VR Pediatric® Injection** *see* Alprostadil *on page 51*


## Protamine Sulfate (PROE ta meen SUL fate)

**Therapeutic Category** Antidote, Heparin

**Use** Treatment of heparin overdosage; neutralize heparin during surgery or dialysis procedures

**Usual Dosage** Protamine dosage is determined by the dosage of heparin; 1 mg of protamine neutralizes 90 USP units of heparin (lung) and 115 USP units of heparin (intestinal); maximum dose: 50 mg

In the situation of heparin overdosage, since blood heparin concentrations decrease rapidly **after** administration, adjust the protamine dosage depending upon the duration of time since heparin administration as follows:

| Time Elapsed | Dose of Protamine (mg) to Neutralize 100 units of Heparin |
|---|---|
| Immediate | 1-1.5 |
| 30-60 min | 0.5-0.75 |
| >2 h | 0.25-0.375 |

If heparin administered by deep S.C. injection, use 1-1.5 mg protamine per 100 units heparin; this may be done by a portion of the dose (eg, 25-50 mg) given slowly I.V. followed by the remaining portion as a continuous infusion over 8-16 hours (the expected absorption time of the S.C. heparin dose)

**Mechanism of Action** Combines with strongly acidic heparin to form a stable complex (salt) neutralizing the anticoagulant activity of both drugs

**Local Anesthetic/Vasoconstrictor Precautions** No information available to require special precautions

**Effects on Dental Treatment** No effects or complications reported

**Other Adverse Effects**

>10%:
- Cardiovascular: Hypotension, bradycardia
- Respiratory: Dyspnea

1% to 10%: Hematologic: Hemorrhage

<1%:
- Cardiovascular: Flushing, pulmonary hypertension
- Central nervous system: Lassitude
- Gastrointestinal: Nausea, vomiting
- Miscellaneous: Hypersensitivity reactions

**Drug Uptake** Onset of effect: I.V. injection: Heparin neutralization occurs within 5 minutes

**Pregnancy Risk Factor** C

**Generic Available** Yes

**Comments** Heparin rebound associated with anticoagulation and bleeding has been reported to occur occasionally; symptoms typically occur 8-9 hours after protamine administration, but may occur as long as 18 hours later

♦ **Prothazine-DC®** *see* Promethazine and Codeine *on page 848*

♦ **Protilase®** *see* Pancrelipase *on page 763*

## Protirelin (proe TYE re lin)

**U.S. Brand Names** Relefact® TRH Injection; Thypinone® Injection

**Therapeutic Category** Diagnostic Agent, Thyroid Function

**Synonyms** Lopremone; Thyrotropin Releasing Hormone; TRH

**Use** Adjunct in the diagnostic assessment of thyroid function, and an adjunct to other diagnostic procedures in assessment of patients with pituitary or hypothalamic dysfunction; also causes release of prolactin from the pituitary and is used to detect defective control of prolactin secretion.

**Usual Dosage** I.V.:
- Children <6 years: Experience limited, but doses of 7 mcg/kg have been administered
- Children 6-16 years: 7 mcg/kg to a maximum dose of 500 mcg
- Adults: 500 mcg (range 200-500 mcg)

**Mechanism of Action** Increase release of thyroid stimulating hormone from the anterior pituitary

**Local Anesthetic/Vasoconstrictor Precautions** No information available to require special precautions

**Effects on Dental Treatment** >10% of patients experience dry mouth

**Other Adverse Effects**

>10%:
- Cardiovascular: Flushing of face
- Central nervous system: Headache, lightheadedness
- Gastrointestinal: Nausea
- Genitourinary: Urge to urinate

1% to 10%:
- Central nervous system: Anxiety
- Endocrine & metabolic: Breast enlargement and leaking in lactating women
- Gastrointestinal: Bad taste in mouth, gastritis
- Neuromuscular & skeletal: Paresthesia
- Miscellaneous: Sweating

(Continued)

## Protirelin *(Continued)*

<1%:
- Cardiovascular: Severe hypotension
- Ocular: Temporary loss of vision

**Drug Uptake**
- Peak TSH levels: 20-30 minutes
- Duration: TSH returns to baseline after ~3 hours
- Serum half-life, mean plasma: 5 minutes

**Pregnancy Risk Factor** C

**Generic Available** No

♦ **Protostat®** *see* Metronidazole *on page 667*

## Protriptyline (proe TRIP ti leen)

**U.S. Brand Names** Vivactil®

**Canadian Brand Names** Triptil®

**Therapeutic Category** Antidepressant, Tricyclic

**Use** Treatment of various forms of depression, often in conjunction with psychotherapy

**Usual Dosage** Oral:
- Adolescents: 15-20 mg/day
- Adults: 15-60 mg in 3-4 divided doses
- Elderly: 15-20 mg/day

**Mechanism of Action** Increases the synaptic concentration of serotonin and/or norepinephrine in the central nervous system by inhibition of their reuptake by the presynaptic neuronal membrane

**Local Anesthetic/Vasoconstrictor Precautions** No information available to require special precautions

**Effects on Dental Treatment** >10% of patients experience dry mouth; long-term treatment with TCAs such as protriptyline increases the risk of caries by reducing salivation and salivary buffer capacity

**Other Adverse Effects**

>10%:
- Central nervous system: Dizziness, drowsiness, headache
- Gastrointestinal: Constipation, unpleasant taste, weight gain, increased appetite, nausea
- Neuromuscular & skeletal: Weakness

1% to 10%:
- Cardiovascular: Arrhythmias, hypotension
- Central nervous system: Confusion, delirium, hallucinations, nervousness, restlessness, parkinsonian syndrome, insomnia
- Endocrine & metabolic: Sexual dysfunction
- Gastrointestinal: Diarrhea, heartburn
- Genitourinary: Dysuria
- Neuromuscular & skeletal: Fine muscle tremors
- Ocular: Blurred vision, eye pain
- Miscellaneous: Excessive sweating

<1%:
- Central nervous system: Anxiety, seizures
- Dermatologic: Alopecia, photosensitivity
- Endocrine & metabolic: Breast enlargement, galactorrhea, SIADH
- Gastrointestinal: Trouble with gums, decreased lower esophageal sphincter tone may cause GE reflux
- Genitourinary: Testicular swelling
- Hematologic: Agranulocytosis, leukopenia, eosinophilia
- Hepatic: Cholestatic jaundice, elevated liver enzymes
- Ocular: Increased intraocular pressure
- Otic: Tinnitus
- Miscellaneous: Allergic reactions

**Drug Interactions**

Decreased effect: Phenobarbital may increase the metabolism of protriptyline; protriptyline blocks the uptake of guanethidine and thus prevents the hypotensive effect of guanethidine

Increased toxicity: Clonidine causes hypertensive crisis; protriptyline may be additive with or may potentiate the action of other CNS depressants such as sedatives or hypnotics; with MAO inhibitors, hyperpyrexia, hypertension, tachycardia, confusion, and seizures; protriptyline may increase the prothrombin time in patients stabilized on warfarin; protriptyline potentiates the pressor and cardiac effects of sympathomimetic agents such as isoproterenol, epinephrine, etc; cimetidine and methylphenidate may decrease the metabolism of protriptyline

Additive anticholinergic effects seen with other anticholinergic agents

**Drug Uptake**

Maximum antidepressant effect: 2 weeks of continuous therapy is commonly required

Serum half-life: 54-92 hours, averaging 74 hours

Time to peak serum concentration: Oral: Within 24-30 hours

**Pregnancy Risk Factor** C

**Generic Available** No

**Selected Readings**

Boakes AJ, Laurence DR, Teoh PC, et al, "Interactions Between Sympathomimetic Amines and Antidepressant Agents in Man," *Br Med J*, 1973, 1(849):311-5.

Jastak JT and Yagiela JA, "Vasoconstrictors and Local Anesthesia: A Review and Rationale for Use," *J Am Dent Assoc*, 1983, 107(4):623-30.

Larochelle P, Hamet P, and Enjalbert M, "Responses to Tyramine and Norepinephrine After Imipramine and Trazodone," *Clin Pharmacol Ther*, 1979, 26(1):24-30.

Mitchell JR, "Guanethidine and Related Agents. III Antagonism by Drugs Which Inhibit the Norepinephrine Pump in Man," *J Clin Invest*, 1970, 49(8):1596-604.

Rundegren J, van Dijken J, Mörnstad H, et al, "Oral Conditions in Patients Receiving Long-Term Treatment With Cyclic Antidepressant Drugs," *Swed Dent J*, 1985, 9(2):55-64.

Svedmyr N, "The Influence of a Tricyclic Antidepressive Agent (Protriptyline) on Some of the Circulatory Effects of Noradrenaline and Adrenalin in Man," *Life Sci*, 1968, 7(1):77-84.

♦ **Protropin® Injection** *see* Human Growth Hormone *on page 499*

♦ **Provatene® [OTC]** *see* Beta-Carotene *on page 135*

♦ **Proventil®** *see* Albuterol *on page 43*

♦ **Proventil® HFA** *see* Albuterol *on page 43*

♦ **Provera®** *see* Medroxyprogesterone Acetate *on page 623*

♦ **Provigil®** *see* Modafinil *on page 683*

♦ **Proxigel® Oral [OTC]** *see* Carbamide Peroxide *on page 186*

♦ **Prozac®** *see* Fluoxetine *on page 445*

♦ **PRP-D** *see Haemophilus* b Conjugate Vaccine *on page 486*

♦ **Pseudo-Car® DM** *see* Carbinoxamine, Pseudoephedrine, and Dextromethorphan *on page 189*

# Pseudoephedrine (soo doe e FED rin)

**Related Information**

Acetaminophen and Pseudoephedrine *on page 31*

Acetaminophen, Dextromethorphan, and Pseudoephedrine *on page 32*

Diphenhydramine and Pseudoephedrine *on page 339*

Guaifenesin, Pseudoephedrine, and Dextromethorphan *on page 482*

**U.S. Brand Names** Actifed® Allergy Tablet (Day) [OTC]; Afrin® Tablet [OTC]; Cenafed® [OTC]; Children's Silfedrine® [OTC]; Decofed® Syrup [OTC]; Drixoral® Non-Drowsy [OTC]; Efidac/24® [OTC]; Pedia Care® Oral; Sudafed® [OTC]; Sudafed® 12 Hour [OTC]; Triaminic® AM Decongestant Formula [OTC]

**Canadian Brand Names** Balminil® Decongestant; Eltor®; PMS-Pseudoephedrine; Robidrine®

**Therapeutic Category** Adrenergic Agonist Agent; Decongestant

**Use** Temporary symptomatic relief of nasal congestion due to common cold, upper respiratory allergies, and sinusitis; also promotes nasal or sinus drainage

**Usual Dosage** Oral:

Children:

<2 years: 4 mg/kg/day in divided doses every 6 hours

2-5 years: 15 mg every 6 hours; maximum: 60 mg/24 hours

6-12 years: 30 mg every 6 hours; maximum: 120 mg/24 hours

Adults: 30-60 mg every 4-6 hours, sustained release: 120 mg every 12 hours; maximum: 240 mg/24 hours

**Mechanism of Action** Directly stimulates alpha-adrenergic receptors of respiratory mucosa causing vasoconstriction; directly stimulates beta-adrenergic receptors causing bronchial relaxation, increased heart rate and contractility

**Local Anesthetic/Vasoconstrictor Precautions** Use with caution since pseudoephedrine is a sympathomimetic amine which could interact with epinephrine to cause a pressor response

**Effects on Dental Treatment** Up to 10% of patients could experience tachycardia, palpitations, and dry mouth; use vasoconstrictor with caution

**Other Adverse Effects**

>10%:

Cardiovascular: Tachycardia, palpitations, arrhythmias

Central nervous system: Nervousness, transient stimulation, insomnia, excitability, dizziness, drowsiness, headache

Neuromuscular & skeletal: Tremor

1% to 10%:

Gastrointestinal: Dry mouth

Neuromuscular & skeletal: Weakness

Miscellaneous: Sweating

(Continued)

## Pseudoephedrine *(Continued)*

<1%:

Central nervous system: Convulsions, hallucinations
Gastrointestinal: Nausea, vomiting
Genitourinary: Dysuria
Respiratory: Dyspnea

**Drug Interactions** Increased toxicity with MAO inhibitors (hypertensive crisis) sympathomimetics, CNS depressants, alcohol (sedation)

**Drug Uptake**

Onset of decongestant effect: Oral: 15-30 minutes

Duration: 4-6 hours (up to 12 hours with extended release formulation administration)

Serum half-life: 9-16 hours

**Pregnancy Risk Factor** C

**Generic Available** Yes

♦ **Pseudoephedrine, Acetaminophen, and Dextromethorphan** *see* Acetaminophen, Dextromethorphan, and Pseudoephedrine *on page 32*

♦ **Pseudoephedrine and Acetaminophen** *see* Acetaminophen and Pseudoephedrine *on page 31*

♦ **Pseudoephedrine and Azatadine** *see* Azatadine and Pseudoephedrine *on page 112*

♦ **Pseudoephedrine and Chlorpheniramine** *see* Chlorpheniramine and Pseudoephedrine *on page 233*

♦ **Pseudoephedrine and Dexbrompheniramine** *see* Dexbrompheniramine and Pseudoephedrine *on page 309*

## Pseudoephedrine and Dextromethorphan

(soo doe e FED rin & deks troe meth OR fan)

**U.S. Brand Names** Drixoral® Cough & Congestion Liquid Caps [OTC]; Vicks® 44D Cough & Head Congestion; Vicks® 44 Non-Drowsy Cold & Cough Liqui-Caps [OTC]

**Therapeutic Category** Adrenergic Agonist Agent; Antitussive; Decongestant

**Use** Temporary symptomatic relief of nasal congestion due to common cold, upper respiratory allergies, and sinusitis; also promotes nasal or sinus drainage; symptomatic relief of coughs caused by minor viral upper respiratory tract infections or inhaled irritants; most effective for a chronic nonproductive cough

**Usual Dosage** Oral: Adults: One capsule or 5-10 mL every 6 hours

**Local Anesthetic/Vasoconstrictor Precautions** Use with caution since pseudoephedrine is a sympathomimetic amine which could interact with epinephrine to cause a pressor response

**Effects on Dental Treatment** Up to 10% of patients could experience tachycardia, palpitations, and dry mouth; use vasoconstrictor with caution

**Warnings/Precautions** Research on chicken embryos exposed to concentrations of dextromethorphan relative to those typically taken by humans has shown to cause birth defects and fetal death; more study is needed, but it is suggested that pregnant women should be advised not to use dextromethorphan-containing medications

**Generic Available** Yes

♦ **Pseudoephedrine and Guaifenesin** *see* Guaifenesin and Pseudoephedrine *on page 481*

## Pseudoephedrine and Ibuprofen

(soo doe e FED rin & eye byoo PROE fen)

**U.S. Brand Names** Advil® Cold & Sinus Caplets [OTC]; Dimetapp® Sinus Caplets [OTC]; Dristan® Sinus Caplets [OTC]; Motrin® IB Sinus [OTC]; Sine-Aid® IB [OTC]

**Therapeutic Category** Adrenergic Agonist Agent; Analgesic, Non-narcotic; Decongestant

**Use** Temporary symptomatic relief of nasal congestion due to common cold, upper respiratory allergies, and sinusitis; also promotes nasal or sinus drainage; sinus headaches and pains

**Usual Dosage** Oral: Adults: 1-2 caplets every 4-6 hours

**Local Anesthetic/Vasoconstrictor Precautions** Use with caution since pseudoephedrine is a sympathomimetic amine which could interact with epinephrine to cause a pressor response

**Effects on Dental Treatment** Up to 10% of patients could experience tachycardia, palpitations, and dry mouth; use vasoconstrictor with caution

**Generic Available** Yes

♦ **Pseudoephedrine, Dextromethorphan, and Acetaminophen** *see* Acetaminophen, Dextromethorphan, and Pseudoephedrine *on page 32*

- **Pseudoephedrine, Dextromethorphan, and Guaifenesin** *see* Guaifenesin, Pseudoephedrine, and Dextromethorphan *on page 482*
- **Pseudo-Gest Plus® Tablet [OTC]** *see* Chlorpheniramine and Pseudoephedrine *on page 233*
- **Psor-a-set® Soap [OTC]** *see* Salicylic Acid *on page 900*
- **Psorcon™** *see* Diflorasone *on page 327*
- **psoriGel® [OTC]** *see* Coal Tar *on page 270*
- **P&S® Shampoo [OTC]** *see* Salicylic Acid *on page 900*

## Psyllium (SIL i yum)

**U.S. Brand Names** Effer-Syllium® [OTC]; Fiberall® Powder [OTC]; Fiberall® Wafer [OTC]; Hydrocil® [OTC]; Konsyl® [OTC]; Konsyl-D® [OTC]; Metamucil® [OTC]; Metamucil® Instant Mix [OTC]; Modane® Bulk [OTC]; Perdiem® Plain [OTC]; Reguloid® [OTC]; Serutan® [OTC]; Syllact® [OTC]; V-Lax® [OTC]

**Canadian Brand Names** Fibrepur®; Novo-Mucilax; Prodiem® Plain

**Therapeutic Category** Laxative, Bulk-Producing

**Use** Treatment of chronic atonic or spastic constipation and in constipation associated with rectal disorders; management of irritable bowel syndrome

**Usual Dosage** Oral (administer at least 3 hours before or after drugs):

Children 6-11 years: (Approximately ½ adult dosage) ½ to 1 rounded teaspoonful in 4 oz glass of liquid 1-3 times/day

Adults: 1-2 rounded teaspoonfuls or 1-2 packets or 1-2 wafers in 8 oz glass of liquid 1-3 times/day

**Mechanism of Action** Adsorbs water in the intestine to form a viscous liquid which promotes peristalsis and reduces transit time

**Local Anesthetic/Vasoconstrictor Precautions** No information available to require special precautions

**Effects on Dental Treatment** No effects or complications reported

**Other Adverse Effects** 1% to 10%:

Gastrointestinal: Esophageal or bowel obstruction, diarrhea, constipation, abdominal cramps

Respiratory: Bronchospasm, anaphylaxis upon inhalation in susceptible individuals, rhinoconjunctivitis

**Drug Interactions** Decreased effect of warfarin, digitalis, potassium-sparing diuretics, salicylates, tetracyclines, nitrofurantoin

**Drug Uptake**

Onset of action: 12-24 hour, but full effect may take 2-3 days

Absorption: Oral: Generally not absorbed following administration, small amounts of grain extracts present in the preparation have been reportedly absorbed following colonic hydrolysis

**Pregnancy Risk Factor** C

**Generic Available** Yes

- **P.T.E.-4®** *see* Trace Metals *on page 1001*
- **P.T.E.-5®** *see* Trace Metals *on page 1001*
- **Pulmicort Turbuhaler®** *see* Budesonide *on page 155*
- **Pulmozyme®** *see* Dornase Alfa *on page 349*
- **Puralube® Tears Solution [OTC]** *see* Artificial Tears *on page 97*
- **Purge® [OTC]** *see* Castor Oil *on page 196*
- **Puri-Clens™ [OTC]** *see* Methylbenzethonium Chloride *on page 658*
- **Purinethol®** *see* Mercaptopurine *on page 636*
- **P-V-Tussin®** *see* Hydrocodone, Phenylephrine, Pyrilamine, Phenindamine, Chlorpheniramine, and Ammonium Chloride *on page 511*
- **$P_xE_x$® Ophthalmic** *see* Pilocarpine and Epinephrine *on page 804*

## Pyrantel Pamoate (pi RAN tel PAM oh ate)

**U.S. Brand Names** Antiminth® [OTC]; Pin-Rid® [OTC]; Pin-X® [OTC]; Reese's® Pinworm Medicine [OTC]

**Therapeutic Category** Anthelmintic

**Use** Roundworm (*Ascaris lumbricoides*), pinworm (*Enterobius vermicularis*), and hookworm (*Ancylostoma duodenale* and *Necator americanus*) infestations, and trichostrongyliasis

**Usual Dosage** Children and Adults (purgation is not required prior to use): Oral:

Roundworm, pinworm, or trichostrongyliasis: 11 mg/kg administered as a single dose; maximum dose: 1 g. (**Note:** For pinworm infection, dosage should be repeated in 2 weeks and all family members should be treated).

Hookworm: 11 mg/kg administered once daily for 3 days

**Mechanism of Action** Causes the release of acetylcholine and inhibits cholinesterase; acts as a depolarizing neuromuscular blocker, paralyzing the helminths

**Local Anesthetic/Vasoconstrictor Precautions** No information available to require special precautions

(Continued)

## Pyrantel Pamoate *(Continued)*

**Effects on Dental Treatment** No effects or complications reported

**Other Adverse Effects**

1% to 10%: Gastrointestinal: Anorexia, nausea, vomiting, abdominal cramps, diarrhea

<1%:

Central nervous system: Dizziness, drowsiness, insomnia, headache
Dermatologic: Rash
Gastrointestinal: Tenesmus
Hepatic: Liver enzymes (elevated)
Neuromuscular & skeletal: Weakness

**Drug Uptake**

Absorption: Oral: Poor
Time to peak serum concentration: Within 1-3 hours

**Pregnancy Risk Factor** C

**Generic Available** No

**Comments** Purgation is not required prior to use

## Pyrazinamide (peer a ZIN a mide)

**Related Information**

Nonviral Infectious Diseases *on page 1095*

**Canadian Brand Names** PMS-Pyrazinamide; Tebrazid

**Therapeutic Category** Antitubercular Agent

**Use** Adjunctive treatment of tuberculosis in combination with other antituberculosis agents

**Usual Dosage** Oral (calculate dose on ideal body weight rather than total body weight): **Note:** A four-drug regimen (isoniazid, rifampin, pyrazinamide, and either streptomycin or ethambutol) is preferred for the initial, empiric treatment of TB. When the drug susceptibility results are available, the regimen should be altered as appropriate.

**Patients with TB and without HIV infection:**

**OPTION 1:**

Isoniazid resistance rate <4%: Administer daily isoniazid, rifampin, and pyrazinamide for 8 weeks followed by isoniazid and rifampin daily or directly observed therapy (DOT) 2-3 times/week for 16 weeks

If isoniazid resistance rate is not documented, ethambutol or streptomycin should also be administered until susceptibility to isoniazid or rifampin is demonstrated. Continue treatment for at least 6 months or 3 months beyond culture conversion.

**OPTION 2:** Administer daily isoniazid, rifampin, pyrazinamide, and either streptomycin or ethambutol for 2 weeks followed by DOT 2 times/week administration of the same drugs for 6 weeks, and subsequently, with isoniazid and rifampin DOT 2 times/week administration for 16 weeks

**OPTION 3:** Administer isoniazid, rifampin, pyrazinamide, and either ethambutol or streptomycin by DOT 3 times/week for 6 months

**Patients with TB and with HIV infection:**

Administer any of the above OPTIONS 1, 2 or 3, however, treatment should be continued for a total of 9 months and at least 6 months beyond culture conversion

**Note:** Some experts recommend that the duration of therapy should be extended to 9 months for patients with disseminated disease, miliary disease, disease involving the bones or joints, or tuberculosis lymphadenitis

Children and Adults:

Daily therapy: 15-30 mg/kg/day (maximum: 2 g/day)
Directly observed therapy (DOT): Twice weekly: 50-70 mg/kg (maximum: 4 g)
DOT: 3 times/week: 50-70 mg/kg (maximum: 3 g)

Elderly: Start with a lower daily dose (15 mg/kg) and increase as tolerated

**Mechanism of Action** Converted to pyrazinoic acid in susceptible strains of *Mycobacterium* which lowers the pH of the environment

**Local Anesthetic/Vasoconstrictor Precautions** No information available to require special precautions

**Effects on Dental Treatment** No effects or complications reported

**Other Adverse Effects**

1% to 10%:

Central nervous system: Malaise
Gastrointestinal: Nausea, vomiting, anorexia
Neuromuscular & skeletal: Arthralgia, myalgia

<1%:

Central nervous system: Fever

Dermatologic: Skin rash, itching, acne, photosensitivity
Endocrine & metabolic: Gout
Genitourinary: Dysuria
Hematologic: Porphyria, thrombocytopenia
Hepatic: Hepatotoxicity
Renal: Interstitial nephritis

**Drug Interactions** No data reported

**Drug Uptake** Bacteriostatic or bactericidal depending on the drug's concentration at the site of infection

Absorption: Oral: Well absorbed
Serum half-life: 9-10 hours, increased with reduced renal or hepatic function
End-stage renal disease: 9 hours
Time to peak serum concentration: Within 2 hours

**Pregnancy Risk Factor** C

**Generic Available** Yes

## Pyrethrins (pye RE thrins)

**U.S. Brand Names** A-200™ Shampoo [OTC]; Barc® Liquid [OTC]; End Lice® Liquid [OTC]; Lice-Enz® Shampoo [OTC]; Pronto® Shampoo [OTC]; Pyrinex® Pediculicide Shampoo [OTC]; Pyrinyl II® Liquid [OTC]; Pyrinyl Plus® Shampoo [OTC]; R & C® Shampoo [OTC]; RID® Shampoo [OTC]; Tisit® Blue Gel [OTC]; Tisit® Liquid [OTC]; Tisit® Shampoo [OTC]; Triple X® Liquid [OTC]

**Therapeutic Category** Antiparasitic Agent, Topical; Pediculocide

**Use** Treatment of *Pediculus humanus* infestations (head lice, body lice, pubic lice and their eggs)

**Usual Dosage** Application of pyrethrins: Topical:
Apply enough solution to completely wet infested area, including hair
Allow to remain on area for 10 minutes
Wash and rinse with large amounts of warm water
Use fine-toothed comb to remove lice and eggs from hair
Shampoo hair to restore body and luster
Treatment may be repeated if necessary once in a 24-hour period
Repeat treatment in 7-10 days to kill newly hatched lice

**Mechanism of Action** Pyrethrins are derived from flowers that belong to the chrysanthemum family. The mechanism of action on the neuronal membranes of lice is similar to that of DDT. Piperonyl butoxide is usually added to pyrethrin to enhance the product's activity by decreasing the metabolism of pyrethrins in arthropods.

**Local Anesthetic/Vasoconstrictor Precautions** No information available to require special precautions

**Effects on Dental Treatment** No effects or complications reported

**Other Adverse Effects** 1% to 10%: Local: Pruritus, burning, stinging, irritation with repeat use

**Drug Interactions** No data reported

**Drug Uptake**
Onset of action: ~30 minutes
Absorption: Topical into the system is minimal

**Pregnancy Risk Factor** C

**Generic Available** Yes

♦ **Pyridiate®** *see* Phenazopyridine *on page 788*
♦ **Pyridium®** *see* Phenazopyridine *on page 788*

## Pyridoxine (peer i DOKS een)

**U.S. Brand Names** Nestrex®

**Therapeutic Category** Antidote, Cycloserine Toxicity; Antidote, Hydralazine Toxicity; Antidote, Isoniazid Toxicity; Vitamin, Water Soluble

**Use** Prevents and treats vitamin $B_6$ deficiency, pyridoxine-dependent seizures in infants, adjunct to treatment of acute toxicity from isoniazid, cycloserine, or hydralazine overdose

**Usual Dosage**
Recommended daily allowance (RDA):
Children:
1-3 years: 0.9 mg
4-6 years: 1.3 mg
7-10 years: 1.6 mg
Adults:
Male: 1.7-2.0 mg
Female: 1.4-1.6 mg
Dietary deficiency: Oral:
Children: 5-25 mg/24 hours for 3 weeks, then 1.5-2.5 mg/day in multiple vitamin product
(Continued)

## Pyridoxine *(Continued)*

Adults: 10-20 mg/day for 3 weeks

Drug-induced neuritis (eg, isoniazid, hydralazine, penicillamine, cycloserine):

Oral:

Children:

Treatment: 10-50 mg/24 hours

Prophylaxis: 1-2 mg/kg/24 hours

Adults:

Treatment: 100-200 mg/24 hours

Prophylaxis: 25-100 mg/24 hours

Treatment of seizures and/or coma from acute isoniazid toxicity, a dose of pyridoxine hydrochloride equal to the amount of INH ingested can be given I.M./I.V. in divided doses together with other anticonvulsants; if the amount INH ingested is not known, administer 5 g I.V. pyridoxine

Treatment of acute hydralazine toxicity, a pyridoxine dose of 25 mg/kg in divided doses I.M./I.V. has been used

**Mechanism of Action** Precursor to pyridoxal, which functions in the metabolism of proteins, carbohydrates, and fats; pyridoxal also aids in the release of liver and muscle-stored glycogen and in the synthesis of GABA (within the central nervous system) and heme

**Local Anesthetic/Vasoconstrictor Precautions** No information available to require special precautions

**Effects on Dental Treatment** No effects or complications reported

**Other Adverse Effects** <1%:

Central nervous system: Sensory neuropathy, seizures have occurred following I.V. administration of very large doses, headache

Gastrointestinal: Nausea

Endocrine & metabolic: Decreased serum folic acid secretions

Hepatic: Elevated AST

Neuromuscular & skeletal: Paresthesia

Miscellaneous: Allergic reactions have been reported

**Drug Interactions** Decreased serum levels of levodopa, phenobarbital, and phenytoin

**Drug Uptake**

Absorption: Enteral, parenteral: Well absorbed from GI tract

Serum half-life: 15-20 days

**Pregnancy Risk Factor** A (C if dose exceeds RDA recommendation)

**Generic Available** Yes

## Pyrimethamine (peer i METH a meen)

**U.S. Brand Names** Daraprim®

**Therapeutic Category** Antimalarial Agent

**Use** Prophylaxis of malaria due to susceptible strains of plasmodia; used in conjunction with quinine and sulfadiazine for the treatment of uncomplicated attacks of chloroquine-resistant *P. falciparum* malaria; used in conjunction with fast-acting schizonticide to initiate transmission control and suppression cure; synergistic combination with sulfonamide in treatment of toxoplasmosis

**Usual Dosage**

Malaria chemoprophylaxis (for areas where chloroquine-resistant *P. falciparum* exists): Begin prophylaxis 2 weeks before entering endemic area:

Children: 0.5 mg/kg once weekly; not to exceed 25 mg/dose

**or**

Children:

<4 years: 6.25 mg once weekly

4-10 years: 12.5 mg once weekly

Children >10 years and Adults: 25 mg once weekly

Dosage should be continued for all age groups for at least 6-10 weeks after leaving endemic areas

Chloroquine-resistant *P. falciparum* malaria (when used in conjunction with quinine and sulfadiazine):

Children:

<10 kg: 6.25 mg/day once daily for 3 days

10-20 kg: 12.5 mg/day once daily for 3 days

20-40 kg: 25 mg/day once daily for 3 days

Adults: 25 mg twice daily for 3 days

Toxoplasmosis:

Infants for congenital toxoplasmosis: Oral: 1 mg/kg once daily for 6 months with sulfadiazine then every other month with sulfa, alternating with spiramycin.

Children: Loading dose: 2 mg/kg/day divided into 2 equal daily doses for 1-3 days (maximum: 100 mg/day) followed by 1 mg/kg/day divided into 2 doses for 4 weeks; maximum: 25 mg/day

With sulfadiazine or trisulfapyrimidines: 2 mg/kg/day divided every 12 hours for 3 days followed by 1 mg/kg/day once daily or divided twice daily for 4 weeks given with trisulfapyrimidines or sulfadiazine

Adults: 50-75 mg/day together with 1-4 g of a sulfonamide for 1-3 weeks depending on patient's tolerance and response, then reduce dose by 50% and continue for 4-5 weeks **or** 25-50 mg/day for 3-4 weeks

**Mechanism of Action** Inhibits parasitic dihydrofolate reductase, resulting in inhibition of vital tetrahydrofolic acid synthesis

**Local Anesthetic/Vasoconstrictor Precautions** No information available to require special precautions

**Effects on Dental Treatment** Atrophic glossitis has been reported

**Other Adverse Effects**

1% to 10%:

Gastrointestinal: Anorexia, abdominal cramps, vomiting

Hematologic: Megaloblastic anemia, leukopenia, thrombocytopenia, agranulocytosis

<1%:

Central nervous system: Insomnia, lightheadedness, fever, malaise, seizures, depression

Dermatologic: Skin rash, dermatitis, abnormal skin pigmentation

Gastrointestinal: Diarrhea, dry mouth, atrophic glossitis

Hematologic: Pulmonary eosinophilia

**Drug Interactions**

Decreased effect: Pyrimethamine effectiveness decreased by acid

Increased effect: Sulfonamides (synergy), methotrexate, TMP/SMX

**Drug Uptake**

Absorption: Oral: Well absorbed

Serum half-life: 80-95 hours

**Pregnancy Risk Factor** C

**Generic Available** No

- **Pyrinex® Pediculicide Shampoo [OTC]** *see* Pyrethrins *on page 867*
- **Pyrinyl II® Liquid [OTC]** *see* Pyrethrins *on page 867*
- **Pyrinyl Plus® Shampoo [OTC]** *see* Pyrethrins *on page 867*

## Pyrithione Zinc (peer i THYE one zingk)

**U.S. Brand Names** DHS Zinc® [OTC]; Head & Shoulders® [OTC]; Theraplex Z® [OTC]; Zincon® Shampoo [OTC]; ZNP® Bar [OTC]

**Therapeutic Category** Antiseborrheic Agent, Topical

**Use** Relieves the itching, irritation and scalp flaking associated with dandruff and/or seborrheal dermatitis of the scalp

**Usual Dosage** Shampoo hair twice weekly, wet hair, apply to scalp and massage vigorously, rinse and repeat

**Local Anesthetic/Vasoconstrictor Precautions** No information available to require special precautions

**Effects on Dental Treatment** No effects or complications reported

**Generic Available** No

## Quazepam (KWAY ze pam)

**U.S. Brand Names** Doral®

**Therapeutic Category** Benzodiazepine; Hypnotic; Sedative

**Use** Treatment of insomnia; more likely than triazolam to cause daytime sedation and fatigue; is classified as a long-acting benzodiazepine hypnotic (like flurazepam - Dalmane®), this long duration of action may prevent withdrawal symptoms when therapy is discontinued

**Usual Dosage** Adults: Oral: Initial: 15 mg at bedtime, in some patients the dose may be reduced to 7.5 mg after a few nights

**Mechanism of Action** Depresses all levels of the CNS, including the limbic and reticular formation, probably through the increased action of gamma-aminobutyric acid (GABA), which is a major inhibitory neurotransmitter in the brain

**Local Anesthetic/Vasoconstrictor Precautions** No information available to require special precautions

**Effects on Dental Treatment** >10% of patients will experience dry mouth which disappears with cessation of drug therapy

**Other Adverse Effects**

>10%:

Central nervous system: Drowsiness

1% to 10%:

Central nervous system: Headache, fatigue, dizziness

(Continued)

## Quazepam *(Continued)*

Gastrointestinal: Xerostomia, dyspepsia

<1%:

Central nervous system: Slurred speech, irritability
Endocrine & metabolic: Changes in libido
Genitourinary: Urinary retention, incontinence
Hematologic: Leukocytosis, thrombocytosis
Hepatic: Jaundice, increased total bilirubin, increased alkaline phosphatase
Neuromuscular & skeletal: Dysarthria, dystonia
Renal: Increased BUN, increased creatinine

**Drug Interactions** Increased effect/toxicity with CNS depressants (narcotics, alcohol, MAO inhibitors, TCAs, anesthetics, barbiturates, phenothiazines)

**Drug Uptake**

Absorption: Oral: Rapid
Serum half-life:
Parent drug: 25-41 hours
Active metabolite: 40-114 hours

**Pregnancy Risk Factor** X

**Generic Available** No

♦ **Questran®** *see* Cholestyramine Resin *on page 244*

♦ **Questran® Light** *see* Cholestyramine Resin *on page 244*

## Quetiapine (kwe TYE a peen)

**U.S. Brand Names** Seroquel®

**Therapeutic Category** Antipsychotic Agent

**Synonyms** Quetiapine Fumarate

**Use** Management of psychotic disorders; this antipsychotic drug belongs to a new chemical class, the dibenzothiazepine derivatives

**Usual Dosage** Adults: Oral: 25-100 mg 2-3 times/day

**Mechanism of Action** Mechanism of action of quetiapine, as with other antipsychotic drugs, is unknown. However, it has been proposed that this drug's antipsychotic activity is mediated through a combination of dopamine type 2 ($D_2$) and serotonin type 2 ($5HT_2$) antagonism. However, it is an antagonist at multiple neurotransmitter receptors in the brain: serotonin $5HT_{1A}$ and $5HT_2$, dopamine $D_1$ and $D_2$, histamine $H_1$, and adrenergic alpha$_1$- and alpha$_2$-receptors; but appears to have no appreciable affinity at cholinergic muscarinic and benzodiazepine receptors.

Antagonism at receptors other than dopamine and $5HT_2$ with similar receptor affinities may explain some of the other effects of quetiapine. The drug's antagonism of histamine $H_1$ receptors may explain the somnolence observed with it. The drug's antagonism of adrenergic alpha$_1$-receptors may explain the orthostatic hypotension observed with it.

**Local Anesthetic/Vasoconstrictor Precautions** No information available to require special precautions

**Effects on Dental Treatment** No effects or complications reported

**Other Adverse Effects**

Cardiovascular: Postural hypotension (4% to 14%)
Central nervous system: Agitation (6% to 28%), somnolence (6% to 39%), headache (5% to 31%), insomnia (4% to 15%), dizziness (2% to 11%)
Gastrointestinal: Dry mouth (8% to 19%)
Hepatic: Serum ALT increases (5% to 17%)
Miscellaneous: <2%: Tachycardia, dyspepsia, constipation, weight gain, increases in total cholesterol and triglycerides; hypothyroidism developed in a small number of patients. Treatment-related extrapyramidal symptoms were not observed in animal studies and lens changes have been observed in patients receiving long-term therapy.

**Drug Interactions** CYP2D6 and 3A3/4 enzyme substrate

Caution with other centrally acting drugs; avoid alcohol. May enhance effects of antihypertensive agents; may antagonize levodopa, dopamine agonists. Increased clearance when given with phenytoin or thioridazine, caution with other liver enzyme inducers (carbamazepine, barbiturates, rifampin, glucocorticoids); although data is not yet available, caution is advised with inhibitors of cytochrome P-450 (eg, ketoconazole, erythromycin); reduces the clearance of lorazepam.

**Drug Uptake**

Absorption: Accumulation is predictable upon multiple dosing
Serum half-life, mean terminal: ~6 hours

**Pregnancy Risk Factor** C

**Dosage Forms** Tablet, as fumarate: 25 mg, 100 mg, 200 mg

♦ **Quetiapine Fumarate** *see* Quetiapine *on this page*

- **Quibron®** *see* Theophylline and Guaifenesin *on page 973*
- **Quibron®-T** *see* Theophylline *on page 969*
- **Quibron®-T/SR** *see* Theophylline *on page 969*
- **Quinaglute® Dura-Tabs®** *see* Quinidine *on page 873*
- **Quinalan®** *see* Quinidine *on page 873*
- **Quinamm®** *see* Quinine *on page 874*

# Quinapril (KWIN a pril)

**Related Information**

Cardiovascular Diseases *on page 1066*

**U.S. Brand Names** Accupril®

**Therapeutic Category** Angiotensin-Converting Enzyme (ACE) Inhibitor

**Use** Management of hypertension and treatment of congestive heart failure; increase circulation in Raynaud's phenomenon; idiopathic edema

**Unlabeled use:** Hypertensive crisis, diabetic nephropathy, rheumatoid arthritis, diagnosis of anatomic renal artery stenosis, hypertension secondary to scleroderma renal crisis, diagnosis of aldosteronism, idiopathic edema, Bartter's syndrome, postmyocardial infarction for prevention of ventricular failure

**Usual Dosage**

Adults: Oral: Initial: 10 mg once daily, adjust according to blood pressure response at peak and trough blood levels; in general, the normal dosage range is 20-80 mg/day

Elderly: Initial: 2.5-5 mg/day; increase dosage at increments of 2.5-5 mg at 1- to 2-week intervals

**Mechanism of Action** Competitive inhibitor of angiotensin-converting enzyme (ACE); prevents conversion of angiotensin I to angiotensin II, a potent vasoconstrictor; results in lower levels of angiotensin II which causes an increase in plasma renin activity and a reduction in aldosterone secretion; a CNS mechanism may also be involved in hypotensive effect as angiotensin II increases adrenergic outflow from CNS; vasoactive kallikreins may be decreased in conversion to active hormones by ACE inhibitors, thus reducing blood pressure

**Local Anesthetic/Vasoconstrictor Precautions** No information available to require special precautions

**Effects on Dental Treatment** No effects or complications reported

**Drug-Drug Interactions With ACEIs**

| Precipitant Drug | Drug (Category) and Effect | Description |
|---|---|---|
| Antacids | ACE Inhibitors: decreased | Decreased bioavailability of ACEIs. May be more likely with captopril. Separate administration times by 1-2 hours. |
| NSAIDs (indomethacin) | ACEIs: decreased | Reduced hypotensive effects of ACEIs. More prominent in low renin or volume dependent hypertensive patients. |
| Phenothiazines | ACEIs: increased | Pharmacologic effects of ACEIs may be increased. |
| ACEIs | Allopurinol: increased | Higher risk of hypersensitivity reaction possible when given concurrently. Three case reports of Stevens-Johnson syndrome with captopril. |
| ACEIs | Digoxin: increased | Increased plasma digoxin levels. |
| ACEIs | Lithium: increased | Increased serum lithium levels and symptoms of toxicity may occur. |
| ACEIs | Potassium preps/ potassium sparing diuretics increased | Coadministration may result in elevated potassium levels. |

**Other Adverse Effects**

1% to 10%:

Cardiovascular: Hypotension

Central nervous system: Dizziness, headache, fatigue

Gastrointestinal: Diarrhea

Renal: Elevated BUN and serum creatinine

Respiratory: Upper respiratory symptoms, cough

<1%:

Cardiovascular: Chest discomfort, flushing, myocardial infarction, angina pectoris, orthostatic hypotension, rhythm disturbances, tachycardia, peripheral edema, vasculitis, palpitations, syncope

Central nervous system: Fever, malaise, depression, somnolence, insomnia

Dermatologic: Urticaria, pruritus, angioedema

(Continued)

## Quinapril *(Continued)*

Endocrine & metabolic: Gout
Gastrointestinal: Pancreatitis, abdominal pain, anorexia, constipation, flatulence, dry mouth
Hematologic: Neutropenia, bone marrow suppression
Hepatic: Hepatitis
Neuromuscular & skeletal: Arthralgia, shoulder pain
Ocular: Blurred vision
Respiratory: Bronchitis, sinusitis, pharyngeal pain
Miscellaneous: Sweating

**Drug Interactions** See table.

**Drug Uptake**
Serum half-life, elimination:
Quinapril: 0.8 hours
Quinaprilat: 2 hours
Time to peak serum concentration:
Quinapril: 1 hour
Quinaprilat: ~2 hours

**Pregnancy Risk Factor** C (first trimester); D (second and third trimester)

**Generic Available** No

## Quinestrol (kwin ES trole)

**Related Information**
Endocrine Disorders & Pregnancy *on page 1082*

**U.S. Brand Names** Estrovis®

**Therapeutic Category** Estrogen Derivative

**Use** Atrophic vaginitis; hypogonadism; primary ovarian failure; vasomotor symptoms of menopause; prostatic carcinoma; osteoporosis prophylactic

**Usual Dosage** Adults: Female: Oral: 100 mcg once daily for 7 days; followed by 100 mcg/week beginning 2 weeks after inception of treatment; may increase to 200 mcg/week if necessary

**Mechanism of Action** Increases the synthesis of DNA, RNA, and various proteins in target tissues; reduces the release of gonadotropin-releasing hormone from the hypothalamus; reduces FSH and LH release from the pituitary

**Local Anesthetic/Vasoconstrictor Precautions** No information available to require special precautions

**Effects on Dental Treatment** No effects or complications reported

**Other Adverse Effects**
>10%:
Cardiovascular: Peripheral edema
Endocrine & metabolic: Enlargement of breasts (female and male), breast tenderness
Gastrointestinal: Nausea, anorexia, bloating
1% to 10%:
Central nervous system: Headache
Endocrine & metabolic: Increased libido (female), decreased libido (male)
Gastrointestinal: Vomiting, diarrhea
<1%:
Cardiovascular: Hypertension, thromboembolism, myocardial infarction, edema
Central nervous system: Depression, dizziness, anxiety, stroke
Dermatologic: Chloasma, melasma, rash
Endocrine: Breast tumors, amenorrhea, alterations in frequency and flow of menses, decreased glucose tolerance, elevated triglycerides and LDL
Gastrointestinal: GI distress
Hepatic: Cholestatic jaundice
Ocular: Intolerance to contact lenses
Miscellaneous: Increased susceptibility to *Candida* infection

**Drug Interactions** No significant interactions reported

**Drug Uptake**
Onset of therapeutic effect: Commonly within 3 days of treatment
Duration: Can persist for as long as 4 months
Serum half-life: 120 hours

**Pregnancy Risk Factor** X

**Generic Available** No

## Quinethazone (kwin ETH a zone)

**Related Information**
Cardiovascular Diseases *on page 1066*

**U.S. Brand Names** Hydromox®

**Therapeutic Category** Diuretic, Thiazide

**Use** Adjunctive therapy in treatment of edema and hypertension

**Usual Dosage** Adults: Oral: 50-100 mg once daily up to a maximum of 200 mg/day

**Mechanism of Action** Quinethazone is a quinazoline derivative which increases the renal excretion of sodium and chloride and an accompanying volume of water due to inhibition of the tubular mechanism of electrolyte reabsorption.

**Local Anesthetic/Vasoconstrictor Precautions** No information available to require special precautions

**Effects on Dental Treatment** No effects or complications reported

**Other Adverse Effects**

1% to 10%: Endocrine & metabolic: Hypokalemia

<1%:

- Cardiovascular: Hypotension
- Central nervous system: Drowsiness
- Dermatologic: Photosensitivity, rash
- Endocrine & metabolic: Fluid and electrolyte imbalances (hypocalcemia, hypomagnesemia, hyponatremia), hyperglycemia
- Gastrointestinal: Nausea, vomiting, anorexia
- Hematologic: Aplastic anemia, hemolytic anemia, leukopenia, agranulocytosis, thrombocytopenia
- Hepatic: Hepatitis
- Renal: Prerenal azotemia, polyuria, uremia

**Drug Interactions**

Decreased effect of oral hypoglycemics; decreased absorption with cholestyramine and colestipol

Increased effect with furosemide and other loop diuretics

Increased toxicity/levels of lithium

**Drug Uptake**

Onset of action: 2 hours

Duration: 18-24 hours

**Pregnancy Risk Factor** D

**Generic Available** No

♦ **Quinidex® Extentabs®** *see* Quinidine *on this page*

## Quinidine (KWIN i deen)

**Related Information**

Cardiovascular Diseases *on page 1066*

**U.S. Brand Names** Cardioquin®; Quinaglute® Dura-Tabs®; Quinalan®; Quinidex® Extentabs®; Quinora®

**Therapeutic Category** Antiarrhythmic Agent, Class I-A; Antiarrhythmic Agent (Supraventricular & Ventricular)

**Use** Prophylaxis after cardioversion of atrial fibrillation and/or flutter to maintain normal sinus rhythm; also used to prevent reoccurrence of paroxysmal supraventricular tachycardia, paroxysmal A-V junctional rhythm, paroxysmal ventricular tachycardia, paroxysmal atrial fibrillation, and atrial or ventricular premature contractions; also has activity against *Plasmodium falciparum* malaria

**Usual Dosage Dosage expressed in terms of the salt: 267 mg of quinidine gluconate = 200 mg of quinidine sulfate**

Children: Test dose for idiosyncratic reaction (sulfate, oral or gluconate, I.M.): 2 mg/kg or 60 mg/m$^2$

- Oral (quinidine sulfate): 15-60 mg/kg/day in 4-5 divided doses or 6 mg/kg every 4-6 hours; usual 30 mg/kg/day or 900 mg/m$^2$/day given in 5 daily doses
- I.V. **not** recommended (quinidine gluconate): 2-10 mg/kg/dose given at a rate ≤10 mg/minute every 3-6 hours as needed

Adults: Test dose: Oral, I.M.: 200 mg administered several hours before full dosage (to determine possibility of idiosyncratic reaction)

- Oral:
  - Sulfate: 100-600 mg/dose every 4-6 hours; begin at 200 mg/dose and titrate to desired effect (maximum daily dose: 3-4 g)
  - Gluconate: 324-972 mg every 8-12 hours
- I.M.: 400 mg/dose every 4-6 hours
- I.V.: 200-400 mg/dose diluted and given at a rate ≤10 mg/minute

**Mechanism of Action** Class 1A antiarrhythmic agent; depresses phase O of the action potential; decreases myocardial excitability and conduction velocity, and myocardial contractility by decreasing sodium influx during depolarization and potassium efflux in repolarization; also reduces calcium transport across cell membrane

**Local Anesthetic/Vasoconstrictor Precautions** No information available to require special precautions

(Continued)

## Quinidine *(Continued)*

**Effects on Dental Treatment** When taken over a long period of time, the anticholinergic side effects from quinidine can cause a reduction of saliva production or secretion contributing to discomfort and dental disease (ie, caries, oral candidiasis and periodontal disease)

**Other Adverse Effects**

>10%: Gastrointestinal: Bitter taste, diarrhea, anorexia, nausea, vomiting, stomach cramping

1% to 10%:

- Cardiovascular: Hypotension, syncope
- Central nervous system: Lightheadedness, severe headache
- Dermatologic: Skin rash
- Ocular: Blurred vision
- Otic: Tinnitus
- Respiratory: Wheezing

<1%:

- Cardiovascular: Tachycardia, heart block, ventricular fibrillation, vascular collapse
- Central nervous system: Confusion, delirium, fever, vertigo
- Dermatologic: Angioedema
- Hematologic: Anemia, thrombocytopenic purpura, blood dyscrasias
- Otic: Impaired hearing
- Respiratory: Respiratory depression

**Drug Interactions**

Decreased effect: Phenobarbital, phenytoin, and rifampin may decrease quinidine serum concentrations

Increased toxicity:

- Verapamil, amiodarone, alkalinizing agents, and cimetidine may increase quinine serum concentrations
- Quinidine may increase plasma concentration of digoxin, digoxin dosage may need to be reduced (by one-half) when quinidine is initiated
- Beta-blockers (ie, propranolol) + quinine may cause enhanced bradycardia; increased nifedipine plasma concentration
- Quinidine may enhance coumarin anticoagulants

**Drug Uptake**

Serum half-life:

- Children: 2.5-6.7 hours
- Adults: 6-8 hours; increased half-life with elderly, cirrhosis, and congestive heart failure

**Pregnancy Risk Factor** C

**Generic Available** Yes

## Quinine (KWYE nine)

**U.S. Brand Names** Formula Q® [OTC]; Legatrin® [OTC]; M-KYA® [OTC]; Quinamm®; Quiphile®; Q-vel®

**Therapeutic Category** Antimalarial Agent; Muscle Relaxant

**Use** Suppression or treatment of chloroquine-resistant *P. falciparum* malaria; treatment of *Babesia microti* infection; prevention and treatment of nocturnal recumbency leg muscle cramps

**Usual Dosage** Oral:

Children:

- Treatment of chloroquine-resistant malaria: 25 mg/kg/day in divided doses every 8 hours for 3-7 days in conjunction with another agent
- Babesiosis: 25 mg/kg/day, (up to a maximum of 650 mg/dose) divided every 8 hours for 7 days

Adults:

- Treatment of chloroquine-resistant malaria: 650 mg every 8 hours for 3-7 days in conjunction with another agent
- Suppression of malaria: 325 mg twice daily and continued for 6 weeks after exposure
- Babesiosis: 650 mg every 6-8 hours for 7 days
- Leg cramps: 200-300 mg at bedtime

**Mechanism of Action** Depresses oxygen uptake and carbohydrate metabolism; intercalates into DNA, disrupting the parasite's replication and transcription; affects calcium distribution within muscle fibers and decreases the excitability of the motor end-plate region; cardiovascular effects similar to quinidine

**Local Anesthetic/Vasoconstrictor Precautions** No information available to require special precautions

**Effects on Dental Treatment** No effects or complications reported

**Other Adverse Effects**
>10%:
Central nervous system: Severe headache
Gastrointestinal: Nausea, vomiting, diarrhea
Ocular: Blurred vision
Otic: Tinnitus
<1%:
Cardiovascular: Flushing of the skin, anginal symptoms
Central nervous system: Fever
Dermatologic: Rash, pruritus
Endocrine & metabolic: Hypoglycemia
Gastrointestinal: Epigastric pain
Hematologic: Hemolysis, thrombocytopenia
Hepatic: Hepatitis
Ocular: Nightblindness, diplopia, optic atrophy
Otic: Impaired hearing
Miscellaneous: Hypersensitivity reactions

**Drug Interactions**
Decreased effect: Phenobarbital, phenytoin, and rifampin may decrease quinine serum concentrations
Increased toxicity:
Verapamil, amiodarone, alkalizing agents, and cimetidine may increase quinidine serum concentrations
Quinidine may increase plasma concentration of digoxin, digoxin dosage may need to be reduced (by one-half) when quinidine is initiated
Beta-blockers + quinidine may cause enhanced bradycardia
Quinidine may enhance coumarin anticoagulants

**Drug Uptake**
Absorption: Oral: Readily absorbed mainly from the upper small intestine
Serum half-life:
Children: 6-12 hours
Adults: 8-14 hours
Time to peak serum concentration: Within 1-3 hours

**Pregnancy Risk Factor** D
**Generic Available** Yes

♦ **Quinora®** *see* Quinidine *on page 873*
♦ **Quinsana Plus® [OTC]** *see* Tolnaftate *on page 997*
♦ **Quiphile®** *see* Quinine *on previous page*
♦ **Q-vel®** *see* Quinine *on previous page*
♦ **QYS®** *see* Hydroxyzine *on page 518*

## Rabies Immune Globulin (Human)

(RAY beez i MYUN GLOB yoo lin, HYU man)

**Related Information**
Animal and Human Bites Guidelines *on page 1164*

**U.S. Brand Names** Hyperab®; Imogam®

**Therapeutic Category** Immune Globulin

**Use** Part of postexposure prophylaxis of persons with rabies exposure who lack a history or pre-exposure or postexposure prophylaxis with rabies vaccine or a recently documented neutralizing antibody response to previous rabies vaccination; although it is preferable to give RIG with the first dose of vaccine, it can be given up to 8 days after vaccination

**Usual Dosage** Children and Adults: I.M.: 20 units/kg in a single dose (RIG should always be administered in conjunction with rabies vaccine (HDCV)); infiltrate ½ of the dose locally around the wound; give the remainder I.M.

**Mechanism of Action** Rabies immune globulin is a solution of globulins dried from the plasma or serum of selected adult human donors who have been immunized with rabies vaccine and have developed high titers of rabies antibody. It generally contains 10% to 18% of protein of which not less than 80% is monomeric immunoglobulin G.

**Local Anesthetic/Vasoconstrictor Precautions** No information available to require special precautions

**Effects on Dental Treatment** No effects or complications reported

**Other Adverse Effects**
1% to 10%:
Central nervous system: Fever (mild)
Local: Soreness at injection site
<1%:
Dermatologic: Urticaria, angioedema
Neuromuscular & skeletal: Stiffness, soreness of muscles
Miscellaneous: Anaphylactic shock
(Continued)

## Rabies Immune Globulin (Human) *(Continued)*

**Drug Interactions**
Decreased effect: Live vaccines, corticosteroids, immunosuppressive agents; should not be administered within 3 months

**Pregnancy Risk Factor** C

**Generic Available** No

## Rabies Virus Vaccine (RAY beez VYE rus vak SEEN)

**Related Information**
Animal and Human Bites Guidelines *on page 1164*

**U.S. Brand Names** Imovax® Rabies I.D. Vaccine; Imovax® Rabies Vaccine

**Therapeutic Category** Vaccine, Inactivated Virus

**Use** Veterinarians, animal handlers, certain laboratory workers, and persons living in or visiting countries for longer than 1 month where rabies is a constant threat.

Complete pre-exposure prophylaxis does not eliminate the need for additional therapy with rabies vaccine after a rabies exposure. The Food and Drug Administration has not approved the I.D. use of rabies vaccine for postexposure prophylaxis. Recommendations for I.D. use of HDCV are currently being discussed. The decision for postexposure rabies vaccination depends on the species of biting animal, the circumstances of biting incident, and the type of exposure (bite, saliva contamination of wound, and so on). The type of and schedule for postexposure prophylaxis depends upon the person's previous rabies vaccination status or the result of a previous or current serologic test for rabies antibody. For postexposure prophylaxis, rabies vaccine should always be administered I.M., **not** I.D.

**Usual Dosage**

**Pre-exposure prophylaxis:** Two 1 mL doses I.M. 1 week apart, third dose 3 weeks after second. If exposure continues, booster doses can be given every 2 years, or an antibody titer determined and a booster dose given if the titer is inadequate.

**Postexposure prophylaxis:** All postexposure treatment should begin with immediate cleansing of the wound with soap and water

Persons not previously immunized as above: Rabies immune globulin 20 units/kg body weight, half infiltrated at bite site if possible, remainder I.M.; and 5 doses of rabies vaccine, 1 mL I.M., one each on days 0, 3, 7, 14, 28

Persons who have previously received postexposure prophylaxis with rabies vaccine, received a recommended I.M. pre-exposure series of rabies vaccine or have a previously documented rabies antibody titer considered adequate: Two doses of rabies vaccine, 1 mL I.M., one each on days 0 and 3

**Mechanism of Action** Rabies vaccine is an inactivated virus vaccine which promotes immunity by inducing an active immune response. The production of specific antibodies requires about 7-10 days to develop. Rabies immune globulin or antirabies serum, equine (ARS) is given in conjunction with rabies vaccine to provide immune protection until an antibody response can occur.

**Local Anesthetic/Vasoconstrictor Precautions** No information available to require special precautions

**Effects on Dental Treatment** No effects or complications reported

**Other Adverse Effects** >10%:
Central nervous system: Dizziness, malaise, encephalomyelitis, transverse myelitis, fever, pain
Dermatologic: Itching, erythema
Gastrointestinal: Nausea, headache, abdominal pain
Local: Local discomfort, swelling
Neuromuscular & skeletal: Neuroparalytic reactions, myalgia

**Drug Interactions** Decreased effect with immunosuppressive agents, corticosteroids, antimalarial drugs (ie, chloroquine); persons on these drugs should receive RIG (3 doses/1 mL each) by the I.M. route

**Drug Uptake**
Onset of effect: I.M.: Rabies antibody appears in the serum within 7-10 days
Peak effect: Within 30-60 days and persists for at least 1 year

**Pregnancy Risk Factor** C

**Generic Available** No

## Raloxifene (ral OX i feen)

**U.S. Brand Names** Evista®

**Therapeutic Category** Selective Estrogen Receptor Modulator (SERM)

**Synonyms** Keoxifene Hydrochloride; Raloxifene Hydrochloride

**Use** Prevention of osteoporosis in postmenopausal women

**Usual Dosage** Adults: Oral: One tablet daily may be administered any time of the day without regard to meals

**Mechanism of Action** A selective estrogen receptor modulator, meaning that it affects some of the same receptors that estrogen does, but not all, and in some instances, it antagonizes or blocks estrogen; it acts like estrogen to prevent bone loss and improve lipid profiles, but it has the potential to block some estrogen effects such as those that lead to breast cancer and uterine cancer

**Local Anesthetic/Vasoconstrictor Precautions** No information available to require special precautions

**Effects on Dental Treatment** No effects or complications reported

**Drug Interactions** Manufacturer's information states that caution should be used when raloxifene is coadministered with other highly protein-bound drugs such as ibuprofen and naproxen. Raloxifene could displace the NSAID or vice versa leading to increased free active form of the target drug.

**Dosage Forms** Tablet, as hydrochloride: 60 mg

**Comments** The decrease in estrogen-related adverse effects with the selective estrogen-receptor modulators in general and raloxifene in particular should improve compliance and decrease the incidence of cardiovascular events and fractures while not increasing breast cancer

♦ **Raloxifene Hydrochloride** *see* Raloxifene *on previous page*

## Ramipril (ra MI pril)

**Related Information**

Cardiovascular Diseases *on page 1066*

**U.S. Brand Names** Altace™

**Therapeutic Category** Angiotensin-Converting Enzyme (ACE) Inhibitor

**Use** Treatment of hypertension, alone or in combination with thiazide diuretics

**Unlabeled use:** Congestive heart failure

**Usual Dosage** Adults: Oral: 2.5-5 mg once daily, maximum: 20 mg/day

**Mechanism of Action** Ramipril is an angiotensin-converting enzyme (ACE) inhibitor which prevents the formation of angiotensin II from angiotensin I and exhibits pharmacologic effects that are similar to captopril. Ramipril must undergo enzymatic saponification by esterases in the liver to its biologically active metabolite, ramiprilat. The pharmacodynamic effects of ramipril result from the high-affinity, competitive, reversible binding of ramiprilat to angiotensin-converting enzyme thus preventing the formation of the potent vasoconstrictor angiotensin II. This isomerized enzyme-inhibitor complex has a slow rate of dissociation, which results in high potency and a long duration of action; a CNS mechanism may also be involved in the hypotensive effect as angiotensin II increases adrenergic outflow from CNS; vasoactive kallikreins may be decreased in conversion to active hormones by ACE inhibitors, thus reducing blood pressure

**Local Anesthetic/Vasoconstrictor Precautions** No information available to require special precautions

**Effects on Dental Treatment** No effects or complications reported

**Drug-Drug Interactions With ACEIs**

| Precipitant Drug | Drug (Category) and Effect | Description |
|---|---|---|
| Antacids | ACE Inhibitors: decreased | Decreased bioavailability of ACEIs. May be more likely with captopril. Separate administration times by 1-2 hours. |
| NSAIDs (indomethacin) | ACEIs: decreased | Reduced hypotensive effects of ACEIs. More prominent in low renin or volume dependent hypertensive patients. |
| Phenothiazines | ACEIs: increased | Pharmacologic effects of ACEIs may be increased. |
| ACEIs | Allopurinol: increased | Higher risk of hypersensitivity reaction possible when given concurrently. Three case reports of Stevens-Johnson syndrome with captopril. |
| ACEIs | Digoxin: increased | Increased plasma digoxin levels. |
| ACEIs | Lithium: increased | Increased serum lithium levels and symptoms of toxicity may occur. |
| ACEIs | Potassium preps/ potassium sparing diuretics increased | Coadministration may result in elevated potassium levels. |

**Other Adverse Effects**

1% to 10%:

Cardiovascular: Tachycardia, chest pain, palpitations

Central nervous system: Insomnia, headache, dizziness, fatigue, malaise

(Continued)

## Ramipril *(Continued)*

Dermatologic: Rash, pruritus, alopecia
Gastrointestinal: Dysgeusia, abdominal pain, vomiting, nausea, diarrhea, anorexia, constipation, dysgeusia
Neuromuscular & skeletal: Paresthesia
Renal: Oliguria
Respiratory: Transient cough

<1%:
Cardiovascular: Hypotension
Dermatologic: Angioedema
Endocrine & metabolic: Hyperkalemia
Hematologic: Neutropenia, agranulocytosis
Renal: Proteinuria; elevated BUN, serum creatinine

**Drug Interactions** See table.

**Drug Uptake**
Absorption: Well absorbed from GI tract (50% to 60%)
Serum half-life: Ramiprilat: >50 hours
Time to peak serum concentration: ~1 hour

**Pregnancy Risk Factor** C (first trimester); D (second and third trimesters)

**Generic Available** No

♦ **Ramses® [OTC]** *see* Nonoxynol 9 *on page 728*

## Ranitidine Bismuth Citrate (ra NI ti deen BIZ muth SIT rate)

**U.S. Brand Names** Tritec®

**Therapeutic Category** Histamine $H_2$ Antagonist; *H. Pylori* Agent

**Use** Used in combination with clarithromycin for the treatment of active duodenal ulcer associated with *H. pylori* infection; not to be used alone for the treatment of active duodenal ulcer

**Usual Dosage** Adults: Oral: 400 mg twice daily for 4 weeks with clarithromycin 500 mg 3 times/day for first 2 weeks

**Mechanism of Action** As a complex of ranitidine and bismuth citrate, gastric acid secretion is inhibited by histamine-blocking activity at the parietal cell and the structural integrity of *H. pylori* organisms is disrupted; additionally bismuth reduces the adherence of *H. pylori* to epithelial cells of the stomach and may exert a cytoprotectant effect, inhibiting pepsin, as well. Adequate eradication of *Helicobacter pylori* is achieved with the combination of clarithromycin.

**Local Anesthetic/Vasoconstrictor Precautions** No information available to require special precautions

**Effects on Dental Treatment** 60% to 70% of patients will have darkening of the tongue and/or stool; 11% experience taste disturbance

**Other Adverse Effects**

>1%:
Central nervous system: Headache (14%), dizziness (1% to 2%)
Gastrointestinal: Diarrhea (9%), nausea/vomiting (3%), constipation, abdominal pain, gastric upset (<10%)
Miscellaneous: Flu-like symptoms (2%)

<1%:
Dermatologic: Rash, pruritus
Hematologic: Anemia, thrombocytopenia
Hepatic: Elevated LFTs

**Warnings/Precautions** Use in children has not been established

**Drug Interactions** See individual monographs
Increased effect: Optimal antimicrobial effects of ranitidine bismuth citrate occur when the drug is taken with food

**Drug Uptake**
Absorption:
Bismuth: Minimal systemic absorption (≤1%)
Ranitidine: 50% to 60% (dose-dependent)
Serum half-life:
Complex: 5-8 days
Bismuth: 11-28 days
Ranitidine: 3 hours
Time to peak serum concentration:
Bismuth: 1-2 hours
Ranitidine: 0.5-5 hours
Time to peak effect of complex: 1 week

**Pregnancy Risk Factor** C

**Dosage Forms** Tablet: 400 mg (ranitidine 162 mg, trivalent bismuth 128 mg, and citrate 110 mg)

## Ranitidine Hydrochloride (ra NI ti deen hye droe KLOR ide)

**Related Information**

Dental Drug Interactions: Update on Drug Combinations Requiring Special Considerations *on page 1225*

Ranitidine Bismuth Citrate *on previous page*

**U.S. Brand Names** Zantac®; Zantac® 75 [OTC]

**Canadian Brand Names** Apo®-Ranitidine; Novo-Ranidine; Nu-Ranit

**Therapeutic Category** Histamine $H_2$ Antagonist

**Use** Short-term treatment of active duodenal ulcers and benign gastric ulcers; long-term prophylaxis of duodenal ulcer and gastric hypersecretory states, gastroesophageal reflux, recurrent postoperative ulcer, upper GI bleeding, prevention of acid-aspiration pneumonitis during surgery, and prevention of stress-induced ulcers; causes fewer interactions than cimetidine

**Usual Dosage** Giving oral dose at 6 PM may be better than 10 PM bedtime, the highest acid production usually starts at approximately 7 PM, thus giving at 6 PM controls acid secretion better

Children:
- Oral: 1.25-2.5 mg/kg/dose every 12 hours; maximum: 300 mg/day
- I.M., I.V.: 0.75-1.5 mg/kg/dose every 6-8 hours, maximum daily dose: 400 mg
- Continuous infusion: 0.1-0.25 mg/kg/hour (preferred for stress ulcer prophylaxis in patients with concurrent maintenance I.V.s or TPNs)

Adults:
- Short-term treatment of ulceration: 150 mg/dose twice daily or 300 mg at bedtime
- Prophylaxis of recurrent duodenal ulcer: Oral: 150 mg at bedtime
- Gastric hypersecretory conditions:
  - Oral: 150 mg twice daily, up to 6 g/day
  - I.M., I.V.: 50 mg/dose every 6-8 hours (dose not to exceed 400 mg/day)
  - I.V.: 50 mg/dose IVPB every 6-8 hours (dose not to exceed 400 mg/day)

**or**

  - Continuous I.V. infusion: Initial: 50 mg IVPB, followed by 6.25 mg/hour titrated to gastric pH >4.0 for prophylaxis or >7.0 for treatment; **continuous I.V. infusion is preferred in patients with active bleeding**
- Gastric hypersecretory conditions: Doses up to 2.5 mg/kg/hour (220 mg/hour) have been used

**Mechanism of Action** Competitive inhibition of histamine at $H_2$-receptors of the gastric parietal cells, which inhibits gastric acid secretion, gastric volume and hydrogen ion concentration reduced

**Local Anesthetic/Vasoconstrictor Precautions** No information available to require special precautions

**Effects on Dental Treatment** No effects or complications reported

**Other Adverse Effects**

Endocrine & metabolic: Gynecomastia

Hepatic: Hepatitis

Neuromuscular & skeletal: Arthralgias

1% to 10%:
- Central nervous system: Dizziness, sedation, malaise, headache, drowsiness
- Dermatologic: Rash
- Gastrointestinal: Constipation, nausea, vomiting, diarrhea

<1%:
- Cardiovascular: Bradycardia, tachycardia
- Central nervous system: Fever, confusion
- Hematologic: Thrombocytopenia, neutropenia, agranulocytosis
- Respiratory: Bronchospasm

**Drug Interactions**

Decreased effect: Variable effects on warfarin; antacids may decrease absorption of ranitidine; ketoconazole and itraconazole absorptions are decreased

May produce altered serum levels of procainamide and ferrous sulfate

Decreased effect of nondepolarizing muscle relaxants, cefpodoxime, cyanocobalamin (decreased absorption), diazepam, oxaprozin

Decreased toxicity of atropine

Increased toxicity of cyclosporine (increased serum creatinine), gentamicin (neuromuscular blockade), glipizide, glyburide, midazolam (increased concentrations), metoprolol, pentoxifylline, phenytoin, quinidine

**Drug Uptake**

Absorption: Oral: 50% to 60%

Serum half-life:
- Children 3.5-16 years: 1.8-2 hours
- Adults: 2-2.5 hours
- End-stage renal disease: 6-9 hours

(Continued)

## Ranitidine Hydrochloride *(Continued)*

Time to peak serum concentration: Oral: Within 1-3 hours and persisting for 8 hours

**Pregnancy Risk Factor** B

**Generic Available** Yes

- **Raudixin®** *see* Rauwolfia Serpentina *on this page*
- **Rauverid®** *see* Rauwolfia Serpentina *on this page*

## Rauwolfia Serpentina (rah WOOL fee a ser pen TEEN ah)

**U.S. Brand Names** Raudixin®; Rauverid®; Wolfina®

**Therapeutic Category** Antihypertensive Agent; Rauwolfia Alkaloid

**Synonyms** Whole Root Rauwolfia

**Use** Mild essential hypertension; relief of agitated psychotic states

**Usual Dosage** Adults: Oral: 200-400 mg/day in 2 divided doses

**Local Anesthetic/Vasoconstrictor Precautions** No information available to require special precautions

**Effects on Dental Treatment** No effects or complications reported

**Pregnancy Risk Factor** C

**Generic Available** Yes

- **Raxar®** *see* Grepafloxacin *on page 477*
- **R & C® Shampoo [OTC]** *see* Pyrethrins *on page 867*
- **Rea-Lo® [OTC]** *see* Urea *on page 1034*
- **Rebetron™** *see* Interferon Alfa-2b and Ribavirin Combination Pack *on page 541*
- **Recombinant Hirudin** *see* Lepirudin *on page 575*
- **Recombinant Human Interleukin-11** *see* Oprelvekin *on page 743*
- **Recombinant Interleukin-11** *see* Oprelvekin *on page 743*
- **Recombinate®** *see* Antihemophilic Factor (Recombinant) *on page 90*
- **Recombivax HB®** *see* Hepatitis B Vaccine *on page 495*
- **Redutemp® [OTC]** *see* Acetaminophen *on page 27*
- **Reese's® Pinworm Medicine [OTC]** *see* Pyrantel Pamoate *on page 865*
- **Reference Values for Adults** *see page 1238*
- **Refludan®** *see* Lepirudin *on page 575*
- **Refresh® Ophthalmic Solution [OTC]** *see* Artificial Tears *on page 97*
- **Refresh® Plus Ophthalmic Solution [OTC]** *see* Artificial Tears *on page 97*
- **Regitine®** *see* Phentolamine *on page 794*
- **Reglan®** *see* Metoclopramide *on page 664*
- **Regranex®** *see* Becaplermin *on page 122*
- **Regulace® [OTC]** *see* Docusate and Casanthranol *on page 347*
- **Regular (Concentrated) Iletin® II U-500** *see* Insulin Preparations *on page 537*
- **Regular Iletin® I** *see* Insulin Preparations *on page 537*
- **Regular Insulin** *see* Insulin Preparations *on page 537*
- **Regular Purified Pork Insulin** *see* Insulin Preparations *on page 537*
- **Regular Strength Bayer® Enteric 500 Aspirin [OTC]** *see* Aspirin *on page 100*
- **Regulax SS® [OTC]** *see* Docusate *on page 346*
- **Reguloid® [OTC]** *see* Psyllium *on page 865*
- **Relafen®** *see* Nabumetone *on page 695*
- **Relefact® TRH Injection** *see* Protirelin *on page 861*
- **Relief® Ophthalmic Solution** *see* Phenylephrine *on page 795*
- **Remeron®** *see* Mirtazapine *on page 679*
- **Remicade™** *see* Infliximab *on page 535*

## Remifentanil (rem i FEN ta nil)

**U.S. Brand Names** Ultiva™

**Therapeutic Category** Analgesic, Narcotic; General Anesthetic, Intravenous

**Use** Analgesic for use during general anesthesia for continued analgesia

**Usual Dosage** Adults: I.V. continuous infusion:

During induction: 0.5-1 mcg/kg/minute

During maintenance:

- With nitrous oxide (66%): 0.4 mcg/kg/minute (range: 0.1-2 mcg/kg/min)
- With isoflurane: 0.25 mcg/kg/minute (range: 0.05-2 mcg/kg/min)
- With propofol: 0.25 mcg/kg/minute (range: 0.05-2 mcg/kg/min)

Continuation as an analgesic in immediate postoperative period: 0.1 mcg/kg/minute (range: 0.025-0.2 mcg/kg/min)

**Mechanism of Action** Binds with stereospecific mu-opioid receptors at many sites within the CNS, increases pain threshold, alters pain reception, inhibits ascending pain pathways

**Local Anesthetic/Vasoconstrictor Precautions** No information available to require special precautions

**Effects on Dental Treatment** No effects or complications reported

**Other Adverse Effects**

>10%: Gastrointestinal: Nausea, vomiting

1% to 10%:

Cardiovascular: Hypotension, bradycardia, tachycardia, hypertension
Central nervous system: Dizziness, headache, agitation, fever
Dermatologic: Pruritus
Ocular: Visual disturbances
Respiratory: Respiratory depression, apnea, hypoxia
Miscellaneous: Shivering, postoperative pain

**Drug Interactions** Increased effect with CNS depressants

**Drug Uptake** Serum half-life: 10 minutes (dose-dependent)

**Pregnancy Risk Factor** C

♦ **Renacidin®** *see* Citric Acid Bladder Mixture *on page 255*

♦ **Renagel®** *see* Sevelamer *on page 911*

♦ **Renese®** *see* Polythiazide *on page 817*

♦ **Renoquid®** *see* Sulfacytine *on page 940*

♦ **Renormax®** *see* Spirapril *on page 930*

♦ **Rentamine®** *see* Chlorpheniramine, Ephedrine, Phenylephrine, and Carbetapentane *on page 233*

♦ **ReoPro®** *see* Abciximab *on page 24*

## Repaglinide (re PAG li nide)

**U.S. Brand Names** Prandin™

**Therapeutic Category** Hypoglycemic Agent, Oral

**Use** As an adjunct to diet and exercise to lower blood glucose on non-insulin-dependent (Type II) diabetes patients

**Usual Dosage** Oral: Adults: 0.5 - 4.0 mg before each meal; the starting dose in oral hypoglycemic naive individuals or in those with HbA1c levels under 8% is 0.5 mg before each meal. For other patients, the starting dose is 1-2 mg before each meal. The dose can be adjusted (by prescribers) up to 4 mg before each meal. If a meal is skipped, the patient should also skip the repaglinide dose

**Mechanism of Action** Stimulates insulin secretion from the beta cells of the pancreas by binding to sites on the beta cell. Prandin is minimally excreted by the kidney, which may be an advantage for patients (often elderly) who often suffer from decreased kidney function.

**Local Anesthetic/Vasoconstrictor Precautions** No information available to require special precautions

**Effects on Dental Treatment** No effects or complications reported

**Other Adverse Effects**

>10%:

Central nervous system: Headache
Endocrine & metabolic: Hyperglycemia, hypoglycemia, related symptoms

1% to 10%:

Cardiovascular: Chest pain
Gastrointestinal: Nausea, epigastric fullness, heartburn, constipation, diarrhea, anorexia, tooth disorder
Genitourinary: Urinary tract infection
Neuromuscular: Arthralgia, back pain, paresthesia
Miscellaneous: Allergy

**Drug Interactions** CYP3A4 enzyme substrate

Decreased effect: Drugs that induce cytochrome P-450 3A4 may increase metabolism of repaglinide (troglitazone rifampin, barbiturates, carbamazepine). Certain drugs (thiazides, diuretics, corticosteroids, phenothiazines, thyroid products, estrogens, oral contraceptives, phenytoin, nicotinic acid, sympathomimetics, calcium channel blockers, isoniazid) tend to produce hyperglycemia and may lead to loss of glycemic control.

Increased effect: Agents that inhibit cytochrome P-450 3A4 (ketoconazole, miconazole) and antibacterial agents (erythromycin) may increase repaglinide concentrations

Increased toxicity: Since this agent is highly protein bound, the toxic potential is increased when given concomitantly with other highly protein bound drugs (ie, phenylbutazone, oral anticoagulants, hydantoins, salicylates, NSAIDs, sulfonamides) - increase hypoglycemic effect

**Drug Uptake** Absorption: Rapidly and completely from the GI tract with peak plasma drug levels within 1 hour

(Continued)

## Repaglinide *(Continued)*

**Pregnancy Risk Factor** C

**Dosage Forms** Tablet: 0.5 mg

**Comments** Known as NovoNorm™ elsewhere

- ♦ **Repan®** *see* Butalbital Compound *on page 163*
- ♦ **Repan®** *see* Butalbital Compound and Acetaminophen *on page 164*
- ♦ **Reposans-10®** *see* Chlordiazepoxide *on page 224*
- ♦ **Requip™** *see* Ropinirole *on page 895*
- ♦ **Resaid®** *see* Chlorpheniramine and Phenylpropanolamine *on page 233*
- ♦ **Rescaps-D® S.R. Capsule** *see* Caramiphen and Phenylpropanolamine *on page 184*
- ♦ **Rescon Liquid [OTC]** *see* Chlorpheniramine and Phenylpropanolamine *on page 233*
- ♦ **Rescriptor®** *see* Delavirdine *on page 302*

## Reserpine (re SER peen)

**Related Information**

Cardiovascular Diseases *on page 1066*

**U.S. Brand Names** Serpalan®; Serpasil®

**Canadian Brand Names** Novo-Reserpine

**Therapeutic Category** Alpha-Adrenergic Blockers - Peripheral-Acting (Alpha$_1$-Blockers)

**Use** Management of mild to moderate hypertension

**Unlabeled use:** Management of tardive dyskinesia

**Usual Dosage** Oral (full antihypertensive effects may take as long as 3 weeks):

Children: 0.01-0.02 mg/kg/24 hours divided every 12 hours; maximum dose: 0.25 mg/day

Adults: 0.1-0.25 mg/day in 1-2 doses; initial: 0.5 mg/day for 1-2 weeks; maintenance: reduce to 0.1-0.25 mg/day

Elderly: Initial: 0.05 mg once daily, increasing by 0.05 mg every week as necessary

**Mechanism of Action** Reduces blood pressure via depletion of sympathetic biogenic amines (norepinephrine and dopamine); this also commonly results in sedative effects

**Local Anesthetic/Vasoconstrictor Precautions** No information available to require special precautions

**Effects on Dental Treatment** >10% of patients experience dry mouth

**Other Adverse Effects**

>10%:

Central nervous system: Dizziness

Gastrointestinal: Anorexia, diarrhea, nausea, vomiting

Respiratory: Nasal congestion

1% to 10%:

Cardiovascular: Peripheral edema, arrhythmias, bradycardia, chest pain

Central nervous system: Headache

Gastrointestinal: Black stools, bloody vomit

Genitourinary: Impotence

<1%:

Cardiovascular: Hypotension

Central nervous system: Drowsiness, fatigue, mental depression, parkinsonism

Dermatologic: Skin rash

Endocrine & metabolic: Sodium and water retention

Gastrointestinal: Elevated gastric acid secretion

Genitourinary: Dysuria

Neuromuscular & skeletal: Trembling of hands/fingers

**Drug Interactions**

Decreased effect of indirect-acting sympathomimetics

Increased effect/toxicity of MAO inhibitors, direct-acting sympathomimetics, and tricyclic antidepressants

**Drug Uptake**

Onset of antihypertensive effect: Within 3-6 days

Duration: 2-6 weeks

Absorption: Oral: ~40%

Serum half-life: 50-100 hours

**Pregnancy Risk Factor** C

**Generic Available** Yes

- ♦ **Reserpine and Chlorothiazide** *see* Chlorothiazide and Reserpine *on page 230*

- **Reserpine and Hydrochlorothiazide** *see* Hydrochlorothiazide and Reserpine *on page 504*
- **Respa-1st®** *see* Guaifenesin and Pseudoephedrine *on page 481*
- **Respa-DM®** *see* Guaifenesin and Dextromethorphan *on page 479*
- **Respa-GF®** *see* Guaifenesin *on page 478*
- **Respaire®-60 SR** *see* Guaifenesin and Pseudoephedrine *on page 481*
- **Respaire®-120 SR** *see* Guaifenesin and Pseudoephedrine *on page 481*
- **Respbid®** *see* Theophylline *on page 969*
- **Respiratory Diseases** *see page 1079*
- **Restoril®** *see* Temazepam *on page 955*
- **Retavase™** *see* Reteplase *on this page*

## Reteplase (RE ta plase)

**U.S. Brand Names** Retavase™

**Therapeutic Category** Thrombolytic Agent

**Use** Management of acute myocardial infarction

**Usual Dosage**

Children: Not recommended

Adults: 10 units I.V. over 2 minutes, followed by a second dose 30 minutes later of 10 units I.V. over 2 minutes

Withhold second dose if serious bleeding or anaphylaxis occurs

**Mechanism of Action** Reteplase is a nonglycosylated form of tPA produced by recombinant DNA technology using *E. coli*; it initiates local fibrinolysis by binding to fibrin in a thrombus (clot) and converts entrapped plasminogen to plasmin

**Local Anesthetic/Vasoconstrictor Precautions** No information available to require special precautions

**Effects on Dental Treatment** No effects or complications reported

**Other Adverse Effects**

>10%:

Cardiovascular: Hypotension, arrhythmias, trauma arrhythmias

Hematologic: Bleeding

1% to 10%: Hematologic: Anemia, genitourinary bleeding, gastrointestinal bleeding, injection site bleeding

<1%:

Central nervous system: Intracranial hemorrhage

Miscellaneous: Allergic reactions, anaphylaxis

**Drug Interactions** Increased effect: Anticoagulants, aspirin, ticlopidine, dipyridamole, abciximab and heparin are at least additive

**Drug Uptake**

Onset: 30-90 minutes

Serum half-life: 13-16 minutes

**Pregnancy Risk Factor** C

**Generic Available** No

- **Retin-A™ Micro Topical** *see* Tretinoin, Topical *on page 1009*
- **Retin-A™ Topical** *see* Tretinoin, Topical *on page 1009*
- **Retrovir®** *see* Zidovudine *on page 1058*
- **Revex®** *see* Nalmefene *on page 700*
- **Rēv-Eyes™** *see* Dapiprazole *on page 297*
- **ReVia® Oral** *see* Naltrexone *on page 702*
- **Rexigen Forte®** *see* Phendimetrazine *on page 788*
- **Rezulin®** *see* Troglitazone *on page 1027*
- **R-Gel® [OTC]** *see* Capsaicin *on page 181*
- **R-Gen®** *see* Iodinated Glycerol *on page 545*
- **R-Gene®** *see* Arginine *on page 94*
- **rGM-CSF** *see* Sargramostim *on page 904*
- **Rheaban® [OTC]** *see* Attapulgite *on page 109*
- **Rheomacrodex®** *see* Dextran *on page 311*
- **Rheumatoid Arthritis and Osteoarthritis** *see page 1092*
- **Rheumatrex®** *see* Methotrexate *on page 651*
- **rhIL-11** *see* Oprelvekin *on page 743*
- **Rhinall® Nasal Solution [OTC]** *see* Phenylephrine *on page 795*
- **Rhinatate® Tablet** *see* Chlorpheniramine, Pyrilamine, and Phenylephrine *on page 238*
- **Rhindecon®** *see* Phenylpropanolamine *on page 797*
- **Rhinocort®** *see* Budesonide *on page 155*
- **Rhinosyn-DMX® [OTC]** *see* Guaifenesin and Dextromethorphan *on page 479*
- **Rhinosyn® Liquid [OTC]** *see* Chlorpheniramine and Pseudoephedrine *on page 233*

- **Rhinosyn-PD® Liquid [OTC]** *see* Chlorpheniramine and Pseudoephedrine *on page 233*
- **Rhinosyn-X® Liquid [OTC]** *see* Guaifenesin, Pseudoephedrine, and Dextromethorphan *on page 482*

## $Rh_o$(D) Immune Globulin (ar aych oh (dee) i MYUN GLOB yoo lin)

**U.S. Brand Names** Gamulin® Rh; HypRho®-D; HypRho®-D Mini-Dose; MICRhoGAM™; Mini-Gamulin® Rh; RhoGAM™

**Therapeutic Category** Immune Globulin

**Use** Prevent isoimmunization in Rh-negative individuals exposed to Rh-positive blood during delivery of an Rh-positive infant, as a result of an abortion, following amniocentesis or abdominal trauma, or following a transfusion accident; to prevent hemolytic disease of the newborn if there is a subsequent pregnancy with an Rh-positive fetus

**Usual Dosage** Adults (administered I.M. to mothers **not** to infant) I.M.:

Obstetrical usage: 1 vial (300 mcg) prevents maternal sensitization if fetal packed red blood cell volume that has entered the circulation is <15 mL; if it is more, give additional vials. The number of vials = RBC volume of the calculated fetomaternal hemorrhage divided by 15 mL

Postpartum prophylaxis: 300 mcg within 72 hours of delivery

Antepartum prophylaxis: 300 mcg at approximately 26-28 weeks gestation; followed by 300 mcg within 72 hours of delivery if infant is Rh-positive

Following miscarriage, abortion, or termination of ectopic pregnancy at up to 13 weeks of gestation: 50 mcg ideally within 3 hours, but may be given up to 72 hours after; if pregnancy has been terminated at 13 or more weeks of gestation, administer 300 mcg

**Mechanism of Action** Suppresses the immune response and antibody formation of Rh-negative individuals to Rh-positive red blood cells

**Local Anesthetic/Vasoconstrictor Precautions** No information available to require special precautions

**Effects on Dental Treatment** No effects or complications reported

**Other Adverse Effects** <1%:

Central nervous system: Lethargy, temperature elevation
Gastrointestinal: Splenomegaly
Hepatic: Elevated bilirubin
Local: Pain at the injection site
Neuromuscular & skeletal: Myalgia

**Drug Uptake** Serum half-life: 23-26 days

**Pregnancy Risk Factor** C

**Generic Available** No

**Comments** Administered I.M. to mothers **not** to infant; will prevent hemolytic disease of newborn in subsequent pregnancy

- **RhoGAM™** *see* $Rh_o$(D) Immune Globulin *on this page*
- ***r*HuEPO-α** *see* Epoetin Alfa *on page 376*
- **Rhulicaine® [OTC]** *see* Benzocaine *on page 128*

## Ribavirin (rye ba VYE rin)

**U.S. Brand Names** Virazole® Aerosol

**Therapeutic Category** Antiviral Agent, Inhalation Therapy

**Synonyms** RTCA; Tribavirin

**Use** Treatment of patients with respiratory syncytial virus (RSV) infections; specially indicated for treatment of severe lower respiratory tract RSV infections in patients with an underlying compromising condition (prematurity, bronchopulmonary dysplasia and other chronic lung conditions, congenital heart disease, immunodeficiency, immunosuppression), and recent transplant recipients; may also be used in other viral infections including influenza A and B and adenovirus

**Usual Dosage** Children and Adults:

Aerosol inhalation: Use with Viratek® small particle aerosol generator (SPAG-2) at a concentration of 20 mg/mL (6 g reconstituted with 300 mL of sterile water without preservatives)

Aerosol only: 12-18 hours/day for 3 days, up to 7 days in length

**Mechanism of Action** Inhibits replication of RNA and DNA viruses; inhibits influenza virus RNA polymerase activity and inhibits the initiation and elongation of RNA fragments resulting in inhibition of viral protein synthesis

**Local Anesthetic/Vasoconstrictor Precautions** No information available to require special precautions

**Effects on Dental Treatment** No effects or complications reported

**Other Adverse Effects**

1% to 10%:

Central nervous system: Fatigue, headache, insomnia

Gastrointestinal: Nausea, anorexia
Hematologic: Anemia

<1%:

Cardiovascular: Hypotension, cardiac arrest, digitalis toxicity
Dermatologic: Rash, skin irritation
Ocular: Conjunctivitis
Respiratory: Mild bronchospasm, worsening of respiratory function, apnea, accumulation of fluid in ventilator tubing

**Drug Uptake**

Absorption: Absorbed systemically from the respiratory tract following nasal and oral inhalation; absorption is dependent upon respiratory factors and method of drug delivery; maximal absorption occurs with the use of the aerosol generator via an endotracheal tube; highest concentrations are found in the respiratory tract and erythrocytes

Serum half-life, plasma:

Children: 6.5-11 hours
Adults: 24 hours, much longer in the erythrocyte (16-40 days), which can be used as a marker for intracellular metabolism

Time to peak serum concentration: Inhalation: Within 60-90 minutes

**Pregnancy Risk Factor** X

**Generic Available** No

**Comments** RSV season is usually December to April; viral shedding period for RSV is usually 3-8 days

## Riboflavin (RYE boe flay vin)

**U.S. Brand Names** Riobin®

**Therapeutic Category** Vitamin, Water Soluble

**Use** Dental and Medical: Prevent riboflavin deficiency and treat ariboflavinosis

**Usual Dosage** Oral:

Riboflavin deficiency:

Children: 2.5-10 mg/day in divided doses
Adults: 5-30 mg/day in divided doses

Recommended daily allowance:

Children: 0.4-1.8 mg
Adults: 1.2-1.7 mg

**Mechanism of Action** Component of flavoprotein enzymes that work together, which are necessary for normal tissue respiration; also needed for activation of pyridoxine and conversion of tryptophan to niacin

**Local Anesthetic/Vasoconstrictor Precautions** No information available to require special precautions

**Effects on Dental Treatment** No effects or complications reported

**Warnings/Precautions** Riboflavin deficiency often occurs in the presence of other B vitamin deficiencies

**Drug Interactions** Decreased absorption with probenecid

**Drug Uptake**

Absorption: Readily via GI tract, however, food increases extent of GI absorption; GI absorption is decreased in patients with hepatitis, cirrhosis, or biliary obstruction

Serum half-life, biologic: 66-84 minutes

**Pregnancy Risk Factor** A (C if dose exceeds RDA recommendation)

**Dosage Forms** Tablet: 25 mg, 50 mg, 100 mg

**Generic Available** Yes

♦ **Rid-A-Pain® [OTC]** *see* Benzocaine *on page 128*
♦ **Ridaura®** *see* Auranofin *on page 109*
♦ **Ridenol® [OTC]** *see* Acetaminophen *on page 27*
♦ **RID® Shampoo [OTC]** *see* Pyrethrins *on page 867*

## Rifabutin (rif a BYOO tin)

**Related Information**

Nonviral Infectious Diseases *on page 1095*
Systemic Viral Diseases *on page 1115*

**U.S. Brand Names** Mycobutin®

**Therapeutic Category** Antibiotic, Miscellaneous; Antitubercular Agent

**Use** Adjunctive therapy for the prevention of disseminated *Mycobacterium avium* complex (MAC) in patients with advanced HIV infection

**Usual Dosage** Oral:

Children: Efficacy and safety of rifabutin have not been established in children; a limited number of HIV-positive children with MAC have been given rifabutin for MAC prophylaxis; doses of 5 mg/kg/day have been useful

Adults: 300 mg once daily; for patients who experience gastrointestinal upset, rifabutin can be administered 150 mg twice daily with food

(Continued)

## Rifabutin *(Continued)*

**Mechanism of Action** Inhibits DNA-dependent RNA polymerase at the beta subunit which prevents chain initiation

**Local Anesthetic/Vasoconstrictor Precautions** No information available to require special precautions

**Effects on Dental Treatment** No effects or complications reported

**Other Adverse Effects**

>10%:

- Dermatologic: Rash
- Genitourinary: Discolored urine
- Hematologic: Neutropenia, leukopenia

1% to 10%:

- Central nervous system: Headache
- Gastrointestinal: Vomiting, nausea, abdominal pain, diarrhea, anorexia, flatulence, eructation
- Hematologic: Anemia, thrombocytopenia
- Neuromuscular & skeletal: Myalgia

<1%:

- Cardiovascular: Chest pain
- Central nervous system: Fever, insomnia
- Gastrointestinal: Dyspepsia, taste perversion

**Drug Interactions** Decreased plasma concentration (due to induction of liver enzymes) of verapamil, methadone, digoxin, cyclosporine, corticosteroids, oral anticoagulants, theophylline, barbiturates, chloramphenicol, ketoconazole, oral contraceptives, quinidine, halothane

**Drug Uptake**

Absorption: Oral: Readily absorbed 53%

Serum half life, terminal: 45 hours (range: 16-69 hours)

Peak serum level: Within 2-4 hours

**Pregnancy Risk Factor** B

**Generic Available** No

♦ **Rifadin®** *see* Rifampin *on this page*

♦ **Rifamate®** *see* Rifampin and Isoniazid *on next page*

## Rifampin (RIF am pin)

**Related Information**

Nonviral Infectious Diseases *on page 1095*

**U.S. Brand Names** Rifadin®; Rimactane®

**Canadian Brand Names** Rifadin®; Rimactane®; Rofact™

**Therapeutic Category** Antibiotic, Miscellaneous; Antitubercular Agent

**Use** Management of active tuberculosis; eliminate meningococci from asymptomatic carriers; prophylaxis of *Haemophilus influenzae* type B infection; used in combination with other anti-infectives in the treatment of staphylococcal infections

**Usual Dosage** I.V. infusion dose is the same as for the oral route

Tuberculosis therapy: Oral:

**Note:** A four-drug regimen (isoniazid, rifampin, pyrazinamide, and either streptomycin or ethambutol) is preferred for the initial, empiric treatment of TB. When the drug susceptibility results are available, the regimen should be altered as appropriate.

**Patients with TB and without HIV infection:**

**OPTION 1:**

Isoniazid resistance rate <4%: Administer daily isoniazid, rifampin, and pyrazinamide for 8 weeks followed by isoniazid and rifampin daily or directly observed therapy (DOT) 2-3 times/week for 16 weeks

If isoniazid resistance rate is not documented, ethambutol or streptomycin should also be administered until susceptibility to isoniazid or rifampin is demonstrated. Continue treatment for at least 6 months or 3 months beyond culture conversion.

**OPTION 2:** Administer daily isoniazid, rifampin, pyrazinamide, and either streptomycin or ethambutol for 2 weeks followed by DOT 2 times/week administration of the same drugs for 6 weeks, and subsequently, with isoniazid and rifampin DOT 2 times/week administration for 16 weeks

**OPTION 3:** Administer isoniazid, rifampin, pyrazinamide, and either ethambutol or streptomycin by DOT 3 times/week for 6 months

**Patients with TB and with HIV infection:**

Administer any of the above OPTIONS 1, 2 or 3, however, treatment should be continued for a total of 9 months and at least 6 months beyond culture conversion

**Note:** Some experts recommend that the duration of therapy should be extended to 9 months for patients with disseminated disease, miliary disease, disease involving the bones or joints, or tuberculosis lymphadenitis

Children <12 years of age: Oral:

Daily therapy: 10-20 mg/kg/day in divided doses every 12-24 hours (maximum: 600 mg/day)

Directly observed therapy (DOT): Twice weekly: 10-20 mg/kg (maximum: 600 mg)

DOT: 3 times/week: 10-20 mg/kg (maximum: 600 mg)

Adults: Oral:

Daily therapy: 10 mg/kg/day (maximum: 600 mg/day)

Directly observed therapy (DOT): Twice weekly: 10 mg/kg (maximum: 600 mg)

DOT: 3 times/week: 10 mg/kg (maximum: 600 mg)

*H. influenzae* prophylaxis: Oral:

Children: 20 mg/kg/day every 24 hours for 4 days, not to exceed 600 mg/dose

Adults: 600 mg every 24 hours for 4 days

Meningococcal prophylaxis: Oral:

<1 month: 10 mg/kg/day in divided doses every 12 hours for 2 days

Children: 20 mg/kg/day in divided doses every 12 hours for 2 days

Adults: 600 mg every 12 hours for 2 days

Nasal carriers of *Staphylococcus aureus*: Oral:

Children: 15 mg/kg/day divided every 12 hours for 5-10 days in combination with other antibiotics

Adults: 600 mg/day for 5-10 days in combination with other antibiotics

Synergy for *Staphylococcus aureus* infections: Oral: Adults: 300-600 mg twice daily with other antibiotics

**Mechanism of Action** Inhibits bacterial RNA synthesis by binding to the beta subunit of DNA-dependent RNA polymerase, blocking RNA transcription

**Local Anesthetic/Vasoconstrictor Precautions** No information available to require special precautions

**Effects on Dental Treatment** No effects or complications reported

**Other Adverse Effects**

1% to 10%:

Gastrointestinal: Diarrhea, stomach cramps, discoloration of feces, saliva, sputum

Genitourinary: Discoloration of urine

Ocular: Discoloration of tears (reddish orange)

Miscellaneous: Discoloration of sweat, fungal overgrowth

<1%:

Central nervous system: Drowsiness, fatigue, ataxia, confusion, fever, headache

Dermatologic: Rash, pruritus

Gastrointestinal: Nausea, vomiting, stomatitis

Hematologic: Eosinophilia, blood dyscrasias (leukopenia, thrombocytopenia)

Hepatic: Hepatitis

Local: Irritation at the I.V. site

Renal: Renal failure

Miscellaneous: Flu-like syndrome

**Drug Interactions** Inducer of both Cytochrome P-450 3A and cytochrome P-450 2D6

Decreased effect: Rifampin induces liver enzymes which may decrease the plasma concentration of verapamil, methadone, digoxin, cyclosporine, corticosteroids, oral anticoagulants, theophylline, barbiturates, chloramphenicol, ketoconazole, oral contraceptives, quinidine, halothane, ketoconazole

**Drug Uptake**

Absorption: Oral: Well absorbed

Serum half-life: 3-4 hours, prolonged with hepatic impairment

Time to peak serum concentration: Oral: 2-4 hours and persisting for up to 24 hours; food may delay or slightly reduce

**Pregnancy Risk Factor** C

**Generic Available** No

## Rifampin and Isoniazid (RIF am pin & eye soe NYE a zid)

**U.S. Brand Names** Rifamate®

**Therapeutic Category** Antibiotic, Miscellaneous; Antitubercular Agent

**Use** Management of active tuberculosis; see individual monographs for additional information

**Usual Dosage** Oral: 2 capsules/day

(Continued)

## Rifampin and Isoniazid *(Continued)*

**Local Anesthetic/Vasoconstrictor Precautions** No information available to require special precautions

**Effects on Dental Treatment** No effects or complications reported

**Pregnancy Risk Factor** C

**Generic Available** No

## Rifampin, Isoniazid, and Pyrazinamide

(RIF am pin, eye soe NYE a zid, & peer a ZIN a mide)

**U.S. Brand Names** Rifater®

**Therapeutic Category** Antibiotic, Miscellaneous; Antitubercular Agent

**Use** Management of active tuberculosis

**Local Anesthetic/Vasoconstrictor Precautions** No information available to require special precautions

**Effects on Dental Treatment** No effects or complications reported

**Pregnancy Risk Factor** C

**Generic Available** No

## Rifapentine (RIF a pen teen)

**U.S. Brand Names** Priftin®

**Therapeutic Category** Antitubercular Agent

**Use** Treatment of pulmonary tuberculosis (indication is based on the 6-month follow-up treatment outcome observed in controlled clinical trial). Rifapentine must always be used in conjunction with at least one other antituberculosis drug to which the isolate is susceptible; it may also be necessary to add a third agent (either streptomycin or ethambutol) until susceptibility is known.

**Usual Dosage**

Children: No dosing information available

Adults: **Rifapentine should not be used alone**; initial phase should include a 3- to 4-drug regimen

Intensive phase of short-term therapy (initial 2 months): 600 mg (four 150 mg tablets) given twice weekly (at an interval not less than 72 hours); following the intensive phase, treatment should continue with rifapentine 600 mg once weekly for 4 months in combination with INH or appropriate agent for susceptible organisms

**Mechanism of Action** Inhibits DNA-dependent RNA polymerase in susceptible strains of *Mycobacterium tuberculosis* (but not in mammalian cells). Rifapentine is bactericidal against both intracellular and extracellular MTB organisms. Strains which are resistant to other rifamycins including rifampin are likely to be resistant to rifapentine. Cross-resistance does not appear between rifapentine and other nonrifamycin antimycobacterial agents.

**Local Anesthetic/Vasoconstrictor Precautions** No information available to require special precautions

**Effects on Dental Treatment** No effects or complications reported

**Other Adverse Effects**

>10%: Endocrine & metabolic: Hyperuricemia (most likely due to pyrazinamide from initiation phase combination therapy)

1% to 10%:

Cardiovascular: Hypertension

Central nervous system: Headache, dizziness

Dermatologic: Rash, pruritus, acne

Gastrointestinal: Anorexia, nausea, vomiting, dyspepsia, diarrhea

Genitourinary: Pyuria, proteinuria, hematuria, urinary casts

Hematologic: Neutropenia, lymphopenia, anemia, leukopenia, thrombocytosis

Hepatic: Increased ALT, AST

Neuromuscular & skeletal: Arthralgia, pain

Respiratory: Hemoptysis

<1%:

Cardiovascular: Peripheral edema

Central nervous system: Aggressive reaction, fatigue

Dermatologic: Urticaria, skin discoloration

Endocrine & metabolic: Hyperkalemia, hypovolemia, increased alkaline phosphatase, increased LDH

Gastrointestinal: Constipation, esophagitis, gastritis, pancreatitis

Hematologic: Thrombocytopenia, neutrophilia, leukocytosis, purpura, hematoma

Hepatic: Bilirubinemia, hepatitis

Neuromuscular & skeletal: Gout, arthrosis

**Drug Interactions** Rifapentine is an inducer of cytochrome P-450 3A4 and P-450 2C8/9. Rifapentine may increase the metabolism of coadministered drugs that are metabolized by these enzymes. Enzymes are induced within 4 days after the first dose and returned to baseline 14 days after discontinuation of rifapentine. The magnitude of enzyme induction is dose and frequency dependent.

Rifampin has been shown to accelerate the metabolism and may reduce activity of the following drugs (therefore, rifapentine may also do the same): Phenytoin, disopyramide, mexiletine, quinidine, tocainide, chloramphenicol, clarithromycin, dapsone, doxycycline, fluoroquinolones, warfarin, fluconazole, itraconazole, ketoconazole, barbiturates, benzodiazepines, beta-blockers, diltiazem, nifedipine, verapamil, corticosteroids, cardiac glycoside preparations, clofibrate, oral or other systemic hormonal contraceptives, haloperidol, HIV protease inhibitors, sulfonylureas, cyclosporine, tacrolimus, levothyroxine, methadone, progestins, quinine, delavirdine, zidovudine, sildenafil, theophylline, amitriptyline, and nortriptyline.

Rifapentine should be used with extreme caution, if at all, in patients who are also taking protease inhibitors

Patients using oral or other systemic hormonal contraceptives should be advised to change to nonhormonal methods of birth control when receiving concomitant rifapentine.

Rifapentine metabolism is mediated by esterase activity, therefore, there is minimal potential for rifapentine metabolism to be affected by other drug therapy.

**Drug Uptake**

Absorption: Food increases AUC and $C_{max}$ by 43% and 44% respectively.

Half-life: Rifapentine: 14-17 hours; 25-desacetyl rifapentine: 13 hours

Bioavailability: ~70%

Time to peak serum concentration: 5-6 hours

**Pregnancy Risk Factor** C

**Dosage Forms** Tablet, film-coated: 150 mg

♦ **Rifater®** *see* Rifampin, Isoniazid, and Pyrazinamide *on previous page*

♦ **rIL-11** *see* Oprelvekin *on page 743*

♦ **Rilutek®** *see* Riluzole *on this page*

## Riluzole (RIL yoo zole)

**U.S. Brand Names** Rilutek®

**Therapeutic Category** Amyotrophic Lateral Sclerosis (ALS) Agent

**Use** Amyotrophic lateral sclerosis (ALS): Treatment of patients with ALS; riluzole can extend survival or time to tracheostomy

**Usual Dosage** Adults: Oral: 50 mg every 12 hours; no increased benefit can be expected from higher daily doses, but adverse events are increased

**Mechanism of Action** Inhibitory effect on glutamate release, inactivation of voltage-dependent sodium channels; and ability to interfere with intracellular events that follow transmitter binding at excitatory amino acid receptors

**Local Anesthetic/Vasoconstrictor Precautions** No information available to require special precautions

**Effects on Dental Treatment** No effects or complications reported

**Other Adverse Effects** >10%:

Gastrointestinal: Nausea, abdominal pain, constipation

Hepatic: ALT (SGPT) elevations

**Drug Interactions** Cytochrome P-450 1A2 (CYP 1A2) substrate

Decreased effect: Drugs that induce CYP 1A2 (eg, cigarette smoke, charbroiled food, rifampin, omeprazole) could increase the rate of riluzole elimination

Increased toxicity: Inhibitors of CYP 1A2 (eg, caffeine, theophylline, amitriptyline, quinolones) could decrease the rate of riluzole elimination

**Drug Uptake**

Absorption: Well absorbed (90%); a high fat meal decreases absorption of riluzole (decreasing AUC by 20% and peak blood levels by 45%)

Bioavailability: Oral: Absolute (50%)

**Pregnancy Risk Factor** C

**Dosage Forms** Tablet: 50 mg

**Generic Available** No

♦ **Rimactane®** *see* Rifampin *on page 886*

## Rimantadine (ri MAN ta deen)

**Related Information**

Systemic Viral Diseases *on page 1115*

**U.S. Brand Names** Flumadine®

**Therapeutic Category** Antiviral Agent, Oral

**Use** Prophylaxis (adults and children >1 year) and treatment (adults) of influenza A viral infection

(Continued)

## Rimantadine *(Continued)*

**Usual Dosage** Oral:

Prophylaxis:

Children <10 years: 5 mg/kg give once daily; maximum: 150 mg

Children >10 years and Adults: 100 mg twice daily; decrease to 100 mg/day in elderly or in patients with severe hepatic or renal impairment ($Cl_{cr}$ ≤10 mL/minute)

Treatment: Adults: 100 mg twice daily; decrease to 100 mg/day in elderly or in patients with severe hepatic or renal impairment ($Cl_{cr}$ ≤10 mL/minute)

**Mechanism of Action** Exerts its inhibitory effect on three antigenic subtypes of influenza A virus (H1N1, H2N2, H3N2) early in the viral replicative cycle, possibly inhibiting the uncoating process; it has no activity against influenza B virus and is 2- to 8-fold more active than amantadine

**Local Anesthetic/Vasoconstrictor Precautions** No information available to require special precautions

**Effects on Dental Treatment** No effects or complications reported

**Other Adverse Effects** 1% to 10%:

Cardiovascular: Orthostatic hypotension, edema

Central nervous system: Dizziness, confusion, headache, insomnia, difficulty in concentrating, anxiety, restlessness, irritability, hallucinations; incidence of CNS side effects may be less than that associated with amantadine

Gastrointestinal: Nausea, vomiting, dry mouth, abdominal pain, anorexia

Genitourinary: Urinary retention

**Drug Interactions**

Acetaminophen: Reduction in AUC and peak concentration of rimantadine

Aspirin: Peak plasma and AUC concentrations of rimantadine are reduced

Cimetidine: Rimantadine clearance is decreased (~16%)

**Drug Uptake**

Absorption: Tablet and syrup formulations are equally absorbed; $T_{max}$: 6 hours

Serum half-life: 25.4 hours (increased in elderly)

**Pregnancy Risk Factor** C

**Generic Available** No

## Rimexolone (ri MEKS oh lone)

**U.S. Brand Names** Vexol®

**Therapeutic Category** Anti-inflammatory Agent, Ophthalmic; Corticosteroid, Ophthalmic

**Use** Treatment of inflammation after ocular surgery and the treatment of anterior uveitis

**Usual Dosage** Adults: Ophthalmic: Instill 1 drop in conjunctival sac 2-4 times/day up to every 4 hours; may use every 1-2 hours during first 1-2 days

**Mechanism of Action** Decreases inflammation by suppression of migration of polymorphonuclear leukocytes and reversal of increased capillary permeability

**Local Anesthetic/Vasoconstrictor Precautions** No information available to require special precautions

**Effects on Dental Treatment** No effects or complications reported

**Other Adverse Effects**

1% to 10%: Ocular: Temporary mild blurred vision

<1%: Ocular: Stinging, burning eyes, corneal thinning, increased intraocular pressure, glaucoma, damage to the optic nerve, defects in visual activity, cataracts, secondary ocular infection

**Drug Uptake** Absorption: Through aqueous humor

**Pregnancy Risk Factor** C

**Generic Available** No

- **Riobin®** *see* Riboflavin *on page 885*
- **Riopan® [OTC]** *see* Magaldrate *on page 610*
- **Riopan Plus® [OTC]** *see* Magaldrate and Simethicone *on page 610*

## Risedronate (ris ED roe nate)

**U.S. Brand Names** Actonel®

**Therapeutic Category** Bisphosphonate Derivative

**Use** FDA approved: Treatment of Paget's disease of bone in patients who meet at least one of the following criteria: 1) serum alkaline phosphatase ≥2 times the upper limit of normal; 2) symptomatic; 3) to induce remission in those who are at risk for future complications

**Unlabeled use:** Prevention of bone loss in postmenopausal women (5 mg/day cyclically for 2 years then 1 year off therapy)

**Usual Dosage** Adults: Oral: 30 mg once daily for 2 months; retreatment may be considered (following post-treatment observation of ≥2 months) if relapse occurs or if treatment fails to normalize serum alkaline phosphatase. For retreatment, the dose and duration of therapy are the same as for initial treatment. No data available on more than one course of treatment.

**Local Anesthetic/Vasoconstrictor Precautions** No information available to require special precautions

**Effects on Dental Treatment** No effects or complications reported

**Other Adverse Effects**

>10%:

Central nervous system: Headache (18%)
Dermatologic: Rash (11.5%)
Gastrointestinal: Abdominal pain (11.5%), diarrhea (19.7%)
Neuromuscular & skeletal: Arthralgia (32.8%)

1% to 10%:

Cardiovascular: Chest pain (6.6%), edema (8.2%)
Central nervous system: Dizziness (6.6%)
Gastrointestinal: Belching (3.3%), colitis (3.3%), constipation (6.6%), nausea (9.8%)
Neuromuscular & skeletal: Bone pain (4.9%), leg cramps (3.3%), myasthenia (3.3%), asthenia (4.9%)
Ocular: Amblyopia (3.3%), dry eyes (3.3%)
Otic: Tinnitus (3.3%)
Respiratory: Bronchitis (3.3%), sinusitis (4.9%)
Miscellaneous: Flu-like syndrome (9.8%), neoplasm (3.3%)

<1%: Ocular: Bilateral iritis

**Contraindications** Hypersensitivity to bisphosphonates or any component of the product; hypocalcemia

**Drug Interactions** Decreased effect: Calcium supplements and antacids interfere with the absorption of risedronate

**Pregnancy Risk Factor** C

**Dosage Forms** Tablet: 30 mg

**Generic Available** No

♦ **Risperdal®** *see* Risperidone *on this page*

## Risperidone (ris PER i done)

**U.S. Brand Names** Risperdal®

**Therapeutic Category** Antipsychotic Agent

**Use** Management of psychotic disorders (eg, schizophrenia); nonpsychotic symptoms associated with dementia in elderly

**Usual Dosage** Recommended starting dose: 1 mg twice daily; slowly increase to the optimum range of 4-8 mg/day; daily dosages >10 mg does not appear to confer any additional benefit, and the incidence of extrapyramidal reactions is higher than with lower doses

**Mechanism of Action** Risperidone is a benzisoxazole derivative, mixed serotonin-dopamine antagonist; binds to 5-$HT_2$ receptors in the CNS and in the periphery with a very high affinity; binds to dopamine-$D_2$ receptors with less affinity. The binding affinity to the dopamine-$D_2$ receptor is 20 times lower than the 5-$HT_2$ affinity. The addition of serotonin antagonism to dopamine antagonism (classic neuroleptic mechanism) is thought to improve negative symptoms of psychoses and reduce the incidence of extrapyramidal side effects.

**Local Anesthetic/Vasoconstrictor Precautions** No information available to require special precautions

**Effects on Dental Treatment** Up to 10% of dental patients will experience significant dry mouth and orthostatic hypotension. These effects disappear with cessation of drug therapy.

**Other Adverse Effects**

1% to 10%:

Cardiovascular: Hypotension (especially orthostatic), tachycardia, arrhythmias, abnormal T waves with prolonged ventricular repolarization; EKG changes, syncope
Central nervous system: Sedation (occurs at daily doses ≥20 mg/day), headache, dizziness, restlessness, anxiety, extrapyramidal reactions, dystonic reactions, pseudoparkinson signs and symptoms, tardive dyskinesia, neuroleptic malignant syndrome, altered central temperature regulation
Dermatologic: Photosensitivity (rare)
Endocrine & metabolic: Amenorrhea, galactorrhea, gynecomastia, sexual dysfunction (up to 60%)
Gastrointestinal: Constipation, adynamic ileus, GI upset, dry mouth (problem for denture user), nausea and anorexia, weight gain
Genitourinary: Urinary retention, overflow incontinence, priapism
Hematologic: Agranulocytosis, leukopenia (usually in patients with large doses for prolonged periods)
Hepatic: Cholestatic jaundice

(Continued)

## Risperidone *(Continued)*

Ocular: Blurred vision, retinal pigmentation, decreased visual acuity (may be irreversible)

<1%: Central nervous system: Seizures

**Drug Interactions** May antagonize effects of levodopa; carbamazepine decreases risperidone serum concentrations; clozapine decreases clearance of risperidone

**Drug Uptake**

Absorption: Oral: Rapid

Serum half-life: 24 hours (risperidone and its active metabolite)

Time to peak: Peak plasma concentrations within 1 hour

**Pregnancy Risk Factor** C

**Generic Available** No

- **Ritalin®** *see* Methylphenidate *on page 660*
- **Ritalin-SR®** *see* Methylphenidate *on page 660*

## Ritodrine (RI toe dreen)

**U.S. Brand Names** Yutopar®

**Therapeutic Category** Adrenergic Agonist Agent; Beta$_2$-Adrenergic Agonist Agent

**Use** Inhibits uterine contraction in preterm labor

**Usual Dosage** Adults:

I.V.: 50-100 mcg/minute; increase by 50 mcg/minute every 10 minutes; continue for 12 hours after contractions have stopped

Oral: Start 30 minutes before stopping I.V. infusion; 10 mg every 2 hours for 24 hours, then 10-20 mg every 4-6 hours up to 120 mg/day

**Mechanism of Action** Tocolysis due to its uterine beta$_2$-adrenergic receptor stimulating effects; this agent's beta$_2$ effects can also cause bronchial relaxation and vascular smooth muscle stimulation

**Local Anesthetic/Vasoconstrictor Precautions** No information available to require special precautions

**Effects on Dental Treatment** No effects or complications reported

**Other Adverse Effects**

>10%:

Cardiovascular: Increases in maternal and fetal heart rates and maternal hypertension, palpitations

Endocrine & metabolic: Temporary hyperglycemia

Gastrointestinal: Nausea, vomiting

Neuromuscular & skeletal: Tremor

1% to 10%:

Cardiovascular: Chest pain

Central nervous system: Nervousness, anxiety, restlessness

<1%:

Endocrine & metabolic: Ketoacidosis

Hepatic: Impaired liver function

Miscellaneous: Anaphylactic shock

**Drug Interactions**

Decreased effect with beta-blockers

Increased effect/toxicity with meperidine, sympathomimetics, diazoxide, magnesium, betamethasone (pulmonary edema), potassium-depleting diuretics, general anesthetics

**Drug Uptake**

Absorption: Oral: Rapid

Serum half-life: 15 hours

Time to peak serum concentration: Within 0.5-1 hour

**Pregnancy Risk Factor** B

**Generic Available** No

## Ritonavir (rye TON a veer)

**Related Information**

HIV Infection and AIDS *on page 1085*

Systemic Viral Diseases *on page 1115*

**U.S. Brand Names** Norvir®

**Therapeutic Category** Antiviral Agent, Oral; Protease Inhibitor

**Use** Treatment of HIV, especially advanced cases; usually is used as part of triple or double therapy with other nucleoside and protease inhibitors

**Usual Dosage** Adults: Oral: 600 mg twice daily with meals

**Mechanism of Action** As a protease inhibitor, ritonavir prevents cleavage of protein precursors essential for HIV infection of new cells and viral replication. Saquinavir- and zidovudine-resistant HIV isolates are generally susceptible to ritonavir. Used in combination therapy, resistance to ritonavir develops slowly; strains resistant to ritonavir are cross-resistant to indinavir and saquinavir.

**Local Anesthetic/Vasoconstrictor Precautions** No information available to require special precautions

**Effects on Dental Treatment** No effects or complications reported

**Other Adverse Effects**

1% to 10%:

- Gastrointestinal: Nausea, vomiting, diarrhea, dysgeusia
- Neuromuscular & skeletal: Circumoral and peripheral paresthesias, weakness

<1%:

- Central nervous system: Headache, confusion
- Endocrine & metabolic: Elevated triglycerides, cholesterol
- Hepatic: Elevated LFTs

**Contraindications** Hypersensitivity to ritonavir or any of its components; avoid use with astemizole, terfenadine, and rifabutin

**Warnings/Precautions** Use caution in patients with hepatic insufficiency; safety and efficacy have not been established in children <16 years of age; use caution with benzodiazepines, antiarrhythmics (flecainide, encainide, bepridil, amiodarone, quinidine) and certain analgesics (meperidine, piroxicam, propoxyphene)

**Drug Interactions**

Decreased effect: Concurrent use of rifampin, rifabutin, dexamethasone, and many anticonvulsants lowers serum concentration of ritonavir

Increased toxicity: Ketoconazole increases ritonavir's plasma levels; ritonavir may decrease metabolism of astemizole and result in rare but serious cardiac arrhythmias; enhanced cardiac effects when administered with flecainide, encainide, quinidine, amiodarone, bepridil. Increased toxic effects also possible with coadministration with cisapride and benzodiazepines.

Clarithromycin produces small increases in ritonavir serum concentrations that are unlikely to produce toxicity. Ritonavir significantly increases clarithromycin concentrations. The clinical significance of this effect is unknown. Erythromycin is likely to interact similarly.

**Drug Uptake**

Absorption: Well absorbed; $T_{max}$: 2-4 hours

Half-life: 3-5 hours

**Pregnancy Risk Factor** B

**Dosage Forms**

Capsule: 100 mg

Solution: 80 mg/mL (240 mL)

**Generic Available** No

**Selected Readings**

Ouellet D, Hsu A, Granneman GR, et al, "Pharmacokinetic Interaction Between Ritonavir and Clarithromycin," *Clin Pharmacol Ther*, 1998, 64(4):355-62.

♦ **Rituxan®** *see* Rituximab *on this page*

## Rituximab (ri TUK si mab)

**U.S. Brand Names** Rituxan®

**Therapeutic Category** Antineoplastic Agent, Miscellaneous

**Synonyms** C2B8

**Use** Treatment of patients with relapsed or refractory low-grade or follicular, CD20 positive, B-cell non-Hodgkin's lymphoma

**Usual Dosage** Adults: I.V.: 375 mg/m$^2$ given as an I.V. infusion once weekly for 4 doses (days 1, 8, 15, and 22); may be administered in an outpatient setting; DO NOT ADMINISTER AS AN INTRAVENOUS PUSH OR BOLUS

**Mechanism of Action** Binds specifically to the antigen CD20 (human B-lymphocyte-restricted differentiation antigen, Bp35), a hydrophobic transmembrane protein with a molecular weight of approximately 35 kD located on pre-B and mature B lymphocytes. The antigen is also expressed on > 90% of B-cell non-Hodgkin's lymphomas (NHL) but is not found on hematopoietic stem cells, pro-B cells, normal plasma cells or other normal tissues. CD20 regulates an early step(s) in the activation process for cell cycle initiation and differentiation, and possibly functions as a calcium ion channel. CD20 is not shed from the cell surface and does not internalize upon antibody binding. Free CD20 antigen is not found in the circulation.

**Local Anesthetic/Vasoconstrictor Precautions** No information available to require special precautions

**Effects on Dental Treatment** No effects or complications reported

**Warnings/Precautions** DO NOT ADMINISTER AS AN INTRAVENOUS PUSH OR BOLUS. Associated with hypersensitivity reactions which may respond to adjustments in the infusion rate. Hypotension, bronchospasm, and angioedema have occurred in association with infusion as part of an infusion-related symptom complex. Infusion should be interrupted for severe reactions and can be resumed at a 50% reduction in rate (eg, from 100 mg/hour to 50 mg/hour) when symptoms have completely resolved. Treatment of these symptoms with diphenhydramine and acetaminophen is recommended; additional treatment with bronchodilators or I.V. saline may be indicated. In most cases, patients who have experienced nonlife-threatening reactions have been able to complete the full course of therapy.

**Drug Uptake**

Absorption: I.V.: Immediate and results in a rapid and sustained depletion of circulating and tissue-based B-cells

Half-life, mean serum: 59.8 hours after the first infusion and 174 hours after the fourth infusion

Duration: Detectable in the serum of patients 3-6 months after completion of treatment. B-cell recovery began ~6 months following completion of treatment. Median B-cell levels returned to normal by 12 months following completion of treatment.

**Pregnancy Risk Factor** C

(Continued)

## Rituximab *(Continued)*

**Dosage Forms** Injection: 100 mg (10 mL); 500 mg (10 mL)

## Rizatriptan (rye za TRIP tan)

**U.S. Brand Names** Maxalt®; Maxalt-MLT™

**Therapeutic Category** Antimigraine Agent; Serotonin Agonist

**Use** Acute treatment of migraine with or without aura

**Usual Dosage** Oral: 5-10 mg, repeat after 2 hours if significant relief is not attained; maximum: 30 mg in a 24-hour period (Use 5 mg dose in patients receiving propranolol with a maximum of 15 mg in 24 hours)

**Mechanism of Action** Selective agonist for serotonin ($5\text{-}HT_{1D}$ receptor) in cranial arteries to cause vasoconstriction and reduce sterile inflammation associated with antidromic neuronal transmission correlating with relief of migraine

**Local Anesthetic/Vasoconstrictor Precautions** No information available to require special precautions

**Effects on Dental Treatment** No effects or complications reported

**Other Adverse Effects**

>1%:

- Cardiovascular: Systolic/diastolic blood pressure increases (5-10 mm Hg), chest pain (5%)
- Central nervous system: Dizziness, drowsiness (13% to 30%)
- Dermatologic: Skin flushing
- Endocrine & metabolic: Mild increase in growth hormone, hot flashes
- Gastrointestinal: Nausea, vomiting, abdominal pain (<5%)
- Respiratory: Dyspnea

<1%:

- Cardiovascular: Syncope, EKG changes
- Neuromuscular & skeletal: Neck pain/stiffness
- Miscellaneous: Chills, heat sensitivity, facial edema, hangover, tachycardia, palpitation, bradycardia, muscle weakness, myalgia, arthralgia, decreased mental activity, neurological/psychiatric abnormalities, nasopharyngeal irritation, blurred vision, tinnitus, dry eyes, eye pain, diaphoresis, pruritus, polyuria

**Drug Interactions**

Use within 24 hours of another selective $5\text{-}HT_1$ agonist or ergot-containing drug should be avoided due to possible additive vasoconstriction

Propranolol: Plasma concentration of rizatriptan increased 70%

SSRIs: Rarely, concurrent use results in weakness and incoordination; monitor closely

MAO inhibitors and nonselective MAO inhibitors increase concentration of rizatriptan

**Drug Uptake**

Onset of action: Within 30 minutes

Duration: 14-16 hours

Half-life: 2-3 hours

Time to peak concentration: 1-1.5 hours

**Pregnancy Risk Factor** C

**Dosage Forms** Tablet, as benzoate:

Maxalt®: 5 mg, 10 mg

Maxalt-MLT™ (orally disintegrating): 5 mg, 10 mg

**Generic Available** No

**RMS® Rectal** *see* Morphine Sulfate *on page 688*

**Robafen® AC** *see* Guaifenesin and Codeine *on page 478*

**Robafen® CF [OTC]** *see* Guaifenesin, Phenylpropanolamine, and Dextromethorphan *on page 481*

**Robafen DM® [OTC]** *see* Guaifenesin and Dextromethorphan *on page 479*

**Robaxin®** *see* Methocarbamol *on page 649*

**Robaxisal®** *see* Methocarbamol and Aspirin *on page 650*

**Robicillin® VK** *see* Penicillin V Potassium *on page 776*

**Robinul®** *see* Glycopyrrolate *on page 473*

**Robitussin® [OTC]** *see* Guaifenesin *on page 478*

**Robitussin® A-C** *see* Guaifenesin and Codeine *on page 478*

**Robitussin-CF® [OTC]** *see* Guaifenesin, Phenylpropanolamine, and Dextromethorphan *on page 481*

**Robitussin® Cough Calmers [OTC]** *see* Dextromethorphan *on page 314*

**Robitussin®-DAC** *see* Guaifenesin, Pseudoephedrine, and Codeine *on page 482*

**Robitussin®-DM [OTC]** *see* Guaifenesin and Dextromethorphan *on page 479*

**Robitussin-PE® [OTC]** *see* Guaifenesin and Pseudoephedrine *on page 481*

**Robitussin® Pediatric [OTC]** *see* Dextromethorphan *on page 314*

**Robitussin® Severe Congestion Liqui-Gels® [OTC]** *see* Guaifenesin and Pseudoephedrine *on page 481*

**Rocaltrol®** *see* Calcitriol *on page 170*

**Rocephin®** *see* Ceftriaxone *on page 209*

## Rocky Mountain Spotted Fever Vaccine

(ROK ee MOUN ten SPOT ted FEE ver vak SEEN)

**Therapeutic Category** Vaccine, Live Bacteria

**Local Anesthetic/Vasoconstrictor Precautions** No information available to require special precautions

**Effects on Dental Treatment** No effects or complications reported

**Generic Available** No

## Rofecoxib (roe fe COX ib)

**U.S. Brand Names** Vioxx®

**Therapeutic Category** Selective Cyclooxygenase-2 Inhibitor

**Use** Relief of the signs and symptoms of osteoarthritis; management of acute pain in adults; treatment of primary dysmenorrhea

**Usual Dosage** Adults: Oral:

Osteoarthritis: 12.5 mg once daily; may be increased to a maximum of 25 mg once daily

Acute pain, including dental pain, and management of dysmenorrhea: 50 mg once daily as needed (use for longer than 5 days is not recommended)

**Mechanism of Action** Inhibits prostaglandin synthesis by decreasing the activity of the enzyme, cyclo-oxygenase-2 (COX-2), which results in decreased formation of prostaglandin precursors. Rofecoxib does not inhibit cyclo-oxygenase-1 (COX-1) at therapeutic concentrations.

**Local Anesthetic/Vasoconstrictor Precautions** No information available to require special precautions

**Effects on Dental Treatment** In models of postoperative dental pain, rofecoxib was effective against dental pain rated as moderate to severe. The analgesic efficacy of a single 50 mg dose of rofecoxib was apparently similar to 400 mg of ibuprofen or 550 mg of naproxen sodium. The onset of analgesia for postoperative dental pain with a single 50 mg dose of rofecoxib was 45 minutes.

Platelets: Bleeding time was not altered after a single dose of 500 mg or 1000 mg of rofecoxib. In addition, according to the manufacturer, multiple doses of rofecoxib 12.5 mg, 25 mg, and up to 375 mg administered daily up to 12 days, had no effect on bleeding time relative to placebo. However, according to the manufacturer, rofecoxib may increase the INR in patients receiving warfarin (see Drug Interactions).

**Other Adverse Effects** 2% to 10%:

Cardiovascular: Peripheral edema (3.7%), hypertension (3.5%)

Central nervous system: Headache (4.7%), dizziness (3%)

Gastrointestinal: Diarrhea (6.5%), nausea (5.2%), heartburn (4.2%), epigastric discomfort (3.8%), dyspepsia (3.5%), abdominal pain (3.4%)

Genitourinary: Urinary tract infection (2.8%)

Neuromuscular & skeletal: Back pain (2.5%), weakness (2.2%)

Respiratory: Upper respiratory infection (8.5%), bronchitis (2.0%), sinusitis (2.7%)

Miscellaneous: Flu-like syndrome (2.9%)

**Warnings/Precautions** Gastrointestinal irritation, ulceration, bleeding, and perforation may occur with NSAIDs (it is unclear whether rofecoxib is associated with rates of these events which are similar to nonselective NSAIDs). Use with caution in patients with a history of GI disease (bleeding or ulcers), decreased renal function, hepatic disease, congestive heart failure, hypertension, or asthma. Anaphylactoid reactions may occur, even with no prior exposure to rofecoxib.

**Drug Interactions** May be a mild inducer of cytochrome P-450 isoenzyme 3A4 (CYP3A4)

Increased effect: Cimetidine increases AUC of rofecoxib by 23%. Rofecoxib may increase plasma concentrations of methotrexate and lithium. Rofecoxib may be used with low-dose aspirin, however rates of gastrointestinal bleeding may be increased with coadministration. Rofecoxib may increase the INR in patients receiving warfarin and may increase the risk of bleeding complications.

Decreased effects: Efficacy of thiazide diuretics, loop diuretics (furosemide) or ACE-inhibitors may be diminished by rofecoxib. Rifampin reduces the serum concentration of rofecoxib by approximately 50%. Antacids may reduce rofecoxib absorption.

**Drug Uptake**

Onset: 45 minutes; Duration: >24 hours

Half-life: 17 hours; Time to peak: 2-3 hours

**Pregnancy Risk Factor** C (D after 34-weeks gestation or close to delivery)

**Dosage Forms**

Suspension, oral: 12.5 mg/5 mL, 25 mg/5 mL

Tablets: 12.5 mg, 25 mg

**Roferon-A®** *see* Interferon Alfa-2a *on page 538*

**Rogaine® [OTC]** *see* Minoxidil *on page 678*

**Rolaids® [OTC]** *see* Dihydroxyaluminum Sodium Carbonate *on page 334*

**Rolaids® Calcium Rich [OTC]** *see* Calcium Carbonate *on page 172*

**Rolatuss® Plain Liquid** *see* Chlorpheniramine and Phenylephrine *on page 232*

**Romazicon™** *see* Flumazenil *on page 438*

**Rondamine®-DM Drops** *see* Carbinoxamine, Pseudoephedrine, and Dextromethorphan *on page 189*

**Rondec®** *see* Carbinoxamine and Pseudoephedrine *on page 188*

**Rondec®-DM** *see* Carbinoxamine, Pseudoephedrine, and Dextromethorphan *on page 189*

## Ropinirole (roe PIN i role)

**U.S. Brand Names** Requip™

**Therapeutic Category** Anti-Parkinson's Agent

**Synonyms** Ropinirole Hydrochloride

**Use** Treatment of idiopathic Parkinson's disease; in patients with early Parkinson's disease who were not receiving concomitant levodopa therapy as well as in patients with advanced disease on concomitant levodopa

(Continued)

## Ropinirole *(Continued)*

**Usual Dosage** Adults: Oral: Dosage should be increased to achieve a maximum therapeutic effect, balanced against the principal side effects of nausea, dizziness, somnolence, and dyskinesia

Recommended starting dose: 0.25 mg 3 times/day; based on individual patient response, the dosage should be titrated with weekly increments

Week 1: 0.25 mg 3 times/day; total daily dose: 0.75 mg

Week 2: 0.5 mg 3 times/day; total daily dose: 1.5 mg

Week 3: 0.75 mg 3 times/day; total daily dose: 2.25 mg

Week 4: 1 mg 3 times/day; total daily dose: 3 mg

After week 4, if necessary, daily dosage may be increased by 1.5 mg/day on a weekly basis up to a dose of 9 mg/day, then by up to 3 mg/day weekly to a total of 24 mg/day

**Mechanism of Action** Ropinirole has a high relative *in vitro* specificity and full intrinsic activity at the $D_2$ and $D_3$ dopamine receptor subtypes, binding with higher affinity to $D_3$ than to $D_2$ or $D_4$ receptor subtypes; relevance of $D_3$ receptor binding in Parkinson's disease is unknown. Ropinirole has moderate *in vitro* affinity for opioid receptors. Ropinirole and its metabolites have negligible *in vitro* affinity for dopamine $D_1$, 5-$HT_1$, 5-$HT_2$, benzodiazepine, GABA, muscarinic, $alpha_1$-, $alpha_2$-, and beta-adrenoreceptors. Although precise mechanism of action of ropinirole is unknown, it is believed to be due to stimulation of postsynaptic dopamine $D_2$-type receptors within the caudate-putamen in the brain. Ropinirole caused decreases in systolic and diastolic blood pressure at doses above 0.25 mg. The mechanism of ropinirole-induced postural hypotension is believed to be due to $D_2$-mediated blunting of the noradrenergic response to standing and subsequent decrease in peripheral vascular resistance.

**Local Anesthetic/Vasoconstrictor Precautions** No information available to require special precautions

**Effects on Dental Treatment** Up to 2% of patients may experience increased salivation, dry mouth

**Other Adverse Effects**

Early Parkinson's disease:

Cardiovascular: Syncope, dependent/leg edema, orthostatic symptoms

Central nervous system: Dizziness, somnolence (40%), headache, fatigue, pain, confusion, hallucinations

Gastrointestinal: Nausea (60%), dyspepsia, constipation, abdominal pain

Genitourinary: Urinary tract infections

Neuromuscular & skeletal: Asthenia

Ocular: Abnormal vision

Respiratory: Pharyngitis

Miscellaneous: Viral infection, diaphoresis (increased)

Advanced Parkinson's disease (with levodopa):

Cardiovascular: Hypotension (2%), syncope (3%)

Central nervous system: Dizziness (26%), aggravated parkinsonism, somnolence, headache (17%), insomnia, hallucinations, confusion (9%), pain (5%), paresis (3%), amnesia (5%), anxiety (6%), abnormal dreaming (3%)

Gastrointestinal: Nausea (30%), abdominal pain (9%), vomiting (7%), constipation (6%), diarrhea (5%), dysphagia (2%), flatulence (2%), xerostomia, weight loss (2%)

Genitourinary: Urinary tract infections

Neuromuscular & skeletal: Dyskinesias (34%), falls (10%), hypokinesia (5%), paresthesia (5%), tremor (6%), arthralgia (7%), arthritis (3%)

Respiratory: Upper respiratory tract infection

Miscellaneous: Injury, increased diaphoresis (7%), viral infection, increased drug level (7%)

Endocrine & metabolic: Hypoglycemia, increased LDH, hyperphosphatemia, hyperuricemia, diabetes mellitus, hypokalemia, hypercholesterolemia, hyperkalemia, acidosis, hyponatremia, dehydration, hypochloremia

Gastrointestinal: Weight increase

Hepatic: Increased alkaline phosphatase

Neuromuscular & skeletal: Increased CPK

Renal: Elevated BUN, glycosuria

Miscellaneous: Thirst, increased lactate dehydrogenase (LDH)

**Drug Uptake**

Absorption: Not affected by food; $T_{max}$ increased by 2.5 hours when drug taken with a meal; absolute bioavailability was 55%, indicating first-pass effect; relative bioavailability from tablet compared to oral solution is 85%

Serum half-life, elimination: ~6 hours; Time to peak concentration: ~1-2 hours

**Pregnancy Risk Factor** C

**Dosage Forms** Tablet: 0.25 mg, 0.5 mg, 1 mg, 2 mg, 5 mg

**Dietary Considerations** Ropinirole can be taken with or without food

## Ropivacaine (roe PIV a kane)

**U.S. Brand Names** Naropin™

**Therapeutic Category** Local Anesthetic, Injectable

**Use** Local anesthetic (injectable) for use in surgery, postoperative pain management, and obstetrical procedures when local or regional anesthesia is needed. It can be administered via local infiltration, epidural block and epidural infusion, or intermittent bolus.

**Usual Dosage** Ropivacaine dose varies with procedure, onset and the depth of anesthesia desired, vascularity of tissues, the duration of anesthesia, and the condition of the patient

Adults:
- Lumbar epidural for surgery: 15-30 mL of 0.5% to 1%
- Lumbar epidural block for cesarean section: 20-30 mL of 0.5%
- Thoracic epidural block for postoperative pain relief: 5-15 mL of 0.5%
- Major nerve block: 35-50 mL dose of 0.5% (175-250 mg)
- Field block: 1-40 mL dose of 0.5% (5-200 mg)
- Lumbar epidural for labor pain: Initial: 10-20 mL 0.2%; continuous infusion dose: 6-14 mL/hour of 0.2% with incremental injections of 10-15 mL/hour of 0.2% solution

**Mechanism of Action** Local anesthetics bind selectively to the intracellular surface of sodium channels to block influx of sodium into the axon. As a result, depolarization necessary for action potential propagation and subsequent nerve function is prevented. The block at the sodium channel is reversible. When drug diffuses away from the axon, sodium channel function is restored and nerve propagation returns.

**Local Anesthetic/Vasoconstrictor Precautions** No information available to require special precautions

**Effects on Dental Treatment** No effects or complications reported

**Other Adverse Effects**

>10% (dose and route related):
- Cardiovascular: Hypotension, bradycardia
- Gastrointestinal: Nausea, vomiting
- Neuromuscular & skeletal: Back pain
- Miscellaneous: Shivering

1% to 10% (dose related):
- Cardiovascular: Hypertension, tachycardia, bradycardia
- Central nervous system: Headache, dizziness, anxiety, lightheadedness
- Gastrointestinal: Vomiting
- Neuromuscular & skeletal: Hypoesthesia, paresthesia, circumoral paresthesia
- Otic: Tinnitus
- Respiratory: Apnea

**Drug Interactions**

Increased effect: Other local anesthetics or agents structurally related to the amide-type anesthetics

Increased toxicity (possible but not yet reported): Drugs that decrease cytochrome P-450 1A enzyme function

**Drug Uptake**

Duration of action (dependent on dose and route administered): 3-15 hours generally

Half-life:
- Epidural: 5-7 hours
- I.V.: 2.4 hours

**Pregnancy Risk Factor** B

**Dosage Forms**

Infusion, as hydrochloride: 2 mg/mL (100 mL, 200 mL)

Injection, as hydrochloride (single dose): 2 mg/mL (20 mL); 5 mg/mL (30 mL); 7.5 mg/mL (10 mL, 20 mL); 10 mg/mL (10 mL, 20 mL)

**Generic Available** No

**Comments** Not available with vasoconstrictor (epinephrine) and not available in dental (1.8 mL) carpules

♦ **RotaShield®** *see* Rotavirus Vaccine *on this page*

## Rotavirus Vaccine

**U.S. Brand Names** RotaShield®

**Therapeutic Category** Vaccine

**Use** Prevention of gastroenteritis caused by the rotavirus serotypes responsible for the majority of disease in infants and children in the U.S. (serotypes G 1,2,3 and 4)

**Usual Dosage For oral administration only**

Children: Three 2.5 mL doses are administered. The recommended schedule for immunization is at 2, 4, and 6 months of age. The first dose may be administered as early as 6 weeks of age, with subsequent doses at least 3 weeks apart. The third dose has been administered to infants up to 33 weeks of age with no increase in adverse reactions. Initiation of vaccination after the age of 6 months is not currently recommended due to an increased risk of fever. RotaShield® does not diminish the efficacy of OPV, DTP, or Hib when administered concurrently. Repeat dosing of vaccine is not recommended if an infant should regurgitate a dose.

Adults: Not approved for administration to adults

(Continued)

## Rotavirus Vaccine *(Continued)*

Reconstitute lyophilized vaccine by adding diluent from Dispette®, then withdraw reconstituted solution back into Dispette® (may reuse cap to store until administration). Must be administered within 60 minutes of reconstitution if stored at room temperature, or within 4 hours of reconstitution if refrigerated. Place tip of Dispette® into the infant's mouth and slowly squeeze out contents.

**Mechanism of Action** Rotavirus is presumed to be transmitted via the oral-fecal route, causing infection of cells in the small intestine. Rotavirus vaccine includes a rhesus virus and three rhesus-human reassortment viruses. The live virus vaccine stimulates production of IgG and IgA antibodies which cross-react with human serotypes. The four serotypes which cause the majority of infections in humans are neutralized by these antibodies.

**Local Anesthetic/Vasoconstrictor Precautions** No information available to require special precautions

**Effects on Dental Treatment** No effects or complications reported

**Other Adverse Effects**

>10%: Central nervous system: Fever (>38°C to <39°C) (11% to 21%), decreased appetite (11% to 17%), irritability (36% to 41%), decreased activity (10% to 20%)

1% to 10%: Central nervous system: Fever (≥39°C) (1% to 2%)

The incidence of fever is greater when administered to infants >6 months of age. The highest incidence of adverse effects was associated with the first dose of the vaccine. By the third dose, there were no significant differences in the incidence of adverse effects between vaccine and placebo.

**Drug Interactions** No drug interactions have been reported. No data have been reported with respect to administration of orally or intravenously administered immune globulin-containing products.

**Pregnancy Risk Factor** C

**Dosage Forms** Powder, lyophilized, for oral solution: 2.5 mL diluent (Dispette®); specialized diluent contains citric acid and sodium bicarbonate

- **Rowasa®** *see* Mesalamine *on page 638*
- **Roxanol™ Oral** *see* Morphine Sulfate *on page 688*
- **Roxanol Rescudose®** *see* Morphine Sulfate *on page 688*
- **Roxanol SR™ Oral** *see* Morphine Sulfate *on page 688*
- **Roxicet® 5/500** *see* Oxycodone and Acetaminophen *on page 751*
- **Roxicodon** [illegible] *see* Oxycodone *on page 750*
- **Roxilox®** *see* Oxycodone and Acetaminophen *on page 751*
- **Roxiprin®** *see* Oxycodone and Aspirin *on page 753*
- **R-Tannamine® Tablet** *see* Chlorpheniramine, Pyrilamine, and Phenylephrine *on page 238*
- **R-Tannate® Tablet** *see* Chlorpheniramine, Pyrilamine, and Phenylephrine *on page 238*
- **RTCA** *see* Ribavirin *on page 884*
- **Rubella and Measles Vaccines, Combined** *see* Measles and Rubella Vaccines, Combined *on page 618*

## Rubella and Mumps Vaccines, Combined

(rue BEL a & mumpz vak SEENS, kom BINED)

**U.S. Brand Names** Biavax® II

**Therapeutic Category** Vaccine, Live Virus

**Use** Promote active immunity to rubella and mumps by inducing production of antibodies

**Usual Dosage** Children >12 months and Adults: 1 vial in outer aspect of the upper arm; children vaccinated before 12 months of age should be revaccinated

**Local Anesthetic/Vasoconstrictor Precautions** No information available to require special precautions

**Effects on Dental Treatment** No effects or complications reported

**Other Adverse Effects** 1% to 10%:

Central nervous system: Febrile seizures, fever
Local: Burning, stinging
Neuromuscular & skeletal: Soreness
Miscellaneous: Allergic reactions

**Pregnancy Risk Factor** X

**Dosage Forms** Injection (mixture of 2 viruses):

1. Wistar RA 27/3 strain of rubella virus
2. Jeryl Lynn (B level) mumps strain grown cell cultures of chick embryo

**Generic Available** No

**Comments** Federal law requires that the date of administration, the vaccine manufacturer, lot number of vaccine, and the administering person's name, title and address be entered into the patient's permanent medical record

♦ **Rubella, Measles and Mumps Vaccines, Combined** *see* Measles, Mumps, and Rubella Vaccines, Combined *on page 618*

## Rubella Virus Vaccine, Live (rue BEL a VYE rus vak SEEN, live)

**U.S. Brand Names** Meruvax® II

**Therapeutic Category** Vaccine, Live Virus

**Synonyms** German Measles Vaccine

**Use** Provide vaccine-induced immunity to rubella

**Usual Dosage** Children ≥12 months and Adults: S.C.: 0.5 mL in outer aspect of upper arm; children vaccinated before 12 months of age should be revaccinated

**Mechanism of Action** Rubella vaccine is a live attenuated vaccine that contains the Wistar Institute RA 27/3 strain, which is adapted to and propagated in human diploid cell culture. It is the only strain of rubella vaccine marketed in the U.S. Antibody titers after immunization last 6 years without significant decline; 90% of those vaccinated have protection for at least 15 years.

**Local Anesthetic/Vasoconstrictor Precautions** No information available to require special precautions

**Effects on Dental Treatment** No effects or complications reported

**Other Adverse Effects**

>10%:
- Dermatologic: Erythema, urticaria, rash
- Local: Tenderness
- Neuromuscular & skeletal: Arthralgias

1% to 10%:
- Central nervous system: Malaise, fever, headache
- Gastrointestinal: Sore throat
- Miscellaneous: Lymphadenopathy

<1%:
- Ocular: Optic neuritis
- Miscellaneous: Hypersensitivity, allergic reactions to the vaccine

**Drug Uptake**

Onset of effect: Antibodies to the vaccine are detectable within 2-4 weeks following immunization

Duration: Protection against both clinical rubella and asymptomatic viremia is probably life-long. Vaccine-induced antibody levels have been shown to persist for at least 10 years without substantial decline. If the present pattern continues, it will provide a basis for the expectation that immunity following vaccination will be permanent. However, continued surveillance will be required to demonstrate this point.

**Pregnancy Risk Factor** X

**Generic Available** No

**Comments** Federal law requires that the date of administration, the vaccine manufacturer, lot number of vaccine, and the administering person's name, title and address be entered into the patient's permanent record

♦ **Rubeola Vaccine** *see* Measles Virus Vaccine, Live *on page 619*

♦ **Rubex®** *see* Doxorubicin *on page 353*

♦ **Rubidomycin Hydrochloride** *see* Daunorubicin Hydrochloride *on page 299*

♦ **Rum-K®** *see* Potassium Chloride *on page 822*

♦ **Ru-Tuss®** *see* Chlorpheniramine, Phenylephrine, Phenylpropanolamine, and Belladonna Alkaloids *on page 236*

♦ **Ru-Tuss® DE** *see* Guaifenesin and Pseudoephedrine *on page 481*

♦ **Ru-Tuss® Expectorant [OTC]** *see* Guaifenesin, Pseudoephedrine, and Dextromethorphan *on page 482*

♦ **Ru-Tuss® Liquid** *see* Chlorpheniramine and Phenylephrine *on page 232*

♦ **Ru-Vert-M®** *see* Meclizine *on page 620*

♦ **Rymed®** *see* Guaifenesin and Pseudoephedrine *on page 481*

♦ **Rymed-TR®** *see* Guaifenesin and Phenylpropanolamine *on page 480*

♦ **Ryna-C® Liquid** *see* Chlorpheniramine, Pseudoephedrine, and Codeine *on page 237*

♦ **Ryna-CX®** *see* Guaifenesin, Pseudoephedrine, and Codeine *on page 482*

♦ **Ryna® Liquid [OTC]** *see* Chlorpheniramine and Pseudoephedrine *on page 233*

♦ **Rynatan® Pediatric Suspension** *see* Chlorpheniramine, Pyrilamine, and Phenylephrine *on page 238*

♦ **Rynatan® Tablet** *see* Chlorpheniramine, Pyrilamine, and Phenylephrine *on page 238*

- **Rynatuss® Pediatric Suspension** *see* Chlorpheniramine, Ephedrine, Phenylephrine, and Carbetapentane *on page 233*
- **Rythmol®** *see* Propafenone *on page 850*
- **S-2®** *see* Epinephrine, Racemic *on page 375*
- **Sabin Vaccine** *see* Poliovirus Vaccine, Live, Trivalent, Oral *on page 813*
- **Safe Tussin® 30 [OTC]** *see* Guaifenesin and Dextromethorphan *on page 479*
- **Safe Writing Practices** *see page 1276*
- **Saizen® Injection** *see* Human Growth Hormone *on page 499*
- **Sal-Acid® Plaster [OTC]** *see* Salicylic Acid *on this page*
- **Salactic® Film [OTC]** *see* Salicylic Acid *on this page*
- **Salagen®** *see* Pilocarpine (Dental) *on page 804*
- **Saleto-200® [OTC]** *see* Ibuprofen *on page 522*
- **Saleto-400®** *see* Ibuprofen *on page 522*
- **Saleto-600®** *see* Ibuprofen *on page 522*
- **Saleto-800®** *see* Ibuprofen *on page 522*
- **Salflex®** *see* Salsalate *on page 902*
- **Salgesic®** *see* Salsalate *on page 902*


## Salicylic Acid (sal i SIL ik AS id)

**U.S. Brand Names** Clear Away® Disc [OTC]; Compound W® [OTC]; Dr Scholl's® Disk [OTC]; Dr Scholl's® Wart Remover [OTC]; DuoFilm® [OTC]; DuoPlant® Gel [OTC]; Freezone® Solution [OTC]; Gordofilm® Liquid; Mediplast® Plaster [OTC]; Mosco® Liquid [OTC]; Occlusal®-HP Liquid; Off-Ezy® Wart Remover [OTC]; Panscol® [OTC]; Psor-a-set® Soap [OTC]; P&S® Shampoo [OTC]; Sal-Acid® Plaster [OTC]; Salactic® Film [OTC]; Sal-Plant® Gel [OTC]; Trans-Ver-Sal® AdultPatch [OTC]; Trans-Ver-Sal® PediaPatch [OTC]; Trans-Ver-Sal® PlantarPatch [OTC]; Wart-Off® [OTC]

**Canadian Brand Names** Acnex®; Acnomel®; Trans-Planta®; Trans-Ver-Sal®

**Therapeutic Category** Keratolytic Agent

**Use** Topically for its keratolytic effect in controlling seborrheic dermatitis or psoriasis of body and scalp, dandruff, and other scaling dermatoses; also used to remove warts, corns, and calluses

**Usual Dosage**

Lotion, cream, gel: Apply a thin layer to affected area once or twice daily

Plaster: Cut to size that covers the corn or callus, apply and leave in place for 48 hours; do not exceed 5 applications over a 14-day period

Solution: Apply a thin layer directly to wart using brush applicator once daily as directed for 1 week or until wart is removed

**Mechanism of Action** Produces desquamation of hyperkeratotic epithelium via dissolution of the intercellular cement which causes the cornified tissue to swell, soften, macerate, and desquamate. Salicylic acid is keratolytic at concentrations of 3% to 6%; it becomes destructive to tissue at concentrations >6%. Concentrations of 6% to 60% are used to remove corns and warts and in the treatment of psoriasis and other hyperkeratotic disorders.

**Local Anesthetic/Vasoconstrictor Precautions** No information available to require special precautions

**Effects on Dental Treatment** No effects or complications reported

**Other Adverse Effects**

>10%: Local: Burning and irritation at site of exposure on normal tissue

1% to 10%:

Central nervous system: Dizziness, mental confusion, headache

Otic: Tinnitus

Respiratory: Hyperventilation

**Drug Interactions** No data reported

**Drug Uptake**

Absorption: Absorbed percutaneously, but systemic toxicity is unlikely with normal use

Time to peak serum concentration: Topical: Within 5 hours of application with occlusion

**Pregnancy Risk Factor** C

**Generic Available** Yes


- **Salicylic Acid and Benzoic Acid** *see* Benzoic Acid and Salicylic Acid *on page 130*


## Salicylic Acid and Lactic Acid (sal i SIL ik AS id & LAK tik AS id)

**U.S. Brand Names** Duofilm® Solution

**Therapeutic Category** Keratolytic Agent

**Synonyms** Lactic Acid and Salicylic Acid

**Use** Treatment of benign epithelial tumors such as warts

**Usual Dosage** Apply a thin layer directly to wart once daily (may be useful to apply at bedtime and wash off in morning)

**Local Anesthetic/Vasoconstrictor Precautions** No information available to require special precautions

**Effects on Dental Treatment** No effects or complications reported

**Pregnancy Risk Factor** C

**Generic Available** Yes

**Comments** Protect normal skin tissue with a ring of petrolatum surrounding the affected area; prior to application, soak affected area in hot water for at least 5 minutes; dry thoroughly with a clean towel

- ♦ **Salicylic Acid and Podophyllin** *see* Podophyllin and Salicylic Acid *on page 812*

## Salicylic Acid and Propylene Glycol

(sal i SIL ik AS id & PROE pi leen GLYE cole)

**U.S. Brand Names** Keralyt® Gel

**Therapeutic Category** Keratolytic Agent

**Synonyms** Propylene Glycol and Salicylic Acid

**Use** Removal of excessive keratin in hyperkeratotic skin disorders, including various ichthyosis, keratosis palmaris and plantaris and psoriasis; may be used to remove excessive keratin in dorsal and plantar hyperkeratotic lesions

**Usual Dosage** Apply to area at night after soaking region for at least 5 minutes to hydrate area, and place under occlusion; medication is washed off in morning

**Local Anesthetic/Vasoconstrictor Precautions** No information available to require special precautions

**Effects on Dental Treatment** No effects or complications reported

**Pregnancy Risk Factor** C

**Generic Available** No

- ♦ **Salicylic Acid and Sulfur** *see* Sulfur and Salicylic Acid *on page 947*
- ♦ **SalineX® [OTC]** *see* Sodium Chloride *on page 920*
- ♦ **Salivart® Solution [OTC]** *see* Saliva Substitute *on this page*

## Saliva Substitute (sa LYE va SUB stee tute)

**Related Information**

Patients Undergoing Cancer Therapy *on page 1154*

Products for Xerostomia *on page 1260*

**U.S. Brand Names** Entertainer's Secret® Spray [OTC]; Moi-Stir® Solution [OTC]; Moi-Stir® Swabsticks [OTC]; Mouthkote® Solution [OTC]; Optimoist® Solution [OTC]; Salivart® Solution [OTC]; Salix® Lozenge [OTC]

**Therapeutic Category** Gastrointestinal Agent, Miscellaneous; Saliva Substitute

**Use** Relief of dry mouth and throat in xerostomia

**Usual Dosage** Use as needed

**Local Anesthetic/Vasoconstrictor Precautions** No information available to require special precautions

**Effects on Dental Treatment** No effects or complications reported

**Dosage Forms**

Lozenge: 100s

Solution: 60 mL, 75 mL, 120 mL, 180 mL, 240 mL

Swabstix: 3s

**Generic Available** Yes

- ♦ **Salix® Lozenge [OTC]** *see* Saliva Substitute *on this page*
- ♦ **Salk Vaccine** *see* Poliovirus Vaccine, Inactivated *on page 813*

## Salmeterol (sal ME te role)

**Related Information**

Respiratory Diseases *on page 1079*

**U.S. Brand Names** Serevent®; Serevent® Diskus®

**Therapeutic Category** Adrenergic Agonist Agent; Antiasthmatic; $Beta_2$-Adrenergic Agonist Agent; Bronchodilator

**Use** Maintenance treatment of asthma and in prevention of bronchospasm in patients >12 years of age with reversible obstructive airway disease, including patients with symptoms of nocturnal asthma, who require regular treatment with inhaled, short-acting $beta_2$ agonists; prevention of exercise-induced bronchospasm in patients ≥4 years of age

**Usual Dosage**

Inhalation: 42 mcg (2 puffs) twice daily (12 hours apart) for maintenance and prevention of symptoms of asthma

(Continued)

## Salmeterol *(Continued)*

Prevention of exercise-induced asthma ≥4 years of age:

Serevent®: 42 mcg (2 puffs) 30-60 minutes prior to exercise; additional doses should not be used for 12 hours

Serevent® Diskus®: One inhalation (50 mcg) at least 30 minutes before exercise; additional doses should not be used for 12 hours

Maintenance of bronchodilatation and prevention of symptoms of asthma: Children ≥4 years and Adults: Serevent® Diskus®: One inhalation (50 mcg) twice daily (morning and evening) approximately 12 hours apart

**Mechanism of Action** Relaxes bronchial smooth muscle by selective action on $beta_2$-receptors with little effect on heart rate; because salmeterol acts locally in the lung, therapeutic effect is not predicted by plasma levels

**Local Anesthetic/Vasoconstrictor Precautions** No information available to require special precautions

**Effects on Dental Treatment** No effects or complications reported

**Other Adverse Effects**

>10%:

Central nervous system: Headache

Respiratory: Pharyngitis

1% to 10%:

Cardiovascular: Tachycardia, palpitations, elevation or depression of blood pressure, cardiac arrhythmias

Central nervous system: Nervousness, CNS stimulation, hyperactivity, insomnia, malaise, dizziness

Gastrointestinal: GI upset, diarrhea, nausea

Neuromuscular & skeletal: Tremors (may be more common in the elderly), myalgias, back pain, arthralgia

Respiratory: Upper respiratory infection, cough, bronchitis

<1%: Miscellaneous: Immediate hypersensitivity reactions (rash, urticaria, bronchospasm)

**Drug Interactions** Vascular system effects of salmeterol may be potentiated by MAO inhibitors and tricyclic antidepressants

**Drug Uptake**

Onset of action: 5-20 minutes (average 10 minutes)

Duration: 12 hours

Serum half-life: 3-4 hours

**Pregnancy Risk Factor** C

**Dosage Forms**

Aerosol, oral, as xinafoate: 21 mcg/spray [60 inhalations] (6.5 g), [120 inhalations] (13 g)

Powder, for inhalation: 50 mcg (contains lactose)

**Generic Available** No

♦ **Salmonine® Injection** *see* Calcitonin *on page 169*

♦ **Sal-Plant® Gel [OTC]** *see* Salicylic Acid *on page 900*

## Salsalate (SAL sa late)

**Related Information**

Rheumatoid Arthritis and Osteoarthritis *on page 1092*

**U.S. Brand Names** Argesic®-SA; Artha-G®; Disalcid®; Marthritic®; Mono-Gesic®; Salflex®; Salgesic®; Salsitab®

**Therapeutic Category** Analgesic, Non-narcotic; Anti-inflammatory Agent; Antipyretic; Nonsteroidal Anti-inflammatory Drug (NSAID), Oral; Salicylate

**Use** Treatment of minor pain or fever; arthritis

**Usual Dosage** Adults: Oral: 3 g/day in 2-3 divided doses

**Mechanism of Action** Inhibits prostaglandin synthesis, acts on the hypothalamus heat-regulating center to reduce fever, blocks prostaglandin synthetase action which prevents formation of the platelet-aggregating substance thromboxane $A_2$

**Local Anesthetic/Vasoconstrictor Precautions** No information available to require special precautions

**Effects on Dental Treatment** NSAID formulations are known to reversibly decrease platelet aggregation via mechanisms different than observed with aspirin. The dentist should be aware of the potential of abnormal coagulation. Caution should also be exercised in the use of NSAIDs in patients already on anticoagulant therapy with drugs such as warfarin (Coumadin®).

**Other Adverse Effects**

>10%: Gastrointestinal: Nausea, heartburn, stomach pains, dyspepsia, epigastric discomfort

1% to 10%:

Central nervous system: Fatigue

Dermatologic: Skin rash
Gastrointestinal: Gastrointestinal ulceration
Hematologic: Hemolytic anemia
Neuromuscular & skeletal: Weakness
Respiratory: Dyspnea
Miscellaneous: Anaphylactic shock

<1%:
Central nervous system: Insomnia, nervousness, jitters
Hematologic: Leukopenia, thrombocytopenia, iron deficiency anemia, does not appear to inhibit platelet aggregation, occult bleeding
Hepatic: Hepatotoxicity
Renal: Impaired renal function
Respiratory: Bronchospasm

**Drug Interactions**
Decreased effect with urinary alkalinizers, antacids, corticosteroids; decreased effect of uricosurics, spironolactone
Increased effect/toxicity of oral anticoagulants, hypoglycemics, methotrexate

**Drug Uptake**
Onset of action: Therapeutic effects occur within 3-4 days of continuous dosing
Absorption: Oral: Completely from the small intestine
Serum half-life: 7-8 hours

**Pregnancy Risk Factor** C
**Generic Available** Yes

- **Salsitab®** *see* Salsalate *on previous page*
- **Salt** *see* Sodium Chloride *on page 920*
- **Saluron®** *see* Hydroflumethiazide *on page 512*
- **Salutensin®** *see* Hydroflumethiazide and Reserpine *on page 513*
- **Sandimmune® Injection** *see* Cyclosporine *on page 288*
- **Sandimmune® Oral** *see* Cyclosporine *on page 288*
- **Sandoglobulin®** *see* Immune Globulin, Intravenous *on page 531*
- **Sandostatin®** *see* Octreotide Acetate *on page 736*
- **Sandostatin LAR®** *see* Octreotide Acetate *on page 736*
- **Sani-Supp® Suppository [OTC]** *see* Glycerin *on page 472*
- **Sanorex®** *see* Mazindol *on page 617*
- **Sansert®** *see* Methysergide *on page 663*
- **Santyl®** *see* Collagenase *on page 276*

## Saquinavir (sa KWIN a veer)

**Related Information**
HIV Infection and AIDS *on page 1085*
Systemic Viral Diseases *on page 1115*

**U.S. Brand Names** Invirase®

**Therapeutic Category** Antiviral Agent, Oral

**Use** Treatment of advanced HIV infection, used in combination with older nucleoside analog medications

**Usual Dosage** Oral: 600 mg 3 times/day within 2 hours after a full meal; use in combination with a nucleoside analog (AZT or ddC)

**Mechanism of Action** As an inhibitor of HIV protease, saquinavir prevents the cleavage of viral polyprotein precursors which are needed to generate functional proteins in and maturation of HIV-infected cells

**Local Anesthetic/Vasoconstrictor Precautions** No information available to require special precautions

**Effects on Dental Treatment** No effects or complications reported

**Other Adverse Effects**
1% to 10%:
Dermatologic: Rash
Endocrine & metabolic: Hyperglycemia, elevated CPK
Gastrointestinal: Diarrhea, abdominal discomfort, nausea, abdominal pain, buccal mucosa, ulceration
Neuromuscular & skeletal: Paresthesia, weakness

<1%:
Central nervous system: Headache, confusion, seizures, ataxia, pain
Dermatologic: Stevens-Johnson syndrome
Endocrine & metabolic: Hypoglycemia, hyper- and hypokalemia, low serum amylase
Gastrointestinal: Upper quadrant abdominal pain
Hematologic: Acute myeloblastic leukemia, hemolytic anemia, thrombocytopenia
Hepatic: Jaundice, ascites, exacerbation of chronic liver disease, elevated LFTs, altered AST, ALT, bilirubin, Hgb

(Continued)

## Saquinavir *(Continued)*

Local: Thrombophlebitis

**Drug Interactions**

Decreased effect: Rifampin may decrease saquinavir's plasma levels and AUC by 40% to 80%; other enzyme inducers may induce saquinavir's metabolism (eg, phenobarbital, phenytoin, dexamethasone, carbamazepine)

Increased effect: Ketoconazole significantly increases plasma levels and AUC of saquinavir; as a known, although not potent inhibitor of the cytochrome P-450 system, saquinavir may decrease the metabolism of astemizole (and result in rare but serious cardiac arrhythmias); other drugs which may have increased adverse effects if coadministered with saquinavir include calcium channel blockers, clindamycin, dapsone, quinidine, and triazolam

**Drug Uptake** Absorption: Incomplete; food, especially high fat diets, may increase the absorption and oral bioavailability of saquinavir by five-fold

**Pregnancy Risk Factor** B

**Dosage Forms** Capsule, as mesylate: 200 mg

**Generic Available** No

## Sargramostim (sar GRAM oh stim)

**U.S. Brand Names** Leukine™

**Therapeutic Category** Colony Stimulating Factor

**Synonyms** GM-CSF; Granulocyte-Macrophage Colony Stimulating Factor; rGM-CSF

**Use** Myeloid reconstitution after autologous bone marrow transplantation; to accelerate myeloid recovery in patients with non-Hodgkin's lymphoma, Hodgkin's lymphoma, and acute lymphoblastic leukemia undergoing autologous BMT; following induction chemotherapy in patients with acute myelogenous leukemia to shorten time to neutrophil recovery

**Usual Dosage** All orders should be scheduled between 8 AM and 10 AM daily

Children and Adults: I.V. infusion over ≥2 hours or S.C.

**Bone marrow transplantation failure or engraftment delay:** I.V.: 250 mcg/m²/day for 14 days. The dose can be repeated after 7 days off therapy if engraftment has not occurred. If engraftment still has not occurred, a third course of 500 mcg/m²/day for 14 days may be tried after another 7 days off therapy. If there is still no engraftment, it is unlikely that further dose escalation be beneficial.

**Myeloid reconstitution after autologous bone marrow transplant:** I.V.: 250 mcg/m²/day to begin 2-4 hours after the marrow infusion on day 0 of autologous bone marrow transplant or ≥24 hours after chemotherapy or 12 hours after last dose of radiotherapy. If significant adverse effects or "first dose" reaction is seen at this dose, discontinue the drug until toxicity resolves, then restart at a reduced dose of 125 mcg/m²/day.

**Length of therapy:** Bone marrow transplant patients: GM-CSF should be administered daily for up to 30 days or until the ANC has reached 1000/mm³ for 3 consecutive days following the expected chemotherapy-induced neutrophil-nadir

**Cancer chemotherapy recovery:** I.V.: 3-15 mcg/kg/day for 14-21 days; maximum daily dose is 15 mcg/kg/day due to dose-related adverse effects; **discontinue therapy** if the ANC count is >20,000/mm³

Excessive blood counts return to normal or baseline levels within 3-7 days following cessation of therapy

**Mechanism of Action** Stimulates proliferation, differentiation and functional activity of neutrophils, eosinophils, monocytes, and macrophages; see table.

| Proliferation/Differentiation | G-CSF (Filgrastim) | GM-CSF (Sargramostim) |
|---|---|---|
| Neutrophils | Yes | Yes |
| Eosinophils | No | Yes |
| Macrophages | No | Yes |
| Neutrophil migration | Enhanced | Inhibited |

**Local Anesthetic/Vasoconstrictor Precautions** No information available to require special precautions

**Effects on Dental Treatment** No effects or complications reported

**Other Adverse Effects**

>10%:

Cardiovascular: Tachycardia

Central nervous system: Neutropenic fever

Dermatologic: Alopecia

Gastrointestinal: Nausea, vomiting, diarrhea, mucositis

Hematologic: Thrombocytopenia
Neuromuscular & skeletal: Skeletal pain

1% to 10%:
Cardiovascular: Chest pain, peripheral edema
Central nervous system: Headache
Dermatologic: Skin rash
Endocrine & metabolic: Fluid retention
Gastrointestinal: Anorexia, stomatitis, sore throat, constipation
Hematologic: Leukocytosis, capillary leak syndrome
Local: Pain at injection site
Neuromuscular & skeletal: Weakness
Respiratory: Dyspnea, cough

<1%:
Cardiovascular: Transient supraventricular arrhythmia, pericarditis
Local: Thrombophlebitis
Miscellaneous: Anaphylactic reaction

**Drug Uptake**
Onset of action: Increase in WBC in 7-14 days
Duration: WBC will return to baseline within 1 week after discontinuing drug
Serum half-life: 2 hours
Time to peak serum concentration: S.C.: Within 1-2 hours

**Pregnancy Risk Factor** C

**Generic Available** No

**Comments** Has been demonstrated to accelerate myeloid engraftment in autologous bone marrow transplant, decrease median duration of antibiotic administration, reduce the median duration of infectious episodes, and shorten the median duration of hospitalization, no difference in relapse rate or survival or disease response has been found in placebo-controlled trials. Safety and efficacy of GM-CSF given simultaneously with cytotoxic chemotherapy have not been established. Concurrent treatment may increase myelosuppression. Precaution should be exercised in the usage of GM-CSF in any malignancy with myeloid characteristics. GM-CSF can potentially act as a growth factor for any tumor type, particularly myeloid malignancies. Tumors of nonhematopoietic origin may have surface receptors for GM-CSF.

◆ **Sarna [OTC]** *see* Camphor, Menthol, and Phenol *on page 179*
◆ **Sastid® Plain Therapeutic Shampoo and Acne Wash [OTC]** *see* Sulfur and Salicylic Acid *on page 947*
◆ **Scabene®** *see* Lindane *on page 592*
◆ **Scleromate™** *see* Morrhuate Sodium *on page 689*
◆ **Scopace® Tablet** *see* Scopolamine *on this page*

## Scopolamine (skoe POL a meen)

**U.S. Brand Names** Isopto® Hyoscine Ophthalmic; Scopace® Tablet; Transderm Scop® Patch

**Therapeutic Category** Anticholinergic Agent; Anticholinergic Agent, Ophthalmic; Anticholinergic Agent, Transdermal; Ophthalmic Agent, Mydriatic

**Use** Preoperative medication to produce amnesia and decrease salivation and respiratory secretions; to produce cycloplegia and mydriasis; treatment of iridocyclitis, prevention of nausea and vomiting by motion; produces more CNS depression, mydriasis, and cycloplegia but less effective in preventing reflex bradycardia and effecting the intestines than atropine

**Usual Dosage**
Preoperatively:
Children: I.M., S.C.: 6 mcg/kg/dose (maximum: 0.3 mg/dose) or 0.2 mg/m² may be repeated every 6-8 hours **or** alternatively:
4-7 months: 0.1 mg
7 months to 3 years: 0.15 mg
3-8 years: 0.2 mg
8-12 years: 0.3 mg
Adults: I.M., I.V., S.C.: 0.3-0.65 mg; may be repeated every 4-6 hours

Motion sickness: Transdermal: Children >12 years and Adults: Apply 1 disc behind the ear at least 4 hours prior to exposure and every 3 days as needed; effective if applied as soon as 2-3 hours before anticipated need, best if 12 hours before

Ophthalmic:
Refraction:
Children: Instill 1 drop of 0.25% to eye(s) twice daily for 2 days before procedure
Adults: Instill 1-2 drops of 0.25% to eye(s) 1 hour before procedure
Iridocyclitis:
Children: Instill 1 drop of 0.25% to eye(s) up to 3 times/day

(Continued)

## Scopolamine *(Continued)*

Adults: Instill 1-2 drops of 0.25% to eye(s) up to 4 times/day

**Mechanism of Action** Blocks the action of acetylcholine at parasympathetic sites in smooth muscle, secretory glands and the CNS; increases cardiac output, dries secretions, antagonizes histamine and serotonin

**Local Anesthetic/Vasoconstrictor Precautions** No information available to require special precautions

**Effects on Dental Treatment** >10% of patients medicated with scopolamine patch (Transderm Scop) will experience significant dry mouth. This will disappear with cessation of drug therapy.

**Other Adverse Effects**

Ophthalmic:

>10%: Ocular: Blurred vision, photophobia

1% to 10%:

Ocular: Local irritation, increased intraocular pressure
Respiratory: Congestion

<1%:

Cardiovascular: Vascular congestion, edema
Central nervous system: Drowsiness
Dermatologic: Eczematoid dermatitis
Ocular: Follicular conjunctivitis
Miscellaneous: Exudate

Systemic:

>10%:

Dermatologic: Dry skin
Gastrointestinal: Constipation
Local: Irritation at injection site
Respiratory: Dry nose, throat
Miscellaneous: Decreased sweating

1% to 10%:

Dermatologic: Photosensitivity
Endocrine & metabolic: Decreased flow of breast milk
Gastrointestinal: Dysphagia

<1%:

Cardiovascular: Orthostatic hypotension, ventricular fibrillation, tachycardia, palpitations
Central nervous system: Confusion, headache, loss of memory, ataxia, fatigue
Dermatologic: Skin rash
Gastrointestinal: Bloated feeling, nausea, vomiting
Genitourinary: Dysuria
Neuromuscular & skeletal: Weakness
Ocular: Increased intraocular pain, blurred vision

**Note:** Systemic adverse effects have been reported following ophthalmic administration

**Drug Interactions**

Increased toxicity: Anticholinergics, such as scopolamine, may potentiate the CNS effects of amantadine; may potentiate the anticholinergic effects of amitriptyline and haloperidol

Decreased effects of other drugs: Anticholinergics, such as scopolamine, slow gastric emptying. This effects has reduced the rate of GI absorption of acetaminophen, levodopa, and potassium chloride wax-matrix preparations.

**Drug Uptake**

Onset of effect:

Oral, I.M.: 0.5-1 hour
I.V.: 10 minutes

Duration of effect:

Oral, I.M.: 4-6 hours
I.V.: 2 hours

Absorption: Well absorbed by all routes of administration

**Pregnancy Risk Factor** C

**Generic Available** Yes

♦ **Scopolamine and Phenylephrine** *see* Phenylephrine and Scopolamine *on page 796*

♦ **Scot-Tussin® [OTC]** *see* Guaifenesin *on page 478*

♦ **Scot-Tussin DM® Cough Chasers [OTC]** *see* Dextromethorphan *on page 314*

♦ **Scot-Tussin® Senior Clear [OTC]** *see* Guaifenesin and Dextromethorphan *on page 479*

♦ **SeaMist® [OTC]** *see* Sodium Chloride *on page 920*

♦ **Sebizon® Topical Lotion** *see* Sulfacetamide Sodium *on page 939*

♦ **Sebulex® [OTC]** *see* Sulfur and Salicylic Acid *on page 947*

## Secobarbital (see koe BAR bi tal)

**U.S. Brand Names** Seconal™

**Canadian Brand Names** Novo-Secobarb

**Therapeutic Category** Barbiturate; Hypnotic; Sedative

**Use** Short-term treatment of insomnia and as preanesthetic agent

**Usual Dosage** Hypnotic:

Children: I.M.: 3-5 mg/kg/dose; maximum: 100 mg/dose

Adults:

- Oral: 100 mg at bedtime
- I.M.: 100-200 mg/dose
- I.V.: 50-250 mg/dose

**Mechanism of Action** Interferes with transmission of impulses from the thalamus to the cortex of the brain resulting in an imbalance in central inhibitory and facilitatory mechanisms

**Local Anesthetic/Vasoconstrictor Precautions** No information available to require special precautions

**Effects on Dental Treatment** No effects or complications reported

**Other Adverse Effects**

>10%:

- Central nervous system: Dizziness, lightheadedness, drowsiness, "hangover" effect
- Local: Pain at injection site

1% to 10%:

- Central nervous system: Confusion, mental depression, unusual excitement, nervousness, faint feeling, headache, insomnia, nightmares
- Gastrointestinal: Constipation, nausea, vomiting

<1%:

- Cardiovascular: Hypotension
- Central nervous system: Hallucinations
- Dermatologic: Skin rash, exfoliative dermatitis, Stevens-Johnson syndrome
- Hematologic: Megaloblastic anemia, thrombocytopenia, agranulocytosis
- Local: Thrombophlebitis
- Respiratory: Respiratory depression

**Drug Interactions**

Decreased effect of betamethasone and other corticosteroids, tricyclic antidepressants (TCAs), chloramphenicol, estrogens, cyclophosphamide, oral anticoagulants, doxycycline, theophylline

Increased effect/toxicity with CNS depressants, chloramphenicol, chlorpropamide

**Drug Uptake**

Onset of hypnosis:

- Oral: Within 1-3 minutes
- I.V. injection: Within 15-30 minutes

Duration: ~15 minutes

Absorption: Oral: Well absorbed (90%)

Serum half-life: 25 hours

Time to peak serum concentration: Within 2-4 hours

**Pregnancy Risk Factor** D

**Dosage Forms**

Capsule: 100 mg

Injection, as sodium: 50 mg/mL (2 mL)

**Generic Available** Yes

♦ **Secobarbital and Amobarbital** *see* Amobarbital and Secobarbital *on page 74*

♦ **Seconal™** *see* Secobarbital *on this page*

♦ **Secran®** *see* Vitamins, Multiple *on page 1051*

## Secretin (SEE kre tin)

**U.S. Brand Names** Secretin-Ferring Injection

**Therapeutic Category** Diagnostic Agent, Pancreatic Exocrine Insufficiency; Diagnostic Agent, Zollinger-Ellison Syndrome and Pancreatic Exocrine Disease

**Use** Diagnosis of Zollinger-Ellison syndrome, chronic pancreatic dysfunction, and some hepatobiliary diseases such as obstructive jaundice resulting from cancer or stones in the biliary tract

**Usual Dosage** Potency of secretin is expressed in terms of clinical units (CU).

I.V.:

Pancreatic function: 1 CU/kg slow I.V. injection over 1 minute

Zollinger-Ellison: 2 CU/kg slow I.V. injection over 1 minute

(Continued)

## Secretin *(Continued)*

**Mechanism of Action** Hormone normally secreted by duodenal mucosa and upper jejunal mucosa which increases the volume and bicarbonate content of pancreatic juice; stimulates the flow of hepatic bile with a high bicarbonate concentration, stimulates gastrin release in patients with Zollinger-Ellison syndrome

**Local Anesthetic/Vasoconstrictor Precautions** No information available to require special precautions

**Effects on Dental Treatment** No effects or complications reported

**Other Adverse Effects** <1%:

Cardiovascular: Venous spasm, syncope

Miscellaneous: Hypersensitivity reactions

**Drug Uptake**

Inactivated by proteolytic enzymes if administered orally

Peak output of pancreatic secretions: Within 30 minutes

Duration of action: At least 2 hours

**Pregnancy Risk Factor** Not established

**Generic Available** No

**Comments** Potency of secretin is expressed in terms of clinical units

- ♦ **Secretin-Ferring Injection** *see* Secretin *on previous page*
- ♦ **Sectral®** *see* Acebutolol *on page 26*
- ♦ **Sedapap-10®** *see* Butalbital Compound *on page 163*
- ♦ **Sedapap-10®** *see* Butalbital Compound and Acetaminophen *on page 164*

## Selegiline (seh LEDGE ah leen)

**U.S. Brand Names** Eldepryl®

**Canadian Brand Names** Apo®-Selegiline; Novo-Selegiline

**Therapeutic Category** Anti-Parkinson's Agent

**Use** Adjunct in the management of parkinsonian patients in which levodopa/carbidopa therapy is deteriorating

**Unlabeled use:** Early Parkinson's disease

Investigational use: Alzheimer's disease

Selegiline is also being studied in Alzheimer's disease. Small studies have shown some improvement in behavioral and cognitive performance in patients, however, further study is needed.

**Usual Dosage** Oral:

Adults: 5 mg twice daily with breakfast and lunch or 10 mg in the morning

Elderly: Initial: 5 mg in the morning, may increase to a total of 10 mg/day

**Mechanism of Action** Potent monoamine oxidase (MAO) type-B inhibitor; MAO-B plays a major role in the metabolism of dopamine; selegiline may also increase dopaminergic activity by interfering with dopamine reuptake at the synapse

**Local Anesthetic/Vasoconstrictor Precautions** Selegiline in doses of 10 mg a day or less does not inhibit type-A MAO. Therefore, there are no precautions with the use of vasoconstrictors.

**Effects on Dental Treatment** >10% of patients experience dry mouth; anticholinergic side effects can cause a reduction of saliva production or secretion contributing to discomfort and dental disease (ie, caries, oral candidiasis and periodontal disease)

**Other Adverse Effects**

>10%:

Central nervous system: Mood changes, dyskinesias, dizziness

Gastrointestinal: Nausea, vomiting, abdominal pain

1% to 10%:

Cardiovascular: Orthostatic hypotension, arrhythmias, hypertension

Central nervous system: Hallucinations, confusion, depression, insomnia, agitation, loss of balance

Neuromuscular & skeletal: Increased involuntary movements, bradykinesia, muscle twitches

Miscellaneous: Bruxism

**Drug Interactions** Meperidine in combination with selegiline has caused agitation and delirium; it may be prudent to avoid other opioids as well

**Drug Uptake**

Onset of therapeutic effects: Within 1 hour

Duration: 24-72 hours

Serum half-life: 9 minutes

**Pregnancy Risk Factor** C

**Dosage Forms** Capsule, as hydrochloride: 5 mg

**Generic Available** No

- ♦ **Selenium** *see* Trace Metals *on page 1001*

## Selenium Sulfide (se LEE nee um)

**U.S. Brand Names** Exsel®; Selsun®; Selsun Blue® [OTC]; Selsun Gold® for Women [OTC]

**Canadian Brand Names** Versel®

**Therapeutic Category** Shampoos

**Use** Treatment of itching and flaking of the scalp associated with dandruff, to control scalp seborrheic dermatitis; treatment of tinea versicolor

**Usual Dosage** Topical:

Dandruff, seborrhea: Massage 5-10 mL into wet scalp, leave on scalp 2-3 minutes, rinse thoroughly, and repeat application; shampoo twice weekly for 2 weeks initially, then use once every 1-4 weeks as indicated depending upon control

Tinea versicolor: Apply the 2.5% lotion to affected area and lather with small amounts of water; leave on skin for 10 minutes, then rinse thoroughly; apply every day for 7 days

**Mechanism of Action** May block the enzymes involved in growth of epithelial tissue

**Local Anesthetic/Vasoconstrictor Precautions** No information available to require special precautions

**Effects on Dental Treatment** No effects or complications reported

**Other Adverse Effects**

>10%: Dermatologic: Unusual dryness or oiliness of scalp

1% to 10%:

- Central nervous system: Lethargy
- Dermatologic: Alopecia, hair discoloration
- Gastrointestinal: Vomiting following long-term use on damaged skin, abdominal pain, garlic breath
- Local: Irritation
- Neuromuscular & skeletal: Tremors
- Miscellaneous: Perspiration

**Drug Interactions** No data reported

**Drug Uptake** Absorption: Topical: Not absorbed through intact skin, but can be absorbed through damaged skin

**Pregnancy Risk Factor** C

**Generic Available** Yes

- ♦ **Sele-Pak®** *see* Trace Metals *on page 1001*
- ♦ **Selepen®** *see* Trace Metals *on page 1001*
- ♦ **Selsun®** *see* Selenium Sulfide *on this page*
- ♦ **Selsun Blue® [OTC]** *see* Selenium Sulfide *on this page*
- ♦ **Selsun Gold® for Women [OTC]** *see* Selenium Sulfide *on this page*
- ♦ **Semicid® [OTC]** *see* Nonoxynol 9 *on page 728*
- ♦ **Semprex®-D** *see* Acrivastine and Pseudoephedrine *on page 37*
- ♦ **Senexon® [OTC]** *see* Senna *on this page*

## Senna (SEN na)

**U.S. Brand Names** Black Draught® [OTC]; Senexon® [OTC]; Senna-Gen® [OTC]; Senokot® [OTC]; Senolax® [OTC]; X-Prep® Liquid [OTC]

**Therapeutic Category** Laxative, Stimulant

**Use** Short-term treatment of constipation; evacuate the colon for bowel or rectal examinations

**Usual Dosage**

Children: Oral:

- >6 years: 10-20 mg/kg/dose at bedtime; maximum daily dose: 872 mg
- 6-12 years, >27 kg: 1 tablet at bedtime, up to 4 tablets/day **or** 1/2 teaspoonful of granules (326 mg/tsp) at bedtime (up to 2 teaspoonfuls/day)

Liquid:

- 2-5 years: 5-10 mL at bedtime
- 6-15 years: 10-15 mL at bedtime

Suppository: 1/2 at bedtime

Syrup:

- 1 month to 1 year: 1.25-2.5 mL at bedtime up to 5 mL/day
- 1-5 years: 2.5-5 mL at bedtime up to 10 mL/day
- 5-10 years: 5-10 mL at bedtime up to 20 mL/day

Adults:

- Granules (326 mg/teaspoon): 1 teaspoonful at bedtime, not to exceed 2 teaspoonfuls twice daily
- Liquid: 15-30 mL with meals and at bedtime
- Suppository: 1 at bedtime, may repeat once in 2 hours
- Syrup: 2-3 teaspoonfuls at bedtime, not to exceed 30 mL/day
- Tablet: 187 mg: 2 tablets at bedtime, not to exceed 8 tablets/day

(Continued)

## Senna *(Continued)*

Tablet: 374 mg: 1 at bedtime, up to 4/day; 600 mg: 2 tablets at bedtime, up to 3 tablets/day

**Local Anesthetic/Vasoconstrictor Precautions** No information available to require special precautions

**Effects on Dental Treatment** No effects or complications reported

**Other Adverse Effects** 1% to 10%: Gastrointestinal: Nausea, vomiting, diarrhea, abdominal cramps

**Pregnancy Risk Factor** C

**Generic Available** Yes

**Comments** Some patients will experience considerable gripping

- **Senna-Gen® [OTC]** *see* Senna *on previous page*
- **Senokot® [OTC]** *see* Senna *on previous page*
- **Senolax® [OTC]** *see* Senna *on previous page*
- **Sensorcaine®** *see* Bupivacaine *on page 157*
- **Sensorcaine®-MPF** *see* Bupivacaine *on page 157*
- **Sensorcaine® MPF** *see* Bupivacaine and Epinephrine *on page 158*
- **Septa® Topical Ointment [OTC]** *see* Bacitracin, Neomycin, and Polymyxin B *on page 118*
- **Septisol®** *see* Hexachlorophene *on page 496*
- **Septra®** *see* Trimethoprim and Sulfamethoxazole *on page 1021*
- **Septra® DS** *see* Trimethoprim and Sulfamethoxazole *on page 1021*
- **Ser-Ap-Es®** *see* Hydralazine, Hydrochlorothiazide, and Reserpine *on page 503*
- **Serax®** *see* Oxazepam *on page 748*
- **Serentil®** *see* Mesoridazine *on page 639*
- **Serevent®** *see* Salmeterol *on page 901*
- **Serevent® Diskus®** *see* Salmeterol *on page 901*

## Sermorelin Acetate (ser moe REL in AS e tate )

**U.S. Brand Names** Geref® Injection

**Therapeutic Category** Diagnostic Agent, Pituitary Function

**Use** Evaluate ability of the somatotroph of the pituitary gland to secrete growth hormone

**Usual Dosage** I.V.: In a single dose in the morning following an overnight fast:

Children or subjects <50 kg: Draw venous blood samples for GH determinations 15 minutes before and immediately prior to administration, then administer 1 mcg/kg followed by a 3 mL normal saline flush, draw blood samples again for GH determinations

Adults or subjects >50 kg: Determine the number of ampules needed based on a dose of 1 mcg/kg, draw venous blood samples for GH determinations 15 minutes before and immediately prior to administration, then administer 1 mcg/kg followed by a 3 mL normal saline flush, draw blood samples again for GH determinations

**Local Anesthetic/Vasoconstrictor Precautions** No information available to require special precautions

**Effects on Dental Treatment** No effects or complications reported

**Other Adverse Effects** 1% to 10%:

Cardiovascular: Transient flushing of the face, tightness in the chest
Central nervous system: Headache
Gastrointestinal: Nausea, vomiting
Local: Pain, redness, and/or swelling at the injection site

**Pregnancy Risk Factor** C

**Generic Available** No

- **Seromycin® Pulvules®** *see* Cycloserine *on page 287*
- **Serophene®** *see* Clomiphene *on page 263*
- **Seroquel®** *see* Quetiapine *on page 870*
- **Serostim® Injection** *see* Human Growth Hormone *on page 499*
- **Serpalan®** *see* Reserpine *on page 882*
- **Serpasil®** *see* Reserpine *on page 882*

## Sertraline (SER tra leen)

**Related Information**

Vasoconstrictor Interactions With Antidepressants *on page 1277*

**U.S. Brand Names** Zoloft™

**Therapeutic Category** Antidepressant, Selective Serotonin Reuptake Inhibitor

**Use** Treatment of major depression; also being studied for use in obesity and obsessive-compulsive disorder

**Usual Dosage** Oral:

Adults: Start with 50 mg/day in the morning and increase by 50 mg/day increments every 2-3 days if tolerated to 100 mg/day; additional increases may be necessary; maximum dose: 200 mg/day. If somnolence is noted, give at bedtime.

Elderly: Start treatment with 25 mg/day in the morning and increase by 25 mg/day increments every 2-3 days if tolerated to 75-100 mg/day; additional increases may be necessary; maximum dose: 200 mg/day

**Mechanism of Action** Antidepressant with selective inhibitory effects on presynaptic serotonin (5-HT) reuptake

**Local Anesthetic/Vasoconstrictor Precautions** Although caution should be used in patients taking tricyclic antidepressants, no interactions have been reported with vasoconstrictor and sertraline, a nontricyclic antidepressant which acts to increase serotonin

**Effects on Dental Treatment** No effects or complications reported

**Other Adverse Effects**

1% to 10%: In clinical trials, dizziness and nausea were two most frequent side effects that led to discontinuation of therapy

Cardiovascular: Palpitations

Central nervous system: Insomnia, agitation, dizziness, headache, somnolence, nervousness, fatigue, pain

Dermatologic: Dermatological reactions, sweating

Endocrine & metabolic: Sexual dysfunction in men

Gastrointestinal: Dry mouth, diarrhea or loose stools, nausea, constipation

Genitourinary: Micturition disorders

Neuromuscular & skeletal: Tremors

Ocular: Visual difficulty

Otic: Tinnitus

**Drug Interactions** All serotonin reuptake inhibitors are capable of inhibiting cytochrome P-450 IID6 isoenzyme enzyme system.

Increased/decreased effect of lithium (both increases and decreases level has been reported)

Increased toxicity of diazepam, trazodone via decreased clearance; increased toxicity with MAO inhibitors (hyperpyrexia, tremors, seizures, delirium, coma)

**Drug Uptake**

Absorption: Slow

Serum half-life:

Parent: 24 hours

Metabolites: 66 hours

**Pregnancy Risk Factor** C

**Dosage Forms** Tablet, as hydrochloride: 25 mg, 50 mg, 100 mg

**Generic Available** No

♦ **Serutan® [OTC]** *see* Psyllium *on page 865*

♦ **Serzone®** *see* Nefazodone *on page 707*

## Sevelamer

**U.S. Brand Names** Renagel®

**Therapeutic Category** Phosphate Binder

**Use** Reduction of serum phosphorous in patients with end-stage renal disease

**Usual Dosage** Adults: Oral: 2-4 capsules 3 times/day with meals; the initial dose may be based on serum phosphorous:

(Phosphorous: Initial Dose)

>6.0 mg/dL and <7.5 mg/dL: 2 capsules 3 times/day

>7.5 mg/dL and <9.0 mg/dL: 3 capsules 3 times/day

≥9.0 mg/dL: 4 capsules 3 times/day

Dosage should be adjusted based on serum phosphorous concentration, with a goal of lowering to <6.0 mg/dL; maximum daily dose studied was 30 capsules/day.

**Mechanism of Action** Sevalamer (a polymeric compound) binds phosphate within the intestinal lumen, limiting absorption and decreasing serum phosphate concentrations without altering calcium, aluminum, or bicarbonate concentrations

**Local Anesthetic/Vasoconstrictor Precautions** No information available to require special precautions

**Effects on Dental Treatment** No effects or complications reported

**Other Adverse Effects**

>10%:

Cardiovascular: Hypotension (11%), thrombosis (10%)

Central nervous system: Headache (10%)

Endocrine and metabolic: Decreased absorption of vitamins D, E, K and folic acid

Gastrointestinal: Diarrhea (16%), dyspepsia (5% to 11%), vomiting (12%)

(Continued)

## Sevelamer *(Continued)*

Neuromuscular and skeletal: Pain (13%)
Miscellaneous: Infection (15%)

1% to 10%:
Cardiovascular: Hypertension (9%)
Gastrointestinal: Nausea (7%), flatulence (4%), diarrhea (4%), constipation (2%)
Respiratory: Cough (4%)

**Drug Interactions** No formal drug interaction studies have been undertaken. Sevelamer may bind to some drugs in the gastrointestinal tract and decrease their absorption. When changes in absorption of oral medications may have significant clinical consequences (such as antiarrhythmic and antiseizure medications), these medications should be taken at least 1 hour before or 3 hours after a dose of sevelamer.

**Drug Uptake** Absorption: Not absorbed systemically

**Pregnancy Risk Factor** C

**Dosage Forms** Capsule: 403 mg

♦ **Shur-Seal® [OTC]** *see* Nonoxynol 9 *on page 728*

## Sibutramine (si BYOO tra meen)

**U.S. Brand Names** Meridia™

**Therapeutic Category** Anorexiant

**Synonyms** Sibutramine Hydrochloride

**Use** Management of obesity, including weight loss and maintenance of weight loss, and should be used in conjunction with a reduced calorie diet

**Restrictions** C-IV

**Usual Dosage** Adults ≥16 years: Initial: 10 mg once daily; after 4 weeks may titrate up to 15 mg once daily as needed and tolerated

**Mechanism of Action** A monoamine uptake inhibitor antidepressant; although it has little or no action on monoamine oxidase, sibutramine blocks the neuronal uptake of norepinephrine and, to a lesser extent, serotonin and dopamine; see Additional Information

**Local Anesthetic/Vasoconstrictor Precautions** No information available to require special precautions

**Effects on Dental Treatment** No effects or complications reported

**Drug Interactions** Concurrent use with meperidine may increase the risk of serotonin syndrome; this syndrome includes fever, sweating, agitation, and restlessness

**Dosage Forms** Capsule: 5 mg, 10 mg, 15 mg

**Comments** The mechanism of action of sibutramine is thought to be different from the "fen" drugs. Sibutramine works to suppress the appetite by inhibiting the reuptake of norepinephrine and serotonin. Unlike dexfenfluramine and fenfluramine, it is not a serotonin releaser. Sibutramine is closer chemically to the widely used antidepressants such as fluoxetine (Prozac®). The FDA approved sibutramine over the objections of its own advisory panel, who called the drug too risky. FDA reported that the drug causes blood pressure to increase, generally by a small amount, though in some patients the increases were higher. It is now recommended that patients taking sibutramine have their blood pressure evaluated regularly.

**Selected Readings**

Colchamiro R, "FDA Clears Obesity Drug," *Am Druggist*, 1998, 12.

♦ **Sibutramine Hydrochloride** *see* Sibutramine *on this page*

♦ **Silace-C® [OTC]** *see* Docusate and Casanthranol *on page 347*

♦ **Siladryl® Oral [OTC]** *see* Diphenhydramine *on page 338*

♦ **Silafed® Syrup [OTC]** *see* Triprolidine and Pseudoephedrine *on page 1025*

♦ **Silaminic® Cold Syrup [OTC]** *see* Chlorpheniramine and Phenylpropanolamine *on page 233*

♦ **Silaminic® Expectorant [OTC]** *see* Guaifenesin and Phenylpropanolamine *on page 480*

## Sildenafil (sil DEN a fil)

**U.S. Brand Names** Viagra®

**Therapeutic Category** Phosphodiesterase (Type 5) Enzyme Inhibitor

**Use** Effective in most men with erectile dysfunction (ED), the medical term for impotence, which is associated with a broad range of physical or psychological medical conditions.

**Usual Dosage** Adults: Oral: 50 mg taken one hour before sexual activity; individuals may need more (100 mg) or less (25 mg) and dosing should be determined by a physician depending on effectiveness and side effects. The drug should not be used more than once a day.

**Mechanism of Action** Does not directly cause penile erections, but affects the response to sexual stimulation. The physiologic mechanism of erection of the penis involves release of nitric oxide (NO) in the corpus cavernosum during sexual stimulation. NO then activates the enzyme guanylate cyclase, which results in increased levels of cyclic guanosine monophosphate (cGMP), producing smooth muscle relaxation and inflow of blood to the corpus cavernosum. Sildenafil enhances the effect of NO by inhibiting phosphodiesterase type 5 (PDE5), which is responsible for degradation of cGMP in the corpus cavernosum; when sexual stimulation causes local release of NO, inhibition of PDE5 by sidenafil causes increased levels of cGMP in the corpus cavernosum, resulting in smooth muscle relaxation and inflow of blood to the corpus cavernosum; at recommended doses, it has no effect in the absence of sexual stimulation.

**Local Anesthetic/Vasoconstrictor Precautions** No information available to require special precautions

**Effects on Dental Treatment** No effects or complications reported

**Other Adverse Effects**

>10%:

- Central nervous system: Headache
- Cardiovascular: Flushing

1% to 10%:

- Central nervous system: Dizziness
- Dermatologic: Rash
- Gastrointestinal: Dyspepsia, diarrhea
- Genitourinary: Urinary tract infection
- Ocular: Abnormal vision
- Respiratory: Nasal congestion

**Drug Interactions** Erythromycin administration produces a large increase in sildenafil plasma concentrations. Increased side effects are possible. Erythromycin inhibits the first-pass and systemic metabolism (CYP3A4) of sildenafil, resulting in elevated plasma concentrations and a prolonged half-life.

Twenty-four male subjects received a single 100 mg dose on day 1. On days 2 through 6 subjects received erythromycin (500 mg orally twice daily) or placebo. On day 6 all subjects were given a single 100 mg dose of sildenafil. In the erythromycin group, the area under the concentration curve of sildenafil increased 158% and the peak plasma concentration increased by 108%. Half-life was prolonged from 3.5 hours to 4.1 hours. Increases in sildenafil concentrations could result in increased side effects such as headache, abnormal vision, or flushing. Clarithromycin would be likely to affect sildenafil in a similar manner. Noninhibiting macrolides such as azithromycin or dirithromycin would be unlikely to alter the plasma concentration of sildenafil.

Data from the package insert (1998) indicated the following. When a single 100 mg dose of sildenafil was administered with erythromycin, a specific CYP3A4 inhibitor, at steady state (500 mg bid for 5 days), there was a 182% increase in sildenafil systemic exposure (AUC). Stronger CYP3A4 inhibitors such as ketoconazole and itraconazole would be expected to have still greater effects. Data from patients in clinical trials indicated a reduction in sildenafil clearance when it was coadministered with CYP3A4 inhibitors such as erythromycin and ketoconazole.

**Drug Uptake**

Half-life: 4 hours

Metabolism: Hepatic microsomal isoenzymes (CYP3A4 [major] and CYP2C9 [minor route])

**Pregnancy Risk Factor** B

**Selected Readings**

"Erythromycin (E-Mycin®) and Sildenafil (Viagra®)," in *Hansten and Horn's Drug Interactions Analysis and Management*, Seattle, WA: Applied Therapeutics, Inc, 1998, 2:3N109.

- ♦ **Sildicon-E® [OTC]** *see* Guaifenesin and Phenylpropanolamine *on page 480*
- ♦ **Silphen® Cough [OTC]** *see* Diphenhydramine *on page 338*
- ♦ **Silphen DM® [OTC]** *see* Dextromethorphan *on page 314*
- ♦ **Siltussin® [OTC]** *see* Guaifenesin *on page 478*
- ♦ **Siltussin-CF® [OTC]** *see* Guaifenesin, Phenylpropanolamine, and Dextromethorphan *on page 481*
- ♦ **Siltussin DM® [OTC]** *see* Guaifenesin and Dextromethorphan *on page 479*
- ♦ **Silvadene®** *see* Silver Sulfadiazine *on next page*

## Silver Nitrate (SIL ver NYE trate)

**Therapeutic Category** Ophthalmic Agent, Miscellaneous; Topical Skin Product

**Synonyms** $AgNO_3$

**Use** Prevention of gonococcal ophthalmia neonatorum; cauterization of wounds and sluggish ulcers, removal of granulation tissue and warts

(Continued)

## Silver Nitrate *(Continued)*

**Usual Dosage**

Children and Adults:

Ointment: Apply in an apertured pad on affected area or lesion for approximately 5 days

Sticks: Apply to mucous membranes and other moist skin surfaces only on area to be treated 2-3 times/week for 2-3 weeks

Topical solution: Apply a cotton applicator dipped in solution on the affected area 2-3 times/week for 2-3 weeks

**Mechanism of Action** Free silver ions precipitate bacterial proteins by combining with chloride in tissue forming silver chloride; coagulates cellular protein to form an eschar; silver ions or salts or colloidal silver preparations can inhibit the growth of both gram-positive and gram-negative bacteria. This germicidal action is attributed to the precipitation of bacterial proteins by liberated silver ions. Silver nitrate coagulates cellular protein to form an eschar, and this mode of action is the postulated mechanism for control of benign hematuria, rhinitis, and recurrent pneumothorax.

**Local Anesthetic/Vasoconstrictor Precautions** No information available to require special precautions

**Effects on Dental Treatment** No effects or complications reported

**Other Adverse Effects**

>10%:

Local: Burning and skin irritation

Ocular: Chemical conjunctivitis

1% to 10%:

Dermatologic: Staining of the skin

Hematologic: Methemoglobinemia

Ocular: Cauterization of the cornea, blindness

**Drug Uptake** Absorption: Because silver ions readily combine with protein, there is minimal GI and cutaneous absorption of the 0.5% and 1% preparations

**Pregnancy Risk Factor** C

**Generic Available** Yes

**Comments** Applicators are **not** for ophthalmic use

## Silver Protein, Mild (SIL ver PRO teen mild)

**U.S. Brand Names** Argyrol® S.S. 20%

**Therapeutic Category** Antibiotic, Topical

**Use** Stain and coagulate mucus in eye surgery which is then removed by irrigation; eye infections

**Usual Dosage**

Preop in eye surgery: Place 2-3 drops into eye(s), then rinse out with sterile irrigating solution

Eye infections: 1-3 drops into the affected eye(s) every 3-4 hours for several days

**Local Anesthetic/Vasoconstrictor Precautions** No information available to require special precautions

**Effects on Dental Treatment** No effects or complications reported

**Pregnancy Risk Factor** C

**Generic Available** No

## Silver Sulfadiazine (SIL ver sul fa DYE a zeen)

**U.S. Brand Names** Silvadene®; SSD® AF; SSD® Cream; Thermazene®

**Canadian Brand Names** Dermazin™; Flamazine®

**Therapeutic Category** Antibacterial, Topical

**Use** Prevention and treatment of infection in second and third degree burns

**Usual Dosage** Children and Adults: Topical: Apply once or twice daily with a sterile-gloved hand; apply to a thickness of $^1/_{16}$"; burned area should be covered with cream at all times

**Mechanism of Action** Acts upon the bacterial cell wall and cell membrane. Bactericidal for many gram-negative and gram-positive bacteria and is effective against yeast. Active against *Pseudomonas aeruginosa*, *Pseudomonas maltophilia*, *Enterobacteriae* species, *Klebsiella* species, *Serratia* species, *Escherichia coli*, *Proteus mirabilis*, *Morganella morganii*, *Providencia rettgeri*, *Proteus vulgaris*, *Providencia* species, *Citrobacter* species, *Acinetobacter calcoaceticus*, *Staphylococcus aureus*, *Staphylococcus epidermidis*, *Enterococcus* species, *Candida albicans*, *Corynebacterium diphtheriae*, and *Clostridium perfringens*

**Local Anesthetic/Vasoconstrictor Precautions** No information available to require special precautions

**Effects on Dental Treatment** No effects or complications reported

**Other Adverse Effects**

>10%: Local: Pain, burning

1% to 10%:
Dermatologic: Itching, rash, erythema multiforme, skin discoloration
Hematologic: Hemolytic anemia, leukopenia, agranulocytosis, aplastic anemia
Hepatic: Hepatitis
Renal: Interstitial nephritis
Miscellaneous: Allergic reactions may be related to sulfa component
<1%: Dermatologic: Photosensitivity

**Drug Interactions** Decreased effect: Topical proteolytic enzymes are inactivated

**Drug Uptake**
Absorption: Significant percutaneous absorption of sulfadiazine can occur especially when applied to extensive burns
Serum half-life: 10 hours and is prolonged in patients with renal insufficiency
Time to peak serum concentration: Within 3-11 days of continuous therapy

**Pregnancy Risk Factor** C

**Generic Available** Yes

## Simethicone (sye METH i kone)

**U.S. Brand Names** Degas® [OTC]; Flatulex® [OTC]; Gas Relief®; Gas-X® [OTC]; Maalox® Anti-Gas® [OTC]; Mylanta® Gas® [OTC]; Mylicon® [OTC]; Phazyme® [OTC]; SonoRx®

**Canadian Brand Names** Ovol®

**Therapeutic Category** Antiflatulent

**Use** Relieves flatulence and functional gastric bloating, and postoperative gas pains

**Usual Dosage** Oral:
Children <12 years: 40 mg 4 times/day
Children >12 years and Adults: 40-120 mg after meals and at bedtime as needed, not to exceed 500 mg/day

**Mechanism of Action** Decreases the surface tension of gas bubbles thereby disperses and prevents gas pockets in the GI system

**Local Anesthetic/Vasoconstrictor Precautions** No information available to require special precautions

**Effects on Dental Treatment** No effects or complications reported

**Other Adverse Effects** No data reported

**Drug Interactions** No data reported

**Pregnancy Risk Factor** C

**Generic Available** Yes: Tablet


- **Simethicone and Calcium Carbonate** *see* Calcium Carbonate and Simethicone *on page 173*
- **Simethicone and Magaldrate** *see* Magaldrate and Simethicone *on page 610*
- **Simron® [OTC]** *see* Ferrous Gluconate *on page 427*
- **Simulect®** *see* Basiliximab *on page 120*


## Simvastatin (SIM va stat in)

**Related Information**
Cardiovascular Diseases *on page 1066*

**U.S. Brand Names** Zocor™

**Therapeutic Category** HMG-CoA Reductase Inhibitor; Lipid Lowering Drugs

**Use** Adjunct to dietary therapy to decrease elevated serum total and LDL cholesterol concentrations in primary hypercholesterolemia; treatment of patients with homozygous familial hypercholesterolemia

**Usual Dosage** Adults: Oral: Start with 5-10 mg/day as a single bedtime dose; if LDL is ≤190 mg/dL start with 5 mg; if LDL >190 mg/dL, start with 10 mg/day; increase every 4 weeks as needed; maximum dose: 40 mg/day

**Mechanism of Action** Simvastatin is a methylated derivative of lovastatin that acts by competitively inhibiting 3 hydroxy 3 methylglutaryl coenzyme A reductase (HMG CoA reductase), the enzyme that catalyzes the rate-limiting step in cholesterol biosynthesis

**Local Anesthetic/Vasoconstrictor Precautions** No information available to require special precautions

**Effects on Dental Treatment** No effects or complications reported

**Other Adverse Effects**
1% to 10%:
Central nervous system: Headache, dizziness
Dermatologic: Rash
Gastrointestinal: Flatulence, abdominal cramps, diarrhea, constipation, nausea, dyspepsia, heartburn
Neuromuscular & skeletal: Myalgia, elevated creatine phosphokinase (CPK)
<1%:
Gastrointestinal: Dysgeusia
Ocular: Lenticular opacities, blurred vision
(Continued)

## Simvastatin *(Continued)*

**Drug Interactions**

Increased effect of warfarin, erythromycin, niacin

Increased toxicity of cyclosporin, gemfibrozil

Concurrent use of erythromycin and HMG-CoA reductase inhibitors may result in rhabdomyolysis

**Drug Uptake**

Absorption: Oral: Although 85% is absorbed following administration, <5% reaches the general circulation due to an extensive first-pass effect

Time to peak concentrations: 1.3-2.4 hours

**Pregnancy Risk Factor** X

**Dosage Forms** Tablet: 5 mg, 10 mg, 20 mg, 40 mg

**Generic Available** No

- **Sinarest® 12 Hour Nasal Solution** *see* Oxymetazoline *on page 755*
- **Sinarest® Nasal Solution [OTC]** *see* Phenylephrine *on page 795*
- **Sinarest®, No Drowsiness [OTC]** *see* Acetaminophen and Pseudoephedrine *on page 31*

## Sincalide (SIN ka lide)

**U.S. Brand Names** Kinevac®

**Therapeutic Category** Diagnostic Agent, Gallbladder Function

**Synonyms** C8-CCK; OP-CCK

**Use** Postevacuation cholecystography; gallbladder bile sampling; stimulate pancreatic secretion for analysis

**Usual Dosage** Adults: I.V.:

Contraction of gallbladder: 0.02 mcg/kg over 30 seconds to 1 minute, may repeat in 15 minutes a 0.04 mcg/kg dose

Pancreatic function: 0.02 mcg/kg over 30 minutes administered after secretin

**Mechanism of Action** Stimulates contraction of the gallbladder and simultaneous relaxation of the sphincter of Oddi, inhibits gastric emptying, and increases intestinal motility. Graded doses have been shown to produce graded decreases in small intestinal transit time, thought to be mediated by acetylcholine.

**Local Anesthetic/Vasoconstrictor Precautions** No information available to require special precautions

**Effects on Dental Treatment** No effects or complications reported

**Other Adverse Effects** 1% to 10%:

Cardiovascular: Flushing

Central nervous system: Dizziness

Gastrointestinal: Nausea, abdominal pain, urge to defecate

**Drug Uptake**

Onset of action: Contraction of the gallbladder occurs within 5-15 minutes

Duration: ~1 hour

**Pregnancy Risk Factor** B

**Generic Available** No

**Comments** Preparation of solution: To reconstitute, add 5 mL sterile water for injection to the vial; the solution may be kept at room temperature; use within 24 hours after reconstitution; delivers 1 mcg/mL

- **Sine-Aid® IB [OTC]** *see* Pseudoephedrine and Ibuprofen *on page 864*
- **Sine-Aid®, Maximum Strength [OTC]** *see* Acetaminophen and Pseudoephedrine *on page 31*
- **Sinemet®** *see* Levodopa and Carbidopa *on page 582*
- **Sine-Off® Maximum Strength No Drowsiness Formula [OTC]** *see* Acetaminophen and Pseudoephedrine *on page 31*
- **Sinequan®** *see* Doxepin *on page 351*
- **Sinex® Long-Acting [OTC]** *see* Oxymetazoline *on page 755*
- **Singulair®** *see* Montelukast *on page 687*
- **Sinubid®** *see* Phenyltoloxamine, Phenylpropanolamine, and Acetaminophen *on page 798*
- **Sinufed® Timecelles®** *see* Guaifenesin and Pseudoephedrine *on page 481*
- **Sinumist®-SR Capsulets®** *see* Guaifenesin *on page 478*
- **Sinupan®** *see* Guaifenesin and Phenylephrine *on page 480*
- **Sinus Excedrin® Extra Strength [OTC]** *see* Acetaminophen and Pseudoephedrine *on page 31*
- **Sinus-Relief® [OTC]** *see* Acetaminophen and Pseudoephedrine *on page 31*
- **Sinutab® Tablets [OTC]** *see* Acetaminophen, Chlorpheniramine, and Pseudoephedrine *on page 32*
- **Sinutab® Without Drowsiness [OTC]** *see* Acetaminophen and Pseudoephedrine *on page 31*
- **SK and F 104864** *see* Topotecan *on page 999*

- **Skelaxin®** *see* Metaxalone *on page 643*
- **Skelid®** *see* Tiludronate *on page 986*
- **SKF 104864** *see* Topotecan *on page 999*
- **SKF 104864-A** *see* Topotecan *on page 999*

## Skin Test Antigens, Multiple (skin test AN tee gens, MUL ti pul)

**U.S. Brand Names** Multitest CMI®

**Therapeutic Category** Diagnostic Agent, Skin Test

**Use** Detection of nonresponsiveness to antigens by means of delayed hypersensitivity skin testing

**Usual Dosage** Select only test sites that permit sufficient surface area and subcutaneous tissue to allow adequate penetration of all eight points, avoid hairy areas

Press loaded unit into the skin with sufficient pressure to puncture the skin and allow adequate penetration of all points, maintain firm contact for at least 5 seconds, during application the device should not be "rocked" back and forth and side to side without removing any of the test heads from the skin sites

If adequate pressure is applied it will be possible to observe:

1. The puncture marks of the nine tines on each of the eight test heads
2. An imprint of the circular platform surrounding each test head
3. Residual antigen and glycerin at each of the eight sites

If any of the above three criteria are not fully followed, the test results may not be reliable

Reading should be done in good light, read the test sites at both 24 and 48 hours, the largest reaction recorded from the two readings at each test site should be used; if two readings are not possible, a single 48 hour is recommended

A positive reaction from any of the seven delayed hypersensitivity skin test antigens is **induration ≥2 mm** providing there is no induration at the negative control site; the size of the induration reactions with this test may be smaller than those obtained with other intradermal procedures

**Local Anesthetic/Vasoconstrictor Precautions** No information available to require special precautions

**Effects on Dental Treatment** No effects or complications reported

**Other Adverse Effects** 1% to 10%: Local: Irritation

**Pregnancy Risk Factor** C

**Generic Available** No

**Comments** Contains disposable plastic applicator consisting of eight sterile test heads preloaded with the following seven delayed hypersensitivity skin test antigens and glycerin negative control for percutaneous administration

Test Head No. 1 = Tetanus toxoid antigen
Test Head No. 2 = Diphtheria toxoid antigen
Test Head No. 3 = *Streptococcus* antigen
Test Head No. 4 = Tuberculin, old
Test Head No. 5 = Glycerin negative control
Test Head No. 6 = *Candida* antigen
Test Head No. 7 = *Trichophyton* antigen
Test Head No. 8 = *Proteus* antigen

- **Sleep-eze 3® Oral [OTC]** *see* Diphenhydramine *on page 338*
- **Sleepinal® [OTC]** *see* Diphenhydramine *on page 338*
- **Sleepwell 2-nite® [OTC]** *see* Diphenhydramine *on page 338*
- **Slim-Mint® [OTC]** *see* Benzocaine *on page 128*
- **Slo-bid™** *see* Theophylline *on page 969*
- **Slo-Niacin® [OTC]** *see* Niacin *on page 715*
- **Slo-Phyllin®** *see* Theophylline *on page 969*
- **Slo-Phyllin GG®** *see* Theophylline and Guaifenesin *on page 973*
- **Slow FE® [OTC]** *see* Ferrous Sulfate *on page 427*
- **Slow-K®** *see* Potassium Chloride *on page 822*
- **Slow-Mag® [OTC]** *see* Magnesium Chloride *on page 610*
- **SMZ-TMP** *see* Trimethoprim and Sulfamethoxazole *on page 1021*
- **Snaplets-EX® [OTC]** *see* Guaifenesin and Phenylpropanolamine *on page 480*
- **Sodium Acid Carbonate** *see* Sodium Bicarbonate *on next page*

## Sodium Ascorbate (SOW dee um a SKOR bate)

**U.S. Brand Names** Cenolate®

**Therapeutic Category** Urinary Acidifying Agent; Vitamin, Water Soluble

**Use** Dental and Medical: Prevention and treatment of scurvy and to acidify urine

(Continued)

## Sodium Ascorbate *(Continued)*

**Usual Dosage** Oral, I.V.:
Children:
Scurvy: 100-300 mg/day in divided doses for at least 2 weeks
Urinary acidification: 500 mg every 6-8 hours
Dietary supplement: 35-45 mg/day
Adults:
Scurvy: 100-250 mg 1-2 times/day for at least 2 weeks
Urinary acidification: 4-12 g/day in divided doses
Dietary supplement: 50-60 mg/day
Prevention and treatment of cold: 1-3 g/day

**Local Anesthetic/Vasoconstrictor Precautions** No information available to require special precautions

**Effects on Dental Treatment** No effects or complications reported

**Other Adverse Effects** 1% to 10%:
Cardiovascular: Hypotension with rapid I.V. administration
Gastrointestinal: Diarrhea
Local: Soreness at injection site
Renal: Precipitation of cystine, oxalate, or urate renal stones

**Contraindications** Large doses during pregnancy

**Warnings/Precautions** Use with caution in diabetics, patients with renal calculi, and those on sodium-restricted diets

**Drug Interactions** No data reported

**Drug Uptake**
Therapeutic serum levels: 0.4-1.5 mg/dL
Time to peak serum concentration: Oral: Within 2-3 hours

**Pregnancy Risk Factor** C

**Breast-feeding Considerations** No data reported

**Dosage Forms**
Crystals: 1020 mg per 1/4 teaspoonful [ascorbic acid 900 mg]
Injection: 250 mg/mL [ascorbic acid 222 mg/mL] (30 mL); 562.5 mg/mL [ascorbic acid 500 mg/mL] (1 mL, 2 mL)
Tablet: 585 mg [ascorbic acid 500 mg]

**Generic Available** Yes

♦ **Sodium Benzoate and Caffeine** *see* Caffeine and Sodium Benzoate *on page 168*

## Sodium Bicarbonate (SOW dee um bye KAR bun ate)

**U.S. Brand Names** Neut® Injection

**Therapeutic Category** Alkalinizing Agent; Antacid; Electrolyte Supplement

**Synonyms** Baking Soda; $NaHCO_3$; Sodium Acid Carbonate; Sodium Hydrogen Carbonate

**Use** Management of metabolic acidosis; antacid; alkalinize urine; stabilization of acid base status in cardiac arrest (see precautions) and treatment of life-threatening hyperkalemia

**Usual Dosage**
Cardiac arrest: **Routine use of $NaHCO_3$ is not recommended and should be given only after adequate alveolar ventilation has been established and effective cardiac compressions are provided**
Infants and Children: I.V.: 0.5-1 mEq/kg/dose repeated every 10 minutes or as indicated by arterial blood gases; rate of infusion should not exceed 10 mEq/minute; neonates and children $<2$ years of age should receive 4.2% (0.5 mEq/mL) solution
Adults: I.V.: Initial: 1 mEq/kg/dose one time; maintenance: 0.5 mEq/kg/dose every 10 minutes or as indicated by arterial blood gases
Metabolic acidosis: Dosage should be based on the following formula if blood gases and pH measurements are available:
Infants and Children:
$HCO_3^-$(mEq) = 0.3 x weight (kg) x base deficit (mEq/L) **or**
$HCO_3^-$(mEq) = 0.5 x weight (kg) x [24 - serum $HCO_3^-$ (mEq/L)]
Adults:
$HCO_3^-$(mEq) = 0.2 x weight (kg) x base deficit (mEq/L) **or**
$HCO_3^-$(mEq) = 0.5 x weight (kg) x [24 - serum $HCO_3^-$ (mEq/L)]
If acid-base status is not available: Dose for older Children and Adults: 2-5 mEq/kg I.V. infusion over 4-8 hours; subsequent doses should be based on patient's acid-base status
Chronic renal failure: Oral: Initiate when plasma $HCO_3^-$ <15 mEq/L
Children: 1-3 mEq/kg/day
Adults: Start with 20-36 mEq/day in divided doses, titrate to bicarbonate level of 18-20 mEq/L

Renal tubular acidosis: Oral:
- Distal:
  - Children: 2-3 mEq/kg/day
  - Adults: 0.5-2 mEq/kg/day in 4-5 divided doses
- Proximal: Children: Initial: 5-10 mEq/kg/day; maintenance: Increase as required to maintain serum bicarbonate in the normal range

Urine alkalinization: Oral:
- Children: 1-10 mEq (84-840 mg)/kg/day in divided doses every 4-6 hours; dose should be titrated to desired urinary pH
- Adults: Initial: 48 mEq (4 g), then 12-24 mEq (1-2 g) every 4 hours; dose should be titrated to desired urinary pH; doses up to 16 g/day (200 mEq) in patients <60 years and 8 g (100 mEq) in patients >60 years

Antacid: Adults: Oral: 325 mg to 2 g 1-4 times/day

**Mechanism of Action** Dissociates to provide bicarbonate ion which neutralizes hydrogen ion concentration and raises blood and urinary pH

**Local Anesthetic/Vasoconstrictor Precautions** No information available to require special precautions

**Effects on Dental Treatment** No effects or complications reported

**Other Adverse Effects**

>10%: Gastrointestinal: Belching, gastric distension, flatulence

1% to 10%:
- Cardiovascular: Edema, cerebral hemorrhage, aggravation of congestive heart failure
- Central nervous system: Tetany, intracranial acidosis
- Endocrine & metabolic: Metabolic alkalosis, hypernatremia, hypokalemia, hypocalcemia, hyperosmolality
- Respiratory: Pulmonary edema
- Miscellaneous: Increased affinity of hemoglobin for oxygen-reduced pH in myocardial tissue necrosis when extravasated

**Warnings/Precautions** Rapid administration in neonates and children <2 years of age has led to hypernatremia, decreased CSF pressure and intracranial hemorrhage. **Use of I.V. $NaHCO_3$ should be reserved for documented metabolic acidosis and for hyperkalemia-induced cardiac arrest.** Routine use in cardiac arrest is not recommended. Avoid extravasation, tissue necrosis can occur due to the hypertonicity of $NaHCO_3$. May cause sodium retention especially if renal function is impaired; not to be used in treatment of peptic ulcer; use with caution in patients with CHF, edema, cirrhosis, or renal failure. Not the antacid of choice for the elderly because of sodium content and potential for systemic alkalosis.

**Drug Interactions**

Decreased effect/levels of lithium, chlorpropamide, salicylates due to urinary alkalinization

Increased toxicity/levels of amphetamines, ephedrine, pseudoephedrine, flecainide, quinidine, quinine due to urinary alkalinization

**Drug Uptake**

Oral:
- Onset of action: Rapid
- Duration: 8-10 minutes

I.V.:
- Onset of action: 15 minutes
- Duration: 1-2 hours

Absorption: Oral: Well absorbed

**Pregnancy Risk Factor** C

**Dosage Forms**

Injection: 4% [40 mg/mL = 2.4 mEq/5 mL] (5 mL); 4.2% [42 mg/mL = 5 mEq/10 mL] (10 mL); 7.5% [75 mg/mL = 8.92 mEq/10 mL] (10 mL, 50 mL); 8.4% [84 mg/mL = 10 mEq/10 mL] (10 mL, 50 mL)

Powder: 120 g, 480 g

Tablet: 300 mg [3.6 mEq]; 325 mg [3.8 mEq]; 520 mg [6.3 mEq]; 600 mg [7.3 mEq]; 650 mg [7.6 mEq]

**Dietary Considerations** Oral product should be administered 1-3 hours after meals; concurrent doses with iron may decrease iron absorption

**Generic Available** Yes

**Comments**

Sodium content of injection 50 mL, 8.4% = 1150 mg = 50 mEq; each 6 mg of $NaHCO_3$ contains 12 mEq sodium; 1 mEq $NaHCO_3$ = 84 mg

Each 84 mg of sodium bicarbonate provides 1 mEq of sodium and bicarbonate ions; each gram of sodium bicarbonate provides 12 mEq of sodium and bicarbonate ions

♦ **Sodium Cellulose Phosphate** *see* Cellulose Sodium Phosphate *on page 214*

## Sodium Chloride (SOW dee um KLOR ide)

**U.S. Brand Names** Adsorbonac® Ophthalmic [OTC]; Afrin® Saline Mist [OTC]; AK-NaCl® [OTC]; Ayr® Saline [OTC]; Breathe Free® [OTC]; Dristan® Saline Spray [OTC]; HuMist® Nasal Mist [OTC]; Muro 128® Ophthalmic [OTC]; Muroptic-5® [OTC]; NāSal™ [OTC]; Nasal Moist® [OTC]; Ocean Nasal Mist [OTC]; Pretz® [OTC]; SalineX® [OTC]; SeaMist® [OTC]

**Therapeutic Category** Electrolyte Supplement; Lubricant, Ocular

**Synonyms** NaCl; Normal Saline; Salt

**Use** Prevention of muscle cramps and heat prostration; restoration of sodium ion in hyponatremia; restore moisture to nasal membranes; reduction of corneal edema

**Usual Dosage**

Newborn electrolyte requirement:

Premature: 2-8 mEq/kg/24 hours

Term:

0-48 hours: 0-2 mEq/kg/24 hours

>48 hours: 1-4 mEq/kg/24 hours

Children: I.V.: Hypertonic solutions (>0.9%) should only be used for the initial treatment of acute serious symptomatic hyponatremia; maintenance: 3-4 mEq/kg/day; maximum: 100-150 mEq/day; dosage varies widely depending on clinical condition

Replacement: Determined by laboratory determinations mEq

Sodium deficiency (mEq/kg) = [% dehydration (L/kg)/100 x 70 (mEq/L)] + [0.6 (L/kg) x (140 - serum sodium) (mEq/L)]

Nasal: Use as often as needed

Adults:

GU irrigant: 1-3 L/day by intermittent irrigation

Heat cramps: Oral: 0.5-1 g with full glass of water, up to 4.8 g/day

Replacement I.V.: Determined by laboratory determinations mEq

Sodium deficiency (mEq/kg) = [% dehydration (L/kg)/100 x 70 (mEq/L)] + [0.6 (L/kg) x (140 - serum sodium) (mEq/L)]

To correct acute, serious hyponatremia: mEq sodium = [desired sodium (mEq/L) - actual sodium (mEq/L)] x [0.6 x wt (kg)]; for acute correction use 125 mEq/L as the desired serum sodium; acutely correct serum sodium in 5 mEq/L/dose increments; more gradual correction in increments of 10 mEq/L/day is indicated in the asymptomatic patient

Chloride maintenance electrolyte requirement in parenteral nutrition: 2-4 mEq/kg/24 hours or 25-40 mEq/1000 kcals/24 hours; maximum: 100-150 mEq/24 hours

Sodium maintenance electrolyte requirement in parenteral nutrition: 3-4 mEq/kg/24 hours or 25-40 mEq/1000 kcals/24 hours; maximum: 100-150 mEq/24 hours. See table.

**Approximate Deficits of Water and Electrolytes in Moderately Severe Dehydration**

| Condition | Water (mL/kg) | Sodium (mEq/kg) |
|---|---|---|
| Fasting and thirsting | 100-120 | 5-7 |
| Diarrhea | | |
| isonatremic | 100-120 | 8-10 |
| hypernatremic | 100-120 | 2-4 |
| hyponatremic | 100-120 | 10-12 |
| Pyloric stenosis | 100-120 | 8-10 |
| Diabetic acidosis | 100-120 | 9-10 |

*A **negative** deficit indicates total body **excess** prior to treatment.

Adapted from Behrman RE, Kleigman RM, Nelson WE, et al, eds, *Nelson Textbook of Pediatrics*, 14th ed, WB Saunders Co, 1992.

Ophthalmic:

Ointment: Apply once daily or more often

Solution: Instill 1-2 drops into affected eye(s) every 3-4 hours

Abortifacient: 20% (250 mL) administered by transabdominal intra-amniotic instillation

**Mechanism of Action** Principal extracellular cation; functions in fluid and electrolyte balance, osmotic pressure control, and water distribution

**Local Anesthetic/Vasoconstrictor Precautions** No information available to require special precautions

**Effects on Dental Treatment** No effects or complications reported

**Other Adverse Effects** 1% to 10%:
Cardiovascular: Thrombosis, hypervolemia
Endocrine & metabolic: Hypernatremia, dilution of serum electrolytes, overhydration, hypokalemia
Local: Phlebitis
Respiratory: Pulmonary edema
Miscellaneous: Congestive conditions, extravasation

**Warnings/Precautions** Use with caution in patients with congestive heart failure, renal insufficiency, liver cirrhosis, hypertension, edema; sodium toxicity is almost exclusively related to how fast a sodium deficit is corrected; both rate and magnitude are extremely important

**Drug Interactions** Decreased levels of lithium

**Drug Uptake**
Absorption: Oral, I.V.: Rapid
Distribution: Widely distributed

**Pregnancy Risk Factor** C

**Dosage Forms**
Drops, nasal: 0.9% with dropper
Injection: 0.2% (3 mL); 0.45% (3 mL, 5 mL, 500 mL, 1000 mL); 0.9% (1 mL, 2 mL, 3 mL, 4 mL, 5 mL, 10 mL, 20 mL, 25 mL, 30 mL, 50 mL, 100 mL, 130 mL, 150 mL, 250 mL, 500 mL, 1000 mL); 3% (500 mL); 5% (500 mL); 20% (250 mL); 23.4% (30 mL, 100 mL)
Injection:
  Admixtures: 50 mEq (20 mL); 100 mEq (40 mL); 625 mEq (250 mL)
  Bacteriostatic: 0.9% (30 mL)
  Concentrated: 14.6% (20 mL, 40 mL, 200 mL); 23.4% (10 mL, 20 mL, 30 mL)
Irrigation: 0.45% (500 mL, 1000 mL, 1500 mL); 0.9% (250 mL, 500 mL, 1000 mL, 1500 mL, 2000 mL, 3000 mL, 4000 mL)
Ointment, ophthalmic (Muro 128®): 5% (3.5 g)
Solution:
  Irrigation: 0.9% (1000 mL, 2000 mL)
  Nasal: 0.4% (15 mL, 50 mL); 0.6% (15 mL); 0.65% (20 mL, 45 mL, 50 mL)
  Ophthalmic (Adsorbonac®): 2% (15 mL); 5% (15 mL, 30 mL)
Tablet: 650 mg, 1 g, 2.25 g
Tablet:
  Enteric coated: 1 g
  Slow release: 600 mg

**Generic Available** Yes

## Sodium Citrate and Citric Acid

(SOW dee um SIT rate & SI trik AS id)

**U.S. Brand Names** Bicitra®; Oracit®

**Canadian Brand Names** PMS-Dicitrate™

**Therapeutic Category** Alkalinizing Agent

**Synonyms** Modified Shohl's Solution

**Use** Treatment of chronic metabolic acidosis; alkalinizing agent in conditions where long-term maintenance of an alkaline urine is desirable

**Usual Dosage** Oral:
Infants and Children: 2-3 mEq/kg/day in divided doses 3-4 times/day **or** 5-15 mL with water after meals and at bedtime
Adults: 15-30 mL with water after meals and at bedtime

**Local Anesthetic/Vasoconstrictor Precautions** No information available to require special precautions

**Effects on Dental Treatment** No effects or complications reported

**Other Adverse Effects**
1% to 10%:
  Central nervous system: Tetany
  Endocrine & metabolic: Metabolic alkalosis, hyperkalemia
  Gastrointestinal: Diarrhea, nausea, vomiting

**Warnings/Precautions** Conversion to bicarbonate may be impaired in patients with hepatic failure, in shock, or who are severely ill

**Drug Interactions**
Decreased effect/levels of lithium, chlorpropamide, salicylates due to urinary alkalinization
Increased toxicity/levels of amphetamines, ephedrine, pseudoephedrine, flecainide, quinidine, quinine due to urinary alkalinization

**Pregnancy Risk Factor** C

**Dosage Forms** Solution, oral:
Bicitra®: Sodium citrate 500 mg and citric acid 334 mg per 5 mL (15 mL unit dose, 480 mL)
Oracit®: Sodium citrate 490 mg and citric acid 640 mg per 5 mL

(Continued)

## Sodium Citrate and Citric Acid *(Continued)*

Polycitra®: Sodium citrate 500 mg and citric acid 334 mg with potassium citrate 550 mg per 5 mL

**Dietary Considerations** Should be administered after meals to avoid laxative effect

**Generic Available** No

**Comments** 1 mL of Bicitra® contains 1 mEq of sodium and the equivalent of 1 mEq of bicarbonate

## Sodium Citrate and Potassium Citrate Mixture

(SOW dee um SIT rate & poe TASS ee um SIT rate MIKS chur)

**U.S. Brand Names** Polycitra®

**Therapeutic Category** Alkalinizing Agent

**Use** Conditions where long-term maintenance of an alkaline urine is desirable as in control and dissolution of uric acid and cystine calculi of the urinary tract

**Usual Dosage** Oral:

Children: 5-15 mL diluted in water after meals and at bedtime

Adults: 15-30 mL diluted in water after meals and at bedtime

**Local Anesthetic/Vasoconstrictor Precautions** No information available to require special precautions

**Effects on Dental Treatment** No effects or complications reported

**Pregnancy Risk Factor** Not established

**Dosage Forms** Syrup: Sodium citrate 500 mg, potassium citrate 550 mg, with citric acid 334 mg per 5 mL [sodium 1 mEq, potassium 1 mEq, bicarbonate 2 mEq]

**Dietary Considerations** Should be administered after meals

**Generic Available** Yes

♦ **Sodium Cromoglycate** *see* Cromolyn Sodium *on page 281*

♦ **Sodium Edetate** *see* Edetate Disodium *on page 363*

♦ **Sodium Fluoride** *see* Fluoride *on page 441*

## Sodium Hyaluronate (SOW dee um hye al yoor ON nate)

**U.S. Brand Names** AMO Vitrax®; Amvisc®; Amvisc® Plus; Healon®; Healon® GV

**Therapeutic Category** Ophthalmic Agent, Viscoelastic

**Synonyms** Hyaluronic Acid

**Use** Surgical aid in cataract extraction, intraocular implantation, corneal transplant, glaucoma filtration, and retinal attachment surgery

**Usual Dosage** Depends upon procedure (slowly introduce a sufficient quantity into eye)

**Mechanism of Action** Functions as a tissue lubricant and is thought to play an important role in modulating the interactions between adjacent tissues. Sodium hyaluronate is a polysaccharide which is distributed widely in the extracellular matrix of connective tissue in man. (Vitreous and aqueous humor of the eye, synovial fluid, skin, and umbilical cord.) Sodium hyaluronate forms a viscoelastic solution in water (at physiological pH and ionic strength) which makes it suitable for aqueous and vitreous humor in ophthalmic surgery.

**Local Anesthetic/Vasoconstrictor Precautions** No information available to require special precautions

**Effects on Dental Treatment** No effects or complications reported

**Other Adverse Effects** 1% to 10%: Ocular: Corneal edema, corneal decompensation, transient postoperative increase in intraocular pressure, postoperative inflammatory reactions (iritis, hypopyon)

**Drug Uptake** Absorption: Following intravitreous injection, diffusion occurs slowly

**Pregnancy Risk Factor** C

**Generic Available** No

**Comments** Bring drug to room temperature before instillation into eye

♦ **Sodium Hyaluronate-Chrondroitin Sulfate** *see* Chondroitin Sulfate-Sodium Hyaluronate *on page 246*

♦ **Sodium Hydrogen Carbonate** *see* Sodium Bicarbonate *on page 918*

## Sodium Hypochlorite Solution

(SOW dee um hye poe KLOR ite soe LOO shun)

**Therapeutic Category** Disinfectant, Antibacterial (Topical)

**Synonyms** Dakin's Solution; Modified Dakin's Solution

**Use** Treatment of athlete's foot (0.5%); wound irrigation (0.5%); disinfect utensils and equipment (5%)

**Usual Dosage** Topical irrigation

**Local Anesthetic/Vasoconstrictor Precautions** No information available to require special precautions

**Effects on Dental Treatment** No effects or complications reported

**Other Adverse Effects** 1% to 10%: Dissolves blood clots, delays clotting, irritating to skin

**Contraindications** Hypersensitivity

**Warnings/Precautions** For external use only; avoid eye or mucous membrane contact; do not use on open wounds

**Pregnancy Risk Factor** C

**Dosage Forms**

Solution: 5% (4000 mL)

Solution (modified Dakin's solution):

Full strength: 0.5% (1000 mL)

Half strength: 0.25% (1000 mL)

Quarter strength: 0.125% (1000 mL)

**Generic Available** Yes

♦ **Sodium P.A.S.** *see* Aminosalicylate Sodium *on page 65*

♦ **Sodium-PCA and Lactic Acid** *see* Lactic Acid and Sodium-PCA *on page 570*

## Sodium Phenylbutyrate (SOW dee um fen il BYOO ti rate)

**U.S. Brand Names** Buphenyl®

**Therapeutic Category** Miscellaneous Product

**Synonyms** Ammonapse

**Use** Adjunctive therapy in the chronic management of patients with urea cycle disorder involving deficiencies of carbamoylphosphate synthetase, ornithine transcarbamylase, or argininosuccinic acid synthetase

**Usual Dosage**

Powder: Patients weighing <20 kg: 450-600 mg/kg/day or 9.9-13 g/m²/day, administered in equally divided amounts with each meal or feeding, four to six times daily; safety and efficacy of doses >20 g/day has not been established

Tablet: Children >20 kg and Adults: 450-600 mg/kg/day or 9.9-13 mg/m²/day, administered in equally divided amounts with each meal; safety and efficacy of doses >20 g/day have not been established

**Mechanism of Action** Sodium phenylbutyrate is a prodrug that, when given orally, is rapidly converted to phenylacetate, which is in turn conjugated with glutamine to form the active compound phenylacetyglutamine; phenylacetyglutamine serves as a substitute for urea and is excreted in the urine whereby it carries with it 2 moles of nitrogen per mole of phenylacetyglutamine and can thereby assist in the clearance of nitrogenous waste in patients with urea cycle disorders

**Local Anesthetic/Vasoconstrictor Precautions** No information available to require special precautions

**Effects on Dental Treatment** No effects or complications reported

**Other Adverse Effects**

>10%: Endocrine & metabolic: Amenorrhea, menstrual dysfunction

1% to 10%:

Gastrointestinal: Anorexia, abnormal taste

Miscellaneous: Offensive body odor

**Warnings/Precautions** Since no studies have been conducted in pregnant women, sodium phenylbutyrate should be used cautiously during pregnancy; each 1 gram of drug contains 125 mg of sodium and, therefore, should be used cautiously, if at all, in patients who must maintain a low sodium intake

**Dosage Forms**

Powder: 3.2 g [sodium phenylbutyrate 3 g] per teaspoon (500 mL, 950 mL); 9.1 g [sodium phenylbutyrate 8.6 g] per **tablespoon** (500 mL, 950 mL)

Tablet: 500 mg

**Generic Available** No

## Sodium Phosphates (SOW dee um FOS fates)

**U.S. Brand Names** Fleet® Enema [OTC]; Fleet® Phospho®-Soda [OTC]

**Therapeutic Category** Electrolyte Supplement, Parenteral; Laxative, Saline; Phosphate Salt; Sodium Salt

**Use** Source of phosphate in large volume I.V. fluids; short-term treatment of constipation (oral/rectal) and to evacuate the colon for rectal and bowel exams; treatment and prevention of hypophosphatemia

**Usual Dosage**

Normal requirements elemental phosphorus: Oral:

0-6 months: 240 mg

6-12 months: 360 mg

1-10 years: 800 mg

>10 years: 1200 mg

Pregnancy lactation: Additional 400 mg/day

Adults RDA: 800 mg

(Continued)

## Sodium Phosphates *(Continued)*

I.V. doses should be incorporated into the patient's maintenance I.V. fluids whenever possible; intermittent I.V. infusion should be reserved for severe depletion situations and requires continuous EKG monitoring. It is difficult to determine total body phosphorus deficit due to redistribution into intracellular compartment or bone tissue; (it is recommended that repletion of severe hypophosphatemia (<1 mg/dL in adults) be done via I.V. route since large dose of oral phosphate may cause diarrhea and intestinal absorption may be unreliable). The following dosages are empiric guidelines. **Note:** Doses listed as mmol of phosphate.

Severe hypophosphatemia: I.V.:
- Children:
  - Low dose: 0.08 mmol/kg over 6 hours; use if recent losses and uncomplicated
  - Intermediate dose: 0.16-0.24 mmol/kg over 4-6 hours; use if phosphorus level 0.5-1 mg/dL
  - High dose: 0.36 mmol/kg over 6 hours; use if serum phosphorus <0.5 mg/dL
- Adults: 0.15-0.3 mmol/kg/dose over 12 hours, may repeat as needed to achieve desired serum level
- Maintenance:
  - Children: 0.5-1.5 mmol/kg/24 hours I.V. or 2-3 mmol/kg/24 hours orally in divided doses
  - Adults: 50-70 mmol/24 hours I.V. or 50-150 mmol/24 hours orally in divided doses

Phosphate maintenance electrolyte requirement in parenteral nutrition: 2 mmol/kg/24 hours or 35 mmol/kcal/24 hours; maximum: 15-30 mmol/24 hours

Laxative (Fleet®): Rectal:
- Children 2-12 years: Contents of one 2.25 oz pediatric enema, may repeat
- Children ≥12 years and Adults: Contents of one 4.5 oz enema as a single dose, may repeat

Laxative (Fleet® Phospho®-Soda): Oral:
- Children 5-9 years: 5 mL as a single dose
- Children 10-12 years: 10 mL as a single dose
- Children ≥12 years and Adults: 20-30 mL as a single dose

**Mechanism of Action** As a laxative, exerts osmotic effect in the small intestine by drawing water into the lumen of the gut, producing distention and promoting peristalsis and evacuation of the bowel; phosphorous participates in bone deposition, calcium metabolism, utilization of B complex vitamins, and as a buffer in acid-base equilibrium

**Local Anesthetic/Vasoconstrictor Precautions** No information available to require special precautions

**Effects on Dental Treatment** No effects or complications reported

**Other Adverse Effects** 1% to 10%:
- Cardiovascular: Edema, hypotension
- Endocrine & metabolic: Hypocalcemia, hypernatremia, hyperphosphatemia, calcium phosphate precipitation
- Gastrointestinal: Nausea, vomiting, diarrhea
- Renal: Acute renal failure

**Drug Interactions** Do not give with magnesium- and aluminum-containing antacids or sucralfate which can bind with phosphate

**Drug Uptake**
- Onset of action:
  - Cathartic: 3-6 hours
  - Rectal: 2-5 minutes
- Absorption: Oral: ~1% to 20%

**Pregnancy Risk Factor** C

**Generic Available** Yes

## Sodium Salicylate (SOW dee um sa LIS i late)

**U.S. Brand Names** Uracel®

**Therapeutic Category** Analgesic, Non-narcotic

**Use** Treatment of minor pain or fever; arthritis

**Usual Dosage** Adults: Oral: 325-650 mg every 4 hours

**Mechanism of Action** Inhibits prostaglandin synthesis, acts on the hypothalamus heat-regulating center to reduce fever; decreases pain receptor sensitivity. Other proposed mechanisms of action for salicylate anti-inflammatory action are lysosomal stabilization, kinin and leukotriene production, alteration of chemotactic factors, and inhibition of neutrophil activation. This latter mechanism may be the most significant pharmacologic action to reduce inflammation.

**Local Anesthetic/Vasoconstrictor Precautions** No information available to require special precautions

**Effects on Dental Treatment** No effects or complications reported

**Other Adverse Effects** 1% to 10%:

Dermatologic: Rash, urticaria

Gastrointestinal: Nausea, vomiting, GI distress, GI ulcers, GI bleeding

Hematologic: Platelet inhibition

Hepatic: Hepatotoxicity

Respiratory: Bronchospasm/wheezing

**Drug Interactions** Ammonium chloride, vitamin C (high dose), methionine, antacids, urinary alkalinizers, carbonic anhydrase inhibitors, corticosteroids, nizatidine, alcohol, ACE inhibitors, beta-blockers, loop diuretics, methotrexate, probenecid, sulfinpyrazine, spironolactone, sulfonylureas

**Drug Uptake**

Absorption: From the stomach and small intestine

Serum half-life, aspirin: 15-20 minutes; metabolic pathways are saturable such that salicylates half-life is dose-dependent ranging from 3 hours at lower doses (300-600 mg), 5-6 hours (after 1 g) and 15-30 hours with higher doses; in therapeutic anti-inflammatory doses, half-lives generally range from 6-12 hours

**Pregnancy Risk Factor** C

**Dosage Forms** Tablet, enteric coated: 325 mg, 650 mg

**Generic Available** Yes

**Comments** Sodium content of 1 g: 6.25 mEq; less effective than an equal dose of aspirin in reducing pain or fever; patients hypersensitive to aspirin may be able to tolerate

♦ **Sodium Sulamyd® Ophthalmic** *see* Sulfacetamide Sodium *on page 939*

♦ **Sodium Sulfacetamide and Sulfur** *see* Sulfur and Sulfacetamide Sodium *on page 947*

## Sodium Tetradecyl (SOW dee um tetra DEK il)

**U.S. Brand Names** Sotradecol® Injection

**Therapeutic Category** Sclerosing Agent

**Use** Treatment of small, uncomplicated varicose veins of the lower extremities; endoscopic sclerotherapy in the management of bleeding esophageal varices

**Usual Dosage** I.V.: Test dose: 0.5 mL given several hours prior to administration of larger dose; 0.5-2 mL in each vein, maximum: 10 mL per treatment session; 3% solution reserved for large varices

**Mechanism of Action** Acts by irritation of the vein intimal endothelium

**Local Anesthetic/Vasoconstrictor Precautions** No information available to require special precautions

**Effects on Dental Treatment** No effects or complications reported

**Other Adverse Effects**

1% to 10%:

Central nervous system: Headache

Dermatologic: Urticaria

Gastrointestinal: Mucosal lesions, nausea, vomiting

Local: Discoloration at the site of injection, pain, ulceration at the site, sloughing and tissue necrosis following extravasation

Respiratory: Pulmonary edema

<1%:

Gastrointestinal: Esophageal perforation

Respiratory: Asthma

**Pregnancy Risk Factor** C

**Dosage Forms** Injection, as sulfate: 1% [10 mg/mL] (2 mL); 3% [30 mg/mL] (2 mL)

**Generic Available** Yes

## Sodium Thiosulfate (SOW dee um thye oh SUL fate)

**U.S. Brand Names** Tinver® Lotion

**Therapeutic Category** Antidote, Cyanide; Antifungal Agent, Topical

**Use**

Parenteral: Used alone or with sodium nitrite or amyl nitrite in cyanide poisoning or arsenic poisoning; reduce the risk of nephrotoxicity associated with cisplatin therapy; local infiltration (in diluted form) of selected chemotherapy extravasation

Topical: Treatment of tinea versicolor

**Usual Dosage**

Cyanide and nitroprusside antidote: I.V.:

Children <25 kg: 50 mg/kg after receiving 4.5-10 mg/kg sodium nitrite; a half dose of each may be repeated if necessary

(Continued)

## Sodium Thiosulfate *(Continued)*

Children >25 kg and Adults: 12.5 g after 300 mg of sodium nitrite; a half dose of each may be repeated if necessary

Cyanide poisoning: I.V.: Dose should be based on determination as with nitrite, at rate of 2.5-5 mL/minute to maximum of 50 mL. See table.

**Variation of Sodium Nitrite and Sodium Thiosulfate Dose With Hemoglobin Concentration***

| Hemoglobin (g/dL) | Initial Dose Sodium Nitrite (mg/kg) | Initial Dose Sodium Nitrite 3% (mL/kg) | Initial Dose Sodium Thiosulfate 25% (mL/kg) |
|---|---|---|---|
| 7 | 5.8 | 0.19 | 0.95 |
| 8 | 6.6 | 0.22 | 1.10 |
| 9 | 7.5 | 0.25 | 1.25 |
| 10 | 8.3 | 0.27 | 1.35 |
| 11 | 9.1 | 0.30 | 1.50 |
| 12 | 10.0 | 0.33 | 1.65 |
| 13 | 10.8 | 0.36 | 1.80 |
| 14 | 11.6 | 0.39 | 1.95 |

*Adapted from Berlin DM Jr, "The Treatment of Cyanide Poisoning in Children," *Pediatrics*, 1970, 46:793.

Cisplatin rescue should be given before or during cisplatin administration: I.V. infusion (in sterile water): 12 g/m$^2$ over 6 hours or 9 g/m$^2$ I.V. push followed by 1.2 g/m$^2$ continuous infusion for 6 hours

Arsenic poisoning: I.V.: 1 mL first day, 2 mL second day, 3 mL third day, 4 mL fourth day, 5 mL on alternate days thereafter

Children and Adults: Topical: 20% to 25% solution: Apply a thin layer to affected areas twice daily

**Mechanism of Action**

Cyanide toxicity: Increases the rate of detoxification of cyanide by the enzyme rhodanese by providing an extra sulfur

Cisplatin toxicity: Complexes with cisplatin to form a compound that is nontoxic to either normal or cancerous cells

**Local Anesthetic/Vasoconstrictor Precautions** No information available to require special precautions

**Effects on Dental Treatment** No effects or complications reported

**Other Adverse Effects** 1% to 10%:

Cardiovascular: Hypotension

Central nervous system: Coma, CNS depression secondary to thiocyanate intoxication, psychosis, confusion

Dermatologic: Contact dermatitis

Local: Irritation

Neuromuscular & skeletal: Weakness

Otic: Tinnitus

**Drug Uptake**

Serum half-life: 0.65 hour

**Pregnancy Risk Factor** C

**Generic Available** Yes

**Comments** White, odorless crystals or powder with a salty taste; normal body burden: 1.5 mg/kg

- **Solaquin® [OTC]** *see* Hydroquinone *on page 514*
- **Solaquin Forte®** *see* Hydroquinone *on page 514*
- **Solarcaine® [OTC]** *see* Benzocaine *on page 128*
- **Solatene®** *see* Beta-Carotene *on page 135*
- **Solfoton®** *see* Phenobarbital *on page 790*
- **Solganal®** *see* Aurothioglucose *on page 110*
- **Solu-Cortef®** *see* Hydrocortisone *on page 511*
- **Solu-Medrol®** *see* Methylprednisolone *on page 661*
- **Solurex L.A.®** *see* Dexamethasone *on page 308*
- **Soma®** *see* Carisoprodol *on page 191*
- **Soma® Compound** *see* Carisoprodol *on page 191*
- **Soma® Compound** *see* Carisoprodol and Aspirin *on page 192*

- **Soma® Compound w/Codeine** *see* Carisoprodol, Aspirin, and Codeine *on page 192*
- **Sominex® Oral [OTC]** *see* Diphenhydramine *on page 338*
- **SonoRx®** *see* Simethicone *on page 915*

## Sorbitol (SOR bi tole)

**Therapeutic Category** Genitourinary Irrigant

**Use** Genitourinary irrigant in transurethral prostatic resection or other transurethral resection or other transurethral surgical procedures; diuretic; humectant; sweetening agent; hyperosmotic laxative; facilitate the passage of sodium polystyrene sulfonate through the intestinal tract

**Usual Dosage** Hyperosmotic laxative (as single dose, at infrequent intervals):

Children 2-11 years:
- Oral: 2 mL/kg (as 70% solution)
- Rectal enema: 30-60 mL as 25% to 30% solution

Children >12 years and Adults:
- Oral: 30-150 mL (as 70% solution)
- Rectal enema: 120 mL as 25% to 30% solution
- Adjunct to sodium polystyrene sulfonate: 15 mL as 70% solution orally until diarrhea occurs (10-20 mL/2 hours) or 20-100 mL as an oral vehicle for the sodium polystyrene sulfonate resin

When administered with charcoal:
- Oral:
  - Children: 4.3 mL/kg of 35% sorbitol with 1 g/kg of activated charcoal
  - Adults: 4.3 mL/kg of 70% sorbitol with 1 g/kg of activated charcoal every 4 hours until first stool containing charcoal is passed
- Topical: 3% to 3.3% as transurethral surgical procedure irrigation

**Mechanism of Action** A polyalcoholic sugar with osmotic cathartic actions

**Local Anesthetic/Vasoconstrictor Precautions** No information available to require special precautions

**Effects on Dental Treatment** No effects or complications reported

**Other Adverse Effects**

1% to 10%:
- Cardiovascular: Edema
- Endocrine & metabolic: Fluid and electrolyte losses, lactic acidosis
- Gastrointestinal: Diarrhea, nausea, vomiting, abdominal discomfort, xerostomia

**Contraindications** Anuria

**Warnings/Precautions** Use with caution in patients with severe cardiopulmonary or renal impairment and in patients unable to metabolize sorbitol

**Drug Uptake**

Onset of action: About 0.25-1 hour

Absorption: Oral, rectal: Poor

**Dosage Forms**

Solution: 70%

Solution, genitourinary irrigation: 3% (1500 mL, 3000 mL); 3.3% (2000 mL)

**Generic Available** Yes

- **Sorbitrate®** *see* Isosorbide Dinitrate *on page 555*

## Sotalol (SOE ta lole)

**Related Information**

Cardiovascular Diseases *on page 1066*

**U.S. Brand Names** Betapace®

**Canadian Brand Names** Sotacor®

**Therapeutic Category** Antianginal Agent; Antiarrhythmic Agent, Class II; Antiarrhythmic Agent, Class III; Antiarrhythmic Agent (Supraventricular & Ventricular); Beta-adrenergic Blocker, Cardioselective

**Use** Treatment of documented ventricular arrhythmias, such as sustained ventricular tachycardia, that in the judgment of the physician are life-threatening

**Unlabeled use:** Supraventricular arrhythmias

**Usual Dosage** Sotalol should be initiated and doses increased in a hospital with facilities for cardiac rhythm monitoring and assessment. Proarrhythmic events can occur after initiation of therapy and with each upward dosage adjustment.

Children (oral): The safety and efficacy of sotalol in children have not been established

Supraventricular arrhythmias: 2-4 mg/kg/24 hours was given in 2 equal doses every 12 hours to 18 infants (≤2 months of age). All infants, except one with chaotic atrial tachycardia, were successful controlled with sotalol. Ten infants discontinued therapy between the ages of 7-18 months when it was no longer necessary. Median duration of treatment was 12.8 months.

(Continued)

## Sotalol *(Continued)*

Adults (oral):

Initial: 80 mg twice daily

Dose may be increased (gradually allowing 2-3 days between dosing increments in order to attain steady-state plasma concentrations and to allow monitoring of Q-T intervals) to 240-320 mg/day

Most patients respond to a total daily dose of 160-320 mg/day in 2-3 divided doses

Some patients, with life-threatening refractory ventricular arrhythmias, may require doses as high as 480-640 mg/day; however, these doses should only be prescribed when the potential benefit outweighs the increased of adverse events

Elderly patients: Age does not significantly alter the pharmacokinetics of sotalol, but impaired renal function in elderly patients can increase the terminal half-life, resulting in increased drug accumulation

**Mechanism of Action**

Beta-blocker which contains both beta-adrenoreceptor-blocking (Vaughan Williams Class II) and cardiac action potential duration prolongation (Vaughan Williams Class III) properties

Class II effects: Increased sinus cycle length, slowed heart rate, decreased A-V nodal conduction, and increased A-V nodal refractoriness

Class III effects: Prolongation of the atrial and ventricular monophasic action potentials, and effective refractory prolongation of atrial muscle, ventricular muscle, and atrioventricular accessory pathways in both the antegrade and retrograde directions

Sotalol is a racemic mixture of *d*- and *L*-sotalol; both isomers have similar Class III antiarrhythmic effects while the *L*-isomer is responsible for virtually all of the beta-blocking activity

Sotalol has both $beta_1$- and $beta_2$-receptor blocking activity

The beta-blocking effect of sotalol is a noncardioselective [half maximal at about 80 mg/day and maximal at doses of 320-640 mg/day]. Significant beta blockade occurs at oral doses as low as 25 mg/day.

The Class III effects are seen only at oral doses of ≥160 mg/day

**Local Anesthetic/Vasoconstrictor Precautions** Use with caution; epinephrine has interacted with nonselective beta-blockers to result in initial hypertensive episode followed by bradycardia

**Effects on Dental Treatment** Noncardioselective beta-blockers (ie, propranolol, nadolol) enhance the pressor response to epinephrine, resulting in hypertension and bradycardia. Many nonsteroidal anti-inflammatory drugs such as ibuprofen and indomethacin can reduce the hypotensive effect of beta-blockers after 3 or more weeks of therapy with the NSAID. Short-term NSAID use (ie, 3 days) requires no special precautions in patients taking beta-blockers.

**Other Adverse Effects**

>10%:

Cardiovascular: Bradycardia

Central nervous system: Mental depression

Endocrine & metabolic: Decreased sexual ability

1% to 10%:

Cardiovascular: Congestive heart failure

Central nervous system: Mental confusion, hallucinations, reduced peripheral circulation, anxiety, dizziness, drowsiness, nightmares, insomnia, fatigue

Dermatologic: Itching

Gastrointestinal: Constipation, diarrhea, nausea, vomiting, stomach discomfort

Neuromuscular & skeletal: Weakness

Respiratory: Dyspnea

<1%:

Cardiovascular: Chest pain, hypotension (especially with higher doses), Raynaud's phenomenon

Dermatologic: Skin rash; red, crusted skin

Hematologic: Leukopenia

Local: Phlebitis, skin necrosis after extravasation

Miscellaneous: Sweating, cold extremities

**Drug Interactions** Class Ia antiarrhythmics, such as quinidine, have the potential to prolong refractoriness of sotalol; sotalol should be administered with caution with calcium-blocking drugs because of possible additional effects on A-V conduction

**Drug Uptake**

Onset of action: Rapid, 1-2 hours

Peak effect: 2.5-4 hours

Absorption: Decreased 20% to 30% by meals compared to fasting

Serum half-life: 12 hours

**Pregnancy Risk Factor** B

**Dosage Forms** Tablet, as hydrochloride: 80 mg, 120 mg, 160 mg, 240 mg

**Generic Available** No

- **Sotradecol® Injection** *see* Sodium Tetradecyl *on page 925*
- **Soyacal®** *see* Fat Emulsion *on page 419*
- **Soyalac® [OTC]** *see* Enteral Nutritional Products *on page 371*
- **Span-FF® [OTC]** *see* Ferrous Fumarate *on page 426*

## Sparfloxacin (spar FLOKS a sin)

**U.S. Brand Names** Zagam®

**Therapeutic Category** Antibiotic, Quinolone

**Use** Treatment of adult patients with community acquired pneumonia caused by susceptible strains of *Chlamydia pneumoniae*, *Haemophilus influenzae*, *Haemophilus parainfluenzae*, *Moraxella catarrhalis*, *Mycoplasma pneumoniae*, or *Streptococcus pneumoniae* and acute bacterial exacerbations of acute bronchitis caused by susceptible strains of *Chlamydia pneumoniae*, *Enterobacter cloacae*, *Haemophilus influenzae*, *Haemophilus parainfluenzae*, *Klebsiella pneumoniae*, *Moraxella catarrhalis*, *Staphylococcus aureus*, or *Streptococcus pneumoniae*

**Usual Dosage** Adults: Oral:

Loading dose: 2 tablets (400 mg) on day 1

Maintenance: 1 tablet (200 mg) daily for 10 additional days (total 11 tablets)

**Mechanism of Action** Inhibits DNA-gyrase in susceptible organisms; inhibits relaxation of supercoiled DNA and promotes breakage of double-stranded DNA

**Local Anesthetic/Vasoconstrictor Precautions** No information available to require special precautions

**Effects on Dental Treatment** No effects or complications reported

**Other Adverse Effects**

>1%:

Central nervous system: Insomnia, agitation, sleep disorders, anxiety, delirium

Gastrointestinal: Diarrhea, abdominal pain, vomiting

Hematologic: Leukopenia, eosinophilia, anemia

Hepatic: Increased LFTs

<1%:

Dermatologic: Photosensitivity, rash

Neuromuscular & skeletal: Myalgia, arthralgia

**Warnings/Precautions** Not recommended in children <18 years of age, other quinolones have caused transient arthropathy in children; CNS stimulation may occur (tremor, restlessness, confusion, and very rarely hallucinations or seizures); use with caution in patients with known or suspected CNS disorder or renal dysfunction; prolonged use may result in superinfection; if an allergic reaction (itching, urticaria, dyspnea, pharyngeal or facial edema, loss of consciousness, tingling, cardiovascular collapse) occurs, discontinue the drug immediately; use caution to avoid possible photosensitivity reactions during and for several days following fluoroquinolone therapy; pseudomembranous colitis may occur and should be considered in patients who present with diarrhea

**Drug Interactions**

Decreased effect: Decreased absorption with antacids containing aluminum, magnesium, and/or calcium (by up to 98% if given at the same time); phenytoin serum levels may be reduced by quinolones; antineoplastic agents may also decrease serum levels of fluoroquinolones

Increased toxicity/serum levels: Quinolones cause increased levels of caffeine, warfarin, azlocillin, cyclosporine, and theophylline (although one study indicates that sparfloxacin may not affect theophylline metabolism), azlocillin, cimetidine, and probenecid increase quinolone levels; an increased incidence of seizures may occur with foscarnet

**Drug Uptake**

Absorption: Slow and erratic

Serum half-life: 16 hours

Time to peak serum concentration: 3-5 hours

**Pregnancy Risk Factor** C

**Dosage Forms** Tablet: 200 mg

**Generic Available** No

- **Sparine®** *see* Promazine *on page 846*
- **Spasmolin®** *see* Hyoscyamine, Atropine, Scopolamine, and Phenobarbital *on page 520*
- **Spec-T® [OTC]** *see* Benzocaine *on page 128*
- **Spectazole™** *see* Econazole *on page 362*

## Spectinomycin (spek ti noe MYE sin)

**Related Information**

Nonviral Infectious Diseases *on page 1095*

**U.S. Brand Names** Trobicin®

**Therapeutic Category** Antibiotic, Miscellaneous

**Use** Treatment of uncomplicated gonorrhea (ineffective against syphilis)

**Usual Dosage** I.M.:

Children:

<45 kg: 40 mg/kg/dose 1 time

≥45 kg: See adult dose

Children >8 years who are allergic to PCNS/cephalosporins may be treated with oral tetracycline

Adults:

Uncomplicated urethral endocervical or rectal gonorrhea: 2 g deep I.M. or 4 g where antibiotic resistance is prevalent 1 time; 4 g (10 mL) dose should be given as two 5 mL injections, followed by doxycycline 100 mg twice daily for 7 days

Disseminated gonococcal infection: 2 g every 12 hours

**Mechanism of Action** A bacteriostatic antibiotic that selectively binds to the 30s subunits of ribosomes, and thereby inhibiting bacterial protein synthesis

**Local Anesthetic/Vasoconstrictor Precautions** No information available to require special precautions

**Effects on Dental Treatment** No effects or complications reported

**Other Adverse Effects** <1%:

Central nervous system: Dizziness, headache, chills

Dermatologic: Urticaria, rash, pruritus

Gastrointestinal: Nausea, vomiting

Local: Pain at injection site

**Drug Interactions** No data reported

**Drug Uptake**

Duration of action: Up to 8 hours

Serum half-life: 1.7 hours

Time to peak serum concentration: Within 1 hour

**Pregnancy Risk Factor** B

**Generic Available** No

♦ **Spectrobid®** *see* Bacampicillin *on page 116*

## Spirapril (SPYE ra pril)

**Related Information**

Cardiovascular Diseases *on page 1066*

**U.S. Brand Names** Renormax®

**Therapeutic Category** Angiotensin-Converting Enzyme (ACE) Inhibitor

**Use** Management of mild to severe hypertension

**Usual Dosage** Adults: Oral: 12-48 mg once daily

**Mechanism of Action** Angiotensin-converting enzyme inhibitor; inhibits renin-angiotensin system

**Local Anesthetic/Vasoconstrictor Precautions** No information available to require special precautions

**Effects on Dental Treatment** No effects or complications reported

**Other Adverse Effects**

Cardiovascular: Hypotension (orthostatic)

Central nervous system: Headache, dizziness, migraine headache (exacerbation of), hypoesthesia

Dermatologic: Skin rash

Gastrointestinal: Nausea, diarrhea, vomiting

Neuromuscular & skeletal: Back pain

Ocular: Conjunctivitis

Respiratory: Cough

**Warnings/Precautions** Use with caution in patients with previous hypersensitivity to other ACE inhibitors, pregnancy, renal/hepatic insufficiency, hyperkalemia, autoimmune disease

**Drug Uptake**

Absorption: Oral: 53% to 60% (delayed by high fat meals)

Serum half-life: 1-2 hours

**Pregnancy Risk Factor** C (first trimester); D (second and third trimesters)

**Dosage Forms** Tablet: 3 mg, 6 mg, 12 mg, 24 mg

**Generic Available** No

♦ **Spironazide®** *see* Hydrochlorothiazide and Spironolactone *on page 504*

## Spironolactone (speer on oh LAK tone)

**Related Information**

Cardiovascular Diseases *on page 1066*

**U.S. Brand Names** Aldactone®

**Canadian Brand Names** Novo-Spiroton

**Therapeutic Category** Diuretic, Potassium Sparing

**Use** Management of edema associated with excessive aldosterone excretion; hypertension; primary hyperaldosteronism; hypokalemia; treatment of hirsutism; cirrhosis of liver accompanied by edema or ascites

**Usual Dosage** Administration with food increases absorption. To reduce delay in onset of effect, a loading dose of 2 or 3 times the daily dose may be administered on the first day of therapy. Oral:

Children:

Diuretic, hypertension: 1.5-3.5 mg/kg/day in divided doses every 6-24 hours

Diagnosis of primary aldosteronism: 125-375 mg/m$^2$/day in divided doses

Vaso-occlusive disease: 7.5 mg/kg/day in divided doses twice daily (not FDA approved)

Adults:

Edema, hypertension, hypokalemia: 25-200 mg/day in 1-2 divided doses

Diagnosis of primary aldosteronism: 100-400 mg/day in 1-2 divided doses

Elderly: Initial: 25-50 mg/day in 1-2 divided doses, increasing by 25-50 mg every 5 days as needed

**Mechanism of Action** Competes with aldosterone for receptor sites in the distal renal tubules, increasing sodium chloride and water excretion while conserving potassium and hydrogen ions; may block the effect of aldosterone on arteriolar smooth muscle as well

**Local Anesthetic/Vasoconstrictor Precautions** No information available to require special precautions

**Effects on Dental Treatment** No effects or complications reported

**Other Adverse Effects**

1% to 10%:

Cardiovascular: Hypotension, edema, bradycardia, congestive heart failure

Central nervous system: Dizziness, fatigue, headache

Dermatologic: Rash

Gastrointestinal: Nausea, constipation

Respiratory: Dyspnea

<1%:

Cardiovascular: Flushing

Endocrine & metabolic: Hyperkalemia, dehydration, hyponatremia, gynecomastia, hyperchloremia, metabolic acidosis, postmenopausal bleeding

Genitourinary: Inability to achieve or maintain an erection

**Drug Interactions** Spironolactone potentiates the effects of other diuretics and antihypertensives; spironolactone has been shown to increase the half-life of digoxin; this may result in increased serum digoxin levels and digoxin toxicity

**Drug Uptake**

Serum half-life: 78-84 minutes

Time to peak serum concentration: Within 1-3 hours (primarily as the active metabolite)

**Pregnancy Risk Factor** D

**Dosage Forms** Tablet: 25 mg, 50 mg, 100 mg

**Generic Available** Yes


- ♦ **Spironolactone and Hydrochlorothiazide** *see* Hydrochlorothiazide and Spironolactone *on page 504*
- ♦ **Spirozide®** *see* Hydrochlorothiazide and Spironolactone *on page 504*
- ♦ **Sporanox®** *see* Itraconazole *on page 559*
- ♦ **Sportscreme® [OTC]** *see* Triethanolamine Salicylate *on page 1016*
- ♦ **S-P-T** *see* Thyroid *on page 982*
- ♦ **SRC® Expectorant** *see* Hydrocodone, Pseudoephedrine, and Guaifenesin *on page 511*
- ♦ **SSD® AF** *see* Silver Sulfadiazine *on page 914*
- ♦ **SSD® Cream** *see* Silver Sulfadiazine *on page 914*
- ♦ **SSKI®** *see* Potassium Iodide *on page 824*
- ♦ **Stadol®** *see* Butorphanol *on page 167*
- ♦ **Stadol® NS** *see* Butorphanol *on page 167*
- ♦ **Stagesic® [5/500]** *see* Hydrocodone and Acetaminophen *on page 505*
- ♦ **Stahist®** *see* Chlorpheniramine, Phenylephrine, Phenylpropanolamine, and Belladonna Alkaloids *on page 236*
- ♦ **Stannous Fluoride** *see* Fluoride *on page 441*

## Stanozolol (stan OH zoe lole)

**U.S. Brand Names** Winstrol®

**Therapeutic Category** Anabolic Steroid

**Use** Prophylactic use against hereditary angioedema

**Usual Dosage**

Children: Acute attacks:

<6 years: 1 mg/day

6-12 years: 2 mg/day

Adults: Oral: Initial: 2 mg 3 times/day, may then reduce to a maintenance dose of 2 mg/day or 2 mg every other day after 1-3 months

**Mechanism of Action** Synthetic testosterone derivative with similar androgenic and anabolic actions

**Local Anesthetic/Vasoconstrictor Precautions** No information available to require special precautions

**Effects on Dental Treatment** No effects or complications reported

**Other Adverse Effects**

**Male:**

Postpubertal:

>10%:

Dermatologic: Acne

Endocrine & metabolic: Gynecomastia

Genitourinary: Bladder irritability, priapism

1% to 10%:

Central nervous system: Insomnia, chills

Endocrine & metabolic: Decreased libido,

Gastrointestinal: Nausea, diarrhea

Genitourinary: Prostatic hypertrophy (elderly)

Hematologic: Iron deficiency anemia, suppression of clotting factors

Hepatic: Hepatic dysfunction

<1%: Hepatic: Hepatic necrosis, hepatocellular carcinoma

Prepubertal:

>10%:

Dermatologic: Acne

Endocrine & metabolic: Virilism

1% to 10%:

Central nervous system: Chills, insomnia

Dermatologic: Hyperpigmentation

Gastrointestinal: Diarrhea, nausea

Hematologic: Iron deficiency anemia, suppression of clotting

<1%: Hepatic: Hepatic necrosis, hepatocellular carcinoma

**Female:**

>10%: Endocrine & metabolic: Virilism

1% to 10%:

Central nervous system: Chills, insomnia

Endocrine & metabolic: Hypercalcemia

Gastrointestinal: Nausea, diarrhea

Hematologic: Iron deficiency anemia, suppression of clotting factors

Hepatic: Hepatic dysfunction

<1%: Hepatic: Hepatic necrosis, hepatocellular carcinoma

**Drug Interactions** Stanozolol enhances the hypoprothrombinemic effects of oral anticoagulants; enhances the hypoglycemic effects of insulin and sulfonylureas (oral hypoglycemics)

**Pregnancy Risk Factor** X

**Dosage Forms** Tablet: 2 mg

**Generic Available** No

♦ **Staphcillin®** *see* Methicillin *on page 648*

♦ **Staticin® Topical** *see* Erythromycin, Topical *on page 386*

## Stavudine (STAV yoo deen)

**Related Information**

HIV Infection and AIDS *on page 1085*

Systemic Viral Diseases *on page 1115*

**U.S. Brand Names** Zerit®

**Therapeutic Category** Antiviral Agent, Oral; Antiviral Agent, Parenteral

**Use** For the treatment of adults with advanced HIV infection who are intolerant to approved therapies with proven clinical benefit or who have experienced significant clinical or immunologic deterioration while receiving these therapies, or for whom such therapies are contraindicated

**Usual Dosage** Adults: Oral:

≥60 kg: 40 mg every 12 hours

<60 kg: 30 mg every 12 hours

Dose may be cut in half if symptoms of peripheral neuropathy occur

**Mechanism of Action** Inhibits reverse transcriptase of the human immunodeficiency virus (HIV)

**Local Anesthetic/Vasoconstrictor Precautions** No information available to require special precautions

**Effects on Dental Treatment** No effects or complications reported

**Other Adverse Effects**

>10%: Neuromuscular & skeletal: Peripheral neuropathy

1% to 10%:

Central nervous system: Headache, chills/fever, malaise, insomnia, anxiety, depression

Gastrointestinal: Nausea, vomiting, diarrhea, pancreatitis, abdominal pain

Neuromuscular & skeletal: Myalgia, back pain, weakness

**Drug Interactions** No data reported

**Drug Uptake**

Peak serum level: 1 hour after administration

Serum half-life: 1-1.6 hours

**Pregnancy Risk Factor** C

**Dosage Forms**

Capsule: 15 mg, 20 mg, 30 mg, 40 mg

Powder for oral solution: 1 mg/mL (200 mL)

**Generic Available** No


- **Stelazine®** *see* Trifluoperazine *on page 1016*
- **Stemex®** *see* Paramethasone Acetate *on page 765*
- **Sterapred®** *see* Prednisone *on page 833*
- **Stilphostrol®** *see* Diethylstilbestrol *on page 326*
- **Stimate™** *see* Desmopressin Acetate *on page 306*
- **St Joseph® Adult Chewable Aspirin [OTC]** *see* Aspirin *on page 100*
- **St. Joseph® Cough Suppressant [OTC]** *see* Dextromethorphan *on page 314*
- **St. Joseph® Measured Dose Nasal Solution [OTC]** *see* Phenylephrine *on page 795*
- **Stop® [OTC]** *see* Fluoride *on page 441*
- **Streptase®** *see* Streptokinase *on this page*


## Streptokinase (strep toe KYE nase)

**Related Information**

Cardiovascular Diseases *on page 1066*

**U.S. Brand Names** Kabikinase®; Streptase®

**Therapeutic Category** Thrombolytic Agent

**Use** Thrombolytic agent used in treatment of recent severe or massive deep vein thrombosis, pulmonary emboli, myocardial infarction, and occluded arteriovenous cannulas

**Usual Dosage** I.V.:

Children: Safety and efficacy not established; limited studies have used 3500-4000 units/kg over 30 minutes followed by 1000-1500 units/kg/hour

Clotted catheter: 25,000 units, clamp for 2 hours then aspirate contents and flush with normal saline

Adults: Antibodies to streptokinase remain for at least 3-6 months after initial dose: Administration requires the use of an infusion pump

An intradermal skin test of 100 units has been suggested to predict allergic response to streptokinase. If a positive reaction is not seen after 15-20 minutes, a therapeutic dose may be administered.

**Guidelines for acute myocardial infarction** (AMI): 1.5 million units over 60 minutes

Administration:

Dilute two 750,000 unit vials of streptokinase with 5 mL dextrose 5% in water ($D_5W$) each, gently swirl to dissolve

Add this dose of the 1.5 million units to 150 mL $D_5W$

This should be infused over 60 minutes; an in-line filter ≥0.45 micron should be used

Monitor for the first few hours for signs of anaphylaxis or allergic reaction. **Infusion should be slowed if lowering of 25 mm Hg in blood pressure or terminated if asthmatic symptoms appear.**

Begin heparin 5000-10,000 unit bolus followed by 1000 units/hour approximately 3-4 hours after completion of streptokinase infusion or when PTT is <100 seconds

**Guidelines for acute pulmonary embolism** (APE): 3 million unit dose over 24 hours

(Continued)

## Streptokinase *(Continued)*

Administration:

Dilute four 750,000 unit vials of streptokinase with 5 mL dextrose 5% in water ($D_5W$) each, gently swirl to dissolve

Add this dose of 3 million units to 250 mL $D_5W$, an in-line filter ≥0.45 micron should be used

Administer 250,000 units (23 mL) over 30 minutes followed by 100,000 units/hour (9 mL/hour) for 24 hours

Monitor for the first few hours for signs of anaphylaxis or allergic reaction. **Infusion should be slowed if blood pressure is lowered by 25 mm Hg or if asthmatic symptoms appear.**

Begin heparin 1000 units/hour about 3-4 hours after completion of streptokinase infusion or when PTT is <100 seconds

Monitor PT, PTT, and fibrinogen levels during therapy

Thromboses: 250,000 units to start, then 100,000 units/hour for 24-72 hours depending on location

Cannula occlusion: 250,000 units into cannula, clamp for 2 hours, then aspirate contents and flush with normal saline

**Mechanism of Action** Activates the conversion of plasminogen to plasmin by forming a complex, exposing plasminogen-activating site, and cleaving a peptide bond that converts plasminogen to plasmin; plasmin degrades fibrin, fibrinogen and other procoagulant proteins into soluble fragments; effective both outside and within the formed thrombus/embolus

**Local Anesthetic/Vasoconstrictor Precautions** No information available to require special precautions

**Effects on Dental Treatment** No effects or complications reported

**Other Adverse Effects**

>10%:

Cardiovascular: Hypotension, arrhythmias, trauma arrhythmias, cerebral hemorrhage

Dermatologic: Angioneurotic edema

Hematologic: Surface bleeding, internal bleeding

Ocular: Periorbital swelling

Respiratory: Bronchospasm

Miscellaneous: Anaphylaxis

<1%:

Cardiovascular: Flushing

Central nervous system: Headache, chills, fever

Dermatologic: Rash, itching

Gastrointestinal: Nausea, vomiting

Hematologic: Anemia

Neuromuscular & skeletal: Musculoskeletal pain

Ocular: Eye hemorrhage

Respiratory: Epistaxis

Miscellaneous: Sweating

**Drug Interactions**

Antifibrinolytic agents (aminocaproic acid) cause decreased effectiveness of streptokinase

Anticoagulants, antiplatelet agents cause increased risk of bleeding of streptokinase

**Drug Uptake**

Onset of action: Activation of plasminogen occurs almost immediately

Duration: Fibrinolytic effects last only a few hours, while anticoagulant effects can persist for 12-24 hours

Serum half-life: 83 minutes

**Pregnancy Risk Factor** C

**Dosage Forms** Powder for injection: 250,000 units (5 mL, 6.5 mL); 600,000 units (5 mL); 750,000 units (6 mL, 6.5 mL); 1,500,000 units (6.5 mL, 10 mL, 50 mL)

**Generic Available** No

## Streptomycin (strep toe MYE sin)

**Related Information**

Nonviral Infectious Diseases *on page 1095*

**Therapeutic Category** Antibiotic, Aminoglycoside; Antitubercular Agent

**Use** Combination therapy of active tuberculosis; used in combination with other agents for treatment of streptococcal or enterococcal endocarditis, mycobacterial infections, plague, tularemia, and brucellosis. Streptomycin is indicated for persons from endemic areas of drug-resistant *Mycobacterium tuberculosis* or who are HIV infected.

**Usual Dosage** Intramuscular (may also be given intravenous piggyback):

Tuberculosis therapy: **Note:** A four-drug regimen (isoniazid, rifampin, pyrazinamide and either streptomycin or ethambutol) is preferred for the initial, empiric treatment of TB. When the drug susceptibility results are available, the regimen should be altered as appropriate.

**Patients with TB and without HIV infection:**

**OPTION 1:**

Isoniazid resistance rate <4%: Administer daily isoniazid, rifampin, and pyrazinamide for 8 weeks followed by isoniazid and rifampin daily or directly observed therapy (DOT) 2-3 times/week for 16 weeks

If isoniazid resistance rate is not documented, ethambutol or streptomycin should also be administered until susceptibility to isoniazid or rifampin is demonstrated. Continue treatment for at least 6 months or 3 months beyond culture conversion.

**OPTION 2:** Administer daily isoniazid, rifampin, pyrazinamide, and either streptomycin or ethambutol for 2 weeks followed by DOT 2 times/week administration of the same drugs for 6 weeks, and subsequently, with isoniazid and rifampin DOT 2 times/week administration for 16 weeks

**OPTION 3:** Administer isoniazid, rifampin, pyrazinamide, and either ethambutol or streptomycin by DOT 3 times/week for 6 months

**Patients with TB and with HIV infection:** Administer any of the above OPTIONS 1, 2 or 3, however, treatment should be continued for a total of 9 months and at least 6 months beyond culture conversion

**Note:** Some experts recommend that the duration of therapy should be extended to 9 months for patients with disseminated disease, miliary disease, disease involving the bones or joints, or tuberculosis lymphadenitis

Children:

Daily therapy: 20-30 mg/kg/day (maximum: 1 g/day)

Directly observed therapy (DOT): Twice weekly: 25-30 mg/kg (maximum: 1.5 g)

DOT: 3 times/week: 25-30 mg/kg (maximum: 1 g)

Adults:

Daily therapy: 15 mg/kg/day (maximum: 1 g)

Directly observed therapy (DOT): Twice weekly: 25-30 mg/kg (maximum: 1.5 g)

DOT: 3 times/week: 25-30 mg/kg (maximum: 1 g)

Enterococcal endocarditis: 1 g every 12 hours for 2 weeks, 500 mg every 12 hours for 4 weeks in combination with penicillin

Streptococcal endocarditis: 1 g every 12 hours for 1 week, 500 mg every 12 hours for 1 week

Tularemia: 1-2 g/day in divided doses for 7-10 days or until patient is afebrile for 5-7 days

Plague: 2-4 g/day in divided doses until the patient is afebrile for at least 3 days

Elderly: 10 mg/kg/day, not to exceed 750 mg/day; dosing interval should be adjusted for renal function; some authors suggest not to give more than 5 days/week or give as 20-25 mg/kg/dose twice weekly

**Mechanism of Action** Inhibits bacterial protein synthesis by binding directly to the 30S ribosomal subunits causing faulty peptide sequence to form in the protein chain

**Local Anesthetic/Vasoconstrictor Precautions** No information available to require special precautions

**Effects on Dental Treatment** No effects or complications reported

**Other Adverse Effects**

1% to 10%:

Neuromuscular & skeletal: Neuromuscular blockade

Otic: Ototoxicity (auditory), ototoxicity (vestibular)

Renal: Nephrotoxicity

<1%:

Cardiovascular: Hypotension

Central nervous system: Drug fever, headache, drowsiness

Dermatologic: Skin rash

Gastrointestinal: Nausea, vomiting

Hematologic: Eosinophilia, anemia

Neuromuscular & skeletal: Paresthesia, tremor, arthralgia, weakness

Respiratory: Dyspnea

**Drug Interactions**

Concurrent use of amphotericin, loop diuretics may increase nephrotoxicity of streptomycin

**Drug Uptake**

Absorption: Oral: Absorbed poorly; usually given parenterally

Serum half-life: Adults: 2-4.7 hours, prolonged with renal impairment

Time to peak serum concentration: Within 1 hour

**Pregnancy Risk Factor** D

(Continued)

## Streptomycin *(Continued)*

**Generic Available** Yes

## Streptozocin (strep toe ZOE sin)

**U.S. Brand Names** Zanosar®

**Therapeutic Category** Antineoplastic Agent, Alkylating Agent (Nitrosourea)

**Use** Treat metastatic islet cell carcinoma of the pancreas, carcinoid tumor and syndrome, Hodgkin's disease, palliative treatment of colorectal cancer

**Usual Dosage** I.V. (refer to individual protocols): Children and Adults: 500 mg/m$^2$ for 5 days every 4-6 weeks until optimal benefit or toxicity occurs or may be given in single dose 1000 mg/m$^2$ at weekly intervals for 2 doses, then increased to 1500 mg/m$^2$; usual course of therapy: 4-6 weeks

**Mechanism of Action** Interferes with the normal function of DNA by alkylation and cross-linking the strands of DNA, and by possible protein modification

**Local Anesthetic/Vasoconstrictor Precautions** No information available to require special precautions

**Effects on Dental Treatment** No effects or complications reported

**Other Adverse Effects**

>10%:

Endocrine & metabolic: Hypoalbuminemia, hypophosphatemia

Gastrointestinal: Nausea and vomiting in all patients usually 1-4 hours after infusion; diarrhea in 10% of patients

Emetic potential: High (>90%)

Hepatic: Elevated LFTs

Renal: Renal dysfunction occurs in 65% of patients; proteinuria, decreased $Cl_{cr}$, elevated BUN, renal tubular acidosis; be careful with patients on other nephrotoxic agents; nephrotoxicity (25% to 75% of patients)

1% to 10%:

Endocrine & metabolic: Hypoglycemia is seen in 6% of patients; may be prevented with the administration of nicotinamide

Gastrointestinal: Diarrhea

Local: Pain at injection site

<1%:

Central nervous system: Confusion, lethargy, depression

Hematologic: Leukopenia, thrombocytopenia

Myelosuppressive: WBC: Mild; Platelets: Mild; Onset (days): 7; Nadir (days): 14; Recovery (days): 21

Hepatic: Liver dysfunction

Secondary malignancy

**Drug Interactions**

Phenytoin results in negation of streptozocin cytotoxicity

Doxorubicin prolongs half-life of streptozocin and thus prolongs leukopenia and thrombocytopenia

**Drug Uptake** Serum half-life: 35-40 minutes

**Pregnancy Risk Factor** C

**Generic Available** No

- **Stresstabs® 600 Advanced Formula Tablets [OTC]** *see* Vitamins, Multiple *on page 1051*
- **Stromectol®** *see* Ivermectin *on page 560*
- **Stuartnatal® 1 + 1** *see* Vitamins, Multiple *on page 1051*
- **Stuart Prenatal® [OTC]** *see* Vitamins, Multiple *on page 1051*
- **Sublimaze® Injection** *see* Fentanyl *on page 424*

## Sucralfate (soo KRAL fate)

**Related Information**

Patients Undergoing Cancer Therapy *on page 1154*

**U.S. Brand Names** Carafate®

**Canadian Brand Names** Novo-Sucralate; Sulcrate®; Sulcrate® Suspension Plus

**Therapeutic Category** Gastrointestinal Agent, Miscellaneous

**Use** Short-term management of duodenal ulcers

**Unlabeled uses:** Gastric ulcers; maintenance of duodenal ulcers; suspension may be used topically for treatment of stomatitis due to cancer chemotherapy and other causes of esophageal and gastric erosions; GERD, esophagitis, treatment of NSAID mucosal damage, prevention of stress ulcers, postschlerotherapy for esophageal variceal bleeding.

**Usual Dosage** Oral:

Children: Dose not established, doses of 40-80 mg/kg/day divided every 6 hours have been used

Stomatitis: 2.5-5 mL (1 g/10 mL suspension), swish and spit or swish and swallow 4 times/day

Adults:

Stress ulcer prophylaxis: 1 g 4 times/day

Stress ulcer treatment: 1 g every 4 hours

Duodenal ulcer:

Treatment: 1 g 4 times/day, 1 hour before meals or food and at bedtime for 4-8 weeks, or alternatively 2 g twice daily; treatment is recommended for 4-8 weeks in adults, the elderly will require 12 weeks

Maintenance: Prophylaxis: 1 g twice daily

Stomatitis: 1 g/10 mL suspension, swish and spit or swish and swallow 4 times/day

**Mechanism of Action** Forms a complex by binding with positively charged proteins in exudates, forming a viscous paste-like, adhesive substance, when combined with gastric acid adheres to the damaged mucosal area. This selectively forms a protective coating that protects the lining against peptic acid, pepsin, and bile salts.

**Local Anesthetic/Vasoconstrictor Precautions** No information available to require special precautions

**Effects on Dental Treatment** No effects or complications reported

**Other Adverse Effects**

1% to 10%: Gastrointestinal: Constipation

<1%:

Central nervous system: Dizziness, sleepiness, vertigo

Dermatologic: Rash, pruritus

Gastrointestinal: Diarrhea, nausea, gastric discomfort, indigestion, dry mouth

Neuromuscular & skeletal: Back pain

**Drug Interactions** Decreased effect:

Digoxin, phenytoin, theophylline, ciprofloxacin, itraconazole; because of the potential for sucralfate to alter the absorption of some drugs, separate administration (2 hours before or after) should be considered when alterations in bioavailability are believed to be critical

Antacids/cimetidine/ranitidine: Do not administer concomitantly with sucralfate; these types of drugs reduce acidity; sucralfate requires gastric acid for it's mechanism of action (ie, to form a gel in the stomach as a protective barrier)

**Drug Uptake**

Onset of action: Paste formation and ulcer adhesion occur within 1-2 hours

Duration: Up to 6 hours

Absorption: Oral: <5%

**Pregnancy Risk Factor** B

**Dosage Forms**

Suspension, oral: 1 g/10 mL (420 mL)

Tablet: 1 g

**Generic Available** Yes

- **Sucrets® Cough Calmers [OTC]** *see* Dextromethorphan *on page 314*
- **Sucrets® Sore Throat [OTC]** *see* Hexylresorcinol *on page 497*
- **Sudafed® [OTC]** *see* Pseudoephedrine *on page 863*
- **Sudafed® 12 Hour [OTC]** *see* Pseudoephedrine *on page 863*
- **Sudafed® Cold & Cough Liquid Caps [OTC]** *see* Guaifenesin, Pseudoephedrine, and Dextromethorphan *on page 482*
- **Sudafed® Plus® Liquid [OTC]** *see* Chlorpheniramine and Pseudoephedrine *on page 233*
- **Sudafed® Plus® Tablet [OTC]** *see* Chlorpheniramine and Pseudoephedrine *on page 233*
- **Sudafed® Severe Cold [OTC]** *see* Acetaminophen, Dextromethorphan, and Pseudoephedrine *on page 32*
- **Sufenta®** *see* Sufentanil *on this page*

## Sufentanil (soo FEN ta nil)

**Related Information**

Narcotic Agonists *on page 1223*

**U.S. Brand Names** Sufenta®

**Therapeutic Category** Analgesic, Narcotic

**Use** Analgesic supplement in maintenance of balanced general anesthesia

**Usual Dosage**

Children <12 years: 10-25 mcg/kg with 100% $O_2$, maintenance: 25-50 mcg as needed

Adults: Dose should be based on body weight. **Note:** In obese patients (ie, >20% above ideal body weight), use lean body weight to determine dosage.

1-2 mcg/kg with $NO_2/O_2$ for endotracheal intubation; maintenance: 10-25 mcg as needed

2-8 mcg/kg with $NO_2/O_2$ more complicated major surgical procedures; maintenance: 10-50 mcg as needed

(Continued)

## Sufentanil *(Continued)*

8-30 mcg/kg with 100% $O_2$ and muscle relaxant produces sleep; at doses ≥8 mcg/kg maintains a deep level of anesthesia; maintenance: 10-50 mcg as needed

**Mechanism of Action** Binds to opiate receptors in the CNS causing inhibition of ascending pain pathways, altering the perception of and response to pain; ultra-short-acting narcotic

**Local Anesthetic/Vasoconstrictor Precautions** No information available to require special precautions

**Effects on Dental Treatment** No effects or complications reported

**Other Adverse Effects**

>10%:
- Cardiovascular: Bradycardia, hypotension
- Central nervous system: Drowsiness
- Gastrointestinal: Nausea, vomiting
- Respiratory: Respiratory depression

1% to 10%:
- Cardiovascular: Cardiac arrhythmias, orthostatic hypotension
- Central nervous system: Confusion, CNS depression
- Gastrointestinal: Biliary spasm
- Ocular: Blurred vision

<1%:
- Cardiovascular: Circulatory depression
- Central nervous system: Convulsions, dysesthesia, paradoxical CNS excitation or delirium; mental depression, dizziness
- Dermatologic: Skin rash, urticaria, itching
- Gastrointestinal: Biliary spasm
- Genitourinary: Urinary tract spasm
- Respiratory: Laryngospasm, bronchospasm
- Miscellaneous: Cold, clammy skin; physical and psychological dependence with prolonged use

**Drug Interactions** Increased effect/toxicity with CNS depressants, beta-blockers

**Drug Uptake**

Onset of action: 1-3 minutes

Duration: Dose dependent

**Pregnancy Risk Factor** C

**Dosage Forms** Injection, as citrate: 50 mcg/mL (1 mL, 2 mL, 5 mL)

**Generic Available** Yes

♦ **Sugar-Free Liquid Pharmaceuticals** *see page 1261*

♦ **Sular®** *see* Nisoldipine *on page 723*

## Sulconazole (sul KON a zole)

**U.S. Brand Names** Exelderm®

**Therapeutic Category** Antifungal Agent, Topical

**Use** Treatment of superficial fungal infections of the skin, including tinea cruris (jock itch), tinea corporis (ringworm), tinea versicolor, and possibly tinea pedis (athlete's foot - cream only)

**Usual Dosage** Adults: Topical: Apply a small amount to the affected area and gently massage once or twice daily for 3 weeks (tinea cruris, tinea corporis, tinea versicolor) to 4 weeks (tinea pedis).

**Mechanism of Action** Substituted imidazole derivative which inhibits metabolic reactions necessary for the synthesis of ergosterol, an essential membrane component. The end result is usually fungistatic; however, sulconazole may act as a fungicide in *Candida albicans* and parapsilosis during certain growth phases.

**Local Anesthetic/Vasoconstrictor Precautions** No information available to require special precautions

**Effects on Dental Treatment** No effects or complications reported

**Other Adverse Effects** 1% to 10%: Local: Itching, burning, stinging, redness

**Drug Interactions** No data reported

**Drug Uptake** Absorption: Topical: About 8.7% absorbed percutaneously

**Pregnancy Risk Factor** C

**Dosage Forms**

Cream, as nitrate: 1% (15 g, 30 g, 60 g)

Solution, as nitrate, topical: 1% (30 mL)

**Generic Available** No

♦ **Sulf-10® Ophthalmic** *see* Sulfacetamide Sodium *on next page*

## Sulfabenzamide, Sulfacetamide, and Sulfathiazole

(sul fa BENZ a mide, sul fa SEE ta mide & sul fa THYE a zole)

**U.S. Brand Names** Femguard®; Gyne-Sulf®; Sulfa-Gyn®; Sulfa-Trip®; Sultrin™; Trysul®; V.V.S.®

**Therapeutic Category** Antibiotic, Vaginal

**Use** Treatment of *Haemophilus vaginalis* vaginitis

**Usual Dosage** Adults:

Cream: Insert one applicatorful in vagina twice daily for 4-6 days; dosage may then be decreased to ½ to ¼ of an applicatorful twice daily

Tablet: Insert one intravaginally twice daily for 10 days

**Mechanism of Action** Interferes with microbial folic acid synthesis and growth via inhibition of para-aminobenzoic acid metabolism

**Local Anesthetic/Vasoconstrictor Precautions** No information available to require special precautions

**Effects on Dental Treatment** No effects or complications reported

**Other Adverse Effects**

>10%:

Dermatologic: Pruritus, urticaria

Local: Irritation

<1%:

Dermatologic: Stevens-Johnson syndrome

Miscellaneous: Allergic reactions

**Drug Interactions** No data reported

**Drug Uptake** Absorption: Absorption from the vagina is variable and unreliable

**Pregnancy Risk Factor** C

**Generic Available** Yes

## Sulfacetamide Sodium (sul fa SEE ta mide SOW dee um)

**U.S. Brand Names** AK-Sulf® Ophthalmic; Bleph®-10 Ophthalmic; Cetamide® Ophthalmic; Isopto® Cetamide® Ophthalmic; Klaron® Lotion; Ocusulf-10® Ophthalmic; Sebizon® Topical Lotion; Sodium Sulamyd® Ophthalmic; Sulf-10® Ophthalmic

**Therapeutic Category** Antibiotic, Ophthalmic

**Use** Treatment and prophylaxis of conjunctivitis due to susceptible organisms; corneal ulcers; adjunctive treatment with systemic sulfonamides for therapy of trachoma; topical application in scaling dermatosis (seborrheic); bacterial infections of the skin

**Usual Dosage**

Children >2 months and Adults: Ophthalmic:

Ointment: Apply to lower conjunctival sac 1-4 times/day and at bedtime

Solution: Instill 1-3 drops several times daily up to every 2-3 hours in lower conjunctival sac during waking hours and less frequently at night

Children >12 years and Adults: Topical:

Seborrheic dermatitis: Apply at bedtime and allow to remain overnight; in severe cases, may apply twice daily

Secondary cutaneous bacterial infections: Apply 2-4 times/day until infection clears

**Mechanism of Action** Interferes with bacterial growth by inhibiting bacterial folic acid synthesis through competitive antagonism of PABA

**Local Anesthetic/Vasoconstrictor Precautions** No information available to require special precautions

**Effects on Dental Treatment** No effects or complications reported

**Other Adverse Effects**

1% to 10%: Local: Irritation, stinging, burning

<1%:

Central nervous system: Headache, browache

Dermatologic: Stevens-Johnson syndrome, exfoliative dermatitis, toxic epidermal necrolysis

Ocular: Blurred vision

Miscellaneous: Hypersensitivity reactions

**Drug Interactions** Decreased effect: Silver, gentamicin (antagonism)

**Drug Uptake**

Serum half-life: 7-13 hours

**Pregnancy Risk Factor** C

**Generic Available** Yes

## Sulfacetamide Sodium and Fluorometholone

(sul fa SEE ta mide SOW dee um & flure oh METH oh lone)

**U.S. Brand Names** FML-S® Ophthalmic Suspension

**Therapeutic Category** Antibiotic, Ophthalmic; Anti-inflammatory Agent, Ophthalmic

(Continued)

## Sulfacetamide Sodium and Fluorometholone *(Continued)*

**Use** Steroid-responsive inflammatory ocular conditions where infection is present or there is a risk of infection

**Local Anesthetic/Vasoconstrictor Precautions** No information available to require special precautions

**Effects on Dental Treatment** No effects or complications reported

**Pregnancy Risk Factor** C

**Generic Available** Yes

## Sulfacetamide Sodium and Phenylephrine

(sul fa SEE ta mide SOW dee um & fen il EF rin)

**U.S. Brand Names** Vasosulf® Ophthalmic

**Therapeutic Category** Antibiotic, Ophthalmic; Ophthalmic Agent, Vasoconstrictor

**Usual Dosage** Instill 1 or 2 drops into the lower conjunctival sac(s) every 2 or 3 hours during the day, less often at night

**Local Anesthetic/Vasoconstrictor Precautions** No information available to require special precautions

**Effects on Dental Treatment** No effects or complications reported

**Pregnancy Risk Factor** C

**Generic Available** Yes

## Sulfacetamide Sodium and Prednisolone

(sul fa SEE ta mide SOW dee um & pred NIS oh lone)

**U.S. Brand Names** AK-Cide® Ophthalmic; Blephamide® Ophthalmic; Cetapred® Ophthalmic; Isopto® Cetapred® Ophthalmic; Metimyd® Ophthalmic; Vasocidin® Ophthalmic

**Therapeutic Category** Antibiotic, Ophthalmic; Corticosteroid, Ophthalmic

**Use** Steroid-responsive inflammatory ocular conditions where infection is present or there is a risk of infection; ophthalmic suspension may be used as an otic preparation

**Usual Dosage** Children >2 months and Adults: Ophthalmic:
- Ointment: Apply to lower conjunctival sac 1-4 times/day
- Solution: Instill 1-3 drops every 2-3 hours while awake

**Mechanism of Action** Interferes with bacterial growth by inhibiting bacterial folic acid synthesis through competitive antagonism of PABA; decreases inflammation by suppression of migration of polymorphonuclear leukocytes and reversal of increased capillary permeability; suppresses the immune system by reducing activity and volume of the lymphatic system

**Local Anesthetic/Vasoconstrictor Precautions** No information available to require special precautions

**Effects on Dental Treatment** No effects or complications reported

**Other Adverse Effects**

1% to 10%: Local: Burning, stinging

<1%:
- Central nervous system: Vertigo, seizures, psychoses, pseudotumor cerebri, headache
- Dermatologic: Stevens-Johnson syndrome, skin atrophy
- Endocrine & metabolic: Cushing's syndrome, pituitary-adrenal axis suppression, growth suppression
- Gastrointestinal: Peptic ulcer, nausea, vomiting
- Neuromuscular & skeletal: Muscle weakness, osteoporosis, fractures
- Ocular: Cataracts, glaucoma

**Drug Interactions** Decreased effect: Silver, gentamicin, vaccines, toxoids

**Pregnancy Risk Factor** C

**Generic Available** Yes

♦ **Sulfacetamide Sodium and Sulfur** *see* Sulfur and Sulfacetamide Sodium *on page 947*

♦ **Sulfacet-R® Topical** *see* Sulfur and Sulfacetamide Sodium *on page 947*

## Sulfacytine (sul fa SYE teen)

**U.S. Brand Names** Renoquid®

**Therapeutic Category** Antibiotic, Sulfonamide Derivative

**Use** Treatment of urinary tract infections

**Usual Dosage** Adults: Oral: Initial: 500 mg, then 250 mg every 4 hours for 10 days

**Local Anesthetic/Vasoconstrictor Precautions** No information available to require special precautions

**Effects on Dental Treatment** No effects or complications reported

**Other Adverse Effects**

>10%:

Central nervous system: Fever, dizziness, headache

Dermatologic: Itching, skin rash, photosensitivity

Gastrointestinal: Anorexia, nausea, vomiting, diarrhea

1% to 10%:

Dermatologic: Stevens-Johnson syndrome, Lyell's syndrome

Hematologic: Granulocytopenia, leukopenia, thrombocytopenia, aplastic anemia, hemolytic anemia

Hepatic: Hepatitis

<1%:

Endocrine & metabolic: Thyroid function disturbance

Genitourinary: Crystalluria

Hepatic: Jaundice

Renal: Hematuria, interstitial nephritis, acute nephropathy

Miscellaneous: Serum sickness-like reactions

**Pregnancy Risk Factor** B (D at term)

**Generic Available** No

## Sulfadiazine (sul fa DYE a zeen)

**U.S. Brand Names** Microsulfon®

**Canadian Brand Names** Coptin®

**Therapeutic Category** Antibiotic, Sulfonamide Derivative

**Use** Treatment of urinary tract infections and nocardiosis, rheumatic fever prophylaxis; adjunctive treatment in toxoplasmosis; uncomplicated attack of malaria

**Usual Dosage** Oral:

Congenital toxoplasmosis:

Newborns and Children <2 months: 100 mg/kg/day divided every 6 hours in conjunction with pyrimethamine 1 mg/kg/day once daily and supplemental folinic acid 5 mg every 3 days for 6 months

Children >2 months: 25-50 mg/kg/dose 4 times/day

Toxoplasmosis:

Children: 120-150 mg/kg/day, maximum dose: 6 g/day; divided every 6 hours in conjunction with pyrimethamine 2 mg/kg/day divided every 12 hours for 3 days followed by 1 mg/kg/day once daily (maximum: 25 mg/day) with supplemental folinic acid

Adults: 2-8 g/day divided every 6 hours in conjunction with pyrimethamine 25 mg/day and with supplemental folinic acid

**Mechanism of Action** Interferes with bacterial growth by inhibiting bacterial folic acid synthesis through competitive antagonism of PABA

**Local Anesthetic/Vasoconstrictor Precautions** No information available to require special precautions

**Effects on Dental Treatment** No effects or complications reported

**Other Adverse Effects**

>10%:

Central nervous system: Fever, dizziness, headache

Dermatologic: Itching, skin rash, photosensitivity

Gastrointestinal: Anorexia, nausea, vomiting, diarrhea

1% to 10%:

Dermatologic: Lyell's syndrome, Stevens-Johnson syndrome

Hematologic: Granulocytopenia, leukopenia, thrombocytopenia, aplastic anemia, hemolytic anemia

Hepatic: Hepatitis

<1%:

Endocrine & metabolic: Thyroid function disturbance

Genitourinary: Crystalluria

Hepatic: Jaundice

Renal: Interstitial nephritis, acute nephropathy, hematuria

Miscellaneous: Serum sickness-like reactions

**Drug Interactions** Decreased effect with PABA or PABA metabolites of drugs (eg, procaine, proparacaine, tetracaine, sunscreens); decreased effect of oral anticoagulants and oral hypoglycemic agents

**Drug Uptake**

Absorption: Oral: Well absorbed

Serum half-life: 10 hours

Time to peak serum concentration: Within 3-6 hours

**Pregnancy Risk Factor** B (D at term)

**Generic Available** Yes

## Sulfadiazine, Sulfamethazine, and Sulfamerazine

(sul fa DYE a zeen sul fa METH a zeen & sul fa MER a zeen)

**Therapeutic Category** Antibiotic, Sulfonamide Derivative; Antibiotic, Vaginal

**Synonyms** Multiple Sulfonamides; Trisulfapyrimidines

**Use** Treatment of toxoplasmosis

**Usual Dosage** Adults: Oral: 2-4 g to start, then 2-4 g/day in 3-6 divided doses

**Mechanism of Action** Interferes with microbial folic acid synthesis and growth via inhibition of para-aminobenzoic acid metabolism

**Local Anesthetic/Vasoconstrictor Precautions** No information available to require special precautions

**Effects on Dental Treatment** No effects or complications reported

**Pregnancy Risk Factor** B (D at term)

**Generic Available** No

## Sulfadoxine and Pyrimethamine

(sul fa DOKS een & peer i METH a meen)

**U.S. Brand Names** Fansidar®

**Therapeutic Category** Antimalarial Agent

**Use** Treatment of *Plasmodium falciparum* malaria in patients in whom chloroquine resistance is suspected; malaria prophylaxis for travelers to areas where chloroquine-resistant malaria is endemic

**Usual Dosage** Children and Adults: Oral:

Treatment of acute attack of malaria: A single dose of the following number of Fansidar® tablets is used in sequence with quinine or alone:

- 2-11 months: 1/4 tablet
- 1-3 years: 1/2 tablet
- 4-8 years: 1 tablet
- 9-14 years: 2 tablets
- >14 years: 2-3 tablets

Malaria prophylaxis:

The first dose of Fansidar® should be taken 1-2 days before departure to an endemic area (CDC recommends that therapy be initiated 1-2 weeks before such travel), administration should be continued during the stay and for 4-6 weeks after return. Dose = pyrimethamine 0.5 mg/kg/dose and sulfadoxine 10 mg/kg/dose up to a maximum of 25 mg pyrimethamine and 500 mg sulfadoxine/dose weekly.

- 2-11 months: 1/8 tablet weekly **or** 1/4 tablet once every 2 weeks
- 1-3 years: 1/4 tablet once weekly **or** 1/2 tablet once every 2 weeks
- 4-8 years: 1/2 tablet once weekly **or** 1 tablet once every 2 weeks
- 9-14 years: 3/4 tablet once weekly **or** 1 1/2 tablets once every 2 weeks
- >14 years: 1 tablet once weekly **or** 2 tablets once every 2 weeks

**Mechanism of Action** Sulfadoxine interferes with bacterial folic acid synthesis and growth via competitive inhibition of para-aminiobenzoic acid; pyrimethamine inhibits microbial dihydrofolate reductase, resulting in inhibition of tetrahydrofolic acid synthesis

**Local Anesthetic/Vasoconstrictor Precautions** No information available to require special precautions

**Effects on Dental Treatment** No effects or complications reported

**Other Adverse Effects**

>10%:

- Central nervous system: Ataxia, seizures, headache
- Dermatologic: Photosensitivity
- Gastrointestinal: Atrophic glossitis, vomiting, gastritis
- Hematologic: Megaloblastic anemia, leukopenia, thrombocytopenia, pancytopenia
- Neuromuscular & skeletal: Tremors
- Miscellaneous: Hypersensitivity

1% to 10%:

- Dermatologic: Stevens-Johnson syndrome
- Hepatic: Hepatitis

<1%:

- Dermatologic: Erythema multiforme, toxic epidermal necrolysis, rash
- Endocrine & metabolic: Thyroid function dysfunction
- Gastrointestinal: Anorexia, glossitis
- Genitourinary: Crystalluria
- Hepatic: Hepatic necrosis
- Respiratory: Respiratory failure

**Drug Interactions**

Decreased effect with PABA or PABA metabolites of local anesthetics

Increased toxicity with methotrexate, other sulfonamides, co-trimoxazole

**Drug Uptake**
Absorption: Oral: Well absorbed
Serum half-life:
Pyrimethamine: 80-95 hours
Sulfadoxine: 5-8 days
Time to peak serum concentration: Within 2-8 hours
**Pregnancy Risk Factor** C
**Generic Available** No

- **Sulfa-Gyn®** *see* Sulfabenzamide, Sulfacetamide, and Sulfathiazole *on page 939*
- **Sulfalax® [OTC]** *see* Docusate *on page 346*
- **Sulfamethoprim®** *see* Trimethoprim and Sulfamethoxazole *on page 1021*

## Sulfamethoxazole (sul fa meth OKS a zole)

**U.S. Brand Names** Gantanol®; Urobak®
**Canadian Brand Names** Apo®-Sulfamethoxazole
**Therapeutic Category** Antibiotic, Sulfonamide Derivative
**Use** Treatment of urinary tract infections, nocardiosis, toxoplasmosis, acute otitis media, and acute exacerbations of chronic bronchitis due to susceptible organisms
**Usual Dosage** Oral:
Children >2 months: 50-60 mg/kg as single dose followed by 50-60 mg/kg/day divided every 12 hours; maximum: 3 g/24 hours or 75 mg/kg/day
Adults: 2 g stat, 1 g 2-3 times/day; maximum: 3 g/24 hours
**Mechanism of Action** Interferes with bacterial growth by inhibiting bacterial folic acid synthesis through competitive antagonism of PABA
**Local Anesthetic/Vasoconstrictor Precautions** No information available to require special precautions
**Effects on Dental Treatment** No effects or complications reported
**Other Adverse Effects**
>10%:
Central nervous system: Fever, dizziness, headache
Dermatologic: Itching, skin rash, photosensitivity
Gastrointestinal: Anorexia, nausea, vomiting, diarrhea
1% to 10%:
Dermatologic: Lyell's syndrome, Stevens-Johnson syndrome
Hematologic: Granulocytopenia, leukopenia, thrombocytopenia, aplastic anemia, hemolytic anemia
Hepatic: Hepatitis
<1%:
Cardiovascular: Vasculitis
Endocrine & metabolic: Thyroid function disturbance
Genitourinary: Crystalluria
Hepatic: Jaundice
Renal: Hematuria, acute nephropathy, interstitial nephritis
Miscellaneous: Serum sickness-like reactions
**Drug Interactions**
Decreased effect with PABA or PABA metabolites of drugs (ie, procaine, proparacaine, tetracaine)
Increased effect of oral anticoagulants, oral hypoglycemic agents, and methotrexate
**Drug Uptake**
Absorption: Oral: 90%
Serum half-life: 9-12 hours, prolonged with renal impairment
Time to peak serum concentration: Within 3-4 hours
**Pregnancy Risk Factor** B (D at term)
**Generic Available** Yes: Tablet

## Sulfamethoxazole and Phenazopyridine

(sul fa meth OKS a zole & fen az oh PEER i deen)
**U.S. Brand Names** Azo Gantanol®
**Therapeutic Category** Antibiotic, Sulfonamide Derivative
**Use** Treatment of urinary tract infections complicated with pain
**Usual Dosage** Oral: 4 tablets to start, then 2 tablets twice daily for up to 2 days, then switch to sulfamethoxazole only
**Local Anesthetic/Vasoconstrictor Precautions** No information available to require special precautions
**Effects on Dental Treatment** No effects or complications reported
**Other Adverse Effects**
Central nervous system: Confusion, depression, hallucinations, ataxia, seizures, fever, kernicterus in neonates
(Continued)

## Sulfamethoxazole and Phenazopyridine *(Continued)*

Dermatologic: Rash, erythema multiforme, Stevens-Johnson syndrome, epidermal necrolysis
Gastrointestinal: Nausea, vomiting, glossitis, stomatitis, diarrhea, pseudomembranous colitis
Hematologic: Thrombocytopenia, megaloblastic anemia, granulocytopenia, aplastic anemia, hemolysis (with G-6-PD deficiency)
Hepatic: Serum sickness, hepatitis
Renal & genitourinary: Interstitial nephritis

**Drug Interactions** Warfarin, methotrexate

**Pregnancy Risk Factor** B (D at term)

**Generic Available** Yes

- **Sulfamethoxazole and Trimethoprim** *see* Trimethoprim and Sulfamethoxazole *on page 1021*
- **Sulfamylon®** *see* Mafenide *on page 609*

## Sulfanilamide (sul fa NIL a mide)

**U.S. Brand Names** AVC™ Cream; AVC™ Suppository; Vagitrol®

**Therapeutic Category** Antifungal Agent, Vaginal

**Use** Treatment of vulvovaginitis caused by *Candida albicans*

**Usual Dosage** Adults: Female: Insert one applicatorful intravaginally once or twice daily continued through 1 complete menstrual cycle or insert one suppository intravaginally once or twice daily for 30 days

**Mechanism of Action** Interferes with microbial folic acid synthesis and growth via inhibition of para-aminiobenzoic acid metabolism

**Local Anesthetic/Vasoconstrictor Precautions** No information available to require special precautions

**Effects on Dental Treatment** No effects or complications reported

**Other Adverse Effects**

1% to 10%:
Central nervous system: Kernicterus
Dermatologic: Itching, skin rash, exfoliative dermatitis, Stevens-Johnson syndrome
Gastrointestinal: Nausea, vomiting
Hematologic: Agranulocytosis, hemolytic anemia in patients with severe G-6-PD deficiency
Hepatic: Hepatic toxicity
Local: Burning, irritation
Renal: Crystalluria

<1%: Genitourinary: Irritation of penis of sexual partner

**Drug Interactions** No data reported

**Pregnancy Risk Factor** B (D at term)

**Dosage Forms**

Cream, vaginal (AVC™, Vagitrol®): 15% [150 mg/g] (120 g with applicator)
Suppository, vaginal (AVC™): 1.05 g (16s)

**Generic Available** No

## Sulfasalazine (sul fa SAL a zeen)

**U.S. Brand Names** Azulfidine®; Azulfidine® EN-tabs®

**Canadian Brand Names** Apo®-Sulfasalazine; PMS-Sulfasalazine; Salazopyrin®; Salazopyrin EN-Tabs®; S.A.S™

**Therapeutic Category** 5-Aminosalicylic Acid Derivative; Anti-inflammatory Agent

**Use** Management of ulcerative colitis

**Usual Dosage** Oral:

Children >2 years: 40-60 mg/kg/day in 3-6 divided doses, not to exceed 6 g/day; maintenance dose: 20-30 mg/kg/day in 4 divided doses; not to exceed 2 g/day
Adults: 1 g 3-4 times/day, 2 g/day maintenance in divided doses; not to exceed 6 g/day

**Mechanism of Action** May be related to the immunosuppressant properties that have been observed in animal and *in vitro* models, to its affinity for connective tissue, and/or to the relatively high concentration it reaches in serous fluids, the liver and intestinal walls, as demonstrated in autoradiographic studies in animals; sulfasalazine (SS) has also been described as a highly efficient vehicle for carrying its principal metabolites, 5-aminosalicylic acid (5-ASA) and sulfapyridine (SP), to the colon, where a local action for both of them has been postulated; recent clinical studies utilizing rectal administration of SS, SP and 5-ASA have indicated that the major therapeutic action may reside in the 5-ASA moiety

**Local Anesthetic/Vasoconstrictor Precautions** No information available to require special precautions

**Effects on Dental Treatment** No effects or complications reported

**Other Adverse Effects**

>10%:

Central nervous system: Fever, dizziness, headache
Dermatologic: Itching, skin rash, photosensitivity
Gastrointestinal: Anorexia, nausea, vomiting, diarrhea
Genitourinary: Reversible oligospermia

1% to 10%:

Dermatologic: Lyell's syndrome, Stevens-Johnson syndrome
Hematologic: Granulocytopenia, leukopenia, thrombocytopenia, aplastic anemia, hemolytic anemia
Hepatic: Hepatitis

<1%:

Endocrine & metabolic: Thyroid function disturbance
Genitourinary: Crystalluria
Hepatic: Jaundice
Renal: Interstitial nephritis, acute nephropathy, hematuria
Miscellaneous: Serum sickness-like reactions

**Drug Interactions**

Decreased effect with iron, digoxin and PABA or PABA metabolites of drugs (ie, procaine, proparacaine, tetracaine)

Decreased effect of oral anticoagulants, methotrexate, and oral hypoglycemic agents

**Drug Uptake**

Absorption: 10% to 15% of dose is absorbed as unchanged drug from the small intestine

Serum half-life: 5.7-10 hours

**Pregnancy Risk Factor** B (D at term)

**Generic Available** Yes

♦ **Sulfatrim®** *see* Trimethoprim and Sulfamethoxazole *on page 1021*
♦ **Sulfatrim® DS** *see* Trimethoprim and Sulfamethoxazole *on page 1021*
♦ **Sulfa-Trip®** *see* Sulfabenzamide, Sulfacetamide, and Sulfathiazole *on page 939*

## Sulfinpyrazone (sul fin PEER a zone)

**U.S. Brand Names** Anturane®

**Canadian Brand Names** Antazone®; Anturan®; Apo®-Sulfinpyrazone; Novo-Pyrazone; Nu-Sulfinpyrazone

**Therapeutic Category** Uric Acid Lowering Agent

**Use** Treatment of chronic gouty arthritis and intermittent gouty arthritis

**Unlabeled use:** To decrease the incidence of sudden death postmyocardial infarction

**Usual Dosage** Adults: Oral: 100-200 mg twice daily; maximum daily dose: 800 mg

**Mechanism of Action** Acts by increasing the urinary excretion of uric acid, thereby decreasing blood urate levels; this effect is therapeutically useful in treating patients with acute intermittent gout, chronic tophaceous gout, and acts to promote resorption of tophi; also has antithrombic and platelet inhibitory effects

**Local Anesthetic/Vasoconstrictor Precautions** No information available to require special precautions

**Effects on Dental Treatment** No effects or complications reported

**Other Adverse Effects**

>10%: Gastrointestinal: Nausea, vomiting, stomach pain

1% to 10%: Dermatologic: Dermatitis, skin rash

<1%:

Cardiovascular: Flushing
Central nervous system: Dizziness, headache
Dermatologic: Rash
Hematologic: Anemia, leukopenia, increased bleeding time (decreased platelet aggregation)
Hepatic: Hepatic necrosis
Renal: Nephrotic syndrome, polyuria, uric acid stones

**Drug Interactions**

Decreased effect/levels of theophylline, verapamil; decreased uricosuric activity with salicylates, niacins

Increased effect of oral hypoglycemics and anticoagulants

Risk of acetaminophen hepatotoxicity is increased, but therapeutic effects may be reduced

**Drug Uptake**

Absorption: Complete and rapid

Serum half-life, elimination: 2.7-6 hours

(Continued)

## Sulfinpyrazone *(Continued)*

Time to peak serum concentration: 1.6 hours

**Pregnancy Risk Factor** C

**Generic Available** Yes

## Sulfisoxazole (sul fi SOKS a zole)

**U.S. Brand Names** Gantrisin®

**Canadian Brand Names** Novo-Soxazole; Sulfizole®

**Therapeutic Category** Antibiotic, Sulfonamide Derivative

**Use** Treatment of urinary tract infections, otitis media, *Chlamydia*; nocardiosis; treatment of acute pelvic inflammatory disease in prepubertal children; often used in combination with trimethoprim

**Usual Dosage**

Oral (not for use in patients <2 months of age):

Children >2 months: 75 mg/kg stat, followed by 120-150 mg/kg/day in divided doses every 4-6 hours; not to exceed 6 g/day

Pelvic inflammatory disease: 100 mg/kg/day in divided doses every 6 hours; used in combination with ceftriaxone

*Chlamydia trachomatis*: 100 mg/kg/day in divided doses every 6 hours

Adults: 2-4 g stat, 4-8 g/day in divided doses every 4-6 hours

Pelvic inflammatory disease: 500 mg every 6 hours for 21 days; used in combination with ceftriaxone

*Chlamydia trachomatis*: 500 mg every 6 hours for 10 days

Elderly: 2 g stat, then 2-8 g/day in divided doses every 6 hours

Ophthalmic: Children and Adults:

Solution: Instill 1-2 drops to affected eye every 2-3 hours

Ointment: Apply small amount to affected eye 1-3 times/day and at bedtime

**Mechanism of Action** Interferes with bacterial growth by inhibiting bacterial folic acid synthesis through competitive antagonism of PABA

**Local Anesthetic/Vasoconstrictor Precautions** No information available to require special precautions

**Effects on Dental Treatment** No effects or complications reported

**Other Adverse Effects**

>10%:

Central nervous system: Fever, dizziness, headache

Dermatologic: Itching, skin rash, photosensitivity

Gastrointestinal: Anorexia, nausea, vomiting, diarrhea

1% to 10%:

Dermatologic: Lyell's syndrome, Stevens-Johnson syndrome

Hematologic: Granulocytopenia, leukopenia, thrombocytopenia, aplastic anemia, hemolytic anemia

Hepatic: Hepatitis

<1%:

Endocrine & metabolic: Thyroid function disturbance

Genitourinary: Crystalluria

Hepatic: Jaundice

Renal: Interstitial nephritis, acute nephropathy, hematuria

Miscellaneous: Serum sickness-like reactions

**Drug Interactions**

Decreased effect with PABA or PABA metabolites of drugs (ie, procaine, proparacaine, tetracaine), thiopental

Increased effect of oral anticoagulants, methotrexate and oral hypoglycemic agents

**Drug Uptake**

Absorption: Sulfisoxazole acetyl is hydrolyzed in the GI tract to sulfisoxazole which is readily absorbed

Serum half-life: 4-7 hours, prolonged with renal impairment

Time to peak serum concentration: Within 2-3 hours

**Pregnancy Risk Factor** B (D at term)

**Generic Available** Yes

## Sulfisoxazole and Phenazopyridine

(sul fi SOKS a zole & fen az oh PEER i deen)

**U.S. Brand Names** Azo Gantrisin®

**Therapeutic Category** Antibiotic, Sulfonamide Derivative; Local Anesthetic, Urinary

**Use** Treatment of urinary tract infections and nocardiosis

**Usual Dosage** Adults: Oral: 4-6 tablets to start, then 2 tablets 4 times/day for 2 days, then continue with sulfisoxazole only

**Mechanism of Action** Interferes with bacterial growth by inhibiting bacterial folic acid synthesis through competitive antagonism of PABA; phenazopyridine exerts local anesthetic or analgesic action on urinary tract mucosa through an unknown mechanism

**Local Anesthetic/Vasoconstrictor Precautions** No information available to require special precautions

**Effects on Dental Treatment** No effects or complications reported

**Other Adverse Effects**

>10%:

Central nervous system: Fever, dizziness, headache

Dermatologic: Itching, skin rash, photosensitivity

Gastrointestinal: Anorexia, nausea, vomiting, diarrhea

1% to 10%:

Dermatologic: Lyell's syndrome, Stevens-Johnson syndrome

Hematologic: Granulocytopenia, leukopenia, thrombocytopenia, aplastic anemia, hemolytic anemia

Hepatic: Hepatitis

<1%:

Endocrine & metabolic: Thyroid function disturbance

Genitourinary: Crystalluria

Hepatic: Jaundice

Renal: Hematuria, acute nephropathy, interstitial nephritis

Miscellaneous: Serum sickness-like reactions

**Drug Interactions**

Decreased effect with PABA or PABA metabolites of drugs (ie, procaine, proparacaine, tetracaine), thiopental

Increased effect of oral anticoagulants, methotrexate and oral hypoglycemic agents

**Drug Uptake**

Absorption: Sulfisoxazole acetyl is hydrolyzed in the GI tract to sulfisoxazole which is readily absorbed

Serum half-life: 4-7 hours, prolonged with renal impairment

Time to peak serum concentration: Within 2-3 hours

**Pregnancy Risk Factor** B (D at term)

**Generic Available** Yes

♦ **Sulfoxaprim®** *see* Trimethoprim and Sulfamethoxazole *on page 1021*

♦ **Sulfoxaprim® DS** *see* Trimethoprim and Sulfamethoxazole *on page 1021*

## Sulfur and Salicylic Acid (SUL fur & sal i SIL ik AS id)

**U.S. Brand Names** Aveeno® Cleansing Bar [OTC]; Fostex® [OTC]; Pernox® [OTC]; Sastid® Plain Therapeutic Shampoo and Acne Wash [OTC]; Sebulex® [OTC]

**Therapeutic Category** Antiseborrheic Agent, Topical

**Synonyms** Salicylic Acid and Sulfur

**Use** Therapeutic shampoo for dandruff and seborrheal dermatitis; acne skin cleanser

**Usual Dosage** Children and Adults:

Shampoo: Initial: Use daily or every other day; 1-2 treatments/week will usually maintain control

Soap: Use daily or every other day

**Local Anesthetic/Vasoconstrictor Precautions** No information available to require special precautions

**Effects on Dental Treatment** No effects or complications reported

**Other Adverse Effects** Local: Topical preparations containing 2% to 5% sulfur generally are well tolerated, local irritation may occur, concentration >15% is very irritating to the skin, higher concentration (eg, 10% or higher) may cause systemic toxicity (eg, headache, vomiting, muscle cramps, dizziness, collapse)

**Pregnancy Risk Factor** C

**Generic Available** Yes

**Comments** For external use only

## Sulfur and Sulfacetamide Sodium

(SUL fur & sul fa SEE ta mide SOW dee um)

**U.S. Brand Names** Novacet® Topical; Sulfacet-R® Topical

**Therapeutic Category** Acne Products

**Synonyms** Sodium Sulfacetamide and Sulfur; Sulfacetamide Sodium and Sulfur

**Use** Aid in the treatment of acne vulgaris, acne rosacea and seborrheic dermatitis

**Usual Dosage** Topical: Apply in a thin film 1-3 times/day

**Local Anesthetic/Vasoconstrictor Precautions** No information available to require special precautions

**Effects on Dental Treatment** No effects or complications reported

**Generic Available** Yes

## Sulindac (sul IN dak)

**Related Information**

Rheumatoid Arthritis and Osteoarthritis *on page 1092*
Temporomandibular Dysfunction (TMD) *on page 1149*

**U.S. Brand Names** Clinoril®

**Canadian Brand Names** Apo®-Sulin; Novo-Sundac

**Therapeutic Category** Analgesic, Non-narcotic; Anti-inflammatory Agent; Nonsteroidal Anti-inflammatory Drug (NSAID), Oral

**Use** Management of inflammatory disease, rheumatoid disorders; acute gouty arthritis; structurally similar to indomethacin but acts like aspirin; safest NSAID for use in mild renal impairment

**Usual Dosage** Maximum therapeutic response may not be realized for up to 3 weeks. Oral:

Children: Dose not established

Adults: 150-200 mg twice daily or 300-400 mg once daily; not to exceed 400 mg/day

**Mechanism of Action** Inhibits prostaglandin synthesis by decreasing the activity of the enzyme, cyclo-oxygenase, which results in decreased formation of prostaglandin precursors

**Local Anesthetic/Vasoconstrictor Precautions** No information available to require special precautions

**Effects on Dental Treatment** NSAID formulations are known to reversibly decrease platelet aggregation via mechanisms different than observed with aspirin. The dentist should be aware of the potential of abnormal coagulation. Caution should also be exercised in the use of NSAIDs in patients already on anticoagulant therapy with drugs such as warfarin (Coumadin®).

**Other Adverse Effects**

>10%:

- Central nervous system: Dizziness
- Dermatologic: Skin rash
- Gastrointestinal: Abdominal cramps, heartburn, indigestion, nausea

1% to 10%:

- Central nervous system: Headache, nervousness
- Dermatologic: Itching
- Endocrine & metabolic: Fluid retention
- Gastrointestinal: Vomiting
- Otic: Tinnitus

<1%:

- Cardiovascular: Congestive heart failure, hypertension, arrhythmias, tachycardia
- Central nervous system: Confusion, hallucinations, aseptic meningitis, mental depression, drowsiness, insomnia
- Dermatologic: Urticaria, erythema multiforme, toxic epidermal necrolysis, Stevens-Johnson syndrome, angioedema
- Endocrine & metabolic: Polydipsia, hot flashes
- Gastrointestinal: Gastritis, GI ulceration
- Genitourinary: Cystitis
- Hematologic: Agranulocytosis, anemia, hemolytic anemia, bone marrow suppression, leukopenia, thrombocytopenia
- Hepatic: Hepatitis
- Neuromuscular & skeletal: Peripheral neuropathy
- Ocular: Toxic amblyopia, blurred vision, conjunctivitis, dry eyes
- Otic: Decreased hearing
- Renal: Polyuria, acute renal failure
- Respiratory: Allergic rhinitis, dyspnea, epistaxis

**Drug Interactions**

Decreased effect: Aspirin may decrease sulindac serum concentrations

Increased toxicity: Sulindac may increase digoxin, methotrexate, and lithium serum concentrations; other nonsteroidal anti-inflammatories may increase adverse gastrointestinal effects of sulindac

**Drug Uptake**

Absorption: 90%

Serum half-life:

- Parent drug: 7 hours
- Active metabolite: 18 hours

**Pregnancy Risk Factor** B (D at term)

**Dosage Forms** Tablet: 150 mg, 200 mg

**Generic Available** Yes

♦ **Sultrin™** *see* Sulfabenzamide, Sulfacetamide, and Sulfathiazole *on page 939*

♦ **Sumacal® [OTC]** *see* Glucose Polymers *on page 470*

## Sumatriptan Succinate (SOO ma trip tan SUKS i nate)

**U.S. Brand Names** Imitrex®

**Therapeutic Category** Antimigraine Agent; Serotonin Agonist

**Use** Acute treatment of migraine with or without aura

**Unlabeled use:** Cluster headaches

**Usual Dosage** Adults:

Oral: 25 mg (taken with fluids); maximum recommended dose is 100 mg. If a satisfactory response has not been obtained at 2 hours, a second dose of up to 100 mg may be given. Efficacy of this second dose has not been examined. If a headache returns, additional doses may be taken at intervals of at least 2 hours up to a daily maximum of 300 mg. There is no evidence that an initial dose of 100 mg provides substantially greater relief than 25 mg.

Intranasal: Single dose of 5, 10, or 20 mg administered in one nostril; a 10 mg dose may be achieved by administration of a single 5 mg dose in each nostril; if headache returns, the dose may be repeated once after 2 hours, not to exceed a total daily dose of 40 mg

S.C.: 6 mg; a second injection may be administered at least 1 hour after the initial dose, but not more than two injections in a 24-hour period

**Mechanism of Action** Selective agonist for serotonin ($5HT_{1-D}$ receptor) in cranial arteries to cause vasoconstriction and reduces sterile inflammation associated with antidromic neuronal transmission correlating with relief of migraine

**Local Anesthetic/Vasoconstrictor Precautions** No information available to require special precautions

**Effects on Dental Treatment** No effects or complications reported

**Other Adverse Effects**

>10%:

- Central nervous system: Dizziness
- Endocrine & metabolic: Hot flashes
- Local: Injection site reaction

1% to 10%:

- Cardiovascular: Tightness in chest
- Central nervous system: Burning sensation, drowsiness, headache
- Gastrointestinal: Abdominal discomfort, mouth discomfort, jaw discomfort
- Neuromuscular & skeletal: Myalgia, neck pain, weakness, numbness
- Miscellaneous: Sweating

<1%:

- Dermatologic: Skin rashes
- Endocrine & metabolic: Polydipsia, dehydration, dysmenorrhea
- Gastrointestinal: Thirst
- Genitourinary: Dysuria
- Renal: Renal calculus
- Respiratory: Dyspnea
- Miscellaneous: Hiccups

**Drug Interactions** MAO-A inhibitors cause two-fold increase in the area under the sumatriptan plasma concentration-time curve; no effect seen with MAO-B inhibitor

**Drug Uptake** After S.C. administration:

Serum half-life, terminal: 115 minutes

Time to peak serum concentration: 5-20 minutes

**Pregnancy Risk Factor** C

**Dosage Forms**

Injection: 12 mg/mL (0.5 mL, 2 mL)

Spray, nasal: 5 mg (100 mcL); 20 mg (100 mcL)

Tablet: 25 mg, 50 mg

**Generic Available** No

♦ **Sumycin®** *see* Tetracycline *on page 965*
♦ **Sunscreen, PABA-Free** *see* Methoxycinnamate and Oxybenzone *on page 656*
♦ **SuperChar® [OTC]** *see* Charcoal *on page 219*
♦ **Supprelin™** *see* Histrelin *on page 498*
♦ **Suppress® [OTC]** *see* Dextromethorphan *on page 314*
♦ **Suprax®** *see* Cefixime *on page 201*

## Suprofen (soo PROE fen)

**U.S. Brand Names** Profenal®

**Therapeutic Category** Nonsteroidal Anti-inflammatory Drug (NSAID), Ophthalmic

**Use** Inhibition of intraoperative miosis

**Usual Dosage** Adults: On day of surgery, instill 2 drops in conjunctival sac at 3, 2, and 1 hour prior to surgery; or 2 drops in sac every 4 hours, while awake, the day preceding surgery

(Continued)

## Suprofen *(Continued)*

**Mechanism of Action** Inhibits prostaglandin synthesis

**Local Anesthetic/Vasoconstrictor Precautions** No information available to require special precautions

**Effects on Dental Treatment** NSAID formulations are known to reversibly decrease platelet aggregation via mechanisms different than observed with aspirin. The dentist should be aware of the potential of abnormal coagulation. Caution should also be exercised in the use of NSAIDs in patients already on anticoagulant therapy with drugs such as warfarin (Coumadin®).

**Other Adverse Effects**

1% to 10%: Topical: Transient burning or stinging, redness, iritis

<1%:

Systemic: Chemosis, photophobia

Topical: Discomfort, pain, punctate epithelial staining

**Drug Interactions** Decreased effect: When used concurrently with suprofen, acetylcholine chloride and carbachol ophthalmic preparations may be ineffective

**Drug Uptake**

Half-life, elimination: 2-4 hours

Time to peak serum concentration: ~1 hour

**Pregnancy Risk Factor** C

**Generic Available** No

- **Surbex® [OTC]** *see* Vitamin B Complex *on page 1050*
- **Surbex-T® Filmtabs® [OTC]** *see* Vitamin B Complex With Vitamin C *on page 1050*
- **Surbex® with C Filmtabs® [OTC]** *see* Vitamin B Complex With Vitamin C *on page 1050*
- **Surfak® [OTC]** *see* Docusate *on page 346*
- **Surgicel®** *see* Cellulose, Oxidized *on page 213*
- **Surgicel® Absorbable Hemostat** *see* Cellulose, Oxidized Regenerated *on page 213*
- **Surmontil®** *see* Trimipramine *on page 1023*
- **Survanta®** *see* Beractant *on page 135*
- **Sus-Phrine®** *see* Epinephrine (Dental) *on page 374*
- **Sustaire®** *see* Theophylline *on page 969*
- **Sustiva™** *see* Efavirenz *on page 364*
- **Sween® Cream [OTC]** *see* Methylbenzethonium Chloride *on page 658*
- **Swim-Ear® Otic [OTC]** *see* Boric Acid *on page 147*
- **Syllact® [OTC]** *see* Psyllium *on page 865*
- **Symmetrel®** *see* Amantadine *on page 57*
- **Synacol® CF [OTC]** *see* Guaifenesin and Dextromethorphan *on page 479*
- **Synagis®** *see* Palivizumab *on page 761*
- **Synalar®** *see* Fluocinolone *on page 440*
- **Synalar-HP®** *see* Fluocinolone *on page 440*
- **Synalgos®-DC** *see* Dihydrocodeine Compound *on page 331*
- **Synarel®** *see* Nafarelin *on page 697*
- **Synemol®** *see* Fluocinolone *on page 440*
- **Synthetic Lung Surfactant** *see* Colfosceril Palmitate *on page 275*
- **Synthroid®** *see* Levothyroxine *on page 585*
- **Syntocinon®** *see* Oxytocin *on page 759*
- **Syracol-CF® [OTC]** *see* Guaifenesin and Dextromethorphan *on page 479*
- **Systemic Viral Diseases** *see page 1115*
- **Tac™-3** *see* Triamcinolone *on page 1010*
- **Tac™-40** *see* Triamcinolone *on page 1010*
- **TACE®** *see* Chlorotrianisene *on page 230*

## Tacrine (TAK reen)

**U.S. Brand Names** Cognex®

**Therapeutic Category** Cholinergic Agent

**Use** Treatment of mild to moderate dementia of the Alzheimer's type

**Usual Dosage** Adults: Initial: 10 mg 4 times/day; may increase by 40 mg/day adjusted every 6 weeks; maximum: 160 mg/day; best administered separate from meal times; see table.

Patients with clinical jaundice confirmed by elevated total bilirubin (>3 mg/dL) should not be rechallenged with tacrine

**Dose Adjustment Based Upon Transaminase Elevations**

| ALT | Regimen |
|---|---|
| ≤3 x ULN* | Continue titration |
| >3 to ≤5 x ULN | Decrease dose by 40 mg/day, resume when ALT returns to normal |
| >5 x ULN | Stop treatment, may rechallenge upon return of ALT to normal |

*ULN = upper limit of normal.

**Mechanism of Action** A deficiency of cortical acetylcholine is believed to account for some of the clinical manifestations of mild to moderate dementia. Tacrine probably acts by elevating acetylcholine concentrations in the cortical areas by slowing the degradation of acetylcholine released by still intact cholinergic neurons.

**Local Anesthetic/Vasoconstrictor Precautions** No information available to require special precautions

**Effects on Dental Treatment** No effects or complications reported

**Other Adverse Effects** 1% to 10%:

Gastrointestinal: Diarrhea, nausea, abdominal discomfort, anorexia
Renal: Polyuria
Miscellaneous: Sweating, ataxia

**Warnings/Precautions** The use of tacrine has been associated with elevations in serum transaminases; serum transaminases (specifically ALT) must be monitored throughout therapy; use extreme caution in patients with current evidence of a history of abnormal liver function tests; use caution in patients with bladder outlet obstruction, asthma, and sick-sinus syndrome (tacrine may cause bradycardia). Also, patients with cardiovascular disease, asthma, or peptic ulcer should use cautiously.

**Drug Interactions**

Cholinergic drugs: Increased cholinergic effects such as diarrhea and abdominal discomfort seen when tacrine is combined with other cholinergics such as bethanechol
Anticholinergics: Tacrine may inhibit the therapeutic effects of anticholinergics, and anticholinergics may inhibit the effects of tacrine
Cigarette smoking: Tobacco appears to significantly reduce the plasma concentrations of tacrine
Cimetidine (Tagamet®) increases tacrine plasma levels
Enoxacin (Penetrex) may be a potent inhibitor of liver metabolism of tacrine
Fluvoxamine (Luvox®) markedly increases tacrine plasma levels and may increase tacrine adverse effects
Levodopa: Tacrine may inhibit the effects of levodopa in patients with parkinsonism
Propranolol: Both tacrine and propranolol can slow heart rate; additive bradycardia is a possibility
Theophylline: Tacrine can markedly increase theophylline plasma levels which can lead to theophylline toxicity

**Drug Uptake**

Peak plasma concentrations: 1-2 hours
Plasma bound: 55%
Serum half-life, elimination: 2-4 hours, steady-state achieved in 24-36 hours

**Pregnancy Risk Factor** C

**Dosage Forms** Capsule, as hydrochloride: 10 mg, 20 mg, 30 mg, 40 mg

**Generic Available** No

## Tacrolimus (ta KROE li mus)

**U.S. Brand Names** Prograf®

**Therapeutic Category** Immunosuppressant Agent

**Use** Potent immunosuppressive drug used in liver, kidney, heart, lung, or small bowel transplant recipients

**Usual Dosage**

Children:
- I.V. continuous infusion: 0.1 mg/kg/day
- Oral: 0.3 mg/kg/day

Adults:
- I.V. continuous infusion: Initial (at least 6 hours after transplantation): 0.05-0.1 mg/kg/day
- Oral (within 2-3 days): 0.15-0.3 mg/kg/day in divided doses every 12 hours; give 8-12 hours after discontinuation of the I.V. infusion; may gradually adjust (decrease) maintenance dose via pharmacokinetic monitoring

**Mechanism of Action** Suppressed humoral immunity (inhibits T-lymphocyte activation); produced by the fungus streptomyces tsukubaensis

(Continued)

## Tacrolimus *(Continued)*

**Local Anesthetic/Vasoconstrictor Precautions** No information available to require special precautions

**Effects on Dental Treatment** No effects or complications reported

**Other Adverse Effects**

>10%:
- Cardiovascular: Hypertension, peripheral edema
- Central nervous system: Headache, insomnia, pain, fever
- Dermatologic: Pruritus
- Endocrine & metabolic: Hypo-/hyperkalemia, hyperglycemia, hypomagnesemia
- Gastrointestinal: Diarrhea, nausea, anorexia, vomiting, abdominal pain
- Hematologic: Anemia, leukocytosis
- Hepatic: LFT abnormalities, ascites
- Neuromuscular & skeletal: Tremors, paresthesias, back pain, weakness
- Renal: Nephrotoxicity, elevated creatinine and BUN
- Respiratory: Pleural effusion, atelectasis, dyspnea

1% to 10%:
- Dermatologic: Rash
- Gastrointestinal: Constipation
- Genitourinary: Urinary tract infection
- Hematologic: Thrombocytopenia
- Renal: Oliguria

**Drug Interactions**

Antacids: Tacrolimus absorption impaired (separate administration by at least 2 hours)

Nephrotoxic antibiotics potentially increase tacrolimus associated nephrotoxicity; amphotericin B potentially increases tacrolimus associated nephrotoxicity

Agents which may increase tacrolimus plasma concentrations and consequently its effect and toxicity include erythromycin, clarithromycin, clotrimazole, fluconazole, itraconazole, ketoconazole, diltiazem, nicardipine, verapamil, bromocriptine, cimetidine, danazol, metoclopramide, methylprednisolone, cyclosporine (synergistic immunosuppression)

Agents which may decrease tacrolimus plasma concentrations and consequently its effect include rifampin, rifabutin, phenytoin, phenobarbital, and carbamazepine

**Drug Uptake**

Absorption: Better in small bowel patients with a closed stoma; unlike cyclosporine, clamping of the T-tube in liver transplant patients does not alter trough concentrations or AUC; food within 15 minutes of administration decreases absorption (27%); $T_{max}$: 0.5-4 hours

Serum half-life, elimination: 12 hours (range: 4-40 hours, twice as fast in children)

**Pregnancy Risk Factor** C; because FK-506 does cross into breast milk, breast feeding is not advised while tacrolimus therapy is ongoing

**Generic Available** No


- ♦ **Tagamet®** *see* Cimetidine *on page 249*
- ♦ **Tagamet® HB [OTC]** *see* Cimetidine *on page 249*
- ♦ **Talacen®** *see* Pentazocine Compound *on page 780*
- ♦ **Talwin®** *see* Pentazocine *on page 779*
- ♦ **Talwin® Compound** *see* Pentazocine Compound *on page 780*
- ♦ **Talwin® NX** *see* Pentazocine *on page 779*
- ♦ **Tambocor™** *see* Flecainide *on page 433*
- ♦ **Tamine® [OTC]** *see* Brompheniramine and Phenylpropanolamine *on page 153*


## Tamoxifen (ta MOKS i fen)

**U.S. Brand Names** Nolvadex®

**Canadian Brand Names** Alpha-Tamoxifen®; Apo®-Tamox; Novo-Tamoxifen; Tamofen®; Tamone®

**Therapeutic Category** Antineoplastic Agent, Hormone (Antiestrogen)

**Use** Palliative or adjunctive treatment of advanced breast cancer; reduce the occurrence of contralateral breast cancer in patients receiving adjuvant tamoxifen therapy for breast cancer; reduce the incidence of breast cancer in women at high risk for breast cancer

**Unlabeled use:** Treatment of mastalgia, gynecomastia, male breast cancer, and pancreatic carcinoma. Studies have shown tamoxifen to be effective in the treatment of primary breast cancer in elderly women. Comparative studies with other antineoplastic agents in elderly women with breast cancer had more favorable survival rates with tamoxifen. Initiation of hormone therapy rather than chemotherapy is justified for elderly patients with metastatic breast cancer who are responsive.

**Usual Dosage** Oral (**refer to individual protocols**):

Adults: 10-20 mg twice daily in the morning and evening

High-dose therapy is under investigation

**Mechanism of Action** Competitively binds to estrogen receptors on tumors and other tissue targets, producing a nuclear complex that decreases DNA synthesis and inhibits estrogen effects; nonsteroidal agent with potent antiestrogenic properties which compete with estrogen for binding sites in breast and other tissues; cells accumulate in the $G_0$ and $G_1$ phases; therefore, tamoxifen is cytostatic rather than cytocidal.

**Local Anesthetic/Vasoconstrictor Precautions** No information available to require special precautions

**Effects on Dental Treatment** No effects or complications reported

**Other Adverse Effects**

>10%:

Gastrointestinal: Little to mild nausea (10%), vomiting, weight gain

General: Flushing, increased bone and tumor pain and local disease flare shortly after starting therapy; this will subside rapidly, but patients should be aware of this since many may discontinue the drug due to the side effects; skin rash, hepatotoxicity

Hematologic: Myelosuppressive, transient thrombocytopenia occurs in ~24% of patients receiving 10-20 mg/day; platelet counts return to normal within several weeks in spite of continued administration; leukopenia has also been reported and does resolve during continued therapy; anemia has also been reported

1% to 10%:

Cardiovascular: Thromboembolism; tamoxifen has been associated with the occurrence of venous thrombosis and pulmonary embolism; arterial thrombosis has also been described in a few case reports

Central nervous system: Lightheadedness, depression, dizziness, headache, lassitude, mental confusion

Dermatologic: Rash

Endocrine & metabolic: Hypercalcemia may occur in patients with bone metastases; galactorrhea and vitamin deficiency, menstrual irregularities

Genitourinary: Vaginal bleeding or discharge, endometriosis, priapism, possible endometrial cancer

Neuromuscular & skeletal: Weakness

Ocular: Ophthalmologic effects (visual acuity changes, cataracts, or retinopathy), corneal opacities

**Drug Interactions** Increased toxicity:

Allopurinol results in exacerbation of allopurinol-induced hepatotoxicity

Cyclosporine may result in increased cyclosporine serum levels

Warfarin results in significant enhancement of the anticoagulant effects of warfarin; has been speculated that a decrease in antitumor effect of tamoxifen may also occur due to alterations in the percentage of active tamoxifen metabolites

**Drug Uptake**

Absorption: Well absorbed from GI tract

Serum half-life: 7 days

Time to peak serum concentration: Oral: Within 4-7 hours

**Pregnancy Risk Factor** D

**Dosage Forms** Tablet, as citrate: 10 mg, 20 mg

**Generic Available** Yes

## Tamsulosin (tam SOO loe sin)

**U.S. Brand Names** Flomax®

**Therapeutic Category** Alpha-Adrenergic Blocking Agent

**Synonyms** Tamsulosin Hydrochloride

**Use** Treatment of signs and symptoms of benign prostatic hyperplasia (BPH)

**Usual Dosage** Oral: Adults: 0.4 mg once daily ~30 minutes after the same meal each day

**Mechanism of Action** An antagonist of $alpha_{1A}$ adrenoceptors in the prostate. Three subtypes identified: $alpha_{1A}$, $alpha_{1B}$, $alpha_{1D}$ have distribution that differs between human organs and tissue. Approximately 70% of the $alpha_1$-receptors in human prostate are of $alpha_{1A}$ subtype. The symptoms associated with benign prostatic hyperplasia (BPH) are related to bladder outlet obstruction, which is comprised of two underlying components: static and dynamic. Static is related to an increase in prostate size, partially caused by a proliferation of smooth muscle cells in the prostatic stroma. Severity of BPH symptoms and the degree of urethral obstruction do not correlate well with the size of the prostate. Dynamic is a function of an increase in smooth muscle tone in the prostate and bladder neck leading to constriction of the bladder outlet. Smooth muscle tone is mediated by

(Continued)

## Tamsulosin *(Continued)*

the sympathetic nervous stimulation of $alpha_1$ adrenoceptors, which are abundant in the prostate, prostatic capsule, prostatic urethra, and bladder neck. Blockade of these adrenoceptors can cause smooth muscles in the bladder neck and prostate to relax, resulting in an improvement in urine flow rate and a reduction in symptoms of BPH.

**Local Anesthetic/Vasoconstrictor Precautions** No information available to require special precautions

**Effects on Dental Treatment** No effects or complications reported

**Drug Uptake**

Absorption: >90%

Peak concentrations:

$C_{max}$: Fasting: 40% to 70% increase

$T_{max}$:

Fasting: 4-5 hours

With food: 6-7 hours

Half-life:

Healthy volunteers: 9-13 hours

Target population: 14-15 hours

**Dosage Forms** Capsule, as hydrochloride: 0.4 mg

- **Tamsulosin Hydrochloride** *see* Tamsulosin *on previous page*
- **Tanac® [OTC]** *see* Benzocaine *on page 128*
- **Tanoral® Tablet** *see* Chlorpheniramine, Pyrilamine, and Phenylephrine *on page 238*
- **Tao®** *see* Troleandomycin *on page 1028*
- **Tapazole®** *see* Methimazole *on page 648*
- **Taractan®** *see* Chlorprothixene *on page 240*
- **Tarka®** *see* Trandolapril and Verapamil *on page 1004*
- **Tasmar®** *see* Tolcapone *on page 995*
- **Tavist®** *see* Clemastine *on page 257*
- **Tavist®-1 [OTC]** *see* Clemastine *on page 257*
- **Tavist-D®** *see* Clemastine and Phenylpropanolamine *on page 258*
- **Taxol®** *see* Paclitaxel *on page 760*
- **Taxotere®** *see* Docetaxel *on page 346*

## Tazarotene (taz AR oh teen)

**U.S. Brand Names** Tazorac®

**Therapeutic Category** Keratolytic Agent

**Use** Topical treatment of facial acne fulgaris; topical treatment of stable plaque psoriasis of up to 20% body surface area involvement

**Usual Dosage** Children >12 years and Adults: Topical:

Acne: Cleanse the face gently. After the skin is dry, apply a thin film of tazarotene (2 mg/cm²) once daily, in the evening, to the skin where the acne lesions appear. Use enough to cover the entire affected area. Tazarotene was investigated ≤12 weeks during clinical trials for acne.

Psoriasis: Apply tazarotene once daily, in the evening, to psoriatic lesions using enough (2 mg/cm²) to cover only the lesion with a thin film to no more than 20% of body surface area. If a bath or shower is taken prior to application, dry the skin before applying the gel. Because unaffected skin may be more susceptible to irritation, avoid application of tazarotene to these areas. Tazarotene was investigated for up to 12 months during clinical trials for psoriasis.

**Local Anesthetic/Vasoconstrictor Precautions** No information available to require special precautions

**Effects on Dental Treatment** No effects or complications reported

**Pregnancy Risk Factor** X

**Dosage Forms** Gel: 0.05% (30 g, 100 g); 0.1% (30 g, 100 g)

- **Tazicef®** *see* Ceftazidime *on page 207*
- **Tazidime®** *see* Ceftazidime *on page 207*
- **Tazorac®** *see* Tazarotene *on this page*
- **3TC** *see* Lamivudine *on page 571*
- **Tear Drop® Solution [OTC]** *see* Artificial Tears *on page 97*
- **TearGard® Ophthalmic Solution [OTC]** *see* Artificial Tears *on page 97*
- **Teargen® Ophthalmic Solution [OTC]** *see* Artificial Tears *on page 97*
- **Tearisol® Solution [OTC]** *see* Artificial Tears *on page 97*
- **Tears Naturale® Free Solution [OTC]** *see* Artificial Tears *on page 97*
- **Tears Naturale® II Solution [OTC]** *see* Artificial Tears *on page 97*
- **Tears Naturale® Solution [OTC]** *see* Artificial Tears *on page 97*
- **Tears Plus® Solution [OTC]** *see* Artificial Tears *on page 97*

- **Tears Renewed® Solution [OTC]** *see* Artificial Tears *on page 97*
- **Tebamide®** *see* Trimethobenzamide *on page 1020*
- **Teczem®** *see* Enalapril and Diltiazem *on page 368*
- **Tedral®** *see* Theophylline, Ephedrine, and Phenobarbital *on page 974*
- **Tegison®** *see* Etretinate *on page 416*
- **Tegopen®** *see* Cloxacillin *on page 268*
- **Tegretol®** *see* Carbamazepine *on page 185*
- **Tegretol®-XR** *see* Carbamazepine *on page 185*
- **Telachlor®** *see* Chlorpheniramine *on page 231*
- **Teladar®** *see* Betamethasone *on page 136*
- **Teldrin® [OTC]** *see* Chlorpheniramine *on page 231*


## Telmisartan

**U.S. Brand Names** Micardis®

**Therapeutic Category** Angiotensin II Antagonist

**Use** Treatment of hypertension; may be used alone or in combination with other antihypertensive agents

**Usual Dosage** Adults: Oral: Initial: 40 mg once daily; usual maintenance dose range: 20-80 mg/day. Patients with volume depletion should be initiated on the lower dosage with close supervision.

**Mechanism of Action** Telmisartan is a nonpeptide angiotensin receptor antagonist. Angiotensin II acts as a vasoconstrictor. In addition to causing direct vasoconstriction, angiotensin II also stimulates the release of aldosterone. Once aldosterone is released, sodium as well as water are reabsorbed. The end result is an elevation in blood pressure. Telmisartan binds to the AT1 angiotensin II receptor. This binding prevents angiotensin II from binding to the receptor thereby blocking the vasoconstriction and the aldosterone secreting effects of angiotensin II.

**Local Anesthetic/Vasoconstrictor Precautions** No information available to require special precautions

**Effects on Dental Treatment** No effects or complications reported

**Other Adverse Effects**

1% to 10%:

- Cardiovascular: Hypertension (1%), chest pain (1%), peripheral edema (1%)
- Central nervous system: Headache (1%), dizziness (1%), pain (1%), fatigue (1%)
- Gastrointestinal: Diarrhea (3%), dyspepsia (1%), nausea (1%), abdominal pain (1%)
- Genitourinary: Urinary tract infection (1%)
- Neuromuscular & skeletal: Back pain (3%), myalgia (1%)
- Respiratory: Upper respiratory infection (7%), sinusitis (3%), pharyngitis (1%), cough (1.6%)
- Miscellaneous: Flu-like syndrome (1%)

<1%: Angioedema, allergic reaction, elevated liver enzymes, decrease in hemoglobin, increased serum creatinine and BUN, impotence, sweating, flushing, fever, malaise, palpitations, angina, tachycardia, abnormal EKG, insomnia, anxiety, nervousness, migraine, vertigo, depression, somnolence, paresthesia, involuntary muscle contractions, constipation, flatulence, dry mouth, hemorrhoids, gastroenteritis, enteritis, reflux, toothache, gout, hypercholesterolemia, diabetes mellitus, arthritis, arthralgia, leg cramps, fungal infection, abscess, otitis media, asthma, dyspnea, bronchitis, rhinitis, epistaxis, dermatitis, eczema, pruritus, rash, frequent urination, cystitis, abnormal vision, conjunctivitis, tinnitus, earache, cerebrovascular disorder

**Drug Interactions** May increase serum digoxin concentrations; telmisartan is not metabolized by cytochrome P-450. Telmisartan decreased the trough concentrations of warfarin during concurrent therapy, however INR was not changed.

**Drug Uptake**

- Onset of action: 1-2 hours
- Duration: Up to 24 hours
- Half-life, terminal: ~24 hours
- Time to peak: 0.5-1 hour

**Pregnancy Risk Factor** C (1st trimester); D (2nd & 3rd trimester)

## Temazepam (te MAZ e pam)

**U.S. Brand Names** Restoril®

**Canadian Brand Names** Apo®-Temazepam

**Therapeutic Category** Benzodiazepine; Hypnotic; Sedative

**Use** Treatment of anxiety and as an adjunct in the treatment of depression; also may be used in the management of panic attacks; transient insomnia and sleep latency

(Continued)

## Temazepam *(Continued)*

**Usual Dosage** Adults: Oral: 15-30 mg at bedtime; 15 mg in elderly or debilitated patients

**Mechanism of Action** Benzodiazepine anxiolytic sedative that produces CNS depression at the subcortical level, except at high doses, whereby it works at the cortical level; causes minimal change in REM sleep patterns

**Local Anesthetic/Vasoconstrictor Precautions** No information available to require special precautions

**Effects on Dental Treatment** >10% of patients will exhibit significant dry mouth; normal salivary flow returns with cessation of drug therapy

**Other Adverse Effects**

1% to 10%:

Central nervous system: Drowsiness, headache, fatigue, nervousness, lethargy, dizziness, "hangover" feeling, anxiety, depression, euphoria, confusion, nightmares, vertigo

Gastrointestinal: Nausea, xerostomia, diarrhea, abdominal discomfort

Neuromuscular & skeletal: Weakness

Ocular: Blurred vision

<1%:

Cardiovascular: Palpitations

Central nervous system: Ataxia, amnesia, hallucinations

Gastrointestinal: Anorexia, vomiting

Neuromuscular & skeletal: Backache, tremor

Ocular: Burning

Respiratory: Dyspnea

Miscellaneous: Diaphoresis

**Warnings/Precautions** Safety and efficacy in children <18 years of age have not been established; do not use in pregnant women; may cause drug dependency; avoid abrupt discontinuance in patients with prolonged therapy or seizure disorders; use with caution in patients receiving other CNS depressants, in patients with hepatic dysfunction, and the elderly

**Drug Interactions** Increased effect of CNS depressants; contraindicated with alcohol

**Drug Uptake**

Serum half-life: 9.5-12.4 hours

Time to peak serum concentration: Within 2-3 hours

**Pregnancy Risk Factor** X

**Dosage Forms** Capsule: 7.5 mg, 15 mg, 30 mg

**Generic Available** Yes

♦ **Temazin® Cold Syrup [OTC]** *see* Chlorpheniramine and Phenylpropanolamine *on page 233*

♦ **Temovate®** *see* Clobetasol *on page 260*

♦ **Temporomandibular Dysfunction (TMD)** *see page 1149*

♦ **Tempra® [OTC]** *see* Acetaminophen *on page 27*

♦ **Tenex®** *see* Guanfacine *on page 485*

## Teniposide (ten i POE side)

**U.S. Brand Names** Vumon Injection

**Therapeutic Category** Antineoplastic Agent, Miscellaneous

**Synonyms** EPT; VM-26

**Use** Treatment of Hodgkin's and non-Hodgkin's lymphomas, acute lymphocytic leukemia, bladder carcinoma and neuroblastoma

**Usual Dosage** I.V.:

Children: 130 mg/m$^2$/week, increasing to 150 mg/m$^2$ after 3 weeks and up to 180 mg/m$^2$ after 6 weeks

Adults: 50-180 mg/m$^2$ once or twice weekly for 4-6 weeks or 20-60 mg/m$^2$/day for 5 days

Acute lymphoblastic leukemia (ALL): 165 mg/m$^2$ twice weekly for 8-9 doses **or** 250 mg/m$^2$ weekly for 4-8 weeks

Small cell lung cancer: 80-90 mg/m$^2$/day for 5 days

**Mechanism of Action** Inhibits mitotic activity; inhibits cells from entering mitosis

**Local Anesthetic/Vasoconstrictor Precautions** No information available to require special precautions

**Effects on Dental Treatment** No effects or complications reported

**Other Adverse Effects**

>10%:

Gastrointestinal: Mucositis, nausea, vomiting, diarrhea

Hematologic: Myelosuppression, leukopenia, neutropenia, thrombocytopenia

Miscellaneous: Infection

1% to 10%:
- Cardiovascular: Hypotension
- Central nervous system: Fever
- Dermatologic: Alopecia, rash
- Hematologic: Hemorrhage
- Miscellaneous: Hypersensitivity

<1%:
- Endocrine & metabolic: Metabolic abnormalities
- Hepatic: Hepatic dysfunction
- Neuromuscular & skeletal: Peripheral neurotoxicity
- Renal: Renal dysfunction

**Drug Interactions** Increased toxicity:

Methotrexate: Alteration of MTX transport has been found as a slow efflux of MTX and its polyglutamated form out of the cell, leading to intercellular accumulation of MTX

Sodium salicylate, sulfamethizole, tolbutamide: displace teniposide from protein-binding sites - could cause substantial increases in free drug levels, resulting in potentiation of toxicity

**Drug Uptake** Serum half-life: 5 hours

**Pregnancy Risk Factor** D

**Generic Available** No


- ♦ **Ten-K®** *see* Potassium Chloride *on page 822*
- ♦ **Tenoretic®** *see* Atenolol and Chlorthalidone *on page 106*
- ♦ **Tenormin®** *see* Atenolol *on page 105*
- ♦ **Tenuate®** *see* Diethylpropion *on page 325*
- ♦ **Tenuate® Dospan®** *see* Diethylpropion *on page 325*
- ♦ **Terak® Ophthalmic Ointment** *see* Oxytetracycline and Polymyxin B *on page 759*
- ♦ **Terazol®** *see* Terconazole *on page 959*


## Terazosin (ter AY zoe sin)

**Related Information**

Cardiovascular Diseases *on page 1066*

**U.S. Brand Names** Hytrin®

**Therapeutic Category** Alpha-Adrenergic Blockers - Peripheral-Acting (Alpha$_1$-Blockers)

**Use** Management of mild to moderate hypertension; considered a step 2 drug in stepped approach to hypertension; benign prostate hypertrophy

**Usual Dosage** Adults: Oral:

Hypertension: Initial: 1 mg at bedtime; slowly increase dose to achieve desired blood pressure, up to 20 mg/day; usual dose: 1-5 mg/day

Dosage reduction may be needed when adding a diuretic or other antihypertensive agent; if drug is discontinued for greater than several days, consider beginning with initial dose and retitrate as needed; dosage may be given on a twice daily regimen if response is diminished at 24 hours and hypotensive is observed at 2-4 hours following a dose

Benign prostatic hypertrophy: Initial: 1 mg at bedtime, increasing as needed; most patients require 10 mg day; if no response after 4-6 weeks of 10 mg/day, may increase to 20 mg/day

**Mechanism of Action** Alpha$_1$-specific blocking agent with minimal alpha$_2$ effects; this allows peripheral postsynaptic blockade, with the resultant decrease in arterial tone, while preserving the negative feedback loop which is mediated by the peripheral presynaptic alpha$_2$-receptors; terazosin relaxes the smooth muscle of the bladder neck, thus reducing bladder outlet obstruction

**Local Anesthetic/Vasoconstrictor Precautions** No information available to require special precautions

**Effects on Dental Treatment** Up to 10% of patients could experience dry mouth

**Other Adverse Effects**

>10%:
- Cardiovascular: Orthostatic hypotension
- Central nervous system: Dizziness, lightheadedness, drowsiness, headache, malaise

1% to 10%:
- Cardiovascular: Edema, palpitations
- Central nervous system: Fatigue, nervousness
- Gastrointestinal: Dry mouth
- Genitourinary: Urinary incontinence

<1%:
- Cardiovascular: Angina
- Central nervous system: Nightmares, hypothermia
- Dermatologic: Rash

(Continued)

## Terazosin *(Continued)*

Endocrine & metabolic: Sexual dysfunction
Gastrointestinal: Nausea
Genitourinary: Priapism
Renal: Polyuria
Respiratory: Dyspnea, nasal congestion

**Drug Interactions** Increased hypotensive effect with diuretics and antihypertensive medications (especially beta-blockers)

**Drug Uptake**
Absorption: Oral: Rapid
Serum half-life: 9.2-12 hours
Time to peak serum concentration: Within 1 hour

**Pregnancy Risk Factor** C

**Dosage Forms**
Capsule: 1 mg, 2 mg, 5 mg, 10 mg
Tablet: 1 mg, 2 mg, 5 mg, 10 mg

**Generic Available** No

## Terbinafine (TER bin a feen, TOP i kal)

**U.S. Brand Names** Lamisil®

**Therapeutic Category** Antifungal Agent, Topical

**Use** Topical antifungal for the treatment of tinea pedis (athlete's foot), tinea cruris (jock itch), and tinea corporis (ring worm)

**Unlabeled use:** Cutaneous candidiasis and pityriasis versicolor

**Usual Dosage** Adults: Topical:
Athlete's foot: Apply to affected area twice daily for at least 1 week, not to exceed 4 weeks
Ringworm and jock itch: Apply to affected area once or twice daily for at least 1 week, not to exceed 4 weeks

**Mechanism of Action** Synthetic alkylamine derivative which inhibits squalene epoxidases which is a key enzyme in sterol biosynthesis in fungi to result in a deficiency in ergosterol within fungal cell wall and result in fungal cell death

**Local Anesthetic/Vasoconstrictor Precautions** No information available to require special precautions

**Effects on Dental Treatment** No effects or complications reported

**Other Adverse Effects** 1% to 10%:
Dermatologic: Pruritus, contact dermatitis
Local: Irritation, stinging

**Drug Interactions** No data reported

**Drug Uptake** Absorption: Topical: Limited

**Pregnancy Risk Factor** B

**Generic Available** No

## Terbinafine, Oral (TER bin a feen, OR al)

**U.S. Brand Names** Lamisil® Oral

**Therapeutic Category** Antifungal Agent

**Use** Treatment of onychomycosis infections of the toenail or fingernail

**Usual Dosage** Adults: Oral:
Fingernail onychomycosis: 250 mg once daily for 6 weeks
Toenail onychomycosis: 250 mg once daily for 12 weeks

**Mechanism of Action** Terbinafine is a synthetic allylamine derivative which inhibits squalene epoxidase which is a key enzyme in sterol biosynthesis in fungi. The resulting deficiency in ergosterol within the cell wall causes fungi death.

**Local Anesthetic/Vasoconstrictor Precautions** No information available to require special precautions

**Effects on Dental Treatment** No effects or complications reported

**Other Adverse Effects**
>10%:
Central nervous system: Headache
1% to 10%:
Dermatologic: Rash, pruritus, urticaria
Gastrointestinal: Diarrhea, dyspepsia, abdominal pain, nausea, flatulence, abnormal taste
Hepatic: Elevated liver enzyme ≥2 times upper limit of normal range
Ocular: Visual disturbance

**Drug Interactions**
Decreases clearance of I.V. administered caffeine
Increases clearance of cyclosporine by 15%
Terbinafine clearance increased by rifampin (100%), cimetidine (33%)
Terbinafine clearance decreased by terfenadine (16%)

Terbinafine clearance unaffected by cyclosporine

**Drug Uptake**

Absorption: Oral: >70%

Serum half-life: 200-400 hours

**Pregnancy Risk Factor** B

**Dosage Forms** Tablet: 250 mg

**Generic Available** No

## Terbutaline (ter BYOO ta leen)

**Related Information**

Respiratory Diseases *on page 1079*

**U.S. Brand Names** Brethaire®; Brethine®; Bricanyl®

**Therapeutic Category** Adrenergic Agonist Agent; Antiasthmatic; $Beta_2$-Adrenergic Agonist Agent; Bronchodilator

**Use** Bronchodilator in reversible airway obstruction and bronchial asthma

**Usual Dosage**

Children <12 years:

Oral: Initial: 0.05 mg/kg/dose 3 times/day, increased gradually as required; maximum: 0.15 mg/kg/dose 3-4 times/day or a total of 5 mg/24 hours

S.C.: 0.005-0.01 mg/kg/dose to a maximum of 0.3 mg/dose every 15-20 minutes for 3 doses

Nebulization: 0.01-0.03 mg/kg/dose every 4-6 hours

Inhalation: 1-2 inhalations every 4-6 hours

Children >12 years and Adults:

Oral:

12-15 years: 2.5 mg every 6 hours 3 times/day; not to exceed 7.5 mg in 24 hours

>15 years: 5 mg/dose every 6 hours 3 times/day; if side effects occur, reduce dose to 2.5 mg every 6 hours; not to exceed 15 mg in 24 hours

S.C.: 0.25 mg/dose repeated in 15-30 minutes for one time only; a total dose of 0.5 mg should not be exceeded within a 4-hour period

Nebulization: 0.01-0.03 mg/kg/dose every 4-6 hours

Inhalation: 2 inhalations every 4-6 hours; wait 1 minute between inhalations

**Mechanism of Action** Relaxes bronchial smooth muscle by action on $beta_2$-receptors with less effect on heart rate

**Local Anesthetic/Vasoconstrictor Precautions** No information available to require special precautions

**Effects on Dental Treatment** No effects or complications reported

**Other Adverse Effects**

>10%:

Central nervous system: Nervousness, restlessness

Neuromuscular & skeletal: Trembling

1% to 10%:

Cardiovascular: Tachycardia, hypertension

Central nervous system: Dizziness, drowsiness, headache, insomnia

Gastrointestinal: Dry mouth, nausea, vomiting, bad taste in mouth

Neuromuscular & skeletal: Muscle cramps, weakness

Miscellaneous: Sweating

<1%:

Cardiovascular: Chest pain, arrhythmias

Respiratory: Paradoxical bronchospasm

**Drug Interactions**

Decreased effect with beta-blockers

Increased toxicity with MAO inhibitors, tricyclic antidepressants (TCAs)

**Drug Uptake**

Onset of action:

Oral: 30-45 minutes

S.C.: Within 6-15 minutes

Serum half-life: 11-16 hours

**Pregnancy Risk Factor** B

**Dosage Forms**

Aerosol, oral, as sulfate: 0.2 mg/actuation (10.5 g)

Injection, as sulfate: 1 mg/mL (1 mL)

Tablet, as sulfate: 2.5 mg, 5 mg

**Generic Available** No

## Terconazole (ter KONE a zole)

**U.S. Brand Names** Terazol®

**Therapeutic Category** Antifungal Agent, Vaginal

**Use** Local treatment of vulvovaginal candidiasis

(Continued)

## Terconazole *(Continued)*

**Usual Dosage** Adults: Female: Insert 1 applicatorful intravaginally at bedtime for 7 consecutive days

**Mechanism of Action** Triazole ketal antifungal agent; involves inhibition of fungal cytochrome P-450. Specifically, terconazole inhibits cytochrome P-450-dependent 14-alpha-demethylase which results in accumulation of membrane disturbing 14-alpha-demethylsterols and ergosterol depletion.

**Local Anesthetic/Vasoconstrictor Precautions** No information available to require special precautions

**Effects on Dental Treatment** No effects or complications reported

**Other Adverse Effects** 1% to 10%: Genitourinary: Vulvar/vaginal burning

**Drug Interactions** No data reported

**Drug Uptake** Absorption: Extent of systemic absorption after vaginal administration may be dependent on the presence of a uterus; 5% to 8% in women who had a hysterectomy versus 12% to 16% in nonhysterectomy women

**Pregnancy Risk Factor** C

**Dosage Forms**

Cream, vaginal: 0.4% (45 g); 0.8% (20 g)

Suppository, vaginal: 80 mg (3s)

**Generic Available** No

## Terpin Hydrate (TER pin HYE drate)

**Therapeutic Category** Expectorant

**Use** Symptomatic relief of cough

**Local Anesthetic/Vasoconstrictor Precautions** No information available to require special precautions

**Effects on Dental Treatment** No effects or complications reported

**Dosage Forms** Elixir: 85 mg/5 mL (120 mL)

**Generic Available** Yes

## Terpin Hydrate and Codeine (TER pin HYE drate & KOE deen)

**Therapeutic Category** Cough Preparation; Expectorant

**Synonyms** ETH and C

**Use** Symptomatic relief of cough

**Usual Dosage** Based on codeine content

Adults: 10-20 mg/dose every 4-6 hours as needed

Children (not recommended): 1-1.5 mg/kg/24 hours divided every 4 hours; maximum: 30 mg/24 hours

2-6 years: 1.25-2.5 mL every 4-6 hours as needed

6-12 years: 2.5-5 mL every 4-6 hours as needed

**Local Anesthetic/Vasoconstrictor Precautions** No information available to require special precautions

**Effects on Dental Treatment** No effects or complications reported

**Pregnancy Risk Factor** C

**Generic Available** Yes

- **Terra-Cortril® Ophthalmic Suspension** *see* Oxytetracycline and Hydrocortisone *on page 759*
- **Terramycin® I.M. Injection** *see* Oxytetracycline *on page 758*
- **Terramycin® Ophthalmic Ointment** *see* Oxytetracycline and Polymyxin B *on page 759*
- **Terramycin® Oral** *see* Oxytetracycline *on page 758*
- **Terramycin® w/Polymyxin B Ophthalmic Ointment** *see* Oxytetracycline and Polymyxin B *on page 759*
- **Tesamone® Injection** *see* Testosterone *on next page*
- **Teslac®** *see* Testolactone *on this page*
- **TESPA** *see* Thiotepa *on page 979*
- **Tessalon® Perles** *see* Benzonatate *on page 130*
- **Testoderm® Transdermal System** *see* Testosterone *on next page*

## Testolactone (tes toe LAK tone)

**U.S. Brand Names** Teslac®

**Therapeutic Category** Androgen

**Use** Palliative treatment of advanced disseminated breast carcinoma

**Usual Dosage** Adults: Female: Oral: 250 mg 4 times/day for at least 3 months; desired response may take as long as 3 months

**Mechanism of Action** Testolactone is a synthetic testosterone derivative without significant androgen activity. The drug inhibits steroid aromatase activity, thereby blocking the production of estradiol and estrone from androgen precursors such as testosterone and androstenedione. Unfortunately, the enzymatic block provided by testolactone is transient and is usually limited to a period of 3 months.

**Local Anesthetic/Vasoconstrictor Precautions** No information available to require special precautions

**Effects on Dental Treatment** No effects or complications reported

**Other Adverse Effects** 1% to 10%:

Cardiovascular: Edema
Dermatologic: Maculopapular rash
Endocrine & metabolic: Hypercalcemia
Gastrointestinal: Anorexia, diarrhea, nausea, swelling of tongue
Neuromuscular & skeletal: Paresthesias, peripheral neuropathies

**Drug Interactions** No data reported

**Drug Uptake** Absorption: Oral: Absorbed well

**Pregnancy Risk Factor** C

**Dosage Forms** Tablet: 50 mg

**Generic Available** No

♦ **Testopel® Pellet** *see* Testosterone *on this page*

## Testosterone (tes TOS ter one)

**U.S. Brand Names** Androderm® Transdermal System; Andro-L.A.® Injection; Andropository® Injection; Delatest® Injection; Delatestryl® Injection; depAndro® Injection; Depotest® Injection; Depo®-Testosterone Injection; Duratest® Injection; Durathate® Injection; Everone® Injection; Histerone® Injection; Tesamone® Injection; Testoderm® Transdermal System; Testopel® Pellet

**Therapeutic Category** Androgen

**Use** Androgen replacement therapy in the treatment of delayed male puberty; postpartum breast pain and engorgement; inoperable breast cancer; male hypogonadism

**Usual Dosage**

Delayed puberty: Males: Children: I.M.: 40-50 mg/m²/dose (cypionate or enanthate) monthly for 6 months
Initiation of pubertal growth: 40-50 mg/m²/dose (cypionate or enanthate) monthly until the growth rate falls to prepubertal levels (~5 cm/year)
During terminal growth phase: 100 mg/m²/dose (cypionate or enanthate) monthly until growth ceases
Maintenance virilizing dose: 100 mg/m²/dose (cypionate or enanthate) twice monthly or 50-400 mg/dose every 2-4 weeks
Inoperable breast cancer: Adults: I.M.: 200-400 mg every 2-4 weeks
Hypogonadism: Males: Adults:
I.M.:
Testosterone or testosterone propionate: 10-25 mg 2-3 times/week
Testosterone cypionate or enanthate: 50-400 mg every 2-4 weeks
Postpubertal cryptorchism: Testosterone or testosterone propionate: 10-25 mg 2-3 times/week
Topical: Initial: 6 mg/day system applied daily applied on scrotal skin. If scrotal area is inadequate, start with a 4 mg/day system. Transdermal system should be worn for 22-24 hours. Determine total serum testosterone after 3-4 weeks of daily application. If patients have not achieved desired results after 6-8 weeks of therapy, another form of testosterone replacement therapy should be considered.

**Mechanism of Action** Principal endogenous androgen responsible for promoting the growth and development of the male sex organs and maintaining secondary sex characteristics in androgen-deficient males

**Local Anesthetic/Vasoconstrictor Precautions** No information available to require special precautions

**Effects on Dental Treatment** No effects or complications reported

**Other Adverse Effects**

>10%:
Dermatologic: Acne
Endocrine & metabolic: Menstrual problems (amenorrhea), virilism, breast soreness
Genitourinary: Epididymitis, priapism, bladder irritability

1% to 10%:
Cardiovascular: Flushing, edema
Central nervous system: Excitation, aggressive behavior, sleeplessness, anxiety, mental depression, headache
Dermatologic: Hirsutism (increase in pubic hair growth)
Gastrointestinal: Nausea, vomiting, GI irritation
Genitourinary: Prostatic hypertrophy, prostatic carcinoma, impotence, testicular atrophy
Hepatic: Hepatic dysfunction

(Continued)

## Testosterone *(Continued)*

<1%:

Endocrine & metabolic: Gynecomastia, hypercalcemia, hypoglycemia
Hematologic: Leukopenia, suppression of clotting factors, polycythemia
Hepatic: Cholestatic hepatitis, hepatic necrosis
Miscellaneous: Hypersensitivity reactions

**Drug Interactions** Increased toxicity: Effects of oral anticoagulants may be enhanced

**Drug Uptake**

Duration of effect: Based upon the route of administration and which testosterone ester is used; the cypionate and enanthate esters have the longest duration, up to 2-4 weeks after I.M. administration

Serum half-life: 10-100 minutes

**Pregnancy Risk Factor** X

**Dosage Forms**

Injection:

Aqueous suspension: 25 mg/mL (10 mL, 30 mL); 50 mg/mL (10 mL, 30 mL); 100 mg/mL (10 mL, 30 mL)
In oil, as cypionate: 100 mg/mL (1 mL, 10 mL); 200 mg/mL (1 mL, 10 mL)
In oil, as enanthate: 100 mg/mL (5 mL, 10 mL); 200 mg/mL (5 mL, 10 mL)
In oil, as propionate: 50 mg/mL (10 mL, 30 mL); 100 mg/mL (10 mL, 30 mL)

Pellet: 75 mg (1 pellet per vial)

Transdermal system:

Androderm®: 2.5 mg/day
Testoderm®: 4 mg/day; 6 mg/day

**Generic Available** Yes

♦ **Testosterone and Estradiol** *see* Estradiol and Testosterone *on page 389*

♦ **Testred®** *see* Methyltestosterone *on page 662*

## Tetanus Immune Globulin (Human)

(TET a nus i MYUN GLOB yoo lin HYU man)

**Related Information**

Animal and Human Bites Guidelines *on page 1164*

**U.S. Brand Names** Hyper-Tet®

**Therapeutic Category** Immune Globulin

**Synonyms** TIG

**Use** Passive immunization against tetanus; tetanus immune globulin is preferred over tetanus antitoxin for treatment of active tetanus; part of the management of an unclean, nonminor wound in a person whose history of previous receipt of tetanus toxoid is unknown or who has received less than three doses of tetanus toxoid

**Usual Dosage** I.M.:

Prophylaxis of tetanus:

Children: 4 units/kg; some recommend administering 250 units to small children
Adults: 250 units

Treatment of tetanus:

Children: 500-3000 units; some should infiltrate locally around the wound
Adults: 3000-6000 units

**Tetanus Prophylaxis in Wound Management**

| Number of Prior Tetanus Toxoid Doses | Clean, Minor Wounds | | All Other Wounds | |
|---|---|---|---|---|
| | Td* | TIG† | Td* | TIG† |
| Unknown or <3 | Yes | No | Yes | Yes |
| ≥3‡ | No# | No | No¶ | No |

Adapted from Report of the Committee on Infectious Diseases, American Academy of Pediatrics, Elk Grove Village, IL: American Academy of Pediatrics, 1986.

*Adult tetanus and diphtheria toxoids; use pediatric preparations (DT or DTP) if the patient is <7 years old.

†Tetanus immune globulin.

‡If only three doses of fluid tetanus toxoid have been received, a fourth dose of toxoid, preferably an adsorbed toxoid, should be given.

#Yes, if >10 years since last dose.

¶Yes, if >5 years since last dose.

**Mechanism of Action** Passive immunity toward tetanus

**Local Anesthetic/Vasoconstrictor Precautions** No information available to require special precautions

**Effects on Dental Treatment** No effects or complications reported

**Other Adverse Effects**
>10%: Local: Pain, tenderness, erythema at injection site
1% to 10%:
Central nervous system: Fever (mild)
Dermatologic: Urticaria, angioedema
Neuromuscular & skeletal: Muscle stiffness
Miscellaneous: Anaphylaxis reaction
<1%: Local: Sensitization to repeated injections
**Drug Uptake** Absorption: Well absorbed
**Pregnancy Risk Factor** C
**Generic Available** No
**Comments** Tetanus immune globulin is preferred over tetanus antitoxin for treatment of active tetanus

## Tetanus Toxoid, Adsorbed (TET a nus TOKS oyd, ad SORBED)

**Therapeutic Category** Toxoid
**Use** Active immunization against tetanus
**Usual Dosage** Adults: I.M.:
Primary immunization: 0.5 mL; repeat 0.5 mL at 4-8 weeks after first dose and at 6-12 months after second dose
Routine booster doses are recommended only every 5-10 years
**Mechanism of Action** Tetanus toxoid preparations contain the toxin produced by virulent tetanus bacilli (detoxified growth products of *Clostridium tetani*). The toxin has been modified by treatment with formaldehyde so that is has lost toxicity but still retains ability to act as antigen and produce active immunity.
**Local Anesthetic/Vasoconstrictor Precautions** No information available to require special precautions
**Effects on Dental Treatment** No effects or complications reported
**Other Adverse Effects**
>10%: Local: Induration/redness at injection site
1% to 10%:
Central nervous system: Chills, fever
Local: Sterile abscess at injection site
Miscellaneous: Allergic reaction
<1%:
Central nervous system: Fever >103°F, malaise, neurological disturbances
Local: Blistering at injection site
Miscellaneous: Arthus-type hypersensitivity reactions have occurred rarely in patients >25 years of age and who have received multiple booster doses
**Drug Uptake** Duration of immunization following primary immunization: ~10 years
**Pregnancy Risk Factor** C
**Generic Available** No
**Comments** Routine booster doses are recommended only every 10 years

## Tetanus Toxoid, Fluid (TET a nus TOKS oyd FLOO id)

**Therapeutic Category** Toxoid
**Synonyms** Tetanus Toxoid Plain
**Use** Active immunization against tetanus in adults and children
**Usual Dosage**
Anergy testing: Intradermal: 0.1 mL
Primary immunization (**Note:** Td, TD, DTaP/DTwP are recommended): Adults: Inject 3 doses of 0.5 mL I.M. or S.C. at 4- to 8-week intervals; give fourth dose 6-12 months after third dose
Booster doses: I.M., S.C.: 0.5 mL every 10 years
**Mechanism of Action** Tetanus toxoid preparations contain the toxin produced by virulent tetanus bacilli (detoxified growth products of *Clostridium tetani*). The toxin has been modified by treatment with formaldehyde so that is has lost toxicity but still retains ability to act as antigen and produce active immunity.
**Local Anesthetic/Vasoconstrictor Precautions** No information available to require special precautions
**Effects on Dental Treatment** No effects or complications reported
**Other Adverse Effects**
>10%: Local: Induration/redness at injection site
1% to 10%:
Central nervous system: Chills, fever
Local: Sterile abscess at injection site
Miscellaneous: Allergic reaction
<1%:
Central nervous system: Fever >103°F, malaise, neurological disturbances
Local: Blistering at injection site
(Continued)

## Tetanus Toxoid, Fluid *(Continued)*

Miscellaneous: Arthus-type hypersensitivity reactions

**Pregnancy Risk Factor** C

**Generic Available** No

**Comments** Tetanus Toxoid, Adsorbed is preferred for all basic immunizing and recall reactions because of more persistent antitoxin titer induction

♦ **Tetanus Toxoid Plain** *see* Tetanus Toxoid, Fluid *on previous page*

## Tetracaine (TET ra kane)

**Related Information**

Mouth Pain, Cold Sore, Canker Sore Products *on page 1253*

Oral Nonviral Soft Tissue Ulcerations or Erosions *on page 1141*

Oral Pain *on page 1122*

**U.S. Brand Names** Pontocaine®; Viractin® [OTC]

**Canadian Brand Names** Ametop™; Supracaine®

**Therapeutic Category** Dental/Local Anesthetics; Local Anesthetic, Injectable; Local Anesthetic, Oral; Local Anesthetic, Topical

**Use**

Dental: Ester-type local anesthetic topically applied to nose and throat for various diagnostic procedures

Medical: Spinal anesthesia; local anesthesia in the eye for various diagnostic and examination purposes

**Usual Dosage** Children and Adults: Topical: Applied as a 1% or 2% cream to affected areas 3-4 times/day as needed

**Mechanism of Action** Local anesthetics bind selectively to the intracellular surface of sodium channels to block influx of sodium into the axon. As a result, depolarization necessary for action potential propagation and subsequent nerve function is prevented. The block at the sodium channel is reversible. When drug diffuses away from the axon, sodium channel function is restored and nerve propagation returns.

**Local Anesthetic/Vasoconstrictor Precautions** No information available to require special precautions

**Effects on Dental Treatment** No effects or complications reported

**Other Adverse Effects** 1% to 10%: Dermatologic: Contact dermatitis, burning, stinging, angioedema

**Contraindications** Hypersensitivity to tetracaine or any component; ophthalmic secondary bacterial infection, patients with liver disease, CNS disease, meningitis (if used for epidural or spinal anesthesia), myasthenia gravis

**Warnings/Precautions** No pediatric dosage recommendations

**Drug Interactions** No data reported

**Drug Uptake**

Onset: Rapid

Duration of action: Topical: 1.5-3 hours

**Pregnancy Risk Factor** C

**Breast-feeding Considerations** No data reported

**Dosage Forms**

Cream: 1%

Cream (Viractin®): 2% (4 g)

Gel (Viractin®): 2% (4 g)

**Generic Available** Yes

## Tetracaine and Dextrose (TET ra kane & DEKS trose)

**Related Information**

Oral Pain *on page 1122*

**U.S. Brand Names** Pontocaine® With Dextrose Injection

**Therapeutic Category** Dental/Local Anesthetics; Local Anesthetic, Injectable

**Use** Spinal anesthesia (saddle block)

**Usual Dosage** Dose varies with procedure, depth of anesthesia, duration desired and physical condition of patient

**Local Anesthetic/Vasoconstrictor Precautions** No information available to require special precautions

**Effects on Dental Treatment** No effects or complications reported

**Pregnancy Risk Factor** C

**Generic Available** Yes

♦ **Tetracaine Hydrochloride, Benzocaine Butyl Aminobenzoate and Benzalkonium Chloride** *see* Benzocaine, Butyl Aminobenzoate, Tetracaine, and Benzalkonium Chloride *on page 129*

## Tetracycline (tet ra SYE kleen)

**Related Information**

Dental Drug Interactions: Update on Drug Combinations Requiring Special Considerations *on page 1225*
Oral Bacterial Infections *on page 1128*
Oral Nonviral Soft Tissue Ulcerations or Erosions *on page 1141*
Periodontal Diseases *on page 1132*

**U.S. Brand Names** Achromycin®; Achromycin® V; Sumycin®; Tetracyn®

**Canadian Brand Names** Apo®-Tetra; Novo-Tetra; Nu-Tetra

**Therapeutic Category** Acne Products; Antibiotic, Ophthalmic; Antibiotic, Tetracycline Derivative; Antibiotic, Topical

**Use**

Dental: Treatment of periodontitis associated with presence of *Actinobacillus actinomycetemcomitans* (AA). As adjunctive therapy in recurrent aphthous ulcers

Medical: In medicine for treatment of susceptible bacterial infections of both gram-positive and gram-negative organisms; also some unusual organisms including *Mycoplasma*, *Chlamydia*, and *Rickettsia*; may also be used for acne, exacerbations of chronic bronchitis, and treatment of gonorrhea and syphilis in patients that are allergic to penicillin

**Usual Dosage** Adults: 250 mg every 6 hours until improvement (usually 10 days or more)

**Mechanism of Action** Inhibits bacterial protein synthesis by binding with the 30S and possibly the 50S ribosomal subunit(s) of susceptible bacteria; may also cause alterations in the cytoplasmic membrane

**Local Anesthetic/Vasoconstrictor Precautions** No information available to require special precautions

**Effects on Dental Treatment** Opportunistic "superinfection" with *Candida albicans*; tetracycline's are not recommended for use during pregnancy or in children ≤8 years of age since they have been reported to cause enamel hypoplasia and permanent teeth discoloration. The use of tetracycline's should only be used in these patients if other agents are contraindicated or alternative antimicrobials will not eradicate the organism. Long-term use associated with oral candidiasis.

**Other Adverse Effects**

>10%: Gastrointestinal: Discoloration of teeth and enamel hypoplasia (infants)

1% to 10%:

- Dermatologic: Photosensitivity
- Gastrointestinal: Nausea, diarrhea

**Contraindications** Hypersensitivity to tetracycline or any component; do not administer to children ≤8 years of age

**Warnings/Precautions** Use of tetracyclines during tooth development may cause permanent discoloration of the teeth and enamel, hypoplasia and retardation of skeletal development and bone growth with risk being the greatest for children <4 years of age and those receiving high doses; use with caution in patients with renal or hepatic impairment and in pregnancy; dosage modification required in patients with renal impairment; pseudotumor cerebri has been reported with tetracycline use; outdated drug can cause nephropathy.

**Drug Interactions** Dairy products; calcium, magnesium or aluminum-containing antacids, iron, zinc, cimetidine causes decreased tetracycline absorption; methoxyflurane anesthesia when concurrent with tetracycline may cause fatal nephrotoxicity; warfarin with tetracyclines leads to increased anticoagulation; penicillin-tetracycline combination counteracts antibiotic effects of each; decreased effect of oral contraceptives

**Drug Uptake**

Absorption: Oral: 75%
Serum half-life: Normal renal function: 8-11 hours
Time to peak serum concentration: Oral: Within 2-4 hours

**Pregnancy Risk Factor** D; B (topical)

**Breast-feeding Considerations** May be taken while breast-feeding

**Dosage Forms**

Capsule: 100 mg, 250 mg, 500 mg
Suspension, oral: 125 mg/5 mL (60 mL, 480 mL)
Tablet: 250 mg, 500 mg

**Dietary Considerations** Should be taken 1 hour before or 2 hours after meals with adequate amounts of fluid; food decreases absorption; avoid taking antacids, iron, dairy products, or milk formulas within 3 hours of tetracyclines; decreases absorption of magnesium, zinc, calcium, iron, and amino acids

**Generic Available** Yes

**Comments** *Helicobacter pylori*: Clinically effective treatment regimens include triple therapy with amoxicillin or tetracycline, metronidazole, and bismuth subsalicylate; amoxicillin, metronidazole, and $H_2$ receptor antagonist; or double therapy

(Continued)

## Tetracycline *(Continued)*

with amoxicillin and omeprazole. Adult dose of tetracycline against *H. pylori*: 250 mg 3 times/day to 500 mg 4 times/day

**Selected Readings**

Gordon JM and Walker CB, "Current Status of Systemic Antibiotic Usage in Destructive Periodontal Disease," *J Periodontol*, 1993, 64(8 Suppl): 760-71.

Rams TE and Slots J, "Antibiotics in Periodontal Therapy: An Update," *Compendium*, 1992, 13(12):1130, 1132, 1134.

Seymour RA and Heasman PA, "Tetracyclines in the Management of Periodontal Diseases. A Review," *J Clin Periodontol*, 1995, 22(1):22-35.

Seymour RA and Heasman PA, "Pharmacological Control of Periodontal Disease. II. Antimicrobial Agents," *J Dent*, 1995, 23(1):5-14

## Tetracycline Periodontal Fibers

(tet ra SYE kleen per ee oh DON tal FYE bers)

**Related Information**

Dental Drug Interactions: Update on Drug Combinations Requiring Special Considerations *on page 1225*

**U.S. Brand Names** Actisite®

**Therapeutic Category** Antibacterial, Dental

**Use**

Dental: Treatment of adult periodontitis; as an adjunct to scaling and root planing for the reduction of pocket depth and bleeding on probing in selected patients with adult periodontitis

Medical: No data reported

**Usual Dosage**

Children: Has not been established

Adults: Insert fiber to fill the periodontal pocket; each fiber contains 12.7 mg of tetracycline in 23 cm (9 inches) and provides continuous release of drug for 10 days; fibers are to be secured in pocket with cyanoacrylate adhesive and left in place for 10 days

**Mechanism of Action** Tetracycline is an antibiotic which inhibits growth of susceptible microorganisms. Tetracycline binds primarily to the 30S subunits of bacterial ribosomes, and appears to prevent access of aminoacyl tRNA to the acceptor site on the mRNA-ribosome complex. The fiber releases tetracycline into the periodontal site at a rate of 2 mcg/cm/hour.

**Local Anesthetic/Vasoconstrictor Precautions** No information available to require special precautions

**Effects on Dental Treatment** 1% to 10% of patients experience gingival inflammation, pain in mouth, glossitis, candidiasis, staining of tongue

**Other Adverse Effects** 1% to 10%:

Dermatologic: Local erythema following removal

Miscellaneous: Discomfort from fiber placement

**Contraindications** Known hypersensitivity to tetracyclines

**Warnings/Precautions** Use of tetracyclines is not recommended during pregnancy because of interference with fetal bone and dental development

**Drug Interactions** No data reported

**Drug Uptake**

The fiber releases tetracycline at a rate of 2 mcg/cm/hour

Tissue fluid concentrations:

- Gingival fluid: ~1590 mcg/mL of tetracycline per site over 10 days
- Plasma: During fiber treatment of up to 11 teeth, the tetracycline plasma concentration was below any detectable levels (<0.1 mcg/mL)
  - Oral: 500 mg of tetracycline produces a peak plasma level of 3-4 mcg/mL
- Saliva: ~50.7 mcg/mL of tetracycline immediately after fiber treatment of 9 teeth

**Pregnancy Risk Factor** C

**Breast-feeding Considerations** It is not known whether tetracycline from periodontal fibers is distributed into human breast milk

**Dosage Forms** Fibers 23 cm (9") in length; 12.7 mg of tetracycline hydrochloride per fiber

**Dietary Considerations** No data reported

**Generic Available** No

**Comments** A number of different facultative and obligate anaerobic bacteria have been found to be causative factors in periodontal disease. These include *Actinobacillus actinomycetemcomitans* (AA), *Fusobacterium nucleatum*, and *Porphyromonas gingivalis*. These bacteria are sensitive to tetracyclines at similar concentrations as those released from the tetracycline-impregnated fibers. Placement of tetracycline periodontal fibers into gingival pockets decreases inflammation, edema, pocket depth, and bleeding upon probing.

**Selected Readings**


Baer PN, "Actisite (Tetracycline Hydrochloride Periodontal Fiber): A Critique," *Periodontal Clin Investig*, 1994, 16(2):5-7.

Greenstein G, "Treating Periodontal Diseases With Tetracycline-Impregnanted Fibers: Data and Controversies," *Compend Contin Educ Dent*, 1995, 16(5)448-55.

Kerry G, "Tetracycline-Loaded Fibers as Adjunctive Treatment in Periodontal Disease," *J Am Dent Assoc*, 1994, 125(9):1199-203.

Michalowicz BS, Pihlstrom BL, Drisko CL, et al, "Evaluation of Periodontal Treatments Using Controlled-Release Tetracycline Fibers: Maintenance Response," *J Periodontol*, 1995, 66(8):708-15.

Mombelli A, Lehmann B, Tonetti M, et al, "Clinical Response to Local Delivery of Tetracycline in Relation to Overall and Local Periodontal Conditions," *J Clin Periodontol*, 1997, 24(7):470-77.

Vandekerckhove BN, Quirynen M, and van Steenberghe D, "The Use of Tetracycline-Containing Controlled-Release Fibers in the Treatment of Refractory Periodontitis," *J Periodontol*, 1997, 68(4):353-61.


♦ **Tetracyn®** *see* Tetracycline *on page 965*

## Tetrahydrozoline (tet ra hye DROZ a leen)

**U.S. Brand Names** Collyrium Fresh® Ophthalmic [OTC]; Eyesine® Ophthalmic [OTC]; Geneye® Ophthalmic [OTC]; Mallazine® Eye Drops [OTC]; Murine® Plus Ophthalmic [OTC]; Optigene® Ophthalmic [OTC]; Tetrasine® Extra Ophthalmic [OTC]; Tetrasine® Ophthalmic [OTC]; Tyzine® Nasal; Visine® Extra Ophthalmic [OTC]

**Therapeutic Category** Adrenergic Agonist Agent; Adrenergic Agonist Agent, Ophthalmic; Nasal Agent, Vasoconstrictor; Ophthalmic Agent, Vasoconstrictor

**Use** Symptomatic relief of nasal congestion and conjunctival congestion

**Usual Dosage**

Nasal congestion: Intranasal:

Children 2-6 years: Instill 2-3 drops of 0.05% solution every 4-6 hours as needed, no more frequent than every 3 hours

Children >6 years and Adults: Instill 2-4 drops or 3-4 sprays of 0.1% solution every 3-4 hours as needed, no more frequent than every 3 hours

Conjunctival congestion: Ophthalmic: Adults: Instill 1-2 drops in each eye 2-4 times/day

**Mechanism of Action** Stimulates alpha-adrenergic receptors in the arterioles of the conjunctiva and the nasal mucosa to produce vasoconstriction

**Local Anesthetic/Vasoconstrictor Precautions** No information available to require special precautions

**Effects on Dental Treatment** No effects or complications reported

**Other Adverse Effects**

>10%:

Local: Transient stinging

Respiratory: Sneezing

1% to 10%:

Cardiovascular: Tachycardia, palpitations, hypertension, heart rate

Central nervous system: Headache

Neuromuscular & skeletal: Tremor

Ocular: Blurred vision

**Drug Interactions** Increased toxicity: MAO inhibitors can cause an exaggerated adrenergic response if taken concurrently or within 21 days of discontinuing MAO inhibitor; beta-blockers can cause hypertensive episodes and increased risk of intracranial hemorrhage; anesthetics

**Drug Uptake**

Onset of decongestant effect: Intranasal: Within 4-8 hours

Duration: Ophthalmic vasoconstriction: 2-3 hours

**Pregnancy Risk Factor** C

**Dosage Forms** Solution, as hydrochloride:

Nasal: 0.05% (15 mL), 0.1% (30 mL, 473 mL)

Ophthalmic: 0.05% (15 mL)

**Generic Available** Yes

♦ **Tetrasine® Extra Ophthalmic [OTC]** *see* Tetrahydrozoline *on this page*

♦ **Tetrasine® Ophthalmic [OTC]** *see* Tetrahydrozoline *on this page*

♦ **Teveten®** *see* Eprosartan *on page 378*

♦ **TG** *see* Thioguanine *on page 977*

♦ **6-TG** *see* Thioguanine *on page 977*

♦ **T/Gel® [OTC]** *see* Coal Tar *on page 270*

♦ **T-Gen®** *see* Trimethobenzamide *on page 1020*

♦ **T-Gesic® [5/500]** *see* Hydrocodone and Acetaminophen *on page 505*

## Thalidomide (tha LI doe mide)

**Related Information**

HIV Infection and AIDS *on page 1085*

Oral Nonviral Soft Tissue Ulcerations or Erosions *on page 1141*

(Continued)

## Thalidomide *(Continued)*

**U.S. Brand Names** Thalomid®

**Therapeutic Category** Immunosuppressant Agent

**Use** FDA-approved:

Acute treatment of cutaneous manifestations of moderate to severe erythema nodosum leprosum (ENL)

Maintenance therapy for suppression of cutaneous manifestations of ENL recurrence

**Investigational:** Treatment or prevention of graft-versus-host reactions after bone marrow transplantation; in aphthous ulceration in HIV-positive patients; Langerhans cell histiocytosis, Behçet's syndrome; hypnotic agent; also may be effective in rheumatoid arthritis, discoid lupus, and erythema multiforme; useful in type 2 lepra reactions, but not type 1; can assist in healing mouth ulcers in AIDS patients.

**Restrictions** Thalidomide is approved for marketing only under a special distribution program. This program, called the "System for Thalidomide Education and Prescribing Safety" (STEPS), has been approved by the FDA. Prescribing and dispensing of thalidomide is restricted to prescribers and pharmacists registered with the program.

**Usual Dosage**

Cutaneous ENL:

- Initiate dosing at 100-300 mg/day taken once daily at bedtime (at least 1 hour after evening meal)
- Patients weighing <50 kg: Initiate at lower dose
- Severe cutaneous reaction or previously requiring high dose may be initiated at 400 mg/day; doses may be divided, but taken 1 hour after meals
- Dosing should continue until active reaction subsides (usually at least 2 weeks), then tapered in 50 mg decrements every 2-4 weeks
- Patients who flare during tapering or with a history or requiring prolonged maintenance should be maintained on the minimum dosage necessary to control the reaction. Efforts to taper should be repeated every 3-6 months.

Behçet's syndrome: 100-400 mg/day

Graft-versus-host reactions:

- Children: 3 mg/kg 4 times/day
- Adults: 100-1600 mg/day; usual initial dose: 200 mg 4 times/day for use up to 700 days

AIDS-related aphthous stomatitis: 200 mg twice daily for 5 days, then 200 mg/day for up to 8 weeks

Discoid lupus erythematosus: 100-400 mg/day; maintenance dose: 25-50 mg

**Mechanism of Action** A derivative of glutethimide; mode of action for immunosuppression is unclear; inhibition of neutrophil chemotaxis and decreased monocyte phagocytosis may occur; may cause 50% to 80% reduction of tumor necrosis factor - alpha

**Local Anesthetic/Vasoconstrictor Precautions** No information available to require special precautions

**Effects on Dental Treatment** 1% to 10% of patients may experience moniliasis, tooth pain; in HIV-seropositive patients, oral moniliasis was seen in 6.3% to 11.1% of patients; aphthous stomatitis has been reported

**Other Adverse Effects**

Controlled clinical trials: ENL:

>10%:

- Central nervous system: Somnolence (37.5%), headache (12.5%)
- Dermatologic: Rash (20.8%)

1% to 10%:

- Cardiovascular: Peripheral edema
- Central nervous system: Dizziness (4.2%), vertigo (8.3%), chills, malaise (8.3%)
- Dermatologic: Dermatitis (fungal) (4.2%), nail disorder (4.2%), pruritus (8.3%), rash (maculopapular) (4.2%)
- Gastrointestinal (4.2%): Constipation, diarrhea, nausea, abdominal pain
- Genitourinary: Impotence (8.2%)
- Neuromuscular & skeletal: Asthenia (8.3%), pain (8.3%), back pain (4.2%), neck pain (4.2%), neck rigidity (4.2%), tremor (4.2%)
- Respiratory (4.2%): Pharyngitis, rhinitis, sinusitis

HIV-seropositive:

General: An increased viral load has been noted in patients treated with thalidomide. This is of uncertain clinical significance - see monitoring

>10%:

- Central nervous system: Somnolence (36% to 37%), dizziness (18.7% to 19.4%), fever (19.4% to 21.9%), headache (16.7% to 18.7%)

Dermatologic: Rash (25%), maculopapular rash (16.7% to 18.7%), acne (3.1% to 11.1%)
Gastrointestinal: AST increase (2.8% to 12.5%), diarrhea (11.1% to 18.7%), nausea (≤12.5%)
Hematologic: Leukopenia (16.7% to 25%), anemia (5.6% to 12.5%)
Neuromuscular & skeletal: Paresthesia (5.6% to 15.6%), weakness (5.6% to 21.9%)
Miscellaneous: Diaphoresis (≤12.5%), lymphadenopathy (5.6% to 12.5%)

1% to 10%:
Cardiovascular: Peripheral edema (3.1% to 8.3%)
Central nervous system: Nervousness (2.8% to 9.4%), insomnia (≤9.4%), agitation (≤9.4%), chills (≤9.4%)
Dermatologic: Dermatitis (fungal) (5.6% to 9.4%), nail disorder (≤3.1%), pruritus (2.8% to 6.3%)
Gastrointestinal: Anorexia (2.8% to 9.4%), constipation (2.8% to 9.4%), xerostomia (8.3% to 9.4%), flatulence (8.3% to 9.4%), multiple abnormalities LFTs (≤9.4%), abdominal pain (2.8% to 3.1%)
Neuromuscular & skeletal: Back pain (≤5%), pain (≤3.1%)
Respiratory: Pharyngitis (6.3% to 8.3%), sinusitis (3.1% to 8.3%)
Miscellaneous: Accidental injury (≤5.6%), infection (6.3% to 8.3%)

Literature reports of other adverse reactions: Bradycardia, orthostatic hypotension, Raynaud's syndrome, hangover effect, migraine, erythema nodosum, petechiae, purpura, amenorrhea, galactorrhea, gynecomastia, menorrhagia, hypomagnesemia, hypothyroidism, myxedema, Hodgkin's disease, dyspnea, carpal tunnel, dysesthesia, foot-drop, CML, lymphopenia, pancytopenia, bile duct obstruction, stomach ulcer, acute renal failure, enuresis, oliguria, diplopia, nystagmus, lymphedema, suicide attempt

**Contraindications** Pregnancy or women in childbearing years, neuropathy (peripheral), thalidomide hypersensitivity

**Warnings/Precautions** Liver, hepatic, neurological disorders, constipation, congestive heart failure, hypertension; see Patient Information

**Drug Interactions** Other medications known to cause peripheral neuropathy should be used with caution in patients receiving thalidomide; thalidomide may enhance the sedative activity of other drugs such as ethanol, barbiturates, reserpine, and chlorpromazine

**Drug Uptake**
Serum half-life: 8.7 hours
Peak plasma levels: 2-6 hours

**Pregnancy Risk Factor** X

Embryotoxic with limb defects noted from the 27th to 40th gestational day of exposure; all cases of phocomelia occur from the 27th to 42nd gestational day; fetal cardiac, gastrointestinal, and genitourinary tract abnormalities have also been described

Even a single dose of thalidomide taken during pregnancy can cause severe defects or fetal death. Mortality at or shortly after birth may be as high as 40%. It is not known if thalidomide is excreted in human milk. A decision should be made to discontinue nursing or the drug.

**Dosage Forms** Capsule: 50 mg (boxes contain 6 prescription packs of 14 capsules each)

**Selected Readings**

Jacobson JM, Greenspan JS, Spritzler J, et al, "Thalidomide for the Treatment of Oral Aphthous Ulcers in Patients With Human Immunodeficiency Virus Infection," *N Engl J Med*, 1997, 336:1487-93.

♦ **Thalitone®** *see* Chlorthalidone *on page 242*
♦ **Thalomid®** *see* Thalidomide *on page 967*
♦ **THAM-E® Injection** *see* Tromethamine *on page 1029*
♦ **THAM® Injection** *see* Tromethamine *on page 1029*
♦ **Theo-24®** *see* Theophylline *on this page*
♦ **Theobid®** *see* Theophylline *on this page*
♦ **Theochron®** *see* Theophylline *on this page*
♦ **Theoclear® L.A.** *see* Theophylline *on this page*
♦ **Theo-Dur®** *see* Theophylline *on this page*
♦ **Theolair™** *see* Theophylline *on this page*

## Theophylline (thee OF i lin)

**Related Information**

Aminophylline *on page 63*
Dental Drug Interactions: Update on Drug Combinations Requiring Special Considerations *on page 1225*
Respiratory Diseases *on page 1079*
(Continued)

## Theophylline *(Continued)*

**U.S. Brand Names** Aerolate III®; Aerolate JR®; Aerolate SR® S; Aquaphyllin®; Asmalix®; Elixophyllin®; Quibron®-T; Quibron®-T/SR; Respbid®; Slo-bid™; Slo-Phyllin®; Sustaire®; Theo-24®; Theobid®; Theochron®; Theoclear® L.A.; Theo-Dur®; Theolair™; Theospan®-SR; Theovent®; Theo-X®; Uni-Dur®; Uniphyl®

**Canadian Brand Names** Apo®-Theo LA; Phyllocontin®; Pulmophylline

**Therapeutic Category** Antiasthmatic; Bronchodilator; Theophylline Derivative

**Use** Bronchodilator in reversible airway obstruction due to asthma, chronic bronchitis, and emphysema; for neonatal apnea/bradycardia

**Usual Dosage** Use ideal body weight for obese patients

I.V.: Initial: Maintenance infusion rates:

Children:

6 weeks to 6 months: 0.5 mg/kg/hour

6 months to 1 year: 0.6-0.7 mg/kg/hour

Children >1 year and Adults:

**Treatment of acute bronchospasm**: I.V.: Loading dose (in patients not currently receiving aminophylline or theophylline): 6 mg/kg (based on aminophylline) given I.V. over 20-30 minutes; administration rate should not exceed 25 mg/minute (aminophylline). See table.

**Approximate I.V. Theophylline Dosage for Treatment of Acute Bronchospasm**

| Group | Dosage for next 12 h* | Dosage after 12 h* |
|---|---|---|
| Infants 6 wk to 6 mo | 0.5 mg/kg/h | |
| Children 6 mo to 1 y | 0.6-0.7 mg/kg/h | |
| Children 1-9 y | 0.95 mg/kg/h (1.2 mg/kg/h) | 0.79 mg/kg/h (1 mg/kg/h) |
| Children 9-16 y and young adult smokers | 0.79 mg/kg/h (1 mg/kg/h) | 0.63 mg/kg/h (0.8 mg/kg/h) |
| Healthy, nonsmoking adults | 0.55 mg/kg/h (0.7 mg/kg/h) | 0.39 mg/kg/h (0.5 mg/kg/h) |
| Older patients and patients with cor pulmonale | 0.47 mg/kg/h (0.6 mg/kg/h) | 0.24 mg/kg/h (0.3 mg/kg/h) |
| Patients with congestive heart failure or liver failure | 0.39 mg/kg/h (0.5 mg/kg/h) | 0.08-0.16 mg/kg/h (0.1-0.2 mg/kg/h) |

*Equivalent hydrous aminophylline dosage indicated in parentheses.

**Maintenance Dose for Acute Symptoms**

| Population Group | Oral Theophylline (mg/kg/day) | I.V. Aminophylline |
|---|---|---|
| Premature infant or newborn - 6 wk (for apnea/ bradycardia) | 4 | 5 mg/kg/day |
| 6 wk - 6 mo | 10 | 12 mg/kg/day or continuous I.V. infusion* |
| Infants 6 mo-1 y | 12-18 | 15 mg/kg/day or continuous I.V. infusion* |
| Children 1-9 y | 20-24 | 1 mg/kg/hour |
| Children 9-12 y, and adolescent daily smokers of cigarettes or marijuana, and otherwise healthy adult smokers <50 y | 16 | 0.9 mg/kg/hour |
| Adolescents 12-16 y (nonsmokers) | 13 | 0.7 mg/kg/hour |
| Otherwise healthy nonsmoking adults (including elderly patients) | 10 (not to exceed 900 mg/day) | 0.5 mg/kg/hour |
| Cardiac decompensation, cor pulmonale and/or liver dysfunction | 5 (not to exceed 400 mg/day) | 0.25 mg/kg/hour |

*For continuous I.V. infusion divide total daily dose by 24 = mg/kg/hour.

**Approximate I.V. maintenance dosages are based upon continuous infusions**; bolus dosing (often used in children <6 months of age) may be determined by multiplying the hourly infusion rate by 24 hours and dividing by the desired number of doses/day; see table.

Dosage should be adjusted according to serum level measurements during the first 12- to 24-hour period; see table.

### Dosage Adjustment After Serum Theophylline Measurement

| Serum Theophylline | | Guidelines |
|---|---|---|
| Within normal limits | 10-20 mcg/mL | Maintain dosage if tolerated. Recheck serum theophylline concentration at 6- to 12-month intervals.* |
| Too high | 20-25 mcg/mL | Decrease doses by about 10%. Recheck serum theophylline concentration after 3 days and then at 6- to 12-month intervals.* |
| | 25-30 mcg/mL | Skip next dose and decrease subsequent doses by about 25%. Recheck serum theophylline. |
| | >30 mcg/mL | Skip next 2 doses and decrease subsequent doses by 50%. Recheck serum theophylline. |
| Too low | 7.5-10 mcg/mL | Increase dose by about 25%.† Recheck serum theophylline concentration after 3 days and then at 6- to 12-month intervals.* |
| | 5-7.5 mcg/mL | Increase dose by about 25% to the nearest dose increment† and recheck serum theophylline for guidance in further dosage adjustment (another increase will probably be needed, but this provides a safety check). |

From Weinberger M and Hendeles L,"Practical Guide to Using Theophylline," *J Resp Dis*, 1981, 2:12-27.

*Finer adjustments in dosage may be needed for some patients.

†Dividing the daily dose into 3 doses administered at 8-hour intervals may be indicated if symptoms occur repeatedly at the end of a dosing interval.

**Oral theophylline:** Initial dosage recommendation: Loading dose (to achieve a serum level of about 10 mcg/mL; loading doses should be given using a rapidly absorbed oral product **not** a sustained release product):

If no theophylline has been administered in the previous 24 hours: 4-6 mg/kg theophylline

If theophylline has been administered in the previous 24 hours: administer ½ loading dose or 2-3 mg/kg theophylline can be given in emergencies when serum levels are not available

On the average, for every 1 mg/kg theophylline given, blood levels will rise 2 mcg/mL

Ideally, defer the loading dose if a serum theophylline concentration can be obtained rapidly. However, if this is not possible, exercise clinical judgment. If the patient is not experiencing theophylline toxicity, this is unlikely to result in dangerous adverse effects.

See table.

### Oral Theophylline Dosage for Bronchial Asthma*

| Age | Initial 3 Days | Second 3 Days | Steady-State Maintenance |
|---|---|---|---|
| <1 y | 0.2 x (age in weeks) + 5 | | 0.3 x (age in weeks) + 8 |
| 1-9 y | 16 up to a maximum of 400 mg/24 h | 20 | 22 |
| 9-12 y | 16 up to a maximum of 400 mg/24 h | 16 up to a maximum of 600 mg/24 h | 20 up to a maximum of 800 mg/24 h |
| 12-16 y | 16 up to a maximum of 400 mg/24 h | 16 up to a maximum of 600 mg/24 h | 18 up to a maximum of 900 mg/24 h |
| Adults | 400 mg/24 h | 600 mg/24 h | 900 mg/24 h |

*Dose in mg/kg/24 hours of theophylline.

(Continued)

## Theophylline *(Continued)*

**Increasing dose:** The dosage may be increased in approximately 25% increments at 2- to 3-day intervals so long as the drug is tolerated or until the maximum dose is reached

**Maintenance dose:** In children and healthy adults, a slow-release product can be used; the total daily dose can be divided every 8-12 hours

**Mechanism of Action** Causes bronchodilatation, diuresis, CNS and cardiac stimulation, and gastric acid secretion by blocking phosphodiesterase which increases tissue concentrations of cyclic adenine monophosphate (cAMP) which in turn promotes catecholamine stimulation of lipolysis, glycogenolysis, and gluconeogenesis and induces release of epinephrine from adrenal medulla cells

**Local Anesthetic/Vasoconstrictor Precautions** No information available to require special precautions

**Effects on Dental Treatment** Prescribe erythromycin products with caution to patients taking theophylline products. Erythromycin will delay the normal metabolic inactivation of theophyllines leading to increased blood levels; this has resulted in nausea, vomiting and CNS restlessness. Azithromycin does not cause these effects in combination with theophylline products.

**Other Adverse Effects** See table.

| Theophylline Serum Levels (mcg/mL)* | Adverse Reactions |
|---|---|
| 15-25 | GI upset, diarrhea, N/V, abdominal pain, nervousness, headache, insomnia, agitation, dizziness, muscle cramp, tremor |
| 25-35 | Tachycardia, occasional PVC |
| >35 | Ventricular tachycardia, frequent PVC, seizure |

*Adverse effects do not necessarily occur according to serum levels. Arrhythmia and seizure can occur without seeing the other adverse effects.

**Uncommon at serum theophylline concentrations ≤20 mcg/mL**

1% to 10%:

Cardiovascular: Tachycardia

Central nervous system: Nervousness, restlessness

Gastrointestinal: Nausea, vomiting

**Factors Reported to Affect Theophylline Serum Levels**

| Decreased Theophylline Level | Increased Theophylline Level |
|---|---|
| Smoking (cigarettes, marijuana) | Hepatic cirrhosis |
| High protein/low carbohydrate diet | Cor pulmonale |
| Charcoal | CHF |
| Phenytoin | Fever/viral illness |
| Phenobarbital | Propranolol |
| Carbamazepine | Allopurinol (>600 mg/d) |
| Rifampin | Erythromycin |
| I.V. isoproterenol | Cimetidine |
| Aminoglutethimide | Troleandomycin |
| Barbiturates | Ciprofloxacin |
| Hydantoins | Oral contraceptives |
| Ketoconazole | Beta blockers |
| Sulfinpyrazone | Calcium channel blockers |
| Isoniazid | Corticosteroids |
| Loop diuretics | Disulfiram |
| Sympathomimetics | Ephedrine |
| | Influenza virus vaccine |
| | Interferon |
| | Macrolides |
| | Mexiletine |
| | Quinolones |
| | Thiabendazole |
| | Thyroid hormones |
| | Carbamazepine |
| | Isoniazid |
| | Loop diuretics |

<1%:
- Central nervous system: Insomnia, irritability, seizures
- Dermatologic: Skin rash
- Gastrointestinal: Gastric irritation
- Neuromuscular & skeletal: Tremor
- Miscellaneous: Allergic reactions

**Drug Interactions** Decreased effect/increased toxicity: Changes in diet may affect the elimination of theophylline; charcoal-broiled foods may increase elimination, reducing half-life by 50%; see table for factors affecting serum levels.

**Drug Uptake**

Absorption: Oral: Up to 100% absorbed depending upon formulation used

Half-life: Highly variable and dependent upon age, liver function, cardiac function, lung disease, and smoking history

**Pregnancy Risk Factor** C

**Dosage Forms**

Capsule:
- Immediate release (Elixophyllin®): 100 mg, 200 mg
- Timed release:
  - 8-12 hours (Aerolate®): 65 mg [III]; 130 mg [JR], 260 mg [SR]
  - 8-12 hours (Slo-bid™): 50 mg, 75 mg, 100 mg, 125 mg, 200 mg, 300 mg
  - 8-12 hours (Slo-Phyllin® Gyrocaps®): 60 mg, 125 mg, 250 mg
  - 12 hours (Theobid® Duracaps®): 260 mg
  - 12 hours (Theoclear® L.A.): 130 mg, 260 mg
  - 12 hours (Theospan®-SR): 130 mg, 260 mg
  - 12 hours (Theovent®): 125 mg, 250 mg
  - 24 hours (Theo-24®): 100 mg, 200 mg, 300 mg

Elixir (Asmalix®, Elixomin®, Elixophyllin®): 80 mg/15 mL (15 mL, 30 mL, 480 mL, 4000 mL)

Infusion, in $D_5W$: 0.4 mg/mL (1000 mL); 0.8 mg/mL (500 mL, 1000 mL); 1.6 mg/mL (250 mL, 500 mL); 2 mg/mL (100 mL); 3.2 mg/mL (250 mL); 4 mg/mL (50 mL, 100 mL);

Solution, oral:
- Theolair™: 80 mg/15 mL (15 mL, 18.75 mL, 30 mL, 480 mL)

Syrup:
- Aquaphyllin®, Slo-Phyllin®, Theoclear-80®, Theostat-80®: 80 mg/15 mL (15 mL, 30 mL, 500 mL)
- Accurbron®: 150 mg/15 mL (480 mL)

Tablet: Immediate release:
- Slo-Phyllin®: 100 mg, 200 mg
- Theolair™: 125 mg, 250 mg
- Quibron®-T: 300 mg

Tablet:
- Controlled release (Theo-X®): 100 mg, 200 mg, 300 mg
- Timed release:
  - 12-24 hours: 100 mg, 200 mg, 300 mg, 450 mg
  - 8-12 hours (Quibron®-T/SR): 300 mg
  - 8-12 hours (Respbid®): 250 mg, 500 mg
  - 8-12 hours (Sustaire®): 100 mg, 300 mg
  - 8-12 hours (T-Phyl®): 200 mg
  - 12-24 hours (Theochron®): 100 mg, 200 mg, 300 mg
  - 8-24 hour: 100 mg, 200 mg, 300 mg
  - 8-24 hours (Theo-Dur®): 100 mg, 200 mg, 300 mg, 450 mg
  - 8-24 hours (Theo-Sav®): 100 mg, 200 mg, 300 mg
  - 24 hours (Theolair™-SR): 200 mg, 250 mg, 300 mg, 500 mg
  - 24 hours (Uni-Dur®): 400 mg, 600 mg
  - 24 hours (Uniphyl®): 400 mg

**Generic Available** Yes

## Theophylline and Guaifenesin (thee OF i lin & gwye FEN e sin)

**U.S. Brand Names** Bronchial®; Glycerol-T®; Quibron®; Slo-Phyllin GG®

**Therapeutic Category** Antiasthmatic; Bronchodilator; Expectorant; Theophylline Derivative

**Use** Symptomatic treatment of bronchospasm associated with bronchial asthma, chronic bronchitis and pulmonary emphysema

**Usual Dosage** Adults: Oral: 16 mg/kg/day or 400 mg theophylline/day, in divided doses, every 6-8 hours

**Local Anesthetic/Vasoconstrictor Precautions** No information available to require special precautions

**Effects on Dental Treatment** Do not prescribe any erythromycin product to patients taking theophylline products. Erythromycin will delay the normal metabolic inactivation of theophyllines leading to increased blood levels; this has resulted in nausea, vomiting and CNS restlessness

(Continued)

## Theophylline and Guaifenesin *(Continued)*

**Pregnancy Risk Factor** C

**Dosage Forms**

Capsule: Theophylline 150 mg and guaifenesin 90 mg; theophylline 300 mg and guaifenesin 180 mg

Elixir: Theophylline 150 mg and guaifenesin 90 mg per 15 mL (480 mL)

**Generic Available** Yes

## Theophylline, Ephedrine, and Hydroxyzine

(thee OF i lin, e FED rin, & hye DROKS i zeen)

**U.S. Brand Names** Hydrophed®; Marax®

**Therapeutic Category** Antiasthmatic; Bronchodilator; Theophylline Derivative

**Use** Possibly effective for controlling bronchospastic disorders

**Usual Dosage**

Children:

2-5 years: ½ tablet 2-4 times/day or 2.5 mL 3-4 times/day

>5 years: ½ tablet 2-4 times/day or 5 mL 3-4 times/day

Adults: 1 tablet 2-4 times/day

**Local Anesthetic/Vasoconstrictor Precautions** Use vasoconstrictors with caution since ephedrine may enhance cardiostimulation and vasopressor effects of sympathomimetics

**Effects on Dental Treatment** Prescribe erythromycin products with caution to patients taking theophylline products. Erythromycin will delay the normal metabolic inactivation of theophyllines leading to increased blood levels; this has resulted in nausea, vomiting and CNS restlessness

**Pregnancy Risk Factor** C

**Dosage Forms**

Syrup, dye free: Theophylline 32.5 mg, ephedrine 6.25 mg, and hydroxyzine 2.5 mg per 5 mL

Tablet: Theophylline 130 mg, ephedrine 25 mg, and hydroxyzine 10 mg

**Generic Available** Yes

## Theophylline, Ephedrine, and Phenobarbital

(thee OF i lin, e FED rin, & fee noe BAR bi tal)

**U.S. Brand Names** Tedral®

**Therapeutic Category** Antiasthmatic; Bronchodilator; Theophylline Derivative

**Synonyms** Ephedrine, Theophylline and Phenobarbital

**Use** Prevention and symptomatic treatment of bronchial asthma; relief of asthmatic bronchitis and other bronchospastic disorders

**Usual Dosage**

Children >60 lb: 1 tablet or 5 mL every 4 hours

Adults: 1-2 tablets or 10-20 mL every 4 hours

**Local Anesthetic/Vasoconstrictor Precautions** Use vasoconstrictors with caution since ephedrine may enhance cardiostimulation and vasopressor effects of sympathomimetics

**Effects on Dental Treatment** Prescribe erythromycin products with caution to patients taking theophylline products. Erythromycin will delay the normal metabolic inactivation of theophyllines leading to increased blood levels; this has resulted in nausea, vomiting and CNS restlessness

**Pregnancy Risk Factor** D

**Dosage Forms**

Suspension: Theophylline 65 mg, ephedrine sulfate 12 mg, and phenobarbital 4 mg per 5 mL

Tablet: Theophylline 118 mg, ephedrine sulfate 25 mg, and phenobarbital 11 mg; theophylline 130 mg, ephedrine sulfate 24 mg, and phenobarbital 8 mg

**Generic Available** Yes


- **Theophylline Ethylenediamine** *see* Aminophylline *on page 63*
- **Theospan®-SR** *see* Theophylline *on page 969*
- **Theovent®** *see* Theophylline *on page 969*
- **Theo-X®** *see* Theophylline *on page 969*
- **Therabid® [OTC]** *see* Vitamins, Multiple *on page 1051*
- **Thera-Combex® H-P Kapseals® [OTC]** *see* Vitamin B Complex With Vitamin C *on page 1050*
- **TheraCys®** *see* BCG Vaccine *on page 121*
- **Theraflu® Non-Drowsy Formula Maximum Strength [OTC]** *see* Acetaminophen, Dextromethorphan, and Pseudoephedrine *on page 32*
- **Thera-Flur®** *see* Fluoride *on page 441*
- **Thera-Flur-N®** *see* Fluoride *on page 441*
- **Theragran® [OTC]** *see* Vitamins, Multiple *on page 1051*

♦ **Theragran® Hematinic®** *see* Vitamins, Multiple *on page 1051*
♦ **Theragran® Liquid [OTC]** *see* Vitamins, Multiple *on page 1051*
♦ **Theragran-M® [OTC]** *see* Vitamins, Multiple *on page 1051*
♦ **Thera-Hist® Syrup [OTC]** *see* Chlorpheniramine and Phenylpropanolamine *on page 233*
♦ **Theramin® Expectorant [OTC]** *see* Guaifenesin and Phenylpropanolamine *on page 480*
♦ **Therapeutic Multivitamins** *see* Vitamins, Multiple *on page 1051*
♦ **Theraplex Z® [OTC]** *see* Pyrithione Zinc *on page 869*
♦ **Thermazene®** *see* Silver Sulfadiazine *on page 914*
♦ **Theroxide® Wash [OTC]** *see* Benzoyl Peroxide *on page 130*

## Thiabendazole (thye a BEN da zole)

**U.S. Brand Names** Mintezol®

**Therapeutic Category** Anthelmintic

**Use** Treatment of strongyloidiasis, cutaneous larva migrans, visceral larva migrans, dracunculiasis, trichinosis, and mixed helminthic infections

**Usual Dosage** Purgation is not required prior to use; drinking of fruit juice aids in expulsion of worms by removing the mucous to which the intestinal tapeworms attach themselves.

Children and Adults: Oral: 50 mg/kg/day divided every 12 hours; maximum dose: 3 g/day
- Strongyloidiasis: For 2 consecutive days
- Cutaneous larva migrans: For 2-5 consecutive days
- Visceral larva migrans: For 5-7 consecutive days
- Trichinosis: For 2-4 consecutive days
- Dracunculosis: 50-75 mg/kg/day divided every 12 hours for 3 days

**Mechanism of Action** Inhibits helminth-specific mitochondrial fumarate reductase

**Local Anesthetic/Vasoconstrictor Precautions** No information available to require special precautions

**Effects on Dental Treatment** No effects or complications reported

**Other Adverse Effects**

>10%:
- Central nervous system: Seizures, hallucinations, delirium, dizziness, drowsiness, headache
- Gastrointestinal: Anorexia, diarrhea, nausea, vomiting, drying of mucous membranes
- Neuromuscular & skeletal: Numbness
- Otic: Tinnitus

1% to 10%: Dermatologic: Skin rash, Stevens-Johnson syndrome

<1%:
- Central nervous system: Chills
- Genitourinary: Malodor of urine
- Hematologic: Leukopenia
- Hepatic: Hepatotoxicity
- Ocular: Blurred or yellow vision
- Renal: Nephrotoxicity
- Miscellaneous: Lymphadenopathy, hypersensitivity reactions

**Drug Interactions** Increased levels of theophylline and other xanthines

**Drug Uptake**

Absorption: Rapid and nearly complete

Time to peak serum concentration: Within 1-2 hours

**Pregnancy Risk Factor** C

**Generic Available** No

## Thiamine (THYE a min)

**U.S. Brand Names** Betalin®S; Biamine®

**Canadian Brand Names** Betaxin®; Bewon®

**Therapeutic Category** Vitamin, Water Soluble

**Use** Treatment of thiamine deficiency including beriberi, Wernicke's encephalopathy syndrome, and peripheral neuritis associated with pellagra, alcoholic patients with altered sensorium; various genetic metabolic disorders

**Usual Dosage**

Recommended daily allowance:
- <6 months: 0.3 mg
- 6 months to 1 year: 0.4 mg
- 1-3 years: 0.7 mg
- 4-6 years: 0.9 mg
- 7-10 years: 1 mg
- 11-14 years: 1.1-1.3 mg

(Continued)

## Thiamine *(Continued)*

>14 years: 1-1.5 mg

Thiamine deficiency (beriberi):

Children: 10-25 mg/dose I.M. or I.V. daily (if critically ill), or 10-50 mg/dose orally every day for 2 weeks, then 5-10 mg/dose orally daily for 1 month

Adults: 5-30 mg/dose I.M. or I.V. 3 times/day (if critically ill); then orally 5-30 mg/day in single or divided doses 3 times/day for 1 month

Wenicke's encephalopathy: Adults: Initial: 100 mg I.V., then 50-100 mg/day I.M. or I.V. until consuming a regular, balanced diet

Dietary supplement (depends on caloric or carbohydrate content of the diet):

Children: 0.5-1 mg/day

Adults: 1-2 mg/day

**Note:** The above doses can be found in multivitamin preparations

Metabolic disorders: Oral: Adults: 10-20 mg/day (dosages up to 4 g/day in divided doses have been used)

**Mechanism of Action** An essential coenzyme in carbohydrate metabolism by combining with adenosine triphosphate to form thiamine pyrophosphate

**Local Anesthetic/Vasoconstrictor Precautions** No information available to require special precautions

**Effects on Dental Treatment** No effects or complications reported

**Other Adverse Effects** <1%:

Cardiovascular: Cardiovascular collapse and death

Dermatologic: Rash, angioedema

Neuromuscular & skeletal: Paresthesia

Miscellaneous: Feeling of warmth

**Drug Interactions** No data reported

**Drug Uptake** Absorption:

Oral: Adequate

I.M.: Rapid and complete

**Pregnancy Risk Factor** A (C if dose exceeds RDA recommendation)

**Generic Available** Yes

## Thiethylperazine (thye eth il PER a zeen)

**U.S. Brand Names** Norzine®

**Therapeutic Category** Antiemetic

**Use** Relief of nausea and vomiting

**Unlabeled use:** Treatment of vertigo

**Usual Dosage** Children >12 years and Adults:

Oral, I.M., rectal: 10 mg 1-3 times/day as needed

I.V. and S.C. routes of administration are not recommended

**Mechanism of Action** Blocks postsynaptic mesolimbic dopaminergic receptors in the brain; exhibits a strong alpha-adrenergic blocking effect and depresses the release of hypothalamic and hypophyseal hormones; acts directly on chemoreceptor trigger zone and vomiting center

**Local Anesthetic/Vasoconstrictor Precautions** No information available to require special precautions

**Effects on Dental Treatment** >10% of patients will experience dry mouth

**Other Adverse Effects**

>10%:

Central nervous system: Drowsiness, dizziness

Respiratory: Dry nose

1% to 10%:

Cardiovascular: Tachycardia, orthostatic hypotension

Central nervous system: Confusion, convulsions, extrapyramidal effects, tardive dyskinesia, fever, headache

Hematologic: Agranulocytosis

Hepatic: Cholestatic jaundice

Otic: Tinnitus

**Drug Interactions** Increased effect/toxicity with CNS depressants (eg, anesthetics, opiates, tranquilizers, alcohol), lithium, atropine, epinephrine, MAO inhibitors, TCAs

**Drug Uptake**

Onset of antiemetic effect: Within 30 minutes

Duration of action: ~4 hours

**Pregnancy Risk Factor** X

**Generic Available** No

## Thimerosal (thye MER oh sal)

**U.S. Brand Names** Aeroaid® [OTC]; Mersol® [OTC]; Merthiolate® [OTC]

**Therapeutic Category** Antibacterial, Topical

**Use** Organomercurial antiseptic with sustained bacteriostatic and fungistatic activity

**Usual Dosage** Apply 1-3 times/day

**Local Anesthetic/Vasoconstrictor Precautions** No information available to require special precautions

**Effects on Dental Treatment** No effects or complications reported

**Generic Available** Yes

## Thioguanine (thye oh GWAH neen)

**Therapeutic Category** Antineoplastic Agent, Antimetabolite

**Synonyms** 2-Amino-6-Mercaptopurine; TG; 6-TG; 6-Thioguanine; Tioguanine

**Use** Remission induction in acute myelogenous (nonlymphocytic) leukemia; treatment of chronic myelogenous leukemia and acute lymphocytic leukemia

**Usual Dosage** Total daily dose can be given at one time; offers little advantage over mercaptopurine; is sometimes ordered as 6-thioguanine, with 6 being part of the drug name and not some kind of unit or strength

Oral (refer to individual protocols):
- Children <3 years: Combination drug therapy for acute nonlymphocytic leukemia: 3.3 mg/kg/day in divided doses twice daily for 4 days
- Children and Adults: 2-3 mg/kg/day calculated to nearest 20 mg or 75-200 mg/m²/day in 1-2 divided doses for 5-7 days or until remission is attained

**Mechanism of Action** Purine analog that is incorporated into DNA and RNA resulting in the blockage of synthesis and metabolism of purine nucleotides

**Local Anesthetic/Vasoconstrictor Precautions** No information available to require special precautions

**Effects on Dental Treatment** No effects or complications reported

**Other Adverse Effects**

1% to 10%:
- Dermatologic: Skin rash
- Endocrine & metabolic: Hyperuricemia
- Gastrointestinal: Mild nausea or vomiting, anorexia, stomatitis, diarrhea
  - Emetic potential: Low (<10%)
- Neuromuscular: Unsteady gait

<1%:
- Central nervous system: Neurotoxicity
- Dermatologic: Photosensitivity
- Hepatic: Hepatitis, jaundice, veno-occlusive hepatic disease

**Drug Uptake**
- Absorption: Oral: 30%
- Serum half-life, terminal: 11 hours
- Time to peak serum concentration: Within 8 hours

**Pregnancy Risk Factor** D

**Generic Available** No

♦ **6-Thioguanine** *see* Thioguanine *on this page*
♦ **Thiola™** *see* Tiopronin *on page 988*

## Thiopental (thye oh PEN tal)

**U.S. Brand Names** Pentothal® Sodium

**Therapeutic Category** Barbiturate; General Anesthetic, Intravenous; Sedative

**Use** Induction of anesthesia; adjunct for intubation in head injury patients; control of convulsive states; treatment of elevated intracranial pressure

**Usual Dosage** I.V.:

Induction anesthesia:
- Children 1-12 years: 5-6 mg/kg
- Adults: 3-5 mg/kg

Maintenance anesthesia:
- Children: 1 mg/kg as needed
- Adults: 25-100 mg as needed

Increased intracranial pressure: Children and Adults: 1.5-5 mg/kg/dose; repeat as needed to control intracranial pressure

Seizures:
- Children: 2-3 mg/kg/dose, repeat as needed
- Adults: 75-250 mg/dose, repeat as needed

**Rectal administration:** (Patient should be NPO for no less than 3 hours prior to administration)

**Suggested initial doses of thiopental rectal suspension are:**
- <3 months: 15 mg/kg/dose
- >3 months: 25 mg/kg/dose

(Continued)

## Thiopental *(Continued)*

**Note:** The age of a premature infant should be adjusted to reflect the age that the infant would have been if full-term (eg, an infant, now age 4 months, who was 2 months premature should be considered to be a 2-month old infant).

Doses should be rounded downward to the nearest 50 mg increment to allow for accurate measurement of the dose

Inactive or debilitated patients and patients recently medicated with other sedatives, (eg, chloral hydrate, meperidine, chlorpromazine, and promethazine), may require smaller doses than usual

**If the patient is not sedated within 15-20 minutes, a single repeat dose of thiopental can be given. The single repeat doses are:**

<3 months: <7.5 mg/kg/dose

>3 months: 15 mg/kg/dose

Adults weighing >90 kg should not receive >3 g as a total dose (initial plus repeat doses)

Children weighing >34 kg should not receive >1 g as a total dose (initial plus repeat doses)

Neither adults nor children should receive more than one course of thiopental rectal suspension (initial dose plus repeat dose) per 24-hour period

**Mechanism of Action** Interferes with transmission of impulses from the thalamus to the cortex of the brain resulting in an imbalance in central inhibitory and facilitatory mechanisms

**Local Anesthetic/Vasoconstrictor Precautions** No information available to require special precautions

**Effects on Dental Treatment** No effects or complications reported

**Other Adverse Effects**

>10%: Local: Pain on I.M. injection

1% to 10%: Gastrointestinal: Cramping, diarrhea, rectal bleeding

<1%:

Cardiovascular: Hypotension, peripheral vascular collapse, myocardial depression, cardiac arrhythmias

Central nervous system: Seizures, headache, emergence delirium, prolonged somnolence and recovery, anxiety

Dermatologic: Erythema, pruritus, urticaria

Gastrointestinal: Nausea, vomiting

Hematologic: Hemolytic anemia

Local: Thrombophlebitis

Neuromuscular & skeletal: Tremor, involuntary muscle movement, twitching, rigidity, radial nerve palsy

Respiratory: Respiratory depression, coughing, circulatory depression, rhinitis, apnea, laryngospasm, bronchospasm, sneezing, dyspnea

Miscellaneous: Hiccups, anaphylactic reactions

**Drug Interactions** Increased toxicity with CNS depressants (especially narcotic analgesics and phenothiazines), salicylates, sulfisoxazole

**Drug Uptake**

Onset of action: I.V.: Anesthesia occurs in 30-60 seconds

Duration: 5-30 minutes

Serum half-life: 3-11.5 hours, decreased in children vs adults

**Pregnancy Risk Factor** C

**Dosage Forms**

Injection, as sodium: 250 mg, 400 mg, 500 mg, 1 g, 2.5 g, 5 g

Suspension, rectal, as sodium: 400 mg/g (2 g)

**Generic Available** Yes

♦ **Thiophosphoramide** *see* Thiotepa *on next page*

## Thioridazine (thye oh RID a zeen)

**U.S. Brand Names** Mellaril®; Mellaril-S®

**Canadian Brand Names** Apo®-Thioridazine; Novo-Ridazine; PMS-Thioridazine

**Therapeutic Category** Antipsychotic Agent; Phenothiazine Derivative

**Use** Management of manifestations of psychotic disorders; depressive neurosis; alcohol withdrawal; dementia in elderly; behavioral problems in children

**Usual Dosage** Oral:

Children >2 years: Range: 0.5-3 mg/kg/day in 2-3 divided doses; usual: 1 mg/kg/day; maximum: 3 mg/kg/day

Behavior problems: Initial: 10 mg 2-3 times/day, increase gradually

Severe psychoses: Initial: 25 mg 2-3 times/day, increase gradually

Adults:

Psychoses: Initial: 50-100 mg 3 times/day with gradual increments as needed and tolerated; maximum: 800 mg/day in 2-4 divided doses; if >65 years, initial dose: 10 mg 3 times/day

Depressive disorders, dementia: Initial: 25 mg 3 times/day; maintenance dose: 20-200 mg/day

**Mechanism of Action** Blocks postsynaptic mesolimbic dopaminergic receptors in the brain; exhibits a strong alpha-adrenergic blocking effect and depresses the release of hypothalamic and hypophyseal hormones

**Local Anesthetic/Vasoconstrictor Precautions** Most pharmacology textbooks state that in presence of phenothiazines, systemic doses of epinephrine paradoxically decrease the blood pressure. This is the so called "epinephrine reversal" phenomenon. This has never been observed when epinephrine is given by infiltration as part of the anesthesia procedure.

**Effects on Dental Treatment** Significant hypotension may occur, especially when the drug is administered parenterally; orthostatic hypotension is due to alpha-receptor blockade, the elderly are at greater risk for orthostatic hypotension

Tardive dyskinesia; Prevalence rate may be 40% in elderly; development of the syndrome and the irreversible nature are proportional to duration and total cumulative dose over time

Extrapyramidal reactions are more common in elderly with up to 50% developing these reactions after 60 years of age; drug-induced **Parkinson's syndrome** occurs often; **Akathisia** is the most common extrapyramidal reaction in elderly

Increased confusion, memory loss, psychotic behavior, and agitation frequently occur as a consequence of anticholinergic effects

Antipsychotic associated sedation in nonpsychotic patients is extremely unpleasant due to feelings of depersonalization, derealization, and dysphoria

**Other Adverse Effects**

>10%:

Central nervous system: Pseudoparkinsonism, akathisia, dystonias, tardive dyskinesia (persistent), dizziness

Cardiovascular: Hypotension, orthostatic hypotension

Gastrointestinal: Constipation

Ocular: Pigmentary retinopathy

Respiratory: Basal congestion

Miscellaneous: Decreased sweating

1% to 10%:

Dermatologic: Photosensitivity, skin rash

Endocrine & metabolic: Changes in menstrual cycle, changes in libido, pain in breasts

Gastrointestinal: Weight gain, nausea, vomiting, stomach pain

Genitourinary: Dysuria, ejaculatory disturbances

Neuromuscular & skeletal: Trembling of fingers

<1%:

Central nervous system: Neuroleptic malignant syndrome (NMS), impairment of temperature regulation, lowering of seizures threshold

Dermatologic: Discoloration of skin (blue-gray)

Endocrine & metabolic: Galactorrhea

Genitourinary: Priapism

Hematologic: Agranulocytosis, leukopenia

Hepatic: Cholestatic jaundice, hepatotoxicity

Ocular: Cornea and lens changes

**Drug Interactions**

Decreased effect with anticholinergics

Decreased effect of guanethidine

Increased toxicity with CNS depressants, lithium (rare), tricyclic antidepressants (cardiotoxicity), propranolol, pindolol

**Drug Uptake**

Duration of action: 4-5 days

Serum half-life: 21-25 hours

Time to peak serum concentration: Within 1 hour

**Pregnancy Risk Factor** C

**Generic Available** Yes

## Thiotepa (thye oh TEP a)

**Therapeutic Category** Antineoplastic Agent, Alkylating Agent

**Synonyms** TESPA; Thiophosphoramide; Triethylenethiophosphoramide; TSPA

**Use** Treatment of superficial tumors of the bladder; palliative treatment of adenocarcinoma of breast or ovary; lymphomas and sarcomas; meningeal neoplasms;

(Continued)

## Thiotepa *(Continued)*

control pleural, pericardial or peritoneal effusions caused by metastatic tumors; high-dose regimens with autologous bone marrow transplantation

**Usual Dosage** Refer to individual protocols. Dosing must be based on the clinical and hematologic response of the patient.

Children: Sarcomas: I.V.: 25-65 mg/m² as a single dose every 21 days
Adults:
- I.M., I.V., S.C.: 30-60 mg/m² once per week
- I.V. doses of 0.3-0.4 mg/kg by rapid I.V. administration every 1-4 weeks, or 0.2 mg/kg or 6-8 mg/m²/day for 4-5 days every 2-4 weeks
- High-dose therapy for bone marrow transplant: I.V.: 500 mg/m²; up to 900 mg/m²
- I.M. doses of 15-30 mg in various schedules have been given
- Intracavitary: 0.6-0.8 mg/kg
- Intrapericardial dose: Usually 15-30 mg

**Mechanism of Action** Alkylating agent that reacts with DNA phosphate groups to produce cross-linking of DNA strands leading to inhibition of DNA, RNA, and protein synthesis; mechanism of action has not been explored as thoroughly as the other alkylating agents, it is presumed that the aziridine rings open and react as nitrogen mustard; reactivity is enhanced at a lower pH

**Local Anesthetic/Vasoconstrictor Precautions** No information available to require special precautions

**Effects on Dental Treatment** No effects or complications reported

**Other Adverse Effects**

Carcinogenesis: Like other alkylating agents, this drug is carcinogenic

>10%: Local: Pain at injection site
- Hematologic: Dose-limiting toxicity which is dose-related and cumulative; moderate to severe leukopenia and severe thrombocytopenia have occurred. Anemia and pancytopenia may become fatal, so careful hematologic monitoring is required; intravesical administration may cause bone marrow suppression as well.
  - Myelosuppressive: WBC: Moderate; Platelets: Severe; Onset (days): 7-10; Nadir (days): 14; Recovery (days): 28

1% to 10%:
- Central nervous system: Dizziness, fever, headache
- Dermatologic: Alopecia, rash, pruritus
- Endocrine & metabolic: Hyperuricemia
- Gastrointestinal: Stomatitis
  - Emetic potential: Low (<10%); nausea and vomiting rarely occur
- Renal: Hematuria

<1%:
- Gastrointestinal: Tightness of the throat, anorexia
- Genitourinary: Hemorrhagic cystitis
- Miscellaneous: Allergic reactions

**Drug Uptake**

Absorption: Following intracavitary instillation, the drug is unreliably absorbed (10% to 100%) through the bladder mucosa; variable I.M. absorption

Serum half-life, terminal: 109 minutes with dose-dependent clearance

**Pregnancy Risk Factor** D

**Generic Available** No

## Thiothixene (thye oh THIKS een)

**U.S. Brand Names** Navane®

**Therapeutic Category** Antipsychotic Agent; Phenothiazine Derivative

**Use** Management of psychotic disorders

**Usual Dosage**

Children <12 years: Oral: 0.25 mg/kg/24 hours in divided doses (dose not well established)

Children >12 years and Adults: Mild to moderate psychosis:
- Oral: 2 mg 3 times/day, up to 20-30 mg/day; more severe psychosis: Initial: 5 mg 2 times/day, may increase gradually, if necessary; maximum: 60 mg/day
- I.M.: 4 mg 2-4 times/day, increase dose gradually; usual: 16-20 mg/day; maximum: 30 mg/day; change to oral dose as soon as able

**Mechanism of Action** Elicits antipsychotic activity by postsynaptic blockade of CNS dopamine receptors resulting in inhibition of dopamine-mediated effects; also has alpha-adrenergic blocking activity

**Local Anesthetic/Vasoconstrictor Precautions** Most pharmacology textbooks state that in presence of phenothiazines, systemic doses of epinephrine paradoxically decrease the blood pressure. This is the so called "epinephrine reversal" phenomenon. This has never been observed when epinephrine is given by infiltration as part of the anesthesia procedure.

**Effects on Dental Treatment** Significant hypotension may occur, especially when the drug is administered parenterally; orthostatic hypotension is due to alpha-receptor blockade, the elderly are at greater risk for orthostatic hypotension

Tardive dyskinesia: Prevalence rate may be 40% in elderly; development of the syndrome and the irreversible nature are proportional to duration and total cumulative dose over time

Extrapyramidal reactions are more common in elderly with up to 50% developing these reactions after 60 years of age; drug-induced **Parkinson's syndrome** occurs often; **Akathisia** is the most common extrapyramidal reaction in elderly

Increased confusion, memory loss, psychotic behavior, and agitation frequently occur as a consequence of anticholinergic effects

Antipsychotic associated sedation in nonpsychotic patients is extremely unpleasant due to feelings of depersonalization, derealization, and dysphoria

**Other Adverse Effects**

>10%:

Cardiovascular: Hypotension, orthostatic hypotension
Central nervous system: Pseudoparkinsonism, akathisia, dystonias, tardive dyskinesia (persistent), dizziness
Gastrointestinal: Constipation
Ocular: Pigmentary retinopathy
Respiratory: Nasal congestion
Miscellaneous: Decreased sweating

1% to 10%:

Dermatologic: Photosensitivity, skin rash
Endocrine & metabolic: Changes in menstrual cycle, changes in libido, pain in breasts
Gastrointestinal: Weight gain, nausea, vomiting, stomach pain
Genitourinary: Dysuria, ejaculatory disturbances
Neuromuscular & skeletal: Trembling of fingers

<1%:

Central nervous system: Neuroleptic malignant syndrome (NMS), impairment of temperature regulation, lowering of seizures threshold
Endocrine & metabolic: Galactorrhea
Dermatologic: Discoloration of skin (blue-gray)
Genitourinary: Priapism
Hematologic: Agranulocytosis, leukopenia
Hepatic: Cholestatic jaundice, hepatotoxicity
Ocular: Fornea and lens changes

**Drug Interactions**

Decreased effect of guanethidine; decreased effect with anticholinergics
Increased toxicity with CNS depressants, anticholinergics, alcohol

**Drug Uptake** Serum half-life: >24 hours with chronic use

**Pregnancy Risk Factor** C

**Generic Available** Yes

♦ **Thorazine®** *see* Chlorpromazine *on page 238*

♦ **Thrombate III™** *see* Antithrombin III *on page 92*

♦ **Thrombinar®** *see* Thrombin, Topical *on this page*

## Thrombin, Topical (THROM bin, TOP i kal)

**U.S. Brand Names** Thrombinar®; Thrombogen®; Thrombostat®

**Therapeutic Category** Hemostatic Agent

**Use** Dental & Medical: Hemostasis whenever minor bleeding from capillaries and small venules is accessible

**Usual Dosage** Use 1000-2000 units/mL of solution where bleeding is profuse; apply powder directly to the site of bleeding or on oozing surfaces; use 100 units/mL for bleeding from skin or mucosal surfaces

**Mechanism of Action** Catalyzes the conversion of fibrinogen to fibrin

**Local Anesthetic/Vasoconstrictor Precautions** No information available to require special precautions

**Effects on Dental Treatment** No effects or complications reported

**Other Adverse Effects** 1% to 10%:

Central nervous system: Fever
Miscellaneous: Allergic type reaction

**Contraindications** Hypersensitivity to thrombin or any component

**Warnings/Precautions** Do not inject, for topical use only

**Drug Interactions** No data reported

(Continued)

## Thrombin, Topical *(Continued)*

**Pregnancy Risk Factor** C

**Breast-feeding Considerations** No data reported

**Dosage Forms** Powder: 1000 units, 5000 units, 10,000 units, 20,000 units, 50,000 units

**Generic Available** No

**Comments** Topical thrombin is not to be used in conjunction with oxidized cellulose

- **Thrombogen®** *see* Thrombin, Topical *on previous page*
- **Thrombostat®** *see* Thrombin, Topical *on previous page*
- **Thypinone® Injection** *see* Protirelin *on page 861*
- **Thyrar®** *see* Thyroid *on this page*
- **Thyro-Block®** *see* Potassium Iodide *on page 824*

## Thyroid (THYE royd)

**Related Information**

Endocrine Disorders & Pregnancy *on page 1082*

**U.S. Brand Names** Armour® Thyroid; S-P-T; Thyrar®; Thyroid Strong®

**Therapeutic Category** Thyroid Product

**Use** Replacement or supplemental therapy in hypothyroidism; pituitary TSH suppressants (thyroid nodules, thyroiditis, multinodular goiter, thyroid cancer), thyrotoxicosis, diagnostic suppression tests

**Usual Dosage** Oral:

Children: See table.

**Recommended Pediatric Dosage for Congenital Hypothyroidism**

| Age | Daily Dose (mg) | Daily Dose/kg (mg) |
|---|---|---|
| 0-6 mo | 15-30 | 4.8-6 |
| 6-12 mo | 30-45 | 3.6-4.8 |
| 1-5 y | 45-60 | 3-3.6 |
| 6-12 y | 60-90 | 2.4-3 |
| >12 y | >90 | 1.2-1.8 |

Adults: Initial: 15-30 mg; increase with 15 mg increments every 2-4 weeks; use 15 mg in patients with cardiovascular disease or myxedema. Maintenance dose: Usually 60-120 mg/day; monitor TSH and clinical symptoms.

Thyroid cancer: Requires larger amounts than replacement therapy

**Mechanism of Action** The primary active compound is $T_3$ (triiodothyronine), which may be converted from $T_4$ (thyroxine) and then circulates throughout the body to influence growth and maturation of various tissues; exact mechanism of action is unknown; however, it is believed the thyroid hormone exerts its many metabolic effects through control of DNA transcription and protein synthesis; involved in normal metabolism, growth, and development; promotes gluconeogenesis, increases utilization and mobilization of glycogen stores and stimulates protein synthesis, increases basal metabolic rate

**Local Anesthetic/Vasoconstrictor Precautions** No precautions with vasoconstrictor are necessary if patient is well controlled with thyroid preparations

**Effects on Dental Treatment** No effects or complications reported

**Other Adverse Effects** <1%:

Cardiovascular: Palpitations, tachycardia, cardiac arrhythmias, chest pain

Central nervous system: Nervousness, headache, insomnia, fever, clumsiness

Dermatologic: Alopecia

Endocrine & metabolic: Changes in menstrual cycle

Gastrointestinal: Weight loss, increased appetite, diarrhea, abdominal cramps, vomiting, constipation

Neuromuscular & skeletal: Excessive bone loss with overtreatment (excess thyroid replacement), tremor, hand tremors, myalgia

Respiratory: Dyspnea

Miscellaneous: Heat intolerance, sweating

**Drug Interactions**

Decreased effect:

Thyroid hormones increase the therapeutic need for oral hypoglycemics or insulin

Cholestyramine can bind thyroid and reduce its absorption

Increased toxicity: Thyroid may potentiate the hypoprothrombinemic effect of oral anticoagulants

**Drug Uptake**

Absorption: $T_4$ is 48% to 79% absorbed; $T_3$ is 95% absorbed; desiccated thyroid contains thyroxine, liothyronine, and iodine (primarily bound); following absorption thyroxine is largely converted to liothyronine

Serum half-life:

Liothyronine: 1-2 days

Thyroxine: 6-7 days

**Pregnancy Risk Factor** A

**Dosage Forms**

Capsule, pork source in soybean oil (S-P-T): 60 mg, 120 mg, 180 mg, 300 mg

Tablet:

Armour® Thyroid: 15 mg, 30 mg, 60 mg, 90 mg, 120 mg, 180 mg, 240 mg, 300 mg

Thyrar® (bovine source): 30 mg, 60 mg, 120 mg

Thyroid Strong® (60 mg is equivalent to 90 mg thyroid USP):

Regular: 30 mg, 60 mg, 120 mg

Sugar coated: 30 mg, 60 mg, 120 mg, 180 mg

Thyroid USP: 15 mg, 30 mg, 60 mg, 120 mg, 180 mg, 300 mg

**Generic Available** Yes

♦ **Thyroid Strong®** *see* Thyroid *on previous page*

♦ **Thyrolar®** *see* Liotrix *on page 593*

## Thyrotropin (thye roe TROE pin)

**U.S. Brand Names** Thytropar®

**Therapeutic Category** Diagnostic Agent, Hypothyroidism; Diagnostic Agent, Thyroid Function

**Use** Diagnostic aid to differentiate thyroid failure; diagnosis of decreased thyroid reserve, to differentiate between primary and secondary hypothyroidism and between primary hypothyroidism and euthyroidism in patients receiving thyroid replacement

**Usual Dosage** Adults: I.M., S.C.: 10 units/day for 1-3 days; follow by a radioiodine study 24 hours past last injection, no response in thyroid failure, substantial response in pituitary failure

**Mechanism of Action** Stimulates formation and secretion of thyroid hormone, increases uptake of iodine by thyroid gland

**Local Anesthetic/Vasoconstrictor Precautions** No information available to require special precautions

**Effects on Dental Treatment** No effects or complications reported

**Other Adverse Effects** <1%:

Cardiovascular: Tachycardia

Central nervous system: Fever, headache

Endocrine & metabolic: Menstrual irregularities

Gastrointestinal: Nausea, vomiting, increased bowel motility

Miscellaneous: Anaphylaxis with repeated administration

**Drug Interactions** No data reported

**Drug Uptake** Serum half-life: 35 minutes, dependent upon thyroid state

**Pregnancy Risk Factor** C

**Dosage Forms** Injection: 10 units

**Generic Available** No

♦ **Thyrotropin Releasing Hormone** *see* Protirelin *on page 861*

♦ **Thytropar®** *see* Thyrotropin *on this page*

## Tiagabine (tye AJ a bene)

**U.S. Brand Names** Gabitril®

**Therapeutic Category** Anticonvulsant, Miscellaneous

**Synonyms** Tiagabine Hydrochloride

**Use** Adjunctive therapy in adults and children 12 years and older in the treatment of partial seizures

**Usual Dosage** Children >12 years and Adults: Oral: Starting dose: 4 mg once daily; the total daily dose may be increased in 4 mg increments beginning the second week of therapy; thereafter, the daily dose may be increased by 4-8 mg/day until clinical response is achieved, up to a maximum of 32 mg/day; the total daily dose at higher levels should be given in divided doses 2-4 times/day

**Mechanism of Action** The exact mechanism by which tiagabine exerts antiseizure activity is not definitively known; however, *in vitro* experiments demonstrate that it enhances the activity of gamma aminobutyric acid (GABA), the major neuroinhibitory transmitter in the nervous system; it is thought that binding to the GABA uptake carrier inhibits the uptake of GABA into presynaptic neurons, allowing an increased amount of GABA to be available to postsynaptic

(Continued)

## Tiagabine *(Continued)*

neurons; based on *in vitro* studies, tiagabine does not inhibit the uptake of dopamine, norepinephrine, serotonin, glutamate or choline

**Local Anesthetic/Vasoconstrictor Precautions** No information available to require special precautions

**Effects on Dental Treatment** No effects or complications reported

**Other Adverse Effects** All adverse effects are dose related

Central nervous system: Dizziness, headache, somnolence, CNS depression, memory disturbance, ataxia

Neuromuscular & skeletal: Tremors, weakness

**Contraindications** Patients who have demonstrated hypersensitivity to the drug or any of its agreements

**Warnings/Precautions** Anticonvulsants should not be discontinued abruptly because of the possibility of increasing seizure frequency; clinical studies were carried out that demonstrated an increase in seizure frequency upon abrupt withdrawal; tiagabine should be withdrawn gradually to minimize the potential of increased seizure frequency, unless safety concerns require a more rapid withdrawal

**Drug Interactions** The clearance of tiagabine is affected by the coadministration of hepatic enzyme inducing anti-epilepsy drugs; tiagabine is cleared more rapidly in patients who have been treated with carbamazepine, phenytoin, primidone and phenobarbital than in patients who have not received these drugs

**Drug Uptake**

Absorption: Rapid (within 1 hour); food prolongs absorption

Serum half-life: 6.7 hours

**Dosage Forms** Tablet: 4 mg, 12 mg, 16 mg, 20 mg

**Selected Readings**

Patsalos PN and Sander JW, "Newer Antiepileptic Drugs: Towards an Improved Risk-Benefit Ratio," *Drug Saf*, 1994, 11(1):37-67.

- **Tiagabine Hydrochloride** *see* Tiagabine *on previous page*
- **Tiamate®** *see* Diltiazem *on page 334*
- **Tiazac™** *see* Diltiazem *on page 334*
- **Ticar®** *see* Ticarcillin *on this page*

## Ticarcillin (tye kar SIL in)

**U.S. Brand Names** Ticar®

**Therapeutic Category** Antibiotic, Penicillin

**Use** Treatment of susceptible infections such as septicemia, acute and chronic respiratory tract infections, skin and soft tissue infections, and urinary tract infections due to susceptible strains of *Pseudomonas*, *Proteus*, and *Escherichia coli* and *Enterobacter*, normally used with other antibiotics (ie, aminoglycosides)

**Usual Dosage** Ticarcillin is generally given I.M. only for the treatment of uncomplicated urinary tract infections

Children: I.V.: Serious Infections:200-300 mg/kg/day in divided doses every 4-6 hours; doses as high as 400 mg/kg/day divided every 4 hours have been used in acute pulmonary exacerbations of cystic fibrosis

Maximum dose: 24 g/day

Urinary tract infections: I.M., I.V.: 50-100 mg/kg/day in divided doses every 6-8 hours

Adults: I.V.: 1-4 g every 4-6 hours

**Mechanism of Action** Interferes with bacterial cell wall synthesis during active multiplication, causing cell wall death and resultant bactericidal activity against susceptible bacteria

**Local Anesthetic/Vasoconstrictor Precautions** No information available to require special precautions

**Effects on Dental Treatment** Prolonged use of penicillins may lead to development of oral candidiasis

**Other Adverse Effects** <1%:

Central nervous system: Convulsions, confusion, drowsiness, fever

Dermatologic: Rash

Endocrine & metabolic: Electrolyte imbalance

Hematologic: Hemolytic anemia, positive Coombs' reaction

Local: Thrombophlebitis

Neuromuscular & skeletal: Myoclonus

Renal: Acute interstitial nephritis

Miscellaneous: Hypersensitivity reactions, anaphylaxis, Jarisch-Herxheimer reaction

**Drug Interactions**

Decreased effect: Tetracyclines cause decreased ticarcillin effectiveness

Increased effect:
Probenecid causes increased ticarcillin levels
Neuromuscular blockers cause increased duration of blockade
Aminoglycosides cause synergistic efficacy

**Drug Uptake**
Absorption: I.M.: 86%
Serum half-life, adults: 1-1.3 hours, prolonged with renal impairment and/or hepatic impairment
Peak serum levels: I.M.: Within 30-75 minutes

**Pregnancy Risk Factor** B

**Generic Available** No

## Ticarcillin and Clavulanate Potassium

(tye kar SIL in & klav yoo LAN ate poe TASS ee um)

**U.S. Brand Names** Timentin®

**Therapeutic Category** Antibiotic, Penicillin

**Use** Treatment of infections of lower respiratory tract, urinary tract, skin and skin structures, bone and joint, and septicemia caused by susceptible organisms. Clavulanate expands activity of ticarcillin to include beta-lactamase producing strains of *S. aureus*, *H. influenzae*, *Enterobacteriaceae*, *Klebsiella*, *Citrobacter*, and *Serratia*

**Usual Dosage** I.V.:
Children: 200-300 mg of ticarcillin component/kg/day in divided doses every 4-6 hours
Adults: 3.1 g (ticarcillin 3 g plus clavulanic acid 0.1 g) every 4-6 hours; maximum: 18-24 g/day
Urinary tract infections: 3.1 g every 6-8 hours

**Mechanism of Action** Ticarcillin interferes with bacterial cell wall synthesis during active multiplication, causing cell wall death and resultant bactericidal activity against susceptible bacteria; clavulanic acid prevents degradation of ticarcillin by binding to the active site on beta-lactamase

**Local Anesthetic/Vasoconstrictor Precautions** No information available to require special precautions

**Effects on Dental Treatment** Prolonged use of penicillins may lead to development of oral candidiasis

**Other Adverse Effects** <1%:
Central nervous system: Convulsions, confusion, drowsiness, fever
Dermatologic: Rash
Endocrine & metabolic: Electrolyte imbalance
Hematologic: Hemolytic anemia, positive Coombs' reaction
Local: Thrombophlebitis
Neuromuscular & skeletal: Myoclonus
Renal: Acute interstitial nephritis
Miscellaneous: Hypersensitivity reactions, anaphylaxis, Jarisch-Herxheimer reaction

**Drug Interactions**
Decreased effect: Tetracyclines cause decreased penicillin effectiveness; aminoglycosides cause physical inactivation of aminoglycosides in the presence of high concentrations of ticarcillin and potential toxicity in patients with mild-moderate renal dysfunction
Increased effect:
Probenecid causes increased penicillin levels
Neuromuscular blockers causes increased duration of blockade
Aminoglycosides cause synergistic efficacy

**Drug Uptake** Serum half-life:
Clavulanate: 66-90 minutes
Ticarcillin: 66-72 minutes in patients with normal renal function; clavulanic acid does not affect the clearance of ticarcillin

**Pregnancy Risk Factor** B

**Generic Available** No

- **TICE® BCG** *see* BCG Vaccine *on page 121*
- **Ticlid®** *see* Ticlopidine *on this page*

## Ticlopidine (tye KLOE pi deen)

**Related Information**
Cardiovascular Diseases *on page 1066*

**U.S. Brand Names** Ticlid®

**Therapeutic Category** Platelet Aggregation Inhibitor

**Use** Platelet aggregation inhibitor that reduces the risk of thrombotic stroke in patients who have had a stroke or stroke precursors
(Continued)

## Ticlopidine *(Continued)*

**Unlabeled use**: Protection of aortocoronary bypass grafts, diabetic microangiopathy, ischemic heart disease, prevention of postoperative DVT, reduction of graft loss following renal transplant

**Usual Dosage** Adults: Oral: 1 tablet twice daily with food

**Mechanism of Action** Ticlopidine is an inhibitor of platelet function with a mechanism which is different from other antiplatelet drugs. The drug significantly increases bleeding time. This effect may not be solely related to ticlopidine's effect on platelets. The prolongation of the bleeding time caused by ticlopidine is further increased by the addition of aspirin in *ex vivo* experiments. Although many metabolites of ticlopidine have been found, none have been shown to account for *in vivo* activity.

**Local Anesthetic/Vasoconstrictor Precautions** No information available to require special precautions

**Effects on Dental Treatment** No effects or complications reported

**Other Adverse Effects**

1% to 10%: Dermatologic: Skin rash

<1%:

- Dermatologic: Bruising
- Gastrointestinal: Diarrhea, nausea, vomiting, GI pain
- Hematologic: Neutropenia, thrombocytopenia
- Hepatic: Elevated liver function tests
- Otic: Tinnitus
- Renal: Hematuria
- Respiratory: Epistaxis

**Drug Interactions**

Decreased effect with antacids (decreased absorption), corticosteroids; decreased effect of digoxin, cyclosporine

Increased effect/toxicity of aspirin, anticoagulants, antipyrine, theophylline, cimetidine (increased levels), NSAIDs

**Drug Uptake**

Onset of action: Within 6 hours

Serum half-life, elimination: 24 hours

**Pregnancy Risk Factor** B

**Generic Available** No


- ♦ **Ticon®** *see* Trimethobenzamide *on page 1020*
- ♦ **TIG** *see* Tetanus Immune Globulin (Human) *on page 962*
- ♦ **Tigan®** *see* Trimethobenzamide *on page 1020*
- ♦ **Tilade® Inhalation Aerosol** *see* Nedocromil Sodium *on page 707*


## Tiludronate (tye LOO droe nate)

**U.S. Brand Names** Skelid®

**Therapeutic Category** Bisphosphonate Derivative

**Synonyms** Tiludronate Disodium

**Use** Paget's disease of the bone

**Usual Dosage** Adults: Oral: 400 mg (2 tablets) [tiludronic acid] daily

**Mechanism of Action** Inhibition of normal and abnormal bone resorption. Inhibits osteoclasts through at least two mechanisms: disruption of the cytoskeletal ring structure, possibly by inhibition of protein-tyrosine-phosphatase, thus leading to the detachment of osteoclasts from the bone surface area and the inhibition of the osteoclast proton pump.

**Local Anesthetic/Vasoconstrictor Precautions** No information available to require special precautions

**Effects on Dental Treatment** No effects or complications reported

**Drug Uptake** Peak plasma concentrations: Within 2 hours

**Dosage Forms** Tablet, as disodium: 240 mg [tiludronic acid 200 mg]; dosage is expressed in terms of tiludronic acid.


- ♦ **Tiludronate Disodium** *see* Tiludronate *on this page*
- ♦ **Timentin®** *see* Ticarcillin and Clavulanate Potassium *on previous page*


## Timolol (TYE moe lole)

**Related Information**

Cardiovascular Diseases *on page 1066*

**U.S. Brand Names** Betimol® Ophthalmic; Blocadren® Oral; Timoptic® Ophthalmic; Timoptic-XE® Ophthalmic

**Canadian Brand Names** Apo®-Timol; Apo®-Timop; Gen-Timolol; Novo-Timol; Nu-Timolol

**Therapeutic Category** Antianginal Agent; Antiglaucoma Agent; Beta-adrenergic Blocker, Noncardioselective; Beta-Adrenergic Blocker, Ophthalmic

**Use** Ophthalmic dosage form used to treat elevated intraocular pressure such as glaucoma or ocular hypertension; orally for treatment of hypertension and angina and reduce mortality following myocardial infarction and prophylaxis of migraine

**Usual Dosage**

Children and Adults: Ophthalmic: Initial: 0.25% solution, instill 1 drop twice daily; increase to 0.5% solution if response not adequate; decrease to 1 drop/day if controlled; do not exceed 1 drop twice daily of 0.5% solution

Adults: Oral:

Hypertension: Initial: 10 mg twice daily, increase gradually every 7 days, usual dosage: 20-40 mg/day in 2 divided doses; maximum: 60 mg/day

Prevention of myocardial infarction: 10 mg twice daily initiated within 1-4 weeks after infarction

Migraine headache: Initial: 10 mg twice daily, increase to maximum of 30 mg/day

**Mechanism of Action** Blocks both $beta_1$- and $beta_2$-adrenergic receptors, reduces intraocular pressure by reducing aqueous humor production or possibly outflow; reduces blood pressure by blocking adrenergic receptors and decreasing sympathetic outflow, produces a negative chronotropic and inotropic activity through an unknown mechanism

**Local Anesthetic/Vasoconstrictor Precautions** No information available to require special precautions

**Effects on Dental Treatment** No effects or complications reported

**Other Adverse Effects**

Ophthalmic:

1% to 10%:

Dermatologic: Alopecia

Ocular: Burning, stinging of eyes

<1%:

Dermatologic: Skin rash

Ocular: Blepharitis, conjunctivitis, keratitis, vision disturbances

Oral:

>10%: Endocrine & metabolic: Decreased sexual ability

1% to 10%:

Cardiovascular: Bradycardia, arrhythmia, reduced peripheral circulation

Central nervous system: Dizziness, itching, fatigue

Neuromuscular & skeletal: Weakness

Respiratory: Dyspnea

<1%:

Cardiovascular: Chest pain, congestive heart failure

Central nervous system: Hallucinations, mental depression, anxiety, nightmares

Dermatologic: Skin rashes

Gastrointestinal: Diarrhea, nausea, vomiting, stomach discomfort

Neuromuscular & skeletal: Numbness in toes and fingers

Ocular: Dry sore eyes

**Drug Interactions** No data reported with ophthalmic preparation

**Drug Uptake**

Onset of hypotensive effect: Oral: Within 15-45 minutes

Peak effect: Within 0.5-2.5 hours

Duration of action: ~4 hours; intraocular effects persist for 24 hours after ophthalmic instillation

Serum half-life: 2-2.7 hours; prolonged with reduced renal function

**Pregnancy Risk Factor** C

**Generic Available** Yes

- **Timoptic® Ophthalmic** *see* Timolol *on previous page*
- **Timoptic-XE® Ophthalmic** *see* Timolol *on previous page*
- **Tinactin® [OTC]** *see* Tolnaftate *on page 997*
- **Tinactin® for Jock Itch [OTC]** *see* Tolnaftate *on page 997*
- **TinBen® [OTC]** *see* Benzoin *on page 130*
- **TinCoBen® [OTC]** *see* Benzoin *on page 130*
- **Tindal®** *see* Acetophenazine *on page 35*
- **Tine Test** *see* Tuberculin Purified Protein Derivative *on page 1031*
- **Tine Test PPD** *see* Tuberculin Purified Protein Derivative *on page 1031*
- **Ting® [OTC]** *see* Tolnaftate *on page 997*
- **Tinver® Lotion** *see* Sodium Thiosulfate *on page 925*

## Tioconazole (tye oh KONE a zole)

**U.S. Brand Names** Vagistat®

**Therapeutic Category** Antifungal Agent, Vaginal

**Use** Local treatment of vulvovaginal candidiasis

(Continued)

## Tioconazole *(Continued)*

**Usual Dosage** Adults: Vaginal: Insert 1 applicatorful in vagina, just prior to bedtime, as a single dose

**Mechanism of Action** A 1-substituted imidazole derivative with a broad antifungal spectrum against a wide variety of dermatophytes and yeasts, usually at a concentration of ≤6.25 mg/L; has been demonstrated to be at least as active *in vitro* as other imidazole antifungals. *In vitro*, tioconazole has been demonstrated 2-8 times as potent as miconazole against common dermal pathogens including *Trichophyton mentagrophytes*, *T. rubrum*, *T. erinacei*, *T. tonsurans*, *Microsporum canis*, *Microsporum gypseum*, and *Candida albicans*. Both agents appear to be similarly effective against *Epidermophyton floccosum*.

**Local Anesthetic/Vasoconstrictor Precautions** No information available to require special precautions

**Effects on Dental Treatment** No effects or complications reported

**Other Adverse Effects**

1% to 10%: Genitourinary: Vulvar/vaginal burning

<1%:

- Genitourinary: Vulvar itching, soreness, swelling, or discharge
- Renal: Polyuria

**Drug Interactions** No data reported

**Drug Uptake**

Absorption: Intravaginal: Following application small amounts of drug are absorbed systemically (25%) within 2-8 hours

Serum half-life: 21-24 hours

**Pregnancy Risk Factor** C

**Generic Available** No

♦ **Tioguanine** *see* Thioguanine *on page 977*

## Tiopronin (tye oh PROE nin)

**U.S. Brand Names** Thiola™

**Therapeutic Category** Urinary Tract Product

**Use** Prevention of kidney stone (cystine) formation in patients with severe homozygous cystinuric who have urinary cystine >500 mg/day who are resistant to treatment with high fluid intake, alkali, and diet modification, or who have had adverse reactions to penicillamine

**Usual Dosage** Adults: Initial dose is 800 mg/day, average dose is 1000 mg/day

**Local Anesthetic/Vasoconstrictor Precautions** No information available to require special precautions

**Effects on Dental Treatment** No effects or complications reported

**Pregnancy Risk Factor** C

**Generic Available** No

## Tirofiban (tye roe FYE ban)

**Related Information**

Cardiovascular Diseases *on page 1066*

**U.S. Brand Names** Aggrastat®

**Therapeutic Category** Platelet Aggregation Inhibitor

**Synonyms** Tirofiban Hydrochloride

**Use** In combination with heparin, is indicated for the treatment of acute coronary syndrome, including patients who are to be managed medically and those undergoing PTCA or atherectomy. In this setting, it has been shown to decrease the rate of a combined endpoint of death, new myocardial infarction or refractory ischemia/repeat cardiac procedure.

**Usual Dosage** Adults: I.V.: Initial rate of 0.4 mcg/kg/minute for 30 minutes and then continued at 0.1 mcg/kg/minute; dosing should be continued through angiography and for 12-24 hours after angioplasty or atherectomy

**Mechanism of Action** A reversible antagonist of fibrinogen binding to the GP IIb/IIIa receptor, the major platelet surface receptor involved in platelet aggregation. When administered intravenously, it inhibits *ex vivo* platelet aggregation in a dose- and concentration-dependent manner. When given according to the recommended regimen, >90% inhibition is attained by the end of the 30-minute infusion. Platelet aggregation inhibition is reversible following cessation of the infusion.

**Local Anesthetic/Vasoconstrictor Precautions** No information available to require special precautions

**Effects on Dental Treatment** No effects or complications reported

**Other Adverse Effects** Bleeding is the major drug-related adverse effect. TIMI criteria are used to classify these events: Major bleeding: 1.4% to 2.2%, minor bleeding: 10.5% to 12.0%, transfusion required: 4.0% to 4.3%.

>1%: Nonbleeding adverse events:
- Cardiovascular: Bradycardia (4%), coronary artery dissection (5%), edema (2%)
- Central nervous system: Dizziness (3%), fever (>1%), headache (>1%), vasovagal reaction (2%)
- Gastrointestinal: Nausea (>1%)
- Genitourinary: Pelvic pain (6%)
- Hematologic: Thrombocytopenia: <90,000/mm$^3$ (1.5%), <50,000/mm$^3$ (0.3%)
- Neuromuscular & skeletal: Leg pain (3%)
- Miscellaneous: Diaphoresis (2%)

<1%:
- Central nervous system: Intracranial bleeding (0.0% to 0.1%)
- Gastrointestinal: GI bleeding (0.1% to 0.2%)
- Genitourinary: Retroperitoneal bleeding (0.0% to 0.6%), GU bleeding (0.0% to 0.1%)

**Drug Interactions** Use with aspirin and heparin is associated with an increase in bleeding over aspirin and heparin alone. Caution when used with other drugs which affect hemostasis - thrombolytics, oral anticoagulants, nonsteroidal anti-inflammatory drugs, dipyridamole, ticlopidine and clopidogrel. Avoid concomitant use of other IIb/IIIa antagonists; levothyroxine and omeprazole increase tirofiban clearance; however, the clinical significance of this interaction remains to be demonstrated.

**Pregnancy Risk Factor** B

**Dosage Forms** Injection: 50 mcg/mL (500 mL); 250 mcg/mL (50 mL)

**Generic Available** No

- ♦ **Tirofiban Hydrochloride** *see* Tirofiban *on previous page*
- ♦ **Ti-Screen® [OTC]** *see* Methoxycinnamate and Oxybenzone *on page 656*
- ♦ **Tisit® Blue Gel [OTC]** *see* Pyrethrins *on page 867*
- ♦ **Tisit® Liquid [OTC]** *see* Pyrethrins *on page 867*
- ♦ **Tisit® Shampoo [OTC]** *see* Pyrethrins *on page 867*
- ♦ **Titralac® Plus Liquid [OTC]** *see* Calcium Carbonate and Simethicone *on page 173*

## Tizanidine (tye ZAN i deen)

**U.S. Brand Names** Zanaflex®

**Therapeutic Category** Alpha$_2$-Adrenergic Agonist Agent

**Use** Intermittent management of increased muscle tone associated with spasticity (eg, multiple sclerosis, spinal cord injury)

**Usual Dosage**

Adults: 2-4 mg 3 times/day
- Usual initial dose: 4 mg, may increase by 2-4 mg as needed for satisfactory reduction of muscle tone every 6-8 hours to a maximum of three doses in any 24-hour period
- Maximum dose: 36 mg/day

**Mechanism of Action** An alpha$_2$-adrenergic agonist agent which decreases excitatory input to alpha motor neurons; an imidazole derivative chemically-related to clonidine, which acts as a centrally acting muscle relaxant with alpha$_2$-adrenergic agonist properties; acts on the level of the spinal cord

**Local Anesthetic/Vasoconstrictor Precautions** No information available to require special precautions

**Effects on Dental Treatment** >10% of patients medicated with tizanidine will experience significant dry mouth; this will disappear with cessation of drug therapy

**Other Adverse Effects**

>10%:
- Cardiovascular: Hypotension
- Central nervous system: Sedation, daytime drowsiness, somnolence
- Gastrointestinal: Xerostomia

1% to 10%:
- Cardiovascular: Bradycardia, syncope
- Central nervous system: Fatigue, dizziness, anxiety, nervousness, insomnia
- Dermatologic: Pruritus, skin rash
- Gastrointestinal: Nausea, vomiting, dyspepsia, constipation, diarrhea
- Hepatic: Elevation of liver enzymes
- Neuromuscular & skeletal: Muscle weakness, tremor

<1%:
- Cardiovascular: Palpitations, ventricular extrasystoles
- Central nervous system: Psychotic-like symptoms, visual hallucinations, delusions
- Hepatic: Hepatic failure

(Continued)

## Tizanidine *(Continued)*

**Warnings/Precautions** Reduce dose in patients with liver or renal disease; use with caution in patients with hypotension or cardiac disease

**Drug Interactions**

Increased effect: Oral contraceptives

Increased toxicity: Additive hypotensive effects may be seen with diuretics, other alpha adrenergic agonists, or antihypertensives; CNS depression with alcohol, baclofen or other CNS depressants

**Drug Uptake**

Duration: 3-6 hours

Serum half-life: 4-8 hours

Time to peak serum concentration: 1-5 hours

**Pregnancy Risk Factor** C

**Generic Available** No

- **TMP-SMZ** *see* Trimethoprim and Sulfamethoxazole *on page 1021*
- **TOBI™ Inhalation Solution** *see* Tobramycin *on this page*
- **TobraDex®** *see* Tobramycin and Dexamethasone *on next page*

## Tobramycin (toe bra MYE sin)

**U.S. Brand Names** AKTob® Ophthalmic; Nebcin® Injection; TOBI™ Inhalation Solution; Tobrex® Ophthalmic

**Therapeutic Category** Antibiotic, Aminoglycoside; Antibiotic, Ophthalmic

**Use** Treatment of documented or suspected *Pseudomonas aeruginosa* infection; infection with a nonpseudomonal enteric bacillus which is more sensitive to tobramycin than gentamicin based on susceptibility tests; empiric therapy in cystic fibrosis and immunocompromised patients; topically used to treat superficial ophthalmic infections caused by susceptible bacteria; inhaled version used for improving lung function and controlling *Pseudomonas aeruginosa* infections in people with cystic fibrosis (CF)

**Usual Dosage** Individualization is critical because of the low therapeutic index

**Use of ideal body weight (IBW) for determining the mg/kg/dose appears to be more accurate than dosing on the basis of total body weight (TBW)**

In morbid obesity, dosage requirement may best be estimated using a dosing weight of IBW + 0.4 (TBW - IBW)

Initial and periodic peak and trough plasma drug levels should be determined, particularly in critically ill patients with serious infections or in disease states known to significantly alter aminoglycoside pharmacokinetics (eg, cystic fibrosis, burns, or major surgery); 2-3 serum level measurements should be obtained after the initial dose to measure the half-life in order to determine the frequency of subsequent doses

Once daily dosing: Higher peak serum drug concentration to MIC ratios, demonstrated aminoglycoside postantibiotic effect, decreased renal cortex drug uptake, and improved cost-time efficiency are supportive reasons for the use of once daily dosing regimens for aminoglycosides. Current research indicates these regimens to be as effective for nonlife-threatening infections, with no higher incidence of nephrotoxicity, than those requiring multiple daily doses. Doses are determined by calculating the entire day's dose via usual multiple dose calculation techniques and administering this quantity as a single dose. Doses are then adjusted to maintain mean serum concentrations above the MIC(s) of the causative organism(s). (Example: 2.5-5 mg/kg as a single dose; expected $Cp_{max}$: 10-20 mcg/mL and $Cp_{min}$: <1 mcg/mL). Further research is needed for universal recommendation in all patient populations and gram-negative disease; exceptions may include those with known high clearance (eg, children, patients with cystic fibrosis, or burns who may require shorter dosage intervals) and patients with renal function impairment for whom longer than conventional dosage intervals are usually required.

Children <5 years: I.M., I.V.: 2.5 mg/kg/dose every 8 hours

Children >5 years: 1.5-2.5 mg/kg/dose every 8 hours

**Note:** Some patients may require larger or more frequent doses if serum levels document the need (ie, cystic fibrosis or febrile granulocytopenic patients).

Adults: I.M., I.V.:

Severe life-threatening infections: 2-2.5 mg/kg/dose

Urinary tract infection: 1.5 mg/kg/dose

Synergy (for gram-positive infections): 1 mg/kg/dose

Children and Adults: Ophthalmic: Instill 1-2 drops of solution every 4 hours; apply ointment 2-3 times/day; for severe infections apply ointment every 3-4 hours, or solution 2 drops every 30-60 minutes initially, then reduce to less frequent intervals

Children and Adults: Inhalation: Inhaled twice daily and requires about 10-15 minutes per treatment. The TOBI™ treatment regimen consists of repeated cycles of 28-days on drug, followed by 28-days off drug.

**Mechanism of Action** Interferes with bacterial protein synthesis by binding to 30S and 50S ribosomal subunits resulting in a defective bacterial cell membrane

**Local Anesthetic/Vasoconstrictor Precautions** No information available to require special precautions

**Effects on Dental Treatment** No effects or complications reported

**Other Adverse Effects**

1% to 10%:

- Renal: Nephrotoxicity
- Neuromuscular & skeletal: Neurotoxicity (neuromuscular blockade)
- Otic: Ototoxicity (auditory), ototoxicity (vestibular)

<1%:

- Cardiovascular: Hypotension
- Central nervous system: Drug fever, headache, drowsiness
- Dermatologic: Skin rash
- Gastrointestinal: Nausea, vomiting
- Hematologic: Eosinophilia anemia
- Neuromuscular & skeletal: Paresthesia, tremor, arthralgia, weakness
- Ocular: Lacrimation, itching, edema of the eyelid, keratitis
- Respiratory: Dyspnea

**Drug Interactions**

Increased effect: Extended spectrum penicillins (synergistic)

Increased toxicity:

- Neuromuscular blockers increase neuromuscular blockade
- Amphotericin B, cephalosporins, loop diuretics cause increased risk of nephrotoxicity

**Drug Uptake**

Absorption: I.M.: Rapid and complete

Serum half-life:

- Adults: 2-3 hours, directly dependent upon glomerular filtration rate
- Adults with impaired renal function: 5-70 hours

Time to peak serum concentration:

- I.M.: Within 30-60 minutes
- I.V.: Within 30 minutes

**Pregnancy Risk Factor** C

**Generic Available** Yes

## Tobramycin and Dexamethasone

(toe bra MYE sin & deks a METH a sone)

**U.S. Brand Names** TobraDex®

**Therapeutic Category** Antibiotic, Ophthalmic; Corticosteroid, Ophthalmic

**Use** Treatment of external ocular infection caused by susceptible gram-negative bacteria and steroid responsive inflammatory conditions of the palpebral and bulbar conjunctiva, lid, cornea, and anterior segment of the globe

**Usual Dosage** Children and Adults: Ophthalmic: Instill 1-2 drops of solution every 4 hours; apply ointment 2-3 times/day; for severe infections apply ointment every 3-4 hours, or solution 2 drops every 30-60 minutes initially, then reduce to less frequent intervals

**Mechanism of Action** Refer to individual monographs for Dexamethasone and Tobramycin

**Local Anesthetic/Vasoconstrictor Precautions** No information available to require special precautions

**Effects on Dental Treatment** No effects or complications reported

**Other Adverse Effects** 1% to 10%:

- Dermatologic: Allergic contact dermatitis, delayed wound healing
- Ocular: Lacrimation, itching, edema of eyelid, keratitis, increased intraocular pressure, glaucoma, cataract formation

**Drug Interactions** Refer to individual monographs for Tobramycin and Dexamethasone

**Drug Uptake**

Absorption: Absorbed into the aqueous humor

Time to peak serum concentration: 1-2 hours after instillation in the cornea and aqueous humor

**Pregnancy Risk Factor** B

**Generic Available** No

♦ **Tobrex® Ophthalmic** *see* Tobramycin *on previous page*

## Tocainide (toe KAY nide)

**Related Information**

Cardiovascular Diseases *on page 1066*

**U.S. Brand Names** Tonocard®

**Therapeutic Category** Antiarrhythmic Agent, Class I-B; Antiarrhythmic Agent (Supraventricular & Ventricular)

**Use** Suppress and prevent symptomatic life-threatening ventricular arrhythmias

**Unlabeled use:** Trigeminal neuralgia

**Usual Dosage** Adults: Oral: 1200-1800 mg/day in 3 divided doses, up to 2400 mg/day

**Mechanism of Action** Class 1B antiarrhythmic agent; suppresses automaticity of conduction tissue, by increasing electrical stimulation threshold of ventricle, HIS-Purkinje system, and spontaneous depolarization of the ventricles during diastole by a direct action on the tissues; blocks both the initiation and conduction of nerve impulses by decreasing the neuronal membrane's permeability to sodium ions, which results in inhibition of depolarization with resultant blockade of conduction

**Local Anesthetic/Vasoconstrictor Precautions** No information available to require special precautions

**Effects on Dental Treatment** No effects or complications reported

**Other Adverse Effects**

>10%:

- Central nervous system: Nervousness, confusion, ataxia, dizziness
- Gastrointestinal: Nausea, anorexia
- Neuromuscular & skeletal: Tremor

1% to 10%:

- Cardiovascular: Hypotension, tachycardia
- Dermatologic: Skin rash
- Gastrointestinal: Vomiting, diarrhea
- Neuromuscular & skeletal: Arthralgia, myalgia, paresthesia
- Ocular: Blurred vision

<1%:

- Cardiovascular: Bradycardia, palpitations
- Hematologic: Agranulocytosis, anemia, leukopenia, neutropenia
- Respiratory: Respiratory arrest
- Miscellaneous: Sweating

**Drug Interactions**

Decreased plasma levels: Phenobarbital, phenytoin, rifampin, and other hepatic enzyme inducers, cimetidine and drugs which make the urine acidic

Increased effect of tocainide, allopurinol

Increased toxicity/levels of caffeine and theophylline

**Drug Uptake**

Absorption: Oral: Extensive, 99% to 100%

Serum half-life: 11-14 hours, prolonged with renal and hepatic impairment with half-life increased to 23-27 hours

Time to peak: Peak serum levels occur within 30-160 minutes

**Pregnancy Risk Factor** C

**Generic Available** No

## Tocophersolan (toe kof er SOE lan)

**U.S. Brand Names** Liqui-E®

**Therapeutic Category** Vitamin, Fat Soluble

**Synonyms** TPGS

**Use** Treatment of vitamin E deficiency resulting from malabsorption due to prolonged cholestatic hepatobiliary disease

**Usual Dosage** Dietary supplement: Oral: 15 mg (400 units) every day

**Local Anesthetic/Vasoconstrictor Precautions** No information available to require special precautions

**Effects on Dental Treatment** No effects or complications reported

**Pregnancy Risk Factor** A/C

**Generic Available** No

**Comments** Studies indicate that TPGS is absorbed better than fat soluble forms of vitamin E in patients with impaired digestion and absorption and when coadministered with cyclosporin to transplant recipients it improves cyclosporin absorption. Due to these findings, this product has a valuable role in the liver transplant patient population.

- ♦ **Tofranil®** *see* Imipramine *on page 528*
- ♦ **Tofranil-PM®** *see* Imipramine *on page 528*

## Tolazamide (tole AZ a mide)

**Related Information**

Endocrine Disorders & Pregnancy *on page 1082*

**U.S. Brand Names** Tolinase®

**Therapeutic Category** Antidiabetic Agent; Hypoglycemic Agent, Oral; Sulfonylurea Agent

**Use** Adjunct to diet for the management of mild to moderately severe, stable, noninsulin-dependent (type II) diabetes mellitus

**Usual Dosage** Oral (doses >1000 mg/day normally do not improve diabetic control):

Adults: Initial: 100 mg/day, increase at 2- to 4-week intervals; maximum dose: 1000 mg; give as a single or twice daily dose

Conversion from insulin → tolazamide

10 units day = 100 mg/day

20-40 units/day = 250 mg/day

>40 units/day = 250 mg/day and 50% of insulin dose

Doses >500 mg/day should be given in 2 divided doses

**Mechanism of Action** Stimulates insulin release from the pancreatic beta cells; reduces glucose output from the liver; insulin sensitivity is increased at peripheral target sites

**Local Anesthetic/Vasoconstrictor Precautions** No information available to require special precautions

**Effects on Dental Treatment** Use salicylates with caution in patients taking tolazamide because of potential increased hypoglycemia; NSAIDs such as ibuprofen and naproxen may be safely used. Tolazamide-dependent diabetics (noninsulin dependent, Type II) should be appointed for dental treatment in morning in order to minimize chance of stress-induced hypoglycemia.

**Other Adverse Effects**

>10%:

Central nervous system: Headache, dizziness

Gastrointestinal: Anorexia, nausea, vomiting, diarrhea, constipation, heartburn, epigastric fullness

1% to 10%: Dermatologic: Rash, urticaria, photosensitivity

<1%:

Endocrine & metabolic: Hypoglycemia

Hematologic: Aplastic anemia, hemolytic anemia, bone marrow suppression, thrombocytopenia, agranulocytosis

Hepatic: Cholestatic jaundice

Renal: Diuretic effect

**Drug Interactions** Increased toxicity: Monitor patient closely; large number of drugs interact with sulfonylureas including salicylates, anticoagulants, $H_2$ antagonists, tricyclic antidepressants, MAO inhibitors, beta-blockers, thiazides

**Drug Uptake**

Onset of action: Oral: Within 4-6 hours

Duration: 10-24 hours

Serum half-life: 7 hours

**Pregnancy Risk Factor** D

**Dosage Forms** Tablet: 100 mg, 250 mg, 500 mg

**Generic Available** Yes

## Tolazoline (tole AZ oh leen)

**U.S. Brand Names** Priscoline®

**Therapeutic Category** Alpha-Adrenergic Blocking Agent, Parenteral; Vasodilator, Coronary

**Use** Treatment of persistent pulmonary vasoconstriction and hypertension of the newborn (persistent fetal circulation), peripheral vasospastic disorders

**Usual Dosage** Neonates: Initial: I.V.: 1-2 mg/kg over 10-15 minutes via scalp vein or upper extremity; maintenance: 1-2 mg/kg/hour; use lower maintenance doses in patients with decreased renal function. Also used in neonates for acute vasospasm "cath toes" at 0.25 mg/kg/hour (no load); maximum dose: 6-8 mg/kg/hour

**Mechanism of Action** Competitively blocks alpha-adrenergic receptors to produce brief antagonism of circulating epinephrine and norepinephrine; reduces hypertension caused by catecholamines and causes vascular smooth muscle relaxation (direct action); results in peripheral vasodilation and decreased peripheral resistance

**Local Anesthetic/Vasoconstrictor Precautions** No information available to require special precautions

**Effects on Dental Treatment** No effects or complications reported

(Continued)

## Tolazoline *(Continued)*

**Other Adverse Effects**

>10%:

Cardiovascular: Hypotension

Endocrine & metabolic: Hypochloremic alkalosis

Gastrointestinal: GI bleeding, abdominal pain

Hematologic: Thrombocytopenia

Local: Burning at injection site

Renal: Acute renal failure, oliguria

1% to 10%:

Cardiovascular: Peripheral vasodilation, tachycardia

Gastrointestinal: Nausea, diarrhea

Neuromuscular & skeletal: Increased pilomotor activity

<1%:

Cardiovascular: Hypertension, arrhythmias

Hematologic: Increased agranulocytosis, pancytopenia

Ocular: Mydriasis

Respiratory: Pulmonary hemorrhage, increased secretions

**Drug Interactions**

Increased toxicity: Disulfiram reaction may possibly be seen with concomitant ethanol use

**Drug Uptake** Time to peak serum concentration: Within 30 minutes

**Pregnancy Risk Factor** C

**Generic Available** No

## Tolbutamide (tole BYOO ta mide)

**Related Information**

Endocrine Disorders & Pregnancy *on page 1082*

**U.S. Brand Names** Orinase®

**Canadian Brand Names** Apo®-Tolbutamide; Mobenol®; Novo-Butamide

**Therapeutic Category** Antidiabetic Agent; Hypoglycemic Agent, Oral; Sulfonylurea Agent

**Use** Adjunct to diet for the management of mild to moderately severe, stable, noninsulin-dependent (type II) diabetes mellitus

**Usual Dosage** Divided doses may increase gastrointestinal side effects

Adults:

Oral: Initial: 500-1000 mg 1-3 times/day; usual dose should not be more than 2 g/day

I.V. bolus: 1 g over 2-3 minutes

Elderly: Oral: Initial: 250 mg 1-3 times/day; usual: 500-2000 mg; maximum: 3 g/day

**Mechanism of Action** A sulfonylurea hypoglycemic agent; its ability to lower elevated blood glucose levels in patients with functional pancreatic beta cells is similar to the other sulfonylurea agents; stimulates synthesis and release of endogenous insulin from pancreatic islet tissue. The hypoglycemic effect is attributed to an increased sensitivity of insulin receptors and improved peripheral utilization of insulin. Suppression of glucagon secretion may also contribute to the hypoglycemic effects of tolbutamide.

**Local Anesthetic/Vasoconstrictor Precautions** No information available to require special precautions

**Effects on Dental Treatment** Use salicylates with caution in patients taking tolazamide because of potential increased hypoglycemia; NSAIDs such as ibuprofen and naproxen may be safely used. Tolbutamide-dependent diabetics (noninsulin dependent, Type II) should be appointed for dental treatment in morning in order to minimize chance of stress-induced hypoglycemia

**Other Adverse Effects**

>10%:

Central nervous system: Headache, dizziness

Gastrointestinal: Constipation, diarrhea, heartburn, anorexia, epigastric fullness

1% to 10%: Dermatologic: Skin rash, urticaria, photosensitivity

<1%:

Cardiovascular: Venospasm

Endocrine & metabolic: SIADH, hypoglycemia, disulfiram-type reactions

Hematologic: Thrombocytopenia, agranulocytosis, leukopenia, aplastic anemia, hemolytic anemia, bone marrow suppression

Hepatic: Cholestatic jaundice

Local: Thrombophlebitis

Otic: Tinnitus

Miscellaneous: Hypersensitivity reaction

**Drug Interactions** Increased toxicity: Monitor patient closely; large number of drugs interact with sulfonylureas including salicylates, anticoagulants, $H_2$ antagonists, TCA, MAO inhibitors, beta-blockers, thiazides

**Drug Uptake**

Peak hypoglycemic action:
- Oral: 1-3 hours
- I.V.: 30 minutes

Duration:
- Oral: 6-24 hours
- I.V.: 3 hours

Absorption: Oral: Rapid

Serum half-life: Plasma: 4-25 hours

Time to peak serum concentration: 3-5 hours

**Pregnancy Risk Factor** D

**Dosage Forms**

Injection, diagnostic, as sodium: 1 g (20 mL)

Tablet: 250 mg, 500 mg

**Generic Available** Yes

## Tolcapone (TOLE ka pone)

**U.S. Brand Names** Tasmar®

**Therapeutic Category** Anti-Parkinson's Agent

**Use** Adjunct to levodopa and carbidopa for the treatment of signs and symptoms of idiopathic Parkinson's disease

**Usual Dosage** Adults: Oral: Initial 100 mg 3 times/day, may increase to 200 mg 3 times/day

**Mechanism of Action** Tolcapone is a selective and reversible inhibitor of catechol-o-methyltransferase (COMT)

**Local Anesthetic/Vasoconstrictor Precautions** No information available to require special precautions

**Effects on Dental Treatment** Dopaminergic therapy in Parkinson's disease (ie, treatment with levodopa) is associated with orthostatic hypotension. Tolcapone enhances levodopa bioavailability and may increase the occurrence of hypotension/syncope in the dental patient. The patient should be carefully assisted from the chair and observed for signs of orthostatic hypotension.

**Other Adverse Effects**

>10%:
- Cardiovascular: Orthostasis
- Central nervous system: Sleep disorder, excessive dreaming, headache, dizziness, somnolence, confusion
- Gastrointestinal: Nausea, anorexia, diarrhea
- Neuromuscular & skeletal: Dyskinesia, dystonia, muscle cramps

1% to 10%:
- Cardiovascular: Hypotension, chest pain
- Central nervous system: Hallucination, syncope, fatigue
- Gastrointestinal: Vomiting, constipation, dry mouth, dyspepsia, abdominal pain, flatulence
- Genitourinary: Urine discoloration
- Neuromuscular & skeletal: Hyperkinesia, stiffness, arthritis
- Respiratory: Dyspnea

<1%:
- Cardiovascular: Bradycardia, coronary artery disorder, heart arrest, angina pectoris, myocardial infarct, myocardial ischemia, arteriosclerosis, thrombosis, hypertension, vasodilation
- Central nervous system: Amnesia, extrapyramidal syndrome, manic reaction, cerebrovascular accident, psychosis, delirium, encephalopathy, meningitis
- Dermatologic: Cellulitis
- Endocrine & metabolic: Hypercholesteremia
- Gastrointestinal: Gastrointestinal hemorrhage, colitis, duodenal ulcer
- Hematologic: Uterine hemorrhage, anemia, leukemia, thrombocytopenia, cholecystitis, neuralgia, hemiplegia, hematuria
- Hepatic: Fatal liver injury
- Neuromuscular & skeletal: Myoclonus
- Respiratory: Bronchitis, epistaxis, hyperventilation
- Miscellaneous: Allergic reaction

**Warnings/Precautions** Due to reports of fatal liver injury associated with use of this drug, the manufacturer is advising that tolcapone be reserved for use only in patients who do not have severe movement abnormalities and who do not respond to or who are not appropriate candidates for other available treatments.

(Continued)

## Tolcapone *(Continued)*

It is not recommended that patients receive tolcapone concomitantly with nonselective MAO inhibitors. Selegiline is a selective MAO-B inhibitor and can be taken with tolcapone.

**Drug Interactions** CYP3A4 and CYP2A6 enzyme substrate; COMT inhibition could slow the metabolism of methyldopa, dobutamine, apomorphine, and isoproterenol

**Drug Uptake**

Absorption: Rapid with $T_{max}$ at 2 hours
Serum half-life: 2-3 hours

**Dosage Forms** Tablet: 100 mg, 200 mg

- **Tolectin®** *see* Tolmetin *on this page*
- **Tolectin® DS** *see* Tolmetin *on this page*
- **Tolinase®** *see* Tolazamide *on page 993*

## Tolmetin (TOLE met in)

**Related Information**

Rheumatoid Arthritis and Osteoarthritis *on page 1092*

**U.S. Brand Names** Tolectin®; Tolectin® DS

**Canadian Brand Names** Novo-Tolmetin

**Therapeutic Category** Analgesic, Non-narcotic; Nonsteroidal Anti-inflammatory Drug (NSAID), Oral

**Use** Treatment of rheumatoid arthritis and osteoarthritis, juvenile rheumatoid arthritis

**Usual Dosage** Oral:

Children ≥2 years:
- Anti-inflammatory: Initial: 20 mg/kg/day in 3 divided doses, then 15-30 mg/kg/day in 3 divided doses
- Analgesic: 5-7 mg/kg/dose every 6-8 hours

Adults: 400 mg 3 times/day; usual dose: 600 mg to 1.8 g/day; maximum: 2 g/day

**Mechanism of Action** Inhibits prostaglandin synthesis by decreasing the activity of the enzyme, cyclo-oxygenase, which results in decreased formation of prostaglandin precursors

**Local Anesthetic/Vasoconstrictor Precautions** No information available to require special precautions

**Effects on Dental Treatment** NSAID formulations are known to reversibly decrease platelet aggregation via mechanisms different than observed with aspirin. The dentist should be aware of the potential of abnormal coagulation. Caution should also be exercised in the use of NSAIDs in patients already on anticoagulant therapy with drugs such as warfarin (Coumadin®).

**Other Adverse Effects**

>10%:
- Central nervous system: Dizziness
- Dermatologic: Skin rash
- Gastrointestinal: Abdominal cramps, heartburn, indigestion, nausea

1% to 10%:
- Central nervous system: Headache, nervousness
- Dermatologic: Itching
- Endocrine & metabolic: Fluid retention
- Gastrointestinal: Vomiting
- Otic: Tinnitus

<1%:
- Cardiovascular: Congestive heart failure, hypertension, arrhythmias, tachycardia
- Central nervous system: Confusion, hallucinations, aseptic meningitis, mental depression, drowsiness, insomnia
- Dermatologic: Urticaria, erythema multiforme, toxic epidermal necrolysis, Stevens-Johnson syndrome, angioedema
- Endocrine & metabolism: Polydipsia, hot flashes
- Gastrointestinal: Gastritis, GI ulceration
- Genitourinary: Cystitis
- Hematologic: Agranulocytosis, anemia, hemolytic anemia, bone marrow suppression, leukopenia, thrombocytopenia
- Hepatic: Hepatitis
- Neuromuscular & skeletal: Peripheral neuropathy
- Ocular: Toxic amblyopia, blurred vision, conjunctivitis, dry eyes
- Otic: Decreased hearing
- Renal: Polyuria, acute renal failure
- Respiratory: Allergic rhinitis, dyspnea, epistaxis

**Drug Interactions**

Decreased effect with aspirin; decreased effect of thiazides, furosemide

Increased toxicity of digoxin, methotrexate, cyclosporine, lithium, insulin, sulfonylureas, potassium-sparing diuretics, aspirin

**Drug Uptake**

Absorption: Oral: Well absorbed

Time to peak serum concentration: Within 30-60 minutes

**Pregnancy Risk Factor** C (D if used in the 3rd trimester or near delivery)

**Dosage Forms**

Capsule, as sodium (Tolectin® DS): 400 mg

Tablet, as sodium (Tolectin®): 200 mg, 600 mg

**Generic Available** Yes

## Tolnaftate (tole NAF tate)

**U.S. Brand Names** Absorbine® Antifungal [OTC]; Absorbine® Jock Itch [OTC]; Absorbine Jr.® Antifungal [OTC]; Aftate® for Athlete's Foot [OTC]; Aftate® for Jock Itch [OTC]; Blis-To-Sol® [OTC]; Breezee® Mist Antifungal [OTC]; Dr Scholl's Athlete's Foot [OTC]; Dr Scholl's Maximum Strength Tritin [OTC]; Genaspor® [OTC]; NP-27® [OTC]; Quinsana Plus® [OTC]; Tinactin® [OTC]; Tinactin® for Jock Itch [OTC]; Ting® [OTC]; Zeasorb-AF® Powder [OTC]

**Canadian Brand Names** Pitrex®; Tinaderm®

**Therapeutic Category** Antifungal Agent, Topical

**Use** Treatment of tinea pedis, tinea cruris, tinea corporis, tinea manuum, tinea versicolor infections

**Usual Dosage** Children and Adults: Topical: Wash and dry affected area; apply 1-3 drops of solution or a small amount of cream or powder and rub into the affected areas 2-3 times/day for 2-4 weeks

**Mechanism of Action** Distorts the hyphae and stunts mycelial growth in susceptible fungi

**Local Anesthetic/Vasoconstrictor Precautions** No information available to require special precautions

**Effects on Dental Treatment** No effects or complications reported

**Other Adverse Effects** 1% to 10%:

Dermatologic: Pruritus, contact dermatitis

Local: Irritation, stinging

**Drug Interactions** No data reported

**Drug Uptake** Onset of action: Response may be seen 24-72 hours after initiation of therapy

**Pregnancy Risk Factor** C

**Generic Available** Yes

## Tolterodine (tole TER oh dine)

**U.S. Brand Names** Detrol™

**Therapeutic Category** Anticholinergic Agent

**Use** Treatment of patients with an overactive bladder with symptoms of urinary frequency, urgency, or urge incontinence

**Usual Dosage** Adults: Oral: Initial: 2 mg twice daily. The dose may be lowered to 1 mg twice daily based on individual response and tolerability.

Dosing adjustment in patients concurrently taking cytochrome P-450 3A4 inhibitors: 1 mg twice daily

**Mechanism of Action** Tolterodine is a competitive antagonist of muscarinic receptors. In animal models, tolterodine demonstrates selectivity for urinary bladder receptors over salivary receptors. Urinary bladder contraction is mediated by muscarinic receptors. Tolterodine increases residual urine volume and decreases detrusor muscle pressure.

**Local Anesthetic/Vasoconstrictor Precautions** No information available to require special precautions

**Effects on Dental Treatment** The anticholinergic effects of tolterodine are selective for the urinary bladder rather than salivary glands; xerostomia should not be significant

**Other Adverse Effects**

>10%: Central nervous system: Headache

1% to 10%:

- Cardiovascular: Chest pain, hypertension (1.5%)
- Central nervous system: Vertigo (8.6%), nervousness (1.1%), somnolence (3.0%)
- Dermatologic: Pruritus (1.3%), rash (1.9%), dry skin (1.7%)
- Gastrointestinal: Abdominal pain (7.6%), constipation (6.5%), diarrhea (4.0%), dyspepsia (5.9%), flatulence (1.3%), nausea (4.2%), vomiting (1.7%), weight gain (1.5%)

(Continued)

## Tolterodine *(Continued)*

Genitourinary: Dysuria (2.5%), polyuria (1.1%), urinary retention (1.7%), urinary tract infection (5.5%)
Neuromuscular & skeletal: Back pain, falling (1.3%), paresthesia (1.1%)
Ocular: Vision abnormalities (4.7%), dry eyes (3.8%)
Respiratory: Bronchitis (2.1%), cough (2.1%), pharyngitis (1.5%), rhinitis (1.1%), sinusitis (1.1%), upper respiratory infection (5.9%)
Miscellaneous: Flu-like symptoms (4.4%), infection (2.1%)

**Drug Interactions** Cytochrome P-450 3A4 substrate; cytochrome P-450 2D6 substrate

Increased toxicity: Macrolide antibiotics/azole antifungal agents may inhibit the metabolism of tolterodine. Doses of tolterodine >1 mg twice daily should not be exceeded.

Fluoxetine, which inhibits cytochrome P-450 2D6, increases concentration 4.8 times. Other drugs which inhibit this isoenzyme may also interact. Studies with inhibitors of cytochrome isoenzyme 3A4 have not been performed.

**Drug Uptake** Time to peak serum concentration: 1-2 hours

**Pregnancy Risk Factor** C

**Dosage Forms** Tablet, as tartrate: 1 mg, 2 mg

**Generic Available** No

- **Tolu-Sed® DM [OTC]** *see* Guaifenesin and Dextromethorphan *on page 479*
- **Tonocard®** *see* Tocainide *on page 992*
- **Topamax®** *see* Topiramate *on this page*
- **Topicort®** *see* Desoximetasone *on page 307*
- **Topicort®-LP** *see* Desoximetasone *on page 307*

## Topiramate (toe PYE ra mate)

**U.S. Brand Names** Topamax®

**Therapeutic Category** Anticonvulsant, Miscellaneous

**Use** Adjunctive therapy for partial onset seizures in adults

**Usual Dosage** Adults: Initial: 50 mg/day; titrate by 50 mg/day at 1-week intervals to target dose of 200 mg twice daily; usual maximum dose: 1600 mg/day

**Mechanism of Action** Mechanism is not fully understood, it is thought to decrease seizure frequency by blocking sodium channels in neurons, enhancing GABA activity, and by blocking glutamate activity

**Local Anesthetic/Vasoconstrictor Precautions** No information available to require special precautions

**Effects on Dental Treatment** Up to 10% of patients may experience gingivitis and dry mouth

**Other Adverse Effects**

>10%:
Central nervous system: Fatigue, dizziness, ataxia, somnolence, psychomotor slowing, nervousness, memory difficulties, speech problems
Gastrointestinal: Nausea
Neuromuscular & skeletal: Paresthesia, tremor
Ocular: Nystagmus
Respiratory: Upper respiratory infections

1% to 10%:
Cardiovascular: Chest pain, edema
Central nervous system: Language problems, abnormal coordination, confusion, depression, difficulty concentrating, hypoesthesia
Endocrine & metabolic: Hot flashes
Gastrointestinal: Dyspepsia, abdominal pain, anorexia, constipation, xerostomia, gingivitis, weight loss
Neuromuscular & skeletal: Myalgia, weakness, back pain, leg pain, rigors
Otic: Decreased hearing
Renal: Nephrolithiasis
Respiratory: Pharyngitis, sinusitis, epistaxis
Miscellaneous: Flu-like symptoms

**Warnings/Precautions** Avoid abrupt withdrawal of topiramate therapy, withdraw slowly to minimize the potential of increased seizure frequency; the risk of kidney stones is about 2-4 times that of the untreated population; the risk of this event may be reduced by increasing fluid intake; use cautiously in patients with hepatic or renal impairment, during pregnancy, or in nursing mothers.

**Drug Interactions**

Decreased effect: Phenytoin can decrease topiramate levels by as much as 48%, carbamazepine reduces it by 40% and valproic acid reduces topiramate by 14%; digoxin levels and norethindrone blood levels are decreased when coadministered with topiramate

Increased toxicity: Concomitant administration with other CNS depressants will increase its sedative effects; coadministration with other carbonic anhydrase inhibitors may increase the chance of nephrolithiasis

**Drug Uptake**

Absorption: Good; unaffected by food

Serum half-life: Mean: 21 hours in adults

Time to peak serum concentration: ~2-4 hours

**Pregnancy Risk Factor** C

**Dosage Forms**

Capsule, sprinkles: 15 mg, 25 mg, 50 mg

Tablet: 25 mg, 100 mg, 200 mg

**Generic Available** No

- **TOPO** *see* Topotecan *on this page*
- **Toposar® Injection** *see* Etoposide *on page 414*

## Topotecan (toe poe TEE kan)

**U.S. Brand Names** Hycamtin™

**Therapeutic Category** Antineoplastic Agent, Antibiotic

**Synonyms** Hycamptamine; SK and F 104864; SKF 104864; SKF 104864-A; TOPO; TPT

**Use** Treatment of ovarian cancer after failure of first-line chemotherapy; treatment of small cell lung cancer sensitive disease after failure of first-line chemotherapy

**Usual Dosage**

Children: A phase I study in pediatric patients by CCSG determined the recommended phase II dose to be 5.5 mg/mm$^2$ as a 24-hour continuous infusion

Adults: Most phase II studies currently utilize topotecan at 1.5-2.0 mg/mm$^2$/day for 5 days, repeated every 21-28 days. Alternative dosing regimens evaluated in phase I studies have included 21-day continuous infusion (recommended phase II dose: 0.53-0.7 mg/mm$^2$/day) and weekly 24-hour infusions (recommended phase II dose: 1.5 mg/mm$^2$/week).

Dose modifications: Dosage modification may be required for toxicity

**Mechanism of Action** Topotecan (TPT), like other camptothecin (CPT) analogues, is a potent inhibitor of topoisomerase I. Structure-activity studies have revealed a direct relationship between the ability of CPT analogues to inhibit topoisomerase I catalytic activity and their potency as cytotoxic agents.

**Local Anesthetic/Vasoconstrictor Precautions** No information available to require special precautions

**Effects on Dental Treatment** No effects or complications reported

**Other Adverse Effects**

>10%:

- Central nervous system: Headache
- Dermatologic: Alopecia
- Gastrointestinal: Nausea, vomiting, diarrhea
- Hematologic: Neutropenia
- Respiratory: Dyspnea

1% to 10%:

- Central nervous system: Fatigue
- Gastrointestinal: Constipation, abdominal pain
- Hepatic: AST and ALT elevations, bilirubin elevation
- Neuromuscular & skeletal: Paresthesia

<1%:

- Gastrointestinal: Stomatitis
- Neuromuscular & skeletal: Arthralgia, myalgia

**Drug Interactions** Concurrent administration of topotecan (TPT) and G-CSF in clinical trials results in severe myelosuppression. Concurrent *in vitro* exposure to TPT and the topoisomerase II inhibitor etoposide results in no altered effect; sequential exposure results in potentiation. Concurrent exposure to TPT and 5-azacytidine results in potentiation both *in vitro* and *in vivo*.

**Drug Uptake** Serum half-life: 3 hours

**Pregnancy Risk Factor** D

**Generic Available** No

**Comments** Constituted vial: When constituted with 2 mL of sterile water for injection, USP, each mL contains topotecan 2.5 mg and mannitol 50 mg with a pH of approximately 3.5. Final infusion preparation: Topotecan constituted solution should be further diluted in 5% dextrose injection. Topotecan should NOT be diluted in buffered solutions.

- **Toprol XL® [Succinate]** *see* Metoprolol *on page 666*
- **TOPV** *see* Poliovirus Vaccine, Live, Trivalent, Oral *on page 813*
- **Toradol® Injection** *see* Ketorolac Tromethamine *on page 566*
- **Toradol® Oral** *see* Ketorolac Tromethamine *on page 566*

## Toremifene (TORE em i feen)

**U.S. Brand Names** Fareston®

**Therapeutic Category** Antineoplastic Agent, Miscellaneous

**Synonyms** FC1157a; Toremifene Butyrate

**Use** Treatment of advanced breast cancer; management of desmoid tumors and endometrial carcinoma

**Usual Dosage** Refer to individual protocols
60-240 mg/day
200-300 mg/day
60 mg for 3 days, then 20 mg/day

**Mechanism of Action** At low doses, toremifene inhibits tumor growth by depleting cytosolic estrogen receptors. At higher doses, it acts on estrogen receptors. The exact mechanism of action is not clear, but may involve effects on calcium channels, calmodulin, and/or protein kinase C.

**Local Anesthetic/Vasoconstrictor Precautions** No information available to require special precautions

**Effects on Dental Treatment** No effects or complications reported

**Other Adverse Effects**

>10%:
- Central nervous system: Dizziness or vertigo (12%), anxiety, depression, fatigue, headache, insomnia, irritability, lethargy
- Endocrine & metabolic: Hot flashes
- Gastrointestinal: Nausea and vomiting (40%)
- Hematologic: Decreased antithrombin III levels
- Neuromuscular & skeletal: Tremors
- Miscellaneous: Sweating

1% to 10%:
- Dermatologic: Rash, pruritus, urticaria
- Gastrointestinal: Abdominal discomfort, anorexia, constipation, diarrhea, increased appetite
- Genitourinary: Vaginal bleeding and discharge (3% to 8%)
- Hematologic: Anemia
- Neuromuscular & skeletal: Bone pain (3%)
- Ocular: Dry eyes (3%)

<1%: Endocrine & metabolic: Hypercalcemia

**Contraindications** Hypersensitivity to toremifene or any component

**Warnings/Precautions** Toremifene should be used cautiously in patients with anemia or hepatic failure

**Drug Uptake**
Serum half-life: Elimination:
N-desmethyltoremifene: 6 days
4-hydroxytoremifene: 5 days
Time to peak serum concentration: 1.5-4.5 hours

**Dosage Forms** Tablet: 10 mg, 20 mg, 60 mg, 200 mg

**Generic Available** No

**Selected Readings**

Gams R, "Phase III Trials of Toremifene vs Tamoxifen," *Oncology*, 1997, 11(5 Suppl 4): 23-8.
Hamm JT, "Phase I and II Studies of Toremifene," *Oncology*, 1997, 11(5 Suppl 4):19-22.
Holli K, "Evolving Role of Troemifene in the Adjuvant Setting," *Oncology*, 1997, 11(5 Suppl 4):48-51.
Kangas L, "Review of the Pharmacological Properties of Toremifene," *J Steroid Biochem*, 1990, 36(3):191-5.
Pyrhönen S, Valavaara R, Modig H, et al, "Comparison of Toremifene and Tamoxifen in Postmenopausal Patients With Advanced Breast Cancer: A Randomized Double-Blind, the "Nordic" Phase III Study," *Br J Cancer*, 1997, 76(2):270-7.
Williams GM and Jeffrey AM, "Safety Assessment of Tamoxifen and Toremifene," *Oncology*, 1997, 11(5 Suppl 4):41-7.

♦ **Toremifene Butyrate** *see* Toremifene *on this page*

♦ **Tornalate®** *see* Bitolterol *on page 145*

## Torsemide (TOR se mide)

**Related Information**
Cardiovascular Diseases *on page 1066*

**U.S. Brand Names** Demadex®

**Therapeutic Category** Diuretic, Loop

**Use** Management of edema associated with congestive heart failure and hepatic or renal disease; used alone or in combination with antihypertensives in treatment of hypertension; I.V. form is indicated when rapid onset is desired

**Usual Dosage** Adults: Oral, I.V.:
Congestive heart failure: 10-20 mg once daily; may increase gradually for chronic treatment by doubling dose until the diuretic response is apparent (for acute treatment, I.V. dose may be repeated every 2 hours with double the dose as needed)

Chronic renal failure: 20 mg once daily; increase as described above

Hepatic cirrhosis: 5-10 mg once daily with an aldosterone antagonist or a potassium-sparing diuretic; increase as described above

Hypertension: 5 mg once daily; increase to 10 mg after 4-6 weeks if an adequate hypotensive response is not apparent; if still not effective, an additional antihypertensive agent may be added

**Mechanism of Action** Inhibits reabsorption of sodium and chloride in the ascending loop of Henle and distal renal tubule, interfering with the chloride-binding cotransport system, thus causing increased excretion of water, sodium, chloride, magnesium, and calcium; does not alter GFR, renal plasma flow, or acid-base balance

**Local Anesthetic/Vasoconstrictor Precautions** No information available to require special precautions

**Effects on Dental Treatment** No effects or complications reported

**Other Adverse Effects**

>10%: Cardiovascular: Orthostatic hypotension

1% to 10%:

- Central nervous system: Headache, dizziness, vertigo
- Dermatologic: Photosensitivity, urticaria
- Endocrine & metabolic: Electrolyte imbalance, dehydration, hyperuricemia
- Gastrointestinal: Diarrhea, loss of appetite, stomach cramps or pain, pancreatitis
- Ocular: Blurred vision

<1%:

- Dermatologic: Skin rash
- Endocrine & metabolic: Gout
- Gastrointestinal: Nausea
- Hepatic: Hepatic dysfunction
- Hematologic: Agranulocytosis, leukopenia, anemia, thrombocytopenia
- Local: Redness at injection site
- Otic: Ototoxicity
- Renal: Nephrocalcinosis, prerenal azotemia, interstitial nephritis

**Drug Interactions**

Aminoglycosides: Ototoxicity may be increased; anticoagulant activity is enhanced

Beta-blockers: Plasma concentrations of beta-blockers may be increased

Cisplatin: Ototoxicity may be increased

Digitalis: Arrhythmias may occur with diuretic-induced electrolyte disturbances

Lithium: Plasma concentrations of lithium may be increased

NSAIDs: Torsemide efficacy may be decreased

Probenecid: Torsemide action may be reduced

Salicylates: Diuretic action may be impaired in patients with cirrhosis and ascites

Sulfonylureas: Glucose tolerance may be decreased

Thiazides: Synergistic effects may result

**Drug Uptake**

Onset of diuresis: 30-60 minutes

Peak effect: 1-4 hours

Duration: ~6 hours

Absorption: Oral: Rapid

Serum half-life: 2-4; 7-8 hours in cirrhosis (dose modification appears unnecessary)

**Pregnancy Risk Factor** B

**Generic Available** No

- ♦ **Totacillin®** *see* Ampicillin *on page 81*
- ♦ **Totacillin®-N** *see* Ampicillin *on page 81*
- ♦ **Touro Ex®** *see* Guaifenesin *on page 478*
- ♦ **Touro LA®** *see* Guaifenesin and Pseudoephedrine *on page 481*
- ♦ **TPGS** *see* Tocophersolan *on page 992*
- ♦ **TPT** *see* Topotecan *on page 999*
- ♦ **Trace-4®** *see* Trace Metals *on this page*

## Trace Metals (trase MET als)

**U.S. Brand Names** Chroma-Pak®; Iodopen®; Molypen®; M.T.E.-4®; M.T.E.-5®; M.T.E.-6®; Multe-pak-4®; Multe-pak-5®; Neotrace-4®; PedtE-PAK-4®; Pedtrace-4®; P.T.E.-4®; P.T.E.-5®; Sele-Pak®; Selepen®; Trace-4®; Zinca-Pak®

**Therapeutic Category** Trace Element, Parenteral

**Synonyms** Chromium; Copper; Iodine; Manganese; Molybdenum; Neonatal Trace Metals; Selenium; Zinc

**Use** Prevent and correct trace metal deficiencies

**Usual Dosage** See table.

(Continued)

## Trace Metals *(Continued)*

**Recommended Daily Parenteral Dosage**

| | Infants | Children | Adults |
|---|---|---|---|
| Chromium[1] | 0.2 mcg/kg | 0.2 mcg/kg (max 5 mcg) | 10-15 mcg |
| Copper[2] | 20 mcg/kg | 20 mcg/kg (max 300 mcg) | 0.5-1.5 mg |
| Manganese[2,3] | 1 mcg/kg | 1 mcg/kg (max 50 mcg) | 150-800 mcg |
| Molybdenum[1,4] | 0.25 mcg/kg | 0.25 mcg/kg (max 5 mcg) | 20-120 mcg |
| Selenium[1,4] | 2 mcg/kg | 2 mcg/kg (max 30 mcg) | 20-40 mcg |
| Zinc<br>preterm<br>term <3 mo<br>term >3 mo | <br>400 mcg/kg<br>250 mcg/kg<br>100 mcg/kg | 50 mcg/kg (max 5 mg) | 2.5-4 mg |

[1]Omit in patients with renal dysfunction.

[2]Omit in patients with obstructive jaundice.

[3]Current available commercial products are not in appropriate ratios to maintain this recommendation — doses of up to 10 mcg/kg have been used.

[4]Indicated for use in long-term parenteral nutrition patients.

**Local Anesthetic/Vasoconstrictor Precautions** No information available to require special precautions

**Effects on Dental Treatment** No effects or complications reported

**Pregnancy Risk Factor** C

**Generic Available** Yes

**Comments** Persistent diarrhea or excessive gastrointestinal fluid losses from ostomy sites may grossly increase zinc losses

## Tramadol (TRA ma dole)

**U.S. Brand Names** Ultram®

**Therapeutic Category** Analgesic, Non-narcotic

**Use**

Dental: Relief of moderate to moderately severe dental pain

Medical: Relief of moderate to moderately severe medical pain

**Usual Dosage** Adults: Oral: 50-100 mg every 4-6 hours, not to exceed 400 mg/day

**Mechanism of Action** Binds to μ-opiate receptors in the CNS causing inhibition of ascending pain pathways, altering the perception of and response to pain; also inhibits the reuptake of norepinephrine and serotonin, which also modifies the ascending pain pathway

**Local Anesthetic/Vasoconstrictor Precautions** No information available to require special precautions

**Effects on Dental Treatment** No effects or complications reported

**Other Adverse Effects** >1%:

Central nervous system: Dizziness, somnolence, restlessness

Gastrointestinal: Nausea, constipation

Miscellaneous: Sweating

**Contraindications** Previous hypersensitivity to tramadol or any components; should not be administered in cases of acute intoxication with alcohol, hypnotics, centrally acting analgesics, opioids, or psychotropic drugs

**Warnings/Precautions** Elderly patients and patients with chronic respiratory disorders may be at greater risk of adverse events; liver disease; patients with myxedema, hypothyroidism, or hypoadrenalism should use tramadol with caution and at reduced dosages; not recommended during pregnancy or in nursing mothers

**Drug Interactions** Carbamazepine decreases half-life by 33% to 50%; increased toxicity with monoamine oxidase inhibitors (seizures); quinidine inhibits cytochrome CYP2D6, thereby increasing tramadol serum concentrations; cimetidine increases tramadol half-life by 20% to 25%

**Drug Uptake**

Absorption: Oral: ~75%

Onset of action: ~1 hour

Serum half-life, elimination: 6 hours

Time to peak serum concentration: 2 hours

**Pregnancy Risk Factor** C

**Breast-feeding Considerations** No data reported

**Dosage Forms** Tablet, as hydrochloride: 50 mg

**Generic Available** No

**Comments** Literature reports suggest that the efficacy of tramadol in oral surgery pain is equivalent to the combination of aspirin and codeine. One study (Olson et al 1990) showed acetaminophen and dextropropoxyphene combination to be superior to tramadol and another study (Mehlisch et al, 1990) showed tramadol to be superior to acetaminophen and dextropropoxyphene combination. Tramadol appears to be at least equal to if not better than codeine alone. Seizures have been reported with the use of tramadol.

**Selected Readings**


Collins M, Young I, Sweeney P, et al, "The Effect of Tramadol on Dento-Alveolar Surgical Pain," *Br J Oral Maxillofac Surg*, 1997, 35(1):54-8.

Kahn LH, Alderfer RJ, and Graham DJ, "Seizures Reported With Tramadol," *JAMA*, 1997, 278(20):1661.

Lewis KS and Han NH, "Tramadol: A New Centrally Acting Analgesic," *Am J Health Syst Pharm*, 1997, 54(6):643-52.

Mehlisch DR, Minn F, and Brown P, "Tramadol Hydrochloride: Efficacy Compared to Codeine Sulfate, Acetaminophen With Dextropropoxyphene and Placebo in Dental Extraction Pain," *Clin Pharmacol Ther*, 1992.

Olson NZ, Sunshine A, O'Neill, et al, *Tramadol Hydrochloride: Oral Efficacy in Postoperative Pain*, American Pain Society 9th Annual Scientific Meeting, St Louis, MO, October, 1990.

Sunshine A, "New Clinical Experience With Tramadol," *Drugs*, 1994, 47(Suppl 1):8-18.

Sunshine A, Olson NZ, Zighelboim I, et al, "Analgesic Oral Efficacy of Tramadol Hydrochloride in Postoperative Pain," *Clin Pharmacol Ther*, 1992; 51(6):740-6.

Voorhees F, Leibold DG, Stumpf, et al, "Tramadol Hydrochloride: Efficacy Compared to Codeine Sulfate, Aspirin With Codeine Phosphate, and Placebo in Dental Extraction Pain," *Clin Pharmacol Ther*, 1992, 51:122.

Wynn RL, "Tramadol (Ultram) – A New Kind of Analgesic," *Gen Dent*, 1996, 44(3):216-8,220.


♦ **Trandate®** *see* Labetalol *on page 568*

## Trandolapril (tran DOE la pril)

**U.S. Brand Names** Mavik®

**Therapeutic Category** Angiotensin-Converting Enzyme (ACE) Inhibitor

**Use** Management of hypertension alone or in combination with other antihypertensive agents

**Usual Dosage** Adults:

Non-African-American patients: 0.5-1 mg for those not receiving diuretics; increase dose at 0.5-1 mg increments at 1- to 2-week intervals; maximum dose: 4 mg/day

African-American patients: Initiate doses of 1-2 mg; maximum dose: 4 mg/day

**Mechanism of Action** Trandolapril is an angiotensin-converting enzyme (ACE) inhibitor which prevents the formation of angiotensin II from angiotensin I. Trandolapril must undergo enzymatic hydrolysis, mainly in liver, to its biologically active metabolite, trandolaprilat. A CNS mechanism may also be involved in the hypotensive effect as angiotensin II increases adrenergic outflow from the CNS. Vasoactive kallikrein's may be decreased in conversion to active hormones by ACE inhibitors, thus, reducing blood pressure.

**Local Anesthetic/Vasoconstrictor Precautions** No information available to require special precautions

**Effects on Dental Treatment** No effects or complications reported

**Other Adverse Effects**

Cardiovascular: Tachycardia, chest pain, palpitations, orthostatic blood pressure changes, syncope, heart failure, hypotension, cardiogenic shock

Central nervous system: Headache, fatigue, dizziness, malaise, vertigo, drowsiness, ataxia, nervousness, insomnia, fever

Dermatologic: Rash, pruritus, alopecia, exfoliative dermatitis, urticaria, photosensitivity, angioedema

Endocrine & metabolic: Hyperkalemia, decreased libido

Gastrointestinal: Dysgeusia, abdominal pain, nausea, vomiting, diarrhea, anorexia, constipation, dry mouth, dysgeusia, glossitis

Genitourinary: Impotence

Hematologic: Neutropenia, agranulocytosis

Hepatic: Hepatitis

Neuromuscular & skeletal: Arthritis, arthralgia, myalgia, paresthesias

Ocular: Blurred vision

Otic: Tinnitus

Renal: Oliguria, Elevated BUN, elevated serum creatinine, proteinuria, worsening renal failure

Respiratory: Chest pain, chronic cough (nonproductive, persistent - more frequent in women)

Miscellaneous: Sweating

**Warnings/Precautions** Neutropenia, agranulocytosis, angioedema, decreased renal function (hypertension, renal artery stenosis, CHF), hepatic dysfunction

(Continued)

## Trandolapril *(Continued)*

(elimination, activation), proteinuria, first-dose hypotension (hypovolemia, CHF, dehydrated patients at risk, eg, diuretic use, elderly), elderly (due to renal function changes); use with caution and modify dosage in patients with renal impairment; use with caution in patients with collagen vascular disease, CHF, hypovolemia, valvular stenosis, hyperkalemia (>5.7 mEq/L), anesthesia

**Drug Interactions**

ACE inhibitors (trandolapril) and potassium-sparing diuretics → additive hyperkalemic effect

ACE inhibitors (trandolapril) and indomethacin or nonsteroidal anti-inflammatory agents → reduced antihypertensive response to ACE inhibitors (trandolapril)

Allopurinol and trandolapril → neutropenia

Antacids and ACE inhibitors → ↓ absorption of ACE inhibitors

Phenothiazines and ACE inhibitors → ↑ ACE inhibitor effect

Probenecid and ACE inhibitors (trandolapril) → ↑ ACE inhibitors (trandolapril) levels

Rifampin and ACE inhibitors (trandolapril) → ↓ ACE inhibitor effect

Digoxin and ACE inhibitors → ↑ serum digoxin levels

Lithium and ACE inhibitors → ↑ lithium serum levels

Tetracycline and ACE inhibitors (trandolapril) → ↓ tetracycline absorption (up to 37%)

Food decreases trandolapril absorption; rate, but not extent, of ramipril and fosinopril is reduced by concomitant administration with food; food does not reduce absorption of enalapril, lisinopril, or benazepril; trandolapril has a decreased rate and extent (25% to 30%) of absorption when taken with a high fat meal

**Drug Uptake**

Absorption: Rapid

Half-life: 24 hours

**Pregnancy Risk Factor** C (first trimester); D (second & third trimester)

**Generic Available** No

**Comments** Patients taking diuretics are at risk for developing hypotension on initial dosing; to prevent this, discontinue diuretics 2-3 days prior to initiating trandolapril; may restart diuretics if blood pressure is not controlled by trandolapril alone

**Selected Readings**

Bevan EG, McInnes GT, Aldigier JC, et al, "Effect of Renal Function on the Pharmacokinetics and Pharmacodynamics of Trandolapril," *Br J Clin Pharmacol*, 1993, 35(2):128-35.

Conen H and Brunner HR, "Pharmacologic Profile of Trandolapril, A New Angiotensin-Converting Enzyme Inhibitor," *Am J Heart*, 1993, 125(5 Pt 2):1524-31.

Zannad F, "Trandolapril. How Does It Differ From Other Angiotensin-Converting Enzyme Inhibitors?" *Drugs*, 1993, 46(Suppl 2):172-81.

## Trandolapril and Verapamil (tran DOE la pril & ver AP a mil)

**U.S. Brand Names** Tarka®

**Therapeutic Category** Antihypertensive Agent, Combination

**Use** Combination drug for the treatment of hypertension

**Usual Dosage** Dose is individualized

**Local Anesthetic/Vasoconstrictor Precautions** No information available to require special precautions

**Effects on Dental Treatment** No effects or complications reported

**Dosage Forms** Tablet:

Trandolapril 1 mg and verapamil hydrochloride 240 mg

Trandolapril 2 mg and verapamil hydrochloride 180 mg

Trandolapril 2 mg and verapamil hydrochloride 240 mg

Trandolapril 4 mg and verapamil hydrochloride 240 mg

**Generic Available** No

## Tranexamic Acid (tran eks AM ik AS id)

**U.S. Brand Names** Cyklokapron® Injection; Cyklokapron® Oral

**Therapeutic Category** Antihemophilic Agent

**Use** Short-term use (2-8 days) in hemophilia patients during and following tooth extraction to reduce or prevent hemorrhage

**Usual Dosage** Children and Adults: I.V.: 10 mg/kg immediately before surgery, then 25 mg/kg/dose orally 3-4 times/day for 2-8 days

Alternatively:

Oral: 25 mg/kg 3-4 times/day beginning 1 day prior to surgery

I.V.: 10 mg/kg 3-4 times/day in patients who are unable to take oral

**Mechanism of Action** Forms a reversible complex that displaces plasminogen from fibrin resulting in inhibition of fibrinolysis; it also inhibits the proteolytic activity of plasmin

**Local Anesthetic/Vasoconstrictor Precautions** No information available to require special precautions

**Effects on Dental Treatment** No effects or complications reported

**Other Adverse Effects**

>10%: Gastrointestinal: Nausea, diarrhea, vomiting

1% to 10%:

Cardiovascular: Hypotension, thrombosis

Ocular: Blurred vision

<1%: Endocrine & metabolic: Unusual menstrual discomfort

**Drug Uptake** Serum half-life: 2-10 hours

**Pregnancy Risk Factor** B

**Generic Available** No

**Comments** Antifibrinolytic drugs are useful for the control of bleeding after dental extractions in patients with hemophilia because the oral mucosa and saliva are rich in plasminogen activators. In a clinical trial, tranexamic acid reduced recurrent bleeding and the amount of clotting-factor-replacement therapy needed. In adults, the oral dose was 20-25 mg/kg tranexamic acid every 8 hours until the dental sockets were completely healed. Mouthwashes containing tranexamic acid are effective for preventing oral bleeding in patients with hemophilia and in patients requiring dental extraction while receiving long-term oral anticoagulant therapy.

**Selected Readings**

Forbes CD, Barr RD, Reid G, et al, "Tranexamic Acid in Control of Haemorrhage After Dental Extraction in Haemophilia and Christmas Disease," *BMJ*, 1972, 2:311-3.

Mannuccio PM, "Hemostatic Drugs," *N Eng J Med*, 1998, 339:245-53.

Sindet-Pedersen S, "Distribution of Tranexamic Acid to Plasma and Salivar After Oral Administration and Mouth Rinsing: A Pharmacokinetic Study," *J Clin Pharmacol*, 1987, 27:1005-8.

Sindet-Pedersen S, Ramstron G, Bernvil S, et al, "Hemostatic Effect of Tranexamic Acid Mouthwash in Anticoagulant-Treated Patients Undergoing Oral Surgery," *N Eng J Med*, 1989, 320:840-3.

♦ **Transdermal-NTG®** *see* Nitroglycerin *on page 725*
♦ **Transderm-Nitro®** *see* Nitroglycerin *on page 725*
♦ **Transderm Scop® Patch** *see* Scopolamine *on page 905*
♦ **Trans-Ver-Sal® AdultPatch [OTC]** *see* Salicylic Acid *on page 900*
♦ **Trans-Ver-Sal® PediaPatch [OTC]** *see* Salicylic Acid *on page 900*
♦ **Trans-Ver-Sal® PlantarPatch [OTC]** *see* Salicylic Acid *on page 900*
♦ **Tranxene®** *see* Clorazepate *on page 267*

## Tranylcypromine (tran il SIP roe meen)

**U.S. Brand Names** Parnate®

**Therapeutic Category** Antidepressant, Monoamine Oxidase Inhibitor

**Use** Symptomatic treatment of depressed patients refractory to or intolerant to tricyclic antidepressants or electroconvulsive therapy; has a more rapid onset of therapeutic effect than other MAO inhibitors, but causes more severe hypertensive reactions

**Usual Dosage** Adults: Oral: 10 mg twice daily, increase by 10 mg increments at 1- to 3-week intervals; maximum: 60 mg/day

**Mechanism of Action** Inhibits the enzymes monoamine oxidase A and B which are responsible for the intraneuronal metabolism of norepinephrine and serotonin and increasing their availability to postsynaptic neurons; decreased firing rate of the locus ceruleus, reducing norepinephrine concentration in the brain; agonist effects of serotonin

**Local Anesthetic/Vasoconstrictor Precautions** Attempts should be made to avoid use of vasoconstrictor due to possibility of hypertensive episodes with monoamine oxidase inhibitors

**Effects on Dental Treatment** Orthostatic hypotension in >10% of patients; meperidine should be avoided as an analgesic due to toxic reactions with MAO inhibitors

**Other Adverse Effects**

1% to 10%: Cardiovascular: Orthostatic hypotension

<1%:

Cardiovascular: Edema, hypertensive crises

Central nervous system: Drowsiness, hyperexcitability, headache

Dermatologic: Skin rash, photosensitivity

Gastrointestinal: Dry mouth, constipation

Genitourinary: Urinary retention

Hepatic: Hepatitis

Ocular: Blurred vision

**Drug Interactions**

Decreased effect of antihypertensives

Increased toxicity with disulfiram (seizures), fluoxetine and other serotonin-active agents (eg, paroxetine, sertraline), tricyclic antidepressants (cardiovascular instability), meperidine (cardiovascular instability), phenothiazine (hypertensive

(Continued)

## Tranylcypromine *(Continued)*

crisis), sympathomimetics (hypertensive crisis), sumatriptan (hypothetical), CNS depressants, levodopa (hypertensive crisis), tyramine-containing foods (eg, aged foods), dextroamphetamine (psychosis)

**Drug Uptake**

Onset of action: 2-3 weeks are required of continued dosing to obtain full therapeutic effect

Serum half-life: 90-190 minutes

Time to peak serum concentration: Within 2 hours

**Pregnancy Risk Factor** C

**Generic Available** No

## Trastuzumab

**U.S. Brand Names** Herceptin®

**Therapeutic Category** Antineoplastic Agent; Monoclonal Antibody

**Use** Treatment of patients with metastatic breast cancer whose tumors overexpress the HER2 protein

**Usual Dosage** Adults: I.V.:

Loading dose: 4 mg/kg over 90 minutes; do not administer as an I.V. bolus or I.V. push

Maintenance dose: 2 mg/kg once weekly (may be infused over 30 minutes if prior infusions are well tolerated)

**Mechanism of Action** Trastuzumab is a monoclonal antibody which binds to the extracellular domain of the human epidermal growth factor receptor 2 protein (HER2). It mediates antibody-dependent cellular cytotoxicity against cells which overproduce HER2.

**Local Anesthetic/Vasoconstrictor Precautions** No information available to require special precautions

**Effects on Dental Treatment** Stomatitis occurs in <1% of patients

**Other Adverse Effects** The most common reactions were infusion-associated, occurring in up to 40% of patients consisting primarily of fever and/or chills which were mild to moderate in severity. These may be treated with acetaminophen, diphenhydramine, and meperidine with or without reduction of the infusion rate.

>10%:

- Central nervous system: Pain (47%), fever (36%), chills (32%), headache (26%)
- Dermatologic: Rash (18%)
- Gastrointestinal: Nausea (33%), diarrhea (25%), vomiting (23%), abdominal pain (22%), anorexia (14%)
- Neuromuscular & skeletal: Weakness (42%), back pain (22%)
- Respiratory: Cough (26%), dyspnea (22%), rhinitis (14%), pharyngitis (12%)
- Miscellaneous: Infection (20%)

1% to 10%:

- Cardiovascular: Peripheral edema (10%), congestive heart failure (7%), tachycardia (5%)
- Central nervous system: Insomnia (14%), dizziness (13%), depression (6%)
- Dermatologic: Herpes simplex (2%), acne (2%)
- Gastrointestinal: Nausea and vomiting (8%)
- Genitourinary: Urinary tract infection (5%)
- Hematologic: Anemia (4%), leukopenia (3%)
- Neuromuscular & skeletal: Bone pain (7%), arthralgia (6%), paresthesia (9%), peripheral neuritis (2%), neuropathy (1%)
- Respiratory: Sinusitis (9%)
- Miscellaneous: Flu syndrome (10%), accidental injury (6%), allergic reaction (3%)

<1%: Cellulitis, anaphylactoid reaction, ascites, hydrocephalus, radiation injury, deafness, amblyopia, vascular thrombosis, pericardial effusion, cardiac arrest, hypotension, syncope, hemorrhage, shock, arrhythmia, hepatic failure, gastroenteritis, hematemesis, ileus, intestinal obstruction, colitis, esophageal ulcer, stomatitis, pancreatitis, hepatitis, hypothyroidism, pancytopenia, acute leukemia, coagulopathy, lymphangitis

**Drug Interactions** Increased effect: Paclitaxel may result in a decrease in clearance of trastuzumab, increasing serum concentrations

**Drug Uptake** Serum half-life: Mean: 5.8 days (range: 1-32 days)

**Pregnancy Risk Factor** B

**Dosage Forms** Powder for injection: 440 mg

♦ **Trasylol®** *see* Aprotinin *on page 93*

## Trazodone (TRAZ oh done)

**Related Information**

Vasoconstrictor Interactions With Antidepressants *on page 1277*

**U.S. Brand Names** Desyrel®

**Therapeutic Category** Antidepressant, Miscellaneous

**Use** Treatment of depression

**Usual Dosage** Oral: Therapeutic effects may take up to 4 weeks to occur; therapy is normally maintained for several months after optimum response is reached to prevent recurrence of depression

Children 6-18 years: Initial: 1.5-2 mg/kg/day in divided doses; increase gradually every 3-4 days as needed; maximum: 6 mg/kg/day in 3 divided doses

Adolescents: Initial: 25-50 mg/day; increase to 100-150 mg/day in divided doses

Adults: Initial: 150 mg/day in 3 divided doses (may increase by 50 mg/day every 3-7 days); maximum: 600 mg/day

Elderly: 25-50 mg at bedtime with 25-50 mg/day dose increase every 3 days for inpatients and weekly for outpatients, if tolerated; usual dose: 75-150 mg/day

**Mechanism of Action** Inhibits reuptake of serotonin and norepinephrine by the presynaptic neuronal membrane and desensitization of adenyl cyclase, down regulation of beta-adrenergic receptors, and down regulation of serotonin receptors

**Local Anesthetic/Vasoconstrictor Precautions** No information available to require special precautions

**Effects on Dental Treatment** >10% of patients will experience dry mouth; trazodone elicits anticholinergic effects, but occur much less frequently than with tricyclic antidepressants; more than 10% of patients will have significant dry mouth especially in the elderly which could contribute to periodontal diseases and oral discomfort

**Other Adverse Effects**

>10%:

Central nervous system: Dizziness, headache, confusion

Gastrointestinal: Nausea, bad taste in mouth

Neuromuscular & skeletal: Muscle tremors

1% to 10%:

Gastrointestinal: Diarrhea, constipation

Neuromuscular & skeletal: Weakness

Ocular: Blurred vision

<1%:

Cardiovascular: Hypotension, tachycardia, bradycardia

Central nervous system: Agitation, seizures, extrapyramidal reactions

Dermatologic: Skin rash

Genitourinary: Prolonged priapism, urinary retention

Hepatic: Hepatitis

**Drug Interactions**

Decreased effect: Clonidine, methyldopa, anticoagulants

Increased toxicity: Fluoxetine; increased effect/toxicity of phenytoin, CNS depressants, MAO inhibitors; digoxin serum levels increase

**Drug Uptake**

Onset of effect: Therapeutic effects take 1-3 weeks to appear

Serum half-life: 4-7.5 hours, 2 compartment kinetics

Time to peak serum concentration: Within 30-100 minutes, prolonged in the presence of food (up to 2.5 hours)

**Pregnancy Risk Factor** C

**Generic Available** Yes

♦ **Trecator®-SC** *see* Ethionamide *on page 408*

♦ **Trental®** *see* Pentoxifylline *on page 783*

## Tretinoin, Oral (TRET i noyn, oral)

**U.S. Brand Names** Vesanoid®

**Therapeutic Category** Antineoplastic Agent, Miscellaneous

**Synonyms** All-*trans*-Retinoic Acid

**Use** Acute promyelocytic leukemia (APL): Induction of remission in patients with APL, French American British (FAB) classification M3 (including the M3 variant), characterized by the presence of the t(15;17) translocation or the presence of the PML/RARα gene who are refractory to or who have relapsed from anthracycline chemotherapy, or for whom anthracycline-based chemotherapy is contraindicated. Tretinoin is for the induction of remission only. All patients should receive an accepted form of remission consolidation or maintenance therapy for APL after completion of induction therapy with tretinoin.

(Continued)

## Tretinoin, Oral *(Continued)*

**Usual Dosage** Oral:

Children: There are limited clinical data on the pediatric use of tretinoin. Of 15 pediatric patients (age range: 1-16 years) treated with tretinoin, the incidence of complete remission was 67%. Safety and efficacy in pediatric patients <1 year of age have not been established. Some pediatric patients experience severe headache and pseudotumor cerebri, requiring analgesic treatment and lumbar puncture for relief. Increased caution is recommended. Consider dose reduction in children experiencing serious or intolerable toxicity; however, the efficacy and safety of tretinoin at doses <45 mg/m²/day have not been evaluated.

Adults: 45 mg/m²/day administered as two evenly divided doses until complete remission is documented. Discontinue therapy 30 days after achievement of complete remission or after 90 days of treatment, whichever occurs first. If after initiation of treatment the presence of the t(15;17) translocation is not confirmed by cytogenetics or by polymerase chain reaction studies and the patient has not responded to tretinoin, consider alternative therapy.

**Note:** Tretinoin is for the induction of remission only. Optimal consolidation or maintenance regimens have not been determined. All patients should therefore receive a standard consolidation or maintenance chemotherapy regimen for APL after induction therapy with tretinoin unless otherwise contraindicated.

**Mechanism of Action** Retinoid that induces maturation of acute promyelocytic leukemia (APL) cells in cultures; induces cytodifferentiation and decreased proliferation of APL cells

**Local Anesthetic/Vasoconstrictor Precautions** No information available to require special precautions

**Effects on Dental Treatment** <1% of patients may have bleeding gums, dry mouth

**Other Adverse Effects** Virtually all patients experience some drug-related toxicity, especially headache, fever, weakness and fatigue. These adverse effects are seldom permanent or irreversible nor do they usually require therapy interruption

>10%:

- Cardiovascular: Arrhythmias, flushing, hypotension, hypertension, peripheral edema, chest discomfort, edema
- Central nervous system: Dizziness, anxiety, insomnia, depression, confusion, malaise, pain
- Dermatologic: Burning, redness, cheilitis, inflammation of lips, dry skin, pruritus, photosensitivity
- Endocrine & metabolic: Increased serum concentration of triglycerides
- Gastrointestinal: GI hemorrhage, abdominal pain, other GI disorders, diarrhea, constipation, dyspepsia, abdominal distention, weight gain or loss, anorexia, xerostomia
- Hematologic: Hemorrhage, disseminated intravascular coagulation
- Local: Phlebitis, injection site reactions
- Neuromuscular & skeletal: Bone pain, arthralgia, myalgia, paresthesia
- Ocular: Itching of eye
- Renal: Renal insufficiency
- Respiratory: Upper respiratory tract disorders, dyspnea, respiratory insufficiency, pleural effusion, pneumonia, rales, expiratory wheezing, dry nose
- Miscellaneous: Infections, shivering

1% to 10%:

- Cardiovascular: Cardiac failure, cardiac arrest, myocardial infarction, enlarged heart, heart murmur, ischemia, stroke, myocarditis, pericarditis, pulmonary hypertension, secondary cardiomyopathy, cerebral hemorrhage, pallor
- Central nervous system: Intracranial hypertension, agitation, hallucination, agnosia, aphasia, cerebellar edema, cerebellar disorders, convulsions, coma, CNS depression, encephalopathy, hypotaxia, no light reflex, neurologic reaction, spinal cord disorder, unconsciousness, dementia, forgetfulness, somnolence, slow speech, hypothermia
- Dermatologic: Skin peeling on hands or soles of feet, rash, cellulitis
- Endocrine & metabolic: Fluid imbalance, acidosis
- Gastrointestinal: Hepatosplenomegaly, ulcer, unspecified liver disorder
- Genitourinary: Dysuria, polyuria, enlarged prostate
- Hepatic: Ascites, hepatitis
- Neuromuscular & skeletal: Tremor, leg weakness, hyporeflexia, dysarthria, facial paralysis, hemiplegia, flank pain, asterixis, abnormal gait
- Ocular: Dry eyes, photophobia
- Renal: Acute renal failure, renal tubular necrosis

Respiratory: Lower respiratory tract disorders, pulmonary infiltration, bronchial asthma, pulmonary/larynx edema, unspecified pulmonary disease

Miscellaneous: Face edema, lymph disorders

**Warnings/Precautions** **Not to be used in women of childbearing potential** unless woman is capable of complying with effective contraceptive measures; therapy is normally begun on the second or third day of next normal menstrual period; two reliable methods of effective contraception must be used during therapy and for 1 month after discontinuation of therapy, unless abstinence is the chosen method. Within one week prior to the institution of tretinoin therapy, the patient should have blood or urine collected for a serum or urine pregnancy test with a sensitivity of at least 50 mIU/L. When possible, delay tretinoin therapy until a negative result from this test is obtained. When a delay is not possible, place the patient on two reliable forms of contraception. Repeat pregnancy testing and contraception counseling monthly throughout the period of treatment.

**Drug Interactions** Metabolized by the hepatic cytochrome P-450 system: All drugs that induce or inhibit this system would be expected to interact with tretinoin cytochrome P-450 2C9 substrate

Increased toxicity: Ketoconazole increases the mean plasma AUC of tretinoin

**Drug Uptake**

Serum half-life, terminal: Parent drug: 0.5-2 hours

Time to peak serum concentration: Within 1-2 hours

**Pregnancy Risk Factor** D

**Dosage Forms** Capsule: 10 mg

**Generic Available** No

## Tretinoin, Topical (TRET i noyn, TOP i kal)

**U.S. Brand Names** Avita® Topical; Retin-A™ Micro Topical; Retin-A™ Topical

**Canadian Brand Names** Retisol-A®; Stieva-A®; Stieva-A® Forte

**Therapeutic Category** Acne Products; Retinoic Acid Derivative; Vitamin, Topical

**Use** Treatment of acne vulgaris, photodamaged skin, and some skin cancers

**Usual Dosage** Children >12 years and Adults: Topical: Apply once daily before retiring; if stinging or irritation develops, decrease frequency of application. Relapses normally occur within 3-6 weeks after stopping medication.

**Mechanism of Action** Keratinocytes in the sebaceous follicle become less adherent which allows for easy removal; decreases microcomedone formation

**Local Anesthetic/Vasoconstrictor Precautions** No information available to require special precautions

**Effects on Dental Treatment** No effects or complications reported

**Other Adverse Effects** 1% to 10%:

Cardiovascular: Edema

Dermatologic: Excessive dryness, erythema, scaling of the skin, hyperpigmentation or hypopigmentation, photosensitivity, initial acne flare-up

Local: Stinging, blistering

**Drug Interactions** Increased toxicity: Sulfur, benzoyl peroxide, salicylic acid, resorcinol (potentiates adverse reactions seen with tretinoin)

**Drug Uptake** Absorption: Topical: Minimum absorption occurs

**Pregnancy Risk Factor** C

**Dosage Forms**

Cream:

Avita®: 0.025% (20 g, 45 g)

Retin-A™: 0.025% (20 g, 45 g); 0.05% (20 g, 45 g); 0.1% (20 g, 45 g)

Gel, topical (Retin-A™): 0.01% (15 g, 45 g); 0.025% (15 g, 45 g)

Gel, topical (Retin-A™ Micro): 0.1% (20 g, 45 g)

Liquid, topical (Retin-A™): 0.05% (28 mL)

**Generic Available** No

♦ **TRH** *see* Protirelin *on page 861*

♦ **Triacet™** *see* Triamcinolone *on next page*

## Triacetin (trye a SEE tin)

**U.S. Brand Names** Ony-Clear® Nail

**Therapeutic Category** Antifungal Agent, Topical

**Synonyms** Glycerol Triacetate

**Use** Fungistat for athlete's foot and other superficial fungal infections

**Usual Dosage** Apply twice daily, cleanse areas with dilute alcohol or mild soap and water before application; continue treatment for 7 days after symptoms have disappeared

**Local Anesthetic/Vasoconstrictor Precautions** No information available to require special precautions

**Effects on Dental Treatment** No effects or complications reported

(Continued)

## Triacetin *(Continued)*

**Generic Available** No

♦ **Triacin-C®** *see* Triprolidine, Pseudoephedrine, and Codeine *on page 1026*

♦ **Triam-A®** *see* Triamcinolone *on this page*

## Triamcinolone (trye am SIN oh lone)

**Related Information**

Corticosteroid Equivalencies Comparison *on page 1221*
Corticosteroids, Topical Comparison *on page 1222*
Oral Nonviral Soft Tissue Ulcerations or Erosions *on page 1141*
Respiratory Diseases *on page 1079*

**U.S. Brand Names** Amcort®; Aristocort®; Aristocort® A; Aristocort® Forte; Aristocort® Intralesional; Aristospan® Intra-Articular; Aristospan® Intralesional; Atolone®; Azmacort™; Delta-Tritex®; Flutex®; Kenacort®; Kenaject-40®; Kenalog®; Kenalog-10®; Kenalog-40®; Kenalog® H; Kenalog® in Orabase®; Kenonel®; Nasacort®; Nasacort® AQ; Tac™-3; Tac™-40; Triacet™; Triam-A®; Triam Forte®; Triderm®; Tri-Kort®; Trilog®; Trilone®; Tristoject®

**Therapeutic Category** Anti-inflammatory Agent; Corticosteroid, Inhalant; Corticosteroid, Systemic; Corticosteroid, Topical (Medium Potency)

**Synonyms** Triamcinolone Acetonide, Aerosol; Triamcinolone Acetonide, Parenteral; Triamcinolone Diacetate, Oral; Triamcinolone Diacetate, Parenteral; Triamcinolone Hexacetonide; Triamcinolone, Oral

**Use** Severe swelling or immunosuppression; nasal spray for symptoms of seasonal and perennial allergic rhinitis

**Usual Dosage** In general, single I.M. dose of 4-7 times oral dose will control patient from 4-7 days up to 3-4 weeks.

Children 6-12 years:
- Oral inhalation: 1-2 inhalations 3-4 times/day, not to exceed 12 inhalations/day
- I.M. (acetonide or hexacetonide): 0.03-0.2 mg/kg at 1- to 7-day intervals
- Intra-articular, intrabursal, or tendon-sheath injection: 2.5-15 mg, repeated as needed

Children >12 years and Adults:
- Intranasal: 2 sprays in each nostril once daily; may increase after 4-7 days up to 4 sprays once daily or 1 spray 4 times/day in each nostril
- Topical: Apply a thin film 2-3 times/day
- Oral: 4-48 mg/day
- I.M.: Acetonide or hexacetonide: 60 mg (of 40 mg/mL), additional 20-100 mg doses (usual: 40-80 mg) may be given when signs and symptoms recur, best at 6-week intervals to minimize HPA suppression
- Oral inhalation: 2 inhalations 3-4 times/day, not to exceed 16 inhalations/day
- Intra-articular (hexacetonide): 2-20 mg every 3-4 weeks as hexacetonide salt
- Intralesional (use 10 mg/mL) (diacetate or acetonide): 1 mg/injection site, may be repeated one or more times/week depending upon patients response; maximum; 30 mg at any one time; may use multiple injections if they are more than 1 cm apart
- Intra-articular, intrasynovial, and soft-tissue injection (use 10 mg/mL or 40 mg/mL) (diacetate or acetonide): 2.5-40 mg depending upon location, size of joints, and degree of inflammation; repeat when signs and symptoms recur
- Sublesional (as acetonide): Up to 1 mg per injection site and may be repeated one or more times weekly; multiple sites may be injected if they are 1 cm or more apart, not to exceed 30 mg
- See table.

**Triamcinolone Dosing**

| | Acetonide | Diacetate | Hexacetonide |
|---|---|---|---|
| Intrasynovial | 2.5-40 mg | 5-40 mg | |
| Intralesional | 2.5-40 mg | 5-48 mg | Up to 0.5 mg/sq inch affected area |
| Sublesional | 1-30 mg | | |
| Systemic I.M. | 2.5-60 mg/d | ~40 mg/wk | 20-100 mg |
| Intra-articular | | 5-40 mg | 2-20 mg average |
| large joints | 5-15 mg | | 10-20 mg |
| small joints | 2.5-5 mg | | 2-6 mg |
| Tendon sheaths | 10-40 mg | | |
| Intradermal | 1 mg/site | | |

**Mechanism of Action** Decreases inflammation by suppression of migration of polymorphonuclear leukocytes and reversal of increased capillary permeability;

suppresses the immune system by reducing activity and volume of the lymphatic system; suppresses adrenal function at high doses

**Local Anesthetic/Vasoconstrictor Precautions** No information available to require special precautions

**Effects on Dental Treatment** No effects or complications reported

**Other Adverse Effects**

>10%:
- Central nervous system: Insomnia, nervousness
- Gastrointestinal: Increased appetite, indigestion

1% to 10%:
- Dermatologic: Hirsutism
- Endocrine & metabolic: Diabetes mellitus
- Neuromuscular & skeletal: Arthralgia
- Ocular: Cataracts
- Respiratory: Epistaxis

<1%:
- Central nervous system: Seizures, mood swings, headache, delirium, hallucinations, euphoria
- Dermatologic: Skin atrophy, bruising, hyperpigmentation, acne
- Endocrine & metabolic: Amenorrhea, sodium and water retention, Cushing's syndrome, hyperglycemia
- Gastrointestinal: Abdominal distention, ulcerative esophagitis, pancreatitis
- Hematologic: Bone growth suppression
- Neuromuscular & skeletal: Muscle wasting
- Miscellaneous: Hypersensitivity reactions

**Drug Uptake**

Duration of action: Oral: 8-12 hours
Absorption: Topical: Systemic absorption may occur
Serum half-life, biologic: 18-36 hours
Time to peak: I.M.: Within 8-10 hours

**Pregnancy Risk Factor** C

**Generic Available** Yes

**Comments** Triamcinolone 16 mg is equivalent to cortisone 100 mg (no mineralocorticoid activity)

♦ **Triamcinolone Acetonide, Aerosol** *see* Triamcinolone *on previous page*

## Triamcinolone Acetonide Dental Paste

(trye am SIN oh lone a SEE toe nide DEN tal paste)

**U.S. Brand Names** Kenalog® in Orabase®

**Canadian Brand Names** Oracort

**Therapeutic Category** Anti-inflammatory Agent

**Use**

Dental: For adjunctive treatment and for the temporary relief of symptoms associated with oral inflammatory lesions and ulcerative lesions resulting from trauma
Medical: Localized inflammation responsive to steroids

**Usual Dosage** Press a small dab (about 1/4 inch) to the lesion until a thin film develops. A larger quantity may be required for coverage of some lesions. For optimal results use only enough to coat the lesion with a thin film.

**Mechanism of Action** Decreases inflammation by suppression of migration of polymorphonuclear leukocytes and reversal of increased capillary permeability; suppresses the immune system by reducing activity and volume of the lymphatic system; suppresses adrenal function at high doses

**Local Anesthetic/Vasoconstrictor Precautions** No information available to require special precautions

**Effects on Dental Treatment** No effects or complications reported

**Other Adverse Effects** No data reported

**Contraindications** Known hypersensitivity to triamcinolone; contraindicated in the presence of fungal, viral, or bacterial infections of the mouth or throat

**Warnings/Precautions** Patients with tuberculosis, peptic ulcer or diabetes mellitus should not be treated with any corticosteroid preparation without the advice of the patient's physician. Normal immune responses of the oral tissues are depressed in patients receiving topical corticosteroid therapy. Virulent strains of oral microorganisms may multiply without producing the usual warning symptoms of oral infections. The small amount of steroid released from the topical preparation makes systemic effects very unlikely. If local irritation or sensitization should develop, the preparation should be discontinued. If significant regeneration or repair of oral tissues has not occurred in seven days, re-evaluation of the etiology of the oral lesion is advised.

**Drug Interactions** No data reported

**Drug Uptake**

Absorption: Topical: Systemic absorption may occur
(Continued)

## Triamcinolone Acetonide Dental Paste *(Continued)*

Serum half-life: Biological: 18-36 hours

**Pregnancy Risk Factor** C

**Breast-feeding Considerations** No data reported

**Dosage Forms** Tubes: 5 g; each g provides 1 mg (0.1%) triamcinolone in emollient dental paste containing gelatin, pectin, and carboxymethylcellulose sodium in a polyethylene and mineral oil gel base

**Generic Available** Yes

**Comments** When applying to tissues, attempts to spread this preparation may result in a granular, gritty sensation and cause it to crumble. This preparation should be applied at bedtime to permit steroid contact with the lesion throughout the night.

- **Triamcinolone Acetonide, Parenteral** *see* Triamcinolone *on page 1010*
- **Triamcinolone Diacetate, Oral** *see* Triamcinolone *on page 1010*
- **Triamcinolone Diacetate, Parenteral** *see* Triamcinolone *on page 1010*
- **Triamcinolone Hexacetonide** *see* Triamcinolone *on page 1010*
- **Triamcinolone, Oral** *see* Triamcinolone *on page 1010*
- **Triam Forte®** *see* Triamcinolone *on page 1010*
- **Triaminic® Allergy Tablet [OTC]** *see* Chlorpheniramine and Phenylpropanolamine *on page 233*
- **Triaminic® AM Decongestant Formula [OTC]** *see* Pseudoephedrine *on page 863*
- **Triaminic® Cold Tablet [OTC]** *see* Chlorpheniramine and Phenylpropanolamine *on page 233*
- **Triaminic® Expectorant [OTC]** *see* Guaifenesin and Phenylpropanolamine *on page 480*
- **Triaminicol® Multi-Symptom Cold Syrup [OTC]** *see* Chlorpheniramine, Phenylpropanolamine, and Dextromethorphan *on page 236*
- **Triaminic® Oral Infant Drops** *see* Pheniramine, Phenylpropanolamine, and Pyrilamine *on page 790*
- **Triaminic® Syrup [OTC]** *see* Chlorpheniramine and Phenylpropanolamine *on page 233*

## Triamterene (trye AM ter een)

**Related Information**

Cardiovascular Diseases *on page 1066*

**U.S. Brand Names** Dyrenium®

**Therapeutic Category** Diuretic, Potassium Sparing

**Use** Alone or in combination with other diuretics to treat edema and hypertension; decreases potassium excretion caused by kaliuretic diuretics

**Usual Dosage** Oral:

Children: 2-4 mg/kg/day in 1-2 divided doses; maximum: 300 mg/day

Adults: 100-300 mg/day in 1-2 divided doses; maximum dose: 300 mg/day

**Mechanism of Action** Competes with aldosterone for receptor sites in the distal renal tubules, increasing sodium, chloride, and water excretion while conserving potassium and hydrogen ions; may block the effect of aldosterone on arteriolar smooth muscle as well

**Local Anesthetic/Vasoconstrictor Precautions** No information available to require special precautions

**Effects on Dental Treatment** No effects or complications reported

**Other Adverse Effects**

1% to 10%:

Cardiovascular: Hypotension, edema, congestive heart failure, bradycardia

Central nervous system: Dizziness, headache, fatigue

Dermatologic: Rash

Gastrointestinal: Constipation, nausea

Respiratory: Dyspnea

<1%:

Cardiovascular: Flushing

Endocrine & metabolic: Hyperkalemia, dehydration, hyponatremia, gynecomastia, hyperchloremic, metabolic acidosis, postmenopausal bleeding

Genitourinary: Inability to achieve or maintain an erection

**Drug Interactions**

Increased risk of hyperkalemia if given together with amiloride, spironolactone, angiotensin-converting enzyme (ACE) inhibitors

Increased toxicity of amantadine (possibly by decreasing its renal excretion)

**Drug Uptake**

Onset of action: Diuresis occurs within 2-4 hours

Duration: 7-9 hours

Absorption: Oral: Unreliable

**Pregnancy Risk Factor** D
**Dosage Forms** Capsule: 50 mg, 100 mg
**Generic Available** No

- ♦ **Triapin®** *see* Butalbital Compound *on page 163*
- ♦ **Triapin®** *see* Butalbital Compound and Acetaminophen *on page 164*
- ♦ **Triavil®** *see* Amitriptyline and Perphenazine *on page 69*

## Triazolam (trye AY zoe lam)

**Related Information**

Dental Drug Interactions: Update on Drug Combinations Requiring Special Considerations *on page 1225*
Patients Requiring Sedation *on page 1152*

**U.S. Brand Names** Halcion®
**Canadian Brand Names** Apo®-Triazo; Gen-Triazolam; Novo-Triolam; Nu-Triazo
**Therapeutic Category** Benzodiazepine; Hypnotic; Sedative
**Use**

Dental: Oral premedication before dental procedures
Medical: Short-term treatment of insomnia

**Restrictions** C-IV; Refillable up to 5 times in 6 months
**Usual Dosage** Oral:

Children <18 years: Dosage not established
Adults: 0.25 mg taken the evening before oral surgery; or 0.25 mg 1 hour before procedure

**Mechanism of Action** Depresses all levels of the CNS, including the limbic and reticular formation, probably through the increased action of gamma-aminobutyric acid (GABA), which is a major inhibitory neurotransmitter in the brain
**Local Anesthetic/Vasoconstrictor Precautions** No information available to require special precautions
**Effects on Dental Treatment** No effects or complications reported
**Other Adverse Effects**

>10%: Central nervous system: Drowsiness
1% to 10%:
Central nervous system: Headache, dizziness, nervousness, lightheadedness, coordination disorders, ataxia
Gastrointestinal: Nausea, vomiting
<1%:
Cardiovascular: Tachycardia, chest pain
Central nervous system: Euphoria, tiredness, confusion, memory impairment, depression, insomnia, dreams/nightmares, amnesia
Dermatologic: Dermatitis
Gastrointestinal: Constipation, taste alteration, diarrhea, xerostomia
Ocular: Visual disturbances
Otic: Tinnitus

**Contraindications** Hypersensitivity to triazolam, or any component, cross-sensitivity with other benzodiazepines may occur; severe uncontrolled pain; pre-existing CNS depression; narrow-angle glaucoma; not to be used in pregnancy or lactation
**Warnings/Precautions** May cause drug dependency; avoid abrupt discontinuance in patients with prolonged therapy or seizure disorders; not considered a drug of choice in the elderly
**Drug Interactions** Decreased effect with phenytoin, phenobarbital; increased effect/toxicity with CNS depressants, cimetidine, erythromycin
**Drug Uptake**

Onset of hypnotic effect: Within 15-30 minutes
Duration: 6-7 hours
Serum half-life: 1.7-5 hours
Time to peak serum concentration: Oral: ~2 hours

**Pregnancy Risk Factor** X
**Breast-feeding Considerations** No data reported
**Dosage Forms** Tablet: 0.125 mg, 0.25 mg
**Dietary Considerations** No data reported
**Generic Available** Yes
**Comments** Triazolam (0.25 mg) 1 hour prior to dental procedure has been used as an oral pre-op sedative
**Selected Readings**

Berthold CW, Dionne RA, and Corey SE, "Comparison of Sublingually and Orally Administered Triazolam for Premedication Before Oral Surgery," *Oral Surg Oral Med Oral Pathol Oral Radiol Endod*, 1997, 84(2):119-24.
Berthold CW, Schneider A, and Dionne RA, "Using Triazolam to Reduce Dental Anxiety," *J Am Dent Assoc*, 1993, 124(11):58-64.

(Continued)

## Triazolam *(Continued)*

Kaufman E, Hargreaves KM, and Dionne RA, "Comparison of Oral Triazolam and Nitrous Oxide With Placebo and Intravenous Diazepam for Outpatient Premedication," *Oral Surg Oral Med Oral Pathol*, 1993, 75(2):156-64.
Kurzrock M, "Triazolam and Dental Anxiety," *J Am Dent Assoc*, 1994, 125(4):358, 360.
Lieblich SE and Horswell B, "Attenuation of Anxiety in Ambulatory Oral Surgery Patients With Oral Triazolam," *J Oral Maxillofac Surg*, 1991, 49(8):792-7.
Milgrom P, Quarnstrom FC, Longley A, et al, "The Efficacy and Memory Effects of Oral Triazolam Premedication in Highly Anxious Dental Patients," *Anesth Prog*, 1994, 41(3):70-6.

♦ **Triban®** *see* Trimethobenzamide *on page 1020*
♦ **Tribavirin** *see* Ribavirin *on page 884*
♦ **Tri-Chlor®** *see* Trichloroacetic Acid *on this page*

## Trichlormethiazide (trye klor meth EYE a zide)

**Related Information**
Cardiovascular Diseases *on page 1066*

**U.S. Brand Names** Metahydrin®; Naqua®

**Therapeutic Category** Diuretic, Thiazide

**Use** Management of mild to moderate hypertension; treatment of edema in congestive heart failure and nephrotic syndrome

**Usual Dosage** Oral:
Children >6 months: 0.07 mg/kg/24 hours or 2 $mg/m^2$/24 hours
Adults: 1-4 mg/day

**Mechanism of Action** The diuretic mechanism of action of the thiazides is primarily inhibition of sodium, chloride, and water reabsorption in the renal distal tubules, thereby producing diuresis with a resultant reduction in plasma volume. The antihypertensive mechanism of action of the thiazides is unknown. It is known that doses of thiazides produce greater reduction in blood pressure than equivalent diuretic doses of loop diuretics. There has been speculation that the thiazides may have some influence on vascular tone mediated through sodium depletion, but this remains to be proven.

**Local Anesthetic/Vasoconstrictor Precautions** No information available to require special precautions

**Effects on Dental Treatment** No effects or complications reported

**Other Adverse Effects**
1% to 10%: Endocrine & metabolic: Hypokalemia
<1%:
- Cardiovascular: Hypotension
- Dermatologic: Photosensitivity
- Endocrine & metabolic: Fluid and electrolyte imbalances (hypocalcemia, hypomagnesemia, hyponatremia); hyperglycemia
- Hematologic: Rarely blood dyscrasias
- Renal: Prerenal azotemia

**Drug Interactions**
Decreased effect of oral hypoglycemics; decreased absorption with cholestyramine and colestipol
Increased effect with furosemide and other loop diuretics
Increased toxicity/levels of lithium

**Drug Uptake**
Onset of of diuretic effect: Within 2 hours
Peak: 4 hours
Duration: 12-24 hours

**Pregnancy Risk Factor** D

**Generic Available** Yes

## Trichloroacetic Acid (trye klor oh a SEE tik AS id)

**U.S. Brand Names** Tri-Chlor®

**Therapeutic Category** Keratolytic Agent

**Use** Debride callous tissue

**Usual Dosage** Apply to verruca, cover with bandage for 5-6 days, remove verruca, reapply as needed

**Local Anesthetic/Vasoconstrictor Precautions** No information available to require special precautions

**Effects on Dental Treatment** No effects or complications reported

**Generic Available** Yes

♦ **Tri-Clear® Expectorant [OTC]** *see* Guaifenesin and Phenylpropanolamine *on page 480*

## Triclosan and Fluoride

**Related Information**
Periodontal Diseases *on page 1132*

**U.S. Brand Names** Colgate Total® Toothpaste

**Therapeutic Category** Antibacterial, Dental; Mineral, Oral; Mineral, Oral Topical

**Use** Anticavity, antigingivitis, antiplaque toothpaste

**Usual Dosage** Brush teeth thoroughly after each meal or at least twice daily

**Mechanism of Action** Triclosan is an antibacterial agent which helps to prevent gingivitis with regular use. Fluoride promotes remineralization of decalcified enamel, inhibits the cariogenic microbial process in dental plaque, and increases tooth resistance to acid dissolution

**Local Anesthetic/Vasoconstrictor Precautions** No information available

**Effects on Dental Treatment** No effects

**Other Adverse Effects** No data reported

**Warnings/Precautions** Antigingivitis and antiplaque effects have not been determined in children less than 6 years of age. If an amount greater than used for brushing is swallowed, seek professional assistance of contact a poison control center immediately

**Pregnancy Risk Factor** No data reported

**Breast-feeding Considerations** No data reported

**Dosage Forms** Toothpaste, in 4.2 oz (119g) tube (contains triclosan 0.30% and sodium fluoride 0.24%)

**Dietary Considerations** No data reported

**Comments** It has been shown that stannous fluoride and triclosan when formulated into a toothpaste vehicle provide plaque inhibitory effects. To provide a longer retention time of the triclosan in plaque, a polymer has been added to the toothpaste vehicle. The polymer is known as PVM/MA which stands for polyvinylmethyl ether/maleic acid copolymer, and is listed as an inactive ingredient (PVM/MA Copolymer) on the manufacturer's label. Studies have reported that the retention of triclosan in plaque (exceeding the minimal inhibitory concentration) after polymer application was 14 hours after brushing. On-going studies are evaluating the effects of triclosan/copolymer on alveolar bone loss. Rosling et al. have reported that the daily use of Colgate Total® reduced (1) the frequency of deep periodontal pockets and (2) the number of sites that exhibited additional probing attachment and bone loss.

**Selected Readings**

Binney A, Addy M, Owens J, et al, "A Comparison of Triclosan and Stannous Fluoride Toothpastes for Inhibition of Plaque Growth," *J Clin Periodontol*, 1997, 24:166-70.

Ellwood RP, Worthington HV, Blinkhorn AS, et al, "Effect of a Triclosan/Copolymer Dentifrice on the Incidence of Periodontal Attachment Loss in Adolescents," *J Clin Periodontol*, 1998, 25(5):363-7.

Mandel ID, "The New Toothpastes," *J Calif Dent Assoc*, 1998, 26(3):186-90.

Rosling B, Wannfors B, Volpe AR, et a, "The Use of a Triclosan/Copolymer Dentifrice May Retard the Progression of Periodontitis," *J Clin Periodontol*, 1997, 24:873-80.

♦ **Tricor**® *see* Fenofibrate *on page 422*

♦ **Triderm**® *see* Triamcinolone *on page 1010*

♦ **Tridesilon**® *see* Desonide *on page 307*

## Tridihexethyl (trye dye heks ETH il)

**U.S. Brand Names** Pathilon®

**Therapeutic Category** Anticholinergic Agent; Antispasmodic Agent, Gastrointestinal

**Use** Adjunctive therapy in peptic ulcer treatment

**Usual Dosage** Adults: Oral: 1-2 tablets 3-4 times/day before meals and 2 tablets at bedtime

**Local Anesthetic/Vasoconstrictor Precautions** No information available to require special precautions

**Effects on Dental Treatment** >10% of patients experience dry mouth

**Other Adverse Effects**

>10%:
- Dermatologic: Dry skin
- Gastrointestinal: Constipation, dry throat
- Respiratory: Dry nose
- Miscellaneous: Decreased sweating

1% to 10%: Gastrointestinal: Dysphagia

<1%:
- Dermatologic: Rash
- Cardiovascular: Tachycardia
- Central nervous system: Confusion, headache, loss of memory, nausea, fatigue, drowsiness, nervousness, insomnia
- Gastrointestinal: Bloated feeling, vomiting
- Genitourinary: Urinary retention
- Neuromuscular & skeletal: Weakness
- Ocular: Increased intraocular pressure, blurred vision

**Pregnancy Risk Factor** C

(Continued)

## Tridihexethyl *(Continued)*

**Generic Available** No

- **Tridil®** *see* Nitroglycerin *on page 725*
- **Tridione®** *see* Trimethadione *on page 1019*

## Triethanolamine Polypeptide Oleate-Condensate

(trye eth a NOLE a meen pol i PEP tide OH lee ate-KON den sate)

**U.S. Brand Names** Cerumenex®

**Therapeutic Category** Otic Agent, Cerumenolytic

**Use** Removal of ear wax (cerumen)

**Usual Dosage** Children and Adults: Otic: Fill ear canal, insert cotton plug; allow to remain 15-30 minutes; flush ear with lukewarm water as a single treatment; if a second application is needed for unusually hard impactions, repeat the procedure

**Mechanism of Action** Emulsifies and disperses accumulated cerumen

**Local Anesthetic/Vasoconstrictor Precautions** No information available to require special precautions

**Effects on Dental Treatment** No effects or complications reported

**Other Adverse Effects** <1%: Dermatologic: Mild erythema and pruritus, severe eczematoid reactions, localized dermatitis

**Drug Interactions** No data reported

**Drug Uptake** Onset of effect: Produces slight disintegration of very hard ear wax by 24 hours

**Pregnancy Risk Factor** C

**Dosage Forms** Solution, otic: 6 mL, 12 mL

**Generic Available** No

## Triethanolamine Salicylate (trye eth a NOLE a meen sa LIS i late)

**U.S. Brand Names** Myoflex® [OTC]; Sportscreme® [OTC]

**Therapeutic Category** Analgesic, Topical

**Use** Relief of pain of muscular aches, rheumatism, neuralgia, sprains, arthritis on intact skin

**Usual Dosage** Apply to area as needed

**Local Anesthetic/Vasoconstrictor Precautions** No information available to require special precautions

**Effects on Dental Treatment** No effects or complications reported

**Other Adverse Effects** 1% to 10%:

Central nervous system: Confusion, drowsiness
Gastrointestinal: Nausea, vomiting, diarrhea
Respiratory: Hyperventilation

**Generic Available** No

- **Triethylenethiophosphoramide** *see* Thiotepa *on page 979*
- **Trifed-C®** *see* Triprolidine, Pseudoephedrine, and Codeine *on page 1026*

## Trifluoperazine (trye floo oh PER a zeen)

**U.S. Brand Names** Stelazine®

**Therapeutic Category** Antipsychotic Agent; Phenothiazine Derivative

**Use** Treatment of psychoses and management of nonpsychotic anxiety

**Usual Dosage**

Children 6-12 years: Psychoses:

- Oral: Hospitalized or well supervised patients: Initial: 1 mg 1-2 times/day, gradually increase until symptoms are controlled or adverse effects become troublesome; maximum: 15 mg/day
- I.M.: 1 mg twice daily

Adults:

- Psychoses:
  - Outpatients: Oral: 1-2 mg twice daily
  - Hospitalized or well supervised patients: Initial: 2-5 mg twice daily with optimum response in the 15-20 mg/day range; do not exceed 40 mg/day
  - I.M.: 1-2 mg every 4-6 hours as needed up to 10 mg/24 hours maximum
- Nonpsychotic anxiety: Oral: 1-2 mg twice daily; maximum: 6 mg/day; therapy for anxiety should not exceed 12 weeks; do not exceed 6 mg/day for longer than 12 weeks when treating anxiety; agitation, jitteriness, or insomnia may be confused with original neurotic or psychotic symptoms

**Mechanism of Action** Blocks postsynaptic mesolimbic dopaminergic receptors in the brain; exhibits a strong alpha-adrenergic blocking effect and depresses the release of hypothalamic and hypophyseal hormones

**Local Anesthetic/Vasoconstrictor Precautions** Most pharmacology textbooks state that in presence of phenothiazines, systemic doses of epinephrine paradoxically decrease the blood pressure. This is the so called "epinephrine reversal" phenomenon. This has never been observed when epinephrine is given by infiltration as part of the anesthesia procedure.

**Effects on Dental Treatment** Significant hypotension may occur, especially when the drug is administered parenterally; orthostatic hypotension is due to alpha-receptor blockade, the elderly are at greater risk for orthostatic hypotension

Tardive dyskinesia: Prevalence rate may be 40% in elderly; development of the syndrome and the irreversible nature are proportional to duration and total cumulative dose over time

Extrapyramidal reactions are more common in elderly with up to 50% developing these reactions after 60 years of age; drug-induced **Parkinson's syndrome** occurs often; **Akathisia** is the most common extrapyramidal reaction in elderly

Increased confusion, memory loss, psychotic behavior, and agitation frequently occur as a consequence of anticholinergic effects

Antipsychotic associated sedation in nonpsychotic patients is extremely unpleasant due to feelings of depersonalization, derealization, and dysphoria

**Other Adverse Effects**

>10%:
- Cardiovascular: Hypotension, orthostatic hypotension
- Central nervous system: Pseudoparkinsonism, akathisia, dystonias, tardive dyskinesia (persistent), dizziness
- Gastrointestinal: Constipation
- Ocular: Pigmentary retinopathy
- Respiratory: Nasal congestion
- Miscellaneous: Decreased sweating

1% to 10%:
- Dermatologic: Photosensitivity, skin rash
- Endocrine & metabolic: Changes in menstrual cycle, changes in libido, pain in breasts
- Gastrointestinal: Weight gain, nausea, vomiting, stomach pain
- Genitourinary: Dysuria, ejaculatory disturbances
- Neuromuscular & skeletal: Trembling of fingers

<1%:
- Central nervous system: Neuroleptic malignant syndrome (NMS), impairment of temperature regulation, lowering of seizures threshold
- Dermatologic: Discoloration of skin (blue-gray)
- Endocrine & metabolic: Galactorrhea
- Genitourinary: Priapism
- Hematologic: Agranulocytosis, leukopenia
- Hepatic: Cholestatic jaundice, hepatotoxicity
- Ocular: Cornea and lens changes

**Drug Interactions**

Decreased effect of anticonvulsants (increases requirements), guanethidine, anticoagulants; decreased effect with anticholinergics

Increased effect/toxicity with CNS depressants, metrizamide (increased seizures), propranolol, lithium (rare encephalopathy)

**Drug Uptake** Serum half-life: >24 hours with chronic use

**Pregnancy Risk Factor** C

**Generic Available** Yes

## Triflupromazine (trye floo PROE ma zeen)

**U.S. Brand Names** Vesprin®

**Therapeutic Category** Phenothiazine Derivative

**Use** Treatment of psychoses, nausea, vomiting, and intractable hiccups

**Usual Dosage**

Children: I.M.: 0.2-0.25 mg/kg

Adults:
- I.M.: 5-15 mg every 4 hours
- I.V.: 1 mg

**Local Anesthetic/Vasoconstrictor Precautions** Most pharmacology textbooks state that in presence of phenothiazines, systemic doses of epinephrine paradoxically decrease the blood pressure. This is the so called "epinephrine reversal" phenomenon. This has never been observed when epinephrine is given by infiltration as part of the anesthesia procedure.

**Effects on Dental Treatment** Significant hypotension may occur, especially when the drug is administered parenterally; orthostatic hypotension is due to alpha-receptor blockade, the elderly are at greater risk for orthostatic hypotension

(Continued)

## Triflupromazine *(Continued)*

Tardive dyskinesia: Prevalence rate may be 40% in elderly; development of the syndrome and the irreversible nature are proportional to duration and total cumulative dose over time

Extrapyramidal reactions are more common in elderly with up to 50% developing these reactions after 60 years of age; drug-induced **Parkinson's syndrome** occurs often; **Akathisia** is the most common extrapyramidal reaction in elderly

Increased confusion, memory loss, psychotic behavior, and agitation frequently occur as a consequence of anticholinergic effects

Antipsychotic associated sedation in nonpsychotic patients is extremely unpleasant due to feelings of depersonalization, derealization, and dysphoria

**Pregnancy Risk Factor** C

**Generic Available** No

## Trifluridine (trye FLURE i deen)

**Related Information**

Systemic Viral Diseases *on page 1115*

**U.S. Brand Names** Viroptic®

**Therapeutic Category** Antiviral Agent, Ophthalmic

**Use** Treatment of primary keratoconjunctivitis and recurrent epithelial keratitis caused by herpes simplex virus types I and II

**Usual Dosage** Adults: Instill 1 drop into affected eye every 2 hours while awake, to a maximum of 9 drops/day, until re-epithelialization of corneal ulcer occurs; then use 1 drop every 4 hours for another 7 days; do **not** exceed 21 days of treatment; if improvement has not taken place in 7-14 days, consider another form of therapy

**Mechanism of Action** Interferes with viral replication by incorporating into viral DNA in place of thymidine, inhibiting thymidylate synthetase resulting in the formation of defective proteins

**Local Anesthetic/Vasoconstrictor Precautions** No information available to require special precautions

**Effects on Dental Treatment** No effects or complications reported

**Other Adverse Effects**

1% to 10%: Ocular: Burning, stinging

<1%:

- Cardiovascular: Hyperemia
- Ocular: Palpebral edema, epithelial keratopathy, keratitis, stromal edema, increased intraocular pressure
- Miscellaneous: Hypersensitivity reactions

**Drug Interactions** No data reported

**Drug Uptake** Absorption: Ophthalmic instillation: Systemic absorption is negligible, while corneal penetration is adequate

**Pregnancy Risk Factor** C

**Generic Available** No

♦ **Triglycerides, Medium Chain** *see* Medium Chain Triglycerides *on page 622*

♦ **Trihexy**® *see* Trihexyphenidyl *on this page*

## Trihexyphenidyl (trye heks ee FEN i dil)

**U.S. Brand Names** Artane®; Trihexy®

**Canadian Brand Names** Apo®-Trihex; Novo-Hexidyl; PMS-Trihexyphenidyl; Trihexyphen®

**Therapeutic Category** Anticholinergic Agent; Anti-Parkinson's Agent

**Use** Adjunctive treatment of Parkinson's disease; also used in treatment of drug-induced extrapyramidal effects and acute dystonic reactions

**Usual Dosage** Adults: Oral: Initial: 1-2 mg/day, increase by 2 mg increments at intervals of 3-5 days; usual dose: 5-15 mg/day in 3-4 divided doses

**Mechanism of Action** Thought to act by blocking excess acetylcholine at cerebral synapses; many of its effects are due to its pharmacologic similarities with atropine

**Local Anesthetic/Vasoconstrictor Precautions** No information available to require special precautions

**Effects on Dental Treatment** >10% of patients experience significant dry mouth; normal salivary flow will resume with cessation of drug therapy. Prolonged xerostomia may contribute to development of caries, periodontal disease, oral candidiasis and discomfort

**Other Adverse Effects**

>10%:

- Dermatologic: Dry skin
- Gastrointestinal: Constipation

Respiratory: Dry nose, throat
Miscellaneous: Decreased sweating

1% to 10%:
Endocrine & metabolic: Decreased flow of breast milk
Gastrointestinal: Dysphagia
Ocular: Photosensitivity

<1%:
Cardiovascular: Orthostatic hypotension, ventricular fibrillation, tachycardia, palpitations
Central nervous system: Confusion, drowsiness, headache, loss of memory, fatigue, ataxia
Dermatologic: Skin rash
Gastrointestinal: Bloated feeling, nausea, vomiting
Genitourinary: Dysuria
Neuromuscular & skeletal: Weakness
Ocular: Increased intraocular pain, blurred vision

**Drug Interactions**
Decreased effect of levodopa
Increased toxicity with narcotic analgesics, phenothiazines, TCAs, quinidine, levodopa, anticholinergics

**Drug Uptake**
Peak effect: Within 1 hour
Serum half-life: 3.3-4.1 hours
Time to peak serum concentration: Within 1-1.5 hours

**Pregnancy Risk Factor** C

**Dosage Forms**
Capsule, as hydrochloride, sustained release: 5 mg
Elixir, as hydrochloride: 2 mg/5 mL (480 mL)
Tablet, as hydrochloride: 2 mg, 5 mg

**Generic Available** Yes: Tablet


- ♦ **Tri-K®** *see* Potassium Acetate, Potassium Bicarbonate, and Potassium Citrate *on page 819*
- ♦ **Tri-Kort®** *see* Triamcinolone *on page 1010*
- ♦ **Trilafon®** *see* Perphenazine *on page 786*
- ♦ **Tri-Levlen®** *see* Ethinyl Estradiol and Levonorgestrel *on page 402*
- ♦ **Trilisate®** *see* Choline Magnesium Trisalicylate *on page 244*
- ♦ **Trilog®** *see* Triamcinolone *on page 1010*
- ♦ **Trilone®** *see* Triamcinolone *on page 1010*
- ♦ **Trimazide®** *see* Trimethobenzamide *on next page*


## Trimethadione (trye meth a DYE one)

**U.S. Brand Names** Tridione®

**Therapeutic Category** Anticonvulsant, Oxazolidinedione

**Synonyms** Troxidone

**Use** Control absence (petit mal) seizures refractory to other drugs

**Usual Dosage** Oral:
Children: Initial: 25-50 mg/kg/24 hours in 3-4 equally divided doses every 6-8 hours
Adults: Initial: 900 mg/day in 3-4 equally divided doses, increase by 300 mg/day at weekly intervals until therapeutic results or toxic symptoms appear

**Local Anesthetic/Vasoconstrictor Precautions** No information available to require special precautions

**Effects on Dental Treatment** No effects or complications reported

**Other Adverse Effects**

>10%:
Central nervous system: Dizziness, drowsiness, sedation, headache
Ocular: Diplopia, photophobia

1% to 10%:
Central nervous system: Insomnia
Dermatologic: Alopecia
Gastrointestinal: Anorexia, stomach upset
Miscellaneous: Hiccups

<1%:
Dermatologic: Exfoliative dermatitis
Hematologic: Aplastic anemia, agranulocytosis, thrombocytopenia, exacerbation of porphyria
Hepatic: Hepatitis
Neuromuscular & skeletal: Myasthenia gravis syndrome
Miscellaneous: Systemic lupus erythematosus (SLE), nephrosis

**Pregnancy Risk Factor** D

**Generic Available** No

## Trimethaphan Camsylate (Discontinued 4/96)

(trye METH a fan KAM si late)

**U.S. Brand Names** Arfonad®

**Therapeutic Category** Adrenergic Blocking Agent; Anticholinergic Agent; Ganglionic Blocking Agent

**Use** Immediate and temporary reduction of blood pressure in patients with hypertensive emergencies; controlled hypotension during surgery

**Usual Dosage** Administration requires the use of an infusion pump

Severe hypertension and hypertensive emergencies: I.V.:

Children: 50-150 mcg/kg/minute; dilute 150 mg x weight (kg) to 250 mL in $D_5W$ then dose in mcg/kg/minute = 10 x infusion rate in mL/hour

Adults: Initial rate: 0.5-1 mg/minute; titrate dose to the desired effect

Hypertension due to acute dissecting aneurysms: Initial rate: 1-2 mg/minute, adjusting as needed to keep systolic blood pressure of 100-120 mm Hg

Controlled hypotension during surgery: Initial rate: 3-4 mg/minute adjusted to maintain blood pressure at a desirable level; usual dosage needed 0.3-6 mg/minute

**Mechanism of Action** Blocks transmission in both adrenergic and cholinergic ganglia by blocking stimulation from presynaptic receptors to postsynaptic receptors mediated by acetylcholine; possesses direct peripheral vasodilatory activity and is a weak histamine releaser

**Local Anesthetic/Vasoconstrictor Precautions** No information available to require special precautions

**Effects on Dental Treatment** No effects or complications reported

**Other Adverse Effects** 1% to 10%:

Cardiovascular: Hypotension (especially orthostatic), tachycardia
Central nervous system: Restlessness
Dermatologic: Itching, urticaria
Endocrine & metabolic: Sodium and water retention
Gastrointestinal: Anorexia, nausea, vomiting, dry mouth, adynamic ileus
Genitourinary: Urinary retention
Neuromuscular & skeletal: Weakness
Ocular: Mydriasis, cycloplegia
Respiratory: Apnea, respiratory arrest

**Drug Interactions** Increased effect:

Anesthetics, procainamide, diuretics, and other hypotensive agents may increase hypotensive effects of trimethaphan

Effects of tubocurarine and succinylcholine may be prolonged by trimethaphan

**Pregnancy Risk Factor** C

**Generic Available** No

## Trimethobenzamide (trye meth oh BEN za mide)

**U.S. Brand Names** Arrestin®; Pediatric Triban®; Tebamide®; T-Gen®; Ticon®; Tigan®; Triban®; Trimazide®

**Therapeutic Category** Antiemetic

**Use** Control of nausea and vomiting (especially for long-term antiemetic therapy); less effective than phenothiazines but may be associated with fewer side effects

**Usual Dosage** Rectal use is contraindicated in neonates and premature infants

Children:

Rectal: <14 kg: 100 mg 3-4 times/day
Oral, rectal: 14-40 kg: 100-200 mg 3-4 times/day

Adults:

Oral: 250 mg 3-4 times/day
I.M., rectal: 200 mg 3-4 times/day

**Mechanism of Action** Acts centrally to inhibit the medullary chemoreceptor trigger zone

**Local Anesthetic/Vasoconstrictor Precautions** No information available to require special precautions

**Effects on Dental Treatment** No effects or complications reported

**Other Adverse Effects**

>10%: Central nervous system: Drowsiness

1% to 10%:

Cardiovascular: Hypotension
Central nervous system: Dizziness, headache
Gastrointestinal: Diarrhea
Neuromuscular & skeletal: muscle cramps

<1%:

Central nervous system: Mental depression, convulsions, opisthotonus
Dermatologic: Hypersensitivity skin reactions
Hematologic: Blood dyscrasias
Hepatic: Hepatic impairment

**Drug Interactions** Antagonism of oral anticoagulants may occur

**Drug Uptake**

Onset of antiemetic effect:

Oral: Within 10-40 minutes

I.M.: Within 15-35 minutes

Duration: 3-4 hours

Absorption: Rectal: ~60%

**Pregnancy Risk Factor** C

**Generic Available** No

## Trimethoprim (trye METH oh prim)

**U.S. Brand Names** Proloprim®; Trimpex®

**Therapeutic Category** Antibiotic, Miscellaneous

**Use** Treatment of urinary tract infections; acute otitis media in children; acute exacerbations of chronic bronchitis in adults; in combination with other agents for treatment of toxoplasmosis, *Pneumocystis carinii*

**Usual Dosage** Oral:

Children: 4 mg/kg/day in divided doses every 12 hours

Adults: 100 mg every 12 hours or 200 mg every 24 hours

**Mechanism of Action** Inhibits folic acid reduction to tetrahydrofolate, and thereby inhibits microbial growth

**Local Anesthetic/Vasoconstrictor Precautions** No information available to require special precautions

**Effects on Dental Treatment** No effects or complications reported

**Other Adverse Effects**

>10%: Dermatologic: Rash, pruritus

1% to 10%: Hematologic: Megaloblastic anemia

<1%:

Central nervous system: Fever

Dermatologic: Exfoliative dermatitis

Gastrointestinal: Nausea, vomiting, epigastric distress

Hepatic: Cholestatic jaundice, elevated LFTs

Hematologic: Thrombocytopenia, neutropenia, leukopenia

Renal: Elevated BUN and serum creatinine

**Drug Interactions** Increased effect/toxicity/levels of phenytoin

**Drug Uptake**

Absorption: Oral: Readily and extensive

Serum half-life: 8-14 hours, prolonged with renal impairment

Time to peak serum concentration: Within 1-4 hours

**Pregnancy Risk Factor** C

**Generic Available** Yes

## Trimethoprim and Polymyxin B

(trye METH oh prim & pol i MIKS in bee)

**U.S. Brand Names** Polytrim® Ophthalmic

**Therapeutic Category** Antibiotic, Ophthalmic

**Synonyms** Polymyxin B and Trimethoprim

**Use** Treatment of surface ocular bacterial conjunctivitis and blepharoconjunctivitis

**Usual Dosage** Instill 1-2 drops in eye(s) every 4-6 hours

**Local Anesthetic/Vasoconstrictor Precautions** No information available to require special precautions

**Effects on Dental Treatment** No effects or complications reported

**Other Adverse Effects** 1% to 10%: Local: Burning, stinging, itching, increased redness

**Generic Available** No

## Trimethoprim and Sulfamethoxazole

(trye METH oh prim & sul fa meth OKS a zole)

**Related Information**

Animal and Human Bites Guidelines *on page 1164*

**U.S. Brand Names** Bactrim™; Bactrim™ DS; Cotrim®; Cotrim® DS; Septra®; Septra® DS; Sulfamethoprim®; Sulfatrim®; Sulfatrim® DS; Sulfoxaprim®; Sulfoxaprim® DS; Trisulfam®; Uroplus® DS; Uroplus® SS

**Canadian Brand Names** Apo®-Sulfatrim; Novo-Trimel; Nu-Cotrimox; Pro-Trin®; Roubac®; Trisulfa®; Trisulfa-S®

**Therapeutic Category** Antibiotic, Sulfonamide Derivative

**Synonyms** Co-trimoxazole; SMZ-TMP; Sulfamethoxazole and Trimethoprim; TMP-SMZ

(Continued)

## Trimethoprim and Sulfamethoxazole *(Continued)*

**Use**

Oral treatment of urinary tract infections; acute otitis media in children; acute exacerbations of chronic bronchitis in adults; prophylaxis of *Pneumocystis carinii* pneumonitis (PCP)

I.V. treatment of documented PCP, empiric treatment of PCP in immune compromised patients; treatment of documented or suspected shigellosis, typhoid fever, *Nocardia asteroides* infection, or other infections caused by susceptible bacterial

**Usual Dosage** Dosage recommendations are based on the trimethoprim component

Children >2 months:
- Mild to moderate infections: Oral, I.V.: 8 mg TMP/kg/day in divided doses every 12 hours
- Serious infection/*Pneumocystis*: I.V.: 20 mg TMP/kg/day in divided doses every 6 hours
- Urinary tract infection prophylaxis: Oral: 2 mg TMP/kg/dose daily
- Prophylaxis of *Pneumocystis*: Oral, I.V.: 10 mg TMP/kg/day or 150 mg TMP/$m^2$/day in divided doses every 12 hours for 3 days/week; dose should not exceed 320 mg trimethoprim and 1600 mg sulfamethoxazole 3 days/week

Adults:
- Urinary tract infection/chronic bronchitis: Oral: 1 double strength tablet every 12 hours for 10-14 days
- Sepsis: I.V.: 20 TMP/kg/day divided every 6 hours
- *Pneumocystis carinii*:
  - Prophylaxis: Oral, I.V.: 10 mg TMP/kg/day divided every 12 hours for 3 days/week
  - Treatment: I.V.: 20 mg TMP/kg/day divided every 6 hours

**Mechanism of Action** Sulfamethoxazole interferes with bacterial folic acid synthesis and growth via inhibition of dihydrofolic acid formation from para-aminobenzoic acid; trimethoprim inhibits dihydrofolic acid reduction to tetrahydrofolate resulting in sequential inhibition of enzymes of the folic acid pathway

**Local Anesthetic/Vasoconstrictor Precautions** No information available to require special precautions

**Effects on Dental Treatment** No effects or complications reported

**Other Adverse Effects**

>10%:
- Dermatologic: Allergic skin reactions including rashes and urticaria, photosensitivity
- Gastrointestinal: Nausea, vomiting, anorexia

1% to 10%:
- Dermatologic: Stevens-Johnson syndrome, toxic epidermal necrolysis
- Hematologic: Blood dyscrasias
- Hepatic: Hepatitis

<1%:
- Central nervous system: Confusion, depression, hallucinations, seizures, fever, ataxia, kernicterus in neonates
- Dermatologic: Erythema multiforme
- Gastrointestinal: Stomatitis, diarrhea, pseudomembranous colitis
- Hematologic: Thrombocytopenia, megaloblastic anemia, granulocytopenia, aplastic anemia, hemolysis (with G-6-PD deficiency)
- Renal: Interstitial nephritis
- Miscellaneous: Serum sickness

**Drug Interactions** Co-trimoxazole causes:
- Decreased effect: Cyclosporines
- Increased effect: Sulfonylureas and oral anticoagulants
- Increased toxicity: Phenytoin, cyclosporines (nephrotoxicity), methotrexate (displaced from binding sites)

**Drug Uptake**
- Absorption: Oral: 90% to 100%
- Serum half-life:
  - SMX: 9 hours
  - TMP: 6-17 hours, both are prolonged in renal failure
- Time to peak serum concentration: Within 1-4 hours

**Pregnancy Risk Factor** C

**Dosage Forms** The 5:1 ratio (SMX to TMP) remains constant in all dosage forms:
- Injection: Sulfamethoxazole 80 mg and trimethoprim 16 mg per mL (5 mL, 10 mL, 20 mL, 30 mL, 50 mL)
- Suspension, oral: Sulfamethoxazole 200 mg and trimethoprim 40 mg per 5 mL (20 mL, 100 mL, 150 mL, 200 mL, 480 mL)

Tablet: Sulfamethoxazole 400 mg and trimethoprim 80 mg
Tablet, double strength: Sulfamethoxazole 800 mg and trimethoprim 160 mg

**Generic Available** Yes

## Trimetrexate Glucuronate (tri me TREKS ate gloo KYOOR oh nate)

**U.S. Brand Names** Neutrexin®

**Therapeutic Category** Antibiotic, Miscellaneous

**Use** Alternative therapy for the treatment of moderate-to-severe *Pneumocystis carinii* pneumonia (PCP) in immunocompromised patients, including patients with acquired immunodeficiency syndrome (AIDS), who are intolerant of, or are refractory to, co-trimoxazole therapy or for whom co-trimoxazole and pentamidine are contraindicated (concurrent folinic acid (leucovorin) must always be administered)

**Usual Dosage** Adults: I.V.: 45 mg/m$^2$ once daily over 60 minutes for 21 days; it is necessary to reduce the dose in patients with liver dysfunction, although no specific recommendations exist

**Mechanism of Action** Exerts an antimicrobial effect through potent inhibition of the enzyme dihydrofolate reductase (DHFR)

**Local Anesthetic/Vasoconstrictor Precautions** No information available to require special precautions

**Effects on Dental Treatment** No effects or complications reported

**Other Adverse Effects** 1% to 10%:
- Central nervous system: Seizures, fever
- Dermatologic: Rash
- Gastrointestinal: Stomatitis, nausea, vomiting
- Hematologic: Neutropenia, thrombocytopenia, anemia
- Hepatic: Elevated liver function tests
- Neuromuscular & skeletal: Peripheral neuropathy
- Renal: Elevated serum creatinine
- Miscellaneous: Flu-like illness, hypersensitivity reactions

**Drug Interactions**
- Decreased effect of pneumococcal vaccine
- Increased toxicity (infection rates) of yellow fever vaccine

**Drug Uptake** Serum half-life: 15-17 hours

**Pregnancy Risk Factor** D

**Generic Available** No

## Trimipramine (trye MI pra meen)

**U.S. Brand Names** Surmontil®

**Canadian Brand Names** Apo®-Trimip; Novo-Tripramine; Nu-Trimipramine; Rhotrimine®

**Therapeutic Category** Antidepressant, Tricyclic

**Use** Treatment of various forms of depression, often in conjunction with psychotherapy

**Usual Dosage** Adults: Oral: 50-150 mg/day as a single bedtime dose up to a maximum of 200 mg/day outpatient and 300 mg/day inpatient

**Mechanism of Action** Increases the synaptic concentration of serotonin and/or norepinephrine in the central nervous system by inhibition of their reuptake by the presynaptic neuronal membrane

**Local Anesthetic/Vasoconstrictor Precautions** Use with caution; epinephrine, norepinephrine and levonordefrin have been shown to have an increased pressor response in combination with TCAs

**Effects on Dental Treatment** >10% of patients experience dry mouth; long-term treatment with TCAs such as trimipramine increases the risk of caries by reducing salivation and salivary buffer capacity

**Other Adverse Effects**

>10%:
- Central nervous system: Dizziness, drowsiness, headache
- Gastrointestinal: Constipation, increased appetite, nausea, unpleasant taste, weight gain
- Neuromuscular & skeletal: Weakness

1% to 10%:
- Cardiovascular: Arrhythmias, hypotension
- Central nervous system: Confusion, delirium, hallucinations, nervousness, restlessness, parkinsonian syndrome, insomnia
- Endocrine & metabolic: Sexual dysfunction
- Gastrointestinal: Diarrhea, heartburn
- Genitourinary: Dysuria
- Neuromuscular & skeletal: Fine muscle tremors
- Ocular: Blurred vision, eye pain
- Miscellaneous: Excessive sweating

(Continued)

## Trimipramine *(Continued)*

<1%:

Central nervous system: Anxiety, seizures
Dermatologic: Alopecia, photosensitivity
Endocrine & metabolic: Breast enlargement, galactorrhea, SIADH
Gastrointestinal: Trouble with gums, decreased lower esophageal sphincter tone may cause GE reflux
Genitourinary: Testicular swelling
Hematologic: Agranulocytosis, leukopenia, eosinophilia
Hepatic: Cholestatic jaundice, elevated liver enzymes
Ocular: Increased intraocular pressure
Otic: Tinnitus
Miscellaneous: Allergic reactions

**Drug Interactions**

Decreased effect of guanethidine, clonidine; decreased effect with barbiturates, carbamazepine, phenytoin

Increased effect/toxicity with MAO inhibitors (hyperpyretic crises), CNS depressants, alcohol (CNS depression), methylphenidate (increased levels), cimetidine (decreased clearance), anticholinergics

**Drug Uptake**

Therapeutic plasma levels: Oral: Occurs within 6 hours
Serum half-life: 20-26 hours

**Pregnancy Risk Factor** C

**Generic Available** Yes

- **Trimox®** *see* Amoxicillin *on page 76*
- **Trimpex®** *see* Trimethoprim *on page 1021*
- **Trinalin®** *see* Azatadine and Pseudoephedrine *on page 112*
- **Tri-Nefrin® Extra Strength Tablet [OTC]** *see* Chlorpheniramine and Phenylpropanolamine *on page 233*
- **Tri-Norinyl®** *see* Ethinyl Estradiol and Norethindrone *on page 404*
- **Triofed® Syrup [OTC]** *see* Triprolidine and Pseudoephedrine *on next page*
- **Triostat™** *see* Liothyronine *on page 592*
- **Triotann® Tablet** *see* Chlorpheniramine, Pyrilamine, and Phenylephrine *on page 238*

## Trioxsalen (trye OKS a len)

**U.S. Brand Names** Trisoralen®

**Therapeutic Category** Psoralen

**Use** In conjunction with controlled exposure to ultraviolet light or sunlight for repigmentation of idiopathic vitiligo; increasing tolerance to sunlight with albinism; enhance pigmentation

**Usual Dosage** Children >12 years and Adults: Oral: 10 mg/day as a single dose, 2-4 hours before controlled exposure to UVA (for 15-35 minutes) or sunlight; do not continue for longer than 14 days

**Mechanism of Action** Psoralens are thought to form covalent bonds with pyrimidine bases in DNA which inhibit the synthesis of DNA. This reaction involves excitation of the trioxsalen molecule by radiation in the long-wave ultraviolet light (UVA) resulting in transference of energy to the trioxsalen molecule producing an excited state. Binding of trioxsalen to DNA occurs only in the presence of ultraviolet light. The increase in skin pigmentation produced by trioxsalen and UVA radiation involves multiple changes in melanocytes and interaction between melanocytes and keratinocytes. In general, melanogenesis is stimulated but the size and distribution of melanocytes is unchanged.

**Local Anesthetic/Vasoconstrictor Precautions** No information available to require special precautions

**Effects on Dental Treatment** No effects or complications reported

**Other Adverse Effects**

>10%:

Dermatologic: Itching
Gastrointestinal: Nausea

1% to 10%:

Central nervous system: Dizziness, headache, mental depression, insomnia, nervousness
Dermatologic: Severe burns from excessive sunlight or ultraviolet exposure
Gastrointestinal: Gastric discomfort

**Drug Interactions** No data reported

**Drug Uptake**

Peak photosensitivity: 2 hours
Duration: Skin sensitivity to light remains for 8-12 hours
Absorption: Rapid

Serum half-life, elimination: ~2 hours

**Pregnancy Risk Factor** C

**Generic Available** No

## Tripelennamine (tri pel EN a meen)

**U.S. Brand Names** PBZ®; PBZ-SR®

**Therapeutic Category** Antihistamine

**Use** Perennial and seasonal allergic rhinitis and other allergic symptoms including urticaria

**Usual Dosage** Oral:

Children: 5 mg/kg/day in 4-6 divided doses, up to 300 mg/day maximum

Adults: 25-50 mg every 4-6 hours, extended release tablets 100 mg morning and evening up to 100 mg every 8 hours

**Mechanism of Action** Competes with histamine for $H_1$-receptor sites on effector cells in the gastrointestinal tract, blood vessels, and respiratory tract

**Local Anesthetic/Vasoconstrictor Precautions** No information available to require special precautions

**Effects on Dental Treatment** Chronic use of antihistamines will inhibit salivary flow, particularly in elderly patients; this may contribute to periodontal disease and oral discomfort

**Other Adverse Effects**

>10%:

- Central nervous system: Slight to moderate drowsiness
- Respiratory: Thickening of bronchial secretions

1% to 10%:

- Central nervous system: Headache, fatigue, nervousness, dizziness
- Gastrointestinal: Appetite increase, weight gain, nausea, diarrhea, abdominal pain, dry mouth
- Neuromuscular & skeletal: Arthralgia
- Respiratory: Pharyngitis

<1%:

- Cardiovascular: Edema, palpitations, hypotension
- Central nervous system: Depression, sedation, paradoxical excitement, insomnia
- Dermatologic: Angioedema, photosensitivity, rash
- Genitourinary: Urinary retention
- Hepatic: Hepatitis
- Neuromuscular & skeletal: Myalgia, paresthesia, tremor
- Ocular: Blurred vision
- Respiratory: Bronchospasm, epistaxis

**Drug Interactions** Increased effect/toxicity with alcohol, CNS depressants, MAO inhibitors

**Drug Uptake**

Onset of antihistaminic effect: Within 15-30 minutes

Duration: 4-6 hours (up to 8 hours with PBZ-SR®)

**Pregnancy Risk Factor** B

**Generic Available** Yes


- ♦ **Triphasil®** *see* Ethinyl Estradiol and Levonorgestrel *on page 402*
- ♦ **Tri-Phen-Chlor®** *see* Chlorpheniramine, Phenyltoloxamine, Phenylpropanolamine, and Phenylephrine *on page 237*
- ♦ **Triphenyl® Expectorant [OTC]** *see* Guaifenesin and Phenylpropanolamine *on page 480*
- ♦ **Triphenyl® Syrup [OTC]** *see* Chlorpheniramine and Phenylpropanolamine *on page 233*
- ♦ **Triple Antibiotic® Topical** *see* Bacitracin, Neomycin, and Polymyxin B *on page 118*
- ♦ **Triple X® Liquid [OTC]** *see* Pyrethrins *on page 867*
- ♦ **Triposed® Syrup [OTC]** *see* Triprolidine and Pseudoephedrine *on this page*
- ♦ **Triposed® Tablet [OTC]** *see* Triprolidine and Pseudoephedrine *on this page*


## Triprolidine and Pseudoephedrine

(trye PROE li deen & soo doe e FED rin)

**U.S. Brand Names** Actagen® Syrup [OTC]; Actagen® Tablet [OTC]; Allercon® Tablet [OTC]; Allerfrin® Syrup [OTC]; Allerfrin® Tablet [OTC]; Allerphed® Syrup [OTC]; Aprodine® Syrup [OTC]; Aprodine® Tablet [OTC]; Cenafed® Plus Tablet [OTC]; Genac® Tablet [OTC]; Silafed® Syrup [OTC]; Triofed® Syrup [OTC]; Triposed® Syrup [OTC]; Triposed® Tablet [OTC]

**Therapeutic Category** Antihistamine/Decongestant Combination

**Use** Temporary relief of nasal congestion, decongest sinus openings, running nose, sneezing, itching of nose or throat and itchy, watery eyes due to common cold, hay fever, or other upper respiratory allergies

(Continued)

## Triprolidine and Pseudoephedrine *(Continued)*

**Usual Dosage** Oral:

Children:

Syrup:

4 months to 2 years: 1.25 mL 3-4 times/day

2-4 years: 2.5 mL 3-4 times/day

4-6 years: 3.75 mL 3-4 times/day

6-12 years: 5 mL every 4-6 hours; do not exceed 4 doses in 24 hours

Tablet: ½ every 4-6 hours; do not exceed 4 doses in 24 hours

Children >12 years and Adults:

Syrup: 10 mL every 4-6 hours; do not exceed 4 doses in 24 hours

Tablet: 1 every 4-6 hours; do not exceed 4 doses in 24 hours

**Mechanism of Action** Refer to Pseudoephedrine monograph

Triprolidine is a member of the propylamine (alkylamine) chemical class of $H_1$-antagonist antihistamines. As such, it is considered to be relatively less sedating than traditional antihistamines of the ethanolamine, phenothiazine, and ethylenediamine classes of antihistamines. Triprolidine has a shorter half-life and duration of action than most of the other alkylamine antihistamines. Like all $H_1$-antagonist antihistamines, the mechanism of action of triprolidine is believed to involve competitive blockade of $H_1$-receptor sites resulting in the inability of histamine to combine with its receptor sites and exert its usual effects on target cells. Antihistamines do not interrupt any effects of histamine which have already occurred. Therefore, these agents are used more successfully in the prevention rather than the treatment of histamine-induced reactions.

**Local Anesthetic/Vasoconstrictor Precautions** Use with caution since pseudoephedrine is a sympathomimetic amine which could interact with epinephrine to cause a pressor response

**Effects on Dental Treatment** Chronic use of antihistamines will inhibit salivary flow, particularly in elderly patients; this may contribute to periodontal disease and oral discomfort

**Other Adverse Effects**

>10%:

Cardiovascular: Tachycardia

Central nervous system: Slight to moderate drowsiness, nervousness, insomnia, transient stimulation

Respiratory: Thickening of bronchial secretions

1% to 10%:

Central nervous system: Headache, fatigue, dizziness

Gastrointestinal: Appetite increase, weight gain, nausea, diarrhea, abdominal pain, dry mouth

Genitourinary: Dysuria

Neuromuscular & skeletal: Arthralgia, weakness

Respiratory: Pharyngitis

Miscellaneous: Sweating

<1%:

Central nervous system: Depression, hallucinations, convulsions, paradoxical excitement, sedation

Cardiovascular: Edema, palpitations, hypotension

Dermatologic: Angioedema, rash, photosensitivity

Genitourinary: Urinary retention

Hepatic: Hepatitis

Neuromuscular & skeletal: Myalgia, paresthesia, tremor

Ocular: Blurred vision

Respiratory: Bronchospasm, dyspnea, epistaxis

**Drug Interactions**

Decreased effect of guanethidine, reserpine, methyldopa

Increased toxicity with MAO inhibitors (hypertensive crisis), sympathomimetics, CNS depressants, alcohol (sedation)

**Pregnancy Risk Factor** C

**Generic Available** Yes

## Triprolidine, Pseudoephedrine, and Codeine

(trye PROE li deen, soo doe e FED rin, & KOE deen)

**U.S. Brand Names** Actagen-C®; Actifed® With Codeine; Allerfrin® w/Codeine; Aprodine® w/C; Triacin-C®; Trifed-C®

**Therapeutic Category** Antihistamine/Decongestant Combination; Cough Preparation

**Use** Symptomatic relief of cough

**Usual Dosage** Oral:

Children:

2-6 years: 2.5 mL 4 times/day

7-12 years: 5 mL 4 times/day
Children >12 years and Adults: 10 mL 4 times/day

**Local Anesthetic/Vasoconstrictor Precautions** Use with caution since pseudoephedrine is a sympathomimetic amine which could interact with epinephrine to cause a pressor response

**Effects on Dental Treatment** Up to 10% of patients could experience tachycardia, palpitations, and dry mouth; use vasoconstrictor with caution

**Pregnancy Risk Factor** C

**Generic Available** Yes


- ♦ **TripTone® Caplets® [OTC]** *see* Dimenhydrinate *on page 335*
- ♦ **Tris Buffer** *see* Tromethamine *on page 1029*
- ♦ **Tris(hydroxymethyl)aminomethane** *see* Tromethamine *on page 1029*
- ♦ **Trisoralen®** *see* Trioxsalen *on page 1024*
- ♦ **Tri-Statin® II Topical** *see* Nystatin and Triamcinolone *on page 735*
- ♦ **Tristoject®** *see* Triamcinolone *on page 1010*
- ♦ **Trisulfam®** *see* Trimethoprim and Sulfamethoxazole *on page 1021*
- ♦ **Trisulfapyrimidines** *see* Sulfadiazine, Sulfamethazine, and Sulfamerazine *on page 942*
- ♦ **Tri-Tannate® Plus** *see* Chlorpheniramine, Ephedrine, Phenylephrine, and Carbetapentane *on page 233*
- ♦ **Tri-Tannate® Tablet** *see* Chlorpheniramine, Pyrilamine, and Phenylephrine *on page 238*
- ♦ **Tritec®** *see* Ranitidine Bismuth Citrate *on page 878*
- ♦ **Tri-Vi-Flor®** *see* Vitamins, Multiple *on page 1051*
- ♦ **Trobicin®** *see* Spectinomycin *on page 930*
- ♦ **Trocaine® [OTC]** *see* Benzocaine *on page 128*
- ♦ **Trocal® [OTC]** *see* Dextromethorphan *on page 314*


## Troglitazone (TROE gli to zone)

**U.S. Brand Names** Rezulin®

**Therapeutic Category** Antidiabetic Agent; Hypoglycemic Agent, Oral

**Use** Use in patients with type II diabetes currently on insulin therapy whose hyperglycemia is not controlled ($HbA_{1c}$ >8.5%) despite insulin therapy of over 30 units/day given as multiple infections

**Usual Dosage** Oral (take with meals):

Adults:

Continue the current insulin dose upon initiation of troglitazone therapy.

Initiate therapy at 200 mg once daily in patients on insulin therapy. For patients not responding adequately, increase the dose after 2-4 weeks. The usual dose is 400 mg/day; maximum recommended dose: 600 mg/day.

It is recommended that the insulin dose be decreased by 10% to 25% when fasting plasma glucose concentrations decrease to <120 mg/dL in patients receiving concomitant insulin and troglitazone. Individualize further adjustments based on glucose-lowering response.

Elderly: Steady-state pharmacokinetics of troglitazone and metabolites in healthy elderly subjects were comparable to those seen in young adults

**Mechanism of Action** Thiazolidinedione antidiabetic agent that lowers blood glucose by improving target cell response to insulin, without increasing pancreatic insulin secretion. It has a unique mechanism of action that is dependent on the presence of insulin for activity. Troglitazone decreases hepatic glucose output and increases insulin-dependent glucose disposal in skeletal muscle and possible liver and adipose tissue.

**Local Anesthetic/Vasoconstrictor Precautions** No information available to require special precautions

**Effects on Dental Treatment** Troglitazone-dependent diabetics should be appointed for dental treatment in morning in order to minimize chance of stress-induced hypoglycemia

**Other Adverse Effects**

>10%:

Central nervous system: Headache, pain
Miscellaneous: Infection

1% to 10%:

Cardiovascular: Peripheral edema
Central nervous system: Dizziness
Gastrointestinal: Nausea, diarrhea, pharyngitis
Genitourinary: Urinary tract infection
Neuromuscular & skeletal: Neck pain, weakness
Respiratory: Rhinitis

**Warnings/Precautions** Patients with New York Heart Association (NYHA) Class III and IV cardiac status were not studied during clinical trials. Heart enlargement

(Continued)

## Troglitazone *(Continued)*

without microscopic changes has been observed in rodents at exposures exceeding 14 times the AUC of the 400 mg human dose. Caution is advised during the administration of troglitazone to patients with NYHA Class III or IV cardiac status.

During all clinical studies, a total of 20 troglitazone-treated patients were withdrawn from treatment because of liver function test abnormalities. Two of the 20 patients developed reversible jaundice. Both had liver biopsies that were consistent with an idiosyncratic drug reaction.

Because of its mechanism of action, troglitazone is active only in the presence of insulin. Therefore, do not use in type I diabetes or for the treatment of diabetic ketoacidosis.

Patients receiving troglitazone in combination with insulin may be at risk for hypoglycemia, and a reduction in the dose of insulin may be necessary. Hypoglycemia has not been observed during the administration of troglitazone as monotherapy and would not be expected based on the mechanism of action.

Across all clinical studies, hemoglobin declined by 3% to 4% in troglitazone-treated patients compared with 1% to 2% with placebo. White blood cell counts also declined slightly in troglitazone-treated patients compared with those treated with placebo. These changes occurred within the first 4-8 weeks of therapy. Levels stabilized and remained unchanged for ≤ 2 years of continuing therapy. These changes may be due to the dilutional effects of increased plasma volume and have not been associated with any significant hematologic clinical effects.

**Drug Interactions** Cytochrome P-450 3A4 Enzyme Inducer

Decreased effects:

- Cholestyramine: Concomitant administration of cholestyramine with troglitazone reduces the absorption of troglitazone by 70%; COADMINISTRATION OF CHOLESTYRAMINE AND TROGLITAZONE IS NOT RECOMMENDED.
- Oral contraceptives: Administration of troglitazone with an oral contraceptive containing ethinyl estradiol and norethindrone reduced the plasma concentrations of both by 30%. These changes could result in loss of contraception.

Increased toxicity: Sulfonylureas (glyburide): Coadministration of troglitazone with glyburide may further decrease plasma glucose levels

**Drug Uptake**

Half-life, plasma elimination: 16-34 hours

Time to peak plasma concentrations: 2-3 hours

**Pregnancy Risk Factor** B

**Dosage Forms** Tablet: 200 mg, 400 mg

**Dietary Considerations** Food increases absorption by 30% to 85%

**Generic Available** No

## Troleandomycin (troe lee an doe MYE sin)

**U.S. Brand Names** Tao®

**Therapeutic Category** Antibiotic, Macrolide

**Use** Adjunct in the treatment of corticosteroid-dependent asthma due to its steroid-sparing properties; antibiotic with spectrum of activity similar to erythromycin

**Usual Dosage** Oral:

Children 7-13 years: 25-40 mg/kg/day divided every 6 hours (125-250 mg every 6 hours)

- Adjunct in corticosteroid-dependent asthma: 14 mg/kg/day in divided doses every 6-12 hours not to exceed 250 mg every 6 hours; dose is tapered to once daily then alternate day dosing

Children >13 years and adults: 250-500 mg 4 times/day

**Mechanism of Action** Decreases methylprednisolone clearance from a linear first order decline to a nonlinear decline in plasma concentration. Tao® also has an undefined action independent of its effects on steroid elimination. Inhibits RNA-dependent protein synthesis at the chain elongation step; binds to the 50S ribosomal subunit resulting in blockage of transpeptidation.

**Local Anesthetic/Vasoconstrictor Precautions** No information available to require special precautions

**Effects on Dental Treatment** No effects or complications reported

**Other Adverse Effects**

>10%: Gastrointestinal: Abdominal cramping and discomfort

1% to 10%:

- Dermatologic: Urticaria, skin rashes
- Gastrointestinal: Nausea, vomiting, diarrhea

<1%:

- Dermatologic: Rectal burning
- Hepatic: Cholestatic jaundice

**Drug Interactions** Increased effect/toxicity/levels of astemizole, carbamazepine, ergot alkaloids, methylprednisolone, terfenadine, theophylline, and triazolam

**Drug Uptake**

Time to peak serum concentration: Within 2 hours

**Pregnancy Risk Factor** C

**Generic Available** No

## Tromethamine (troe METH a meen)

**U.S. Brand Names** THAM-E® Injection; THAM® Injection

**Therapeutic Category** Alkalinizing Agent, Parenteral

**Synonyms** Tris Buffer; Tris(hydroxymethyl)aminomethane

**Use** Correction of metabolic acidosis associated with cardiac bypass surgery or cardiac arrest; to correct excess acidity of stored blood that is preserved with acid citrate dextrose (ACD); to prime the pump-oxygenator during cardiac bypass surgery; indicated in severe metabolic acidosis in patients in whom sodium or carbon dioxide elimination is restricted [eg, infants needing alkalinization after receiving maximum sodium bicarbonate (8-10 mEq/kg/24 hours)]

**Usual Dosage** Dose depends on buffer base deficit; when deficit is known: tromethamine (mL of 0.3 M solution) = body weight (kg) x base deficit (mEq/L); when base deficit is not known: 3-6 mL/kg/dose I.V. (1-2 mEq/kg/dose)

Metabolic acidosis with cardiac arrest:

- I.V.: 3.5-6 mL/kg (1-2 mEq/kg/dose) into large peripheral vein; 500-1000 mL if needed in adults
- I.V. continuous drip: Infuse slowly by syringe pump over 3-6 hours

Excess acidity of acid citrate dextrose priming blood: 14-70 mL of 0.3 molar solution added to each 500 mL of blood

**Mechanism of Action** Acts as a proton acceptor, which combines with hydrogen ions to form bicarbonate buffer, to correct acidosis

**Local Anesthetic/Vasoconstrictor Precautions** No information available to require special precautions

**Effects on Dental Treatment** No effects or complications reported

**Other Adverse Effects**

1% to 10%:

- Cardiovascular: Venospasm
- Local: Tissue irritation, necrosis with extravasation

<1%:

- Endocrine & metabolic: Hyperkalemia, hypoglycemia, hyperosmolality of serum
- Hematologic: Increased blood coagulation time
- Hepatic: Liver cell destruction from direct contact with THAM®
- Respiratory: Apnea, respiratory depression

**Drug Uptake**

Absorption: 30% of dose is not ionized

**Pregnancy Risk Factor** C

**Generic Available** No

**Comments** 1 mM = 120 mg = 3.3 mL = 1 mEq of THAM®

- ♦ **Tronolane® [OTC]** *see* Pramoxine *on page 828*
- ♦ **Tropicacyl®** *see* Tropicamide *on this page*

## Tropicamide (troe PIK a mide)

**U.S. Brand Names** Mydriacyl®; Opticyl®; Tropicacyl®

**Therapeutic Category** Ophthalmic Agent, Mydriatic

**Synonyms** Bistropamide

**Use** Short-acting mydriatic used in diagnostic procedures; as well as preoperatively and postoperatively; treatment of some cases of acute iritis, iridocyclitis, and keratitis

**Usual Dosage** Children and Adults (individuals with heavily pigmented eyes may require larger doses):

Cycloplegia: Instill 1-2 drops (1%); may repeat in 5 minutes

Exam must be performed within 30 minutes after the repeat dose; if the patient is not examined within 20-30 minutes, instill an additional drop

Mydriasis: Instill 1-2 drops (0.5%) 15-20 minutes before exam; may repeat every 30 minutes as needed

**Mechanism of Action** Prevents the sphincter muscle of the iris and the muscle of the ciliary body from responding to cholinergic stimulation

**Local Anesthetic/Vasoconstrictor Precautions** No information available to require special precautions

**Effects on Dental Treatment** No effects or complications reported

(Continued)

## Tropicamide *(Continued)*

**Other Adverse Effects** 1% to 10%:

Cardiovascular: Tachycardia, vascular congestion, edema, parasympathetic stimulations

Central nervous system: Drowsiness, headache

Dermatologic: Eczematoid dermatitis

Gastrointestinal: Dryness of the mouth

Local: Transient stinging

Ocular: Blurred vision, photophobia with or without corneal staining, increased intraocular pressure, follicular conjunctivitis

**Drug Uptake**

Onset of mydriasis: ~20-40 minutes

Duration: ~6-7 hours

Onset of cycloplegia: Within 30 minutes

Duration: <6 hours

**Pregnancy Risk Factor** C

**Generic Available** Yes

## Trovafloxacin/Alatrofloxacin

**U.S. Brand Names** Trovan™

**Therapeutic Category** Antibiotic, Quinolone

**Synonyms** CP-99,219-27

**Use** Treatment of pneumonia, bronchitis, meningitis, uncomplicated urinary tract, and skin and soft tissue infections

**Usual Dosage** Adults:

Oral: 100-200 mg/day; total duration of therapy and dose depend on indication

I.V. (alatrofloxacin): 300 mg followed by 200 mg/day

**Mechanism of Action** Trovafloxacin is a unique fluoroquinolone antibiotic with *in vitro* activity against atypical, Gram-negative, Gram-positive including penicillin-resistant pneumococci, intracellular and anaerobic pathogens. It is a fluoroquinolone with a 2-4-difluorophenyl substituent at the N-1 position and a fused pyrolidine substituent at the 7 position.

**Local Anesthetic/Vasoconstrictor Precautions** No information available to require special precautions

**Effects on Dental Treatment** No effects or complications reported

**Other Adverse Effects** The most frequent adverse effect is mild dizziness in about 10% of patients; other symptoms include nausea, headache, vomiting, vaginitis, and diarrhea

**Drug Interactions**

Decreased trovafloxacin absorption: Sucralfate, ferrous sulfate, antacids, omeprazole

No effect by trovafloxacin: Theophylline, warfarin, digoxin

**Drug Uptake**

Protein binding: ~70%

Serum half-life: ~10 hours

Peak plasma concentration: 0.3-10.1 mg/L

Time to peak plasma concentration: 1-3 hours

**Pregnancy Risk Factor** C

**Dosage Forms**

Injection, as mesylate (alatrofloxacin): 5 mg/mL (40 mL, 60 mL)

Tablet, as mesylate (trovafloxacin): 100 mg, 200 mg

**Comments** *In vitro* trovafloxacin was more active than sparfloxacin, ofloxacin, ciprofloxacin, ceftriaxone, erythromycin and vancomycin against *S. pneumoniae.* It was also more active against penicillin-resistant strains than ceftriaxone, erythromycin or vancomycin. Trovafloxacin is very effective in bronchitis and pneumonia. It has good activity against resistant organisms, and penetration of the cerebral spinal fluid giving potential in the treatment of central nervous system infections.

♦ **Trovan™** *see* Trovafloxacin/Alatrofloxacin *on this page*

♦ **Troxidone** *see* Trimethadione *on page 1019*

♦ **Truphylline®** *see* Aminophylline *on page 63*

♦ **Trusopt®** *see* Dorzolamide *on page 350*

## Trypsin, Balsam Peru, and Castor Oil

(TRIP sin, BAL sam pe RUE, & KAS tor oyl)

**U.S. Brand Names** Granulex

**Therapeutic Category** Enzyme, Topical Debridement; Protectant, Topical; Topical Skin Product

**Use** Treatment of decubitus ulcers, varicose ulcers, debridement of eschar, dehiscent wounds and sunburn

**Usual Dosage** Apply a minimum of twice daily or as often as necessary

**Local Anesthetic/Vasoconstrictor Precautions** No information available to require special precautions

**Effects on Dental Treatment** No effects or complications reported

**Generic Available** No

- **Trysul®** *see* Sulfabenzamide, Sulfacetamide, and Sulfathiazole *on page 939*
- **TSPA** *see* Thiotepa *on page 979*
- **TST** *see* Tuberculin Purified Protein Derivative *on this page*
- **T-Stat® Topical** *see* Erythromycin, Topical *on page 386*

## Tuberculin Purified Protein Derivative

(too BER kyoo lin PURE eh fide PRO teen dah RIV ah tiv)

**U.S. Brand Names** Aplisol®; Aplitest®; Tine Test PPD; Tubersol®

**Therapeutic Category** Diagnostic Agent, Skin Test

**Synonyms** Mantoux; PPD; Tine Test; TST; Tuberculin Skin Test

**Use** Skin test in diagnosis of tuberculosis, to aid in assessment of cell-mediated immunity; routine tuberculin testing is recommended at 12 months of age and at every 1-2 years thereafter, before the measles vaccination

**Usual Dosage** Children and Adults: Intradermal: 0.1 mL about 4" below elbow; use 1/4" to 1/2" or 26- or 27-gauge needle; significant reactions are ≥5 mm in diameter

Interpretation of induration of tuberculin skin test injections: Positive: ≥10 mm; inconclusive: 5-9 mm; negative: <5 mm

Interpretation of induration of Tine test injections: Positive: >2 mm and vesiculation present; inconclusive: <2 mm (give patient Mantoux test of 5 TU/0.1 mL - base decisions on results of Mantoux test); negative: <2 mm or erythema of any size (no need for retesting unless person is a contact of a patient with tuberculosis or there is clinical evidence suggestive of the disease)

**Mechanism of Action** Tuberculosis results in individuals becoming sensitized to certain antigenic components of the *M. tuberculosis* organism. Culture extracts called tuberculins are contained in tuberculin skin test preparations. Upon intracutaneous injection of these culture extracts, a classic delayed (cellular) hypersensitivity reaction occurs. This reaction is characteristic of a delayed course (peak occurs >24 hours after injection, induration of the skin secondary to cell infiltration, and occasional vesiculation and necrosis). Delayed hypersensitivity reactions to tuberculin may indicate infection with a variety of nontuberculosis mycobacteria, or vaccination with the live attenuated mycobacterial strain of *M. bovis* vaccine, BCG, in addition to previous natural infection with *M. tuberculosis.*

**Local Anesthetic/Vasoconstrictor Precautions** No information available to require special precautions

**Effects on Dental Treatment** No effects or complications reported

**Other Adverse Effects** 1% to 10%:

Central nervous system: Pain

Gastrointestinal: Ulceration

Dermatologic: Vesiculation

Miscellaneous: Necrosis

**Drug Uptake**

Onset of action: Delayed hypersensitivity reactions to tuberculin usually occur within 5-6 hours following injection

Peak effect: Become maximal at 48-72 hours

Duration: Reactions subside over a few days

**Pregnancy Risk Factor** C

**Generic Available** Yes

**Comments** Test dose: 0.1 mL intracutaneously; examine site at 48-72 hours after administration; whenever tuberculin is administered, a record should be made of the administration technique (Mantoux method, disposable multiple-puncture device), tuberculin used (OT or PPD), manufacturer and lot number of tuberculin used, date of administration, date of test reading, and the size of the reaction in millimeters (mm).

- **Tuberculin Skin Test** *see* Tuberculin Purified Protein Derivative *on this page*
- **Tubersol®** *see* Tuberculin Purified Protein Derivative *on this page*
- **Tuinal®** *see* Amobarbital and Secobarbital *on page 74*
- **Tums® [OTC]** *see* Calcium Carbonate *on page 172*
- **Tums® E-X Extra Strength Tablet [OTC]** *see* Calcium Carbonate *on page 172*
- **Tums® Extra Strength Liquid [OTC]** *see* Calcium Carbonate *on page 172*
- **Tusibron® [OTC]** *see* Guaifenesin *on page 478*
- **Tusibron-DM® [OTC]** *see* Guaifenesin and Dextromethorphan *on page 479*
- **Tussafed® Drops** *see* Carbinoxamine, Pseudoephedrine, and Dextromethorphan *on page 189*

- ♦ **Tussafin® Expectorant** *see* Hydrocodone, Pseudoephedrine, and Guaifenesin *on page 511*
- ♦ **Tuss-Allergine® Modified T.D. Capsule** *see* Caramiphen and Phenylpropanolamine *on page 184*
- ♦ **Tussar® SF Syrup** *see* Guaifenesin, Pseudoephedrine, and Codeine *on page 482*
- ♦ **Tuss-DM® [OTC]** *see* Guaifenesin and Dextromethorphan *on page 479*
- ♦ **Tussigon®** *see* Hydrocodone and Homatropine *on page 508*
- ♦ **Tussionex®** *see* Hydrocodone and Chlorpheniramine *on page 508*
- ♦ **Tussi-Organidin® DM NR** *see* Guaifenesin and Dextromethorphan *on page 479*
- ♦ **Tussi-Organidin® NR** *see* Guaifenesin and Codeine *on page 478*
- ♦ **Tuss-LA®** *see* Guaifenesin and Pseudoephedrine *on page 481*
- ♦ **Tussogest® Extended Release Capsule** *see* Caramiphen and Phenylpropanolamine *on page 184*
- ♦ **Tusstat® Syrup** *see* Diphenhydramine *on page 338*
- ♦ **Twice-A-Day® Nasal [OTC]** *see* Oxymetazoline *on page 755*
- ♦ **Twilite® Oral [OTC]** *see* Diphenhydramine *on page 338*
- ♦ **Twin-K®** *see* Potassium Citrate and Potassium Gluconate *on page 823*
- ♦ **Two-Dyne®** *see* Butalbital Compound *on page 163*
- ♦ **Two-Dyne®** *see* Butalbital Compound and Acetaminophen *on page 164*
- ♦ **Tylenol® [OTC]** *see* Acetaminophen *on page 27*
- ♦ **Tylenol® Cold Effervescent Medication Tablet [OTC]** *see* Chlorpheniramine, Phenylpropanolamine, and Acetaminophen *on page 236*
- ♦ **Tylenol® Cold No Drowsiness [OTC]** *see* Acetaminophen, Dextromethorphan, and Pseudoephedrine *on page 32*
- ♦ **Tylenol® Extended Relief [OTC]** *see* Acetaminophen *on page 27*
- ♦ **Tylenol® Flu Maximum Strength [OTC]** *see* Acetaminophen, Dextromethorphan, and Pseudoephedrine *on page 32*
- ♦ **Tylenol® Sinus, Maximum Strength [OTC]** *see* Acetaminophen and Pseudoephedrine *on page 31*
- ♦ **Tylenol® With Codeine** *see* Acetaminophen and Codeine *on page 28*
- ♦ **Tylox®** *see* Oxycodone and Acetaminophen *on page 751*
- ♦ **Typhim Vi®** *see* Typhoid Vaccine *on this page*


## Typhoid Vaccine (TYE foid vak SEEN)

**U.S. Brand Names** Typhim Vi®; Vivotif Berna™ Oral

**Therapeutic Category** Vaccine, Inactivated Bacteria

**Synonyms** Typhoid Vaccine Live Oral Ty21a

**Use** Promotes active immunity to typhoid fever for patients exposed to typhoid carrier or foreign travel to typhoid fever endemic area

**Usual Dosage**

S.C.:

Children 6 months to 10 years: 0.25 mL; repeat in ≥4 weeks (total immunization is 2 doses)

Children >10 years and Adults: 0.5 mL; repeat dose in ≥4 weeks (total immunization is 2 doses)

Booster: 0.25 mL every 3 years for children 6 months to 10 years and 0.5 mL every 3 years for children >10 years and adults

Oral: Adults:

Primary immunization: 1 capsule on alternate days (day 1, 3, 5, and 7)

Booster immunization: Repeat full course of primary immunization every 5 years

**Mechanism of Action** Virulent strains of *Salmonella typhi* cause disease by penetrating the intestinal mucosa and entering the systemic circulation via the lymphatic vasculature. One possible mechanism of conferring immunity may be the provocation of a local immune response in the intestinal tract induced by oral ingesting of a live strain with subsequent aborted infection. The ability of *Salmonella typhi* to produce clinical disease (and to elicit an immune response) is dependent on the bacteria having a complete lipopolysaccharide. The live attenuate Ty21a strain lacks the enzyme UDP-4-galactose epimerase so that lipopolysaccharide is only synthesized under conditions that induce bacterial autolysis. Thus, the strain remains avirulent despite the production of sufficient lipopolysaccharide to evoke a protective immune response. Despite low levels of lipopolysaccharide synthesis, cells lyse before gaining a virulent phenotype due to the intracellular accumulation of metabolic intermediates.

**Local Anesthetic/Vasoconstrictor Precautions** No information available to require special precautions

**Effects on Dental Treatment** No effects or complications reported

**Other Adverse Effects**
Oral:
1% to 10%:
Dermatologic: Skin rash
Gastrointestinal: Abdominal discomfort, stomach cramps, diarrhea, nausea, vomiting
<1%: Miscellaneous: Anaphylactic reaction
Injection: >10%:
Dermatologic: Erythema
Local: Tenderness, induration
Neuromuscular & skeletal: Myalgia

**Drug Uptake**
Oral:
Onset of immunity to *Salmonella typhi*: Within about 1 week
Duration: ~5 years
Parenteral: Duration of immunity: ~3 years

**Pregnancy Risk Factor** C

**Generic Available** Yes: Injection only

**Comments** Inactivated bacteria vaccine; federal law requires that the date of administration, the vaccine manufacturer, lot number of vaccine, and the administering person's name, title and address be entered into the patient's permanent medical record

- **Typhoid Vaccine Live Oral Ty21a** *see* Typhoid Vaccine *on previous page*
- **Tyzine® Nasal** *see* Tetrahydrozoline *on page 967*
- **U-90152S** *see* Delavirdine *on page 302*
- **UAD Otic®** *see* Neomycin, Polymyxin B, and Hydrocortisone *on page 712*
- **UCB-P071** *see* Cetirizine *on page 218*
- **ULR-LA®** *see* Guaifenesin and Phenylpropanolamine *on page 480*
- **Ultiva™** *see* Remifentanil *on page 880*
- **Ultram®** *see* Tramadol *on page 1002*
- **Ultra Mide®** *see* Urea *on next page*
- **Ultrase® MT12** *see* Pancrelipase *on page 763*
- **Ultrase® MT20** *see* Pancrelipase *on page 763*
- **Ultra Tears® Solution [OTC]** *see* Artificial Tears *on page 97*
- **Ultravate™** *see* Halobetasol *on page 488*
- **Unasyn®** *see* Ampicillin and Sulbactam *on page 83*

## Undecylenic Acid and Derivatives

(un de sil EN ik AS id & dah RIV ah tivs)

**U.S. Brand Names** Caldesene® Topical [OTC]; Fungoid® AF Topical Solution [OTC]; Pedi-Pro Topical [OTC]

**Therapeutic Category** Antifungal Agent, Topical

**Synonyms** Zinc Undecylenate

**Use** Treatment of athlete's foot (tinea pedis), ringworm (except nails and scalp), prickly heat, jock itch (tinea cruris), diaper rash and other minor skin irritations due to superficial dermatophytes

**Usual Dosage** Children and Adults: Topical: Apply as needed twice daily after cleansing the affected area for 2-4 weeks

**Local Anesthetic/Vasoconstrictor Precautions** No information available to require special precautions

**Effects on Dental Treatment** No effects or complications reported

**Other Adverse Effects** 1% to 10%: Dermatologic: Skin irritation, sensitization

**Generic Available** Yes

**Comments** Ointment should be applied at night, powder may be applied during the day or used alone when a drying effect is needed

- **Unguentine® [OTC]** *see* Benzocaine *on page 128*
- **Uni-Ace® [OTC]** *see* Acetaminophen *on page 27*
- **Uni-Bent® Cough Syrup** *see* Diphenhydramine *on page 338*
- **Unicap® [OTC]** *see* Vitamins, Multiple *on page 1051*
- **Uni-Decon®** *see* Chlorpheniramine, Phenyltoloxamine, Phenylpropanolamine, and Phenylephrine *on page 237*
- **Uni-Dur®** *see* Theophylline *on page 969*
- **Unipen®** *see* Nafcillin *on page 698*
- **Uniphyl®** *see* Theophylline *on page 969*
- **Uniretic™** *see* Moexipril and Hydrochlorothiazide *on page 685*
- **Unitrol® [OTC]** *see* Phenylpropanolamine *on page 797*
- **Uni-tussin® [OTC]** *see* Guaifenesin *on page 478*
- **Uni-tussin® DM [OTC]** *see* Guaifenesin and Dextromethorphan *on page 479*

- ♦ **Univasc®** *see* Moexipril *on page 684*
- ♦ **Unna's Boot** *see* Zinc Gelatin *on page 1061*
- ♦ **Unna's Paste** *see* Zinc Gelatin *on page 1061*
- ♦ **Uracel®** *see* Sodium Salicylate *on page 924*


## Urea (yoor EE a)

**U.S. Brand Names** Amino-Cerv™ Vaginal Cream; Aquacare® [OTC]; Carmol® [OTC]; Nutraplus® [OTC]; Rea-Lo® [OTC]; Ultra Mide®; Ureacin®-20 [OTC]; Ureacin®-40; Ureaphil®

**Canadian Brand Names** Onyvul®; Uremol™; Urisec®; Velvelan®

**Therapeutic Category** Diuretic, Osmotic; Topical Skin Product

**Use** Reduces intracranial pressure and intraocular pressure; topically promotes hydration and removal of excess keratin in hyperkeratotic conditions and dry skin; mild cervicitis

**Usual Dosage**

Children: I.V. slow infusion:

- <2 years: 0.1-0.5 g/kg
- >2 years: 0.5-1.5 g/kg

Adults:

- I.V. infusion: 1-1.5 g/kg by slow infusion (1-2½ hours); maximum: 120 g/24 hours
- Topical: Apply 1-3 times/day
- Vaginal: Insert 1 applicatorful in vagina at bedtime for 2-4 weeks

**Mechanism of Action** Elevates plasma osmolality by inhibiting tubular reabsorption of water, thus enhancing the flow of water into extracellular fluid

**Local Anesthetic/Vasoconstrictor Precautions** No information available to require special precautions

**Effects on Dental Treatment** No effects or complications reported

**Other Adverse Effects**

>10%: Gastrointestinal: Nausea, vomiting

1% to 10%:

- Central nervous system: Headache
- Local: Transient stinging, local irritation, tissue necrosis from extravasation of I.V. preparation

<1%: Endocrine & metabolic: Electrolyte imbalance

**Drug Interactions** Decreased effect/toxicity/levels of lithium

**Drug Uptake**

Onset of therapeutic effect: I.V.: Maximum effects within 1-2 hours

Duration: 3-6 hours (diuresis can continue for up to 10 hours)

Serum half-life: 1 hour

**Pregnancy Risk Factor** C

**Generic Available** Yes

## Urea and Hydrocortisone (yoor EE a & hye droe KOR ti sone)

**U.S. Brand Names** Carmol-HC® Topical

**Therapeutic Category** Corticosteroid, Topical (Low Potency); Topical Skin Product

**Synonyms** Hydrocortisone and Urea

**Use** Inflammation of corticosteroid-responsive dermatoses

**Usual Dosage** Apply thin film and rub in well 1-4 times/day

**Local Anesthetic/Vasoconstrictor Precautions** No information available to require special precautions

**Effects on Dental Treatment** No effects or complications reported

**Pregnancy Risk Factor** C

**Generic Available** No


- ♦ **Ureacin®-20 [OTC]** *see* Urea *on this page*
- ♦ **Ureacin®-40** *see* Urea *on this page*
- ♦ **Ureaphil®** *see* Urea *on this page*
- ♦ **Urecholine®** *see* Bethanechol *on page 139*
- ♦ **Urex®** *see* Methenamine *on page 647*
- ♦ **Urised®** *see* Methenamine *on page 647*
- ♦ **Urispas®** *see* Flavoxate *on page 432*
- ♦ **Urobak®** *see* Sulfamethoxazole *on page 943*
- ♦ **Urocit®-K** *see* Potassium Citrate *on page 823*
- ♦ **Urodine®** *see* Phenazopyridine *on page 788*


## Urofollitropin (yoor oh fol li TROE pin)

**U.S. Brand Names** Fertinex® Injection; Metrodin® Injection

**Therapeutic Category** Ovulation Stimulator

**Use** Induction of ovulation in patients with polycystic ovarian disease and to stimulate the development of multiple oocytes

**Usual Dosage** Adults: Female: S.C.: 75 units/day for 7-12 days, used with hCG may repeat course of treatment 2 more times

**Mechanism of Action** Preparation of follicle-stimulating hormone 75 IU with <1 IU of luteinizing hormone (LH) which is isolated from the urine of postmenopausal women. Follicle-stimulating hormone plays a role in the development of follicles. Elevated FSH levels early in the normal menstrual cycle are thought to play a significant role in recruiting a cohort of follicles for maturation. A single follicle is enriched with FSH receptors and becomes dominant over the rest of the recruited follicles. The increased number of FSH receptors allows it to grow despite declining FSH levels. This dominant follicle secretes low levels of estrogen and inhibin which further reduces pituitary FSH output. The ovarian stroma, under the influence of luteinizing hormone, produces androgens which the dominant follicle uses as precursors for estrogens.

**Local Anesthetic/Vasoconstrictor Precautions** No information available to require special precautions

**Effects on Dental Treatment** No effects or complications reported

**Other Adverse Effects**

>10%:
- Endocrine & metabolic: Ovarian enlargement
- Local: Swelling at injection site, pain

1% to 10%:
- Cardiovascular: Arterial thromboembolism
- Central nervous system: Fever, chills
- Dermatologic: Rash
- Gastrointestinal: Nausea, vomiting, abdominal pain, diarrhea
- Miscellaneous: Hyperstimulation syndrome

**Drug Interactions** No data reported

**Drug Uptake**

Serum half-life, elimination: 3.9 hours and 70.4 hours (FSH has two half-lives)

**Pregnancy Risk Factor** X

**Generic Available** No

♦ **Urogesic®** *see* Phenazopyridine *on page 788*

## Urokinase (yoor oh KIN ase)

**Related Information**

Cardiovascular Diseases *on page 1066*

**U.S. Brand Names** Abbokinase®

**Therapeutic Category** Thrombolytic Agent

**Use** Thrombolytic agent used in treatment of recent severe or massive deep vein thrombosis, pulmonary emboli, myocardial infarction, and occluded arteriovenous cannulas; more expensive than streptokinase; not useful on thrombi over 1 week old

**Usual Dosage**

Children and Adults: Deep vein thrombosis: I.V.: Loading: 4400 units/kg over 10 minutes, then 4400 units/kg/hour for 12 hours

Adults:

Myocardial infarction: Intracoronary: 750,000 units over 2 hours (6000 units/minute over up to 2 hours)

Occluded I.V. catheters:

5000 units (use only Abbokinase® Open Cath) in each lumen over 1-2 minutes, leave in lumen for 1-4 hours, then aspirate; may repeat with 10,000 units in each lumen if 5000 units fails to clear the catheter; **do not infuse into the patient**; volume to instill into catheter is equal to the volume of the catheter

I.V. infusion: 200 units/kg/hour in each lumen for 12-48 hours at a rate of at least 20 mL/hour

Dialysis patients: 5000 units is administered in each lumen over 1-2 minutes; leave urokinase in lumen for 1-2 days, then aspirate

Clot lysis (large vessel thrombi): Loading: I.V.: 4400 units/kg over 10 minutes, increase to 6000 units/kg/hour; maintenance: 4400-6000 units/kg/hour adjusted to achieve clot lysis or patency of affected vessel; doses up to 50,000 units/kg/hour have been used. **Note:** Therapy should be initiated as soon as possible after diagnosis of thrombi and continued until clot is dissolved (usually 24-72 hours).

Acute pulmonary embolism: Three treatment alternatives: 3 million unit dosage

Alternative 1: 12-hour infusion: 4400 units/kg (2000 units/lb) bolus over 10 minutes followed by 4400 units/kg/hour (2000 units/lb); begin heparin 1000 units/hour approximately 3-4 hours after completion of urokinase infusion or when PTT is <100 seconds

(Continued)

## Urokinase *(Continued)*

Alternative 2: 2-hour infusion: 1 million unit bolus over 10 minutes followed by 2 million units over 110 minutes; begin heparin 1000 units/hour approximately 3-4 hours after completion of urokinase infusion or when PTT is <100 seconds

Alternative 3: Bolus dose only: 15,000 units/kg over 10 minutes; begin heparin 1000 units/hour approximately 3-4 hours after completion of urokinase infusion or when PTT is <100 seconds

**Mechanism of Action** Promotes thrombolysis by directly activating plasminogen to plasmin, which degrades fibrin, fibrinogen, and other procoagulant plasma proteins

**Local Anesthetic/Vasoconstrictor Precautions** No information available to require special precautions

**Effects on Dental Treatment** No effects or complications reported

**Other Adverse Effects**

>10%:
- Cardiovascular: Hypotension, arrhythmias
- Dermatologic: Angioneurotic edema
- Hematologic: Bleeding at sites of percutaneous trauma
- Ocular: Periorbital swelling
- Respiratory: Bronchospasm
- Miscellaneous: Anaphylaxis

<1%:
- Central nervous system: Headache, chills
- Dermatologic: Rash
- Gastrointestinal: Nausea, vomiting
- Hematologic: Anemia
- Ocular: Eye hemorrhage
- Respiratory: Epistaxis
- Miscellaneous: Sweating

**Drug Interactions** Increased toxicity (increased bleeding) with anticoagulants, antiplatelet drugs, aspirin, indomethacin, dextran

**Drug Uptake**

Onset of action: I.V.: Fibrinolysis occurs rapidly

Duration: 4 or more hours

Serum half-life: 10-20 minutes

**Pregnancy Risk Factor** B

**Generic Available** No

- ♦ **Uro-KP-Neutral®** *see* Potassium Phosphate and Sodium Phosphate *on page 826*
- ♦ **Uroplus® DS** *see* Trimethoprim and Sulfamethoxazole *on page 1021*
- ♦ **Uroplus® SS** *see* Trimethoprim and Sulfamethoxazole *on page 1021*
- ♦ **Ursodeoxycholic Acid** *see* Ursodiol *on this page*

## Ursodiol (ER soe dye ole)

**U.S. Brand Names** Actigall™

**Therapeutic Category** Gallstone Dissolution Agent

**Synonyms** Ursodeoxycholic Acid

**Use** Gallbladder stone dissolution

**Usual Dosage** Adults: Oral: 8-10 mg/kg/day in 2-3 divided doses; use beyond 24 months is not established; obtain ultrasound images at 6-month intervals for the first year of therapy; 30% of patients have stone recurrence after dissolution

**Mechanism of Action** Decreases the cholesterol content of bile and bile stones by reducing the secretion of cholesterol from the liver and the fractional reabsorption of cholesterol by the intestines

**Local Anesthetic/Vasoconstrictor Precautions** No information available to require special precautions

**Effects on Dental Treatment** No effects or complications reported

**Other Adverse Effects**

1% to 10%: Gastrointestinal: Diarrhea

<1%:
- Central nervous system: Fatigue, headache
- Dermatologic: Rash, pruritus
- Gastrointestinal: Nausea, vomiting, dyspepsia, metallic taste, abdominal pain, biliary pain, constipation

**Drug Uptake** Serum half-life: 100 hours

**Pregnancy Risk Factor** B

**Generic Available** No

**Comments** Use beyond 24 months is not established; obtain ultrasound images at 6-month intervals for the first year of therapy; 30% of patients have stone recurrence after dissolution

- **Utimox**® *see* Amoxicillin *on page 76*
- **Vagistat**® *see* Tioconazole *on page 987*
- **Vagitrol**® *see* Sulfanilamide *on page 944*

## Valacyclovir (val ay SYE kloe veer)

**Related Information**

Systemic Viral Diseases *on page 1115*

**U.S. Brand Names** Valtrex®

**Therapeutic Category** Antiviral Agent, Oral

**Use** Treatment of herpes zoster (shingles) in immunocompetent patients; episodic treatment of recurrent genital herpes in immunocompetent patients; for first episode genital herpes

**Usual Dosage** Oral: Adults:

Shingles: 1 g 3 times/day for 7 days

Genital herpes: 500 mg twice daily

**Mechanism of Action** Valacyclovir, the L-valyl ester of acyclovir, is rapidly converted to acyclovir before it exerts its antiviral activity against HSV-1, HSV-2, or VZV. It is most active against HSV-1 and least against VZV due to its varied affinity for thymidine kinase. Thymidine kinase converts it into acyclovir monophosphate; this is then converted into the diphosphate and triphosphate forms. Acyclovir triphosphate inhibits replication of herpes viral DNA via competitive inhibition of herpes viral DNA polymerase, incorporation and termination of the growing viral DNA chain, and inactivation of the viral DNA polymerase.

**Local Anesthetic/Vasoconstrictor Precautions** No information available to require special precautions

**Effects on Dental Treatment** No effects or complications reported

**Other Adverse Effects**

>10%: Gastrointestinal: Nausea

1% to 10%:

Central nervous system: Headache, dizziness

Gastrointestinal: Diarrhea, constipation, abdominal pain, anorexia

Neuromuscular & skeletal: Weakness

**Drug Interactions** Decreased toxicity: Cimetidine and/or probenecid has decreased the rate but not the extent of valacyclovir conversion to acyclovir

**Drug Uptake**

Absorption: Rapid and converted to acyclovir and L-valine by first-pass/hepatic metabolism

Serum half-life: Normal renal function: 2.5-3.3 hours

**Pregnancy Risk Factor** B

**Dosage Forms** Caplets: 500 mg

**Generic Available** No

- **Valergen® Injection** *see* Estradiol *on page 387*
- **Valertest No.1® Injection** *see* Estradiol and Testosterone *on page 389*
- **Valisone®** *see* Betamethasone *on page 136*
- **Valium® Injection** *see* Diazepam *on page 316*
- **Valium® Oral** *see* Diazepam *on page 316*
- **Valpin® 50** *see* Anisotropine *on page 87*

## Valproic Acid and Derivatives

(val PROE ik AS id & dah RIV ah tives)

**U.S. Brand Names** Depacon®; Depakene®; Depakote®

**Canadian Brand Names** Deproic

**Therapeutic Category** Anticonvulsant, Miscellaneous

**Use** Management of simple and complex absence seizures; mixed seizure types; myoclonic and generalized tonic-clonic (grand mal) seizures; may be effective in partial seizures and infantile spasms

**Usual Dosage** Children and Adults:

Oral: Initial: 10-15 mg/kg/day in 1-3 divided doses; increase by 5-10 mg/kg/day at weekly intervals until therapeutic levels are achieved; maintenance: 30-60 mg/kg/day in 2-3 divided doses

Children receiving more than 1 anticonvulsant (ie, polytherapy) may require doses up to 100 mg/kg/day in 3-4 divided doses

Rectal: Dilute syrup 1:1 with water for use as a retention enema; loading dose: 17-20 mg/kg one time; maintenance: 10-15 mg/kg/dose every 8 hours

**Mechanism of Action** Causes increased availability of gamma-aminobutyric acid (GABA), an inhibitory neurotransmitter, to brain neurons or may enhance the action of GABA or mimic its action at postsynaptic receptor sites

(Continued)

## Valproic Acid and Derivatives *(Continued)*

**Local Anesthetic/Vasoconstrictor Precautions** No information available to require special precautions

**Effects on Dental Treatment** No effects or complications reported

**Other Adverse Effects**

1% to 10%:

Endocrine & metabolic: Change in menstrual cycle

Gastrointestinal: Abdominal cramps, anorexia, diarrhea, nausea, vomiting, weight gain

<1%:

Central nervous system: Drowsiness, ataxia, irritability, confusion, restlessness, hyperactivity, headache, malaise

Dermatologic: Alopecia, erythema multiforme

Endocrine & metabolic: Hyperammonemia

Gastrointestinal: Pancreatitis

Hematologic: Thrombocytopenia, prolongation of bleeding time

Hepatic: Transient elevated liver enzymes, liver failure

Neuromuscular & skeletal: Tremor

Ocular: Nystagmus, spots before eyes

**Drug Interactions**

Carbamazepine decreases the plasma concentrations of valproic acid

Cholestyramine decreases the gastrointestinal absorption of valproic acid

Erythromycin - in one patient, valproic acid plasma levels increased after erythromycin resulting in symptoms of valproic acid toxicity

Clozapine - valproic acid decreases the plasma concentrations of clozapine

Felbamate decreases the plasma levels of valproic acid

Isoniazid - valproic acid plasma levels have increased after isoniazid

Lamotrigine - valproic acid inhibits the metabolism of lamotrigine; lamotrigine stimulates the metabolism of valproic acid resulting in lower plasma concentrations

Phenobarbital - valproic acid increases the plasma levels of phenobarbital; phenobarbital toxicity (excessive sedation) may occur in some patients

Primidone - valproic acid may increase the plasma levels of phenobarbital that is produced from primidone; excessive phenobarbital response may occur

Other - alcohol and CNS depressants may potentiate the depressant effects of valproic acid; valproic acid may increase the risk of bleeding in patients receiving anticoagulants (ie, warfarin) and antithrombotics (ie, aspirin)

**Drug Uptake**

Serum half-life: Adults: 8-17 hours

Time to peak serum concentration: Within 1-4 hours; 3-5 hours after divalproex (enteric coated)

**Pregnancy Risk Factor** D

**Generic Available** Yes

**Selected Readings**

Redington K, Wells C, and Petito F, "Erythromycin and Valproic Acid Interaction," *Ann Intern Med*, 1992, 116(10):877-8.

## Valrubicin

**U.S. Brand Names** Valstar™

**Therapeutic Category** Antineoplastic Agent

**Use** Intravesical therapy of BCG-refractory carcinoma *in situ* of the urinary bladder

**Usual Dosage** Adults: Intravesical: 800 mg once weekly for 6 weeks; no specific dosing adjustment is necessary in elderly

**Mechanism of Action** Blocks function of DNA topoisomerase II; inhibits DNA synthesis, causes extensive chromosomal damage, and arrests cell development

**Local Anesthetic/Vasoconstrictor Precautions** No information available to require special precautions

**Effects on Dental Treatment** No effects or complications reported

**Other Adverse Effects**

>10%: Genitourinary: Frequency (61%), dysuria (56%), urgency (57%), bladder spasm (31%), hematuria (29%), bladder pain (28%), urinary incontinence (22%), cystitis (15%), urinary tract infection (15%)

1% to 10%:

Cardiovascular: Chest pain (2%), vasodilation (2%), peripheral edema (1%)

Central nervous system: Headache (4%), malaise (4%), dizziness (3%), fever (2%)

Dermatologic: Rash (3%)

Endocrine & metabolic: Hyperglycemia (1%)

Gastrointestinal: Abdominal pain (5%), nausea (5%), diarrhea (3%), vomiting (2%), flatulence (1%)

Genitourinary: Nocturia (7%), burning symptoms (5%), urinary retention (4%), urethral pain (3%), pelvic pain (1%), hematuria (microscopic) (3%)
Hematologic: Anemia (2%)
Neuromuscular & skeletal: Weakness (4%), back pain (3%), myalgia (1%)
Respiratory: Pneumonia (1%)

<1%: Tenesmus, pruritus, taste disturbance, skin irritation, decreased urine flow, urethritis

**Drug Interactions** No specific drug interactions studies have been performed; the systemic exposure to valrubicin is negligible, and interactions are unlikely

**Drug Uptake** Absorption: Well absorbed into bladder tissue, negligible systemic absorption. Trauma to mucosa may increase absorption, and perforation greatly increases absorption with significant systemic myelotoxicity.

**Pregnancy Risk Factor** C

**Dosage Forms** Injection: 200 mg/5mL

## Valsartan (val SAR tan)

**U.S. Brand Names** Diovan™

**Therapeutic Category** Angiotensin II Antagonist

**Use** Treatment of hypertension alone or in combination with other antihypertensives

**Usual Dosage** Adults: 80 mg/day; may be increased to 160 mg if needed (maximal effects observed in 4-6 weeks)

**Mechanism of Action** As a prodrug, valsartan produces direct antagonism of the angiotensin II (AT2) receptors, unlike the angiotensin-converting enzyme inhibitors. It displaces angiotensin II from the AT1 receptor and produces its blood pressure lowering effects by antagonizing AT1-induced vasoconstriction, aldosterone release, catecholamine release, arginine vasopressin release, water intake, and hypertrophic responses. This action results in more efficient blockade of the cardiovascular effects of angiotensin II and fewer side effects than the ACE inhibitors.

**Local Anesthetic/Vasoconstrictor Precautions** No information available to require special precautions

**Effects on Dental Treatment** No effects or complications reported

**Other Adverse Effects** Similar incidence to placebo; independent of race, age, and gender

>1%:

Central nervous system: Headache, dizziness, drowsiness, ataxia
Endocrine & metabolic: Decreased libido
Gastrointestinal: Diarrhea, abdominal pain, nausea, abnormal taste
Genitourinary: Polyuria
Hematologic: Neutropenia
Hepatic: Increased LFTs
Neuromuscular & skeletal: Arthralgia
Respiratory: Cough, upper respiratory infection, rhinitis, sinusitis, pharyngitis

<1%:

Hematologic: Anemia
Renal: Increased Cr

**Warnings/Precautions** Use extreme caution with concurrent administration of potassium-sparing diuretics or potassium supplements, in patients with mild-moderate hepatic dysfunction (adjust dose), in those who may be sodium/water depleted (eg, on high-dose diuretics), and in the elderly; avoid use in patients with congestive heart failure, unilateral renal artery stenosis, aortic/mitral valve stenosis, coronary artery disease, or hypertrophic cardiomyopathy, if possible

**Drug Interactions**

Decreased effect: Phenobarbital, ketoconazole, troleandomycin, sulfaphenazole
Increased effect: Cimetidine, moxonidine

**Drug Uptake**

Serum half-life: 9 hours
Time to peak serum concentration: 2 hours (maximal effect: 4-6 hours)

**Pregnancy Risk Factor** C, first trimester. D, second and third trimesters

♦ **Valstar™** *see* Valrubicin *on previous page*
♦ **Valtrex®** *see* Valacyclovir *on page 1037*
♦ **Vancenase®** *see* Beclomethasone *on page 122*
♦ **Vancenase® AQ** *see* Beclomethasone *on page 122*
♦ **Vanceril®** *see* Beclomethasone *on page 122*
♦ **Vancocin®** *see* Vancomycin *on this page*
♦ **Vancoled®** *see* Vancomycin *on this page*

## Vancomycin (van koe MYE sin)

**Related Information**

Cardiovascular Diseases *on page 1066*

(Continued)

## Vancomycin *(Continued)*

**U.S. Brand Names** Lyphocin®; Vancocin®; Vancoled®

**Canadian Brand Names** Vancocin® CP

**Therapeutic Category** Antibiotic, Miscellaneous

**Use**

Treatment of patients with the following infections or conditions:

- Infections due to documented or suspected methicillin-resistant *S. aureus* or beta-lactam resistant coagulase negative *Staphylococcus*
- Serious or life-threatening infections (ie, endocarditis, meningitis) due to documented or suspected staphylococcal or streptococcal infections in patients who are allergic to penicillins and/or cephalosporins
- Empiric therapy of infections associated with gram-positive organisms; used orally for staphylococcal enterocolitis or for antibiotic-associated pseudomembranous colitis produced by *C. difficile*

**Usual Dosage** Initial dosage recommendation: I.V.:

Infants >1 month and Children with staphylococcal central nervous system infection: 60 mg/kg/day in divided doses every 6 hours

Adults with normal renal function: 1 g every 12 hours

**Antibiotic lock technique (for catheter infections):** 2 mg/mL in SWI/NS or $D_5W$; instill 3-5 mL into catheter port as a flush solution instead of heparin lock (**Note:** Do not mix with any other solutions)

Intrathecal: Vancomycin is available as a powder for injection and may be diluted to 1-5 mg/mL concentration in preservative-free 0.9% sodium chloride for administration into the CSF

- Children: 5-20 mg/day
- Adults: 20 mg/day

Oral: Pseudomembranous colitis produced by *C. difficile*:

- Children: 40 mg/kg/day in divided doses every 6-8 hours, added to fluids
- Adults: 125 mg 4 times/day

**Mechanism of Action** Inhibits bacterial cell wall synthesis by blocking glycopeptide polymerization through binding tightly to D-alanyl-D-alanine portion of cell wall precursor

**Local Anesthetic/Vasoconstrictor Precautions** No information available to require special precautions

**Effects on Dental Treatment** No effects or complications reported

**Other Adverse Effects**

>10%: Cardiovascular: Hypotension accompanied by flushing and erythematous rash on face and upper body (red neck or red man syndrome)

1% to 10%:

- Central nervous system: Chills, drug fever
- Hematologic: Eosinophilia

**Contraindications** Hypersensitivity to vancomycin or any component; avoid in patients with previous severe hearing loss

**Warnings/Precautions** Use with caution in patients with renal impairment or those receiving other nephrotoxic or ototoxic drugs; dosage modification required in patients with impaired renal function (especially elderly)

**Drug Interactions** Increased toxicity with general anesthetic agents

**Drug Uptake**

Serum half-life (biphasic):

- Children >3 years: 2.2-3 hours
- Adults: 5-11 hours, prolonged significantly with reduced renal function

Time to peak serum concentration: I.V.: Within 45-65 minutes

**Pregnancy Risk Factor** C

**Breast-feeding Considerations** No data reported

**Dosage Forms**

- Capsule, as hydrochloride: 125 mg, 250 mg
- Powder for oral solution, as hydrochloride: 1 g, 10 g
- Powder for injection, as hydrochloride: 500 mg, 1 g, 2 g, 5 g, 10 g

**Generic Available** Yes


- ♦ **Vanoxide® [OTC]** *see* Benzoyl Peroxide *on page 130*
- ♦ **Vanoxide-HC®** *see* Benzoyl Peroxide and Hydrocortisone *on page 131*
- ♦ **Van R Gingibraid®** *see* Epinephrine, Racemic and Aluminum Potassium Sulfate *on page 375*
- ♦ **Vansil™** *see* Oxamniquine *on page 746*
- ♦ **Vantin®** *see* Cefpodoxime *on page 205*
- ♦ **Vaponefrin®** *see* Epinephrine, Racemic *on page 375*

## Varicella-Zoster Immune Globulin (Human)

(var i SEL a- ZOS ter i MYUN GLOB yoo lin HYU man)

**Therapeutic Category** Immune Globulin

**Synonyms** VZIG

**Use** Passive immunization of susceptible immunodeficient patients after exposure to varicella; most effective if begun within 96 hours of exposure

**VZIG supplies are limited, restrict administration to those meeting the following criteria:**

**One of the following underlying illnesses or conditions:**

- Neoplastic disease (eg, leukemia or lymphoma)
- Congenital or acquired immunodeficiency
- Immunosuppressive therapy with steroids, antimetabolites or other immunosuppressive treatment regimens
- Newborn of mother who had onset of chickenpox within 5 days before delivery or within 48 hours after delivery
- Premature (≥28 weeks gestation) whose mother has no history of chickenpox
- Premature (<28 weeks gestation or ≤1000 g VZIG) regardless of maternal history

**One of the following types of exposure to chickenpox or zoster patient(s):**

- Continuous household contact
- Playmate contact (>1 hour play indoors)
- Hospital contact (in same 2-4 bedroom or adjacent beds in a large ward or prolonged face-to-face contact with an infectious staff member or patient)
- Susceptible to varicella-zoster

Age of <15 years; administer to immunocompromised adolescents and adults and to other older patients on an individual basis

An acceptable alternative to VZIG prophylaxis is to treat varicella, if it occurs, with high-dose I.V. acyclovir

**Usual Dosage** High risk susceptible patients who are exposed again more than 3 weeks after a prior dose of VZIG should receive another full dose; there is no evidence VZIG modifies established varicella-zoster infections.

I.M.: Administer by deep injection in the gluteal muscle or in another large muscle mass. Inject 125 units/10 kg (22 lb); maximum dose: 625 units (5 vials); minimum dose: 125 units; do not give fractional doses. Do not inject I.V. See table.

**VZIG Dose Based on Weight**

| Weight of Patient | | Dose | |
|---|---|---|---|
| kg | lb | Units | No. of Vials |
| 0-10 | 0-22 | 125 | 1 |
| 10.1-20 | 22.1-44 | 250 | 2 |
| 20.1-30 | 44.1-66 | 375 | 3 |
| 30.1-40 | 66.1-88 | 500 | 4 |
| >40 | >88 | 625 | 5 |

**Mechanism of Action** The exact mechanism has not been clarified but the antibodies in varicella-zoster immune globulin most likely neutralize the varicella-zoster virus and prevent its pathological actions

**Local Anesthetic/Vasoconstrictor Precautions** No information available to require special precautions

**Effects on Dental Treatment** No effects or complications reported

**Other Adverse Effects**

1% to 10%: Local: Discomfort at the site of injection (pain, redness, swelling)

<1%:

- Central nervous system: Headache, malaise
- Dermatologic: Rash, angioedema
- Gastrointestinal: GI symptoms
- Respiratory: Respiratory symptoms
- Miscellaneous: Anaphylactic shock

**Pregnancy Risk Factor** C

**Generic Available** No

**Comments** Should be administered within 96 hours of exposure

- ♦ **Vascor®** *see* Bepridil *on page 134*
- ♦ **Vaseretic® 5-12.5** *see* Enalapril and Hydrochlorothiazide *on page 369*
- ♦ **Vaseretic® 10-25** *see* Enalapril and Hydrochlorothiazide *on page 369*
- ♦ **Vasocidin® Ophthalmic** *see* Sulfacetamide Sodium and Prednisolone *on page 940*
- ♦ **VasoClear® Ophthalmic [OTC]** *see* Naphazoline *on page 703*

- **Vasocon-A® [OTC] Ophthalmic** *see* Naphazoline and Antazoline *on page 704*
- **Vasocon Regular® Ophthalmic** *see* Naphazoline *on page 703*
- **Vasoconstrictor Interactions With Antidepressants** *see page 1277*
- **Vasodilan®** *see* Isoxsuprine *on page 558*

# Vasopressin (vay soe PRES in)

**U.S. Brand Names** Pitressin®

**Canadian Brand Names** Pressyn®

**Therapeutic Category** Antidiuretic Hormone Analog; Hormone, Posterior Pituitary

**Use** Treatment of diabetes insipidus; prevention and treatment of postoperative abdominal distention; differential diagnosis of diabetes insipidus

**Unlabeled use:** Adjunct in the treatment of GI hemorrhage and esophageal varices

**Usual Dosage**

Diabetes insipidus (highly variable dosage; titrated based on serum and urine sodium and osmolality in addition to fluid balance and urine output):
- Children: I.M., S.C.: 2.5-10 units 2-4 times/day as needed
- Adults:
  - I.M., S.C.: 5-10 units 2-4 times/day as needed (dosage range 5-60 units/day)
  - Intranasal: Administer on cotton pledget or nasal spray

Abdominal distention: Adults: I.M.: 5 mg stat, 10 mg every 3-4 hours

GI hemorrhage: Children and Adults: Continuous I.V. infusion: 0.5 milliunit/kg/hour (0.0005 unit/kg/hour); double dosage as needed every 30 minutes to a maximum of 10 milliunits/kg/hour
- Children: 0.01 units/kg/minute; continue at same dosage (if bleeding stops) for 12 hours, then taper off over 24-48 hours
- Adults: I.V.: Initial: 0.2-0.4 unit/minute, then titrate dose as needed; if bleeding stops, continue at same dose for 12 hours, taper off over 24-48 hours

**Mechanism of Action** Increases cyclic adenosine monophosphate (cAMP) which increases water permeability at the renal tubule resulting in decreased urine volume and increased osmolality; causes peristalsis by directly stimulating the smooth muscle in the GI tract

**Local Anesthetic/Vasoconstrictor Precautions** No information available to require special precautions

**Effects on Dental Treatment** No effects or complications reported

**Other Adverse Effects**

1% to 10%:
- Cardiovascular: Hypertension, bradycardia, arrhythmias, venous thrombosis, vasoconstriction with higher doses, angina, circumoral pallor
- Central nervous system: Pounding in the head, fever, vertigo
- Dermatologic: Urticaria
- Gastrointestinal: Flatulence, abdominal cramps, nausea, vomiting
- Neuromuscular & skeletal: Tremor
- Miscellaneous: Sweating

<1%:
- Cardiovascular: Myocardial infarction
- Endocrine & metabolic: Water intoxication
- Miscellaneous: Allergic reaction

**Drug Interactions**

Decreased effect: Lithium, epinephrine, demeclocycline, heparin, and alcohol block antidiuretic activity to varying degrees

Increased effect: Chlorpropamide, phenformin, urea and fludrocortisone potentiate antidiuretic response

**Drug Uptake**

Nasal:
- Onset of action: 1 hour
- Duration: 3-8 hours
- Serum half-life: 15 minutes

Parenteral: Duration of action: I.M., S.C.: 2-8 hours

Absorption: Destroyed by trypsin in GI tract, must be administered parenterally or intranasally

**Pregnancy Risk Factor** B

**Generic Available** Yes

- **Vasosulf® Ophthalmic** *see* Sulfacetamide Sodium and Phenylephrine *on page 940*
- **Vasotec®** *see* Enalapril *on page 366*
- **V-Cillin K®** *see* Penicillin V Potassium *on page 776*
- **VCR** *see* Vincristine *on page 1046*

♦ **V-Dec-M®** *see* Guaifenesin and Pseudoephedrine *on page 481*
♦ **Veetids®** *see* Penicillin V Potassium *on page 776*
♦ **Velban®** *see* Vinblastine *on page 1046*
♦ **Velosef®** *see* Cephradine *on page 217*
♦ **Velosulin® Human** *see* Insulin Preparations *on page 537*

## Venlafaxine (VEN la faks een)

**Related Information**
Vasoconstrictor Interactions With Antidepressants *on page 1277*

**U.S. Brand Names** Effexor®

**Therapeutic Category** Antidepressant, Miscellaneous

**Use** Treatment of depression in adults; has demonstrated effectiveness for obsessive-compulsive disorder, although it has not been approved for this indication

**Usual Dosage** Adults: Oral: 75 mg/day, administered in 2 or 3 divided doses, taken with food; dose may be increased in 75 mg/day increments at intervals of at least 4 days, up to 225-375 mg/day

**Mechanism of Action** Venlafaxine and its active metabolite o-desmethylvenlafaxine (ODV) are potent inhibitors of neuronal serotonin and norepinephrine reuptake and weak inhibitors of dopamine reuptake; causes beta-receptor down regulation and reduces adenylcyclase coupled beta-adrenergic systems in the brain

**Local Anesthetic/Vasoconstrictor Precautions** No information available to require special precautions

**Effects on Dental Treatment** >10% of patients experience significant dry mouth which may contribute to oral discomfort, especially in older patients

**Other Adverse Effects**

≥10%:
- Central nervous system: Headache, somnolence, dizziness, insomnia, nervousness
- Gastrointestinal: Nausea, constipation
- Genitourinary: Abnormal ejaculation
- Neuromuscular & skeletal: Neck pain, weakness
- Miscellaneous: Sweating

1% to 10%:
- Cardiovascular: Palpitations, hypertension, sinus tachycardia
- Central nervous system: Anxiety
- Gastrointestinal: Weight loss, anorexia, vomiting, diarrhea, dysphagia
- Genitourinary: Impotence
- Neuromuscular & skeletal: Tremor
- Ocular: Blurred vision

<1%:
- Central nervous system: Seizures
- Otic: Ear pain

**Drug Interactions** Increased toxicity: Cimetidine, MAO inhibitors (hyperpyrexic crisis); tricyclic antidepressants (TCAs), fluoxetine, sertraline, phenothiazine, class 1C antiarrhythmics, warfarin; venlafaxine is a weak inhibitor of cytochrome P-450-2D6, which is responsible for metabolizing antipsychotics, antiarrhythmics, TCAs, and beta-blockers. Therefore, interactions with these agents are possible, however, less likely than with more potent enzyme inhibitors.

**Drug Uptake**
Absorption: Oral: 92% to 100%
Serum half-life: 3-7 hours (venlafaxine) and 11-13 hours (ODV)

**Pregnancy Risk Factor** C

**Generic Available** No

♦ **Venoglobulin®-I** *see* Immune Globulin, Intravenous *on page 531*
♦ **Venoglobulin®-S** *see* Immune Globulin, Intravenous *on page 531*
♦ **Ventolin®** *see* Albuterol *on page 43*
♦ **Ventolin® Rotocaps®** *see* Albuterol *on page 43*
♦ **VePesid® Injection** *see* Etoposide *on page 414*
♦ **VePesid® Oral** *see* Etoposide *on page 414*

## Verapamil (ver AP a mil)

**Related Information**
Calcium Channel Blockers & Gingival Hyperplasia *on page 1204*
Cardiovascular Diseases *on page 1066*

**U.S. Brand Names** Calan®; Calan® SR; Covera-HS®; Isoptin®; Isoptin® SR; Verelan®

**Canadian Brand Names** Apo®-Verap; Novo-Veramil; Nu-Verap

**Therapeutic Category** Antianginal Agent; Antiarrhythmic Agent, Class IV; Antiarrhythmic Agent (Supraventricular & Ventricular); Calcium Channel Blocker

(Continued)

## Verapamil *(Continued)*

**Use** Orally used for treatment of angina pectoris (vasospastic, chronic stable, unstable) and hypertension; I.V. for supraventricular tachyarrhythmias (PSVT, atrial fibrillation, atrial flutter)

**Usual Dosage**

Children: SVT:

I.V.:

<1 year: 0.1-0.2 mg/kg over 2 minutes; repeat every 30 minutes as needed

1-16 years: 0.1-0.3 mg/kg over 2 minutes; maximum: 5 mg/dose, may repeat dose in 15 minutes if adequate response not achieved; maximum for second dose: 10 mg/dose

Oral (dose not well established):

1-5 years: 4-8 mg/kg/day in 3 divided doses **or** 40-80 mg every 8 hours

>5 years: 80 mg every 6-8 hours

Adults:

SVT: I.V.: 5-10 mg (approximately 0.075-0.15 mg/kg), second dose of 10 mg (~0.15 mg/kg) may be given 15-30 minutes after the initial dose if patient tolerates, but does not respond to initial dose

Angina: Oral: Initial dose: 80-120 mg twice daily (elderly or small stature: 40 mg twice daily); range: 240-480 mg/day in 3-4 divided doses

Hypertension: Usual dose is 80 mg 3 times/day or 240 mg/day (sustained release); range 240-480 mg/day (no evidence of additional benefit in doses >360 mg/day)

**Mechanism of Action** Inhibits calcium ion from entering the "slow channels" or select voltage-sensitive areas of vascular smooth muscle and myocardium during depolarization; produces a relaxation of coronary vascular smooth muscle and coronary vasodilation; increases myocardial oxygen delivery in patients with vasospastic angina; slows automaticity and conduction of A-V node.

**Local Anesthetic/Vasoconstrictor Precautions** No information available to require special precautions

**Effects on Dental Treatment** Calcium channel blockers (CCB) have been reported to cause gingival hyperplasia (GH). Verapamil induced GH has appeared 11 months or more after subjects took daily doses of 240-360 mg. The severity of hyperplastic syndrome does not seem to be dose-dependent. Gingivectomy is only successful if CCB therapy is discontinued. GH regresses markedly one week after CCB discontinuance with all symptoms resolving in 2 months. If a patient must continue CCB therapy, begin a program of professional cleaning and patient plaque control to minimize severity and growth rate of gingival tissue.

**Other Adverse Effects**

1% to 10%:

Cardiovascular: Bradycardia; first, second, or third degree A-V block; congestive heart failure; hypotension; peripheral edema

Central nervous system: Dizziness, lightheadedness, nausea, fatigue

Dermatologic: Skin rash

Gastrointestinal: Constipation

Neuromuscular & skeletal: Weakness

<1%:

Cardiovascular: Chest pain, hypotension (excessive), tachycardia, flushing

Endocrine & metabolic: Galactorrhea

Gastrointestinal: Gingival hyperplasia

**Drug Interactions**

$H_2$-blockers (such as cimetidine) cause increased plasma levels of verapamil

Beta-blockers cause increased cardiac depressant effects on A-V conduction in combination with verapamil

Verapamil may cause increases in blood levels of the following drugs: Carbamazepine, cyclosporin, digitalis, quinidine, and theophylline; toxicities to all the above drugs could result

**Drug Uptake**

Oral (nonsustained tablets):

Peak effect: 2 hours

Duration: 6-8 hours

I.V.:

Peak effect: 1-5 minutes

Duration: 10-20 minutes

Serum half-life:

Infants: 4.4-6.9 hours

Adults: Single dose: 2-8 hours, increased up to 12 hours with multiple dosing; increased half-life with hepatic cirrhosis

**Pregnancy Risk Factor** C

**Generic Available** Yes

**Selected Readings**

Wynn RL, "Update on Calcium Channel Blocker Induced Gingival Hyperplasia," *Gen Dent*, 1995, 43(3):218-22.

- **Verazinc® [OTC]** *see* Zinc Supplements *on page 1062*
- **Verazinc® Oral [OTC]** *see* Zinc Sulfate *on page 1062*
- **Vercyte®** *see* Pipobroman *on page 809*
- **Verelan®** *see* Verapamil *on page 1043*
- **Vergon® [OTC]** *see* Meclizine *on page 620*
- **Vermizine®** *see* Piperazine *on page 808*
- **Vermox®** *see* Mebendazole *on page 619*
- **Verr-Canth™** *see* Cantharidin *on page 180*
- **Verrex-C&M®** *see* Podophyllin and Salicylic Acid *on page 812*
- **Versacaps®** *see* Guaifenesin and Pseudoephedrine *on page 481*
- **Versed® Injection** *see* Midazolam *on page 674*
- **Versed® Syrup** *see* Midazolam *on page 674*
- **Vesanoid®** *see* Tretinoin, Oral *on page 1007*
- **Vesprin®** *see* Triflupromazine *on page 1017*
- **Vexol®** *see* Rimexolone *on page 890*
- **Viagra®** *see* Sildenafil *on page 912*
- **Vibramycin®** *see* Doxycycline *on page 355*
- **Vibra-Tabs®** *see* Doxycycline *on page 355*
- **Vicks® 44D Cough & Head Congestion** *see* Pseudoephedrine and Dextromethorphan *on page 864*
- **Vicks® 44E [OTC]** *see* Guaifenesin and Dextromethorphan *on page 479*
- **Vicks® 44 Non-Drowsy Cold & Cough Liqui-Caps [OTC]** *see* Pseudoephedrine and Dextromethorphan *on page 864*
- **Vicks Children's Chloraseptic® [OTC]** *see* Benzocaine *on page 128*
- **Vicks Chloraseptic® Sore Throat [OTC]** *see* Benzocaine *on page 128*
- **Vicks® DayQuil® Allergy Relief 4 Hour Tablet [OTC]** *see* Brompheniramine and Phenylpropanolamine *on page 153*
- **Vicks® DayQuil® Sinus Pressure & Congestion Relief [OTC]** *see* Guaifenesin and Phenylpropanolamine *on page 480*
- **Vicks Formula 44® [OTC]** *see* Dextromethorphan *on page 314*
- **Vicks Formula 44® Pediatric Formula [OTC]** *see* Dextromethorphan *on page 314*
- **Vicks® Pediatric Formula 44E [OTC]** *see* Guaifenesin and Dextromethorphan *on page 479*
- **Vicks Sinex® Nasal Solution [OTC]** *see* Phenylephrine *on page 795*
- **Vicodin® [5/500]** *see* Hydrocodone and Acetaminophen *on page 505*
- **Vicodin® ES [7.5/750]** *see* Hydrocodone and Acetaminophen *on page 505*
- **Vicodin® HP** *see* Hydrocodone and Acetaminophen *on page 505*
- **Vicon-C® [OTC]** *see* Vitamin B Complex With Vitamin C *on page 1050*
- **Vicon Forte®** *see* Vitamins, Multiple *on page 1051*
- **Vicon® Plus [OTC]** *see* Vitamins, Multiple *on page 1051*
- **Vicoprofen®** *see* Hydrocodone and Ibuprofen *on page 509*

## Vidarabine (vye DARE a been)

**Related Information**

Oral Viral Infections *on page 1137*
Systemic Viral Diseases *on page 1115*

**U.S. Brand Names** Vira-A®

**Therapeutic Category** Antiviral Agent, Ophthalmic

**Use** Treatment of acute keratoconjunctivitis and epithelial keratitis due to herpes simplex virus; herpes simplex conjunctivitis

**Usual Dosage** Children and Adults: Ophthalmic: Keratoconjunctivitis: Place 1/2" of ointment in lower conjunctival sac 5 times/day every 3 hours while awake until complete re-epithelialization has occurred, then twice daily for an additional 7 days

**Mechanism of Action** Inhibits viral DNA synthesis by blocking DNA polymerase

**Local Anesthetic/Vasoconstrictor Precautions** No information available to require special precautions

**Effects on Dental Treatment** No effects or complications reported

**Other Adverse Effects** Ocular: Burning, lacrimation, keratitis, photophobia, foreign body sensation, uveitis

**Drug Interactions** No data reported

**Pregnancy Risk Factor** C

**Generic Available** No

- **Vi-Daylin® [OTC]** *see* Vitamins, Multiple *on page 1051*

- **Vi-Daylin/F®** *see* Vitamins, Multiple *on page 1051*
- **Videx®** *see* Didanosine *on page 323*

## Vinblastine (vin BLAS teen)

**U.S. Brand Names** Alkaban-AQ®; Velban®

**Therapeutic Category** Antineoplastic Agent, Mitotic Inhibitor

**Synonyms** Vincaleukoblastine; VLB

**Use** Palliative treatment of Hodgkin's disease; advanced testicular germinal-cell cancers; non-Hodgkin's lymphoma, histiocytosis, and choriocarcinoma

**Usual Dosage Refer to individual protocols.** Varies depending upon clinical and hematological response. Give at intervals of at least 7 days and only after leukocyte count has returned to at least 4000/mm$^3$; maintenance therapy should be titrated according to leukocyte count. Dosage should be reduced in patients with recent exposure to radiation therapy or chemotherapy; single doses in these patients should not exceed 5.5 mg/m$^2$.

Children and Adults: I.V.: 4-20 mg/m$^2$ (0.1-0.5 mg/kg) every 7-10 days **or** 5-day continuous infusion of 1.4-1.8 mg/m$^2$/day **or** 0.1-0.5 mg/kg/week

**Mechanism of Action** VLB binds to tubulin and inhibits microtubule formation, therefore, arresting the cell at metaphase by disrupting the formation of the mitotic spindle; it is specific for the M and S phases; binds to microtubular protein of the mitotic spindle causing metaphase arrest

**Local Anesthetic/Vasoconstrictor Precautions** No information available to require special precautions

**Effects on Dental Treatment** No effects or complications reported

**Other Adverse Effects**

>10%:

Dermatologic: Alopecia

Hematologic: May cause severe bone marrow suppression and is the dose-limiting toxicity of vinblastine (unlike vincristine); severe granulocytopenia and thrombocytopenia may occur following the administration of vinblastine and nadir 7-10 days after treatment

1% to 10%:

Cardiovascular: Tachycardia, orthostatic hypotension

Central nervous system: Depression, malaise, seizures, headache

Dermatologic: Rash, photosensitivity

Endocrine & metabolic: Hyperuricemia

Gastrointestinal: Paralytic ileus, stomatitis, nausea and vomiting are most common and are easily controlled with standard antiemetics; constipation, diarrhea, abdominal cramps, anorexia, metallic taste

Emetic potential: Moderate (30% to 60%)

Genitourinary: Urinary retention

Local: Extravasation: Vinblastine is a vesicant and can cause tissue irritation and necrosis if infiltrated; if extravasation occurs, follow institutional policy, which may include hyaluronidase and hot compresses

Neuromuscular & skeletal: Jaw pain, weakness, myalgia; vinblastine rarely produces neurotoxicity at clinical doses; however, neurotoxicity may be seen, especially at high doses; if it occurs, symptoms are similar to vincristine toxicity: peripheral neuropathy, loss of deep tendon reflexes, and GI symptoms

<1%:

Central nervous system: Neurotoxicity, pain

Dermatologic: Dermatitis

Gastrointestinal: Hemorrhagic colitis

Neuromuscular & skeletal: Numbness, myalgia

Respiratory: Bronchospasm

**Drug Uptake**

Absorption: Not reliably absorbed from the GI tract and must be given I.V.

Serum half-life (biphasic):

Initial 0.164 hours

Terminal: 25 hours

**Pregnancy Risk Factor** D

**Generic Available** Yes

- **Vincaleukoblastine** *see* Vinblastine *on this page*
- **Vincasar® PFS™ Injection** *see* Vincristine *on this page*

## Vincristine (vin KRIS teen)

**U.S. Brand Names** Oncovin® Injection; Vincasar® PFS™ Injection

**Therapeutic Category** Antineoplastic Agent, Mitotic Inhibitor

**Synonyms** LCR; Leurocristine; VCR

**Use** Treatment of leukemias, Hodgkin's disease, neuroblastoma, malignant lymphomas, Wilms' tumor, and rhabdomyosarcoma

**Usual Dosage** Refer to individual protocols as dosages vary with protocol used. Adjustments are made depending upon clinical and hematological response and upon adverse reactions

Children: I.V. (maximum single dose: 2 mg):
- ≤10 kg or BSA <1 m$^2$: 0.05 mg/kg once weekly
- 2 mg/m$^2$; may repeat every week

Adults: I.V.: 0.4-1.4 mg/m$^2$ (up to 2 mg maximum); may repeat every week

**Mechanism of Action** Binds to microtubular protein of the mitotic spindle causing metaphase arrest; cell-cycle phase specific in the M and S phases

**Local Anesthetic/Vasoconstrictor Precautions** No information available to require special precautions

**Effects on Dental Treatment** No effects or complications reported

**Other Adverse Effects**

>10%:
- Dermatologic: Alopecia: Occurs in 20% to 70% of patients
- Local: Extravasation: Vincristine is a vesicant and can cause tissue irritation and necrosis if infiltrated; if extravasation occurs, follow institutional policy, which may include hyaluronidase and hot compresses

1% to 10%:
- Cardiovascular: Hypotension (orthostatic)
- Central nervous system: Neurotoxicity, seizures, CNS depression, cranial nerve paralysis
- Dermatologic: Skin rash
- Endocrine & metabolic: Hyperuricemia, SIADH
- Gastrointestinal: Weight loss, paralytic ileus, constipation and possible paralytic ileus secondary to neurologic toxicity; oral ulceration, nausea, diarrhea, vomiting, bloating, abdominal cramps, anorexia, metallic taste
- Local: Phlebitis
- Hematologic: Occasionally mild leukopenia and thrombocytopenia may occur
- Neuromuscular & skeletal: Numbness, motor difficulties, jaw pain, leg pain, myalgias, cramping, weakness

<1%:
- Cardiovascular: Hypertension, hypotension
- Central nervous system: Headache, fever; alterations in mental status such as depression, confusion, or insomnia. Cranial nerve palsies, headaches, jaw pain, optic atrophy with blindness have been reported. Intrathecal administration of vincristine has uniformly caused death, vincristine should **never** be administered by this route. Neurologic effects of vincristine may be additive with those of other neurotoxic agents and spinal cord irradiation.
- Dermatologic: Photophobia, rash
- Endocrine & metabolic: SIADH: Rarely occurs, but may be related to the neurologic toxicity; may cause symptomatic hyponatremia with seizures; the increase in serum ADH concentration usually subsides within 2-3 days after onset
- Gastrointestinal: Stomatitis, weight loss; constipation, paralytic ileus, and urinary tract disturbances may occur. All patients should be on a prophylactic bowel management regimen.
- Neuromuscular & skeletal: Peripheral neuropathy: Frequently the dose-limiting toxicity of vincristine. Most frequent in patients >40 years of age; occurs usually after an average of 3 weekly doses, but may occur after just one dose. Manifested as loss of the deep tendon reflexes in the lower extremities, tingling, pain, paresthesias of the fingers and toes (stocking glove sensation), and "foot drop" or "wrist drop".

**Drug Uptake**

Absorption: Oral: Poor

Serum half-life: Terminal: 24 hours

**Pregnancy Risk Factor** D

**Generic Available** Yes

## Vinorelbine (vi NOR el been)

**U.S. Brand Names** Navelbine®

**Therapeutic Category** Antineoplastic Agent, Mitotic Inhibitor

**Use** Treatment of nonsmall cell lung cancer (as a single agent or in combination with cisplatin)

**Unlabeled use:** Breast cancer, ovarian carcinoma (cisplatin-resistant), Hodgkin's disease

**Usual Dosage** Varies depending upon clinical and hematological response (refer to individual protocols)

Adults: I.V.: 30 mg/m$^2$ every 7 days

**Mechanism of Action** Semisynthetic *Vinca* alkaloid which binds to tubulin and inhibits microtubule formation, therefore, arresting the cell at metaphase by

(Continued)

## Vinorelbine *(Continued)*

disrupting the formation of the mitotic spindle; it is specific for the M and S phases; binds to microtubular protein of the mitotic spindle causing metaphase arrest

**Local Anesthetic/Vasoconstrictor Precautions** No information available to require special precautions

**Effects on Dental Treatment** No effects or complications reported

**Other Adverse Effects**

1% to 10%:

Cardiovascular: Chest pain

Central nervous system: Fatigue

Endocrine & metabolic: SIADH

Gastrointestinal: Nausea, vomiting, constipation

Genitourinary: Hemorrhagic cystitis

Hematologic: Neutropenia, leukopenia (nadir 7-8 days with recovery by days 15-17), anemia

Hepatic: Transient elevation in liver enzymes

Local: Phlebitis at sight of infusion, vesicant with extravasation

Neuromuscular & skeletal: Decreased deep tendon reflexes, tumor pain, jaw pain, parasthesia

Respiratory: Acute reversible dyspnea, hypoxemia, interstitial pulmonary infiltrates

<1%:

Cardiovascular: Myocardial infarction

Dermatologic: Alopecia

Hematologic: Thrombocytopenia

**Drug Uptake**

Absorption: Not reliably absorbed from the GI tract and must be given I.V.

Serum half-life (triphasic): Terminal: 27.7-43.6 hours

**Pregnancy Risk Factor** D

**Generic Available** No

- **Vioform® [OTC]** *see* Clioquinol *on page 260*
- **Viokase®** *see* Pancrelipase *on page 763*
- **Vioxx®** *see* Rofecoxib *on page 895*
- **Vira-A®** *see* Vidarabine *on page 1045*
- **Viracept®** *see* Nelfinavir *on page 708*
- **Viractin® [OTC]** *see* Tetracaine *on page 964*
- **Viramune®** *see* Nevirapine *on page 715*
- **Virazole® Aerosol** *see* Ribavirin *on page 884*
- **Virilon®** *see* Methyltestosterone *on page 662*
- **Viroptic®** *see* Trifluridine *on page 1018*
- **Viscoat®** *see* Chondroitin Sulfate-Sodium Hyaluronate *on page 246*
- **Visine® Extra Ophthalmic [OTC]** *see* Tetrahydrozoline *on page 967*
- **Visine® L.R. Ophthalmic [OTC]** *see* Oxymetazoline *on page 755*
- **Visken®** *see* Pindolol *on page 806*
- **Vistacon®** *see* Hydroxyzine *on page 518*
- **Vistaject-25®** *see* Hydroxyzine *on page 518*
- **Vistaject-50®** *see* Hydroxyzine *on page 518*
- **Vistaquel®** *see* Hydroxyzine *on page 518*
- **Vistaril®** *see* Hydroxyzine *on page 518*
- **Vistazine®** *see* Hydroxyzine *on page 518*
- **Vistide®** *see* Cidofovir *on page 248*
- **Vita-C® [OTC]** *see* Ascorbic Acid *on page 97*
- **VitaCarn® Oral** *see* Levocarnitine *on page 580*
- **Vital HN® [OTC]** *see* Enteral Nutritional Products *on page 371*

## Vitamin A (VYE ta min aye)

**U.S. Brand Names** Aquasol® A [OTC]

**Therapeutic Category** Vitamin, Fat Soluble

**Use** Dental and Medical: Treatment and prevention of vitamin A deficiency

**Usual Dosage**

RDA:

<1 year: 375 mcg

1-3 years: 400 mcg

4-6 years: 500 mcg*

7-10 years: 700 mcg*

>10 years: 800-1000 mcg*

Male: 1000 mcg

Female: 800 mcg

*mcg retinol equivalent (0.3 mcg retinol = 1 unit vitamin A)

Vitamin A supplementation in measles (recommendation of the World Health Organization): Children: Oral: Give as a single dose; repeat the next day and at 4 weeks for children with ophthalmologic evidence of vitamin A deficiency:
- 6 months to 1 year: 100,000 units
- >1 year: 200,000 units

**Note:** Use of vitamin A in measles is recommended only for patients 6 months to 2 years of age hospitalized with measles and its complications **or** patients >6 months of age who have any of the following risk factors and who are not already receiving vitamin A: immunodeficiency, ophthalmologic evidence of vitamin A deficiency including night blindness, Bitot's spots or evidence of xerophthalmia, impaired intestinal absorption, moderate to severe malnutrition including that associated with eating disorders, or recent immigration from areas where high mortality rates from measles have been observed

**Note:** Monitor patients closely; dosages >25,000 units/kg have been associated with toxicity

Severe deficiency with xerophthalmia: Oral:
- Children 1-8 years: 5000-10,000 units/kg/day for 5 days or until recovery occurs
- Children >8 years and Adults: 500,000 units/day for 3 days, then 50,000 units/day for 14 days, then 10,000-20,000 units/day for 2 months

Deficiency (without corneal changes): Oral:
- Children 1-8 years: 200,000 units every 4-6 months
- Children >8 years and Adults: 100,000 units/day for 3 days then 50,000 units/day for 14 days

Malabsorption syndrome (prophylaxis): Children >8 years and Adults: Oral: 10,000-50,000 units/day of water miscible product

Dietary supplement: Oral:
- Children:
  - 6 months to 3 years: 1500-2000 units/day
  - 4-6 years: 2500 units/day
  - 7-10 years: 3300-3500 units/day
- Children >10 years and Adults: 4000-5000 units/day

**Mechanism of Action** Needed for bone development, growth, visual adaptation to darkness, testicular and ovarian function, and as a cofactor in many biochemical processes

**Local Anesthetic/Vasoconstrictor Precautions** No information available to require special precautions

**Effects on Dental Treatment** No effects or complications reported

**Other Adverse Effects** 1% to 10%:
- Central nervous system: Irritability, vertigo, lethargy, malaise, fever, headache
- Dermatologic: Drying or cracking of skin
- Endocrine & metabolic: Hypercalcemia
- Gastrointestinal: Weight loss
- Ocular: Visual changes
- Miscellaneous: Hypervitaminosis A

**Contraindications** Hypervitaminosis A, hypersensitivity to vitamin A or any component

**Warnings/Precautions** Evaluate other sources of vitamin A while receiving this product; patients receiving >25,000 units/day should be closely monitored for toxicity

**Drug Interactions**
- Decreased effect: Cholestyramine decreases absorption of vitamin A; neomycin and mineral oil may also interfere with vitamin A absorption
- Increased toxicity: Retinoids may have additive adverse effects

**Drug Uptake** Absorption: Vitamin A in dosages **not** exceeding physiologic replacement is well absorbed after oral administration; water miscible preparations are absorbed more rapidly than oil preparations; large oral doses, conditions of fat malabsorption, low protein intake, or hepatic or pancreatic disease reduces oral absorption

**Pregnancy Risk Factor** A (X if dose exceeds RDA recommendation)

**Dosage Forms**
- Capsule: 10,000 units [OTC], 25,000 units, 50,000 units
- Drops, oral (water miscible) [OTC]: 5000 units/0.1 mL (30 mL)
- Injection: 50,000 units/mL (2 mL)
- Tablet [OTC]: 5000 units

**Generic Available** Yes

## Vitamin A and Vitamin D (VYE ta min aye & VYE ta min dee)

**U.S. Brand Names** A and D™ Ointment [OTC]

**Therapeutic Category** Protectant, Topical; Topical Skin Product

(Continued)

## Vitamin A and Vitamin D *(Continued)*

**Use** Temporary relief of discomfort due to chapped skin, diaper rash, minor burns, abrasions, as well as irritations associated with ostomy skin care

**Usual Dosage** Topical: Apply locally with gentle massage as needed

**Local Anesthetic/Vasoconstrictor Precautions** No information available to require special precautions

**Effects on Dental Treatment** No effects or complications reported

**Other Adverse Effects** Irritation

**Pregnancy Risk Factor** B

**Generic Available** Yes

♦ **Vitamin $B_5$** *see* Pantothenic Acid *on page 764*

## Vitamin B Complex (VYE ta min bee KOM pleks)

**U.S. Brand Names** Apatate® [OTC]; Gevrabon® [OTC]; Lederplex® [OTC]; Lipovite® [OTC]; Mega B® [OTC]; Megaton™ [OTC]; Mucoplex® [OTC]; NeoVadrin® B Complex [OTC]; Orexin® [OTC]; Surbex® [OTC]

**Therapeutic Category** Vitamin, Water Soluble

**Use** Supportive nutritional supplementation in conditions in which water-soluble vitamins are required like GI disorders, chronic alcoholism, pregnancy, severe burns, and recovery from surgery

**Usual Dosage** Dosage is usually 1 tablet or capsule/day; please refer to package insert

**Local Anesthetic/Vasoconstrictor Precautions** No information available to require special precautions

**Effects on Dental Treatment** No effects or complications reported

**Generic Available** Yes

## Vitamin B Complex With Vitamin C

(VYE ta min bee KOM pleks with VYE ta min see)

**U.S. Brand Names** Allbee® With C [OTC]; Surbex-T® Filmtabs® [OTC]; Surbex® with C Filmtabs® [OTC]; Thera-Combex® H-P Kapseals® [OTC]; Vicon-C® [OTC]

**Therapeutic Category** Vitamin, Water Soluble

**Use** Supportive nutritional supplementation in conditions in which water-soluble vitamins are required like GI disorders, chronic alcoholism, pregnancy, severe burns, and recovery from surgery

**Usual Dosage** Adults: Oral: 1 every day

**Local Anesthetic/Vasoconstrictor Precautions** No information available to require special precautions

**Effects on Dental Treatment** No effects or complications reported

**Generic Available** Yes

## Vitamin B Complex With Vitamin C and Folic Acid

(VYE ta min bee KOM pleks with VYE ta min see & FOE lik AS id)

**U.S. Brand Names** Berocca®; Nephrocaps® [OTC]

**Therapeutic Category** Vitamin, Water Soluble

**Use** Supportive nutritional supplementation in conditions in which water-soluble vitamins are required like GI disorders, chronic alcoholism, pregnancy, severe burns, and recovery from surgery

**Usual Dosage** Adults: Oral: 1 every day

**Local Anesthetic/Vasoconstrictor Precautions** No information available to require special precautions

**Effects on Dental Treatment** No effects or complications reported

**Generic Available** Yes

## Vitamin E (VYE ta min ee)

**U.S. Brand Names** Amino-Opti-E® [OTC]; Aquasol E® [OTC]; E-Complex-600® [OTC]; E-Vitamin® [OTC]; Vita-Plus® E Softgels® [OTC]; Vitec® [OTC]; Vite E® Creme [OTC]

**Therapeutic Category** Vitamin, Fat Soluble

**Use** Dental and Medical: Prevention and treatment of hemolytic anemia secondary to vitamin E deficiency, dietary supplement

**Usual Dosage** One unit of vitamin E = 1 mg *dl*-alpha-tocopherol acetate. Oral:

Vitamin E deficiency:

- Children (with malabsorption syndrome): 1 unit/kg/day of water miscible vitamin E (to raise plasma tocopherol concentrations to the normal range within 2 months and to maintain normal plasma concentrations)
- Adults: 60-75 units/day

Prevention of vitamin E deficiency:

- Adults: 30 units/day

Prevention of retinopathy of prematurity or BPD secondary to $O_2$ therapy: (American Academy of Pediatrics considers this use investigational and routine use is not recommended):

Retinopathy prophylaxis: 15-30 units/kg/day to maintain plasma levels between 1.5-2 μg/mL (may need as high as 100 units/kg/day)

Cystic fibrosis, beta-thalassemia, sickle cell anemia may require higher daily maintenance doses:

Cystic fibrosis: 100-400 units/day

Beta-thalassemia: 750 units/day

Sickle cell: 450 units/day

Recommended daily allowance:

Children:

1-3 years: 6 mg (9 units)

4-10 years: 7 mg (10.5 units)

Children >11 years and Adults:

Male: 10 mg (15 units)

Female: 8 mg (12 units)

Topical: Apply a thin layer over affected area

**Mechanism of Action** Prevents oxidation of vitamin A and C; protects polyunsaturated fatty acids in membranes from attack by free radicals and protects red blood cells against hemolysis

**Local Anesthetic/Vasoconstrictor Precautions** No information available to require special precautions

**Effects on Dental Treatment** No effects or complications reported

**Other Adverse Effects** <1%:

Central nervous system: Headache

Dermatologic: Contact dermatitis with topical preparation

Gastrointestinal: Nausea, diarrhea, intestinal cramps

Genitourinary: Gonadal dysfunction

Neuromuscular & skeletal: Weakness

Ocular: Blurred vision

**Contraindications** Hypersensitivity to drug or any components

**Warnings/Precautions** May induce vitamin K deficiency; necrotizing enterocolitis has been associated with oral administration of large dosages (eg, >200 units/day) of a hyperosmolar vitamin E preparation in low birth weight infants

**Drug Interactions**

Decreased absorption with mineral oil

Delayed absorption of iron

Increased effect of oral anticoagulants

**Drug Uptake**

Absorption: Oral: Depends upon the presence of bile; absorption is reduced in conditions of malabsorption, in low birth weight premature infants, and as dosage increases; water miscible preparations are better absorbed than oil preparations

**Pregnancy Risk Factor** A (C if dose exceeds RDA recommendation)

**Dosage Forms**

Capsule: 100 units, 200 units, 330 mg, 400 units, 500 units, 600 units, 1000 units

Capsule, water miscible: 73.5 mg, 147 mg, 165 mg, 330 mg, 400 units

Cream: 50 mg/g (15 g, 30 g, 60 g, 75 g, 120 g, 454 g)

Drops, oral: 50 mg/mL (12 mL, 30 mL)

Liquid, topical: 10 mL, 15 mL, 30 mL, 60 mL

Lotion: 120 mL

Oil: 15 mL, 30 mL, 60 mL

Ointment, topical: 30 mg/g (45 g, 60 g)

Tablet: 200 units, 400 units

**Generic Available** Yes

- **Vitamin, Multiple, Prenatal** *see* Vitamins, Multiple *on this page*
- **Vitamin, Multiple, Therapeutic** *see* Vitamins, Multiple *on this page*
- **Vitamin, Multiple With Iron** *see* Vitamins, Multiple *on this page*

## Vitamins, Multiple (VYE ta mins MUL ti pul)

**U.S. Brand Names** Adeflor®; Allbee® With C; Becotin® Pulvules®; Cefol® Filmtab®; Chromagen® OB [OTC]; Eldercaps® [OTC]; Filibon® [OTC]; Florvite®; LKV-Drops® [OTC]; Multi Vit® Drops [OTC]; M.V.I.®; M.V.I.®-12; M.V.I.® Concentrate; M.V.I.® Pediatric; Natabec® [OTC]; Natabec® FA [OTC]; Natabec® Rx; Natalins® [OTC]; Natalins® Rx; NeoVadrin® [OTC]; Niferex®-PN; Poly-Vi-Flor®; Poly-Vi-Sol® [OTC]; Pramet® FA; Pramilet® FA; Prenavite® [OTC]; Secran®; Stresstabs® 600 Advanced Formula Tablets [OTC]; Stuartnatal® 1 + 1; Stuart Prenatal® [OTC]; Therabid® [OTC]; Theragran® [OTC]; Theragran® Hematinic®; Theragran® Liquid [OTC]; Theragran-M® [OTC]; Tri-Vi-Flor®; Unicap® [OTC]; Vicon Forte®; Vicon® Plus [OTC]; Vi-Daylin® [OTC]; Vi-Daylin/F®

(Continued)

## Multivitamin Products Available

| Product | Content Given Per | A IU | D IU | E IU | C mg | FA mg | $B_1$ mg | $B_2$ mg | $B_3$ mg | $B_6$ mg | $B_{12}$ mcg | Other |
|---|---|---|---|---|---|---|---|---|---|---|---|---|
| Theragran® | 5 mL liquid | 10,000 | 400 | | 200 | | 10 | 10 | 100 | 4.1 | 5 | $B_5$ 21.4 mg |
| Vi-Daylin® | 1 mL drops | 1500 | 400 | 4.1 | 35 | | 0.5 | 0.6 | 8 | 0.4 | 1.5 | Alcohol <0.5% |
| Vi-Daylin® Iron | 1 mL | 1500 | 400 | 4.1 | 35 | | 0.5 | 0.6 | 8 | 0.4 | | Fe 10 mg |
| Albee® with C | tablet | | | | 300 | | 15 | 10.2 | | 5 | | Niacinamide 50 mg, pantothenic acid 10 mg |
| Vitamin B complex | tablet | | | | | 400 mcg | 1.5 | 1.7 | | 2 | 6 | Niacinamide 20 mg |
| Hexavitamin | cap/tab | 5000 | 400 | | 75 | | 2 | 3 | 20 | | | |
| Iberet-Folic-500® | tablet | | | | 500 | 0.8 | 6 | 6 | 30 | 5 | 25 | $B_5$ 10 mg, Fe 105 mg |
| Stuartnatal® 1+1 | tablet | 4000 | 400 | 11 | 120 | 1 | 1.5 | 3 | 20 | 10 | 12 | Cu, Zn 25 mg, Fe 65 mg, Ca 200 mg |
| Theragran-M® | tablet | 5000 | 400 | 30 | 90 | 0.4 | 3 | 3.4 | 30 | 3 | 9 | Cl, Cr, I, K, $B_5$ 10 mg, Mg, Mn, Mo, P, Se, Zn 15 mg, Fe 27 mg, biotin 30 mcg, beta-carotene 1250 IU |
| Vi-Daylin® | tablet | 2500 | 400 | 15 | 60 | 0.3 | 1.05 | 1.2 | 13.5 | 1.05 | 4.5 | |
| M.V.I.®-12 injection | 5 mL | 3300 | 200 | 10 | 100 | 0.4 | 3 | 3.6 | 40 | 4 | 5 | $B_5$ 15 mg, biotin 60 mcg |
| M.V.I.®-12 unit vial | 20 mL | | | | | | | | | | | |
| M.V.I.® pediatric powder | 5 mL | 2300 | 400 | 7 | 80 | 0.14 | 1.2 | 1.4 | 17 | 1 | 1 | $B_5$ 5 mg, biotin 20 mcg, vitamin K 200 mcg |

## Vitamins, Multiple *(Continued)*

**Therapeutic Category** Vitamin

**Synonyms** B Complex; B Complex With C; Children's Vitamins; Hexavitamin; Multiple Vitamins; Multivitamins/Fluoride; Parenteral Multiple Vitamin; Prenatal Vitamins; Therapeutic Multivitamins; Vitamin, Multiple, Prenatal; Vitamin, Multiple, Therapeutic; Vitamin, Multiple With Iron

**Use** Dental and Medical: Dietary supplement

**Usual Dosage**

Infants 1.5-3 kg: I.V.: 3.25 mL/24 hours (M.V.I.® Pediatric)

Children:

Oral:

≤2 years: Drops: 1 mL/day (premature infants may get 0.5-1 mL/day)

>2 years: Chew 1 tablet/day

≥4 years: 5 mL/day liquid

I.V.: >3 kg and <11 years: 5 mL/24 hours (M.V.I.® Pediatric)

Adults:

Oral: 1 tablet/day or 5 mL/day liquid

I.V.: >11 years: 5 mL of vials 1 and 2 (M.V.I.®-12)/one TPN bag/day

I.V. solutions: 10 mL/24 hours (M.V.I.®-12)

**Local Anesthetic/Vasoconstrictor Precautions** No information available to require special precautions

**Effects on Dental Treatment** No effects or complications reported

**Other Adverse Effects** 1% to 10%: Miscellaneous: Hypervitaminosis; refer to individual vitamin entries for individual reactions

**Contraindications** Hypersensitivity to product components

**Warnings/Precautions** RDA values are not requirements, but are recommended daily intakes of certain essential nutrients; periodic dental exams should be performed to check for dental fluorosis; use with caution in patients with severe renal or liver failure

**Drug Interactions** No data reported

**Pregnancy Risk Factor** A (C if used in doses above RDA recommendation)

**Dosage Forms** See table.

**Generic Available** Yes

- **Vitaneed™ [OTC]** *see* Enteral Nutritional Products *on page 371*
- **Vita-Plus® E Softgels® [OTC]** *see* Vitamin E *on page 1050*
- **Vitec® [OTC]** *see* Vitamin E *on page 1050*
- **Vite E® Creme [OTC]** *see* Vitamin E *on page 1050*
- **Vitrasert®** *see* Ganciclovir *on page 462*
- **Vitravene®** *see* Fomivirsen *on page 454*
- **Vivactil®** *see* Protriptyline *on page 862*
- **Viva-Drops® Solution [OTC]** *see* Artificial Tears *on page 97*
- **Vivelle™ Transdermal** *see* Estradiol *on page 387*
- **Vivonex® [OTC]** *see* Enteral Nutritional Products *on page 371*
- **Vivonex® T.E.N. [OTC]** *see* Enteral Nutritional Products *on page 371*
- **Vivotif Berna™ Oral** *see* Typhoid Vaccine *on page 1032*
- **V-Lax® [OTC]** *see* Psyllium *on page 865*
- **VLB** *see* Vinblastine *on page 1046*
- **VM-26** *see* Teniposide *on page 956*
- **Volmax®** *see* Albuterol *on page 43*
- **Voltaren® Ophthalmic** *see* Diclofenac *on page 320*
- **Voltaren® Oral** *see* Diclofenac *on page 320*
- **Voltaren-XR® Oral** *see* Diclofenac *on page 320*
- **Vontrol®** *see* Diphenidol *on page 340*
- **VōSol® HC Otic** *see* Acetic Acid, Propylene Glycol Diacetate, and Hydrocortisone *on page 34*
- **Vumon Injection** *see* Teniposide *on page 956*
- **V.V.S.®** *see* Sulfabenzamide, Sulfacetamide, and Sulfathiazole *on page 939*
- **Vytone® Topical** *see* Iodoquinol and Hydrocortisone *on page 547*
- **VZIG** *see* Varicella-Zoster Immune Globulin (Human) *on page 1041*

## Warfarin (WAR far in)

**Related Information**

Cardiovascular Diseases *on page 1066*

Dental Drug Interactions: Update on Drug Combinations Requiring Special Considerations *on page 1225*

Dicumarol *on page 322*

**U.S. Brand Names** Coumadin®

**Canadian Brand Names** Warfilone®

## Warfarin *(Continued)*

**Therapeutic Category** Anticoagulant (Warfarin-like)

**Use** Prophylaxis and treatment of venous thrombosis, pulmonary embolism and thromboembolic disorders; atrial fibrillation with risk of embolism and as an adjunct in the prophylaxis of systemic embolism after myocardial infarction

**Unlabeled use:** Prevention of recurrent transient ischemic attacks and to reduce risk of recurrent myocardial infarction

**Usual Dosage**

Oral:

Children: 0.05-0.34 mg/kg/day; children <12 months of age may require doses at or near the high end of this range; consistent anticoagulation may be difficult to maintain in children <5 years of age

Adults: 5-15 mg/day for 2-5 days, then adjust dose according to results of prothrombin time; usual maintenance dose ranges from 2-10 mg/day

I.V. (administer as a slow bolus injection): 2-5 mg/day

**Mechanism of Action** Interferes with hepatic synthesis of vitamin K-dependent coagulation factors (II, VII, IX, X)

**Drugs Which Increase Bleeding Tendency With Warfarin**

| Inhibit Platelet Aggregation | Inhibit Procoagulant Factors | Ulcerogenic Drugs |
|---|---|---|
| Cephalosporins<br>Dipyridamole<br>Indomethacin<br>Oxyphenbutazone<br>Penicillin, parenteral<br>Phenylbutazone<br>Salicylates<br>Sulfinpyrazone | Antimetabolites<br>Quinidine<br>Quinine<br>Salicylates | Adrenal corticosteroids<br>Indomethacin<br>Oxyphenbutazone<br>Phenylbutazone<br>Potassium products<br>Salicylates |

Use of these agents with oral anticoagulants may increase the chances of hemorrhage.

**Drugs and Mechanisms Which Decrease Anticoagulant Effects of Warfarin**

| Induction of Enzymes | | Increased Procoagulant Factors | Decreased Drug Absorption | Other |
|---|---|---|---|---|
| Barbiturates<br>Carbamazepine<br>Glutethimide<br>Griseofulvin | Nafcillin<br>Phenytoin<br>Rifampin | Estrogens<br>Oral contraceptives<br>Vitamin K (including nutritional supplements) | Aluminum hydroxide<br>Cholestyramine*<br>Colestipol* | Ethchlorvynol<br>Griseofulvin<br>Spironolactone†<br>Sucralfate |

Decreased anticoagulant effect may occur when these drugs are administered with oral anticoagulants.

*Cholestyramine and colestipol may increase the anticoagulant effect by binding vitamin K in the gut; yet, the decreased drug absorption appears to be of more concern.

†Diuretic-induced hemoconcentration with subsequent concentration of clotting factors has been reported to decrease the effects of oral anticoagulants.

**Drugs and Mechanisms Which Enhance Anticoagulant Effects of Warfarin**

| Decrease Vitamin K | Displace Anticoagulant | Inhibit Metabolism | Other |
|---|---|---|---|
| Oral antibiotics<br>Can ↑ or ↓ an INR<br>Check an INR 3 days after a patient begins antibiotics to see the INR value and adjust the warfarin dose accordingly | Chloral hydrate<br>Clofibrate<br>Diazoxide<br>Ethacrynic acid<br>Miconazole<br>Nalidixic acid<br>Phenylbutazone<br>Salicylates<br>Sulfonamides<br>Sulfonylureas<br>Triclofos | Acetaminophen<br>Alcohol<br>(acute ingestion)*<br>Allopurinol<br>Amiodarone<br>Chloramphenicol<br>Chlorpropamide<br>Cimetidine<br>Co-trimoxazole<br>Disulfiram<br>Metronidazole<br>Phenylbutazone<br>Phenytoin<br>Propoxyphene<br>Sulfinpyrazone<br>Sulfonamides<br>Tolbutamide | Acetaminophen<br>Anabolic steroids<br>Clofibrate<br>Danazol<br>Erythromycin<br>Gemfibrozil<br>Glucagon<br>Influenza vaccine<br>Ketoconazole<br>Propranolol<br>Ranitidine<br>Sulindac<br>Thyroid drugs |

* The hypoprothrombinemic effect of oral anticoagulants has been reported to be both increased and decreased during chronic and excessive alcohol ingestion. Data are insufficient to predict the direction of this interaction in alcoholic patients.

**Local Anesthetic/Vasoconstrictor Precautions** No information available to require special precautions

**Effects on Dental Treatment** Signs of warfarin overdose may first appear as bleeding from gingival tissue; consultation with prescribing physician is advisable prior to surgery to determine temporary dose reduction or withdrawal of medication

**Other Adverse Effects**

1% to 10%:

Dermatologic: Skin lesions, alopecia, skin necrosis

Gastrointestinal: Anorexia, nausea, vomiting, stomach cramps, diarrhea

Hematologic: Hemorrhage; leukopenia, unrecognized bleeding sites (eg, colon cancer) may be uncovered by anticoagulation

Respiratory: Hemoptysis

<1%:

Central nervous system: Fever

Dermatologic: Skin rash, discolored toes (blue or purple)

Gastrointestinal: Mouth ulcers

Hematologic: Agranulocytosis

Hepatic: Hepatotoxicity

Renal: Renal damage

**Drug Interactions** See tables.

**Drug Uptake**

Onset of anticoagulation effect: Oral: Within 36-72 hours

Absorption: Oral: Rapid

Serum half-life: 42 hours, highly variable among individuals

**Pregnancy Risk Factor** D

**Generic Available** Yes: Tablet


- **Wart-Off® [OTC]** *see* Salicylic Acid *on page 900*
- **4-Way® Long Acting Nasal Solution [OTC]** *see* Oxymetazoline *on page 755*
- **Wellbutrin®** *see* Bupropion *on page 160*
- **Wellbutrin® SR** *see* Bupropion *on page 160*
- **Wellcovorin®** *see* Leucovorin *on page 577*
- **Whitfield's Ointment [OTC]** *see* Benzoic Acid and Salicylic Acid *on page 130*
- **Whole Root Rauwolfia** *see* Rauwolfia Serpentina *on page 880*
- **Wigraine®** *see* Ergotamine *on page 382*
- **40 Winks® [OTC]** *see* Diphenhydramine *on page 338*
- **Winstrol®** *see* Stanozolol *on page 932*
- **Wolfina®** *see* Rauwolfia Serpentina *on page 880*
- **WR2721** *see* Amifostine *on page 59*
- **Wycillin®** *see* Penicillin G Procaine *on page 775*
- **Wydase® Injection** *see* Hyaluronidase *on page 501*
- **Wygesic®** *see* Propoxyphene and Acetaminophen *on page 855*
- **Wymox®** *see* Amoxicillin *on page 76*
- **Wytensin®** *see* Guanabenz *on page 483*
- **Xalatan®** *see* Latanoprost *on page 574*
- **Xanax®** *see* Alprazolam *on page 50*
- **Xeloda™** *see* Capecitabine *on page 180*
- **X-Prep® Liquid [OTC]** *see* Senna *on page 909*
- **X-seb® T [OTC]** *see* Coal Tar and Salicylic Acid *on page 270*
- **Xylocaine®** *see* Lidocaine *on page 586*
- **Xylocaine® With Epinephrine** *see* Lidocaine and Epinephrine *on page 587*


## Xylometazoline (zye loe met AZ oh leen)

**U.S. Brand Names** Otrivin® [OTC]

**Therapeutic Category** Adrenergic Agonist Agent; Nasal Agent, Vasoconstrictor

**Use** Symptomatic relief of nasal and nasopharyngeal mucosal congestion

**Usual Dosage**

Children 2-12 years: Instill 2-3 drops (0.05%) in each nostril every 8-10 hours

Children >12 years and Adults: Instill 2-3 drops or sprays (0.1%) in each nostril every 8-10 hours

**Mechanism of Action** Stimulates alpha-adrenergic receptors in the arterioles of the conjunctiva and the nasal mucosa to produce vasoconstriction

(Continued)

## Xylometazoline *(Continued)*

**Local Anesthetic/Vasoconstrictor Precautions** No information available to require special precautions

**Effects on Dental Treatment** No effects or complications reported

**Other Adverse Effects** 1% to 10%:

Cardiovascular: Palpitations
Central nervous system: Drowsiness, dizziness, seizures, headache
Ocular: Blurred vision, ocular irritation, photophobia
Miscellaneous: Sweating

**Drug Interactions** No data reported

**Drug Uptake**

Onset of action: Intranasal: Local vasoconstriction occurs within 5-10 minutes
Duration: 5-6 hours

**Pregnancy Risk Factor** C

**Generic Available** Yes

- **Yellow Mercuric Oxide** *see* Mercuric Oxide *on page 637*
- **Yocon®** *see* Yohimbine *on this page*
- **Yodoxin®** *see* Iodoquinol *on page 546*

## Yohimbine (yo HIM bine)

**U.S. Brand Names** Aphrodyne™; Dayto Himbin®; Yocon®; Yohimex™

**Therapeutic Category** Impotency Agent

**Use** No FDA sanctioned indications

**Usual Dosage** Adults: Oral: Impotence: 5.4 mg 3 times/day

**Mechanism of Action** Derived from the bark of the yohimbe tree (Pausingstalia yohimbe), this indole alkaloid produces an alpha$_2$-adrenergic blockade; also is a weak MAO inhibitor; parasympathetic tone is also decreased

**Local Anesthetic/Vasoconstrictor Precautions** No information available to require special precautions

**Effects on Dental Treatment** No effects or complications reported

**Other Adverse Effects**

Cardiovascular: Tachycardia, bradycardia, hypertension, hypotension (orthostatic), flushing, shock, sinus tachycardia, vasodilation, sinus bradycardia
Central nervous system: Anxiety, mania, hallucinations, irritability, dizziness, psychosis, insomnia, headache, panic attacks
Gastrointestinal: Nausea, vomiting, anorexia
Hematologic: Neutropenia, agranulocytosis
Neuromuscular & skeletal: Tremors, paresthesia
Ocular: Lacrimation, mydriasis
Respiratory: Bronchospasm, sinusitis
Miscellaneous: Antidiuretic action, salivation, diaphoresis

**Drug Interactions** Antidepressants, other mood-modifying drugs

**Drug Uptake**

Absorption: Oral: 33%
Half-life: 0.6 hour

**Generic Available** Yes

- **Yohimex™** *see* Yohimbine *on this page*
- **Yutopar®** *see* Ritodrine *on page 892*

## Zafirlukast (za FIR loo kast)

**U.S. Brand Names** Accolate®

**Therapeutic Category** Leukotriene Receptor Antagonist

**Use** Prophylaxis and chronic treatment of asthma in adults and children ≥12 years of age

**Usual Dosage** Oral:

Children <12 years: Safety and effectiveness has not been established
Adults: 20 mg twice daily
Elderly: The mean dose (mg/kg) normalized AUC and $C_{max}$ increase and plasma clearance decreases with increasing age. In patients >65 years of age, there is an 2-3 fold greater $C_{max}$ and AUC compared to younger adults

**Mechanism of Action** Zafirlukast is a selectively and competitive leukotriene-receptor antagonist (LTRA) of leukotriene D4 and E4 (LTD4 and LTE4), components of slow-reacting substance of anaphylaxis (SRSA). Cysteinyl leukotriene production and receptor occupation have been correlated with the pathophysiology of asthma, including airway edema, smooth muscle constriction and altered cellular activity associated with the inflammatory process, which contribute to the signs and symptoms of asthma.

**Local Anesthetic/Vasoconstrictor Precautions** No information available to require special precautions

**Effects on Dental Treatment** No effects or complications reported

**Other Adverse Effects**

>10%: Central nervous system: Headache (12.9%)

1% to 10%:

Central nervous system: Dizziness, pain, fever

Gastrointestinal: Nausea, diarrhea, abdominal pain, vomiting, dyspepsia

Neuromuscular & skeletal: Myalgia, weakness

**Drug Interactions** Cytochrome P-450 2C9 and 3A4 isoenzyme inhibitor

Decreased effect:

Erythromycin: Coadministration of a single dose of zafirlukast with erythromycin to steady state results in decreased mean plasma levels of zafirlukast by 40% due to a decrease in zafirlukast bioavailability.

Theophylline: Coadministration of zafirlukast at steady state with a single dose of liquid theophylline preparations results in decreased mean plasma levels of zafirlukast by 30%, but no effects on plasma theophylline levels were observed.

Increased effect: Aspirin: Coadministration of zafirlukast with aspirin results in mean increased plasma levels of zafirlukast by 45%

Increased toxicity: Warfarin: Coadministration of zafirlukast with warfarin results in a clinically significant increase in prothrombin time (PT). Closely monitor prothrombin times of patients on oral warfarin anticoagulant therapy and zafirlukast, and adjust anticoagulant dose accordingly.

**Drug Uptake**

Absorption: Food reduces bioavailability by 40%

Serum half-life: 10 hours

Time to peak serum concentration: 3 hours

**Pregnancy Risk Factor** B

**Dosage Forms** Tablet: 20 mg

♦ **Zagam®** *see* Sparfloxacin *on page 929*

## Zalcitabine (zal SITE a been)

**Related Information**

HIV Infection and AIDS *on page 1085*

Systemic Viral Diseases *on page 1115*

**U.S. Brand Names** Hivid®

**Therapeutic Category** Antiviral Agent, Oral

**Use** The FDA has approved zalcitabine for use in the treatment of HIV infections only in combination with zidovudine in adult patients with advanced HIV disease demonstrating a significant clinical or immunological deterioration

**Usual Dosage** Safety and efficacy in children <13 years of age have not been established

Adults: Monotherapy: 0.75 mg every 8 hours (2.25 mg total daily dose)

Combination therapy: 0.75 mg every 8 hours, given together with 200 mg of zidovudine (ie, total daily dose: 2.25 mg of zalcitabine and 600 mg of zidovudine); if zalcitabine is permanently discontinued or interrupted due to toxicities, decrease zidovudine dose to 100 mg every 4 hours

**Mechanism of Action**

Purine nucleoside analogue, zalcitabine or 2',3'-dideoxycitidine (ddC) has been found to have *in vitro* activity and is reported to be successful against HIV in short term clinical trials

Intracellularly, ddc is converted to active metabolite ddCTP; lack the presence of the 3'-hydroxyl group necessary for phosphodiester linkages during DNA replication. As a result viral replication is prematurely terminated. ddCTP acts as a competitor for binding sites on the HIV-RNA dependent DNA polymerase (reverse transcriptase) to further contribute to inhibition of viral replication.

**Local Anesthetic/Vasoconstrictor Precautions** No information available to require special precautions

**Effects on Dental Treatment** Oral ulceration in >10% of patients

**Other Adverse Effects**

>10%: Gastrointestinal: Oral ulcers

1% to 10%:

Cardiovascular: Chest pain

Central nervous system: Headache, dizziness, fatigue

Dermatologic: Rash, pruritus

Gastrointestinal: Nausea, dysphagia, anorexia, abdominal pain, vomiting, diarrhea, weight loss

Neuromuscular & skeletal: Myalgia, foot pain

Respiratory: Pharyngitis

<1%:

Cardiovascular: Edema, hypertension, palpitations, syncope, atrial fibrillation, tachycardia, heart racing

(Continued)

## Zalcitabine *(Continued)*

Central nervous system: Night sweats, fever, pain, malaise
Endocrine & metabolic: Hyperglycemia, hypocalcemia
Gastrointestinal: Constipation, pancreatitis
Hepatic: Jaundice, hepatitis
Neuromuscular & skeletal: Myositis, peripheral neuropathy, weakness
Respiratory: Epistaxis

**Drug Interactions** Increased toxicity:

Amphotericin, foscarnet, and aminoglycosides may potentiate the risk of developing peripheral neuropathy or other toxicities associated with zalcitabine by interfering with the renal elimination of zalcitabine

Other drugs associated with peripheral neuropathy include chloramphenicol, cisplatin, dapsone, disulfiram, ethionamide, glutethimide, gold hydralazine, iodoquinol, isoniazid, metronidazole, nitrofurantoin, phenytoin, ribavirin, and vincristine

Concomitant use of zalcitabine with didanosine is not recommended

**Drug Uptake**

Absorption: Food decreases absorption by 39%
Serum half-life: 2.9 hours

**Pregnancy Risk Factor** C

**Generic Available** No


- **Zanaflex®** *see* Tizanidine *on page 989*
- **Zanosar®** *see* Streptozocin *on page 936*
- **Zantac®** *see* Ranitidine Hydrochloride *on page 879*
- **Zantac® 75 [OTC]** *see* Ranitidine Hydrochloride *on page 879*
- **Zantryl®** *see* Phentermine *on page 793*
- **Zarontin®** *see* Ethosuximide *on page 409*
- **Zaroxolyn®** *see* Metolazone *on page 665*
- **Zeasorb-AF® Powder [OTC]** *see* Miconazole *on page 672*
- **Zeasorb-AF® Powder [OTC]** *see* Tolnaftate *on page 997*
- **Zebeta®** *see* Bisoprolol *on page 143*
- **Zefazone®** *see* Cefmetazole *on page 202*
- **Zemplar™** *see* Paricalcitol *on page 766*
- **Zenapax®** *see* Dacliximab *on page 293*
- **Zephiran® [OTC]** *see* Benzalkonium Chloride *on page 128*
- **Zephrex®** *see* Guaifenesin and Pseudoephedrine *on page 481*
- **Zephrex LA®** *see* Guaifenesin and Pseudoephedrine *on page 481*
- **Zerit®** *see* Stavudine *on page 932*
- **Zestoretic®** *see* Lisinopril and Hydrochlorothiazide *on page 596*
- **Zestril®** *see* Lisinopril *on page 594*
- **Zetar® [OTC]** *see* Coal Tar *on page 270*
- **Ziac™** *see* Bisoprolol and Hydrochlorothiazide *on page 144*
- **Ziagen®** *see* Abacavir *on page 24*


## Zidovudine (zye DOE vyoo deen)

**Related Information**

HIV Infection and AIDS *on page 1085*
Systemic Viral Diseases *on page 1115*
Zidovudine and Lamivudine *on next page*

**U.S. Brand Names** Retrovir®

**Canadian Brand Names** Apo®-Zidovudine; Novo-AZT

**Therapeutic Category** Antiviral Agent, Oral; Antiviral Agent, Parenteral

**Use** Management of patients with HIV infections who have had at least one episode of *Pneumocystis carinii* pneumonia or who have CD4 cell counts of ≤500/mm³; patients who have HIV-related symptoms or who are asymptomatic with abnormal laboratory values indicating HIV-related immunosuppression; does not reduce risk of transmitting HIV infections

**Usual Dosage**

Prevention of maternal-fetal HIV transmission:

Neonatal: Oral: 2 mg/kg/dose every 6 hours for 6 weeks beginning 8-12 hours after birth; infants unable to receive oral dosing may receive 1.5 mg/kg I.V. infused over 30 minutes every 6 hours

Maternal (>14 weeks gestation): Oral: 100 mg 5 times/day until the start of labor; during labor and delivery, administer zidovudine I.V. at 2 mg/kg over 1 hour followed by a continuous I.V. infusion of 1 mg/kg/hour until the umbilical cord is clamped

Asymptomatic/symptomatic HIV infection:
Children 3 months to 12 years:
Oral: 90-180 mg/m²/dose every 6 hours; maximum: 200 mg every 6 hours
I.V.: 1-2 mg/kg/dose (infused over 1 hour) administered every 4 hours around-the-clock (6 doses/day)

Adults:
Asymptomatic HIV infection: Oral: 100 mg every 4 hours while awake (500 mg/day)
Symptomatic HIV infection
Oral: Initial: 200 mg every 4 hours (1200 mg/day), then after 1 month, 100 mg every 4 hours (600 mg/day)
I.V.: 1-2 mg/kg/dose (infused over 1 hour) administered every 4 hours around-the-clock (6 doses/day)
**Patients should receive I.V. therapy only until oral therapy can be administered**
Combination therapy with zalcitabine: Oral: 200 mg with zalcitabine 0.75 mg every 8 hours

**Mechanism of Action** Zidovudine is a thymidine analog which interferes with the HIV viral RNA dependent DNA polymerase resulting in inhibition of viral replication

**Local Anesthetic/Vasoconstrictor Precautions** No information available to require special precautions

**Effects on Dental Treatment** No effects or complications reported

**Other Adverse Effects**
>10%:
Central nervous system: Severe headache, insomnia
Gastrointestinal: Nausea
Hematologic: Anemia, leukopenia, neutropenia
1% to 10%:
Dermatologic: Rash, hyperpigmentation of nails (bluish-brown)
Hematologic: Changes in platelet count
<1%:
Central nervous system: Neurotoxicity, confusion, mania, seizures
Gastrointestinal: Anorexia
Hematologic: Bone marrow suppression, granulocytopenia, thrombocytopenia, pancytopenia
Hepatic: Hepatotoxicity, cholestatic jaundice
Local: Tenderness
Neuromuscular & skeletal: Myopathy, weakness

**Drug Interactions** Increased toxicity: Coadministration with drugs that are nephrotoxic (amphotericin B), cytotoxic (flucytosine, vincristine, vinblastine, doxorubicin, interferon), inhibit glucuronidation or excretion (acetaminophen, cimetidine, indomethacin, lorazepam, probenecid, aspirin), or interfere with RBC/WBC number or function (acyclovir, ganciclovir, pentamidine, dapsone)

**Drug Uptake**
Absorption: Oral: Well absorbed (66% to 70%)
Serum half-life: Terminal: 60 minutes
Time to peak serum concentration: Within 30-90 minutes

**Pregnancy Risk Factor** C

**Generic Available** No

## Zidovudine and Lamivudine

**Related Information**
HIV Infection and AIDS *on page 1085*

**U.S. Brand Names** Combivir®

**Therapeutic Category** Antiviral Agent, Oral

**Synonyms** AZT + 3TC

**Use** Treatment of HIV infection when therapy is warranted based on clinical and/or immunological evidence of disease progression. Combivir® given twice daily, provides an alternative regimen to lamivudine 150 mg twice daily plus zidovudine 600 mg/day in divided doses; this drug form reduces capsule/tablet intake for these two drugs to 2 per day instead of up to 8.

**Usual Dosage** Children >12 years and Adults: Oral: One tablet twice daily

**Mechanism of Action** The combination of zidovudine and lamivudine are believed to act synergistically to inhibit reverse transcriptase via DNA chain termination after incorporation of the nucleoside analogue as well as to delay the emergence of mutations conferring resistance

**Local Anesthetic/Vasoconstrictor Precautions** No information available to require special precautions

**Effects on Dental Treatment** No effects or complications reported

**Other Adverse Effects** See individual agents

(Continued)

## Zidovudine and Lamivudine *(Continued)*

**Drug Interactions** See individual agents

**Drug Uptake** Half-life: Zidovudine: 0.5-3 hours; lamivudine: 5-7 hours

**Dosage Forms** Tablet: Zidovudine 300 mg and lamivudine 150 mg

- **Zilactin-B® Medicated [OTC]** *see* Benzocaine *on page 128*

## Zileuton (zye LOO ton)

**U.S. Brand Names** Zyflo™

**Therapeutic Category** 5-Lipoxygenase Inhibitor

**Use** Prophylaxis and chronic treatment of asthma in adults and children ≥12 years of age

**Usual Dosage** Oral:

Adults: 600 mg 4 times/day with meals and at bedtime

Elderly: Zileuton pharmacokinetics were similar in healthy elderly subjects (>65 years) compared with healthy younger adults (18-40 years)

**Mechanism of Action** Specific inhibitor of 5-lipoxygenase and thus inhibits leukotriene (LTB1, LTC1, LTD1 and LTE1) formation. Leukotrienes are substances that induce numerous biological effects including augmentation of neutrophil and eosinophil migration, neutrophil and monocyte aggregation, leukocyte adhesion, increased capillary permeability and smooth muscle contraction.

**Local Anesthetic/Vasoconstrictor Precautions** No information available to require special precautions

**Effects on Dental Treatment** No effects or complications reported

**Other Adverse Effects**

>10%:

Central nervous system: Headache (24.6%)

Hepatic: ALT elevation (12%)

1% to 10%:

Cardiovascular: Chest pain

Central nervous system: Pain, dizziness, fever, insomnia, malaise, nervousness, somnolence

Gastrointestinal: Dyspepsia, nausea, abdominal pain, constipation, flatulence

Hematologic: Low white blood cell count

Neuromuscular & skeletal: Myalgia, arthralgia, weakness

Ocular: Conjunctivitis

**Warnings/Precautions** Elevations of one or more liver function tests may occur during therapy. These laboratory abnormalities may progress, remain unchanged or resolve with continued therapy. Use with caution in patients who consume substantial quantities of alcohol or have a past history of liver disease. Zileuton is not indicated for use in the reversal of bronchospasm in acute asthma attacks, including status asthmaticus. Zileuton can be continued during acute exacerbations of asthma.

**Drug Interactions** Cytochrome P-450 1A2, 2C9 and 3A4 enzyme substrate

Increased toxicity:

Propranolol: Doubling of propranolol AUC and consequent increased beta-blocker activity

Terfenadine: Decrease in clearance of terfenadine leading to increase in AUC

Theophylline: Doubling of serum theophylline concentrations - reduce theophylline dose and monitor serum theophylline concentrations closely.

Warfarin: Clinically significant increases in prothrombin time (PT) - monitor PT closely

**Drug Uptake**

Absorption: Oral: Rapidly absorbed

Serum half-life: 2.5 hours

Time to peak serum concentration: 1.7 hours

**Pregnancy Risk Factor** C

**Generic Available** No

- **Zinacef®** *see* Cefuroxime *on page 210*
- **Zinc** *see* Trace Metals *on page 1001*
- **Zinc Acetate** *see* Zinc Supplements *on page 1062*
- **Zinca-Pak®** *see* Trace Metals *on page 1001*
- **Zincate®** *see* Zinc Supplements *on page 1062*
- **Zincate® Oral** *see* Zinc Sulfate *on page 1062*

## Zinc Chloride (zingk KLOR ide)

**Therapeutic Category** Trace Element, Parenteral

**Use** Cofactor for replacement therapy to different enzymes helps maintain normal growth rates, normal skin hydration and senses of taste and smell

**Usual Dosage** Clinical response may not occur for up to 6-8 weeks

Supplemental to I.V. solutions:
Premature Infants <1500 g, up to 3 kg: 300 mcg/kg/day
Full-term Infants and Children ≤5 years: 100 mcg/kg/day
Adults:
Stable with fluid loss from small bowel: 12.2 mg zinc/liter TPN or 17.1 mg zinc/kg (added to 1000 mL I.V. fluids) of stool or ileostomy output
Metabolically stable: 2.5-4 mg/day, add 2 mg/day for acute catabolic states

**Local Anesthetic/Vasoconstrictor Precautions** No information available to require special precautions

**Effects on Dental Treatment** No effects or complications reported

**Other Adverse Effects** <1%:
Cardiovascular: Hypotension
Gastrointestinal: Indigestion, nausea, vomiting
Hematologic: Neutropenia, leukopenia
Hepatic: Jaundice
Respiratory: Pulmonary edema

**Pregnancy Risk Factor** C

**Generic Available** Yes

**Comments** Clinical response may not occur for up to 6-8 weeks

♦ **Zincfrin® Ophthalmic [OTC]** *see* Phenylephrine and Zinc Sulfate *on page 797*

## Zinc Gelatin (zingk JEL ah tin)

**U.S. Brand Names** Gelucast®

**Therapeutic Category** Protectant, Topical

**Synonyms** Dome Paste Bandage; Unna's Boot; Unna's Paste; Zinc Gelatin Boot

**Use** Protectant and to support varicosities and similar lesions of the lower limbs

**Usual Dosage** Apply externally as an occlusive boot

**Local Anesthetic/Vasoconstrictor Precautions** No information available to require special precautions

**Effects on Dental Treatment** No effects or complications reported

**Other Adverse Effects** 1% to 10%: Local: Irritation

**Dosage Forms** Bandage: 3" x 10 yards, 4" x 10 yards

**Generic Available** Yes

♦ **Zinc Gelatin Boot** *see* Zinc Gelatin *on this page*
♦ **Zincon® Shampoo [OTC]** *see* Pyrithione Zinc *on page 869*

## Zinc Oxide (zingk OKS ide)

**Therapeutic Category** Topical Skin Product

**Synonyms** Base Ointment; Lassar's Zinc Paste

**Use** Protective coating for mild skin irritations and abrasions; soothing and protective ointment to promote healing of chapped skin, diaper rash

**Usual Dosage** Children and Adults: Topical: Apply as required for affected areas several times daily

**Mechanism of Action** Mild astringent with weak antiseptic properties

**Local Anesthetic/Vasoconstrictor Precautions** No information available to require special precautions

**Effects on Dental Treatment** No effects or complications reported

**Other Adverse Effects** 1% to 10%:
Dermatologic: Skin sensitivity
Local: Irritation

**Generic Available** Yes

## Zinc Oxide, Cod Liver Oil, and Talc

(zingk OKS ide, kod LIV er oyl, & talk)

**U.S. Brand Names** Desitin® Topical [OTC]

**Therapeutic Category** Protectant, Topical

**Use** Relief of diaper rash, superficial wounds and burns, and other minor skin irritations

**Usual Dosage** Topical: Apply thin layer as needed

**Local Anesthetic/Vasoconstrictor Precautions** No information available to require special precautions

**Effects on Dental Treatment** No effects or complications reported

**Other Adverse Effects** 1% to 10%: Local: Skin sensitivity, irritation

**Dosage Forms** Ointment, topical: Zinc oxide, cod liver oil and talc in a petrolatum and lanolin base (30 g, 60 g, 120 g, 240 g, 270 g)

**Generic Available** Yes

## Zinc Sulfate (zingk SUL fate)

**U.S. Brand Names** Eye-Sed® Ophthalmic [OTC]; Orazinc® Oral [OTC]; Verazinc® Oral [OTC]; Zincate® Oral

**Therapeutic Category** Electrolyte Supplement

**Use** Zinc supplement (oral and parenteral); may improve wound healing in those who are deficient

**Usual Dosage**

RDA: Oral:

Birth to 6 months: 3 mg elemental zinc/day
6-12 months: 5 mg elemental zinc/day
1-10 years: 10 mg elemental zinc/day
≥11 years: 15 mg elemental zinc/day

Zinc deficiency: Oral:

Infants and Children: 0.5-1 mg elemental zinc/kg/day divided 1-3 times/day; somewhat larger quantities may be needed if there is impaired intestinal absorption or an excessive loss of zinc

Adults: 110-220 mg zinc sulfate (25-50 mg elemental zinc)/dose 3 times/day

**Local Anesthetic/Vasoconstrictor Precautions** No information available to require special precautions

**Effects on Dental Treatment** No effects or complications reported

**Pregnancy Risk Factor** C

**Dosage Forms**

Capsule: 110 mg [elemental zinc 25 mg]; 220 mg [elemental zinc 50 mg]
Injection: 1 mg/mL (10 mL, 30 mL); 4 mg/mL (10 mL); 5 mg/mL (5 mL, 10 mL, 50 mL)
Tablet: 66 mg [elemental zinc 15 mg]; 200 mg [elemental zinc 46 mg]

**Dietary Considerations** May be administered with food if GI upset occurs; avoid foods high in calcium or phosphorus

**Generic Available** Yes

♦ **Zinc Sulfate** *see* Zinc Supplements *on this page*

## Zinc Supplements (zink)

**U.S. Brand Names** Eye-Sed® [OTC]; Orazinc® [OTC]; Verazinc® [OTC]; Zincate®

**Therapeutic Category** Mineral, Oral; Mineral, Parenteral; Trace Element

**Synonyms** Zinc Acetate; Zinc Sulfate

**Use** Cofactor for replacement therapy to different enzymes helps maintain normal growth rates, normal skin hydration and senses of taste and smell; zinc supplement (oral and parenteral); may improve wound healing in those who are deficient. May be useful to promote wound healing in patients with pressure sores.

**Usual Dosage** Clinical response may not occur for up to 6-8 weeks

Zinc sulfate:

RDA: Oral:

Birth to 6 months: 3 mg elemental zinc/day
6-12 months: 5 mg elemental zinc/day
1-10 years: 10 mg elemental zinc/day (44 mg zinc sulfate)
≥11 years: 15 mg elemental zinc/day (65 mg zinc sulfate)

Zinc deficiency: Oral:

Infants and Children: 0.5-1 mg elemental zinc/kg/day divided 1-3 times/day; somewhat larger quantities may be needed if there is impaired intestinal absorption or an excessive loss of zinc

Adults: 110-220 mg zinc sulfate (25-50 mg elemental zinc)/dose 3 times/day

Parenteral: TPN: I.V. infusion (chloride or sulfate): Supplemental to I.V. solutions (clinical response may not occur for up to 6-8 weeks):

Premature Infants <1500 g, up to 3 kg: 300 mcg/kg/day
Full-term Infants and Children ≤5 years: 100 mcg/kg/day

**or**

Premature Infants: 400 mcg/kg/day
Term <3 months: 250 mcg/kg/day
Term >3 months: 100 mcg/kg/day
Children: 50 mcg/kg/day
Adults:

Stable with fluid loss from small bowel: 12.2 mg zinc/liter TPN or 17.1 mg zinc/kg (added to 1000 mL I.V. fluids) of stool or ileostomy output

Metabolically stable: 2.5-4 mg/day, add 2 mg/day for acute catabolic states

**Mechanism of Action** Provides for normal growth and tissue repair, is a cofactor for more than 70 enzymes; ophthalmic astringent and weak antiseptic due to precipitation of protein and clearing mucus from outer surface of the eye

**Local Anesthetic/Vasoconstrictor Precautions** No information available to require special precautions

**Effects on Dental Treatment** No effects or complications reported

**Other Adverse Effects** <1%:
Cardiovascular: Hypotension
Gastrointestinal: Indigestion, nausea, vomiting
Hematologic: Neutropenia, leukopenia
Hepatic: Jaundice
Respiratory: Pulmonary edema

**Drug Interactions**
Decreased effect of zinc with dairy products; bran products and iron reduce absorption of zinc from GI tract
Zinc appears to inhibit the absorption of ciprofloxacin and tetracyclines by binding in GI tract. The absorption of doxycycline (Vibramycin®) is not affected by zinc.

**Pregnancy Risk Factor** C

- **Zinc Undecylenate** *see* Undecylenic Acid and Derivatives *on page 1033*
- **Zinecard®** *see* Dexrazoxane *on page 310*
- **Zithromax™** *see* Azithromycin *on page 114*
- **ZNP® Bar [OTC]** *see* Pyrithione Zinc *on page 869*
- **Zocor™** *see* Simvastatin *on page 915*
- **Zofran®** *see* Ondansetron *on page 740*
- **Zoladex® Implant** *see* Goserelin *on page 475*
- **Zolicef®** *see* Cefazolin *on page 199*

## Zolmitriptan (zohl mi TRIP tan)

**U.S. Brand Names** Zomig®
**Therapeutic Category** Antimigraine Agent; Serotonin Agonist
**Synonyms** 311C90
**Use** Acute treatment of adult migraine, with or without auras.
**Usual Dosage** Adults: Oral: Single doses of 1, 2.5 or 5 mg are effective in reducing symptoms of a migraine attack. Patients should be started at a dose of 2.5 mg or lower since the incidence of side effects increases somewhat with dose. If the headache returns, the dose may be repeated after 2 hours but NOT TO EXCEED 10 mg within a 24-hour period.
**Mechanism of Action** A selective 5-hydroxytryptamine (5-HT 1B/1D) receptor agonist. The drug binds tightly and specifically to this receptor. The current theory of migraine headaches suggests that symptoms are due to local cranial vasodilation or to the release of sensory neuropeptides through nerve endings in the trigeminal system. The activity of zolmitriptan can most likely be attributed to its agonist effects at the 5-HT 1B/1D receptors in intracranial blood vessels and sensory nerves, which results in cranial vessel constriction and the inhibition of pro-inflammatory neuropeptide release.
**Local Anesthetic/Vasoconstrictor Precautions** No information available to require special precautions
**Effects on Dental Treatment** No effects or complications reported
**Drug Uptake** Half-life: 2.5-3 hours
**Dosage Forms** Tablet: 2.5 mg, 5 mg
**Comments** Not intended for the prophylactic therapy of migraine or for use in the management of hemiplegic or basilar migraine. The safety and effectiveness of zolmitriptan for the treatment of cluster headache, have not been confirmed.

- **Zoloft™** *see* Sertraline *on page 910*

## Zolpidem (zole PI dem)

**U.S. Brand Names** Ambien™
**Therapeutic Category** Hypnotic; Sedative
**Use** Short-term treatment of insomnia
**Usual Dosage** Duration of therapy should be limited to 7-10 days
Adults: Oral: 10 mg immediately before bedtime; maximum dose: 10 mg
Elderly: 5 mg immediately before bedtime
**Mechanism of Action** Structurally dissimilar to benzodiazepine, however, has much or all of its actions explained by its effects on benzodiazepine (BZD) receptors, especially the omega-1 receptor; retains hypnotic and much of the anxiolytic properties of the BZD, but has reduced effects on skeletal muscle and seizure threshold.
**Local Anesthetic/Vasoconstrictor Precautions** No information available to require special precautions
**Effects on Dental Treatment** No effects or complications reported
**Other Adverse Effects**
1% to 10%:
Central nervous system: Headache, drowsiness, dizziness
Gastrointestinal: Nausea, diarrhea
Neuromuscular & skeletal: Myalgia
(Continued)

## Zolpidem *(Continued)*

<1%:

Central nervous system: Amnesia, confusion
Gastrointestinal: Vomiting
Neuromuscular & skeletal: Falls, tremor

**Drug Interactions** Increased effect/toxicity with alcohol, CNS depressants

**Drug Uptake**

Onset of action: 30 minutes
Duration: 6-8 hours
Absorption: Rapid
Serum half-life: 2-2.6 hours, in cirrhosis increased to 9.9 hours

**Pregnancy Risk Factor** B

**Dosage Forms** Tablet, as tartrate: 5 mg, 10 mg

**Generic Available** No

- **Zomig®** *see* Zolmitriptan *on previous page*
- **Zone-A Forte®** *see* Pramoxine and Hydrocortisone *on page 828*
- **ZORprin®** *see* Aspirin *on page 100*
- **Zostrix® [OTC]** *see* Capsaicin *on page 181*
- **Zostrix®-HP [OTC]** *see* Capsaicin *on page 181*
- **Zosyn™** *see* Piperacillin and Tazobactam Sodium *on page 808*
- **Zovia®** *see* Ethinyl Estradiol and Ethynodiol Diacetate *on page 400*
- **Zovirax®** *see* Acyclovir *on page 38*
- **Z-PAKS™** *see* Azithromycin *on page 114*
- **Zyban™** *see* Bupropion *on page 160*
- **Zydone® [5/500]** *see* Hydrocodone and Acetaminophen *on page 505*
- **Zyflo™** *see* Zileuton *on page 1060*
- **Zyloprim®** *see* Allopurinol *on page 48*
- **Zymase®** *see* Pancrelipase *on page 763*
- **Zyprexa™** *see* Olanzapine *on page 738*
- **Zyrtec®** *see* Cetirizine *on page 218*

# ORAL MEDICINE TOPICS

## PART I.

## DENTAL MANAGEMENT AND THERAPEUTIC CONSIDERATIONS IN MEDICALLY COMPROMISED PATIENTS

This section focuses on common medical conditions and their associated drug therapies with which the dentist must be familiar. Patient profiles with commonly associated drug regimens are described.

### TABLE OF CONTENTS

# CARDIOVASCULAR DISEASES

Cardiovascular disease is the most prevalent human disease affecting over 60 million Americans and this group of diseases accounts for more than 50% of all deaths in the United States. Surgical and pharmacologic therapy have resulted in many cardiovascular patients living healthy and profitable lives. Consequently, patients presenting to the dental office may require treatment planning modifications related to the medical management of their cardiovascular disease. For the purposes of this text, we will cover ischemic heart disease including angina pectoris and myocardial infarction, cardiac arrhythmias, congestive heart failure, and hypertension.

## ISCHEMIC HEART DISEASE

Any long-term decrease in the delivery of oxygen to the heart muscle can lead to the condition ischemic heart disease. Often arteriosclerosis and atherosclerosis result in a narrowing of the coronary vessels' lumina and are the most common causes of vascular ischemic heart disease. Other causes such as previous infarct, mitral valve regurgitation, and ruptured septa may also lead to ischemia in the heart muscle. The two most common major conditions that result from ischemic heart disease are angina pectoris and myocardial infarction. Sudden death, a third category, can likewise result from ischemia.

To the physician, the most common presenting sign or symptom of ischemic heart disease is chest pain. This chest pain can be of a transient nature as in angina pectoris or the result of a myocardial infarction. It is now believed that sudden death represents a separate occurrence that essentially involves the development of a lethal cardiac arrhythmia or coronary artery spasm leading to an acute shutdown of the heart muscle blood supply. Risk factors in patients for coronary atherosclerosis include cigarette smoking, elevated blood lipids, hypertension, as well as diabetes mellitus, age, and gender (male).

Lipid-lowering and cholesterol-lowering drugs including atorvastatin, cholestyramine, colestipol, fluvastatin, gemfibrozil, lovastatin, nicotinic acid, pravastatin, probucol, and simvastatin (seen in the following list) have become standard treatments for patients with developing atherosclerosis in an attempt to lower blood cholesterol and thereby, indirectly reduce the risk of ischemia heart disease.

**Lipid-Lowering Drugs**

Cholestyramine Resin (Prevalite®, Questran®) *on page 244*
Clofibrate (Atromid-S®) *on page 262*
Colestipol (Colestid®) *on page 274*
Dextrothyroxine (Choloxin®) *on page 314*
Fenofibrate (Lipidil®, Tricor®) *on page 422*
Gemfibrozil (Lopid®) *on page 465*
Niacin (Nicotinic Acid) *on page 715*
Probucol (Lorelco®) *on page 840*

**HMG-CoA Reductase Inhibitors**

Atorvastatin (Lipitor®) *on page 106*
Cerivastatin (Baycol®) *on page 217*
Fluvastatin (Lescol®) *on page 451*
Lovastatin (Mevacor®) *on page 605*
Pravastatin (Pravachol®) *on page 828*
Simvastatin (Zocor™) *on page 915*

## ANGINA PECTORIS

Angina pectoris is a symptomatic manifestation of ischemic heart disease characterized by thoracic pain resulting from oxygen deprivation to the heart muscle. Often metabolites build up in the vessels and the muscle tissue leading to the pain. Occasionally, the pain can radiate to the left arm or to the jaw. The pain is often midsternal and usually described as an extreme pressure sensation, not unlike an elephant sitting on one's chest (which we have all undoubtedly experienced). Three forms of angina pectoris are usually recognized. Stable angina includes chest pain that predictably is precipitated by overexertion, cold, or overactivity. Unstable angina pectoris usually is defined as a recent change in pattern of occurrence, usually a decreased threshold of stimulus and an unpredictable response to the major drug of choice, nitroglycerin. Prinzmetal's angina or variant angina often occurs due to spasm in a single large coronary artery and may have a cardiac dysrhythmia associated with it. Regardless of the type of angina pectoris, treatment includes control of risk factors, reducing oxygen demand to the myocardium, and increasing coronary blood flow.

The most common antianginal drugs fall into three categories. Nitrates are first-line drugs in the management of angina and include oral nitrate tablets or capsules. Nitrates can also be available as transcutaneous patches and are available in solution for I.V. administration. Beta-adrenergic blockers, the second category, are often used when a patient's angina responds poorly to nitrates.

Calcium channel blockers are also indicated for angina related to coronary vessel spasm with or without atherosclerosis. These drugs inhibit calcium ion passage through the slow channels of cell membranes. They tend to be used alone or in combination with nitrates and beta-blockers.

Selected antianginal drugs include:

**Nitrates**

Erythrityl Tetranitrate (Cardilate®) *on page 383*
Isosorbide Dinitrate (Dilitrate®-SR; Isordil®; Sorbitrate®) *on page 555*
Isosorbide Mononitrate (Imdur®; Ismo™; Monoket®) *on page 556*
Nitroglycerin (various products) *on page 725*
Pentaerythritol Tetranitrate (Duotrate®; Peritrate®) *on page 777*

**Beta-Adrenergic Blockers**

Atenolol (Tenormin®) *on page 105*
Betaxolol (Betoptic®, Kerlone®) *on page 138*
Bisoprolol (Zebeta®) *on page 143*
Carteolol (Cartrol®; Ocupress®) *on page 194*
Nadolol (Corgard®) *on page 696*
Propranolol (Betachron E-R®; Inderal®) *on page 857*
Sotalol (Betapace®) *on page 927*
Timolol (Blocadren®) *on page 986*

**Calcium Channel Blockers**

Amlodipine (Norvasc®) *on page 71*
Bepridil (Vascor®) *on page 134*
Diltiazem (Cardizem®, Dilacor™ XR) *on page 334*
Nicardipine (Cardene®) *on page 717*
Nifedipine (Adalat®; Procardia®) *on page 720*
Verapamil (Calan®; Covera-HS®; Isoptin®; Verelan®) *on page 1043*

The dental management of the patient with angina pectoris may include: sedation techniques for complicated procedures (see "Patients Requiring Sedation" *on page 1152*), to limit the extent of procedures, and to limit the use of local anesthesia containing 1:100,000 epinephrine to two carpules. Anesthesia without vasoconstrictor might also be selected. The appropriate use of vasoconstrictor in anesthesia, however, should be weighed against the necessity to maximize anesthesia. Please see "Management of Office Emergencies" *on page 1174*. Complete history and appropriate referral and consultation with the patient's physician for those patients who are known to be at risk for angina pectoris is recommended.

# MYOCARDIAL INFARCTION

Myocardial infarction is the leading cause of death in the United States. It is an acute irreversible ischemic event that produces an area of myocardial necrosis in the heart tissue. If a patient has a previous history of myocardial infarction, he/she may be taking a variety of drugs (ie, antihypertensives, lipid lowering drugs, ACE inhibitors, and antianginal medications) to not only prevent a second infarct, but to treat the long-term associated ischemic heart disease. Postmyocardial infarction patients are often taking anticoagulants such as warfarin and antiplatelet agents such as aspirin. Consultation with the prescribing physician by the dentist is necessary prior to invasive procedures. Temporary dose reduction may allow the dentist to proceed with most procedures.

Aspirin (various products) *on page 100*
Warfarin (Coumadin®) *on page 1053*

Thrombolytic drugs, that might dissolve hemostatic plugs, may also be given on a short-term basis immediately following an infarct and include:

Alteplase (Activase®) *on page 52*
Anistreplase (Eminase®) *on page 87*

## CARDIOVASCULAR DISEASES *(Continued)*

Streptokinase (Kabikinase®; Streptase®) *on page 933*
Urokinase (Abbokinase®) *on page 1035*

Alteplase is also currently in use for acute myocardial infarction. Following myocardial infarction and rehabilitation, outpatients may be placed on anticoagulants (such as coumadin), diuretics, beta-adrenergic blockers, ACE inhibitors to reduce blood pressure, and calcium-channel blockers. Depending on the presence or absence of continued angina pectoris, patients may also be taking nitrates, beta-blockers, or calcium-channel blockers as indicated for treatment of angina.

## BETA-ADRENERGIC BLOCKING AGENTS CATEGORIZED ACCORDING TO SPECIFIC PROPERTIES

### Alpha-Adrenergic Blocking Activity

Labetalol (Normodyne®, Trandate®) *on page 568*

### Intrinsic Sympathomimetic Activity

Acebutolol (Sectral®) *on page 26*
Pindolol (Visken®) *on page 806*

### Long Duration of Action and Fewer CNS Effects

Acebutolol (Sectral®) *on page 26*
Atenolol (Tenormin®) *on page 105*
Betaxolol (Kerlone®) *on page 138*
Nadolol (Corgard®) *on page 696*

### Beta$_1$-Receptor Selectivity

Acebutolol (Sectral®) *on page 26*
Atenolol (Tenormin®) *on page 105*
Metoprolol (Lopressor®, Toprol XL®) *on page 666*

### Non-Selective (blocks both beta$_1$ and beta$_2$ receptors)

Betaxolol (Kerlone®) *on page 138*
Labetalol (Normodyne®, Trandate®) *on page 568*
Nadolol (Corgard®) *on page 696*
Pindolol (Visken®) *on page 806*
Propranolol (Inderal®) *on page 857*
Timolol (Blocadren®) *on page 986*

## ARRHYTHMIAS

Abnormal cardiac rhythm can develop spontaneously and survivors of a myocardial infarction are often left with an arrhythmia. An arrhythmia is any alteration or disturbance in the normal rate, rhythm, or conduction through the cardiac tissue. This is known as a cardiac arrhythmia. Abnormalities in rhythm can occur in either the atria or the ventricles. Various valvular deformities, drug effects, and chemical derangements can initiate arrhythmias. These arrhythmias can be a slowing of the heart rate (<60 beats/minute) as defined in bradycardia or tachycardia resulting in a rapid heart beat (usually >150 beats/minute). The dentist will encounter a variety of treatments for management of arrhythmias. Usually, underlying causes such as reduced cardiac output, hypertension, and irregular ventricular beats will require treatment. Pacemaker therapy is also sometimes used. Indwelling pacemakers may require supplementation with antibiotics, and consultation with the physician is certainly appropriate. Sinus tachycardia is often treated with drugs such as:

Propranolol (Betachron ER®; Inderal®) *on page 857*
Quinidine (Cardioquin®; Quinaglute®; Quinalan®; Quinidex®; Quinora®) *on page 873*

Beta-blockers are often used to slow cardiac rate and diazepam may be helpful when anxiety is a contributing factor in arrhythmia. When atrial flutter and atrial fibrillation are diagnosed, digitalis preparations such as digitoxin and digoxin are the drugs of choice.

Digitoxin (Crystodigin®) *on page 328*
Digoxin (Lanoxin®) *on page 329*

## ANTICOAGULANT THERAPY

Patients postmyocardial infarction and those with atrial fibrillation are also frequently placed on anticoagulants such as Coumadin®. (See Myocardial Infarction Section on previous page.)

Large numbers of patients are receiving oral anticoagulation therapy. The dental clinician is often faced with the decision as to how to manage these patients prior to invasive dental procedures. Key factors regarding the patient receiving anticoagulant therapy include: what is the bleeding risk of the procedure planned? what are the clotting risks (ie, can the medication management be safely altered)? and what is the patient's current anticoagulant therapy level in terms of bleeding measurements (ie, laboratory evaluations) and their prognosis?

Most patients receiving anticoagulant therapy are on one of two regimens. Warfarin, under the name Coumadin®, is the most common long-term outpatient anticoagulant given. Many patients, however, are also on aspirin products to achieve some level of anticoagulation. The mechanisms of the action of these two drugs are different and it is important that the clinician be aware of the appropriate tests and the appropriate time relative to treatment selection.

Partial thromboplastin time and bleeding time (IVY) are appropriate measures for platelet dysfunction. Aspirin, ticlopidine (Ticlid®), and other new drugs, such as Clopidogrel (Plavix®), are actually considered antiplatelet drugs, whereas oral Coumadin® is considered an oral anticoagulant. Aspirin works by inhibiting cyclo-oxygenase which is an enzyme involved in the platelet system associated with clot formation. As little as one aspirin (300 mg dose) can result in an alteration in this enzyme pathway. Although aspirin is cleared from the circulation very quickly (within 15-30 minutes), the effect on the life of the platelet may last for up to 7-10 days. Therefore, the clinician planning an invasive procedure on patients with antiplatelet therapy may wish to consider a change prior to one week before the invasive treatment.

The effects of Coumadin® on the coagulation within patients, occur by way of the vitamin K-dependent clotting mechanism and are generally monitored by measuring the prothrombin time known as the PT. Often to prevent venous thrombosis, a patient will be maintained at approximately 1.5 times their normal prothrombin time. Other anticoagulant goals such as prevention of arterial thromboembolism, as in patients with artificial heart valves, may require 2-2.5 times the normal prothrombin time. It is important for the clinician to obtain not only the accurate PT but also the International Normalized Ratio (INR) for the patient. This ratio is calculated by dividing the patient's PT by the mean normal PT for the laboratory, which is determined by using the International Sensitivity Index (ISI) to adjust for the lab's reagents.

The response to oral anticoagulants varies greatly in patients and should be monitored regularly. The dental clinician planning an invasive procedure should consider not only what the patient can tell them from a historical point-of-view, but also when the last monitoring test was performed. In general, most dental procedures can be performed in patients that are 1.5 times normal or less. Some textbooks even suggest that 2 times normal would pose little risk in most dental patients and procedures, but these values may be misleading unless the INR is also determined. When in doubt, the prudent dental clinician would consult with the patients physician and obtain current prothrombin time in order to evaluate fully and plan for his patients. The clinician is referred to the excellent review: Herman WW, Konzelman JL, and Sutley SH, "Current Perspectives on Dental Patients Receiving Coumadin Anticoagulant Therapy," *J Am Dent Assoc*, 1997, 128:327-35.

### Coumadin®-like Anticoagulants

Dicumarol *on page 322*
Warfarin (Coumadin®) *on page 1053*

### Platelet Aggregation Inhibitors

Aspirin (various products) *on page 100*
Clopidogrel (Plavix®) *on page 266*
Eptifibatide (Integrillin®) *on page 379*
Ticlopidine (Ticlid®) *on page 985*
Tirofiban (Aggrastat®) *on page 988*

### Other

Lepirudin (Refludan®) *on page 575*

## CARDIOVASCULAR DISEASES *(Continued)*

The basis for anticoagulation therapy is that mitral stenosis may be the result of the long-term arrhythmia and there is concern over the possibility of stroke. Ventricular dysrhythmias are often treated with drugs such as quinidine, procainamide, lidocaine, beta-adrenergic agents, and calcium channel blockers. Quinidine is used for selected arrhythmias. Lidocaine is often used when there are ventricular dysrhythmias. Procainamide (Pronestyl®) or flecainide (Tambocor®) are alternative agents.

Over the past three decades, there has been an increasing use of drugs that relate to the clotting mechanism in patients. These drugs have included the widespread use of aspirin as well as an increasing use of the anticoagulant found in warfarin or Coumadin®. Also, there has been increasing evidence that more patients have a gastrointestinal sensitivity to aspirin. Therefore, alternative analgesics such as acetaminophen and the NSAID products have expanded in utilization tremendously. These factors resulted in numerous potential drug interactions that, until now, have been thought to be quite innocuous. The use of acetaminophen, which is primarily for analgesic and antipyretic properties, has increased dramatically. The drug is available as an over-the-counter medication for a wide range of nonspecific conditions and, in fact, in the United States, acetaminophen is the most frequently ingested medication.

Regarding dental management patients that are already taking warfarin, the use of analgesics is implicated as a potential source of drug interaction. In a recent article by Hayek in *JAMA*, it was found that patients taking warfarin for anticoagulation identified the use of dangerously elevated INRs and the fact was discovered that they concomitantly had been taking acetaminophen (not necessarily with their physician's recommendation). The study of the international normalized ratio (INR) in these patients has indicated that additional factors independently influence the INR as well as the potential interaction with acetaminophen. These factors included advanced malignancy, patients who did not take their warfarin properly (therefore, took more than was necessary), changes in oral intake of liquids or solids, acute diarrhea leading to dehydration, alcohol consumption, and vitamin K intake. The mechanisms of these augmenting factors for enhancement of the INR are that the cytochrome P450 system, present in the liver, is also affected by changes in metabolism associated with these factors. For instance, the metabolism of alcohol in the liver alters its ability to manage the CYP450 enzyme system necessary for warfarin, therefore, enhancing its presence and potentially increasing the half-life of warfarin. As oral intake of nutrients declines in patients with either diarrhea or reduced intake of liquids and/or solids, absorption of vitamin K is reduced and the vitamin K dependent system of metabolism of warfarin changes, therefore increasing warfarin blood levels. These factors, along with the liver metabolism of acetaminophen, have resulted in the increased concern that patients, who may be taking acetaminophen as an analgesic or for other reasons, may be at risk for enhancing or elevating, inadvertently, their anticoagulation effect of warfarin. The dentist should be aware of this potential interaction in prescribing any drug containing acetaminophen or in recommending that a patient use an analgesic for relief of even mild pain on a prolonged basis. Therefore, the dentist must be concerned with these factors and is referred to the discussion in the Pain Management Chapter of this text for more consideration (adapted from *JAMA*, March 4, 1998, Vol 279, No 9).

Acetaminophen *on page 27*

# CLASSIFICATION OF ANTIARRHYTHMIC DRUGS

**Supraventricular**

Digitoxin (digitalis) (Crystodigin®) *on page 328*
Digoxin (Lanoxin®) *on page 329*

**Supraventricular and Ventricular**

Acebutolol (Sectral®) *on page 26*
Adenosine (Adenocard®) *on page 40*
Amiodarone (Cordarone®) *on page 66*
Atenolol (Tenormin®) *on page 105*
Bepridil (Vascor®) *on page 134*
Bisoprolol (Zebeta®) *on page 143*
Bretylium (Bretylol®) *on page 148*
Diltiazem (Cardizem®; Dilacor™ XR) *on page 334*
Disopyramide (Norpace®) *on page 343*
Encainide (Enkaid®) *on page 369*
Flecainide (Tambocor®) *on page 433*

Lidocaine (Xylocaine®) *on page 586*
Mexiletine (Mexitil®) *on page 669*
Moricizine (Ethmozine®) *on page 687*
Nicardipine (Cardene®) *on page 717*
Phenytoin (Dilantin®) *on page 799*
Procainamide (Pronestyl®) *on page 840*
Propafenone (Rythmol®) *on page 850*
Propranolol (Inderal®) *on page 857*
Quinidine (Cardioquin®; Quinaglute®; Quinalan®; Quinidex®; Quinora®) *on page 873*
Sotalol (Betapace®) *on page 927*
Tocainide (Tonocard®) *on page 992*
Verapamil (Calan®, Isoptin®) *on page 1043*

Treatment of arrhythmias often can result in oral manifestations including oral ulcerations with drugs such as procainamide, lupus-like lesions, as well as xerostomia.

## CONGESTIVE HEART FAILURE

Congestive heart failure is a clinical disease that occurs when the heart muscle gradually fails to deliver adequate oxygenated blood to the tissues. The chronically failing heart will attempt to compensate by three physiologic mechanisms: enlargement, increased heart rate, or dilatation. As the congestive heart failure becomes more profound, myocardial contractility diminishes and sodium and water retention increase leading to edema in the peripheral extremities. Edema is commonly seen in the patient with congestive heart failure. The failure of the heart may be right sided, left sided, or both. The treatment of congestive heart failure is usually rest with increased oxygenation.

The long-term treatment is to attempt to increase the strength and efficiency of the heart contractions, to avoid arrhythmias, and to reduce retention of water and sodium. Digitalis is one of the primary drugs used in treatment of congestive heart failure. It is usually prescribed in small doses and is coupled with diuretics and/or angiotensin-converting enzyme (ACE) inhibitors to decrease water retention. Nitrates and hydralazine are often given to patients with acute heart failure. The dentist may find that the patient is well compensated; however, treatment of CHF represents a complicated pharmacologic pattern necessary to be analyzed. Consultation with the managing physician regarding the patient's stability is recommended. Clinical signs of congestive heart failure might include distended neck veins, peripheral edema, and a ruddy complexion. Beta-blockers are now being approved for CHF, as well as hypertension

Digitoxin (Crystodigin®) *on page 328*
Digoxin (Lanoxin®) *on page 329*

**Angiotensin-Converting Enzyme Inhibitors**

Captopril (Capoten®) *on page 182*
Enalapril (Vasotec®) *on page 366*
Fosinopril (Monopril®) *on page 457*
Lisinopril (Prinivil®) *on page 594*
Quinapril (Accupril®) *on page 871*
Ramipril (Altace™) *on page 877*
Trandolapril (Mavik®) *on page 1003*

**Combined Alpha- and Beta-Adrenergic Blocking Agent**

Carvedilol (Coreg®) *on page 195*

**Direct-Acting Vasodilators**

Hydralazine (Apresoline®) *on page 501*

**Nitrates**

Erythrityl Tetranitrate (Cardilate®) *on page 383*
Isosorbide Dinitrate (Dilitrate®-SR, Isordil®, Sorbitrate®) *on page 555*
Isosorbide Mononitrate (Imdur®; Ismo™; Monoket®) *on page 556*
Nitroglycerin (various products) *on page 725*
Pentaerythritol Tetranitrate (Duotrate®; Peritrate®) *on page 777*

## HYPERTENSION

Hypertension is defined as (1) systolic blood pressure (SBP) of 140 mm of mercury or greater; (2) and/or diastolic blood pressure (DBP) of 90 mm of mercury or greater; (3) and/or the fact that the patient is taking antihypertension medications regardless of what their pressure readings are. The overall goal in identifying and treating patients

## CARDIOVASCULAR DISEASES *(Continued)*

with sustained elevated high blood pressure is to reduce the risk of cardiovascular-associated morbidity and mortality. Positive relationships between systolic blood pressure, diastolic blood pressure, and cardiovascular risk have been known for many years.

### CLASSIFICATION OF BLOOD PRESSURE FOR ADULTS ≥18 YEARS OF AGE*

**Table 1.**

| Average DBP mm Hg | Average SBP mm Hg | | | |
|---|---|---|---|---|
| | <120 | 120-129 | 130-139 | ≥140 |
| <80 | Optimal* | Normal | High Normal | High |
| 80-84 | Normal | Normal | High Normal | High |
| 85-89 | High Normal | High Normal | High Normal | High |
| ≥90 | High | High | High | High |

*Optimal blood pressure, with regard to cardiovascular risk, is SBP <120 mm Hg and DBP <80 mm Hg. However, unusually low readings should be evaluated for clinical significance.

Adapted from the *Joint National Committee Report*, October, 1992.

**Table 2.**

| Category | Systolic (mm Hg) | | Diastolic (mm Hg) |
|---|---|---|---|
| Optimal† | <120 | and | <80 |
| Normal | <130 | and | <85 |
| High-Normal | 130-139 | or | 85-89 |
| Hypertension‡ | | | |
| Stage 1 | 140-159 | or | 90-99 |
| Stage 2 | 160-179 | or | 100-109 |
| Stage 3 | ≥180 | or | ≥110 |

*Not taking antihypertensive drugs and not acutely ill. When systolic and diastolic blood pressures fall into different categories, the higher category should be selected to classify the individual's blood pressure status. For example, 160/92 mm Hg should be classified as stage 2 hypertension, and 174/120 mm Hg should be classified as stage 3 hypertension. Isolated systolic hypertension is defined as SBP of 140 mm Hg or greater and DBP below 90 mm Hg and staged appropriately (ie, 170/82 mm Hg is defined as stage 2 isolated systolic hypertension). In addition to classifying stages of hypertension on the basis of average blood pressure levels, clinicians should specify presence or absence of target organ disease and additional risk factors. The specificity is important for risk classification and treatment (see table 5).

†Optimal blood pressure with respect to cardiovascular risk is below 120/80 mm Hg. However, unusually low readings should be evaluated for clinical significance.

‡Based on the average of two or more readings taken at each of two or more visits after an initial screening.

Recently, a 6th Report of the Joint National Committee on Prevention, Detection, Evaluation and Treatment of High Blood Pressure was released in the winter of 1998 in the NIH publication #98-4080 by the National Institutes of Health. In these new recommendations, several classifications, schemes, and strategies for treatment have not only been clarified, but they have been updated to reflect trends in therapeutics. The initial referral criteria have changed, combining two of the higher levels of blood pressure into one. The table indicates the various stages of high blood pressure ranging from optimal to stage 3 hypertension. Once the patient's blood pressure has been classified, a management scheme called "risk stratification and treatment" is applied. This scheme combines the actual blood pressure measurement with other risk factors that have been shown to impact directly and indirectly on the prognosis of the patient, and therefore, the necessity for intervention via therapeutics. Basically, this risk stratification identifies the patient into an A, B, or C category of risk and then when coupling that with the patient's actual blood pressure helps the practicing physician to determine an action plan. Other clarifications in the 6th National Report include a clarification of the complications often seen in African-American individuals when taking beta-blockers. Therefore, many of these patients may be found to be on other drug therapies such as ACE inhibitors. Also, clarification has been provided for the drugs of choice of the average older individual in order to control blood pressure. These drugs usually include, but are not limited, to diuretics and beta-blockers or in combination. Lastly, the referral scheme has changed subtly in that the higher risk categories are now referred based on clinical situation. Also, some suggestions regarding the use of drugs in pregnant individuals where high blood pressure has been identified has not been made more clear. The physician may, therefore, have patients who are pregnant and who are suffering from elevated blood pressure on a variety of drug alternatives. These are outlines in the associated tables. The 6th Report of the Joint National Committee also has cited specific known drug interactions commonly seen with antihypertension therapy. Although these interactions are not numerous, the dentist would most likely be interested in the changes in efficacy of beta-blockers when used in combination with NSAIDs.

**Table 3.**
**RECOMMENDATIONS FOR FOLLOW-UP BASED ON INITIAL BLOOD PRESSURE MEASUREMENTS FOR ADULTS**

| Initial Blood Pressure (mm Hg)* | | Follow-Up Recommended† |
|---|---|---|
| **Systolic** | **Diastolic** | |
| <130 | <85 | Recheck in 2 years |
| 130-139 | 85-89 | Recheck in 1 year‡ |
| 140-159 | 90-99 | Confirm within 2 months‡ |
| 160-179 | 100-109 | Evaluate or refer to source of care within 1 month |
| ≥180 | ≥110 | Evaluate or refer to source of care immediately or within 1 week depending on clinical situation |

*If systolic and diastolic categories are different, follow recommendations for shorter time follow-up (eg, 160/86 mm Hg should be evaluated or referred to source of care within 1 month).

†Modify the scheduling of follow-up according to reliable information about past blood pressure measurements, other cardiovascular risk factors, or target organ disease.

‡Provide advice about Lifestyle modifications.

**Table 4.**
**COMPONENTS OF CARDIOVASCULAR RISK STRATIFICATION IN PATIENTS WITH HYPERTENSION**

| |
|---|
| **Major Risk Factors** |
| Smoking |
| Dyslipidemia |
| Diabetes mellitus |
| Age >60 years |
| Sex (men and postmenopausal women) |
| Family history of cardiovascular disease: women <65 years of age or men <age 55 |
| **Target Organ Damage/Clinical Cardiovascular Disease** |
| Heart diseases |
| Left ventricular hypertrophy |
| Angina/prior myocardial infarction |
| Prior coronary revascularization |
| Heart failure |
| Stroke or transient ischemic attack |
| Nephropathy |
| Peripheral arterial disease |
| Retinopathy |

**Table 5.**
**FOLLOW-UP CRITERIA FOR FIRST-OCCASION MEASUREMENT IN ADULTS ≥18 YEARS OR OLDER**

| Systolic | Diastolic | Follow-Up Recommended |
|---|---|---|
| <130 | <85 | Recheck within 2 years |
| 130-139 | 85-89 | Recheck within 1 year |
| 140-159 | 90-99 | Confirm within 2 months |
| 160-179 | 100-109 | Evaluate or refer to source of care within 1 month |
| ≥180 | ≥110 | Evaluate or refer to source of care immediately or within 1 week depending on clinical situation |

If systolic and diastolic categories are different, follow the shorter time follow-up (Source: *JNC* VI 11/97).

## CARDIOVASCULAR DISEASES *(Continued)*

### Table 6.
### ANTIHYPERTENSIVE DRUGS USED IN PREGNANCY*

The Report of the NHBPEP Working Group on High Blood Pressure in Pregnancy permits continuation of drug therapy in women with chronic hypertension (except for ACE inhibitors). In addition, angiotensin II receptor blockers should not be used during pregnancy. In women with chronic hypertension with diastolic levels of 100 mm Hg or greater (lower when end organ damage or underlying renal disease is present) and in women with acute hypertension when levels are 105 mm Hg or greater, the following agents are suggested.

| Suggested Drug | Comments |
|---|---|
| Central alpha-agonists | Methyldopa (C) is the drug of choice recommended by the NHBPEP Working Group |
| Beta-blockers | Atenolol (C) and metoprolol (C) appear to be safe and effective in late pregnancy. Labetalol (C) also appears to be effective (alpha- and beta-blockers) |
| Calcium antagonists | Potential synergism with magnesium sulfate may lead to precipitous hypotension (C) |
| ACE inhibitors, angiotensin II receptor blockers | Fetal abnormalities, including death, can be caused, and these drugs should not be used in pregnancy (D) |
| Diuretics | Diuretics (C) are recommended for chronic hypertension if prescribed before gestation or if patients appear to be salt-sensitive. They are not recommended in pre-eclampsia. |
| Direct vasodilators | Hydralazine (C) is the parenteral drug of choice based on its long history of safety and efficacy (C) |

*Adapted from Sibai and Lindheimer. There are several other antihypertensive drugs for which there are very limited data. The U.S. Food and Drug Administration classifies pregnancy risk as follows: C - adverse effects in animals; no controlled trials in humans; use if risk appears justified. D - positive evidence of fetal risk
ACE: Angiotensin-converting enzyme.

### Table 7.
### CAUSES OF INADEQUATE RESPONSIVENESS TO THERAPY

- Pseudoresistance
  - "White-coat hypertension"' or office elevations
  - Pseudohypertension in older patients
  - Use of regular cuff on very obese arm
- Nonadherence to therapy
- Volume overload
  - Excess salt intake
  - Progressive renal damage (nephrosclerosis)
  - Fluid retention from reduction of blood pressure
  - Inadequate diuretic therapy
- Drug-related causes
  - Doses too low
  - Wrong type of diuretic
  - Inappropriate combinations
  - Rapid inactivation (eg, hydralazine)
  - Drug actions and interactions
    - Sympathomimetics
    - Nasal decongestants
    - Appetite suppressants
    - Cocaine and other illicit drugs
    - Caffeine
    - Oral contraceptives
    - Adrenal steroids
    - Licorice (as may be found in chewing tobacco)
    - Cyclosporine, tacrolimus
    - Erythropoietin
    - Antidepressants
    - Nonsteroidal anti-inflammatory drugs
- Associate Conditions
  - Smoking
  - Increasing obesity
  - Sleep apnea
  - Insulin resistance/hyperinsulinemia

Ethanol intake of more than 1 oz (30 mL) per day
Anxiety-induced hyperventilation or panic attacks
Chronic pain
Intense vasoconstriction
Organic brain syndrome (eg, memory deficit)

Identifiable causes of hypertension

**Table 8.**
**RISK STRATIFICATION AND TREATMENT**

| Blood Pressure Stage (mm Hg) | Risk Group A* | Risk Group B† | Risk Group C‡ |
|---|---|---|---|
| High-normal (130-139/85-89) | Lifestyle modification | Lifestyle modification | Drug therapy# |
| Stage 1 (140-159/90-99) | Lifestyle modification (up to 12 months) | Lifestyle modification§ (up to 6 months) | Drug therapy |
| Stages 2 and 3 (≥160/≥100) | Drug therapy | Drug therapy | Drug therapy |

For example, a patient with diabetes and a blood pressure of 142/94 mm Hg plus left ventricular hypertrophy should be classified as having stage 1 hypertension with target organ disease (left ventricular hypertrophy) and with another major risk factor (diabetes). This patient would be categorized as Stage 1, Risk Group C, and recommended for immediate initiation of pharmacologic treatment.

*No risk factors; no TOD/CCD (indicates target organ disease/clinical cardiovascular disease)
†At least 1 risk factor, not including diabetes; no TOD/CCD
‡TOD/CCD and/or diabetes, with or without other risk factors
#For those with heart failure, renal insufficiency, or diabetes
§For patients with multiple risk factors, clinicians should consider drugs as initial therapy plus Lifestyle modifications

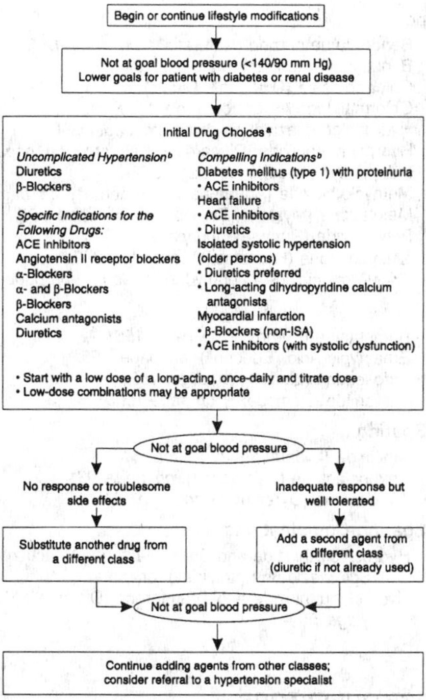


[a] Unless contraindicated. ACE indicates angiotensin-converting enzyme; ISA, intrinsic sympathomimetic activity.
[b] Based on randomized controlled trials.

Adapted from The Sixth Report of the Joint National Committee on Prevention, Detection, Evaluation, and Treatment of High Blood Pressure (JNC VI), Archives of Internal Medicine. 1997, 157:2413-46.

## CARDIOVASCULAR DISEASES *(Continued)*

Generally, peripheral vascular resistance, intravascular fluid volume, and cardiac output determine the blood pressure of a patient. Selection of therapies for patients being treated for prolonged elevated blood pressure is generally dependent upon the severity of the condition, age, and the pharmacological stability related to other cardiac diseases. Nonpharmacologic management of the patient with elevated sustained blood pressure begins with diet restriction, avoidance of fatty foods, an exercise program, reduction in sodium intake, and cessation of smoking. If there is an inadequate response, pharmacologic management usually begins with a diuretic or a beta-adrenergic receptor blocker.

ACE inhibitors, calcium channel blockers, alpha-adrenergic blockers are very popular as early treatment modalities and data on these agents reducing long-term morbidity and mortality are now being published. If there is an inadequate response to these drugs, practitioners often increase drug dosage, substitute another drug, or add a second agent from a different class. If there is still inadequate response, a second or third agent can be added, along with a diuretic if one has not already been utilized. Different combinations of drugs are often used in treating African-American patients.

When given in combination, these drugs can create not only side effects including xerostomia and oral ulcerations, but profound reduction in blood pressure. The newer drug classifications Angiotensin Receptor Antagonists and T-type Calcium Channel Blockers are having new drugs approved regularly and are showing promise as alternative therapies.

# CLASSIFICATION OF ANTIHYPERTENSIVES

## DIURETICS

### Thiazide-Type

- Bendroflumethiazide (Naturetin®) *on page 127*
- Benzthiazide (Exna®) *on page 132*
- Chlorothiazide (Diurigen®, Diuril®) *on page 229*
- Chlorthalidone (Hygroton®) *on page 242*
- Hydrochlorothiazide (Esidrix®) *on page 503*
- Hydroflumethiazide (Diucardin®; Saluron®) *on page 512*
- Indapamide (Lozol®) *on page 532*
- Methyclothiazide (Aquatensen®, Enduron®) *on page 657*
- Metolazone (Mykrox®, Zaroxolyn®) *on page 665*
- Polythiazide (Renese®) *on page 817*
- Quinethazone (Hydromox®) *on page 872*
- Trichlormethiazide (Metahydrin®; Naqua®) *on page 1014*

### Loop

- Bumetanide (Bumex®) *on page 156*
- Ethacrynic Acid (Edecrin®) *on page 395*
- Furosemide (Lasix®) *on page 460*
- Torsemide (Demadex®) *on page 1000*

### Potassium-Sparing

- Amiloride (Midamor®) *on page 61*
- Spironolactone (Aldactone®) *on page 931*
- Triamterene (Dyrenium®) *on page 1012*

### Potassium-Sparing Combinations

- Hydrochlorothiazide and Spironolactone (Aldactazide®; Alazide®; Spironazide®; Spirozide®) *on page 504*
- Hydrochlorothiazide and Triamterene (Dyazide®; Maxzide®) *on page 504*

## ADRENERGIC INHIBITORS

### Noncardioselective Beta-Adrenergic Blockers

- Carteolol (Cartrol®, Ocupress®) *on page 194*
- Carvedilol (Coreg®) *on page 195*

Nadolol (Corgard®) *on page 696*
Penbutolol (Levatol®) *on page 771*
Pindolol (Visken®) *on page 806*
Propranolol (Inderal®) *on page 857*
Timolol (Blocadren®) *on page 986*

**Cardioselective Beta-Adrenergic Blockers**

Acebutolol (Sectral®) *on page 26*
Atenolol (Tenormin®) *on page 105*
Betaxolol (Kerlone®) *on page 138*
Bisoprolol (Zebeta™) *on page 143*
Metoprolol (Lopressor®, Toprol XL®) *on page 666*
Sotalol (Betapace®) *on page 927*

**Combined Alpha- and Beta-Adrenergic Blockers**

Carvedilol (Coreg®) *on page 195*
Labetalol (Normodyne®, Trandate®) *on page 568*

**Alpha-Adrenergic Blockers - Peripheral-Acting (Alpha$_1$-Blockers)**

Doxazosin (Cardura®) *on page 351*
Guanadrel (Hylorel®) *on page 483*
Guanethidine (Ismelin®) *on page 484*
Prazosin (Minipress®) *on page 830*
Reserpine (Serpalan®, Serpasil®) *on page 882*
Terazosin (Hytrin®) *on page 957*

**Alpha-Adrenergic Blockers - Central-Acting (Alpha$_2$-Agonists)**

Clonidine (Catapres®) *on page 265*
Guanabenz (Wytensin®) *on page 483*
Guanfacine (Tenex®) *on page 485*
Methyldopa (Aldomet®) *on page 658*

## VASODILATORS

**Direct-Acting**

Hydralazine (Apresoline®) *on page 501*
Minoxidil (Loniten®) *on page 678*

**Angiotensin-Converting Enzyme Inhibitors**

Benazepril (Lotensin®) *on page 125*
Captopril (Capoten®) *on page 182*
Enalapril (Vasotec®) *on page 366*
Fosinopril (Monopril®) *on page 457*
Lisinopril (Prinivil®) *on page 594*
Moexipril (Univasc®) *on page 684*
Quinapril (Accupril®) *on page 871*
Ramipril (Altace™) *on page 877*
Spirapril (Renormax®) *on page 930*
Trandolapril (Mavik®) *on page 1003*

**Angiotensin-Converting Enzyme Inhibitors Combinations**

Captopril and Hydrochlorothiazide (Capozide®) *on page 183*
Enalapril and Hydrochlorothiazide (Vasoretic®) *on page 369*
Lisinopril and Hydrochlorothiazide (Prinzide®; Zestoretic®) *on page 596*

**Calcium Channel Blockers**

Amlodipine (Norvasc®) *on page 71*
Bepridil (Vascor®) *on page 134*
Diltiazem (Cardizem®, Dilacor™ XR) *on page 334*
Felodipine (Plendil®) *on page 421*
Isradipine (DynaCirc®) *on page 558*
Nicardipine (Cardene®) *on page 717*
Nifedipine (Adalat®, Procardia®) *on page 720*
Nisoldipine (Sular™) *on page 723*
Verapamil (Calan®, Isoptin®) *on page 1043*

**T-Type Calcium Channel Blockers**

Mibefradil (Posicor®) *on page 671*

**Angiotensin Receptor Antagonists**

Eprosartan (Teveten®) *on page 378*
Irbesartan (Avapro®) *on page 548*
Losartan (Cozaar®) *on page 603*
Valsartan (Diovan®) *on page 1039*

## CARDIOVASCULAR DISEASES *(Continued)*

The most common oral side effects of the management of the hypertensive patient are related to the antihypertensive drug therapy. A dry sore mouth can be caused by diuretics and central-acting adrenergic inhibitors. Occasionally, lichenoid reactions can occur in patients taking quinidine and methyldopa. The thiazides are occasionally also implicated. Lupus-like face rashes can be seen in patients taking calcium channel blockers as well as documented gingival hyperplasia in Appendix; see listing below.

Calcium Channel Blockers & Gingival Hyperplasia *on page 1204*

# RESPIRATORY DISEASES

Diseases of the respiratory system put dental patients at increased risk in the dental office because of their decreased pulmonary reserve, the medications they may be taking, drug interactions between these medications, medications the dentist may prescribe, and in some patients with infectious respiratory diseases, a risk of disease transmission.

The respiratory system consists of the nasal cavity, the nasopharynx, the trachea, and the components of the lung including, of course, the bronchi, the bronchioles, and the alveoli. The diseases that affect the lungs and the respiratory system can be separated by location of affected tissue. Diseases that affect the lower respiratory tract are often chronic, although infections can also occur. Three major diseases that affect the lower respiratory tract are often encountered in the medical history for dental patients. These include chronic bronchitis, emphysema, and asthma. Diseases that affect the upper respiratory tract are usually of the infectious nature and include sinusitis and the common cold. The upper respiratory tract infections may also include a wide variety of nonspecific infections, most of which are also caused by viruses. Influenza produces upper respiratory type symptoms and is often caused by orthomyxoviruses. Herpangina is caused by the Coxsackie type viruses and results in upper respiratory infections in addition to pharyngitis or sore throat. One serious condition, known as croup, has been associated with *Haemophilus influenzae* infections. Other more serious infections might include respiratory syncytial virus, adenoviruses, and parainfluenza viruses.

The respiratory symptoms that are often encountered in both upper respiratory and lower respiratory disorders include cough, dyspnea (difficulty in breathing), the production of sputum, hemoptysis (coughing up blood), a wheeze, and occasionally chest pain. One additional symptom, orthopnea (difficulty in breathing when lying down) is often used by the dentist to assist in evaluating the patient with the condition, pulmonary edema. This condition results from either respiratory disease or congestive heart failure.

No effective drug treatments are available for the management of many of the upper respiratory tract viral infections. However, amantadine (sold under the brand name Symmetrel®) is a synthetic drug given orally (200 mg/day) and has been found to be effective against some strains of influenza. Treatment other than for influenza includes supportive care products available over the counter. These might include antihistamines for symptomatic relief of the upper respiratory congestion, antibiotics to combat secondary bacterial infections, and in severe cases, fluids when patients have become dehydrated during the illness (see Therapeutic Category Index for selection). The treatment of herpangina may include management of the painful ulcerations of the oropharynx. The dentist may become involved in managing these lesions in a similar way to those seen in other acute viral infections (see Viral Infection section).

## SINUSITIS

Sinusitis also represents an upper respiratory infection that often comes under the purview of the practicing dentist. Acute sinusitis characterized by nasal obstruction, fever, chills, and midface head pain may be encountered by the dentist and discovered as part of a differential work-up for other facial or dental pain. Chronic sinusitis may likewise produce similar dental symptoms. Dental drugs of choice may include ephedrine or nasal drops, antihistamines, and analgesics. These drugs sometimes require supplementation with antibiotics. Most commonly, broad spectrum antibiotics, such as ampicillin, are prescribed. These are often combined with antral lavage to re-establish drainage from the sinus area. Surgical intervention such as a Caldwell-Luc procedure opening into the sinus is rarely necessary and many of the second generation antibiotics such as cephalosporins are used successfully in treating the acute and chronic sinusitis patient (see "Antibiotic Prophylaxis" *on page 1097*).

## LOWER RESPIRATORY DISEASES

Lower respiratory tract diseases, including asthma, chronic bronchitis, and emphysema are often identified in dental patients. Asthma is an intermittent respiratory disorder that produces recurrent bronchial smooth muscle spasm, inflammation, swelling of the bronchial mucosa, and hypersecretion of mucus. The incidence of childhood asthma appears to be increasing and may be related to the presence of pollutants such as sulfur dioxide and indoor cigarette smoke. The end result is widespread narrowing of the airways and decreased ventilation with increased

## RESPIRATORY DISEASES *(Continued)*

airway resistance, especially to expiration. Asthmatic patients often suffer from asthmatic attacks when stimulated by respiratory tract infections, exercise, and cold air. Medications such as aspirin and some nonsteroidal anti-inflammatory agents as well as cholinergic and beta-adrenergic blocking drugs, can also trigger asthmatic attacks in addition to chemicals, smoke, and emotional anxiety.

The classical chronic obstructive pulmonary diseases (COPD) of chronic bronchitis and emphysema are both characterized by chronic airflow obstructions during normal ventilatory efforts. They often occur in combination in the same patient and their treatment is similar. One common finding is that the patient is often a smoker. The dentist can play a role in reinforcement of smoking cessation in patients with chronic respiratory diseases.

Treatments include a variety of drugs depending on the severity of the symptoms and the respiratory compromise upon full respiratory evaluation. Patients who are having acute and chronic obstructive pulmonary attacks may be susceptible to infection and antibiotics such as penicillin, ampicillin, tetracycline, or trimethoprim-sulfamethoxazole are often used to eradicate susceptible infective organisms. Corticosteroids, as well as a wide variety of respiratory stimulants, are available in inhalant and/or oral forms. In patients using inhalant medication, oral candidiasis is occasionally encountered.

Amantadine (Symmetrel®) *on page 57*
Analgesics *on page 1283*
Antibiotics *on page 1287*
Antihistamines *on page 1293*
Decongestants *on page 1303*
Epinephrine (Dental) (Sus-Phrine®) *on page 374*

## SPECIFIC DRUGS USED IN THE TREATMENT OF CHRONIC RESPIRATORY CONDITIONS

### Beta$_2$-Selective

Albuterol (Proventil®,Ventolin®) *on page 43*
Bitolterol (Tornalate®) *on page 145*
Isoetharine (Bronkosol®, Bronkometer®) *on page 551*
Metaproterenol (Alupent®) *on page 642*
Pirbuterol (Maxair™) *on page 809*
Salmeterol (Serevent®) *on page 901*
Terbutaline (Brethine®, Brethaire®) *on page 959*

### Methylxanthines

Aminophylline (Somophylline®) *on page 63*
Oxtriphylline (Choledyl®) *on page 749*
Theophylline (Theo-Dur®, Slo-Bid®) *on page 969*

### Mast Cell Stabilizer

Cromolyn Sodium (Intal®) *on page 281*
Nedocromil Sodium (Tilade®) *on page 707*

### Corticosteroids

Beclomethasone (Beclovent®, Vanceril®) *on page 122*
Dexamethasone (Decadron® phosphate Respihaler®) *on page 308*
Flunisolide (AeroBid®; Nasarel®) *on page 439*
Fluticasone (Flovent®) *on page 450*
Mometasone Furoate (Nasonex®) *on page 686*
Prednisone (Deltasone®; Liquid Pred®; Meticorten®; Prednicen-M®; Sterapred®) *on page 833*
Triamcinolone (Azmacort™) *on page 1010*

### Anticholinergics

Ipratropium (Atrovent®) *on page 547*

### Leukotriene Receptor Antagonists

Montelukast (Singulair®) *on page 687*
Zafirlukast (Accolate®) *on page 1056*

### 5-Lipoxygenase Inhibitors

Zileuton (Zyflo®) *on page 1060*

Other respiratory diseases include tuberculosis and sarcoidosis which are considered to be restrictive granulomatous respiratory diseases. Tuberculosis is covered in "Nonviral Infectious Diseases" *on page 1095*. Sarcoidosis is a condition that at one time was thought to be similar to tuberculosis, however, it is a multisystem disorder of unknown origin which has as a characteristic lymphocytic and mononuclear phagocytic accumulation in epithelioid granulomas within the lung. It occurs worldwide but shows a slight increased prevalence in temperate climates. The treatment of sarcoidosis is usually one that corresponds to its usually benign course, however, many patients are placed on corticosteroids at the level of 40-60 mg of prednisone daily. This treatment is continued for a protracted period of time. As in any disease requiring steroid therapy, consideration of adrenal suppression is necessary. Alteration of steroid dosage prior to stressful dental procedures may be necessary, usually increasing the steroid dosage prior to and during the stressful procedures and then gradually returning the patient to the original dosage over several days. Even in the absence of evidence of adrenal suppression, consultation with the prescribing physician for appropriate dosing and timing of procedures is advisable.

Prednisone *on page 833*

# RELATIVE POTENCY OF ENDOGENOUS AND SYNTHETIC CORTICOSTEROIDS

| Agent | Equivalent Dose (mg) |
|---|---|
| **Short-Acting (8-12 h)** | |
| Cortisol | 20 |
| Cortisone | 25 |
| **Intermediate-Acting (18-36 h)** | |
| Prednisolone | 5 |
| Prednisone | 5 |
| Methylprednisolone | 4 |
| Triamcinolone | 4 |
| **Long-Acting (36-54 h)** | |
| Betamethasone | 0.75 |
| Dexamethasone | 0.75 |

Potential drug interactions for the respiratory disease patient exist. An acute sensitivity to aspirin-containing drugs and some of the nonsteroidal anti-inflammatory drugs is a threat for the asthmatic patient. Barbiturates and narcotics may occasionally precipitate asthmatic attacks as well. Erythromycin, clarithromycin, and ketoconazole are contraindicated in patients who are taking theophylline due to potential enhancement of theophylline toxicity. Patients that are taking steroid preparations as part of their respiratory therapy may require alteration in dosing prior to stressful dental procedures. The physician should be consulted.

Barbiturates *on page 1299*
Clarithromycin *on page 256*
Erythromycin *on page 383*
Ketoconazole *on page 564*

# ENDOCRINE DISORDERS & PREGNANCY

The human endocrine system manages metabolism and homeostasis. Numerous glandular tissues produce hormones that act in broad reactions with tissues throughout the body. Cells in various organ systems may be sensitive to the hormone, or they release, in reaction to the hormone, a second hormone that acts directly on another organ. Diseases of the endocrine system may have importance in dentistry. For the purposes of this section, we will limit our discussion to diseases of the thyroid tissues, diabetes mellitus, and conditions requiring the administration of synthetic hormones, and pregnancy.

## THYROID

Thyroid diseases can be classified into conditions that cause the thyroid to be overactive (hyperthyroidism) and those that cause the thyroid to be underactive (hypothyroidism). Clinical signs and symptoms associated with hyperthyroidism may include goiter, heat intolerance, tremor, weight loss, diarrhea, and hyperactivity. Thyroid hormone production can be tested by TSH levels and additional screens may include radioactive iodine uptake or a pre-$T_4$ (tetraiodothyronine, thyroxine) assay or iodine index or total serum $T_3$ (triiodothyronine). The results of thyroid function tests may be altered by ingestion of antithyroid drugs such as propylthiouracil, estrogen-containing drugs, and organic and inorganic iodides. When a diagnosis of hyperthyroidism has been made, treatment usually begins with antithyroid drugs which may include propranolol coupled with radioactive iodides as well as surgical procedures to reduce thyroid tissue. Generally, the beta-blockers are used to control cardiovascular effects of excessive $T_4$. Propylthiouracil or methimazole are the most common antithyroid drugs used. The dentist should be aware that epinephrine is definitely contraindicated in patients with uncontrolled hyperthyroidism.

Diseases and conditions associated with hypothyroidism may include bradycardia, drowsiness, cold intolerance, thick dry skin, and constipation. Treatment of hypothyroidism is generally with replacement thyroid hormone until a euthyroid state is achieved. Various preparations are available, the most common is levothyroxine, commonly known as Synthroid® or Levothroid® and is generally the drug of choice for thyroid replacement therapy.

**Drugs to Treat Hypothyroidism**

Levothyroxine (Levothroid®, Levoxyl®, Synthroid®) *on page 585*
Liothyronine (Cytomel®, Triostat™) *on page 592*
Liotrix (Thyrolar®) *on page 593*
Thyroid (Armour® Thyroid, S-P-T, Thyrar®, Thyroid Strong®) *on page 982*

**Drugs to Treat Hyperthyroidism**

Methimazole (Tapazole®) *on page 648*
Potassium Iodide (Pima®, SSKI®, Thyro-Block®) *on page 824*
Propranolol (Betachron E-R®, Inderal®) *on page 857*
Propylthiouracil *on page 859*

## DIABETES

Diabetes mellitus refers to a condition of prolonged hyperglycemia associated with either abnormal production or lack of production of insulin. Commonly known as Type 1 diabetes, insulin-dependent diabetes (IDDM) is a condition where there are absent or deficient levels of circulating insulin therefore triggering tissue reactions associated with prolonged hyperglycemia. The kidney's attempt to excrete the excess glucose and the organs that do not receive adequate glucose essentially are damaged. Small vessels and arterial vessels in the eye, kidney, and brain are usually at the greatest risk. Generally, blood sugar levels between 70-120 mg/dL are considered to be normal. Inadequate insulin levels allow glucose to rise to greater than the renal threshold which is 180 mg/dL, and such elevations prolonged lead to organ damage.

The goals of treatment of the diabetic are to maintain metabolic control of the blood glucose levels and to reduce the morbid effects of periodic hyperglycemia. Insulin therapy is the primary mechanism to attain management of consistent insulin levels. Insulin preparations are categorized according to their duration of action. Generally, NPH or intermediate-acting insulin and long-acting insulin can be used in combination with short-acting or regular insulin to maintain levels consistent throughout the day.

In Type 2 or noninsulin-dependent diabetes (NIDDM), the receptor for insulin in the tissues is generally down regulated and the glucose, therefore, is not utilized at an appropriate rate. There is perhaps a stronger genetic basis for noninsulin-dependent diabetes than for Type 1. Treatment of the diabetes Type 2 patient is generally directed toward early nonpharmacologic intervention, mainly weight reduction, moderate exercise, and lower plasma-glucose concentrations. Oral hypoglycemic agents as seen in the list below are often used to maintain blood sugar levels. Often 30% of Type 2 diabetics require insulin as well as oral hypoglycemics in order to manage their diabetes. Generally, the two classes of oral hypoglycemics are the sulfonylureas and the biguanides. The sulfonylureas are prescribed more frequently and they stimulate beta cell production of insulin, increased glucose utilization, and tend to normalize glucose metabolism in the liver. The uncontrolled diabetic may represent a challenge to the dental practitioner.

Insulin Preparations (various products) *on page 537*

**TYPES OF INSULIN**

| Type | Action | Duration (h) |
|---|---|---|
| Regular | Rapid | 5-7 |
| Semilente | Rapid | 10-14 |
| Lispro | Rapid | 3.5 h |
| NPH | Intermediate | 18-24 |
| Lente | Intermediate | 14-20 |
| Ultralente | Prolonged | >36 |

**Oral Hypoglycemic Agents**

Acarbose (Precose®) *on page 25*
Acetohexamide (Dymelor®) *on page 34*
Chlorpropamide (Diabinese®) *on page 240*
Glimepiride (Amaryl®) *on page 468*
Glipizide (Glucotrol®) *on page 469*
Glyburide (Diaβeta; Glynase™, PresTab™, Micronase®) *on page 471*
Metformin (Glucophage®) *on page 643*
Miglitol (Glyset®) *on page 676*
Repaglinide (Prandin®) *on page 881*
Tolazamide (Tolinase®) *on page 993*
Tolbutamide (Orinase®) *on page 994*
Troglitazone (Rezulin®)*on page 1027*

**Adjunct Therapy**

Cisapride (Propulsid®) *on page 251*
Metoclopramide (Clopra®, Maxolon®, Octamide®, Reglan®) *on page 664*

Oral manifestations of uncontrolled diabetes might include abnormal neutrophil function resulting in a poor response to periodontal pathogens. Increased risk of gingivitis and periodontitis in these patients is common. Candidiasis is a frequent occurrence. Denture sore mouth may be more prominent and poor wound healing following extractions may be one of the complications encountered.

## HORMONAL THERAPY

Two uses of hormonal supplementation include oral contraceptives and estrogen replacement therapy. Drugs used for contraception interfere with fertility by inhibiting release of follicle stimulating hormone, luteinizing hormone, and by preventing ovulation. There are few oral side effects; however, moderate gingivitis, similar to that seen during pregnancy, has been reported. The dentist should be aware that decreased effect of oral contraceptives has been reported with most antibiotics. See individual monographs for specific details. Drugs commonly encountered include:

Estradiol (various products) *on page 387*
Ethinyl Estradiol and Ethynodiol Diacetate (Demulen®) *on page 400*

## ENDOCRINE DISORDERS & PREGNANCY *(Continued)*

Ethinyl Estradiol and Levonorgestrel (Levlen®, Nordette®, Levora®, Tri-Levlen®, Triphasil™) *on page 402*
Ethinyl Estradiol and Norethindrone (Ortho-Novum™, Ortho-Novum™ 1/35) *on page 404*
Levonorgestrel (Norplant®) *on page 584*
Medroxyprogesterone Acetate (Amen®, Curretab®, Cycrin®, Depo-Provera®, Provera®) *on page 623*
Mestranol and Norethindrone (Ortho-Novum™ 1/50) *on page 639*
Mestranol and Norethynodrel (Enovid®) *on page 641*
Norethindrone (Aygestin®, Micronor®, Nor-Q.D.®) *on page 730*
Norgestrel (Ovrette®) *on page 731*

Estrogens or derivatives are usually prescribed as replacement therapy following menopause or cyclic irregularities and to inhibit osteoporosis. The following list of drugs may interact with antidepressants and barbiturates. New tissue-specific estrogens like Evista® may help with the problem of osteoporosis.

Chlorotrianisene (TACE®) *on page 230*
Estrogens, Conjugated (Premarin®) *on page 391*
Estrogens, Esterified (Estratab®, Menest®) *on page 392*
Estrogens and Medroxyprogesterone (Prempro®) *on page 390*
Estrogens and Methyltestosterone (Estratest®, Premarin®) *on page 391*
Estrone (Aquest®, Kestrone®) *on page 393*
Estropipate (Ogen®, Ortho-Est®) *on page 394*
Ethinyl Estradiol (Estinyl®) *on page 399*
Quinestrol (Estrovis®) *on page 872*
Raloxifene (Evista®) *on page 876*

## PREGNANCY

Normal endocrine and physiologic functions are altered during pregnancy. Endogenous estrogens and progesterone increase and placental hormones are secreted. Thyroid stimulating hormone and growth hormone also increase. Cardiovascular changes can result and increased blood volume can lead to blood pressure elevations and transient heart murmurs. Generally, in a normal pregnancy, oral gingival changes will be limited to gingivitis. Alteration of treatment plans might include limiting administration of all drugs to emergency procedures only during the first and third trimesters and medical consultation regarding the patients' status for all elective procedures. Limiting dental care throughout pregnancy to preventive procedures is not unreasonable.

# HIV INFECTION AND AIDS

Human immunodeficiency virus (HIV) represents agents HIV-1 and HIV-2 that produce a devastating systemic disease. The virus causes disease by leading to elevated risk of infections in patients and, from our experience over the last 18 years, there clearly are oral manifestations associated with these patients. Also, there has been a revolution in infection control in our dental offices over the last two decades due to our expanding knowledge of this infectious agent. Infection control practices (see "Infectious Disease Information" *on page 1232*) have been elevated to include all of the infectious agents with which dentists often come into contact. These might include in addition to HIV, hepatitis viruses (of which the serotypes include A, B, C, D, E, F, and G) , the herpes viruses; sexually transmitted diseases such as syphilis, gonorrhea, papillomavirus, all of which are covered elsewhere in this book.

Acquired immunodeficiency syndrome (AIDS) has been recognized since early 1981 as a unique clinical syndrome manifest by opportunistic infections or by neoplasms complicating the underlying defect in the cellular immune system. These defects are now known to be brought on by infection and pathogenesis with human immunodeficiency virus 1 or 2 (HIV-1 is the predominant serotype identified). The major cellular defect brought on by infection with HIV is a depletion of T-cells, primarily the sub-type, T-helper cells, known as CD4+ cells. Over these years, our knowledge regarding HIV infection and the oral manifestations often associated with patients with HIV or AIDS, has increased dramatically. Populations of individuals known to be at high risk of HIV transmission include homosexuals, intravenous drug abuse patients, transfusion recipients, patients with other sexually transmitted diseases, and patients practicing promiscuous sex.

The definitions of AIDS have also evolved over this period of time. The natural history of HIV infection along with some of the oral manifestations can be reviewed in Table 1. The risk of developing these opportunistic infections increases as the patient progresses to AIDS.

**Table 1.**
**NATURAL HISTORY OF HIV INFECTION/ORAL MANIFESTATIONS**

| Time From Transmission (Average) | Observation | CD4 Cell Count |
|---|---|---|
| 0 | Viral transmissions | Normal: 1000 (±500/mm$^3$) |
| 2-4 weeks | Self-limited infectious mononucleosis-like illness with fever, rash, leukopenia, mucocutaneous ulcerations (mouth, genitals, etc), thrush | Transient decrease |
| 6-12 weeks | Seroconversion (rarely requires ≥3 months for seroconversion) | Normal |
| 0-8 years | Healthy/asymptomatic HIV infection; peripheral/persistent generalized lymphadenopathy; HPV, thrush, OHL; RAU, periodontal diseases, salivary gland diseases; dermatitis | ≥500/mm$^3$ gradual reduction with average decrease of 50-80/mm$^3$/ year |
| 4-8 years | Early symptomatic HIV infection previously called (AIDS-related complex): Thrush, vaginal candidiasis (persistent, frequent and/or severe), cervical dysplasia/CA Hodgkin's lymphoma, B-cell lymphoma, oral hairy leukoplakia, salivary gland diseases, ITP, xerostomia, dermatitis, shingles; RAU, herpes simplex, HPV, bacterial infections, periodontal diseases, molluscum contagiosum, other physical symptoms: fever, weight loss, fatigue | ≥300-500/mm$^3$ |
| 6-10 years | AIDS: Wasting syndrome, *Candida* esophagitis, Kaposi's sarcoma, HIV-associated dementia, disseminated *M. avium*, Hodgkin's or B-cell lymphoma, herpes simplex >30 days; PCP; cryptococcal meningitis, other systemic fungal infections; CMV | <200/mm$^3$ |

Natural history indicates course of HIV infection in absence of antiretroviral treatment. Adapted from Bartlett JG, "A Guide to HIV Care from the AIDS Care Program of the Johns Hopkins Medical Institutions," 2nd ed.

PCP - *Pneumocystis carinii* pneumonia; ITP - idiopathic thrombocytopenia purpura; HPV - human papilloma virus; OHL - oral hairy leukoplakia; RAU - recurrent aphthous ulcer

## HIV INFECTION AND AIDS *(Continued)*

Patients with HIV infection and/or AIDS are seen in dental offices throughout the country. In general, it is the dentist's obligation to treat HIV individuals including patients of record and other patients who may seek treatment when the office is accepting new patients. These patients are protected under the Americans with Disabilities Act and the dentist has an obligation as described. Two excellent publications, one by the American Dental Association and the other by the American Academy of Oral Medicine, outline the dentist's responsibility as well as a very detailed explanation of dental management protocols for HIV patients. These protocols, however, are evolving just as our knowledge of HIV has evolved. New drugs and their interactions (see Dental Drug Interactions *on page 1225* in Appendix) present the dentist with continuous need for updates regarding the appropriate management of HIV patients. Diagnostic tests, including determining viral load in combination with the CD4 status, now are used to modify a patient's treatment in ways that allow them to remain relatively illness-free for longer periods of time. This places more of a responsibility on the dental practice team to be aware of drug changes, of new drugs, and of the appropriate oral management in such patients.

Our knowledge of AIDS allows us to properly treat these patients while protecting ourselves, our staff, and other patients in the office. All types of infectious disease require consistent practices in our dental offices known as Universal Precautions (see Infectious Disease Information *on page 1232* in Appendix). The office team that utilizes these precautions appropriately is well protected against passage of infectious agents. These agents include sexually transmitted disease agents, the highly virulent hepatitis viruses, and the less virulent but always worrisome HIV. In general, an office that is practicing universal precautions is one that is considered safe for patients and staff. Throughout this spectrum, HIV is placed somewhere in the middle in terms of infection risk in the dental office. Other sexually transmitted diseases and infectious diseases such as tuberculosis represent a greater threat to the dentist than HIV itself. However, due to the grave danger of HIV infection, many of our precautions have been instituted to assist the dentist in protecting himself, his staff, and other patients in situations where the office may be involved in treating a patient that is HIV positive.

As in the management of all medically compromised patients, the appropriate care of HIV patients begins with a complete and thorough history. This history must allow the dentist to identify risk factors in the development of HIV as well as identify those patients known to be HIV positive. Knowledge of all medications prescribed to patients at risk is also important.

The current antiretroviral therapy used to treat patients with HIV infection and/or AIDS includes three primary classifications of drugs. These are the nucleoside analogs, protease inhibitors, and the non-nucleoside/nucleotide analogs (analogs refers to chemicals that can substitute competitively for naturally produced cell components such as found in DNA, RNA, or proteins). The newest drugs include several nucleoside analogs, abacavir (Ziagen®), subprotease inhibitors, amprenavir, and several non-nucleoside analogs, efavirenz (Sustiva®) and adefovir (Preveon®). Finding the perfect "cocktail" of anti-HIV medications still eludes clinicians. This is partly due to the fact that therapies are still too novel and the patient's years too few to study. Numerous recently published studies have indicated that combinations of drugs are far better than individual drug therapy. Several of these studies have looked at two drug combinations particularly between nucleoside analogs in combination with protease inhibitors. The newer drugs (non-nucleoside analogs) have added the possibility of a triple cocktail. Recently several studies indicated that this three-drug combination may be the best in managing HIV infection.

When HIV was first discovered, the efforts for monitoring HIV infection focused on the CD4 blood levels and the ratios between the helper cells, suppressor cells within the patient's immune system. These markers were used to indicate success or failure of drug therapies as patients moved through HIV pathogenesis toward AIDS. More recently, however, the advent of protease inhibitors has allowed clinicians to monitor the actual presence of viral RNA within the patient and the term viral load has become the focus of therapy monitoring. The availability of better therapies and our rapidly expanding knowledge of molecular biology of the HIV virus have created new opportunities to control the AIDS epidemic. Cases can be monitored quite closely looking at the number of copy units or virions within the patient's bloodstream as an indication in combination with other infections and/or declining or increasing CD4 numbers to establish prognostic values for the patient's success. Long-term survival of patients infected with HIV has been accomplished by monitoring and adjusting therapy to these numbers.

Comprehensive coordinated approaches, that have been advocated by researchers, have sought to establish national standards for HIV reporting, greater access to effective newly approved medications, improved access to individual physicians treating HIV patients, and continued protection of patient's privacy. These goals allow the reporting of studies that suggest that combination therapies, some of which have been tried in less controlled individual patient treatments, may prove useful in larger populations of HIV-infected individuals. As these studies are reported, the dental clinician should be aware that patients' drug therapies change rapidly, various combinations may be tried, and the side effects and interactions as described in the chapter on drug interactions and the CYP system will also emerge. The dentist must be aware of these potential interactions with seemingly innocuous drugs such as clarithromycin, erythromycin, and some of the sedative drugs that a dentist may utilize in their practice as well as some of the analgesics. These drug interactions may be the most important part of monitoring that the dentist provides in helping to manage a situation. Some of the antiviral drugs more commonly used for HIV, AIDS, Asymptomatic, CD4 <500, and the newer drugs (ie, protease inhibitors, nucleoside analogs, and non-nucleoside nucleotide analogs) are listed in Table 2.

**Table 2.**
**CATEGORIES OF ANTIRETROVIRAL DRUGS**

| Nucleoside Analogs | Protease Inhibitors | Non-Nucleoside/ Nucleotide Analogs |
|---|---|---|
| Zidovudine (Retrovir®, AZT, SDV) | Saquinavir (Invirase®) | Nevirapine (Viramune®) |
| Didanosine (Videx®, ddi) | Ritonavir (Norvir®) | Delavirdine (Rescriptor®) |
| Zalcitabine (HIVID®, ddc) | Indinavir (Crixivan®) | Efavirenz (Sustiva®) |
| Stavudine (Zerit®, d4T) | Nelfinavir (Viracept®) | Adefovir (Preveon®) |
| Lamivudine (Epivir®) | Amprenavir (141W94)* | |
| Abacavir (Ziagen®) | | |

*FDA approval pending.

The presence of other infections is an important part of the health history. Appropriate medical consultation may be mandated after a health history in order to accomplish a complete evaluation of the patients at risk. Uniformity in the taking of a history from a patient is the dentist's best plan for all patients so that no selectivity or discrimination can be implicated.

An appropriate review of symptoms may also identify oral and systemic conditions that may be present in aggressive HIV disease. Medical physical examination may reveal pre-existing or developing intra- or extra-oral signs/symptoms of progressive disease. Aggressive herpes simplex, herpes zoster, papillomavirus, Kaposi's sarcoma or lymphoma are among the disorders that might be identified. In addition to these, intra-oral examination may raise suspicion regarding fungal infections, angular cheilitis, squamous cell carcinoma, and recurrent aphthous ulcers. The dentist should be vigilant in all patients regardless of HIV risk.

It will always be up to the dental practitioner to determine whether testing for HIV should be recommended following the history and physical examination of a new patient. Because of the severe psychological implications of learning of HIV positivity for a patient, the dentist should be aware that there are appropriate referral sites where psychological counseling and appropriate discrete testing for the patient is available. The dentist's office should have these sites available for referral should the patient be interested. Candid discussions, however, with the patient regarding risk factors and/or other signs or symptoms in their history and physical condition that may indicate a higher HIV risk than the normal population, should be an area the dentist feels comfortable in broaching with any new patient. Oftentimes, it is appropriate to recommend testing for other infectious diseases should risk factors be present. For example, testing for hepatitis B may be appropriate for the patient and along with this the dentist could recommend that the patient consider HIV testing. Because of the legal issues involved, anonymity for HIV testing may be appropriate and it is always up to the patient to follow the doctor's recommendations.

## HIV INFECTION AND AIDS *(Continued)*

When a patient has either given a positive history of knowing that they are HIV positive or it has been determined after referral for consultation, the dentist should be aware of the AIDS-defining illnesses. Of course, current medical status and drug therapy that the patient may be undergoing is of equal importance. The dentist, through medical consultation and regular follow-up with the patient's physician, should be made aware of the CD4 count (Table 3), the viral load, and the drugs that the patient is taking. The presence of other AIDS-defining illnesses as well as complications, such as higher risk of endocarditis and the risk of other systemic infections such as tuberculosis, are extremely important for the dentist. These may make an impact on the dental treatment plan in terms of the selection of preprocedural antibiotics or the use of oral medications to treat opportunistic infections in or around the oral cavity.

**Table 3.**
**CD4+ LYMPHOCYTE COUNT AND PERCENTAGE AS RELATED TO THE RISK OF OPPORTUNISTIC INFECTION**

| CD4+ Cells/mm$^3$ | CD4+ Percentage* | Risk of Opportunistic Infection |
|---|---|---|
| >600 | 32-60 | No increased risk |
| 400-500 | <29 | Initial immune suppression |
| 200-400 | 14-28 | Appearance of opportunistic infections, some may be major |
| <200 | <14 | Severe immune suppression. AIDS diagnosis. Major opportunistic infections. Although variable, prognosis for surviving more than 3 years is poor. |
| <50 | — | Although variable, prognosis for surviving more than 1 year is poor |

*Several studies have suggested that the CD4+ percentage demonstrates less variability between measurements, as compared to the absolute CD4+ cell count. CD4+ percentages may therefore give a clearer impression of the course of disease.

Adapted from Glick M and Silverman S, "Dental Management of HIV-Infected Patients," *J Am Dent Assoc* (Supplement to Reviewers), 1995.

AIDS-defining illnesses such as candidiasis, recurrent pneumonia, or lymphoma are clearly important to the dentist. Chemotherapy that might be being given to the patient for treatment for any or all of these disorders can have implications in terms of the patient's response to simple dental procedures.

Drug therapies have become complex in the treatment of HIV/AIDS. Because of the moderate successes with protease inhibitors and the drug combination therapies, more patients are living longer and receiving more dental care throughout their lives. Drug therapies are often tailored to the current CD4 count in combination with the viral load. In general, patients with high CD4 counts are usually at lower risk for complications in the dental office than patients with low CD4 counts. However, the presence of a high viral load with or without a stable CD4 count may be indicative or a more rapid progression of the HIV/AIDS disease process than had previously been thought. Patients with a high viral load and a declining CD4 count are considered to have the greatest risk and the poorest prognosis of all the groups.

Other organ damage, such as liver compromise potentially leading to bleeding disorders, can be found as the disease progresses to AIDS. Liver dysfunction may be related to pre-existing hepatic diseases due to previous infection with a hepatitis virus such as hepatitis B or other drug toxicities associated with the treatment of AIDS. The dentist must have available current prothrombin and partial thromboplastin times (PT and PTT) in order to accurately evaluate any risk of bleeding abnormality. Platelet count and liver function studies are also important. Potential drug interactions include some antibiotics, as well as any anticoagulating drugs, which may be contraindicated in such patients. It may be necessary to avoid nonsteroidal anti-inflammatory drugs as well as aspirin. (See the introductory text "Pharmacology of Drug Metabolism and Interactions" *on page 12*).

The use of preprocedural antibiotics is another issue in the HIV patient. As the absolute neutrophil count declines during the progression of AIDS, the use of antibiotics as a preprocedural step prior to dental care may be necessary. If protracted treatment plans are necessary, the dentist should receive updated information as the patient receives such from their physician. It is always important that the dentist have current CD4 counts, viral load assay, as well as liver function studies, AST and ALT, and bleeding indicators including platelet count, PT, and PTT. If any other existing conditions such as cardiac involvement or joint prostheses are involved, antibiotic coverage may also be necessary. However, these determinations are no different than in the non-HIV population and this subject is covered in "Preprocedural Antibiotic

Prophylaxis Guidelines for Dental Patients" *on page 1097*. See Table 4 for normal blood values as general guidelines for provision of dental care.

**Table 4.**
**NORMAL BLOOD VALUES**

| Test | Range of Normal Values |
|---|---|
| **Complete blood count (CBC)** | |
| White blood cells | 4,500-11,000 |
| Red blood cells (male) | 4.6-6.2 x $10^6$ µL |
| Red blood cells (female) | 4.2-5.4 x $10^6$ µL |
| Platelets | 150,000-450,000 |
| Hematocrit (male) | 40% to 54% |
| Hematocrit (female) | 38% to 47% |
| Hemoglobin (male) | 13.5-18 g/dL |
| Hemoglobin (female) | 12-16 g/dL |
| Mean corpuscular volume (MCV) | 80-96 $µm^3$ |
| Mean corpuscular hemoglobin (MCH) | 27-31 pg |
| Mean corpuscular hemoglobin concentration (MCHC) | 32% to 36% |
| **Differential white blood cell count (%)** | |
| Segmented neutrophils | 56 |
| Bands | 3.0 |
| Eosinophils | 2.7 |
| Basophils | 0.3 |
| Lymphocytes | 34.0 |
| Monocytes | 4.0 |
| **Hemostasis** | |
| Bleeding time (BT) | 2-8 minutes |
| Prothrombin time (PT) | 10-13 seconds |
| Activated partial thromboplastin time (aPTT) | 25-35 seconds |
| **Serum chemistry** | |
| Glucose (fasting) | 70-110 mg/dL |
| Blood urea nitrogen (BUN) | 8-23 mg/dL |
| Creatinine (male) | 0.1-0.4 mg/dL |
| Creatinine (female) | 0.2-0.7 mg/dL |
| Bilirubin, indirect (unconjugated) | 0.3 mg/dL |
| Bilirubin, direct (conjugated) | 0.1-1 mg/dL |
| Calcium | 9.2-11 mg/dL |
| Magnesium | 1.8-3 mg/dL |
| Phosphorus | 2.3-4.7 mg/dL |
| **Serum electrolytes** | |
| Sodium ($Na^+$) | 136-142 mEq/L |
| Potassium ($K^+$) | 3.8-5 mEq/L |
| Chloride ($Cl^-$) | 95-103 mEq/L |
| Bicarbonate ($HCO_3^-$) | 21-28 mmol/L |
| **Serum enzymes** | |
| Alkaline phosphatase | 20-130 IU/L |
| Alanine aminotransferase (ALT) (formerly called SGPT) | 4-36 units/L |
| Aspartate aminotransferase (AST) (formerly called SGOT) | 8-33 units/L |
| Amylase | 16-120 Somogyi units/dL |
| Creatine kinase (CK) (male) | 55-170 units/L |
| Creatine kinase (CK) (female) | 30-135 units/L |

The consideration of current blood values is important in long-term care of any medically compromised patient and in particular the HIV-positive patient. Preventive dental care is likewise valuable in these patients, however, the dentist's approach should be no different than as with all patients. See Table 5 for oral lesions commonly associated with HIV disease and a brief description of their usual treatment. The clinician is referred to other sections of the text for more detailed descriptions of these common oral lesions. Other important parts of the text that may be useful for the dentist include the Office Protocol for Universal Precautions *on page 1232* and the Frequently Asked Questions at the end of this chapter. The clinician should also be aware that several of the protease inhibitors have now been associated with drug interactions. Some of these drug interactions include therapies that the dentist may be utilizing. The basis for these drug interactions with the protease inhibitors is the inhibition of cytochrome P-450

## HIV INFECTION AND AIDS *(Continued)*

isoforms which are important in the normal liver function and metabolism of drugs. A detailed description of the mechanisms of inhibition can be found in the section "Pharmacology of Drug Metabolism and Interactions" *on page 12*, as well as a table illustrating some of the known drug interactions with antiviral therapy and drugs commonly prescribed in the dental office. The metabolism of these drugs could be affected by the patient's antiviral therapy. Please see the section on selected references for more information on management of HIV patients.

**Table 5.**
**ORAL LESIONS COMMONLY SEEN IN HIV/AIDS**

| Condition | Management |
|---|---|
| Oral candidiasis | See "Oral Fungal Infections" *on page 1134* |
| Angular cheilitis | See "Oral Fungal Infections" *on page 1134* |
| Oral hairy leukoplakia | See "Systemic Viral Diseases" *on page 1115* |
| Periodontal diseases<br>Linear gingivitis<br>Ulcerative periodontitis | See "Oral Bacterial Infections" *on page 1128* |
| Herpes simplex | Acyclovir - see "Systemic Viral Diseases" *on page 1115* |
| Herpes zoster | Acyclovir - see "Systemic Viral Diseases" *on page 1115* |
| Chronic aphthous ulceration | Palliation / Thalidomide (Thalomid®) |
| Salivary gland disease | Referral |
| Human papillomavirus | Laser / Surgical excision |
| Kaposi's sarcoma | See "Antibiotic Prophylaxis" *on page 1097*; Biopsy / Laser |
| Kaposi's lymphoma | Biopsy / Referral |
| Tuberculosis | Referral |

Dapsone (Avlosulfon®) *on page 298*
Delavirdine (Rescriptor™) *on page 302*
Didanosine (Videx®) *on page 323*
Indinavir (Crixivan®) *on page 533*
Lamivudine (Epivir®) *on page 571*
Nelfinavir (Viracept®) *on page 708*
Ritonavir (Norvir®) *on page 892*
Stavudine (Zerit®) *on page 932*
Thalidomide (Thalomid®) *on page 967*
Zalcitabine (Hivid®) *on page 1057*
Zidovudine (Retrovir®) *on page 1058*
Zidovudine and Lamivudine (Combivir®) *on page 1059*

## FREQUENTLY ASKED QUESTIONS

*How does one get AIDS, aside from having unprotected sex?*

Our current knowledge about the immunodeficiency virus is that it is carried via semen, contaminated needles, blood products, transfusion products, if indeed the transfusion products have not been tested, and potentially in other fluids of the body. Patients at highest risk would include I.V. drug abuse patients, patients receiving multiple transfusions with blood that has not been screened for HIV, or patients practicing unprotected sex with multiple partners where the history of the partner may not be as clear as the patient would like.

*Are patients safe from AIDS or HIV infection when they present to the dentist office?*

Our current knowledge indicates that the answer is an unequivocal yes. The patient is protected because the dental offices are practicing universal precautions using antimicrobial hand-washing agents, gloves, face masks, eye protection, special clothing, aerosol control, and instrument soaking and autoclaving. All of these procedures stop the potential transmission to a new patient as well as allow for easy disposal of contaminated office supplies for elimination of microbes by an antimicrobial technique should they be contaminated through the treatment of another patient. These precautions are mandated by the OSHA requirements and are covered in Universal Precautions in the Appendix.

*What is the most common opportunistic infection that HIV-positive patients suffer that may be important in dentistry?*

The most common opportunistic infection important to dentistry is oral candidiasis. This disease can present as white plaques, red areas, or angular cheilitis occurring at the corners of the mouth. Management of such lesions is appropriate by the dentist and is described in this handbook (see Oral Fungal Infections *on page 1134*). Other oral complications would include HIV-associated periodontal disease, as well as the other conditions outlined in Table 5. Of great concern to the dentist is the risk of tuberculosis. In many HIV-positive patients, tuberculosis has become a serious life-threatening opportunistic infection. The dentist should be aware that appropriate referral for anyone showing such respiratory signs and symptoms would be prudent.

*Can one patient infect another through unprotected sex if the other patient has tested negative for HIV?*

Yes, there is always the possibility that a sexual partner may be in the early window of time when plasma viremia is not at a detectable level. The antibody response to that plasma viremia may be slightly delayed and diagnostic testing may not indicate HIV positivity. This window of time represents a period when the patient may be infectious but yet not show up on normal diagnostic testing.

*Can HIV be passed by oral fluids?*

As our knowledge about HIV has evolved, we have thought that HIV is inactivated in saliva by an agent possibly associated with secretory leukocyte protease inhibitors known as SLPI. There is, however, a current resurgence in our interest in oral transmission because of some research that indicates that in moderate to advanced periodontal lesions or in other oral lesions where there is tissue damage, then the presence of a serous exudate may increase the risk of transmission. The dentist should be aware of this ongoing research and attempt to renew knowledge regularly so that any future breakthroughs will be noted.

# RHEUMATOID ARTHRITIS AND OSTEOARTHRITIS

Arthritis and its variations represent the most common chronic musculoskeletal disorders of man. The conditions can essentially be divided into rheumatoid, osteoarthritic, and polyarthritic presentations. Differences in age of onset and joint involvement exist and it is now currently believed that the diagnosis of each may be less clear than previously thought. These autoinflammatory diseases have now been shown to affect young and old alike. Criteria for a diagnosis of rheumatoid arthritis include a positive serologic test for rheumatoid factor, subcutaneous nodules, affected joints on opposite sides of the body, and clear radiographic changes. The hematologic picture includes moderate normocytic hypochromic anemia, mild leukocytosis, and mild thrombocytopenia. During acute inflammatory periods, C-reactive protein is elevated and IgG and IgM (rheumatoid factors) can be detected. Osteoarthritis lacks these diagnostic features.

Other systemic conditions, such as systemic lupus erythematosus and Sjögren's syndrome, are often found simultaneously with some of the arthritic conditions. The treatment of arthritis includes the use of slow-acting and rapid-acting anti-inflammatory agents ranging from the gold salts to aspirin (see following listings). Long-term usage of these drugs can lead to numerous adverse effects including bone marrow suppression, platelet suppression, and oral ulcerations. The dentist should be aware that steroids (usually prednisone) are often prescribed along with the listed drugs and are often used in dosages sufficient to induce adrenal suppression. Adjustment of dosing prior to invasive dental procedures may be indicated along with consultation with the managing physician. Alteration of steroid dosage prior to stressful dental procedures may be necessary, usually increasing the steroid dosage prior to and during the stressful procedures and then gradually returning the patient to the original dosage over several days. Even in the absence of evidence of adrenal suppression, consultation with the prescribing physician for appropriate dosing and timing of procedures is advisable.

**Gold Salts**

Auranofin (Ridaura®) *on page 109*
Aurothioglucose (Solganol®) *on page 110*

**Metabolic Inhibitor**

Leflunomide (Arava®) *on page 574*
Methotrexate *on page 651*

**Immunomodulator**

Etanercept (Enbrel®) *on page 395*

**Nonsteroidal Anti-inflammatory Agents**

Aminosalicylate Sodium (Sodium P.A.S.) *on page 65*
Choline Magnesium Trisalicylate (Trilisate®) *on page 244*
Choline Salicylate (Arthropan®) *on page 245*
Diclofenac (Cataflam®, Voltaren®) *on page 320*
Diflunisal (Dolobid®) *on page 327*
Etodolac (Lodine®) *on page 413*
Fenoprofen (Nalfon®) *on page 424*
Flurbiprofen (Ansaid®) *on page 448*
Ibuprofen (various products) *on page 522*
Indomethacin (Indocin®) *on page 534*
Ketoprofen (Orudis®) *on page 565*
Ketorolac (Toradol®) *on page 566*
Magnesium Salicylate (Doan's®, Magan®, Mobidin®) *on page 613*
Meclofenamate (Meclomen®) *on page 621*
Mefenamic Acid (Ponstel®) *on page 624*
Nabumetone (Relafen®) *on page 695*
Naproxen (Naprosyn®) *on page 705*
Oxaprozin (Daypro™) *on page 747*
Oxyphenbutazone *on page 757*
Piroxicam (Feldene®) *on page 810*
Salsalate (various products) *on page 902*
Sulindac (Clinoril®) *on page 948*

Tolmetin (Tolectin®) *on page 996*

**COX-2 Inhibitor NSAID**

Celecoxib (Celebrex®) *on page 211*

**Combination NSAID Product to Prevent GI Distress**

Diclofenac and Misoprostol (Arthrotec®) *on page 321*

**Salicylates**

Aspirin (various products) *on page 100*
Choline Magnesium Trisalicylate (Trilisate®) *on page 244*
Salsalate (Argesic®-SA, Artha-G®, Disalcid®, Marthritic® Mono-Gesic®, Salflex®, Salgesic®, Salsitab®) *on page 902*

**Other**

Hydroxychloroquine (Plaquenil®) *on page 515*
Prednisone (various products) *on page 833*

## ANTI-INFLAMMATORY AGENTS USED IN THE TREATMENT OF RHEUMATOID ARTHRITIS AND OSTEOARTHRITIS

| Drug | Adverse Effects |
|---|---|
| **SLOW-ACTING** | |
| **GOLD SALTS** | |
| Aurothioglucose I.M. parenteral injection (Myochrysine®); Auranofin (Ridaura®) | GI intolerance, diarrhea; leukopenia, thrombocytopenia, and/or anemia; skin and oral eruptions; possible nephrotoxicity and hepatotoxicity |
| **METABOLIC INHIBITOR** | |
| Leflunomide (Arava®) | Diarrhea, respiratory tract infection |
| Methotrexate | Oral ulcerations, leukopenia |
| **IMMUNOMODULATOR** | |
| Etanercept (Enbrel®) | Headache, respiratory tract infection, positive ANA |
| **OTHER** | |
| Hydroxychloroquine (Plaquenil®) | Usually mild and reversible; ophthalmic complications |
| Prednisone | Insomnia, nervousness, indigestion, increased appetite |
| **RAPID-ACTING** | |
| **SALICYLATES** | |
| Aspirin | Inhibition of platelet aggregation; gastrointestinal (GI) irritation, ulceration, and bleeding; tinnitus; teratogenicity |
| Choline magnesium salicylate (Trilisate®) | GI irritation and ulceration, weakness, skin rash, hemolytic anemia, troubled breathing |
| Salsalate | |
| **OTHER NONSTEROIDAL ANTI-INFLAMMATORY DRUGS** | |
| Diclofenac (Cataflam®, Voltaren®); Diflunisal (Dolobid®); Etodolac (Lodine®); Fenoprofen calcium (Nalfon®); Flurbiprofen sodium (Ansaid®); Ibuprofen (Motrin®); Indomethacin (Indocin®); Ketoprofen (Orudis®); Ketorolac tromethamine (Toradol®); Meclofenamate (Meclomen®); Nabumetone (Relafen®); Naproxen (Naprosyn®); Oxaprozin (Daypro™); Phenylbutazone; Piroxicam (Feldene®); Salsalate (Argesic®-SA, Artha-G®, Disalcid®, Mono-Gesic®, Salflex®, Salgesic®, Salsitab®); Sulindac (Clinoril®); Tolmetin (Tolectin®) | GI irritation, ulceration, and bleeding; inhibition of platelet aggregation; displacement of protein-bound drugs (eg, oral anticoagulants, sulfonamides, and sulfonylureas); headache; vertigo; mucocutaneous rash or ulceration; parotid enlargement |

## RHEUMATOID ARTHRITIS AND OSTEOARTHRITIS *(Continued)*

### ANTI-INFLAMMATORY AGENTS USED IN THE TREATMENT OF RHEUMATOID ARTHRITIS AND OSTEOARTHRITIS *(continued)*

| Drug | Adverse Effects |
|---|---|
| **COX-2 INHIBITOR NSAID** | |
| Celecoxib (Celebrex®) | Headache, dyspepsia, upper respiratory tract infection, sinusitis |
| **COMBINATION NSAID PRODUCT TO PREVENT GI DISTRESS** | |
| Diclofenac and Misoprostol (Arthrotec®) | Inhibition of platelet aggregation; displacement of protein-bound drugs (eg, oral anticoagulants, sulfonamides, and sulfonylureas); headache; vertigo; mucocutaneous rash or ulceration; parotid enlargement; diarrhea |

# NONVIRAL INFECTIOUS DISEASES

Nonviral infectious diseases are numerous. For the purposes of this text, discussion will be limited to tuberculosis, gonorrhea, and syphilis.

## TUBERCULOSIS

Tuberculosis is caused by the organism *Mycobacterium tuberculosis* as well as a variety of other mycobacteria including *M. bovis*, *M. avium-intracellulare*, and *M. kansasii*. Diagnosis of tuberculosis can be made from a skin test and a positive chest x-ray as well as acid-fast smears of cultures from respiratory secretions. Nucleic acid probes and polymerase chain reaction (PCR) to identify nucleic acid of *M. tuberculosis* have recently become useful.

The treatment of tuberculosis is based on the general principle that multiple drugs should reduce infectivity within 2 weeks and that failures in therapy may be due to noncompliance with the long-term regimens necessary. General treatment regimens last 6-12 months.

Isoniazid-resistant and multidrug-resistant mycobacterial infections have become an increasingly significant problem in recent years. TB as an opportunistic disease in HIV-positive patients has also risen. Combination drug therapy has always been popular in TB management and the advent of new antibiotics has not diminished this need.

### ANTITUBERCULOSIS DRUGS

**Bactericidal Agents**

Capreomycin (Capastat®) *on page 181*
*Isoniazid (INH™, Laniazid®, Nydrazid®) *on page 552*
Kanamycin (Kantrex®) *on page 561*
*Pyrazinamide *on page 866*
Rifabutin (Mycobutin®) *on page 885*
*Rifampin (Rifadin®, Rimactane®) *on page 886*
*Streptomycin *on page 934*

**Bacteriostatic Agents**

Cycloserine (Seromycin® Pulvules®) *on page 287*
*Ethambutol (Myambutol®) *on page 396*
Ethionamide (Trecator®-SC) *on page 408*
Para-Aminosalicylate Sodium *on page 765*

*Drugs of Choice

## SEXUALLY TRANSMITTED DISEASES

Sexually transmitted diseases (STDs) represent a group of infectious diseases that include bacterial, fungal, and viral etiologies. Several related infections are covered elsewhere. Gonorrhea and syphilis will be covered here.

The management of a patient with a STD begins with identification. Paramount to the correct management of patients with a history of gonorrhea or syphilis is when the condition was diagnosed, how and with what agent it was treated, did the condition recur, and are there any residual signs and symptoms potentially indicating active or recurrent disease. With universal precautions, the patient with *Neisseria gonorrhoea* or *Treponema pallidum* infection pose little threat to the dentist; however, diagnosis of oral lesions may be problematic. Gonococcal pharyngitis, primary syphilitic lesions (chancre), secondary syphilitic lesions (mucous patch), and tertiary lesions (gumma) may be identified by the dentist.

**Drugs used in treatment of gonorrhea/syphilis include:**

Cefixime (Suprax®) *on page 201*
Ceftriaxone (Rocephin®) *on page 209*
Ciprofloxacin (Cipro™) *on page 250*
Doxycycline (alternate) (Doryx®, Doxy®, Doxychel®, Vibramycin®, Vibra-Tabs®) *on page 355*
Ofloxacin (Floxin®, Ocuflox™) *on page 737*
Penicillin G Benzathine (Bicillin® L-A; Permapen®) *on page 773*
Penicillin G, Parenteral, Aqueous (Pfizerpen®) *on page 775*
Spectinomycin (alternate) (Trobicin®) *on page 930*

## NONVIRAL INFECTIOUS DISEASES *(Continued)*

The drugs listed above are often used alone or in stepped regimens, particularly when there is concomitant *Chlamydia* infection or when there is evidence of disseminated disease. The proper treatment for syphilis depends on the state of the disease.

**Current treatment regimens for syphilis include:**

| | |
|---|---|
| 1°, 2°, early latent (<1 y) | Benzathine penicillin G<br>I.M.: 2-4 million units x 1 (alternate doxycycline) |
| Latent (>1 y), gumma, or cardiovascular | As above but once weekly for 3 weeks |
| Neurosyphilis | Aqueous penicillin G<br>I.V.: 12-24 million units/day for 14 days |

# ANTIBIOTIC PROPHYLAXIS

# PREPROCEDURAL GUIDELINES FOR DENTAL PATIENTS

## INTRODUCTION

In dental practice the clinician is often confronted with a decision to prescribe antibiotics. The focus of this chapter is on the use of antibiotics as a preprocedural treatment in the prevention of adverse infectious sequelae in the two most commonly encountered situations: prevention of endocarditis and prosthetic implants.

The criteria for preprocedural decisions begins with patient evaluation. An accurate and complete medical history is always the initial basis for any prescriptive treatments on the part of the dentist. These prescriptive treatments can include ordering appropriate laboratory tests, referral to the patient's physician for consultation, or immediate decision to prescribe preprocedural antibiotics. The dentist should also be aware that antibiotic coverage of the patient might be appropriate due to diseases that are covered elsewhere in this text, such as human immunodeficiency virus, cavernous thrombosis, undiagnosed or uncontrolled diabetes, lupus, renal failure, and periods of neutropenia as are often associated with cancer chemotherapy. In these instances, medical consultation is almost always necessary in making antibiotic decisions in order to tailor the treatment and dosing to the individual patient's needs.

All tables or figures in this chapter were adapted from the ADA Advisory Statement: "Antibiotic Prophylaxis for Dental Patients With Total Joint Replacement," *J Am Dent Assoc*, 1997, 128:1004-8 or from Dajani AS, Taubert KA, Wilson W, et al, "Prevention of Bacterial Endocarditis. Recommendations by the American Heart Association," *JAMA*, 1997, 7(22):1794-801.

## PREVENTION OF BACTERIAL ENDOCARDITIS

Guidelines for the prevention of bacterial endocarditis have been updated by the American Heart Association with approval by the Council of Scientific Affairs of the American Dental Association.[1] These guidelines supercede those issued and published in 1990.[2] They were developed to more clearly define the situations of antibiotic use, to reduce costs to the patient, to reduce gastrointestinal adverse effects, and to improve patient compliance. Highlights of the current recommendations are shown in Table 1 and the specific antibiotic regimens are listed in Table 2 and further illustrated in Figure 1 found at the end of this chapter. Amoxicillin at a dose of 2 g 1 hour before the procedure is the suggested regimen for standard general prophylaxis. A follow-up dose is no longer necessary. This dose of amoxicillin is lower than the previous dosing regimen of 3 g 1 hour before the procedure and then 1.5 g 6 hours after the initial dose. Dajani, et al,[1] stated that the 2 g dose of amoxicillin resulted in adequate serum levels for several hours. They also stated that a second dose is not necessary, both because of a prolonged serum level of amoxicillin above the minimal inhibitory concentration for oral streptococci and an inhibitory activity of 6-14 hours by amoxicillin against streptococci.[3,4] The new pediatric dose is 50 mg/kg orally 1 hour before the procedure and not to exceed the adult dose. Amoxicillin is an amino-type penicillin with an extended spectrum of antibacterial action compared to penicillin VK. Amoxicillin is available in capsules (500 mg), liquid suspension (250 mg/5 mL) and chewable tablets (250 mg). The approximate retail cost of a 500 mg generic capsule is $1.80. The pharmacology of amoxicillin as a dental antibiotic has been reviewed previously in *General Dentistry*.[5]

## ANTIBIOTIC PROPHYLAXIS *(Continued)*

**Table 1.**
**HIGHLIGHTS OF THE NEWEST GUIDELINES FOR ENDOCARDITIS PREVENTION**

| No. | Change From Old Guidelines |
|---|---|
| 1. | Oral initial dosing for amoxicillin reduced to 2 g |
| 2. | Follow-up antibiotic dose is no longer recommended |
| 3. | Erythromycin is no longer recommended for penicillin-allergic patients |
| 4. | Clindamycin and other alternatives have been recommended to replace the erythromycin regimens |
| 5. | Clearer guidelines for prophylaxis decisions for patients with mitral valve prolapse have been developed |

For individuals unable to take oral medications, intramuscular or intravenous ampicillin is recommended for both adults and children (Table 2). It is to be given 30 minutes before the procedure at the same doses used for the oral amoxicillin medication. Ampicillin is also an amino-type penicillin having an antibacterial spectrum similar to amoxicillin. Ampicillin is not absorbed from the gastrointestinal tract as effectively as amoxicillin and, therefore, is not recommended for oral use.

**Table 2.**
**PROPHYLACTIC REGIMENS FOR BACTERIAL ENDOCARDITIS FOR DENTAL PROCEDURES**

| Situation | Agent | Regimen* |
|---|---|---|
| Standard general prophylaxis | Amoxicillin *on page 76* | Adults: 2 g orally 1 hour before procedure<br>Children: 50 mg/kg orally 1 hour before procedure |
| Unable to take oral medications | Ampicillin *on page 81* | Adults: 2 g I.M. or I.V. within 30 min before procedure<br>Children: 50 mg/kg I.M. or I.V. within 30 min before procedure |
| Allergic to penicillin | Clindamycin *on page 258*<br>or | Adults: 600 mg orally 1 hour before procedure<br>Children: 20 mg/kg orally 1 hour before procedure |
| | Cephalexin *on page 214*<br>or<br>Cefadroxil *on page 198* | Adults: 2 g orally 1 hour before procedure<br>Children: 50 mg/kg orally 1 hour before procedure |
| | Azithromycin *on page 114*<br>or<br>Clarithromycin *on page 256* | Adults: 500 mg orally 1 hour before procedure<br>Children: 15 mg/kg orally 1 hour before procedure |
| Allergic to penicillin and unable to take oral medications | Clindamycin *on page 258*<br>or | Adults: 600 mg I.V. within 30 min before procedure<br>Children: 20 mg/kg I.V. within 30 min before procedure |
| | Cefazolin *on page 199* | Adults: 1 g I.M. or I.V. within 30 min before procedure<br>Children: 25 mg/kg I.M. or I.V. within 30 min before procedure |

*Total children's dose should not exceed adult dose.

**Note:** Cephalosporins should not be used in individuals with immediate-type hypersensitivity reaction (urticaria, angioedema, or anaphylaxis) to penicillins

Individuals who are allergic to the penicillins such as amoxicillin or ampicillin should be treated with an alternate antibiotic. The new guidelines have suggested a number of alternate agents including clindamycin, cephalosporins, azithromycin, and clarithromycin. Clindamycin (Cleocin®) occupies an important niche in dentistry as a useful and effective antibiotic and it was a recommended alternative agent for the prevention of bacterial endocarditis in the previous guidelines.[2] In the new guidelines, the oral adult dose is 600 mg 1 hour before the procedure. A follow-up dose is not necessary. Clindamycin is available as 300 mg capsules; thus 2 capsules will provide the recommended dose. The children's oral dose for clindamycin is 20 mg/kg 1 hour before the procedure. Clindamycin is available as pediatric-flavored granules for oral solution. When reconstituted with water, each bottle yields a solution containing 75 mg/5 mL. Intravenous clindamycin is recommended in adults and children who are allergic to penicillin and unable to take oral medications. Refer to Table 2 for the intravenous doses of clindamycin.

Clindamycin was developed in the 1960s as a semisynthetic derivative of lincomycin which was found in the soil organism, *Streptomyces lincolnensis*, near Lincoln, Nebraska. It is commercially available as the hydrochloride salt to improve solubility in the gastrointestinal tract. Clindamycin is antibacterial against most aerobic gram-positive cocci including staphylococci and streptococci, and against many types of anaerobic gram-negative and gram-positive organisms. It has been used over the years in dentistry as an alternative to penicillin and erythromycins for the treatment of oral-facial infections. For a review, see Wynn and Bergman.[6]

The mechanism of antibacterial action of clindamycin is the same as erythromycin. It inhibits protein synthesis in susceptible bacteria resulting in the inhibition of bacterial growth and replication. Following oral administration of a single dose of clindamycin (150 mg, 300 mg, or 600 mg) on an empty stomach, 90% of the dose is rapidly absorbed into the bloodstream and peak serum concentrations are attained within 45-80 minutes. Administration with food does not markedly impair absorption into the bloodstream. Clindamycin serum levels exceed the minimum inhibitory concentration (MIC) for bacterial growth for at least 6 hours after the recommended dose of 600 mg. The serum half-life is 2-3 hours.

Adverse effects of clindamycin after a single dose are virtually nonexistent. Although it is estimated that 1% of patients taking clindamycin will develop symptoms of pseudomembranous colitis, these symptoms usually develop after 9-14 days of clindamycin therapy. These symptoms have never been reported in patients taking an acute dose for the prevention of endocarditis.

In lieu of clindamycin, penicillin-allergic individuals may receive cephalexin (Keflex®) or cefadroxil (Duricef®) provided that they have not had an immediate-type sensitivity reaction such as anaphylaxis, urticaria, or angioedema to penicillins. These antibiotics are first-generation cephalosporins having an antibacterial spectrum of action similar to amoxicillin and ampicillin. They elicit a bactericidal action by inhibiting cell wall synthesis in susceptible bacteria. The recommended adult prophylaxis dose for either of these drugs is 2 g 1 hour before the procedure. Again, no follow-up dose is needed. Cephalexin is supplied as 500 mg capsules and 500 mg tablets. Cefadroxil is supplied as 500 mg capsules and 1 g tablets. The children's oral dose for cephalexin and cefadroxil is 50 mg/kg 1 hour before the procedure. Both antibiotics are available in the form of oral suspension at concentrations of 125 mg, 250 mg, and 500 mg/5 mL.

For those individuals (adults and children) allergic to penicillin and unable to take oral medicines, parenteral cefazolin (Ancef®) may be used provided that they do not have the sensitivities described previously and footnoted in Table 2. Cefazolin is also a first-generation cephalosporin. Please note that the parenteral cefazolin can be given I.M. or I.V. Refer to Table 2 for the adult and children's doses of parenteral cefazolin.

Azithromycin (Zithromax®) and clarithromycin (Biaxin™) are members of the erythromycin-class of antibiotics known as the macrolides. The pharmacology of these drugs has been reviewed previously in *General Dentistry*.[7] The erythromycins have been available for use in dentistry and medicine since the mid 1950s. Azithromycin and clarithromycin represent the first additions to this class in over 40 years. The adult prophylactic dose for either drug is 500 mg 1 hour before the procedure with no follow-up dose. Azithromycin is well absorbed from the gastrointestinal tract and is extensively taken up from the circulation into tissues with a slow release from those tissues. It reaches peak serum levels in 2-4 hours. The serum half-life of azithromycin is 68 hours. Although the erythromycin family of drugs are known to inhibit the hepatic metabolism of theophylline and carbamazepine to enhance their effects, azithromycin has not been shown to affect the liver metabolism of these drugs.[8,9] Azithromycin is available under the brand name of Zithromax® and is not available generically as of this report. It is supplied as 250 mg capsules at a cost of $406 per 50 capsules.

Clarithromycin achieves peak plasma concentrations in 3 hours and maintains effective serum concentrations over a 12-hour period. Reports indicate that clarithromycin probably interacts with theophylline and carbamazepine by elevating the plasma concentrations of the two drugs.[7] Clarithromycin is available under the brand name of Biaxin® and is not available generically as of this report. Clarithromycin is supplied as 250 mg and 500 mg tablets at a cost of approximately $300 per 100 tablets. The pediatric prophylactic dose of azithromycin and clarithromycin is 15 mg/kg orally 1 hour before the procedure. Clarithromycin (Biaxin®) is available as powder for reconstitution to final concentrations of 125 mg and 500 mg per 5 mL. Azithromycin (Zithromax®) for oral suspension is supplied as single-dose packets containing 1 g of drug in each packet.

## ANTIBIOTIC PROPHYLAXIS *(Continued)*

Amoxicillin (Amoxil®, Biomox®, Larotid®, Polymox®, Trimox®, Utimox®, Wymox®) *on page 76*

Ampicillin (Amcill®, Marcillin®, Omnipen®, Polycillin®, Principen®, Totacillin®) *on page 81*

Azithromycin (Zithromax™) *on page 114*

Cefadroxil (Duricef®, Ultracef®) *on page 198*

Cefazolin (Ancef®) *on page 199*

Cephalexin (Keflex®) *on page 214*

Clarithromycin (Biaxin™) *on page 256*

Clindamycin (Cleocin®) *on page 258*

### Clinical Considerations for Dentistry

See Algorithm Figure 1 at the end of this chapter

The clinician should review carefully those detailed dental procedures in Table 3 to determine those treatment conditions where prophylaxis is, or is not, recommended. In general, in patients with cardiac conditions where prophylaxis is recommended (Table 4), invasive dental procedures where bleeding is likely to be induced from hard or soft tissues (Table 3) should be preceded by antibiotic coverage (Table 2). Clearly, the production of significant bacteremia during a dental procedure is the major risk factor. Patients with a suspicious history of a cardiac condition who are in need of an immediate dental procedure should be prophylaxed with an appropriate antibiotic prior to the procedure(s) until medical evaluation has been completed and the risk level determined. If unanticipated bleeding develops during a procedure in an at-risk patient, appropriate antibiotics should be given immediately. The efficacy of this action is based on animal studies and is possibly effective up to 2 hours after the bacteremia.[10]

**Table 3.**
**DENTAL PROCEDURES AND PREPROCEDURAL ANTIBIOTICS**

| **Endocarditis or Prosthesis Prophylaxis Recommended Due to Likely Significant Bacteremia** |
|---|
| Dental extractions |
| Periodontal procedures including surgery, subgingival placement of antibiotic fibers/strips, scaling and root planing, probing, recall maintenance |
| Dental implant placement and reimplantation of avulsed teeth |
| Endodontic (root canal) instrumentation or surgery only beyond the apex |
| Initial placement of orthodontic bands but not brackets |
| Intraligamentary local anesthetic injections |
| Prophylactic cleaning of teeth or implants where bleeding is anticipated |
| **Endocarditis Prophylaxis Not Recommended Due to Usually Insignificant Bacteremia** |
| Restorative dentistry (operative and prosthodontic) with or without retraction cord** |
| Local anesthetic injections (nonintraligamentary) |
| Intracanal endodontic treatment; postplacement and build-up* |
| Placement of rubber dam* |
| Postoperative suture removal |
| Placement of removable prosthodontic/orthodontic appliances |
| Oral impressions* |
| Fluoride treatments |
| Taking of oral radiographs |
| Orthodontic appliance adjustment |
| Shedding of primary teeth |
| **In general, the presence of moderate to severe gingival inflammation may elevate these procedures to a higher risk of bacteremia.** |

*Prophylaxis is recommended for patients with high- and moderate-risk cardiac as well as high-risk prosthesis conditions

This includes restoration of decayed teeth and replacement of missing teeth

**Clinical judgment may indicate antibiotic use in any circumstances that may create significant bleeding.

Patients with moderate to advanced gingival inflammatory disease and/or periodontitis should be considered at greater risk of bacteremia. However, the ongoing daily risk of self-induced bacteremia in these patients is currently thought to be minimal as compared to the bacteremia during dental procedures. The clinician may wish to consider the use of a preprocedural antimicrobial rinse in addition to antibiotic prophylaxis and, of course, efforts should always focus on improving periodontal health during dental care. If a series of dental procedures is planned, the clinician must judge whether an interval between procedures, requiring prophylaxis, should be scheduled. The literature supports 9- to 14-day intervals as ideal to minimize the risk of emergence of resistant organisms.[11,12] Since serum levels of the standard amoxicillin dose may be adequate for 6-14 hours depending on the specific organism challenge, the clinician may have to consider the efficacy of a second dose if multiple procedures are planned over the course of a single day.

**Table 4.**
**CARDIAC CONDITIONS PREDISPOSING TO ENDOCARDITIS**

| **Endocarditis Prophylaxis Recommended** |
|---|
| High-Risk Category |
| Prosthetic cardiac valves, including bioprosthetic and homograft valves |
| Previous bacterial endocarditis |
| Complex cyanotic congenital heart disease (eg, single ventricle states, transposition of the great arteries, tetralogy of Fallot) |
| Surgically constructed systemic pulmonary shunts or conduits |
| Moderate-Risk Category |
| Most other congenital cardiac malformations (other than above and below) |
| Acquired valvar dysfunction (eg, rheumatic heart disease) |
| Hypertrophic cardiomyopathy |
| Mitral valve prolapse with valvar regurgitation and/or thickened leaflets* |
| **Endocarditis Prophylaxis Not Recommended** |
| Negligible-Risk Category (no greater risk than the general population) |
| Isolated secundum atrial septal defect |
| Surgical repair of atrial septal defect, ventricular septal defect, or patent ductus arteriosus (without residual defects beyond 6 mo) |
| Previous coronary artery bypass graft surgery |
| Mitral valve prolapse without valvar regurgitation |
| Physiologic, functional, or innocent heart murmurs |
| Previous Kawasaki disease without valvar dysfunction |
| Previous rheumatic fever without valvar dysfunction |
| Cardiac pacemakers (intravascular and epicardial) and implanted defibrillators |
| ****Specific risk for patients with a history of fenfluramine or dexfenfluramine (fen-phen or Redux®) use, has not been determined. Such patients should have medical evaluation for potential cardiac damage, as currently recommended by the FDA.** |

For patients with suspected or confirmed mitral valve prolapse (MVP), the risk of infection as well as other complications such as tachycardia, syncope, congestive heart failure, or progressive regurgitation are variable. The risk depends on age and severity of MVP. The decision to recommend prophylaxis in such patients is oftentimes controversial but it is generally agreed that the determination of regurgitation is the most predictive (see Algorithm Figure 2 at the end of this chapter). Therefore, patients with MVP with mitral regurgitation require prophylaxis. If the regurgitation is undetermined and the patient is in need of an immediate procedure, then prophylaxis should be given in any case and the patient referred for further evaluation. If echocardiographic or Doppler studies demonstrate regurgitation, then prophylaxis would be recommended routinely. If no regurgitation can be demonstrated by these studies, then MVP alone does not require prophylaxis.

## NEW ISSUES REGARDING PREVENTION OF ENDOCARDITIS

Strom, et al,[13] in a recent report published in the *Annals of Internal Medicine* showed that dental treatment does not seem to be a risk factor for infective endocarditis, even in patients predisposed to endocarditis due to valvular abnormalities. This was a large-scale population based case-control study done in 54 Philadelphia area hospitals from 1988-1990. This study is to be taken seriously because (1) of its magnitude and scale, having evaluated a large number of patients from hospitals within the Delaware Valley Case Control Network, and (2) for the potential impact that these findings may have on the dental profession in that they were unable to demonstrate any independent risk for endocarditis attributed to prior dental treatment. The methods used for the study and the results of their findings are further explained in Table 5.

## ANTIBIOTIC PROPHYLAXIS *(Continued)*

**Table 5.**
**SUMMARY OF THE STUDY BY STROM, ET AL,[13] CALLING FOR RECONSIDERATION OF THE POLICIES FOR ANTIBIOTIC PROPHYLAXIS IN DENTAL PATIENTS***

The study identified hospitalized patients having infective endocarditis from 54 hospitals within the Delaware Valley Case-Control Network. Persons with community-acquired infective endocarditis not associated with intravenous drugs were compared with similar numbers of community residents, matched by age, sex, and neighborhood residence. Information on demographic characteristics, host risk factors, and dental treatment was obtained in order to quantitate the risk for endocarditis from dental treatment and from cardiac abnormalities. Quantitation of risk involved statistical analyses of frequencies and cross-tabulations between case-control status and potential risk factors.

**Results**

The study identified 287 case patients having infective endocarditis. Of the 287 identified, 273 completed the required interviews; 104 on the case patients had pre-existing valvular heart disease.

**Infecting Organisms:** 272 (95%) of 287 had multiple positive blood cultures.

**Dental Risk Factors:** No individual dental procedure was significantly associated with infective endocarditis except tooth extraction in the 2 months before hospital admission (performed in 6 case patients and 0 controls).

**Risk in Persons Infected with Dental Flora:** Negative results when analyses of case patients infected with dental flora were compared to controls.

**Risk of Dental Treatment in Persons with Known Cardiac Valvular Abnormalities:** Among case patients and controls with known cardiac abnormalities – the target of antibiotic prophylaxis – the risk of infective endocarditis was not increased by dental treatment.

**Risk in Persons with Known Cardiac Valvular Abnormalities and Infection with Dental Flora:** The study found no significant increased risk from dental treatment.

**Cardiac Risk Factors:** A patient-reported history of any cardiac valvular abnormality was highly associated with infective endocarditis.

*Text of the complete report may be accessed at: http://www.acponline.org/journals/annals/15nov98/endoedit.htm.

The report by Strom, et al,[13] comes on the heels of two previous studies by van der Meer, et al,[15,16] which have shown no link between dental procedures and endocarditis. It is also consistent with a number of commentaries challenging the values of the dental preprocedural use of antibiotics to prevent endocarditis.[17,18,19,20] As a result, Strom, et al,[13] have called for a reconsideration of the policies for administering antibiotic prophylaxis to patients with cardiac abnormalities undergoing dental treatment.

In an editorial in the same issue of *Annals of Internal Medicine*, Durack[21] suggested a scale back on prophylaxis against endocarditis before dental treatment. He suggested that prophylaxis should not be recommended for most dental procedures except extractions and gingival surgery (including implant placement), and not recommended for most underlying cardiac conditions except prosthetic valves and previous endocarditis. And when any one or more of these four risk factors are present, prophylaxis should follow the guidelines of the American Heart Association.[1] Durack has also suggested that mitral valve prolapse (MVP) not be included among the underlying conditions for prophylaxis. Although a significant number of cases of endocarditis do occur in patients with mitral valve prolapse, the denominator of susceptible persons is large and the risk encountered by an individual patient with MVP is lower than that for patients with prosthetic valves, previous endocarditis, or both. Furthermore, the prognosis for cure of viridans streptococcal endocarditis in a patient with MVP is good. In support of this statement, Durack cites the studies by Clemens and Ransohoff[18] and Bor and Himmelstein.[19] Durack emphasized that his proposed changes could eliminate most of the prophylactic doses currently given to dental patients.

## PROPOSED CHANGES IN THE CONTEXT OF THE CURRENT AHA RECOMMENDATIONS

The recent recommendations by the American Heart Association[1] represent an attempt to scale back the dosing of antibiotics with a continued emphasis on the use of oral rather than parenteral medications. Recommendations for the prevention of endocarditis have been evolving since the first AHA pronouncement in 1955. (See review by Little[22]). There have been nine major revisions since 1955. Many of the changes were driven from reports showing that antibiotics could prevent experimental endocarditis.[23,24] The most recent change[1] included the elimination of some parenteral regimens and the elimination of a second follow-up dose. The current regimen is undoubtedly the most simple and convenient to date. If history holds true, the regimen will again be modified as authorities and experts evaluate evolving data from the studies described above, and as they take into consideration the commentaries such as that of Durack[21] and others.[17,18,19,20]

In the editorial, Durack balances the discussion by describing both the problems that could occur if there was a significant scale back of antibiotic use and the benefits to be achieved. Durack agrees that, occasionally, dental procedures cause endocarditis and cites two cases from the 1930s.[25,26] However, his argument is that although a direct relationship occurs, this happens too rarely to justify the routine use of antibiotic prophylaxis.

One of the problems of a scale back is that new cases of endocarditis may occur. Durack[21] states, however, that if promptly treated, endocarditis after dental treatment has a reasonably good prognosis. Also, malpractice claims have been generated in the past relative to the issue of antibiotic prophylaxis[27] and a curtailing of prophylaxis before dental treatment would certainly improve the atmosphere for continued claims, unless of course the suggested changes are endorsed by the American Heart Association.

Durack lists a number of benefits to be gained with a scale back. One obvious benefit is a reduction in antibiotic use. Ironically, with the new recommendations by the AHA, although the numbers of patients exposed to antibiotics probably has not changed, the initial dose of the antibiotic has been reduced and the follow-up dose has been eliminated. Another benefit is the fewer side effects of drugs to be expected. Unless there is allergic response however, amoxicillin at 2 g dose is virtually side-effect free. We are unaware of any report of an allergic reaction or anaphylaxis in patients taking a simple dose of oral amoxicillin who claimed to have no penicillin allergies. In addition, a single dose of amoxicillin causes less gastrointestinal effects.[28] Also, clindamycin has never been shown to induce pseudomembranous colitis after a single dose of 600 mg. A third benefit suggested was the added convenience for the patient. We think there is little inconvenience to taking a single dose of antibiotic (eg, 4 tablets of amoxicillin). Two additional benefits expressed by Durack were that there would be less work for the healthcare providers, and there would be lower costs of third-party payers.

We feel, as Durack does, that a key argument for reassessing the regimens for prophylaxis is the development of antibiotic-induced bacterial resistance. Viridans streptococci have been reported to become more resistant to antibiotics.[29] Also, Durack alerts the reader to the fact that viridans streptococci have the potential to accept resistance genes from passing bacteria and to donate them to other bacteria in the oral cavity. This has occurred in the case of resistant pneumococci.[30] We agree that the case against ill-considered use of unnecessary antibiotics is strong in view of the emergent bacterial resistance problem. Recently, the Centers for Disease Control (CDC) has reported a strain of *Staphylococcus aureus* resistant to vancomycin, the antibiotic considered as the last line of defense against this pathogen. The implication of this finding is the possibility of continued development of resistant bacterial pathogens due to the unnecessary exposure of patients to antibiotics.

We feel that prudent use of antibiotics is mandatory, but a comprehensive scale back of prophylaxis for endocarditis may not be warranted. Each patient must be evaluated with a full history designed to identify cardiac conditions. If the history is only suggestive of a high-risk condition, then medical evaluation is necessary before determining the need for preprocedural antibiotics. Only when a dental emergency exists in such a patient should antibiotics be given prior to this confirmation. If dentists proceed with inadequate history or follow-up medical evaluation, then antibiotics could be appropriate. We believe that strict adherence to accepted history and referral guidelines will further curtail unnecessary use of preprocedural antibiotics. The AHA has listed those cardiac conditions associated with endocarditis in which prophylaxis has been recommended. Table 6 lists these conditions in comparison with those suggested by Durack. The AHA has also recommended those dental procedures considered to be invasive and which require antibiotic prophylaxis. Table 7 lists these procedures in comparison with those suggested by Durack.

## ANTIBIOTIC PROPHYLAXIS *(Continued)*

**Table 6.**
**COMPARISONS OF THE CARDIAC RISKS RECOMMENDED BY THE AHA[1] AND THOSE SUGGESTED BY DURACK[21] IN WHICH PROPHYLAXIS IS RECOMMENDED**

| | |
|---|---|
| AHA: | High risk |
| | Prosthetic cardiac valves, including bioprosthetic and homograft valves |
| | Previous bacterial endocarditis |
| | Complex cyanotic congenital heart disease (eg, single ventricle states, transposition of the great arteries, tetralogy of Fallot) |
| | Surgically constructed systemic pulmonary shunts or conduits |
| AHA: | Moderate risk |
| | Most other congenital cardiac malformations (other than above and those mentioned in the negligible risk category in reference 1) |
| | Acquired valvar dysfunction (eg, rheumatic heart disease) |
| | Hypertrophic cardiac myopathy |
| | Mitral valve prolapse with valvar regurgitation and/or thickened leaflets |
| Durack*: | Prophylaxis "not recommended" for most underlying cardiac conditions except prosthetic valves and previous endocarditis. |

*Text of the complete report may be accessed at: http://www.acponline.org/journals/annals/15nov98/endoedit.htm

**Table 7.**
**COMPARISONS OF THE DENTAL PROCEDURES RECOMMENDED BY THE AHA[1] AND THOSE SUGGESTED BY DURACK[21] IN WHICH PROPHYLAXIS IS RECOMMENDED**

| |
|---|
| AHA recommendations: |
| Dental extractions |
| Periodontal procedures including surgery, scaling, and root planing, probing, recall maintenance |
| Dental implant placement; reimplantation of avulased teeth |
| Endodontic (root canal) instrumentation or surgery only beyond apex |
| Subgingival placement of antibiotic fibers or strips |
| Initial placement of orthodontic bands but not brackets |
| Intraligamentary local anesthetic injections |
| Prophylactic cleaning of teeth or implants where bleeding is anticipated |
| Durack recommendations*: |
| Prophylaxis not recommended for most dental procedures except extractions and gingival surgery including implant placement |

*Text of the complete report may be accessed at: http://www.acponline.org/journals/annals/15nov98/endoedit.htm

## SEEKING THE BEST POSSIBLE OUTCOMES FOR OUTPATIENTS

The rationale for prophylaxis is based on four assumptions.

1. Patients with acquired or congenital heart disease are at increased risk of developing endocarditis[31]
2. The risk of endocarditis is increased following procedures that cause bacteria; bacteremia after dental and oral procedures occurs in 18% to 95% of cases[32]
3. Certain healthcare procedures cause bacteremia with organisms that can cause endocarditis (dental and oral procedures are included)
4. Most cases of endocarditis are caused by bacteria that are usually sensitive to antibiotics.

Experts agree that only a small number of cases of bacterial endocarditis are associated with medical or dental procedures and that there is limited evidence to suggest antibiotic regimens are effective in humans.[32] Also, no prospective study has proven that prophylaxis is effective against endocarditis.[32] In a retrospective survey of 533 patients with valvular prostheses who underwent 677 dental or surgical procedures, 6 cases of endocarditis occurred in 229 patients who received no antibiotics as compared with none in 304 patients who received antibiotic prophylaxis. According to Durack,[33] a prospective trial powerful enough to establish or disprove the efficacy of prophylaxis would require the random assignment of 6000 or more patients, all with cardiac disease, to receive an antibiotic or placebo before undergoing dental procedures. The assumption, therefore, is that this definitive type of study will never occur.

Chenoweth and Burket[32] agree that prophylaxis against endocarditis has not been proven to be effective or cost-beneficial in prospective studies and it probably never will be proven.

In the update of the recommendations for antibiotic prophylaxis,[1] the AHA agreed that there are currently no randomized or carefully controlled human trials in patients with underlying structural heart disease to definitively establish that antibiotic prophylaxis provides protection against development of endocarditis during a bacteremia-inducing procedure. Most cases of endocarditis are not attributable to any invasive procedure. However, antibiotic prophylaxis is warranted because of the previous established rationale described above.

Although AHA states that the guidelines are only recommendations and should not be considered as a standard of care statement, it is clear that they have become a standard of care based on the potential legal implications for optimal prevention during invasive dental procedures.[22] Little[22] also reiterated that only a small number of cases of bacterial endocarditis are associated with medical or dental procedures and that there is limited evidence to suggest that these regimens are effective in humans.

Of course Strom, et al[13] and Durack[21] are not suggesting that the practitioner unilaterally start to scale back on antibiotic coverage. We believe, however, that their arguments should be seriously considered in future updating of AHA recommendations. Until then, the clinician should be sensitized to arguments in favor of scale back and consider the following in those situations suggesting antibiotic prophylaxis.

1. Carefully ascertain by history the degree to which the underlying condition creates a risk of endocarditis. Consult with the physician when in doubt. Please consider only those cardiac conditions recommended by the AHA and listed in Table 6. They were developed from opinions voiced by national and international experts at endocarditis meetings around the world.
2. Ascertain the apparent risk of bacteremia with the dental procedure. If significant bleeding is not anticipated, please do not premedicate. We feel that the dental procedures recommended by the AHA and listed in Table 7 are associated with high potential for bacteremia. Specific patient characteristics, such as severe periodontal inflammation, may justify the clinician considering some normally low-risk procedures to be more significant.
3. In patients where endocarditis prophylaxis has been determined to be necessary, the dentist should make every effort to combine procedures on a given day, so as to minimize the number of episodes of preprocedural antibiotic use.
4. Try to restrict the alternate drug to clindamycin in those patients allergic to penicillin. Other regimens should only be designed in consultation with the physician. For example, a single dose of clindamycin would only be truly contraindicated in patients with active colitis at the time or in patients that had previously demonstrated adverse GI or other reactions to clindamycin. In designing any alternative regimens, the clinician should be reminded that cephalosporins can demonstrate cross-allergenicity in patients allergic to penicillin that had a type I hypersensitivity reaction.
5. Try to educate the patient on our efforts as a profession to restrict overexposure of the population to antibiotics.

We feel that by adhering to the above principles, overuse of antibiotics will be reduced, and the potential for development of antibiotic-induced bacterial resistance due to overexposure with antibiotics in the cardiac patient undergoing invasive dental treatment will be minimized.

## PREPROCEDURAL ANTIBIOTICS FOR PROSTHETIC IMPLANTS

A significant number of dental patients have had total joint replacements or other implanted prosthetic devices.[34] Prior to performing dental procedures that might induce bacteremia, the dentist must consider the use of antibiotic prophylaxis in these patients. Until recently, only the American Heart Association had taken a formal stance on implanted devices by suggesting guidelines for the use of antibiotic prophylaxis in patients with prosthetic heart valves.[1,2] These guidelines and the recent guidelines for prevention of bacterial endocarditis have been published in *General Dentistry.*[37]

The use of antibiotics in patients with other prosthetic devices, including total joint replacements has remained controversial because of several issues. Late infections of implanted prosthetic devices have rarely been associated with microbial organisms of oral origin.[36] Secondly, since late infections in such patients are often not reported, data is lacking to substantiate or refute this potential.[37] Also, there is general acceptance that patients with acute infections at distant sites such as the oral cavity may be at greater

## ANTIBIOTIC PROPHYLAXIS *(Continued)*

risk of infection of an implanted prosthetic device. Periodontal disease has been implicated as a distant site infection.[36] Since antibiotics are associated with allergies and other adverse reactions, and because the frequent use of antibiotics may lead to emergence of resistant organisms,[34] any perceived benefit of antibiotic prophylaxis must always be weighed against known risks of toxicity, allergy, or potential microbial resistance.

Recently, an advisory group made up of representatives from the American Dental Association and the American Academy of Orthopedic Surgeons published a statement in the *Journal of the American Dental Association* on the use of antibiotics prior to dental procedures in patients with total joint replacements.[38] The statement concluded that antibiotic prophylaxis should not be prescribed routinely for most dental patients with total joint replacements or for any patients with pins, plates, and screws. However, in an attempt to base the guidelines on available scientific evidence, the advisory group stated that certain patients may be potential risks for joint infection thus justifying the use of prophylactic antibiotics. Those conditions considered by the advisory group to be associated with potential elevated risk of joint infections are listed in Table 8.[39,43] The dentist should carefully review the patient's history to ensure identification of those medical problems leading to potential elevated risks of joint infections as listed in Table 8. Where appropriate, medical consultation with the patient's internist or orthopedist may be prudent to assist in this determination. The orthopedist should be queried specifically, as to the status of the joint prosthesis itself.

**Table 8.**
**PATIENTS WITH POTENTIAL ELEVATED RISK OF JOINT INFECTION**

| |
|---|
| Inflammatory arthropathies: Rheumatoid arthritis, systemic lupus erythematosus |
| Disease-, drug-, or radiation-induced immunosuppression |
| Insulin-dependent diabetes |
| First 2 years following joint replacement |
| Previous prosthetic joint infections |
| Patients with acute infections at a distant site |
| Hemophilia |

Patients who present with elevated risks of joint infections, in which the dentist is going to perform any procedures associated with a high risk of bacteremia, need to receive preprocedural antibiotics. Those dental procedures associated with high risk of bacteremia are listed in Table 3. Patients undergoing dental procedures involving low risk of bacteremia, probably do not require premedication even though the patient may be in the category of elevated risk of joint infections. Patients with an acute oral infection or moderate to severe gingival inflammation and/or periodontitis must be considered at higher risk for bacteremia during dental procedures than those without active dental disease. In these patients, as in all patients, the dental clinician should aggressively treat these oral conditions striving for optimum oral health. The listing of low bacteremia risks in Table 3 may need to be reconsidered, depending on the patient's oral health.

## ANTIBIOTIC REGIMENS

The antibiotic prophylaxis regimens as suggested by the advisory panel are listed in Table 9. These regimens are not exactly the same as those listed in Table 2 (for prevention of endocarditis) and must be reviewed carefully to avoid confusion. Cephalexin, cephradine, or amoxicillin may be used in patients not allergic to penicillin. The selected antibiotic is given as a single 2 g dose 1 hour before the procedure. A follow-up dose is not recommended. Cephalexin (Keflex®) and amoxicillin have been described earlier in this chapter. Cephradine (Velosef®) is a first-generation cephalosporin-type antibiotic effective against anaerobic bacteria and aerobic gram-positive bacteria. It is used in medicine predominantly to treat infections of the bones and joints, infections of the lower respiratory tract, urinary tract, and skin and soft tissues.

Parenteral cefazolin (Ancef®) or ampicillin are the recommended antibiotics for those patients unable to take oral medications; see Table 9 for doses. Cefazolin is a first-generation cephalosporin effective against anaerobes and aerobic gram-positive bacteria. Ampicillin is an aminopenicillin described earlier. For patients allergic to penicillin, clindamycin is the recommended antibiotic of choice. Clindamycin is active against aerobic and anaerobic streptococci, most staphylococci, the *Bacteroides*, and the *Actinomyces* families of bacteria. The recommended oral and parenteral doses of clindamycin in the joint prosthetic patient are listed in Table 9.

**Table 9.**
**ANTIBIOTIC REGIMENS FOR PATIENTS WITH PROSTHETIC IMPLANTS**

| |
|---|
| Patients not allergic to penicillin: Cephalexin, cephradine, or amoxicillin |
| 2 g orally 1 hour prior to dental procedure |
| Patients not allergic to penicillin and unable to take oral medications: Cefazolin or ampicillin |
| Cefazolin 1 g or ampicillin 2 g I.M. or I.V. 1 hour prior to the procedure |
| Patients allergic to penicillin: Clindamycin |
| 600 mg orally 1 hour prior to dental procedure |
| Patients allergic to penicillin and unable to take oral medications: Clindamycin |
| 600 mg I.V. 1 hour prior to the procedure |

Amoxicillin (Amoxil®, Biomox®, Larotid®, Polymox®, Trimox®, Utimox®, Wymox®) *on page 76*
Ampicillin (Amcill®, Marcillin®, Omnipen®, Polycillin®, Principen®, Totacillin®) *on page 81*
Cefazolin (Ancef®) *on page 199*
Cephalexin (Keflex®) *on page 214*
Cephradine (Velosef®) *on page 217*
Clindamycin (Cleocin®) *on page 258*

**Clinical Considerations for Dentistry**

See Algorithm Figure 3 at the end of this chapter.

The frequency of postinsertion infections in patients who have undergone total joint replacement or prosthetic device placement is variable. The most common cause of infection with all devices is found to be from contamination at the time of surgical insertions.[39,44] The presence of an acute distant infection at a site other than the joint, however, appears to be a risk factor for late infection of these devices. The rationale by the American Dental Association and the American Academy of Orthopedic Surgeons in their advisory statement[38] has been to provide guidelines to minimize the use of antibiotics to the first 2 years following total joint replacement. As more data are collected, these recommendations may be revised. However, it is thought to be prudent for the dental clinician to fully evaluate all patients with respect to history and or physical findings prior to determining the risk.

If a procedure considered to be low risk for bacteremia is performed in a patient at risk for joint complications, and inadvertent bleeding occurs, then an appropriate antibiotic should be given immediately. Although this is not ideal, animal studies suggest that it may be useful.[10] Likewise, in patients where concern exists over joint complications and a medical consultation cannot be immediately obtained, the patient should be treated as though antibiotic coverage is necessary until such time that an appropriate consultation can be completed. The presence of an acute oral infection, in addition to any preexisting dental conditions, may increase the risk of late infection at the prosthetic joint. Even though most late joint infections are caused by *Staphylococcus* sp, the risk of bacteremia involving another organism, predominant in an acute infection, may increase the risk of joint infection.[34,39,44-46]

The dentist may also need to consider the question of multiple procedures over a period of time. Procedures planned over a period of several days would best be rescheduled at intervals of 9-14 days. The risk of emergence of resistant organisms in patients receiving multiple short-term doses of antibiotics has been shown to be greater than those receiving antibiotics over longer intervals of time.[11,12]

# FREQUENTLY ASKED QUESTIONS

*Can erythromycin still be used to prevent bacterial endocarditis in dental patients?*

If the clinician has successfully used erythromycin in the past, this form of prophylaxis can be continued using the regimen included in the recommendation of 1990.[2] Erythromycin has, however, been excluded for the vast majority of patients due to gastric upset.

*If the patient is presently taking antibiotics for some other ailment, is prophylaxis still necessary?*

If a patient is already taking antibiotics for another condition, prophylaxis should be accomplished with a drug from another class. For example, in the patient who is not allergic to penicillin who is taking erythromycin for a medical condition such as mycoplasma infection, amoxicillin would be the drug of choice for prophylaxis. Also, in the penicillin-allergic patient taking clindamycin, prophylaxis would best be

## ANTIBIOTIC PROPHYLAXIS *(Continued)*

accomplished with azithromycin or clarithromycin. The new guidelines[1] restated the position that doses of antibiotics for prevention of recurrence of rheumatic fever are thought to be inadequate to prevent bacterial endocarditis and prophylaxis should be accomplished with the full dose of a drug from another class.

*Can clindamycin be used safely in patients with gastrointestinal disorders?*

If a patient has a history of inflammatory bowel disease and is allergic to penicillin, azithromycin or clarithromycin should be selected over clindamycin. In patients with a negative history of inflammatory bowel disease, clindamycin has not been shown to induce colitis following a single-dose administration.

*Why do the suggested drug regimens for patients with joint prostheses resemble so closely the regimens for the prevention of bacterial endocarditis?*

Bacteremia is the predisposing risk factor for the development of endocarditis in those patients at risk due to a cardiac condition. Likewise, the potential of bacteremia during dental procedures is considered to be the risk factor in some late joint prostheses infections, even though this risk is presumed to be much lower.

*How do we determine those patients who have had joint replacement complications?*

Patients who have had complications during the initial placement of a total joint would be those who had infection following placement, those with recurrent pain, or those who have had previous joint replacement failures. If the patient reports even minor complications, a medical consultation with the orthopedist would be the most appropriate action for the dentist.

*Is prophylaxis required in patients with pins, screws, or plates often used in orthopedic repairs?*

There is currently no evidence supporting use of antibiotics following the placement of pins, plates, or screws. Breast implants, dental implants, and implanted lenses in the eye following cataract surgery are also all thought to be at minimal risk for infection following dental procedures. Therefore, no antibiotic prophylaxis is recommended in these situations. There is, however, some evidence indicating elevated risk of infection following some types of penile implants and some vascular access devices, used during chemotherapy.[34] It is recommended that the dentist discuss such patients with the physician prior to determining the need for antibiotics.

*What should I do if medical consultation results in a recommendation that differs from the published guidelines endorsed by the American Dental Association?*

The dentist is ultimately responsible for treatment recommendations. Ideally, by communicating with the physician, a consensus can be achieved that is either in agreement with the guidelines or is based on other established medical reasoning.

*What is the best antibiotic modality for treating dental infections?*

Penicillin is still the drug of choice for treatment of infections in and around the oral cavity. Phenoxy-methyl penicillin (Pen VK®) has long been the most commonly selected antibiotic. In penicillin-allergic individuals, erythromycin may be an appropriate consideration. If another drug is sought, clindamycin prescribed 300 mg as a loading dose followed by 150 mg 4 times a day would be an appropriate regimen for a dental infection. In general, if there is no response to Pen VK®, then Augmentin® may be a good alternative in the nonpenicillin-allergic patient because of its slightly altered spectrum. Recommendations would include that the patient should take the drug with food.

*Is there cross-allergenicity between the cephalosporins and penicillin?*

The incidence of cross-allergenicity is 5% to 8% in the overall population. If a patient has demonstrated a Type I hypersensitivity reaction to penicillin, namely urticaria or anaphylaxis, then this incidence would increase to 20%.

*Is there definitely an interaction between contraception agents and antibiotics?*

There are well founded interactions between contraceptives and antibiotics. The best instructions that a patient could be given by their dentist are that should an antibiotic be necessary and the dentist is aware that the patient is on contraceptives, and if the patient is using chemical contraceptives, the patient should seriously consider additional means of contraception during the antibiotic management.

*Are antibiotics necessary in diabetic patients?*

In the management of diabetes, control of the diabetic status is the key factor relative to all morbidity issues. If a patient is well controlled, then antibiotics will likely not be necessary. However, in patients where the control is questionable or where they have recently been given a different drug regimen for their diabetes or if they are being titrated to an appropriate level of either insulin or oral hypoglycemic agents during these periods of time, the dentist might consider preprocedural antibiotics to be efficacious.

*Do nonsteroidal anti-inflammatory drugs interfere with blood pressure medication?*

At the current time there is no clear evidence that NSAIDs interfere with any of the blood pressure medications that are currently in use.

*Is a patient who has taken phentermine at risk for cardiac problems just like a patient who took "fen-phen"?*

No, there is often confusion with these drug names. "Fen-phen" referred to a combined use of fenfluramine and phentermine and it is this combination that has led to the FDA statement (see Table 4). The single drug phentermine has not been implicated in this current concern over cardiac complications.

## ANTIBIOTIC PROPHYLAXIS *(Continued)*

### Figure 1
### Preprocedural Dental Action Plan for Patients With a History Indicative of Elevated Endocarditis Risk

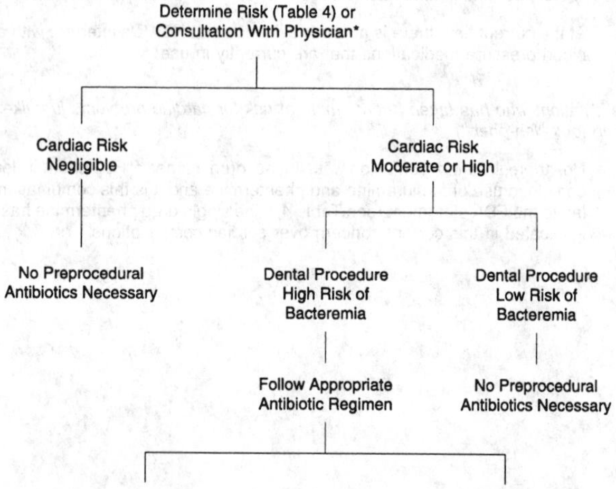


**Allergic to Penicillin**

| | | |
|---|---|---|
| Oral: | Clindamycin | 600 mg (20 mg/kg) 1 h prior |
| | Cephalexin | 2 g (50 mg/kg) 1 h prior |
| | Cefadroxil | 2 g (50 mg/kg) 1 h prior |
| | Azithromycin | 500 mg (15 mg/kg) 1 h prior |
| | Clarithromycin | 500 mg (15 mg/kg) 1 h prior |
| I.V.: | Clindamycin | 600 mg (20 mg/kg) 30 min prior |
| I.M. or I.V.: | Cefazolin | 1 g (25 mg/kg) 30 min prior |

**Not Allergic to Penicillin**

| | |
|---|---|
| Oral: | Amoxicillin 2 g (50 mg/kg) 1 h prior |
| I.M. or I.V.: | Ampicillin 2 g (50 mg/kg) 30 min prior |

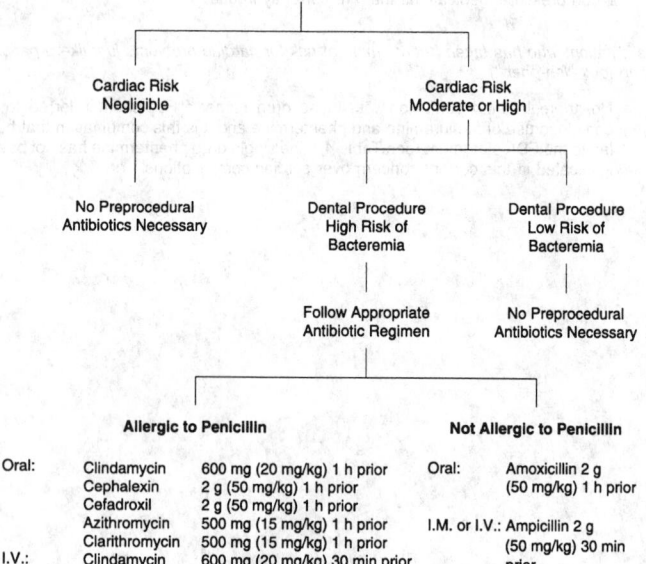

Child dosages are parentheses and should never exceed adult dose. Cephalosporins should be avoided in patients with previous Type I hypersensitivity reactions to penicillin due to some evidence of cross allergenicity.

* For Emergency Dental Care the clinician should attempt phone consultation. If unable to contact patient's physician or determine risk, the patient should be treated as though there is moderate or high risk of cardiac complication and follow the algorithm.

**Figure 2**
**Patient With Suspected Mitral Valve Prolapse**

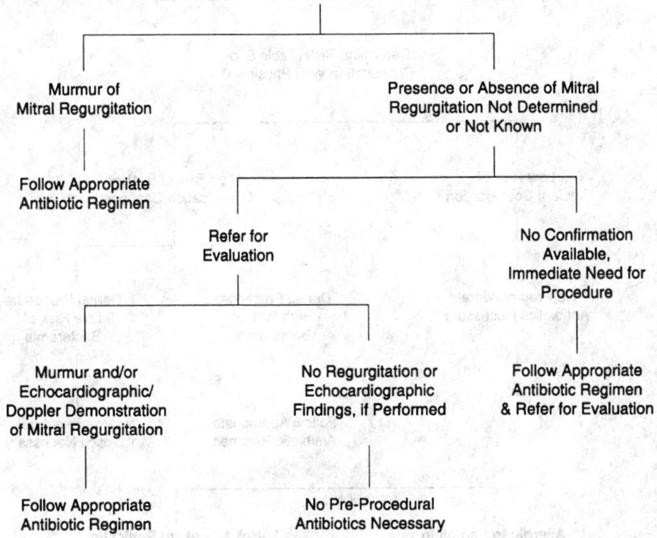

## ANTIBIOTIC PROPHYLAXIS *(Continued)*

**Figure 3**
**Preprocedural Dental Action Plan for Patients With Prosthetic Implants**

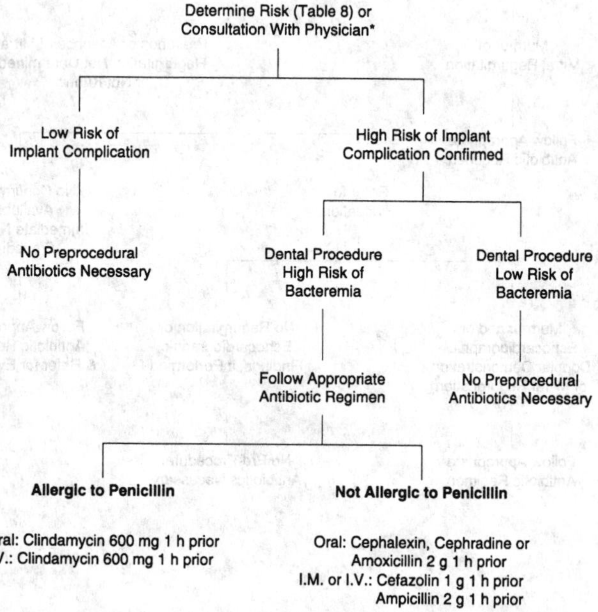


Cephalosporins should be avoided in patients with previous Type I hypersensitivity reactions to penicillin due to some evidence of cross allergenicity.

*For Emergency Dental Care the clinician should attempt phone consultation. If unable to contact patient's physician or determine risk, the patient should be treated as though there is high risk of implant complication and follow the algorithm.

## REFERENCES


1. Dajani AS, Taubert KA, Wilson W, et al, "Prevention of Bacterial Endocarditis. Recommendations by the American Heart Association," *JAMA*, 1997, 277(22):1794-801.
2. Dajani AS, Bisno AI, Chung KJ, et al, "Prevention of Bacterial Endocarditis. Recommendations by the American Heart Association," *JAMA*, 1990, 264(22): 2919-22.
3. Dajani AS, Bawdon RE, and Berry MC, "Oral Amoxicillin as Prophylaxis for Endocarditis: What Is the Optimal Dose?" *Clin Infect Dis*, 1994, 18(2):157-60.
4. Fluckiger U, Francioli P, Blaser J, et al, "Role of Amoxicillin Serum Levels for Successful Prophylaxis of Experimental Endocarditis Due to Tolerant Streptococci," *J Infect Dis*, 1994, 169(6):1397-400.
5. Wynn RL, "Amoxicillin Update," *Gen Dent*, 1991, 39(5):322, 324, 326.
6. Wynn RL and Bergman SA, "Antibiotics and Their Use in the Treatment of Orofacial Infections, Part I," *Gen Dent*, 1994, 42(5): 398, 400, 402.
7. Wynn RL, "New Erythromycins," *Gen Dent*, 1996, 44(4):304-7.
8. Clauzel AM, Visier S, and Michel FB, "Efficacy and Safety of Azithromycin in Lower Respiratory Tract Infections," *Eur Respir J*, 1990, 3(Suppl 10):89S.
9. Rapeport WG, Dewland PM, Muirhead DC, et al, "Lack of Interaction Between Azithromycin and Carbamazepine," *Br J Clin Pharmacol*, 1992, 30:551P.
10. Berney P and Francioli P, "Successful Prophylaxis of Experimental Streptococcal Endocarditis With Single-Dose Amoxicillin Administered After Bacterial Challenge," *J Infect Dis*, 1990, 161(2):281-5.
11. Leviner E, Tzukert AA, Benoliel R, et al, "Development Resistant Oral Viridans Streptococci After Administration of Prophylactic Antibiotics: Time Management in the Dental Treatment of Patients Susceptible to Infective Endocarditis," *Oral Surg Oral Med Oral Pathol*, 1987, 64(4):417-20.
12. Simmons NA, Cawson RA, Clark CA, et al, "Prophylaxis of Infective Endocarditis," *Lancet*, 1986, 1(8492):1267.
13. Strom BL, Abrutyn E, Berlin JA, et al, "Dental and Cardiac Risk Factors for Infective Endocarditis. A Population-Based, Case-Control Study," *Ann Intern Med*, 1998, 129(10):761-9.
14. Strom BL, Abrutyn E, Berlin JA, et al, "Prophylactic Antibiotics to Prevent Infective Endocarditis? Relative Risks Re-Assessed," *J Investig Med*, 1996, 44:229.
15. van der Meer JT, Thompson J, Valkenburg HA, et al, "Epidemiology of Bacterial Endocarditis in the Netherlands. II. Antecedent Procedures and Use of Prophylaxis," *Arch Intern Med*, 1992, 152(9):1869-73.
16. van der Meer JT, Van Wijk W, Thompson J, et al, "Efficacy of Antibiotic Prophylaxis for Prevention of Native-Valve Endocarditis," *Lancet*, 1992, 339(8786):135-9.
17. Gutheroth WG, "How Important Are Dental Procedures as a Cause of Infective Endocarditis?" *Am J Cardiol*, 1984, 54(7):797-801.
18. Clemens JD and Ransohoff DF, "A Quantitative Assessment of Pre-Dental Antibiotic Prophylaxis for Patients With Mitral-Valve Prolapse," *J Chron Dis*, 1984, 37(7):531-44.
19. Bor DH and Himmelstein DU, "Endocarditis Prophylaxis for Patients With Mitral Valve Prolapse. A Quantitative Analysis," *Am J Med*, 1984, 76(4):711-7.
20. Pallasch TJ, "A Critical Appraisal of Antibiotic Prophylaxis," *Int Dent J*, 1989, 39(3):183-96.
21. Durack DT, "Antibiotics for Prevention of Endocarditis During Dentistry: Time to Scale Back?" *Ann Intern Med*, 1998, 129(10):829-31.
22. Little J, "The American Heart Association's Guidelines for the Prevention of Bacterial Endocarditis: A Critical Review," *Gen Dent*, 1998, 46:508-15.
23. Moreillon P, Francioli P, Overholser D, et al, "Mechanisms of Successful Amoxicillin Prophylaxis of Experimental Endocarditis Due to *Streptococcus Intermedius*," *J Infect Dis*, 1986, 154(5):801-7.
24. Malinverni R, Francioli PB, and Glauser MP, "Comparison of Single and Multiple Doses of Prophylactic Antibiotics in Experimental Streptococcal Endocarditis," *Circulation*, 1987, 76(2):376-82.
25. Sale L, "Some Tragic Results Following Extraction of Teeth. II." *J Am Dent Assoc*, 1939, 26:1647-51.
26. Okell CC and Elliott SD, "Bacteriaemia and Oral Sepsis With Special Reference to the Etiology of Subacute Endocarditis," *Lancet*, 1935, 2:869-72.
27. Martin MV, Butterworth ML, and Longman LP, "Infective Endocarditis and the Dental Practitioner: A Review of 53 Cases Involving Litigation," *Br Dent J*, 1997, 182(12):465-8.
28. "Risks for and Prevention of Infective Endocarditis," *Cardiology Clinics - Diagnosis and Management of Infective Endocarditis*, Child JS, ed, Philadelphia, PA: WB Saunders Co, 1996, 14:327-43.
29. Doern GV, Ferraro MJ, Brueggemann AB, et al, "Emergence of High Rates of Antimicrobial Resistance Among Viridans Group Streptococci in the United States," *Antimicrob Agents Chemother*, 1996, 40(4):891-4.

## ANTIBIOTIC PROPHYLAXIS *(Continued)*


30. Dowson CG, Coffey TJ, Kell C, et al, "Evolution of Penicillin Resistance in *Streptococcus pneumoniae*, the Role of *Streptococcus mitis* in the Formation of a Low Affinity PBP2B in *S. pneumoniae*," *Mol Microbiol*, 1993, (3): 635-43.
31. Steckelberg JM and Wilson WR, "Risk Factors for Infective Endocarditis" *Infect Dis Clin N Am*, 1993, 7(1):9-19.
32. Chenoweth CE and Burket JS, "Antimicrobial Prophylaxis: Principles and Practice," *Formulary*, 1997, 32:692-708.
33. Durack DT, "Prevention of Infective Endocarditis," *N Engl J Med*, 1995, 332(1):38-44.
34. Little JW, Falace DA, Miller CS, et al, "Prosthetic Implants," *Dental Management of the Medically Compromised Patient*, 5th ed, Mosby, St Louis: MO, 1997, 602-17.
35. Wynn RL, Meiller TF, and Crossley HL, "New Guidelines for the Prevention of Bacterial Endocarditis. American Heart Association," *Gen Dent*, 1997, 45(5):426-8, 430-4.
36. Bartzokas CA, Johnson R, Jane M, et al, "Relation Between Mouth and Haematogenous Infection in Total Joint Replacements," *BMJ*, 1994, 309(6953):506-8.
37. Hopkins CC, "Recognition of Endemic and Epidemic Prosthetic Device Infections: The Role of Surveillance, the Hospital Infection Control Practitioner, and the Hospital Epidemiologist," *Infect Dis Clin North Am*, 1989, 3(2):211-20.
38. "Advisory Statement. Antibiotic Prophylaxis for Dental Patients With Total Joint Replacement. American Dental Association; American Academy of Orthopaedic Surgeons," *J Am Dent Assoc*, 1997, 128(7):1004-8.
39. Ching DW, Gould IM, Rennie JA, et al, "Prevention of Late Haematogenous Infection in Major Prosthetic Joints," *J Antimicrob Chemother*, 1989, 23(5):676-80.
40. Brause BD, "Infections Associated With Prosthetic Joints," *Clin Rheum Dis*, 1986, 12(2):523-36.
41. Johnson DP and Bannister GC, "The Outcome of Infected Arthroplasty of the Knee," *J Bone Joint Surg (Br)*, 1986, 68(2):289-91.
42. Jacobson JJ, Millard HD, Plezia R, et al, "Dental Treatment and Late Prosthetic Joint Infections," *Oral Surg Oral Med Oral Pathol*, 1986, 61(4):413-7.
43. Jacobson JJ, Patel B, Asher G, et al, "Oral Staphylococcus in Older Subjects With Rheumatoid Arthritis," *J Am Geriatr Soc*, 1997, 45(5):590-3.
44. Hanssen AD, Osmon DR, and Nelson CL, "Prevention of Deep Prosthetic Joint Infection," *J Bone Joint Surg*, 1996, 78:458-71.
45. Skiest DJ and Coykendall AL, "Prosthetic Hip Infection Related to a Dental Procedure Despite Antibiotic Prophylaxis," *Oral Surg Oral Med Oral Pathol Oral Radiol Endod*, 1995, 79(5):661-3.
46. Wahl M, "Myths of Dental-Induced Prosthetic Joint Infections," *Clin Infect Dis*, 1995, 20(5):1420-5.

# SYSTEMIC VIRAL DISEASES

## HEPATITIS

The hepatitis viruses are a group of DNA and RNA viruses that produce symptoms associated with inflammation of the liver. Currently, hepatitis A through G have been identified by immunological testing; however, hepatitis A through E have received most attention in terms of disease identification. Recently, however, there has been increased interest in hepatitis viruses F and G, particularly as relate to healthcare professionals. Our knowledge is expanding rapidly in this area and the clinician should be alert to changes in the literature that might update their knowledge. Hepatitis F, for instance, remains a diagnosis of exclusion effectively being non-A, B, C, D, E, or G. Whereas, hepatitis G has serologic testing available, however, not commercially at this time. Research evaluations of various antibody and RT-PCR tests for hepatitis G are under development at this time.

Signs and symptoms of viral hepatitis in general are quite variable. Patients infected may range from asymptomatic to experiencing flu-like symptoms only. In addition, fever, nausea, joint muscle pain, jaundice, and hepatomegaly along with abdominal pain can result from infection with one of the hepatitis viruses. The virus also can create an acute or chronic infection. Usually following these early symptoms or the asymptomatic period, the patient may recover or may go on to develop chronic liver dysfunction. Liver dysfunction may be represented primarily by changes in liver function tests known as LFTs and these primarily include aspartate aminotransferase known as AST and alanine aminotransferase known as ALT. In addition, for A, B, C, D, and E there are serologic tests for either antigen, antibody, or both. Of hepatitis A through G, five forms have both acute and chronic forms whereas A and E appear to only create acute disease. There are differences in the way clinicians may approach a known postexposure to one of the hepatitis viruses. In many instances, gamma globulin may be used, however, the indications for gamma globulin as a drug limit their use to several of the viruses only. The dental clinician should be aware that the gastroenterologist may choose to give gamma globulin off-label.

Hepatitis A virus is an enteric virus that is a member of the Picornavirus family along with Coxsackie viruses and poliovirus. Previously known as infectious hepatitis, hepatitis A has been detected in humans for centuries. It causes acute hepatitis, often transmitted by oral-fecal contamination and having an incubation period of approximately 30 days. Typically, constitutional symptoms are present and jaundice may occur. Drug therapy that the dentist may encounter in a patient being treated for hepatitis A would primarily include immunoglobulin.

Hepatitis B virus is previously known as serum hepatitis and has particular trophism for liver cells. Hepatitis B virus causes both acute and chronic disease in susceptible patients. The incubation period is often long and the diagnosis might be made by serologic markers even in the absence of symptoms. No drug therapy for acute hepatitis B is known; however, chronic hepatitis has recently been successfully treated with alfa-interferon. There are vaccines available for hepatitis A and B. Hepatitis C virus was described in 1988 and has been formerly classified as non-A/non-B. It is clear that hepatitis C represents a high percentage of the transfusion-associated hepatitis that is seen. Treatment of acute hepatitis C infection is generally supportive. Interferon Alfa-2a therapy has been used with some success recently and interferon-alfa may be beneficial with hepatitis C related chronic hepatitis. Hepatitis D is previously known as the delta agent and is a virus that is incomplete in that it requires previous infection with hepatitis B in order to be manifested. Currently, no antiviral therapy is effective against hepatitis D. Hepatitis E virus is an RNA virus that represents a proportion of the previously classified non-A/non-B diagnoses. There is currently no antiviral therapy against hepatitis E.

Hepatitis F, as was mentioned, remains a diagnosis of exclusion. There are no known immunological tests available for identification of hepatitis F at present and currently the Centers for Disease Control have not come out with specific guidelines or recommendations. It is thought, however, that hepatitis F is a bloodborne virus and it has been used as a diagnosis in several cases of post-transfusion hepatitis. Hepatitis G virus (HGV), is the newest hepatitis and is also assumed to be a bloodborne virus. Similar in family to hepatitis C, it is thought to occur concomitantly with hepatitis C and appears to be even more prevalent in some blood donors than hepatitis C. Occupational transmission of HGV is currently under study (see the references for updated information) and currently there are no specific CDC recommendations for postexposure to an HGV individual as the testing for identification remains experimental.

## SYSTEMIC VIRAL DISEASES *(Continued)*

### PRE-EXPOSURE PROPHYLAXIS FOR HEPATITIS B

| |
|---|
| Health care workers* |
| Special patient groups (eg. adolescents, infants born to $HB_sAg$–positive mothers, military personnel, etc) |
| Hemodialysis patients† |
| Recipients of certain blood products‡ |
| Lifestyle factors |
| Homosexual and bisexual men |
| Intravenous drug abusers |
| Heterosexually active persons with multiple sexual partners or recently acquired sexually transmitted diseases |
| Environmental factors |
| Household and sexual contacts of HBV carriers |
| Prison inmates |
| Clients and staff of institutions for the mentally handicapped |
| Residents, immigrants and refugees from areas with endemic HBV infection |
| International travelers at increased risk of acquiring HBV infection |

*The risk of hepatitis B virus (HBV) infection for health care workers varies both between hospitals and within hospitals. Hepatitis B vaccination is recommended for all health care workers with blood exposure.

†Hemodialysis patients often respond poorly to hepatitis B vaccination; higher vaccine doses or increased number of doses are required. A special formulation of one vaccine is now available for such persons (Recombivax HB®, 40 mcg/mL). The anti-$HB_s$ (antibody to hepatitis B surface antigen) response of such persons should be tested after they are vaccinated, and those who have not responded should be revaccinated with 1-3 additional doses.

Patients with chronic renal disease should be vaccinated as early as possible, ideally before they require hemodialysis. In addition, their anti- $HB_s$ levels should be monitored at 6- to 12-month intervals to assess the need for revaccination.

‡Patients with hemophilia should be immunized subcutaneously, not intramuscularly.

## POSTEXPOSURE PROPHYLAXIS FOR HEPATITIS B*

| Exposure | Hepatitis B Immune Globulin | Hepatitis B Vaccine |
|---|---|---|
| Perinatal | 0.5 mL I.M. within 12 h of birth | 0.5 mL† I.M. within 12 h of birth (no later than 7 d), and at 1 and 6 mo‡; test for $HB_sAg$ and anti-$HB_s$ at 12-15 mo |
| Sexual | 0.06 mL/kg I.M. within 14 d of sexual contact; a second dose should be given if the index patient remains $HB_sAg$-positive after 3 mo and hepatitis B vaccine was not given initially | 1 mL I.M. at 0, 1, and 6 mo for homosexual and bisexual men and regular sexual contacts of persons with acute and chronic hepatitis B |
| **Percutaneous; exposed person unvaccinated** | | |
| Source known $HB_sAg$-positive | 0.06 mL/kg I.M. within 24 h | 1 mL I.M. within 7 d, and at 1 and 6 mo§ |
| Source known, $HB_sAg$ status not known | Test source for $HB_sAg$; if source is positive, give exposed person 0.06 mL/kg I.M. once within 7 d | 1 mL I.M. within 7 d, and at 1 and 6 mo§ |
| Source not tested or unknown | Nothing required | 1 mL I.M. within 7 d, and at 1 and 6 mo |
| **Percutaneous; exposed person vaccinated** | | |
| Source known $HB_sAg$-positive | Test exposed person for anti-$HB_s$¶. If titer is protective, nothing is required; if titer is not protective, give 0.06 mL/kg within 24 h. | Review vaccination status# |
| Source known, $HB_sAg$ status not known | Test source for $HB_sAg$ and exposed person for anti-$HB_s$. If source is $HB_sAg$-negative, or if source is $HB_sAg$-positive but anti-$HB_s$ titer is protective, nothing is required. If source is $HB_sAg$-positive and anti-$HB_s$ titer is not protective or if exposed person is a known nonresponder, give 0.06 mL/kg I.M. within 24 h. A second dose of hepatitis B immune globulin can be given 1 mo later if a booster dose of hepatitis B vaccine is not given. | Review vaccination status# |
| Source not tested or unknown | Test exposed person for anti-$HB_s$. If anti-$HB_s$ titer is protective, nothing is required. If anti-$HB_s$ titer is not protective, 0.06 mL/kg may be given along with a booster dose of hepatitis B vaccine. | Review vaccination status# |

*$HB_sAg$ = hepatitis B surface antigen; anti-$HB_s$ = antibody to hepatitis B surface antigen; I.M. = intramuscularly; SRU = standard ratio units.

†Each 0.5 mL dose of plasma-derived hepatitis B vaccine contains 10 mcg of $HB_sAg$; each 0.5 mL dose of recombinant hepatitis B vaccine contains 5 mcg or 10 mcg of $HB_sAg$.

‡If hepatitis B immune globulin and hepatitis B vaccine are given simultaneously, they should be given at separate sites.

§If hepatitis B vaccine is not given, a second dose of hepatitis B immune globulin should be given 1 month later.

¶Anti-$HB_s$ titers <10 SRU by radioimmunoassay or negative by enzyme immunoassay indicate lack of protection. Testing the exposed person for anti-$HB_s$ is not necessary if a protective level of antibody has been shown within the previous 24 months.

#If the exposed person has not completed a three-dose series of hepatitis B vaccine, the series should be completed. Test the exposed person for anti-$HB_s$. If the antibody level is protective, nothing is required. If an adequate antibody response in the past is shown on retesting to have declined to an inadequate level, a booster dose (1 mL) of hepatitis B vaccine should be given. If the exposed person has inadequate antibody or is a known nonresponder to vaccination, a booster dose can be given along with one dose of hepatitis B immune globulin.

## SYSTEMIC VIRAL DISEASES *(Continued)*

### TYPES OF HEPATITIS VIRUS

| Features | A | B | C | D | E | F | G |
|---|---|---|---|---|---|---|---|
| **Incubation Period** | 2-6 wks | 8-24 wks | 2-52 wks | 3-13 wks | 3-6 wks | Unknown | Unknown |
| **Onset** | Abrupt | Insidious | Insidious | Abrupt | Abrupt | Insidious | Insidious |
| **Symptoms** | | | | | | | |
| Jaundice | Adults: 70% to 80%; Children: 10% | 25% | 25% | Varies | Unknown | Unknown | Unknown |
| Asymptomatic Patients | Adults: 50%; Children: Most | ~75% | ~75% | Rare | Rare | Common | Common |
| **Routes of Transmission** | | | | | | | |
| Fecal/Oral | Yes | No | No | No | Yes | Unknown | Unknown |
| Parenteral | Rare | Yes | Yes | Yes | No | | |
| Sexual | No | Yes | Possible | Yes | No | | |
| Perinatal | No | Yes | Possible | Possible | No | | |
| Water/Food | Yes | No | No | No | Yes | | |
| **Sequelae** (% of patients) | | | | | | | |
| Chronic state | No | Adults: 6% to 10%; Children: 25% to 50%; Infants: 70% to 90% | >75% | 10% to 15% | No | Unknown | Likely |
| **Case-Fatality Rate** | 0.6% | 1.4% | 1% to 2% | 30% | 1% to 2%; Pregnant women: 20% | Unknown | Unknown |

Hepatitis A Vaccine (Havrix®) *on page 494*
Hepatitis B Immune Globulin (H-BIG®, HyperHep®) *on page 494*
Hepatitis B Vaccine (Engerix-B®, Recombivax HB®) *on page 495*
Immune Globulin, Intramuscular (Gamastan®, Gammar®) *on page 530*
Immune Globulin, Intravenous (Gamimune® N, Gammagard®, Gammagard® S/D, Gammar®-P, Polygam®, Polygam® S/D, Sandoglobulin®, Venoglobulin®-I, Venoglobulin®-S) *on page 531*
Interferon Alfa-2a (Roferon-A®) *on page 538*
Interferon Alfa-2b (Intron® A) *on page 540*

## HERPES

The herpes viruses not only represent a topic of specific interest to the dentist due to oral manifestations, but are widespread as systemic infections. Herpes simplex virus is also of interest because of its central nervous system infections and its relationship as one of the viral infections commonly found in AIDS patients. Oral herpes infections will be covered elsewhere. Treatment of herpes simplex primary infection includes acyclovir. Ganciclovir is an alternative drug and foscarnet is also occasionally used. Epstein-Barr virus is a member of the herpesvirus family and produces syndromes important in dentistry, including infectious mononucleosis with the commonly found oral pharyngitis and petechial hemorrhages, as well as being the causative agent of Burkitt's lymphoma. The relationship between Epstein-Barr virus to oral hairy leukoplakia in AIDS patients has not been shown to be one of cause and effect; however, the presence of Epstein-Barr in these lesions is consistent. Currently, there is no accepted treatment for Epstein-Barr virus, although acyclovir has been shown in *in vitro* studies to have some efficacy. Varicella-zoster virus is another member of the herpesvirus family and is the causative agent of two clinical entities, chickenpox and shingles or herpes zoster. Oral manifestations of both chickenpox and herpes zoster include vesicular eruptions often leading to confluent mucosal ulcerations. Acyclovir is the drug of choice for treatment of herpes zoster infections.

There are other herpes viruses that produce disease in man and animals. These viruses have no specific treatment, therefore, incidence is thought to be less common than those mentioned and the specific treatment is not determined at present. The role of some of these viruses in concomitant infection with the HIV and other coinfection viruses is still under study.

# ANTIVIRALS

## ANTIVIRAL AGENTS OF ESTABLISHED THERAPEUTIC EFFECTIVENESS

| Viral Infection | Drug |
|---|---|
| Cytomegalovirus | |
| Retinitis | Ganciclovir<br>Foscarnet |
| Pneumonia | Ganciclovir |
| Hepatitis viruses | |
| Chronic hepatitis C | Interferon Alfa-2a |
| Chronic hepatitis B | Interferon Alfa-2b |
| Herpes simplex virus | |
| Orofacial herpes | |
| First episode | Acyclovir |
| Recurrence | Acyclovir<br>Penciclovir |
| Genital herpes | |
| First episode | Acyclovir |
| Recurrence | Acyclovir |
| Suppression | Acyclovir |
| Encephalitis | Acyclovir |
| Mucocutaneous disease in immunocompromised | Acyclovir |
| Neonatal | Acyclovir |
| Keratoconjunctivitis | Trifluridine<br>Vidarabine |
| Influenza A virus | Amantadine<br>Rimantadine |
| Papillomavirus | |
| Condyloma acuminatum | Interferon Alfa-2b<br>Imiquimod (Aldara®):<br>(use for oral lesions is under study) |
| Respiratory syncytial virus | Ribavirin |
| Varicella-zoster virus | |
| Varicella in normal children | Acyclovir |
| Varicella in immunocompromised | Acyclovir |
| Herpes zoster in immunocompromised | Acyclovir |
| Herpes zoster in normal hosts | Acyclovir<br>Famciclovir |

Acyclovir (Zovirax®) *on page 38*
Amantadine (Symmetrel®) *on page 57*
Atovaquone (Mepron™) *on page 107*
Cidofovir (Vistide®) *on page 248*
Famciclovir (Famvir™) *on page 418*
Foscarnet (Foscavir®) *on page 455*
Ganciclovir (Cytovene®, Vitrasert®) *on page 462*
Hepatitis B Immune Globulin (H-BIG®, HyperHep®) *on page 494*
Imiquimod (Aldara®) *on page 530*
Immune Globulin, Intramuscular (Gamastan®, Gammar®) *on page 530*
Interferon Alfa-2a (Roferon-A®) *on page 538*
Interferon Alfa-2b (Intron® A) *on page 540*
Interferon Alfa-N3 (Alferon® N) *on page 543*
Penciclovir (Denavir®) *on page 771*
Rifabutin (Mycobutin®) *on page 885*
Rimantadine (Flumadine®) *on page 889*
Trifluridine (Viroptic®) *on page 1018*
Valacyclovir (Valtrex®) *on page 1037*
Vidarabine (Vira-A®) *on page 1045*

# PART II. DENTAL MANAGEMENT AND THERAPEUTIC CONSIDERATIONS IN PATIENTS WITH SPECIFIC ORAL CONDITIONS AND OTHER MEDICINE TOPICS

This second part of the text focuses on therapies the dentist may choose to prescribe for patients suffering from oral disease or are in need of special care. Some overlap between these sections has resulted from systemic conditions that have oral manifestations and vice-versa. Cross-references to the descriptions and the monographs for individual drugs described elsewhere in this handbook allow for easy retrieval of information. Example prescriptions of selected drug therapies for each condition are presented so that the clinician can evaluate alternate approaches to treatment. Seldom is there a single drug of choice.

Those drug prescriptions listed represent prototype drugs and popular prescriptions and are examples only. The therapeutic index is available for cross-referencing if alternatives and additional drugs are sought.

## TABLE OF CONTENTS

# ORAL PAIN

## PAIN PREVENTION

For the dental patient, the prevention of pain aids in relieving anxiety and reduces the probability of stress during dental care. For the practitioner, dental procedures can be accomplished more efficiently in a "painless" situation. Appropriate selection and use of local anesthetics is one of the foundations for success in this arena. Local anesthetics listed below include drugs for the most commonly confronted dental procedures. Ester anesthetics are no longer available in dose form for dental injections, and historically had a higher incidence of allergic manifestations due to the formation of the metabolic by-product, para-aminobenzoic acid. The amides have an almost negligible allergic rate, however, at least one well documented case of amide allergy was reported by Seng, et al.

The potential interaction between acetaminophen and warfarin has been recently raised in the literature. The cytochrome P450 system of drug metabolism for these vitamin K dependent metabolic pathways has raised the possibility that prolonged use of acetaminophen may inadvertently enhance, to dangerous levels, the anticoagulation effect of warfarin. As monitored by the INR, the effects of these drugs may be one and one-half to two times greater than as expected from the warfarin dosage alone. This potential interaction could be of importance in selecting an analgesic/antipyretic drug for the dental patient.

### LOCAL ANESTHETICS

Bupivacaine (Marcaine®, Sensorcaine® MPF) *on page 157*

Bupivacaine and Epinephrine (Marcaine® with Epinephrine; Sensorcaine®) *on page 158*

Chloroprocaine (Nesacaine®) *on page 226*

Etidocaine With Epinephrine (Duranest® with Epinephrine) *on page 411*

Lidocaine and Epinephrine (Octocaine® 50; Octocaine® 100; Xylocaine® with Epinephrine) *on page 587*

Lidocaine (Dilocaine®, Duo-Trach®, Nervocaine®, Octocaine®, Xylocaine®) *on page 586*

Lidocaine Transoral (Dentipatch®) *on page 590*

Mepivacaine Dental Anesthetic (Carbocaine® 3%; Isocaine® 3%; Polocaine® 3%) *on page 634*

Mepivacaine and Levonordefrin (Carbocaine® 2% with Neo-Cobefrin®, Isocaine® 2%; Polocaine® 2%) *on page 632*

Prilocaine (Citanest® Plain 4%) *on page 835*

Prilocaine With Epinephrine (Citanest Forte® with Epinephrine) *on page 836*

Ropivacaine (Naropin®) *on page 896*

Tetracaine (Pontocaine®, Viractin®) *on page 964*

Tetracaine and Dextrose (Pontocaine® with Dextrose Injection) *on page 964*

The selection of a vasoconstrictor with the local anesthetic must be based on the length of the procedure to be performed, the patient's medical status (epinephrine is contraindicated in patients with uncontrolled hyperthyroidism), and the need for hemorrhage control. The following table lists some of the common drugs with their duration of action. Transoral patches with lidocaine are now available (Dentipatch®) and the new long-acting amide injectable, Ropivacaine (Naropin®) may be useful for postoperative pain management.

**DENTAL ANESTHETICS**
**(Average Duration by Route)**

| Product | Infiltration | Inferior Alveolar Block |
|---|---|---|
| Marcaine® HCl 0.5% with epinephrine 1:200,000 (bupivacaine and epinephrine) | 60 minutes | 5-7 hours |
| Carbocaine® HCl 3% (mepivacaine) | 20 minutes | 40 minutes |
| Carbocaine® HCl 2% with Neo-Cobefrin® 1:20,000 (mepivacaine HCl and levonordefrin) | 50 minutes | 60-75 minutes |
| Duranest® Injection (etidocaine) | 5-10 hours | 5-10 hours |
| Citanest® Plain 4% (prilocaine) | 20 minutes | 2.5 hours |
| Citanest Forte® with Epinephrine (prilocaine with epinephrine) | 2.25 hours | 3 hours |
| Lidocaine HCl 2% and epinephrine 1:100,000 (lidocaine and epinephrine) | 60 minutes | 90 minutes |

The use of preinjection topical anesthetics can assist in pain prevention (see also "Oral Viral Infections" *on page 1137* and "Oral Nonviral Soft Tissue Ulcerations or Erosions" *on page 1141*). Some clinicians are also using EMLA® (eutectic mixture of local anesthetic with lidocaine and prilocaine) as a topical. Skin patch available by Astra not currently approved for oral use.

Benzocaine (Hurricaine®, Numzident®, various other products) *on page 128*

Lidocaine (Dilocaine®, Duo-Trach®, Nervocaine®, Octocaine®, Xylocaine®) *on page 586*

Lidocaine Transoral (Dentipatch®) *on page 590*

Tetracaine (Pontocaine®, Viractin®) *on page 964*

## PAIN MANAGEMENT

The patient with existing acute or chronic oral pain requires appropriate treatment and sensitivity on the part of the dentist, all for the purpose of achieving relief from the oral source of pain. Pain can be divided into mild, moderate, and severe levels and requires a subjective assessment by the dentist based on knowledge of the dental procedures to be performed, the presenting signs and symptoms of the patient, and the realization that most dental procedures are invasive often leading to pain once the patient has left the dental office. The practitioner must be aware that the treatment of the source of the pain is usually the best management. If infection is present, treatment of the infection will directly alleviate the patient's discomfort. However, a patient who is not in pain tends to heal better and it is wise to adequately cover the patient for any residual or recurrent discomfort suffered. Likewise, many of the procedures that the dentist performs have pain associated with them. Much of this pain occurs after leaving the dentist office due to an inflammatory process or a healing process that has been initiated. It is difficult to assign specific pain levels (mild, moderate, or severe) for specific procedures; however, the dentist should use his or her prescribing capacity judiciously so that overmedication is avoided.

The following categories of drugs and appropriate example prescriptions for each follow. These include management of mild pain with aspirin products, acetaminophen, and some of the nonsteroidal noninflammatory agents. Management of moderate pain includes codeine, Vicodin®, Vicodin ES®, Lorcet® 10/650; and Motrin® in the 800 mg dosage. Severe pain may require treatment with Percodan®, Percocet®, or Demerol®. All prescription pain preparations should be closely monitored for efficacy and discontinued if the pain persists or requires a higher level formulation.

The chronic pain patient represents a particular challenge for the practitioner. Some additional drugs that may be useful in managing the patient with chronic pain are covered in the temporomandibular dysfunction section of this text. It is always incumbent on the practitioner to reevaluate the diagnosis, source of pain, and treatment, whenever prolonged use of analgesics (narcotic or non-narcotic) is contemplated. Drugs such as Dilaudid® are not recommended for management of dental pain in most states.

Narcotic analgesics can be used on a short-term basis or intermittently in combination with non-narcotic therapy in the chronic pain patient. Judicious prescribing,

## ORAL PAIN *(Continued)*

monitoring, and maintenance by the practitioner is imperative, particularly whenever considering the use of a narcotic analgesic due to the abuse and addiction liabilities.

## MILD PAIN

Acetaminophen (various products) *on page 27*

Aspirin (various products) *on page 100*

Diflunisal (Dolobid®) *on page 327*

Ibuprofen (various products) *on page 522*

Ketoprofen (Actron®, Orudis®, Orudis KT®, Oruvail®) *on page 565*

Naproxen (Aleve®, Anaprox®, Naprosyn®) *on page 705*

## OVER-THE-COUNTER PRESCRIPTION EXAMPLES

**Rx**

Aspirin 325 mg

Disp

Sig: Take 2-3 tablets every 4 hours

**Rx**

Ibuprofen 200 mg

Disp

Sig: Take 2-3 tablets every 4 hours, up to 3200 mg (16 tablets)/day

**Note:** Ibuprofen is available over-the-counter as Motrin IB®, Advil®, Nuprin®, and many other brands in 200 mg tablets.

**Note:** NSAIDs should never be taken together, nor should they be combined with aspirin. NSAIDs have anti-inflammatory effects as well as analgesics. An allergy to aspirin constitutes a contradiction to all the new NSAIDs. Aspirin and the NSAIDs may increase post-treatment bleeding.

**Rx**

Acetaminophen 325 mg

Disp

Sig: Take 2-3 tablets every 4 hours

Products include: Tylenol®, Datril®, Anacin® 3, and many others

**Note:** Acetaminophen can be given if patient has allergy, bleeding problems, or stomach upset secondary to aspirin or NSAIDs.

**Rx**

Aleve® 220 mg

Disp

Sig: 1-2 tablets every 8 hours

Ingredient: Naproxen

**Rx**

Orudis KT® 12.5 mg

Disp

Sig: 1-2 tablets every 8 hours

Ingredient: Ketoprofen

## PRESCRIPTION ONLY EXAMPLES

**Rx**

Ketoprofen 25 mg

Disp

Sig: 1-2 tablets every 8 hours

**Rx**

Dolobid® 500 mg

Disp 16 tablets

Sig: Take 2 tablets initially, then 1 tablet every 8-12 hours for pain

Ingredient: Diflunisal

# MODERATE/MODERATELY SEVERE PAIN

Aspirin and Codeine (Empirin® with Codeine) *on page 102*

Dihydrocodeine Compound (Synalgos® DC) *on page 331*

Hydrocodone and Acetaminophen (Lortab®, Vicodin®, various products) *on page 505*

Ibuprofen (various products) *on page 522*

A new class of NSAIDs has been approved and indicated in the treatment of arthritis, COX-2 inhibitors (celecoxib, Celebrex®; rofecoxib, Vioxx®). Rofecoxib (Vioxx®) is indicated for use in short-term oral pain management. Celecoxib is currently not indicated for use in short-term oral pain management.

The following is a guideline to use when prescribing codeine with either aspirin or acetaminophen (Tylenol®):

Codeine No. 2 = codeine 15 mg

Codeine No. 3 = codeine 30 mg

Codeine No. 4 = codeine 60 mg

Example: ASA No. 3 = aspirin 325 mg + codeine 30 mg

## PRESCRIPTION EXAMPLES

**Rx**

Motrin® 800 mg*

Disp 16 tablets

Sig: Take 1 tablet 3 times/day

Ingredient: Ibuprofen

**Note:** For more severe pain, Motrin® (800 mg) can be given up to 4 times/day.

***Note:** Also available as 600 mg

## ORAL PAIN *(Continued)*

> **Rx**
>
> Tylenol® No. 3*
>
> Disp 16 (sixteen) tablets
>
> Sig: Take 1 tablet every 4 hours as needed for pain

Ingredients: Acetaminophen and codeine

***Note:** Also available as #2 and #4

> **Rx**
>
> Synalgos® DC
>
> Disp 16 (sixteen) capsules
>
> Sig: Take 1 capsule every 4 hours as needed for pain

Ingredients: Dihydrocodeine 16 mg, aspirin 356.4 mg, and caffeine 30 mg

> **Rx**
>
> Vicodin®
>
> Disp 16 (sixteen) tablets
>
> Sig: Take 1 tablet every 4 hours for pain

Ingredients: Hydrocodone 5 mg and acetaminophen 500 mg

**Note:** Available as Vicodin ES® for use 1 tablet every 8-12 hours

> **Rx**
>
> Lortab® 5 mg*
>
> Disp 16 (sixteen) tablets
>
> Sig: Take 1 or 2 tablets every 4 hours for pain (do not exceed 8 tablets in 24 hours)

Ingredients: Hydrocodone 5 mg and acetaminophen 500 mg

***Note:** Available under other brand names with varying dosages and strengths

## SEVERE PAIN

Hydrocodone and Ibuprofen (Vicoprofen®) *on page 509*

Meperidine (Demerol®) *on page 629*

Oxycodone (OxyContin®, OxyIR®, Roxicodone™) *on page 750*

Oxycodone and Acetaminophen (Percocet®, Roxicet®, Roxilox®, Tylox®) *on page 751*

Oxycodone and Aspirin (Codoxy®, Percodan®, Roxiprin®) *on page 753*

### PRESCRIPTION EXAMPLES

> **Rx**
>
> Vicoprofen®
>
> Disp 16 (sixteen) tablets
>
> Sig: Take 1-2 tablets every 4-6 hours for pain — No Refills

Ingredients: Hydrocodone 7.5 mg and ibuprofen 200 mg

**Rx**

Demerol® 50 mg*

Disp 16 (sixteen) tablets

Sig: Take 1 tablet every 4 hours for pain — No Refills

Ingredients: Meperidine

*Triplicate prescription required in some states

**Rx**

Roxicodone™ 5 mg

Disp 24 tablets

Sig: Take 1 tablet every 6 hours for pain — No Refills

Ingredients: Oxycodone

Some formulations available as controlled release

**Rx**

Percodan®*

Disp 16 (sixteen) tablets

Sig: Take 1 tablet every 4 hours for pain — No Refills

Ingredients: Oxycodone 4.88 mg and aspirin 325 mg

*Triplicate prescription required in some states

**Rx**

Percocet® tablets or Tylox® capsules*

Disp 16 (sixteen) tablets or capsules

Sig: Take 1 tablet every 4 hours for pain — No Refills

Ingredients: Oxycodone 5 mg and acetaminophen 325 mg
(Tylox® contains acetaminophen 500 mg)

*Triplicate prescription required in some states

# ORAL BACTERIAL INFECTIONS

Dental infection can occur for any number of reasons, primarily involving pulpal and periodontal infections. Secondary infections of the soft tissues as well as sinus infections pose special treatment challenges. The drugs of choice in treating most oral infections have been selected because of their efficacy in providing adequate blood levels for delivery to the oral tissues and their proven usefulness in managing dental infections. Penicillin and erythromycin remain the two primary drugs for treatment of dental infections of pulpal origin. The management of soft tissue infections may require the use of additional drugs.

## SINUS INFECTION TREATMENT

Sinus infections represent a common condition which may present with confounding dental complaints. Treatment is sometimes instituted by the dentist, but due to the often chronic and recurrent nature of sinus infections, early involvement of an otolaryngologist is advised. These infections may require antibiotics of varying spectrum as well as requiring the management of sinus congestion. Although amoxicillin is usually adequate, many otolaryngologists go directly to Augmentin®. Second generation cephalosporins and clarithromycin are sometimes used depending on the chronicity of the problem.

Amoxicillin and Clavulanate Potassium (Augmentin®) *on page 77*
Amoxicillin Trihydrate (various products) *on page 76*
Ceftibuten (Cedax®) *on page 207*
Chlorpheniramine (Chlor-Trimeton®, various products) *on page 231*
Clarithromycin (Biaxin™) *on page 256*
Loratadine and Pseudoephedrine (Claritin-D®) *on page 601*
Oxymetazoline (Afrin®, various products) *on page 755*
Pseudoephedrine (Sudafed®, various products) *on page 863*

## PRESCRIPTION EXAMPLES

**Rx**

Amoxicillin 500 mg
Disp 21 capsules
Sig: Take 1 capsule 3 times/day

**Rx**

Augmentin® 500
Disp 30 tablets
Sig: Take 1 tablet 3 times/day

Ingredients: Amoxicillin 500 mg and clavulanate potassium 125 mg

The selected antibiotic should be used with a nasal decongestant and possibly an antihistamine.

**Rx**

Afrin® Nasal Spray (OTC)
Disp 15 mL
Sig: Spray 1 time in each nostril every 6-8 hours for no more than 3 days

Ingredient: Oxymetazoline

**OR**

**Rx**

Sudafed® 60 mg tablets (OTC)
Disp 30 tablets
Sig: Take 1 tablet every 4-6 hours as needed for congestion

Ingredient: Pseudoephedrine

**Rx**

Chlor-Trimeton® 4 mg (OTC)
Disp 14 tablets
Sig: Take 1 tablet 2 times/day

Ingredient: Chlorpheniramine

# PULPAL AND PERIODONTAL INFECTIONS

Regardless of the condition to be treated, consideration should always be given to managing and monitoring the course of the infection with observations at 24 and 72 hours to ensure efficacy of the drug selected. Due to the usual multiorganism etiology of most pulpal and periodontal dental infections, culture and sensitivity studies may not be pertinent. Penicillin, clindamycin, and erythromycin are first-line drugs of choice for most dental infections. Some periodontal infections respond well to tetracyclines and metronidazole. Although culturing oral infections is not always necessary, a complete listing of the spectrum of antibiotics available can be found in the Appendix. Oral antimicrobial rinses may be useful in periodontal infections.

## THE CLINICIAN AND PULPAL INFECTIONS

The clinician should be aware that the management of oral infections may require the use of a loading dose of the drug usually in the case of penicillin VK one gram instead of the 500 mg constant dose or the use of 300 mg of clindamycin prior to the onset of the regular regimen as outlined. The clinician should also be aware that some infections may be refractory to this initial therapy and broader spectrum antibiotics such as Augmentin® may be necessary to assist in the management of the acute infection.

Common Oral-Facial Infections and Antibiotics for Treatment *on page 1268*

Amoxicillin and Clavulanate Potassium (Augmentin®) *on page 77*
Amoxicillin Trihydrate (various products) *on page 76*
Cephalexin (Biocef®, Cefanex®, Keflet®, Keflex®, Keftab®) *on page 214*
Chlorhexidine (Peridex®, PerioGard®) *on page 225*
Clindamycin (Cleocin®) *on page 258*
Dicloxacillin (Dycill®, Dynapen®, Pathocil®) *on page 321*
Erythromycin (various products) *on page 383*
Metronidazole (Flagyl®, MetroGel®, Protostat®) *on page 667*
Mouthwash, Antiseptic (Listerine®) *on page 690*
Penicillin V Potassium (various products) *on page 776*
Tetracycline (Achromycin®, Sumycin®, Tetracyn®) *on page 965*

**Note:** Often penicillins are prescribed with a double or triple loading dose initially, then followed by the course described below.

## PRESCRIPTION EXAMPLES

**Rx**

Penicillin V potassium 500 mg
Disp 28 tablets
Sig: Take 1 tablet 4 times/day

**Rx**

Augmentin® 500 mg
Disp 28 tablets
Sig: Take 1 tablet 4 times/day

## ORAL BACTERIAL INFECTIONS *(Continued)*

**Rx**

Erythromycin base 250 mg

Disp 28 (enteric coated) tablets

Sig: Take 1 tablet 4 times/day

**Rx**

Cephalexin 250 mg

Disp 28 capsules

Sig: Take 1 capsule 4 times/day

**Rx**

Dicloxacillin 250 mg

Disp 28 capsules

Sig: Take 2 capsules once every 6 hours

**Rx**

Clindamycin 300 mg (Cleocin®)

Disp 14 capsules

Sig: Take 1 capsule every 6 hours

**Rx**

Metronidazole 250 mg (Flagyl®)

Disp 40 tablets

Sig: Take 1 tablet 4 times/day

**Rx**

Chlorhexidine Gluconate 0.12% (Peridex® and PerioGard®)

Disp 1 bottle

Sig: 20 mL for 30 seconds 3 times/day

**Rx**

Listerine® (OTC)

Disp 1 bottle

Sig: 20 mL for 30 seconds twice daily

## FREQUENTLY ASKED QUESTIONS

*What is the best antibiotic modality for treating dental infections?*

Penicillin is still the drug of choice for treatment of infections in and around the oral cavity. Phenoxy-methyl penicillin (Pen VK®) long has been the most commonly selected antibiotic. In penicillin-allergic individuals, erythromycin may be an appropriate consideration. If another drug is sought, clindamycin prescribed 300 mg as a loading dose followed by 150 mg 4 times/day would be an appropriate regimen for a dental infection. In general, if there is no response to Pen VK®, then Augmentin® may be a good alternative in the nonpenicillin-allergic patient because of its slightly altered spectrum. Recommendations would include that the patient should take the drug with food.

*Is there cross-allergenicity between the cephalosporins and penicillin?*

The incidence of cross-allergenicity is 5% to 8% in the overall population. If a patient has demonstrated a Type I hypersensitivity reaction to penicillin, namely urticaria or anaphylaxis, then this incidence would increase to 20%.

*Is there definitely an interaction between contraception agents and antibiotics?*

There are well founded interactions between contraceptives and antibiotics. The best instructions that a patient could be given by their dentist are that should an antibiotic be necessary and the dentist is aware that the patient is on contraceptives, and if the patient is using chemical contraceptives, the patient should seriously consider additional means of contraception during the antibiotic management.

*Are antibiotics necessary in diabetic patients?*

In the management of diabetes, control of the diabetic status is the key factor relative to all morbidity issues. If a patient is well controlled, then antibiotics will likely not be necessary. However, in patients where the control is questionable or where they have recently been given a different drug regimen for their diabetes or if they are being titrated to an appropriate level of either insulin or oral hypoglycemic agents during these periods of time, the dentist might consider preprocedural antibiotics to be efficacious.

*Do nonsteroidal anti-inflammatory drugs interfere with blood pressure medication?*

At the current time there is no clear evidence that NSAIDs interfere with any of the blood pressure medications that are currently in usage.

# PERIODONTAL DISEASES

Periodontal diseases are common to mankind affecting, according to some epidemiologic studies, greater than 80% of the worldwide population. The conditions refer primarily to diseases that are caused by accumulations of dental plaque and the subsequent immune response of the host to the bacteria and toxins present in this plaque. Although most of the organisms that have been implicated in advanced periodontal diseases are anaerobic in nature, some aerobes contribute by either co-aggregation with the anaerobic species or direct involvement with specific disease types.

Periodontal condition, as a group of diseases, affects the soft tissues supporting the teeth (ie, gingiva) leading to the term gingivitis or inflammation of gingival structures and those conditions that affect the bone and ligament supporting the teeth (ie, periodontitis) resulting from the infection and/or inflammation of these structures. Diseases of the periodontia can be further subdivided into various types including adult periodontitis, early onset periodontitis, prepubertal periodontitis, and rapidly progressing periodontitis. In addition, specific conditions associated with predisposing immunodeficiency disease, such as those found in HIV-infected patients, create further subclassifications of the periodontal diseases, some of which are covered in those chapters associated with those conditions.

It is well accepted that control of most periodontal diseases requires, at the very minimum, appropriate mechanical cleansing of the dentition and the supporting structures by the patient. These efforts include brushing, some type of interdental cleaning, preferably with either floss or other aids, as well as appropriate sulcular cleaning usually with a brush.

Following appropriate dental treatment by the general dental practitioner and/or the periodontist, aids to these efforts by the patient might include the use of chemical agents to assist in the control of the periodontal diseases, or to prevent periodontal diseases. There are many available chemical agents on the market, only some of which are approved by the American Dental Association. Several have been tested utilizing guidelines published in 1986 by the American Dental Association for assessment of agents that claim efficacy in the management of periodontal diseases. These chemical agents include chlorhexidine (Peridex®, PerioGard®), which are bisbiguanides and benzalkonium chloride, which is a quarternary compound. Chlorhexidine, in various concentrations, has shown efficacy in reducing plaque and gingivitis in patients with short-term utilization. Some side effects include staining of the dentition which is reversible by dental prophylaxis. Chlorhexidine demonstrates the concept of substantivity, indicating that after its use, it has a continued effect in reducing the ability of plaque to form. It has been shown to be useful in a variety of periodontal conditions including acute necrotizing ulcerative gingivitis and healing studies. Some disturbances in taste and accumulation of calculus have been reported, however, chlorhexidine is the most applicable chemical agent of the bisbiguanides that has been studied to date.

Other chemical agents available as mouthwashes include the phenol compound Listerine Antiseptic®. These compounds are primarily restricted to prototype agents; the first to be approved by the ADA being Listerine Antiseptic®. Listerine Antiseptic® has been shown to be effective against plaque and gingivitis in long-term studies and comparable to chlorhexidine in these long-term investigations. However, chlorhexidine performs better than Listerine Antiseptic® in short-term investigations. Triclosan, the chemical agent found in the toothpaste Total®, has been recently approved by the FDA and is an aid in the prevention of gingivitis. Antiplaque activity of triclosan is enhanced with the addition of zinc citrate and there are no serious side effects to the use of triclosan. Sanguinarine is a principle herbal extract used for antiplaque activity. It is an alkyloid from the plant *Sanguinaria canalensis* and has some antimicrobial properties perhaps due to its enzyme activity. Zinc citrate and zinc chloride have often been added to toothpastes as well as enzymes such as mucinase, mutanase, and dextrinase which have demonstrated varying results in studies. Some commercial anionic surfactants are available on the market which include aminoalcohols and the agent Plax® which essentially is comprised of sodium thiosulfate as a surfactant. Recent studies have shown Plax® to have some efficacy when it is added to triclosan.

Long-term use of prescription medications, including antibiotics, is seldom recommended and is not in any way a substitute for general dental/periodontal therapies. As adjunctive therapy, however, benefit has been shown and the new formulations of doxycycline (Periostat® and Atridox®), are recommended for long-term or repetitive treatments. It should be noted that the manufacturer's claims indicate that Periostat® functions as a collagenase inhibitor not as an antibiotic at recommended low doses for long-term therapy. Atridox®, however, functions as an antibiotic and is not recommended for constant long-term therapy, but rather in repetitive applications as necessary. Prescription medications used in efforts to treat periodontal diseases have historically included the use of antibiotics such as tetracycline although complications with use with young patients have often precluded their prescription. Doxycycline is often preferred to tetracycline in low doses. This broad-spectrum bacteriostatic agent has shown efficacy against a wide variety of bacterial organisms found in periodontal disease.

The drug metronidazole is a nitromidazole. It is an agent that was originally used in treatment of protozoan infections and some anaerobic bacteria. It is bactericidal and has a good absorption and distribution throughout the body. The studies using metronidazole have suggested that it has a variety of uses in periodontal treatment and can be used as adjunct in both acute necrotizing ulcerative gingivitis and has specific efficacy against spirochetes, bacteria, and some *Porphyromonas* species. Clindamycin is a derivative of vancomycin and has been useful in treatment of supporative periodontal lesions. However, long-term use is precluded by its complicating toxicities associated with colitis and gastrointestinal problems.

Research has also shown that various combination therapies of metronidazole and tetracycline for juvenile periodontitis and metronidazole with amoxicillin for rapidly progressive disease can be useful. The use of other prescription drugs including nonsteroidal anti-inflammatory, as well as other antibacterial agents, have been under study. Effects on prostaglandins of NSAIDS may indirectly slow periodontal disease progression. New research is currently underway in this regard. Perhaps, in combination therapy with some of the antibiotics, these drugs may assist in reducing the patient's immune response or inflammatory response to the presence of disease-causing bacteria.

Of greatest interest has been the improvement in technology for delivery of chemical agents to the periodontally-diseased site. These systems include biodegradable gelatins and biodegradable chips that can be placed under the gingiva and deliver antibacterial agents directly to the site as an adjunct to periodontal treatment. The initial therapy of mechanical debridement by the periodontal therapist is essential prior to using any chemical agent, and the dentist should be aware that the development of newer agents does not substitute for appropriate periodontal therapy and maintenance. The trade names of the gelatin chips and subgingival delivery systems include Periochip®, Atridox®, and Periostat®.

In addition to the periodontal therapy, consideration of the patient's pre-existing or developing medical conditions are important in the management of the periodontal patient. Several diseases illustrate these points most acutely. The reader is referred to the chapters on Diabetes, Cardiovascular Disease, Pregnancy, Respiratory Disease, HIV, and Cancer Chemotherapy. It has long been accepted that uncontrolled diabetes may predispose to periodontal lesions. Now, under current investigation is the hypothesis that pre-existing periodontal diseases may make it more difficult for a diabetic patient to come under control. In addition, the inflammatory response and immune challenge that is ongoing in periodontal disease appears to be implicated in the development of coronary artery disease as well as an increased risk of myocardial infarction and/or stroke. The accumulation of intra-arterial plaques appears enhanced by the presence of the inflammatory response often seen systemically in patients suffering with periodontal disease. The American Heart Association is currently considering recommendations regarding antibiotic prophylaxis in patients with cardiovascular disease. In addition, the clinician is referred to the section on preprocedural antibiotics in the text for a consideration of antibiotic usage in patients that may be at risk for infective endocarditis. Other conditions including pregnancy and respiratory diseases such as COPD, HIV, and cancer therapy must be considered in the overall view of periodontal diseases. The reader is referred to the sections within the text.

Listerine Antiseptic® *on page 690*
Chlorhexidine (Peridex®, PerioGard®, Periochip®) *on page 225*
Metronidazole *on page 667*
Benzalkonium chloride *on page 128*
Tetracycline *on page 965*
Doxycycline (Periostat®, Atridox®) *on page 356*
Amoxicillin *on page 76*
Clindamycin *on page 258*
NSAIDs see Pain Management Chapter *on page 1122*
Triclosan and Fluorides (Total®) *on page 1014*

# ORAL FUNGAL INFECTIONS

Oral fungal infections can result from alteration in oral flora, immunosuppression, and underlying systemic diseases that may allow the overgrowth of these opportunistic organisms. These systemic conditions might include diabetes, long-term xerostomia, adrenal suppression, anemia, and chemotherapy-induced myelosuppression for the management of cancer. Drugs of choice in treating fungal infections are amphotericin B, ciclopirox olamine, clotrimazole, itraconazole, ketoconazole, fluconazole, naftifine hydrochloride, nystatin, and oxiconazole. Patients being treated for fungal skin infections may also be using topical antifungal preparations coupled with a steroid such as triamcinolone. Clinical presentation might include pseudomembranous, atrophic, and hyperkeratotic forms. Fungus has also been implicated in denture stomatitis and symptomatic geographic tongue.

Nystatin (Mycostatin®) is effective topically in the treatment of candidal infections of the skin and mucous membrane. The drug is extremely well tolerated and appears to be nonsensitizing. In persons with denture stomatitis in which monilial organisms play at least a contributory role, it is important to soak the prosthesis overnight in a nystatin suspension. Nystatin ointment can be placed in the denture during the daytime much like a denture adhesive. Medication should be continued for at least 48 hours after disappearance of clinical signs in order to prevent relapse. Patients must be re-evaluated after 14 days of therapy. Predisposing systemic factors must be reconsidered if the oral fungal infection persists. Topical applications rely on contact of the drug with the lesions. Therefore, 4-5 times daily with a dissolving troche or pastille is appropriate. Concern over the presence of sugar in the troches and pastilles has led practitioners to sometimes prescribe the vaginal suppository formulation.

Amphotericin B (Fungizone®) *on page 79*
Clotrimazole (Mycelex®) troches *on page 267*
Fluconazole (Diflucan®) *on page 434*
Itraconazole (Sporanox®) *on page 559*
Ketoconazole (Nizoral®) *on page 564*
Nystatin (Mycostatin®) ointment or cream *on page 734*
Nystatin (Mycostatin®) oral suspension *on page 734*
Nystatin (Mycostatin®) pastilles *on page 734*
Nystatin (Mycostatin®) powder *on page 734*
Nystatin and Triamcinolone (Mycolog®) cream *on page 735*

**Note:** Consider Peridex® oral rinse, or Listerine® antiseptic oral rinse for long-term control in immunosuppressed patients.

## PRESCRIPTION EXAMPLES

**Rx**

Mycostatin® pastilles

Disp 70 pastilles

Sig: Dissolve 1 tablet in mouth until gone, 4-5 times/day for 14 days

Ingredients: 200,000 units of nystatin per tablet

Special indications: Pastille is more effective than oral suspension due to prolonged contact

**Rx**

Mycostatin® oral suspension

Disp 60 mL (2 oz)

Sig: Use 1 teaspoonful 4-5 times/day; rinse and hold in mouth as long as possible before swallowing or spitting out (2 minutes); do not eat or drink for 30 minutes following application

Ingredients: Nystatin 100,000 units/mL; vehicle contains 50% sucrose and not more than 1% alcohol

**Rx**

Mycostatin® ointment or cream

Disp 15 g or 30 g tube

Sig: Apply liberally to affected areas 4-5 times/day; do not eat or drink for 30 minutes after application

**Note:** Denture wearers should apply to dentures prior to each insertion; for edentulous patients, we can also prescribe Mycostatin® powder (15 g) to be sprinkled on denture

Ingredients:

Cream: 100,000 units nystatin per g, aqueous vanishing cream base

Ointment: 100,000 units nystatin per g, polyethylene and mineral oil gel base

**OR**

**Rx**

Mycelex® troche 10 mg

Disp 70 tablets

Sig: Dissolve 1 tablet in mouth 5 times/day

Ingredients: Clotrimazole

**Note:** Tablets contain sucrose, risk of caries with prolonged use (>3 months); care must be exercised in diabetic patients

**Rx**

Fungizone® oral suspension

Disp 50 mL

Sig: 1 mL, swish and swallow 4 times/day between meals

## MANAGEMENT OF FUNGAL INFECTIONS REQUIRING SYSTEMIC MEDICATION

If the patient is refractory to topical treatment, consideration of a systemic route might include Diflucan® or Nizoral®. Also, when the patient cannot tolerate topical therapy, ketoconazole (Nizoral®) is an effective, well tolerated, systematic drug for mucocutaneous candidiasis. Concern over liver function and possible drug interactions must be considered.

### PRESCRIPTION EXAMPLES

**Rx**

Nizoral® 200 mg

Disp 10 or 28 tablets

Sig: Take 1 tablet daily for 10-14 days

Ingredients: Ketoconazole

**Note:** To be used if *Candida* infection does not respond to mycostatin; potential for liver toxicity; liver function should be monitored with long-term use (>3 weeks)

**Rx**

Diflucan® 100 mg

Disp 15 tablets

Sig: Take 2 tablets the first day and 1 tablet a day for 10-14 days

Ingredients: Fluconazole

**ORAL FUNGAL INFECTIONS** *(Continued)*

## MANAGEMENT OF ANGULAR CHEILITIS

Angular cheilitis may represent the clinical manifestation of a multitude of etiologic factors. Cheilitis-like lesions may result from local habits, from a decrease in the intermaxillary space, or from nutritional deficiency. More commonly, angular cheilitis represents a mixed infection coupled with an inflammatory response involving *Candida albicans* and other organisms. The drug of choice is now formulated to contain nystatin and triamcinolone and the effect is excellent.

## PRESCRIPTION EXAMPLE

**Rx**

Mycolog® cream

Disp 15 g tube

Sig: Apply to affected area after each meal and before bedtime

# ORAL VIRAL INFECTIONS

Oral viral infections are most commonly caused by herpes simplex viruses and Coxsackie viruses. Oral pharyngeal infections and upper respiratory infections are commonly caused by the Coxsackie group A viruses. Soft tissue viral infections, on the other hand, are most often caused by the herpes simplex viruses. Herpes zoster or varicella-zoster virus, which is one of the herpes family of viruses, can likewise cause similar viral eruptions involving the mucosa.

The diagnosis of an acute viral infection is one that begins by ruling out bacterial etiology and having an awareness of the presenting signs and symptoms associated with viral infection. Acute onset and vesicular eruption on the soft tissues generally favors a diagnosis of viral infection. Unfortunately, vesicles do not remain for a great length of time in the oral cavity; therefore, the short-lived vesicles rupture leaving ulcerated bases as the only indication of their presence. These ulcers, however, are generally small in size and only when left unmanaged do they coalesce to form larger, irregular ulcerations. Distinction should be made between the commonly occurring intraoral ulcers (aphthous ulcerations) which do not have a viral etiology and the lesions associated with intraoral herpes. The management of an oral viral infection may be palliative for the most part; however, with the advent of acyclovir we now have a drug that can assist us in managing primary and secondary infection. Human *Papillomavirus* is implicated in a number of oral lesions, the most common of which is *Condyloma acuminatum.* Recently, Aldara® has been approved for genital warts; oral use is under study.

It should be noted that herpes can present as, a primary infection (gingivostomatitis), recurrent lip lesions (herpes labialis), and intraoral ulcers (recurrent intraoral herpes), three primary forms involving the oral and perioral tissues. Primary infection is one that is generally a systemic infection that leads to acute gingivostomatitis involving multiple tissues of the buccal mucosa, lips, tongue, floor of the mouth, and the gingiva. Treatment of primary infections utilizes acyclovir in combination with supportive care. Dyclonine 0.5%, a topical anesthetic used in combination with Benadryl® 0.5% in a saline vehicle, are found to be effective oral rinses in the symptomatic treatment of primary herpetic gingivostomatitis. Other agents available for symptomatic and supportive treatment include commercially available elixir of Benadryl®, Xylocaine® viscous, Ora-Jel® (OTC), Camphophenique® (OTC), and antibiotics to prevent secondary infections. Systemic supportive therapy should include forced fluids, high concentration protein, vitamin and mineral food supplements, and rest.

**Antivirals**

Acyclovir (Zovirax®) *on page 38*
Imiquimod (Aldara®) *on page 530*
Nelfinavir (Viracept®) *on page 708*
Penciclovir (Denavir®) *on page 771*
Vidarabine (Vira-A®) *on page 1045*

**Supportive Therapy**

Diphenhydramine (Benadryl®, various products) *on page 338*
Dyclonine (Dyclone®) *on page 360*
Lidocaine (Xylocaine®) *on page 586*

**Antibiotics for Prevention of Secondary Bacterial Infection**

Erythromycin (various products) *on page 383*
Penicillin V Potassium (various products) *on page 776*

## PRIMARY INFECTION

### PRESCRIPTION EXAMPLE

**Rx**

Zovirax® 200 mg

Disp 70 capsules

Sig: Take 1 capsule every 4 hours (maximum: 5/day) for 2 weeks

Ingredient: Acyclovir

## ORAL VIRAL INFECTIONS *(Continued)*

## SUPPORTIVE CARE FOR PAIN AND PREVENTION OF SECONDARY INFECTION

Primary infections often become secondarily infected with bacteria, requiring antibiotics. Dietary supplement may be necessary. Options are presented due to variability in patient compliance and response.

## PRESCRIPTION EXAMPLE

**Rx**

Benadryl® powder 0.5% with dyclonine 0.5% in saline

Disp 8 oz

Sig: Rinse with 1 teaspoonful every 2 hours

Ingredient: Diphenhydramine and dyclonine

**Rx**

Benadryl® elixir 12.5 mg/5 mL

Disp 4 oz bottle

Sig: Rinse with 1 teaspoonful for 2 minutes before each meal

Ingredient: Diphenhydramine

**Rx**

Benadryl® elixir 12.5 mg/5 mL with Kaopectate®, 50% mixture by volume

Disp 8 oz

Sig: Rinse with 1 teaspoonful every 2 hours

Ingredients: Diphenhydramine and attapulgite

**Rx**

Xylocaine® viscous 2%

Disp 450 mL bottle

Sig: Swish with 1 tablespoon 4 times/day and spit out

Ingredient: Lidocaine

**Rx**

Penicillin V 250 mg tablets

Disp 40 tablets

Sig: 1 tablet 4 times/day

**Rx**

Erythromycin 250 mg tablets

Disp 40 tablets

Sig: 1 tablet 4 times/day

**Rx**

Meritene®

Disp 1 lb can (plain, chocolate, eggnog flavors)

Sig: Take 3 servings daily; prepare as indicated on can

Ingredients: Protein-vitamin-mineral food supplement

## RECURRENT HERPETIC INFECTIONS

Following this primary infection, the herpesvirus remains latent until such time as it has the opportunity to recur. The etiology of this latent period and the degree of viral shedding present during latency is currently under study; however, it is thought that some trigger in the mucosa or the skin causes the virus to begin to replicate. This process may involve Langerhans cells which are immunocompetent antigen-presenting cells resident in all epidermal surfaces. The virus replication then leads to eruptions in tissues surrounding the mouth. The most common form of recurrence is the lip lesion or herpes labialis, however, intraoral recurrent herpes also occurs with some frequency. Prevention of recurrences has been attempted with drugs such as Lysine® (500-1000 mg/day). Response has been variable. Pain management during intraoral recurrences can be utilized as in primary infections.

Water-soluble bioflavonoid-ascorbic acid complex, now available as Peridin-C®, may be helpful in reducing the signs and symptoms associated with recurrent herpes simplex virus infections. As with all agents used, the therapy is more effective when instituted in the early prodromal stage of the disease process.

### PRESCRIPTION EXAMPLE

Rx

Citrus bioflavonoids and ascorbic acid tablets 400 mg (Peridin-C®)

Disp 10 tablets

Sig: Take 2 tablets at once, then 1 tablet tid for 3 days

## PREVENTION

Where a recurrence is usually precipitated by exposure to sunlight, the lesion may be prevented by the application to the area of a sunscreen, with a high skin protection factor (SPF) in the range of 10-15.

### PRESCRIPTION EXAMPLE

Rx

PreSun® (OTC) 15 sunscreen lotion

Disp 4 fluid oz

Sig: Apply to susceptible area 1 hour before sun exposure

## TREATMENT

Vidarabine (Vira-A®) possesses antiviral activity against herpes simplex types 1 and 2. The ophthalmic ointment may be used topically to treat recurrent mucosal and skin lesions. In the 3% strength, it does not penetrate well on the skin lesions thereby providing questionable relief of symptoms. If recommended, its use should be closely monitored. Penciclovir, an active metabolite of famciclovir, has been recently approved in a cream for treatment of recurrent herpes lesions. The drug is to be released in the near future; prescribing information will be available at that time.

### PRESCRIPTION EXAMPLES

Rx

Vira-A® ophthalmic ointment 3%

Disp 3.5 g tube

Sig: Apply to affected area 4 times/day

Ingredient: Vidarabine

## ORAL VIRAL INFECTIONS *(Continued)*

| Rx |
| --- |
| Zovirax® ointment 5% (3%) |
| Disp 15 g |
| Sig: Apply thin layer to lesions 6 times/day for 7 days |

Ingredient: Acyclovir

| Rx |
| --- |
| Zovirax® 200 mg |
| Disp 70 capsules |
| Sig: Take 1 capsule every 4 hours (maximum: 5/day) for 2 weeks |

Ingredient: Acyclovir

# ORAL NONVIRAL SOFT TISSUE ULCERATIONS OR EROSIONS

## RECURRENT APHTHOUS STOMATITIS

Kenalog® in Orabase is indicated for the temporary relief of symptoms associated with infrequent recurrences of minor aphthous lesions and ulcerative lesions resulting from trauma. More severe forms of recurrent aphthous stomatitis may be treated with an oral suspension of tetracycline. The agent appears to reduce the duration of symptoms and decrease the rate of recurrence by reducing secondary bacterial infection. Its use is contraindicated during the last half of pregnancy, infancy, and childhood to the age of 8 years. *Lactobacillus acidophilus* preparations (Bacid®, Lactinex®) are occasionally effective for reducing the frequency and severity of the lesions. Patients with long-standing history of recurrent aphthous stomatitis should be evaluated for iron, folic acid, and vitamin $B_{12}$ deficiencies. Regular use of Listerine® antiseptic has been shown in clinical trials to reduce the severity, duration, and frequency of aphthous stomatitis. Chlorhexidine oral rinses 20 mL x 30 sec bid or tid have also demonstrated efficacy in reducing the duration of aphthae. With both of these products, however, patient intolerance of the burning from the alcohol content is of concern. Viractin® has been approved for symptomatic relief. Immunocompromised patients such as those with AIDS may have severe ulcer recurrences and the drug thalidomide has been approved for these patients.

Amlexanox (Aphthasol®) *on page 70*
Attapulgite (Diasorb®, Kaopectate®, Rheaban®) *on page 109*
Chlorhexidine (Peridex®, PerioGard®) *on page 225*
Clobetasol (Temovate®) *on page 260*
Dexamethasone (Decadron®) *on page 308*
Diphenhydramine (Benadryl®, various products) *on page 338*
Fluocinonide (Lidex®) ointment with Orabase *on page 440*
*Lactobacillus acidophilus* and *Lactobacillus bulgaricus* (Bacid®, Lactinex®) *on page 570*
Metronidazole (Flagyl®) *on page 667*
Mouthwash, Antiseptic (Listerine®) *on page 690*
Prednisone (various products) *on page 833*
Tetracaine (Pontocaine®, Viractin®) *on page 964*
Tetracycline liquid *on page 965*
Thalidomide (Thalomid®) *on page 967*
Triamcinolone (Kenalog®) Acetonide Dental Paste *on page 1011*

## PRESCRIPTION EXAMPLES

**Rx**

Listerine® antiseptic (OTC)
20 mL x 30 sec bid

**Rx**

Peridex® oral rinse
Disp 1 bottle
Sig: 20 mL x 30 sec tid

**Rx**

PerioGard® oral rinse
Disp 1 bottle
Sig: 20 mL x 30 sec tid

## ORAL NONVIRAL SOFT TISSUE ULCERATIONS OR EROSIONS *(Continued)*

**Rx**

Tetracycline capsules 250 mg

Disp 40 capsules

Sig: Suspend contents of 1 capsule in a teaspoonful of water; rinse for 2 minutes 4 times/day and swallow

**Note:** This comes as liquid 125 mg/5 mL which is convenient to use

Sig: Swish 5 mL for 2 minutes 4 times/day

**Rx**

Kenalog® in Orabase 0.1%

Disp 5 g tube

Sig: Coat the lesion with a film after each meal and at bedtime

## BURNING TONGUE SYNDROME, GEOGRAPHIC TONGUE, MILD FORMS OF ORAL LICHEN PLANUS

Elixir of Benadryl®, a potent antihistamine, is used in the oral cavity primarily as a mild topical anesthetic agent for the symptomatic relief of certain allergic deficiencies which should be ruled out as possible etiologies for the oral condition under treatment. It is often used alone as well as in solutions with agents such as Kaopectate® or Maalox® to assist in coating the oral mucosa. Benadryl® can also be used in capsule form.

### PRESCRIPTION EXAMPLE

**Rx**

Benadryl® elixir 12.5 mg/5 mL

Disp 4 oz bottle

Sig: Rinse with 1 teaspoonful for 2 minutes before each meal and swallow

Ingredient: Diphenhydramine

## EROSIVE LICHEN PLANUS AND MAJOR APHTHAE

Elixir of dexamethasone (Decadron®), a potent anti-inflammatory agent, is used topically in the management of acute episodes of erosive lichen planus and major aphthae. Continued supervision of the patient during treatment is essential.

### PRESCRIPTION EXAMPLE

**Rx**

Decadron® elixir 0.5 mg/5 mL

Disp 100 mL bottle

Sig: Rinse with 1 teaspoonful for 2 minutes 4 times/day; do not swallow

Ingredient: Dexamethasone

For severe cases and when the oropharynx is involved, some practitioners have the patient swallow after a 2-minute rinse.

| | |
|---|---|
| Allergy | Benadryl® |
| Aphthous | Benadryl®/Maalox® (compounded prescription)<br>Benadryl®/Kaopectate® (compounded prescription)<br>Lidex® in Orabase (compounded prescription)<br>Kenalog® in Orabase<br>Tetracycline mouth rinse |
| Oral inflammatory disease | Lidex® in Orabase (compounded prescription)<br>Kenalog® in Orabase<br>Prednisone<br>Temovate® cream |

The use of long-term steroids is always of concern due to possible adrenal suppression. If systemic steroids are contemplated for a protracted time, medical consultation is advisable.

## PRESCRIPTION EXAMPLES

**Rx**

Benadryl® 50 mg

Disp 16 capsules

Sig: 3-4 times/day

Ingredient: Diphenhydramine hydrochloride

Special considerations: Use 3-4 times/day for 4 days depending on the duration of the allergic reaction; may cause drowsiness

**Rx**

Benadryl® syrup (mix 50/50) with Kaopectate®*

Disp 8 oz total

Sig: Use 2 teaspoons as rinse as needed to relieve pain or burning (use after meals)

***Note:** Benadryl can be mixed with Maalox® if constipation is a problem

**Rx**

Kenalog® in Orabase®

Disp 5 mg

Sig: Apply thin layer to affected area 3 times/day

**Rx**

Lidex® ointment mixed 50/50 with Orabase®

Disp 30 g total

Sig: Apply thin layer to oral lesions 4-6 times/day

Ingredient: Fluocinonide 0.05%

**Note:** To be used for oral inflammatory lesions that do not respond to Kenalog® in Orabase®

Ingredient: Triamcinolone acetonide

## ORAL NONVIRAL SOFT TISSUE ULCERATIONS OR EROSIONS *(Continued)*

**Systemic steroids may be considered:**

**Rx**

Prednisone 5 mg

Disp 60 tablets

Sig: Take 4 tablets in morning and 4 tablets at noon for 4 days; then decrease the total number of tablets by 1 each day until down to zero

**Caution:** Take medication with food

**For a high potency corticosteroid:**

**Rx**

Temovate® cream 0.05%

Disp 15 g tube

Sig: Apply locally 4-6 times/day

**And for secondary infections:**

**Rx**

Tetracycline liquid 125 mg/5 mL

Disp 100 mL

Sig: Rinse 1 tablespoonful in mouth 4 times/day then spit out; do not eat or drink for 30 minutes after using

**Note:** Tetracycline rinse is effective in approximately 33% of the patients with aphthous ulcers

## NECROTIZING ULCERATING PERIODONTITIS (HIV Periodontal Disease)

### Initial Treatment (In-Office)

Betadine rinse *on page 827*
Ensure patient has no iodine allergies
Gentle debridement

### At-Home

**Listerine® rinses**

Peridex® rinse *on page 225*
Metronidazole (Flagyl®) 7-10 days *on page 667*

### Follow-Up Therapy

Proper dental cleaning including scaling and root planing (repeat as needed)

Continue Peridex® rinse (indefinite) *on page 225*
Listerine® antiseptic rinse (20 mL for 30 seconds twice daily)

# DENTIN HYPERSENSITIVITY; HIGH CARIES INDEX; XEROSTOMIA

## DENTIN HYPERSENSITIVITY

Suggested steps in resolving dentin hypersensitivity (a thorough exam had ruled any other source for the problem).

**Treatment Steps**

- Home treatment with a desensitizing toothpaste containing potassium nitrate (used to brush teeth as well as a thin layer applied, each night for 2 weeks)
- If needed, in office potassium oxalate (Protect® by Butler) and/or in office fluoride iontophoresis
- If sensitivity is still not tolerable to the patient, consider pumice then dentin adhesive and unfilled resin or composite restoration overlaying a glass ionomer base

**Home Products: All contain nitrate as active ingredient**

Promise®
Denquel®
Sensodyne®

Dentifrice Products *on page 1242*

## ANTICARIES AGENTS

Fluoride gel 0.4%, rinse 0.05% *on page 441*

New toothpastes with triclosan such as Colgate Total® show promise for combined treatment/prevention of caries, plaque, and gingivitis.

## FLUORIDE GELS

Oral Rinse Products *on page 1257*

Used for the prevention of demineralization of the tooth structure secondary to xerostomia. For patients with long-term or permanent xerostomia, daily application is accomplished using custom gel applicator trays. Patients with porcelain crowns should use a neutral pH fluoride.

1.1% neutral pH sodium fluoride
Thera-Flur-N® or Prevident®
0.4% stannous fluoride
Gel-Kam® unflavored

## REMINERALIZING GEL

In addition to fluoride gel to remineralize enamel breakdown in severely xerostomic patients, applicator trays may be used.

Revive®

**Note:** Many preparations are available over-the-counter so prescriptions sometimes are not required. If caries is severe, use fluoride gel in custom tray once daily as long as needed (years).

## ANTIPLAQUE AGENTS

### PRESCRIPTION EXAMPLES

**Rx**

Listerine® antiseptic (OTC)
20 mL for 30 seconds twice daily

**Rx**

Peridex® oral rinse 0.12%
Disp 3 times 16 oz
Sig: ½ oz, swish for 30 seconds 2-3 times/day

## DENTIN HYPERSENSITIVITY; HIGH CARIES INDEX; XEROSTOMIA *(Continued)*

**Rx**

PerioGard® oral rinse

Disp 3 times 16 oz

Sig: ½ oz, swish for 30 seconds 2-3 times/day

Ingredient: Chlorhexidine

Peridex may:

- Stain teeth yellow to brown (can be removed with dental cleaning)
- Alter taste (temporary)
- Increase the deposition of calculus (reversible)

Chlorhexidine (Peridex®) *on page 225*

## XEROSTOMIA

Dry mouth associated with radiation therapy, drug therapy, aging, and Sjögren's disease may be managed by rinsing with a solution of sodium carboxymethylcellulose. It is a nonirritating agent that moistens and lubricates the oral tissues and may be used for prolonged periods of time without adverse effects. Salagen® was recently indicated for these patients. For dentulous patients, fluoride and electrolytes have been added to this solution to reduce caries susceptibility (Xero-Lube®). Consideration of alternative medical drug regimens in consult with the physician may assist in management. Numerous patients being treated for anxiety or depression are often susceptible to chronic xerostomia due to medications selected; see table on following page.

Pilocarpine (Dental) (Salagen®) *on page 804*

Saliva Substitute (Moi-Stir®; MouthKote®; Optimoist®; Salivart®; Xero-Lube®) *on page 901*

## OTHER DRUGS IMPLICATED IN XEROSTOMIA

| >10% | 1% to 10% |
|---|---|
| Alprazolam | Acrivastine and Pseudoephedrine |
| Amitriptyline hydrochloride | Albuterol |
| Amoxapine | Amantadine hydrochloride |
| Anisotropine methylbromide | Amphetamine sulfate |
| Atropine sulfate | Astemizole |
| Belladonna and Opium | Azatadine maleate |
| Benztropine mesylate | Beclomethasone dipropionate |
| Bupropion | Bepridil hydrochloride |
| Chlordiazepoxide | Bitolterol mesylate |
| Clomipramine hydrochloride | Brompheniramine maleate |
| Clonazepam | Carbinoxamine and Pseudoephedrine |
| Clonidine | Chlorpheniramine maleate |
| Clorazepate dipotassium | Clemastine fumarate |
| Cyclobenzaprine | Clozapine |
| Desipramine hydrochloride | Cromolyn sodium |
| Diazepam | Cyproheptadine hydrochloride |
| Dicyclomine hydrochloride | Dexchlorpheniramine maleate |
| Diphenoxylate and Atropine | Dextroamphetamine sulfate |
| Doxepin hydrochloride | Dimenhydrinate |
| Ergotamine | Diphenhydramine hydrochloride |
| Estazolam | Disopyramide phosphate |
| Flavoxate | Doxazosin |
| Flurazepam hydrochloride | Dronabinol |
| Glycopyrrolate | Ephedrine sulfate |
| Guanabenz acetate | Flumazenil |
| Guanfacine hydrochloride | Fluvoxamine |
| Hyoscyamine sulfate | Gabapentin |
| Interferon Alfa-2a | Guaifenesin and Codeine |
| Interferon Alfa-2b | Guanadrel sulfate |
| Interferon Alfa-N3 | Guanethidine sulfate |
| Ipratropium bromide | Hydroxyzine |
| Isoproterenol | Hyoscyamine, Atropine, Scopolamine, and Phenobarbital |
| Isotretinoin | Imipramine |
| Loratadine | Isoetharine |
| Lorazepam | Levocabastine hydrochloride |
| Loxapine | Levodopa |
| Maprotiline hydrochloride | Levodopa and Carbidopa |
| Methscopolamine bromide | Levorphanol tartrate |
| Molindone hydrochloride | Meclizine hydrochloride |
| Nabilone | Meperidine hydrochloride |
| Nefazodone | Methadone hydrochloride |
| Oxybutynin chloride | Methamphetamine hydrochloride |
| Oxazepam | Methyldopa |
| Paroxetine | Metoclopramide |
| Phenelzine sulfate | Morphine sulfate |
| Prochlorperazine | Nortriptyline hydrochloride |
| Propafenone hydrochloride | Ondansetron |
| Protriptyline hydrochloride | Oxycodone and Acetaminophen |
| Quazepam | Oxycodone and Aspirin |
| Reserpine | Pentazocine |
| Selegiline hydrochloride | Phenylpropanolamine hydrochloride |
| Temazepam | Prazosin hydrochloride |
| Thiethylperazine maleate | Promethazine hydrochloride |
| Trihexyphenidyl hydrochloride | Propoxyphene |
| Trimipramine maleate | Pseudoephedrine |
| Venlafaxine | Risperidone |
| | Sertraline hydrochloride |
| | Terazosin |
| | Terbutaline sulfate |

## DENTIN HYPERSENSITIVITY; HIGH CARIES INDEX; XEROSTOMIA *(Continued)*

## PRESCRIPTION EXAMPLES

**Rx**

Sodium carboxymethylcellulose (Baker) 0.5% aqueous solution

Disp 8 oz

Sig: Use as a rinse frequently as needed to relieve symptoms of dry mouth

**Rx**

Xero-Lube®*

Disp 1 bottle

Sig: Apply several drops or sprays to mouth as necessary for dryness

**Note:** Consider topical treatment in custom trays for those patients with severe xerostomia

***Note:** Alternatives: Moi-Stir®; MouthKote®; Optimoist®; Salivart®

Systemic stimulation of saliva has been achieved in some patients using pilocarpine.

**Rx**

Salagen® 5 mg

Disp 120 tablets

Sig: 1 tablet 3-4 times/day, not top exceed 30 mg/day

**Note:** Patients should be treated for a minimum of 90 days to achieve clinical effects.

# TEMPOROMANDIBULAR DYSFUNCTION (TMD)

Temporomandibular dysfunction comprises a broad spectrum of signs and symptoms. Although TMD presents in patterns, diagnosis is often difficult. Evaluation and treatment is time-intensive and no single therapy or drug regimen has been shown to be universally beneficial.

The thorough diagnostician should perform a screening examination for the temporomandibular joint on all patients. Ideally, a base line maximum mandibular opening along with lateral and protrusive movement evaluation should be performed. Secondly, the joint area should be palpated and an adequate exam of the muscles of mastication and the muscles of the neck and shoulders should be made. These muscle would include the elevators of the mandible (masseter, internal pterygoid, and temporalis); the depressors of the mandible (including the external pterygoid and digastric); etrusive muscles (including the temporalis and digastric), and protrusive muscles (including the external and internal pterygoids). These muscles also account for lateral movement of the mandible. The clinician should also be alert to indicators of dysfunction, primarily a history of pain with jaw function, chronic history of joint noise (although this can often be misinterpreted), pain in the muscles of the neck, limited jaw movement, pain in the actual muscles of mastication, and headache or even earache. The signs and symptoms are extremely variable and the clinician should be alert for any or all of these areas of interest. Because of the complexity of both evaluation and diagnosis, the general dentist often finds it too time consuming to spend the countless hours evaluating and treating the temporomandibular dysfunction patient. Therefore, oral medicine specialists trained in temporomandibular evaluation and treatment often accept referrals for the management of these complicated patients.

The Oral Medicine specialist in TMD management, the physical therapist interested in head and neck pain, and the Oral and Maxillofacial surgeon will all work together with the referring general dentist to accomplish successful patient treatment. Table 1 lists the wide variety of treatment alternatives available to the team. Depending on the diagnosis, one or more of the therapies might be selected. For organic diseases of the joint not responding to nonsurgical approaches, a wide variety of surgical techniques are available (Table 2).

## ACUTE TMD

Acute TMD oftentimes presents alone or as an episode during a chronic pattern of signs and symptoms. Trauma such as a blow to the chin or the side of the face can result in acute TMD. Occasionally, similar symptoms will follow a lengthy wide open mouth dental procedure.

The condition usually presents as continuous deep pain in the TMJ. If edema is present in the joint, the condyle sometimes can be displaced which will cause abnormal occlusion of the posterior teeth on the affected side. The diagnosis is usually based on the history and clinical presentation. Management of the patient includes:

1. Restriction of all mandibular movement to function in a pain-free range of motion
2. Soft diet
3. NSAIDs (eg, Anaprox® DS 1 tablet every 12 hours for 7-10 days)
4. Moist heat applications to the affected area for 15-20 minutes, 4-6 times/day

Additional therapies could include referral to a physical therapist for ultrasound therapy 2-4 times/week and a single injection of steroid in the joint space. A team approach with an oral maxillofacial surgeon for this procedure may be helpful. Spray and stretch with Fluori-methane® is often helpful for rapid relief of trismus.

Dichlorodifluoromethane and Trichloromonofluoromethane (Fluori-methane®) *on page 319*

## CHRONIC TMD

Following diagnosis which is often problematic, the most common therapeutic modalities include:

- Explaining the problem to the patient
- Recommending a soft diet:
  - avoid chewing gum, salads, biting into large sandwiches, biting into hard fruit
  - diet should consist of soft foods such as eggs, yogurt, casseroles, soup, ground meat

## TEMPOROMANDIBULAR DYSFUNCTION (TMD) *(Continued)*

- Reducing stress; moist heat application 4-6 times daily for 15-20 minutes coupled with a monitored exercise program will be beneficial. Usually, working with a physical therapist is ideal.
- Medications include analgesics, anti-inflammatories, tranquilizers, and muscle relaxants

# MEDICATION OPTIONS

Most commonly used medication (NSAIDs):

Aminosalicylate Sodium (Sodium P.A.S.) *on page 65*
Choline Magnesium Trisalicylate (Trilisate®) *on page 244*
Choline Salicylate (Arthropan®) *on page 245*
Diclofenac (Cataflam®, Voltaren®) *on page 320*
Diflunisal (Dolobid®) *on page 327*
Etodolac (Lodine®) *on page 413*
Fenoprofen (Nalfon®) *on page 424*
Flurbiprofen (Ansaid®) *on page 448*
Ibuprofen (various products) *on page 522*
Indomethacin (Indocin®) *on page 534*
Ketoprofen (Orudis®) *on page 565*
Ketorolac (Toradol®) *on page 566*
Magnesium Salicylate (Doan's®, Magan®, Mobidin®) *on page 613*
Meclofenamate (Meclomen®) *on page 621*
Mefenamic Acid (Ponstel®) *on page 624*
Nabumetone (Relafen®) *on page 695*
Naproxen (Naprosyn®) *on page 705*
Oxaprozin (Daypro™) *on page 747*
Oxyphenbutazone *on page 757*
Piroxicam (Feldene®) *on page 810*
Salsalate (various products) *on page 902*
Sulindac (Clinoril®) *on page 948*
Tolmetin (Tolectin®) *on page 996*

Tranquilizers and muscle relaxants when used appropriately can provide excellent adjunctive therapy. These drugs should be primarily used for a short period of time to manage acute pain. In low dosages, amitriptyline is often used to treat chronic pain and occasionally migraine headache.

Common minor tranquilizers include:

Alprazolam (Xanax®) *on page 50*

Diazepam (Valium®) *on page 316*

Lorazepam (Ativan®) *on page 602*

Common muscle relaxants include:

Chlorzoxazone (Parafon® Forte DSC) *on page 242*

Methocarbamol (Robaxin®) *on page 649*

Orphenadrine (Norgesic® Forte) *on page 744*

Cyclobenzaprine (Flexeril®) *on page 284*

Muscle relaxants and tranquilizers should generally be prescribed with an analgesic or NSAID to relieve pain as well

Narcotic analgesics can be used on a short-term basis or intermittently in combination with non-narcotic therapy in the chronic pain patient. Judicious prescribing, monitoring, and maintenance by the practitioner is imperative whenever considering the use of narcotic analgesics due to the abuse and addiction liabilities.

**Table 1.**
**TMD - NONSURGICAL THERAPIES**

1. Moist heat and cold spray
2. Injections in muscle trigger areas (procaine)
3. Exercises (passive, active)
4. Medications
   a. Muscle relaxants
   b. Minerals
   c. Multiple vitamins (Ca, $B_6$, $B_{12}$)
5. Orthopedic craniomandibular repositioning appliance (splints)
6. Biofeedback, acupuncture
7. Physiotherapy: TMJ muscle therapy
8. Myofunctional therapy
9. TENS (transcutaneous electrical neural stimulation), Myo-Monitor
10. Dental therapy
    a. Equilibration (coronoplasty)
    b. Restoring occlusion to proper vertical dimension of maxilla to mandible by orthodontics, dental restorative procedures, orthognathic surgery, permanent splint, or any combination of these

**Table 2.**
**TMD - SURGICAL THERAPIES**

1. Cortisone injection into joint (with local anesthetic)
2. Bony and/or fibrous ankylosis: requires surgery (osteoarthrotomy with prosthetic appliance)
3. Chronic subluxation: requires surgery, depending on problem (possibly eminectomy and/or prosthetic implant)
4. Osteoarthritis: requires surgery, depending on problem
   a. Arthroplasty with implant
   b. Meniscectomy with implant
   c. Arthroplasty with repair of disc and/or implant
   d. Implant with Silastic insert
5. Rheumatoid arthritis
   a. Arthroplasty with implant with Silastic insert
   b. "Total" TMJ replacement
6. Tumors: require osteoarthrotomy — removal of tumor and restoring of joint when possible
7. Chronic disc displacement: requires repair of disc and possible removal of bone from condyle

# PATIENTS REQUIRING SEDATION

Anxiety constitutes the most frequently found psychiatric problem in the general population. Anxiety can range from simple phobias to severe debilitating anxiety disorders. Functional results of this anxiety can, therefore, range from simple avoidance of dental procedures to panic attacks when confronting stressful situations such as seen in some patients regarding dental visits. Many patients claim to be anxious over dental care when in reality they simply have not been managed with modern techniques of local anesthesia, the availability of sedation, or the caring dental practitioner.

The dentist may detect anxiety in patients during the treatment planning evaluation phase of the care. The anxious person may appear overly alert, may lean forward in the dental chair during conversation or may appear concerned over time, possibly using this as a guise to require that they cut short their dental visit. Anxious persons may also show signs of being nervous by demonstrating sweating, tension in their muscles including their temporomandibular musculature, or they may complain of being tired due to an inability to obtain an adequate night's sleep.

The management of such patients requires a methodical approach to relaxing the patient, discussing their dental needs, and then planning, along with the patient the best way to accomplish dental treatment in the presence of their fears, both real or imagined. Consideration may be given to sedation to assist with managing the patient. This sedation can be oral or parenteral, or inhalation in the case of nitrous oxide. The dentist must be adequately trained in administering the sedative of choice, as well as in monitoring the patient during the sedated procedures. Numerous medications are available to achieve the level of sedation usually necessary in the dental office: Valium®, Ativan®, Xanax®, Vistaril®, Serax®, and BuSpar® represent a few. BuSpar® is soon to be available as a transdermal patch. These oral sedatives can be given prior to dental visits as outlined in the following prescriptions. They have the advantage of allowing the patient a good night's sleep prior to the day of the procedures and providing on the spot sedation during the procedures. Nitrous oxide represents an in the office administered sedative that is relatively safe, but requires additional training and carefully planned monitoring protocols of any auxiliary personnel during the inhalation procedures. Both the oral and the inhalation techniques can, however, be applied in a very useful manner to manage the anxious patient in the dental office.

Alprazolam (Xanax®) *on page 50*
Buspirone (BuSpar®) *on page 161*
Diazepam (Valium®) *on page 316*
Hexobarbital (Pre-Sed®) *on page 497*
Hydroxyzine (Vistaril®, various products) *on page 518*
Lorazepam (Ativan®) *on page 602*
Nitrous Oxide *on page 727*
Oxazepam (Serax®) *on page 748*
Triazolam (Halcion®) *on page 1013*

## PRESCRIPTION EXAMPLES

**Rx**

Valium® 5 mg*

Disp 6 (six) tablets

Sig: Take 1 tablet in evening before going to bed and 1 tablet 1 hour before your appointment

Ingredient: Diazepam

***Note:** Also available as 2 mg and 10 mg

**Rx**

Ativan® 1 mg*

Disp 4 (four) tablets

Sig: Take 2 tablets in evening before going to bed and take 2 tablets 1 hour before your appointment

Ingredient: Lorazepam

***Note:** Also available as 0.5 mg and 2 mg

**Rx**

Xanax® 0.5 mg

Disp 4 (four) tablets

Sig: Take 1 tablet in evening before going to bed and 1 tablet 1 hour before your appointment

Ingredient: Alprazolam

**Rx**

Pre-Sed® 260 mg

Disp 6 (six) tablets

Sig: Take 1 tablet* 1 hour prior to dental appointment

Ingredient: Hexobarbital
*Dose may be 2 tablets 1 hour prior

**Rx**

Vistaril® 25 mg

Disp 16 capsules

Sig: Take 2 capsules in evening before going to bed and 2 capsules 1 hour before your appointment

Ingredient: Hydroxyzine

**Rx**

Halcion® 0.25 mg

Disp 4 (four) tablets

Sig: Take 1 tablet in evening before going to bed and 1 tablet 1 hour before your appointment

Ingredient: Triazolam

**Rx**

Serax® 10 mg

Disp 2 (two) capsules

Sig: Take 1 capsule before bed and 1 capsule 30 minutes before your appointment.

Ingredient: Oxazepam

# PATIENTS UNDERGOING CANCER THERAPY

The statistics released by the American Cancer Society for projections of cancer trends in 1998 are indeed encouraging. Due to re-evaluation of the incidence of prostate cancer diagnoses, as well as decreases in other cancer categories, there has been a 9% decrease in the adjusted estimate for cancer rates. As healthcare practitioners, the reduction in cancer occurrence cannot be thought to be an end in itself. Other efforts in early detection and identification by the dental team as well as the management of oral complications associated with cancer treatment as outlined in this chapter are ever important for the dental practitioner. Treatment projections for new cancer cases also have shown signs of improvement. Although prostate cancer still leads as the site diagnosed by sex for the most prevalence, there have been reductions in lung and bronchial cancer and the success in treating prostate cancer as measured by estimated cancer deaths is also down.

The dental management recommendations for patients undergoing chemotherapy, bone marrow transplantation, and/or radiation therapy for the treatment of cancer are based primarily on clinical observations. The following protocols will provide a conservative, consistent approach to the dental management of patients undergoing chemotherapy or bone marrow transplantation. Many of the cancer chemotherapy drugs produce oral side effects including mucositis, oral ulceration, dry mouth, acute infections, and taste aberrations. Cancer drugs include antibiotics, alkylating agents, antimetabolites, DNA inhibitors, hormones, and cytokines (see "Cancer Chemotherapy Regimens" *on page 1205*).

## DENTAL PROTOCOL

All patients undergoing chemotherapy or bone marrow transplantation for malignant disease should have the following baseline:

A. Panoramic radiograph
B. Dental consultation and examination
C. Dental prophylaxis and cleaning (if the neutrophil count is $>1500/mm^3$ and the platelet count is $>50,000/mm^3$
   - Prophylaxis and cleaning will be deferred if the patient's neutrophil count is <1500 and the platelet count is <50,000. Oral hygiene recommendations will be made.

D. Oral Hygiene. Patients should be encouraged to follow normal hygiene procedures. Addition of a chlorhexidine mouth rinse such as Peridex® or PerioGard® is usually helpful. If patient develops oral mucositis, tolerance of such alcohol-based products may be limited.
E. If the patient develops mucositis, bacterial, viral, and fungal cultures should be obtained. Sucralfate suspension in either a pharmacy prepared form or Carafate® suspension as well as Benadryl® or Xylocaine® viscous can assist in helping the patient to tolerate food. Patients may also require systemic analgesics for pain relief depending on the presence of mucositis. Positive fungal cultures may require a nystatin swish and swallow prescription.
F. The determination of performing dental procedures must be based on the goal of preventing infection during periods of neutropenia. Timing of procedures must be coordinated with the patient's hematologic status.
G. If oral surgery is required, at least 7-10 days of healing should be allowed before the anticipated date of bone marrow suppression (eg, ANC of $<1000/mm^3$ and/or platelet count of $50,000/mm^3$).
H. Daily use of topical fluorides is recommended for those who have received radiation therapy to the head-neck region involving salivary glands. Any patients with prolonged xerostomia subsequent to graft versus host disease and/or chemotherapy can also be considered for fluoride supplement. Use the fluoride-containing mouthwashes (Act®, Fluorigard®, etc) each night before going to sleep; swish, hold 1-2 minutes, spit out or use prescription fluorides (gels or rinses); apply them daily for 3-4 minutes as directed; if the mouth is sore (mucositis), use flavorless/colorless gels (Thera-Flur®, Gel-Kam®). Improvement in salivary flow following radiation therapy to the head and neck has been noted with Salagen®. See "Oral Rinse Products" *on page 1257*.

Benzonatate (Tessalon® Perles) *on page 130*

Chlorhexidine (Peridex®, PerioGard®) *on page 225*

Diphenhydramine (Benadryl® elixir) *on page 338*

Lidocaine (Xylocaine®) *on page 586*

Pilocarpine (Dental) (Salagen®) *on page 804*

Povidone-Iodine (Betadine®) *on page 827*

Sucralfate (Carafate®) *on page 936*

## PRESCRIPTION EXAMPLES

**Rx**

Peridex® or PerioGard® oral rinse

Disp 3 bottles

Sig: 20 mL x 30 sec tid; swish and expectorate

Ingredient: Chlorhexidine

**Rx**

Xylocaine® viscous 2%

Disp 450 mL bottles

Sig: Swish with 1 tablespoonful 4 times/day

Ingredient: Lidocaine

**Rx**

Betadine® mouthwash 0.8%

Disp 6 oz bottle

Sig: Rinse with 1 tablespoonful 4 times/day; do not swallow

Ingredient: Povidone-Iodine

**Rx**

Mycostatin® oral suspension 100,000 units/mL

Disp 60 mL bottle

Sig: 2 mL 4 times/day; hold in mouth for 2 minutes and swallow

Ingredient: Nystatin

When the oral mucous membranes are especially sensitive, nystatin "popsicles" can be made by adding 2 mL of nystatin oral suspension to the water in ice cube trays. Tessalon Perles® have been used ad lib to provide relief in painful mucositis.

**Rx**

Tessalon Perles®

Disp 50

Sig: Squeeze contents of capsule and apply to lesion

Ingredient: Benzonatate

# ORAL CARE PRODUCTS

## BACTERIAL PLAQUE CONTROL

Patients should use an extra soft bristle toothbrush and dental floss for removal of plaque. Sponge/foam sticks and lemon-glycerine swabs do not adequately remove bacterial plaque.

## PATIENTS UNDERGOING CANCER THERAPY *(Continued)*

### PRESCRIPTION EXAMPLE

**Rx**

Ultra Suave® toothbrush

Biotene Supersoft® toothbrush

Chlorhexidine 0.12% (Peridex® or other preparations available in Canada and Europe) may be used to assist with bacterial plaque control.

### SALIVA SUBSTITUTES

Carboxymethylcellulose or mucopolysaccharide*-based sprays for temporary relief from xerostomia include:

Moi-Stir® *on page 901*
*Mouth-Kote® *on page 901*
Optimoist® *on page 901*
Salivart® *on page 901*

### FLUORIDE GELS

Oral Rinse Products *on page 1257*

Used for the prevention of demineralization of the tooth structure secondary to xerostomia. For patients with long-term or permanent xerostomia, daily application is accomplished using custom gel applicator trays. Patients with porcelain crowns should use a neutral pH fluoride.

1.1% neutral pH sodium fluoride
Thera-Flur-N® or PreviDent® *on page 441*
0.4% stannous fluoride
Gel-Kam® unflavored *on page 441*

### REMINERALIZING GEL

In addition to fluoride gel to remineralize enamel breakdown in severely xerostomic patients, applicator trays may be used.

Revive®

### ORAL AND LIP MOISTURIZERS/LUBRICANTS

Mouth Pain, Cold Sore, Canker Sore Products *on page 1253*

Water-based gels should first be used to provide moisture to dry oral tissues.

Surgi-Lube®
K-Y Jelly®
Oral Balance®
Mouth Moisturizer®

## PALLIATION OF PAIN

Mouth Pain, Cold Sore, Canker Sore Products *on page 1253*

Palliative pain preparations should be monitored for efficacy.

- For relief of pain associated with isolated ulcerations, topical anesthetic and protective preparations may be used.
  - Orabase-B® with 20% benzocaine *on page 128*
  - Oratect Gel® with 15% benzocaine and protective film *on page 128*
- For generalized oral pain:
  - Chloraseptic Spray® (OTC) anesthetic spray without alcohol *on page 791*
  - Ulcer-Ease® anesthetic/analgesic mouthrinse
  - Xylocaine® 2% viscous *on page 586*

May anesthetize swallowing mechanism and cause aspiration of food; caution patient against using too close to eating; lack of sensation may also allow patient to damage intact mucosa

Tantum Mouthrinse® (benzydamine hydrochloride); available only in Canada and Europe; may be diluted as required

## PATIENT PREPARED PALLIATIVE MIXTURES

Coating agents:

Maalox® *on page 56*

Mylanta® *on page 56*

Gelusil® *on page 56*

Kaopectate® *on page 109*

These products can be mixed with Benadryl® elixir 50:50

Diphenhydramine (Benadryl®) *on page 338*

Mouth Pain, Cold Sore, Canker Sore Products *on page 1253*

Topical anesthetics (diphenhydramine chloride)

Benadryl® elixir or Benylin® cough syrup *on page 338*

Choose product with lowest alcohol and sucrose contents; ask pharmacist for assistance

## PHARMACY PREPARATIONS

A Pharmacist may also prepare the following solutions for relief of generalized oral pain:

**Benadryl-Lidocaine Solution**

Diphenhydramine injectable 1.5 mL (50 mg/mL) *on page 338*

Xylocaine viscous 2% (45 mL) *on page 586*

Magnesium aluminum hydroxide solution (45 mL)

Swish and hold 1 teaspoonful in mouth for 30 seconds

Do not use too close to eating

**Rx**

Carafate suspension 1 g/10 mL

Disp 420 mL

Sig: Swish and hold 1 teaspoonful in mouth for 30 seconds

# CHEMICAL DEPENDENCY AND SMOKING CESSATION

## INTRODUCTION

As long as history has been recorded, every society has used drugs that alter mood, thought, and feeling. In addition, pharmacological advances sometimes have been paralleled by physical as well as unfortunate behavioral dependence on agents initially consumed for therapeutic purposes.

In 1986, the American Dental Association passed a policy statement recognizing chemical dependency as a disease. In recognizing this disease, the Association mandated that dentists have a responsibility to include questions relating to a history of chemical dependency or more broadly substance abused in their health history questionnaire. A positive response may require the dentist to alter the treatment plan for the patient's dental care. This includes patients who are actively abusing alcohol, drugs, or patients who are in recovery. The use and abuse of drugs is not a topic that is usually found in the dental curriculum. Information about substance abuse is usually gleaned from newspapers, magazines, or just hearsay.

This chapter reviews street drugs, where they come from, signs and symptoms of the drug abuser, and some of the dental implications of treating patients actively using or in recovery from these substances. There are many books devoted to this topic that provide greater detail. The intent is to provide an overview of some of the most prevalent drugs, how patients abusing these drugs may influence dental treatment, and how to recognize some signs and symptoms of use and withdrawal.

Street drugs, like other drugs, can come from various sources. They may be derived from natural sources (ie, morphine and codeine). They may be semisynthetic, that is a natural product is chemically modified to produce another molecule (ie, morphine conversion to heroin). Street drugs may also be synthetic with no natural origin.

## BENZODIAZEPINES AND OTHER NONALCOHOL SEDATIVES

Benzodiazepines are the most commonly prescribed drugs worldwide. These drugs are used mainly for treatment of anxiety disorders and, in some instances, insomnia. Even though they are used in high quantities throughout the world, intentional abuse is not that common. These drugs, however, have the ability to induce a strong physical dependency on the use of the medication. As tolerance builds up to the drug, the physical dependency increases dramatically. Unlike the street drugs where addiction is a primary consideration, the overuse of benzodiazepine lies in its ability to induce this physical dependency. When these drugs are taken for several weeks, there is relatively little tolerance induced. However, after several months, the proportion of patients who become tolerant increases and reducing the dose or stopping the medication produces severe withdrawal symptoms.

| Benzodiazepine Withdrawal Symptoms |
|---|
| Craving for benzodiazepines<br>Irritability<br>Anxiety<br>Sleep disturbances |

It is extremely difficult for the physician to distinguish between the withdrawal symptoms and the reappearance of the myriad anxiety symptoms that cause the drug to be prescribed initially. Many patients increase their dose over time because tolerance develops to at least the sedative effects of the drug. The antianxiety benefits of the benzodiazepines continue to occur long after tolerance to the sedating effects. Patients often take these drugs for many years with relatively few ill effects other than the risk of withdrawal. The dentist should be keenly aware of the signs and symptoms and the historical pattern in patients taking benzodiazepines.

## BARBITURATES AND NON-BENZODIAZEPINE SEDATIVES

The use of barbiturates as sedative medications has declined over the years due to the increased safety and efficacy of benzodiazepines. Abuse problems with barbiturates resemble those with the benzodiazepines in many ways. Drugs in this category are frequently prescribed as hypnotics for patients complaining of insomnia. The physician should, therefore, be aware of the problems that can develop when the hypnotic agent is withdrawn. The underlying problem that has lead to the insomnia is not treated directly by the use of barbiturates and the patient seeking a sleep medication may have altered ability to sleep normally because of the medication. The withdrawal symptoms for the barbiturates are similar to the benzodiazepine sedatives.

## ALCOHOL

The chronic use of alcohol as well as that of other sedatives is associated with the development of depression. The risk of suicide among alcoholics is one of the highest of any diagnostic category. Cognitive deficits have been reported in alcoholics tested while sober. These deficits usually improve after weeks to months of abstinence. More severe recent memory impairment is associated with specific brain damage caused by nutritional deficiencies common in alcoholics.

Alcohol is toxic to many organ systems. As a result, the medical complications of alcohol abuse and dependence include liver disease, cardiovascular disease, endocrine and gastrointestinal effects, and malnutrition, in addition to CNS dysfunctions. Ethanol readily crosses the placental barrier, producing the *fetal alcohol syndrome*, a major cause of mental retardation.

| Alcohol Withdrawal Syndrome Signs and Symptoms |
|---|
| Alcohol craving |
| Tremor, irritability |
| Nausea |
| Sleep disturbance |
| Tachycardia |
| Hypertension |
| Sweating |
| Perceptual distortion |
| Seizures (12-48 hours after last drink) |
| Delirium tremens (rare in uncomplicated withdrawal): |
| Severe agitation |
| Confusion |
| Visual hallucinations |
| Fever, profuse sweating |
| Tachycardia |
| Nausea, diarrhea |
| Dilated pupils |

## NICOTINE

Cigarette (nicotine) addiction is influenced by multiple variables. Nicotine itself produces reinforcement; users compare nicotine to stimulants such as cocaine or amphetamine, although its effects are of lower magnitude.

Nicotine is absorbed readily through the skin, mucous membranes, and of course, through the lungs. The pulmonary route produces discernible central nervous system effects in as little as 7 seconds. Thus, each puff produces some discrete reinforcement. With 10 puffs per cigarette, the 1 pack per day smoker reinforces the habit 200 times daily. The timing, setting, situation, and preparation all become associated repetitively with the effects of nicotine.

Nicotine has both stimulant and depressant actions. The smoker feels alert, yet there is some muscle relaxation. Nicotine activates the nucleus accumbens reward system in the brain. Increased extracellular dopamine has been found in this region after nicotine injections in rats. Nicotine affects other systems as well, including the release of endogenous opioids and glucocorticoids.

| Nicotine Withdrawal Syndrome Signs and Symptoms |
|---|
| Irritability, impatience, hostility |
| Anxiety |
| Dysphoric or depressed mood |
| Difficulty concentrating |
| Restlessness |
| Decreased heart rate |
| Increased appetite or weight gain |

Medications to assist users in breaking a nicotine habit are available.

## CHEMICAL DEPENDENCY AND SMOKING CESSATION *(Continued)*

Bupropion (Zyban®) *on page 160*

Nicotine (Habitrol®, Nicoderm®, Nicorette® (polacrilex gum - OTC), Nicotrol® (OTC), ProStep®) *on page 718*

## SMOKING CESSATION PRODUCTS

Several years ago, the journal *Science* stated that about 80% of smokers say they want to quit, but each year fewer than 1 in 10 actually succeed. Nicotine transdermal delivery preparations (or nicotine patches) were approved by the U.S. Food and Drug Administration in 1992 as aids to smoking cessation for the relief of nicotine withdrawal symptoms. Four preparations were approved simultaneously: Habitrol®, Nicoderm®, Nicotrol®, and ProStep®. These products differ in how much nicotine is released and whether they provide a 24-hour or 16-hour release time.

Studies are still being reported on the effectiveness of nicotine patches on smoking cessation. Most previous studies had good entry criteria including definition of the Fagerstrom score. Dr Fred Cowan of Oregon Health Sciences University described these Fagerstrom criteria in a previous report on nicotine substitutes in AGD *Impact*. Abstinence of smoking cessation has usually been assessed by self-report, measurement of carbon monoxide in breath, and plasma or urine nicotine products.

In numerous protocols, percentages of study subjects who abstained from smoking after 3-10 weeks of patch treatment with nicotine compared to placebo, have never exceeded 40%. After the initial assessment, six studies continued to follow the study subjects through 24-52 weeks of patch treatment. The results were even poorer with less than 25% sustained success. A review of these and additional studies, reveals some general conclusions regarding the effectiveness of nicotine patches in smoking cessation. In every study, many smokers abstained after treatment with placebo patches; nicotine treatment was initially more effective than placebo; and improved abstinence rates were more marked in the short term (10 weeks) than in the long term (52 weeks). Subjects undergoing smoking cessation trails tended to gain weight irrespective of whether placebo or nicotine patches were worn. Patients often favor the nicotine polacrilex gum (Nicorette®) which releases nicotine into the blood stream via the oral mucosa.

Data are now available from smoking cessation studies carried out in general medical practices. The effectiveness of nicotine patch substitution under these conditions is similar to the results described above. Most patch systems and gum are now available as over-the-counter products; only Habitrol® remains prescription. Practitioners and patients should remain skeptical since these aids appear to work best only when supplemented with psychological counseling and a single-minded effort on the part of the patient. New products such as Zyban® are now also being marketed as smoking cessation aids. These drugs are norepinephrine serotonin reuptake inhibitors and their action directly affects the craving for tobacco.

## OPIATES

The opiates are most often called narcotics. The most common opiate found on the street is heroin. Heroin is the diacetyl derivative of morphine which is extracted from opium. Although commercial production of morphine involves extraction from the dried opium plant which grows in many parts of the world, some areas still harvest opium by making slits in the unripened seed pod. The pod secretes a white, viscous material which upon contact with the air turns a blackish-brown color. It is this off-white material that is called opium. The opium is then dried and smoked or processed to yield morphine and codeine. Actually, the raw opium contains several chemicals that are used medicinally or commercially. Much (it has been estimated that 50%) of the morphine is converted chemically into heroin which finds its way into the United States and then on the street. Heroin is a Schedule I drug and as such has no acceptable use in the United States today. In fact, possession is a violation of the Controlled Substances Act of 1970. The majority of the heroin found on the streets is from Southeast Asia and can be as concentrated as 100%.

The heroin user goes through many phases once the drug has been administered. When administered intravenously, the user initially feels a "rush" often described as an "orgasmic rush". This initial feeling is most likely due to the release of histamine resulting in cutaneous vasodilation, itching, and a flushed appearance. Shortly after this "rush" the user becomes euphoric. This euphoric stage often called "stoned" or being "high" lasts approximately 3-4 hours. During this stage, the user is lethargic, slow to react to stimuli, speech is slurred, pain reaction threshold is elevated, exhibits xerostomia, slowed heart rate, and the pupils may be constricted. Following the "high", the abuser is "straight" for about 2 hours, with no tell-tale signs of abuse. Approximately 6-8 hours following the last injection of heroin, the user begins to experience a runny nose, lacrimation, and abdominal muscle cramps as they begin the withdrawal from the drug. During this stage and the one that follows, the person may become agitated as they develop anxiety about where they are going to get their next "hit". The withdrawal signs and symptoms become more intense. For the next 3 days, the abuser begins to sweat profusely in combination with cutaneous vasoconstriction. The skin becomes cold and clammy, hence the term "cold turkey". Tachycardia, pupillary dilation, diarrhea, and salivation occur for the 3 days following the last injection. Withdrawal signs and symptoms may last longer than the average of 3 days or they may be more abrupt.

**Opioid Withdrawal Signs and Symptoms**

| Symptoms | Signs |
|---|---|
| **Regular Withdrawal** | |
| Craving for opioids | Pupillary dilation |
| Restlessness, irritability | Sweating |
| Increased sensitivity to pain | Piloerection ("gooseflesh") |
| Nausea, cramps | Tachycardia |
| Muscle aches | Vomiting, diarrhea |
| Dysphoric mood | Increased blood pressure |
| Insomnia, anxiety | Yawning |
| | Fever |
| **Protracted Withdrawal** | |
| Anxiety<br>Insomnia<br>Drug craving | Cyclic changes in weight, pupil size, respiratory center sensitivity |

Many of these patients who have been abusing opiates for any length of time will exhibit multiple carious lesions, particularly class V lesions. This increased caries rate is probably a result of the heroin-induced xerostomia, high intake of sweets, and lack of daily oral hygiene. Patients who are recovering from heroin or any opiate addiction should not be given any kind of opiate analgesic, whether it be for sedation or as a postoperative analgesic because of the increased chance of relapse. The nonsteroidal anti-inflammatory drugs (NSAIDs) should be used to control any postoperative discomfort. Patients who admit to a past history of intravenous heroin use or any intravenous drug for that matter, are at higher risk for subacute bacterial endocarditis (SBE), HIV disease, and hepatitis but with the exception of postoperative analgesia should present no special problem for dental care.

# MARIJUANA

The number one most abused illegal drug by high school students today is marijuana. Marijuana is a plant that grows throughout the world, but is particularly suited for a warm, humid environment. There are three species of plant but the two most frequently cited are *Cannabis sativa* and *Cannabis indica*. All species possess a female and male plant. Although approximately 450 chemicals have been isolated from the plant, the major psychoactive ingredient is delta-9-tetrahydrocannabinol (THC). Of these 450 chemicals, there are about 23 psychoactive chemicals, THC being the most abundant. The highest concentration of THC is found in the bud of the female plant. The concentration of THC varies according to growing conditions and location on the plant but has increased from about 2% to 3% in marijuana sold in the 50s to about 30% sold on the streets today. Marijuana can be smoked in cigarettes (joints), pipes, water pipes (bongs), or baked in brownies, cakes, etc, and then ingested. However, smoking marijuana is more efficient and the "high" has a quicker onset. Marijuana is a Schedule I drug but has been promoted as a medicinal for the treatment of glaucoma, for increasing appetite in patients who have HIV disease, and to prevent the nausea associated with cancer chemotherapy. In response to this request, the FDA approved dronabinol (Marinol®), a synthetic THC and placed this drug in Schedule II to be prescribed by physicians for the indicated medical conditions.

Dronabinol (Marinol®) *on page 358*

An individual under the influence of marijuana may exhibit no signs or symptoms of intoxication. The pharmacologic effects are dose-dependent and depend to a large extent on the set and setting of the intoxicated individual. As the dose of THC increases, the person experiences euphoria or a state of well-being, often referred to as "mellowing out". Everything becomes comical, problems disappear, and their appetite for snack foods increases. This is called the "munchies". The marijuana produces time and spatial distortion, which contribute, as the dose increases, to a dysphoria characterized by paranoia and fear. Although there has never been a death reported from marijuana overdose, certainly the higher doses may produce such bizarre circumstances as to increase the chances of accidental death. THC is fat soluble. Daily

## CHEMICAL DEPENDENCY AND SMOKING CESSATION *(Continued)*

consumption of marijuana will result in THC being stored in body fat which will result in detectable amounts of THC being found in the urine for as long as 60 days in some cases.

| Marijuana Withdrawal Syndrome Signs and Symptoms |
|---|
| Restlessness |
| Irritability |
| Mild agitation |
| Insomnia |
| Restlessness |
| Sleep EEG disturbance |
| Nausea, cramping |

Because of anxiety associated with dental visits, marijuana would be the most likely drug, after alcohol, to be used when coming to the dental office. But, unlike alcohol, marijuana may not produce any detectable odor on the breath nor any signs of intoxication. Fortunately, local anesthetics, analgesics, and antibiotics used by the general dentist do not interact with marijuana. The major concern with the marijuana intoxicated patient is a failure to follow directions while in the chair, and the inability to follow postoperative instructions.

## COCAINE

Cocaine, referred to on the street as "snow", "nose candy", "girl", and many other euphemisms, has created an epidemic. This drug is like no other local anesthetic. Known for about the last two thousand years, cocaine has been used and abused by politicians, scientists, farmers, warriors, and of course, on the street. Cocaine is derived from the leaves of a plant called *Erythroxylon coca* which grows in South America. Ninety percent of the world's supply of cocaine originates in Peru, Bolivia, and Colombia. At last estimate, the United States consumes 75% of the world's supply. The plant grows to a height of approximately four feet and produces a red berry. Farmers go through the fields stripping the leaves from the plant three times a year. During the working day the farmers chew the coca leaves to suppress appetite and fight the fatigue of working the fields. The leaves are transported to a laboratory site where the cocaine is extracted by a process called maceration. It takes approximately 7-8 pounds of leaves to produce one ounce of cocaine.

On the streets of the United States, cocaine can be found in two forms. One form is as the hydrochloride salt. In this form, the cocaine can be "snorted" or it can be dissolved in water and injected intravenously. The other form of cocaine is as the free base. The free base form can be smoked. The free base form is sometimes referred to as "crack", "rock", or "free base". It is called crack because it cracks or pops when large pieces are smoked. It is called rock because it is so hard and difficult to break into smaller pieces. The most popular method of administration of cocaine is "snorting." In this method, small amounts of cocaine hydrochloride are divided into segments or "lines". The person uses any straw-like device to inhale one or more lines of the cocaine into their nose. Although the cocaine does not reach the lungs, enough cocaine is absorbed through the nasal mucosa to provide a "high" within 3-5 minutes. Rock or crack on the other hand is heated and inhaled from any device available. This form of cocaine does reach the lungs and provides a much faster onset of action as well as a more intense stimulation. There are dangers to the user with any form of cocaine. Undoubtedly the most dangerous form, though, is the intravenous route.

| Cocaine Withdrawal Signs and Symptoms |
|---|
| Dysphoria, depression |
| Sleepiness, fatigue |
| Cocaine craving |
| Bradycardia |

The cocaine user, regardless of how the cocaine was administered, presents the potential of a life-threatening situation in the dental operatory. The patient under the influence of cocaine could be compared to a car going 100 miles per hour. Blood pressure is elevated and heart rate is likely increased. The use of a local anesthetic with epinephrine in such a patient may result in a medical emergency. Such patients can be identified by their jitteriness, irritability, talkativeness, tremors, and short abrupt speech patterns. These same signs and symptoms may also be seen in a normal dental patient with preoperative dental anxiety; therefore, the dentist must be particularly alert in order to identify the potential cocaine abuser. If a patient is suspected, they should never be given a local anesthetic with vasoconstrictor for fear of exacerbating the cocaine-induced sympathetic response. Life-threatening episodes of cardiac arrhythmias and hypertensive crises have been reported when local anesthetic with vasoconstrictor was administered to a patient under the influence of cocaine. No local anesthetic used by any dentist can interfere with, nor test positive for cocaine in any urine testing screen. Therefore, the dentist needn't be concerned with any false drug use accusations associated with dental anesthesia.

## PSYCHEDELIC AGENTS

Perceptual distortions that include hallucinations, illusions, and disorders of thinking such as paranoia can be produced by toxic doses of many drugs. These phenomena also may be seen during toxic withdrawal from sedatives such as alcohol. There are, however, certain drugs that have as their primary effect the production of perception, thought, or mood disturbances at low doses with minimal effects on memory and orientation. These are commonly called *hallucinogenic drugs*, but their use does not always result in frank hallucinations.

**LSD:** LSD is the most potent hallucinogenic drug and produces significant psychedelic effects with a total dose of as little as 25-50 mcg. This drug is over 3000 times more potent than mescaline. LSD is sold on the illicit market in a variety of forms. A popular contemporary system involves postage stamp-sized papers impregnated with varying doses of LSD (50-300 mcg or more). A majority of street samples sold as LSD actually contain LSD. In contrast, the samples of mushrooms and other botanicals sold as sources of psilocybin and other psychedelics have a low probability of containing the advertised hallucinogenics.

**Phencyclidine (PCP):** PCP deserves special mention because of its widespread availability and because its pharmacological effects are different from LSD. PCP was originally developed as an anesthetic in the 1950s and later abandoned because of a high frequency of postoperative delirium with hallucinations. It was classed as a dissociative anesthetic because, in the anesthetized state, the patient remains conscious with staring gaze, flat facies, and rigid muscles. It was discovered as a drug of abuse in the 1970s, first in an oral form and then in a smoked version enabling a better control over the dose.

## INHALANTS

Anesthetic gases such as nitrous oxide or halothane are sometimes used as intoxicants by medical personnel. Nitrous oxide also is abused by food service employees because it is supplied for use as a propellant in disposable aluminum minitanks for whipping cream canisters. Nitrous oxide produces euphoria and analgesia and then loss of consciousness. Compulsive use and chronic toxicity rarely are reported, but there are obvious risks of overdose associated with the abuse of this anesthetic. Chronic use has been reported to cause peripheral neuropathy.

The dental team should be alert to the signs and symptoms of drug abuse and withdrawal. Further reading is recommended.

# ANIMAL AND HUMAN BITES GUIDELINES

The dentist is often confronted with early management of animal and human bites. The following protocols may assist in appropriate care and referral.

## WOUND MANAGEMENT

**Irrigation:** Critically important; irrigate all penetration wounds using 20 mL syringe, 19-gauge needle and >250 mL 1% povidone iodine solution. This method will reduce wound infection by a factor of 20. When there is high risk of rabies, use viricidal 1% benzalkonium chloride in addition to the 1% povidone iodine. Irrigate wound with normal saline after antiseptic irrigation.

**Debridement:** Remove all crushed or devitalized tissue remaining after irrigation; minimize removal on face and over thin skin areas or anywhere you would create a worse situation than the bite itself already has; do not extend puncture wounds surgically — rather, manage them with irrigation and antibiotics.

**Suturing:** Close most dog bites if <8 hours (<12 hours on face); do not routinely close puncture wounds, or deep or severe bites on the hands or feet, as these are at highest risk for infection. Cat and human bites should not be sutured unless cosmetically important. Wound edge freshening, where feasible, reduces infection; minimize sutures in the wound and use monofilament on the surface.

**Immobilization:** Critical in all hand wounds; important for infected extremities.

**Hospitalization/I.V. Antibiotics:** Admit for I.V. antibiotics all significant human bites to the hand, especially closed fist injuries, and bites involving penetration of the bone or joint (a high index of suspicion is needed). Consider I.V. antibiotics for significant established wound infections with cellulitis or lymphangitis, any infected bite on the hand, any infected cat bite, and any infection in an immunocompromised or asplenic patient. Outpatient treatment with I.V. antibiotics may be possible in selected cases by consulting with infectious disease.

## LABORATORY ASSESSMENT

**Gram's Stain:** Not useful prior to onset of clinically apparent infection; examination of purulent material may show a predominant organism in established infection, aiding antibiotic selection; not warranted unless results will change your treatment.

**Culture:** Not useful or cost-effective prior to onset of clinically apparent infection.

**X-ray:** Whenever you suspect bony involvement, especially in craniofacial dog bites in very small children or severe bite/crush in an extremity; cat bites with their long needle like teeth may cause osteomyelitis or a septic joint, especially in the hand or wrist.

## IMMUNIZATIONS

**Tetanus:** All bite wounds are contaminated. If not immunized in last 5 years, or if not current in a child, give DPT, DT, Td, or TT as indicated. For absent or incomplete primary immunization, give 250 units tetanus immune globulin (TIG) in addition.

**Rabies:** In the U.S. 30,000 persons are treated each year in an attempt to prevent 1-5 cases. Domestic animals should be quarantined for 10 days to prove need for prophylaxis. High risk animal bites (85% of cases = bat, skunk, raccoon) usually receive treatment consisting of:

- human rabies immune globulin (HRIG): 20 units/kg I.M. (unless previously immunized with HDCV)
- human diploid cell vaccine (HDCV): 1 mL I.M. on days 0, 3, 7, 14, and 28 (unless previously immunized with HDCV - then give only first 2 doses)

Rabies Immune Globulin, Human *on page 875*
Rabies Virus Vaccine *on page 876*
Tetanus Immune Globulin, Human *on page 962*

# BITE WOUNDS AND PROPHYLACTIC ANTIBIOTICS

**Parenteral vs Oral:** If warranted, consider an initial I.V. dose to rapidly establish effective serum levels, especially if high risk, delayed treatment, or if patient reliability is poor.

**Dog Bite:**

1. Rarely get infected (~5%)
2. Infecting organisms: Staph coag negative, staph coag positive, alpha strep, diphtheroids, beta strep, *Pseudomonas aeruginosa*, gamma strep, *Pasteurella multocida*
3. Prophylactic antibiotics are seldom indicated. Consider for high risk wounds such as distal extremity puncture wounds, severe crush injury, bites occurring in cosmetically sensitive areas (eg, face), or in immunocompromised or asplenic patients.

**Cat Bite:**

1. Often get infected (~25% to 50%)
2. Infecting organisms: *Pasteurella multocida* (first 24 hours), coag positive staph, anaerobic cocci (after first 24 hours)
3. Prophylactic antibiotics are indicated in all cases.

**Human Bite:**

1. Intermediate infection rate (~15% to 20%)
2. Infecting organisms: Coag positive staph $\alpha$, $\beta$, $\gamma$ strep, *Haemophilus*, *Eikenella corrodens*, anaerobic streptococci, *Fusobacterium*, *Veillonella*, bacteroides.
3. Prophylactic antibiotics are indicated in almost all cases except superficial injuries.

Amoxicillin (various products) *on page 76*
Amoxicillin and Clavulanate Potassium (Augmentin®) *on page 77*
Cefazolin (Ancef®; Kefzol®; Zolicef®) *on page 199*
Cefotetan (Cefotan®) *on page 204*
Ceftriaxone (Rocephin®) *on page 209*
Clindamycin (Cleocin®) *on page 258*
Doxycycline (various products) *on page 355*
Imipenem/Cilastatin (Primaxin®) *on page 527*
Trimethoprim and Sulfamethoxazole (various products) *on page 1021*

## ANIMAL AND HUMAN BITES GUIDELINES *(Continued)*

### BITE WOUND ANTIBIOTIC REGIMENS

| | Dog Bite | Cat Bite | Human Bite |
|---|---|---|---|
| **Prophylactic Antibiotics** | | | |
| Prophylaxis | No routine prophylaxis, consider if involves face or hand, or immunosuppressed or asplenic patients | Routine prophylaxis | Routine prophylaxis |
| Prophylactic antibiotic | Amoxicillin | Amoxicillin | Amoxicillin |
| Penicillin allergy | Doxycycline if >10 y or co-trimoxazole | Doxycycline if >10 y or co-trimoxazole | Doxycycline if >10 y or erythromycin and cephalexin* |
| **Outpatient Oral Antibiotic Treatment** (mild to moderate infection) | | | |
| Established infection | Amoxicillin and clavulanic acid | Amoxicillin and clavulanic acid | Amoxicillin and clavulanic acid |
| Penicillin allergy (mild infection only) | Doxycycline if >10 y | Doxycycline if >10 y | Cephalexin* or clindamycin |
| **Outpatient Parenteral Antibiotic Treatment** (moderate infections — single drug regimens) | | | |
| | Ceftriaxone | Ceftriaxone | Cefotetan |
| **Inpatient Parenteral Antibiotic Treatment** | | | |
| Established infection | Ampicillin + cefazolin | Ampicillin + cefazolin | Ampicillin + clindamycin |
| Penicillin allergy | Cefazolin* | Ceftriaxone* | Cefotetan* or imipenem |
| **Duration of Prophylactic and Treatment Regimens** | | | |
| Prophylaxis: 5 days | | | |
| Treatment: 10-14 days | | | |

*Contraindicated if history of immediate hypersensitivity reaction (anaphylaxis) to penicillin.

# NATURAL PRODUCTS, HERBALS, AND DIETARY SUPPLEMENTS

Medical problem: " I have a toothache."
2000 BC response: "Here, eat this root."
1000 AD: "That root is heathen; here, say this prayer."
1850 AD: "That prayer is superstitious; here, drink this potion."
1940 AD: "That potion is snake oil; here, swallow this pill."
1985 AD: "That pill is ineffective; here, take this new antibiotic."
2000 AD: "That antibiotic is artificial; here, eat this root."
Adapted from an anonymous Internet communication.

## INTRODUCTION

For centuries, Eastern and Western civilizations have attributed a large number of medical uses to plants and herbs. Over time, modern scientific methodologies have emerged from some of these remedies. Conversely, some of these agents have fallen into less popularity as more medical knowledge has evolved. In spite of this dichotomy, herbal and natural therapies for treatment of common medical ailments have become exceedingly popular. In America, people consistently seek out natural products that may be able to offset some perceived ailment or may assist in the prevention of an ailment. One area that has consistently drawn patients interested in herbal or natural remedies has been the area of weight loss. There are numerous systemic considerations when some of the natural products that have been attributed weight loss powers are utilized. Many of these products are sold under the blanket of dietary supplements and, therefore, avoid some of the more stringent Food and Drug Administration legislation. In 1994, that legislation was modified to include herbs, vitamins, minerals, and amino acids that may be taken as dietary supplements and that information must be available to patients taking them. The real concern, however, lies in the fact that health claims need not be approved by the FDA, but the advertisements must include a disclaimer saying that the product has not yet been fully evaluated. Claims of medicinal use/value are often drawn from popular use, not necessarily from scientific studies. The safety, however, when these agents are taken in combination with other prescription drugs is of concern and medical risk might result. Many of these natural products may have real medicinal value but caution on the part of the dental clinician is prudent. It is impossible within this chapter to cover all of the popular natural products. The chapter, therefore, has been limited to brief reviews of some of the most popular dietary supplements, herbs, and natural remedies currently being used by patients you might treat and what we know about the effects of some of these agents on the body's various systems. An extensive reading list is provided.

## TOP 20 MOST POPULAR NATURAL PRODUCTS

### ALFALFA

Alfalfa has been touted as a natural laxative, an antifungal, a liver detoxifier, a diuretic, and a food additive useful in treating kidney stones and urinary infections. Alfalfa is an important animal feed worldwide and its chemical constituents are well known. However, studies have concluded that alfalfa contains nothing of significant therapeutic value in the amounts generally recommended. The seed contains L-canabanine which has been implicated in pancytopenia in humans and may induce systemic lupus in monkeys. Allergic reactions have been provoked in some users.

### ALOE VERA

Products derived from this plant have been used for centuries. Aloe is popularly used as a cure-all and it has been advertised for use in treating acne, burns, and minor wounds. Although the FDA does not recognize the uses of aloe for the treatment of any specific condition, there is evidence to suggest that fresh aloe gel is an effective agent in wound healing. Data to support these claims are inconclusive, however, and the use of aloe by patients should not interfere with dental care.

### BILBERRY

Bilberry, also known as blueberry, is recommended by herbalists for use in connection with vascular and blood disorders and in treating varicose veins, thromboses, diarrhea, and angina. Preliminary studies have indicated that bilberry may have some benefit in aiding visual acuity, however, there is little clinical evidence to support the widespread usage. Potential interactions with over-the-counter prescription medications are unknown at this time.

## NATURAL PRODUCTS, HERBALS, AND DIETARY SUPPLEMENTS *(Continued)*

### CAYENNE

Most cooks know of the chemical cayenne that is the active ingredient in chili pepper and lends itself to the strong taste of this herb. Cayenne has been known for many years to stimulate digestion and to promote sweating; sometimes assisting, therefore, in reducing fever. Cayenne contains an ingredient known as capsaicin which is the active ingredient in many over-the-counter and prescription forms of cream to treat arthritis. Capsaicin appears to alter the action of the compound associated with pain, the mechanism of which has not been completely studied.

### CHAMOMILE

This agent is often found in the form of dried leaves that can be used to create a tea. The tea is taken internally and has been recommended by naturalists as a cure for stomach pain, menstrual discomfort, and stress. Chamomile teas appear to have some unknown mechanism of immune activation, perhaps due to the presence of flavonoids in the compound.

### CRANBERRY

Cranberry has been used for centuries as an agent to assist in treatment of urinary tract infections. Cranberry juices contain pH-altering chemical which may be of use in treating these infections. It is now thought that the cranberry actually prevents bacteria from adhering to the lining of the bladder and urinary tract. Again, this agent is rich in flavonoids, citric acids, and vitamin C.

### ECHINACEA

Echinacea is reported to have uses for treatment of colds, flu, bacterial and fungal infections, and even cancer. AIDS patients are sometimes advised by their peers to take echinacea. To date, pharmacological components and their actions on the human body are unclear. However, complex polysaccharides are found in the agent and seem to hold some promise as compounds for immunostimulation. In general, echinacea appears to be relatively safe but clinical information is lacking.

### EPHEDRA

Also known as ma-huang, ephedra has been used in China for more than 4000 years to treat symptoms of upper respiratory infections and asthma. Ephedra can be used as a nasal decongestant and has recently gained new popularity as a weight loss product. This agent, when used in combination with St John's Wort, apparently has effects on serotonin levels similar to the drug fenfluramine which was recently taken off the market. This combination of drugs has been known as natural fen-phen. Ephedra has also been recommended as an aphrodisiac.

### FEVERFEW

Feverfew has a long history of use in traditional and cult medicine as a treatment for fever, headache, and menstrual irregularities. More recently, it has been suggested for migraine headaches, arthritis, and insect bites. The dentist should be aware that patients may self-medicate with feverfew in an effort to treat migraine headaches. One study of commercially available feverfew products has found that there is a lactone present that appears to have some activity. However, there are no long-term toxicology studies to indicate or refute this claim.

### GARLIC

Garlic and related products have been used for thousands of years. It is generally considered by herbalists and naturalists as a cure-all. When garlic is crushed, it produces allicin which possesses some antibiotic, antiplatelet, anticholesterol properties. In addition, other sulfur-containing compounds are found in garlic and these produce some antithrombotic properties. For the most part, the consumption of moderate amounts of garlic is harmless. Large doses, however, are likely to stimulate heartburn and gastric or intestinal disorders.

### GINGER

Ginger has been taken for centuries due to its calming effects on an upset stomach. The stem of the rhizome from a tropical plant has been used to make the ginger root. Today it is widely used for morning sickness, seasickness, and motion sickness. Ginger may have some effect on cholesterol levels although further study is necessary. The presence of essential oils in ginger may be the active ingredients in this agent.

### GINKGO BILOBA

Ginkgo supplements are claimed by herbalists to help with the aging process and with mental acuity. The most popular of these agents is used as an extract to promote improved blood flow to a portion of the body. Clinical research has not proven that these claims are or are not true.

### GINSENG

Ginseng is commonly used as a substance to support general good health and has also been marketed in some countries as an aphrodisiac. As with the majority of herbal agents, there are few clinical studies. However, commercial products vary widely and the clinician may be aware that ginseng could produce some side effects.

### GREEN TEA

Green tea has been widely used in Asia to treat numerous ailments. This tea is derived from leaves and delicate leaf buds of an evergreen bush. It is thought that green tea has some antioxidant effect, as well as containing compounds and flavonoids as with many of the other herbs.

### KAVA

Kava is one of the most popular herbs on today's market. It is extracted from a root and is used to promote sleep and relaxation in anxious patients. This agent appears to be extremely safe, however, the full effect of the active ingredient know as kavalactones, is unknown. They appear to have an effect on the neural transmitter activity in the central nervous system.

### LICORICE

Licorice has been used for centuries to treat intestinal disorders and stomach distress. There appears to be some activity of licorice on patients who suffer from mild preulcerous conditions in the GI tract. Again, the flavonoids appear to be an active component.

### PSYLLIUM

Psyllium has been used by herbalists and natural product advocates to promote regular intestinal function, primarily as an agent to assist in constipation and in GI distress.

### ST JOHN'S WORT

St John's wort has become popular in the treatment of depression, anxiety, and even in AIDS. While some of the constituents seem to show a minimal amount of antidepressant activity, other components may suggest that St John's wort is ineffective in treating these illnesses.

### SAW PALMETTO

Saw palmetto was an official drug used for a variety of ailments, mainly associated with urogenital disorders. It has actually been shown to have some efficacy in managing benign prostate hypertrophy. The drug, however, has not yet passed any of the rigid FDA requirements prior to being able to substantiate this claim.

### VALERIAN

Valerian has, for centuries, made claims of being a natural tranquilizer, a relaxant for pain and muscle spasms, as well as promoting restful sleep. The dentist should be aware that some patients may be drawn to use valerian in an effort to reduce TMD dysfunction or muscle pain.

Herbalists have often used these natural products singularly or in combination to achieve a therapeutic effect. Some of the natural agents have been combined for assisted weight loss or for reduction of more serious ailments such as high blood pressure or cardiovascular disease. One such combination recommends ephedra and St John's wort as a "natural fen-phen". These agents are not directly related to fenfluramine, but are thought to also act on serotonin levels in the brain. The dentist should be aware that there are some known interactions of these agents with drug therapies that the dentist may be using. However, our knowledge is extremely limited in this extent. The dentist is referred for additional readings so that a personal opinion can be formed.

# EFFECTS ON VARIOUS SYSTEMS

## CENTRAL NERVOUS SYSTEM

**(Aconite, Ginseng, Xanthine derivatives)**

Aconite and hawthorn have potentially sedating effects, and aconite also contains various alkaloids and traces of ephedrine. Some documented central nervous system (CNS) effects of aconite include sedation, vertigo, and incoordination. Hawthorn has been reported to exert a depressive effect on the CNS leading to sedation.

# NATURAL PRODUCTS, HERBALS, AND DIETARY SUPPLEMENTS *(Continued)*

Ginseng, ma-huang, and xanthine derivatives can exert a stimulant effect on the central nervous system. Some of the CNS effects of ginseng include nervousness, insomnia, and euphoria. The action of ma-huang is due to the presence of ephedrine and pseudoephedrine. Ma-huang exerts a stimulant action on the CNS similar to decongestant/weight loss products (Dexatrim®, etc) thus causing nervousness, insomnia, and anxiety. Kola nut, green tea, guarana, and yerba mate contain varying amounts of caffeine, a xanthine derivative. Stimulant properties exerted by these herbs are expected to be comparable to those of caffeine, including insomnia, nervousness, and anxiety.

Products containing aconite and hawthorn should be used with caution in patients with known history of depression, vertigo, or syncope. Ginseng or xanthine derivatives should be avoided in patients with history of insomnia or anxiety. Use of natural products with these components may contribute to a worsening of a patient's pre-existing medical condition. Patients taking CNS-active medications should avoid or use extreme caution when using preparations containing any of the above components. These components may interact directly or indirectly with CNS-active medications causing an increase or decrease in overall effect.

## CARDIOVASCULAR SYSTEM

### CONGESTIVE HEART FAILURE

**(Diuretics, Xanthine derivatives, Licorice, Ginseng, Aconite)**

*Alisma plantago*, bearberry (*Arctostaphylos uva-ursi*), buchu (*Barosma betulina*), couch grass, dandelion, horsetail rush, juniper, licorice, and xanthine derivatives exert varying degrees of diuretic action. Many patients with congestive heart failure (CHF) are already taking a diuretic medication. By taking products containing one or more of these components, patients already on diuretic medications may increase their risk for dehydration.

Ginseng and licorice can potentially worsen congestive heart failure and edema by causing fluid retention. Aconite has varying effects on the heart that itself could lead to heart failure. Patients with CHF should be advised to consult with their healthcare provider before using products containing any of these components.

### HYPERTENSION/HYPOTENSION

**(Diuretics, Ginkgo biloba, Ginseng, Hawthorn, Ma-huang, Xanthine derivatives)**

The stimulant properties of ginseng and ma-huang could worsen pre-existing hypertension. Elevated blood pressure has been reported as a side effect of ginseng. Although ma-huang contains ephedrine, a known vasoconstrictor, ma-huang's effect on blood pressure varies between individuals. Ma-huang can cause hypotension or hypertension. Due to its unpredictable effects, patients with pre-existing hypertension should use caution when using natural products containing ma-huang. Providers should caution patients with labile hypertension against the use of ginseng.

The diuretic effect of xanthine derivatives and other diuretic components could increase the effects of antihypertensive medications, increasing the risk for hypotension. Hawthorn and ginkgo biloba can cause vasodilation increasing the hypotensive effects of antihypertensive medication. Patients susceptible to hypotension or patients taking antihypertensive medication should use caution when taking products containing xanthine derivatives or diuretics. Patients with pre-existing hypertension or hypotension who wish to use products containing these components should be closely monitored by a healthcare professional for changes in blood pressure control.

### ARRHYTHMIAS

**(Ginseng)**

It has been reported that ginseng may increase the risk of arrhythmias, although it is unclear whether this effect is due to the actual ingredient (ginseng) or other possible impurities. Patients at risk for arrhythmias should be cautioned against the use of products containing ginseng without first consulting with their healthcare provider.

# GASTROINTESTINAL SYSTEM

## PEPTIC ULCER DISEASE

### (Betaine Hydrochloride, White Willow)

Betaine hydrochloride is a source of hydrochloric acid. The acid released from betaine hydrochloride could aggravate an existing ulcer. White willow, like aspirin, contains salicylates.

Aspirin has been known to induce gastric damage by direct irritation on the gastric mucosa and by an indirect systemic effect. As a result, patients with a history of peptic ulcer disease or gastritis are informed to avoid use of aspirin and other salicylate derivatives. These precautions should also apply to white willow. Patients with a history of peptic ulcer disease or gastritis should not use products containing white willow or betaine hydrochloride as either could exacerbate ulcers.

## INFLAMMATORY BOWEL DISEASE

### (Cascara Sagrada, Senna, Dandelion)

Cascara sagrada and senna are stimulant laxatives. Their laxative effect is exerted by stimulation of peristalsis in the colon and by inhibition of water and electrolyte secretion. The laxative effect produced by these herbs could induce an exacerbation of inflammatory bowel disease. Patients with a history of inflammatory bowel disease should avoid using products containing cascara sagrada or senna, and use caution when taking products containing dandelion which may also have a laxative effect.

## OBSTRUCTION/ILEUS

### (Glucomannan, Kelp, Psyllium)

Glucomannan, kelp, and psyllium act as bulk laxatives. In the presence of water, bulk laxatives swell or form a viscous solution adding extra bulk in the gastrointestinal tract. The resulting mass is thought to stimulate peristalsis. In the presence of an ileus, these laxatives could cause an obstruction.

If sufficient water is not consumed when taking a bulk laxative, a semisolid mass can form resulting in an obstruction. Any patient who wishes to take a natural product containing kelp, psyllium, or glucomannan should drink sufficient water to decrease the risk of obstruction. This may be of concern in particular disease states such as CHF or other cases where excess fluid intake may influence the existing disease presentation. Patients with a suspected obstruction or ileus should avoid using products containing kelp, psyllium, or glucomannan without consent of their primary healthcare provider.

# HEMATOLOGIC SYSTEM

## ANTICOAGULATION THERAPY & COAGULATION DISORDERS

### (Horsetail Rush, Ginseng, Ginkgo Biloba, Guarana, White Willow)

Horsetail rush, ginseng, ginkgo biloba, guarana, and white willow can potentially affect platelet aggregation and bleeding time. Ginkgo biloba, ginseng, guarana, and white willow inhibit platelet aggregation resulting in an increase in bleeding time. Horsetail rush, on the other hand, may decrease bleeding time. Patients with coagulation disorders or patients on anticoagulation therapy may be sensitive to the effects on coagulation by these components and should, therefore, avoid use of products containing any of these components.

# ENDOCRINE SYSTEM

## DIABETES MELLITUS

### (Chromium, Glucomannan, Ginseng, Hawthorn, Ma-huang, Periploca, Spirulina)

Ma-huang and spirulina both may increase glucose levels. This could cause a decrease in glucose control, thereby, increasing a patient's risk for hyperglycemia. Patients with diabetes or glucose intolerance should avoid using ma-huang and spirulina containing products.

Chromium, ginseng, glucomannan, periploca (*gymneme sylvestre*), and hawthorn should be used with caution in patients being treated for diabetes. These ingredients may reduce glucose levels increasing the risk for hypoglycemia in patients who are already taking a hypoglycemic agent. Patients with diabetes who wish to use products containing these ingredients should be closely monitored for fluctuations in blood glucose levels.

## NATURAL PRODUCTS, HERBALS, AND DIETARY SUPPLEMENTS *(Continued)*

## OTHER

### PHENYLKETONURIA

### (Aspartame, Spirulina)

Patients with phenylketonuria should not use products containing aspartame or spirulina. Aspartame, a common artificial sweetener, is metabolized to phenylalanine, while spirulina contains phenylalanine.

### GOUT

### (Diuretics, White Willow)

Patients with a history of gout should avoid using natural products containing components with diuretic action or white willow. By increasing urine output, ingredients with diuretic action may concentrate uric acid in the blood increasing the risk of gout in these patients. White willow, like aspirin, may inhibit excretion of urate resulting in an increase in uric acid concentration. The increase in urate levels could cause precipitation of uric acid resulting in an exacerbation of gout.

**SELECTED NATURAL PRODUCTS SOLD FOR WEIGHT LOSS**

| Product (Distributor) | Other Ingredients |
|---|---|
| 24 hour Diet Herbal Tea® (GNC) | Papaya (carcia papaya), moon daisy (leucanthemum vulgare), parsley (petroselinum hortense), citrus peel (citrus aurantium), spices, natural flavor, althaea |
| 24 hour Diet Shake® (GNC) | Soy protein isolate, sodium/calcium caseinate, whey, corn syrup solids, fiber blend, Dutch cocoa, herbal blend (dahlulin, chickweed, schizandra, L-selenomethionate, inosine, CoQ10), sunflower oil, calcium blend |
| 24 hour Diet Shake | Potassium chloride, natural/artificial flavors, magnesium oxide, soy lecithin, vitamin C, vitamin E, d-alpha tocopherol, vitamin A palmitate, niacinamide, zinc oxide, iron, copper gluconate, d-calcium panthenate |
| 24 hour Diet Shake | Vitamin $D_3$, pyridoxine hydrochloride, riboflavin, thiamine mononitrate, cyanocobalamin, folate, biotin, potassium iodide |
| 24 hour Dietgel: Energy for Dieters® (GNC) | Cayenne powder, cranberry concentrate, gotu kola |
| Chroma Plus Slim® (Richardson Labs) | L-carnitine USP, choline bitartrate, inositol, DL-methionine, potassium chloride, pantothenic acid, vitamin $B_6$, peppermint, bromelain |
| Chroma Slim for Men® (Richardson Labs) | L-carnitine USP, choline bitartrate, inositol, DL-methionine, pantothenic acid, vitamin $B_6$, peppermint, saw palmetto berries, cayenne, mustard seed powder, cinnamon, ginger root extract |
| Chroma Slim Plus Complete® (Richardson Labs) | Hydroxycitric acid, vanadyl sulfate, CoQ10, inositol, folate, potassium chloride, magnesium oxide, $B_5$ (cal d-pantothenate), niacin, whole food blend, mustard seed, cayenne |
| Citralean® (Advanced Research) | Hydroxycitric acid, vanadyl sulfate |
| Diet Fuel: Thermogenic Formula® (Twin Lab) | Hydroxycitric acid, L-carnitine, potassium phosphate, magnesium phosphate, citrus, bioflavonoids, ginger root powder, cayenne powder |
| Diet Max: Fat Control® (Kal, Inc) | Lotus leaf, cinnamon bark, stephania, rhaponticum, L-carnitine tartrate, niacin, choline bitartrate, pantothenic acid, vitamin $B_6$, capsicum powder, mustard powder, magnesium oxide/citrate, potassium citrate |

## SELECTED NATURAL PRODUCTS SOLD FOR WEIGHT LOSS *(continued)*

| Product (Distributor) | Other Ingredients |
|---|---|
| Diet Max: Sweet Balance® (Kal, Inc) | Bittermelon, bay leaf powder, cinnamon powder, niacin, magnesium citrate/oxide, medium chain triglycerides, lecithin, oleic acid, natural mixed tocopherols |
| Excel: Fat Burner Formula® (Human Energy Co) | Garcinia cambogia, (hydroxycitric acid), cayenne |
| Fat Burners® (Action Labs, Inc) | Choline, inositol, methionine, vitamin $B_6$, bromelain (pineapple), potassium citrate, calcium ascorbate, L-carnitine, pantothine, corn silk, alfalfa |
| Fat Fighters® (Only Natural, Inc) | Oat bran, rice brain, apple pectin, carrot fiber, beef fiber, L-acidophilus, lecithin, choline bitartrate, inositol, L-carnitine, aloe vera, bromelain, CoQ10, calcium carbonate, magnesium hydroxide, potassium citrate |
| Ginseng Trim Maxx® (Body Breakthrough) | Locust plant (cassia augustifolia), gynostermma (pentaphyllum), lycii berry leaf |
| Metabo Lift Thermogenic Formula® (Twin Lab) | Cayenne |
| Slim Max® (USA Sports Labs) | Potassium, L-carnitine complex, vitamin $B_6$, bromelain |
| Super Diet Max With Chromium® (Natural Max Co) | Mustard seed powder, garcinia cambogia, schizandra extract |
| Super Dieters Tea® (Laci Le Beau) | Citrus reticulate (orange peel), carcia papaya, lonicera japonica (honeysuckle), chrysanthemum officinalis (German chamomile), spice, natural flavor, althaea officinalis |
| Thermachrome 5000 | L-carnitine, ginger, boron proteinate, gotu kola, saw palmetto |
| Ultra Lean Herbal® (Schiff) | Garcinia cambogia extract, cayenne, iodine, potassium (glycerophosphate), magnesium (glycinate), cellulose, vegetable stearates |
| Ultra Lean Tablet® (Schiff) | Cayenne, iodine, potassium (glycerophosphate), magnesium (glycinate), vanadyl sulfate, cellulose, vegetable stearates, brindall berry extract (garcinia cambogia) |

Adapted from Mistry MG and Mays DA, "Precautions Against Global Use of Natural Products for Weight Loss: A Review of Active Ingredients and Issues Concerning Concomitant Disease States," *Therapeutic Perspectives*, 1996, 10(1):2.

# DENTAL OFFICE EMERGENCIES

Protocols should be established for most Office Emergencies. Recognition and rapid diagnosis lead to appropriate management. Major drugs discussed under the various headings are listed below.

Ammonia Spirit, Aromatic *on page 72*
Atropine *on page 108*
Dexamethasone (Decadron®) *on page 308*
Diazepam (Valium®) *on page 316*
Diphenhydramine (Benadryl®) *on page 338*
Epinephrine *on page 374*
Hydrocortisone *on page 511*
Isoproterenol *on page 553*
Naloxone (Narcan®) *on page 701*
Meperidine (Demerol®) *on page 629*
Methohexital (Brevital®) *on page 651*
Morphine *on page 688*
Theophylline *on page 969*

## SYNCOPE (Fainting)

**Cause:** Decreased circulation of blood to the brain

**Symptoms:**

- Pallor
- Anxiety
- Nausea
- Diaphoresis
- Rapid pulse (tachycardia)
- Loss of consciousness
- Decreased blood pressure
- Dilatation of pupils

**Treatment:**

- Place patient in supine position, with feet slightly elevated
- Maintain airway
- Monitor vital signs
- Administer oxygen
- Place crushed ammonia carpule under nose
- Apply cold compress to face and neck
- Reassure and comfort patient

## POSTURAL HYPOTENSION - ORTHOSTATIC HYPOTENSION (Syncope in Moving From the Supine to Upright Position)

**Treatment:**

- Place patient in supine position
- Maintain airway; check breathing
- Oxygen (as needed)
- Monitor vital signs
- Reposition patient slowly, after stable

## AIRWAY OBSTRUCTION

**Cause:** Foreign body in larynx and pharynx

**Symptoms:**

- Choking
- Gagging
- Violent expiratory effort
- Substernal notch retraction
- Cyanosis
- Labored breathing
- Rapid pulse initially, then decreased pulse
- Cardiac arrest

**Treatment:**

- Place patient in supine position
- Tilt head backward
- Clear airway manually of debris (suction oral cavity)
- Check for respiratory sounds; ventilate if necessary
- Administer oxygen
- Perform Heimlich maneuver, if needed
- Place oropharyngeal or nasopharyngeal airway, if obstruction is visible, try to dislodge
- Perform cricothyrotomy, if unable to clear airway
- If foreign body passes, refer immediately for radiographic examination
- Child: Small child may be held upside down and four sharp blows delivered between shoulder blades

## HYPERVENTILATION SYNDROME

**Cause:** Excessive loss of carbon dioxide, producing respiratory alkalosis

**Symptoms:**

- Rapid, shallow breathing
- Confusion
- Vertigo (dizziness)
- Paresthesia (numbness or tingling of extremities)
- Carpo-pedal spasm

**Treatment:**

- Position patient semi-reclining
- Calm and reassure patient vocally
- Instruct patient to breathe carbon dioxide enriched air through rebreathing bag
- Do **not** administer oxygen
- Administer medication to calm patient, if needed

## BRONCHIAL ASTHMA

**Cause:** Spasm and constriction of the bronchi

**Symptoms:**

- Labored breathing
- Wheezing
- Anxiety
- Cyanosis

**Treatment:**

- Position patient semi-reclining
- Administer bronchodilator-mistometer
- Administer oxygen
- Administer parenteral medications:
  - Adult: I.M. epinephrine 1:1000 0.3 mL, repeat if necessary
  - Children: I.M. epinephrine 1:1000 0.1 mL, repeat if necessary
- I.V. medication optional:
  - Aminophylline: 250 mg (slowly)
  - Hydrocortisone sodium succinate: 100 mg

## DENTAL OFFICE EMERGENCIES *(Continued)*

## DRUG OVERDOSE

### LOCAL ANESTHETIC

**Cause:** Drug overdose

**Symptoms:** Excitement of central nervous system followed by depression

- Apprehension
- Anxiety
- Restlessness
- Confusion
- Tremors
- Rapid breathing
- Rapid heart rate

**Treatment:**

Mild Reaction:

- Administer oxygen, if needed
- Monitor vital signs
- Administer anticonvulsant drug, if needed (ie, Valium® - I.V.)
- Medical consult, if necessary

Severe Reaction:

- Place patient in supine position
- Suction mouth and throat
- Manage seizures
- Provide basic life support
- Monitor vital signs
- Administer anticonvulsant drug, if needed
- Manage postseizure depression

### EPINEPHRINE OVERDOSE

**Treatment:**

- Position patient semi-reclining
- Monitor vital signs
- Administer oxygen, if necessary (except during hyperventilation syndrome)
- Reassure patient

### SEDATIVE-HYPNOTIC OVERDOSE

**Treatment:**

- Place patient in supine position
- Maintain airway
- Monitor vital signs
- Administer oxygen and artificially ventilate, if necessary
- Administer Vasoxyl®, 20 mg I.V., for low blood pressure

### NARCOTIC-ANALGESIC OVERDOSE

**Treatment:**

- Place patient in supine position
- Maintain airway
- Check ventilation
- Artificial ventilation and oxygen, as needed
- Administer Narcan® (naloxone) 0.4 mg I.M. or I.V.

## DRUG REACTIONS - ALLERGY

### URTICARIA OR PRURITUS

**Cause:** Allergy

**Symptoms:**

- Urticaria: Red eruption of face, neck, hands, and arms

- Pruritus: Itching of above areas

**Treatment:**

Immediate:

- Administer epinephrine 0.3 mL of 1:1000 I.M. or I.V.
- Administer antihistamine
- Prescribe for oral antihistamine
- Withdraw drug in question

Delayed:

- Administer Benadryl® (diphenhydramine hydrochloride) 50 mg orally or I.M. every 6-8 hours
- If severe, administer Benadryl® 10-50 mg I.V. initially
- Withdraw drug in question

### ANGIONEUROTIC EDEMA

**Cause:** Allergic reaction

**Symptoms:**

- Single localized sealing of lips, eyelids, cheeks, pharynx, and larynx
- Pruritus, urticaria, hoarseness, stridor, cyanosis

**Treatment:**

- Administer Benadryl® 10-50 mg I.M. or I.V.
- Administer epinephrine 0.2-0.5 mL, 1:1000 I.M. or S.C.
- Inject Solu-Cortef® 100 mg I.M. or Decadron® 4 mg I.V.
- Administer oxygen
- Give aminophylline 250 mg I.V., slowly
- Withdraw drug in question

## ANAPHYLACTIC SHOCK

**Cause:** Allergic reaction

**Symptoms:**

- Progressive respiratory and circulatory failure
- Itching of nose and hands
- Flushed face
- Feeling of substernal depression
- Labored breathing, stridor
- Coughing
- Sudden hypotension
- Cyanosis
- Loss of consciousness
- Incontinence

**Treatment:**

- Place patient in supine position
- Clear airway
- Monitor vital signs
- Administer oxygen and ventilate manually, if necessary
- Administer aqueous epinephrine 1:1000, 0.2-0.5 mL I.M. or S.C. (Children: 0.125-0.25 mL I.V.)
- Give Decadron® 4 mg I.V., if necessary
- Start I.V. fluids (1000 mL or 500 mL of $D_5W$ or Ringer's lactate)
- Give aminophylline 250 mg I.V. very slowly
- Apply tourniquet to injection site (if injection is in extremity)
- Transfer patient to hospital

## SEIZURE DISORDERS

**Cause:**

- Intermittent disorder of nervous system caused by sudden discharge of cerebral neurons
- Idiosyncracy to drug

**Symptoms:**

- Excitement, tremor, followed by clonic-tonic convulsions

## DENTAL OFFICE EMERGENCIES *(Continued)*

- Trance-like state

**Treatment:**
- Place patient on floor
- Loosen clothing and ensure safety of patient
- Maintain airway
- Administer Valium® 5-20 mg I.V. or Brevital® I.V. (Children: 5 mg I.V.) until cessation of seizure
- Be prepared for postseizure depression; support respiration

## CEREBRAL VASCULAR ACCIDENTS

**Cause:** Obstruction of blood vessel of brain

**Symptoms:**
- Weakness
- Confusion
- Headache
- Dizziness
- Dysphagia
- Vital signs usually satisfactory
- Aphasia
- Nausea
- Paralysis
- Loss of consciousness

**Treatment:**

Transient Ischemic Attack
- Monitor vital signs
- Obtain medical consult with physician

CVA (Conscious Patient)
- Position patient semi-reclining
- Monitor vital signs
- Seek medical assistance

CVA (Unconscious Patient)
- Place patient in supine position
- Record vital signs
- Provide basic life support
- Transfer to hospital

## RESPIRATORY ARREST

**Cause:**
- Respiratory obstruction
- Drug overdose
- Allergic reaction
- Cessation of breathing

**Symptoms:**
- Change in pattern of breathing to possible cessation of respirations
- Patient unable to breathe
- Cyanosis

**Treatment:**
- Place patient in supine position with firm back support
- Maintain airway
- Give oxygen and artificially ventilate
- Administer Narcan® 1 mL if due to narcotic depression
- Give CPR, if necessary
- Transfer to hospital

## ANGINA PECTORIS

**Cause:**
- Insufficient blood supply to cardiac muscle

- May be precipitated by stress and anxiety

**Symptoms:**

- Pain in chest
- Vital signs satisfactory
- Patient history of angina; pain persists 3-5 minutes

**Treatment:**

- Position patient semi-reclining
- Administer oxygen
- Administer nitroglycerin 1/150 gr sublingually (may be repeated in 5 minutes)
- Reassure patient
- If history of angina or pain does not subside, suspect myocardial infarction

## MYOCARDIAL INFARCTION

**Cause:** Occlusion of coronary vessels

**Symptoms:**

- Severe pain in chest which may radiate to neck, shoulder, and jaws
- Palpitations, tachycardia
- Dyspnea
- Cyanosis
- Diaphoresis
- Weakness
- Feeling of impending doom
- Pulse thready

**Treatment:**

- Position patient semi-reclining with firm back support
- Administer oxygen
- Reassure patient
- Inject morphine sulfate 10-15 mg I.M. or Demerol® 75-100 mg for pain
- Start I.V. fluids 1000 $D_5W$ or Ringer's lactate
- Transfer to hospital

**Management of Special Complications**

- Arrhythmias: Do not administer drugs unless EKG is on site
- Sudden death: Administer CPR
- Transfer to hospital; accompany patient in ambulance

## CARDIAC ARREST

A sudden emergency due to either actual standstill (asystole) or ventricular fibrillation with ineffective contractions; respiratory arrest may follow

**Signs & symptoms:**

- Collapse of blood pressure
- Dilated pupils
- Ashen skin
- No peripheral pulse
- Possible loss of respiration

## DENTAL OFFICE EMERGENCIES *(Continued)*

- No heart sounds

**Treatment:** CPR

- Slap anterior left chest briskly, only if you witness the arrest
- Place patient in supine position with firm back support
- Make sure airway is open; suction mouth and pharynx; intubate, if necessary
- Closed chest cardiac massage 60/minute (CPR - adult)
- Give oxygen under positive pressure with AMBU resuscitator up to 8 L/minute
- If no AMBU or tracheal tube available, give 4 breaths (mouth to mouth); then start closed chest cardiac compression (60/minute)
- Start I.V. sodium bicarbonate I.V. 44.6 mEq (children: half the dose)
- Monitor EKG
- If in ventricular fibrillation: Defibrillate 200-400 watt/second (start at 200, if no result, move up to higher voltage)
- Keep patient warm
- Epinephrine 0.5 mL I.V. 1:1000 in 10 mL of saline
- Repeat sodium bicarbonate unless blood is pH normal
- May need other drugs (ie, $CaCl_2$, atropine, etc)

Transvenous pacemaker may be needed to reinitiate heartbeat
Possible open chest massage (very few indications and may not be any more effective than closed massage)

## INSULIN SHOCK

**Cause:** Hypoglycemia or hyperinsulinism

**Symptoms:**

- Nervousness
- Confusion
- Profuse sweating
- Sudden onset
- Drooling from mouth
- Full and bounding pulse
- Convulsions
- Moist, pale skin
- Coma

**Treatment:**

- Administer oral sugar with orange juice
- If unconscious, administer 50% dextrose I.V.

## DIABETIC ACIDOSIS

**Cause:** Hyperglycemia, insufficient insulin in the body to metabolize carbohydrates and fats, acidosis

**Symptoms:**

- Gradual onset
- Dry, flushed skin
- Dry mouth, intense thirst
- Exaggerated respirations (Kussmaul)
- Confusion
- Disoriented
- Stuporous
- Sweet breath
- Coma

**Treatment:**

- Call for medical assistance
- Position patient semi-reclining
- Maintain airway, administer oxygen
- Start I.V. and administer lactated Ringer's
- Keep warm
- Administer basic life support
- Transfer to hospital

## ADRENAL INSUFFICIENCY

**Cause:** Insufficient corticosteroid output during a stimulus such as a stressful dental situation or infection

**Symptoms:**

- Weakness
- Pallor
- Cardiovascular attack
- Perspiration
- Thready, rapid pulse

**Treatment:**

- Administer oxygen
- Send for medical assistance
- Administer Decadron® 4 mg I.V. to adults, 1-4 mg I.V. to children

# SUGGESTED READINGS

## ANTIBIOTIC PROPHYLAXIS

See listing at the back of the chapter.

## CANCER

American Cancer Society, *Cancer Facts and Figures* 1995, Atlanta, GA.

American Cancer Society, *Cancer Manual,* 8th ed, American Cancer Society, Boston, MA Division, 1990.

Barasch A, Gofa A, Krutchkoff DJ, et al, "Squamous Cell Carcinoma of the Gingiva. A Case Series Analysis," *Oral Surg Oral Med Oral Pathol Oral Radiol Endod,*, 1995, 80(2):183-7.

Carl W, "Oral Complications of Local and Systemic Cancer Treatment," *Curr Opin Oncol,* 1995, 7(4):320-4.

Chambers MS, Toth BB, Martin JW, et al, "Oral and Dental Management of the Cancer Patient: Prevention and Treatment of Complications," *Support Care Cancer,* 1995, 3(3):168-75.

Hobson RS and Clark JD, "Management of the Orthodontic Patient 'At Risk' From Infective Endocarditis," *Br Dent J,* 1995, 179(2):48.

Jullien JA, Downer MC, Zakrzewska JM, et al, "Evaluation of a Screening Test for the Early Detection of Oral Cancer and Precancer," *Community Dent Health,* 1995, 12(1):3-7.

Messer NC, Yant WR, and Archer RD, "Developing Provider Partnerships in the Detection of Oral Cancer and the Prevention of Smokeless Tobacco Use," *Md Med J,* 1995, 44(10):788-91.

National Institutes of Health, Consensus Development Conference on Oral Complications of Cancer Therapies: Diagnosis, Prevention, and Treatment. NCI Monograph No. 9 U.S. Public Health Service, Washington, DC: U.S. Government Printing Office, 1990.

National Institutes of Health, Consensus Development Conference on Oral Complications of Cancer Therapies: Diagnosis, Prevention, and Treatment. (Final Conference Statement and Recommendations), *J Am Dent Assoc,* 1989, 119(1):179-83.

Partridge M and Langdon JD, "Oral Cancer: A Serious and Growing Problem," *Ann R Coll Surg Engl,* 1995, 77(5):321-2.

Peterson DE and Sonis ST, eds, *Oral Complications of Cancer Chemotherapy,* Boston, MA: Martinus and Nijhoff, 1983.

Peterson DE, Elias EG, and Sonis ST, eds, *Head and Neck Management of the Cancer Patient,* Boston, MA: Martinus and Nijhoff Publishers, 1986.

Sandmann BJ, Sokol SA, and Buck GW, "Formulation and Stability of an Oral Mouthwash to Treat Symptoms of Mucositis," *Int Pharm Abstracts,* 1996, 33(1).

Shaffer J and Wexler LF, "Reducing Low-Density Lipoprotein Cholesterol Levels in an Ambulatory Care System. Results of Multidisciplinary Collaborative Practice Lipid Clinic Compared With Traditional Physician-Based Care," *Arch Int Med,* 1995, 155(21):2330-5.

Silverman S, *Oral Cancer,* 3rd ed, Atlanta, GA: American Cancer Society, 1990.

Takinami S, Yahata H, Kanoshima A, et al, "Hepatocellular Carcinoma Metastatic to the Mandible," *Oral Surg Oral Med Oral Pathol Oral Radiol Endod,* 1995, 79(5):649-54.

Vigneswaran N, Tilashalski K, Rodu B, et al, "Tobacco Use and Cancer. A Reappraisal," *Oral Surg Oral Med Oral Pathol Oral Radiol Endod,* 1995, 80(2):178-82.

## CARDIOVASCULAR

American Dental Association: *ADA Oral Health Care Guidelines: Patients With Cardiovascular Disease,* Chicago, IL: American Dental Association, 1989.

American Heart Association, *Textbook of Advanced Cardiac Life Support,* 2nd ed, American Heart Association, Dallas, TX, 1990.

Assael LA, "Acute Cardiac Care in Dental Practice," *Dent Clin N Am,* 1995, 39(3):555-65.

Dajani AS, Bisno AL, Chung KJ, et al, "Prevention of Bacterial Endocarditis. Recommendations by the American Heart Association," *JAMA,* 1990, 264(22):2919-22.

Giuliani ER, Gersh BJ, McGoon MD, et al, *Mayo Clinic Practice of Cardiology,* 3rd ed, St Louis, MO: Mosby-Year Book, Inc, 1996, 1698-814.

Gorgia H, et al, "Prevention of Tolerance to Hemodynamic Effects of Nitrates With Concomitant Use of Hydralazine in Patients With Chronic Heart Failure," *J Am Coll Cardiol,* 1995, 26(1):1575-80.

Grey AB, Stapleton JP, Evans MC, et al, "The Effect of the Anti-Estrogen Tamoxifen on Cardiovascular Risk Factors in Normal Postmenopausal Women," *J Clin Endocrinol Metab,* 1995, 80(11):3191-5.

Henning RJ and Grenvik A, *Critical Care Cardiology,* New York, NY: Churchill Livingston, 1989, 233.

Kerpen SJ, Kerpen HO, and Sachs SA, "Mitral Valve Prolapse: A Significant Cardiac Defect in the Development of Infective Endocarditis," *Spec Care Dentist,* 1984, 4(4):158-9.

McDonald CC, Alexander FE, Whyte BW, et al, "Cardiac and Vascular Morbidity in Women Receiving Adjuvant Tamoxifen for Breast Cancer in a Randomised Trial. The Scottish Cancer Trials Breast Group," *BMJ,* 1995, 311(7011):977-80.

Murgatroyd FD and Camm AJ, "Atrial Arrhythmias," *Lancet,* 1993, 341(8856):1317-22.

Naegeli B, Osswald S, Deola M, et al, "Intermittent Pacemaker Dysfunction Caused by Digital Mobile Telephones," *J Am Coll Cardiol,* 1996, 27(6):1471-7.

Pabor M, et al , "Risk of Gastrointestinal Haemorrhage With Calcium Antagonists in Hypertensive Persons Over 67 Years Old," *Lancet,* 1996, 347(20):1061-5.

Pieper SJ and Stanton MS, "Narrow QRS Complex Tachycardias," *Mayo Clin Proc,* 1995, 70(4):371-5.

Pritchett EL, "Management of Atrial Fibrillation," *N Engl J Med,* 1992, 326(19):1264-71.

*Textbook of Advanced Cardiac Life Support,* 2nd ed, Dallas, TX: American Heart Association, 1990.

The Fifth Report of the Joint National Committee on Detection, Evaluation, and Treatment of High Blood Pressure (JNC V), *Arch Intern Med,* 1993, 153(2):154-83.

Tierney LM, McPhee SJ, Papadakis MA, et al, *Current Medical Diagnosis and Treatment,* East Norwalk, CT: Appleton & Lange, 1993.

Williams GH, "Hypertensive Vascular Disease," *Harrison's Principles in Internal Medicine,* 13th ed, Isselbacher KJ, et al, eds, New York, NY: McGraw-Hill, 1994, 1116-31.

## CHEMICAL DEPENDENCY AND SMOKING CESSATION

Abelin T, et al, "Controlled Trial of Transdermal Nicotine Patch in Tobacco Withdrawal," *Lancet,* 1989, 1(1):7-10.

Alterman AI, Droba M, Antelo RE, et al, "Amantadine May Facilitate Detoxification of Cocaine Addicts," *Drug Alcohol Depend,* 1992, 31(1):19-29.

Benowitz NL, Porchet H, Sheiner L, et al, "Nicotine Absorption and Cardiovascular Effects With Smokeless Tobacco Use: Comparison With Cigarettes and Nicotine Gum," *Clin Pharmacol Ther,* 1988, 44(1):23-8.

Buchkremer G, Bents H, Horstmann M, et al, "Combination of Behavioral Smoking Cessation and Transdermal Nicotine Substitution," *Addict Behav,* 1989, 14(2):229-38.

## SUGGESTED READINGS *(Continued)*


Ciancio SG, ed, *ADA Guide to Dental Therapeutics,* 1st ed, Chicago, IL: ADA Publishing Co, 1998.

Cowan FF, "Dentists Prescribe Nicotine Substitutes, in Just the Right Dose," *AGD Impact,* 1993, 12(2):11.

Daughton DM, Heatley SA, Prendergast JJ, et al, "Effect of Transdermal Nicotine Delivery as an Adjunct to Low-Intervention Smoking Cessation Therapy," *Arch Int Med,* 1991, 151(4):749-52.

DSM IV, *Diagnostic and Statistical Manual of Mental Disorders,* 4th ed, Washington DC: American Psychiatric Association, 1994.

Fagerstrom KO, "Measuring Degree of Physical Dependence to Tobacco Smoking With Reference to Individualization of Treatment," *Addict Behav,* 1978, 3(3-4):235-41.

Fiester S, Goldstein M, Resnick M, et al, "Practice Guideline for the Treatment of Patients With Nicotine Dependence," *Am J Psych,* 1996, 15(10):Supplement 31.

Gariti P, Auriacombe M, Incmikoski R, et al, "A Randomized Double-Blind Study of Neuroelectric Therapy in Opiate and Cocaine Detoxification," *J Subst Abuse,* 1992, 4(3):299-308.

Henningfield JE, "Nicotine Medications for Smoking Cessation," *N Engl J Med,* 1995, 333(18):1196-203.

Herkenham MA, "Localization of Cannabinoid Receptors in Brain: Relationship to Motor and Reward Systems," *Biological Basis of Substance Abuse,* Korenman SG and Barchas JD, eds, New York, NY: Oxford University Press, 1993, 187-200.

Higgins ST, Budney AJ, Bickel WK, et al, "Outpatient Behavioral Treatment for Cocaine Dependence: One-Year Outcome," Problems of Drug Dependence Symposium, College. 1994.

Hurt RD, Finlayson RE, Morse RM, et al, "Nicotine-Replacement Therapy With Use of a Transdermal Nicotine Patch - A Randomized Double-Blind Placebo Controlled Trial," *Mayo Clin Proc,* 1990, 65(12):1529-37.

Kreek MJ, "Rationale for Maintenance Pharmacotherapy of Opiate Dependence," O'Brien CP and Barchas JD, eds, *Addictive States,* New York, NY: Raven Press, 1992, 205-30.

Krumpe P, "Efficacy of Transdermal Nicotine Administration as an Adjunct for Smoking Cessation in Heavily Nicotine Addicted Smokers," *Am Rev Respir Dis,* 1989, 139(1):A377.

Leshner AI, "Molecular Mechanisms of Cocaine Addiction," *N Engl J Med,* 1996, 335(2):128-9.

Li Wan Po A, "Transdermal Nicotine in Smoking Cessation: A Meta-analysis" *Eur J Clin Pharmacol,* 1993, 45(6):519-28.

Mendelson JH and Mello NK, "Management of Cocaine Abuse and Dependence," *N Engl J Med,* 1996, 334(15):965-72.

Mulligan SC, Masterson JG, Devane JG, et al, "Clinical and Pharmacokinetic Properties of a Transdermal Nicotine Patch," *Clin Pharmacol Ther,* 1990, 47(3):331-7.

Nowak R, "Nicotine Scrutinized as FDA Seeks to Regulate Cigarettes," *Science,* 1994, 263(5153):1555-6.

O'Brien CP, "Drug Addiction and Drug Abuse," *The Pharmacological Basis of Therapeutics,* 9th ed, Molinoff PB and Ruddon R, eds, New York, NY: McGraw-Hill, 1996, 557-77.

O'Brien CP, "Treatment of Alcoholism as a Chronic Disorder," *Toward a Molecular Basis of Alcohol Use and Abuse,* Jansson B, Jornvall H, Rydberg U, et al, eds, Basel, Switzerland: Birkhauser Verlag, 1994, Vol 71, EXS, 349-59.

Ostrowski DJ and DeNelsky GY, "Pharmacologic Management of Patients Using Smoking Cessation Aids," *Dental Clin North Am,* 1996, 40(3):779-801.

Rose JE, Levin ED, Behm FM, et al, "Transdermal Nicotine Facilitates Smoking Cessation," *Clin Pharmacol Ther,* 1990, 47(3):323-30.

Sachs DPL, et al, "Effectiveness of a 16-Hour Transdermal Nicotine Patch in a Medical Practice Setting Without Intensive Group Counseling," *Arch Intern Med,* 1993, 153(1):1881-90.

Schneider NG, Olmstead R, Nilsson F, et al, "Efficacy of a Nicotine Inhaler in Smoking Cessation: A Double-Blind, Placebo-Controlled Trial," *Addiction,* 1996, 91(9):1293-306.

Self DW, Barnhart WJ, Lehman DA, et al, "Opposite Modulation of Cocaine-Seeking Behavior by D1- and D2-Like Dopamine Receptor Agonists," *Science,* 1996, 271(5255):1586-9.

The Smoking Cessation Clinical Practice Guideline Panel and Staff, The Agency for Health Care Policy and Research Smoking Cessation Clinical Practice Guideline, *JAMA,* 1996, 275(1):1270-80.

Tonnesen P, Norregaard J, Simonsen K, et al, "A Double-Blind Trial of a 16-Hour Transdermal Nicotine Patch in Smoking Cessation," *N Engl J Med,* 1991, 325(5):311-5.

Transdermal Nicotine Group, "Transdermal Nicotine for Smoking Cessation. Six-Month Results From Two Multicenter Controlled Clinical Trials," *JAMA,* 1991, 266(22):3133-8.

## DIAGNOSIS AND MANAGEMENT OF PAIN

Beckett D, "Topical Guanethidine Relieves Dental Hypersensitivity and Pain," *J R Soc Med,* 1995, 88(1):60.

Berthold CW, Schneider A, and Dionne RA, "Using Triazolam to Reduce Dental Anxiety," *J Am Dent Assoc,* 1993, 124(11):58-64.

Brown RS, Hinderstein B, Reynolds DC, et al, "Using Anesthetic Localization to Diagnose Oral and Dental Pain," *J Am Dent Assoc,* 1995, 126(5):633-4, 637-41.

Coderre TJ, Katz J, Vaccarino AL, et al, "Contribution of Central Neuroplasticity to Pathological Pain: Review of Clinical and Experimental Evidence," *Pain,* 1993, 52(3):259-85.

Delcanho RE and Graff-Radford SB, "Chronic Paroxysmal Hemicrania Presenting as Toothache," *J Orofacial Pain,* 1993, 7:300.

Denson DD and Katz JA, "Nonsteroidal Anti-inflammatory Agents," *Practical Management of Pain,* 2nd ed, PP Raj, ed, St Louis, MO: Mosby Year Book, 1992.

Forbes JA, Butterworth GA, Burchfield WH, et al, "Evaluation of Ketorolac, Aspirin, and an Acetaminophen-Codeine Combination in Postoperative Oral Surgery Pain," *Pharmacotherapy,* 1990, 10(6 Pt 2):77S-93S.

Graff-Radford SB, "Headache Problems That Can Present as Toothache," *Dent Clin North Am,* 1991, 35(1):155-70.

Harvey M and Elliott M, "Transcutaneous Electrical Nerve Stimulation (TENS) for Pain Management During Cavity Preparations in Pediatric Patients," *ASDC J Dent Child,* 1995, 62(1):49-51.

Henry G, "Postoperative Pain Experience With Flurbiprofen and Acetaminophen With Codeine," *J Dent Res,* 1992, 71:952.

Jaffe JH and Martin WR, "Opioid Analgesic and Antagonists," *The Pharmacological Basis of Therapeutics,* 8th ed, Gilman AG, Rall TW, Nies AD, et al, eds, New York, NY: Maxwell Pergamon MacMillan Publishing, 1990.

Kalso E and Vainio A, "Morphine and Oxycodone Hydrochloride in the Management of Cancer Pain," *Clin Pharmacol Ther,* 1990, 47(5):639-46.

Lee AG, "A Case Report. Jaw Claudication: A Sign of Giant Cell Arteritis," *J Am Dent Assoc,* 1995, 126(7):1028-9.

McQuay H, Carroll D, Jadad AR, et al, "Anticonvulsant Drugs for Management of Pain: A Systemic Review," *BMJ,* 1995, 311(7012):1047-52.

## SUGGESTED READINGS *(Continued)*


Olin BR, Hebel SK, Connell SI, et al, *Drug Facts and Comparisons,* 1993, St Louis, MO: Facts and Comparisons, Inc.

Pendeville PE, Van Boven MJ, Contreras V, et al, "Ketorolac Tromethamine for Postoperative Analgesia in Oral Surgery," *Acta Anaesthesiol Belg,* 1995, 46(1):25-30.

Robertson S, Goodell H, and Wolff HG, "The Teeth as a Source of Headache and Other Pain," *Arch Neurol Psychiatry,* 1947, 57:277.

Sandler NA, Ziccardi V, and Ochs M, "Differential Diagnosis of Jaw Pain in the Elderly," *J Am Dent Assoc* 1995, 126(9):1263-72.

Scully C, Eveson JW, and Porter SR, "Munchausen's Syndrome: Oral Presentations," *Br Dent J,* 1995, 178(2):65-7.

Seng GF, Kraus K, Cartwright G, et al, "Confirmed Allergic Reactions to Amide Local Anesthetics," *Gen Dent,* 1996, 44(1):52-4.

Ship JA, Grushka M, Lipton JA, et al, "Burning Mouth Syndrome: An Update" *J Am Dent Assoc,* 1995, 126(7):842-53.

Wright EF and Schiffman EL, "Treatment Alternatives for Patients With Masticatory Myofascial Pain," *J Am Dent Assoc,* 1995, 126(7):1030-9.


## HIV INFECTION AND AIDS


Borrow P, Lewicki H, Hahn BH, et al, "Virus-Specific CD8+ Cytotoxic T-Lymphocyte Activity Associated With Control of Viremia in Primary Human Immunodeficiency Virus Type I Infection," *J Virol,* 1994, 68(9):6103-9.

Brookmeyer R and Gail MH, "AIDS Epidemiology: A Quantitative Approach," New York, NY: Oxford Press, 1994.

Center for Disease Control (CDC), CfDC. "Update: AIDS Cases in Males Who Have Sex With Males," *MMWR Morb Mortal Wkly Rep,* 1995, 44(29):401-2.

Center for Disease Control (CDC), CfDC. "First 500,000 AIDS Cases," *MMWR Morb Mortal Wkly Rep,* 1995, 44(46):849-53.

Center for Disease Control (CDC), CfDC. "Update: HIV Exposures in HCWs," *MMWR Morb Mortal Wkly Rep,* 1995, 44(50):929.

Center for Disease Control (CDC), CfDCaP. "Recommended Infection-Control Practices for Dentistry," *MMWR Morb Mortal Wkly Rep,* 1993, 42(RR-8).

Center for Disease Control (CDC), CfDCaP. "Revised Classification System for HIV Infection and Expanded Surveillance Case Definition for AIDS Among Adolescents and Adults," *MMWR Morb Mortal Wkly Rep,* 1993, 41(RR-17).

Council on Dental Materials I, and Equipment, Therapeutics CoD, Research CoD, Practice CoD, "Infection Control Recommendations for the Dental Office and the Dental Laboratory," *J Am Dent Assoc,* 1992, 123(8).

El-Sadr W, Oleske JM, Agins BD, et al, "Evaluation and Management of Early HIV Infection," Agency for Health Care Policy and Research, Public Health Service, US Department of Health and Human Services, 1994 Clinical Practice Guideline No. 7, ACHPR Publication No. 94-0572, Rockville, MD.

Glick M, *Dental Management of Patients With HIV,* Chicago, IL: Quintessence Publishing Co, 1994.

Glick M and Silverman S, "Dental Management of HIV-Infected Patients," *J Am Dent Assoc* (Supplement to Reviewers), 1995.

Glick M, *Clinicians Guide to Treatment of HIV-Infected Patients,* Academy of Oral Medicine, 1996.

Greenspan D, Greenspan JS, Schiodt M, et al, *AIDS and the Mouth,* Munksgaard, Copenhagen, 1990.

Greenspan JS and Greenspan D, "Oral Manifestations of HIV Infection," *The Proceedings of the Second International Workshop,* Chicago, IL: Quintessence Publishing Co, 1995.

"Oral Health Care for Adults With HIV Infection," New York, NY: AIDS Institute, New York State Department of Health, 1993.

Little JW, Melnick SL, Rhame FS, et al, "Prevalence of Oral Lesions in Symptomatic and Asymptomatic HIV Patients," *Gen Dent*, 1994, 42(5):446-50.

Silverman S, *Color Atlas of Oral Manifestations of AIDS*, 2nd ed, St Louis, MO: Mosby, 1996.

Travers K, Souleymane M, Mrlink R, et al, "Natural Protection Against HIV-1 Provided by HIV-2," *Science*, 1995, 268(5219):1833.

Weiss R, "The Virus and Its Target Cells," Broder S, Merigan T, Bolognesis D, eds, *Textbook of AIDS Medicine*, Baltimore, MD: Williams & Wilkins, 1994.

Zeitlen S and Shaha A, "Parotid Manifestations of HIV Infection," *J Surg Oncol*, 1991, 47(4):230-2.

## NATURAL PRODUCTS, HERBALS, AND DIETARY SUPPLEMENTS

*1995 Martindale - The Extra Pharmacopoeia*, Vol 86, Roy Pharm Soc, GB, 1996.

Castleman M, *The Healing Herbs: The Ultimate Guide to the Curative Power of Nature's Medicines*, Rodale Press, Emmaus, 1991.

Lust J, *The Herb Book*, New York, NY: Benedict Lust Publications, 1974.

Mistry MG and Mays DA, "Precautions Against Global Use of Natural Products for Weight Loss: A Review of Active Ingredients and Issues Concerning Concomitant Disease States," *Therapeutic Perspectives*, 1996, 10(1):2.

Murray M and Pizzorno J, *Encyclopedia of Natural Medicine*, Prima Publishing, 1991.

Olin BR, Hebel SK, Connell SI, et al, *Drug Facts and Comparisons*, St Louis, MO: Facts and Comparisons, Inc, 1993.

Polunin M and Robbins C, *The Natural Pharmacy*, New York, NY: MacMillan Publishing, 1992.

Tyler VF, *The Honest Herbal: A Sensible Guide to the Use of Herbs and Related Remedies*, Birmingham, AL: The Hawthorn Press, Inc, 1993.

## ORAL INFECTIONS

Baron EJ and Finegold SM, eds, "Gram-Negative Cocci (*Neisseria* and *Branhamella*)," Bailey and Scott's Diagnostic Microbiology, St Louis, MO: Mosby Year Book, 1990.

Borssen E and Sundquist G, "Actinomycosis of Infected Dental Root Canals," *Oral Surg Oral Med Oral Pathol*, 1981, 51(1):643-7.

1993 Sexually Transmitted Diseases Treatment Guidelines, Centers for Disease Control and Prevention, *MMWR Morb Mortal Wkly Rep*, 1993, 42(RR-14):1-102.

Chow AW, "Infections of the Oral Cavity, Neck, and Head," *Principles and Practice of Infectious Diseases*, 4th ed, Mandell GL, Bennett JE, Dolin R, eds, New York, NY: Churchill Livingstone, 1995, 593-605.

Crockett DN, O'Grady JF, and Reade PC, "*Candida* Species and *Candida albicans* Morphotypes in Erythematous Candidiasis, "*Oral Surg Oral Med Oral Pathol*, 1992, 73(5):559-63.

Dajani A, Taubert K, Ferrieri P, et al, "Treatment of Acute Streptococcal Pharyngitis and Prevention of Rheumatic Fever: A Statement for Health Professionals," *Pediatrics*, 1995, 96(4):758-64.

Diz Dios P, Ocampo Hermida A, Miralles Alvarez C, et al, "Fluconazole-Resistant Oral Candidiasis in HIV-Infected Patients," *AIDS*, 1995, 9(7):809-10.

Dobson RL, "Antimicrobial Therapy for Cutaneous Infections," *J Am Acad Dermatol*, 1990, 22(5):871-3.

Ferris DG, Litaker MS, Woodward L, et al, "Treatment of Bacterial Vaginosis: A Comparison of Oral Metronidazole, Metronidazole Vaginal Gel, and Clindamycin Vaginal Cream," *J Fam Pract*, 1995, 41(5):443-9.

## SUGGESTED READINGS *(Continued)*


Fox RI, Luppi M, Kang HI, et al, "Reactivation of Epstein-Barr Virus in Sjögren's Syndrome," *Springer Semin Immunopathol,* 1991, 13(2):217-31.

Giunta JL and Fiumara NJ, "Facts About Gonorrhea and Dentistry," *Oral Surg Oral Med Oral Pathol,* 1986, 62(5):529-31.

Goldberg MH and Topazian R, "Odontogenic Infections and Deep Facial Space Infections of Dental Origin," *Oral and Maxillofacial Infections,* 3rd ed, Philadelphia, PA: WB Saunders, 1994, 232-6.

Goulden V and Goodfield MJ, "Treatment of Childhood Dermatophyte Infections With Oral Terbinafine," *Pediatr Dermatol,* 1995, 12(1):53-4.

"Cefadroxil in the Management of Facial Cellulitis of Odontogenic Origin," *Oral Surg Oral Med Oral Pathol,* 1991, 71(4):496-8.

Hook EW 3d and Marra CM, "Acquired Syphilis in Adults," *N Engl J Med,* 1992, 326(16):1060-9.

Larsen PE, "Alveolar Osteitis After Surgical Removal of Impacted Mandibular Third Molars. Identification of the Patient at Risk," *Oral Surg Oral Med Oral Pathol,* 1992, 73(4):393-7.

Lewis MA, Parkhurst CL, Douglas CW, et al, "Prevalence of Penicillin Resistant Bacteria in Acute Suppurative Oral Infection," *J Antimicrob Chemother,* 1995, 35(6):785-91.

Musher DM, Hamill RJ, and Baughn RE, "Effect of Human Immunodeficiency Virus (HIV) Infection on the Course of Syphilis and on the Response to Treatment," *Ann Intern Med,* 1990, 113(11):872-81.

Muzyka BC and Glick M, "A Review of Oral Fungal Infections and Appropriate Therapy," *J Am Dent Assoc,* 1995, 126(1):63-72.

Namavar F, Roosendaal R, Kuipers EJ, et al, "Presence of *Helicobacter pylori* in the Oral Cavity, Oesophagus, Stomach and Faeces of Patients With Gastritis," *Eur J Clin Microbiol Infect Dis* 1995, 14(4):234-7.

Nguyen AM, el-Zaatari FA, and Graham DY, "*Helicobacter pylori* in the Oral Cavity. A Critical Review of the Literature," *Oral Surg Oral Med Oral Pathol Oral Radiol Endod,* 1995, 79(6):705-9.

Pogrel MA, "Complications of Third Molar Surgery," *J Oral Maxillofac Surg,* 1990, 2(1):441-8.

Schiodt M, "HIV-Associated Salivary Gland Disease: A Review," *Oral Surg Oral Med Oral Pathol,* 1992, 73(2):164-7.

Sjögren U, Figdor L, Spangberg, et al, "The Antimicrobial Effect of Calcium Hydroxide as a Short-Term Intracanal Dressing," *Int Endod,* 1991, 24(3):119-24.

Talal N, Dauphinee MJ, Dang H, et al, "Detection of Serum Antibodies to Retroviral Proteins in Patients With Primary Sjögren's Syndrome (Autoimmune Exocrinopathy)," *Arthritis Rheum,* 1990, 33(6):774-81.

Torabinejad M, Kettering JD, McGraw JC, et al, "Factors Associated With Endodontic Interappointment Emergencies of Teeth With Necrotic Pulps," *J Endod,* 1988, 14(5):261-6.

Walton R and Fouad A, "Endodontic Interappointment Flare-Ups: A Prospective Study of Incidence and Related Factors," *J Endod,* 1992, 18(4):172-7.

Wheeler TT, Alberts MA, Dolan TA, et al, "Dental, Visual, Auditory and Olfactory Complications in Paget's Disease of Bone," *J Am Geriatr Soc,* 1995, 43(12):1384-91.

Williams JW Jr, Holleman DR Jr, Samsa GP, et al, "Randomized Controlled Trial of 3 vs 10 Days of Trimethoprim/Sulfamethoxazole for Acute Maxillary Sinusitis," *JAMA,* 1995, 273(13):1015-21.

Wormser GP, "Lyme Disease: Insights Into the Use of Antimicrobials for Prevention and Treatment in the Context of Experience With Other Spirochetal Infections," *Mt Sinai J Med,* 1995, 62(3):188-95.

## ORAL LEUKOPLAKIA

Barker JN, Mitra RS, Griffiths CE, et al, "Keratinocytes as Initiators of Inflammation," *Lancet,* 1991, 337(8735):211-4.

Belton CM and Eversole LR, "Oral Hairy Leukoplakia: Ultrastructural Features," *J Oral Pathol,* 1986, 15(9):493-9.

Boehncke WH, Kellner I, Konter U, et al, "Differential Expression of Adhesion Molecules on Infiltrating Cells in Inflammatory Dermatoses," *J Am Acad Dermatol,* 1992, 26(6):907-13.

Chou MJ and Daniels TE, "Langerhans Cells Expressing HLA-DQ, HLA-DR, and T6 Antigens in Normal Oral Mucosa and Lichen Planus," *J Oral Pathol Med,* 1989, 18(10):573-6.

Corso B, Eversole LR, and Hutt-Fletcher L, "Hairy Leukoplakia: Epstein-Barr Virus Receptors on Oral Keratinocyte Plasma Membranes," *Oral Surg Oral Med Oral Pathol,* 1989, 67(4):416-21.

Eisen D, Ellis CN, Duell EA, et al, "Effect of Topical Cyclosporine Rinse on Oral Lichen Planus. A Double-Blind Analysis," *N Engl J Med,* 1990, 323(5):290-4.

Greenspan D, Greenspan JS, Overby G, et al, "Risk Factors for Rapid Progression From Hairy Leukoplakia to AIDS: A Nested Case-Control Study, *J Acquir Immune Defic Syndr,* 1991, 4(7):652-8.

Regezi JA, Stewart JC, Lloyd RV, et al, "Immunohistochemical Staining of Langerhans Cells and Macrophages in Oral Lichen Planus," *Oral Surg Oral Med Oral Pathol,* 1985, 60(4):396-402.

Sciubba JJ, "Oral Leukoplakia," *Crit Rev Oral Biol Med,* 1995, 6(2):147-60.

## ORAL SOFT TISSUE DISEASES

Anhalt GJ, "Pemphigoid: Bullous and Cicatricial," *Dermatol Clin,* 1990, 8(4):701-16.

Berk MA and Lorincz AL, "The Treatment of Bullous Pemphigoid With Tetracycline and Niacinamide. A Preliminary Report," *Arch Dermatol,* 1986, 122(6):670-4.

Den Besten P and Giambro N, "Treatment of Fluorosed and White-Spot Human Enamel With Calcium Sucrose Phosphate *in vitro,*"*Pediatr Dent* 1995, 17(5):340-5.

Firth NA and Reade PC, "Angiotensin-Converting Enzyme Inhibitors Implicated in Oral Mucosal Lichenoid Reactions," *Oral Surg Oral Med Oral Pathol,* 1989, 67(1):41-4.

Fritz KA and Weston WL, "Topical Glucocorticosteroids," *Ann Allergy,* 1983, 50(2):68-76.

Gallant C and Kenny P, "Oral Glucocorticoids and Their Complications. A Review," *J Am Acad Dermatol,* 1986, 14(2):161-77.

Goupil MT, "Occupational Health and Safety Emergencies," *Dent Clin North Am,* 1995, 39(3):637-47.

Grady D, Ernster VL, Stillman L, et al, "Smokeless Tobacco Use Prevents Aphthous Stomatitis," *Oral Surg Oral Med Oral Pathol,* 1992, 74(4):463-5.

Hamuryudan V, Yurdakul S, Serdaroglu S, et al, "Topical Alpha Interferon in the Treatment of Oral Ulcers in Behcet's Syndrome: A Preliminary Report," *Clin Exp Rheumatol,* 1990, 8(1):51-4.

Hoover CI, Olson JA, and Greenspan JS, "Humoral Responses and Cross-Reactivity to Viridans Streptococci in Recurrent Aphthous Ulceration," *J Dent Res,* 1986, 65(8):1101-4.

Jungell P, "Oral Lichen Planus: A Review," *Int J Oral Maxillofac Surg,* 1991, 20(3):129-35.

Lindemann RA, Riviere GR, and Sapp JP, "Oral Mucosal Antigen Reactivity During Exacerbation and Remission Phases of Recurrent Aphthous Ulceration," *Oral Surg Oral Med Oral Pathol,* 1985, 60(3):281-4.

MacPhail LA, Greenspan D, Greenspan JS, et al, "Recurrent Aphthous Ulcers in Association With HIV Infection. Diagnosis and Treatment," *Oral Surg Oral Med Oral Pathol,* 1992, 73(3):283-8.

## SUGGESTED READINGS *(Continued)*

Meiller TF, Kutcher MJ, Overholser CD, et al, "Effect of an Antimicrobial Mouthrinse on Recurrent Aphthous Ulcerations," *Oral Surg Oral Med Oral Pathol,* 1991, 72(4):425-9.

Moncarz V, Ulmansky M, and Lustmann J, "Lichen Planus: Exploring Its Malignant Potential," *J Am Dent Assoc,* 1993, 124(3):102-8.

Pederson A, Klausen B, Hougen P, et al, "T-Lymphocyte Subsets in Recurrent Aphthous Ulceration," *J Oral Pathol Med,* 1989, 18(1):59-60.

Porter SR, Scully C, and Flint S, "Hematological Status in Recurrent Aphthous Stomatitis Compared With Other Oral Disease," *Oral Surg Oral Med Oral Pathol,* 1988, 66(1):41-4.

Porter SR, Scully C, and Midda M, "Adult Linear Immunoglobulin, A Disease Manifesting as Desquamative Gingivitis," *Oral Surg Oral Med Oral Pathol,* 1990, 70(4):450-3.

Rodu B and Mattingly G, "Oral Mucosal Ulcers: Diagnosis and Management," *J Am Dent Assoc,* 1992, 123(10):83-6.

Rothman KJ, "Teratogenicity of High Vitamin A Intake," *N Engl J Med,* 1995, 333(21):1414-5.

Savage NW, "Oral Ulceration. Assessment of Treatment of Commonly Encountered Oral Ulcerative Disease," *Aust Fam Physician,* 1988, 17(4):247-50.

Schiodt M, Holmstrup P, Dabelsteen E, et al, "Deposits of Immunoglobulins, Complement, and Fibrinogen in Oral Lupus Erythematosus, Lichen Planus, and Leukoplakia," *Oral Surg Oral Med Oral Pathol,* 1981, 51(6):603-8.

Scully C and Porter S, "Recurrent Aphthous Stomatitis: Current Concepts of Etiology, Pathogenesis, and Management," *J Oral Pathol Med,* 1989, 18(1):21-7.

Shiohara T, Moriya N, Mochizuki T, et al, "Lichenoid Tissue Reaction (LTR) Induced by Local Transfer of Ia-Reactive T-cell Clones: LTR by Epidermal Invasion of Cytotoxic Lymphokine-Producing Autoreactive T Cells," *J Invest Dermatol,* 1987, 89(1):8-14.

Shohat-Zabarski R, Kalderon S, Klein T, et al, "Close Association of HLA-B51 in Persons With Recurrent Aphthous Stomatitis," *Oral Surg Oral Med Oral Pathol,* 1992, 74(4):455-8.

Van Dis ML and Vincent SD, "Diagnosis and Management of Autoimmune and Idiopathic Mucosal Diseases," *Dent Clin North Am,* 1992, 36(4):897-917.

Vincent SD and Lilly GE, "Clinical, Historic, and Therapeutic Features of Aphthous Stomatitis. Literature Review and Open Clinical Trial Employing Steroids," *Oral Surg, Oral Med, Oral Pathol,* 1992, 74(1):79-86.

## ORAL VIRAL DISEASES

Ades AE, Peckham CS, Dale GE, et al, "Prevalence of Antibodies to Herpes Simplex Virus Types 1 and 2 in Pregnant Women, and Estimated Rates of Infection," *J Epidemiol Community Health,* 1989, 43(1):53-60.

Amsterdam JD, Maislin G, and Rybakowski J, "A Possible Antiviral Action of Lithium Carbonate in Herpes Simplex Virus Infections," *Biol Psychiatry,* 1990, 27(4):447-53.

Balfour HH, Rotbart HA, Feldman S, et al, "Acyclovir Treatment of Varicella in Otherwise Healthy Adolescents. The Collaborative Acyclovir Varicella Study Group," *J Pediatr,* 1992, 120(4):627-33.

Carey WD and Patel G, "Viral Hepatitis in the 1990s, Part III, Hepatitis C, Hepatitis E, and Other Viruses," *Cleve Clin J Med,* 1992, 59(6):595-601.

Chang Y, et al, "Identification of Herpesvirus-Like DNA Sequences in AIDS-Associated Kaposi's Sarcoma," *Science,* 1994, 266(5192):1865-9.

Corey L and Spear PG, "Infections With Herpes Simplex Viruses," *N Engl J Med,* 1986, 314(11):686-91, 749-57.

Dolin R, "Antiviral Chemotherapy and Chemoprophylaxis," *Science,* 1985, 227(4692):1296-303.

Ficarra G and Shillitoe EJ, "HIV-Related Infections of the Oral Cavity," *Oral Biol Med,* 1992, 3(3):207-31.

Fiddian AP and Ivanyi L, "Topical Acyclovir in the Management of Recurrent *Herpes labialis,*" *Br J Dermatol* 1983, 109(3):321-6.

Gupta S, Govindarajan S, Cassidy WM, et al, "Acute Delta Hepatitis: Serological Diagnosis With Particular Reference to Hepatitis Delta Virus RNA," *Am J Gastroenterol,* 1991, 86(9):1227-31.

Huff JC, Bean B, Balfour HH Jr, et al, "Therapy of Herpes Zoster With Oral Acyclovir ," *Am J Med,* 1988, 85(2A):84-9.

Johnson RJ, Gretch DR, and Yamabe H, "Membranoproliferative Glomerulonephritis Associated With Hepatitis C Virus Infection," *N Engl J Med,* 1993, 328(7):505-6.

Markowitz M, et al, "A Preliminary Study of Ritonavir, an Inhibitor of HIV-1 Protease, to Treat HIV-1 Infection," *N Engl J Med,* 1995, 333(23):1534-9.

McCreary C, Bergin C, Pilkington R, et al, "Clinical Parameters Associated With Recalcitrant Oral Candidiasis in HIV Infection: A Preliminary Study," *Int J STD AIDS,* 1995, 6(3):204-7.

Robinson WS, "Hepatitis B Virus and Hepatitis D Virus," *Principles and Practice of Infectious Disease,* 4th ed, 1995, New York, NY: Churchill Livingstone. 1995.

Roizman B and Sears AE, "An Inquiry Into the Mechanisms of Herpes Simplex Virus Latency," *Annu Rev in Microbiol,* 1987, 41:543-71.

Rooney JF, Bryson Y, Mannix ML, et al, "Prevention of Ultraviolet Light-Induced *Herpes labialis* by Sunscreen," *Lancet* 1991, 338(8780):1419-22.

Snijders PJ, Schulten EA, Mullink H, et al, "Detection of Human Papillomavirus and Epstein-Barr Virus DNA Sequences in Oral Mucosa of HIV-Infected Patients by the Polymerase Chain Reaction," *Am J Pathol,* 1990, 137(3):659-66.

Spruance SL, Stewart JC, Rowe NH, et al, "Treatment of Recurrent Herpes Simplex Labialis With Oral Acyclovir," *J Infect Dis,* 1990, 161(2):185-90.

Whitley RJ, Soong SJ, Dolin R, et al, "Early Vidarabine Therapy to Control the Complications of Herpes Zoster in Immunosuppressed Patients," *N Engl J Med,* 1982, 307(16):971-5.

## PERIODONTAL DISEASE

Beck J, Garcia R, Heiss G, et al, "Periodontal Disease and Cardiovascular Disease," *J Periodontol,* 1996, 67(Suppl 10):S1123-7.

Bollen CM and Quirynen M, "Microbiological Response to Mechanical Treatment in Combination With Adjunctive Therapy. A Review of the Literature," *J Periodontol,* 1996, 67(11):1143-58.

Brecx M, Netuschil L, Reichart B, et al, "Efficacy of Listerine®, Meridol®, and Chlorhexidine Mouthrinses on Plaque, Gingivitis, and Plaque Bacteria Vitality," *J Clin Periodontol,* 1990, 17(1):292-7.

Briner WW, Grossman E, Buckner RY, et al, "Effect of Chlorhexidine Gluconate Mouthrinse on Plaque Bacteria," *J Periodontol Res,* 1986, 21(Suppl 16):S44-52.

Ciancio SG, Mather BS, and Burnell HL, "Clinical Evaluation of a Quaternary Ammonium Compound Containing Mouthrinse," *J Periodontol,* 1975, 46(1):397-401.

Ciancio SG, "Medications at Risk Factors for Periodontal Disease," *J Periodontol,* 1996, 67(Suppl 10):S1055-9.

Committee on Research, Science and Therapy of the American Academy of Periodontology, "Tobacco Use and the Periodontal Patient," *J Periodontol,* 1996, 67(1):51-6.

Committee on Research, Science and Therapy of the American Academy of Periodontology, "Diabetes and Periodontal Disease," *J Periodontol,* 1996, 67(2):166-76.

## SUGGESTED READINGS *(Continued)*


Committee on Research, Science and Therapy of the American Academy of Periodontology, "Periodontal Management of Patients With Cardiovascular Diseases," *J Periodontol,* 1996, 67(6):627-35.

Crout RJ, Lee HM, Schroeder K, et al, "The Cyclic Regimen of Low-Dose Doxycycline for Adult Periodontitis. A Preliminary Study," *J Periodontol,* 1996, 67(5):506-14.

DePaola LG, Overholser CD, Meiller TF, et al, "Chemotherapeutic Inhibition of Supragingival Dental Plaque and Gingivitis Development," *J Clin Periodontol,* 1989, 16(1):311-5.

Genco RJ, "Current View of Risk Factors for Periodontal Diseases," *J Periodontol,* 1996, 67(Suppl 10):S1041-9.

Grassi M, Williams AC, Winkler JR, et al, "Management of HIV-Associated Periodontal Disease," *Oral Manifestation of AIDS,* Robertson PB and Greenspan JS, eds, Littleton, MA: PSG Publishing, 1988, 119-30.

Heaseman PA, Benn DK, Kelly PJ, et al, "The Use of Topical Flurbiprofen as an Adjunct to Nonsurgical Management of Periodontal Disease," *J Clin Periodontol,* 1993, 20(1):457-64.

Hitzig C, Charbit Y, Bitton C, et al, "Topical Metronidazole as an Adjunct to Subgingival Debridement in the Treatment of Chronic Periodontitis," *J Clin Periodontol,* 1994, 21(2):146-51.

Howell TH and Williams RC, "Nonsteroidal Anti-Inflammatory Drugs as Inhibitors of Periodontal Disease Progression," *Crit Rev Oral Biol Med,* 1993, 4(2):177-96.

Kjaerheim V, Skaare A, Barkvoll P, et al, "Antiplaque, Antibacterial, and Anti-Inflammatory Properties of Triclosan Mouthrinses in Combination With Zinc Citrate or Polyvinylmethylether Maleic Acid (PVM-MA) Copolymer," *Eur J Oral Sci,* 1996, 104(5-6):529-34.

Loesche WJ, Giordano J, Soehren S, et al, "Nonsurgical Treatment of Patients With Periodontal Disease," *Oral Surg, Oral Med Oral Pathol,* 1996, 81(5):533-43.

Michalowicz BS, Pihlstrom BL, Drisko CL, et al, "Evaluation of Periodontal Treatments Using Controlled-Release Tetracycline Fibers: Maintenance Response," *J Periodontol,* 1995, 66(8):708-15.

Miller LS, Manwell MA, Newbold D, et al, "The Relationship Between Reduction in Periodontal Inflammation and Diabetes Control. A Report of 9 Cases," *J Periodontol,* 1992, 63(1):843-8.

Misra DN, "Interaction of Chlorhexidine Digluconate With and Adsorption of Chlorhexidine on Hydroxyapatite," *J Biomed Mat Res,* 1994, 28(11):1375-81.

Moran J, Addy M, and Newcombe R, "A Clinical Trial to Assess the Efficacy of Sanguinarine-Zinc Mouthrinse (Viadent®) Compared With Chlorhexidine Mouthrinse (Corsodyl®)," *J Clin Periodontol,* 1988, 15(1):612-6.

Overholser CD, Meiller TF, DePaola LG, et al, "Comparative Effects of 2 Chemotherapeutic Mouthrinses on the Development of Supragingival Dental Plaque and Gingivitis," *J Clin Periodontol,* 1990, 17(1):575-9.

Palomo F, Wantland L, Sanchez A, et al, "The Effect of Three Commercially Available Dentifrices Containing Triclosan on Supragingival Plaque Formation and Gingivitis: A Six Month Clinical Study," *Int Dent J,* 1994, 44(l Suppl 1):75-81.

Pavici MJ, van Winkelhoff AJ, Steures NH, et al, "Microbiological and Clinical Effects of Metronidazole and Amoxicillin in *Actinobacillus actinomycetemcomitans*-Associated Periodontitis. A 2-Year Evaluation," *J Clin Periodontol,* 1994, 21(2):107-12.

Ross NM, Mankodi SM, Mostler KL, et al, "Effects of Rinsing Time on Antiplaque-Antigingivitis Efficacy of Listerine®, *J Clin Periodontol,* 1993, 20(1):279-81.

Sastrowijoto SH, Van der Veiden U, Van Steenburgen TJ, et al, "Improved Metabolic Control, Clinical Periodontal Status and Subgingival Microbiology in

Insulin-Dependent Diabetes Mellitus. A Prospective Study," *J Clin Periodontol*, 1990, 17(1):233-42.

Seymour RA and Heasman PA, "Tetracyclines in the Management of Periodontal Diseases. A Review," *J Clin Periodontol*, 1995, 22(1):22-35.

Seymour RA and Heasman PA, "Pharmacological Control of Periodontal Disease. II. Antimicrobial Agents," *J Dent*, 1995, 23(1):5-14.

Southard GL, Boulware RT, Walbourn DR, et al, "Sanguinarine, A New Antiplaque Agent: Retention and Plaque Specificity," *J Am Dent Assoc*, 1984, 108(1):338-41.

U.S. Food and Drug Administration Center for Drug Evaluation and Research, Drug Approvals for July 1997, available from: URL:http://www.fda.gov/cder/da/da0797.htm, 1997.

Wahlin YB, "Effects of Chlorhexidine Mouthrinse on Oral Health in Patients With Acute Leukemia," *Oral Surg Oral Med Oral Pathol*, 1989, 68(1):279-87.

Wynn RL, Meiller TF, and Crossley HL, *Drug Information Handbook for Dentistry*, 3rd ed, Cleveland, OH: Lexi-Comp, Inc, 1997.

## PERIODONTOLOGY

Barak S, Engelberg IS, and Hiss J, "Gingival Hyperplasia Caused by Nifedipine. Histopathologic Findings," *J Periodontol*, 1987, 58(9):639-42.

Carson HG and Rainone AD, "Occult Periodontal Disease With Heat Sensitivity: A Different Diagnostic Problem," *Gen Dent*, 1992, 23(3):191-5.

Checchi L, Trombelli L, and Nonato M, "Postoperative Infections and Tetracycline Prophylaxis in Periodontal Surgery: A Retrospective Study," *Quintessence Int*, 1992, 23(3):191-5.

Creath CJ, Steinmetz S, and Roebuck R, "A Case Report. Gingival Swelling Due to a Fingernail-Biting Habit," *J Am Dent Assoc*, 1995, 126(7):1019-21.

Crow HC and Ship JA, "Are Gingival and Periodontal Conditions Related to Salivary Gland Flow Rates in Healthy Individuals?" *J Am Dent Assoc*, 1995, 126(11):1514-20.

Dens F, Boute P, Otten J, et al, "Dental Caries, Gingival Health, and Oral Hygiene of Long-Term Survivors of Paediatric Malignant Diseases," *Arch Dis Child*, 1995, 72(2):129-32.

Harel-Raviv M, Ekler M, Lalani K, et al, "Nifedipine-Induced Gingival Hyperplasia. A Comprehensive Review and Analysis," *Oral Surg Oral Med Oral Pathol*, 1995, 79(6):715-22.

Holt RD, Wilson M, and Musa S, "Mycoplasmas in Plaque and Saliva of Children and Their Relationship to Gingivitis," *J Periodontol*, 1995, 66(2):97-101.

Lareau DE, Herzberg MC, and Nelson RD, "Human Neutrophil Migration Under Agarose to Bacteria Associated With the Development of Gingivitis," *J Periodontol*, 1984, 55(9):540-9.

Listgarten MA, "Pathogenesis of Periodontitis," *J Clin Periodontol*, 1986, 13(5):418-30.

Listgarten MA, Lindhe J, and Hellden L, "Effect of Tetracycline and/or Scaling on Human Periodontal Disease. Clinical, Microbiological, and Histological Observations," *J Clin Periodontol*, 1978, 5(4):246-71.

Loesche WJ, Syed SA, Laughon BE, et al, "The Bacteriology of Acute Necrotizing Ulcerative Gingivitis," *J Periodontol*, 1982, 53(4):223-30.

McLoughlin P, Newman L, and Brown A, "Oral Squamous Cell Carcinoma Arising in Phenytoin-Induced Hyperplasia," *Br Dent J*, 1995, 178(5):183-4.

Moghadam BK and Gier RE, "Common and Less Common Gingival Overgrowth Conditions," *Cutis*, 1995, 56(1):46-8.

Mombelli A, Buser D, Lang NP, et al, "Suspected Periodontopathogens in Erupting Third Molar Sites of Periodontally Healthy Individuals," *J Clin Periodontol*, 1990, 17(1):48-54.

## SUGGESTED READINGS *(Continued)*


Moore LV, Moore WE, Cato EP, et al, "Bacteriology of Human Gingivitis," *J Dent Res,* 1987, 66(5):989-95.

Navazesh M and Mulligan R, "Systemic Dissemination as a Result of Oral Infection in Individuals 50 Years of Age and Older," *Spec Care Dentist,* 1995, 15(1):11-9.

Nery EB, Edson RG, Lee KK, et al, "Prevalence of Nifedipine-Induced Gingival Hyperplasia," *J Periodontol,* 1995, 66(7):572-8.

Nickoloff BJ, Griffiths CE, and Barker JN, "The Role of Adhesion Molecules, Chemotactic Factors, and Cytokines in Inflammatory and Neoplastic Skin Disease," *J Invest Dermatol,* 1990, 94(Suppl 6):151S-7S.

Pinson M, Hoffman WH, Garnick JJ, et al, "Periodontal Disease and Type I Diabetes Mellitus in Children and Adolescents," *J Clin Periodontol,* 1995, 22(2):118-23.

Preber H and Bergstrom J, "Effect of Cigarette Smoking on Periodontal Healing Following Surgical Therapy," *J Clin Periodontol,* 1990, 17(5):324-8.

Ramfjord SP and Ash MM, "Periodontology and Periodontics: Modern Theory and Practice," St Louis, MO: Ishryalar Euro-America, 1989.

Ramsdale DR, Morris JL, and Hardy P,"Gingival Hyperplasia With Nifedipine," *Br Heart J,* 1995, 73(2):115.

Ransier A, Epstein JB, Lunn R, et al, "A Combined Analysis of a Toothbrush, Foam Brush, and a Chlorhexidine-Soaked Foam Brush in Maintaining Oral Hygiene," *Cancer Nurs,* 1995, 18(5):393-6.

Robertson PB and Greenspan JS, *Perspectives on Oral Manifestations of AIDS: Diagnosis and Management of HIV-Associated Infection,* Littleton, MA: PSG Publishing Co, 1988.

Wahlstrom E, Zamora JU, and Teichman S, "Improvement in Cyclosporine-Associated Gingival Hyperplasia With Azithromycin Therapy," *N Engl J Med,* 1995, 332(11):753-4.


## RESPIRATORY DISEASES


"Asthma Mortality and Hospitalization Among Children and Young Adults - United States, 1980-1993," *Morb Mortal Wkly Rep,* 1996, 45(17):350-3.

Barnes PF and Barrows SA, "Tuberculosis in the 1990s," *Ann Intern Med,* 1993, 119(5):400-10.

Snider DE, Jr and Roper WL, "The New Tuberculosis," *N Engl J Med,* 1992, 326(10):703-5.

Cohen C, Krutchkoff D, and Eisenberg E, "Systemic Sarcoidosis: Report of Two Cases With Oral Lesions," *J Oral Surg,* 1981, 39(8):613-8.

DeLuke DM and Sciubba JJ, "Oral Manifestations of Sarvoidosis: Report of a Case Masquerading as a Neoplasm," *Oral Surg Oral Med Oral Pathol,* 1985, 59(2):184-8.

Drosos AA, Constantopoulos SH, Psychos D, et al, "The Forgotten Cause of Sicca Complex: Sarcoidosis," *J Rheumatol,* 1989, 16(12):1548-51.

Egman DH and Christiani DC, *Respiratory Disorders in Occupational Health: Recognizing and Preventing Work-Related Disease,* 2nd ed, Levy BS and Wegman DH, eds, Boston, MA: Little-Brown, 1988, 319-44.

Frieden TR, Sterling T, Pablos-Mendez A, et al, "The Emergence of Drug Resistant Tuberculosis in New York City," *N Engl J Med,* 1993, 328(8):521-6.

Murciano D, Auclair MH, Pariente R, et al, "A Randomized Controlled Trial of Theophylline in Patients With Severe Chronic Obstructive Pulmonary Disease," *N Engl J Med,* 1989, 320(23):1521-5.

Bass JB, Farer LS, Hopewell PC, et al, "Treatment of Tuberculosis and Tuberculosis Infection in Adults and Children. American Thoracic Society and the Centers for Disease Control and Prevention," *Am J Respir Crit Care Med,* 1994, 149(5):1359-74.

## TEMPOROMANDIBULAR DYSFUNCTION

Becker IM, "Occlusion as a Causative Factor in TMD. Scientific Basis to Occlusal Therapy, *NY State Dent J,* 1995, 61(9):54-7.

Bell WE, et al, *Temporomandibular Disorders: Classification Diagnosis, Management,* 3rd ed, Chicago, IL: Year Book Medical Publishers, 1990.

Bloch M, Riba H, Redensky D, et al, "Cranio-Mandibular Disorder in Children," *NY State Dent J,* 1995, 61(3):48-50.

Canavan D and Gratt BM, "Electronic Thermography for the Assessment of Mild and Moderate Temporomandibular Joint Dysfunction," *Oral Surg Oral Med Oral Pathol Oral Radiol Endod,* 1995, 79(6):778-86.

Carlson CR, Okeson JP, Falace DA, et al, "Comparison of Psychologic and Physiologic Functioning Between Patients With Masticatory Muscle Pain and Matched Controls," *J Orofacial Pain,* 1993, 7(1):15-22.

Clark GT and Takeuchi H, "Temporomandibular Dysfunction, Chromic Orofacial Pain and Oral Motor Disorders in the 21st Century," *J Calif Dent Assoc,* 1995, 23(4):44-6, 48-50.

Clayton JA, "Occlusion and Prosthodontics," *Dent Clin North Am,* 1995, 39(2):313-33.

Dos Santos J Jr, "Supportive Conservative Therapies for Temporomandibular Disorders," *Dent Clin North Am,* 1995, 39(2):459-77.

Kai S, Kai H, Nakayama E, et al, "Clinical Symptoms of Open Lock Position of the Condyle. Relation to Anterior Dislocation of the Temporomandibular Joint," *Oral Surg Oral Med Oral Pathol,* 1992, 74(2):143-8.

Lund JP, Donga R, Widmer CG, et al, "The Pain-Adaptation Model: A Discussion of the Relationship Between Chronic Musculoskeletal Pain and Motor Activity," *Can J Physiol Pharmacol,* 1991, 69(5):683-94.

Okeson JP, "Occlusion and Functional Disorders of the Masticatory System," *Dent Clin North Am,* 1995, 39(2):285-300.

Okeson JP, *The Management of Temporomandibular Disorders and Occlusion,* 3rd ed, St Louis, MO: Mosby Year Book, 1993.

Quinn JH, "Mandibular Exercises to Control Bruxism and Deviation Problems," *Cranio,* 1995, 13(1):30-4.

Schiffman E, Haley D, Baker C, et al, "Diagnostic Criteria for Screening Headache Patients for Temporomandibular Disorders," *Headache,* 1995, 35(3):121-4.

"Temporomandibular Disorder Prosthodontics: Treatment and Management Goals. Report of the Committee on Temporomandibular Disorders of the American College of Prosthodontics," *J Prosthodontology,* 1995, 4(1):58-64.

Widmark G, Kahnberg KE, Haraldson T, et al, "Evaluation of TMJ Surgery in Cases Not Responding to Conservative Treatment," *Cranio,* 1995, 13(1):44-9.

# APPENDIX TABLE OF CONTENTS

# COMMON SYMBOLS & ABBREVIATIONS

| | |
|---|---|
| µg | microgram |
| °C | degrees Celsius (Centigrade) |
| < | less than |
| > | greater than |
| ≤ | less than or equal to |
| ≥ | greater than or equal to |
| ABG | arterial blood gas |
| ACE | angiotensin-converting enzyme |
| ACLS | adult cardiac life support |
| ADH | antidiuretic hormone |
| AED | antiepileptic drug |
| ALL | acute lymphoblastic leukemia |
| ALT | alanine aminotransferase (was SGPT) |
| AML | acute myeloblastic leukemia |
| ANA | antinuclear antibodies |
| ANC | absolute neutrophil count |
| ANL | acute nonlymphoblastic leukemia |
| APTT | activated partial thromboplastin time |
| ASA (class I-IV) | classification of surgical patients according to their baseline health (eg, healthy ASA I and II or increased severity of illness ASA III or IV) |
| AST | aspartate aminotransferase (was SGOT) |
| A-V | atrial-ventricular |
| BMT | bone marrow transplant |
| BUN | blood urea nitrogen |
| cAMP | cyclic adenosine monophosphate |
| CBC | complete blood count |
| CHF | congestive heart failure |
| CI | cardiac index |
| $Cl_{cr}$ | creatinine clearance |
| CNS | central nervous system |
| COPD | chronic obstructive pulmonary disease |
| CSF | cerebral spinal fluid |
| CT | computed tomography |
| CVA | cerebral vascular accident |
| CVP | central venous pressure |
| d | day |
| $D_5W$ | dextrose 5% in water |
| $D_5/_{0.45}$ NaCl | dextrose 5% in sodium chloride 0.45% |
| $D_{10}W$ | dextrose 10% in water |
| DIC | disseminated intravascular coagulation |
| DNA | deoxyribonucleic acid |
| DVT | deep vein thrombosis |
| EEG | electroencephalogram |
| EKG | electrocardiogram |
| ESR | erythrocyte sedimentation rate |
| E.T. | endotracheal |
| $FEV_1$ | forced expiratory volume |
| FVC | forced vital capacity |
| g | gram |
| G-6-PD | glucose-6-phosphate dehydrogenase |
| GA | gestational age |
| GABA | gamma-aminobutyric acid |
| GE | gastroesophageal |
| GI | gastrointestinal |
| GU | genitourinary |
| h | hour |
| HIV | human immunodeficiency virus |
| HPLC | high performance liquid chromatography |
| IBW | ideal body weight |
| ICP | intracranial pressure |
| IgG | immune globulin G |
| I.M. | intramuscular |
| INR | international normalized ratio |
| I.O. | intraosseous |
| I.V. | intravenous |
| IVH | intraventricular hemorrhage |

*(continued)*

| | |
|---|---|
| IVP | intravenous push |
| I & O | input and output |
| IOP | intraocular pressure |
| I.T. | intrathecal |
| JRA | juvenile rheumatoid arthritis |
| kg | kilogram |
| L | liter |
| LDH | lactate dehydrogenase |
| LE | lupus erythematosus |
| LP | lumbar puncture |
| MAO | monoamine oxidase |
| MAP | mean arterial pressure |
| mcg | microgram |
| mg | milligram |
| MI | myocardial infarction |
| μmol | micromole |
| min | minute |
| mL | milliliter |
| mo | month |
| mOsm | milliosmoles |
| MRI | magnetic resonance image |
| ND | nasoduodenal |
| ng | nanogram |
| NG | nasogastric |
| NMDA | n-methyl-d-aspartate |
| nmol | nanomole |
| NPO | nothing per os (nothing by mouth) |
| NSAID | nonsteroidal anti-inflammatory drug |
| O.R. | operating room |
| OTC | over-the-counter (nonprescription) |
| PALS | pediatric advanced life support |
| PCA | postconceptional age |
| PCP | *Pneumocystis carinii* pneumonia |
| PCWP | pulmonary capillary wedge pressure |
| PDA | patent ductus arteriosus |
| PNA | postnatal age |
| PSVT | paroxysmal supraventricular tachycardia |
| PT | prothrombin time |
| PTT | partial thromboplastin time |
| PUD | peptic ulcer disease |
| PVC | premature ventricular contraction |
| qsad | add an amount sufficient to equal |
| RAP | right atrial pressure |
| RIA | radioimmunoassay |
| RNA | ribonucleic acid |
| S-A | sino-atrial |
| S.C. | subcutaneous |
| $S_{cr}$ | serum creatinine |
| SIADH | syndrome of inappropriate antidiuretic hormone |
| S.L. | sublingual |
| SLE | systemic lupus erythematosus |
| SVR | systemic vascular resistance |
| SVT | supraventricular tachycardia |
| SWI | sterile water for injection |
| TT | thrombin time |
| UTI | urinary tract infection |
| $V_d$ | volume of distribution |
| $V_{dss}$ | volume of distribution at steady-state |
| y | year |

*Other than drug synonyms

# APOTHECARY/METRIC EQUIVALENTS

## Approximate Liquid Measures

Basic equivalent: 1 fluid ounce = 30 mL

Examples:

| | | | |
|---|---|---|---|
| 1 gallon | 3800 mL | 1 gallon | 128 fluid ounces |
| 1 quart | 960 mL | 1 quart | 32 fluid ounces |
| 1 pint | 480 mL | 1 pint | 16 fluid ounces |
| 8 fluid oz | 240 mL | 15 minims | 1 mL |
| 4 fluid oz | 120 mL | 10 minims | 0.6 mL |

## Approximate Household Equivalents

| | | | |
|---|---|---|---|
| 1 teaspoonful | 5 mL | 1 tablespoonful | 15 mL |

## Weights

Basic equivalents:

| | | | |
|---|---|---|---|
| 1 oz | 30 g | 15 gr | 1 g |

Examples:

| | | | |
|---|---|---|---|
| 4 oz | 120 g | 1 gr | 60 mg |
| 2 oz | 60 g | 1/100 gr | 600 mcg |
| 10 gr | 600 mg | 1/150 gr | 400 mcg |
| 7½ gr | 500 mg | 1/200 gr | 300 mcg |
| 16 oz | 1 lb | | |

## Metric Conversions

Basic equivalents:

| | | | |
|---|---|---|---|
| 1 g | 1000 mg | 1 mg | 1000 mcg |

Examples:

| | | | |
|---|---|---|---|
| 5 g | 5000 mg | 5 mg | 5000 mcg |
| 0.5 g | 500 mg | 0.5 g | 500 mcg |
| 0.05 g | 50 mg | 0.05 mg | 50 mcg |

## Exact Equivalents

| | | | |
|---|---|---|---|
| 1 g | = 15.43 gr | 0.1 mg | = 1/600 gr |
| 1 mL | = 16.23 minims | 0.12 mg | = 1/500 gr |
| 1 minim | = 0.06 mL | 0.15 mg | = 1/400 gr |
| 1 gr | = 64.8 mg | 0.2 mg | = 1/300 gr |
| 1 pint (pt) | = 473.2 mL | 0.3 mg | = 1/200 gr |
| 1 oz | = 28.35 g | 0.4 mg | = 1/150 gr |
| 1 lb | = 453.6 g | 0.5 mg | = 1/120 gr |
| 1 kg | = 2.2 lbs | 0.6 mg | = 1/100 gr |
| 1 qt | = 946.4 mL | 0.8 mg | = 1/80 gr |
| | | 1 mg | = 1/65 gr |

## Solids*

| | |
|---|---|
| ¼ grain | = 15 mg |
| ½ grain | = 30 mg |
| 1 grain | = 60 mg |
| 1½ grains | = 100 mg |
| 5 grains | = 300 mg |
| 10 grains | = 600 mg |

*Use exact equivalents for compounding and calculations requiring a high degree of accuracy.

# POUNDS-KILOGRAMS CONVERSION

**1 pound = 0.45359 kilograms**
**1 kilogram = 2.2 pounds**

| lb | = kg | lb | = kg | lb | = kg |
|---|---|---|---|---|---|
| 1 | 0.45 | 70 | 31.75 | 140 | 63.50 |
| 5 | 2.27 | 75 | 34.02 | 145 | 65.77 |
| 10 | 4.54 | 80 | 36.29 | 150 | 68.04 |
| 15 | 6.80 | 85 | 38.56 | 155 | 70.31 |
| 20 | 9.07 | 90 | 40.82 | 160 | 72.58 |
| 25 | 11.34 | 95 | 43.09 | 165 | 74.84 |
| 30 | 13.61 | 100 | 45.36 | 170 | 77.11 |
| 35 | 15.88 | 105 | 47.63 | 175 | 79.38 |
| 40 | 18.14 | 110 | 49.90 | 180 | 81.65 |
| 45 | 20.41 | 115 | 52.16 | 185 | 83.92 |
| 50 | 22.68 | 120 | 54.43 | 190 | 86.18 |
| 55 | 24.95 | 125 | 56.70 | 195 | 88.45 |
| 60 | 27.22 | 130 | 58.91 | 200 | 90.72 |
| 65 | 29.48 | 135 | 61.24 | | |

# TEMPERATURE CONVERSION

**Celsius to Fahrenheit = (°C x 9/5) + 32 = °F**
**Fahrenheit to Celsius = (°F - 32) x 5/9 = °C**

| °C | = °F | °C | = °F | °C | = °F |
|---|---|---|---|---|---|
| 100.0 | 212.0 | 39.0 | 102.2 | 36.8 | 98.2 |
| 50.0 | 122.0 | 38.8 | 101.8 | 36.6 | 97.9 |
| 41.0 | 105.8 | 38.6 | 101.5 | 36.4 | 97.5 |
| 40.8 | 105.4 | 38.4 | 101.1 | 36.2 | 97.2 |
| 40.6 | 105.1 | 38.2 | 100.8 | 36.0 | 96.8 |
| 40.4 | 104.7 | 38.0 | 100.4 | 35.8 | 96.4 |
| 40.2 | 104.4 | 37.8 | 100.1 | 35.6 | 96.1 |
| 40.0 | 104.0 | 37.6 | 99.7 | 35.4 | 95.7 |
| 39.8 | 103.6 | 37.4 | 99.3 | 35.2 | 95.4 |
| 39.6 | 103.3 | 37.2 | 99.0 | 35.0 | 95.0 |
| 39.4 | 102.9 | 37.0 | 98.6 | 0 | 32.0 |
| 39.2 | 102.6 | | | | |

# BODY SURFACE AREA OF ADULTS AND CHILDREN

## Calculating Body Surface Area in Children

In a child of average size, find weight and corresponding surface area on the boxed scale to the left; or, use the nomogram to the right. Lay a straightedge on the correct height and weight points for the child, then read the intersecting point on the surface area scale.

**FOR CHILDREN OF NORMAL HEIGHT AND WEIGHT**

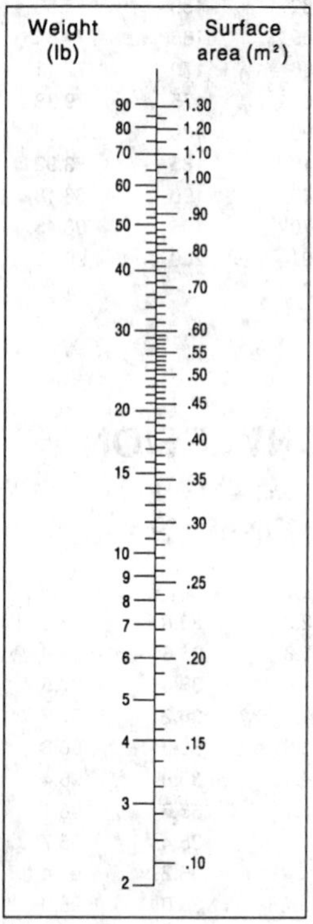


**NOMOGRAM**

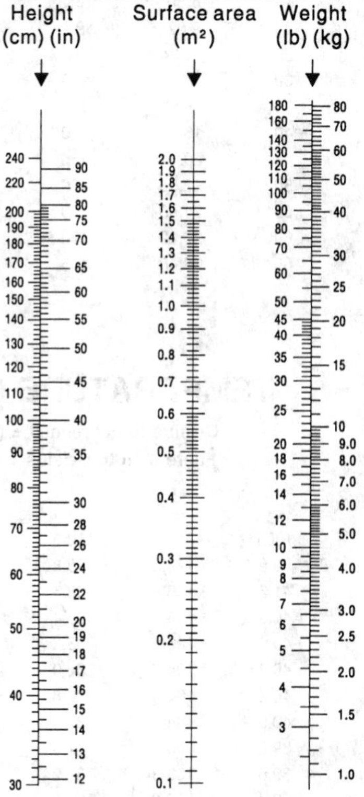


**BODY SURFACE AREA FORMULA (Adult and Pediatric)**

$$BSA\ (m^2) = \sqrt{\frac{Ht\ (in) \times Wt\ (lb)}{3131}} \quad \text{or, in metric: } BSA\ (m^2) = \sqrt{\frac{Ht\ (cm) \times Wt\ (kg)}{3600}}$$

**References**

Lam TK and Leung DT, "More on Simplified Calculation of Body Surface Area," *N Engl J Med*, 1988, 318(17):1130 (Letter).

Mosteller RD, "Simplified Calculation of Body Surface Area", *N Engl J Med*, 1987, 317(17):1098 (Letter).

# AVERAGE WEIGHTS AND SURFACE AREAS

## Average Weight and Surface Area of Preterm Infants, Term Infants, and Children

| Age | Average Weight (kg)* | Approximate Surface Area ($m^2$) |
|---|---|---|
| **Weeks Gestation** | | |
| 26 | 0.9-1 | 0.1 |
| 30 | 1.3-1.5 | 0.12 |
| 32 | 1.6-2 | 0.15 |
| 38 | 2.9-3 | 0.2 |
| 40 (term infant at birth) | 3.1-4 | 0.25 |
| **Months** | | |
| 3 | 5 | 0.29 |
| 6 | 7 | 0.38 |
| 9 | 8 | 0.42 |
| **Year** | | |
| 1 | 10 | 0.49 |
| 2 | 12 | 0.55 |
| 3 | 15 | 0.64 |
| 4 | 17 | 0.74 |
| 5 | 18 | 0.76 |
| 6 | 20 | 0.82 |
| 7 | 23 | 0.90 |
| 8 | 25 | 0.95 |
| 9 | 28 | 1.06 |
| 10 | 33 | 1.18 |
| 11 | 35 | 1.23 |
| 12 | 40 | 1.34 |
| **Adult** | 70 | 1.73 |

*Weights from age 3 months and older are rounded off to the nearest kilogram.

# CALCIUM CHANNEL BLOCKERS & GINGIVAL HYPERPLASIA

| Generic Preparation | FDA Approval | Cases Cited in Literature | Common Name |
|---|---|---|---|
| Amlodipine | 1992 | 3 | Norvasc® |
| Bepridil | 1993 | 0 | Vascor® |
| Diltiazem | 1982 | >20 | Cardizem®; Dilacor® |
| Felodipine | 1992 | 1 | Plendil® |
| Isradipine | 1991 | 1 | DynaCirc® |
| Nicardipine | 1989 | 0 | Cardene® |
| Nifedipine | 1982 | >120 | Adalat®; Procardia® |
| Nimodipine | 1989 | 0 | Nimotop® |
| Nisoldipine | 1995 | 0 | Sular® |
| Nitrendipine* | | 1 | Baypress® |
| Verapamil | 1982 | 7 | Calan®; Isoptin®; Verelan® |

*Not yet approved for use in the United States.

## SOME GENERAL OBSERVATIONS OF CCB-INDUCED GH

Most of the reported cases listed in the Calcium Channel Blockers and Gingival Hyperplasia table have involved patients >50 years of age taking CCBs chronically for postmyocardial infarction syndrome, angina pain, essential hypertension, and Raynaud's syndrome. Nifedipine-induced GH has appeared between 1 and 9 months after a daily dose of 30-100 mg, verapamil-induced GH has appeared at 11 months or more after a daily dose of 240-360 mg, and diltiazem-induced GH has appeared between 1 and 24 months after a daily dose of 60-135 mg. As with phenytoin, there does not seem to be a dose-dependent effect of CCBs on the severity of the hyperplastic syndrome. Discontinuance of the CCB usually results in complete disappearance or marked regression of symptoms, with symptoms reappearing upon remedication. The time required after drug discontinuance for marked regression of GH has been one week. Complete disappearance of all symptoms usually takes two months. If gingivectomy is performed and the drug retained or resumed, the hyperplasia will usually recur. Only when the medication is discontinued or a switch to a non-CCB occurs will the gingivectomy usually be successful. One study of Nishikawa[1], et al, showed that if nifedipine could not be discontinued, hyperplasia did not recur after gingivectomy when extensive plaque control was carried out. If the CCB is changed to another class of cardiovascular agent, the gingival hyperplasia will probably regress and disappear. A switch to another CCB, however, will probably result in continued hyperplasia. For example, Giustiniani[2], et al, reported disappearance of symptoms within 15 days after discontinuance of verapamil, with the reoccurrence of symptoms after resumption with diltiazem. The reader is referred to the review of 1991[3] for descriptive clinical and histological findings of CCB-induced GH.

1. Nishikawa SI, Tada H, Hamasaki A, et al, "Nifedipine-Induced Gingival Hyperplasia: A Clinical and In Vitro Study," *J Periodontol*, 1991, 62(1):30-5.
2. Giustiniani S, Robestelli della Cuna F, and Marienei M, "Hyperplastic Gingivitis During Diltiazem Therapy," *Int J Cardiol*, 1987, 15(2):247-9.
3. Wynn RL, "Calcium Channel Blockers and Gingival Hyperplasia," *Gen Dent*, 1991, 240-3.

# CANCER CHEMOTHERAPY REGIMENS

## ADULT REGIMENS

### Breast Cancer

**AC**

Doxorubicin (Adriamycin®), I.V., 45 mg/m², day 1
Cyclophosphamide, I.V., 500 mg/m², day 1

Repeat cycle every 21 days

**ACe**

Doxorubicin (Adriamycin®), I.V., 40 mg/m², day 1
Cyclophosphamide, P.O., 200 mg/m²/day, days 1-3 or 3-6

Repeat cycle every 21-28 days

**CAF**

Cyclophosphamide, P.O., 100 mg/m², days 1-14
Doxorubicin (Adriamycin®), I.V., 30 mg/m², days 1 & 8
Fluorouracil, I.V., 400-500 mg/m², days 1 & 8

Repeat cycle every 28 days

**or**

Cyclophosphamide, I.V., 500 mg/m², day 1
Doxorubicin (Adriamycin®), I.V., 50 mg/m², day 1
Fluorouracil, I.V., 500 mg/m², day 1

Repeat cycle every 21 days

**CFM**

Cyclophosphamide, I.V., 500 mg/m², day 1
Fluorouracil, I.V., 500 mg/m², day 1
Mitoxantrone, I.V., 10 mg/m², day 1

Repeat cycle every 21 days

**CFPT**

Cyclophosphamide, I.V., 150 mg/m², days 1-5
Fluorouracil, I.V., 300 mg/m², days 1-5
Prednisone, P.O., 10 mg tid, days 1-7
Tamoxifen, P.O., 10 mg bid, days 1-42

Repeat cycle every 42 days

**CMF**

Cyclophosphamide, P.O., 100 mg/m², days 1-14
Methotrexate, I.V., 40 mg/m², days 1 & 8
Fluorouracil, I.V., 600 mg/m², days 1 & 8

Repeat cycle every 28 days

**or**

Cyclophosphamide, I.V., 600 mg/m², days 1 & 8
Methotrexate, I.V., 40-60 mg/m², days 1 & 8
Fluorouracil, I.V., 400-600 mg/m², days 1 & 8

Repeat cycle every 28 days

**CMFP**

Cyclophosphamide, P.O., 100 mg/m², days 1-14
Methotrexate, I.V., 40-60 mg/m², days 1 & 8
Fluorouracil, I.V., 600-700 mg/m², days 1 & 8
Prednisone, P.O., 40 mg (first 3 cycles only), days 1-14

Repeat cycle every 28 days

**CMFVP (Cooper's)**

Cyclophosphamide, P.O., 2-2.5 mg/kg/day for 9 months
Methotrexate, I.V., 0.7 mg/kg/wk for 8 weeks then every other week for 7 months
Fluorouracil, I.V., 12 mg/kg/wk for 8 weeks then every other week for 7 months
Vincristine, I.V., 0.035 mg/kg (max: 2 mg/wk) for 5 weeks then once monthly
Prednisone, P.O., 0.75 mg/kg/day, taper over next 40 days, discontinue, days 1-10

**or**

Cyclophosphamide, I.V., 400 mg/m², day 1
Methotrexate, I.V., 30 mg/m², days 1 & 8
Fluorouracil, I.V., 400 mg/m², days 1 & 8
Vincristine, I.V., 1 mg, days 1 & 8
Prednisone, P.O., 20 mg qid, days 1-7

Repeat cycle every 28 days

**FAC**

Fluorouracil, I.V., 500 mg/m², days 1 & 8
Doxorubicin (Adriamycin®), I.V., 50 mg/m², day 1
Cyclophosphamide, I.V., 500 mg/m², day 1

Repeat cycle every 21 days

## CANCER CHEMOTHERAPY REGIMENS *(Continued)*

**IMF**

Ifosfamide, I.V., 1.5 g/m², days 1 & 8
Mesna, I.V., 20% of ifosfamide dose, give immediately before and 4 and 8 hours after ifosfamide infusion, days 1 & 8
Methotrexate, I.V., 40 mg/m², days 1 & 8
Fluorouracil, I.V., 600 mg/m², days 1 & 8
Repeat cycle every 28 days

**NFL**

Mitoxantrone (Novantrone®), I.V., 12 mg/m², day 1
Fluorouracil, I.V., 350 mg/m², days 1-3, given after leucovorin calcium
Leucovorin calcium, I.V., 300 mg/m², days 1-3
**or**
Mitoxantrone (Novantrone®), I.V., 10 mg/m², day 1
Fluorouracil, I.V., 1000 mg/m² continuous infusion, given after leucovorin calcium, days 1-3
Leucovorin calcium, I.V., 100 mg/m², days 1-3
Repeat cycle every 21 days

**VATH**

Vinblastine, I.V., 4.5 mg/m², day 1
Doxorubicin (Adriamycin®), I.V., 45 mg/m², day 1
Thiotepa, I.V., 12 mg/m², day 1
Fluoxymesterone (Halotestin®), P.O., 30 mg qd, days 1-21
Repeat cycle every 21 days

**Single-Agent Regimens**

Docetaxel, I.V., 60-100 mg/m² over 1 hour; patient must be premedicated with dexamethasone 8 mg bid P.O. for 3 days, start one day before docetaxel; repeat cycle every 3 weeks

Doxorubicin, I.V., 60 mg/m², every 3 weeks
**or**
Doxorubicin, I.V., 20 mg/m², every week
**or**
Doxorubicin, I.V., 20 mg/m² continuous infusion, days 1-3, every 3 weeks

Mitomycin C, I.V., 8-10 mg/m², every 6-8 weeks

Paclitaxel, I.V., 175 mg/m² over 3-24 h, every 21 d
Patient must be premedicated with:
Dexamethasone 20 mg P.O., 12 and 6 h prior
Diphenhydramine 50 mg I.V., 30 min prior
Cimetidine 300 mg I.V., or ranitidine 50 mg I.V., 30 min prior

Vinblastine, I.V., 12 mg/m², every 3-4 weeks

Vinorelbine, I.V., 30 mg/m², days 1 and 8; repeat cycle every 3 weeks

### Colon Cancer

**F-CL**

Fluorouracil, I.V., 375 mg/m², days 1-5
Leucovorin calcium, I.V., 200 mg/m², days 1-5
Repeat cycle every 28 days
**or**
Fluorouracil, I.V., 500 mg/m² weekly 1 h after initiating the calcium leucovorin infusion for 6 weeks
Leucovorin calcium, I.V., 500 mg/m², over 2 h, weekly for 6 weeks
Two-week break, then repeat cycle

**FLe**

Fluorouracil, I.V., 450 mg/m² for 5 days, then, after a pause of 4 weeks, 450 mg/m², weekly for 48 weeks
Levamisole, P.O., 50 mg tid for 3 days, repeated every 2 weeks for 1 year

**FMV**

Fluorouracil, I.V., 10 mg/kg/day, days 1-5
Methyl-CCNU, P.O., 175 mg/m², day 1
Vincristine, I.V., 1 mg/m² (max: 2 mg), day 1
Repeat cycle every 35 days

**FU/LV**

Fluorouracil, I.V., 370-400 mg/m²/day, days 1-5
Leucovorin calcium, I.V., 200 mg/m²/day, commence infusion 15 min prior to fluorouracil infusion, days 1-5
Repeat cycle every 21 days
**or**
Fluorouracil, I.V., 1000 mg/m²/day by continuous infusion, days 1-4
Leucovorin calcium, I.V., 200 mg/m²/day, days 1-4
Repeat cycle every 28 days

**Weekly 5FU/LV**

Fluorouracil, I.V., 600 mg/m$^2$ over 1 h given after leucovorin, repeat weekly x 6 then 2-week rest period = 1 cycle, days 1, 8, 15, 22, 29, 36
Leucovorin calcium, I.V., 500 mg/m$^2$ over 2 h, days 1, 8, 15, 22, 29, 36
Repeat cycle every 56 days

**5FU/LDLF**

Fluorouracil, I.V., 425 mg/m$^2$/day, days 1-5
Leucovorin calcium, I.V., 20-25 mg/m$^2$/day, days 1-5
Repeat cycle every 28 days

## Gastric Cancer

**EAP**

Etoposide, I.V., 120 mg/m$^2$, days 4, 5, 6
Doxorubicin (Adriamycin®), I.V., 20 mg/m$^2$, days 1, 7
Cisplatin (Platinol®), I.V., 40 mg/m$^2$, days 2, 8
Repeat cycle every 21 days

**ELF**

Etoposide, I.V., 120 mg/m$^2$, days 1-3
Leucovorin calcium, I.V., 300 mg/m$^2$, days 1-3
Fluorouracil, I.V., 500 mg/m$^2$, days 1-3
Repeat cycle every 21-28 days

**FAM**

Fluorouracil, I.V., 600 mg/m$^2$, days 1, 8, 29, & 36
Doxorubicin (Adriamycin®), I.V., 30 mg/m$^2$, days 1 & 29
Mitomycin C, I.V., 10 mg/m$^2$, day 1
Repeat cycle every 56 days

**FAME**

Fluorouracil, I.V., 350 mg/m$^2$, days 1-5, 36-40
Doxorubicin (Adriamycin®), I.V., 40 mg/m$^2$, days 1 & 36
Methyl-CCNU, P.O., 150 mg/m$^2$, day 1
Repeat cycle every 70 days

**FAMTX**

Methotrexate, IVPB, 1500 mg/m$^2$, day 1
Fluorouracil, IVPB, 1500 mg/m$^2$ 1 h after methotrexate, day 1
Leucovorin calcium, P.O., 15 mg/m$^2$ q6h x 48 h 24 h after methotrexate, day 2
Doxorubicin (Adriamycin®), IVPB, 30 mg/m$^2$, day 15
Repeat cycle every 28 days

**FCE**

Fluorouracil, I.V., 900 mg/m$^2$/day continuous infusion, days 1-5
Cisplatin, I.V., 20 mg/m$^2$, days 1-5
Etoposide, I.V., 90 mg/m$^2$, days 1, 3, & 5
Repeat cycle every 21 days

**PFL**

Cisplatin (Platinol®), I.V., 25 mg/m$^2$ continuous infusion, days 1-5
Fluorouracil, I.V., 800 mg/m$^2$ continuous infusion, days 2-5
Leucovorin calcium, I.V., 500 mg/m$^2$ continuous infusion, days 1-5
Repeat cycle every 28 days

**Single-Agent Regimens**

Irinotecan, I.V., over 90 minutes: 125 mg/m$^2$/week; repeat weekly for 4 weeks, then 2-week rest period

**or**

Irinotecan, I.V. over 30-90 minutes: 350 mg/m$^2$; repeat every 21 days

## Genitourinary Cancer

### Bladder

**CAP**

Cyclophosphamide, I.V., 400 mg/m$^2$, day 1
Doxorubicin (Adriamycin®), I.V., 40 mg/m$^2$, day 1
Cisplatin (Platinol®), I.V., 60 mg/m$^2$, day 1
Repeat cycle every 21 days

**CISCA**

Cisplatin, I.V., 70-100 mg/m$^2$, day 2
Cyclophosphamide, I.V., 650 mg/m$^2$, day 1
Doxorubicin (Adriamycin®), I.V., 50 mg/m$^2$, day 1
Repeat cycle every 21-28 days

**CMV**

Cisplatin, I.V., 100 mg/m$^2$ over 4 h start 12 h after MTX, day 2
Methotrexate, I.V., 30 mg/m$^2$, days 1 & 8
Vinblastine, I.V., 4 mg/m$^2$, days 1 & 8
Repeat cycle every 21 days

## CANCER CHEMOTHERAPY REGIMENS *(Continued)*

**m-PFL**

Methotrexate, I.V., 60 mg/m$^2$, day 1
Cisplatin (Platinol®), I.V., 25 mg/m$^2$ continuous infusion, days 2-6
Fluorouracil, I.V., 800 mg/m$^2$ continuous infusion, days 2-6
Leucovorin calcium, I.V., 500 mg/m$^2$ continuous infusion, days 2-6
Repeat cycle every 28 days for 4 cycles

**MVAC**

Methotrexate, I.V., 30 mg/m$^2$, days 1, 15, 22
Vinblastine, I.V., 3 mg/m$^2$, days 2, 15, 22
Doxorubicin (Adriamycin®), I.V., 30 mg/m$^2$, day 2
Cisplatin, I.V., 70 mg/m$^2$, day 2
Repeat cycle every 28 days

### Prostate

**FL**

Flutamide, P.O., 250 mg tid, days 1-28
Leuprolide acetate, S.C., 1 mg qd, days 1-28
Repeat cycle every 28 days

**or**

Flutamide, P.O., 250 mg tid, days 1-28
Leuprolide acetate depot, I.M., 7.5 mg, day 1
Repeat cycle every 28 days

**FZ**

Flutamide, P.O., 250 mg tid
Goserelin acetate (Zoladex®), S.C., 3.6 mg implant, every 28 days

**L-VAM**

Leuprolide acetate, S.C., 1 mg qd, days 1-28
Vinblastine, I.V., 1.5 mg/m$^2$/day continuous infusion, days 2-7
Doxorubicin (Adriamycin®), I.V., 50 mg/m$^2$ continuous infusion, day 1
Mitomycin C, I.V., 10 mg/m$^2$, day 2
Repeat cycle every 28 days

### Testicular, Induction, Good Risk

**BEP**

Bleomycin, I.V., 30 units, days 2, 9, 16
Etoposide, I.V., 100 mg/m$^2$, days 1-5
Cisplatin (Platinol®), I.V., 20 mg/m$^2$, days 1-5
Repeat cycle every 21 days

**PE**

Cisplatin (Platinol®), I.V., 20 mg/m$^2$, days 1-5
Etoposide, I.V., 100 mg/m$^2$, days 1-5
Repeat cycle every 21 days

**PVB**

Cisplatin (Platinol®), I.V., 20 mg/m$^2$, days 1-5
Vinblastine, I.V., 6 mg/m$^2$, days 1, 2
Bleomycin, I.V., 30 units, weekly
Repeat cycle every 21-28 days

### Testicular, Induction, Poor Risk

**VIP**

Etoposide (VePesid®), I.V., 75 mg/m$^2$, days 1-5
Ifosfamide, I.V., 1.2 g/m$^2$, days 1-5
Cisplatin (Platinol®), I.V., 20 mg/m$^2$, days 1-5
Mesna, I.V., 120 mg/m$^2$ then 1200 mg/m$^2$/day continuous infusion, days 1-5
Repeat cycle every 21 days

**VIP (Einhorn)**

Vinblastine, I.V., 0.11 mg/kg, days 1-2
Ifosfamide, I.V., 1200 mg/m$^2$, days 1-5
Cisplatin (Platinol®), I.V., 20 mg/m$^2$, days 1-5
Mesna, I.V., 120 mg/m$^2$, then 1200 mg/m$^2$/day continuous infusion, days 1-5
Repeat cycle every 21 days

### Testicular, Induction, Salvage

**VAB VI**

Vinblastine, I.V., 4 mg/m$^2$, day 1
Dactinomycin (Actinomycin D), I.V., 1 mg/m$^2$, day 1
Bleomycin, I.V., 30 units push day 1, then 20 units/m$^2$/day continuous infusion, days 1-3
Cisplatin, I.V., 120 mg/m$^2$, day 4
Cyclophosphamide, I.V., 600 mg/m$^2$, day 1
Repeat cycle every 21 days

**VBP (PVB)**

Vinblastine, I.V., 6 mg/m², days 1 & 2
Bleomycin, I.V., 30 units, days 1, 8, 15, (22)
Cisplatin (Platinol®), I.V., 20 mg/m², days 1-5

Repeat cycle every 21-28 days

## Gestational Trophoblastic Cancer

**DMC**

Dactinomycin, I.V., 0.37 mg/m², days 1-5
Methotrexate, I.V., 11 mg/m², days 1-5
Cyclophosphamide, I.V., 110 mg/m², days 1-5

Repeat cycle every 21 days

## Head and Neck Cancer

**CAP**

Cyclophosphamide, I.V., 500 mg/m², day 1
Doxorubicin (Adriamycin®), I.V., 50 mg/m², day 1
Cisplatin (Platinol®), I.V., 50 mg/m², day 1

Repeat cycle every 28 days

**CF**

Cisplatin, I.V., 100 mg/m², day 1
Fluorouracil, I.V., 1000 mg/m²/day continuous infusion, days 1-5

Repeat cycle every 21-28 days

**CF**

Carboplatin, I.V., 400 mg/m², day 1
Fluorouracil, I.V., 1000 mg/m²/day continuous infusion, days 1-5

Repeat cycle every 21-28 days

**COB**

Cisplatin, I.V., 100 mg/m², day 1
Vincristine (Oncovin®), I.V., 1 mg/m², days 2 & 5
Bleomycin, I.V., 30 units/day continuous infusion, days 2-5

Repeat cycle every 21 days

**5-FU HURT**

Hydroxyurea, P.O., 1000 mg q12h x 11 doses; start PM of admission, give 2 hours prior to radiation therapy, days 0-5
Fluorouracil, I.V., 800 mg/m²/day continuous infusion, start AM after admission, days 1-5
Paclitaxel, I.V., 5-25 mg/m²/day continuous infusion, start AM after admission; dose escalation study — refer to protocol, days 1-5
G-CSF, S.C., 5 mcg/kg/day, days 6-12, start ≥12 hours after completion of 5-FU infusion

5-7 cycles may be administered

**MAP**

Mitomycin C, I.V., 8 mg/m², day 1
Doxorubicin (Adriamycin®), I.V., 40 mg/m², day 1
Cisplatin (Platinol®), I.V., 60 mg/m², day 1

Repeat cycle every 28 days

**MBC (MBD)**

Methotrexate, I.M./I.V., 40 mg/m², days 1 & 15
Bleomycin, I.M./I.V., 10 units, days 1, 8, 15
Cisplatin, I.V., 50 mg/m², day 4

Repeat cycle every 21 days

**MF**

Methotrexate, I.V., 125-250 mg/m², day 1
Fluorouracil, I.V., 600 mg/m² beginning 1 h after methotrexate, day 1
Leucovorin calcium, I.V./P.O., 10 mg/m² q6h x 5 doses beginning 24 h after methotrexate

Repeat cycle every 7 days

**PFL**

Cisplatin (Platinol®), I.V., 100 mg/m², day 1
Fluorouracil, I.V., 600-800 mg/m²/day continuous infusion, days 1-5
Leucovorin calcium, I.V., 200-300 mg/m²/day, days 1-5

Repeat cycle every 21 days

**PFL+IFN**

Cisplatin (Platinol®), I.V., 100 mg/m², day 1
Fluorouracil, I.V., 640 mg/m²/day continuous infusion, days 1-5
Leucovorin calcium, P.O., 100 mg q4h, days 1-5
Interferon alfa-2b, S.C., 2 x $10^6$ units/m², days 1-6

**Wayne State**

Cisplatin (Platinol®), I.V., 100 mg/m² over 30 minutes, day 1
Fluorouracil, I.V., 1000 mg/m² continuous infusion, days 1-4 (or 5)

Repeat cycle every 21 days

# CANCER CHEMOTHERAPY REGIMENS *(Continued)*

**Single-Agent Regimens**

Carboplatin, I.V., 300-400 mg/m$^2$, over 2 hours every 21-28 days
Methotrexate, I.V., 40 mg/m$^2$, every week, escalating day 14 by 5 mg/m$^2$/wk as tolerated
Cisplatin I.V., 100 mg/m$^2$, every 28 days divided into 1, 2, or 4 equal doses per month
Vinorelbine, I.V., 25-30 mg/m$^2$, repeat weekly

## Leukemias

### Acute Lymphoblastic, Induction

**DVP**

Daunorubicin, I.V., 45 mg/m$^2$, days 1, 2, 3, 14
Vincristine, I.V., 2 mg/m$^2$ (max: 2 mg), days 1, 8, 15, 22
Prednisone, P.O., 45 mg/m$^2$, days 1-28 (35)

**DVPA**

Daunorubicin, I.V., 50 mg/m$^2$, days 1-3
Vincristine, I.V., 2 mg, days 1, 8, 15, 22
Prednisone, P.O., 60 mg/m$^2$, days 1-28
Asparaginase, I.M., 6000 units/m$^2$, days 17-28

**VAD**

Vincristine, I.V., 0.4 mg continuous infusion, days 1-4
Doxorubicin (Adriamycin®), I.V., 12 mg/m$^2$ continuous infusion, days 1-4
Dexamethasone, P.O., 40 mg, days 1-4, 9-12, 17-20

**VP**

Vincristine, I.V., 2 mg/m$^2$/wk for 4-6 weeks (max: 2 mg)
Prednisone, P.O., 60 mg/m$^2$/day in divided doses for 4 weeks, taper weeks 5-7

**VP-L-Asparaginase**

Vincristine, I.V., 2 mg/m$^2$/wk for 4-6 wk (max: 2 mg)
Prednisone, P.O., 60 mg/m$^2$/day for 4-6 wk, then taper
L-asparaginase, I.V., 10,000 units/m$^2$/day

**no known acronym**

Cyclophosphamide, I.V., 1200 mg/m$^2$, day 1
Daunorubicin, I.V., 45 mg/m$^2$, days 1-3
Prednisone, P.O., 60 mg/m$^2$, days 1-21
Vincristine, I.V., 2 mg/m$^2$, weekly
L-asparaginase, I.V., 6000 units/m$^2$, 3 times/wk

**or**

Pegaspargase, I.M./I.V., 2500 units/m$^2$, every 14 days if patient develops hypersensitivity to native L-asparaginase

### Acute Lymphoblastic, Maintenance

**MM**

Mercaptopurine, P.O., 50-75 mg/m$^2$, days 1-7
Methotrexate, P.O./I.V., 20 mg/m$^2$, day 1

Repeat cycle every 7 days

**MMC (MTX + MP + CTX)***

Methotrexate, I.V., 20 mg/m$^2$/wk
Mercaptopurine, P.O., 50 mg/m$^2$/day
Cyclophosphamide, I.V., 200 mg/m$^2$/wk

*Continue all 3 drugs until relapse of disease or after 3 years of remission.

### Acute Lymphoblastic, Relapse

**AVDP**

Asparaginase, I.V., 15,000 units/m$^2$, days 1-5, 8-12, 15-19, 22-26
Vincristine, I.V., 2 mg/m$^2$ (max: 2 mg), days 8, 15, 22
Daunorubicin, I.V., 30-60 mg/m$^2$, days 8, 15, 22
Prednisone, P.O., 40 mg/m$^2$, days 8-12, 15-19, 22-26

### Acute Myeloid Leukemia

**5+2**

***Induction***
Cytarabine (Ara-C), I.V., 100-200 mg/m$^2$ continuous infusion, days 1-5
Daunorubicin, I.V., 45 mg/m$^2$, days 1-2

**7+3**

***Induction***
Cytarabine, I.V., 100-200 mg/m$^2$/day continuous infusion, days 1-7
Daunorubicin, I.V., 45 mg/m$^2$/day, days 1-3

***Modified 7+3 (considerations in elderly patients)***
Cytarabine, I.V., 100 mg/m$^2$/day continuous infusion, days 1-7
Daunorubicin, I.V., 30 mg/m$^2$/day, days 1-3

**D-3+7**

*Induction*
Daunorubicin, I.V., 45 mg/m$^2$, days 1-3
Cytarabine (Ara-C), I.V., 100-200 mg/m$^2$ continuous infusion, days 1-7

**DAT/DCT**

*Induction*
Daunorubicin, I.V., 60 mg/m$^2$/day, days 1-3
Cytarabine (Ara-C), I.V., 200 mg/m$^2$/day continuous infusion, days 1-5
Thioguanine, P.O., 100 mg/m$^2$ q12h, days 1-5

***Modified DAT (considerations in elderly patients)***
Daunorubicin, I.V., 50 mg/m$^2$, day 1
Cytarabine (Ara-C), S.C., 100 mg/m$^2$/day q12h, days 1-5
Thioguanine, P.O., 100 mg/m$^2$ q12h, days 1-5

**HDAC**

*Induction*
Cytarabine, I.V., 3 g/m$^2$ I.V. over 2-3 h q12h x 12 doses, days 1-6

***Modified (considerations in elderly patients)***
Cytarabine, I.V., 2 g/m$^2$ I.V. over 2-3 h q12h x 12 doses, days 1-6

**HiDAC**

*Consolidation*
Cytarabine (Ara-C), I.V., 3000 mg/m$^2$ q12h, days 1-6

**or**

Cytarabine (Ara-C), I.V., 3000 mg/m$^2$ q12h, days 1, 3, 5

**I-3+7**

*Induction*
Idarubicin, I.V., 12 mg/m$^2$, days 1-3
Cytarabine (Ara-C), I.V., 100 mg/m$^2$ continuous infusion, days 1-7

**IC**

*Induction*
Idarubicin (Idamycin®), I.V., 12 mg/m$^2$/day, days 1-3
Cytarabine, I.V., 100-200 mg/m$^2$/day continuous infusion, days 1-7

**LDAC**

*Considerations in Elderly Patients*
Cytarabine, S.C., 10 mg/m$^2$ bid, days 10-21

**MC**

*Induction*
Mitoxantrone, I.V., 12 mg/m$^2$/day, days 1-3
Cytarabine, I.V., 100-200 mg/m$^2$/day continuous infusion, days 1-7

*Consolidation*
Mitoxantrone, I.V., 12 mg/m$^2$, days 1-2
Cytarabine (Ara-C), I.V., 100 mg/m$^2$ continuous infusion, days 1-5

Repeat cycle every 28 days

**MV**

*Induction*
Mitoxantrone, I.V., 10 mg/m$^2$/day, days 1-5
Etoposide (VePesid®), I.V., 100 mg/m$^2$/day, days 1-3

## Acute Nonlymphoblastic, Consolidation

**CD**

Cytarabine, I.V., 3000 mg/m$^2$ q12h, days 1-6
Daunorubicin, I.V., 30 mg/m$^2$/day, days 7-9

## Chronic Lymphocytic Leukemia

**CHL + PRED**

Chlorambucil, P.O., 0.4 mg/kg/day for 1 day every other week
Prednisone, P.O., 100 mg/day for 2 days every other week; adjust dosage according to blood counts every 2 weeks prior to therapy; increase initial dose of 0.4 mg/kg by 0.1 mg/kg every 2 weeks until toxicity or disease control is achieved

**CVP**

Cyclophosphamide, P.O., 400 mg/m$^2$/day, days 1-5
Vincristine (Oncovin®), I.V., 1.4 mg/m$^2$ (max: 2 mg), day 1
Prednisone, P.O., 100 mg/m$^2$, days 1-5

Repeat cycle every 21 days

**Fludarabine**, I.V., 25-30 mg/m$^2$ over 30 min, days 1-5

Repeat cycle every 28 days

**Cladribine** (2-CdA) for fludarabine resistant, I.V., 0.1 mg/kg/day continuous infusion, days 1-7

Repeat cycle every 28 days

## CANCER CHEMOTHERAPY REGIMENS *(Continued)*

### Lung Cancer

#### Small Cell

**ACE/CAE**

Doxorubicin (Adriamycin®), I.V., 45 mg/m², day 1
Cyclophosphamide, I.V., 1000 mg/m², day 1
Etoposide, I.V., 50 mg/m²/day, days 1-5

Repeat cycle every 21 days

**CAV**

Cyclophosphamide, I.V., 1000 mg/m², day 1
Doxorubicin (Adriamycin®), I.V., 50 mg/m², day 1
Vincristine, I.V., 1.4 mg/m² (max: 2 mg), day 1

Repeat cycle every 3 weeks

**CAVE**

Cyclophosphamide, I.V., 750 mg/m², day 1
Doxorubicin (Adriamycin®), I.V., 50 mg/m², day 1
Vincristine, I.V., 1.4 mg/m² (max: 2 mg), day 1
Etoposide, I.V., 60-100 mg/m², days 1-3

Repeat cycle every 3 weeks

**CHOR***

Cyclophosphamide, I.V., 750 mg/m²/day, days 1 & 22
Doxorubicin (Adriamycin®), I.V., 50 mg/m²/day, days 1 & 22
Vincristine, I.V., 1 mg, days 1, 8, 15, 22
Radiation, total dose 3000 rad, 10 daily fractions over 2 weeks beginning with day 36, days 1, 8, 15, 22

**CMC-High Dose***

Cyclophosphamide, I.V., 1000 mg/m²/day, days 1 & 29
Methotrexate, I.V., 15 mg/m²/day twice weekly for 6 weeks, days 1 & 29
Lomustine (CCNU), P.O., 100 mg/m², day 1

*If disease responds, proceed to maintenance therapy.

**CODE**

Cisplatin, I.V., 25 mg/m², every week for 9 weeks
Vincristine (Oncovin®), I.V., 1 mg/m², weeks 1, 2, 4, 6, 8
Doxorubicin, I.V., 25 mg/m², weeks 1, 3, 5, 7, 9
Etoposide, I.V., 80 mg/m², weeks 1, 3, 5, 7, 9

**COPE**

Cyclophosphamide, I.V., 750 mg/m², day 1
Vincristine (Oncovin®), I.V., 1.4 mg/m² (max: 2 mg), day 3
Cisplatin (Platinol®), I.V., 20 mg/m², days 1-3
Etoposide, I.V., 100 mg/m², days 1-3

Repeat cycle every 21 days

**EC**

Etoposide, I.V., 60-100 mg/m², days 1-3
Carboplatin, I.V., 400 mg/m², day 1

Repeat cycle every 28 days

**EP**

Etoposide, I.V., 75-100 mg/m², days 1-3
Cisplatin (Platinol®), I.V., 75-100 mg/m², day 1

Repeat cycle every 21-28 days

**MICE (ICE)**

Mesna uroprotection, I.V. at 20% of ifosfamide doses given immediately before and at 4 and 8 hours after ifosfamide infusion
Ifosfamide, I.V., 2000 mg/m², days 1-3
Carboplatin, I.V., 300-350 mg/m², day 1
Etoposide, I.V., 60-100 mg/m², days 1-3

**PE**

Cisplatin (Platinol®), I.V., 50 mg/m², day 1
Etoposide, I.V., 60 mg/m², days 1-5

Repeat cycle every 21-28 days

**or**

Cisplatin (Platinol®), I.V., 75 mg/m², day 2
Etoposide, I.V., 125 mg/m², days 1, 3, & 5

Repeat cycle every 28 days

**or**

Cisplatin (Platinol®), I.V., 100 mg/m², day 1
Etoposide, I.V., 100 mg/m², days 1-3

Repeat cycle every 28 days

**POCC**

Procarbazine, P.O., 100 mg/m²/day, days 1-14
Vincristine (Oncovin®), I.V., 2 mg/day (max: 2 mg), days 1 & 8
Cyclophosphamide, I.V., 600 mg/m²/day, days 1 & 8
Lomustine (CCNU), P.O., 60 mg/m², day 1

Repeat cycle every 28 days

**VAC (CAV) (Induction)**

Vincristine, I.V., 2 mg/m², day 1
Doxorubicin (Adriamycin®), I.V., 50 mg/m², day 1
Cyclophosphamide, I.V., 750 mg/m², day 1

Repeat cycle every 21 days x 4 cycles

**VC**

Etoposide (VePesid®), I.V., 100-200 mg/m², days 1-3
Carboplatin, I.V., 50-125 mg/m², days 1-3

Repeat cycle every 28 days

**Single-Agent Regimen**

Etoposide, P.O., 160 mg/m², days 1-5

Repeat cycle every 28 days

or

Etoposide, P.O., 50 mg/m², days 1-21

**Nonsmall Cell**

**CAMP**

Cyclophosphamide, I.V., 300 mg/m², days 1 & 8
Doxorubicin (Adriamycin®), I.V., 20 mg/m², days 1 & 8
Methotrexate, I.V., 15 mg/m², days 1 & 8
Procarbazine, P.O., 100 mg/m², days 1-10

Repeat cycle every 28 days

**CAP**

Cyclophosphamide, I.V., 400 mg/m², day 1
Doxorubicin (Adriamycin®), I.V., 40 mg/m², day 1
Cisplatin (Platinol®), I.V., 60 mg/m², day 1

Repeat cycle every 28 days

**CV**

Cisplatin, I.V., 60-80 mg/m², day 1
Etoposide (VePesid®), I.V., 120 mg/m², days 4, 6, & 8

Repeat cycle every 21-28 days

**CVI**

Carboplatin, I.V., 300 mg/m², day 1
Etoposide (VePesid®), I.V., 60-100 mg/m², day 1
Ifosfamide, I.V., 1.5 g/m², days 1, 3 & 5
Mesna, I.V., 20% of ifosfamide dose, given immediately before and 4 and 8 hours after ifosfamide infusion, days 1, 3 & 5

Repeat cycle every 28 days

**EP**

Etoposide, I.V., 75-100 mg/m², days 1-3
Cisplatin (Platinol®), I.V., 75-100 mg/m², day 1

Repeat cycle every 21-28 days

**FAM**

Fluorouracil, I.V., 600 mg/m², days 1, 8, 28, & 36
Doxorubicin (Adriamycin®), I.V., 30 mg/m², days 1 & 28
Mitomycin C, I.V., 10 mg/m², day 1

Repeat cycle every 56 days

**FOMi***

Fluorouracil, I.V., 300 mg/m²/day, days 1-4
Vincristine (Oncovin®), I.V., 2 mg, day 1
Mitomycin C, I.V., 10 mg/m², day 1

*Repeat at 3-week intervals for 3 courses; thereafter, every 6 weeks.

**FOMi/CAP**

Fluorouracil, I.V., 300 mg/m², days 1-4
Vincristine, I.V., 2 mg, day 1
Mitomycin C, I.V., 10 mg/m², day 1
Cyclophosphamide, I.V., 400 mg/m², day 28
Doxorubicin (Adriamycin®), I.V., 40 mg/m², day 28
Cisplatin, I.V., 40 mg/m², day 28

Repeat cycle every 56 days

**MACC**

Methotrexate, I.V., 40 mg/m², day 1
Doxorubicin (Adriamycin®), I.V., 40 mg/m², day 1
Cyclophosphamide, I.V., 400 mg/m², day 1
Lomustine, P.O., 30 mg/m², day 1

Repeat cycle every 21 days

## CANCER CHEMOTHERAPY REGIMENS *(Continued)*

**MICE (ICE)**

Mesna uroprotection, I.V. at 20% of ifosfamide doses given immediately before and at 4 and 8 hours after ifosfamide infusion
Ifosfamide, I.V., 2000 mg/m$^2$, days 1-3
Carboplatin, I.V., 300-350 mg/m$^2$, day 1
Etoposide, I.V., 60-100 mg/m$^2$, day 1

**MVP**

Mitomycin, I.V., 8 mg/m$^2$, days 1, 29, 71
Vinblastine, I.V., 4.5 mg/m$^2$, days 15, 22, 29, then every 2 weeks
Cisplatin (Platinol®), I.V., 120 mg/m$^2$, days 1, 29, then every 6 weeks

**PFL**

Cisplatin (Platinol®), I.V., 25 mg/m$^2$, days 1-5
Fluorouracil, I.V., 800 mg/m$^2$ continuous infusion, days 2-5
Leucovorin calcium, I.V., 500 mg/m$^2$ continuous infusion, days 1-5

Repeat cycle every 28 days

**Single-Agent Regimen**

Vinorelbine (Navelbine®), I.V., 30 mg/m$^2$, every week

### Lymphoma

#### Hodgkin's

**ABVD**

Doxorubicin (Adriamycin®), I.V., 25 mg/m$^2$, days 1 & 15
Bleomycin, I.V., 10 units/m$^2$, days 1 & 15
Vinblastine, I.V., 6 mg/m$^2$, days 1 & 15
Dacarbazine, I.V., 150 mg/m$^2$, days 1-5

Repeat cycle every 28 days

or

Dacarbazine, I.V., 375 mg/m$^2$, days 1 & 15

**ChlVPP**

Chlorambucil, P.O., 6 mg/m$^2$, days 1-14 (max: 10 mg/day)
Vinblastine, I.V., 6 mg/m$^2$, days 1-8 (max: 10 mg dose)
Procarbazine, P.O., 50 mg/m$^2$, days 1-14 (max: 150 mg/day)
Prednisone, P.O., 40 mg/m$^2$, days 1-14 (25 mg/m$^2$ for children)

**CVPP**

Lomustine (CCNU), P.O., 75 mg/m$^2$, day 1
Vinblastine, I.V., 4 mg/m$^2$, days 1, 8
Procarbazine, P.O., 100 mg/m$^2$, days 1-14
Prednisone, P.O., 30 mg/m$^2$, days 1-14 (cycles 1 & 4 only)

Repeat cycle every 28 days

**DHAP**

Dexamethasone, P.O./I.V., 40 mg, days 1-4
Cytarabine (Ara-C), I.V., 2 g/m$^2$, q12h for 2 doses, day 2
Cisplatin (Platinol®), I.V., 100 mg/m$^2$ continuous infusion, day 1

Repeat cycle every 3-4 weeks

**EVA**

Etoposide, I.V., 100 mg/m$^2$, days 1-3
Vinblastine, I.V., 6 mg/m$^2$, day 1
Doxorubicin (Adriamycin®), I.V., 50 mg/m$^2$, day 1

Repeat cycle every 28 days

**MOPP**

Mechlorethamine, I.V., 6 mg/m$^2$, days 1 & 8
Vincristine (Oncovin®), I.V., 1.4 mg/m$^2$ (max: 2.5 mg), days 1 & 8
Procarbazine, P.O., 100 mg/m$^2$, days 1-14
Prednisone, P.O., 40 mg/m$^2$ (cycles 1 & 4 only), days 1-14

Repeat cycle every 28 days

**MOPP/ABV Hybrid**

Mechlorethamine, I.V., 6 mg/m$^2$, day 1
Vincristine (Oncovin®), I.V., 1.4 mg/m$^2$ (max: 2 mg), day 1
Procarbazine, P.O., 100 mg/m$^2$, days 1-7
Prednisone, P.O., 40 mg/m$^2$, days 1-14
Doxorubicin (Adriamycin®), I.V., 35 mg/m$^2$, day 8
Bleomycin, I.V., 10 units/m$^2$, day 8
Vinblastine, I.V., 6 mg/m$^2$, day 8

Repeat cycle every 28 days

**MVPP**

Mechlorethamine, I.V., 6 mg/m$^2$, days 1 & 8
Vinblastine, I.V., 6 mg/m$^2$, days 1 & 8
Procarbazine, P.O., 100 mg/m$^2$, days 1-14
Prednisone, P.O., 40 mg/m$^2$, days 1-14

Repeat cycle every 42 days

**NOVP**

Mitoxantrone (Novantrone®), I.V., 10 mg/m$^2$, day 1
Vincristine (Oncovin®), I.V., 2 mg, day 8
Vinblastine, I.V., 6 mg/m$^2$, day 1
Prednisone, P.O., 100 mg/m$^2$, days 1-5

Repeat cycle every 21 days

**Stanford V**

Mechlorethamine, I.V., 6 mg/m$^2$, weeks 1, 5, 9
Doxorubicin, I.V., 25 mg/m$^2$, weeks 1, 3, 5, 7, 9, 11
Vinblastine, I.V., 6 mg/m$^2$, weeks 1, 3, 5, 7, 9, 11
Vincristine, I.V., 1.4 mg/m$^2$, weeks 2, 4, 6, 8, 10, 12
Bleomycin, I.V., 5 units/m$^2$, weeks 2, 4, 6, 8, 10, 12
Etoposide, I.V., 60 mg/m$^2$ x 2, weeks 3, 7, 11
Prednisone, P.O., 40 mg/m$^2$, daily, dose tapered over the last 15 days

## Non-Hodgkin's

**BACOP**

Bleomycin, I.V., 5 units/m$^2$, days 15 & 22
Doxorubicin (Adriamycin®), I.V., 25 mg/m$^2$, days 1 & 8
Cyclophosphamide, I.V., 650 mg/m$^2$, days 1 & 8
Vincristine (Oncovin®), I.V., 1.4 mg/m$^2$ (max: 2 mg), days 1 & 8
Prednisone, P.O., 60 mg/m$^2$, days 15-28

Repeat cycle every 28 days

**CHOP**

Cyclophosphamide, I.V., 750 mg/m$^2$, day 1
Doxorubicin (Hydroxydaunomycin), I.V., 50 mg/m$^2$, day 1
Vincristine (Oncovin®), I.V., 1.4 mg/m$^2$ (max: 2 mg), day 1
Prednisone, P.O., 100 mg/m$^2$, days 1-5

Repeat cycle every 21 days

**CHOP-Bleo**

Cyclophosphamide, I.V., 750 mg/m$^2$, day 1
Doxorubicin (Hydroxydaunomycin), I.V., 50 mg/m$^2$, day 1
Vincristine (Oncovin®), I.V., 2 mg, days 1 & 5
Prednisone, P.O., 100 mg, days 1-5
Bleomycin, I.V., 15 units, days 1 & 5

Repeat cycle every 21-28 days

**COMLA**

Cyclophosphamide, I.V., 1500 mg/m$^2$, day 1
Vincristine (Oncovin®), I.V., 1.4 mg/m$^2$ (max: 2.5 mg), days 1, 8, 15
Methotrexate, I.V., 120 mg/m$^2$, days 22, 29, 36, 43, 50, 57, 64, 71
Leucovorin calcium rescue, P.O., 25 mg/m$^2$, q6h for 4 doses, beginning 24 hours after each methotrexate dose
Cytarabine (Ara-C), I.V., 300 mg/m$^2$, days 22, 29, 36, 43, 50, 57, 64, 71

Repeat cycle every 21 days

**COP**

Cyclophosphamide, I.V., 800-1000 mg/m$^2$, day 1
Vincristine (Oncovin®), I.V., 1.4 mg/m$^2$ (max: 2 mg), day 1
Prednisone, P.O., 60 mg/m$^2$, days 1-5

Repeat cycle every 21 days

**COP-BLAM**

Cyclophosphamide, I.V., 400 mg/m$^2$, day 1
Vincristine (Oncovin®), I.V., 1 mg/m$^2$, day 1
Prednisone, P.O., 40 mg/m$^2$, days 1-10
Bleomycin, I.V., 15 mg, day 14
Doxorubicin (Adriamycin®), I.V., 40 mg/m$^2$, day 1
Procarbazine (Matulane®), P.O., 100 mg/m$^2$, days 1-10

**COPP (or "C" MOPP)**

Cyclophosphamide, I.V., 400-650 mg/m$^2$, days 1 & 8
Vincristine (Oncovin®), I.V., 1.4-1.5 mg/m$^2$ (max: 2 mg), days 1 & 8
Procarbazine, P.O., 100 mg/m$^2$, days 1-14
Prednisone, P.O., 40 mg/m$^2$, days 1-14

Repeat cycle every 28 days

**CVP**

Cyclophosphamide, P.O., 400 mg/m$^2$, days 1-5
Vincristine, I.V., 1.4 mg/m$^2$ (max: 2 mg), day 1
Prednisone, P.O., 100 mg/m$^2$, days 1-5

Repeat cycle every 21 days

**DHAP**

Dexamethasone (Decadron®), I.V., 10 mg q6h, days 1-4
Cytarabine (Ara-C), I.V., 2 g/m$^2$ q12h x 2 doses, day 2
Cisplatin (Platinol®), I.V., 100 mg/m$^2$ continuous infusion, day 1

Repeat cycle every 21-28 days

## CANCER CHEMOTHERAPY REGIMENS *(Continued)*

**ESHAP**

Etoposide, I.V., 60 mg/m$^2$, days 1-4
Cisplatin, I.V., 25 mg/m$^2$ continuous infusion, days 1-4
Cytarabine (Ara-C), I.V., 2 g/m$^2$, immediately following completion of etoposide and cisplatin therapy
Methylprednisolone, I.V., 500 mg/day, days 1-4
Repeat cycle every 21-28 days

**IMVP-16**

Ifosfamide, I.V., 4 g/m$^2$ continuous infusion over 24 h, day 1
Mesna, I.V., 800 mg/m$^2$ bolus prior to ifosfamide, then 4 g/m$^2$ continuous infusion over 12 hours concurrent w/ifosfamide; then 2.4 g/m$^2$ continuous infusion over 12 hours after ifosfamide infusion, day 1
Methotrexate, I.V., 30 mg/m$^2$, days 3 & 10
Etoposide (VePesid®), I.V., 100 mg/m$^2$, days 1-3
Repeat cycle every 21-28 days

**MACOP-B**

Methotrexate, I.V., 100 mg/m$^2$ weeks 2, 6, 10
Doxorubicin (Adriamycin®), I.V., 50 mg/m$^2$ weeks 1, 3, 5, 7, 9, 11
Cyclophosphamide, I.V., 350 mg/m$^2$ weeks 1, 3, 5, 7, 9, 11
Vincristine (Oncovin®), I.V., 1.4 mg/m$^2$ (max: 2 mg) weeks 2, 4, 8, 10, 12
Bleomycin, I.V., 10 units/m$^2$, weeks 4, 8, 12
Prednisone, P.O., 75 mg/day tapered over 15 d, days 1-15
Leucovorin calcium, P.O., 15 mg q6h x 6 doses 24 h after methotrexate, weeks 2, 6, 10

**m-BACOD**

Methotrexate, I.V., 200 mg/m$^2$, days 8 & 15
Leucovorin calcium, P.O., 10 mg/m$^2$ q6h x 8 doses beginning 24 h after each methotrexate dose, days 8 & 15
Bleomycin, I.V., 4 units/m$^2$, day 1
Doxorubicin (Adriamycin®), I.V., 45 mg/m$^2$, day 1
Cyclophosphamide, I.V., 600 mg/m$^2$, day 1
Vincristine (Oncovin®), I.V., 1 mg/m$^2$, day 1
Dexamethasone, P.O., 6 mg/m$^2$, days 1-5
Repeat cycle every 21 days

**m-BACOS**

Methotrexate, I.V., 1 g/m$^2$, day 2
Bleomycin, I.V., 10 units/m$^2$, day 1
Doxorubicin (Adriamycin®), I.V., 50 mg/m$^2$ continuous infusion, day 1
Cyclophosphamide, I.V., 750 mg/m$^2$, day 1
Vincristine (Oncovin®), I.V., 1.4 mg/m$^2$ (max: 2 mg), day 1
Leucovorin calcium rescue, P.O., 15 mg q6h for 8 doses, starting 24 hours after methotrexate
Methylprednisolone, I.V., 500 mg, days 1-3
Repeat cycle every 21-25 days

**MINE**

Mesna, I.V., 1.33 g/m$^2$/day concurrent with ifosfamide dose, then 500 mg P.O. 4 hours after each ifosfamide infusion, days 1-3
Ifosfamide, I.V., 1.33 g/m$^2$/day, days 1-3
Mitoxantrone (Novantrone®), I.V., 8 mg/m$^2$, day 1
Etoposide, I.V., 65 mg/m$^2$/day, days 1-3
Repeat cycle every 28 days

**Pro-MACE**

Prednisone, P.O., 60 mg/m$^2$, days 1-14
Methotrexate, I.V., 1.5 g/m$^2$, day 14
Leucovorin calcium, I.V., 50 mg/m$^2$ q6h x 5 doses beginning 24 h after methotrexate dose, day 14
Doxorubicin (Adriamycin®), I.V., 25 mg/m$^2$, days 1 & 8
Cyclophosphamide, I.V., 650 mg/m$^2$, days 1 & 8
Etoposide, I.V., 120 mg/m$^2$, days 1 & 8
Repeat cycle every 28 days

**Pro-MACE-CytaBOM**

Prednisone, P.O., 60 mg/m$^2$, days 1-14
Doxorubicin (Adriamycin®), I.V., 25 mg/m$^2$, day 1
Cyclophosphamide, I.V., 650 mg/m$^2$, day 1
Etoposide, I.V., 120 mg/m$^2$, day 1
Cytarabine, I.V., 300 mg/m$^2$, day 8
Bleomycin, I.V., 5 units/m$^2$, day 8
Vincristine (Oncovin®), I.V., 1.4 mg/m$^2$ (max: 2 mg), day 8
Methotrexate, I.V., 120 mg/m$^2$, day 8
Leucovorin calcium, P.O., 25 mg/m$^2$ q6h x 4 doses, day 9
Repeat cycle every 21 days

## Malignant Melanoma

**BCDT**

Carmustine (BCNU), I.V., 150 mg/m$^2$, day 1
Cisplatin, I.V., 25 mg/m$^2$, days 1-3, 21-23
Dacarbazine, I.V., 220 mg/m$^2$, days 1-3, 21-23
Tamoxifen, P.O., 10 mg bid, days 1-42

**BHD**

Carmustine (BCNU), I.V., 100-150 mg/m$^2$, day 1
Repeat cycle every 42 days

Hydroxyurea, P.O., 1480 mg/m$^2$, days 1-5
Dacarbazine, I.V., 100-150 mg/m$^2$, days 1-5
Repeat cycle every 21 days

**DTIC-ACTD**

Dacarbazine, I.V., 750 mg/m$^2$, day 1
Dactinomycin, I.V., 1 mg/m$^2$, day 1
Repeat cycle every 28 days

**VBC**

Vinblastine, I.V., 6 mg/m$^2$, days 1 & 2
Bleomycin, I.V., 15 units/m$^2$/day continuous infusion, days 1-5
Cisplatin, I.V., 50 mg/m$^2$, day 5
Repeat cycle every 28 days

**VDP**

Vinblastine, I.V., 5 mg/m$^2$, days 1 & 2
Dacarbazine, I.V., 150 mg/m$^2$, days 1-5
Cisplatin (Platinol®), I.V., 75 mg/m$^2$, day 5
Repeat cycle every 21-28 days

### Multiple Myeloma

**AC (DC)**

Doxorubicin (Adriamycin®), I.V., 30 mg/m$^2$, day 1
Carmustine, I.V., 30 mg/m$^2$, day 1
Repeat cycle every 21-28 days

**BCP**

Carmustine (BCNU), I.V., 75 mg/m$^2$, day 1
Cyclophosphamide, I.V., 400 mg/m$^2$, day 1
Prednisone, P.O., 75 mg, days 1-7
Repeat cycle every 28 days

**EDAP**

Etoposide, I.V., 100-200 mg/m$^2$, days 1-4
Dexamethasone, P.O./I.V., 40 mg/m$^2$, days 1-5
Cytarabine (Ara-C), 1000 mg, day 5
Cisplatin (Platinol®), I.V., 20 mg continuous infusion, days 1-4

**MeCP**

Methyl-CCNU, P.O., 100 mg/m$^2$, day 1
Repeat cycle every 56 days

Cyclophosphamide, I.V., 600 mg/m$^2$, day 1
Prednisone, P.O., 40 mg/m$^2$/day, days 1-7
Repeat cycle every 28 days

**MP**

Melphalan, P.O., 8 mg/m$^2$, days 1-4
Prednisone, P.O., 40 mg/m$^2$/day, days 1-7
Repeat cycle every 28 days

**M-2**

Vincristine, I.V., 0.03 mg/kg (max: 2 mg), day 1
Carmustine, I.V., 0.5 mg/kg, day 1
Cyclophosphamide, I.V., 10 mg/kg, day 1
Melphalan, P.O., 0.25 mg/kg, days 1-4
Prednisone, P.O., 1 mg/kg/day, then taper next 14 days, days 1-7
Repeat cycle every 35 days

**VAD**

Vincristine, I.V., 0.4 mg/day continuous infusion, days 1-4
Doxorubicin (Adriamycin®), I.V., 9-10 mg/m$^2$/day continuous infusion, days 1-4
Dexamethasone, P.O., 40 mg, days 1-4, 9-12, 17-20
Repeat cycle every 25-35 days

**VBAP**

Vincristine, I.V., 1 mg, day 1
Carmustine (BCNU), I.V., 30 mg/m$^2$, day 1
Doxorubicin (Adriamycin®), I.V., 30 mg/m$^2$, day 1
Prednisone, P.O., 100 mg, days 1-4
Repeat cycle every 21 days

## CANCER CHEMOTHERAPY REGIMENS *(Continued)*

**VCAP**

Vincristine, I.V., 1 mg, day 1
Cyclophosphamide, P.O., 100 mg/m$^2$, days 1-4
Doxorubicin (Adriamycin®), I.V., 25 mg/m$^2$, day 2
Prednisone, P.O., 60 mg/m$^2$, days 1-4

Repeat cycle every 28 days

**Single-Agent Regimens**

**DEX**

Dexamethasone, 20 mg/m$^2$ every morning for 4 days beginning on days 1, 9, and 17, every 14 days for 3 cycles
Interferon alfa-2b, S.C., 3 million units 3 times/week for maintenance therapy in patients with significant response to initial chemotherapy treatment

### Ovarian Cancer

#### Epithelial

**CC**

Carboplatin, I.V., 300 mg/m$^2$, day 1
Cyclophosphamide, I.V., 600 mg/m$^2$, day 1

Repeat cycle every 28 days

**CDC**

Carboplatin, I.V., 300 mg/m$^2$, day 1
Doxorubicin, I.V., 40 mg/m$^2$, day 1
Cyclophosphamide, I.V., 500 mg/m$^2$, day 1

Repeat cycle every 28 days

**CHAP**

Cyclophosphamide, I.V., 300-500 mg/m$^2$, day 1
Hexamethylmelamine, P.O., 150 mg/m$^2$, days 1-7
Doxorubicin (Adriamycin®), I.V., 30-50 mg/m$^2$, day 1
Cisplatin (Platinol®), I.V., 50 mg/m$^2$, day 1

Repeat cycle every 28 days

**CP**

Cyclophosphamide, I.V., 600 mg/m$^2$, day 1
Cisplatin (Platinol®), I.V., 75-100 mg/m$^2$, day 1

Repeat cycle every 21 days

**PAC (CAP)**

Cisplatin (Platinol®), I.V., 50 mg/m$^2$, day 1
Doxorubicin (Adriamycin®), I.V., 50 mg/m$^2$, day 1
Cyclophosphamide, I.V., 750 mg/m$^2$, day 1

Repeat cycle every 21 days x 8 cycles

**PT**

Cisplatin (Platinol®), I.V., 75 mg/m$^2$ (after Taxol®), day 1
Taxol®, I.V., 135 mg/m$^2$, day 1

Repeat cycle every 21 days

**Single-Agent Regimen**

Paclitaxel, I.V., 135 mg/m$^2$ continuous infusion, over 24 hours
 Patient must be premedicated with:
 Dexamethasone 20 mg P.O., 12 and 6 h prior
 Diphenhydramine 50 mg I.V., 30 min prior
 Cimetidine 300 mg I.V., or ranitidine 50 mg I.V., 30 min prior

#### Germ Cell

**BEP**

Bleomycin, I.V., 30 units, days 2, 9, 16
Etoposide, I.V., 100 mg/m$^2$, days 1-5
Cisplatin (Platinol®), I.V., 20 mg/m$^2$, days 1-5

**VAC**

Vincristine, I.V., 1.2-1.5 mg/m$^2$ (max: 2 mg) weekly for 10-12 weeks, or every 2 weeks for 12 doses
Dactinomycin (Actinomycin D), I.V., 0.3-0.4 mg/m$^2$, days 1-5
Cyclophosphamide, I.V., 150 mg/m$^2$, days 1-5

Repeat every 28 days

### Pancreatic Cancer

**FAM**

Fluorouracil, I.V., 600 mg/m$^2$/wk, weeks 1, 2, 5, 6, 9
Doxorubicin (Adriamycin®), I.V., 30 mg/m$^2$/wk, weeks 1, 5, 9
Mitomycin C, I.V., 10 mg/m$^2$/wk, weeks 1, 9

**FMS (SMF)**

Fluorouracil, I.V., 600 mg/m$^2$, days 1, 8, 29 & 36
Mitomycin C, I.V., 10 mg/m$^2$, day 1
Streptozocin, I.V., 1 g/m$^2$, days 1, 8, 29 & 36

Repeat cycle every 56 days

**SD**

Streptozocin, I.V., 500 mg/m$^2$, days 1-5
Doxorubicin, I.V., 50 mg/m$^2$, days 1 & 22

Repeat cycle every 42 days

## Renal Cancer

**Single-Agent Regimens**

Aldesleukin (rIL-2), various dosing regimens — please refer to the literature
Interferon alfa-2b, various dosing regimens — please refer to the literature
Floxuridine, S.C., 0.1 mg/kg, days 1-14

Repeat cycle every 21 days

Vinblastine, I.V., 1.2 mg/m$^2$ continuous infusion, days 1-4

## Sarcoma

### Bony Sarcoma

**AC**

Doxorubicin (Adriamycin®), I.V., 75-90 mg/m$^2$ 96-h continuous infusion
Cisplatin, I.A./I.V., 90-120 mg/m$^2$, 6 days

Repeat cycle every 28 days

**CYVADIC**

Cyclophosphamide, I.V., 600 mg/m$^2$, day 1
Vincristine, I.V., 1.4 mg/m$^2$ (max: 2 mg) weekly x 6 weeks, then on day 1 of future cycles
Doxorubicin (Adriamycin®), I.V., 15 mg/m$^2$/day continuous infusion, days 1-4
Dacarbazine (DTIC), I.V., 250 mg/m$^2$/day continuous infusion, days 1-4

Repeat cycle every 21-28 days

**HDMTX**

Methotrexate, I.V., 8-12 g/m$^2$
Leucovorin calcium, I.V./P.O., 15-25 mg q6h for at least 10 doses beginning 24 h after methotrexate dose; courses repeated weekly for 2-4 weeks, alternating with various cancer chemotherapy combination regimens

**IMAC**

Ifosfamide, I.V., 1.2 g/m$^2$/day continuous infusion, days 1-5
Mesna, I.V., 400 mg/m$^2$ bolus prior to ifosfamide infusion day 1, then 1.2 g/m$^2$/day continuous infusion days 1-5 concurrent with ifosfamide, then 600 mg/m$^2$ continuous infusion over 12 hours after ifosfamide infusion, days 1-5
Doxorubicin (Adriamycin®), I.V., 15 mg/m$^2$/day continuous infusion, days 2-5
Cisplatin, I.V./I.A., 120 mg/m$^2$ continuous infusion over 24 hours, day 7

Repeat cycle every 28 days

**VAIE**

Vincristine, I.V., 1.5 mg/m$^2$/day, days 1 & 5
Doxorubicin (Adriamycin®), I.V., 20 mg/m$^2$/day continuous infusion, days 1-4
Ifosfamide, I.V., 1800 mg/m$^2$/day, days 1-5
Etoposide, I.V., 50 mg/m$^2$/day, days 1-5

Repeat cycle every 21 days

**VADRIAC — High Dose**

Vincristine, I.V., 1.5 mg/m$^2$/day, days 1 & 5
Cyclophosphamide, I.V., 2.1 g/m$^2$/day, days 1 & 2
Doxorubicin (Adriamycin®), I.V., 25 mg/m$^2$/day continuous infusion, days 1-3

Repeat cycle every 21 days

### Soft-Tissue Sarcoma

**CYADIC**

Cyclophosphamide, I.V., 600 mg/m$^2$, day 1
Doxorubicin (Adriamycin®), I.V., 15 mg/m$^2$/day continuous infusion, days 1-4
Dacarbazine (DTIC), I.V., 250 mg/m$^2$/day continuous infusion, days 1-4

Repeat cycle every 21-28 days

**CYVADIC**

Cyclophosphamide, I.V., 500 mg/m$^2$, day 1
Vincristine, I.V., 1.4 mg/m$^2$ (max: 2 mg), days 1 & 5
Doxorubicin (Adriamycin®), I.V., 50 mg/m$^2$, day 1
Dacarbazine (DTIC), I.V., 250 mg/m$^2$, days 1-5

Repeat cycle every 21 days

**ICE**

Ifosfamide, I.V., 2000 mg/m$^2$, days 1-3
Carboplatin, I.V., 300-600 mg/m$^2$, day 3
Etoposide, I.V., 100 mg/m$^2$, days 1-3

## CANCER CHEMOTHERAPY REGIMENS *(Continued)*

**ID**

Ifosfamide, I.V., 5 g/m² continuous infusion over 24 hours, day 1
Mesna, I.V., 1 g/m² bolus prior to ifosfamide infusion, then 4 g/m² continuous infusion over 32 hours, day 1
Doxorubicin, I.V., 40 mg/m², day 1

Repeat cycle every 21 days

**MAID**

Mesna, I.V., 500 mg/m² bolus 15 min prior to ifosfamide infusion, then q3h x 3, days 1-3
Doxorubicin (Adriamycin®), I.V., 20 mg/m² continuous infusion over 24 h, days 1-3
Ifosfamide, I.V., 2500 mg/m² over 1 h, days 1-3
Dacarbazine*, I.V., 300 mg/m² continuous infusion over 24 h, days 1-3

Repeat cycle every 28 days

*Adriamycin and dacarbazine may be mixed in the same bag.

**VAC**

Vincristine, I.V., 2 mg/m² (max: 2 mg) per week on weeks 1-12
Dactinomycin, I.V., 0.015 mg/kg (max: 0.5 mg) every 3 months for 5-6 courses, days 1-5
Cyclophosphamide, P.O., 2.5 mg/kg/day for 2 years

# CORTICOSTEROID EQUIVALENCIES COMPARISON

| Glucocorticoid | Approximate Equivalent Dose (mg) | Routes of Administration | Relative Anti-inflammatory Potency | Relative Mineralocorticoid Potency | Half-life | |
|---|---|---|---|---|---|---|
| | | | | | Plasma (min) | Biologic (h) |
| **Short-Acting** | | | | | | |
| Cortisone | 25 | P.O., I.M. | 0.8 | 2 | 30 | 8-12 |
| Hydrocortisone | 20 | I.M., I.V. | 1 | 2 | 80-118 | |
| **Intermediate-Acting** | | | | | | |
| Prednisone | 5 | P.O. | 4 | 1 | 60 | 18-36 |
| Prednisolone | 5 | P.O., I.M., I.V., intra-articular, intradermal, soft tissue injection | 4 | 1 | 115-212 | |
| Triamcinolone | 4 | P.O., I.M., intra-articular, intradermal, intrasynovial, soft tissue injection | 5 | 0 | 200+ | |
| Methylprednisolone | 4 | P.O., I.M., I.V. | 5 | 0 | 78-188 | |
| **Long-Acting** | | | | | | |
| Dexamethasone | 0.75 | P.O., I.M., I.V., intra-articular, intradermal, soft tissue injection | 25-30 | 0 | 110-210 | 36-54 |
| Betamethasone | 0.6-0.75 | P.O., I.M., intra-articular, intradermal, intrasynovial, soft tissue injection | 25 | 0 | 300+ | |

# CORTICOSTEROIDS, TOPICAL COMPARISON

| Steroid | | Vehicle |
|---|---|---|
| **Lowest Potency** (may be ineffective for some indications) | | |
| 0.1% | Betamethasone | Cream |
| 0.2% | Betamethasone (Celestone®) | Cream |
| 0.05% | Desonide | Cream |
| 0.04% | Dexamethasone (Hexadrol®)* | Cream |
| 0.1% | Dexamethasone (Decadron® Phosphate, Decaderm®)* | Cream, gel |
| 1% | Hydrocortisone | Cream, ointment, lotion |
| 2.5% | Hydrocortisone | Cream, ointment |
| 0.25% | Methylprednisolone acetate (Medrol®) | Ointment |
| 1% | Methylprednisolone acetate (Medrol®) | Ointment |
| 0.5% | Prednisolone (Meti-Derm®) | Cream |
| **Low Potency** | | |
| 0.01% | Betamethasone valerate (Valisone®, reduced strength) | Cream |
| 0.1% | Clocortolone (Cloderm®) | Cream |
| 0.03% | Flumethasone pivalate (Locorten®) | Cream |
| 0.01% | Fluocinolone acetonide (Synalar®)* | Cream, solution |
| 0.025% | Fluorometholone (Oxylone®) | Cream |
| 0.025% | Flurandrenolide (Cordran®, Cordran® SP)* | Cream, ointment |
| 0.2% | Hydrocortisone valerate (Westcort®) | Cream |
| 0.025% | Triamcinolone acetonide (Kenalog®)* | Cream, ointment |
| **Intermediate Potency** | | |
| 0.025% | Betamethasone benzoate | Cream, gel, lotion |
| 0.1% | Betamethasone valerate (Valisone®)* | Cream, ointment, lotion |
| 0.05% | Desonide (Tridesilon®) | Cream, ointment |
| 0.05% | Desoximetasone (Topicort® LP) | Cream |
| 0.025% | Fluocinolone acetonide* | Cream, ointment |
| 0.05% | Flurandrenolide (Cordran®, Cordran® SP)* | Cream, ointment, lotion |
| 0.025% | Halcinonide (Halog®) | Cream, ointment |
| 0.1% | Triamcinolone acetonide (Kenalog®)* | Cream, ointment |
| **High Potency** | | |
| 0.1% | Amcinonide (Cyclocort®) | Cream, ointment |
| 0.05% | Betamethasone dipropionate (Diprosone®) | Cream, ointment, lotion |
| 0.05% | Clobetasol dipropionate | Cream, ointment |
| 0.25% | Desoximetasone (Topicort®) | Cream |
| 0.05% | Diflorasone diacetate (Florone®, Maxiflor®) | Cream, ointment |
| 0.2% | Fluocinolone (Synalar-HP®) | Cream |
| 0.05% | Fluocinonide (Lidex®)* | Cream, ointment |
| 0.1% | Halcinonide (Halog®) | Cream, ointment, solution |
| 0.5% | Triamcinolone acetonide* | Cream, ointment |

*Fluorinated.

# NARCOTIC AGONISTS

## Comparative Pharmacokinetics

| Drug | Onset (min) | Peak (h) | Duration (h) | t ½ (h) | Average Dosing Interval (h) | | Equianalgesic Doses* (mg) | |
|---|---|---|---|---|---|---|---|---|
| | | | | | | | I.M. | P.O. |
| Alfentanil | Immediate | ND | ND | 1-2 | — | — | ND | NA |
| Buprenorphine | 15 | 1 | 4-8 | 2-3 | | | 0.4 | — |
| Butorphanol | I.M.: 30-60 I.V.: 4-5 | 0.5-1 | 3-5 | 2.5-3.5 | 3 | (3-6) | 2 | — |
| Codeine | P.O.: 30-60 I.M.: 10-30 | 0.5-1 | 4-6 | 3-4 | 3 | (3-6) | 120 | 200 |
| Fentanyl | I.M.: 7-15 I.V.: Immediate | ND | 1-2 | 1.5-6 | 1 | (0.5-2) | 0.1 | NA |
| Hydrocodone | ND | ND | 4-8 | 3.3-4.4 | 6 | (4-8) | ND | ND |
| Hydromorphone | P.O.: 15-30 | 0.5-1 | 4-6 | 2-4 | 4 | (3-6) | 1.5 | 7.5 |
| Levorphanol | P.O.: 10-60 | 0.5-1 | 4-8 | 12-16 | 6 | (6-24) | 2 | 4 |
| Meperidine | P.O./I.M./ S.C.: 10-15 I.V.: ≤5 | 0.5-1 | 2-4 | 3-4 | 3 | (2-4) | 75 | 300 |
| Methadone | P.O.: 30-60 I.V.: 10-20 | 0.5-1 | 4-6 (acute) >8 (chronic) | 15-30 | 8 | (6-12) | 10 | 20 |
| Morphine | P.O.: 15-60 I.V.: ≤5 | P.O./I.M./ S.C.: 0.5-1 I.V.: 0.3 | 3-6 | 2-4 | 4 | (3-6) | 10 | 60# (acute) 30 (chronic) |
| Nalbuphine | I.M.: 30 I.V.: 1-3 | 1 | 3-6 | 5 | | — | 10 | — |
| Naloxone† | 2-5 | 0.5-2 | 0.5-1 | 0.5-1.5 | | — | — | — |
| Oxycodone | P.O.: 10-15 | 0.5-1 | 4-6 | 3-4 | 4 | (3-6) | NA | 30 |
| Oxymorphone | 5-15 | 0.5-1 | 3-6 | | | | 1 | 10‡ |
| Pentazocine | 15-20 | 0.25-1 | 3-4 | 2-3 | 3 | (3-6) | | |
| Propoxyphene | P.O.: 30-60 | 2-2.5 | 4-6 | 3.5-15 | 6 | (4-8) | ND | 130§-200¶ |
| Sufentanil | 1.3-3 | ND | ND | 2.5-3 | — | — | 0.02 | NA |

ND = no data available. NA = not applicable.

*Based on acute, short-term use. Chronic administration may alter pharmacokinetics and decrease the oral parenteral dose ratio. The morphine oral-parenteral ratio decreases to ~1.5-2.5:1 upon chronic dosing.

#Extensive survey data suggest that the relative potency of I.M.:P.O. morphine of 1:6 changes to 1:2-3 with chronic dosing.

†Narcotic antagonist.

‡Rectal.

§HCl salt.

¶Napsylate salt.

## NARCOTIC AGONISTS *(Continued)*

### Comparative Pharmacology

| Drug | Analgesic | Antitussive | Constipation | Respiratory Depression | Sedation | Nausea/ Vomiting |
|---|---|---|---|---|---|---|
| **Phenanthrenes** | | | | | | |
| Codeine | + | +++ | + | + | + | + |
| Hydrocodone | + | +++ | | + | | |
| Hydromorphone | ++ | +++ | + | ++ | + | + |
| Levorphanol | ++ | ++ | ++ | ++ | ++ | + |
| Morphine | ++ | +++ | ++ | ++ | ++ | ++ |
| Oxycodone | ++ | +++ | ++ | ++ | ++ | ++ |
| Oxymorphone | ++ | + | ++ | +++ | | +++ |
| **Phenylpiperidines** | | | | | | |
| Alfentanil | ++ | | | | | |
| Fentanyl | ++ | | | + | | + |
| Meperidine | ++ | + | + | ++ | + | |
| Sufentanil | +++ | | | | | |
| **Diphenylheptanes** | | | | | | |
| Methadone | ++ | ++ | ++ | ++ | + | + |
| Propoxyphene | + | | | + | + | + |
| **Agonist/ Antagonist** | | | | | | |
| Buprenorphine | ++ | N/A | +++ | +++ | ++ | ++ |
| Butorphanol | ++ | N/A | +++ | +++ | ++ | + |
| Dezocine | ++ | | + | ++ | + | ++ |
| Nalbuphine | ++ | N/A | +++ | +++ | ++ | ++ |
| Pentazocine | ++ | N/A | + | ++ | ++ or stimulation | ++ |

# DENTAL DRUG INTERACTIONS: UPDATE ON DRUG COMBINATIONS REQUIRING SPECIAL CONSIDERATIONS

This update discussion includes 16 drug interaction monographs describing clinically important drug combinations requiring special considerations in dental practice. The actions which have resulted from these combinations range from life-threatening adverse effects to attenuation of the therapeutic effects of the interacting drug. The monographs are organized according to the four major groups of drugs used in dentistry: antibiotics, nonsteroidal anti-inflammatory drugs (including aspirin), epinephrine (vasoconstrictors), and narcotic analgesics. An additional monograph on Valium® and alcohol is included.

## ANTIBIOTICS - ORAL CONTRACEPTIVES

### Description of the Interaction

Case reports suggest that antibiotics used in dentistry can reduce the effectiveness of oral contraceptives resulting in breakthrough ovulation and unplanned pregnancies.

### Mechanism

Estrogens, which are components of oral contraceptives, are activated in the intestine by bacteria and reabsorbed into the blood stream as active compounds to inhibit ovulation. Antibiotics reduce the bacteria population in the intestine, which may result in less activated estrogen available to inhibit ovulation.

### Background Reports

Tetracyclines: One report described a woman on an estrogen-type oral contraceptive who became pregnant after a 5-day course of tetracycline[1]. Also, several cases of unintended pregnancy and menstrual irregularities have been reported following concurrent use of tetracyclines and oral contraceptives[2,3].

Penicillins: Ampicillin has been shown to reduce estrogen levels in women not taking oral contraceptives and there are reports of unplanned pregnancies in women taking ampicillin with oral contraceptives[4,5]. Concomitant use of penicillin with estrogen-containing oral contraceptives decreased the efficacy of the contraceptive and increased the incidence of breakthrough bleeding[6,7]. Since amoxicillin is closely related to other penicillins, it may also interact with oral contraceptives.

Cephalosporins: Cephalexin (Keflex®) has been reported to interact with oral contraceptives resulting in an unplanned pregnancy[8].

Erythromycins: Unlike ampicillin and tetracyclines, erythromycins have been implicated in only a few cases of oral contraceptive failure over the last 15 years and it is questionable whether erythromycin was the cause of those reported failures.[9].

### Management

If antibiotics are prescribed to oral contraceptive users, it is suggested that the patients be advised to use additional methods of birth control during both 7 to 10 day dosing, and the two-dose prophylaxis regimens. Any additional method of birth control should be continued through the remaining oral contraceptive cycle.

1. Bacon JF and Shenfield GM, "Pregnancy Attributable to Interaction Between Tetracycline and Oral Contraceptives," *Br Med J*, 1980, 280(6210):293.
2. Orme MLE, "The Clinical Pharmacology of Oral Contraceptive Steroids," *Br J Clin Pharmacol*, 1982, 14:31.
3. Back DJ, Grimmer SF, Orme ML, et al, "Evaluation of Committee on Safety of Medicines Yellow Card Reports on Oral Contraceptive-Drug Interactions With Anticonvulsants and Antibiotics," *Br J Clin Pharmacol*, 1988, 25(5):527-32.
4. Trybuchowski H, "Effect of Ampicillin on the Urinary Output of Steroidal Hormones in Pregnant and Nonpregnant Women," *Clin Chim Acta*, 1973, 45:9-18.
5. Aldercreutz H, Martin F, Lehtinen T, et al, "Effect of Ampicillin Administration on Plasma Conjugated and Unconjugated Estrogen and Progesterone Levels in Pregnancy," *Am J Obstet Gynecol*, 1977, 128(3):266-71.
6. Proudfit CW, "Concurrent Oral Contraceptive and Antibiotic Therapy," *JAMA*, 1981, 246:2076.
7. True RJ, "Interactions Between Antibiotics and Oral Contraceptives," *JAMA*, 1982, 247(10):1408.
8. Bainton R, "Interaction Between Antibiotic Therapy and Contraceptive Medication," *Oral Surg Oral Med Oral Pathol*, 1986, 61(5):453-5.

## TETRACYCLINES - ANTACIDS (Containing Divalent or Trivalent Ions)

### Description of the Interaction

Concomitant therapy with a tetracycline and an antacid containing aluminum, calcium, or magnesium products can reduce serum concentration and the efficacy of the tetracycline.

# DENTAL DRUG INTERACTIONS: UPDATE ON DRUG COMBINATIONS REQUIRING SPECIAL CONSIDERATIONS *(Continued)*

### Mechanism

Aluminum, calcium, and magnesium ions can combine with the tetracycline molecule in the gastrointestinal tract to form a larger ionized molecule unable to be absorbed into the blood stream.

### Background

The interaction between tetracyclines and antacids containing aluminum, calcium, and magnesium is well documented. Foods and dairy products containing calcium will also impair the absorption of tetracyclines. Some reports suggest that doxycycline and minocycline are minimally affected by antacids and dairy products[1,2].

### Management

Tetracyclines should be given as far apart as possible from antacids and dairy products.

1. Welling PG, Koch PA, Lau CC, et al, "Bioavailability of Tetracycline and Doxycycline in Fasted and Nonfasted Subjects," *Antimicrob Agents Chemother*, 1977, 11(3):462-9.
2. "Anti-Infective Drug Interactions," *Drug Interactions and Updates*, Hansten PD and Horn JR, eds, Malvern, PA: Lea and Febiger.

## TETRACYCLINE - PENICILLIN

### Description of the Interaction

Simultaneous tetracycline-penicillin therapy may impair the efficacy of penicillin.

### Mechanism

Penicillin kills bacteria by inhibiting cell wall synthesis. Tetracycline inhibits protein synthesis in bacteria and this action has been shown to antagonize the cell wall inhibiting effect of penicillin.

### Background

Most of the manufacturers product information contains warnings against using tetracyclines and penicillins together.

### Management

Tetracycline-penicillin combination should never be used to treat oral infections. For penicillin two-dose prophylaxis, it would be prudent not to give to patients taking tetracycline. Reappoint if possible.

## ERYTHROMYCIN - PENICILLIN

+ ERYTHROMY
+ LIPITOR (ATORVASTATIN) CHOLES ↓

### Description of the Interaction

Simultaneous erythromycin-penicillin therapy may impair the efficacy of penicillin.

### Mechanism

Penicillin kills bacteria by inhibiting cell wall synthesis. Erythromycin inhibits protein synthesis in bacteria and this action may antagonize the cell wall inhibiting effect of penicillin.

### Background

This interaction has not been sufficiently documented in clinical studies.

### Management

Erythromycin-penicillin combination should not be used to treat oral infections. For penicillin two-dose prophylaxis, it would be prudent not to give to patients taking erythromycin. Reappoint if possible.

## ERYTHROMYCIN - THEOPHYLLINE

### Description of the Interaction

Erythromycins interact with theophylline, a bronchodilator, to result in symptoms suggestive of a relative overdose of theophylline. Resulting symptoms were nausea, vomiting, and seizures.

### Mechanism

A recent study showed that erythromycin forms complexes with a specific enzyme that metabolizes theophylline and that this complex may explain the impairment of theophylline metabolic inactivation resulting in symptoms of theophylline overdose[1].

### Background

An erythromycin regimen of 5 to 20 day daily dosing in theophylline patients caused increased blood levels, a longer half-life and decreased urinary clearance of the theophylline[2]. A more recent review indicated that many patients did not experience any interactions between the two drugs with 8 out of 22 studies reporting no change in theophylline kinetics after erythromycin dosing[3]. The interactions which have occurred have included all formulations of erythromycin. There have been no reported interactions between erythromycin and theophylline when using the prophylaxis dosing schedule.

### Management

Patients taking theophylline and who may be at increased risk for theophylline toxicity should be given erythromycin with caution and only if there is absolutely no alternative to erythromycin. These patients should be monitored closely.

1. Delaforge M and Sartori E, "In Vivo Effects of Erythromycin, Oleandomycin, and Erythralosamine Derivatives on Hepatic Cytochrome P-450," *Biochem Pharmacol*, 1990, 40(2):223-8.
2. Cummins LH, et al, "Erythromycin's Effect on Theophylline Blood Levels. Correspondence," *Pediatrics*, 1977, 59:144-5.
3. Ludden TM, "Pharmacokinetic Interactions of the Macrolide Antibiotics," *Clin Pharmacokinet*, 1985, 10(1):63-79.

## ERYTHROMYCIN - CARBAMAZEPINE (Tegretol®)

### Description of the Interaction

Erythromycin has interacted with carbamazepine (Tegretol®), an antiepileptic, to cause increased blood levels resulting in carbamazepine toxicity[1]. Symptoms were drowsiness, dizziness, nausea, headache, and blurred vision.

### Mechanism

This interaction is suggestive of an inhibition of the hepatic metabolizing enzymes by erythromycin which normally convert carbamazepine to inactive products.

### Background

The increased blood levels of carbamazepine has occurred within one day of concomitant erythromycin therapy[1]. This effect has not been reported with the two-dose erythromycin, prophylaxis regimen.

### Management

Patients taking carbamazepine and who may be at increased risk for carbamazepine toxicity should be given erythromycin with caution and only if there is absolutely no alternative to erythromycin. These patients should be monitored closely.

1. Ludden TM, "Pharmacokinetic Interactions of the Macrolide Antibiotics," *Clin Pharmacokinet*, 1985, 10(1):63.

## ERYTHROMYCIN - TRIAZOLAM (Halcion®)

### Description of the Interaction

Erythromycin has interacted with triazolam (Halcion®), a hypnotic type antianxiety agent, to cause increased blood levels resulting in triazolam toxicity. Resulting effects were psychomotor impairment and memory dysfunction.

### Mechanism

This interaction is suggestive of an inhibition of the hepatic metabolizing enzymes by erythromycin which normally convert triazolam to inactive products.

### Background

Erythromycin has caused significant increases in triazolam blood concentrations within 3 days after 333 mg erythromycin base 3 times/day and triazolam 0.5 mg daily[1].

### Management

Patients taking triazolam should be given erythromycin with caution and only if there is absolutely no alternative to erythromycin. These patients should be closely monitored.

1. Phillips JP, "A Pharmacokinetic Drug Interaction Between Erythromycin and Triazolam," *J Clin Psychopharmacol*, 1986, 6(5):297-9.

## IBUPROFEN (Motrin®, Advil®, Nuprin®) - ORAL ANTICOAGULANTS (Coumarins)

### Description of the Interaction

Bleeding may occur when ibuprofen is administered to patients taking coumarin type anticoagulants.

# DENTAL DRUG INTERACTIONS: UPDATE ON DRUG COMBINATIONS REQUIRING SPECIAL CONSIDERATIONS *(Continued)*

### Mechanism

Inhibition of prostaglandins by ibuprofen results in decreased platelet aggregation and interference with blood clotting, resulting in an enhancement of the anticoagulant effect of coumarins.

### Background

Product information on ibuprofen in the 1995 edition of the *Physicians' Desk Reference* (PDR) states that Motrin® inhibits platelet aggregation, but the effect is quantitatively less and of shorter duration than aspirin. It goes on to state that bleeding has been reported when Motrin® had been administered to patients on coumarin-type anticoagulants and the clinician should use caution in these circumstances. Additional product information on naproxen, diflunisal, and flurbiprofen is listed in the same edition of the PDR. It advises caution when using naproxen with coumarins since interactions have been seen with other NSAIDs of this class; it states that diflunisal, when given with warfarin, resulted in prolongation of prothrombin time; and it states that serious clinical bleeding has been reported in patients taking flurbiprofen together with coumarins. Product information for warfarin (Coumadin®) in the 1995 PDR states that ibuprofen, naproxen, and diflunisal may be responsible for increased prothrombin time response of the warfarin. Flurbiprofen was not mentioned.

### Management

It is suggested that ibuprofen (Motrin®, Advil®, Nuprin®) and other dental NSAIDs such as naproxen (Naprosyn®), naproxen sodium (Anaprox®, Aleve®), diflunisal (Dolobid®), flurbiprofen (ANSAID®), and ketorolac (Toradol® Oral), be used with caution (if at all) in patients taking coumarin-type anticoagulants. Use of other analgesics is preferred.

## IBUPROFEN (Motrin®, Advil®, Nuprin®) - LITHIUM

### Description of the Interaction

Concurrent administration of ibuprofen with lithium produces symptoms of lithium toxicity including nausea, vomiting, slurred speech, and mental confusion.

### Mechanism

Prostaglandins stimulate renal lithium tubular secretion. NSAIDs inhibit prostaglandin-induced renal secretion of lithium, which increases lithium plasma levels and produces symptoms of lithium toxicity.

### Background

Lithium is used for the treatment of acute mania and to prevent recurrent episodes of bipolar (manic-depressive) illness. The therapeutic lithium plasma concentration is extremely narrow (0.8-1.2 mEq/L) and drugs that cause lithium plasma levels to go outside this narrow therapeutic range will result in lithium toxicity. Of the four NSAIDs used in dentistry (ibuprofen, naproxen, diflunisal, and flurbiprofen) the former two have been well documented to interact with lithium. In 1980, Ragheb, et al, reported that a patient taking 2400 mg ibuprofen daily experienced nausea and drowsiness while stabilized on lithium[1]. The lithium plasma level increased from 0.8 to 1.0 mEq/L. Subsequently, in a study of 11 healthy volunteers, Kristoff, et al, observed that 400 mg of ibuprofen 4 times/day combined with 450 mg of lithium carbonate every 12 hours, increased lithium plasma levels within several days[2]. Decreased ability to concentrate, lightheadedness, and fatigue resulted from this interaction.

Ragheb reported that concomitant administration of lithium and ibuprofen (1.8 g/day) in nine patients with bipolar- or schizoid-type disorders resulted in significant increases (average 34%) in lithium plasma concentrations as well as decreases in lithium clearance[3]. Individual variations were observed, with increases in lithium levels ranging from 12% to 66% within 6 days of concomitant administration of ibuprofen. In this study, tremors occurred in three patients as a result of this interaction. Ragheb reported that patients older than 50 years were more susceptible to lithium toxicity. The 1993 edition of the *Physician's Desk Reference* (PDR) (in the monograph for Motrin®) warns that concomitant use of ibuprofen and lithium citrate or carbonate may elevate lithium plasma levels and reduce renal lithium clearance.

In a 1986 study by Ragheb and Powell, concomitant administration of naproxen and lithium has resulted in individual variations in plasma lithium levels (from increases of 0% to 42%[4]. In that study, lithium renal clearance decreased in patients who were taking daily doses of lithium (900 mg) and naproxen (750 mg) for 6 days. The monograph for Naprosyn® in the 1993 PDR cautions that concomitant use of naproxen and lithium could increase lithium plasma concentrations.

Interactions between diflunisal (Dolobid®) and lithium, and flurbiprofen (Ansaid®) and lithium have not been reported. Nor is any potential interaction between these two NSAIDs and lithium mentioned in the PDR. Interestingly, aspirin has been shown to affect plasma lithium levels in healthy subjects[5]. Lack of documentation about diflunisal and flurbiprofen does not mean these agents are safe to use in conjunction with lithium. NSAIDs should be used with caution by dental patients who are taking lithium. Substitution of NSAIDs with acetaminophen preparations may be warranted.

### Management

Extreme caution is necessary in administering NSAIDs to lithium patients; use of analgesics other than NSAIDs is preferred.


1. Ragheb M, Ban TA, Buchanan D, et al, "Interaction of Indomethacin and Ibuprofen With Lithium in Manic Patients Under a Steady-State Lithium Level," *J Clin Psychiatry*, 1980, 41(11):397-8.
2. Kristoff CA, Hayes PE, Barr WH, et al, "Effect of Ibuprofen on Lithium Plasma and Red Blood Cell Concentrations," *Clin Pharm*, 1986, 5(1):51-5.
3. Ragheb M, "Ibuprofen Can Increase Serum Lithium Level in Lithium-Treated Patients," *J Clin Psychiatry*, 1987, 48(4):161-3.
4. Ragheb M and Powell AL, "Lithium Interaction With Sulindac and Naproxen," *J Clin Psychopharmacol*, 1986, 6(3):150-4.
5. Reimann IW, Diener U, and Frolich JC, "Indomethacin But Not Aspirin Increases Plasma Lithium Ion Levels," *Arch Gen Psychiatry*, 1983, 40(3):283-6.


## ASPIRIN - ORAL ANTICOAGULANTS (Coumarins)

### Description of the Interaction

Aspirin increases the risk of bleeding in patients taking oral anticoagulants.

### Mechanism

Small doses of aspirin inhibit platelet function. Larger doses (>3 g/day) elicit a hypoprothrombinemic effect. Aspirin may also displace oral anticoagulants from plasma protein-binding sites. These actions of aspirin all contribute to increase the risk of bleeding in patients taking oral anticoagulants.

### Background

There is much documentation in the literature confirming this interaction. One study using over 500 patients showed that excessive bleeding was about 3 times more common with warfarin (Coumadin®) plus aspirin (500 mg/day) than with warfarin alone[1]. Another study showed enhanced hypoprothrombinemia in warfarin patients during the first few days of aspirin therapy (1 g/day)[2]. There are other reports describing bleeding episodes due to concurrent therapy with aspirin and oral anticoagulants[3,4].

### Management

Patients receiving oral anticoagulants should avoid aspirin and aspirin-containing products.


1. Chesebro JH, Fuster V, Elveback LR, et al, "Trial of Combined Warfarin Therapy Plus Dipyridamole or Aspirin Therapy in Prosthetic Heart Valve Replacement: Danger of Aspirin Compared With Dipyridamole," *Am J Cardiol*, 1983, 51(9):1537-41.
2. Donaldson DR, Sreeharan N, Crow MJ, et al, "Assessment of the Interaction of Warfarin With Aspirin and Dipyridamole," *Thromb Haemost*, 1982, 47(1):77.
3. Starr KJ and Petrie JC, "Drug Interactions in Patients on Long-Term Oral Anticoagulant and Antihypertensive Adrenergic Neuron-Blocking Drugs," *Br Med J*, 1972, 4(833):133-5.
4. Udall JA, "Drug Interference With Warfarin Therapy," *Clin Med*, 1970, 77:20.


## ASPIRIN - PROBENECID (Benemid®)

### Description of the Interaction

Aspirin inhibits the uricosuric action of probenecid.

### Mechanism

Unknown

### Background

The inhibition of probenecid-induced uricosuria by aspirin is dose-dependent. Doses of aspirin of 1 g or less do not appear to affect probenecid uricosuria. Larger doses, however, appear to considerably inhibit uricosuria. Conversely, probenecid appears to inhibit uricosuria following large doses of aspirin. Aspirin does not interfere with the actions of probenecid to inhibit the renal elimination of penicillins.

### Management

It appears prudent to use a nonsalicylate-type analgesic (ie, acetaminophen or NSAID) in patients receiving probenecid as a uricosuric agent (treatment of gouty arthritis).

# DENTAL DRUG INTERACTIONS: UPDATE ON DRUG COMBINATIONS REQUIRING SPECIAL CONSIDERATIONS *(Continued)*

## EPINEPHRINE (Vasoconstrictor) - TRICYCLIC ANTIDEPRESSANTS

### Description of the Interaction

Use of epinephrine as vasoconstrictor in local anesthetic injections may cause a hypertensive interaction in patients taking tricyclic antidepressants.

### Mechanism

Tricyclic antidepressants cause increases of norepinephrine in synaptic areas in the central nervous system and periphery. Epinephrine may add to the effects of norepinephrine resulting in vasoconstriction and transient hypertension.

### Background

There is adequate information in the literature to confirm a hypertensive interaction between epinephrine, norepinephrine, and levonordefrin with TCAs. An I.V. infusion of epinephrine to healthy subjects receiving imipramine resulted in two- to four-fold increases in the pressor response to epinephrine[1,2]. Also cardiac dysrhythmias were reported. Although these effects were seen with I.V. infusions, these reports suggested that caution should certainly be exercised if epinephrine is administered by other routes. I.V. infusions of norepinephrine to healthy subjects receiving imipramine resulted in a four- to eight-fold increase in the pressor response to norepinephrine[1,2] and a later study showed a two-fold increase in pressor response to norepinephrine[3]. Other tricyclics were associated with a three-fold increase in pressor response to norepinephrine[4]. This increased pressor response was probably due to tricyclic antidepressant-induced inhibition of norepinephrine reuptake. Similar effects have been reported with levonordefrin[5].

### Management

The use of epinephrine in patients taking tricyclic type antidepressants is potentially dangerous. Use minimum amounts of vasoconstrictor with caution in patients on tricyclic antidepressants.


1. Boakes AJ, Laurence DR, Teoh PC, et al, "Interactions Between Sympathomimetic Amines and Antidepressant Agents in Man," *Br Med J*, 1973, 1(849):311-5.
2. Svedmyr N, "The Influence of a Tricyclic Antidepressive Agent (Protriptyline) on Some of the Circulatory Effects of Noradrenaline and Adrenaline in Man," *Life Sci*, 1968, 7(1):77-84.
3. Larochelle P, Hamet P, and Enjalbert M, "Response to Tyramine and Norepinephrine After Imipramine and Trazodone," *Clin Pharmacol Ther*, 1979, 26(1):24-30.
4. Mitchell JR, Cavanaugh JH, Arias L, et al, "Guanethidine and Related Agents. III. Antagonism by Drugs Which Inhibit the Norepinephrine Pump in Man," *J Clin Invest*, 1970, 49(8):1596-604.
5. Jastak JT and Yagiela JA, "Vasoconstrictors and Local Anesthesia: A Review and Rationale for Use," *J Am Dent Assoc*, 1983, 107(4):623-30.


## EPINEPHRINE (Vasoconstrictor) - MONOAMINE OXIDASE INHIBITORS

### Description of the Interaction

Use of epinephrine as vasoconstrictor in local anesthetic injections may cause a hypertensive interaction in patients taking monoamine oxidase inhibitors.

### Mechanism

Drugs which inhibit monoamine oxidase cause increases in the concentration of endogenous norepinephrine, serotonin, and dopamine in storage sites throughout the central nervous system. Epinephrine may add to the effects of norepinephrine resulting in vasoconstriction and transient hypertension.

### Background

One study reported on four healthy subjects taking MAOIs and given I.V. epinephrine. There was no significant effect on heart rate or blood pressure[1]. This same study also showed a lack of interaction with norepinephrine and MAOI> Nevertheless, it is advisable that vasoconstrictors be used with caution in these patients. Hansten and Horn[2]report that MAOIs may slightly increase the pressor response to norepinephrine and epinephrine, an action which appeared to be due to receptor sensitivity by the MAOI.

### Management

There is a potential for unexpected increases in blood pressure when using epinephrine vasoconstrictor in patients taking monoamine oxidase inhibitors. Use vasoconstrictor with caution in these patients.


1. Boakes AJ, Laurence DR, Teoh PC, et al, "Interactions Between Sympathomimetic Amines and Antidepressant Agents in Man," *Br Med J*, 1973, 1(849):311-5.

2. Hansten PD and Horn JR, eds, "Monoamine Oxidase Inhibitor Interactions," *Drug Interactions and Updates*, Malvern, PA: Lea and Febiger, 1990, 387-8.

## NARCOTIC ANALGESICS - CIMETIDINE (Tagamet®)

### Description of the Interaction

Cimetidine may increase the adverse effects of narcotic analgesics.

### Mechanism

The hepatic metabolism of narcotic analgesics to inactive products may be inhibited by cimetidine. The central nervous system effects of narcotic analgesics and cimetidine may be additive.

### Background

One study reported that cimetidine, when given to patients taking meperidine (Demerol®), reduced the rate of renal excretion of the narcotic, resulting in increased sedation and an increase in respiratory depression[1]. Additional studies showed that cimetidine may inhibit the liver metabolism of meperidine and fentanyl, another narcotic analgesic thus exacerbating the sedative effects of both of these narcotics[2,3].

### Management

Although the side effects of cimetidine on codeine, hydrocodone, and oxycodone are unknown, it is advised to use caution in prescribing these narcotic analgesics in dental patients taking cimetidine. Ranitidine (Zantac®) is probably less likely to interact with narcotic analgesics.

1. Guay DR, Meatherall RC, Chalmers JL, et al, "Cimetidine Alters Pethidine Disposition in Man," *Br J Clin Pharmacol*, 1984, 18(6):907-14.
2. Knodell RG, Holtzman JL, Crankshaw DL, et al, "Drug Metabolism by Rat and Human Hepatic Microsomes in Response to Interaction With $H_2$-Receptor Antagonists," *Gastroenterology*, 1982, 82(1):84-8.
3. Lee HR, et al, "Effect of Histamine $H_2$-Receptors on Fentanyl Metabolism," *Pharmacologist*, 1982, 24:145.

## BENZODIAZEPINES - Diazepam (Valium®) - ALCOHOL

### Description of the Interaction

Alcohol may enhance the adverse psychomotor effects of benzodiazepines such as Valium®. Combined use may result in dangerous inebriation, ataxia, and respiratory depression.

### Mechanism

Alcohol and benzodiazepines have additive central nervous system depressant activity. Also, alcohol may increase the gastrointestinal absorption of diazepam[1,2] leading to symptoms of diazepam overdose.

### Background

There is much documentation in the literature to confirm the serious interaction between alcohol and benzodiazepines. Many controlled studies have shown that benzodiazepines such as diazepam enhance the detrimental effects of alcohol on simulated driving, reaction times, and other psychomotor skills[3-6].

### Management

Patients receiving benzodiazepines such as diazepam (Valium®) should be warned against taking any alcohol until the benzodiazepine is cleared from the body. This is usually 48-72 hours after the last dose. This interaction has been unpredictable and significant CNS depression and ataxia has occurred with only a single dose of diazepam (5 mg) along with a moderate amount of alcohol.

1. Hayes SL, Pablo G, Radomski T, et al, "Ethanol and Oral Diazepam Absorption," *N Engl J Med*, 1977, 296(4)-186-9.
2. MacLeod SM, Giles HG, Parzalek G, et al, "Diazepam Actions and Plasma Concentrations Following Ethanol Ingestion," *Eur J Clin Pharmacol*, 1977, 11(5):345-9.
3. Linnoila M and Hakkinen S, "Effects of Diazepam and Codeine, Alone and in Combination With Alcohol, on Simulated Driving," *Clin Pharmacol Ther*, 1974, 15(4):368-73.
4. Linnoila M, "Effects of Diazepam, Chlordiazepoxide, Thioridazine, Haloperidol, Flupenthixole, and Alcohol on Psychomotor Skills Related to Driving," *Ann Med Exp Biol Fenn*, 1973, 51(3):125-32.
5. Linnoila M, "Drug Interaction on Psychomotor Skills Related to Driving: Diazepam and Alcohol," *Eur J Clin Pharmacol*, 1973, 5:186.
6. Morland J, Setekleiv J, Haffner JF, et al, "Combined Effects of Diazepam and Ethanol on Psychomotor Functions," *Acta Pharmacol Toxicol*, 1975, 34(1):5-15.

# OCCUPATIONAL EXPOSURE TO BLOODBORNE PATHOGENS (UNIVERSAL PRECAUTIONS)

## OVERVIEW AND REGULATORY CONSIDERATIONS

Every healthcare employee, from nurse to housekeeper, has some (albeit small) risk of exposure to HIV and other viral agents such as hepatitis B and Jakob-Creutzfeldt agent. The incidence of HIV-1 transmission associated with a percutaneous exposure to blood from an HIV-1 infected patient is approximately 0.3% per exposure.[1] In 1989, it was estimated that 12,000 United States healthcare workers acquired hepatitis B annually.[2] An understanding of the appropriate procedures, responsibilities, and risks inherent in the collection and handling of patient specimens is necessary for safe practice and is required by Occupational Safety and Health Administration (OSHA) regulations.

The Occupational Safety and Health Administration published its "Final Rule on Occupational Exposure to Bloodborne Pathogens" in the Federal Register on December 6, 1991. OSHA has chosen to follow the Center for Disease Control (CDC) definition of universal precautions. The Final Rule provides full legal force to universal precautions and requires employers and employees to treat blood and certain body fluids as if they were infectious. The Final Rule mandates that healthcare workers must avoid parenteral contact and must avoid splattering blood or other potentially infectious material on their skin, hair, eyes, mouth, mucous membranes, or on their personal clothing. Hazard abatement strategies must be used to protect the workers. Such plans typically include, but are not limited to, the following:

- safe handling of sharp items ("sharps") and disposal of such into puncture resistant containers
- gloves required for employees handling items soiled with blood or equipment contaminated by blood or other body fluids
- provisions of protective clothing when more extensive contact with blood or body fluids may be anticipated (eg, surgery, autopsy, or deliveries)
- resuscitation equipment to reduce necessity for mouth to mouth resuscitation
- restriction of HIV- or hepatitis B-exposed employees to noninvasive procedures

OSHA has specifically defined the following terms: **Occupational exposure** means reasonably anticipated skin, eye mucous membrane, or parenteral contact with blood or other potentially infectious materials that may result from the performance of an employee's duties. **Other potentially infectious materials** are human body fluids including semen, vaginal secretions, cerebrospinal fluid, synovial fluid, pleural fluid, pericardial fluid, peritoneal fluid, amniotic fluid, saliva in dental procedures, and body fluids that are visibly contaminated with blood, and all body fluids in situations where it is difficult or impossible to differentiate between body fluids; any unfixed tissue or organ (other than intact skin) from a human (living or dead); and HIV-containing cell or tissue cultures, organ cultures, and HIV- or HBV-containing culture medium or other solutions, and blood, organs, or other tissues from experimental animals infected with HIV or HBV. An **exposure incident** involves specific eye, mouth, other mucous membrane, nonintact skin, or parenteral contact with blood or other potentially infectious materials that results from the performance of an employee's duties.[3] It is important to understand that some exposures may go unrecognized despite the strictest precautions.

A written Exposure Control Plan is required. Employers must provide copies of the plan to employees and to OSHA upon request. Compliance with OSHA rules may be accomplished by the following methods.

- **Universal precautions (UPs)** means that all human blood and certain body fluids are treated as if known to be infectious for HIV, HBV, and other bloodborne pathogens. UPs do not apply to feces, nasal secretions, saliva, sputum, sweat, tears, urine, or vomitus unless they contain visible blood.
- **Engineering controls (ECs)** are physical devices which reduce or remove hazards from the workplace by eliminating or minimizing hazards or by isolating the worker from exposure. Engineering control devices include sharps disposal containers, self-resheathing syringes, etc.
- **Work practice controls (WPCs)** are practices and procedures that reduce the likelihood of exposure to hazards by altering the way in which a task is performed. Specific examples are the prohibition of two-handed recapping of needles, prohibition of storing food alongside potentially contaminated material, discouragement of pipetting fluids by mouth, encouraging handwashing after removal of gloves, safe handling of contaminated sharps, and appropriate use of sharps containers.
- **Personal protective equipment (PPE)** is specialized clothing or equipment worn to provide protection from occupational exposure. PPE includes gloves, gowns, laboratory coats (the type and characteristics will depend upon the task and degree of exposure anticipated), face shields or masks, and eye protection. Surgical caps or hoods and/or shoe covers or boots are required in instances in

which gross contamination can reasonably be anticipated (eg, autopsies, orthopedic surgery). If PPE is penetrated by blood or any contaminated material, the item must be removed immediately or as soon as feasible. **The employer must provide and launder or dispose of all PPE at no cost to the employee.** Gloves must be worn when there is a reasonable anticipation of hand contact with potentially infectious material, including a patient's mucous membranes or nonintact skin. Disposable gloves must be changed as soon as possible after they become torn or punctured. Hands must be washed after gloves are removed. OSHA has revised the PPE standards, effective July 5, 1994, to include the requirement that the employer certify in writing that it has conducted a hazard assessment of the workplace to determine whether hazards are present that will necessitate the use of PPE. Also, verification that the employee has received and understood the PPE training is required.[4]

**Housekeeping protocols**: OSHA requires that all bins, cans, and similar receptacles, intended for reuse which have a reasonable likelihood for becoming contaminated, be inspected and decontaminated immediately or as soon as feasible upon visible contamination and on a regularly scheduled basis. Broken glass that may be contaminated must not be picked up directly with the hands. Mechanical means (eg, brush, dust pan, tongs, or forceps) must be used. Broken glass must be placed in a proper sharps container.

Employers are responsible for teaching appropriate clean-up procedures for the work area and personal protective equipment. A 1:10 dilution of household bleach is a popular and effective disinfectant. It is prudent for employers to maintain signatures or initials of employees who have been properly educated. If one does not have written proof of education of universal precautions teaching, then by OSHA standards, such education never happened.

**Pre-exposure and postexposure protocols**: OSHA's Final Rule includes the provision that employees, who are exposed to contamination, be offered the hepatitis B vaccine at no cost to the employee. Employees may decline; however, a declination form must be signed. The employee must be offered free vaccine if he/she changes his/her mind. Vaccination to prevent the transmission of hepatitis B in the healthcare setting is widely regarded as sound practice.[5] In the event of exposure, a confidential medical evaluation and follow-up must be offered at no cost to the employee. Follow-up must include collection and testing of blood from the source individual for HBV and HIV if permitted by state law if a blood sample is available. If a postexposure specimen must be specially drawn, the individual's consent is usually required. Some states may not require consent for testing of patient blood after accidental exposure. One must refer to state and/or local guidelines for proper guidance.

The employee follow-up must also include appropriate postexposure prophylaxis, counseling, and evaluation of reported illnesses. The employee has the right to decline baseline blood collection and/or testing. If the employee gives consent for the collection but not the testing, the sample must be preserved for 90 days in the event that the employee changes his/her mind within that time. Confidentiality related to blood testing must be ensured. **The employer does not have the right to know the results** of the testing of either the source individual or the exposed employee.

## MANAGEMENT OF OCCUPATIONAL EXPOSURE TO HIV IN THE WORKPLACE[6]

1. Likelihood of transmission of HIV-1 from occupational exposure is 0.2% per parenteral exposure (eg, needlestick) to blood from HIV infected patients.
2. Factors that increase risk for occupational transmission include advanced stages of HIV in source patient, hollow bore needle puncture, a poor state of health or inexperience of healthcare worker (HCW).
3. Immediate actions an exposed healthcare worker should take include aggressive first aid at the puncture site (eg, scrubbing site with povidone-iodine solution for 10 minutes) or at mucus membrane site (eg, saline irrigation of eye for 15 minutes). Then immediate reporting to the hospital's occupational medical service. The authors indicate that there is no direct evidence for the efficacy of their recommendations. Other institutions suggest rigorous scrubbing with soap.
4. After first aid is initiated, the healthcare worker should report exposure to a supervisor and to the institution's occupational medical service for evaluation.
5. Occupational medicine should perform a thorough investigation including identifying the HIV and hepatitis B status of the source, type of exposure, volume of inoculum, timing of exposure, extent of injury, appropriateness of first aid, as well as psychological status of the healthcare worker. HIV serologies should be performed on the healthcare worker. HIV risk counselling should begin at this point.
6. All parenteral exposures should be treated equally until they can be evaluated by the occupational medicine service, who will then determine the actual risk of exposure. Follow-up counselling sessions may be necessary.
7. Although the data are not clear, antiviral prophylaxis may be offered to healthcare workers who are parenterally or mucous membrane exposed. If used, antiretroviral prophylaxis should be initiated within 1-2 hours after exposure.

## OCCUPATIONAL EXPOSURE TO BLOODBORNE PATHOGENS (UNIVERSAL PRECAUTIONS) *(Continued)*

8. Counselling regarding risk of exposure, antiviral prophylaxis, plans for follow up, exposure prevention, sexual activity, and providing emotional support and response to concerns are necessary to support the exposed healthcare worker. Follow-up should consist of periodic serologic evaluation and blood chemistries and counts if antiretroviral prophylaxis is initiated. Additional information should be provided to healthcare workers who are pregnant or planning to become pregnant.

## HAZARDOUS COMMUNICATION

Communication regarding the dangers of bloodborne infections through the use of labels, signs, information, and education is required. Storage locations (eg, refrigerators and freezers, waste containers) that are used to store, dispose of, transport, or ship blood or other potentially infectious materials require labels. The label background must be red or bright orange with the biohazard design and the word biohazard in a contrasting color. The label must be part of the container or affixed to the container by permanent means.

Education provided by a qualified and knowledgeable instructor is mandated. The sessions for employees must include:

- accessible copies of the regulation
- general epidemiology of bloodborne diseases
- modes of bloodborne pathogen transmission
- an explanation of the exposure control plan and a means to obtain copies of the written plan
- an explanation of the tasks and activities that may involve exposure
- the use of exposure prevention methods and their limitations (eg, engineering controls, work practices, personal protective equipment)
- information on the types, proper use, location, removal, handling, decontamination, and disposal of personal protective equipment)
- an explanation of the basis for selection of personal protective equipment
- information on the HBV vaccine, including information on its efficacy, safety, and method of administration and the benefits of being vaccinated (ie, the employee must understand that the vaccine and vaccination will be offered free of charge)
- information on the appropriate actions to take and persons to contact in an emergency involving exposure to blood or other potentially infectious materials
- an explanation of the procedure to follow if an exposure incident occurs, including the method of reporting the incident
- information on the postexposure evaluation and follow-up that the employer is required to provide for the employee following an exposure incident
- an explanation of the signs, labels, and color coding
- an interactive question-and-answer period

## RECORD KEEPING

The OSHA Final Rule requires that the employer maintain both education and medical records. The medical records must be kept confidential and be maintained for the duration of employment plus 30 years. They must contain a copy of the employee's HBV vaccination status and postexposure incident information. Education records must be maintained for 3 years from the date the program was given.

OSHA has the authority to conduct inspections without notice. Penalties for cited violation may be assessed as follows.

**Serious violations. In this situation, there is a substantial probability of death or serious physical harm, and the employer knew, or should have known, of the hazard. A violation of this type carries a mandatory penalty of up to $7000 for each violation.**

**Other-than-serious violations**. The violation is unlikely to result in death or serious physical harm. This type of violation carries a discretionary penalty of up to $7000 for each violation.

**Willful violations**. These are violations committed knowingly or intentionally by the employer and have penalties of up to $70,000 per violation with a minimum of $5000 per violation. If an employee dies as a result of a willful violation, the responsible party, if convicted, may receive a personal fine of up to $250,000 and/ or a 6-month jail term. A corporation may be fined $500,000.

Large fines frequently follow visits to laboratories, physicians' offices, and healthcare facilities by OSHA Compliance Safety and Health Offices (CSHOS). Regulations are vigorously enforced. A working knowledge of the final rule and implementation of appropriate policies and practices is imperative for all those involved in the collection and analysis of medical specimens.

Effectiveness of universal precautions in averting exposure to potentially infectious materials has been documented.[7] Compliance with appropriate rules, procedures, and policies, including reporting exposure incidents, is a matter of personal professionalism and prudent self-preservation.

## Footnotes

1. Henderson DK, Fahey BJ, Willy M, et al, "Risk for Occupational Transmission of Human Immunodeficiency Virus Type 1 (HIV-1) Associated With Clinical Exposures. A Prospective Evaluation," *Ann Intern Med*, 1990, 113(10):740-6.
2. Niu MT and Margolis HS, "Moving Into a New Era of Government Regulation: Provisions for Hepatitis B Vaccine in the Workplace, *Clin Lab Manage Rev*, 1989, 3:336-40.
3. Bruning LM, "The Bloodborne Pathogens Final Rule — Understanding the Regulation," *AORN Journal*, 1993, 57(2):439-40.
4. "Rules and Regulations," *Federal Register*, 1994, 59(66):16360-3.
5. Schaffner W, Gardner P, and Gross PA, "Hepatitis B Immunization Strategies: Expanding the Target," *Ann Intern Med*, 1993, 118(4):308-9.
6. Fahey BJ, Beekmann SE, Schmitt JM, et al, "Managing Occupational Exposures to HIV-1 in the Healthcare Workplace," *Infect Control Hosp Epidemiol*, 1993, 14(7):405-12.
7. Wong ES, Stotka JL, Chinchilli VM, et al, "Are Universal Precautions Effective in Reducing the Number of Occupational Exposures Among Healthcare Workers?" *JAMA*, 1991, 265(9):1123-8.

## References

Buehler JW and Ward JW, "A New Definition for AIDS Surveillance," *Ann Intern Med*, 1993, 118(5):390-2.

Brown JW and Blackwell H, "Complying With the New OSHA Regs, Part 1: Teaching Your Staff About Biosafety," *MLO*, 1992, 24(4)24-8. Part 2: "Safety Protocols No Lab Can Ignore," 1992, 24(5):27-9. Part 3: "Compiling Employee Safety Records That Will Satisfy OSHA," 1992, 24(6):45-8.

Department of Labor, Occupational Safety and Health Administration, "Occupational Exposure to Bloodborne Pathogens; Final Rule (29 CFR Part 1910.1030), "*Federal Register*, December 6, 1991, 64004-182.

Gold JW, "HIV-1 Infection: Diagnosis and Management," *Med Clin North Am*, 1992, 76(1):1-18.

"Hepatitis B Virus: A Comprehensive Strategy for Eliminating Transmission in the United States Through Universal Childhood Vaccination," Recommendations of the Immunization Practices Advisory Committee (ACIP), *MMWR Morb Mortal Wkly Rep*, 1991, 40(RR-13):1-25.

"Mortality Attributable to HIV Infection/AIDS — United States", *MMWR Morb Mortal Wkly Rep*, 1991, 40(3):41-4.

National Committee for Clinical Laboratory Standards, "Protection of Laboratory Workers From Infectious Disease Transmitted by Blood, Body Fluids, and Tissue," NCCLS Document M29-T, Villanova, PA: NCCLS, 1989, 9(1).

"Nosocomial Transmission of Hepatitis B Virus Associated With a Spring-Loaded Fingerstick Device — California," *MMWR Morb Mortal Wkly Rep*, 1990, 39(35):610-3.

Polish LB, Shapiro CN, Bauer F, et al, "Nosocomial Transmission of Hepatitis B Virus Associated With the Use of a Spring-Loaded Fingerstick Device," *N Engl J Med*, 1992, 326(11):721-5.

"Recommendations for Preventing Transmission of Human Immunodeficiency Virus and Hepatitis B Virus to Patients During Exposure-Prone Invasive Procedures," *MMWR Morb Mortal Wkly Rep*, 1991, 40(RR-8):1-9.

"Update: Acquired Immunodeficiency Syndrome — United States," *MMWR Morb Mortal Wkly Rep*, 1992, 41(26):463-8.

"Update: Transmission of HIV Infection During an Invasive Dental Procedure — Florida," *MMWR Morb Mortal Wkly Rep*, 1991, 40(2):21-7, 33.

"Update: Universal Precautions for Prevention of Transmission of Human Immunodeficiency Virus, Hepatitis B Virus, and Other Bloodborne Pathogens in Healthcare Settings," *MMWR Morb Mortal Wkly Rep*, 1988, 37(24):377-82, 387-8.

# ORGANISMS ISOLATED IN HEAD & NECK INFECTIONS

| Organisms | Percentage Infections |
|---|---|
| *Alpha hemolytic streptococci* | 41 |
| *Staphylococci aureas* | 27 |
| *Staphylococci epidermidis* | 23 |
| *Bacteroides* sp | 17 |
| *Streptococcus intermedius* | 7 |
| *Klebsiella pneumoniae* | 7 |
| Beta hemolytic streptococci | 7 |
| Non-A, Non-B, Non-D | 7 |
| Group A | 7 |
| Group B | 5 |
| *Peptostreptococcus* sp | 6 |
| Fungi | 6 |
| Mycobacteria tuberculosis | 6 |
| *Actinobacter* | 5 |
| Other anaerobic gram-negative rods | 5 |
| *Proteus* | 3 |
| *Enterobacter* | 3 |
| Anaerobic gram-negative cocci | 3 |
| *Neisseria* | 3 |
| *Bacillus* sp | 3 |
| *Actinomyces* | 3 |
| Other *Klebsiella* sp | 3 |
| *Streptococcus pneumoniae* | 3 |
| *Bifidobacterium* | 3 |
| Microaerophilic streptococci | 3 |
| *Propionibacterium* sp | 3 |
| *Pseudomonas* | 1 |
| *Escherichia coli* | 1 |

# PREDOMINANT CULTIVABLE MICROORGANISMS OF THE ORAL CAVITY

| Type | Predominant Genus or Family |
|---|---|
| Aerobic or Facultative | |
| Gram-positive cocci | *Streptococcus* sp<br>*S. mutans*<br>*S. sanguis*<br>*S. mitior*<br>*S. salivarius* |
| Gram-positive rods | *Lactobacillus* sp<br>*Corynebacterium* sp |
| Gram-negative cocci | *Moraxella* sp |
| Gram-negative rods | *Enterobacteriaceae* sp |
| Anaerobic | |
| Gram-positive cocci | *Peptostreptococcus* sp |
| Gram-positive rods | *Actinomyces* sp<br>*Eubacterium* sp<br>*Lactobacillus* sp<br>*Leptotrichia* sp |
| Gram-negative cocci | *Veillonella* sp |
| Gram-negative rods | *Actinobacillus* sp<br>*Fusobacterium* sp<br>*Prevotella* sp<br>*Porphyromonas* sp<br>*Bacteroides* sp<br>*Campylobacter* sp |
| Spirochetes | *Treponema* sp |
| Fungi | *Candida* sp |

# REFERENCE VALUES FOR ADULTS

## Automated Chemistry (CHEMISTRY A)

| Test | Values | Remarks |
|---|---|---|
| **SERUM PLASMA** | | |
| Acetone | Negative | |
| Albumin | 3.2-5 g/dL | |
| Alcohol, ethyl | Negative | |
| Aldolase | 1.2-7.6 IU/L | |
| Ammonia | 20-70 mcg/dL | Specimen to be placed on ice as soon as collected |
| Amylase | 30-110 units/L | |
| Bilirubin, direct | 0-0.3 mg/dL | |
| Bilirubin, total | 0.1-1.2 mg/dL | |
| Calcium | 8.6-10.3 mg/dL | |
| Calcium, ionized | 2.24-2.46 mEq/L | |
| Chloride | 95-108 mEq/L | |
| Cholesterol, total | ≤220 mg/dL | Fasted blood required – normal value affected by dietary habits<br>This reference range is for a general adult population |
| HDL cholesterol | 40-60 mg/dL | Fasted blood required – normal value affected by dietary habits |
| LDL cholesterol | 65-170 mg/dL | LDLC calculated by Friewald formula... which has certain inaccuracies and is invalid at trig levels >300 mg/dL |
| $CO_2$ | 23-30 mEq/L | |
| Creatine kinase (CK) isoenzymes | | |
| CK-BB | 0% | |
| CK-MB | 0%-3.9% | |
| CK-MM | 96%-100% | |

CK-MB levels must be both ≥4% and 10 IU/L to meet diagnostic criteria for CK-MB positive result consistent with myocardial injury.

| Test | Values | Remarks |
|---|---|---|
| Creatine phosphokinase (CPK) | 8-150 IU/L | |
| Creatinine | 0.5-1.4 mg/dL | |
| Ferritin | 13-300 ng/mL | |
| Folate | 3.6-20 ng/dL | |
| GGT (gamma-glutamyltranspeptidase) | | |
| male | 11-63 IU/L | |
| female | 8-35 IU/L | |
| GLDH | To be determined | |
| Glucose (2-h postprandial) | Up to 140 mg/dL | |
| Glucose, fasting | 60-110 mg/dL | |
| Glucose, nonfasting (2-h postprandial) | 60-140 mg/dL | |
| Hemoglobin $A_{1c}$ | 8 | |
| Hemoglobin, plasma free | <2.5 mg/100 mL | |
| Hemoglobin, total glycosolated (Hb $A_1$) | 4%-8% | |
| Iron | 65-150 mcg/dL | |
| Iron binding capacity, total (TIBC) | 250-420 mcg/dL | |
| Lactic acid | 0.7-2.1 mEq/L | Specimen to be kept on ice and sent to lab as soon as possible |
| Lactate dehydrogenase (LDH) | 56-194 IU/L | |
| Lactate dehydrogenase (LDH) isoenzymes | | |
| $LD_1$ | 20%-34% | |
| $LD_2$ | 29%-41% | |
| $LD_3$ | 15%-25% | |

## Automated Chemistry (CHEMISTRY A) *(continued)*

| Test | Values | Remarks |
|---|---|---|
| $LD_4$ | 1%-12% | |
| $LD_5$ | 1%-15% | |
| Flipped $LD_1/LD_2$ ratios (>1 may be consistent with myocardial injury) particularly when considered in combination with a recent CK-MB positive result | | |
| Lipase | 23-208 units/L | |
| Magnesium | 1.6-2.5 mg/dL | Increased by slight hemolysis |
| Osmolality | 289-308 mOsm/kg | |
| Phosphatase, alkaline | | |
| adults 25-60 y | 33-131 IU/L | |
| adults 61 y or older | 51-153 IU/L | |
| infancy-adolescence | Values range up to 3-5 times higher than adults | |
| Phosphate, inorganic | 2.8-4.2 mg/dL | |
| Potassium | 3.5-5.2 mEq/L | Increased by slight hemolysis |
| Prealbumin | >15 mg/dL | |
| Protein, total | 6.5-7.9 g/dL | |
| SGOT (AST) | <35 IU/L | |
| SGPT (ALT) | <35 IU/L | |
| Sodium | 134-149 mEq/L | |
| Transferrin | >200 mg/dL | |
| Triglycerides | 45-155 mg/dL | Fasted blood required |
| Urea nitrogen (BUN) | 7-20 mg/dL | |
| Uric acid | | |
| male | 2.0-8.0 mg/dL | |
| female | 2.0-7.5 mg/dL | |
| **CEREBROSPINAL FLUID** | | |
| Glucose | 50-70 mg/dL | |
| Protein | | |
| adults and children | 15-45 mg/dL | CSF obtained by lumbar puncture |
| newborn infants | 60-90 mg/dL | |
| On CSF obtained by cisternal puncture: About 25 mg/dL | | |
| On CSF obtained by ventricular puncture: About 10 mg/dL | | |
| **Note:** Bloody specimen gives erroneously high value due to contamination with blood proteins | | |
| **URINE** | | |
| **(24-hour specimen is required for all these tests unless specified)** | | |
| Amylase | 32-641 units/L | The value is in units/L and **not** calculated for total volume |
| Amylase, fluid (random samples) | | Interpretation of value left for physician, depends on the nature of fluid |
| Calcium | Depends upon dietary intake | |
| Creatine | | |
| male | 150 mg/24 h | Higher value on children and during pregnancy |
| female | 250 mg/24 h | |
| Creatinine | 1000-2000 mg/24 h | |
| Creatinine clearance (endogenous) | | |
| male | 85-125 mL/min | A blood sample must accompany urine specimen |
| female | 75-115 mL/min | |
| Glucose | 1 g/24 h | |
| 5-hydroxyindoleacetic acid | 2-8 mg/24 h | |
| Iron | 0.15 mg/24 h | Acid washed container required |

# REFERENCE VALUES FOR ADULTS *(Continued)*

## Automated Chemistry (CHEMISTRY A) *(continued)*

| Test | Values | Remarks |
|---|---|---|
| Magnesium | 146-209 mg/24 h | |
| Osmolality | 500-800 mOsm/kg | With normal fluid intake |
| Oxalate | 10-40 mg/24 h | |
| Phosphate | 400-1300 mg/24 h | |
| Potassium | 25-120 mEq/24 h | Varies with diet; the interpretation of urine electrolytes and osmolality should be left for the physician |
| Sodium | 40-220 mEq/24 h | |
| Porphobilinogen, qualitative | Negative | |
| Porphyrins, qualitative | Negative | |
| Proteins | 0.05-0.1 g/24 h | |
| Salicylate | Negative | |
| Urea clearance | 60-95 mL/min | A blood sample must accompany specimen |
| Urea N | 10-40 g/24 h | Dependent on protein intake |
| Uric acid | 250-750 mg/24 h | Dependent on diet and therapy |
| Urobilinogen | 0.5-3.5 mg/24 h | For qualitative determination on random urine, send sample to urinalysis section in Hematology Lab |
| Xylose absorption test | | |
| children | 16%-33% of ingested xylose | |
| adults | >4 g in 5 h | |
| **FECES** | | |
| Fat, 3-day collection | <5 g/d | Value depends on fat intake of 100 g/d for 3 days preceding and during collection |
| **GASTRIC ACIDITY** | | |
| Acidity, total, 12 h | 10-60 mEq/L | Titrated at pH 7 |

### BLOOD GASES

| | Arterial | Capillary | Venous |
|---|---|---|---|
| pH | 7.35-7.45 | 7.35-7.45 | 7.32-7.42 |
| $pCO_2$ (mm Hg) | 35-45 | 35-45 | 38-52 |
| $pO_2$ (mm Hg) | 70-100 | 60-80 | 24-48 |
| $HCO_3$ (mEq/L) | 19-25 | 19-25 | 19-25 |
| $TCO_2$ (mEq/L) | 19-29 | 19-29 | 23-33 |
| $O_2$ saturation (%) | 90-95 | 90-95 | 40-70 |
| Base excess (mEq/L) | -5 to +5 | -5 to +5 | -5 to +5 |

## HEMATOLOGY
### Complete Blood Count

| Age | Hgb (g/dL) | Hct (%) | RBC (mill/mm³) | RDW |
|---|---|---|---|---|
| 0-3 d | 15.0-20.0 | 45-61 | 4.0-5.9 | <18 |
| 1-2 wk | 12.5-18.5 | 39-57 | 3.6-5.5 | <17 |
| 1-6 mo | 10.0-13.0 | 29-42 | 3.1-4.3 | <16.5 |
| 7 mo to 2 y | 10.5-13.0 | 33-38 | 3.7-4.9 | <16 |
| 2-5 y | 11.5-13.0 | 34-39 | 3.9-5.0 | <15 |
| 5-8 y | 11.5-14.5 | 35-42 | 4.0-4.9 | <15 |
| 13-18 y | 12.0-15.2 | 36-47 | 4.5-5.1 | <14.5 |
| Adult male | 13.5-16.5 | 41-50 | 4.5-5.5 | <14.5 |
| Adult female | 12.0-15.0 | 36-44 | 4.0-4.9 | <14.5 |

| Age | MCV (fL) | MCH (pg) | MCHC (%) | PLTS (x 10³/mm³) |
|---|---|---|---|---|
| 0-3 d | 95-115 | 31-37 | 29-37 | 250-450 |
| 1-2 wk | 86-110 | 28-36 | 28-38 | 250-450 |
| 1-6 mo | 74-96 | 25-35 | 30-36 | 300-700 |
| 7 mo to 2 y | 70-84 | 23-30 | 31-37 | 250-600 |
| 2-5 y | 75-87 | 24-30 | 31-37 | 250-550 |
| 5-8 y | 77-95 | 25-33 | 31-37 | 250-550 |
| 13-18 y | 78-96 | 25-35 | 31-37 | 150-450 |
| Adult male | 80-100 | 26-34 | 31-37 | 150-450 |
| Adult female | 80-100 | 26-34 | 31-37 | 150-450 |

### WBC and Diff

| Age | WBC (x 10³/mm³) | Segs | Bands | Lymphs | Monos |
|---|---|---|---|---|---|
| 0-3 d | 9.0-35.0 | 32-62 | 10-18 | 19-29 | 5-7 |
| 1-2 wk | 5.0-20.0 | 14-34 | 6-14 | 36-45 | 6-10 |
| 1-6 mo | 6.0-17.5 | 13-33 | 4-12 | 41-71 | 4-7 |
| 7 mo to 2 y | 6.0-17.0 | 15-35 | 5-11 | 45-76 | 3-6 |
| 2-5 y | 5.5-15.5 | 23-45 | 5-11 | 35-65 | 3-6 |
| 5-8 y | 5.0-14.5 | 32-54 | 5-11 | 28-48 | 3-6 |
| 13-18 y | 4.5-13.0 | 34-64 | 5-11 | 25-45 | 3-6 |
| Adults | 4.5-11.0 | 35-66 | 5-11 | 24-44 | 3-6 |

| Age | Eosinophils | Basophils | Atypical Lymphs | No. of NRBCs |
|---|---|---|---|---|
| 0-3 d | 0-2 | 0-1 | 0-8 | 0-2 |
| 1-2 wk | 0-2 | 0-1 | 0-8 | 0 |
| 1-6 mo | 0-3 | 0-1 | 0-8 | 0 |
| 7 mo to 2 y | 0-3 | 0-1 | 0-8 | 0 |
| 2-5 y | 0-3 | 0-1 | 0-8 | 0 |
| 5-8 y | 0-3 | 0-1 | 0-8 | 0 |
| 13-18 y | 0-3 | 0-1 | 0-8 | 0 |
| Adults | 0-3 | 0-1 | 0-8 | 0 |

Segs = segmented neutrophils
Bands = band neutrophils
Lymps = lymphocytes
Monos = monocytes

### Erythrocyte Sedimentation Rates and Reticulocyte Counts

| | | |
|---|---|---|
| Sedimentation rate, Westergren | Children | 0-20 mm/hour |
| | Adult male | 0-15 mm/hour |
| | Adult female | 0-20 mm/hour |
| Sedimentation rate, Wintrobe | Children | 0-13 mm/hour |
| | Adult male | 0-10 mm/hour |
| | Adult female | 0-15 mm/hour |
| Reticulocyte count | Newborns | 2%-6% |
| | 1-6 mo | 0%-2.8% |
| | Adults | 0.5%-1.5% |

# DENTIFRICE PRODUCTS

| Product | Abrasive Ingredient | Therapeutic Ingredient | Foaming Agent |
|---|---|---|---|
| Aim AntiTartar Gel Formula with Fluoride | Hydrated silica | Sodium monofluorophosphate 0.79% (fluoride 0.15%) | Sodium lauryl sulfate |
| | **Other Ingredients:** Sorbitol and related polyols, water, glycerin, zinc citrate trihydrate, SD alcohol 38B, flavor, cellulose gum, sodium saccharin, sodium benzoate, blue #1, yellow #10 | | |
| Aim Baking Soda Gel with Fluoride | Hydrated silica | Sodium monofluorophosphate 0.79% (fluoride 0.15%) | Sodium lauryl sulfate |
| | **Other Ingredients:** Sorbitol and related polyols, water, glycerin, SD alcohol 38B, flavor, sodium bicarbonate, cellulose gum, sodium saccharin, sodium benzoate, blue #1, yellow #10 | | |
| Aim Regular Strength Gel with Fluoride | Hydrated silica | Sodium monofluorophosphate 0.79% (fluoride 0.15%) | Sodium lauryl sulfate |
| | **Other Ingredients:** Sorbitol and other related polyols, water, glycerin, SD alcohol 38B, flavor, cellulose gum, sodium saccharin, sodium benzoate, blue #1, yellow #10 | | |
| Aquafresh Baking Soda Toothpaste | Calcium carbonate, hydrated silica | Sodium monofluorophosphate | Sodium lauryl sulfate |
| | **Other Ingredients:** Calcium carrageenan, cellulose gum, colors, flavor, glycerin, PEG-8, sodium benzoate, sodium bicarbonate, sodium saccharin, sorbitol, titanium dioxide, water | | |
| Aquafresh Extra Fresh Toothpaste[a] | Hydrated silica, calcium carbonate | Sodium monofluorophosphate | Sodium lauryl sulfate |
| | **Other Ingredients:** Sorbitol, water, glycerin, PEG-8, titanium dioxide, cellulose gum, flavor, sodium saccharin, sodium benzoate, calcium carrageenan, colors | | |
| Aquafresh for Kids Toothpaste[a] | Hydrated silica, calcium carbonate | Sodium monofluorophosphate | Sodium lauryl sulfate |
| | **Other Ingredients:** Sorbitol, water, glycerin, PEG-8, titanium dioxide, cellulose gum, flavor, sodium saccharin, calcium carrageenan, sodium benzoate, colors | | |
| Aquafresh Sensitive Toothpaste | Hydrated silica | Potassium nitrate, sodium fluoride | Sodium lauryl sulfate |
| | **Other Ingredients:** Colors, flavors, glycerin, sodium benzoate, sodium saccharin, sorbitol, titanium dioxide, water, xanthan gum | | |
| Aquafresh Tartar Control Toothpaste[a] | Hydrated silica | Sodium fluoride | Sodium lauryl sulfate |
| | **Other Ingredients:** Tetrapotassium, pyrophosphate, tetrasodium pyrophosphate, sorbitol, glycerin, PEG-8, flavor, xanthan gum, sodium saccharin, sodium benzoate, D&C red #30 lake, FD&C blue #1, D&C yellow #10, titanium dioxide, water | | |
| Aquafresh Triple Protection Toothpaste[a] | Hydrated silica, calcium carbonate | Sodium monofluorophosphate | Sodium lauryl sulfate |
| | **Other Ingredients:** PEG-8, sorbitol, cellulose gum, sodium benzoate, titanium dioxide, calcium, carrageenan, flavor, sodium saccharin, colors, water | | |
| Aquafresh Whitening Toothpaste | Hydrated silica | Sodium fluoride | Sodium lauryl sulfate |
| | **Other Ingredients:** D&C yellow #10, FD&C blue #1, flavor, glycerin, PEG-8, sodium benzoate, sodium hydroxide, sodium saccharin, sodium tripolyphosphate, sorbitol, titanium dioxide, water, xanthan gum | | |
| Arm & Hammer Dental Care Baking Soda Tartar Control Toothpaste | Sodium bicarbonate | Sodium fluoride | Sodium lauryl sulfate |
| | **Other Ingredients:** Water, glycerin, sodium pyrophosphates, sodium saccharin, PEG-8, flavor blend, sodium phosphates, cellulose gum, sodium lauroyl sarcosinate | | |

| Product | Abrasive Ingredient | Therapeutic Ingredient | Foaming Agent |
|---|---|---|---|
| Arm & Hammer Dental Care Baking Soda Gel | Hydrated silica, sodium bicarbonate | Sodium fluoride | Sodium lauryl sulfate |
| | **Other Ingredients:** Sorbitol, water, glycerin, PEG-8, flavor blend, cellulose gum, sodium lauroyl sarcosinate, sodium saccharin, FD&C blue #1, D&C yellow #10 | | |
| Arm & Hammer Dental Care Baking Soda Tartar Control Gel | Sodium bicarbonate, hydrated silica | Sodium fluoride | Sodium lauryl sulfate |
| | **Other Ingredients:** Water, sorbitol, glycerin, sodium pyrophosphates, PEG-8, flavor, cellulose gum, sodium saccharin, sodium lauroyl sarcosinate, FD&C blue #1, D&C yellow #10 | | |
| Arm & Hammer Dental Care Baking Soda Tooth Powder | Sodium bicarbonate | Sodium fluoride | |
| | **Other Ingredients:** Mint flavor, sodium saccharin, trisodium saccharin, trisodium magnesium oxide, PEG-8 | | |
| Arm & Hammer Dental Care Baking Soda Toothpaste | Sodium bicarbonate | Sodium fluoride | Sodium lauryl sulfate |
| | **Other Ingredients:** Water, glycerin, sodium saccharin, PEG-8, flavor blend, cellulose gum, sodium lauroyl sarcosinate | | |
| Arm & Hammer PerioxiCare Toothpaste | Sodium bicarbonate, silica | Sodium fluoride | Sodium carbonate peroxide, sodium lauryl sulfate |
| | **Other Ingredients:** PEG-8, poloxamer 338, flavor, water, sodium saccharin, sodium lauroyl sarconsinate | | |
| Biotene Antibacterial Dry Mouth Toothpaste | Hydrated silica | Lactoperoxidase (15,000 units), glucose oxidase (10,000 units), lysozyme (16 mg), sodium monofluorophosphate | |
| | **Other Ingredients:** Sorbitol, glycerin, calcium pyrophosphate, xylitol, isoceteth-20, cellulose gum, flavor, sodium benzoate, beta-d-glucose, potassium thiocyanate | | |
| Caffree Anti-Stain Fluoride Toothpaste[a] | | Sodium monofluorophosphate | Sodium lauryl sulfate |
| | **Other Ingredients:** Water, diatomaceous earth, glycerin, sorbitol, aluminum silicate, titanium dioxide, hydroxyethylcellulose, flavor, sodium saccharin, methylparaben, propylparaben | | |
| Close-Up Anti-Plaque Gel | Hydrated silica | Stannous fluoride 0.41% | Sodium lauryl sulfate |
| | **Other Ingredients:** Sorbitol, water, PEG-32, SD alcohol 38B, flavor, zinc citrate trihydrate, cellulose gum, sodium saccharin, sodium benzoate, sodium hydroxide, blue #1 | | |
| Close-Up Crystal Clear Mint Gel | Hydrated silica | Sodium monofluorophosphate 0.79% (fluoride 0.15%) | Sodium lauryl sulfate |
| | **Other Ingredients:** Sorbitol, water, glycerin, SD alcohol 38B, flavor, cellulose gum, sodium saccharin, polysorbate 20, sodium benzoate, sodium chloride, blue #1, mica, red #33, titanium dioxide | | |
| Close-Up Original Gel | Hydrated silica | Sodium monofluorophosphate 0.79% (fluoride 0.15%) | Sodium lauryl sulfate |
| | **Other Ingredients:** Sorbitol, water, glycerin, SD alcohol 38B, flavor, cellulose gum, sodium saccharin, sodium benzoate, sodium chloride, red #33, red #40 | | |
| Close-Up Tartar Control Gel | Hydrated silica | Sodium monofluorophosphate 0.79% (fluoride 0.15%) | Sodium lauryl sulfate |

## DENTIFRICE PRODUCTS *(Continued)*

| Product | Abrasive Ingredient | Therapeutic Ingredient | Foaming Agent |
|---|---|---|---|
| | **Other Ingredients:** Sorbitol and related polyols, water, glycerin, zinc citrate trihydrate, SD alcohol 38B, flavor, cellulose gum, sodium saccharin, sodium benzoate, sodium chloride, red #33, red #40 | | |
| Close-Up with Baking Soda Toothpaste | Hydrated silica | Sodium monofluorophosphate 0.79% (fluoride 0.15%) | Sodium lauryl sulfate |
| | **Other Ingredients:** Sorbitol and related polyols, water, glycerin, SD alcohol 38B, flavor, sodium bicarbonate, cellulose gum, sodium saccharin, sodium benzoate, red #33, red #40, titanium dioxide | | |
| Colgate Baking Soda Gel[a] | Hydrated silica | Sodium fluoride 0.243% | Sodium lauryl sulfate |
| | **Other Ingredients:** Glycerin, PEG-12, cellulose gum, flavor, sodium saccharin, FD&C blue #1, D&C yellow #10 | | |
| Colgate Baking Soda Tartar Control Gel or Toothpaste | Hydrated silica, sodium bicarbonate | Sodium fluoride 0.243% | Sodium lauryl sulfate |
| | **Other Ingredients:** Glycerin, tetrasodium pyrophosphate, PVM/MA copolymer, cellulose gum, flavor, sodium saccharin, sodium hydroxide, titanium dioxide (paste), FD&C blue #1, D& C yellow #10 (gel) | | |
| Colgate Baking Soda Toothpaste[a] | Hydrated silica, sodium bicarbonate | Sodium fluoride 0.243% | Sodium lauryl sulfate |
| | **Other Ingredients:** Glycerin, cellulose gum, flavor, sodium saccharin, titanium dioxide | | |
| Colgate Junior Gel[a] | Hydrated silica | Sodium fluoride 0.243% | Sodium lauryl sulfate |
| | **Other Ingredients:** Sorbitol, PEG-12, flavor, tetrasodium pyrophosphate, cellulose gum, sodium saccharin, mica, titanium dioxide, FD&C blue #1, D&C yellow #10 | | |
| Colgate Micro Cleansing Tartar Control Gel or Toothpaste[a] | Synthetic amorphous silica 27%, hydrated amorphous silica 3% | Sodium fluoride 0.243% | Sodium lauryl sulfate |
| | **Other Ingredients:** Water, sorbitol, glycerin, PEG-12, tetrasodium pyrophosphate, PVM/MA copolymer, cellulose gum, flavor, sodium hydroxide, titanium dioxide (Paste), sodium saccharin, carrageenan, FD&C blue #1 (gel) | | |
| Colgate Peak Toothpaste | Hydrated silica, sodium bicarbonate, precipitated calcium carbonate | | Sodium lauryl sulfate |
| | **Other Ingredients:** Glycerin, cellulose gum, flavor, sodium saccharin, titanium dioxide, sodium benzoate | | |
| Colgate Toothpaste[a] | Dicalcium phosphate dihydrate | Sodium monofluorophosphate 0.76% | Sodium lauryl sulfate |
| | **Other Ingredients:** Glycerin, cellulose gum, tetrasodium pyrophosphate, sodium saccharin, flavor | | |
| Colgate Total Toothpaste[a] | Hydrated silica | Triclosan 0.30%, sodium fluoride 0.24% | Sodium lauryl sulfate |
| | **Other Ingredients:** Water, glycerin, sorbitol, PVM/MA copolymer, cellulose gum, flavor, sodium hydroxide, propylene glycol, carrageenan, sodium saccharin, titanium dioxide | | |
| Colgate Winterfresh Gel[a] | Hydrated silica | Sodium fluoride 0.243% | Sodium lauryl sulfate |
| | **Other Ingredients:** Sorbitol, glycerin, PEG-12, flavor, tetrasodium pyrophosphate, cellulose gum, sodium saccharin, FD&C blue #1 | | |
| Crest Baking Soda Gel or Toothpaste[a] (mint) | Hydrated silica | Sodium fluoride | Sodium lauryl sulfate |

| Product | Abrasive Ingredient | Therapeutic Ingredient | Foaming Agent |
|---|---|---|---|
| | **Other Ingredients:** Sorbitol, water, sodium bicarbonate, glycerin, sodium carbonate, flavor, cellulose gum, sodium saccharin, titanium dioxide (paste), FD&C blue #1 (gel) | | |
| Crest Baking Soda Tartar Control Gel or Toothpaste[a] (mint) | Hydrated silica | Sodium fluoride | Sodium lauryl sulfate |
| | **Other Ingredients:** Water, sodium bicarbonate, glycerin, sorbitol, tetrasodium pyrophosphate, PEG-6, sodium carbonate, flavor, cellulose gum, sodium saccharin, titanium dioxide (paste), FD&C blue #1 (gel) | | |
| Crest Cavity Fighting Gel[a] (cool mint) | Hydrated silica | Sodium fluoride | Sodium lauryl sulfate |
| | **Other Ingredients:** Sorbitol, water, trisodium phosphate, flavor, sodium phosphate, xanthan gum, sodium saccharin, carbomer 956, FD&C blue #1 | | |
| Crest Cavity Fighting Toothpaste[a] (icy mint or regular flavor) | Hydrated silica | Sodium fluoride | Sodium lauryl sulfate |
| | **Other Ingredients:** Sorbitol, water, glycerin, mint, trisodium phosphate, flavor, sodium phosphate, cellulose gum (mint), xanthan gum (regular), sodium saccharin, carbomer 956, titanium dioxide, FD&C blue #1 | | |
| Crest for Kids, Sparkle Fun Gel[a] | Hydrated silica | Sodium fluoride | Sodium lauryl sulfate |
| | **Other Ingredients:** Sorbitol, water, trisodium phosphate, sodium phosphate, xanthan gum, flavor, sodium saccharin, carbomer 956, mica, titanium dioxide, FD&C blue #1 | | |
| Crest Sensitivity Protection Toothpaste[a] (mild mint) | Hydrated silica | Potassium nitrate, sodium fluoride | Sodium lauryl sulfate |
| | **Other Ingredients:** Water, glycerin, sorbitol, trisodium phosphate, cellulose gum, flavor, xanthan gum, sodium saccharin, titanium dioxide | | |
| Crest Tartar Control Gel[a] (fresh mint or smooth mint) | Hydrated silica | Sodium fluoride | Sodium lauryl sulfate |
| | **Other Ingredients:** Water, sorbitol, glycerin, tetrapotassium pyrophosphate, PEG-6, disodium pyrophosphate, tetrasodium pyrophosphate, flavor, xanthan gum, sodium saccharin, carbomer 956, FD&C blue #1, (fresh mint & smooth mint), FD&C yellow #5 (smooth mint) | | |
| Crest Tartar Control Toothpaste[a] (original flavor) | Hydrated silica | Sodium fluoride | Sodium lauryl sulfate |
| | **Other Ingredients:** Water, sorbitol, glycerin, tetrapotassium pyrophosphate, PEG-6, disodium pyrophosphate, tetrasodium pyrophosphate, flavor, xanthan gum, sodium saccharin, carbomer 956, titanium dioxide, FD&C blue #1 | | |
| Dentagard Toothpaste[a] | Hydrated silica | Sodium monofluorophosphate 0.76% | Sodium lauryl sulfate |
| | **Other Ingredients:** Sorbitol, glycerin, PEG-12, flavor, sodium benzoate, titanium dioxide, cellulose gum, sodium saccharin, FD&C red #40 | | |
| Enamelon Toothpaste | Hydrated silica | Sodium fluoride 0.24% | Sodium lauryl sulfate |
| | **Other Ingredients:** Water, glycerin, sorbitol, monoammonium phosphate, calcium sulfate, xanthan gum, flavor, PEG 60, hydrogenated castor oil, sodium saccharin, ammonium chloride, cellulose gum, titanium dioxide, magnesium chloride, methylparaben, propylparaben, FD&C blue #1 | | |
| Gleem Toothpaste | Hydrated silica | Sodium fluoride | Sodium lauryl sulfate |

## DENTIFRICE PRODUCTS *(Continued)*

| Product | Abrasive Ingredient | Therapeutic Ingredient | Foaming Agent |
|---|---|---|---|
| | **Other Ingredients:** Sorbitol, water, trisodium phosphate, flavor, sodium phosphate, xanthan gum, sodium saccharin, carbomer 956, titanium dioxide | | |
| Interplak Toothpaste with Fluoride | Hydrated silica | Sodium fluoride | Sodium lauryl sulfate |
| | **Other Ingredients:** Purified water, poloxamer 407, sorbitol, glycerin, flavor, dibasic sodium phosphate, sodium saccharin, monobasic sodium phosphate, sodium benzoate, D&C yellow #10 | | |
| Mentadent Fluoride Toothpaste with Baking Soda & Peroxide[a] | Hydrated silica, sodium bicarbonate | Sodium fluoride 0.24% (fluoride 0.15%) | Sodium lauryl sulfate, hydrogen peroxide |
| | **Other Ingredients:** Water, sorbitol, glycerin, poloxamer 407, PEG-32, SD alcohol 38B, flavor, cellulose gum, sodium saccharin, phosphoric acid, blue #1, titanium dioxide | | |
| Oragel Gold Toothpaste | Hydrated silica | Potassium nitrate 5%, sodium monofluorophosphate (fluoride 0.20%) | Sodium lauryl sulfate, sodium lauryl inate sincosinate |
| | **Other Ingredients:** Water, glycerin, xanthum gum, sorbitol, flavor, FD&C blue #1 | | |
| Oral-B Sensitive Toothpaste with Fluoride | Hydrated silica | Potassium nitrate 5%, sodium fluoride 0.225% | Sodium lauryl sulfate |
| | **Other Ingredients:** Water, glycerin, cellulose gum, PEG-8, sodium saccharin, methylparaben, propylparaben, flavor | | |
| Oral-B Sesame Street Toothpaste, Bubblegum, or Fruity[a] | Hydrated silica | Sodium fluoride 0.248% | Sodium lauryl sulfate |
| | **Other Ingredients:** Water, sorbitol, glycerin, xanthan gum, acesulfame K, carbomer 980, sodium hydroxide, FD&C red #3, methylparaben, propylparaben | | |
| Oral-B Tooth and Gum Care Toothpaste | Calcium pyrophosphate | Stannous fluoride 0.4% | |
| | **Other Ingredients:** Water, glycerin, sorbitol, PEG-8, sodium saccharin, methylparaben, propylparaben, zinc citrate, flavor, PVM/MA copolymer | | |
| Pearl Drops Baking Soda Whitening Toothpaste Tartar Control | Hydrated silica, sodium bicarbonate | Sodium fluoride | Sodium lauryl sulfate |
| | **Other Ingredients:** Sorbitol, glycerin, tetrapotassium pyrophosphate, tetrasodium pyrophosphate, PEG-12, titanium dioxide, flavor, sodium saccharin, cellulose gum | | |
| Pearl Drops Extra Strength Whitening Toothpaste | Hydrated silica, calcium pyrophosphate, dicalcium phosphate | Sodium monofluorophosphate | Sodium lauryl sulfate |
| | **Other Ingredients:** Sorbitol, glycerin, PEG-12, flavor, titanium dioxide, cellulose gum, trisodium phosphate, sodium phosphate, sodium saccharin | | |
| Pearl Drops Whitening Gel or Paste, Tartar Control w/Fluoride | Hydrated silica | Sodium fluoride | Sodium lauryl sulfate |
| | **Other Ingredients:** Sorbitol, glycerin, tetrapotassium pyrophosphate, tetrasodium pyrophosphate, PEG-12, flavor, titanium dioxide (paste), cellulose gum, sodium saccharin, FD&C blue #1 (gel), FD&C yellow #10 (gel) | | |
| Pearl Drops Whitening Toothpolish Gel | Hydrated silica | Sodium monofluorophosphate | Sodium lauryl sulfate |
| | **Other Ingredients:** Sorbitol, glycerin, PEG-12, flavor, cellulose gum, trisodium phosphate, sodium phosphate, sodium saccharin, FD&C blue #1 | | |

| Product | Abrasive Ingredient | Therapeutic Ingredient | Foaming Agent |
|---|---|---|---|
| Pearl Drops Whitening Toothpolish (regular or spearmint) | Aluminum hydroxide, hydrated silica | Sodium monofluorophosphate | Sodium lauryl sulfate |
| | **Other Ingredients:** Sorbitol, glycerin, PEG-12, flavor, titanium dioxide, cellulose gum, trisodium phosphate, sodium phosphate, sodium saccharin | | |
| Pepsodent Baking Soda Toothpaste | Hydrated silica | Sodium fluoride 0.24% | Sodium lauryl sulfate |
| | **Other Ingredients:** Sorbitol, water, sodium bicarbonate, PEG-32, SD alcohol 38B, flavor, cellulose gum, sodium saccharin, titanium dioxide | | |
| Pepsodent Original Fluoride Toothpaste | Hydrated silica | Sodium monofluorophosphate 0.79% (fluoride 0.15%) | Sodium lauryl sulfate |
| | **Other Ingredients:** Sorbitol and related polyols, water, glycerin, SD alcohol 38B, flavor, cellulose gum, sodium saccharin, sodium benzoate, titanium dioxide | | |
| PeriGel Toothpaste System | Sodium bicarbonate 59% | Sodium fluoride | Hydrogen peroxide 3% |
| Platinum Whitening Toothpaste with Fluoride | | Sodium monofluorophosphate 0.76% | |
| Promise Toothpaste | Silica | Potassium nitrate, sodium monofluorophosphate | Sodium lauryl sulfate |
| | **Other Ingredients:** Water, dicalcium phosphate, hydroxyethylcellulose, flavor, sodium saccharin, methylparaben, propylparaben, D&C yellow #10, FD&C blue #1 | | |
| Pycopay Tooth Powder | Sodium bicarbonate, calcium carbonate, tricalcium phosphate, magnesium carbonate | | |
| | **Other Ingredients:** Sodium chloride, eugenol, methyl salicylate | | |
| Rembrandt Brushing Gel with Peroxide | | Sodium monofluorophosphate | Carbamide peroxide, sodium lauryl sulfate |
| | **Other Ingredients:** Glycerin, sodium citrate, carbomer, titanium dioxide, flavor, triethanolamine | | |
| Rembrandt Whitening Sensitive Toothpaste | | Sodium monofluorophosphate 0.76%, potassium nitrate | Sodium lauryl sulfate |
| | **Other Ingredients:** Dicalcium phosphate dihydrate, glycerin, sorbitol, water, alumina, papain, sodium citrate, flavor, sodium carboxymethylcellulose, sodium saccharin, methylparaben, citric acid, FD&C red #40 | | |
| Rembrandt Whitening Toothpaste (mint or regular) | | Sodium monofluorophosphate 0.76% | Sodium lauryl sulfate |
| | **Other Ingredients:** Dicalcium phosphate dihydrate, water, glycerin, sorbitol, alumina, papain, sodium citrate, flavor, sodium carrageenan, sodium saccharin, methylparaben, citric acid, FD&C blue #1 | | |
| Revelation Toothpowder | Calcium carbonate | | Vegetable soap powder |
| | **Other Ingredients:** Methyl salicylate, menthol | | |
| Sensodyne Baking Soda Toothpaste | Sodium bicarbonate, hydrated silica, silica | Potassium nitrate, sodium fluoride | Sodium lauryl sulfate |
| | **Other Ingredients:** Water, glycerin, sorbitol, flavor, hydroxyethylcellulose, titanium dioxide, sodium saccharin | | |

## DENTIFRICE PRODUCTS *(Continued)*

| Product | Abrasive Ingredient | Therapeutic Ingredient | Foaming Agent |
|---|---|---|---|
| Sensodyne Extra Whitening Toothpaste | Hydrated silica, silica | Potassium nitrate (5%), sodium fluoride (fluoride ion 0.13%) | Sodium lauryl sulfate, calcium peroxide |
| | **Other Ingredients:** Flavor, glycerin, PEG-12, PEG-75, sodium carbonate, sodium saccharin, titanium dioxide, water | | |
| Sensodyne Gel (cool mint) | Hydrated silica, silica | Potassium nitrate, sodium fluoride | |
| | **Other Ingredients:** Water, sorbitol, glycerin, sodium carboxyethylcellulose, sodium methyl cocoyl taurate, flavor, guar gum, sodium saccharin, methylparaben, propylparaben, sodium hydroxide, FD&C blue #1 | | |
| Sensodyne Tartar Control Toothpaste | Hydrated silica, silica | Potassium nitrate (5%), sodium fluoride (fluoride ion 0.13%) | |
| | **Other Ingredients:** Cellulose gum, cocamiopropyl betaine, flavor, glycerin, sodium bicarbonate, sodium saccharin, tetrapotassium pyrophosphate, titanium dioxide, water | | |
| Sensodyne Toothpaste[a] (fresh mint) | Silica | Potassium nitrate, sodium monofluorophosphate | Sodium lauryl sulfate |
| | **Other Ingredients:** Water, dicalcium phosphate dihydrate, glycerin, sorbitol, dicalcium phosphate, hydroxyethylcellulose, flavor, sodium saccharin, methylparaben, propylparaben, D&C yellow #10, FD&C blue #1 | | |
| Sensodyne-SC Toothpaste[a] | Calcium carbonate, silica | Strontium chloride hexahydrate 10% | |
| | **Other Ingredients:** Water, glycerin, sorbitol, hydroxyethylcellulose, sodium methyl cocoyl taurate, flavor, PEG-40, stearate, titanium dioxide, sodium saccharin, methylparaben, propylparaben, D&C red #28 | | |
| Thermodent Toothpaste | Diatomaceous earth, silica | Strontium chloride hexahydrate | Sodium methyl cocoyl taurate |
| | **Other Ingredients:** Sorbitol, glycerin, titanium dioxide, hydroxyethylcellulose, flavor, preservative | | |
| Tom's Natural Baking Soda Toothpaste with Fluoride | Calcium carbonate, sodium bicarbonate | Sodium monofluorophosphate | Sodium lauryl sulfate |
| | **Other Ingredients:** Glycerin, carrageenan, xylitol, peppermint oil | | |
| Tom's Natural Toothpaste for Children with Fluoride | Calcium carbonate, hydrated silica | Sodium monofluorophosphate | Sodium lauryl sulfate |
| | **Other Ingredients:** Glycerin, fruit extracts, carrageenan | | |
| Tom's Natural Toothpaste with Calcium and Fluoride | Calcium carbonate | Sodium monofluorophosphate | Sodium lauryl sulfate |
| | **Other Ingredients:** Glycerin, carrageenan, xylitol, spearmint and peppermint oil | | |
| Tom's Natural Toothpaste with Propolis and Myrrh | Calcium carbonate | | Sodium lauryl sulfate |
| | **Other Ingredients:** Glycerin, carrageenan, oil of spearmint, peppermint, cassia, or fennel, propolis, myrrh | | |
| Toothpaste Booster | | | Hydrogen peroxide, sodium lauryl sulfate |
| | **Other Ingredients:** Deionized water, cornstarch, sorbitol, propylene glycol, carbomer 940, menthol, sodium benzoate, potassium sorbate | | |
| Topol Gel[a] (spearmint) | Hydrated silica | Sodium monofluorophosphate | Sodium lauryl sulfate |

| Product | Abrasive Ingredient | Therapeutic Ingredient | Foaming Agent |
|---|---|---|---|
| | **Other Ingredients:** Sorbitol, deionized water, glycerin, PEG-6, flavor, xanthan gum, sodium saccharin, methylparaben, propylparaben, zirconium silicate, FD&C blue #1, FD&C yellow #5 | | |
| Topol Plus Baking Soda Whitening Gel or Toothpaste | Hydrated silica | Sodium monofluorophosphate | Sodium lauryl sulfate |
| | **Other Ingredients:** Water, sorbitol (gel), glycerin, calcium carbonate (gel), sorbitol, PEG-6, disodium phosphate, flavor, xanthan gum, sodium saccharin, titanium dioxide, methylparaben, propylparaben, FD&C blue #1 (gel) | | |
| Topol Toothpaste[a] (peppermint) | Hydrated silica, sodium bicarbonate | Sodium monofluorophosphate | Sodium lauryl sulfate |
| | **Other Ingredients:** Sorbitol, deionized water, glycerin, PEG-6, flavor, xanthan gum, titanium dioxide, sodium saccharin, methylparaben, propylparaben, zirconium silicate | | |
| Triplex Toothpaste | Hydrated silica, sodium bicarbonate | Sodium fluoride | Calcium peroxide, sodium lauryl sulfate |
| | **Other Ingredients:** Glycerin, sorbitol, urea, flavor, titanium dioxide, carbomer, sodium saccharin, ethyl cellulose, sodium benzoate | | |
| Ultra Brite Baking Soda Toothpaste | Hydrated silica, sodium bicarbonate, alumina | Sodium monofluorophosphate 0.76% | Sodium lauryl sulfate |
| | **Other Ingredients:** Glycerin, tetrasodium pyrophosphate, cellulose gum, flavor, sodium saccharin, titanium dioxide | | |
| Ultra Brite Gel[a] | Hydrated silica | Sodium monofluorophosphate 0.76% | Sodium lauryl sulfate |
| | **Other Ingredients:** Sorbitol, PEG-12, flavor, cellulose gum, sodium saccharin, glycerin, FD&C blue #1, D&C red #33 | | |
| Ultra Brite Toothpaste | Hydrated silica, alumina | Sodium monofluorophosphate 0.76% | Sodium lauryl sulfate |
| | **Other Ingredients:** Glycerin, cellulose gum, carrageenan gum, sodium benzoate, titanium dioxide, sodium saccharin, flavor | | |
| Viadent Fluoride Gel | Hydrated silica | Sodium monofluorophosphate 0.8%, sanguinaria extract 0.075% | Sodium lauryl sulfate |
| | **Other Ingredients:** Sodium saccharin, zinc chloride, teaberry flavor, sodium carboxymethylcellulose, sorbitol | | |
| Viadent Fluoride Toothpaste | Hydrated silica | Sodium monofluorophosphate 0.8%, sanguinaria extract 0.075% | Sodium lauryl sulfate |
| | **Other Ingredients:** Sorbitol, titanium dioxide, carboxymethylcellulose, flavor, sodium saccharin, citric acid, zinc chloride | | |
| Viadent Original Toothpaste | Dicalcium phosphate | Sanguinaria extract 0.075% | Sodium lauryl sulfate |
| | **Other Ingredients:** Glycerin, sorbitol, titanium dioxide, zinc chloride, carrageenan, flavor, sodium saccharin, citric acid | | |

[a]Carries American Dental Association (ADA) seal indicating safety and efficacy.

[b]Topical fluoride rinse

Reprinted with permission from *Handbook of Nonprescription Drugs*, 10th ed, *Product Updates*, Washington, DC, American Pharmaceutical Association, 1995, 265-71.

# DENTURE ADHESIVE PRODUCTS

| Product | Dosage Form | Ingredients |
|---|---|---|
| Confident (Block Drug) | Cream | Carboxymethylcellulose gum 32%, ethylene oxide polymer 13%, petrolatum, liquid petrolatum, propylparaben |
| Corega | Powder | Karaya gum 94.6%, water-soluble ethylene oxide polymer 5%, flavor |
| Dentrol | Liquid | Carboxymethylcellulose sodium, ethylene oxide polymer, mineral oil, polyethylene, flavor, propylparaben |
| Denturite | Liquid, powder | Liquid: Butyl phthalyl butyl glycolate, vinyl acetate, SDA alcohol Powder: Polyethyl methacrylate polymer |
| Effergrip[a] | Cream | Carboxymethylcellulose sodium 24.8%, calcium sodium mixed salt of methyl vinyl ether-maleic anhydride 29.8%, preservatives, red lake blend |
| Ezo Cushions | Pad | Paraffin wax, cotton |
| Fasteeth | Powder | Calcium/zinc poly (vinyl methyl ether maleate), sodium carboxymethylcellulose, cornstarch, silicon dioxide, peppermint oil, rectified |
| Fasteeth Extra Hold | Powder | Calcium/zinc poly (vinyl methyl ether maleate), sodium carboxymethylcellulose, silicon dioxide, peppermint oil, rectified |
| Fixodent | Cream | Calcium/zinc poly (vinyl methyl ether maleate), sodium carboxymethylcellulose, mineral oil, petrolatum, silicon dioxide, color |
| Fixodent Fresh | Cream | Calcium/zinc poly (vinyl methyl ether maleate), sodium carboxymethylcellulose, mineral oil, petrolatum, silicon dioxide, color, peppermint flavor, methyl lactate, menthol |
| Orafix | Cream | Karaya gum 51%, petrolatum 30%, mineral oil 13%, peppermint oil 0.08% |
| Orafix Special[a] | Cream | Gantrez MS955, sodium carboxymethylcellulose type 7H4XF, povidone K-90, white petrolatum, mineral oil, heavy, isopropyl palmitate, isopropyl myristate, flavors, colors |
| Plasti-Liner | Strip | Polyethyl metacrylate polymer, butyl phthalyl butyl glycolate, triacetin |
| Poli-Grip | Cream | Karaya gum 51%, petrolatum 36.7%, liquid petrolatum, magnesium oxide, propylparaben, flavor |
| Poly-Grip Super | Cream | Carboxymethylcellulose sodium, ethylene oxide polymer, petrolatum, mineral oil flavor, propylparaben |
| Poli-Grip Super | Powder | Calcium sodium methyl vinyl ether-maleic copolymer, carboxymethylcellulose sodium, flavor |
| Polident Dentu-Grip | Cream | Carboxymethylcellulose gum 49%, ethylene oxide polymer 21%, flavor |
| Quik-Fix | Liquid, powder | Liquid: Methyl methacrylate monomer, hydroxyethyl metacyclate monomer, colorstable concentrate, triacetin; Powder: Polyethyl methacrylate polymer |

| Product | Dosage Form | Ingredients |
|---|---|---|
| Rigident | Powder | Acacia gum, karaya gum, sodium borate |
| Rigident[a] | Cream | Carboxymethylcellulose sodium, calcium sodium salts of methyl vinyl ether maleic anhydride copolymer, petrolatum, mineral oil, talc, flavor, propylparaben, D&C red #27 aluminum lake |
| Sea-Bond | Pad | Ethylene oxide polymer, sodium alginate |
| Wernet's | Cream | Carboxymethylcellulose gum 32%, petrolatum, mineral oil, ethylene oxide polymer 13%, propylparaben, flavor 0.5% |
| Wernet's | Powder | Karaya gum 94.6%, water-soluble ethylene oxide polymer 5%, flavor 0.4% |

[a]Carries American Dental Association (ADA) seal indicating safety and efficacy.

Reprinted with permission from *Handbook of Nonprescription Drugs*, 10th ed, *Product Updates*, Washington, DC, American Pharmaceutical Association, 1995, 277.

# DENTURE CLEANSER PRODUCTS

| Product | Dosage Form | Ingredients |
|---|---|---|
| Ban-A-Stain** | Liquid | Phosphoric acid 25%, deionized water, imidurea, methylparaben, xanthan gum, alkyl phenoxy polyethoxy ethanol, oil of cassis, FD&C red #40 |
| Complete[a] | Paste | Calcium carbonate, water, glycerin, sorbitol, cellulose gum, sodium lauryl sulfate, silica, flavor, magnesium aluminum silicate, sodium saccharin, methylparaben, propylparaben |
| Dentu-Creme | Paste | Dicalcium phosphate dihydrate, propylene glycol, calcium carbonate, silica, sodium lauryl sulfate, glycerin, hydroxyethylcellulose, flavor, magnesium aluminum silicate, sodium saccharin, methylparaben, propylparaben |
| Efferdent Antibacterial[a] | Tablet | Potassium monopersulfate, sodium perborate monohydrate, sodium carbonate, sodium lauryl sulfoacetate, sodium bicarbonate, citric acid, magnesium stearate, flavor |
| Efferdent, 2 Layer | Tablet | Sodium bicarbonate, sodium carbonate, citric acid, potassium monopersulfate, sodium perborate monohydrate, sodium lauryl sulfoacetate, flavor |
| Polident | Tablet, powder | Potassium monopersulfate, sodium perborate monohydrate, sodium carbonate, surfactant, chelating agents (tablet), proteolytic enzyme (tablet), sodium acid pyrophosphate (powder), sodium bicarbonate, citric acid (tablet), fragrance |
| Rembrandt Daily Denture Renewal | Gel | Citroxain |
| Smokers' Polident | Tablet | Sodium carbonate, potassium monopersulfate, citric acid, sodium bicarbonate, sodium perborate monohydrate, surfactant, chelating agents, proteolytic enzyme, fragrance |

[a]Carries American Dental Association (ADA) seal indicating safety and efficacy.

Reprinted with permission from *Handbook of Nonprescription Drugs*, 10th ed, *Product Updates*, Washington, DC, American Pharmaceutical Association, 1995, 276.

# MOUTH PAIN, COLD SORE, CANKER SORE PRODUCTS

| Product | Anesthetic/ Analgesic | Other Ingredients |
|---|---|---|
| Amosan Powder | | Sodium peroxyborate monohydrate, sodium bitartrate, saccharin, peppermint, menthol, and vanilla flavors |
| Anbesol Baby Gel (grape or original) | Benzocaine 7.5% | Benzoic acid (grape), carbomer 934P, D&C red #33, disodium EDTA, FD&C blue #1 (grape), flavor, glycerin, methylparaben (grape), PEG-8, propylparaben (grape), saccharin, water |
| Anbesol Gel | Benzocaine 6.3%, phenol 0.5%, camphor | Alcohol 70%, carbomer 934P, D&C red #33, D&C yellow #10, FD&C blue #1, FD&C yellow #6, flavor, glycerin |
| Anbesol Liquid | Benzocaine 6.3%, phenol 0.5%, camphor, menthol | Alcohol 70%, glycerin, potassium iodide, povidone iodine |
| Anbesol Maximum Strength Gel | Benzocaine 20% | Alcohol 60%, carbomer 934P, D&C yellow #10, FD&C blue #1, FD&C red #40, flavor, PEG-12, saccharin |
| Anbesol Maximum Strength Liquid | Benzocaine 20% | Alcohol 60%, D&C yellow #10, FD&C blue #1, FD&C red #40, flavor, PEG-8, saccharin |
| Babee Teething Lotion | Benzocaine 2.5%, menthol, camphor | Alcohol 20%, witch hazel |
| Benzodent Denture Analgesic Ointment[a] | Benzocaine 20%, eugenol | 8-hydroxyquinoline sulfate, petrolatum, sodium CMC, color |
| Betadine Mouthwash/ Gargle | | Povidone-iodine 0.5%, alcohol 8.8% |
| Blistex Medicated Lip Ointment | Menthol 0.6%, camphor 0.5%, phenol 0.5% | Allantoin 1% |
| Blistex Lip Medex Ointment | Camphor 1%, menthol 1%, phenol 0.5% | Petrolatum, cocoa butter, flavor, lanolin, mixed waxes, oil of cloves |
| Campho-Phenique Antiseptic Gel | Camphor 10.8%, phenol 4.7% | Eucalyptus oil |
| Campho-Phenique Cold Sore Gel[b] | Camphor 10.8%, phenol 4.7% | Eucalyptus oil |
| Campho-Phenique Liquid | Camphor 10.8%, phenol 4.7% | Eucalyptus oil |
| Chap Stick Medicated Lip Balm (jar or squeeze tube) | Camphor 1%, menthol 0.6%, phenol 0.5% | Petrolatum 60% (jar), petrolatum 67% (squeeze tube), microcrystalline wax, mineral oil, cocoa butter, lanolin, paraffin wax (jar) |
| Chap Stick Medicated Lip Balm Stick | Camphor 1%, menthol 0.6%, phenol 0.5% | Petrolatum 41%, paraffin wax, mineral oil, cocoa butter, 2-octyl dodecanol, arachadyl propionate, polyphenylmethylsiloxane 556, white wax, isopropyl lanolate, carnauba wax, isopropyl myristate, lanolin, fragrance, methylparaben, propylparaben, oleyl alcohol, cetyl alcohol |
| Cold Sore Lotion[b] | Camphor, menthol | Alcohol 85%, gum benzoin 7%, thymol, eucalyptol |
| Curasore Liquid | | Ethyl ether, ethyl alcohol |
| Dent's 3 in 1 Toothache Relief (gel, gum, drops) | Benzocaine 20% | Alcohol 74% (drops), chlorobutanol anhydrous 0.09% (drops), eugenol |

## MOUTH PAIN, COLD SORE, CANKER SORE PRODUCTS
*(Continued)*

| Product | Anesthetic/ Analgesic | Other Ingredients |
|---|---|---|
| Dent's Double-Action Kit (tablets, drops) | Benzocaine 20% (drops) | Denatured alcohol 74%, chlorobutanol 0.09%, acetaminophen 325 mg (tablet), eugenol |
| Dent's Extra Strength Toothache Gum | Benzocaine 20% | Petrolatum, cotton and wax base, beeswax, FD&C red #40 aluminum lake, eugenol |
| Dent's Maxi-Strength Toothache Treatment Drops | Benzocaine 20% | Alcohol 74%, chlorobutanol 0.09%, propylene glycol, FD&C red #40, eugenol |
| Dent-Zel-Ite Oral Mucosal Analgesic Liquid | Benzocaine 5%, camphor | Alcohol 81%, wintergreen, glycerin |
| Dent-Zel-Ite Temporary Dental Filling Liquid | Camphor | Alcohol 55%, sandarac gum, methyl salicylate |
| Dent-Zel-Ite Toothache Relief Drops | Eugenol 85%, camphor | Alcohol 13.5%, wintergreen |
| GargleAid Granular Effervescent | Dyclonine HCl 69 mg | Sucrose, salt, sodium bicarbonate, citric acid, natural lemon flavor, sodium ascorbate |
| HDA Toothache Gel | Benzocaine 6.5% | Clove oil |
| Herpecin-L Stick[b] | | Allantoin, padimate O, titanium dioxide |
| Hurricaine Aerosol (wild cherry) | Benzocaine | Polyethylene glycol, saccharin, flavoring |
| Hurricaine Gel (wild cherry, pina colada, or watermelon) | Benzocaine | Polyethylene glycol, saccharin, flavoring |
| Hurricaine Liquid (wild cherry or pina colada) | Benzocaine | Polyethylene glycol, saccharin, flavoring |
| Isodettes Spray | Phenol 1.4% | Propylene glycol 10%, artificial and sodium hydroxide 0.0047%, natural wild cherry flavor 0.5%, artificial and natural eucalyptus flavor, FD&C red #40, water |
| Kank-A-Professional Strength Liquid[a] | Benzocaine 20%, benzyl alcohol | Benzoin tincture compound 0.5%, cetylpyridinium chloride, ethylcellulose, SD alcohol, dimethyl isosorbide, castor oil, flavor, tannic acid, propylene glycol, saccharin |
| Lip Medex Ointment | Camphor 1.0%, menthol 0.5%, phenol 0.5% | Petrolatum 73.7% |
| Lotion-Jel | Benzocaine | Distilled water, methylparaben, propylparaben, propylene glycol, carbopol 934-P, methyl salicylate, FD&C red #40, 2.2' iminodiethanol |
| Medadyne Liquid | Benzocaine 10%, menthol, camphor | Benzalkonium chloride, tannic acid, flavors, SD alcohol, benzyl alcohol, thymol |
| Mouth Kote-PR Ointment | Benzyl alcohol 3.5%, diphenhydramine 1.25% | PEG 8, cellulose gum, PEG 75, poloxamer 407, yerba santa, flavor |
| Mouth Kote-PR Solution | Diphenhydramine 1.25%, benzyl alcohol 1% | Water, cetylpyridinium chloride, disodium EDTA flavor, sodium benzoate, sodium hydroxide, sodium saccharin, yerba santa |
| Mouth Kote-OR Solution | Benzyl alcohol 1%, menthol | Water, sorbitol, sodium chloride, yerba santa, flavor, poloxamer 407, sodium saccharin, cetylpyridinium chloride, disodium EDTA |

| Product | Anesthetic/ Analgesic | Other Ingredients |
|---|---|---|
| Numzident (Adult Strength) Gel | Benzocaine 10% | PEG 400 47.86%, glycerin 30%, PEG 3350 10%, sodium saccharin 1%, purified water 0.75%, cherry vanilla flavor 0.4% |
| Numzit Teething Gel | Benzocaine 7.5% | PEG 400 66.2%, PEG 3350 26.1%, sodium saccharin 0.036%, clove oil 0.09%, peppermint oil 0.018%, purified water 0.056% |
| Numzit Teething Lotion | Benzocaine 0.2% | Alcohol 12.1%, glycerin 2%, kelgin MV 0.5%, sodium saccharin 0.02%, methylparaben 0.1%, FD&C red #40 0.1%, FD&C blue #1 0.009% |
| Orabase Baby Gel[a] | Benzocaine 7.5% | Glycerin, PEG, carbopol, preservative, sweetener, flavor |
| Orabase Gel | Benzocaine 15% | Ethanol, PEG, hydroxyethyl chloride, tannic acid, salicylic acid, flavor, sodium saccharin |
| Orabase Lip Cream | Benzocaine 5%, menthol 0.5%, camphor, phenol | Allantoin 1%, sodium carboxymethylcellulose, veegum, Tween 80, phenonip, PEG, biopure, talc, kaolin, lanolin, petrolatum, oil of clove, aerosil |
| Orabase Plain Paste[a] | | Pectin, gelatin, carboxymethylcellulose sodium, polyethylene, mineral oil, flavors, preservative, guar, tragacanth |
| Orabase-B with Benzocaine Paste[a] | Benzocaine 20% | Plasticized hydrocarbon gel, guar, carboxymethylcellulose, tragacanth, pectin, preservatives, flavors |
| Orajel Baby Gel | Benzocaine 7.5% | FD&C red #40, flavor, glycerin, polyethylene glycols, sodium saccharin, sorbic acid, sorbitol |
| Orajel Baby Nighttime Formula Gel | Benzocaine 10% | FD&C red #40, flavor, glycerin, polyethylene glycols, sodium saccharin, sorbic acid, sorbitol |
| Orajel Denture Gel | Benzocaine 10%, eugenol | Chlorothymol, FD&C red #40, flavor, polyethylene glycols, purified water, sodium saccharin, sorbic acid |
| Orajel Maximum Strength Gel | Benzocaine 20% | Clove oil, flavor, polyethylene glycols, sodium saccharin, sorbic acid |
| Orajel Mouth-Aid Gel | Benzocaine 20% | Zinc chloride 0.1%, benzalkonium chloride 0.02%. allantoin, carbomer, edetate disodium, peppermint oil, polyethylene glycol, polysorbate 60, propyl gallate, polysorbate 60, glycol, purified water, povidone sodium saccharin propylene, sorbic acid, stearyl alcohol |
| Orajel Mouth-Aid Liquid | Benzocaine 20% | Cetylpyridinium chloride 0.1%, ethylcellulose |
| Orajel Regular Strength Gel | Benzocaine 10% | Clove oil, flavor, polyethylene glycols, sodium saccharin, sorbic acid |
| Orasol Liquid | Benzocaine 6.3%, phenol 0.5% | Alcohol 70% |
| Painalay Sore Throat Gargle & Spray | Phenol 0.5% | |
| Probax Ointment[b] | | Propolis 2%, petrolatum, mineral oil |
| Red Cross Toothache Medication Drops | Eugenol 85% | Sesame oil |
| SensoGARD Gel[b] | Benzocaine 20% | Methylparaben, polycarbophil, polyethylene glycol, propylparaben, sorbitan monooleate |

## MOUTH PAIN, COLD SORE, CANKER SORE PRODUCTS *(Continued)*

| Product | Anesthetic/ Analgesic | Other Ingredients |
|---|---|---|
| Sore Throat Spray (cherry, menthol, or mint) | Phenol 1.4% | |
| Tanac Liquid | Benzocaine 10% | Benzalkonium chloride 0.125%, saccharin |
| Tanac Medicated Gel | Dyclonine HCl 1.0% | Allantoin 0.5% |
| Tanac Roll-On Lotion | Benzocaine 5% | Benzalkonium chloride 0.12%, sodium saccharin, glycerin, polyethylene glycol, tannic acid |
| Tanac Stick | Benzocaine 7.5% | Benzalkonium chloride 0.125% |
| Throtoceptic Pump Spray | Phenol 1.4% | Alum 0.5%, flavor |
| Tisol Solution | Benzyl alcohol 1% | Water, sorbitol, sodium chloride, yerba santa, poloxamer 407, menthol, saccharin, cetylpyridinium chloride, disodium EDTA |
| Vaseline Lip Therapy Ointment | Camphor 0.8%, menthol 0.8%, phenol 0.5% | White petrolatum 92.8%, allantoin 1% |
| Viractin | Tetracaine 2% | |
| Vicks Chloraseptic Advanced Formula Sore Throat Spray | Phenol 1.4% | Colors, flavors, glycerin, purified water, saccharin, sodium |
| Vicks Chloraseptic Sore Throat Spray, Childrens | Phenol 0.5% | FD&C blue #1, FD&C red #40, flavor, glycerin, purified water, saccharin sodium, sorbitol |
| Vicks Chloraseptic Sore Throat Gargle, Menthol | Phenol 1.4% | D&C green #5, D&C yellow #10, FD&C green #3, flavor, glycerin, water, saccharin sodium |
| Zilactin Medicated Gel | Benzyl alcohol 10% | Tannic acid, hydroxypropyl cellulose filmformer |
| Zilactin-L Liquid | Lidocaine 2.5% | |

[a]Carries American Dental Association (ADA) seal indicating safety and efficacy.

[b]For cold sore treatment only.

Reprinted with permission from *Handbook of Nonprescription Drugs*, 10th ed, *Product Updates*, Washington, DC, American Pharmaceutical Association, 1995, 278-81.

# ORAL RINSE PRODUCTS

| Product | Antiseptic | Other Ingredients |
|---|---|---|
| Act[b] | Cetylpyridinium chloride, menthol, methyl salicylate | Sodium fluoride 0.05%, edetate calcium disodium, FD&C green #3, FD&C yellow #5, flavor, glycerin, monobasic sodium phosphate, dibasic sodium phosphate, poloxamer 407, polysorbate-20, potassium sorbate, propylene glycol, sodium benzoate, sodium saccharin, water |
| Act for Kids[ab] | Cetylpyridinium chloride | Sodium fluoride 0.05%, D&C red #33, dibasic sodium phosphate, edetate calcium disodium, flavors, glycerin, monobasic sodium phosphate, poloxamer 407, polysorbate-80, propylene glycol, sodium benzoate, sodium saccharin, water |
| Astring-O-Sol | SD alcohol 38-B, 75.6%, methyl salicylate | Water, myrrh extract, zinc chloride, citric acid |
| Biotene Mouthwash | Lysozyme (6 mg), lactoferrin (6 mg) glucose oxidase (4000 units) | Water, xylitol, hydrogenated starch, propylene glycol, hydroxyethyl cellulose, aloe vera, natural peppermint, poloxamer 407, calcium lactate, zinc gluconate, sodium benzoate, benzoic acid |
| Cankaid | Carbamide peroxide 10% | Citric acid monohydrate, sodium citrate dihydrate, edetate disodium |
| Cepacol Mouthwash/Gargle | Alcohol 14%, cetylpyridinium chloride 0.05% | Edetate disodium, colors, flavors, glycerin, polysorbate 80, saccharin, sodium B phosphate, sodium phosphate, water |
| Cepacol Mouthwash/Gargle, Mint | Alcohol 14.5%, cetylpyridinium chloride 0.5% | Colors, flavors, glucono delta-lactone, glycerin, poloxamer-407, sodium saccharin, sodium gluconate, water |
| Clear Choice | Cetylpyridinium chloride | Glycerin, sodium phosphate, poloxamer 338, flavor, sodium saccharin, domiphen bromide |
| Fluorigard Anti-Cavity Fluoride Rinse[ab] | | Sodium fluoride 0.05% |
| Gly-Oxide[c] | Carbamide peroxide 10% | Citric acid, flavor, glycerin, propylene glycol, sodium stannate, water |
| Lavoris | SD Alcohol 38-B | Water, glycerin, citric acid, poloxamer 407, water, saccharin, clove oil, polysorbate 80, zinc chloride, zinc oxide, sodium hydroxide, flavors, colors |
| Lavoris Crystal Fresh | SD Alcohol 38-B | Purified water, glycerin, poloxamer 407, citric acid, zinc oxide, sodium hydroxide, saccharin, polysorbate 80, flavors |
| Listerine[a] Topical Fluoride Rinse | Alcohol 26.9%, menthol, methyl salicylate, eucalyptol, thymol | |
| Listerine, Coolmint[a] | Alcohol 21.6%, menthol, methyl salicylate, eucalyptol, thymol | Anetmole |

## ORAL RINSE PRODUCTS *(Continued)*

| Product | Antiseptic | Other Ingredients |
|---|---|---|
| Listerine, Freshburst[a] | Alcohol 21.6%, eucalyptol, menthol, methyl salicylate, thymol | Glycerin, benzoic acid, poloxamer 407, sodium saccharin, sodium citrate, FD&C green #3, D&C yellow #10 |
| Listermint with Fluoride | Alcohol 6.65% | Sodium fluoride 0.02%, zinc chloride, glycerin, poloxamer 407, sodium lauryl sulfate, sodium citrate, flavor, sodium saccharin, citric acid, D&C yellow #10, FD&C green #3 |
| Mouth Wash Antiseptic | Alcohol 26.9%, eucalyptol 0.09%, thymol 0.06%, methyl salicylate 0.06%, menthol 0.04% | |
| MouthKote-FR | | Sodium fluoride 0.04%, benzyl alcohol, menthol, water, xylitol, sorbitol, sodium chloride, yerba santa, poloxamer 407, cetylpyridinium chloride, disodium EDTA |
| Orajel Perioseptic[c] | Carbamide peroxide 15% | Citric acid, edetate disodium, propylene glycol, purified water, sodium chloride, sodium, flavor, methylparaben saccharin |
| Oral-B Anti-Cavity Rinse Alcohol Free[b] | Cetylpyridinium chloride monohydrate | Sodium fluoride 0.05%, water, glycerin, cremophor RH40, flavor, methylparaben, sodium saccharin, sodium benzoate, propylparaben, FD&C blue #1 |
| Oral-B Anti-Cavity Rinse[ab] | | Sodium fluoride 0.05%, water, sodium benzoate, potassium sorbate, sodium saccharin, glycerin, PEG-40, FD&C blue #1, phosphoric acid |
| Oral-B Anti-Plaque Rinse | Alcohol 8%, cetylpyridinium chloride | Water, glycerin, sodium saccharin, methylparaben, propylparaben, FD&C blue #1, D&C yellow #10, poloxamer 407 |
| Oral-B Anti-Plaque Rinse Alcohol Free | Cetylpyridinium chloride 0.05% | Water, glycerin, flavor, polysorbate 20, methylparaben, sodium saccharin, propylparaben, sodium benzoate, FD&C blue #1, D&C yellow #10 |
| Peroxyl Hygienic Dental Rinse[c] | Alcohol 5%, hydrogen peroxide 1.5% | Pluronic F108, sorbitol, sodium saccharin, dye, polysorbate 20, mint flavor |
| Peroxyl Oral Spot Treatment Gel[c] | Hydrogen Peroxide 1.5% | Mint flavor, ethyl alcohol 5%, pluronic F108, polysorbate 20, sorbitol, sodium saccharin, dye, pluronic F127 |
| Plax Advanced Formula, Clear Peppermint | Alcohol 8.5% | Water, glycerin, tetrasodium pyrophosphate, benzoic acid, sodium lauryl sulfate, sodium benzoate, polomer 407, flavor, xanthan gum |
| Plax Advanced Formula, Original Flavor | Alcohol 8.5% | Sodium lauryl sulfate, water, glycerin, sodium benzoate, tetrasodium pyrophosphate, benzoic acid, poloxamer 407, saccharin, flavor, xanthan gum |

| Product | Antiseptic | Other Ingredients |
|---|---|---|
| Plax Advanced Formula, Softmint | Alcohol 8.5% | Sodium lauryl sulfate, water, glycerin, sodium benzoate, tetrasodium pyrophosphate, benzoic acid, poloxamer 407, saccharin, flavor, xanthan gum, flavor enhancer, FD&C blue #1, FD&C yellow #5 |
| Scope Baking Soda Clean Mint | SD alcohol 38-F 9.9%, cetylpyridinium chloride, domiphen bromide | Water, sorbitol, sodium bicarbonate, poloxamer 407, polysorbate 80, sodium saccharin, flavor |
| Scope Original, Mint | SD alcohol 38-F 18.9%, cetylpyridinium chloride, domiphen bromide | Purified water, glycerin, sodium saccharin, sodium benzoate, flavor, benzoic acid, FD&C blue #1, FD&C yellow #5 |
| Scope, Peppermint | SD alcohol 38-F 14%, cetylpyridinium chloride, domiphen bromide | Purified water, glycerin, poloxamer 407, sodium saccharin, sodium benzoate, N-ethylmethylcarboxamide, benzoic acid, FD&C blue #1 |
| Targo | | |
| Tech 2000 | Cetylpyridinium chloride | Water, glycerin, poloxamer 407, flavor, FD&C blue #1, FD&C yellow #5, nutritive dextrose or sucrose and/or calcium saccharin |
| Tom's of Maine Mouthwash | Menthol | Water, glycerin, aloe vera juice, witch hazel, poloxamer 335, spearmint oil, ascorbic acid |
| Viadent Oral Rinse | Alcohol 10% | Sanguinaria extract, glycerin, polysorbate 80, flavor, sodium saccharin, poloxamer 237, citric acid, zinc chloride 0.2% |

[a]Carries American Dental Association (ADA) seal indicating safety and efficacy.

[b]Topical fluoride rinse

[c]Oral debriding agent/wound cleanser

Reprinted with permission from *Handbook of Nonprescription Drugs*, 10th ed, *Product Updates*, Washington, DC, American Pharmaceutical Association, 1995, 273-5.

# PRODUCTS FOR XEROSTOMIA

| Product | Dosage Form | Ingredients |
|---|---|---|
| Biotene® | Chewing gum (dental) | Active ingredients: Lactoperioxidase (0.11 units), glucose oxidase (0.15 units)<br>Other ingredients: Sorbitol, gum base, xylitol, hydrogenated glucose syrup, artificial flavor, titanium dioxide, lecithin, resinous glase, BHT, potassium thiocyanate |
| Glandosane | Spray | Sodium carboxymethylcellulose, sorbitol, sodium chloride, potassium chloride, calcium chloride dihydrate, magnesium chloride hexahydrate, dipotassium hydrogen phosphate |
| Moi-Stir 10[a] | Pump spray | Sodium carboxymethylcellulose, potassium chloride, dibasic sodium phosphate, methylparaben, propylparaben |
| Moi-Stir Mouth Moistening | Pump spray | Carboxymethylcellulose |
| Moi-Stir Oral Swabsticks[a] | Swab | Carboxymethylcellulose |
| MouthKote | Spray | Water, xylitol, sorbitol, yerba santa, citric acid, flavor, ascorbic acid, sodium benzoate, sodium saccharin |
| Optimoist | Liquid | Citric acid, calcium phosphate, sodium monofluorophosphate, preservative, sweetener, xylitol, polysorbate 20, flavor, hydroxyethylcellulose, sodium hydroxide |
| OralBalance® | Long-lasting moisturizing gel | Active ingredients (per g): Glucose oxidase (2000 units), lysozyme (5 mg), lactoferrin (5 mg)<br>Other ingredients: Hydrogenated starch, xylitol, hydroxyethylcellulose, glycerate polyhydrate, aloe vera, potassium thiocyanate |
| Salagen® (pilocarpine) | Tablet (Rx only) | Pilocarpine 5 mg |
| Saliva Substitute[a] | Spray | Sorbitol, sodium carboxymethylcellulose, methylparaben |
| Salivart Synthetic Saliva[a] | Aerosol spray | Sorbitol 3%, sodium carboxymethylcellulose 1%, potassium chloride 0.12%, sodium chloride 0.084%, calcium chloride dihydrate, magnesium chloride hexahydrate, potassium phosphate dibasic, nitrogen (as propellant) |

[a]Carries American Dental Association (ADA) seal indicating safety and efficacy.

Adapted with permission from *Handbook of Nonprescription Drugs*, 10th ed, *Product Updates*, Washington, DC, American Pharmaceutical Association, 1995, 272.

# SUGAR-FREE LIQUID PHARMACEUTICALS

The following sugar-free liquid preparations are listed by therapeutic category and alphabetically within each category. Please note that product formulations are subject to change by the manufacturer. Some of these products may contain sorbitol, xylitol, or other sweeteners which may be partially metabolized to provide calories.

**Analgesics**

Acetaminophen Elixir (various)
APAP/APAP Plus
Aspirin/Buffered Aspirin (Medique®)
Bufferin® A/F Nite Time
Children's Anacin-3® Infants Drops
Children's Myapap® Elixir
Children's Panadol® Drops, Liquid, and Chewable Tablets
Children's Tylenol® Chewable Tablets
Conex® Liquid
Conex® With Codeine Liquid
Dolanex® Elixir
Extra Strength Tylenol® PM
Febrol® and Febrol® EX
I-Prin®
Methadone Hydrochloride Intensol
MS-Aid®
Myapap® Drops
No Drowsiness Tylenol®
Pain-Off®
Paregoric USP
Sep-A-Soothe® II
St Joseph® Aspirin-Free Liquid and Drops
Tempra® Chewable Tablets
Tylenol® Drops

**Antacids/Antiflatulents**

Alcalak®
Aldroxicon®
Almag® Suspension
Aludrox® Suspension
Aluminum Hydroxide Suspension
Calglycine® Tablets
Camalox® Suspension
Citrocarbonate® Granules
Creamalin® Suspension
Delcid®
Di-Gel® Liquid (mint, lemon & orange flavored)
Digestamic®
Dimacid®
Gaviscon® Liquid
Gelusil® II
Gelusil® Liquid
Gelusil® Liquid Flavor Pack
Gelusil-M® Liquid
Kolantyl® Gel
Maalox® Plus Suspension
Maalox® Suspension
Maalox® Therapeutic Concentrate
Magnatril® Suspension
Magnesia and Alumina Oral Suspension USP
Mallamint® Chewable Tablets
Marblen® Suspension and Tablets
Medi-Seltzer®/Plus
Milk of Bismuth
Milk of Magnesia USP
Mylanta® Liquid
Mylanta®-II Liquid
Mylicon® Drops
Nephrox® Suspension
Nutrajel®
Nutramag®
Pepto-Bismol® Liquid and Tablets
Phosphaljel® Suspension
Riopan Plus®
Riopan® Suspension
Silain-Gel® Liquid

## SUGAR-FREE LIQUID PHARMACEUTICALS *(Continued)*

Trisogel®
Titralac® Liquid
Titralac® Plus Liquid
WinGel® Liquid and Tablets

**Antiasthmatics**
Aerolate® Liquid
Alupent® Syrup
Choledyl® Pediatric Syrup
Droxine®
Elixophyllin® Elixir
Elixophyllin®-GG Liquid
Lanophyllin® Elixir
Lixolin® Liquid
Lufyllin® Elixir
Metaprel® Syrup
Mucomyst®-10
Mucomyst®-20
Mudrane® GG Elixir
Neothylline® Elixir
Neothylline® G
Organidin® Solution
Slo-Phyllin® 80 Syrup
Somophyllin® Oral Liquid
Somophyllin®-DF Oral Liquid
Tedral® Elixir and Suspension
Theolair™ 80 Syrup
Theolixir®
Theon® Syrup
Theo-Organidin® Elixir
Theophylline Elixir

**Antidepressants**
Sinequan® Oral Concentrate

**Antidiarrheals**
Corrective Mixture With Paregoric
Diasorb® Liquid and Tablets
Di-Gon® II
Diotame®
Donnagel®
Infantol® Pink
Kalicon® Suspension
Kaolin Mixture With Pectin NF
Kaolin-Pectin Suspension
Konsyl® Powder
Lomanate®
Lomotil® Liquid
Paregoric USP (various)
Parepectolin® (various)
Pepto-Bismol®
St Joseph® Antidiarrheal

**Antiepileptics**
Mysoline® Suspension
Paradione® Solution

**Antihistamine-Decongestants**
Actifed® With Codeine
Actifed® Syrup
Actidil® Syrup
Bromphen® Elixir
Dimetane® Decongestant Elixir
Dimetapp® Elixir
Hay-Febrol® Liquid
Isoclor® Liquid and Capsules
Naldecon® Pediatric Drops and Syrup
Naldecon® Syrup
Novahistine® Elixir
Phenergan® Fortis Syrup
Phenergan® Syrup
Rondec® DM Drops
Ryna® Liquid
S-T® Forte® Liquid
Tavist® Syrup
Trind® Liquid
Veltap® Elixir

Vistaril® Oral Suspension

**Anti-Infectives**

Augmentin® Suspension
Furadantin® Oral Suspension
Furoxone® Suspension
Humatin®
Mandelamine® Suspension/Forte®
Minocin® Suspension
Mycifradin® Sulfate Oral Solution
NegGram® Suspension
Proklar® Suspension
Sulfamethoxazole and Trimethoprim Suspension
Vibramycin® Syrup

**Antiparkinsonism Agents**

Artane® Elixir

**Antispasmodics**

Antrocol® Elixir
Spasmophen® Elixir

**Corticosteroids**

Decadron® Elixir
Dexamethasone Solution (Roxane)
Dexamethasone Intensol Solution
Pediapred® Oral Liquid

**Cough Medicines**

Anatuss® With Codeine Syrup
Anatuss® Syrup
Brown Mixture NF (Lannett)
CCP® Caffeine Free
CCP® Cough/Cold Tablets
Cerose-DM®
Chlorgest-HD®
Codagest® Expectorant
Codiclear® DH Syrup
Codimal® DM
Colrex® Compound Elixir
Colrex® Expectorant
Conar® Syrup
Conar® Expectorant Syrup
Conex® Liquid
Conex® With Codeine Syrup
Contac Jr® Liquid
Day-Night Comtrex®
Decoral® Forte®
Dexafed® Cough Syrup
Dimetane®-DC Cough Syrup
Dimetane®-DX Cough Syrup
Entuss® Expectorant Liquid
Fedahist® Expectorant Syrup and Pediatric Drops
Guaificon®-DMS
Histafed® Pediatric Liquid
Hycomine® Syrup and Pediatric Syrup
Lanatuss® Expectorant
Medicon® D
Medi-Synal®
Naldecon-DX® Pediatric Drops and Syrup
Naldecon-DX® Adult Liquid
Non-Drowsy Comtrex®
Noratuss®-II Expectorant and Liquid
Organidin® Solution
Potassium Iodide Solution (various)
Prunicodeine®
Queltuss® Tablets
Robitussin-CF® Liquid
Robitussin® Night Relief Liquid
Rondec®-DM Drops
Rondec®-DM Syrup
Ryna® Liquid
Ryna-C® Liquid
Ryna-CX® Liquid
Scot-Tussin® DM Syrup
Scot-Tussin® Expectorant
Scot-Tussin® DM Cough Chasers
Silexin® Cough Syrup
Sorbutuss®

## SUGAR-FREE LIQUID PHARMACEUTICALS *(Continued)*

S-T® Expectorant, SF/D-F
S-T® Forte®, Sugar-Free
Sudodrin®/Sudodrin® Forte®
Terpin® Hydrate With Codeine Elixir (various)
Toclonol® Expectorant
Toclonol® Expectorant With Codeine
Tolu-Sed® Cough Syrup
Tolu-Sed® DM
Tricodene® Liquid
Trind-DM® Liquid
Tuss-Ornade®
Tussar® SF
Tussionex® Extended Release Suspension
Tussi-Organidin® Liquid
Tussirex® Sugar-Free

**Dental Preparations and Fluoride Preparations**

Cepacol® Mouthwash
Cepastat® Mouthwash and Gargle
Chloraseptic® Mouthwash and Gargle
Fluorigard® Mouthrinse
Fluorinse®
Flura-Drops®
Flura-Loz®
Flura® Tablets
Gel-Kam®
Karigel®
Karigel® N
Luride® Drops
Luride® SF Lozi-Tabs
Luride® 0.25 and 0.5 Lozi-Tabs
Luride® Lozi-Tabs
Pediaflor® Drops
Phos-Flur® Rinse/Supplement
Point-Two® Mouthrinse
Prevident® Disclosing Drops
Thera-Flur® Gel and Drops

**Diagnostic Agents**

Gastrografin®

**Dietary Substitutes**

Co-Salt®

**Iron Preparations/Blood Modifiers**

Amicar® Syrup
Beminal® Stress Plus With Iron
Chel-Iron® Drops
Chel-Iron® Liquid
Geritol® Complete Tablets
Geritonic™ Liquid
Hemo-Vite® Liquid
Iberet® Liquid
Iberet®-500 Liquid
Incremin® With Iron Syrup
Kovitonic® Liquid
Niferex®
Nu-Iron® Elixir
Vita-Plus H® Half Strength, Sugar-Free
Vita-Plus H®, Sugar-Free

**Laxatives**

Agoral® (plain, marshmallow, and raspberry)
Aromatic Cascara Fluidextract USP
Castor Oil
Castor Oil (flavored)
Castor Oil USP
Colace®, Liquid
Cologel®
Disonate™ Liquid
Doxinate® Solution
Emulsoil®
Fiberall® Powder
Haley's MO®
Hydrocil® Instant Powder
Hypaque® Oral Powder
Kondremul®

Kondremul® With Cascara
Konsyl® Powder
Liqui-Doss®
Magnesium Citrate Solution NF
Metamucil® Instant Mix (lemon-lime or orange)
Metamucil® SF Powder
Milk of Magnesia
Milk of Magnesia/Cascara Suspension
Milk of Magnesia/Mineral Oil Emulsion (various)
Milkinol® Liquid
Mineral Oil (various)
Neoloid® Liquid
Nu-LYTELY®
Phospho-Soda®
Sodium Phosphate & Biphosphate Oral Solution USP
Zymenol® Emulsion

**Potassium Products**

Cena-K® Solution
EM-K®-10% Liquid
K-G® Elixir
Kaochlor-Eff® Tablets for Solution
Kaochlor® S-F Solution
Kaon® Elixir (grape and lemon-lime flavor)
Kaon-Cl® 20% Liquid
Kay Ciel® Elixir
Kay Ciel® Powder
Kaylixir®
Klor-Con®/25 Powder
Klor-Con® EF Tablets
Klor-Con® Liquid 20%
Klor-Con® Powder
Klorvess® Effervescent Tablets
Klorvess® Granules
Kolyum® Liquid and Powder
Potachlor® 10% and 20% Liquid
Potasalan® Elixir
Potassine® Liquid
Potassium Chloride Oral Solution USP 5%, 10%, and 20% (various)
Potassium Gluconate Elixir NF
Rum-K® Solution
Tri-K® Liquid
Trikates® Solution

**Sedatives-Tranquilizers-Antipsychotics**

Butabarbital Sodium Elixir
Butisol Sodium® Elixir
Haldol® Concentrate
Loxitane® C Drops
Mellaril® Concentrate
Serentil® Concentrate
Thorazine® Concentrate

**Vitamin Preparations-Nutritionals**

Aquasol A® Drops
BioCal® Tablets
Bugs Bunny™ Chewable Tablets
Bugs Bunny™ Plus Iron Chewable Tablets
Bugs Bunny™ With Extra C Chewable Tablets
Bugs Bunny™ Plus Minerals Chewable Tablets
Calciferol™ Drops
Caltrate® 600 Tablets
Ce-Vi-Sol® Drops
Cod Liver Oil (various)
Decagen® Tablets
DHT™ Intensol Solution (Roxane)
Drisdol® in Propylene Glycol
Flintstones™ Complete Chewable Tablets
Flintstones™ With Extra C Chewable Tablets
Flintstones™ Plus Iron Chewable Tablets
Incremin® With Iron Liquid
Kandium® Drops Tablets
Lanoplex® Elixir
Lycolan® Elixir
Oyst-Cal® 500 Tablets
Pediaflor®
PMS® Relief
Poly-Vi-Flor® Drops

## SUGAR-FREE LIQUID PHARMACEUTICALS *(Continued)*

Poly-Vi-Flor®/Iron Drops
Poly-Vi-Sol® Drops
Poly-Vi-Sol®/Iron Drops
Posture® Tablets
Spiderman™ Children's Chewable Vitamin Tablets
Spiderman™ Children's Plus Iron Tablets
Theragran® Jr Children's Chewable Tablets
Tri-Vi-Flor® Drops
Tri-Vi-Sol® Drops
Tri-Vi-Sol®/Iron Drops
Vi-Daylin® ADC Drops
Vi-Daylin® ADC/Fluoride Drops
Vi-Daylin® ADC Plus Iron Drops
Vi-Daylin® Drops
Vi-Daylin®/Fluoride Drops
Vi-Daylin® Plus Iron Drops
Vitalize®

**Miscellaneous**

Altace™ Capsules
Bicitra® Solution
Cibalith-S® Syrup
Colestid® Granules
Dayto® Himbin® Liquid
Digoxin® Elixir
Duvoid®
Glandosane®
Lipomul®
Lithium Citrate Syrup
Nicorette® Chewing Gum
Polycitra®-K Solution
Polycitra®-LC Solution
Tagamet® Liquid

**References:**

Hill EM, Flaitz CM, and Frost GR, "Sweetener Content of Common Pediatric Oral Liquid Medications," *Am J Hosp Pharm*, 1988, 45(1):135-42.

Kumar A, Rawlings RD, and Beaman DC, "The Mystery Ingredients: Sweeteners, Flavorings, Dyes, and Preservatives in Analgesic/Antipyretic, Antihistamine/Decongestant, Cough and Cold, Antidiarrheal, and Liquid Theophylline Preparations," *Pediatrics*, 1993, 91(5):927-33.

"Sugar Free Products," *Drug Topics Red Book*, 1992, 17-8.

# ALLERGIC SKIN REACTIONS TO DRUGS

Skin eruptions are the most common clinically observed form of drug "allergy." Cutaneous manifestations of hypersensitivity may include pruritus, urticaria, and angioedema; maculopapular, morbilliform, or erythematous rashes; erythema multiforme; eczema; erythema nodosum; photosensitivity reactions; and fixed drug eruptions. The most severe drug-related reactions are exfoliative dermatitis and vesiculobullous eruptions such as the Stevens-Johnson syndrome and toxic epidermal necrolysis (Lyell's syndrome). This table lists the incidence of drugs associated with cutaneous manifestations reported in 22,227 consecutive medical inpatients in the Boston Collaborative Drug Surveillance Program.

| Drug | Reaction per 1000 Recipients |
|---|---|
| Sulfamethoxazole and trimethoprim | 59 |
| Ampicillin | 52 |
| Semisynthetic penicillins | 36 |
| Blood, whole human | 35 |
| Corticotropin | 28 |
| Erythromycin | 23 |
| Sulfisoxazole | 17 |
| Penicillin G | 16 |
| Gentamicin sulfate | 16 |
| Practolol | 16 |
| Cephalosporins | 13 |
| Quinidine | 13 |
| Plasma protein fraction | 12 |
| Dipyrone | 11 |
| Mercurial diuretics | 9.5 |
| Nitrofurantoin | 9.1 |
| Packed RBCs | 8.1 |
| Heparin | 7.7 |
| Chloramphenicol | 6.8 |
| Trimethobenzamide | 6.6 |
| Phenazopyridine | 6.5 |
| Methenamine | 6.4 |
| Nitrazepam | 6.3 |
| Barbiturates | 4.7 |
| Glutethimide | 4.5 |
| Indomethacin | 4.4 |
| Chlordiazepoxide | 4.2 |
| Metoclopramide | 4.0 |
| Diazepam | 3.8 |
| Propoxyphene | 3.4 |
| Isoniazid | 3.0 |
| Guaifenesin and theophylline | 2.9 |
| Nystatin | 2.9 |
| Chlorothiazide | 2.8 |
| Furosemide | 2.6 |
| Isophane insulin suspension | 1.3 |
| Phenytoin | 1.1 |
| Phytonadione | 0.9 |
| Flurazepam | 0.5 |
| Chloral hydrate | 0.2 |

**Reference:**

Patterson R and Anderson J, "Allergic Reactions to Drugs and Biologic Agents," *JAMA*, 1982, 248:2637-45.

# COMMON ORAL-FACIAL INFECTIONS AND ANTIBIOTICS FOR TREATMENT

| Pathogens | Infections | Antibiotics |
|---|---|---|
| Aerobic gram-positive cocci | Cellulitis | Primary |
| | Periapical abscess | |
| | Periodontal abscess | Penicillin VK |
| and | Acute suppurative pulpitis | |
| | Oral-nasal fistulas | Alternates |
| Anaerobes | Pericorinitis | |
| | Osteitis | Erythromycin |
| | Osteomyelitis | |
| | Postsurgical and post-traumatic infection | Clindamycin |

# CONTROLLED SUBSTANCES

### Schedule I = C-I

The drugs and other substances in this schedule have no legal medical uses except research. They have a **high** potential for abuse. They include selected opiates such as heroin, opium derivatives, and hallucinogens.

### Schedule II = C-II

The drugs and other substances in this schedule have legal medical uses and a **high** abuse potential which may lead to severe dependence. They include former "Class A" narcotics, amphetamines, barbiturates, and other drugs.

### Schedule III = C-III

The drugs and other substances in this schedule have legal medical uses and a **lesser** degree of abuse potential which may lead to **moderate** dependence. They include former "Class B" narcotics and other drugs.

### Schedule IV = C-IV

The drugs and other substances in this schedule have legal medial uses and **low** abuse potential which may lead to **moderate** dependence. They include barbiturates, benzodiazepines, propoxyphenes, and other drugs.

### Schedule V = C-V

The drugs and other substances in this schedule have legal medical uses and **low** abuse potential which may lead to **moderate** dependence. They include narcotic cough preparations, diarrhea preparations, and other drugs.

**Note:** These are federal classifications. Your individual state may place a substance into a more restricted category. When this occurs, the more restricted category applies. Consult your state law.

# DRUGS ASSOCIATED WITH ADVERSE HEMATOLOGIC EFFECTS

| Drug | Red Cell Aplasia | Thrombo-cytopenia | Neutro-penia | Pancyto-penia | Hemolysis |
|---|---|---|---|---|---|
| Acetazolamide | | + | + | + | |
| Allopurinol | | | + | | |
| Amiodarone | + | | | | |
| Amphotericin B | | | | + | |
| Amrinone | | ++ | | | |
| Asparaginase | | +++ | +++ | +++ | ++ |
| Barbiturates | | + | | + | |
| Benzocaine | | | | | ++ |
| Captopril | | | ++ | | + |
| Carbamazepine | | ++ | + | | |
| Cephalosporins | | | + | | ++ |
| Chloramphenicol | | + | ++ | +++ | |
| Chlordiazepoxide | | | + | + | |
| Chloroquine | | + | | | |
| Chlorothiazides | | ++ | | | |
| Chlorpropamide | + | ++ | + | ++ | + |
| Chlortetracycline | | | | + | |
| Chlorthalidone | | | + | | |
| Cimetidine | | + | ++ | + | |
| Codeine | | + | | | |
| Colchicine | | | | + | |
| Cyclophosphamide | | +++ | +++ | +++ | + |
| Dapsone | | | | | +++ |
| Desipramine | | ++ | | | |
| Digitalis | | + | | | |
| Digitoxin | | ++ | | | |
| Erythromycin | | + | | | |
| Estrogen | | + | | + | |
| Ethacrynic acid | | | + | | |
| Fluorouracil | | +++ | +++ | +++ | + |
| Furosemide | | + | + | | |
| Gold salts | + | +++ | +++ | +++ | |
| Heparin | | ++ | | + | |
| Ibuprofen | | | + | | + |
| Imipramine | | | ++ | | |
| Indomethacin | | + | ++ | + | |
| Isoniazid | | + | | + | |
| Isosorbide dinitrate | | | | | + |
| Levodopa | | | | | ++ |
| Meperidine | | + | | | |
| Meprobamate | | + | + | + | |
| Methimazole | | | ++ | | |
| Methyldopa | | ++ | | | +++ |
| Methotrexate | | +++ | +++ | +++ | ++ |
| Methylene blue | | | | | + |
| Metronidazole | | | + | | |
| Nalidixic acid | | | | | + |
| Naproxen | | | | + | |
| Nitrofurantoin | | | ++ | | + |
| Nitroglycerine | | + | | | |
| Penicillamine | | ++ | + | | |
| Penicillins | | + | ++ | + | +++ |
| Phenazopyridine | | | | | +++ |
| Phenothiazines | | + | ++ | +++ | + |
| Phenylbutazone | | + | ++ | +++ | + |
| Phenytoin | | ++ | ++ | ++ | + |
| Potassium iodide | | + | | | |
| Prednisone | | + | | | |
| Primaquine | | | | | +++ |
| Procainamide | | | + | | |
| Procarbazine | | + | ++ | ++ | + |
| Propylthiouracil | | + | ++ | + | + |
| Quinidine | | +++ | + | | |
| Quinine | | +++ | + | | |

| Drug | Red Cell Aplasia | Thrombo-cytopenia | Neutro-penia | Pancyto-penia | Hemolysis |
|---|---|---|---|---|---|
| Reserpine | | + | | | |
| Rifampicin | | ++ | + | | +++ |
| Spironolactone | | | + | | |
| Streptomycin | | + | | + | |
| Sulfamethoxazole with trimethoprim | | | + | | |
| Sulfonamides | + | ++ | ++ | ++ | ++ |
| Sulindac | + | + | + | + | |
| Tetracyclines | | + | | | + |
| Thioridazine | | | ++ | | |
| Tolbutamide | | ++ | + | ++ | |
| Triamterene | | | | | + |
| Valproate | + | | | | |
| Vancomycin | | | + | | |

+ = rare or single reports.

++ = occasional reports.

+++ = substantial number of reports.

Adapted from D'Arcy PF and Griffin JP, eds, *Iatrogenic Diseases*, New York, NY: Oxford University Press, 1986, 128-30.

# HERBAL MEDICINES

## CHEMICAL ANALYSIS OF SELECTED PRODUCTS

| Herb | | Main Components | Pharmacological Claim |
|---|---|---|---|
| Latin Name | Chinese Name | | |
| *Ledebouriella seseloides* | Fang feng | Essential oils, alcohol derivatives, organic acids | Dispels "wind", antipyretic, analgesic antibacterial |
| *Potentilla chinensis* | Wei ling cai | Vitamin C, tannin, proteins, Ca++ salts | Antibacterial (antituberculosis) muscle relaxant, removes toxic "heats" |
| *Akebia clematidie* | Chuan mu tong | Aristolochic acid, akebin saponin | Reduces "heat", diuretic, antibacterial myocardial stimulant |
| *Rehmannia glutinosa* | Sheng di huang | Sterol, campesterol, rehmannin, alkaloids | Cardiotonic, diuretic, aids blood coagulation, anti-inflammatory |
| *Paeonia lactiflora* | Chi shao | Glycosides (eg, paeoninflorin), essential oils | Increases leucocyte cell count, removes "heat", eliminates blood stasis |
| *Lophatherum gracile* | Dan zhu ye | Arundoin, cylindrin, frieldelin | Diuretic, removes "heat", reduces "wind", antipyretic, antibacterial |
| *Dictamnus dasycarpus* | Bai xian pi | Dictamnine, alkaloids, psoralen, essential oils | Removes "damp heat", dispels "wind", antifungal |
| *Tribulus terrestris* | Ci ji li | Harmane, harmine | Hypotensive, diuretic, suppresses hyperactivity of liver, promotes blood circulation |
| Glycyrrhiza uralensis | Gan cao | Glycyrrhizin | Strengthens spleen and stomach, removes "heat" and toxins |
| *Schizonepeta tenuifolia* | Jing jie sui | Essential oils, D-methone, Di-limonene | Expels "wind", induces diaphoresis, reduces bleeding time |

# PRESCRIPTION WRITING

Doctor's Name
Address
Phone Number

Patient's Name/Date

Patient's Address/Age

**Rx**

Drug Name/Dosage Size

Disp: Number of tablets, capsules, ounces to be dispensed (roman numerals added as precaution for abused drugs)

Sig: Direction on how drug is to be taken

Doctor's signature

State license number

DEA number (if required)

## PRESCRIPTION REQUIREMENTS

1. Date
2. Full name and address of patient
3. Name and address of prescriber
4. Signature of prescriber

If Class II drug, Drug Enforcement Agency (DEA) number necessary.

If Class II and Class III narcotic, a triplicate prescription form (in the state of California) is necessary and it must be handwritten by the prescriber.

Please turn to appropriate oral medicine chapters for examples of prescriptions.

## ABBREVIATIONS COMMONLY USED IN MEDICAL ORDERS

| Abbreviation | From | Meaning |
|---|---|---|
| $\bar{aa}$, aa | ana | of each |
| ac | ante cibum | before meals or food |
| ad | ad | to, up to |
| a.d. | aurio dextra | right ear |
| ad lib | ad libitum | at pleasure |
| a.l. | aurio laeva | left ear |
| AM | ante meridiem | morning |
| amp | | ampul |
| amt | | amount |
| aq | aqua | water |
| aq. dest. | aqua destillata | distilled water |
| a.s. | aurio sinister | left ear |
| ASAP | | as soon as possible |
| a.u. | aures utrae | each ear |
| bid | bis in die | twice daily |
| bm | | bowel movement |
| bp | | blood pressure |
| BSA | | body surface area |
| c | cong | a gallon |
| $\bar{c}$ | cum | with |
| cal | | calorie |
| cap | capsula | capsule |
| cc | | cubic centimeter |
| cm | | centimeter |
| comp | compositus | compound |
| cont | | continue |
| d | dies | day |

## PRESCRIPTION WRITING *(Continued)*

| Abbreviation | From | Meaning |
|---|---|---|
| d/c | | discontinue |
| dil | dilue | dilute |
| disp | dispensa | dispense |
| div | divide | divide |
| dtd | dentur tales doses | give of such a dose |
| elix, el | elixir | elixir |
| emp | | as directed |
| et | et | and |
| ex aq | | in water |
| f, ft | fac, fiat, fiant | make, let be made |
| FDA | | Food and Drug Administration |
| g | gramma | gram |
| gr | granum | grain |
| gtt | gutta | a drop |
| h | hora | hour |
| hs | hora somni | at bedtime |
| I.M. | | intramuscular |
| I.V. | | intravenous |
| kcal | | kilocalorie |
| kg | | kilogram |
| L | | liter |
| liq | liquor | a liquor, solution |
| mcg | | microgram |
| mEq | | milliequivalent |
| mg | | milligram |
| mixt | mixtura | a mixture |
| mL | | milliliter |
| mm | | millimeter |
| M | misce | mix |
| m. dict | more dictor | as directed |
| NF | | National Formulary |
| no. | numerus | number |
| noc | nocturnal | in the night |
| non rep | non repetatur | do not repeat, no refills |
| NPO | | nothing by mouth |
| O, Oct | octarius | a pint |
| o.d. | oculus dexter | right eye |
| o.l. | oculus laevus | left eye |
| o.s. | oculus sinister | left eye |
| o.u. | oculo uterque | each eye |
| pc, post cib | post cibos | after meals |
| per | | through or by |
| PM | post meridiem | afternoon or evening |
| P.O. | per os | by mouth |
| P.R. | per rectum | rectally |
| prn | pro re nata | as needed |
| pulv | pulvis | a powder |
| q | | every |
| qad | quoque alternis die | every other day |
| qd | | every day |
| qh | quiaque hora | every hour |
| qid | quater in die | four times a day |
| qod | | every other day |
| qs | quantum sufficiat | a sufficient quantity |
| qs ad | | a sufficient quantity to make |
| qty | | quantity |

| Abbreviation | From | Meaning |
|---|---|---|
| qv | quam volueris | as much as you wish |
| Rx | recipe | take, a recipe |
| rep | repetatur | let it be repeated |
| $\bar{s}$ | sine | without |
| sa | secundum artem | according to art |
| sat | sataratus | saturated |
| S.C. | | subcutaneous |
| sig | signa | label, or let it be printed |
| sol | solutio | solution |
| solv | | dissolve |
| $\overline{ss}$ | semis | one-half |
| sos | si opus sit | if there is need |
| stat | statim | at once, immediately |
| supp | suppositorium | suppository |
| syr | syrupus | syrup |
| tab | tabella | tablet |
| tal | | such |
| tid | ter in die | three times a day |
| tr, tinct | tincture | tincture |
| trit | | triturate |
| tsp | | teaspoonful |
| ung | unguentum | ointment |
| USAN | | United States Adopted Names |
| USP | | United States Pharmacopeia |
| u.d., ut dict | ut dictum | as directed |
| v.o. | | verbal order |
| w.a. | | while awake |
| x3 | | 3 times |
| x4 | | 4 times |

# SAFE WRITING PRACTICES

Health professionals and their support personnel frequently produce handwritten copies of information they see in print; therefore, such information is subjected to even greater possibilities for error or misinterpretation on the part of others. Thus, particular care must be given to how drug names and strengths are expressed when creating written healthcare documents.

The following are a few examples of safe writing rules suggested by the Institute for Safe Medication Practices, Inc.*

1. There should be a space between a number and its units as it is easier to read. There should be no periods after the abbreviations mg or mL.

| **Correct** | **Incorrect** |
|---|---|
| 10 mg | 10mg |
| 100 mg | 100mg |

2. Never place a decimal and a zero after a whole number (2 mg is correct and 2.0 mg is **incorrect**). If the decimal point is not seen because it falls on a line or because individuals are working from copies where the decimal point is not seen, this causes a tenfold overdose.
3. Just the opposite is true for numbers less than one. Always place a zero before a naked decimal (0.5 mL is correct, .5 mL is **incorrect**).
4. Never abbreviate the word unit. The handwritten U or u, looks like a 0 (zero), and may cause a tenfold overdose error to be made.
5. IU is not a safe abbreviation for international units. The handwritten IU looks like IV. Write out international units or use int. units.
6. Q.D. is not a safe abbreviation for once daily, as when the Q is followed by a sloppy dot, it looks like QID which means four times daily.
7. O.D. is not a safe abbreviation for once daily, as it is properly interpreted as meaning "right eye" and has caused liquid medications such as saturated solution of potassium iodide and Lugol's solution to be administered incorrectly. There is no safe abbreviation for once daily. It must be written out in full.
8. Do not use chemical names such as 6-mercaptopurine or 6-thioguanine, as sixfold overdoses have been given when these were not recognized as chemical names. The proper names of these drugs are mercaptopurine or thioguanine.
9. Do not abbreviate drug names (5FC, 6MP, 5-ASA, MTX, HCTZ, CPZ, PBZ, etc) as they are misinterpreted and cause error.
10. Do not use the apothecary system or symbols.
11. Do not abbreviate microgram as µg; instead use mcg as there is less likelihood of misinterpretation.
12. When writing an outpatient prescription, write a complete prescription. A complete prescription can prevent the prescriber, the pharmacist, and/or the patient from making a mistake and can eliminate the need for further clarification. The legible prescriptions should contain:
    a. patient's full name
    b. for pediatric or geriatric patients: their age (or weight where applicable)
    c. drug name, dosage form and strength; if a drug is new or rarely prescribed, print this information
    d. number or amount to be dispensed
    e. complete instructions for the patient, including the purpose of the medication
    f. when there are recognized contraindications for a prescribed drug, indicate to the pharmacist that you are aware of this fact (ie, when prescribing a potassium salt for a patient receiving an ACE inhibitor, write "K serum leveling being monitored")

*From "Safe Writing" by Davis NM, PharmD and Cohen MR, MS, Lecturers and Consultants for Safe Medication Practices, 1143 Wright Drive, Huntington Valley, PA 19006. Phone: (215) 947-7566.

# VASOCONSTRICTOR INTERACTIONS WITH ANTIDEPRESSANTS

| Antidepressant | Effects With Epinephrine, Norepinephrine, Levonordefrin | Contraindicated | Recommendation |
|---|---|---|---|
| Bupropion (Wellbutrin®) | No adverse interactions reported | No | No precautions appear to be necessary |
| Fluoxetine (Prozac®) | No adverse interactions reported | No | No precautions appear to be necessary |
| Maprotiline (Ludiomil®) | Potential for inc pressor response | No | Same precaution as TCAs since it has similar pharmacology |
| Paroxetine (Paxil®) | No adverse interactions reported | No | No precautions appear to be necessary |
| Sertraline (Zoloft®) | No adverse interactions reported | No | No precautions appear to be necessary |
| TCAs | epi = inc pressor response; cardiac dysrhythmias; ne = inc pressor response; levo = inc pressor response | No | Potentially dangerous; use minimal amounts with caution in local anesthetics |
| Trazodone (Desyrel®) | No adverse interactions reported | No | No precautions appear to be necessary |
| Venlafaxine (Effexor®) | No adverse interactions reported | No | No precautions appear to be necessary |

Reference: Wynn RL, "Antidepressant Medications", *Gen Dent,* 1992, 40(3):192-7.

# WHAT'S NEW

## New Drugs Introduced or Approved by the FDA in 1998

| Brand Name | Generic Name | Use |
|---|---|---|
| Activelle™ | estradiol and norethindone | Menopause |
| Actonel® | risedronate | Osteoporosis |
| Aggrastat® | tirofiban | Acute coronary syndrome |
| Alrex® | loteprednol | Seasonal allergic conjunctivits |
| Amerge® | naratriptan | Migraine headache |
| Antizol® | fomepizole | Ethylene glycol and methanol poisoning |
| Atacand® | candesartan | Hypertension |
| Azopt® | brinzolamide | Glaucoma |
| Baycol® | cerivastatin | Antihyperlipidemic agent |
| Celebrex® | celecoxib | Rheumatoid arthritis and osteoarthritis |
| Celexa® | citalopram | Depression |
| Colazide® | balsalazide | Acute ulcerative colitis |
| Corlopam® | fenoldapam | Antihypertensive agent |
| Cosopt™ | dorzolamide and timolol | Glaucoma |
| Detrol® | tolterodine | Urinary incontinence |
| Diovan | valsartan and hydrochlorothiazide | Hypertension |
| Emadine® | emedastine | Antihistamine |
| Evista® | faloxifene | Osteoporosis |
| GlucaGen® | glucagon, rDNA | Severe hypoglycemia |
| Halfan® | halofantrine | Antimalarial |
| Infrasurf® | calfactant | Neonatal respiratory distress syndrome |
| Integrillin® | eptifibatide | Acute coronary syndrome |
| LYMErix® | lyme disease vaccine | Lyme disease |
| Lotemax® | loteprednol | Seasonal allergic conjunctivitis |
| Maxalt®/Maxalt® MLT | rizatriptan | Migraine headache |
| Meridia® | sibutramine | Antiobesity agent |
| Micardis® | telmisartan | Hypertension |
| Plavix® | clopidogrel | Reduce atherosclerotic events |
| Prandin® | repaglinide | Antidiabetic |
| Priftin® | rifapentine | Pulmonary TB |
| Provigil® | modafinil | Narcolepsy |
| Refludan® | lepirudin | Heparin-induced thrombocytopenia; anticoagulant |
| Regranex™ | becaplermin | Diabetic foot ulcers |
| Remicade® | infliximab | Crohn's disease |
| Simulect® | basiliximab | Prophylaxis in acute kidney rejection |
| Singulair® | montelukast | Asthma |
| Stemgen® | ancestim | Stimulate peripheral blood progenitor cells |
| Sucraid® | sacrosidase | Sucrase-isomaltase deficiency |
| Synagis® | palivizumab | Respiratory synctial viral infection |
| Tasmar® | tolcapone | Antiparkinson agent |
| Thalomid® | thalidomide | Leprosy |
| Tricor™ | fenofibrate | Antihyperlipidemic |
| Trovan® | trovafloxacin | Antibacterial |
| Viagra™ | sildenafil | Impotence |
| Vitravene™ | fomivirsen | CMV retinis |
| Xeloda™ | capecitabine | Breast cancer |
| Zemplar® | paricalcitol | Hyperparathyroidism |
| Zomig® | zolmitriptan | Antimigraine |

## Pending Drugs or Drugs in Clinical Trials

| Brand Name | Generic Name | Use |
|---|---|---|
| Alredase® | tolrestat | Controlling late complications of diabetes |
| Arkin-Z® | vesnarinone | Congestive heart failure agent |
| Baypress® | nitrendipine | Calcium channel blocker for hypertension |
| Berotec® | fenoterol | Beta-2 agonist for asthma |
| Catatrol® | viloxazine | Bicyclic antidepressant |
| Cipralan® | cifenline succinate | Antiarrhythmic agent |
| Decabid® | indecainide hydrochloride | Antiarrhythmic agent |
| Delaprem® | hexoprenaline sulfate | Tocolytic agent |
| Dirame® | propiram | Opioid analgesic |
| Enable® | tenidap sodium | Arthritis |
| Fareston® | toremifene citrate | Antiestrogen for breast cancer |
| Freedox® | triliazad mesylate | Prevents progressive neuronal degeneration |
| Frisium® | clobazam | Benzodiazepine |
| Gastrozepine® | pirenzepine | Antiulcer drug |
| Inhibace® | cilazapril | ACE inhibitor |
| Isoprinosine® | inosiplex | Immunomodulating drug |
| Lacipil® | lacidipine | Hypertension |
| Maxicam® | isoxicam | NSAID |
| Mentane® | velnacrine | Alzheimer's disease agent |
| Micturin® | terodiline hydrochloride | Agent for urinary incontinence |
| Mogadon® | nitrazepam | Benzodiazepine |
| Motilium® | domperidone | Antiemetic |
| Napa® | acecainide | Antiarrhythmic agent |
| Pindac® | pinacidil | Antihypertensive |
| Prothiaden® | dothiepin hydrochloride | Tricyclic antidepressant |
| Rimadyl® | caprofen | NSAID |
| Roxiam® | remoxipride | Antipsychotic agent |
| Selecor® | celiprolol hydrochloride | Beta-adrenergic blocker |
| Spexil® | trospectomycin | Antibiotic, a spectinomycin analog |
| Targocoid® | teicoplanin | Antibiotic, similar to vancomycin |
| Unicard® | dilevalol | Beta-adrenergic blocker |
| Zaditen® | ketotifen | Antiasthmatic |

# THERAPEUTIC CATEGORY INDEX

## ANALGESIC, NARCOTIC *(Continued)*



## ANALGESIC, NON-NARCOTIC



## ANALGESIC, TOPICAL



## ANALGESIC, URINARY



## ANDROGEN



## ANGIOTENSIN-CONVERTING ENZYME (ACE) INHIBITOR

(Continued)

(Continued)

## CORTICOSTEROID, OTIC



## CORTICOSTEROID, SYSTEMIC



## CORTICOSTEROID, TOPICAL (LOW POTENCY)



## CORTICOSTEROID, TOPICAL (MEDIUM POTENCY)



## CORTICOSTEROID, TOPICAL (MEDIUM/HIGH POTENCY)



## CORTICOSTEROID, TOPICAL (HIGH POTENCY)



## CORTICOSTEROID, TOPICAL (VERY HIGH POTENCY)



## COLD PREPARATION



## COUGH PREPARATION

(Continued)

(Continued)

(Continued)

## VASODILATOR, PERIPHERAL



## VASOPRESSIN ANALOG, SYNTHETIC



## VITAMIN



## VITAMIN A DERIVATIVE



## VITAMIN D ANALOG



## VITAMIN, FAT SOLUBLE



## VITAMIN, TOPICAL



## VITAMIN, WATER SOLUBLE

# ALPHABETICAL INDEX

# NOTES

# Other titles offered by Lexi-Comp . . .

*NEW* titles targeted for future release in print and on CD-ROM will include:

- ***Drug Information for Cardiology***
- ***Drug Information for Cancer***
- ***Drug-Induced Nutrient Depletion Handbook***
- ***Natural Therapeutics Pocket Guide***
- ***Natural Products Information Handbook***

## *DRUG INFORMATION HANDBOOK 6th Edition 98/99*

by Charles Lacy, PharmD; Lora L. Armstrong, BSPharm; Naomi Ingrim, PharmD; and Leonard L. Lance, BSPharm

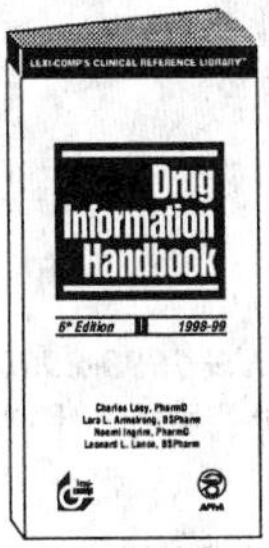


Specifically compiled and designed for the healthcare professional requiring quick access to concisely stated comprehensive data concerning clinical use of medications.

*The Drug Information Handbook* is an ideal portable drug information resource, containing 1100 drug monographs. Each monograph typically provides the reader with up to 29 key points of data concerning clinical use and dosing of the medication. Material provided in the Appendix section is recognized by many users to be, by itself, well worth the purchase of the handbook.

## *DRUG INFORMATION HANDBOOK POCKET 98/99*

by Charles Lacy, PharmD; Lora L. Armstrong, BSPharm; Naomi Ingrim, PharmD; and Leonard L. Lance, BSPharm

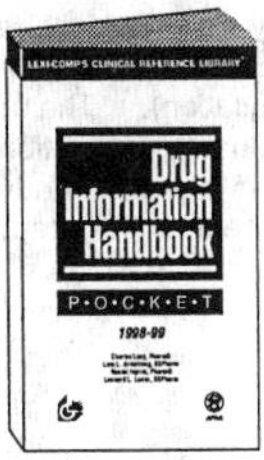


All medications found in the Drug Information Handbook, 6th Edition are included in this abridged pocket edition. It is specifically compiled and designed for the healthcare professional requiring quick access to concisely stated comprehensive data concerning clinical use of medications.

The outstanding cross-referencing allows the user to quickly locate the brand name, generic name, synonym, and related information found in the Appendix making this a useful quick reference for medical professionals at any level of training or experience.

## *PEDIATRIC DOSAGE HANDBOOK 5th Edition 98/99*

by Carol K. Taketomo, PharmD; Jane Hurlburt Hodding, PharmD; and Donna M. Kraus, PharmD

New
More Portable Size!

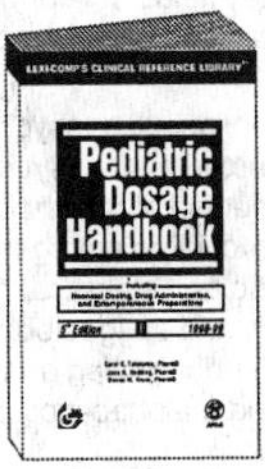


Special considerations must frequently be taken into account when dosing medications for the pediatric patient. This highly regarded quick reference handbook is a compilation of recommended pediatric doses based on current literature as well as the practical experience of the authors and their many colleagues who work every day in the pediatric clinical setting.

*The Pediatric Dosage Handbook* 5th Edition includes neonatal dosing, drug administration, and extemporaneous preparations for 619 medications used in pediatric medicine.

## *DRUG INFORMATION HANDBOOK FOR THE CRIMINAL JUSTICE PROFESSIONAL 98/99*

by Marcelline Burns, PhD; Thomas E. Page, MA; and Jerrold B. Leikin, MD

New!

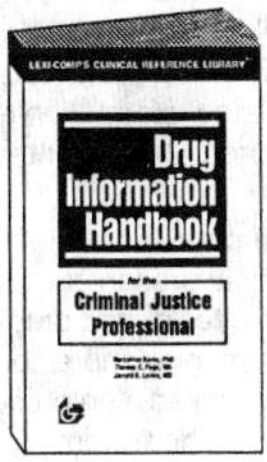


Compiled and designed for police officers, law enforcement officials, and legal professionals who are in need of a reference which relates to information on drugs, chemical substances, and other agents that have abuse and/or impairment potential. This handbook covers over 450 medications, agents, and substances. Each monograph is presented in a consistent format and contains up to 33 fields of information including Scientific Name, Commonly Found In, Abuse Potential, Impairment Potential, Use, When to Admit to Hospital, Mechanism of Toxic Action, Signs & Symptoms of Acute Overdose, Drug Interactions, Warnings/Precautions, and Reference Range. There are many diverse chapter inclusions as well as a glossary of medical terms for the layman along with a slang street drug listing. The appendix contains Chemical, Bacteriologic, and Radiologic Agents - Effects and Treatment; Controlled Substances - Uses and Effects; Medical Examiner Data; Federal Trafficking Penalties, *and much more.*

## *ANESTHESIOLOGY & CRITICAL CARE DRUG HANDBOOK 1999-2000*

by Andrew J. Donnelly, PharmD; Francesca E. Cunningham, PharmD; and Verna L. Baughman, MD

New!

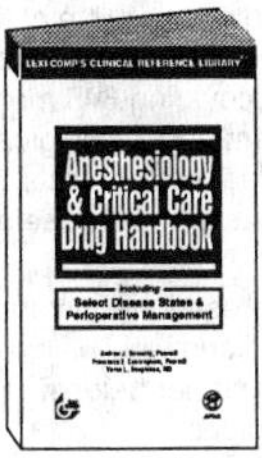


Contains over 512 generic medications with up to 25 fields of information presented in each monograph. It also contains the following Special Issues and Topics: Allergic Reaction, Anesthesia for Cardiac Patients in Noncardiac Surgery, Anesthesia for Obstetric Patients in Nonobstetric Surgery, Anesthesia for Patients With Liver Disease, Chronic Pain Management, Chronic Renal Failure, Conscious Sedation, Perioperative Management of Patients on Antiseizure Medication, Substance Abuse and Anesthesia.

The Appendix contains over 140 pages of useful and valuable information including: Abbreviations & Measurements, Anesthesiology Information, Assessment of Liver & Renal Function, Comparative Drug Charts, Infectious Disease-Prophylaxis & Treatment, Laboratory Values, Therapy Recommendation, Toxicology, *and much more . . .*

## *DRUG INFORMATION HANDBOOK FOR THE ALLIED HEALTH PROFESSIONAL 6th Edition 1999-2000*

by Leonard L. Lance, BSPharm; Charles Lacy, PharmD; and Morton P. Goldman, PharmD

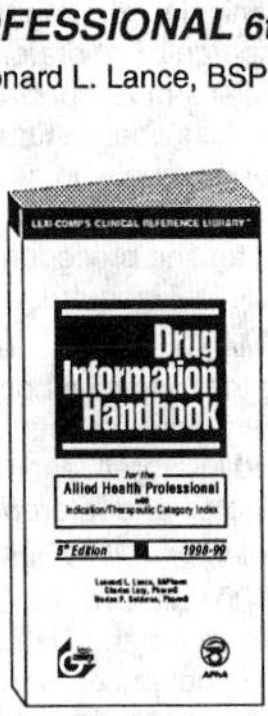


Working with clinical pharmacists, hospital pharmacy and therapeutics committees, and hospital drug information centers, the authors have assisted hundreds of hospitals in developing institution specific formulary reference documentation.

The most current basic drug and medication data from those clinical settings have been reviewed, coalesced, and cross-referenced to create this unique handbook. The handbook offers quick access to abbreviated monographs for 1384 generic drugs.

This is a great tool for physician assistants, medical records personnel, medical transcriptionists and secretaries, pharmacy technicians, and other allied health professionals.

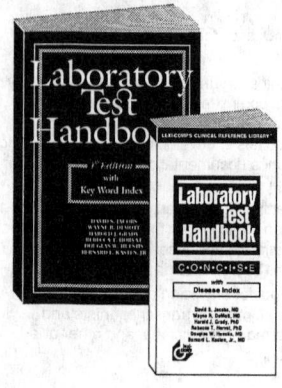

# Lexi-Comp's Clinical Reference Library™ Reply Card

Return this postage-paid card so we can keep you up-to-date on all the latest products, promotions and upgrades.

- [ ] **Please put me on your "Mailing List".**
- [ ] **Please put me on your "Standing Order List" to automatically receive the new edition each year.**

______________________________
Please print name of book

- [ ] **Please send me information on quantity discounts.**

Name (First) ____________ (Last) ____________

Title ______________________________

Company ______________________________

Address ______________________________

City ______________ State/Province ______________

Zip/Postal Code ______________ Country ______________

Telephone: (______) ______________

E-Mail Address ______________________________

**OTHER AREAS OF INTEREST:**

- [ ] Anesthesiology & Critical Care
- [ ] Diagnostic Procedures
- [ ] Drug Information
- [ ] Drug Information for Allied Health
- [ ] Drug Information for Cancer*
- [ ] Drug Information for Cardiology*
- [ ] Drug Information for Dentistry
- [ ] Drug Information for Nursing
- [ ] Drug Information for Psychiatry
- [ ] Geriatric Dosage
- [ ] Natural Products Information*
- [ ] Drug-Induced Nutrient Depletion*
- [ ] Natural Therapeutics*
- [ ] Infectious Diseases
- [ ] Laboratory Test
- [ ] Pediatric Dosage
- [ ] Poisoning & Toxicology

* 1999 targeted release

**ALSO INTERESTED IN THE FOLLOWING:**

- [ ] Lexi-Comp's Formulary/Lab Custom Publishing Service
- [ ] Lexi-Comp's CRL™ on CD-ROM (____Academic____Personal____Institutional)
- [ ] Lexi-Comp's CRL™ on a hand-held device

lexi-comp

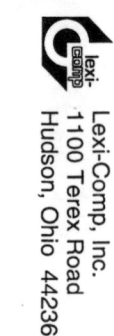

Lexi-Comp, Inc.
1100 Terex Road
Hudson, Ohio 44236-4438

NO POSTAGE
NECESSARY
IF MAILED
IN THE
UNITED STATES

# BUSINESS REPLY MAIL

FIRST-CLASS MAIL PERMIT NO 689 HUDSON, OH

POSTAGE WILL BE PAID BY ADDRESSEE

LEXI-COMP, INC.
Clinical Reference Library™ Reply Card
1100 Terex Road
Hudson, OH 44236-9915